ANTIEPILEPTIC DRUGS
FIFTH EDITION

This book is to be returned on or before
the last date stamped below.

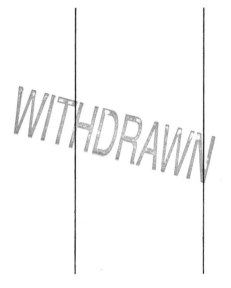

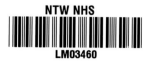

ANTIEPILEPTIC DRUGS

FIFTH EDITION

Editors

RENÉ H. LEVY, PhD

Professor and Chair, Department of Pharmaceutics
Professor of Neurological Surgery
University of Washington Schools of Pharmacy and Medicine
Seattle, Washington

RICHARD H. MATTSON, MD

Professor of Neurology and Director of Medical Studies
Department of Neurology
Yale University School of Medicine and Veterans Affairs Medical Center
West Haven, Connecticut

BRIAN S. MELDRUM, PhD

Professor in Experimental Neurology
Director of Neurology
Institute of Psychiatry
London, England

EMILIO PERUCCA, MD, PhD, FRCP (EDIN)

Professor of Medical Pharmacology
Clinical Pharmacology Unit
Department of Internal Medicine and Therapeutics
University of Pavia; and
Consultant Clinical Pharmacologist
Institute of Neurology, C. Momdino Foundation
Pavia, Italy

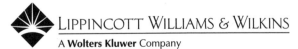

LIPPINCOTT WILLIAMS & WILKINS
A **Wolters Kluwer** Company
Philadelphia • Baltimore • New York • London
Buenos Aires • Hong Kong • Sydney • Tokyo

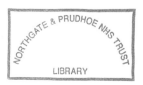

Acquisitions Editor: Anne M. Sydor
Developmental Editor: Raymond E. Reter
Production Editor: Rakesh Rampertab
Manufacturing Manager: Colin I. Warnock
Cover Designer: Mark Lerner
Compositor: Lippincott Williams & Wilkins Desktop Division
Printer: Maple Press

ISBN 0-7817-2321-3

Care has been taken to confirm the accuracy of the information presented and to describe generally accepted practices. However, the authors, editors, and publisher are not responsible for errors or omissions or for any consequences from application of the information in this book and make no warranty, expressed or implied, with respect to the currency, completeness, or accuracy of the contents of the publication. Application of this information in a particular situation remains the professional responsibility of the practitioner.

The authors, editors, and publisher have exerted every effort to ensure that drug selection and dosage set forth in this text are in accordance with current recommendations and practice at the time of publication. However, in view of ongoing research, changes in government regulations, and the constant flow of information relating to drug therapy and drug reactions, the reader is urged to check the package insert for each drug for any change in indications and dosage and for added warnings and precautions. This is particularly important when the recommended agent is a new or infrequently employed drug.

Some drugs and medical devices presented in this publication have Food and Drug Administration (FDA) clearance for limited use in restricted research settings. It is the responsibility of the health care provider to ascertain the FDA status of each drug or device planned for use in their clinical practice.

10 9 8 7 6 5 4 3 2 1

The editors wish to dedicate this edition of the book, *Antiepileptic Drugs*, to the memory of J. Kiffin Penry M.D., who died as a result of longstanding illness (diabetes mellitus). Dr. Penry was one of the primary forces bringing about the concept and publication of this book and served as an editor of all previous four editions.

Dr. Penry came to the NIH in 1965 at the invitation of Dr. Richard Masland to start an Epilepsy Branch following service in the USAF. With characteristic evangelistic zeal he enlisted the cooperation of government, industry, academia, lay organizations and others to be aware of and address the problems of epilepsy from basic science to social needs.

Among the many areas to which he directed attention was the use of available antiepileptic drugs (AEDs). Knowledge of the pharmacology, and pharmacokinetics in particular, was quite limited by practicing physicians and other health care providers. The common practice of prescribing phenobarbital four times daily illustrates the lack of sophistication among this group.

In the late 1960s and early 1970s technological advances in clinical laboratories made possible determination of antiepileptic drug concentrations in the blood and other tissues. Previously, detection and pharmacokinetic studies involved use of radioisotopes and were largely limited to use by academia or industry. The ready availability of detection of quantities of drugs in different tissues led to rapid accumulation of clinical correlative data.

With Dr. Penry's support, a group of interested experts assembled in Warrenton, Virginia, in June 1970 to draft a book that would synthesize and present in one source the available information on the pharmacology of the antiepileptic drugs. Preliminary chapter presentations were given at a symposium sponsored by the National Institutes of Health and held in Phoenix in 1971. The first edition of Antiepileptic Drugs followed this meeting.

Dr. Penry also initiated the Antiepileptic Drug Development (ADD) program in the Epilepsy Branch of NINDS, directed by Dr. Harvey Kupferberg. This team worked closely with the pharmaceutical industry and academe to stimulate new drug discovery and testing. The Epilepsy Branch also established a statistical group that played an important role in educating investigators in conduct of carefully designed controlled clinical trials and in prescribing according to evidence based medicine. Some of the fruition of these efforts is to be found in this edition, which contains sections on eight new AEDs marketed since 1990s.

Dr. Penry also catalyzed the development of Epilepsy Centers with intensive clinical/EEG monitoring, fostered NIH sponsored intramural and extramural epilepsy research and led in fostering international cooperation to develop a classification of seizures and the epilepsies. Last, but not least, he created an educational program after returning to Wake Forest University designed to educate physicians and especially neurologists about the diagnosis and treatment of epilepsy. This program has now been attended by approximately one fifth of all neurologists in the USA.

For these and other pioneering efforts in epilepsy, we wish to dedicate this edition of Antiepileptic Drugs to Dr. Penry.

CONTENTS

CONTRIBUTING AUTHORS

Frank S. Abbott, BSP, MS, PhD Professor and Dean, Faculty of Pharmaceutical Sciences, University of British Columbia, Vancouver, British Columbia, Canada

Fiorenzo Albani, PharmD Research Assistant, Department of Neurological Sciences, University of Bologna, Bologna, Italy

Brian K. Alldredge, PharmD Professor, Department of Clinical Pharmacy and Neurology, University of California, San Francisco, San Francisco, California

Gail D. Anderson, PhD Professor, Department of Pharmacy, University of Washington, Seattle, Washington

Manoj Bajpai, PhD Department of Pharmacokinetics and Drug Metabolism, Amgen Incorporated, Thousand Oaks, California

Agostino Baruzzi, MD Professor of Neurology, Department of Neurological Sciences, University of Bologna, Bologna, Italy

Michel Baulac, MD Hôpital de la Salpetriere, Bat. P. Castaigne, Paris, France

Carl W. Bazil, MD, PhD Assistant Professor, Department of Neurology, Columbia University, New York, New York; and Director, Clinical Anticonvulsant Drug Trials, Comprehensive Epilepsy Center, New York Presbyterian Hospital, New York, New York

Ettore Beghi, MD Chief, Neurophysiological Unit, "San Gerarda" Hospital, Monza, Italy; and Head, Neurological Disorders Laboratory, Institute for Pharmacological Research "Mario Negri," Milan, Italy

Elinor Ben-Menachem, MD, PhD Associate Professor, Department of Clinical Neuroscience, Neurology Section, Sahlgrenska University Hospital, Goteborg, Sweden

Meir Bialer, PhD, MBA David H. Eisenberg Professor of Pharmacy, Department of Pharmaceutics, School of Pharmacy, Faculty of Medicine, The Hebrew University of Jerusalem, Jerusalem, Israel

Victor Biton, MD Director, Arkansas Epilepsy Program, Little Rock, Arkansas

Blaise F. D. Bourgeois, MD Professor of Neurology, Harvard Medical School; and Director, Division of Epilepsy and Clinical Neurophysiology, Children's Hospital Boston, Boston, Massachusetts

Martin J. Brodie, MD Professor of Medicine and Clinical Pharmacology, Department of Medicine and Therapeutics, Glasgow, Scotland, United Kingdom

Thomas R. Browne, MD Professor of Neurology, Department of Neurology, Boston University School of Medicine, Boston, Massachusetts

Joseph Bruni, MD, FRCP(C) Associate Professor, Department of Medicine, University of Toronto; and Consultant Neurologist, Department of Medicine, St. Michael's Hospital, Toronto, Ontario, Canada

Joseph R. Calabrese, MD Professor of Psychiatry, Department of Psychiatry, Case Western Reserve University School of Medicine; and Director, Mood Disorders Program, Department of Psychiatry, University Hospitals of Cleveland, Cleveland, Ohio

Daniel M. Canafax, PharmD Director, Clinical Affairs, Elan Pharmaceuticals, South San Francisco, California

David W. Chadwick, MD Professor of Neurology, Department of Neurological Science, University of Liverpool; and Consultant Neurologist, The Walton Centre for Neurology and Neurosurgery, Liverpool, United Kingdom

Chao Chen, PhD Section Head, Pharmacokinetics, Department of Clinical Pharmacology and Experimental Medicine, GlaxoSmithKline, Greenford, Middlesex, United Kingdom

James C. Cloyd, PharmD Professor and Director, Epilepsy Research and Education Program, College of Pharmacy, University of Minnesota, Minneapolis, Minnesota

Stephen D. Collins, MD, PhD Associate Medical Director, Department of Marketed Products, Abbott Laboratories, Abbott Park, Illinois

Joyce A. Cramer, BS Associate Research Scientist, Yale University School of Medicine, Veterans Affairs Connecticut Health Care System, West Haven, Connecticut

Robert J. DeLorenzo, MD, PhD, MPH George B. Bliley III Professor of Neurology, Department of Neurology, Virginia Commonwealth University, Richmond, Virginia

Marc A. Dichter, MD Department of Neurology, University of Pennsylvania, Philadelphia, Pennsylvania

Maurice Dickins, PhD Senior Scientist, Drug Metabolism and Pharmacokinetics, GlaxoSmithKline, Ware, Hertfordshire, United Kingdom

Dennis R. Doose, PhD Associate Director, Global Clinical Pharmacokinetics and Clinical Pharmacology, Johnson & Johnson Pharmaceutical Research and Development, Raritan, New Jersey

Olivier Dulac, MD Professor, Department of Pediatric Neurology, University of René Descartes, Paris, France

Mervyn J. Eadie, MD, PhD Emeritus Professor, Department of Medicine, University of Queensland; and Honorary Consultant Neurologist, Royal Brisbane Hospital, Brisbane, Queensland, Australia

James A. Ferrendelli, MD Professor and Chairman, Department of Neurology, University of Texas, Houston Medical School; and Chief, Department of Neurology Service, Hermann Hospital, Houston, Texas

Richard W. Fincham, MD Deceased

Jacqueline A. French, MD Professor, Department of Neurology, University of Pennsylvania; and Associate Director, Pennsylvania Epilepsy Center, Department of Neurology, Hospital of the University of Pennsylvania, Philadelphia, Pennsylvania

Buichi Fujitani, PhD Department of International Affairs, Dainippon Pharmaceutical Company, Limited, Osaka, Japan

William R. Garnett, PharmD Professor of Pharmacy and Neurology, Department of Pharmacy, Virginia Commonwealth University, Medical College of Virginia, Richmond, Virginia

Philippe Gelisse, MD Chief of Clinic, Laboratory of Experimental Medicine, Institute of Biology; and Clinical Chief, Epilepsy Unit, Gui de Chauliac Hospital, Montpellier, France

Pierre Genton, MD Neurologist, Centre Saint Paul, Marseille, France

William J. Giardina, PhD Associate Research Fellow, Central Nervous System Diseases Research, Abbott Laboratories, Abbott Park, Illinois

Barry E. Gidal, PharmD Associate Professor, School of Pharmacy and Department of Neurology, University of Wisconsin, Madison, Wisconsin

Tracy A. Glauser, MD Division of Neurology, Children's Hospital Medical Center, Cincinnati, Ohio

John H. Greist, MD Distinguished Senior Scientist, Madison Institute of Medicine; and Clinical Professor of Psychiatry, Department of Psychiatry, University of Wisconsin, Madison, Wisconsin

Houda Hachad, MD Research Associate, Department of Pharmaceutics, University of Washington, Seattle, Washington

Atticus H. Hainsworth, MA, PhD Senior Lecturer in Pharmacology, School of Pharmacy, De Montfort University, Leicester, United Kingdom

Katherine D. Holland, MD, PhD Staff Physician, Department of Neurology, Cleveland Clinic Foundation, Cleveland, Ohio

Gregory L. Holmes, MD Professor of Neurology, Department of Neurology, Harvard Medical School; and Director, Center for Research in Pediatric Epilepsy, Children's Hospital, Boston, Massachusetts

Wayne D. Hooper, PhD Director, Center for Studies in Drug Disposition, University of Queensland, Royal Brisbane Hospital, Queensland, Australia

Svein I. Johannessen, PhD Director of Research, The National Center for Epilepsy, Sandvika, Norway

Reetta Kälviäinen, MD, PhD Head of the Outpatient Clinic, Leader of the Clinical Epilepsy Research Project, Department of Neurology, Kuopio University Hospital and University of Kuopio, Kuopio, Finland

Marc Kamin, MD Director, Clinical Research, Ortho-McNeil Pharmaceutical, Raritan, New Jersey

Roopal M. Karia, MD Fellow and Instructor, Department of Neurology, University of Medicine and Dentistry of New Jersey, Robert Wood Johnson Medical School, New Brunswick, New Jersey

Mary Ann Karolchyk, DO Global Head, Epilepsy Section, Department of Clinical Research and Development, Novartis Pharmaceutical Corporation, Basel, Switzerland

Russell Katz, MD Division of Neuropharmacological Drug Products, Center for Drug Evaluation and Research, United States Food and Drug Administration, Washington, DC

Henrik Klitgaard, PhD Director, Preclinical CNS Research, UCB S.A. Pharma Sector, Braine-l'Alleud, Belgium

Günter Krämer, MD Medical Director, Swiss Epilepsy Center, Zurich, Switzerland

Alan R. Kugler, PhD Pfizer Global Research and Development, Ann Arbor Laboratories, Ann Arbor, Michigan

Harvey J. Kupferberg, MD Epilepsy Branch, National Institute of Neurological Disorders and Stroke, National Institutes of Health, Bethesda, Maryland

Michael J. Leach, PhD Reader in Pharmacology and Drug Development, Department of Chemical and Life Sciences, University of Greenwich, London, United Kingdom

Barbara LeDuc, PhD Massachusetts College of Pharmacy and Applied Sciences, Boston, Massachusetts

Byung In Lee, MD Professor, Department of Neurology, Yonsei University College of Medicine; and Chief, Department of Neurology, Severance Hospital, Seoul, Korea

J. Steven Leeder, PharmD, PhD Associate Professor, Department of Pediatrics and Pharmacology, University of Missouri, Kansas City; and Chief, Section of Developmental Pharmacology and Experimental Therapeutics, Children's Mercy Hospital and Clinics, Kansas City, Missouri

Ilo E. Leppik, MD Director of Research, MINCEP Epilepsy Care, Minneapolis, Minnesota

René H. Levy, PhD Professor and Chair, Department of Pharmaceutics, Professor of Neurological Surgery, University of Washington School of Pharmacy and Medicine, Seattle, Washington

Pierre Loiseau, MD Honorary Professor, Department of Neurology, Bordeaux Medical University, Bordeaux, France

Wolfgang Löscher, PhD Professor and Chairman, Department of Pharmacology, Toxicology and Pharmacy, School of Veterinary Medicine, Hannover, Germany

Robert L. Macdonald, MD, PhD Professor and Chairman, Department of Neurology, Vanderbilt University, Nashville, Tennessee

Doru Georg Margineanu, PhD Senior Scientist, Department of Preclinical CNS Research, UCB S.A. Pharma Sector, Braine-l'Alleud, Belgium

Anthony G. Marson, MD, MRCP Lecturer in Neurology, Department of Neurological Science, University of Liverpool; and Senior Registrar, The Walton Centre for Neurology and Neurosurgery, Liverpool, United Kingdom

Gary G. Mather, PhD, DABT Program Director, Preclinical ADME/Tox, Myriad Pharmaceuticals Inc., Salt Lake City, Utah

Richard H. Mattson, MD Professor of Neurology and Director of Medical Studies, Department of Neurology, Yale University School of Medicine and Veterans Affairs Medical Center, West Haven, Connecticut

Michael J. McLean, MD, PhD Associate Professor, Department of Neurology, Vanderbilt University Medical Center, Nashville, Tennessee

Roberto Michelucci, MD, PhD Deputy Chief, Department of Neurological Sciences, Bellaria Hospital, Bologna, Italy

John W. Miller, MD, PhD Professor, Department of Neurology, University of Washington; and Director, Regional Epilepsy Center, Harborview Medical Center, Seattle, Washington

Francesco Monaco, MD Chief and Professor of Neurology, Department of Neurology, University of Piemonte Orientale "Amedo Avogadro," Novara, Italy

Martha J. Morrell, MD Professor of Clinical Neurology, Department of Neurology, Columbia University, College of Physicians and Surgeons; and Director, Columbia Comprehensive Epilepsy Center, New York, New York

Marco Mula, MD Research Fellow, Department of Neurology, University of Piemonte Orientale "Amedeo Avogadro," Novara, Italy

Richard W. Olsen, PhD Professor, Department of Molecular and Medical Pharmacology, University of California, Los Angeles School of Medicine, Los Angeles, California

Philip N. Patsalos, FRCPath, PhD Senior Lecturer in Clinical Pharmacology, Department of Clinical and Experimental Epilepsy, Institute of Neurology; and Director, Department of Pharmacology and Therapeutics Unit, National Hospital of Neurology and Neurosurgery, London, United Kingdom

Timothy A. Pedley, MD Professor of Neurology, Department of Neurology, Columbia University, New York, New York; and Neurologist-in-Chief, The Neurological Institute of New York, New York Presbyterian Hospital, New York, New York

John M. Pellock, MD Professor, Department of Child Neurology, Virginia Commonwealth University Health Systems; and Chairman, Child Neurology, Medical College of Virginia, Richmond, Virginia

James L. Perhach, PhD, FCP Senior Director, Clinical Pharmacology, Perdue Pharma L.P., Princeton, New Jersey

Emilio Perucca, MD, PhD, FRCP(Edin) Professor of Medical Pharmacology, Clinical Pharmacology Unit, Department of Internal Medicine and Therapeutics, University of Pavia; and Consultant Clinical Pharmacologist, Institute of Neurology, C. Momdino Foundation, Pavia, Italy

Francesco Pisani, MD Associate Professor of Neurology, Department of Neurological Sciences, Psychiatric and Anesthesiological Sciences, University of Messina, Messina, Italy

Asla Pitkänen, MD, PhD Professor of Neurobiology, A.I. Virtanen Institute, University of Kuopio, Kuopio, Finland

Roger J. Porter, MD Vice President, Clinical Pharmacology, Clinical Research and Development, Wyeth-Ayerst Research; and Adjunct Professor of Neurology, University of Pennsylvania, Philadelphia, Pennsylvania

Michael D. Privitera, MD Professor and Vice Chair, Department of Neurology, University of Cincinnati Medical Center, Cincinnati, Ohio

Flavia M. Pryor, RN, BSN Nurse Researcher, Department of Neurology Service, Miami Veterans Affairs Medical Center, Miami, Florida

Isabelle Ragueneau-Majlessi, MD Research Associate, Department of Pharmaceutics, University of Washington, Seattle, Washington

R. Eugene Ramsay, MD Professor of Neurology and Psychiatry, Department of Neurology, University of Miami School of Medicine, Miami, Florida

Andrew D. Randall, MA, PhD Head of Neurophysiology and Neuropharmacology, Department of Neurology, GlaxoSmithKline, Harlow, Essex, United Kingdom

Alan Richens, MD, PhD Emeritus Professor of Pharmacology and Therapeutics, Department of Pharmacology and Therapeutics, University of Wales College of Medicine, Cardiff, United Kingdom

K. Wayne Riggs, PhD Professor, Faculty of Pharmaceutical Sciences, University of British Columbia, Vancouver, British Columbia, Canada

Roberto Riva, MD Research Assistant, Department of Neurological Sciences, University of Bologna, Bologna, Italy

Michael A. Rogawski, MD, PhD Chief, Epilepsy Research Station, National Institute of Neurological Disorders and Stroke, National Institutes of Health, Bethesda, Maryland

Rajesh C. Sachdeo, MD Clinical Professor of Neurology, Department of Neurology, University of Medicine and Dentistry of New Jersey, Robert Wood Johnson Medical School; and Director, Comprehensive Epilepsy Center, Robert Wood University Hospital, New Brunswick, New Jersey

Steven C. Schachter, MD Associate Professor, Department of Neurology, Harvard Medical School; and Director of Clinical Trials, Beth Israel Deaconess Medical Center, Boston, Massachusetts

Richard D. Scheyer, MD Director, Clinical Discover and Human Pharmacology, Aventis Pharmaceuticals, Bridgewater, New Jersey

Bernd Schmidt, MD, PhD Head, Department of Neurology and Psychiatric Clinic, Wittnau Hospital, Wittnau, Germany

Dieter Schmidt, MD Head, Epilepsy Research Group Section, Berlin, Germany

Dorothy D. Schottelius, PhD Research Scientist, Department of Neurology, University of Iowa, Iowa City, Iowa

Masakazu Seino, MD Honorary President, National Epilepsy Center, Shizuoka, Medical Institute of Neurological Diseases, Shizuoka, Japan

Jaymin Shah, PhD Director, Clinical Pharmacology, Elan Pharmaceuticals, South, San Francisco, California

Kent Shellenberger, PhD Vice President, Clinical Affairs, Elan Pharmaceuticals, South San Francisco, California

Melvin D. Shelton, MD, PhD Clinical Trials Section, Mood Disorders Program, Assistant Professor of Psychiatry, Case Western Reserve University School of Medicine, University Hospitals of Cleveland, Cleveland, Ohio

Danny D. Shen, PhD Professor, Department of Pharmacy and Pharmaceutics, University of Washington, Seattle, Washington

Allan L. Sherwin, MD, FRCP(C) Professor of Neurology, Department of Neurology and Neurosurgery, McGill University; and Emeritus Neurologist, Montreal Neurological Hospital and Institute, Montreal, Quebec, Canada

Stephen D. Silberstein, MD, FACP Professor of Neurology, Department of Neurology, Jefferson Medical College; and Director, Jefferson Headache Center, Thomas Jefferson University, Philadelphia, Pennsylvania

R. Duane Sofia, PhD Vice President, Department of Preclinical Research, Wallace Laboratories, Incorporated, Cranbury, New Jersey

Kenneth W. Sommerville, MD Medical Director, Neuroscience, Department of Marketed Products, Clincial Research, Abbott Laboratories, Abbott Park, Illinois

Edoardo Spina, MD, PhD Associate Professor, Section of Pharmacology, Department of Clinical and Experimental Medicine and Pharmacology, University of Messina, Policlinico Universitario, Messina, Italy

James P. Stables, BS(Pharm) Program Director, Anticonvulsant Screening Project, Technology Development Cluster, NINDS, National Institutes of Health, Rockville, Maryland

Alessandro Stefani, MD Diplomate Neuroscienze, University of Tor Vergata, Rome, Italy

Linda J. Stephen, MBChB, MRCGP Honorary Clinical Teacher, Department of Medicine and Therapeutics, University of Glasgow; and Deputy Director, Epilepsy Unit, Western Infirmary, Glasgow, Scotland, United Kingdom

Anthony J. Streeter, PhD Research Fellow, Department of Drug Metabolism, Johnson & Johnson Pharmaceutical Research and Development, Spring House, Pennsylvania

David A. Sun, PhD Research Scientist, Department of Neurology, Virginia Commonwealth University, Medical College of Virginia, Richmond, Virginia

Alan C. Swann, MD Pat R. Rutherford, Jr. Professor and Vice Chair for Research, Department of Psychiatry, University of Texas Health Science Center, Houston, Texas

Carlo Alberto Tassinari, MD Neurological Chief, Department of Neurological Sciences, University of Bologna, Bologna, Italy

Charles P. Taylor, PhD Director, Department of CNS Pharmacology, Pfizer Global Research and Development, Ann Arbor, Michigan

Torbjörn Tomson, MD, PhD Department of Neurology, Karolinska Hospital, Stockholm, Sweden

Michael R. Trimble, MD Professor of Behavioral Neurology, Department of Neurology, Institute of Neurology, London, United Kingdom

Roy E. Twyman, MD Senior Director, Department of Clinical Development, R.W. Johnson Pharmaceutical Research Institute, Raritan, New Jersey

Frank J. E. Vajda, MD, FRACP Professorial Fellow, Department of Medicine, University of Melbourne; and Director, Raoul Wallenberg Australian Center for Clinical Neuropharmacology, St. Vincent's Hospital, Victoria, Australia

H. Steve White, PhD Profesor, Department of Pharmacology and Toxicology; and Director, Anticonvulsant Screening Project, University of Utah, Salt Lake City, Utah

Karen S. Wilcox, PhD Research Assistant Professor, Department of Pharmacology and Toxicology, University of Utah, Salt Lake City, Utah

B. Joe Wilder, MD Associate Professor, Department of Medicine, University of Toronto, Toronto, Ontario, Canada

L. James Willmore, MD Associate Dean and Professor, Department of Neurology and Pharmacology and Physiology, Saint Louis University School of Medicine; and Attending Neurologist, Department of Neurology, Saint Louis University Hospital, Saint Louis, Missouri

Harold H. Wolf Professor, Department of Pharmacology and Toxicology, University of Utah, Salt Lake City

José H. Woodhead, MD Department of Pharmacology and Toxicology, University of Utah, Salt Lake City, Utah

Colleen J. Wurden, PhD Research Associate, Department of Pharmaceutics, University of Washington School of Pharmacy and Medicine, Seattle, Washington

PREFACE

The 5th edition of *Antiepileptic Drugs* embodies the recent unprecedented expansion of the field of epilepsy as a clinical and scientific discipline as well as the concomitant progress achieved in the treatment modalities for this disease. As never before, antiepileptic drugs occupy a place of preeminence in neuropharmacology. Since the last edition, the number of clinically useful agents has continued to increase to the point that some speak of a "plethora" of antiepileptic drugs. This 5th edition includes 16 drugs even when benzodiapines, barbiturates and hydantoins are each counted as "one" drug. Clinicians are now challenged to develop rational therapeutic algorithms that include all the newly available agents. Indeed, as clinical experience accumulates with the "new drugs" of the last edition, particularly gabapentin, lamotrigine and topiramate, the distinction between "old" and "new" drugs is becoming blurred.

The straightforward format that has characterized previous editions has been retained and enhanced. The introductory section on General Principles has been modified with increased emphasis on the contributions and limitations of clinical trials and the importance of patient-related factors in the optimal use of drug therapy. New chapters have been added to discuss the treatment of status epilepticus as well as potential strategies for prevention of epileptogenesis. With respect to the section dealing with individual agents, the 16 drugs have been listed in alphabetical order from benzodiazepines to zonisamide. Presentation of information on each of these compounds has been modified by combining the aspects of chemistry, biotransformation and pharmacokinetics in one chapter and by adding, where appropriate, new chapters reflecting indications outside of epilepsy such as migraine prophylaxis, neuropathic pain and psychiatric disorders. Drugs with limited use (felbamate, primidone, vigabatrin) have been covered in a single chapter. The last section has been reduced in size to include only two drugs in clinical development, with an overview of drugs at earlier stages of development.

Authors who contributed to previous editions have updated their chapters and new authors have been selected on the basis of their expertise. The editors are aware of the potential conflict of interest that could arise when some authors from the pharmaceutical industry were invited to write about a drug marketed by their company. However, this could hardly be avoided, especially for chapters dealing with investigational drugs or areas of research (e.g., new indications) with little information in the public domain.

This edition has been targeted to meet the interests of various audiences. The book should be of special value to all neurologists and physicians involved in the treatment of epilepsy, but also to psychiatrists and to clinicians who manage patients with bipolar disorder, migraine, neuropathic pain and many other conditions in which antiepileptic drugs are increasingly used. The book should also be useful to academicians with an interest in epilepsy, and to pharmacologists, clinical pharmacists, and scientists involved in research and development of new antiepileptic drugs.

The editors wish to express their gratitude to the many distinguished authors who dedicated their invaluable time and expertise to contribute to this book. Special thanks are also due to Brian Rasmussen (University of Washington) and Raymond Reter (Lippincott Williams & Wilkins) for their diligence and heroic efforts in attending to the needs of all contributors and bringing this project to completion. The editors also thank Dr. Anne Sydor (Lippincott Williams & Wilkins) for her leadership and support. We all hope that this work, by facilitating dissemination of up-to-date information on drug therapy, will contribute to our common goal of improving the life of the over 50 million persons who suffer from epilepsy worldwide.

ANTIEPILEPTIC DRUGS

FIFTH EDITION

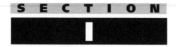

GENERAL PRINCIPLES

GENERAL PRINCIPLES

PRINCIPLES OF ANTIEPILEPTIC DRUG ACTION

MICHAEL A. ROGAWSKI

The ideal antiepileptic drug protects against seizures without adversely affecting the function of the central nervous system and inducing side effects that impair the patient's quality of life. Because seizure activity represents a subtle functional perturbation of the normal physiologic activity of the nervous system, this goal is difficult to attain. Nevertheless, the identification by Merritt and Putnam in 1938 of phenytoin as the first nonsedating anticonvulsant demonstrated that the goal is achievable (1), and in recent years drug screening in animal models has uncovered a wide variety of chemical compounds with excellent anticonvulsant efficacy and a low incidence of side effects.

To exhibit anticonvulsant activity, a drug must act on one or more target molecules in the brain. These targets may include ion channels, neurotransmitter transporters, and neurotransmitter metabolic enzymes. The ultimate effect of these interactions is to modify the bursting properties of neurons and reduce synchronization in neuronal ensembles. In addition, anticonvulsant drugs inhibit the spread of abnormal firing to distant sites (2). Synchronous epileptiform activity in localized neuronal ensembles is associated with interictal spike activity, but is not sufficient for the expression of behavioral seizure activity. Rather, the expression of partial seizures requires the recruitment and synchronization of a large cortical mass, and the ability to interfere with the spread of epileptiform activity is likely to be an essential feature of anticonvulsant drugs that are useful in the treatment of partial seizures. Similarly, generalized seizures, which by definition are associated with bilateral cortical involvement, are believed to result from thalamocortical synchronization (3). Interference with the rhythm-generating mechanisms that underlie this synchronized activity is necessary to abort these seizures.

The mechanisms of action of most antiepileptic drugs is not known with certainty. All drugs—including antiepileptic drugs—have a diversity of actions on biologic systems,

only some of which are related to the desired therapeutic effect. It often is difficult to select from among the many pharmacologic effects of any drug just those that are relevant to its therapeutic activity in epilepsy. This is largely because the fundamental pathophysiology of epilepsy is incompletely understood, and any alteration of the excitability properties of neurons could potentially be relevant to anticonvulsant effects. Moreover, many anticonvulsant drugs appear to act through multiple complementary mechanisms, and indeed this may be an important way in which anticonvulsant drugs that target critical brain excitability systems are able to protect against seizure activity with relatively low central nervous system toxicity (4). Nevertheless, it is convenient to categorize antiepileptic drug actions according to those that involve (a) modulation of voltage-dependent ion channels, (b) enhancement of synaptic inhibition, and (c) inhibition synaptic excitation. Voltage-dependent ion channels (including sodium, calcium, and potassium channels) shape the subthreshold electrical behavior of the neuron, allow it to fire action potentials, regulate its responsiveness to synaptic signals, contribute to the paroxysmal depolarizing shift (the single-cell correlate of the interictal discharge), and ultimately are integral to the generation of seizure discharges. In addition, voltage-dependent ion channels are critical elements in neurotransmitter release, which is required for synaptic transmission. Consequently, they are key targets for anticonvulsants that inhibit epileptic bursting, synchronization, and seizure spread. Synaptic inhibition and excitation are mediated by neurotransmitter-regulated channels; these channels permit synchronization of neural ensembles and allow propagation of the abnormal discharge to local and distant sites. Anticonvulsants that modify excitatory and inhibitory neurotransmission therefore also can suppress bursting and, when they inhibit synaptic excitation, can have prominent effects on seizure spread.

Which ion channels are relevant to the actions of antiepileptic drugs? Studies in animal models have demonstrated that anticonvulsant effects can be achieved by blockade of sodium or calcium channels, and probably also through facilitation of potassium channels (as may be the case for reti-

Michael A. Rogawski, MD, PhD: Chief, Epilepsy Research Section, National Institute of Neurological Disorders and Stroke, National Institutes of Health, Bethesda, Maryland

gabine) (5). Anticonvulsant effects are also well known to be produced by drugs that enhance inhibition mediated by γ-aminobutyric acid type A (GABA_A) receptors (and in some cases, also possibly GABA_B receptors), or through effects on glycine systems, the regionally specific transmitter systems (including monoamines such as catecholamines, serotonin, and histamine, and neuropeptides, including opioid peptides and neuropeptide Y), and the inhibitory neuromodulator adenosine (6–8). In addition, blockade of excitatory amino receptors [including those of the *N*-methyl-D-aspartate (NMDA), α-amino-3-hydroxy-5-methyl-4-isoxazole propionate (AMPA), metabotropic and possibly also kainate types] also can protect against seizures. In principle, it may be possible to prevent the occurrence of seizures by targeting any one or a combination of these systems. In fact, the development of antiepileptic drugs by screening in animal models that are nonbiased with respect to mechanism has uncovered drugs that act by a number of these mechanisms. In many cases, the relevant mechanisms are not shared by other agents. Indeed, it is safe to say that no two marketed drugs works in exactly the same way. This chapter focuses mainly on those molecular targets relevant to the actions of clinically important antiepileptic drugs. Information on additional drug targets of research interest is available (6).

MOLECULAR TARGETS OF ANTIEPILEPTIC DRUGS

Voltage-Gated Sodium Channels

Overview

Brain voltage-gated sodium channels are the molecular targets of a number of chemically diverse antiepileptic drugs.

All of these drugs act by inhibiting ionic current through the channel, but the precise way in which this results in protection against seizures is incompletely understood (9). Nevertheless, the molecular detail through which prototypical sodium channel blocking anticonvulsants such as phenytoin and lamotrigine interact with sodium channels has been extensively characterized.

Voltage-gated sodium channels are responsible for the rising phase of neuronal action potentials. When neurons are depolarized to action potential threshold by an excitatory synaptic input, the sodium channel protein senses the depolarization and within a few hundred microseconds undergoes a conformational change that converts the channel from the closed (deactivated), nonconducting, resting state to the conducting open state that permits sodium flux. Within a few milliseconds, the channel inactivates, terminating the flow of sodium ions. The channel must then be repolarized before it can be activated again by a subsequent depolarization. Brain sodium channels can rapidly cycle through the resting, open, and inactivated states, allowing brain neurons to fire trains of action potentials at high frequency, as is required for normal brain function and for the expression of epileptic activity.

Sodium Channel Structure

The sodium channel from mammalian brain is a complex of α (260 kd), β1(36 kd), and β2 (33 kd) protein subunits (10). The α subunit forms the ion-conducting pore of the channel and also contains the machinery required for voltage-dependent gating. The β subunits are not required for functional activity of the sodium channel, but modulate channel expression and alter the gating properties. α Sub-

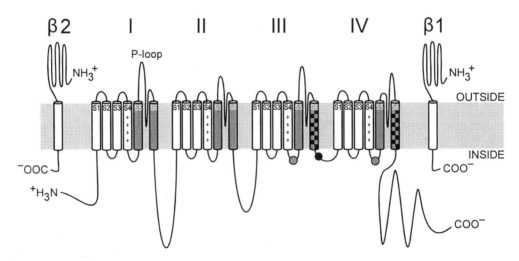

FIGURE 1.1. Primary structures of the subunits of brain type II voltage-gated sodium channels. The main α subunit, consisting of four homologous repeats (I to IV), is shown flanked by the two auxiliary β subunits. Cylinders represent probable α-helical transmembrane segments. Dark gray α-helical segments are believed to form the pore region; P-loops form the outer pore and ion selectivity filter. Plus signs indicate S4 voltage sensors; black circle, inactivation particle in inactivation gate loop ("tethered pore blocker"); and gray circles, sites implicated in forming the receptor for the inactivation gate. IIIS6 and IVS6 (patterned) are regions of modulatory drug binding, including sodium channel blocking anticonvulsants.

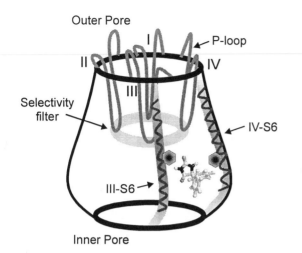

FIGURE 1.2. Schematic illustration of the pore of the voltage-gated sodium channel α-subunit. The S5 and S6 transmembrane α-helical segments from each homologous repeat (I to IV) form the four walls of the pore. The outer pore mouth and ion selectivity filter are formed by reentrant P-loops. The critical α-helical S6 segments in repeat III and IV, which contain the anticonvulsant binding sites (hexagons), are emphasized. A phenytoin molecule is illustrated in association with its binding sites.

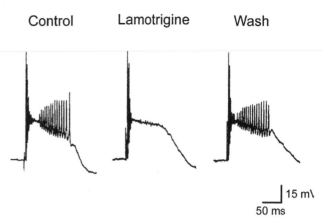

FIGURE 1.3. Lamotrigine (50 μmol/L), a sodium channel blocking anticonvulsant, selectively inhibits epileptiform afterdischarges in CA1 hippocampal neurons without affecting initial action potential responses. The intracellular recording was carried out in a rat hippocampal slice under magnesium-free conditions (to enhance NMDA receptor responses) and in the presence of 20 μmol/L bicuculline (to block GABA$_A$ receptors). Synaptic responses were evoked with Schaffer collateral/commissural fiber stimulation. (From Xie X, Lancaster B, Peakman T, et al. Interaction of the antiepileptic drug lamotrigine with recombinant rat brain type IIA Na$^+$ channels and with native Na$^+$ channels in rat hippocampal neurones. *Pflugers Arch* 1995;430:437–446, with permission.)

units have six α-helical transmembrane segments (S1 to S6) in each of the four homologous domains (I to IV) and a reentrant loop ("P-loop") between transmembrane segments S5 and S6 that dips into the membrane and forms the narrower outer pore and the ion selectivity filter (Figures 1.1 and 1.2). The four subunit-like domains are believed to form a square array in the membrane, with an ion-conducting pore in the center. Each domain contains a number of positively charged amino acid residues in the S4 segment that serve as the voltage sensor that couples membrane depolarization to channel opening and to fast inactivation (11).

Anticonvulsant Modulation of Sodium Channels

Modulation of the gating of brain sodium channels is believed at least in part to account for the anticonvulsant activity of several antiepileptic drugs, including phenytoin, lamotrigine, carbamazepine, oxcarbazepine (12,13), zonisamide (14) and possibly also felbamate (15) and topiramate (16). Antiepileptic agents that act on sodium channels characteristically exhibit protective activity in the maximal electroshock test, a widely used animal model for the screening of anticonvulsant drugs, and they are effective in the treatment of partial and generalized tonic-clonic seizures in humans (9,17,18). These drugs have the unique property that they block high-frequency repetitive spike firing, as is believed to occur during the spread of seizure activity, without affecting ordinary ongoing neural activity (Figure 1.3). This accounts for their ability to protect against seizures without causing a generalized impairment of brain function.

An understanding of the basis by which sodium channel anticonvulsants selectively inhibit high-frequency action potential firing has come from voltage-clamp studies, which allow the kinetic properties of ion channel gating and the voltage dependence of drug action to be characterized in detail. These studies have shown that at hyperpolarized membrane potentials, clinically relevant concentrations of drugs such as phenytoin and lamotrigine produce only a weak block of sodium channels (19,20) (Figure 1.4). However, when the membrane is depolarized, there is a marked increase in the degree of tonic inhibition. For example, the inhibitory potency of phenytoin for recombinant type IIA sodium channels (the predominant form in brain neurons) increases more than 100-fold when the membrane is depolarized from −90 to −60 mV (20) (Figure 1.4B). Moreover, the inhibitory potency is strongly "use-dependent," which means that block accumulates with repetitive activation (Figure 1.4C). These properties of block are explained by preferential binding of the drug to inactivated conformations of the channel. For example, the affinity of phenytoin for inactivated sodium channels is of the order of 7 μmol/L—well within the therapeutic concentration in the cerebrospinal fluid of 4 to 8 μmol/L—whereas its affinity for resting sodium channels is >600 μmol/L (21). Similarly, it is estimated that lamotrigine binds to the inactivated state with an affinity of 7 to 12 μmol/L, which also is within the estimated therapeutic brain concentration range of 10 to 30 μmol/L, whereas the affinity for the resting state is 40- to 200-fold lower (20,22). The effects of these agents at clinically relevant concentrations are mainly on action potential firing; the drug does not directly alter excitatory or

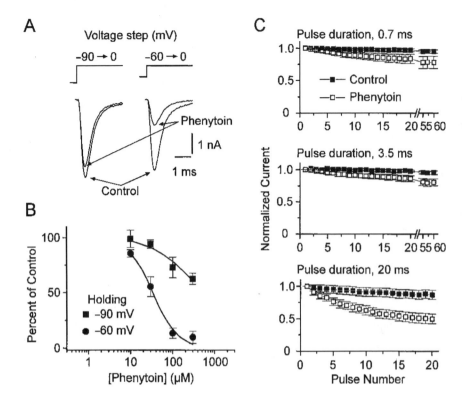

FIGURE 1.4. Voltage-dependent and use-dependent block of human type IIA sodium channels by phenytoin. **A:** Phenytoin (50 μmol/L) inhibits sodium current activated from a holding potential of –60 mV more strongly than from a holding potential of –90 mV. **B:** Concentration–response relationship for phenytoin block of peak sodium current activated from the two holding potentials. There is nearly a 15-fold increase in potency when the current is activated from the more depolarized holding potential. **C:** Accumulation of block with repeated sodium channel activation and inactivation. The extent of use-dependent inhibition increases for longer pulse durations, in which the sodium channels are maintained in the inactivated state for longer times. Currents were normalized to the amplitude of the first pulse in the presence of phenytoin, so that tonic block is not represented. Voltage-clamp recordings are from cloned human brain type IIA α subunits stably expressed in Chinese hamster ovary cells. (From Xie X, Dale TJ, John VH, et al. Electrophysiological and pharmacological properties of the human brain type IIA Na+ channel expressed in a stable mammalian cell line. *Pflugers Arch* 2001;441:425–433, with permission.)

inhibitory synaptic responses. However, the effect on action potentials does ultimately translate into reduced transmitter output at synapses (see later).

In recent years, the mechanism of sodium channel inactivation has been elucidated and this has provided an opportunity to clarify the way in which phenytoin and other sodium channel blocking anticonvulsants appear to promote channel inactivation. The normal predominant (fast) inactivation process results from occlusion of the intracellular mouth of the channel by a short loop of amino acid residues between domains III and IV of the sodium channel α subunit that serves as a "tethered pore blocker" (Figure 1.1). An additional inactivation process referred to as *slow inactivation* begins to come into play with more prolonged depolarizations, such as might occur in association with epileptiform activity. This distinct inactivation mechanism, which is coupled to slow recovery, appears to involve different structural domains of the sodium channel (23), including the outer pore region (24). Phenytoin induces a nonconducting state of the channel that is similar to channel inactivation. This can occur even in sodium channels where fast inactivation has been eliminated by enzymatic removal of the inactivation loop (25). Therefore, phenytoin does not act by stabilizing the normal inactivation state. Rather, phenytoin induces an inactivated state with distinct kinetic properties. Recovery from drug block of the channel occurs much more slowly than does recovery from block by the intrinsic pore blocker (26). This, in part, accounts for phenytoin's unique ability selectively to block high-

frequency firing because, when recovery is slow, block can accumulate during repetitive activation of the channel.

An additional critical feature of phenytoin and lamotrigine block of sodium channels (and one that distinguishes these drugs from local anesthetics) is the slow onset of block. [Rate constants for both phenytoin and lamotrigine are ~10^4 mol/L^{-1} s^{-1} (21,22).] This may result from a strict stereospecific requirement for binding in which only a small fraction of collisions between the drug and the channel acceptor site result in binding (21). However, once binding occurs, it is tight, and unbinding (recovery from block) is slow. Slow binding has two important implications. First, slow binding implies that the time course of sodium currents is not altered in the presence of the drug, and therefore the kinetic properties of action potentials are not perturbed. Second, slow binding means that inhibition of action potentials does not occur with firing induced by synaptic depolarizations of ordinary length. Rather, long depolarizations are required, possibly as long as a few seconds or greater. In focal epilepsies, the cellular events that characterize ictal discharges are sustained depolarizations that evoke intermittent high-frequency bursts of action potentials. Such depolarizations provide the conditions required for drug binding and block. On the other hand, cortical interictal discharges are of shorter duration, and this corresponds with the electroencephalographic concept that such discharges are unaffected by phenytoin. Overall, sodium channel blocking anticonvulsants are expected to have little effect on the physiologic generation of action potentials in well polarized neurons. The voltage- and use-dependent characteristics of block would come into play only during pathologic sustained depolarizing events associated with high-frequency discharges, thus allowing protection against seizures without interfering with normal function.

Anticonvulsant Binding Domain

Studies with mixtures of phenytoin, carbamazepine, and lamotrigine have revealed that these drugs bind to a common recognition site on sodium channels (27). Although these three compounds are structurally dissimilar, they do contain a common motif of two phenyl groups separated by one to two C–C or C–N single bonds (1.5 to 3 Å) (Figure 1.5). These two phenyl groups probably are critical elements in binding. Phenytoin is active in its neutral, uncharged form. Therefore, binding of phenytoin with its receptor on sodium channels is nonionic and involves hydrophobic or induced-dipole interactions. In rat brain type IIA sodium channels, mutations of specific phenylalanine (1764) and tyrosine (1771) residues in the S6 segment of domain IV—a stretch of amino acids that contributes to the inner lining of the channel pore—dramatically reduces the potency for use-dependent block by phenytoin and local anesthetics. This occurs because of decreased drug affinity for the inactivated channel conformation. Thus, transmembrane segment IVS6 likely contributes to the anticonvulsant and local anesthetic receptor. In addition, mutational analysis has revealed that the pore lining residues leucine 1465 and isoleucine 1469 in IIIS6 also form a portion of the high-affinity binding site for sodium channel blocking anticonvulsants (28). The aromatic rings in the anticonvulsant molecules may interact with the aromatic side chains of the critical residues in the IVS6 segment or with the nonpolar side chains of the IIIS6 residues. It is noteworthy that this region of the sodium channel also is implicated in inactivation gating (29). Gating movements of the IIIS6 and IVS6 segments may allow access of the anticonvulsants to their receptor site, which becomes available as the channel opens and increases in affinity as it inactivates.

Differences in Kinetics of Block among Sodium Channel Blocking Anticonvulsants

Although carbamazepine, phenytoin, and lamotrigine interact with sodium channels in a similar fashion at the same binding site, there are quantitative differences in the rate and extent of block. Thus, carbamazepine has approximately threefold lower binding affinity for the inactivated state of the channel (apparent dissociation constant, 25 µmol/L), and the extent of steady-state block at therapeutic concentrations is estimated to be modestly lower (30). However, the binding rate of carbamazepine is approximately five times faster (3.8×10^4 mol/L^{-1} s^{-1}), so that it might be effective in situations where the ictal depolarizations are shorter. In view of the kinetic differences between drugs, the use of combinations of sodium channel blocking anticonvulsants is perhaps not as illogical as it would seem.

Persistent Sodium Current

In addition to effects on the fast sodium current responsible for action potentials, blockade of persistent (noninactivating) sodium currents also may be an important mechanism of anticonvulsant drug action. Persistent sodium current flows through a portion of the same sodium channels that normally give rise to the fast sodium current but temporarily fail to inactivate for an extended period (31). The current carried by the persistent openings is a minute fraction of the fast current. However, this current may play a key role in regulating excitability near firing threshold because it is largely unopposed by other voltage-activated currents in this range of membrane potentials. Moreover, there is evidence that the persistent sodium current con-

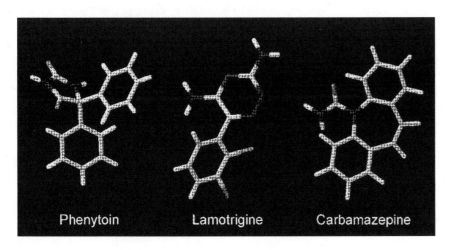

FIGURE 1.5. Comparison of the three-dimensional structures of sodium channel blocking anticonvulsants. The anticonvulsants are structurally dissimilar: phenytoin is a hydantoin (a cyclic ureide); lamotrigine is a dichlorophenyl-triazine; and carbamazepine is a dibenzazepine that is structurally related to the tricyclic antidepressants. The structures are shown to indicate the similar but not superimposable orientations of the phenyl rings (1,2,4-triazine ring in lamotrigine), suggesting the comparable ways in which the drugs may bind to sodium channels.

tributes to the initiation and maintenance of epileptiform activity (32). Several authors have reported that phenytoin (32–34) and topiramate (16) inhibit persistent sodium current at concentrations lower than those that block fast sodium current. The selective reduction of late sodium channel openings may contribute to the ability of these drugs to protect against seizures with minimal interference in normal function.

GABA Systems

Potentiation of inhibitory neurotransmission is a key mechanism of antiepileptic drug action. Although a variety of neurotransmitters, including biogenic amines (e.g., norepinephrine, serotonin) and neuropeptides (e.g., opioid peptides, neuropeptide Y), can mediate inhibition of neuronal excitability through presynaptic or postsynaptic mechanisms, GABA is the major inhibitory neurotransmitter in the forebrain. Neurons that use GABA as their neurotransmitter—mainly interneurons—represent only a small fraction of central nervous system neurons, and in cortical regions critical to epileptogenesis, excitatory synapses may be severalfold more common anatomically than inhibitory ones. However, these inhibitory connections are critically important in restraining the natural tendency of recurrently connected excitatory neurons to transition through positive feedback into synchronized epileptiform discharges.

All clinically relevant antiepileptic drugs that enhance inhibition do so through an action at GABA synapses. GABA acts through fast Cl⁻-permeable ionotropic GABA$_A$ receptors and also through slower metabotropic G-protein–coupled GABA$_B$ receptors. Reduction in the efficacy of synaptic inhibition mediated by GABA$_A$ receptors—for example, with drugs that block GABA$_A$ receptors, like bicuculline and pentylenetetrazol—can lead to seizures. Moreover, rare naturally occurring mutations in the γ subunit of GABA$_A$ receptors have been associated with increased seizure susceptibility in humans (35,36). Conversely, pharmacologic enhancement of GABA$_A$ receptor–mediated synaptic inhibition is an effective anticonvulsant approach. This can occur through a direct action on GABA$_A$ receptors, or indirectly by blockade of the enzymes and transporters responsible for terminating the synaptic actions of GABA. Drugs that act through these mechanisms typically have a broad spectrum of anticonvulsant activity in human seizure disorders, although—with the exception of benzodiazepine receptor agonists—they usually are ineffective in absence seizures.

GABA$_A$ Receptors

Overview

GABA$_A$ receptors are members of the ligand-gated ion channel superfamily, which includes nicotinic acetyl-choline, 5-HT$_3$, and strychnine-sensitive glycine receptors (37,38). Members of this superfamily are heterooligomeric pentamers (Figure 1.6). The protein subunits that constitute the pentamer in GABA$_A$ receptors have a large extracellular amino terminus, four hydrophobic transmembrane domains (M1-4), and a large intracellular domain between M3 and M4. GABA$_A$ receptor subunit proteins are classified into subfamilies termed α, β, γ, δ, ε and θ (Figure 1.7). There are six α subunits, four β subunits (with two splice variants), three γ subunits (with two splice variants), and one each of δ, ε, and θ. In addition, there are two ρ subunits (GABA$_C$ receptors), mainly expressed in the retina, that do not coassemble with other subfamily members and have unique pharmacologic properties. Although more than 2,000 combinations of subunits are theoretically possible, most GABA$_A$ receptors are believed to be composed of α, β, and γ subunits with stoichiometry of 2:2:1. The δ, ε, and θ subunits can replace the γ subunit in some receptor subtypes.

The pharmacology of GABA$_A$ receptors is the best developed and most complex of any of the ligand-gated ion channels. A large number of structurally specific recognition sites for drugs and chemicals have been identified on the receptor–channel complex . However, from the point of view of clinically relevant anticonvulsant drug actions, modulation by benzodiazepine-like agents and barbiturates is of most significance, although felbamate (39) and topiramate (40,41) may also act, in part, through effects on GABA$_A$ receptors. Moreover, there is emerging evidence that neurosteroids—endogenous metabolites of progesterone that act as barbiturate-like modulators of GABA$_A$ receptors—may contribute to hormonal influences on seizure susceptibility (42).

Benzodiazepines

Benzodiazepine receptor agonists, such as diazepam and lorazepam, do not directly activate GABA$_A$ receptors. Rather, they act as positive allosteric modulators to enhance the action of GABA by increasing the frequency of channel openings induced by GABA (43) [and possibly by increasing the single-channel conductance of low-conductance channels (44)]. The sensitivity of GABA$_A$ receptors to benzodiazepines is highly subunit dependent (45). The γ2 subunit is required for full benzodiazepine-positive allosteric modulation. Benzodiazepine activity is reduced when γ2 is replaced by γ1 or γ3, and eliminated if γ is absent or is replaced by δ or ε. The critical nature of the γ2 subunit for benzodiazepine modulation is demonstrated by the nearly complete lack of benzodiazepine activity in γ2 subunit–deficient mice (46).

Benzodiazepine modulation also depends on the α subunit. GABA$_A$ receptors containing the α4 and α6 subunits do not respond to classic benzodiazepines such as diazepam. These subunits have an arginine instead of a histidine at a

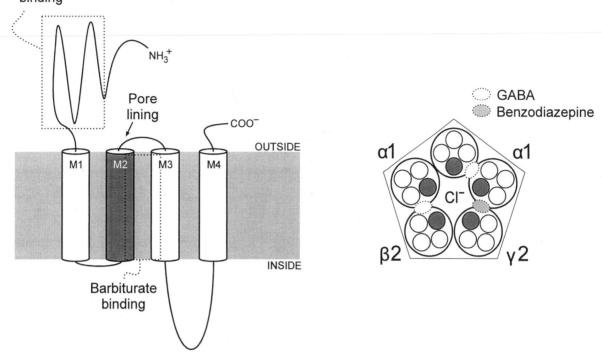

FIGURE 1.6. Left: Primary structure and membrane topology of GABA$_A$ receptor subunits. Residues identified as critical for agonist (GABA) and benzodiazepine binding are in the extracellular amino terminus. The specific residues contributing to binding of the two types of ligands are distinct. Barbiturate binding occurs to the membrane-spanning M2 and M3 segments. **Right:** Schematic illustration of the pentameric structure of GABA$_A$ receptors. Small circles represent membrane-spanning α-helical segments corresponding to those shown in diagram at left. M2 segments form the Cl$^-$ channel pore. Agonist and benzodiazepine binding domains are at homologous positions at subunit interfaces. There are two agonist binding sites and a single benzodiazepine binding site in each GABA$_A$ receptor complex. The α1β2γ2 subunit configuration represents a common GABA$_A$ receptor type.

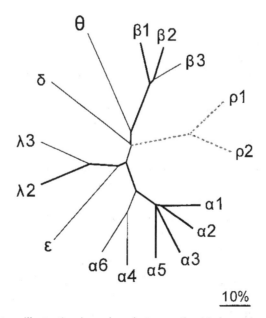

FIGURE 1.7. Radial tree illustrating homology between the 16 cloned human GABA$_A$ receptor subunits. The most abundant subunits in brain are identified by thick line segments. Homomeric receptors composed of ρ subunits, which are expressed primarily in retina, have distinct pharmacologic properties similar to GABA$_C$ receptors as defined by Johnston (167); the extent to which these subunits form heteromeric assemblies with conventional GABA$_A$ receptor subunits is uncertain (168). Homology analysis was produced with ClustalW using NCBI RefSeq records. Scale bar indicates 10% identity.

conserved position, which in the α1 and α2 subunits is position 101. Replacement of this histidine with arginine in the α1 subunit markedly reduces the anticonvulsant (and also sedative and amnestic) activity of diazepam, but does not alter the anxiolytic properties, indicating that the anticonvulsant activity of benzodiazepines in part involves receptors containing the α1 subunit, whereas the anxiolytic actions seem to be mediated by receptors that contain α2, α3, or α5 subunits (47,48). Mutational analysis has further indicated that the benzodiazepine binding pocket of the GABA$_A$ receptor lies at the interface between the α and γ subunits, with residues from each subunit contributing to the benzodiazepine recognition site (49) (Figure 1.6). This site is in a homologous position to the two agonist (GABA) binding sites at the interface between other subunits.

In clinical practice, benzodiazepines have an important role in the acute treatment of status epilepticus. However, two significant limitations largely preclude their use in chronic therapy. The first limitation is the undesirable side effects, including sedation and muscle relaxation, that occur at doses comparable with those that protect against seizures. The second, and probably more important limitation (because side effects tend to diminish in time) relates to the tolerance that develops with chronic use. In animal models, benzodiazepine receptor partial agonists can exhibit anticonvulsant activity without sedative actions (6). These agents also may have reduced tolerance liability. However, in human trials none of these agents has been sufficiently free of side effects and tolerance liability to be clinically useful (50). The development of benzodiazepine receptor ligands that selectively target GABA$_A$ receptor subtypes in a way that confers anticonvulsant activity and avoids these limitations is a goal that has yet to be realized. However, compounds such as AWD 131-138 [1-(4-chlorophenyl)-4-morpholino-imidazolin-2-one], a weak partial benzodiazepine receptor agonist currently in development that seems to lack tolerance liability, may hold promise (51).

Benzodiazepines and Absence Seizures

Hypersynchronous activity in thalamocortical circuits is believed to underlie the 3-Hz spike-and-wave activity characteristic of generalized absence seizures (3,52). The well recognized antiabsence activity of benzodiazepines, such as clonazepam, likely resides in their ability to "desynchronize" these oscillations. Thalamocortical relay neurons and corticothalamic neurons form a mutually excitatory loop whose oscillatory behavior is regulated by inhibitory GABAergic connections to relay neurons from the reticular thalamic nucleus (RTN). In addition to inhibiting relay neurons, RTN neurons send recurrent collaterals to neighboring inhibitory neurons in the RTN. This intranuclear inhibition normally diminishes synchronous firing in the RTN and reduces the inhibitory output below that required for absence seizure activity (53). GABA$_A$ receptors on RTN neurons appear to be highly sensitive to benzodiazepines,

possibly more so than GABA$_A$ receptors on relay neurons. Thus, by selectively enhancing the strength of recurrent inhibition in the RTN, benzodiazepines may promote endogenous antiabsence mechanisms.

Phenobarbital, Felbamate, and Topiramate

Barbiturates, including phenobarbital, also act as positive allosteric modulators of GABA$_A$ receptors, but this occurs in a way distinct from the action of benzodiazepines (Figure 1.8A). GABA-activated chloride channels open in "bursts," interrupted by frequent brief closures. The openings in bursts can be classified into groups with brief, intermediate, and long average durations; longer openings are associated with more prolonged bursts. As the concentration of GABA is increased, the channels open more frequently and enter the longer-lived open states proportionately more often. At clinically relevant concentrations, phenobarbital does not increase the frequency of GABA-induced channel opening, but rather shifts the relative proportion of openings to favor the longest-lived open state associated with prolonged bursting, thus increasing the overall probability that the channel is open (37). In addition, barbiturates have actions on other ion channel systems, including calcium (see later) and sodium channels (54), that likely contribute to their therapeutic activity and may also be a factor in side effects. Apart from their modulatory actions on GABA$_A$ receptors, barbiturates (unlike benzodiazepines) directly activate GABA$_A$ receptors in the absence of GABA (55) (Figure 1.8B). This direct action, which occurs at higher concentrations than the modulatory action, also is likely to contribute to the sedative side effects of phenobarbital. The single-channel conductance of GABA$_A$ receptor channels is similar when the channels are activated by GABA, barbiturates, and the two together, indicating that the structure of the pore is similar when the gate is opened by GABA or barbiturates. However, the macroscopic and single-channel currents directly activated by barbiturates have kinetic properties distinct from barbiturate-potentiated GABA-activated currents (55). Moreover, mutation of a single amino acid in the M2 segment of the β1 subunit eliminates barbiturate potentiation but does not interfere with direct activation (56). Thus, the modulatory and direct actions involve distinct mechanisms.

Felbamate also acts as a weak barbiturate-like positive allosteric modulator of GABA$_A$ receptors (39) (Figure 1.8C). In contrast to barbiturates, felbamate does not activate GABA$_A$ receptor chloride current responses in the absence of GABA, thus perhaps contributing to its lack of sedative side effects. Moreover, both phenobarbital (55,57) and felbamate (39) can block GABA$_A$ receptors at high concentrations. This would be expected to limit the extent of positive modulation (resulting in a partial agonist-like effect), and also could contribute to the reduced tendency of these drugs to produce sedation at anticonvulsant doses (compared with agonists that have greater efficacy, such as

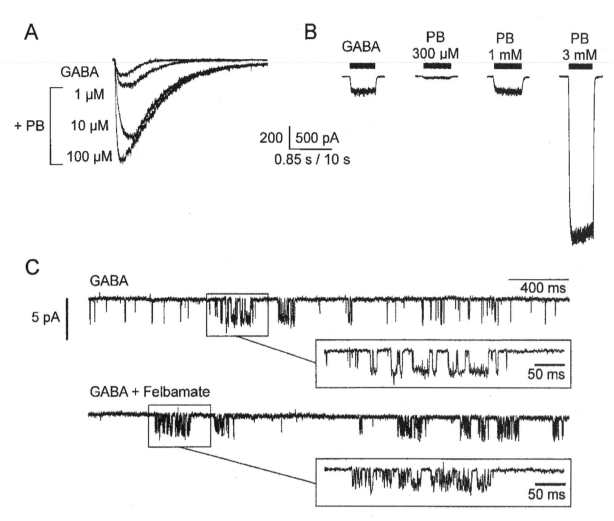

FIGURE 1.8. Modulatory and direct actions of phenobarbital (PB) and felbamate on GABA$_A$ receptors in hippocampal neurons. **A:** PB enhances GABA-activated Cl⁻ current responses. Whole-cell voltage-clamp recording showing family of currents activated by 50 ms-duration pulses of 1 μmol/L GABA. Membrane potential, –50 mV. (From ffrench-Mullen JM, Barker JL, Rogawski MA. Calcium current block by (–)-pentobarbital, phenobarbital, and CHEB but not (+)-pentobarbital in acutely isolated hippocampal CA1 neurons: comparison with effects on GABA-activated Cl⁻ current. *J Neurosci* 1993;13:3211–3221, with permission.) **B:** Whole-cell voltage clamp recording showing direct activation of GABA receptors by high concentrations of PB in the absence of GABA. For comparison, the response to 1 μmol/L GABA is shown. Membrane potential, –60 mV. [From Rho JM, Donevan SD, Rogawski MA. Direct activation of GABA$_A$ receptors by barbiturates in cultured rat hippocampal neurons. *J Physiol (Lond)* 1996;497:509–522, with permission.] **C:** A single GABA$_A$ receptor channel in an outside-out membrane patch activated by 2 μmol/L GABA exhibits brief openings and some flickery bursts (open is downward). Burst openings are more frequent and prolonged in the presence of 3 mmol/L felbamate. Felbamate did not activate GABA$_A$ receptor channels in the absence of GABA. Membrane potential, –80 mV. (From Rho JM, Donevan SD, Rogawski MA. Barbiturate-like actions of the propanediol dicarbamates felbamate and meprobamate. *J Pharmacol Exp Ther* 1997;280:1383–1391, with permission.)

pentobarbital or meprobamate). Topiramate also may act, in part, as an allosteric modulator of GABA receptors, but its complex subunit-specific actions have not been fully characterized (40,41).

GABA Transaminase

The concentration of GABA in the brain is controlled by two pyridoxal-5′-phosphate–dependent enzymes, gluta-

mate decarboxylase (GAD) and GABA transaminase (GABA-T). GAD, a cytosolic enzyme localized to GABAergic neurons, catalyzes the synthesis of GABA, whereas GABA-T catabolizes the conversion of GABA to succinic semialdehyde. The transamination can take place only if α-ketoglutarate is the acceptor of the amine group. Thus, the transamination is coupled to the synthesis of the GABA precursor glutamate: For every molecule of GABA destroyed, one molecule of precursor is formed (Figure 1.9).

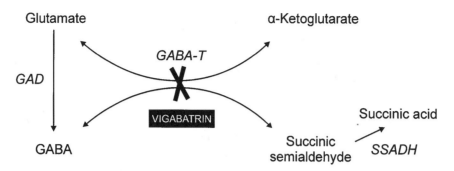

FIGURE 1.9. Metabolism of GABA through the GABA-shunt of the tricarboxylic acid (Krebs) cycle. Degradation of GABA by GABA transaminase (GABA-T; 4-aminobutyrate:2-oxoglutarate aminotransferase) is coupled to the synthesis of the precursor glutamate. Vigabatrin inactivates GABA-T, leading to elevated brain GABA levels. GAD, glutamic acid decarboxylase; SSADH, succinic semialdehyde dehydrogenase.

GABA-T, the product of a single gene, is a mitochondrial enzyme that is expressed widely in brain neurons and glia, and also in peripheral organs (58).

The anticonvulsant vigabatrin (γ-vinyl GABA) is a GABA analog that acts as an irreversible suicide inhibitor of GABA-T (59). The drug initially binds reversibly to the pyridoxal-5′-phosphate cofactor and then irreversibly to the enzyme. Administration of vigabatrin leads to large elevations in brain GABA levels (60–62). The anticonvulsant properties of vigabatrin have been attributed to enhanced GABA-mediated inhibition. Although vigabatrin can cause increased GABA release under some circumstances (63), there is little evidence that it causes a generalized increase in inhibition, and it is not as strongly sedating as GABA receptor modulators such as clonazepam. It has been shown that vigabatrin prevents the fading of inhibitory mechanisms during repetitive stimulation of interneurons and thus preferentially enhances inhibition in a frequency-dependent fashion (64). This effect may occur through a reduction in the sensitivity of the GABA$_B$ receptor mechanisms that normally cause activity-dependent depression of inhibition. Such fading of inhibition is believed to be an important factor that permits focal epileptiform activity to develop into a full-blown seizure (2), and interference with this process could account for the selective suppression of seizures by vigabatrin. An alternative explanation for the anticonvulsant activity of vigabatrin is that it induces a reversal of the GABA transporter, resulting in spontaneous GABA efflux that causes a generalized increase in inhibitory tone (65).

GABA Transporters

The synaptic action of GABA is terminated by its rapid reuptake into presynaptic terminals and surrounding glia by high-affinity plasma membrane GABA transporters (66). The GABA transporters, which are members of the superfamily of 12-membrane-segment transporters, are electrogenic and require Na$^+$ and Cl$^-$ for their activity. Transport of one molecule of GABA involves the cotransport of two Na$^+$ ions and one Cl$^-$ ion. Four GABA transporter proteins have been identified: GAT-1, GAT-2, GAT-3, and BGT-1 (betaine/GABA transporter 1), with distinct regional and cellular localizations in brain (67). GAT-1, the first member of the family to be identified, is the most abundant of the transporters. It is distributed ubiquitously in the nervous system, where it is localized primarily to GABA neurons but also is found in astrocytic processes (68).

In the mid-1970s, the muscimol analog (*R*)-nipecotic acid was identified as a specific GABA uptake inhibitor (69). Nipecotic acid was recognized as having anticonvulsant activity, but only when administered directly into the brain; as a hydrophilic amino acid, it does not effectively penetrate the blood–brain barrier (70). To overcome this problem, a variety of lipophilic analogs were synthesized, including tiagabine, which currently is marketed for the treatment of epilepsy. Tiagabine is a potent and selective competitive inhibitor of GAT-1. The drug binds with high affinity to the transporter, preventing GABA uptake without itself being transported. By slowing the reuptake of synaptically released GABA, tiagabine prolongs inhibitory postsynaptic potentials (71–73) and has a broad spectrum of activity in animal models of epilepsy (74). The prolongation of inhibitory GABA-mediated responses by tiagabine may be enhanced with repetitive activation, as is expected to occur during the synchronous discharge of interneurons associated with epileptic activity. This may minimize the behavioral depression that would accompany indiscriminate enhancement of GABA inhibition. GABA uptake blockers have been identified that affect a broader range of GABA transporters or that specifically inhibit GABA transporters other than GAT-1 (75,76). These compounds also exhibit anticonvulsant activity, but may have different spectrums of activity in animal seizure models.

GABA$_B$ Receptors

Overview

Fast synaptic GABA$_A$ receptor–mediated inhibition often is followed by a slower, late inhibitory response to GABA mediated by metabotropic seven transmembrane domain G-protein–coupled GABA$_B$ receptors (77,78). Presynaptic GABA$_B$ receptors on axon terminals inhibit P/Q and N-type calcium channels, resulting in decreased evoked neurotransmitter release. In contrast, postsynaptic GABA$_B$ receptor activation causes opening of inwardly rectifying potassium channels, leading to membrane hyperpolarization and inhibition of neuronal excitability. In addition, postsynaptic GABA$_B$ receptors negatively coupled to voltage-dependent calcium channels may serve to inhibit calcium channel–dependent burst discharges. Two major human GABA$_B$ receptor genes have been identified: GABA$_{B1}$ (gb1) and GABA$_{B2}$ (gb2), with the GABA$_{B1}$ gene encoding two structurally distinct N-terminal variants, GABA$_{B1a}$ and GABA$_{B1b}$. Functional GABA$_B$ receptors result from heterodimerization of one of the GABA$_{B1}$ variants with GABA$_{B2}$.

Activation of GABA$_B$ receptors with the nonselective agonist baclofen produces anticonvulsant effects in some systems (79,80) and proepileptic effects in others (81). In addition, there are case reports of baclofen-induced convulsive seizures in humans (82), although baclofen in general has little overall effect on seizure frequency (83). The proepileptic effects are believed to occur because of presynaptic, GABA$_B$ receptor–mediated suppression of GABA release from inhibitory interneurons, leading to disinhibition (84). The reduction of inhibition is greater than the suppressive effect on synaptic excitation, so that there is a net increase in excitability.

Gabapentin

Evidence suggests that the anticonvulsant gabapentin may act in part through a specific interaction with postsynaptic GABA$_B$ receptors. Gabapentin, the lipophilic 3-cyclohexyl analog of GABA, was originally synthesized in an attempt to develop a brain-penetrant GABA agonist. In fact, gabapentin is actively transported by the system L transporter, allowing it to enter the brain readily (85). Although gabapentin did not have the expected activity at GABA$_A$ receptors, it has been reported that therapeutically relevant concentrations (15 µmol/L) selectively activate GABA$_{B(1a,2)}$ heterodimers coupled to inwardly rectifying potassium channels (86). In at least some central nervous system regions (including the hippocampus), these GABA$_B$ receptors may be predominantly expressed postsynaptically (78). Thus, the selective action of gabapentin on GABA$_{B(1a,2)}$ receptors to induce potassium channel activation may endow the drug with anticonvulsant activity and eliminate the proconvulsant effects associated with nonselective GABA$_B$ receptor activation. In addition, there may be actions on N- and or P/Q-type voltage-dependent calcium channels coupled to GABA$_{B(1a,2)}$ receptors (87) that could suppress epileptiform burst discharges and, in brain regions with presynaptic GABA$_{B(1a,2)}$ receptors, reduce glutamate release from nerve terminals (88). However, although gabapentin does in fact appear to have baclofen-like actions *in vivo*, these effects are not reversed by GABA$_B$ antagonists, indicating that other mechanisms may be more important (89,90). Alternatives include direct effects on calcium channels (see later) or adenosine triphosphate–sensitive potassium channels (91), or effects on GABA metabolism (92).

GABA$_B$ Receptors in Absence Epilepsy

GABA$_B$ receptors also appear to play a role in generalized absence seizures, with GABA$_B$ agonists such as baclofen increasing the frequency and duration of spike-and-wave discharges in several models of absence seizures (93,94), and GABA$_B$ antagonists exerting strong antiabsence effects (95,96). These pharmacologic observations support the concept that GABA$_B$ receptors are critical to the generation of the 3-Hz rhythmic oscillations in the thalamocortical network that underlie absence seizures (97). GABA$_B$ receptor antagonists represent a potential therapeutic approach in generalized absence. However, because these agents may provoke convulsive seizures, caution is warranted (96).

Calcium Channels

Overview

Voltage-gated calcium channels, like sodium channels, are multisubunit protein complexes that permit ion flux when gated open by membrane depolarization (98). However, there is a larger number of functional calcium channel types with a correspondingly greater diversity of functional roles in neurons. Calcium channels are broadly grouped into high-voltage– and low-voltage–activated families. High-voltage–activated channels—which are further subgrouped as L, R, P/Q, and N types—are largely responsible for the regulation of calcium entry and neurotransmitter release from presynaptic nerve terminals. They represent potential anticonvulsant targets because blockade of these channels inhibits neurotransmitter release (99). However, as yet, there are no practical anticonvulsants that specifically target these channels, with the possible exception of gabapentin, which binds with high affinity to certain calcium channel subunits.

High-voltage activated calcium channels consist minimally of an α1 protein (encoded by one of seven genes) that forms the channel pore and voltage sensor (100). A variety of auxiliary subunits associate with the α1 subunits, including β (four genes), α2δ (three), and γ (six) subunits. The members of the α2δ family include α2δ-1, which is ubiquitously expressed; α2δ-2, which is expressed in brain and heart; and α2δ-3, which is brain specific. α2δ-1 consists of two proteins that are coded by a single gene, the product of which is posttranslationally cleaved from a single polypeptide precursor. The auxiliary subunits serve to enhance incorporation of functional channels in the cell membrane and also allosterically alter their kinetic properties and affect drug modulation.

Gabapentin

There is emerging evidence that among its complex actions gabapentin may act, at least in part, through a selective interaction with voltage-dependent calcium channels. Gabapentin binds with high affinity and specificity to the $\alpha_2\delta$ subunit (101) and can block high-voltage–activated calcium currents in brain (102) and sensory (103) neurons. In addition, the drug appears to suppress glutamate release, possibly through an effect on P/Q-type voltage-dependent calcium channels (88). However, the drug does not affect all calcium currents (104), even those in cells expressing α2δ subunits (105). [α2δ Subunits are ubiquitously coassembled in many voltage-gated calcium channel types and do not determine subgroup type (100); therefore, factors other than α2δ binding must determine P/Q specificity.] Gabapentin has been found to bind only to the α2δ-1 and α2δ-2 subunits, and not to α2δ-3 (106). Moreover, it has nearly threefold higher affinity for α2δ-1, thus providing a possible basis for its cell type specificity. There also is evidence that the β2 subunit interactions may be important for gabapentin actions (105). Nevertheless, the extent to which effects on calcium channels contribute to the anticonvulsant activity of gabapentin remains to be determined.

Lamotrigine

In addition to its actions on voltage-activated sodium channels, lamotrigine also can inhibit high-voltage–activated (N-, P/Q-type) calcium channels (107,108); it does not affect low-voltage–activated T-type calcium channels (109). The importance of calcium channel blockade for lamotrigine's anticonvulsant properties is not well delineated, but this action, along with the sodium channel blockade, could contribute to its effects on neurotransmitter release (see later).

Phenobarbital

Barbiturates are well known to block voltage-activated calcium channels (110). For phenobarbital, block of calcium channels may contribute to the anticonvulsant activity, but effects on GABA$_A$ receptors are likely of greater importance (111).

T-Type Calcium Channels

Low-voltage–activated (T-type) calcium channels are believed to play a role in the regulation of neuronal firing by participating in bursting and intrinsic oscillations (112). In thalamus, these channels are critical to the abnormal oscillatory behavior that underlies generalized absence seizures. The T-type calcium channel family (Ca$_V$T) consists of the α1G, α1H, and α1I subunits, which are ~30% homologous to high-voltage-activated subunits in their putative membrane-spanning regions (113). Thalamic relay neurons express high levels of α1G subunits, whereas thalamic reticular neurons (GABAergic interneurons that modulate and synchronize thalamic output) express high levels of α1I and moderate levels of α1H subunits (114). It has been proposed that the antiabsence seizure activity of ethosuximide is due to blockade of T-type calcium channels in thalamic neurons at clinically relevant concentrations of the drug (115–118). However, this concept has been challenged by Leresche et al. (119), who have proposed that ethosuximide suppresses thalamic bursting mainly by inhibiting a persistent component of the sodium current (I$_{NaP}$) in thalamic neurons without affecting the fast (inactivating) sodium current that constitutes the bulk (97.5%) of the total sodium current. By enhancing the efficacy of bursting and reducing the delay between depolarization and the onset of burst firing, I$_{NaP}$ in thalamic neurons works in concert with the T-type calcium current and plays a pivotal role in burst generation (120). Therefore, it is a plausible target for the action of ethosuximide. More recent studies have suggested that the action of ethosuximide on T-type calcium currents may be more complex than previously thought, with effects on the persistent component of particular importance (118,121,122). Other antiabsence agents also inhibit T-type calcium channels, including the active metabolites of methosuximide (α-methyl-α-phenyl-succinimide) and tridione (dimethadione). Zonisimide may also block T-type calcium channels (123,124).

Glutamate Receptors

NMDA and AMPA Receptors

Ionotropic glutamate receptors of the NMDA and AMPA types are potentially important anticonvulsant targets (6,125–128). These glutamate-gated cation channels mediate the bulk of fast excitatory neurotransmission in the central nervous system (129). Blockade of either of these classes of glutamate receptors is well recognized to protect against seizures in *in vitro* and *in vivo* models. However, no selective glutamate receptor antagonist has proven to be of practical use in epilepsy therapy, largely because agents examined to date have exhibited unacceptable side effects (or were administered at subtherapeutic doses). Nevertheless, weak blockade of excitatory amino acid receptors may be one of a complex of multiple actions through which some clinically useful anticonvulsant drugs protect against seizures, and low-affinity NMDA receptor antagonists have clinical potential (129). In addition, selective AMPA receptor antagonists, such as 2,3-benzodiazepines like talampanel (GYKI 53405; LY 300164), are highly effective anticonvulsants in animal models (131) and have shown promise in early clinical trials.

The best evidence among marketed anticonvulsant drugs for such glutamate receptor blocking actions comes from work with felbamate, which has been shown to inhibit NMDA receptors at clinically relevant concentrations (132). Single-channel recording studies are consistent with a functional channel blocking action of the drug or allosteric effects on channel gating. NMDA receptors in mammalian neurons are heterooligomers formed by coassembly of an obligatory NR1 subunit and at least one type of NR2 subunit (128). Felbamate is modestly more potent as an antagonist of NMDA receptors containing NR2B subunits (133,134). Unlike the NR2A subunit, which is distributed ubiquitously in the central nervous system, expression of the NR2B subunit in the adult is restricted largely to the forebrain (135). It has been proposed that NR2B selectivity could in part contribute to felbamate's low neurobehavioral toxicity in relation to other NMDA receptor antagonists because the drug may target NMDA receptor–mediated synaptic transmission in forebrain areas critical to seizure generation and avoid perturbing nonforebrain structures that could mediate side effects. In addition, NR2B subunits are expressed in high abundance in the immature brain, and this could also account for felbamate's clinical utility in childhood seizure disorders, such as the Lennox-Gastaut syndrome.

Kainate Receptors

The kainate receptors are ionotropic glutamate receptors that share ~40% homology with AMPA receptors and ~20% homology with NMDA receptors (136). Like AMPA and NMDA receptors, kainate receptors are responsible for a portion of glutamate-mediated excitation at some synapses, including those in limbic regions relevant to epilepsy (137). In addition to contributing to postsynaptic excitation, kainate receptors on presynaptic axon terminals serve to modulate glutamate release from excitatory afferents, and they also may have the unique property of suppressing GABA release from inhibitory interneurons, although the exact mechanism for the latter effect is controversial (136,138). The combination of postsynaptic excitation and suppression of inhibition endow kainate receptors with a unique potential to induce epileptic activity. In fact, there is a variety of circumstantial evidence suggesting that kainate receptors may play a role in seizures and epileptogenesis. However, the potential of kainate receptors as antiepileptic drug targets has not been fully explored.

Metabotropic Glutamate Receptors

In addition to its actions on ionotropic NMDA, AMPA, and kainate receptors, synaptically released glutamate also can interact with G-protein–coupled metabotropic glutamate receptors (139). Eight metabotropic glutamate receptors (mGluRs) have been identified to date that are widely distributed in brain. Based on sequence homology, these eight mGluRs are classified into three groups. Group I mGluRs (mGluR1, mGluR5) are positively coupled to phospholipase C and induce hydrolysis of inositol phosphate (PI) and the mobilization of intracellular calcium. Group II mGluRs (mGluR2, mGluR3) and group III mGluRs (mGluR4, mGluR6, mGluR7, mGluR8) are negatively coupled to adenylate cyclase and inhibit the production of cyclic adenosine monophosphate. mGluRs mediate a wide diversity of effects on ion channels, including inhibition of voltage-gated potassium and calcium and nonspecific cation channels (140). In addition, certain group II and III mGluRs, including mGluR2, mGluR4, and mGluR7, are located presynaptically and mediate inhibition of excitatory transmitter release. These diverse actions confer mGluR agonists and antagonists with the capacity both to evoke and inhibit seizures. Indeed, nonselective mGluR agonists and antagonists may have proconvulsant as well as anticonvulsant actions. However, the recent development of selective agents has allowed certain mGluRs to be identified as appropriate anticonvulsant drug targets. Activation of group I mGluRs elicits oscillatory and epileptiform activity *in vitro* (141), and seizure discharges and epileptogenesis in experimental models (142) (as do agonists of other receptors coupled to PI hydrolysis, such as muscarinic cholinergic receptors). Conversely, anticonvulsant effects are often obtained with group II and III mGluR activation (142–144). In contrast to the seizure-inducing properties of group I agonists, group I antagonists, including those that are selective for selective mGluR1 (144,145) and mGluR5 (146), have shown anticonvulsant activity in several seizure models. Among agents targeting mGluRs, group I antagonists seem to have the most clinical potential.

PRESYNAPTIC ACTIONS OF ANTIEPILEPTIC DRUGS

Although blockade of postsynaptic glutamate receptors is not a major factor in the actions of most marketed antiepileptic drugs, effects on other targets—most notably voltage-dependent sodium channels—may indirectly affect glutamate release, thus having the net effect of reducing glutamate-mediated excitatory neurotransmission. In fact, the ultimate way in which sodium channel blocking anticonvulsants protect against seizures may be to a large extent through a reduction in evoked glutamate release. In addition, effects on presynaptic calcium channels and release-regulating receptors such as GABA$_B$ receptors could play a role in the actions of some antiepileptic drugs including, for example, gabapentin (see earlier).

Synaptic glutamate release occurs when presynaptic nerve terminals are invaded by sodium-dependent action potentials. The subsequent activation of high-voltage–activated (N-, P/Q-type) calcium channels in the axon terminal allows calcium entry that evokes the exocytosis of synaptic vesicles containing glutamate. Studies in brain slices and synaptosomes have indicated that sodium channel blocking anticonvulsants, including phenytoin, lamotrigine, carbamazepine, riluzole, and felbamate, can inhibit glutamate release by virtue of their effects on sodium channels (147–149). Although many of these drugs also can block calcium channels (and as a result inhibit release in an inde-

pendent fashion through this mechanism), effects on these channels typically occur at supratherapeutic concentrations, although for some drugs, such as lamotrigine, the interaction with calcium channels may be clinically significant (150–152). Electrophysiologic recordings of synaptic responses demonstrate that sodium and calcium channel blocking anticonvulsants inhibit action potential–dependent synaptic events without affecting action potential–independent ("miniature") synaptic events (Figure 1.10). The latter observation reinforces the concept that these drugs do not block postsynaptic receptors and do not interfere directly with the release machinery, supporting the view that the ultimate way in which they protect against seizures is by indirectly suppressing glutamate release. In

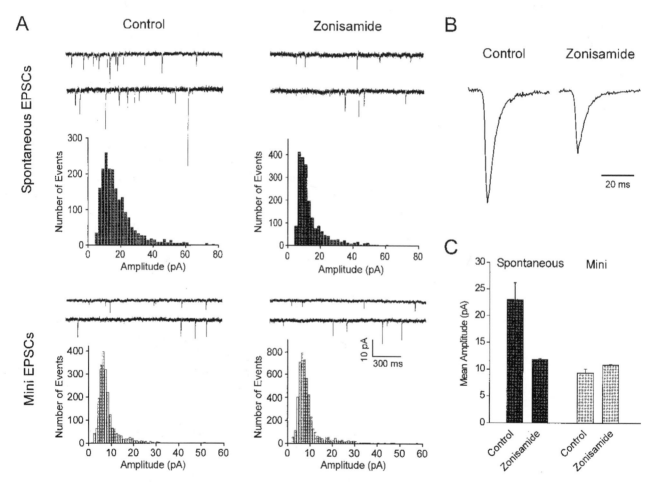

FIGURE 1.10. Sodium channel blocking anticonvulsants suppress action potential–evoked synaptic glutamate release from excitatory terminals. In this series of experiments with zonisamide, whole-cell recordings were made from CA1 hippocampal neurons in brain slices under conditions where GABA$_A$ and NMDA receptors were blocked to isolate fast AMPA receptor–mediated synaptic responses. **A: Top;** the amplitudes of spontaneous action potential–dependent synaptic currents (EPSCs) is reduced in the presence of 20 μmol/L zonisamide. **Bottom:** Miniature (non–action-potential-dependent) EPSCs recorded in the presence of 1 μmol/L tetrodotoxin (to block sodium-dependent action potentials) are unaffected by zonisamide, indicating that the anticonvulsant has a presynaptic action (i.e., affects action potential–evoked glutamate release). **B:** Schematic representation illustrating that zonisamide depresses the mean amplitude of action potential–evoked EPSCs, but does not affect their time course. **C:** Comparison of the effects of zonisamide on the mean amplitudes of spontaneous and miniature EPSCs. Holding potential, −70 mV. (Zhu WJ, Rogawski MA, *unpublished*.)

fact, such drugs may affect GABA release only at relatively higher concentrations as a result of differences in excitation–contraction coupling in glutamatergic and GABAergic neurons (148). However, not all anticonvulsants that inhibit glutamate release do so exclusively through effects on sodium and calcium channels. For example, losigamone may inhibition glutamate release by a mechanism that does not involve sodium channels (153).

ANTIEPILEPTOGENESIS

Currently, antiepileptic drugs are used to reduce or prevent the occurrence of epileptic seizures, and therefore represent symptomatic therapies that do not address the natural course of epilepsy and do not provide a cure. There is no doubt that a preferred approach to therapy would be to prevent the development of epilepsy in those at risk (e.g., in individuals with genetic epilepsies or those with a history of head trauma) or to eliminate seizure susceptibility in those with established epilepsy. In addition, it would be desirable to slow or halt the decline in cognitive functions that many clinicians believe occurs in chronic epilepsy (154). The advent of the kindling model has allowed drugs to be examined for their capacity to interfere with the progressive development of seizure susceptibility (epileptogenesis). In the kindling model, an experimental animal (usually a rodent) subjected to daily, brief deep brain stimulation (usually in the amygdala) progressively develops (usually over the course of 1 week to 10 days) an increased tendency to exhibit a behavioral limbic seizure in response to the stimulation (155). Test agents can be examined for their ability to prevent seizures in fully kindled animals (anticonvulsant action) and also to prevent the development of the enhanced seizure susceptibility (antiepileptogenic action). Kindling also can be induced noninvasively by corneal stimulation (156) or with chemoconvulsants such as pentylenetetrazol (157) and muscarinic cholinergic agonists (158), but the kindled state may not be as persistent and there are important differences in drug sensitivity from the traditional kindling model (159).

NMDA receptor antagonists are the prototypic antiepileptogenic agents. When administered before each kindling stimulation, NMDA antagonists prevent the development of kindling but have little or no effect on the stimulation-evoked afterdischarge (i.e., they do not inhibit the neuronal activation induced by the stimulus), and they also have little or no effect on the expression of kindled seizures in animals that have been kindled in the absence of drug treatment (127,160). Many conventional antiepileptic agents, including phenytoin and carbamazepine, do not prevent epileptogenesis in this model and have only weak activity in protecting against kindled seizures (161). However, some antiepileptic drugs do have antiepileptogenic activity in the kindling model, including valproate (161)

and newer drugs such as levetiracetam (162). In addition, drugs that act primarily on GABA systems, notably tiagabine (163) and vigabatrin (164), as well as phenobarbital (161) and benzodiazepines (165), have antiepileptogenic activity. As yet, the clinical relevance of these observations is uncertain.

MOLECULAR MECHANISMS AND CLINICAL EFFICACY

Pharmacologic studies have demonstrated a wide diversity of molecular targets and mechanisms for antiepileptic drugs. Nevertheless, all antiepileptic drugs appear ultimately to act on ion channel systems, although in some cases the effect is mediated indirectly. The diversity of ion channel targets is remarkable. Structurally novel anticonvulsant compounds—even those that appear similar to older drugs by virtue of their spectrum of actions in animal seizure models—often are found to act on distinct ion channel targets or by new mechanisms. Nonetheless, it is possible to categorize some currently available drugs by mechanism into several broad groups, each with a common spectrum of clinical activities (Table 1.1). Anticonvulsants that act mainly as use- and voltage-dependent *sodium channel blockers*, including phenytoin, carbamazepine, oxcarbazepine, and lamotrigine, are effective in the control of partial and generalized tonic-clonic seizures and are ineffective in the treatment of generalized absence seizures. Agents that *potentiate GABAergic inhibition* by enhancing the synaptic availability of GABA, such as vigabatrin and tiagabine, are effective in partial seizures and may worsen absence seizures. Similarly, barbiturates such as phenobarbital, which augment the function of GABA$_A$ receptors and have additional effects on calcium and other ion channels, are effective in the control of many seizure types but are ineffective in control of absence seizures. In contrast, benzodiazepines, such as diazepam, lorazepam, and clonazepam, which enhance only a subset of GABA$_A$ receptors, are broad-spectrum agents, effective in the treatment of partial, generalized tonic-clonic, generalized absence seizures, and also myoclonic seizures. The specific antiabsence agent ethosuximide seems to act by affecting T-type calcium channels, and possibly also persistent sodium currents. The mechanisms underlying the antiabsence actions of other anticonvulsants, including valproate and lamotrigine, are obscure. Valproate, gabapentin, felbamate, topiramate, zonisamide, and levetiracetam appear to have novel mechanisms (or combinations of mechanisms) of action, possibly affecting calcium channels and glutamate receptors as well as conventional targets, including sodium channels and GABA receptor systems. All of these drugs are effective in the treatment of partial seizures. Topiramate and felbamate probably also are effective in the treatment of absence seizures and other generalized seizure disorders, and are

TABLE 1.1. MOLECULAR TARGETS AND CLINICAL EFFICACY OF ANTIEPILEPTIC DRUGS

Drug	Na$^+$ Channel	Ca^{2+} Channel	GABA$_A$ Receptor	GABA Transaminase	GABA Transporter	GABA$_B$ Receptor	NMDA Receptor	Clinical Efficacy
Phenytoin	I$_{Naf}$, I$_{NaP}$							Partial, GTC
Carbamazepine	▓							Partial, GTC
Oxcarbazepine	▓							Partial, GTC
Lamotrigine	▓	HVA						Partial, GTC, absence[b]
Zonisamide[a]	▓	?T-type						Partial, GTC, myoclonic[b]
Ethosuximide	I$_{NaP}$	T-type						Absence
Phenobarbital			▓					Partial
Benzodiazepines			+ γ2/−α4, α6					Broad spectrum
Vigabatrin				▓				Partial[b]
Tiagabine					▓			Partial
Gabapentin		α2δ				?gb1a-gb2		Partial
Felbamate			▓				▓	Broad spectrum
Topiramate[a]	I$_{Naf}$, I$_{NaP}$		▓					Broad spectrum[b]

GABA, γ-aminobutyric acid; NMDA, *N*-methyl-D-aspartate; I$_{Naf}$, fast sodium current; I$_{NaP}$, persistent sodium current; HVA, high-voltage activated; GTC, generalized tonic-clonic seizures.
[a]Zonisamide and topiramate are weak carbonic anhydrase inhibitors.
[b]Vigabatrin, lamotrigine, zonisamide, and topiramate may be useful in treating infantile spasms.

therefore broad-spectrum agents. Such agents may be useful, along with broad-spectrum agents like valproate and lamotrigine, in the treatment of mixed seizure syndromes, such as the Lennox-Gastaut syndrome.

REFERENCES

1. Merritt HH, Putnam TJ. A new series of anticonvulsant drugs tested by experiments on animals. *Arch Neurol Psychiatry* 1938;39:1003–1015.
2. Dichter MA, Ayala GF. Cellular mechanisms of epilepsy: a status report. *Science* 1987;237:157–164.
3. Avoli M, Rogawski MA, Avanzini G. Generalized epileptic disorders: an update. *Epilepsia* 2001;42:445–457.
4. Rogawski MA. Mechanism-specific pathways for new antiepileptic drug discovery. In: French JA, Leppik IE, Dichter MA, eds. *Antiepileptic drug development*. Philadelphia: Lippincott-Raven, 1998:1–27.
5. Rogawski MA. KCNQ2/KCNQ3 K$^+$ channels and the molecular pathogenesis of epilepsy: implications for therapy. *Trends Neurosci* 2000;23:393–398.
6. Rogawski MA. Epilepsy. In: Pullan L, Patel J, eds. *Neurotherapeutics: emerging strategies*. Totowa, NJ, Humana Press, 1996: 193–273.
7. Vezzani A, Sperk G, Colmers WF. Neuropeptide Y: emerging evidence for a functional role in seizure modulation. *Trends Neurosci* 1999;22:25–30.
8. Weinshenker D, Szot P. Role of catecholamines in seizure susceptibility: new results using genetically engineered mice. *Pharmacol Ther* 2002 (*in press*).
9. Ragsdale DS, Avoli M. Sodium channels as molecular targets for antiepileptic drugs. *Brain Res Brain Res Rev* 1998;26:16–28.
10. Catterall WA. From ionic currents to molecular mechanisms: the structure and function of voltage-gated sodium channels. *Neuron* 2000;26:13–25.
11. Bezanilla F. The voltage sensor in voltage-dependent ion channels. *Physiol Rev* 2000;80:555–592.
12. Schmutz M, Brugger F, Gentsch C, et al. Oxcarbazepine: preclinical anticonvulsant profile and putative mechanisms of action. *Epilepsia* 1994;35[Suppl 5]:S47–50.
13. Ambrósio AF, Silva AP, Malva JO, et al. Inhibition of glutamate release by BIA 2-093 and BIA 2-024, two novel derivatives of carbamazepine, due to blockade of sodium but not calcium channels. *Biochem Pharmacol* 2001;61:1271–1275.
14. Schauf CL. Zonisamide enhances slow sodium inactivation in *Myxicola*. *Brain Res* 1987;413:185–188.
15. Taglialatela M, Ongini E, Brown AM, et al. Felbamate inhibits cloned voltage-dependent Na$^+$ channels from human and rat brain. *Eur J Pharmacol* 1996;316:373–377.
16. Taverna S, Sancini G, Mantegazza M, et al. Inhibition of transient and persistent Na$^+$ current fractions by the new anticonvulsant topiramate. *J Pharmacol Exp Ther* 1999;288:960–968.
17. Rogawski MA, Porter RJ. Antiepileptic drugs: pharmacological mechanisms and clinical efficacy with consideration of promising developmental stage compounds. *Pharmacol Rev* 1990;42: 223–286.
18. White HS, Johnson M, Wolf HH, et al. The early identification of anticonvulsant activity: role of the maximal electroshock and subcutaneous pentylenetetrazol seizure models. *Ital J Neurol Sci* 1995;16:73–77.
19. Ragsdale DS, Scheuer T, Catterall WA. Frequency and voltage-dependent inhibition of type IIA Na$^+$ channels, expressed in mammalian cell line, by local anesthetic, antiarrhythmic, and anticonvulsant drugs. *Mol Pharmacol* 1991;40:756–765.
20. Xie X, Lancaster B, Peakman T, et al. Interaction of the antiepileptic drug lamotrigine with recombinant rat brain type IIA Na$^+$ channels and with native Na$^+$ channels in rat hippocampal neurones. *Pflugers Arch* 1995;430:437–446.
21. Kuo CC, Bean BP. Slow binding of phenytoin to inactivated sodium channels in rat hippocampal neurons. *Mol Pharmacol* 1994;46:716–725.
22. Kuo CC, Lu L. Characterization of lamotrigine inhibition of Na$^+$ channels in rat hippocampal neurones. *Br J Pharmacol* 1997;121:1231–1238.
23. Vedantham V, Cannon S. Slow inactivation does not affect movement of the fast inactivation gate in voltage-gated Na$^+$ channels. *J Gen Physiol* 1998;111:83–93.

24. Ong BH, Tomaselli GF, Balser JR. A structural rearrangement in the sodium channel pore linked to slow inactivation and use dependence. *J Gen Physiol* 2000;116:653–662.
25. Quandt FN. Modification of slow inactivation of single sodium channels by phenytoin in neuroblastoma cells. *Mol Pharmacol* 1988;34:557–565.
26. Kuo CC, Bean BP. Na$^+$ channels must deactivate to recover from inactivation. *Neuron* 1994;12:819–829.
27. Kuo CC. A common anticonvulsant binding site for phenytoin, carbamazepine, and lamotrigine in neuronal Na$^+$ channels. *Mol Pharmacol* 1998;54:712–721.
28. Yarov-Yarovoy V, Brown J, Sharp EM, et al. Molecular determinants of voltage-dependent gating and binding of pore-blocking drugs in transmembrane segment IIIS6 of the Na$^+$ channel α-subunit. *J Biol Chem* 2001;276:20–27.
29. McPhee JC, Ragsdale DS, Scheuer T, et al. A critical role for transmembrane segment IVS6 of the sodium channel α subunit in fast inactivation. *J Biol Chem* 1995;270:12025–12034.
30. Kuo CC, Chen RS, Lu L, et al. Carbamazepine inhibition of neuronal Na$^+$ currents: quantitative distinction from phenytoin and possible therapeutic implications. *Mol Pharmacol* 1997;51: 1077–1083.
31. Taylor CP. Na$^+$ currents that fail to inactivate. *Trends Neurosci* 1993;16:455–460.
32. Segal MM, Douglas AF. Late sodium channel openings underlying epileptiform activity are preferentially diminished by the anticonvulsant phenytoin. *J Neurophysiol* 1997;77:3021–3034.
33. Chao TI, Alzheimer C. Effects of phenytoin on the persistent Na$^+$ current of mammalian CNS neurones. *Neuroreport* 1995;6: 1778–1780.
34. Lampl I, Schwindt P, Crill W. Reduction of cortical pyramidal neuron excitability by the action of phenytoin on persistent Na$^+$ current. *J Pharmacol Exp Ther* 1998;284:228–237.
35. Baulac S, Huberfeld G, Gourfinkel-An I, et al. First genetic evidence of GABA$_A$ receptor dysfunction in epilepsy: a mutation in the γ2-subunit gene. *Nat Genet* 2000;28:46–48.
36. Wallace RH, Marini C, Petrou S, et al. Mutant GABA$_A$ receptor γ2-subunit in childhood absence epilepsy and febrile seizures. *Nat Genet* 2001;28:49–52.
37. Macdonald RL, Olsen RW. GABA$_A$ receptor channels. *Annu Rev Neurosci* 1994;17:569–602.
38. Chebib M, Johnston GAR. GABA-activated ligand gated ion channels: medicinal chemistry and molecular biology. *J Med Chem* 2000;43:1427–1447.
39. Rho JM, Donevan SD, Rogawski MA. Barbiturate-like actions of the propanediol dicarbamates felbamate and meprobamate. *J Pharmacol Exp Ther* 1997;280:1383–1391.
40. White HS, Brown SD, Woodhead JH, et al. Topiramate modulates GABA-evoked currents in murine cortical neurons by a nonbenzodiazepine mechanism. *Epilepsia* 2000;41[Suppl 1]: S17–S20.
41. Gordey M, DeLorey TM, Olsen RW. Differential sensitivity of recombinant GABA$_A$ receptors expressed in *Xenopus* oocytes to modulation by topiramate. *Epilepsia* 2000;41[Suppl 1]: S25–S29.
42. Kokate TG, Banks MK, Magee T, et al. Finasteride, a 5α-reductase inhibitor, blocks the anticonvulsant activity of progesterone in mice. *J Pharmacol Exp Ther* 1999;288:679–684.
43. Rogers CJ, Twyman RE, Macdonald RL. Benzodiazepine and β-carboline regulation of single GABA$_A$ receptor channels of mouse spinal neurones in culture. *J Physiol* 1994;475, 69–82.
44. Eghbali M, Curmi JP, Birnir B, et al. Hippocampal GABA$_A$ channel conductance increased by diazepam. *Nature* 1997;388: 71–75.
45. Barnard EA, Skolnick P, Olsen RW, et al. International Union of Pharmacology—XV—Subtypes of γ-aminobutyric acid$_A$ receptors: classification on the basis of subunit structure and receptor function. *Pharmacol Rev* 1998;50:291–313.
46. Günther U, Benson JA, Benke D, et al. Benzodiazepine-insensitive mice generated by targeted disruption of the γ2 subunit gene of γ-aminobutyric acid type A receptors. *Proc Natl Acad Sci U S A* 1995;92:7749–7753.
47. Rudolph U, Crestani F, Benke D, et al. Benzodiazepine actions mediated by specific γ-aminobutyric acid$_A$ receptor subtypes. *Nature* 1999;401:796–800.
48. McKernan RM, Rosahl TW, Reynolds DS, et al. Sedative but not anxiolytic properties of benzodiazepines are mediated by the GABA$_A$ receptor α$_1$ subtype. *Nat Neurosci* 2000;3:587–592.
49. Sigel E, Buhr A. The benzodiazepine binding site of GABA$_A$ receptors. *Trends Pharmacol Sci* 1997;18:425–429.
50. Korpi ER, Mattila MJ, Wisden W, et al. GABA$_A$-receptor subtypes: clinical efficacy and selectivity of benzodiazepine site ligands. *Ann Med* 1997;29:275–282.
51. Sigel E, Baur R, Netzer R, et al. The antiepileptic drug AWD 131-138 stimulates different recombinant isoforms of the rat GABA$_A$ receptor through the benzodiazepine binding site. *Neurosci Lett* 1998;245:85–88.
52. McCormick DA, Contreras D. On the cellular and network bases of epileptic seizures. *Annu Rev Physiol* 2001;63:815–846.
53. Sohal VS, Huguenard JR. Clonazepam suppresses oscillations in rat thalamic slices. *Neurocomputing* 2001;38:907–913.
54. Kendig JJ. Barbiturates: active form and site of action at node of Ranvier sodium channels. *J Pharmacol Exp Ther* 1981;218: 175–181.
55. Rho JM, Donevan SD, Rogawski MA. Direct activation of GABA$_A$ receptors by barbiturates in cultured rat hippocampal neurons. *J Physiol* 1996;497:509–522.
56. Dalziel JE, Cox GB, Gage PW, et al. Mutant human α$_1$β$_1$(T262Q) GABA$_A$ receptors are directly activated but not modulated by pentobarbital. *Eur J Pharmacol* 1999;385: 283–286.
57. Akk G, Steinbach JH. Activation and block of recombinant GABA$_A$ receptors by pentobarbitone: a single-channel study. *Br J Pharmacol* 2000;130:249–258.
58. Jeon SG, Bahn JH, Jang JS, et al. Human brain GABA transaminase tissue distribution and molecular expression. *Eur J Biochem* 2000;267:5601–5607.
59. De Biase D, Barra D, Bossa F, et al. Chemistry of the inactivation of 4-aminobutyrate aminotransferase by the antiepileptic drug vigabatrin. *J Biol Chem* 1991;266:20056–20061.
60. Riekkinen PJ, Ylinen A, Halonen T, et al. Cerebrospinal fluid GABA and seizure control with vigabatrin. *Br J Clin Pharmacol* 1989;27[Suppl 1]:87S–94S.
61. Löscher W, Horstermann D. Differential effects of vigabatrin, gamma-acetylenic GABA, aminooxyacetic acid, and valproate on levels of various amino acids in rat brain regions and plasma. *Naunyn Schmiedebergs Arch Pharmacol* 1994;349:270–278.
62. Petroff OA, Behar KL, Mattson RH, et al. Human brain γ-aminobutyric acid levels and seizure control following initiation of vigabatrin therapy. *J Neurochem* 1996;67:2399–2404.
63. Gram L, Larsson OM, Johnsen A, et al. Experimental studies of the influence of vigabatrin on the GABA system. *Br J Clin Pharmacol* 1989;27[Suppl 1]:13S–17S.
64. Jackson MF, Esplin B, Čapek R. Reversal of the activity-dependent suppression of GABA-mediated inhibition in hippocampal slices from gamma-vinyl GABA (vigabatrin)-pretreated rats. *Neuropharmacology* 2000;39:65–74.
65. Wu Y, Wang W, Richerson GB. GABA transaminase inhibition induces spontaneous and enhances depolarization-evoked GABA efflux via reversal of the GABA transporter. *J Neurosci* 2001;21:2630–2639.
66. Masson J, Sagn C, Hamon M, et al. Neurotransmitter trans-

porters in the central nervous system. *Pharmacol Rev* 1999;51: 439–464.

67. Ikegaki N, Saito N, Hashima M, et al. Production of specific antibodies against GABA transporter subtypes (GAT1, GAT2, GAT3) and their application to immunocytochemistry. *Brain Res Mol Brain Res* 1994;26:47–54.

68. Minelli A, Brecha NC, Karschin C, et al. GAT-1, a high-affinity GABA plasma membrane transporter, is localized to neurons and astroglia in the cerebral cortex. *J Neurosci* 1995;15: 7734–7746.

69. Krogsgaard-Larsen P, Frolund B, Frydenvang K. GABA uptake inhibitors: design, molecular pharmacology and therapeutic aspects. *Curr Pharm Des* 2000;6:1193–1209.

70. Horton RW, Collins JF, Anlezark GM, et al. Convulsant and anticonvulsant actions in DBA/2 mice of compounds blocking the reuptake of GABA. *Eur J Pharmacol* 1979;59:75–83.

71. Thompson SM, Gahwiler BH. Effects of the GABA uptake inhibitor tiagabine on inhibitory synaptic potentials in rat hippocampal slice cultures. *J Neurophysiol* 1992;67:1698–1701.

72. Engel D, Schmitz D, Gloveli T, et al. Laminar difference in GABA uptake and GAT-1 expression in rat CA1. *J Physiol (Lond)* 1998;512.3:643–649.

73. Jackson MF, Esplin B, Čapek R. Activity-dependent enhancement of hyperpolarizing and depolarizing gamma-aminobutyric acid (GABA) synaptic responses following inhibition of GABA uptake by tiagabine. *Epilepsy Res* 1999;37:25–36.

74. Suzdak PD, Jansen JA. A review of the preclinical pharmacology of tiagabine: a potent and selective anticonvulsant GABA uptake inhibitor. *Epilepsia* 1995;36:612–626.

75. Dalby NO, Thomsen C, Fink-Jensen A, et al. Anticonvulsant properties of two GABA uptake inhibitors NNC 05-2045 and NNC 05-2090, not acting preferentially on GAT1. *Epilepsy Res* 1997;28:51–61

76. Dalby NO. GABA-level increasing and anticonvulsant effects of three different GABA uptake inhibitors. *Neuropharmacology* 2000;39:2399–2407.

77. Couve A, Moss SJ, Menelas N, et al. GABA_B receptors: a new paradigm in G protein signaling. *Mol Cell Neurosci* 2000;16: 296–312.

78. Billinton A, Ige AO, Bolam JP, et al. Advances in the molecular understanding of GABA_B receptors. *Trends Neurosci* 2001;24: 277–282.

79. Ault B, Nadler JV. Anticonvulsant like actions of baclofen in the rat hippocampal slice. *Br J Pharmacol* 1983;78:701–708.

80. Veliskova J, Velisek L, Moshé SL. Age-specific effects of baclofen on pentylenetetrazol-induced seizures in developing rats. *Epilepsia* 1996;37:718–722.

81. Motalli R, Louvel J, Tancredi V, et al. GABA_B receptor activation promotes seizure activity in the juvenile rat hippocampus. *J Neurophysiol* 1999;82:638–647.

82. Kofler M, Kronenberg MF, Rifici C, et al. Epileptic seizures associated with intrathecal baclofen application. *Neurology* 1994;44:25–27.

83. Terrence CF, Fromm GH, Roussan MS. Baclofen: its effect on seizure frequency. *Arch Neurol* 1983;40:28–29.

84. Mott DD, Bragdon AC, Lewis DV, et al. Baclofen has a proepileptic effect in the rat dentate gyrus. *J Pharmacol Exp Ther* 1989;249:721–725.

85. Su TZ, Lunney E, Campbell G, et al. Transport of gabapentin, a gamma-amino acid drug, by system l alpha-amino acid transporters: a comparative study in astrocytes, synaptosomes, and CHO cells. *J Neurochem* 1995;64:2125–2131.

86. Ng GY, Bertrand S, Sullivan R, et al. γ-Aminobutyric acid type B receptors with specific heterodimer composition and postsynaptic actions in hippocampal neurons are targets of anticonvulsant gabapentin action. *Mol Pharmacol* 2001;59:144–152.

87. Bertrand S, Ng GYK, Purisai MG, et al. The anticonvulsant, antihyperalgesic agent gabapentin is an agonist at brain γ-aminobutyric acid type B receptors negatively coupled to voltage-dependent calcium channels. *J Pharmacol Exp Ther* 2001; 298:15–24.

88. Fink K, Meder W, Dooley DJ, et al. Inhibition of neuronal Ca²⁺ influx by gabapentin and subsequent reduction of neurotransmitter release from rat neocortical slices. *Br J Pharmacol* 2000; 130:900–906.

89. Stringer JL, Lorenzo N. The reduction in paired-pulse inhibition in the rat hippocampus by gabapentin is independent of GABA_B receptor activation. *Epilepsy Res* 1999;33:169–176.

90. Patel S, Naeem S, Kesingland A, et al. The effects of GABA_B agonists and gabapentin on mechanical hyperalgesia in models of neuropathic and inflammatory pain in the rat. *Pain* 2001;90: 217–226.

91. Freiman TM, Kukolja J, Heinemeyer J, et al. Modulation of K⁺-evoked [³H]-noradrenaline release from rat and human brain slices by gabapentin: involvement of K_ATP channels. *Naunyn Schmiedebergs Arch Pharmacol* 2001;363:537–542.

92. Taylor CP, Gee NS, Su TZ, et al. A summary of mechanistic hypotheses of gabapentin pharmacology. *Epilepsy Res* 1998;29: 233–249.

93. Marescaux C, Vergnes M., Bernasconi R. GABA_B receptor antagonists: potential new anti-absence drugs. *J Neural Transm Suppl* 1992;35:179–188.

94. Snead OC III. Evidence for GABA_B-mediated mechanisms in experimental generalized absence seizures. *Eur J Pharmacol* 1992; 213:343–349.

95. Hosford DA, Clark S, Cao Z, et al. The role of GABA_B receptor activation in absence seizures of lethargic (*lhlh*) mice. *Science* 1992;257:398–401.

96. Vergnes M, Boehrer A, Simler S, et al. Opposite effects of GABA_B receptor antagonists on absences and convulsive seizures. *Eur J Pharmacol* 1997;332:245–255.

97. Destexhe A. Spike-and-wave oscillations based on the properties of GABA_B receptors. *J Neurosci* 1998;18:9099–9111.

98. Catterall WA. Structure and regulation of voltage-gated Ca²⁺ channels. *Annu Rev Cell Dev Biol* 2000;16:521–555.

99. Turner TJ. Calcium channels coupled to glutamate release. *Prog Brain Res* 1998;116:3–14.

100. Hofmann F, Lacinova L, Klugbauer N. Voltage-dependent calcium channels: from structure to function. *Rev Physiol Biochem Pharmacol* 1999;139:33–87.

101. Gee NS, Brown JP, Dissanayake VUK, et al. The novel anticonvulsant drug, gabapentin (Neurontin) binds to the α₂δ subunit of a calcium channel. *J Biol Chem* 1996;271:5768–5776.

102. Stefani A, Spadoni F, Giacomini P, et al. The effects of gabapentin on different ligand- and voltage-gated currents in isolated cortical neurons. *Epilepsy Res* 2001;43:239–248.

103. Sutton KG, Martin DJ, Pinnock RD, et al. Gabapentin inhibits high-threshold calcium channel currents in cultured rat dorsal root ganglion neurones. *Br J Pharmacol* 2002;43:257–265.

104. Schumacher TB, Beck H, Steinhauser C, et al. Effects of phenytoin, carbamazepine, and gabapentin on calcium channels in hippocampal granule cells from patients with temporal lobe epilepsy. *Epilepsia* 1998;39:355–363.

105. Martin DJ, McClelland D, Herd MB, et al. Gabapentin-mediated inhibition of voltage-activated Ca²⁺ channel currents in cultured sensory neurons is dependent on culture conditions and channel subunit expression. *Neuropharmacology* 2001;42: 353–366.

106. Marais E, Klugbauer N, Hofmann F. Calcium channel α₂δ subunits: structure and gabapentin binding. *Mol Pharmacol* 2001; 59:1243–1248.

107. Stefani A, Spadoni F, Siniscalchi A, et al. Lamotrigine inhibits

Ca^{2+} currents in cortical neurons: functional implications. *Eur J Pharmacol* 1996;307:113–116.

108. Wang S-J, Huang C-C, Hsu K-S, et al. Inhibition of N-type calcium currents by lamotrigine in rat amygdalar neurones. *Neuroreport* 1996;7:3037–3040.

109. Randall A. Physiological activation and pharmacological inhibition of recombinant T-type calcium channels. *Eur J Neurosci* 2000;12[Suppl 11]:146.04.

110. Werz MA, Macdonald RL. Barbiturates decrease voltage-dependent calcium conductance of mouse neurons in dissociated cell culture. *Mol Pharmacol* 1985;28:269–277.

111. ffrench-Mullen JM, Barker JL, Rogawski MA. Calcium current block by (–)-pentobarbital, phenobarbital, and CHEB but not (+)-pentobarbital in acutely isolated hippocampal CA1 neurons: comparison with effects on GABA-activated Cl$^-$ current. *J Neurosci* 1993;13:3211–3221.

112. Huguenard JR. Low-threshold calcium currents in central nervous system neurons. *Annu Rev Physiol* 1996;58:329–358.

113. Perez-Reyes E. Three for T: molecular analysis of the low voltage-activated calcium channel family. *Cell Mol Life Sci* 1999;56:660–669.

114. Talley EM, Cribbs LL, Lee J-H, et al. Differential distribution of three members of a gene family encoding low voltage-activated (T-type) calcium channels. *J Neurosci* 1999;19:1895–1911.

115. Coulter DA, Huguenard JR, Prince DA. Characterization of ethosuximide reduction of low-threshold calcium current in thalamic relay neurons. *Ann Neurol* 1989;25:582–593.

116. Coulter DA, Huguenard JR, Prince DA. Differential effects of petit mal anticonvulsants and convulsants on thalamic neurones: calcium current reduction. *Br J Pharmacol* 1990;100:800–806.

117. Huguenard JR. Neuronal circuitry of thalamocortical epilepsy and mechanisms of antiabsence drug action. *Adv Neurol* 1999;79:991–999.

118. Gomora JC, Daud AN, Weiergraber M, et al. Block of cloned human T-type calcium channels by succinimide antiepileptic drugs. *Mol Pharmacol* 2001;60:1121–1132.

119. Leresche N, Parri HR, Erdemli G, et al. On the action of the anti-absence drug ethosuximide in the rat and cat thalamus. *J Neurosci* 1998;18:4842–4853.

120. Parri HR, Crunelli V. Sodium current in rat and cat thalamocortical neurons: role of a non-inactivating component in tonic and burst firing. *J Neurosci* 1998;18:854–867.

121. Todorovic SM, Lingle CJ. Pharmacological properties of T-type Ca^{2+} current in adult rat sensory neurons: effects of anticonvulsant and anesthetic agents. *J Neurophysiol* 1998;79:240–252.

122. Todorovic SM, Perez-Reyes E, Lingle CJ. Anticonvulsants but not general anesthetics have differential blocking effects on different T-type current variants. *Mol Pharmacol* 2000;58:98–108.

123. Suzuki S, Kawakami K, Nishimura S, et al. Zonisamide blocks T-type calcium channel in cultured neurons of rat cerebral cortex. *Epilepsy Res* 1992;12:21–27.

124. Kito M, Maehara M, Watanabe K. Antiepileptic drugs–calcium current interaction in cultured human neuroblastoma cells. *Seizure* 1994;3:141–149.

125. Rogawski MA. The NMDA receptor, NMDA antagonists and epilepsy therapy: a status report. *Drugs* 1992;44:279–292.

126. Rogawski MA, Donevan SD. AMPA receptors in epilepsy and as targets for antiepileptic drugs. *Adv Neurol* 1999;79:947–963.

127. Chapman AG. Glutamate receptors in epilepsy. *Prog Brain Res* 1998;116:371–383.

128. Löscher W. Pharmacology of glutamate receptor antagonists in the kindling model of epilepsy. *Prog Neurobiol* 1998;54:721–741.

129. Dingledine R, Borges K, Bowie D, et al. The glutamate receptor ion channels. *Pharmacol Rev* 1999;51:7–61.

130. Rogawski MA. Low affinity channel blocking (uncompetitive) NMDA receptor antagonists as therapeutic agents: toward an understanding of their favorable tolerability. *Amino Acids* 2000;19:133–149.

131. Donevan SD, Yamaguchi S, Rogawski MA. Non-N-methyl-D-aspartate receptor antagonism by 3-N-substituted 2,3-benzodiazepines: relationship to anticonvulsant activity. *J Pharmacol Exp Ther* 1994;271:25–29.

132. Subramaniam S, Rho JM, Penix L, et al. Felbamate block of the N-methyl-D-aspartate receptor. *J Pharmacol Exp Ther* 1995;273:878–886.

133. Kleckner NW, Glazewski JC, Chen CC, et al. Subtype-selective antagonism of N-methyl-D-aspartate receptors by felbamate: insights into the mechanism of action. *J Pharmacol Exp Ther* 1999;289:886–894.

134. Harty TP, Rogawski MA. Felbamate block of recombinant N-methyl-D-aspartate receptors: selectivity for the NR2B subunit. *Epilepsy Res* 2000;39:47–55.

135. Mori H, Mishina M. Structure and function of the NMDA receptor channel. *Neuropharmacology* 1995;34:1219–1237.

136. Lerma J, Paternain AV, Rodriguez-Moreno A, et al. Molecular physiology of kainate receptors. *Physiol Rev* 2001;81:971–998.

137. Bleakman D. Kainate receptor pharmacology and physiology. *Cell Mol Life Sci* 1999;56:558–566.

138. Ben-Ari Y, Cossart R. Kainate, a double agent that generates seizures: two decades of progress. *Trends Neurosci* 2000;23:580–587.

139. Conn PJ, Pin JP. Pharmacology and functions of metabotropic glutamate receptors. *Annu Rev Pharmacol Toxicol* 1997;37:205–237.

140. Anwyl R. Metabotropic glutamate receptors: electrophysiological properties and role in plasticity. *Brain Res Brain Res Rev* 1999;29:83–120.

141. Merlin LR, Wong RKS. Role of group I metabotropic glutamate receptors in the patterning of epileptiform activities in vitro. *J Neurophysiol* 1997;78:539–544.

142. Tizzano JP, Griffey KI, Schoepp DD. Induction or protection of limbic seizures in mice by mGluR subtype selective agonists. *Neuropharmacology* 1995;34:1063–1067.

143. Moldrich RX, Talebi A, Beart PM, et al. The mGlu(2/3) agonist 2R,4R-4-aminopyrrolidine-2,4-dicarboxylate, is anti- and proconvulsant in DBA/2 mice. *Neurosci Lett* 2001;299:125–129.

144. Thomsen C, Klitgaard H, Sheardown M, et al. (S)-4-carboxy-3-hydroxyphenylglycine, an antagonist of metabotropic glutamate receptor (mGluR) 1a and an agonist of mGluR2, protects against audiogenic seizures in DBA/2 mice. *J Neurochem* 1994;62:2492–2495.

145. Chapman AG, Yip PK, Yap JS, et al. Anticonvulsant actions of LY 367385 ((+)-2-methyl-4-carboxyphenylglycine) and AIDA ((RS)-1-aminoindan-1,5-dicarboxylic acid). *Eur J Pharmacol* 1999;368:17–24.

146. Chapman AG, Nanan K, Williams M, et al. Anticonvulsant activity of two metabotropic glutamate group I antagonists selective for the mGlu5 receptor: 2-methyl-6-(phenylethynyl)-pyridine (MPEP), and (E)-6-methyl-2-styryl-pyridine (SIB 1893). *Neuropharmacology* 2000;39:1567–1574.

147. Lingamaneni R, Hemmings HC Jr. Effects of anticonvulsants on veratridine- and KCl-evoked glutamate release from rat cortical synaptosomes. *Neurosci Lett* 1999;276:127–130.

148. Prakriya M, Mennerick S. Selective depression of low-release probability excitatory synapses by sodium channel blockers. *Neuron* 2000;26:671–682.

149. Srinivasan J, Richens A, Davies JA. Effects of felbamate on veratridine- and K$^+$-stimulated release of glutamate from mouse cortex. *Eur J Pharmacol* 1996;315:285–288.

150. Stefani A, Spadoni F, Bernardi G. Differential inhibition by riluzole, lamotrigine, and phenytoin of sodium and calcium

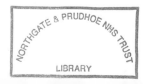

currents in cortical neurons: implications for neuroprotective strategies. *Exp Neurol* 1997;147:115–122.

151. Wang S-J, Huang C-C, Hsu K-S, et al. Presynaptic inhibition of excitatory neurotransmission by lamotrigine in the rat amygdalar neurons. *Synapse* 1996;24:248–255.

152. Wang S-J, Sihra TS, Gean P-W. Lamotrigine inhibition of glutamate release from isolated cerebrocortical nerve terminals (synaptosomes) by suppression of voltage-activated calcium channel activity. *Neuroreport* 2001;12:2255–2258.

153. Jones FA, Davies JA. The anticonvulsant effects of the enantiomers of losigamone. *Br J Pharmacol* 1999;128:1223–1228.

154. Jokeit H, Ebner A. Long term effects of refractory temporal lobe epilepsy on cognitive abilities: a cross sectional study. *J Neurol Neurosurg Psychiatry* 1999;67:44–50.

155. Sato M, Racine RJ, McIntyre DC. Kindling: basic mechanisms and clinical validity. *Electroencephalogr Clin Neurophysiol* 1990; 76:459–472.

156. Matagne A, Klitgaard H. Validation of corneally kindled mice: a sensitive screening model for partial epilepsy in man. *Epilepsy Res* 1998;31:59–71.

157. Mason CR, Cooper RM. A permanent change in convulsive threshold in normal and brain-damaged rats with repeated small doses of pentylenetetrazol. *Epilepsia* 1972;13:663–674.

158. Wasterlain C, Jonec V. Chemical kindling by muscarinic amygdaloid stimulation in the rat. *Brain Res* 1993;271:311–323.

159. Potschka H, Loscher W. Corneal kindling in mice: behavioral and pharmacological differences to conventional kindling. *Epilepsy Res* 1999;37:109–120.

160. Holmes KH, Bilkey DK, Laverty R, et al. The N-methyl-D-aspartate antagonists aminophosphonovalerate and carboxypiperazinephosphonate retard the development and expression of kindled seizures. *Brain Res* 1990;506:227–235.

161. Silver JM, Shin C, McNamara JO. Antiepileptogenic effects of conventional anticonvulsants in the kindling model of epilepsy. *Ann Neurol* 29;356–363.

162. Löscher W, Honack D, Rundfeldt C. Antiepileptogenic effects of the novel anticonvulsant levetiracetam (ucb L059) in the kindling model of temporal lobe epilepsy. *J Pharmacol Exp Ther* 1998;284:474–479.

163. Dalby NO, Nielsen EB. Tiagabine exerts an anti-epileptogenic effect in amygdala kindling epileptogenesis in the rat. *Neurosci Lett* 1997;229:135–137.

164. Shin C, Rigsbee LC, McNamara JO. Anti-seizure and anti-epileptogenic effect of γ-vinyl γ-aminobutyric acid in amygdaloid kindling. *Brain Res* 1986;398:370–374.

165. Schmutz M, Klebs K, Baltzer V. Inhibition or enhancement of kindling evolution by antiepileptics. *J Neural Transm* 1988;72: 245–257.

166. Xie X, Dale TJ, John VH, et al. Electrophysiological and pharmacological properties of the human brain type IIA Na^+ channel expressed in a stable mammalian cell line. *Pflugers Arch* 2001;441:425–433.

167. Johnston GA. GABAc receptors: relatively simple transmitter-gated ion channels? *Trends Pharmacol Sci* 1996;17: 319–323.

168. Zhang D, Pan ZH, Awobuluyi M, et al. Structure and function of GABA$_C$ receptors: a comparison of native versus recombinant receptors. *Trends Pharmacol Sci* 2001;22:121–132.

GENERAL PRINCIPLES

NEUROPHYSIOLOGIC EFFECTS OF ANTIEPILEPTIC DRUGS

CARL W. BAZIL
TIMOTHY A. PEDLEY

Twentieth-century advances in experimental and clinical neurophysiology and in pharmacotherapeutics have revolutionized the diagnosis and treatment of epilepsy. Electroencephalography (EEG) and antiepileptic drugs (AEDs) are inextricably linked in day-to-day practice. Many AEDs have effects on routine EEG and evoked potential recordings, and familiarity with these effects is necessary for accurate test interpretation. At the same time, EEG findings assist in making decisions regarding initiation and withdrawal of AED therapy and, in some cases (e.g., infantile spasms, absence seizures), in determining if the desired therapeutic effect has been achieved.

In this chapter, we review common effects of AEDs on background and interictal EEG activity and on evoked potentials, and we discuss the role of EEG in therapeutic decisions.

ELECTROENCEPHALOGRAPHIC EFFECTS OF ANTIEPILEPTIC DRUGS

The most clinically relevant effects of AEDs are on EEG background activity and on epileptiform discharges. Because of some notable differences, the effects of major agents or classes of agents are considered separately.

Visual Analysis of Electroencephalographic Background Activity

Benzodiazepines

At therapeutic doses, all benzodiazepines increase the amount and prominence of EEG rhythmic fast activity,

Carl W. Bazil, MD, PhD: Assistant Professor, Department of Neurology, Columbia University, New York, New York; and Director, Clinical Anticonvulsant Drug Trials, Comprehensive Epilepsy Center, New York Presbyterian Hospital, New York, New York

Timothy A. Pedley, MD: Professor of Neurology, Department of Neurology, Columbia University, New York, New York; and Neurologist-in-Chief, the Neurological Institute of New York, New York Presbyterian Hospital, New York, New York

usually in the 25- to 35-Hz range (1–4). This effect may be first noticed or most obvious during drowsiness. The voltage of the alpha rhythm usually is correspondingly reduced (4). To some extent, these effects are age and time dependent: EEG changes are more dramatic in younger patients than in older ones, and acute administration results in more prominent beta activity than does chronic use. With a few benzodiazepines (e.g., clonazepam), EEG effects can be dose related (5).

EEG changes related to benzodiazepine intoxication occur sequentially. The rhythmic beta activity increases in voltage and becomes more sustained. This is followed by increasing amounts of slow-frequency activity, which parallel depression of cognitive abilities and increasing lethargy. With onset of coma, the mixture of spindle-like, fast-frequency activity superimposed on continuous slow theta and delta activity resembles EEG patterns seen with barbiturate overdose (6,7).

Barbiturates

At therapeutic doses, barbiturates also entrain faster frequencies into rhythmic patterns, usually in the 18- to 25-Hz range, which are most prominent frontally (6,8,9). As the dosage is raised further and clinical toxicity appears, there is a progression of increasing slow-frequency activity combined with nearly continuous, waxing and waning spindle-like rhythms in the 4- to 12-Hz range ("barbiturate spindles"). Biphasic or triphasic, sharp, slow delta waves may occur (10). Consciousness usually is lost by the time rhythmic or near-rhythmic delta activity predominates with superimposed barbiturate spindles (11). Deep coma is accompanied by a burst-suppression pattern or even electrocerebral inactivity (6,11). This sequence of changes is illustrated in Figure 2.1. With early medical intervention and intensive support, both clinical and EEG features of barbiturate overdose are completely reversible. As the drug is cleared from the system, a reverse sequence of changes is seen (9).

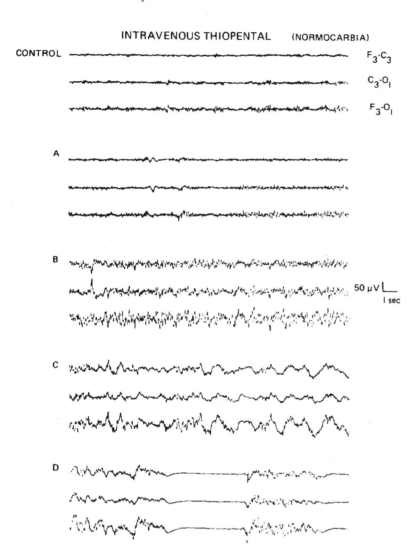

INTRAVENOUS THIOPENTAL   (NORMOCARBIA)

CONTROL ——————————————— F₃-C₃

——————————————— C₃-O₁

——————————————— F₃-O₁

A ———————————————

B

50 μV
1 sec

C

D

FIGURE 2.1. Effect of increasing concentrations of intravenous thiopental on the electroencephalogram. **A:** Increased fast-frequency activity. **B:** Barbiturate spindles of 7 to 10 Hz. **C:** Generalized slow-frequency activity. **D:** Burst-suppression pattern. (From Clark DL, Rosner BS. Neurophysiologic effects of general anesthetics: I. electroencephalogram and sensory evoked responses in man. *Anesthesiology* 1973;38:562–582, with permission.)

Rhythmic fast activity is so typical of acute barbiturate and benzodiazepine administration that its complete absence suggests diffuse underlying organic brain disease (e.g., severe static encephalopathy). Focal or regional asymmetries indicate localized parenchymal dysfunction, which may be due to a chronic epileptogenic focus (12,13) or a cerebral lesion such as porencephalic cyst, tumor, or infarction (6,14). Emergence of EEG fast activity with diazepam has been associated with a good prognosis for seizure control in patients with epilepsy (15).

Phenytoin

Phenytoin usually has no visually discernible effect on the EEG at therapeutic doses, regardless of route of administration (16). No changes were detected during 4 hours of continuous EEG recording in four patients with epilepsy given a 10-mg/kg intravenous (i.v.) dose of phenytoin, even though all patients showed clinical signs of toxicity (17).

At plasma concentrations above 20 μg/mL, phenytoin can slow the mean alpha rhythm frequency slightly, although this is not a consistent effect until there is clinical evidence of drug toxicity (16). This effect may also occur in patients receiving as little as 250 mg of phenytoin i.v. (18). More pronounced symptoms and signs of neurotoxicity are accompanied by progressive EEG changes: increased theta range activity (17), intermittent rhythmic delta activity, and, with severe toxicity (plasma levels >45 μg/mL), high-voltage delta activity (16) (Figure 2.2).

Carbamazepine

Carbamazepine can produce several mild effects on the EEG; these are inconsistent and usually of no clinical consequence. At therapeutic drug concentrations, the most commonly reported changes are mild slowing of the mean alpha rhythm frequency and increased amounts of random theta activity (19,20). Such changes are much more pronounced with toxic doses (6). In a placebo-controlled, dou-

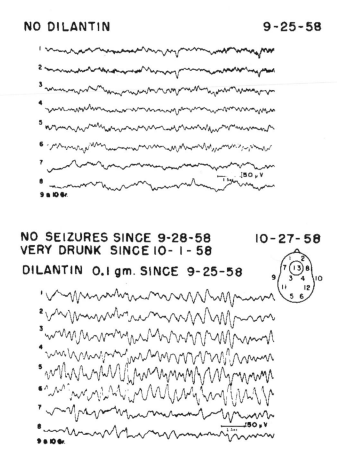

NO DILANTIN   9-25-58

NO SEIZURES SINCE 9-28-58   10-27-58
VERY DRUNK SINCE 10-1-58

DILANTIN 0.1 gm. SINCE 9-25-58

FIGURE 2.2. High-voltage delta activity in a patient with severe phenytoin toxicity. (From Roseman E. Dilantin toxicity: a clinical and electroencephalographic study. *Neurology* 1961;11:912–921, with permission.)

ble-blind trial involving 40 patients with epilepsy, carbamazepine was said to increase theta activity and decrease alpha activity significantly compared with placebo (20), but treated patients also were receiving phenobarbital and phenytoin. Similar EEG effects have been reported in psychiatric patients treated with carbamazepine (21), as well as in patients with epilepsy compared with phenytoin using a randomized, crossover design (22).

Valproate

Several studies of valproate have found no effect on routinely acquired EEG background activity at therapeutic plasma concentrations (23–25). Villarreal et al. (25) studied 25 patients with absence seizures, most of whom had other seizure types and remained on AED polytherapy during the study. Analysis of four channels of EEG recorded using a telemetry system did not detect changes in background activity. Bruni et al. (24) investigated 22 patients with absence seizures before and after 1 year of valproate therapy. Visual review of 6-hour, 16-channel EEG recordings did not reveal changes in background

activity. In contrast, other investigators have reported either slower mean alpha rhythm frequencies (26,27) or increased random theta activity (28), but these effects usually are accompanied by symptoms and signs of clinical toxicity (23).

Newer Anticonvulsants

Much less is known about the EEG effects of the newer AEDs, which include felbamate, gabapentin, lamotrigine, topiramate, tiagabine, levetiracetam, oxcarbazepine, zonisamide, and vigabatrin. In general, because clinical neurotoxicity is less likely to occur with most of these agents, effects on background EEG activity also are less commonly encountered in clinical practice. Only tiagabine has been studied in a published trial; it had no effect on background EEG activity at therapeutic dosages (29). For other drugs, clinical experience and a few published abstracts (30–32) suggest little or no effect on EEG background activity at therapeutic dosages.

Computer-Assisted Analysis of Background Activity

Additional information about the effects of AEDs on EEG background activity has been obtained by using computer-assisted and topographic mapping techniques (33–35). Dumermuth et al. (5) reported a correlation between clonazepam or diazepam blood levels and frontal "beta density." They also found that these drugs decreased the power spectra of frequencies less than 18 Hz. Such quantitative measures are consistent with changes previously described from routine visual inspection of the EEG. Similarly, acute administration of phenobarbital to normal subjects resulted in increased power spectra for frequencies greater than 16 Hz (35), an effect that also would have been predicted from changes described in the routine EEG. Other studies, however, have not found any consistent difference in power spectra between untreated patients with epilepsy and patients treated with either phenobarbital (33) or carbamazepine (33,36).

Beta asymmetries after administration of i.v. thiopental (37) or diazepam (38) have been quantified using spectral analysis.

Patients treated with valproate had less theta activity and less 13- to 19.8-Hz activity than did untreated patients with epilepsy (33). A subgroup analysis showed this to be true only for patients with generalized tonic-clonic seizures; patients with partial seizures showed less delta activity in the valproate-treated group. These results are hard to understand in light of studies of routine EEG that have shown either no effect of valproate on background activity or mild increases in slow-frequency activity. If decreased delta activity were due to suppression of spike–wave discharges by valproate (25,39), this effect should have been seen to an even greater degree in patients with generalized tonic-clonic seizures, which was not the case.

Quantitative effects of phenytoin on EEG activity have been studied in normal volunteers. Oral administration of 100 to 1,000 mg resulted in decreased power in slow-frequency bands and increased power in fast-frequency bands at plasma concentrations above 8 µg/mL (40). The magnitude of the EEG changes paralleled plasma concentrations.

A study of six patients with epilepsy concluded that phenytoin and carbamazepine increase theta and delta power slightly and slow the alpha rhythm when individual patients were compared on or off chronic drug treatment, but these changes varied widely between patients (41). Such effects may represent a physiologic marker of a patient's unique response to pharmacologic cerebral toxicity. It remains to be shown, however, whether these EEG changes correlate with objective measures of impaired cognitive abilities.

Lamotrigine does not affect EEG background activity studied by computerized methods before and after treatment (42), although another quantitative EEG study showed increased beta and decreased theta with lamotrigine, as well as increased alpha and beta frequencies with vigabatrin, and increased beta and theta activities with topiramate (43). Most study patients were comedicated with at least two other agents, and these results therefore must be interpreted cautiously.

EFFECTS OF ANTIEPILEPTIC DRUGS ON EPILEPTIFORM ACTIVITY

With a few notable exceptions, the effect of AEDs on interictal epileptiform activity is variable and inconsistent; routine visual assessment of interictal activity usually does not correlate well with seizure control. In a provocative study, however, Frost et al. (44) offered preliminary evidence that computer-derived measures of interictal spike morphology can be quantified and correlated with seizure control. In a study of 13 children with EEG spike foci and partial seizures, phenobarbital or carbamazepine efficacy was related to decreased spike voltage, decreased spike duration, an increase in the normalized sharpness of the spike, and a decrease in the "composite spike parameter," a computed variable that expressed the relationship among these other basic waveform measures. We are unaware of further studies of this intriguing approach.

So and Gotman (45) studied the effects of high and low AED levels on patterns of ictal discharge in 56 patients with chronically implanted depth electrodes. Reduced drug levels increased seizure frequency and the number of seizures that secondarily generalized. However, low drug levels did not affect the morphology of initial ictal events, duration to contralateral spread, or coherence between discharges.

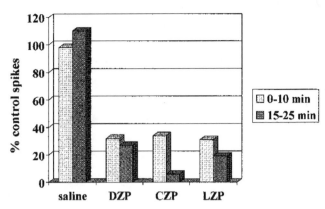

FIGURE 2.3. Reduction in interictal spike count in a group of six epileptic patients after intravenous administration of clonazepam (CZP, 0.5 mg), lorazepam (LZP, 2 mg), diazepam (DZP, 5 mg), or saline as a percentage of preinjection spike counts. (Adapted from Ahmad S, Perucca E, Richens A. The effects of furosemide, mexiletine, (+)propranolol and three benzodiazepine drugs on interictal spike discharges in the electroencephalogram of epileptic patients. *Br J Clin Pharmacol* 1977;4: 683–688, with permission).

The effects of AEDs on EEG epileptiform activity are discussed in the following sections for each major agent or class of agents.

Benzodiazepines

Benzodiazepines are potent AEDs when administered acutely and act rapidly to suppress interictal and ictal EEG discharges. This effect has been demonstrated on both generalized spike–wave activity and focal spike discharges using rectal (46) or i.v. (47–49) diazepam as well as oral or i.v. clonazepam (1,3,47,49). A single i.v. dose of diazepam, 5 mg, or clonazepam, 0.5 mg, administered to 14 epileptic patients in a double-blind, placebo-controlled trial reduced spike discharges to approximately one-third of the baseline rate (diazepam 32% ± 12%; clonazepam 34% ± 11%). A similar but more delayed response was seen with lorazepam (47) (Figure 2.3). Intravenous diazepam aborts or attenuates photoparoxysmal responses (48,50).

Benzodiazepines have been used to help localize the epileptogenic brain region. Intravenous diazepam (50,51) or clonazepam (1) may suppress bilateral spread of epileptiform discharges (secondary bilateral synchrony) without eliminating activity at the focus itself.

Barbiturates

Phenobarbital can reduce the amount of interictal epileptiform activity (52) and sometimes even abolish it completely (53,54). Kellaway et al. (54) monitored 12 children with partial seizures for 24 or 36 hours before and after phenobarbital treatment using computer-assisted visual analysis. In 6 of 11 patients with complete seizure control, no interictal spikes or sharp waves were seen in the posttreatment study.

In the other successfully treated patients, the number of interictal spikes decreased by 20% to 30% after treatment.

In another study, Buchtal et al. (52) found that phenobarbital, at a mean plasma concentration of 10 μg/mL (range, 3 to 22 μg/mL), reduced interictal epileptiform activity by 90% in 11 adult patients with generalized seizures who were selected because of their high rate of spontaneous interictal discharges. Some tolerance to this effect developed, because higher concentrations of phenobarbital were required to produce a similar degree of spike suppression after treatment had been withdrawn for 1 to 2 weeks. A single patient with petit mal epilepsy showed no improvement either clinically or in terms of EEG paroxysms.

Barbiturates can be used to distinguish primary from secondary bilateral synchrony. Lombroso and Erba (55) studied 82 patients with generalized seizures and bilateral spike–wave discharges. In 30 of these patients, administration of i.v. thiopental reduced diffuse spike–wave activity and allowed identification of an EEG focus. This effect was most pronounced in patients with clinical evidence of focal cerebral lesions.

Predictable EEG changes occur during barbiturate withdrawal. Drug-addicted patients showed high-voltage, bisynchronous spike–wave discharges and diffuse slowing during withdrawal (8,56) (Figure 2.4). In patients with partial epilepsy whose barbiturates are discontinued for intensive video/EEG monitoring, withdrawal may be accompanied by generalized epileptiform activity or, rarely, by the apparent appearance of new or additional loci of seizure onset (57). The clinical significance of these newly recognized "foci" is uncertain and must be interpreted in light of other clinical data.

Phenytoin

Most investigators have found that phenytoin treatment does not affect interictal epileptiform discharges (22,58). There are a few reports to the contrary, however. Carrie (59) performed nine overnight EEG studies in a single patient and reported that epileptiform sharp waves increased as the phenytoin level rose and the number of clinical seizures diminished. He speculated that increased interictal activity was a consequence of phenytoin's antiepileptic effect, which had caused "fractionation" of convulsive discharges into interictal abnormalities. On the other hand, two studies have found that epileptiform activity decreased with phenytoin treatment. Buchtal et al. (60) observed that 14 of 27 outpatients and 11 of 12 inpatients with grand mal seizures had reduced amounts of epileptiform activity with phenytoin levels over 10 μg/mL. However, approximately one-sixth of the patients had increased amounts of interictal abnormalities. Interpretation of these results was further confounded by concurrent administration of phenobarbital in some patients. Wilkus and Green (61) found that 3 of 18 patients had fewer epileptiform discharges after 6 months of phenytoin treatment than did

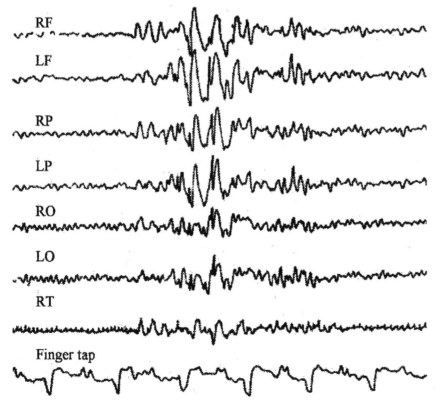

FIGURE 2.4. Electroencephalographic (EEG) changes in acute barbiturate withdrawal. After 52 weeks of treatment with secobarbital, 600 mg daily, the drug was stopped abruptly. These bilaterally synchronous spike–wave discharges appeared within 26 hours and persisted 72 hours after drug withdrawal. The EEG returned to baseline 1 week after withdrawal. (Adapted from Wikler A, Fraser F, Isbell H, et al. Electroencephalograms during cycles of addiction to barbiturates in man. *Electroencephalogr Clin Neurophysiol* 1955;7:1–13, with permission.)

control subjects, but this observation did not correlate with seizure frequency.

Phenytoin withdrawal has been associated with false localization of ictal onset (62).

Carbamazepine

Data regarding the effect of carbamazepine on interictal EEG discharges are conflicting. Most studies have found that carbamazepine either increases the amount of interictal abnormalities or has no effect. Studies by Jongmans (63), Wilkus et al. (22), and Sachdeo and Chokroverty (64) found that carbamazepine increased interictal epileptiform activity, but this was unrelated to seizure control. Wilkus et al. (22) used a randomized, crossover design to compare phenytoin and carbamazepine in 45 patients, most of whom had complex partial seizures. Focal epileptiform discharges increased significantly while patients were taking carbamazepine, but this did not correlate with seizure control. Pryse-Phillips and Jeavons (19) did not find any change in the amount of focal epileptiform activity when all patients were considered together, but 3 of 22 patients had increased epileptiform discharges while on carbamazepine; baseline rates in these patients were reestablished when the drug was stopped. In a double-blind, placebo-controlled trial involving 40 patients with psychomotor epilepsy, 50% of the patients had less, and 38% had more, interictal epileptiform activity while on carbamazepine. These findings, like those of others, did not correlate with seizure control (20). Similarly, Monaco et al. (65) found no consistent effect of carbamazepine on the EEG and no relation between any EEG change and seizure control. Finally, Martins da Silva et al. (58) reported a negative correlation between serum carbamazepine level and interictal epileptiform activity, but their study included only two patients on carbamazepine monotherapy.

Valproate

The effect of valproate on epileptiform activity seems to depend on the type of epilepsy. Valproate clearly reduces generalized spike–wave discharges but probably has little or no effect on focal epileptiform activity.

Valproate suppresses 3-Hz spike–wave activity, and this correlates with control of absence seizures (25,39,66), including attacks present only during hyperventilation (24). Bruni et al. (24) studied patients with absence seizures before and after 1 year of valproate therapy. Fifty-seven percent of patients had the number of spike–wave paroxysms reduced by more than 75%; in one-third of these, spike–wave activity disappeared completely. Valproate was equally effective whether spike–wave paroxysms were of short or long duration. Thus, valproate suppressed over 75% of spike–wave discharges lasting longer than 3

seconds in 62% of patients, and 9 of 21 of these patients had the spike–wave activity eliminated completely. Both Villarreal et al. (25) and Bruni et al. (24) looked at clinical and EEG effects in the same patients at 10 weeks and 1 year after starting valproate treatment. Optimal seizure control was achieved as soon as therapeutic drug levels were achieved, but reductions in the amount of generalized spike–wave activity continued to occur up to 1 year later. Villarreal et al. (25) studied 25 patients with absence seizures treated with valproate. Most of these patients had other seizure types as well and remained on AED polytherapy during the study. Seventy-nine percent of the patients had reduced numbers of spike–wave discharges after introduction of valproate; 45% had spike–wave activity reduced by more than 75%. Reduced numbers of paroxysms lasting longer than 3 seconds correlated with control of absence attacks.

Valproate also suppresses photoparoxysmal responses. In one study, valproate reduced the number of patients showing photoparoxysmal responses by 31% (24). Harding et al. (67) studied 50 patients with photosensitive epilepsy before and during treatment with valproate. Valproate abolished photic-induced epileptiform activity in 27 patients (54%), and 12 patients (24%) were improved as defined by a greater than 75% reduction in the number of flash rates to which the patient was sensitive (the "sensitivity range"). Attenuation of the photoparoxysmal response may persist after an acute valproate dose has been cleared from the blood (68) and up to 3 months after discontinuing chronic therapy (67).

In contrast to the unambiguous effect of valproate on generalized spike–wave activity, studies of focal spike activity have not revealed any consistent changes with treatment. Thus, there are reports of both reduced (23) or unchanged (39) focal epileptiform activity after treatment with valproate.

Ethosuximide

EEG effects of ethosuximide have been less well studied than those of other common AEDs. Reports agree, however, that ethosuximide reduces generalized spike–wave discharges in approximately 50% of treated patients. Sato et al. (66) observed that ethosuximide abolished spike–wave discharges in the 12-hour telemetered EEGs of 6 of 11 patients (55%). Ethosuximide was slightly less effective than valproate in reducing the number of spike–wave discharges lasting 3 seconds or less. Ethosuximide also decreases 3-Hz spike–wave discharges induced by intermittent photic stimulation (67).

Newer Anticonvulsants

Of the newer AEDs, most is known about lamotrigine. Single-dose studies have shown a decrease in both interictal spike activity (69,70) and photoconvulsive responses (69). In patients with refractory absence seizures, lamotrigine can suppress generalized spike–wave discharges (71). In a study of patients with localization related and generalized epilepsy that compared computerized EEG data before and 4 months after addition of lamotrigine, interictal epileptiform discharges were decreased in both frequency (42,72) and duration (42). Rarely, however, lamotrigine has been reported to activate new generalized epileptiform discharges associated with clinical seizures (73).

Felbamate reduces the number of sharp–slow-wave complexes in patients with Lennox-Gastaut syndrome (74). Vigabatrin decreases the frequency of interictal discharges in patients with intractable complex partial seizures, but this is unrelated to its efficacy in controlling seizures (75). In patients participating in a double-blind, add-on study of tiagabine, there was no effect on interictal epileptiform activity (29).

A few of the newer drugs can induce or increase myoclonus. For example, vigabatrin can induce myoclonus and generalized polyspike-and-wave complexes (76). In a double-blind study using a placebo, tiagabine was associated with the disappearance of epileptiform discharges in a few patients (29). Tiagabine also rarely induces new seizure types and can activate new epileptiform discharges (29). Gabapentin does not affect interictal epileptiform activity (72).

EFFECTS OF ANTIEPILEPTIC DRUGS ON SLEEP–WAKE CYCLES

Excessive daytime somnolence and sleep disturbances are common complaints among patients with epilepsy (77). The reasons for this often are unclear because it frequently is difficult to separate the effects of the disorder from those of its treatment. Available data suggest that AEDs affect sleep structure, but it is not now possible to draw a consistent picture of these effects. In some patients, AEDs improve sleep by decreasing the number of microarousals that result from seizure activity (78). Two studies have examined the effects of carbamazepine on normal control subjects (79,80) and found that sleep efficiency was increased and rapid eye movement (REM) density was decreased. A rigorous study of administration of carbamazepine to normal subjects and patients with newly diagnosed epilepsy suggested that reduction in REM by carbamazepine was significant only in patients with epilepsy (72). Drake et al. (81) used ambulatory EEG recordings made in patients' homes to study sleep patterns in 17 patients with focal or generalized epilepsy. Phenytoin, carbamazepine, and valproate each were taken by 5 patients; the other 2 patients took clonazepam. Phenytoin and carbamazepine were associated with decreased total sleep time and significant increases in sleep latency, number of arousals, and periods of wakefulness after sleep onset compared with valproate and clonazepam. Phenytoin increased the amount of stage 1 sleep and decreased stage 2 sleep. Patients taking carbamazepine had significantly less REM sleep than did those taking other drugs. There were no differences among the drugs in the amount of stage 3 or 4 sleep. Interpretation of these data is limited by the heterogeneous patient population and absence of a control or comparison group. Thus, it is not clear whether the observed effects were due solely to AEDs or whether different types of epilepsy affect sleep structure in different ways.

In a somewhat more rigorous study, Wolf et al. (82) used a single-blind protocol to investigate the effects of phenobarbital or phenytoin on sleep in 40 patients with epilepsy. Observations were made before and after therapeutic levels of each drug were achieved. Most of the patients were newly diagnosed and previously untreated; all were on monotherapy during the study. When taking phenobarbital, patients showed significant decreases in sleep latency. More time was spent in stage 2 and less in REM sleep, and interspersed time awake was decreased. Patients on phenytoin fell asleep more rapidly and spent relatively more time in stage 3 or 4 non-REM sleep than in stages 1 or 2. There were no differences between the drugs in the number of awakenings or total amount of REM sleep. Patients with generalized epilepsy tended to have shorter early REM cycles than did patients with focal epilepsy.

A similar study was performed comparing ethosuximide and valproate using a single-blind crossover design (83). Ethosuximide increased stage 1 sleep and decreased the amount of stage 3 or 4 sleep. REM sleep was increased in the early cycles but decreased in the later ones. Valproate's effects were limited to increasing stage 1 sleep and prolonging the first REM phase.

In other reports, phenobarbital has decreased nocturnal arousals, increased stage 2 sleep, and decreased REM periods (82,84,85). Phenytoin has been found to increase the number of arousals and periods of wakefulness (81,82), and also to have no appreciable effect on sleep (86). Information regarding carbamazepine is equally inconsistent. Thus, the drug has been associated with increased arousals, increased episodes of wakefulness, and decreased REM (81), as well as no detectable effects (86). Phenytoin, valproate, and ethosuximide may all increase stage 1 sleep (81,83).

Of the newer AEDs, gabapentin has received the most attention. In patients with epilepsy, gabapentin increased REM and reduced awakenings (87), although it is not clear if this related to improved seizure control. Rao et al. (88) found that gabapentin increased slow-wave sleep in normal control subjects. An add-on study of gabapentin and lamotrigine in patients with epilepsy showed that both drugs increased REM and sleep stability (72), although it is possible that these changes were due to decreased seizure activity (89).

EFFECTS OF ANTIEPILEPTIC DRUGS ON EVOKED POTENTIALS

Many investigators have reported changes in visual evoked potentials (VEPs) in patients with epilepsy using trains of binocular flash stimuli (90) or pattern-reversal stimuli (36,91), but it is difficult to know if observed changes are due to the epileptic disorder or to AEDs. In general, most studies have failed to demonstrate any effect on VEPs by valproate (92) or other antiepileptic agents (93). Martinovic et al. (94) found no differences in pattern-reversal VEPs from untreated patients and patients who were well controlled on valproate or carbamazepine compared with normal control subjects. Treated patients with poor seizure control had prolonged P2 (P100) latencies and N1P2 amplitudes that were not significant. Valproate does, however, affect VEPs in photosensitive patients (90,92,95). Faught and Lee (95) found that the latency of the P2 (P100) component of pattern-reversal VEPs was shorter in patients with photoparoxysmal responses and epilepsy than in control subjects. Latencies increased in patients successfully treated with valproate.

Phenytoin and carbamazepine, but not phenobarbital, valproate, or primidone, prolong interpeak latencies of somatosensory evoked potentials (SSEPs) and brainstem auditory evoked potentials (BAEPs). The magnitude of this effect is related to the plasma drug concentration (36,92, 96–101). Zonisamide does not affect BAEPs or SSEPs at therapeutic dosages (102).

Vigabatrin has been causally linked to both clinical and asymptomatic constriction of the visual fields and other visual abnormalities, especially sensitivity (103–106). Most studies have not found an effect of vigabatrin on VEPs in unselected patients (107) or after brief exposure (108), although some have demonstrated abnormalities with long-term exposure. Krauss et al. (106) studied four patients treated with vigabatrin for 2 to 40 months who experienced symptoms of visual field constriction or blurring. All had evidence of retinal dysfunction on electroretinography (ERG). Two had normal VEPs, one had prolonged VEP latency, and one had normal latencies but decreased P1 amplitude. In another study involving 39 asymptomatic patients who had taken vigabatrin for an average of 52 months (range, 28 to 78 months), 7 (18%) had bilaterally delayed VEPs; 5 of these also had reduced amplitudes (109). The abnormalities did not correlate with severity of clinical symptoms or changes in ERG. In a large study of 201 patients, VEPs were obtained before treatment and again after vigabatrin exposure for up to 24 months (110). There were no consistent changes for the entire group. Although five patients who remained on vigabatrin had prolonged P100 latencies at the end of the study, a similar number had abnormal VEPs before starting the drug. BAEPs and SSEPs do not seem to be affected by vigabatrin (108,110,111). Although vigabatrin can lead to a striking, bilaterally concentric contraction of the visual fields in some patients, the drug does not produce a consistent effect on VEPs. Indeed, VEPs usually are normal even in the presence of a significant visual field defect. In contrast, ERG abnormalities show a high degree of correlation with visual field loss (104,106). Two conclusions emerge: First, the electrophysiologic findings indicate retinal dysfunction, not abnormalities of central white matter, as the origin of the field deficits. Second, VEPs are not a useful screening tool for detecting asymptomatic visual field loss. ERG can detect and quantify retinal dysfunction, and it therefore may be useful in following patients. Both ERG and visual field abnormalities persist, even after the drug is discontinued.

ROLE OF THE ELECTROENCEPHALOGRAM IN TREATMENT DECISIONS

Diagnosis

EEG findings can assist clinicians in determining that a historical paroxysmal event was a seizure. Epileptiform discharges (EEG spikes or sharp waves) are highly correlated with seizure susceptibility (112,113). Unfortunately, this specificity is not matched by a similar degree of sensitivity. In patients with established epilepsy, a single EEG demonstrates specific epileptiform abnormalities in 50% to 59% of cases. Repeated examinations increase the yield of positive findings (112,114), as do sleep and sleep deprivation (77,113). AEDs other than valproate usually do not change these percentages (112).

EEG findings also are helpful in classifying seizures as focal or generalized when clinical information is ambiguous, and in establishing an epilepsy syndrome diagnosis. Such information is important in making rational treatment decisions.

Initiation of Treatment

Although an EEG that shows epileptiform activity often is helpful in diagnostic formulations, treatment decisions require that EEG abnormalities also be characterized in terms of their *epileptogenic* significance, especially their predictive value in calculating risk of further seizures.

Most studies of first unprovoked seizures in adults have reported that the recurrence risk is increased if the EEG is abnormal. van Donselaar et al. (115) performed a prospective study of 165 patients who had had an unprovoked first seizure. All patients had a routine EEG performed after sleep deprivation. If no epileptiform activity was seen, a second EEG was obtained. Seizures recurred within 2 years in 83% of patients whose EEGs showed epileptiform discharges, but in only 12% of patients whose EEGs were normal (Figure 2.5). In patients whose EEGs showed nonepileptiform abnormalities, seizures

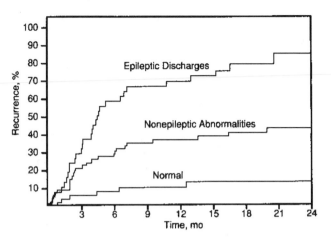

FIGURE 2.5. Cumulative seizure recurrence rates based on electroencephalographic findings in 157 patients with idiopathic first seizures. (From van Donselaar CA, Schimsheimer R, Geerts AT, et al. Value of the electroencephalogram in adult patients with untreated idiopathic first seizure. *Arch Neurol* 1992;49: 231–237, with permission.)

recurred in 41%. None of the patients were treated with AEDs before the second seizure.

Other studies have shown that EEG epileptiform abnormalities increase the risk of recurrence approximately twofold in patients who have had a single unprovoked seizure compared with similar patients with normal EEGs (116,117). A dissenting conclusion was reported by Hopkins et al. (118), who found no relation between EEG findings and risk of recurrence in 408 adult patients. Although their data suggested that fewer patients with abnormal EEGs remained seizure free, especially those with focal epileptiform abnormalities, analysis of recurrence risk at specific time points (3, 12, and 24 months) did not find these differences to be significant.

Children also have a higher risk of seizure recurrence if the EEG is abnormal at the time of a first unprovoked seizure. Camfield et al. (119) studied 168 children with an initial afebrile seizure. Seizures recurred in 68% of children with focal epileptiform discharges but in only 37% of children whose EEGs were normal. Recurrence rates were 45% to 64% in children with other kinds of EEG abnormalities. Other studies have found that any type of EEG abnormality increases the risk of recurrence in children after a first afebrile seizure (116,120).

Discontinuing Antiepileptic Drugs

EEG findings can assist in making decisions about discontinuing AEDs in treated patients whose seizures are in remission. The relation of EEG findings to risk of seizure relapse after drug withdrawal has been studied in both children (121–124) and adults (125–128). In a retrospective study involving 62 adult patients, epileptiform discharges at the time of drug withdrawal were 50% more common in

patients who relapsed, although the finding did not reach statistical significance (128). In a prospective study of 1021 patients, all but 28 had at least one EEG before drug withdrawal. Univariate analysis showed that only patients who had had generalized tonic-clonic seizures and EEGs showing generalized spike–wave abnormalities had a higher risk of seizure relapse; EEG findings were not predictive for other groups (127). In another well designed, prospective investigation, Callaghan et al. (126) studied 92 patients with generalized or complex partial seizures that had been controlled by AEDs for at least 2 years. EEGs were obtained before treatment was started and again before drugs were withdrawn. Patients whose EEGs were normal or improved with treatment had a 94% to 99% reduction in risk of relapse compared with patients whose EEGs were abnormal before treatment and unchanged before withdrawal (Table 2.1). Despite differences among available studies, we conclude that persistent EEG abnormalities increase the risk of seizure relapse after drug withdrawal in adults whose seizures have been in remission for 2 years or more.

There is considerably more agreement regarding EEG findings and seizure relapse in children. Virtually all studies have shown that EEG abnormalities are a major risk factor for seizure relapse after AEDs are discontinued. This association holds regardless of whether the EEG was recorded during the year before AED withdrawal (122), immediately before withdrawal (121,123,124), or after withdrawal (123). The most convincing study is that of Shinnar et al. (124), who prospectively investigated 88 children with afebrile seizures who had been seizure free on AEDs for at least 2 years. EEGs were obtained before drug withdrawal; earlier EEGs were available for comparison in 82 patients. EEG characteristics were strongly predictive of outcome after drug withdrawal: Seizure recurrence was substantially lower in children who had EEGs that were normal or improved at the time drugs were discontinued. Specific EEG features (slow-frequency activity,

TABLE 2.1. ELECTROENCEPHALOGRAPHIC FINDINGS AND RELAPSE RATES

Description	Relapse Rate (%)	No. of Patients Relapsing/ Total
Normal before treatment	35.4	11/31
Abnormal before treatment, normal before withdrawal	11.4	4/35
Abnormal before treatment, abnormal but improved before withdrawal	50.0	2/4
Abnormal before treatment, unchanged before withdrawal	73.7	14/19

From Callaghan N, Garrett A, Goggin T. Withdrawal of anticonvulsant drugs in patients free of seizures for two years. A prospective study. *N Engl J Med* 1988;318:942–946, with permission.

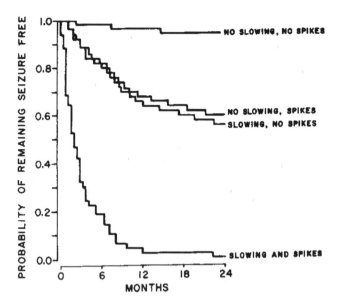

FIGURE 2.6. Effect of slowing and spikes on the probability of remaining free of seizures over time. (From Shinnar S, Vining EPG, Mellits ED, et al. Discontinuing antiepileptic medications in children with epilepsy after two years without seizures: a prospective study. *N Engl J Med* 1985;313:976–980, with permission.)

spikes) were more informative than classification only as normal or abnormal (Figure 2.6).

CONCLUSIONS

Antiepileptic drugs have significant effects on brain physiology as measured by evoked potentials, waking–sleep patterns, and, especially, the EEG. EEG data are helpful in deciding whether to initiate or discontinue treatment. AEDs, especially at toxic levels, often affect EEG background activity, and this may be an important interpretive consideration in some patients. In some circumstances, AEDs may help clarify EEG findings, as in distinguishing primary from secondary bilateral synchrony, or aid in localization of the epileptogenic zone. Whether computer-assisted methods of spike analysis may increase the utility of interictal EEG findings as a gauge of AED efficacy remains to be proved. Finally, AEDs affect waking–sleep cycles and sleep structure, but these associations need further characterization to be clinically useful.

REFERENCES

1. Browne TR. Clonazepam: a review of a new anticonvulsant drug. *Arch Neurol* 1976;33:326–332.
2. Browne TR, Penry JK. Benzodiazepines in the treatment of epilepsy. *Epilepsia* 1973;14:277–310.
3. Fazio C, Manfredini M, Piccinelli A. Treatment of epileptic seizures with clonazepam. *Arch Neurol* 1975;32:304–307.
4. Towler ML. The clinical use of diazepam in anxiety states and depressions. *J Neuropsychiatry* 1962;3[Suppl 1]:68–72.
5. Dumermuth G, Gasser T, Heckeer A, et al. Exploration of EEG components in the beta frequency range. In: Kellaway P, Petersen I, eds. *Qualitative analytic studies in epilepsy.* New York: Raven Press, 1976:533–558.
6. Bauer G. EEG, drug effects and central nervous system poisoning. In: Niedermeyer E, Lopes da Silva FH, eds. *Electroencephalography: basic principles, clinical applications and related fields.* Baltimore: Urban & Schwartzenberg, 1987:567–578.
7. Kurtz D. The EEG in acute and chronic drug intoxication. In: Glaser GH, Redmond A, eds. *Metabolic, endocrine, and toxic diseases. Handbook of electroencephalography and clinical neurophysiology,* vol 15C. Amsterdam: Elsevier, 1976:88–104.
8. Essig CF, Fraser HF. Electroencephalographic changes in man during use and withdrawal of barbiturates in moderate dosage. *Electroencephalogr Clin Neurophysiol* 1958;10:649–656.
9. Prichard JW. Barbiturates: physiological effects I. In: Glaser GH, Penry JK, Woodbury DM, eds. *Antiepileptic drugs: mechanism of action.* New York: Raven Press, 1980:505–522.
10. Kubicki S. Triphasic potentials following a state of deep coma (coma depasse) in patients with intoxication by hypnotics. *Electroencephalogr Clin Neurophysiol* 1967;23:382(abstr).
11. Brazier MAB. The effect of drugs on the electroencephalogram of man. *Clin Pharmacol Ther* 1964;5:102–116.
12. Engel J, Driver MV, Falconer MA. Electrophysiological correlates of pathology and surgical results in temporal lobe epilepsy. *Brain* 1975;98:129–156.
13. Engel J, Rausch R, Lieb JP, et al. Correlation of criteria used for localizing epileptic foci in patients considered for surgical therapy of epilepsy. *Ann Neurol* 1981;9:215–224.
14. Pampiglione G. Induced fast activity in EEG as aid in location of cerebral lesions. *Electroencephalogr Clin Neurophysiol* 1952;4:79–82.
15. Huang ZC, Shen DL. The prognostic significance of diazepam-induced EEG changes in epilepsy: a follow-up study. *Clin Electroencephalogr* 1993;24:179–187.
16. Roseman E. Dilantin toxicity: a clinical and electroencephalographic study. *Neurology* 1961;11:912–921.
17. Nordentoft-Jensen B, Grynderip V. Studies on the metabolism of phenytoin. *Epilepsia* 1966;7:238–245.
18. Riehl J-L, McIntyre HB A quantitative study of the acute effects of diphenylhydantoin on the electroencephalogram of epileptic patients. *Neurology* 1968;18:1107–1112.
19. Pryse-Phillips WEM, Jeavons PM. Effect of carbamazepine (Tegretol) on the electroencephalograph and ward behaviour of patients with chronic epilepsy. *Epilepsia* 1970;11:263–273.
20. Rodin EA, Rim CS, Rennick PM. The effects of carbamazepine on patients with psychomotor epilepsy: results of a double-blind study. *Epilepsia* 1974;15:547–561.
21. Misurec J, Nahunek K, Svestka J, et al. EEG profile of carbamazepine. *Activ Nerv Super* 1985;27:264.
22. Wilkus RJ, Dodrill CB, Troupin AS. Carbamazepine and the electroencephalogram of epileptics: a double-blind study in comparison to phenytoin. *Epilepsia* 1978;19:283–291.
23. Adams DJ, Lüders H, Pippenger C. Sodium valproate in the treatment of intractable seizure disorders: a clinical and electroencephalographic study. *Neurology* 1978;28:152–157.
24. Bruni J, Wilder BJ, Bauman AW, et al. Clinical efficacy and long term effects of valproic acid on spike and wave discharges. *Neurology* 1980;30:42–46.
25. Villarreal HJ, Wilder BJ, Wilmore LJ, et al. Effects of valproic acid on spike and wave discharges in patients with absence seizures. *Neurology* 1978;28:886–891.
26. Miralbel J, Marinier R. Modifications electroencephalo-

graphiques chez des enfants epileptiques traites par le Depakene. *Rev Neurol* 1968;119:313–320.

27. Sackellares JC, Sato S, Dreifuss FE, et al. The effect of valproic acid on the EEG background. In: Wada JA, Penry JK, eds. *Advances in epileptology: Xth epilepsy international symposium.* New York: Raven Press, 1980:132.

28. Gram L, Wulff K, Rasmussen KE, et al. Valproate sodium: a controlled clinical trial including monitoring of drug levels. *Epilepsia* 1977;18:141–148.

29. Kalviainen R, Aikia M, Mervaala E, et al. Long-term cognitive and EEG effects of tiagabine in drug-resistant partial epilepsy. *Epilepsy Res* 1996;25:291–297.

30. Foletti G, Delisle MC, Chardon F, et al. Clinical and EEG effects of lamotrigine as add-on therapy in adults with typical Lennox-Gastaut syndrome unsatisfactorily controlled by current antiepileptic drugs. *Epilepsia* 1999;40[Suppl 2]:166.

31. Salinsky MC, Binder LM, Oken BS, et al. Effects of chronic gabapentin and carbamazepine treatment on EEG, alertness, and cognition in healthy volunteers. *Epilepsia* 2000;41[Suppl 7]:151.

32. Spanedda F, Placidi F, Romigi A, et al. Gabapentin-induced modulation of interictal epileptiform activity related to different vigilance levels. *Epilepsia* 2000;41[Suppl 7]:212.

33. Miyauchi T, Endo K, Yamaguchi T, et al. Computerized analysis of EEG background activity in epileptic patients. *Epilepsia* 1991;32:870–881.

34. Samson-Dollfus D, Senaut J. Analysis of background activity. *Electroencephalogr Clin Neurophysiol Suppl* 1985;37:141–161.

35. Sannita WG, Rapallino MV, Rodriguez G, et al. EEG effects and plasma concentration of phenobarbital in volunteers. *Neuropharmacology* 1980;19:927–930.

36. Mervaala E, Partanen J, Nousianen U, et al. Electrophysiologic effect of gamma-vinyl GABA and carbamazepine. *Epilepsia* 1989;30:189–193.

37. Lieb JF, Sperling MR, Mendius JR, et al. Visual versus computer evaluation of thiopental-induced EEG changes in temporal lobe epilepsy. *Electroencephalogr Clin Neurophysiol* 1986;63:395–407.

38. Gotman J, Gloor P, Quesney LF, et al. Correlations between EEG changes induced by diazepam and the localization of epileptic spikes and seizures. *Electroencephalogr Clin Neurophysiol* 1982;54:614–621.

39. Rowan AJ, Meijer JWA, Binnie CD, et al. Sodium valproate and sodium valproate–ethosuximide combination therapy: intensive monitoring studies. In: Johannesen SI, Morselli P, Pippenger CE, et al., eds. *Antiepileptic drug therapy: advances in drug monitoring.* New York: Raven Press, 1979:161–168.

40. Fink M, Irwin P, Sannita W, et al. Phenytoin: EEG effects and plasma levels in volunteers. *Ther Drug Monit* 1979;1:93–103.

41. Salinsky MC, Oken BS, Morehead L. Intraindividual analysis of antiepileptic drug effects on EEG background rhythms. *Electroencephalogr Clin Neurophysiol* 1994;90:186–193.

42. Marciani MG, Spanedda F, Bassetti MA, et al. Effect of lamotrigine on EEG paroxysmal abnormalities and background activity: a computerized analysis. *Br J Clin Pharmacol* 1996;42:621–627.

43. Neufeld MY, Kogan E, Chistik V, et al. Comparison of the effects of vigabatrin, lamotrigine, and topiramate on quantitative EEGs in patients with epilepsy. *Clin Neuropharmacol* 1999;22:80–86.

44. Frost JD, Kellaway P, Hrachovy RA, et al. Changes in epileptic spike configuration associated with attainment of seizure control. *Ann Neurol* 1986;20:723–726.

45. So N, Gotman J. Changes in seizure activity following anticonvulsant drug withdrawal. *Neurology* 1990;40:407–413.

46. Milligan N, Dhillon S, Oxley J, et al. Absorption of diazepam from the rectum and its effect on interictal spikes in the EEG. *Epilepsia* 1982;23:323–331.

47. Ahmad S, Perucca E, Richens A. The effects of furosemide, mexiletine, (+)propranolol and three benzodiazepine drugs on interictal spike discharges in the electroencephalogram of epileptic patients. *Br J Clin Pharmacol* 1977;4:683–688.

48. Booker HE, Celesia GG. Serum concentrations of diazepam in subjects with epilepsy. *Arch Neurol* 1973;29:191–194.

49. Schmidt D. The influence of antiepileptic drugs on the electroencephalogram: a review of controlled clinical studies. *Electroenceph Clin Neurophysiol Suppl* 1982;36:453–466.

50. Jaffe R, Christoff N. Intravenous diazepam in seizure disorders. *Electroencephalogr Clin Neurophysiol* 1967;23:96(abstr).

51. Laguna JF, Korein J. Diagnostic value of diazepam in electroencephalography. *Arch Neurol* 1972;26:265–271.

52. Buchtal F, Svensmark O, Simonsen H. Relation of EEG and seizures to phenobarbital in serum. *Arch Neurol* 1968;19:567–572.

53. Kellaway P, Carrie JRG. Relationships between quantitative EEG measurements and clinical state in epileptic patients. In: Penry JK, ed. *Epilepsy, the eighth international symposium.* New York: Raven Press, 1977:153–158.

54. Kellaway P, Frost JD, Hrachovy RA. Relationship between clinical state, ictal and interictal EEG discharges and serum drug levels. *Ann Neurol* 1978;4:197(abstr).

55. Lombroso CT, Erba G. Primary and secondary bilateral synchrony in epilepsy. *Arch Neurol* 1970;22:321–334.

56. Wikler A, Fraser F, Isbell H, et al. Electroencephalograms during cycles of addiction to barbiturates in man. *Electroencephalogr Clin Neurophysiol* 1955;7:1–13.

57. Spencer SS, Spencer DD, Williamson PD, et al. Ictal effects of anticonvulsant medication withdrawal in epileptic patients. *Epilepsia* 1981;22:297–307.

58. Martins da Silva A, Aarts JHP, Binnie CD, et al. The circadian distribution of interictal epileptiform EEG activity. *Electroencephalogr Clin Neurophysiol* 1984;58:1–13.

59. Carrie JRG. Computer-assisted EEG sharp transient detection and quantification during overnight recordings in an epileptic patient. In: Kellaway P, Petersen I, eds. *Quantitative analytic studies in epilepsy.* New York: Raven Press, 1976:225–235.

60. Buchtal F, Svensmark O, Schiller PJ. Clinical and electroencephalographic correlations with serum levels of diphenylhydantoin. *Arch Neurol* 1960;2:624–630.

61. Wilkus RJ, Green JR. Electroencephalographic investigations during evaluation of the antiepileptic agent Sulthiame. *Epilepsia* 1974;15:13–25.

62. Engel J, Crandall PH. Falsely localizing ictal onsets with depth EEG telemetry during anticonvulsant withdrawal. *Epilepsia* 1983;24:344–345.

63. Jongmans JWM. Report of the antiepileptic action of Tegretol. *Epilepsia* 1964;5:74–82.

64. Sachdeo R, Chokroverty S. Increasing epileptiform activities in EEG in presence of decreasing clinical seizures after carbamazepine. *Epilepsia* 1985;26:522(abstr).

65. Monaco F, Riccio A, Morselli PL, et al. EEG, seizures, and plasma level correlations in patients on chronic treatment with carbamazepine. *Electroencephalogr Clin Neurophysiol* 1980;48:51P.

66. Sato S, White BG, Penry JK, et al. Valproic acid versus ethosuximide in the treatment of absence seizures. *Neurology* 1982;32:157–163.

67. Harding GFA, Herrick CE, Jeavons PM. A controlled study of the effect of sodium valproate on photosensitive epilepsy and its prognosis. *Epilepsia* 1978;19:555–565.

68. Rowan AJ, Binnie CD, Warfield CA, et al. The delayed effect of sodium valproate on the photoconvulsive response in man. *Epilepsia* 1979;20:61–68.

69. Binnie C, van Emde Boas W, Kasteleijn-Nolste-Trenite DGA, et al. Acute effects of lamotrigine (BW430C) in persons with epilepsy. *Epilepsia* 1986;27:248–254.

70. Jawad S, Oxley J, Yuen WC, et al. The effects of lamotrigine, a novel anticonvulsant on interictal spikes in patients with epilepsy. *Br J Clin Pharmacol* 1986;22:191–193.

71. Buoni S, Grosso S, Fois A. Lamotrigine in typical absence epilepsy. *Brain Dev* 1999;21:303–306.

72. Placidi F, Diomedi M, Scalise A, et al. Effect of anticonvulsants on nocturnal sleep in epilepsy. *Neurology* 2000;54[Suppl 1]:S25–S32.

73. Catania S, Cross H, de Sousa C, et al. Paradoxic reaction to lamotrigine in a child with benign focal epilepsy of childhood with centrotemporal spikes. *Epilepsia* 1999;40:1657–1660.

74. Marciani MG, Spanedda F, Placidi F, et al. Changes of the EEG paroxysmal pattern during felbamate therapy in Lennox-Gastaut syndrome: a case report. *Int J Neurosci* 1998;95:247–253.

75. Ben-Menachem E, Treiman DM. Effect of gamma-vinyl GABA on interictal spikes and sharp waves in patients with intractable complex partial seizures. *Epilepsia* 1989;30:79–83.

76. Marciani MG, Maschio M, Spanedda F, et al. Development of myoclonus in patients with partial epilepsy during treatment with vigabatrin: an electroencephalographic study. *Acta Neurol Scand* 1995;91:1–5.

77. Gibbs EL, Gibbs FA. Diagnostic and localizing value of electroencephalographic studies in sleep. *Res Publ Assoc Nerv Ment Dis* 1947;26:366–376.

78. Wauquier A, Clincke GHC, Declerke AC. Sleep alterations by seizures and anticonvulsants. In: Martins da Silva A, Binnie CD, Meinardi H, eds. *Biorhythms and epilepsy.* New York: Raven Press, 1985:123–135.

79. Gann H, Riemann D, Hohagen F, et al. The influence of carbamazepine on sleep-EEG and the clonidine test in healthy subjects: results of a preliminary study. *Biol Psychiatry* 1994;35:893–896.

80. Riemann D, Gann H, Hohagen F, et al. The effect of carbamazepine on endocrine and sleep variables in a patient with a 48 hour rapid cycling, and healthy controls. *Neuropsychobiology* 1993;27:163–170.

81. Drake ME, Pakalnis A, Bogner JE, et al. Outpatient sleep recording during antiepileptic drug monotherapy. *Clin Electroencephalogr* 1990;21:170–173.

82. Wolf P, Roder-Wanner UU, Brede M. Influence of therapeutic phenobarbital and phenytoin medication on the polygraphic sleep of patients with epilepsy. *Epilepsia* 1984;25:467–475.

83. Wolf P, Roder-Wanner UU, Brede M, et al. Influences of antiepileptic drugs on sleep. In: Martins da Silva A, Binnie CD, Meinardi H, eds. *Biorhythms and epilepsy.* New York: Raven Press, 1985:137–153.

84. Kay DC, Jasinsky DR, Eigenstein RB, et al. Quantified human sleep after phenobarbital. *Clin Pharmacol Ther* 1982;13:221–231.

85. Oswald J. Melancholia and barbiturates: a controlled EEG, body, and eye movement study of sleep. *Br J Psychiatry* 1963;109:66–78.

86. Declerck AC. *Interaction of epilepsy, sleep, and antiepileptics.* Lisse: Swets & Zeitlinger BV, 1983.

87. Placidi F, Diomedi M, Scalise A, et al. Effect of long-term treatment with gabapentin on nocturnal sleep in epilepsy. *Epilepsia* 1997;38[Suppl 8]:179–180.

88. Rao ML, Clarenbach P, Vahlensieck M, et al. Gabapentin aug-

89. ments whole blood serotonin in healthy young men. *J Neural Transm* 1988;73:129–134.

89. Bazil CW, Castro LHM, Walczak TS. Reduction of rapid eye movement sleep by diurnal and nocturnal seizures in temporal lobe epilepsy. *Arch Neurol* 2000; 57:363–368.

90. Faught E, Sutherling WS, Wilkinson EC, et al. Effect of sodium valproate on visual evoked potentials to stimulus trains in patients with photosensitive epilepsy. *Epilepsia* 1980;21:185–186.

91. Mervaala E, Keranen T, Penttila M, et al. Pattern reversal VEP and control SEP latency prolongations in epilepsy. *Epilepsia* 1985;26:441–445.

92. Harding GFA, Alford CA, Powel TE. The effect of sodium valproate on sleep, reaction times, and visual evoked potential in normal subjects. *Epilepsia* 1985;26:597–601.

93. Dravet C, Vigliano P, Santanelli P, et al. Multimodal evoked potentials in chronic epilepsy patients. *Electroencephalogr Clin Neurophysiol* 1989;73:52P.

94. Martinovic Z, Ristanovic D, Dokoc-Ristanovic D, et al. Pattern reversal visual evoked potentials recorded in children with generalized epilepsy. *Clin Electroencephalogr* 1990;21:233–243.

95. Faught E, Lee SI. Pattern-reversal visual evoked potentials in photosensitive epilepsy. *Electroencephalogr Clin Neurophysiol* 1984; 59:125–133.

96. Enoki H, Sanada S, Oka E, et al. Effects of high-dose antiepileptic drugs on event-related potentials in epileptic children. *Epilepsy Res* 1996;25:59–64.

97. Green JB, Walcoff MR, Locke JF. Comparison of phenytoin and phenobarbital effect on far-field auditory and somatosensory evoked potential interpeak latencies. *Epilepsia* 1982;23:417–421.

98. Green JB, Walcoff MR, Locke JF. Phenytoin prolongs far-field somatosensory and auditory evoked potential interpeak latencies. *Neurology* 1982;32:85–88.

99. Hirose G, Kitagawa Y, Chujo T, et al. Acute effects of phenytoin on brainstem auditory evoked potentials: clinical and experimental study. *Neurology* 1986;36:1521–1524.

100. Mervaala E, Keranen T, Tiihonen P, et al. The effects of carbamazepine and sodium valproate on SEPs and BAEPs. *Electroencephalogr Clin Neurophysiol* 1987;68:475–478.

101. Rodin E. Chayasirsobhon S, Klutke G. Brainstem auditory evoked potential readings in patients with epilepsy. *Clin Electroencephalogr* 1982;13:154–161.

102. Kubota F, Ohnishi N, Nakajima M, et al. Effects of zonisamide on BAEP, SSEP, and P300. *Clin Electroencephalogr* 1995;26:120–123.

103. Elke T, Talbot JF, Lawden MC. Severe persistent visual field constriction associated with vigabatrin. *BMJ* 1997;314:180–181.

104. Harding GFA, Wild JM, Robertson KA, et al. Separating the retinal electrophysiologic effects of vigabatrin. *Neurology* 2000; 55:347–352.

105. Hardus P, Verduin WM, Postma G, et al. Concentric contraction of the visual field in patients with temporal lobe epilepsy and its association with the use of vigabatrin medication. *Epilepsia* 2000;41:581–587.

106. Krauss GL, Johnson MA, Miller NR. Vigabatrin-associated retinal cone system dysfunction. *Neurology* 1998;50:614–618.

107. Lawden MC, Eke T, Degg C, et al. Visual field defects associated with vigabatrin therapy. *J Neurol Neurosurg Psychiatry* 1999;67:707–708.

108. Cosi V, Callieco R, Galimberti CA, et al. Effects of vigabatrin (gamma-vinyl-GABA) on visual, brainstem auditory and somatosensory evoked potentials in epileptic patients. *Eur Neurol* 1988;28:42–46.

109. Miller NR, Johnson MA, Paul SR, et al. Visual dysfunction in patients receiving vigabatrin. *Neurology* 1999;53:2082–2087.

110. Maguiere F, Chauvel P, Dewailly J, et al. No effect of long-term vigabatrin treatment on central nervous system conduction in patients with refractory epilepsy: results of a multicenter study of somatosensory and visual evoked potentials. *Epilepsia* 1997; 38:301–308.

111. Ylinen A, Sivenius J, Pitkanen A, et al. γ-Vinyl GABA (vigabatrin) in epilepsy: clinical, neurochemical, and neurophysiologic monitoring in epileptic patients. *Epilepsia* 1992;33:917–922.

112. Ajmone Marsan C, Zivin LS. Factors related to the occurrence of typical paroxysmal abnormalities in the EEG records of epileptic patients. *Epilepsia* 1970;11:361–381.

113. Daly DD. Epilepsy and syncope. In: Daly DD, Pedley TA, eds. *Current practice of clinical electroencephalography*, 2nd ed. New York: Raven Press, 1990:269–334.

114. Salinsky M, Kanter R, Dasheiff R. Effectiveness of multiple EEGs in supporting the diagnosis of epilepsy: an operational curve. *Epilepsia* 1987;28:331–334.

115. van Donselaar CA, Schimsheimer R, Geerts AT, et al. Value of the electroencephalogram in adult patients with untreated idiopathic first seizure. *Arch Neurol* 1992;49:231–237.

116. Annegers JF, Shirts SB, Hauser WA, et al. Risk of recurrence after an initial unprovoked seizure. *Epilepsia* 1986;27:43–50.

117. Hauser WA, Anderson VE, Loewenson RB, et al. Seizure recurrence after first unprovoked seizure. *N Engl J Med* 1982;307: 522–528.

118. Hopkins A, Garman A, Clarke C. The first seizure in adult life: value of clinical features, electroencephalography, and computerized tomographic scanning in prediction of seizure recurrence. *Lancet* 1988;1:721–726.

119. Camfield PR, Camfield CS, Dooley JM, et al. Epilepsy after a first unprovoked seizure in childhood. *Neurology* 1985;35: 1657–1660.

120. Shinnar S, Berg AT, Moshe SL, et al. The risk of recurrence following a first unprovoked seizure in childhood: a prospective study. *Pediatrics* 1990;85:1076–1085.

121. Emerson R, D'Souza BJ, Vining EP, et al. Stopping medication in children with epilepsy: predictors of outcome. *N Engl J Med* 1981;304:1125–1129.

122. Gherpelli JL, Kok F, dal Forno S, et al. Discontinuing medication in epileptic children: a study of risk factors related to recurrence. *Epilepsia* 1992;33:681–686.

123. Matricardi M, Brinciotti M, Bendetti P. Outcome after discontinuation of antiepileptic drug therapy in children with epilepsy. *Epilepsia* 1989;30:582–589.

124. Shinnar S, Vining EPG, Mellits ED, et al. Discontinuing antiepileptic medications in children with epilepsy after two years without seizures: a prospective study. *N Engl J Med* 1985; 313:976–980.

125. Annegers JF, Hauser WA, Elveback LR. Remission of seizures and relapse in patients with epilepsy. *Epilepsia* 1979;20: 729–737.

126. Callaghan N, Garrett A, Goggin T. Withdrawal of anticonvulsant drugs in patients free of seizures for two years: a prospective study. *N Engl J Med* 1988;318:942–946.

127. Medical Research Council Antiepileptic Drug Withdrawal Study Group. Randomised study of antiepileptic drug withdrawal in patients in remission. *Lancet* 1991;337:1175–1180.

128. Overweg J, Binnie CD, Oosting J, et al. Clinical and EEG prediction of seizure recurrence following antiepileptic drug withdrawal. *Epilepsy Res* 1987;1:272–283.

3

GENERAL PRINCIPLES

DISCOVERY AND PRECLINICAL DEVELOPMENT OF ANTIEPILEPTIC DRUGS

H. STEVE WHITE
JOSÉ H. WOODHEAD
KAREN S. WILCOX
JAMES P. STABLES
HARVEY J. KUPFERBERG
HAROLD H. WOLF

In 1974, the National Institute of Neurological Disorders and Stroke established the Anticonvulsant Drug Development (ADD) Program. Since then, this program has been instrumental in stimulating the discovery and development of new chemical entities for the symptomatic treatment of human epilepsy. The ADD Program serves as an excellent example of a successful collaboration between government, the pharmaceutical industry, and academia. Since its inception, this National Institutes of Health (NIH)–sponsored program has accessioned over 24,000 investigational antiepileptic drugs (AEDs) from academic and pharmaceutical chemists worldwide. The initial identification and characterization of their anticonvulsant activity has been established through a contract with the University of Utah Anticonvulsant Screening Project (ASP). The success of this collaboration is exemplified by the worldwide approval of several new AEDs since 1993 and the continued clinical evaluation of numerous other promising candidates.

The long-standing mission of the ASP has been to identify and characterize the anticonvulsant activity of those chemical entities that display a reasonable degree of separation between their anticonvulsant and behaviorally toxic doses. The characterization of a drug's anticonvulsant and behavioral toxicity profile is established using a battery of well defined animal models. Herein lies one of the most frequently discussed issues in the current AED discovery process: What is the most appropriate animal model to use when attempting to screen for efficacy against human epilepsy? The two primary screens of the ASP continue to be the maximal electroshock seizure (MES) test and the subcutaneous pentylenetetrazol (Metrazol; s.c. MET) seizure test. With one exception (i.e., levetiracetam), all of the AEDs approved since 1993 have been found to be active in one or both of these tests. Levetiracetam appears to represent a truly unique compound that is inactive in the traditional MES and s.c. MET tests, yet active in partial and primarily generalized seizure models (1–6). Activity in these models provided the rationale supporting the early clinical evaluation of levetiracetam in patients with epilepsy. In three pivotal trials, levetiracetam was found to be effective as add-on therapy for the management of partial seizures (7–12). In this regard, the identification and development of levetiracetam as an efficacious AED for the treatment of partial seizures demonstrates the need for flexibility when screening for efficacy and the need to incorporate levetiracetam-sensitive models into the early evaluation of an investigational AED.

OVERVIEW OF THE ANTICONVULSANT SCREENING PROJECT TESTING PROTOCOL

The ASP uses a combination of nonmechanistic, mechanistic, and syndrome-specific animal models to identify and characterize the anticonvulsant profile of an investigational AED. The nonmechanistic approach is very well suited for

H. Steve White, MD: Professor, Department of Pharmacology and Toxicology; and Director, Anticonvulsant Screening Project, University of Utah, Salt Lake City, Utah

José H. Woodhead, MD: Department of Pharmacology and Toxicology, University of Utah, Salt Lake City, Utah

Karen S. Wilcox, PhD: Research Assistant Professor, Department of Pharmacology and Toxicology, University of Utah, Salt Lake City, Utah

James P. Stables, BS (Pharm): Program Director, Anticonvulsant Screening Project, Technology Development Cluster, NINDS, National Institute of Health, Rockville, Maryland

Harvey J. Kupferberg, MD: Epilepsy Branch, National Institute of Neurological Disorders and Stroke, National Institutes of Health, Bethesda, Maryland

Harold H. Wolf, MD: Professor, Department of Pharmacology and Toxicology, University of Utah, Salt Lake City, Utah

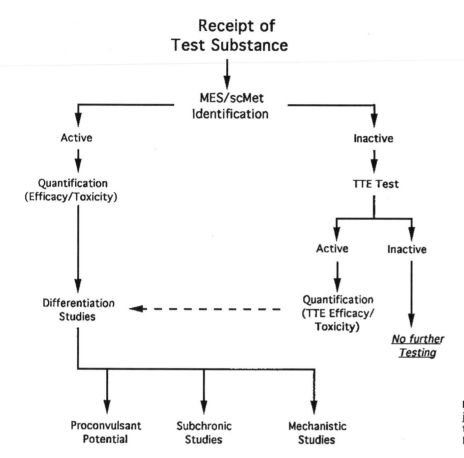

FIGURE 3.1. Anticonvulsant screening project testing paradigm. MES, maximal electroshock seizure; s.c. MET, subcutaneous Metrazol.

the early evaluation of anticonvulsant activity because it assumes that the pharmacodynamic activity of a drug is independent of its mechanism of action. For the most part, the model systems used by the ASP display clear and definable seizure end points and require minimal technical expertise. Furthermore, this approach is ideally suited to the large number of chemically diverse entities that are evaluated annually by the ASP.

The current *in vivo* testing protocol of the ASP has evolved over the last 27 years to include a variety of animal seizure models that have proven to be valuable in identifying clinically effective AEDs (13). On receipt at the laboratories of the ASP, the test substance is subjected to a large number of testing procedures according to the paradigm summarized in Figure 3.1. As shown in Figure 3.1, there are four major phases of the ASP testing protocol: identification, quantification, differentiation, and advanced testing. The specifics of these major phases are outlined in Table 3.1, and the details of many of the anticonvulsant procedures outlined in the table are discussed in the following sections.

MATERIALS AND METHODS

Experimental Animals

Adult male CF No. 1 albino mice (18 to 25 g) and adult male Sprague-Dawley albino rats (100 to 150 g) are used as experimental animals. These particular strains are preferred for anticonvulsant studies because they are docile and easy to handle. Moreover, CF No. 1 mice rarely succumb to induced seizures (14). Animals of the same sex, age, and weight are used to minimize biologic variability (15). The animals are maintained on a 12-hour light/dark cycle and allowed free access to food and water, except during the short time they are removed from their cages for testing. Animals newly received in the laboratory are allowed 24 hours to compensate for the food and water restriction incurred during transit. This is necessary because such restriction increases the severity of MES (16). All animals are maintained and handled in a manner consistent with the recommendations in the U.S. Department of Health, Education and Welfare publication (NIH) No. 8623, *Guide for the Care and Use of Laboratory Animals.* Animals usually are used only once and then disposed of in a humane manner. In those instances where they are used a second time, at least a 1-week interval is allowed for the animal to eliminate the test drug.

Convulsant Chemicals

For tests based on chemically induced convulsions, the convulsant chemical is prepared in a concentration that induces convulsions in more than 97% of animals when injected in

TABLE 3.1. OVERVIEW OF TESTING PROCEDURES[a]

I. Anticonvulsant identification
    a. Mice i.p.
        Dose range: 30,100, and 300 mg/kg
        Tests: MES, s.c. MET, rotorod
        Time of test: ½ and 4 h
    b. Rats p.o. (i.p. at special request)
        Dose: 30 or 50 mg/kg
        Tests: MES (30 mg/kg) or s.c. MET (50 mg/kg) and minimal
           neurotoxicity
        Time of test: ¼, ½, 1, 2, and 4 h
    c. Mice i.p. (compounds inactive in a)
        Dose: 100 mg/kg or < toxic levels
        Test: 6 Hz
        Time of test: ¼, ½, 1, 2, and 4 h
II. Anticonvulsant quantification
    a. Mice i.p.
        TPE: MES, s.c. MET, 6 Hz, rotorod
        ED_{50}: MES, s.c. MET, 6 Hz
        TD_{50}: rotorod
    b. Mice p.o.
        TPE: MES, s.c. MET, rotorod
        ED_{50}: MES, s.c. MET
        TD_{50}: rotorod
    c. Rats p.o.
        TPE: MES, s.c. MET, minimal neurotoxicity
        ED_{50}: MES, s.c. MET
        TD_{50}: minimal neurotoxicity
III. Anticonvulsant differentiation
    a. Mice i.p.
        ED_{50}: s.c. BIC, s.c. PIC
        ED_{50}: Frings AGS
    b. Rats i.p.
        ED_{50}: Expression of hippocampal kindling
        GHB-induced spike-wave seizures
IV. Proconvulsant potential
    a. Mice i.p.
        Timed i.v. infusion of MET
V. Mechanism of action studies
    a. Patch-clamp electrophysiology studies
        Voltage-gated Na^+ channels and receptor-gated ion
           channels (*N*-methyl-D-aspartate, AMPA/kainate, and
           γ-aminobutyric acid)
    b. Recording from synaptically coupled pairs of neurons[a]

MES, maximal electroshock seizure test; s.c. MET, subcutaneous
Metrazol seizure threshold; TTE, threshold tonic extension test;
TPE, time of peak effect; ED_{50}, median effective dose; TD_{50}, median
toxic dose; s.c. BIC, subcutaneous bicuculline test; s.c. PIC,
subcutaneous picrotoxin test; AGS, audiogenic seizure susceptible;
GHB, γ-hydroxybutyrate; i.p., intraperitoneal; p.o., oral; i.v.,
intravenous.
[a]Pair recordings are not routinely conducted at present; however,
ongoing studies are evaluating the potential utility of this test for
differentiating mechanistically novel antiepileptic drugs.

mice in a volume of 0.01 mL/g body weight or in rats in a volume of 0.02 mL/10 g body weight. For mice, MET and picrotoxin (PIC) are dissolved in 0.9% saline sufficient to make a 0.85% and 0.032% solution, respectively. For rats, MET is given in a concentration of 2.82%. Bicuculline (BIC) is dissolved in 1.0 mL of warmed 0.1 N hydrochloric acid with the aid of a micromixer and sufficient 0.9% saline added to make a 0.027% solution. The solution is used within 30 minutes. All chemical convulsants are administered s.c. into a loose fold of skin in the midline of the neck. No other drugs or chemicals are injected in the same s.c. site. The judicious selection of injection sites avoids false-positive results induced by vasoconstrictor substances retarding the absorption of the convulsant agents. Because the doses used in the aforementioned tests induce convulsions in over 97% of animals, it is unnecessary to run control groups simultaneously with the test groups.

Preparation of Test Drugs

Regardless of their water solubility, all drugs are either dissolved or suspended in 0.5% methylcellulose. The test substance is given in a concentration that permits optimal accuracy of dosage without the volume contributing excessively to total body fluid. Thus, the volume used in mice is 0.01 mL/g body weight, and in rats, 0.04 mL/10 g body weight. Test drugs are routinely administered intraperitoneally (i.p.) or orally (p.o.), as indicated in Table 3.1.

Determination of Acute Toxicity

Abnormal neurologic status disclosed by the rotorod test (17) commonly is taken as the end point for minimal behavioral impairment in mice. Abnormal neurologic status disclosed by the positional sense test, muscle tone test, or the gait and stance test is taken as the end point for minimal behavioral impairment in rats. Inability of a rat to perform normally in at least two of these tests indicates that the animal has some neurologic deficit. The names assigned to these tests are those used in the authors' laboratories, and do not necessarily refer to the specific neurologic reflexes involved (18).

Rotorod Test. The rotorod test is used exclusively in mice to assess minimal motor impairment. When a normal mouse is placed on a rod 1 inch in diameter that rotates at a speed of 6 rpm, the mouse can maintain its equilibrium for long periods. Inability of the mouse to maintain its equilibrium in three trials during 1 minute on this rotating rod is used as an indication of such impairment.

Positional Sense Test. If the hind leg of a normal mouse or rat is gently lowered over the edge of a table, the animal will quickly lift its leg back to a normal position. Neurologic deficit is indicated by inability of the animal to correct rapidly such an abnormal position of the limb.

Gait and Stance Test. Neurologic deficit is indicated by a circular or zigzag gait, ataxia, abnormal spread of the legs, abnormal body posture, tremor, hyperactivity, lack of exploratory behavior, somnolence, stupor, catalepsy, and the like.

Muscle Tone Test. Normal animals have a certain amount of skeletal muscle tone that on handling is apparent to the experienced technician. Neurologic deficit is indicated by a loss of skeletal muscle tone characterized by hypotonia or flaccidity.

Anticonvulsant Identification

At present, no single laboratory test, in itself, establishes the presence or absence of anticonvulsant activity or fully predicts the clinical potential of a test substance. In the ASP, three tests are used for the routine identification of anticonvulsant activity: the MES test, the s.c. MET seizure threshold test, and the 6-Hz psychomotor seizure test.

Maximal Electroshock Seizure Test and Subcutaneous Metrazol Seizure Threshold Test

In the MES test, 60-Hz alternating current (mice, 50 mA; rats, 150 mA) is delivered for 0.2 second through corneal electrodes by means of an apparatus similar to that originally designed by Woodbury (19). At the time of administration of the test substance, a drop of 0.5% tetracaine in saline is applied to the eyes of all animals assigned to any electroshock test. Immediately before the placement of corneal electrodes, a drop of electrolyte (saline) is placed on each eye. The animals are restrained by hand and released immediately after stimulation to permit observation of the seizure throughout its entire course. Abolition of the hind limb tonic extensor component is taken as the end point for this test. Tonic extension is considered abolished if the hind limbs are not fully extended at 180° with the plane of the body. Absence of this component suggests that the test substance has the ability to prevent the spread of seizure discharge through neural tissue.

In the s.c. MET test, a convulsive dose (CD_{97}) of MET (85 mg/kg in mice, 56.4 mg/kg in rats) is injected s.c. The animals are placed in isolation cages and observed for the next 30 minutes for the presence or absence of an episode of clonic spasms persisting for at least 5 seconds. Absence of a clonic seizure suggests that the test substance has the ability to raise the seizure threshold.

In identification studies involving mice, the ASP routinely uses the MES and s.c. MET tests. Sixteen mice are randomly divided into three groups of four, eight, and four mice each; each group is then given 30, 100, or 300 mg/kg, respectively, of the test substance i.p. Thirty minutes after administration of the test substance, all animals are subjected to the rotorod test; one animal in the 30 and 300 mg/kg group and three animals in the 100 mg/kg group are then subjected to the MES test, and one animal in each group to the s.c. MET test. Four hours after drug administration, all remaining animals in each group are subjected to the rotorod test; these animals are then subjected to the MES and s.c. MET test as indicated previously. Thus, it requires only 16 mice to cover the dose range of 30, 100, and 300 mg/kg and the periods of 30 minutes and 4 hours.

TABLE 3.2. ANTICONVULSANT IDENTIFICATION IN MICE AFTER INTRAPERITONEAL ADMINISTRATION

		Results[a]	
Test	Dose (mg/kg)	½h	4 h
Toxicity	30	1/4	0/2
	100	7/8	1/4
	300	4/4	0/2
MES	30	0/1	0/1
	100	3/3	0/3
	300	1/1	1/1
s.c. MET	30	0/1	0/1
	100	1/1	0/1
	300	1/1	1/1

MES, maximal electroshock seizure test; s.c. MET, subcutaneous Metrazol seizure threshold test.
[a]Number protected or toxic/number tested.

An example of results obtained with the MES and s.c. MET screening procedures is shown in Table 3.2. As can be seen, these preliminary results suggest that the test substance is effective in toxic doses in the MES and s.c. MET test. Furthermore, they demonstrate that the minimal behaviorally toxic dose is >30 mg/kg but <100 mg/kg. The test substance also appears to have a relatively rapid onset and short duration of action because both the anticonvulsant and neurotoxic effects are greater at 30 minutes than at 4 hours.

In identification studies using rats, 30 mg/kg (MES) or 50 mg/kg (s.c. MET and toxicity) of the test substance is administered orally to 10 groups (5 groups for MES and 5 for s.c. MET) of 4 rats per group. At various times after administration (0.25, 0.5, 1, 2, and 4 hours), animals are evaluated for neurologic deficit and then subjected to the MES or s.c. MET tests. The ratios of animals protected or toxic to animals tested are determined. The initial identification studies in rats provide information as to whether the test substance is active or toxic in a dose of 30 or 50 mg/kg after p.o. administration. It also discloses the time of onset, the approximate time of peak effect (TPE), and the duration of anticonvulsant activity or neurotoxicity. Anticonvulsant identification results obtained in rats with the same test substance described in Table 3.2 are shown in Table 3.3. As can be seen from these data, the test substance is active in rats by the MES test within 15 to 30 minutes after p.o.

TABLE 3.3. ANTICONVULSANT IDENTIFICATION IN RATS AFTER ORAL ADMINISTRATION

		No. Protected or Toxic/No. Tested				
Test	Dose (mg/kg)	¼h	½h	1 h	2 h	4 h
MES	30	4/4	4/4	1/4	1/4	1/4
s.c. MET	50	4/4	4/4	4/4	4/4	4/4
Toxicity	50	0/4	0/4	0/4	0/4	0/4

MES, maximal electroshock seizure test; s.c. MET, subcutaneous Metrazol seizure threshold test.

administration. Similarly, the total duration of action of this compound appears to be quite short; however, additional studies would be necessary to define the duration of action profile. The results summarized in Table 3.3 also suggest that the test compound is active in rats against clonic seizures induced by s.c. MET. In fact, the activity observed after p.o. administration to rats is more impressive than that observed in the mouse identification studies. At the doses tested (30 and 50 mg/kg), no evidence of neurologic deficit (toxicity) is observed. For the test substance profiled in Tables 3.2 and 3.3, the results suggest that further experimental work is justified because the favorable anticonvulsant profile supports possible clinical usefulness in generalized tonic-clonic seizures, complex partial seizures, and perhaps generalized myoclonic seizures (see later for discussion). This particular example also demonstrates the importance of not basing a "go/no-go" decision on the results obtained from one species after one route of administration. In this case, the p.o. rat data clearly are more favorable than those obtained from the mouse after i.p. administration, and provide the framework for additional testing.

The 6-Hz Psychomotor Seizure Test

The MES and s.c. MET tests have become the two most widely used seizure models for the early identification and high-throughput screening of investigational AEDs. These tests, albeit extremely effective in identifying new AEDs that may be useful for the treatment of human generalized tonic-clonic seizures and generalized myoclonic seizures, respectively (20), may miss novel AEDs that may be useful for the treatment of therapy-resistant partial seizures (e.g., levetiracetam). Although ineffective in the traditional MES and s.c. MET tests, levetiracetam has been found to be highly effective [median effective dose (ED_{50}), 19 mg/kg, i.p.] in the 6-Hz seizure model that was originally described in the early 1950s (21,22). In light of the marked sensitivity of levetiracetam to the 6-Hz test, the ASP now routinely screens investigational AEDs found to be inactive in either the MES or s.c. MET tests for their ability to block seizures induced by a low-frequency (6-Hz), long-duration (3-second) stimulus delivered through corneal electrodes.

For this test, 20 mice are pretreated i.p. with 100 mg/kg of the test substance. At varying times (0.25, 0.5, 1, 2, and 4 hours) after treatment, individual mice (4 at each time point) are challenged with sufficient current (32 mA at 6 Hz for 3 seconds) delivered through corneal electrodes to elicit a psychomotor seizure. Typically, the seizure is characterized by a minimal clonic phase that is followed by stereotyped, automatistic behaviors that are not unlike automatistic behaviors of human patients with complex partial seizures. Animals not displaying this behavior (e.g., jaw chomping, whisker movement) are considered protected.

Results are expressed as the number of animals protected out of the number of animals tested over time. Drugs that are

active (i.e., at least two of four animals protected at two or more time points) in the 6-Hz test are evaluated quantitatively, and active compounds may then become candidates for the kindled rat test. Drugs that are found to be active only in the 6-Hz identification test and subsequently found to be active in the kindled rat test represent potentially novel anticonvulsant substances for the treatment of therapy-resistant seizures. Such compounds are worthy of further investigation.

The results from these identification tests (MES and s.c. MET in mice and rats, 6-Hz in mice, and neurologic deficit in mice and rats) provide important preliminary information pertaining to oral bioavailability, species variation, duration of action, toxicity, efficacy, and overall potential of novel anticonvulsant substances.

QUANTIFICATION OF EXPERIMENTAL RESULTS

Anticonvulsant quantification details the ED_{50} by the MES, s.c. MET, or 6-Hz tests; the median toxic dose (TD_{50}) by the rotorod test; the 95% confidence intervals; and protective indices (PI; TD_{50}/ED_{50}). The TPE data provide further insight into the time of onset and the duration of anticonvulsant activity and behavioral impairment. In addition to i.p. studies in mice, anticonvulsant quantification also is conducted in rats after p.o. administration to delineate anticonvulsant activity and behavioral impairment by a different route of administration in another rodent species, and to develop dose information prerequisite to subsequent chronic toxicity studies.

Time of Peak Effect

All quantitative studies are performed at the TPE. To determine the TPE for anticonvulsant activity, five groups of four animals each are administered an appropriate dose of test drug and subjected to the MES, s.c. MET, or 6-Hz test at 0.25, 0.5, 1, 2, or 4 hours. For toxicity determinations, a single group of eight animals is injected and tested for minimal motor impairment at the same time intervals. The time interval showing the greatest animal response is taken as the TPE.

Median Effective or Median Toxic Doses

Eight animals are injected with the dose used in the determination of the TPE and subjected to the respective anticonvulsant or behavioral impairment test. The number of animals responding is recorded and another dose level, usually one-half or double the initial dose, is selected. This procedure is repeated until a minimum of four dose levels has been established with at least two points between the dose level that induces 0% animal response and the dose level that induces 100% animal response.

The various ED_{50}s and TD_{50}s are calculated by a FORTRAN probit analysis program. This program also provides the 95% confidence intervals, the slope of the regression lines, and standard error of the slopes. Reasonable estimates of these values may be determined by the log-probit method of Litchfield and Wilcoxon (23). This statistical treatment provides the kind of data essential for a critical evaluation of anticonvulsant activity and toxicity in structure–activity relationship studies.

ANTICONVULSANT DIFFERENTIATION

After the efficacy of a test substance against MES-, s.c. MET-, or 6-Hz–induced seizures has been quantitated, a battery of tests is used to characterize further the anticonvulsant potential of the substance. Other chemoconvulsants used include the type A γ-aminobutyric acid receptor (GABA$_A$) antagonist BIC and the chloride channel blocker PIC. Ability of a candidate substance to alter seizure threshold also is assessed by the intravenous MET seizure threshold (i.v. MET) test (24). Candidate substances also may be tested for their ability to block the expression of stage 5 seizures in fully kindled animals, to block sound-induced seizures in the genetically susceptible Frings mouse model of reflex epilepsy (25), and to influence spike–wave electrographic seizure profile of the γ-hydroxybutyrate (GHB) model of absence (26).

In contrast to other seizure models, the audiogenic seizure–susceptible mouse model (not detailed later) is of no particular predictive value because it is nondiscriminatory with respect to clinical categories of anticonvulsant drugs (27). Nonetheless, it provides useful information regarding efficacy in a genetically susceptible model. The GHB model (also not described later), like the i.v. MET test, is used in the screening project to ascertain the proconvulsive potential of test substances that exhibit a phenytoin-like anticonvulsant profile in the other models examined, and to differentiate further those compounds that may be potentially useful for the treatment of spike–wave seizures.

Subcutaneous Bicuculline and Picrotoxin Tests

The CD$_{97}$ of BIC (2.70 mg/kg) and PIC (3.15 mg/kg) is injected s.c. at the previously determined TPE for the test substance. The mice are placed in isolation cages and observed for the presence or absence of a clonic seizure. BIC-treated animals are observed for 30 minutes. PIC-treated animals are observed for 45 minutes because of the slower absorption of this convulsant. Absence of a clonic seizure indicates that the substance has the ability to elevate the seizure threshold to chemoconvulsants that act by antagonizing GABA$_A$ receptors and blocking chloride channels, respectively. The activity of substances that exhibit anticonvulsant efficacy in these tests is quantitated by determining ED$_{50}$s, as described previously.

Timed Intravenous Infusion of Metrazol

This test measures the minimal seizure threshold of each animal that has received the ED$_{50}$ of the test substance (24). At the TPE, the convulsant solution (0.5% MET in 0.9% saline containing 10 USP units/mL of heparin sodium) is infused into the tail vein at a constant rate of 0.34 mL/min. The time in seconds from the start of the infusion to the appearance of the first twitch and the onset of clonus is recorded for each experimental and control animal. The times to each end point are converted to milligrams per kilogram of MET for each mouse in the vehicle control and the test drug group (10 mice/group), and the mean doses and standard errors are calculated.

Kindled Rats

None of the tests described thus far is very useful for identifying new drugs that are likely to be useful for the treatment of difficult-to-control seizure types and epilepsy syndromes such as adult complex partial seizures. In recent years, the kindling model has been a useful adjunct to the more traditional anticonvulsant tests for identifying a substance's potential utility for treating complex partial seizures. Kindled seizures provide not only an experimental model of focal seizures, but a means of studying complex brain networks that may contribute to seizure spread and generalization from a focus (28).

Of the various kindling paradigms described in the literature, the rapid hippocampal kindling model of Lothman et al. (28) appears to offer some distinct advantages for the routine screening and evaluation of new anticonvulsant substances. One potentially important advantage of the rapidly recurring hippocampal seizure model is its ability to provide a framework for assessing, in a temporal fashion, drug efficacy in a focal seizure model. Thus, this model has been incorporated into the ASP protocol.

For these studies, the candidate substance is evaluated for its ability to block the kindled motor seizure (seizure scores of 4 and 5) and limbic behavioral seizure (seizure score between 1 and 3) and to effect changes in the electrical afterdischarge duration. The procedures for surgical implantation of a bipolar electrode have been described previously (20). After a 1-week recovery period, animals are kindled to a stage 5 behavioral seizure (20) using a stimulus consisting of a 50-Hz, 10-second train of 1-millisecond, biphasic 200-μA pulses delivered every 30 minutes for 6 hours (12 stimulations per day) on alternating days for a total of 60 stimulations (5 stimulus days). Drug testing usually is initiated after a 1-week stimulus-free period. On each day of a drug trial, animals receive two to three suprathreshold stimulations delivered every 30 minutes before drug treatment. During these control blocks, the stability of the behavioral seizure stage and afterdischarge duration is assessed. Fifteen minutes after the last control block, a single dose of the test substance is administered i.p. After 15 minutes, each rat is then stimulated every 30 minutes for 3 to 4 hours. After each stimulation, individual seizure scores and afterdischarge durations are recorded. The group mean and standard error of the mean are calculated for each parameter. After the last stimulation, animals are allowed 4 to 5 drug- and stimulus-free days between subsequent drug tests.

Using this approach, a drug that reduces the seizure score from 5 to 3 without any effect on afterdischarge duration would be presumed useful against secondarily generalized seizures. In contrast, those drugs that reduce the seizure score from 5 to less than 1, as well as reduce the electrographic afterdischarge, would be anticipated to be effective against focal seizures.

The kindled animal also is an important tool that is used in a limited capacity to identify drugs that prevent or attenuate the development of a seizure focus (i.e., antiepileptic versus anticonvulsant drugs). In an acquisition paradigm, animals begin receiving the test substance before initiation of the kindling process. A parallel control group receives vehicle, and at the TPE individual rats are challenged with the kindling stimulation protocol. On each of the kindling days, dosing always precedes the kindling stimulus. This paradigm is continued until the animals in the vehicle control group become fully kindled. After a 7- to 10-day stimulus- and drug-free period, animals in both groups are challenged with the kindling stimulus. If the seizure score and afterdischarge duration of the drug-treated animals remain significantly lower than in the control group, the treatment would be considered to have delayed or prevented the development of kindling. In addition to expanding the anticonvulsant profile of a candidate substance to its utility in a model of focal seizures, the kindling model is particularly useful for characterizing the anticonvulsant and antiepileptic potential of those "few" drugs that display activity only in the 6-Hz identification test.

MECHANISM OF ACTION STUDIES

One of the goals of the advanced testing conducted by the ASP is to conduct pilot electrophysiologic studies that may identify the molecular mechanism of action of the candidate substance. Although numerous molecular targets exist wherein anticonvulsants may exert an effect, the final common pathway appears to be through modulation of voltage-gated or neurotransmitter-gated ion channels (29–32). Most of the prototype anticonvulsants are thought to exert their primary action by (a) reducing sustained, high-frequency, repetitive firing of action potentials by modulating voltage-dependent sodium (Na^+) channels; (b) enhancing GABA-mediated inhibitory neurotransmission through a receptor-gated chloride channel; or (c) modulating neurotransmitter release and neuronal bursting through an effect on voltage-gated and receptor-gated calcium (Ca^{2+}) channels. In addition, one of the newer anticonvulsant sub-

stances (i.e., retigabine) under clinical development has been found to activate a potassium channel comprising KCNQ2/Q3 potassium channel subunits (33–35). Loss-of-function mutations in this particular channel are thought to provide the basis for human benign familial convulsions (36–38) The common link among the various proposed mechanisms involves the ability of an anticonvulsant to modulate ion channel function. In light of this, the ASP uses the whole-cell patch-clamp technique (39) to assess the effect of promising candidate substances on current flow through voltage-gated and receptor-gated ion channels.

Mouse neuroblastoma cells (N1E-115) are recorded in conditions designed to assess selectively the effect of novel compounds on voltage-gated Na^+ channels. Sodium currents are elicited by brief steps to 0 mV from a variety of holding potentials. The same voltage step paradigms are then performed in the presence of a range of concentrations of the candidate substance. Results from these studies provide information concerning the voltage sensitivity of drugs found to inhibit Na^+ currents.

To assess the effects of the candidate substance on current flow through inhibitory and excitatory receptor-gated ion channels, the whole-cell patch-clamp technique is used to record currents evoked by exogenous application of subsaturating concentrations of GABA, kainate, or N-methyl-D-aspartate (NMDA). The respective ligand-gated currents are induced in cultured murine cortical neurons and agonists are applied either alone or in combination with the candidate substance, thus providing insight into how a compound exerts its anticonvulsant properties.

For some of the more recently developed anticonvulsants (e.g., levetiracetam), it has not been possible to identify the molecular activity contributing to its anticonvulsant action. For others, (e.g., felbamate, topiramate, and zonisamide), their anticonvulsant effect appears to be mediated by more than one molecular action. In this case, it is possible that one or more of a drug's mechanism of action interacts to dampen excitability in the neural networks that underlie seizure generation and propagation in ways that are not immediately obvious by examining individual receptor-gated and voltage-gated ion channels. Thus, to understand better the role that novel anticonvulsants play in modifying circuit behavior, the ASP has begun to examine the effects of anticonvulsants on synaptic transmission between pairs of monosynaptically connected neurons maintained in cell culture (40; Otto et al., personal communication). Inhibitory synapses formed by pairs of neurons in this culture system consist of postsynaptic $GABA_A$ receptors, whereas excitatory synapses have both non-NMDA and NMDA receptors that are colocalized to the synapse. Patch clamping both the presynaptic and postsynaptic neuron of a monosynaptically connected pair of neurons allows for the simultaneous examination of the effect of a compound on a number of presynaptic and postsynaptic neuronal parameters, including input resistance, resting membrane potential, action potential generation, neurotransmitter release, uptake mechanisms, postsynaptic receptor-gated ion channels, presynaptic receptors, and short-term plasticity. Thus, pair recordings represent a powerful paradigm in which to assess the sum total of the actions of an anticonvulsant in a simple neuronal circuit.

EVALUATION OF ANTIEPILEPTIC POTENTIAL

The anticonvulsant potential of a candidate AED usually is assessed by comparing the results obtained with the test substance in well standardized test procedures with those obtained with the established AEDs. For the purpose of dis-

cussion, data for six established and seven second-generation AEDs subjected to several of the previously above described animal models after i.p. and p.o. administration to mice and rats are summarized in Tables 3.4 and 3.5. The $TD_{50}s$ and $ED_{50}s$ provide important information, but they reveal little when viewed alone. For the 13 drugs shown in Table 3.4, the $TD_{50}s$ range from 0.3 to >500 mg/kg. For the active compounds, the $ED_{50}s$ by the MES test range from 5.6 to 263 mg/kg, and those by the s.c. MET test range from 0.02 to 220 mg/kg. Considerably more can be learned from a comparison of PIs, or the TD_{50}/ED_{50} ratio. The PIs, however, are based on the assumption that the slope of the

TABLE 3.4. ANTICONVULSANT PROFILE OF ESTABLISHED AND NEWER AEDs FOLLOWING I.P. ADMINISTRATION TO MICE

Substance	TD_{50} or ED_{50} (mg/kg) and PI[a]						
	TD_{50}	MES	s.c. MET	s.c. BIC	s.c. PIC	AGS	6 Hz[b]
Carbamazepine	45.4 (32.9–54.4)	7.81 (6.32–8.45) PI 5.8	>50	>50	18.2 (23.9–41.6) PI 1.7	11.2 (7.73–16.2) PI 4.1	Max. 75% protection at 40 and 80
Clonazepam	0.26 (0.16–0.42)	25.6 (9.12–65.9) PI 0.01	0.02 (0.016–0.030) PI 13	0.04 (0.02–0.07) PI 6.5	0.07 (0.05–0.10) PI 3.7	0.10 (0.09–0.11) PI 2.6	0.04 (0.03–0.06) PI 6.5
Ethosuximide	341 (290–384)	>500	136 (101–184) PI 2.5	272 (160–657) PI 1.3	226 (193–263) PI 1.5	328 (263–407) PI 1.0	167 (114–223) PI 2.0
Felbamate	220 (134–292)	35.5 (286–407) PI 6.2	126 (72.8–192) PI 1.7	>250	108 (64.6–166) PI 2.0	10.0 (8.19–12.0) PI 22	73.8 (36.3–119) PI 3.0
Gabapentin	>500	78.2 (46.6–127) PI >6.4	47.5 (17.9–86.2) PI >11	>500	>500	91.1 (61.8–129) PI >5.5	—
Lamotrigine	30.0 (24.8–36.2)	7.47 (6.13–9.11) PI 4.0	>40	>40	>40	2.39 (1.62–3.38) PI 13	Max. 50% protection at 20
Levetiracetam	>500	>500	>500	4.70 (0.58–13.4) PI >106	>500	—	19.4 (9.9–36.0) PI >26
Phenobarbital	69.0 (62.8–72.9)	21.8 (15.0–25.5) PI 3.2	13.2 (5.87–15.9) PI 5.2	37.7 (26.5–47.4) PI 1.8	27.5 (20.9–34.8) PI 2.5	—	14.8 (8.9–23.9) PI 4.7
Phenytoin	41.0 (39.4–43.0)	5.64 (4.74–6.45) PI 7.3	>50	>50	>50	3.88 (2.67–5.50) PI 11	Max. 58% protection at 40
Tiagabine	1.29 (0.82–1.85)	>5	0.26 (0.14–0.45) PI 5.0	>10	0.94 (0.50–1.64) PI 1.4	0.13 (0.10–0.16) PI 10	0.66 (0.17–1.23) 2.0
Topiramate	401 (318–535)	33.0 (16.3–58.1) PI 12	>800	>500	>500	4.15 (3.80–4.55) PI 97	>300
Valproic acid	398 (356–445)	263 (237–282) PI 1.5	220 (177–268) PI 1.8	589 (470–765) PI 0.68	270 (186–356) PI 1.5	155 (110–216) PI 2.6	126 (94.5–152) PI 3.2
Zonisamide	134 (113–153)	40.5 (34.5–47.3) PI 3.3	>250	>150	>150	—	97.4 (74.6–136) PI 1.4

TD_{50}, median toxic dose; ED_{50}, median effective dose; MES, maximal electroshock seizure test; s.c. MET, subcutaneous Metrazol seizure threshold; s.c. BIC, subcutaneous bicuculline test; s.c. PIC, subcutaneous picrotoxin test; AGS, audiogenic seizure susceptible.
[a]Protective index (PI) = TD_{50}/ED_{50}. Ranges in parentheses indicate 95% confidence interval.
[b]From Barton et al., *personal communication*.

TABLE 3.5. NEUROTOXICITY AND PROFILE OF ANTICONVULSANT ACTIVITY OF ORALLY ADMINISTERED PROTOTYPE ANTIEPILEPTIC DRUGS IN RATS

Substance	TD$_{50}$ (mg/kg)	MES (mg/kg)	s.c. MET (mg/kg)
Carbamazepine	364 (223–500)	5.35 (3.26–7.62) PI 68[a]	>250
Clonazepam	2.38 (1.43–3.53)	7.86 (5.75–11.6) PI 0.3	0.61 (0.46–0.72) PI 3.9
Ethosuximide	>500	>500	167 (116–237) PI >3.0
Felbamate	>500	25.3 (19.1–30.5) PI >20	>250
Gabapentin	309 (204–450)	14.8 (8.93–21.3) PI 21	>310
Lamotrigine	411 (305–512)	1.26 (0.92–1.56) PI 326	>412
Levetiracetam	>500	>500	Not tested
Phenobarbital	61.1 (43.7–95.9)	9.14 (7.58–11.9) PI 6.7	11.6 (7.74–15.0) PI 5.1
Phenytoin	>1000	28.1 (20.7–35.2) PI >3.6	>500
Tiagabine	86.8 (72.0–104)	Not tested	39.9 (17.6–72.1) PI 2.2
Topiramate	>500	3.27 (2.01–4.98) PI >153	>250
Valproic acid	784 (503–1176)	485 (324–677) PI 1.6	646 (466–869) PI 1.2
Zonisamide	192 (155–242)	21.3 (17.9–25.4) PI 9.0	>300

TD$_{50}$, median toxic dose; MES, maximal electroshock seizure test; s.c. MET, subcutaneous Metrazol seizure threshold.
[a]Protective index (PI) = TD$_{50}$/ED$_{50}$. Ranges in parentheses indicate 95% confidence intervals.

two regression lines (toxicity and anticonvulsant potency) are parallel. If the regression lines are parallel, the calculated PI is the same at any particular point on the regression lines. If the regression lines are not parallel, the PI is valid only at the median effective and toxic level. Above or below this median level, the PI may be either higher or lower. Therefore, in terms of drug tolerability, the calculated PI may be misleading. Ideally, an anticonvulsant drug should be capable of suppressing experimental seizures in all animals at dose levels devoid of even minimal toxic effects. Thus, it is more informative to calculate a "safety ratio" (TD$_3$/ED$_{97}$) for the candidate substance and to compare this with similar ratios for prototype drugs.

Albeit important, a comparative evaluation of a compound based on its PI and safety ratio provides little information about the overall anticonvulsant profile of a candidate drug compared with that of other AEDs tested in the same models. For example, in mice, the anticonvulsant profile of phenytoin, lamotrigine, topiramate, and zonisamide is relatively narrow compared with that of valproic acid, phenobarbital, tiagabine, and felbamate. Interestingly, in mice the anticonvulsant profile of carbamazepine includes activity against MES and PIC, whereas the anticonvulsant profile of gabapentin includes activity in the MES and s.c. MET tests. In addition, all of the sodium channel blockers listed (carbamazepine, phenytoin, and lamotrigine) display less than maximal efficacy in the 6-Hz seizure test.

In contrast, clonazepam and ethosuximide are both active in mice against clonic seizures induced by the chemoconvulsants MET, BIC, and PIC, but are virtually inactive (at nontoxic doses) against tonic extension seizures induced by MES. In contrast to the sodium channel blockers, those AEDs that act by elevating seizure threshold (e.g., clonazepam, ethosuximide, felbamate, phenobarbital, tiagabine, and valproic acid) are fully efficacious in the 6-Hz seizure test.

The anticonvulsant profile of levetiracetam clearly is unique among all of the AEDs listed in Tables 3.4 and 3.5.

As discussed earlier, levetiracetam is inactive in the two traditional screening tests (i.e., MES and s.c. MET); however, levetiracetam displays potent activity in both the s.c. BIC and 6-Hz seizure tests (Table 3.5). Given the clinical utility of levetiracetam in partial seizures, these findings strongly support the inclusion of the s.c. BIC or the 6-Hz seizure test into the initial identification protocol of laboratories evaluating the anticonvulsant activity of investigational AEDs. In the case of levetiracetam, these data provide the rationale for pursuing more advanced testing in other "syndrome-specific" models such as kindling.

An evaluation of an investigational AED in the mouse tests summarized in Table 3.4 usually provides sufficient information to conclude whether a drug possesses anticonvulsant activity after i.p. administration and whether it is likely to have a narrow or broad spectrum of activity. However, it is not clear from these studies if an AED will have activity after p.o. administration. For this purpose, the ASP also evaluates each promising candidate substance in the rat MES and s.c. MET tests after p.o. administration (Table 3.5). Often, drugs are found to be more potent after p.o. administration in the rat MES test (e.g., topiramate) and less potent, or inactive, in the rat s.c. MET test. For example, both gabapentin and felbamate display activity in the mouse s.c. MET test (Table 3.4), yet both are inactive in this test after p.o. administration to rats (Table 3.5). Loss of activity in the rat s.c. MET test is not observed for all drugs active in the mouse s.c. MET test (e.g., clonazepam, ethosuximide, phenobarbital, tiagabine, and valproic acid). From a comparison of the results summarized in Tables 3.4 and 3.5, it appears that activity in the rat s.c. MET test is preserved for those AEDs that also are active in at least one of the other chemoconvulsant mouse models (i.e., s.c. PIC and s.c. BIC). The significance of this observation is not known.

Activity of a test substance in one or more of the electrical and chemical tests described previously provides some insight into the overall anticonvulsant potential of the test substance.

However, a concern voiced recently is that the procedures currently used in the search for novel AEDs are likely to identify "me too" drugs and are unlikely to discover those drugs with different mechanisms of action. In an attempt to address this concern, the ASP evaluates all compounds found to be active in one or more of the initial identification screens for their ability to limit focal and secondarily generalized seizures in the rapid hippocampal kindling model (28). For these studies, the two primary end points (i.e., seizure score and afterdischarge duration) are plotted as a function of time. Because of the relatively short refractory period observed in the hippocampal kindled rat, a time–effect curve can be obtained for each animal. Thus, in a limited number of kindled rats, the duration of action and degree of efficacy against focal or secondarily generalized seizures can be determined quite quickly. Drugs that reduce the seizure score to <1 and significantly attenuate the afterdischarge duration over a prolonged time are considered ideal candidates for further evaluation in this and other models of focal epilepsy.

The correlation between animal models of epilepsy, mechanisms of action, and clinical effectiveness of currently marketed AEDs has been reviewed by Macdonald and Kelly (30) and White (32). Most of the clinically effective AEDs decrease membrane excitability by interacting with ion channels, neurotransmitter receptors, metabolism, or uptake. The only real exception to this generalization is levetiracetam. Very little is known about the precise mechanism through which this AED exerts its effect. The ASP uses standard patch-clamp electrophysiologic techniques to evaluate the ability of an investigational AED to modulate voltage- and receptor-gated ion channels. In addition, the recently implemented pair recording experiments will allow us directly to evaluate the action of AEDs on a number of parameters that are involved in synaptic transmission and plasticity at both excitatory and inhibitory synapses in a simple neural circuit. These studies are conducted in an effort to differentiate the mechanistic profile of the investigational AED from that of the established AEDs. For example, when a drug is demonstrated to possess an anticonvulsant profile that is similar to that of phenytoin and lamotrigine, it would not be surprising to find that it also inhibits voltage-sensitive Na^+ currents. The subsequent demonstration that it lacks activity at the voltage-sensitive Na^+ channel or other molecular sites through which the traditional AEDs are thought to work would be indicative of a novel action. This information, albeit negative, becomes important when attempting to identify the "truly novel" AED. Several of the second-generation AEDs possess rather broad and unique mechanistic profiles compared with the older, established AEDs. For example, felbamate and topiramate are unique among all of the AEDs in that they exert a negative modulatory effect on glutamate currents mediated by the NMDA and α-amino-3-hydroxy-5-methyl-4-isoxazole propionate (AMPA) receptors, respectively. In addition to these activities, both substances also negatively modulate voltage-sensitive Na^+ and Ca^{2+} currents and positively modulate $GABA_A$ receptor function. Topiramate also possesses the ability to inhibit type II and IV carbonic anhydrase. It is likely that the broad mechanistic profile of some of the newer AEDs contributes to their corresponding broad clinical profiles.

The results obtained from the detailed evaluation of a given drug in the battery of seizure and epilepsy models described previously provide the preclinical basis for the clinical evaluation of a candidate antiepileptic substance. Furthermore, they provide some insight into the overall potential clinical utility of a candidate compound. As summarized in Table 3.6, drugs found to be active in the MES

TABLE 3.6. CORRELATION BETWEEN CLINICAL UTILITY AND EFFICACY IN EXPERIMENTAL ANIMAL MODELS OF THE ESTABLISHED AND SECOND-GENERATION ANTIEPILEPTIC DRUGS

Seizure Type	Experimental Model			
	MES (Tonic Extension)	s.c. MET (Clonic Seizures)	Spike-Wave Discharges[a]	Electrical Kindling (Focal Seizures)
Tonic and/or clonic generalized seizures	CBZ, PHT, VPA, PB [FBM, GBP, LTG, TPM, ZNS][b]			
Myoclonic/generalized absence seizures		ESM, VPA, PB[c], BZD [FBM, GBP[c], TGB[c]]		
Generalized absence seizures			ESM, VPA, BZD [LTG, TPM, LVT]	
Partial seizures				CBZ, PHT, VPA, PB, BZD [FBM, GBP, LTG, TPM, TGB, ZNS, LVT]

MES, maximal electroshock seizure test; s.c. MET, subcutaneous Metrazol seizure threshold; BZD, benzodiazepines; CBZ, carbamazepine; ESM, ethosuximide; FBM, felbamate; GBP, gabapentin; LTG, lamotrigine; LVT, levetiracetam; PB, phenobarbital; PHT, phenytoin; TGB, tiagabine; TPM, topiramate; VPA, valproic acid; ZNS, zonisamide.
[a]Data summarized from γ-hydroxybutyrate, GAERS, and *lh/lh* spike-wave models (26,42,47,48).
[b]Drugs in brackets are second-generation antiepileptic drugs.
[c]PB, GBP, and TGB block clonic seizures induced by s.c. MET, but all are inactive against generalized absence seizures.

test are likely to be useful for the management of generalized tonic-clonic seizures; whereas drugs active against fully expressed kindled seizures have all demonstrated activity in clinical trials against partial seizures. In the past, positive results obtained in the s.c. MET seizure test were considered suggestive of potential clinical utility against generalized absence seizures. This interpretation was based largely on the finding that drugs active in the clinic against partial seizures (e.g., ethosuximide, trimethadione, valproic acid, the benzodiazepines) were able to block clonic seizures induced by MET, whereas drugs such as phenytoin and carbamazepine that were ineffective against absence seizures also were inactive in the s.c. MET seizure test. Based on this argument, phenobarbital, gabapentin, and tiagabine should all be effective against spike–wave seizures, and lamotrigine should be inactive against spike–wave seizures. However, clinical experience has demonstrated that this is an invalid prediction. Thus, the barbiturates, gabapentin, and tiagabine all aggravate spike–wave seizure discharge, whereas lamotrigine has been found to be effective against absence seizures. As such, the overall utility of the s.c. MET test in predicting activity against human spike–wave seizures is limited. Before any firm conclusion concerning potential utility against spike–wave seizures is warranted, positive results in the s.c. MET test should be corroborated by positive findings in other models of absence, such as the GHB seizure test, the genetic absence epilepsy in rats from Strasbourg (GAERS) model, and the *lh/lh* mouse (Table 3.6). With this exception, the data obtained in laboratory models correlate reasonably well with the clinical use of these agents and provide a basis for appropriately designed clinical trials that will ultimately determine the overall clinical potential of any given antiepileptic substance.

A further review of the data summarized in Table 3.6 demonstrates the importance of using multiple models in any screening protocol when attempting to identify and characterize the overall potential of a candidate antiepileptic substance. For example, levetiracetam is inactive in the traditional MES and s.c. MET tests, yet it demonstrates excellent efficacy in the GAERS model of primary generalized seizures and in the kindled rat model (1). Likewise, the efficacy of tiagabine and vigabatrin against human partial seizures was not predicted by the MES test, but by the kindled rat model (31,41). Furthermore, as mentioned previously, exacerbation of spike–wave seizures would not have been predicted by the s.c. MET test but by the other models (i.e., GHB, GAERS, and the *lh/lh* mouse), wherein both drugs have been shown to increase spike–wave discharges (42). These examples serve to illustrate the limitations of some of the animal models while emphasizing their overall utility in predicting both clinical efficacy and potential seizure exacerbation. What is clear from this discussion is that there is a need to evaluate each investigational AED in a variety of seizure and epilepsy models. Only then will it be possible to gain a full appreciation of the overall spectrum of activity for a given investigational drug.

THE FUTURE OF ANTIEPILEPTIC DRUG DISCOVERY AND DEVELOPMENT

Since its inception in 1975, the ASP has screened over 24,000 investigational AEDs. In addition to the compounds that have been successfully developed, a number of additional compounds are in various stages of clinical development. Each of these drugs has brought about substantial benefit to the patient population in the form of increased seizure control, increased tolerability, and better safety and pharmacokinetic profiles. Unfortunately for 25% to 40% of patients with epilepsy, there remains a need to identify therapies that will more effectively treat their therapy-resistant seizures. As such, there is a continued need to identify and incorporate more appropriate models of refractory epilepsy into the AED screening process. There are several model systems that could be suggested, including the phenytoin-resistant kindled rat (43); the carbamazepine-resistant kindled rat (44); the 6-Hz psychomotor seizure model (21; Barton et al., personal communication); and the *in vitro* low-magnesium hippocampal slice preparation (45). Unfortunately, it will take the successful clinical development of a drug that is effective for the management of refractory epilepsy before any one of these (or other) model systems is clinically validated. Nonetheless, this should not prevent the community at large from continuing the search for a more effective therapy using the available models. In fact, until there is a validated model, it becomes even more important to characterize and incorporate several of the available models into the drug discovery process, while continuing to identify new models of refractory epilepsy.

There are no known therapies that are capable of modifying the course of acquired epilepsy. Attempts to prevent the development of epilepsy after febrile seizures, traumatic brain injury, and craniotomy with the older, established drugs have been disappointing (46). At the same time, discoveries at the molecular level have provided greater insight into the pathophysiologic process of certain seizure disorders. As such, it may be possible in the not-so-distant future to identify a treatment strategy that slows or halts the progression of epilepsy and prevents the development of epilepsy in susceptible individuals. However, any successful human therapy will necessarily be identified and characterized in a model system that closely approximates human epileptogenesis. There are several potential animal models wherein spontaneous seizures develop secondary to a particular insult or genetic manipulation. If we are to be successful in identifying a novel, disease-modifying therapy in the near future, we must become intentional in our efforts to characterize and incorporate such models of epileptogenesis into our screening protocols.

SUMMARY

In this chapter, the technical procedures used by the NIH-sponsored ASP are described. Special attention has been directed to the order in which these procedures are used and the use of these tests in the detection and quantification of anticonvulsant activity and minimal behavioral toxicity. Data obtained by subjecting six of the prototype AEDs (phenytoin, carbamazepine, ethosuximide, valproate, clonazepam, and phenobarbital) and seven of the second-generation AEDs (felbamate, gabapentin, lamotrigine, levetiracetam, tiagabine, topiramate, and zonisamide) to the anticonvulsant identification and quantification procedures are presented. Attention also is given to the role of anticonvulsant efficacy, acute behavioral toxicity, and protective indices in the evaluation of anticonvulsant potential. Last, the limitations associated with the current approaches are discussed. The rationale and need to broaden the scope of AED screening protocols to include models of therapy resistance and epileptogenesis also is discussed in context with the continuing need to identify more efficacious drugs for the 25% to 40% of patients who remain refractory to the currently available AEDs.

ACKNOWLEDGMENT

This work was supported by contracts (N01-NS-5-23-2, N01-NS-1-2347, N01-NS-4-2361, NO1-NS-9-2328, NO1-NS-4-2311, and NO1-NS-9-2313) from the National Institute of Neurological Disorders and Stroke, National Institutes of Health.

REFERENCES

1. Klitgaard H, Matagne A, Gobert J, et al. Evidence for a unique profile of levetiracetam in rodent models of seizures and epilepsy. *Eur J Pharmacol* 1998;353:191–206.
2. Loscher W, Honack D. Profile of ucb LO59, a novel anticonvulsant drug, in models of partial and generalized epilepsy in mice and rats. *Eur J Pharmacol* 1993;232:147–158.
3. Gower AJ, Hirsch E, Boehrer A, et al. Effects of levetiracetam, a novel antiepileptic drug, on convulsant activity in two genetic rat models of epilepsy. *Epilepsy Res* 1995;22:207–213.
4. Loscher W, Honack D, Rundfeldt C. Antiepileptogenic effects of the novel anticonvulsant levetiracetam (ucb LO59) in the kindling model of temporal lobe epilepsy. *J Pharmacol Exp Ther* 1998;284:474–479.
5. Gower AJ, Noyer M, Verloes R, et al. ucb LO59, a novel anticonvulsant drug: pharmacological profile in animals. *Eur J Pharmacol* 1992;222:193–203.
6. Shorvon SD, Lowenthal A, Janz D, et al. Multicenter double-blind, randomized, placebo-controlled trial of levetiracetam as add-on therapy in patients with refractory partial seizures. *Epilepsia* 2000;41:1179–1186.
7. Chaisewikul R, Privitera MD, Hutton JL, et al. Levetiracetam add-on for drug-resistant localization related (partial) epilepsy (Cochrane Review). *Cochrane Datab Syst Rev* 2001;1: CD001901.
8. Genton P, Gelisse P. Antimyoclonic effect of levetiracetam. *Epilept Disord* 2000;2:209–212.
9. Krauss GL, Bergin A, Kramer RE, et al. Suppression of post-hypoxic and post-encephalitic myoclonus with levetiracetam. *Neurology* 2001;56:411–412.
10. Dooley M, Plosker GL. Levetiracetam: a review of its adjunctive use in the management of partial onset seizures. *Drugs* 2000;60: 871–893.
11. Ben-Menachem E, Falter U. Efficacy and tolerability of levetiracetam 3000 mg/d in patients with refractory partial seizures: a multicenter, double-blind, responder-selected study evaluating monotherapy. European Levetiracetam Study Group. *Epilepsia* 2000;41:1276–1283.
12. Cereghino JJ, Biton V, Abou-Khalil B, et al. Levetiracetam for partial seizures: results of a double-blind, randomized clinical trial. *Neurology* 2000;55:236–242.
13. White HS, Woodhead JH, Franklin MR, et al. General principles: experimental selection, quantification, and evaluation of antiepileptic drugs. In: Levy RH, Mattson RH, Meldrum BS, eds. *Antiepileptic drugs*, 4th ed. New York: Raven Press, 1995: 99–110.
14. Torchiana ML, Stone CA. Post-seizure mortality following electroshock convulsions in certain strains of mice. *Proc Soc Exp Biol Med* 1959;100:290–293.
15. Woolley DE, Timiras PS, Rosenzweig MR, et al. Sex and strain differences in electroshock convulsions of the rat. *Nature* 1961; 190:515–516.
16. Davenport VD, Davenport HW. The relation between starvation, metabolic acidosis and convulsive seizures in rats. *J Nutr* 1948;36:139–152.
17. Dunham MS, Miya TA. A note on a simple apparatus for detecting neurological deficit in rats and mice. *J Am Pharm Assoc Sci Ed* 1957;46:208–209.
18. Swinyard EA. Laboratory evaluation of antiepileptic drugs: review of laboratory methods. *Epilepsia* 1969;10:107–119.
19. Woodbury LA, Davenport VD. Design and use of a new electroshock seizure apparatus, and analysis of factors altering seizure threshold and pattern. *Arch Int Pharmacodyn Ther* 1952;92: 97–104.
20. White HS, Wolf HH, Woodhead JH, et al. The National Institutes of Health Anticonvulsant Drug Development Program: screening for efficacy. *Adv Neurol* 1998;76:29–39.
21. Toman JEP, Everett GM, Richards RM. The search for new drugs against epilepsy. *Tex Rep Biol Med* 1952;10:96–104.
22. Swinyard EA. Electrically induced convulsions. In: Purpura DB, Penry JK, Tower D, et al., eds. *Experimental models of epilepsy*. New York: Raven Press, 1972:443–458.
23. Litchfield JR, Jr., Wilcoxon R. A simplified method of evaluating dose-effect experiments. *J Pharmacol* 1949;96:99–113.
24. Orlof MJ, Williams HL, Pfeiffer CC. Timed intravenous infusion of Metrazol and strychnine for testing anticonvulsant drugs. *Proc Soc Exp Biol Med* 1949;70:254–257.
25. White HS, Patel S, Meldrum BS. Anticonvulsant profile of MDL 27,266: an orally active, broad-spectrum anticonvulsant agent. *Epilepsy Res* 1992;12:217–226.
26. Snead OC. Pharmacological models of generalized absence seizures in rodents. *J Neural Transm Suppl* 1992;35:7–19.
27. Chapman AA, Croucher MJ, Meldrum BS. Evaluation of anticonvulsant drugs in DBA/2 mice with sound-induced seizures. *Arzneimittelforschung* 1984;34:1261–1264.
28. Lothman EW, Salerno RA, Perlin JB, et al. Screening and characterization of antiepileptic drugs with rapidly recurring hippocampal seizures in rats. *Epilepsy Res* 1988;2:366–379.

29. Macdonald RL. Antiepileptic drug actions. *Epilepsia* 1989;30: S19–S28.
30. Macdonald RL, Kelly KM. Antiepileptic drug mechanisms of action. *Epilepsia* 1993;34:S1–S8.
31. Rogawski MA, Porter RJ. Antiepileptic drugs: pharmacological mechanisms and clinical efficacy with consideration of promising developmental stage compounds. *Pharmacol Rev* 1990;42: 223–285.
32. White HS. Comparative anticonvulsant profile and proposed mechanisms of action of the established and newer antiepileptic drugs. In: Pellock JM, Dodson WE, Bourgeois BFD, eds. *Pediatric epilepsy: diagnosis and therapy*, 2nd ed. New York: Demos, 2001:301–316.
33. Hetka R, Rundfeldt C, Heinemann U, et al. Retigabine strongly reduces repetitive firing in rat entorhinal cortex. *Eur J Pharmacol* 1999;386:165–171.
34. Main MJ, Cryan JE, Dupere JR, et al. Modulation of KCNQ2/3 potassium channels by the novel anticonvulsant retigabine. *Mol Pharmacol* 2000;58:253–262.
35. Rundfeldt C, Netzer R. The novel anticonvulsant retigabine activates M-currents in Chinese hamster ovary-cells transfected with human KCNQ2/3 subunits. *Neurosci Lett* 2000;282:73–76.
36. Biervert C, Schroeder BC, Kubisch C, et al. A potassium channel mutation in neonatal human epilepsy. *Science* 1998;279:403–406.
37. Charlier C, Singh NA, Ryan SG, et al. A pore mutation in a novel KQT-like potassium channel gene in an idiopathic epilepsy family. *Nat Genet* 1998;18:53–55.
38. Singh NA, Charlier C, Stauffer D, et al. A novel potassium channel gene, KDNQ2, is mutated in an inherited epilepsy of newborns. *Nat Genet* 1998;18:25–29.
39. Hamill OP, Marty A, Neher E, et al. Improved patch clamp technique for high resolution current recording from cells and cell free membrane patches. *Pflugers Arch* 1981;391:85–100.
40. Wilcox KS, Dichter MA. Paired pulse depression in cultured hippocampal neurons is due to a presynaptic mechanism independent of GABAB autoreceptor activation. *J Neurosci* 1994;14: 1775–1788.
41. Suzdak PD, Jansen JA. A review of the preclinical pharmacology of tiagabine: a potent and selective anticonvulsant GABA uptake inhibitor. *Epilepsia* 1995;36:612–626.
42. Hosford DA, Wang Y. Utility of the lethargic (*lhlh*) mouse model of absence seizures in predicting the effects of lamotrigine, vigabatrin, tiagabine, gabapentin, and topiramate against human absence seizures. *Epilepsia* 1997;38:408–414.
43. Loscher W, Reissmuller E, Ebert U. Anticonvulsant efficacy of gabapentin and levetiracetam in phenytoin-resistant kindled rats. *Epilepsy Res* 2000;40:63–77.
44. Nissinen JPT, Pitkanen A. An animal model of TLE with spontaneous seizures: a new tool for testing the antiepileptic effects of new compounds. *Epilepsia* 2000;41[Suppl 7]:38.
45. Armand V, Rundfeldt C, Heinemann U. Effects of retigabine (D-23129) on different patterns of epileptiform activity induced by low magnesium in rat entorhinal cortex hippocampal slices. *Epilepsia* 2000;41:28–33.
46. Temkin NR. Antiepileptogenesis and seizure prevention trials with antiepileptic drugs: meta-analysis of controlled trials. *Epilepsia* 2001;42:515–524.
47. Marescaux C, Vergnes M. Genetic absence epilepsy in rats from Strasbourg (GAERS). *Ital J Neurol Sci* 1995;16:113–118.
48. Hosford DA, Clark S, Cao Z, et al. The role of GABAB receptor activation in absence seizures of lethargic (lh/lh) mice. *Science* 1992;257:398–401.

4

GENERAL PRINCIPLES

NEW ANTIEPILEPTIC DRUG DEVELOPMENT: MEDICAL PERSPECTIVE

JACQUELINE A. FRENCH
MARC A. DICHTER

This chapter is one of three that address the clinical development of antiepileptic drugs (AEDs). Whereas this one addresses the "medical perspective," the other two address the pharmaceutical and regulatory perspectives. The very fact that these different viewpoints are included is an indication that drug development must satisfy many differing goals. The goal of regulatory authorities is to obtain rigorous scientific evidence that a new AED is safe and effective. The goal of clinicians is to obtain the kind of clinically relevant information about a new AED that will lead to appropriate selection of treatment for their patients, including information about how to use a drug to its maximal advantage, and data that can determine accurate risk assessment. The first priority of the pharmaceutical industry is to obtain drug approval from regulatory bodies, which allows the drug to be marketed and sold. However, the needs of clinicians also must be addressed, if there is to be any demand for the drug once it is available. Clinicians frequently feel that their needs may be subservient to regulatory needs.

Unfortunately, clinical trials leave many clinical questions unanswered. This chapter reviews the ways that information about new AEDs is obtained during the development process. Emphasis is placed on how to interpret regulatory trials in the context of clinical use, and also on sources of information beyond regulatory trials.

HISTORY OF ANTIEPILEPTIC DRUG DEVELOPMENT

Until the middle of the nineteenth century, people with epilepsy were treated with a variety of "home remedies" and superstitious practices, the effectiveness of which is impossible to determine in the modern age. In the 1850s, bromide was introduced as the first true AED, although it was originally proposed as a treatment for epilepsy for the wrong reasons. For the next half-century bromide remained the only drug available, until just after the turn of the twentieth century, when phenobarbital was accidentally discovered to be effective in suppressing seizures. In the late 1930s, the first "rational" plan to discover AEDs was conceived by Tracy Putnam and Houston Merritt, when they developed a model of experimental epilepsy (the maximal electroshock test) and then tested compounds that had chemical structures similar to the barbiturates to find a compound that would suppress seizures while not producing sedation. They discovered phenytoin with this methodology, and within just a few years of their discovery, phenytoin was marketed for the treatment of seizures. Over the next 30 years, a small but steady stream of new antiseizure drugs was discovered and marketed and new animal screening tests were developed to complement the maximal electroshock test. These drugs included ethosuximide, primidone, mesantoin, and carbamazepine. In 1978, sodium valproate, the last of what are now referred to as the *old AEDs* or *conventional AEDs*, was approved for use in the United States, after considerable experience in Europe and considerable pressure on the U.S. Food and Drug Administration (FDA). For the most part, clinical trials of these compounds were not done in the rigorous fashion used today. Monotherapy was not considered a separate issue for approval. Wording in FDA approval statements was broad and inclusive. For example, carbamazepine was approved for "Partial seizures with complex symptomatology (psychomotor, temporal lobe), generalized tonic-clonic seizures and mixed seizure patterns" (1).

In the ensuing 15 years, an intensive AED screening program was developed at the National Institute of Neurological Disorders and Stroke and thousands of new chemical entities were tested in a variety of animal models to look for

Jacqueline A. French, MD: Professor, Department of Neurology, University of Pennsylvania; and Associate Director, Pennsylvania Epilepsy Center, Department of Neurology, Hospital of the University of Pennsylvania, Philadelphia, Pennsylvania

Marc A. Dichter, MD: Department of Neurology, University of Pennsylvania, Philadelphia, Pennsylvania

promising new AEDs. Some clinical trials resulted from these screening tests, but most failed because of either intolerable side effects or lack of demonstrable efficacy.

The "modern era" of new AEDs dawned in 1993 with the approval of the first new AED in 15 years, felbamate. This was followed quickly by a number of new drugs, both in the United States and in Europe, including gabapentin, lamotrigine, topiramate, tiagabine, oxcarbazepine, levetiracetam, and zonisamide. Each of these drugs was first tested as adjunctive therapy in adults with intractable partial seizures, although several were tested in monotherapy trial designs or in pediatric populations almost simultaneously (see pp. 52–53). A number of additional drugs, including some with potentially novel mechanisms of action, were started in clinical trials that did not succeed. Despite the introduction of eight new AEDs, approximately 25% to 35% of adults with partial seizures are not able to become seizure free. Thus, there is a continuing need to develop new drugs that will be effective in the subgroup of patients whose disease remains intractable.

ASSESSMENT OF EFFICACY

As noted previously, many new AEDs have been approved for use in the last several years (2). For the most part, approval has derived from large, well controlled, adjunctive, multicenter trials. These trials, most of similar design, have been an excellent way of determining efficacy to the satisfaction of regulatory bodies. Efficacy can be defined as the ability to reduce seizures in the context of a clinical trial. What these trials are not able to demonstrate is the *effectiveness* of these drugs. Effectiveness is defined as the value of an AED in the environment of use, or, in other words, its ability to benefit patients in clinical practice. Although efficacy and effectiveness are linked, they are not always the same. For example, a drug could demonstrate excellent efficacy, but only when administered in a five-times-per-day schedule. Because most people could not comply with such a schedule, breakthrough seizures would occur as a result of noncompliance, and the drug would not be very effective. Other examples could be given.

Demonstration of Efficacy

In 1962, the Kefauver-Harris amendments to the Federal Food, Drug and Cosmetic Act were passed. This ushered in the modern age of drug testing by requiring that pharmaceuticals be proved efficacious before marketing (3). At the same time, federal agencies were given the authority to decide whether safety and efficacy had been satisfactorily demonstrated. It was after this legislation that clinical trials, as they are now performed, began to emerge.

Two "adequate and well controlled clinical trials," so-called pivotal trials, that demonstrate efficacy must be per-

formed for FDA approval. Although different types of control, including historical control, can be used, placebo control is favored (4). The presence of a placebo control group in most trials to determine efficacy has a significant effect on trial design and subject selection, which is discussed later.

Clinical trials performed for regulatory purposes have several characteristics that make it difficult to extrapolate results to patients in clinical practice. Some of these are discussed in the following sections.

Population

Epilepsy Syndrome

Epilepsy comprises a diverse group of syndromes, each with a unique clinical presentation and frequently different genetics, etiology, and possibly underlying biochemical defect (5). Most regulatory trials are performed in patients with partial epilepsy, demonstrating complex partial seizures, with or without secondary generalization. Subjects also may experience simple partial seizures, but they may or may not be acceptable as a single seizure type for trial enrollment. Partial epilepsy is advantageous because it represents the most common type of epilepsy in adults (6). Also, patients with refractory partial epilepsy are seen at large epilepsy centers, where most efficacy trials are performed. The partial seizure population also is seen as the patients with the greatest unmet need because approximately one-third have uncontrolled seizures despite medical therapy. As a result, many AEDs have been approved for treatment of partial seizures and comparatively few for other types, such as absence, myoclonus, and infantile spasms. Trials in other populations are becoming more common, however. For example, lamotrigine has received approval for use in seizures associated with Lennox-Gastaut syndrome, based on positive clinical trials (7). Topiramate was shown to reduce seizures in a trial in Lennox-Gastaut syndrome (8), as well as in a novel clinical trial of patients with primary generalized tonic-clonic convulsions (9). Large-scale randomized trials of the new drugs have not yet been undertaken in patients with absence seizures or myoclonus.

Seizure Severity

Traditionally, the patients who are enrolled in pivotal trials have very frequent seizures, a long duration of epilepsy, and have failed numerous AEDs before they are recruited. Enrollment criteria usually require a minimum of three to four complex partial or secondarily generalized seizures per month. These criteria ensure that there will be enough measurable seizures during a 3-month trial to obtain a statistically significant result. Commonly, patients experience many more seizures per month than are required by inclusion criteria. Demographic data from several recent pivotal

TABLE 4.1. DEMOGRAPHICS FOR RECENT, RANDOMIZED, PLACEBO-CONTROLLED ADJUNCTIVE TRIALS OF NEW ANTIEPILEPTIC DRUGS

Antiepileptic Drug	Seizure Frequency for Total Population[a] (Median Per Month)	Epilepsy Duration (yr)	Patients Receiving Two or More Background AEDs During Study (%)
Gabapentin (50)	10.8	21 (median)	63
Lamotrigine (51)	13.3	21.3 (mean)	60
Topiramate (52)	11.0	N/A	55
Tiagabine (21)	9.1 (54-mg group)	22.9 (mean)	N/A
Oxcarbazepine (53)	10.0 (2,400-mg group)	N/A	73

AED, antiepileptic drug; N/A, not available.
[a]Unless otherwise noted.

trials are included in Table 4.1. The use of such patients may not demonstrate a new compound's true effectiveness, and it has been hypothesized that our best conventional AEDs might fail such a difficult test (10). Even if the experimental drug can be proved effective in this challenging population, it is unclear whether the results can or should be generalized to the remainder of patients with epilepsy, who, by and large, do not have intractable disease, and have fewer seizures. The effort to conduct trials in patients with less intractable or even new-onset disease has attracted increasing support.

Dose/Titration Selection

Another reason why clinical trials do not necessarily mirror clinical practice is that in trials, patients are titrated to fixed doses, which may either be excessive for that individual, leading to unnecessary toxicity, or too low, leading to suboptimal seizure control. In fact, some of the newer AEDs are being used at doses higher than those that were used in clinical trials, whereas others are used at lower doses. Trial results, as determined by 50% responder rates or percentage seizure reduction rates in recent clinical trials, have been significantly colored by the doses selected for use in the trial. Drugs that are tested at lower doses appear well tolerated, but less effective, whereas drugs tested at higher doses may appear highly effective, but with more toxicity. This appear-

ance is highlighted by the way in which outcomes are statistically calculated in most trials. Patients who are placed on a higher dose than they can tolerate may drop out before the trial is completed. If this occurs, they still may be counted as "responders" if they experienced seizure reduction before dropout, even though the observation period can be short. Table 4.2 shows the highest dose studied in pivotal trials for recently approved AEDs, and the responder rate and the dropout rates at that dose. Also included is the dose now typically considered an average dose for that AED, when used as add-on therapy. In some cases, the dropout rate was higher than the responder rate.

The most confounding aspect of pivotal trials is that they do not allow patients to reach their own "ideal" target dose. All practitioners have experience with patients who are not seizure free when a new AED is initiated, but who eventually can be titrated to a dose that renders them seizure free. Not uncommonly, these patients need to be down-titrated on their concomitant AED medication for higher doses of the new AED to be tolerated. This type of manipulation is not typically accommodated during a clinical trial. Therefore, it is a common belief that clinical trials underrepresent the efficacy of many drugs, even in a population that is difficult to control.

Another variable that clearly colors the results of clinical trials, and the perception of drugs when they are approved, is the selection of titration rates. There are several examples

TABLE 4.2. COMPARISON OF DOSE STUDIED IN ADJUNCTIVE, RANDOMIZED, CONTROLLED TRIALS COMPARED WITH CLINICAL PRACTICE, AND ITS EFFECT ON EFFICACY AND DROPOUT RATES

Antiepileptic Drug	Highest Dose Studied (mg)	Typical Dose Used in Adjunctive Therapy (mg)	% Responder Rate at Highest Dose[a]	Dropout Rate at Highest Dose (%)
Gabapentin (50)	1,800	2,400	26.5 (18)	3.7
Lamotrigine (51)	500	400	34 (16)[b]	13.8
Tiagabine (21)	56	24	29 (25)	16
Levetiracetam (54)	3,000	2,000	39.8 (29.8)	6.9
Topiramate (52)	1,000	400	55 (20)	36
Oxcarbazepine (53)	2,400	1,500	50 (37)	71.6

Responder rate is defined as percentage of patients achieving ≥50% seizure reduction compared with baseline.
[a]Values in parentheses indicate responder rates for placebo.
[b]Based on last 12 weeks of study.

of drugs that may have been titrated too rapidly in clinical trials, leading to a relatively higher dropout rate. One example is lamotrigine. Studies have clearly demonstrated that the incidence of rash is tied to titration rate, as well as background medication (11,12). A very slow titration rate is necessary when lamotrigine is added to valproic acid (12, 13), either alone or in combination with enzyme-inducing AEDs. Unfortunately, this information was not as clear when clinical trials were being performed. The trial that may have been most affected by this was the trial in patients with Lennox-Gastaut syndrome (7). Many patients in this trial were receiving valproic acid, and in retrospect the titration rate was too rapid, leading to a 1% incidence of serious rash. This, in part, led to a black box (serious) warning in FDA labeling when lamotrigine is used in children.

In some instances, rapid titration leads to decreased tolerability because of cognitive or other side effects. This was probably the case for topiramate and zonisamide, both of which are better tolerated when titrated more slowly (14, 15).

The titration rate for pivotal trials may be selected early in drug development, when less information is available. In many cases, the titration rate used in these trials is placed in FDA labeling. Clinicians should be aware that this may not represent the most useful titration rate in all patients. Often, slower titration leads to better tolerability, particularly in patients who are sensitive to drug side effects. On the other hand, a faster titration rate may be safe and effective, and might be considered when a rapid effect is desirable. Unfortunately, rigorously obtained data often are not available to guide the practitioner on the relative risk of rapid titration. One exception to this rule is levetiracetam. A blinded study compared initiation at 1, 2, or 4 g (16). Results indicated that the dropout rates were similar, although side effects were greater in the group started at the highest dose. Of the newer AEDs, only lamotrigine cannot be titrated rapidly owing to safety concerns (13). The others can be rapidly titrated, but an increase in side effects will most likely result.

Serum Levels

It is very frustrating to many clinicians that by the time AEDs are approved, there rarely has been a clear "therapeutic range" established. However, there is a good reason for this. For many AEDs, particularly those that are hepatically metabolized, serum levels are very variable and cannot be predicted by dose (17). As noted previously, patients are randomized to a dose, and not a serum level. The dose that they are randomized to may be too high or too low for them. Also, as noted, overly high or low doses may have been selected for study. In addition, in this very refractory population, even those who achieve a high serum level might not respond (18). Therefore, level–response relationships rarely are established in a randomized, placebo-con-

trolled, dose–response add-on trial (19). In general, the only information that can be obtained is a range of plasma levels achieved in the trials. Optimal serum levels usually are determined by open-label postmarketing investigations in which patients can be titrated to their optimal dose.

Trial Duration

Clinical trials are of short duration. Typically, seizure reduction counts are based on 3 to 4 months of observation. This may be too short to see evidence of the development of tolerance. On the other hand, some drugs may demonstrate an increase in efficacy or a decrease in side effects over time. Increasing efficacy with extended use has been postulated for valproic acid and the vagus nerve stimulator (20). Again, such effects are missed over the typical drug study duration.

Seizure Freedom

Another issue that is difficult to address in controlled clinical trials is the potential for becoming seizure free over the long-term. The goal of epilepsy therapy is a "cure," as manifested by elimination of seizures over years and even decades. Many patients report that introduction of a new AED provides short-term seizure relief, but seizures ultimately recur. This can be devastating, both medically and emotionally. Controlled clinical trials simply are not able to determine how many patients will remain free of seizures. It therefore is critically important to follow patients after randomized, controlled trials have been completed, to determine long-term efficacy. Unfortunately, this is rarely done in a rigorous manner.

Age Extremes

Pivotal trials are performed in the adult population first. For most studies, upper age cutoffs are imposed at 65 to 70 years of age. Lower age cutoffs have been lowered gradually. Whereas the lower cutoff used to be 18 years of age, more recent trials have studied patients as young as 12 years of age (21). Although even younger patients eventually will be tested in randomized, controlled trials leading to a pediatric indication, the elderly rarely are studied in a rigorous manner, despite the high incidence of epilepsy in this age group, with approximately 25% of new cases of epilepsy occurring in elderly people (22). Moreover, the etiologies and pathophysiologic processes are thought to be different in this group, potentially leading to a differentiation in drug response. Also, there are differences in pharmacokinetics and ability to tolerate specific side effects, such as fatigue and cognitive dysfunction, that may distinguish elderly individuals from their younger counterparts (23). Therefore, it is not clear that results from pivotal trials should be generalized to the elderly. One blinded study explored the response to carbamazepine and lamotrigine in a newly diagnosed elderly population, and found that lamotrigine was better tolerated (24). More such studies are needed, and indeed several are ongoing.

Monotherapy versus Polytherapy

Pivotal trials for determining safety and efficacy of new AEDs almost always are designed as adjunct studies. In other words, the drug under investigation is added to any AEDs the subject may already be taking to control his or her seizures. This design allows a placebo control group, which otherwise would be very difficult for such a serious disease. In a recent article, Robert Temple, of the FDA, advocated an add-on study design for "trials...in which omitting standard therapy would generally be unacceptable. Such studies are not directly informative about a drug as monotherapy, but they do provide interpretable evidence of effectiveness in a well-defined setting" (25). In fact, many patients with refractory epilepsy are treated with polytherapy, and it is critically important to determine the effectiveness, safety, and side effect profile in this setting. However, eventually, as less severely ill patients, or even patients with newly diagnosed epilepsy, receive new AEDs, it also is important to obtain information about drug activity in the monotherapy setting. The best way to obtain this information is still controversial, both in the United States and Europe.

The preferred method of demonstrating efficacy in monotherapy would be to compare placebo with active drug. Concerns about patient safety preclude this approach. Several trial designs have been devised that attempt to address safety concerns, but at the same time demonstrate effectiveness of a new drug as monotherapy (26,27). These designs use a "pseudoplacebo" in place of a true placebo. Patients in the pseudoplacebo arm receive some treatment to prevent catastrophic seizures or severe worsening, but not enough to prevent the complex partial seizures that are being evaluated in the study. Previously performed trials of this sort have used low-dose valproic acid or a low dose of the study drug as pseudoplacebo. Two commonly used trial designs use a pseudoplacebo arm. In one, the surgical withdrawal design, the subjects are undergoing medication withdrawal for the purpose of presurgical evaluation. When most or all medication has been eliminated, the experimental AED or placebo/pseudoplacebo is added in a randomized, blinded fashion. The trial ends after subjects have experienced a prespecified number of seizures ("failures") or have gone a certain time (usually 7 to 10 days) without that number of seizures having occurred ("completers"). Analysis is based on how many patients complete in the pseudoplacebo arm compared with the active arm.. These trials now are considered by many experts to be too short to generalize results to the outpatient setting.. A second design is performed in outpatients. Again, patients are randomized to pseudoplacebo or active drug, added on to baseline ther-

apy. Therapeutic failure is determined on the basis of escape criteria, such as doubling of seizure frequency or increase in seizure severity. If more patients receiving pseudoplacebo reach escape criteria compared with those receiving active drug, the drug is determined to be effective in monotherapy. These protocols now are commonly used when a monotherapy indication is sought (28–31).

This trial design, although it provides clear information for regulators, is of little value to clinicians because it does not address improvement when patients convert to monotherapy, but rather compares the patients converting to the study drug with a population that clearly will worsen as a result of being randomized to pseudoplacebo. This provides evidence only that the study drug is better than nothing.

Monotherapy studies also may be performed in newly diagnosed patients. In Europe, studies typically use an active control design, in which a new drug is compared with a standard (32,33). Some studies compare high and low doses. For example, one study in newly diagnosed patients demonstrated that 900 and 1,800 mg of gabapentin were more effective than 300 mg in preventing seizures requiring exit from the study (33). These types of dose-controlled studies in the newly diagnosed are somewhat dangerous. Most newly diagnosed patients who will become seizure free on a given drug appear to do so on relatively low levels of that drug (24). Thus, comparing a low dose with a high dose of a new drug in this population may demonstrate reasonably similar efficacy in both groups, leading to the erroneous conclusion that the drug is not substantially better than placebo, when, in fact, both doses of the study drug may be effective.

Monotherapy trial designs are controversial. Issues have been raised about the ethics of randomizing patients to treatment arms that are known to be suboptimal (pseudoplacebo), and also about the artificial nature of some of the designs, making it difficult to translate results to real-life situations (34–37). There possibly is more dissatisfaction with regulatory trials leading to monotherapy indications than with any other type of industry-sponsored trials. In this arena, only the active-controlled trials performed in Europe provide information useful to clinicians in treating patients. Discussion of the optimal way to perform these trials is ongoing. It is hoped that better solutions will be found in the future, which will provide useful regulatory *and* clinical data.

In a more controversial vein, it can be argued that all of the new (and old) AEDs that have been approved as adjunctive therapies also work in monotherapy, and probably at approximately the same efficacy as drugs that have been more rigorously studied in monotherapy. Thus, one can ask, especially given the ethical issues discussed earlier and the technical difficulties of carrying out monotherapy trials, whether these kinds of trials need to be performed at all. An alternative would be to have AEDs approved for use in partial seizures or primary generalized seizures of a given type without referring to adjunctive or monotherapy. This is especially important because *adjunctive* implies that a given drug will not work by itself, but only as a "helper" to some other form of therapy, and this clearly is not the case for AEDs. The FDA's current position on this issue is that they can approve a drug only for an indication in which there is rigorous proof of its efficacy, and because AEDs can be ethically tested initially only in adjunctive, add-on trials, that is the only indication they can receive from the FDA. This is a major area in which there is a conflict between the regulatory concerns and those of clinicians.

ASSESSMENT OF PHARMACOKINETICS

The behavior of a drug, once it enters the body, depends on it properties of absorption, metabolism, distribution, and elimination. Many AEDs have complex pharmacokinetic properties. Understanding the unique pharmacokinetic characteristics of AEDs is critical to their appropriate use. Most pharmacokinetic characteristics should be thoroughly explored at the time of AED approval. Usually, the first step in obtaining such understanding derives from preclinical investigations. Recently, it has become possible to predict some hepatic metabolic effects *in vitro*. Liver enzyme tests can indicate toxicity and effect on hepatic metabolism, including inhibition of cytochrome P450 enzymes. Liver tests also may help to establish the route of metabolism (e.g., oxidation or glucuronidation) (38). Further information is obtained from early phase 1 and phase 2 trials, which usually include trials specifically aimed at elucidating interactions between AEDs. At this stage, interactions with commonly used medications such as oral contraceptives and warfarin also may be explored (39). By the time large, phase 3, double-blind, placebo-controlled trials begin, most common interactions will have been thoroughly studied. Yet, when AEDs are approved, some pharmacokinetic data still may be lacking. For example, there may be limited data on the behavior of drugs in certain populations, such as the elderly, children, and patients with chronic liver or kidney dysfunction. Pharmacokinetic properties in pregnancy also may be unknown. More important, clinical trials focus on population pharmacokinetics and less on the behavior of a drug in a given individual under clinical conditions. For example, it is very common to down-titrate and ultimately discontinue background AEDs once a new AED is introduced. Because many of the older AEDs either induce or inhibit new AED metabolism (40), changes in serum level of the new AED can be expected. The clinician who is treating such a patient is caught in a dilemma: At what point should the new AED dose be adjusted during down-titration of the background drug, to maintain equivalent serum levels and seizure control? Such questions rarely are addressed in regulatory trials.

ASSESSMENT OF SAFETY AND TOLERABILITY

It can be considered an axiom that no drug is absolutely safe or without side effects. Consequently, AEDs, which often must be taken for years and in relatively high doses, commonly have issues that relate to both tolerability and long-term safety. Both of these are assessed during the development and clinical evaluation of new AEDs, but the ability of short-term studies on limited populations of highly selected individuals to detect all the issues related to either tolerability or safety is severely limited. For the purposes of this discussion, *tolerability* is related to the development of side effects from a drug that are unpleasant and may limit the drug's usefulness, whereas *safety* refers to serious or life-threatening side effects.

AEDs are designed to work on the brain and limit the activity of neurons that are hyperactive during seizures. However, it is imperative that these drugs not interfere with the normal function of the brain. It actually is remarkable that any such compounds can be developed at all, rather than that they all may confer unpleasant side effects in some individuals. Initially, in phase 1 studies, AEDs are tested in a very small number of people who have not been chronically exposed to drugs, and these would likely be those most sensitive to side effects of the drug. Titration rates, dosage, and duration of exposure all affect the likelihood of intolerable side effects. Once the drug gets past this small group of volunteers, it usually is tested on several hundred to a few thousand subjects before it is released. These are patients with intractable epilepsy who typically are on multiple drugs, and who are used to tolerating a variety of side effects while trying to get their seizures under control. In addition, they are highly selected for the clinical trials and often are afforded special medical attention during the clinical trial. Thus, there are reasons why they would be more susceptible to side effects (multiple drugs) as well as less susceptible (experience, enhanced level of care). Typically, at higher doses, and especially during add-on trials, many new AEDs cause some degree of sedation (which may be called *fatigue* or *lethargy*). Sometimes this may decrease as a patient continues to take the medication, a process of growing tolerance. It is hoped that a similar tolerance will not occur to the antiseizure effect of the drug. Other important central nervous system issues of tolerability relate to decreases in cognitive function and changes in affective behavior (e.g., irritability, anxiety). Both of these may be hard to quantitate, especially when specific tests usually are not performed. Other, more easily assessed side effects commonly seen include dizziness, ataxia, diplopia, gastrointestinal symptoms, and headache. It is common for these to be reported during controlled, double-blind studies, and in some cases there is little difference between those on active drug and those on placebo (which is one of the more important aspects of placebo control). In general, if dropout rates are not too high, tolerability issues neither cause the premature termination of a trial nor prevent a successful outcome of a trial and registration of a drug. However, once a drug is approved, a number of additional considerations develop. First, a much larger number of less carefully selected patients are given the drug, and new problems may arise that were not appreciated in the smaller exposure. Second, the drug may be used in patients who have had less experience with AEDs and therefore may be less tolerant. Third, patients stay on the drug for longer periods and new problems with tolerability may be noted, such as excessive weight gain or loss, or hair loss. Fourth, patients may be on other types of drugs that were excluded from the clinical trials (e.g., antibiotics, oral contraceptives, antihypertensives, antidepressants), and tolerability issues may develop based on unanticipated pharmacokinetic or pharmacodynamic interactions.

The most problematic tolerability issue in interpreting clinical trials is distinguishing *phamacodynamic* side effects from those produced by the drug in isolation. Most of the data we have about AEDs derive from adjunctive trials. When AEDs are combined, side effects often are magnified beyond those seen with either drug alone. Often, these pharmacodynamic side effects may be seen with one drug combination, but not others. The magnitude of this problem was highlighted by several monotherapy studies in outpatients. As noted previously, these studies often involve adding a new drug, then removing all background drugs. In such a trial performed with lamotrigine, dizziness occurred in 20% of patients when lamotrigine was used as adjunctive therapy, but in only 7% when background AEDs were withdrawn (28).

Thus, tolerability seen in small clinical trials may not be identical to that seen when a drug becomes available to the larger population of patients with epilepsy, or when the drug is used as monotherapy.

Assessment of Safety

All new chemical entities undergo laboratory (animal) investigation for safety before they are available for testing in humans. These tests include both short-term assessments in multiple species and longer-term assessment for chronic toxicity, especially carcinogenesis (41). In addition, drugs are tested in two species of animals for possible teratogenesis, although it is not clear that for this purpose animal testing can be readily extrapolated to humans. Safety issues then are very carefully monitored during clinical trials and any adverse event, even if apparently unrelated to drug administration, is recorded and reported.

Some potentially serious safety issues are not easily routinely monitored. For example, adverse effects on hormonal status in women or on behavioral states in general may be missed either if they are subtle or take a relatively long exposure to be manifest. Thus, it would not be expected that a propensity to polycystic ovaries or a problem with fertility would be noted in a typical 12- or 24-week exposure to a new AED. Similarly, depression is relatively common in patients with epilepsy, and can be multifactorial, so it is possible that subtle but significant changes in affect could be missed during a brief trial. In general, one sees what one is looking for or, in some cases, things that cannot be ignored. Thus, if trials are not set up to examine specific parameters, safety issues that relate to these conditions could be overlooked. This clearly is not an issue for AEDs alone, but because these drugs are used for prolonged periods in patients who already have a number of associated problems, some types of safety issues may be more problematic.

Perhaps one of the most serious issues in safety assessment relates to the fact that evaluations during brief clinical trials clearly are unable to ascertain serious adverse events that occur only uncommonly or rarely. The recent example of the emergence of very serious safety issues after felbamate was approved is a graphic example of this. In a number of individuals, aplastic anemia or hepatic failure developed, both of which were not seen, or even hinted at, during the clinical trials (42). The combination of felbamate being the first of the new AEDs released and an aggressive and effective marketing campaign resulted in felbamate being taken by more than 100,000 people in the United States within 1 year of approval. These two very serious, and in some cases, fatal, toxic side effects caught the medical community by surprise, but unfortunately emphasize the fact that rare idiosyncratic side effects of any new drug will be detected only after widespread use. Adequate postmarketing surveillance is the only method by which such events will be detected and long-term safety ascertained.

Another issue in the assessment of safety relates to the use of AEDs in the pediatric population. These patients are undergoing profound changes in the brain during their normal development, and it is important that drugs that work on the brain not interfere with these developmental processes. It might take years before adverse effects on these developmental events manifest, and it also would likely take careful, detailed assessments of both cognitive and behavioral performance to detect any problems (43). Unfortunately, an adequate analysis has not been performed on any AED, either "old" or "new." Although gross problems have not been identified, the issue of more subtle changes in general has not been addressed. It would be extremely difficult, and quite impractical, to conduct adequate long-term developmental safety trials during the registration process for drugs that will be used in the pediatric population. On the other hand, it is hard to argue with the importance of such issues. Perhaps, good postmarketing trials could address these issues.

One other major safety issue relates to potential teratogenicity of new AEDs. Most people with epilepsy are young, and half are women. Thus, many people on chronic AED therapy are women who will likely want to become pregnant and have children despite their epilepsy. Data on older AEDs suggest that using one drug in relatively moderate doses does not markedly increase the risk for major fetal malformations over that of offspring of women with epilepsy who are not taking AEDs, in that the risk is still on the order of 4% to 6% (44). Less information is available for the newer AEDs. As mentioned, the validity of preclinical testing is questionable. Fortunately, pregnancy registries have been established in many countries throughout the world to collect data about possible adverse outcomes of pregnancies exposed to AEDs. Over time, these should provide good data about the relative risks of each of the available AEDs.

ALTERNATIVES TO REGULATORY TRIALS

If regulatory trials cannot provide sufficient information to inform the treating physician, what are the alternatives? There have been many attempts to "fill the knowledge gap," each with its own set of problems.

One solution has been to perform a meta-analysis of several trials in an attempt to arrive at comparative efficacy and safety data. Recently, such an analysis was done for many of the new drugs. This study revealed that efficacy rates often paralleled tolerability. In other words, the higher the responder rate, the more tolerability problems existed (2,45). Although this approach has some utility, it suffers from the same problems as do the regulatory trials from which it derives, namely, fixed doses and titration schedules and a refractory patient sample.

What of other solutions? Many studies have been performed that purport to mimic clinical practice. Typically, these trials follow a cohort of patients over a long duration in an open fashion. Variables that typically are assessed include discontinuation rates, adverse events, and percentage seizure freedom (46,47). These trials can definitely provide very important efficacy and safety information, particularly in populations that are not routinely studied in randomized, prospective trials. However, there are drawbacks to this approach, including the absence of a control group, and potential bias with regard to choice of patients that go on each drug.

What would be most useful would be a randomized "use" trial, in which patients are randomized to one of the new drugs, titrated to their ideal dose, and followed over a long period of time. Such trials were common in the 1980s and provided a wealth of data that still is relevant today (48, 49). Some of the European active-controlled monotherapy trials in newly diagnosed patients are performed in this fashion (32,33). A large-scale use trial was initiated recently in Europe. This type of trial should provide clinicians with important information on the effectiveness of the new AEDs.

CONCLUSION

Controlled clinical trials are essential in proving that drugs are safe and effective for use. However, they cannot fully inform the clinician in the use of new AEDs. The typical patient in practice is not treated in the same fashion as a subject in a clinical trial. The need for scientific rigor and a controlled environment in clinical investigation is crucial, but at the same time often introduces a certain rigidity in population selection, titration, dose selection, and manipulation of background drugs that reduces the generalizability of the results. The gaps in knowledge need to be filled by additional studies, which try to address clinical questions in as rigorous a way as possible.

REFERENCES

1. Physicians' Desk Reference, 55th ed. Medical Economics Data Production, Montvale; New Jersey, 2001.
2. Cramer JA, Mattson RH, Scheyer RD, et al. Review of new antiepileptic drugs (AEDs). *Epilepsia* 1998;39:233–234.
3. Kefauver-Harris Drug Amendments Act of 1962. *Federal Register* 1962;21:87–781.
4. Leber PD. Hazards of inference: the active control investigation. *Epilepsia* 1989;30[Suppl 1]:S57–S63; discussion S64–S68.
5. French JA. The art of antiepileptic trial design. *Adv Neurol* 1998; 76:113–123.
6. Hauser WA, Annegers JF, Kurland LT. Prevalence of epilepsy in Rochester, Minnesota: 1940–1980. *Epilepsia* 1991;32:429–445.
7. Motte J, Trevathan E, Arvidsson JF, et al. Lamotrigine for generalized seizures associated with the Lennox-Gastaut syndrome: Lamictal Lennox-Gastaut Study Group. *N Engl J Med* 1997;337: 1807–1812.
8. Sachdeo RC, Glauser TA, Ritter F, et al. A double-blind, randomized trial of topiramate in Lennox-Gastaut syndrome: Topiramate YL Study Group. *Neurology* 1999;52:1882–1887.
9. Biton V, Montouris GD, Ritter F, et al. A randomized, placebo-controlled study of topiramate in primary generalized tonic-clonic seizures: Topiramate YTC Study Group. *Neurology* 1999; 52:1330–1337.
10. Temkin AWN. New AEDs: are the compounds or the studies ineffective? *Epilepsia* 1986;27:644–645.
11. Wallace SJ. Lamotrigine: a clinical overview. *Seizure* 1994;3 [Suppl A]:47–51.
12. Willmore LJ, Messenheimer JA. Adult experience with lamotrigine. *J Child Neurol* 1997;12[Suppl 1]:S16–S18.
13. Messenheimer J, Mullens EL, Giorgi L, et al. Safety review of adult clinical trial experience with lamotrigine. *Drug Saf* 1998; 18:281–296.
14. Biton V, Edwards KR, Montouris GD, et al. Topiramate titration and tolerability. *Ann Pharmacother* 2001;35:173–179.
15. Sander JW. Using topiramate in patients with epilepsy: practical aspects. *Can J Neurol Sci* 1998;25:S16–S18.
16. Betts T, Waegemans T, Crawford P. A multicentre, double-blind, randomized, parallel group study to evaluate the tolerability and efficacy of two oral doses of levetiracetam, 2000 mg daily and 4000 mg daily, without titration in patients with refractory epilepsy. *Seizure* 2000;9:80–87.
17. Perucca E. Is there a role for therapeutic drug monitoring of new anticonvulsants? *Clin Pharmacokinet* 2000;38:191–204.

18. Kilpatrick ES, Forrest G, Brodie MJ. Concentration—effect and concentration—toxicity relations with lamotrigine: a prospective study. *Epilepsia* 1996;37:534–538.
19. Tomson T, Johannessen SI. Therapeutic monitoring of the new antiepileptic drugs. *Eur J Clin Pharmacol* 2000;55:697–705.
20. DeGiorgio CM, Schachter SC, Handforth A, et al. Prospective long-term study of vagus nerve stimulation for the treatment of refractory seizures. *Epilepsia* 2000;41:1195–1200.
21. Uthman BM, Rowan AJ, Ahmann PA, et al. Tiagabine for complex partial seizures: a randomized, add-on, dose- response trial. *Arch Neurol* 1998;55:56–62.
22. Stephen LJ, Brodie MJ. Epilepsy in elderly people. *Lancet* 2000; 355:1441–1446.
23. Rowan AJ. Reflections on the treatment of seizures in the elderly population. *Neurology* 1998;51[Suppl 4]:S28–S33.
24. Brodie MJ, Overstall PW, Giorgi L. Multicentre, double-blind, randomised comparison between lamotrigine and carbamazepine in elderly patients with newly diagnosed epilepsy: the UK Lamotrigine Elderly Study Group. *Epilepsy Res* 1999;37:81–87.
25. Temple R, Ellenberg SS. Placebo-controlled trials and active-control trials in the evaluation of new treatments. Part 1: ethical and scientific issues. *Ann Intern Med* 2000;133:455–463.
26. Pledger GW, Schmidt D. Evaluation of antiepileptic drug efficacy. A review of clinical trial design. *Drugs* 1994;48:498–509.
27. Pledger GW, Kramer LD. Clinical trials of investigational antiepileptic drugs: monotherapy designs. *Epilepsia* 1991;32: 716–721.
28. Gilliam F, Vazquez B, Sackellares JC, et al. An active-control trial of lamotrigine monotherapy for partial seizures. *Neurology* 1998; 51:1018–1025.
29. Sachdeo RC, Reife RA, Lim P, et al. Topiramate monotherapy for partial onset seizures. *Epilepsia* 1997;38:294–300.
30. Beydoun A, Fischer J, Labar DR, et al. Gabapentin monotherapy: II. a 26-week, double-blind, dose-controlled, multicenter study of conversion from polytherapy in outpatients with refractory complex partial or secondarily generalized seizures: the US Gabapentin Study Group 82/83. *Neurology* 1997;49:746–752.
31. Faught E, Sachdeo RC, Remler MP, et al. Felbamate monotherapy for partial-onset seizures: an active-control trial. *Neurology* 1993;43:688–692.
32. Brodie MJ, Richens A, Yuen AW. Double-blind comparison of lamotrigine and carbamazepine in newly diagnosed epilepsy: UK Lamotrigine/Carbamazepine Monotherapy Trial Group. *Lancet* 1995;345:476–479.
33. Chadwick DW, Anhut H, Greiner MJ, et al. A double-blind trial of gabapentin monotherapy for newly diagnosed partial seizures: International Gabapentin Monotherapy Study Group 945-77. *Neurology* 1998;51:1282–1288.
34. Chadwick D. Monotherapy clinical trials of new antiepileptic drugs: design, indications, and controversies. *Epilepsia* 1997;38 [Suppl 9]:S16–S20.
35. French JA. What trials, which designs? *Epilepsia* 1997;38:263–265.
36. Perucca E, Tomson T. Monotherapy trials with the new antiepileptic drugs: study designs, practical relevance and ethical implications. *Epilepsy Res* 1999;33:247–262.
37. Chadwick D, Privitera M. Placebo-controlled studies in neurology: where do they stop? *Neurology* 1999;52:682–685.
38. White HS WJ, Franklin MR, Swinyard EA, Wolf HH. Experimental selection, quantification and evaluation of antiepileptic drugs. In: Levy RH MR, Meldrum BS, eds. *Antiepileptic drugs*. New York: Raven Press, 1995:99–110.
39. Wilbur K, Ensom MH. Pharmacokinetic drug interactions between oral contraceptives and second-generation anticonvulsants. *Clin Pharmacokinet* 2000;38:355–365.
40. French JA, Gidal BE. Antiepileptic drug interactions. *Epilepsia* 2000;41[Suppl 8]:S30–S36.
41. Cereghino J, Kupferberg HS. Preclinical testing. *Epilepsy Res Suppl* 1993;10:19–30.
42. Kaufman DW, Kelly JP, Anderson T, et al. Evaluation of case reports of aplastic anemia among patients treated with felbamate. *Epilepsia* 1997;38:1265–1269.
43. French JA, Leppik I. Testing antiepileptic drugs in children. *J Child Neurol* 1994;9[Suppl 1]:S26–S32.
44. Lindhout D, Omtzigt JG. Pregnancy and the risk of teratogenicity. *Epilepsia* 1992;33[Suppl 4]:S41–S48.
45. Marson AG, Kadir ZA, Hutton JL, et al. The new antiepileptic drugs: a systematic review of their efficacy and tolerability. *Epilepsia* 1997;38:859–880.
46. Lhatoo SD, Wong IC, Polizzi G, et al. Long-term retention rates of lamotrigine, gabapentin, and topiramate in chronic epilepsy. *Epilepsia* 2000;41:1592–1596.
47. Lhatoo SD, Wong IC, Sander JW. Prognostic factors affecting long-term retention of topiramate in patients with chronic epilepsy. *Epilepsia* 2000;41:338–341.
48. Mattson RH, Cramer JA, Collins JF. A comparison of valproate with carbamazepine for the treatment of complex partial seizures and secondarily generalized tonic-clonic seizures in adults: the Department of Veterans Affairs Epilepsy Cooperative Study No. 264 Group. *N Engl J Med* 1992;327:765–771.
49. Mattson RH, Cramer JA, Collins JF, et al. Comparison of carbamazepine, phenobarbital, phenytoin, and primidone in partial and secondarily generalized tonic-clonic seizures. *N Engl J Med* 1985;313:145–151.
50. Gabapentin as add-on therapy in refractory partial epilepsy: a double- blind, placebo-controlled, parallel-group study: the US Gabapentin Study Group No. 5. *Neurology* 1993;43:2292–2298.
51. Matsuo F, Bergen D, Faught E, et al. Placebo-controlled study of the efficacy and safety of lamotrigine in patients with partial seizures: U.S. Lamotrigine Protocol 0.5 Clinical Trial Group. *Neurology* 1993;43:2284–2291.
52. Privitera M, Fincham R, Penry J, et al. Topiramate placebo-controlled dose-ranging trial in refractory partial epilepsy using 600, 800-, and 1,000-mg daily dosages: Topiramate YE Study Group. *Neurology* 1996;46:1678–1683.
53. Barcs G, Walker EB, Elger CE, et al. Oxcarbazepine placebo-controlled, dose-ranging trial in refractory partial epilepsy. *Epilepsia* 2000;41:1597–1607.
54. Cereghino JJ, Biton V, Abou-Khalil B, et al. Levetiracetam for partial seizures: results of a double-blind, randomized clinical trial. *Neurology* 2000;55:236–242.

Antiepileptic Drugs, 5th Edition. Edited by R.H. Levy, R.H. Mattson, B.S. Meldrum, and E. Perucca. Lippincott Williams & Wilkins, Philadelphia © 2002.

GENERAL PRINCIPLES

CLINICAL DEVELOPMENT OF ANTIEPILEPTIC DRUGS: INDUSTRY PERSPECTIVE

ROGER J. PORTER

The major pharmaceutical companies of the world are involved in all aspects of drug development; these large companies are concerned with everything from the conceptual foundations of drug discovery to postmarketing development of additional indications. Antiepileptic drugs have benefited from the Antiepileptic Drug Development (ADD) Program, a program that has been especially effective early in the process, attempting to act as a catalyst to motivate the machinery of industry to "carry the ball" through some of the tricky and expensive stages of early development (1). All this is part of the altruistic effort to hasten the day when the drug will be available to the patients who need it to control their seizures. This chapter concentrates on those factors that typically are the burden of the pharmaceutical company in the development of a new molecule. We assume that the new molecule appears—at least at first—to be efficacious and safe in animals and that the company has chosen to invest its efforts and resources in this molecule; in reality, however, every molecule in the company's pipeline is continuously scrutinized to see if it comes close to its target profile.

THE DEPARTMENTS IN A PHARMACEUTICAL COMPANY

It might be thought that the major effort of a pharmaceutical company is simply to test a drug in humans to see if it is safe and effective. Indeed, this is the single most expensive part of drug development. But before and during the clinical testing, a critical array of other departments make other decisions about the drug. Some of these decisions are relatively routine, but some can decide whether the drug survives to reach the marketplace.

Typically, the departments that are involved with the drug (assuming it is a small molecule) are (a) Discovery, (b)

Roger J. Porter, MD: Vice President, Clinical Pharmacology, Clinical Research and Development, Wyeth-Ayerst Research; and Adjunct Professor of Neurology, University of Pennsylvania, Philadelphia, Pennsylvania

Pharmaceutical Sciences, (c) Drug Safety, (d) Drug Metabolism, (e) Regulatory Affairs, and (f) Clinical Research; in addition, certain departments coordinate projects, such as Project Management, or coordinate information flow, such as Information Management. The roles of only the first six are reviewed in this chapter. These departments have roles that not only are sequential, as listed here, but in most cases parallel to any ongoing clinical work.

Discovery

The Discovery Departments of most large pharmaceutical companies have become quite large because the need for a continuous flow of new compounds is required to maintain the growth rate of the company. In most large companies, the internal discovery efforts are supplemented by a continuous effort to in-license promising compounds and by active interactions or collaborations with academic laboratories and smaller firms (including biotech companies). Critical to the decision for in-licensing are factors such as patent protection, ability of the compound to "fit" into the portfolio of the big company, projected time of development, expected toxicities, timing of competition, and so forth.

Paramount to the decision process is whether the new compound—internal or external—will have an advantage over existing therapy. One of the most important ways that the Discovery Department addresses this issue is continuously to seek compounds with new mechanisms of action (i.e., novel mechanisms or novel targets, or both). An excellent example of an in-licensed compound with a novel mechanism is retigabine. When Wyeth-Ayerst Research first in-licensed the compound, there was good evidence that the drug activated potassium currents in neuronal cells; although we knew that this was a novel approach, we did not know which channels were specifically affected. Later work, in part by Discovery scientists at our partner Asta Medica in Germany, showed that retigabine is an M-channel agonist that is related to a hereditary epilepsy syndrome (2) and to a fundamental excitability current. This additional information may affect the eventual clinical program at later stages. In other words, retigabine was attractive as an in-license candidate in part because of this novel mechanism of action. Later work refined this mechanism and made the drug even more attractive as a potential antiepileptic drug.

One of the typical Discovery activities, when a compound involves receptors or channels, is to characterize the drug against many other potential targets—to analyze the drug's unique characteristics; this permits a full profile of that drug to evaluate potential therapeutic benefits or liabilities. Further, working with drug metabolism, the Discovery team characterizes the metabolites (if any) of the drug to ascertain the level of pharmacologic activity present in each. In addition, the Discovery team may test the drug for other indications to assess activity. Gabapentin is a good example of an antiepileptic drug that has pain as a major secondary indication. These are some of the examples of how the Discovery team "follows along" with the clinical development and assists with the overall progress toward final approval.

Chemical and Pharmaceutical Development

Although early synthesis of small quantities of the drug are performed in the Discovery laboratory, larger quantities soon are required, and Chemical Development is called on to make increasingly larger batches of increasingly pure material. To do this properly requires great knowledge of chemical synthesis and scale-up procedures, if for no other reason than to be efficient and safe in the procedure to be used. The demands for drug substance come from all sides of the organization: Discovery has more tests to run; Drug Safety has to begin work to see if the drug is safe; Drug Metabolism needs to work on the assay of blood and urine levels, and Clinical Research needs drug to mount clinical trials.

As noted previously, besides making the bulk drug (which eventually may be contracted to an outside vendor), Pharmaceutical Development is responsible for the delivery system of the drug to the patient. Unfortunately, this rarely is a simple process. The oral form may require bioavailability enhancement, or it may involve complex multiple drug combinations or delayed release. Pediatric formulations [which may be mandated by the U.S. Food and Drug Administration (FDA)] may necessitate taste masking, solutions, suspensions, sprinkles, or chewables. Parenteral formulations may be needed, although some drugs simply cannot be solubilized sufficiently for intravenous or intramuscular use. All of these efforts must be produced under strict quality control. The product must meet rigid criteria for stability at various temperatures and conditions. All this is to ensure that the eventual marketed product is of the highest possible quality.

Drug Safety

The Drug Safety Department is responsible for the preclinical safety testing and evaluation of the compound. The department provides information to the company about toxicologic risks and sets the stage for introduction into humans. Although animal testing is required, an increasing number of studies are accomplished without using live animals, and every effort is being made to limit such studies and the number of animals used to those that are absolutely necessary to support safe development in humans.

The sophistication and variety of the toxicity studies to be performed are quite remarkable. Typically, the studies begin with general acute, subchronic, and chronic effects of the drug in experimental animals. These may be combined with plasma levels to establish the relationship between the toxic effects and the exposure (3). During this time, a dose–response relationship may be sought if this appears to be clinically relevant, and end points for monitoring adverse effects in animals that also may be helpful in the clinic are determined. Specific areas of interest include carcinogenicity, reproductive and developmental toxicity, genotoxicity, cardiovascular toxicity, immunotoxicity, and neurotoxicity (3).

All of this process is aimed at a continuum of establishing the risk of carrying the compound further into development, even though some of the tests are not completed until just before the clinical program is finished.

Drug Metabolism

The Drug Metabolism Department is responsible for describing what happens to the drug in animals and humans—that is, how the various species modify and eliminate the drug. This includes the classic measurements of absorption, distribution, metabolism, and elimination (ADME). In addition, *in vitro* systems are used to predict the metabolic profile and identify the enzymatic systems that may be involved in metabolism. The department is responsible for creating a sensitive and validated assay for the drug and relevant (active) metabolites in biologic fluids, first for the ADME and animal toxicokinetic studies and later for the studies in humans.

The data derived from these animal studies are used to predict what will happen when the drug is administered to humans (i.e., data such as the degree of absorption, the plasma protein binding, the routes of metabolism, the potential for drug–drug interactions, and the mechanisms of elimination). Toxicokinetic studies combine various doses of the drug with blood sampling and permit scaling for predicting the appropriate starting dose for the first-in-human studies.

Regulatory Affairs

Although not an in-line function of drug development (i.e., this department does not actually handle the compound), Regulatory Affairs is very influential in the flow of the paperwork that creates worldwide approval and eventual marketing. Each company has its group of experts (sometimes combined with clinical research) that orchestrate the complex and numerous submissions to the health agencies in each country.

Clinical Research

After Discovery has chosen the best compound from its series, Chemical and Pharmaceutical Sciences has made and formulated enough pure compound, Drug Safety has done at least the early toxicologic studies, and Drug Metabolism has a sensitive assay in plasma, then Regulatory Affairs can submit a document (which usually contains at least one research protocol from Clinical Research) to the country health authorities to commence clinical investigation. How companies organize their clinical departments varies widely, but the simplest prototype is described here

The first few studies of the new drug typically are carried out by Clinical Pharmacology, a specialized team in each company. The first study usually is a single-dose study, often in human volunteers, with gradually increasing doses to test human tolerability to the compound. If a sufficient safety range of single doses is tolerated, the next study is the multiple-dose study, with gradually increasing doses to evaluate tolerability. Plasma levels are drawn with each dose, and a pharmacokinetic profile is available at the end of these studies. If all goes well in this so-called *phase I*, the drug may then be evaluated for efficacy and safety in patients by the appropriate team of clinical experts in the company, typically designated the Therapeutic Area (TA). Clinical Pharmacology continues

its work throughout development, with studies on the effect of food, age, and sex; it also carries out specialized studies such as dose proportionality, ^{14}C metabolism/disposition, distribution, bioequivalence, and drug interaction studies.

The TA in Clinical Research houses the specialists in the disease area to be studied. These physicians and clinical scientists supplement their own knowledge by making frequent contacts with experts outside the company—usually from academia. These contacts may be as simple as a phone call or as complex as a formal consultants' meeting.

The TA takes the information provided by Clinical Pharmacology and begins cautious studies in humans with the disorder in question. These early clinical efficacy and safety studies are often called *phase II* of development, and usually are designed to accomplish certain goals. First, the drug must continue to be safe in the patient population, just as it was in volunteers. Second, from these studies some estimate of efficacy needs to emerge: Does the drug really do what is intended within its nontoxic range? Third, the appropriate dose must be determined—how much, and how often to dose.

If the drug still looks promising at this stage, and only a tiny percentage of potential drugs screened for initial acting get this far (Figure 5.1), then broader trials, often involving thousands of patients, further test the effectiveness and safety of the drug; this stage is termed *phase III*. The TA is responsible for this very expensive process and for carrying the drug to registration and approval. Every other department noted

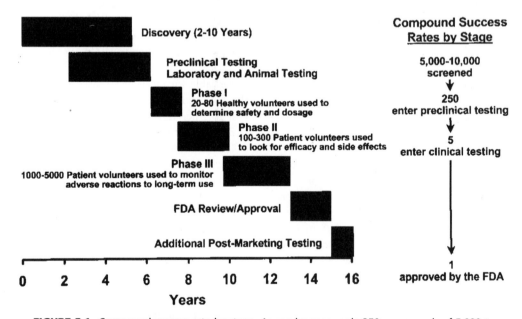

FIGURE 5.1. Compound success rate by stage. As can be seen, only 250 compounds of 5,000 to 10,000 screened enter preclinical testing, and only 5 of these enter the clinic. Only one of these five is approved for marketing. Although this figure emphasizes approval by the U.S. Food and Drug Administration, all large companies now emphasize worldwide registration, and most attempt, insofar as is possible, simultaneous approvals worldwide. (From Pharmaceutical Research and Manufacturers of America. *1999 Industry profile*. Washington, DC: Pharmaceutical Research and Manufacturers of America, 1999, with permission.)

previously remains active in the process right to the end, but the final clinical data in patients are of utmost importance.

CHALLENGES TO THE PHARMACEUTICAL INDUSTRY

Internal Challenges

Many of the internal challenges are inherent in the process of development as reviewed in the preceding section. But some may not be obvious at first glance. The following are some examples of potential challenges at each departmental level:

1. In Discovery, the desired molecule cannot be constructed without making it obviously toxic or obviously insoluble. The talent needed to overcome this problem lies in the medicinal chemists, and every company has an army of these invaluable employees, taking a hypothetical idea that is targeted to a disease and making it a potential reality as a drug.
2. In Pharmaceutical Sciences, the drug cannot be made bioavailable. In spite of the best efforts of talented scientists, some drugs simply cannot achieve a practical portal of entry into humans. Good examples are certain polypeptides, which are enzymatically broken down by the gastrointestinal tract; if practical, these can be given by other routes (e.g., intranasally). But in many cases there is no workable answer and the potential drug is shelved—often forever.
3. In Drug Safety, the drug causes liver enzyme increases in one of two mammalian species, but only at relatively high doses. Because two species usually are tested to ensure an adequate safety margin, a dilemma now is present. Should we move cautiously into humans or should we test yet a third species of nonhuman mammals? Or is the enzyme increase a burden that cannot be overcome?
4. In Drug Metabolism, the drug is found in one nonhuman species to form a potentially carcinogenic metabolite. Should the program be delayed to evaluate this metabolite further? Or do humans not make this metabolite, making the problem moot? Even the potential expense of ascertaining the truth can delay a good drug sufficiently to make it noncompetitive; it may be dropped from the portfolio because of more promising internal competition in other fields or because of the emergence of direct competitors from other companies.
5. In Regulatory Affairs, the Patent Office has determined that a competitor has patented a series of compounds with a similar structure to our drug. It is not clear that our expected patent is comprehensive. The strength of the issue may determine whether to go forward without hesitation or whether negotiation for a license from the competitor may be required. Again, delay in the progress of the drug may push it down the company's priorities—it may be lost or buried by other drugs without so much "baggage," as is the common vernacular in the industry.
6. In Clinical Research, the compound sails through early testing, but in the early efficacy studies of phase II, the effective dose is much higher than expected, and patients are highly variable in their response. Whether to press forward is determined by a host of factors, not the least of which is the expected competitive environment for the drug at time of launch. It may be better to wait for a "backup" compound (if one exists) and end pursuit of the current drug, in spite of the tens of millions of dollars invested thus far.

External Challenges

The external challenges to the pharmaceutical industry are well summarized in the March, 1999 document published by the Pharmaceutical Research and Manufacturers of America (4). Only a few of the relevant issues are included in this portion of the chapter.

Challenges in Research and Development

Only half a century ago, the concepts of sickness and health were quite different from those of today. Parents generally expected that some of their children would die in infancy, and in the pre-antibiotic era, it was more or less expected that some of those who made it through infancy would die of infections such as bacterial pneumonia. Death and disability were still relatively common occurrences at all ages. Expectations about health were tempered by discouraging statistics (5).

In the new millennium, primarily in developed countries, expectations are completely different:

The loss of a child is uniformly tragic and unexpected. Death in middle age is similarly distressing. The vast majority of us live a healthy life and expect to do so into old age, rather naively fearing only accidents in our youth, and cancer and vascular disease as we get older. We expect that children will be born healthy, that infections will disappear with antibiotic treatment, and that artificial hips, heart valves, and knees will replace our natural parts if needed (5).

These optimistic expectations are based on the reality of the health of the majority of people in economically developed countries. Profiting from improved sanitation, safe drinking water, antibiotics, life-style changes, pharmaceuticals—both vaccines and drugs (Figure 5.2)—and many other factors, everyone expects to enjoy life to an old age (5).

These expectations put pressure on all aspects of the health care delivery system. People who are "robbed" of their full lifetime are quick to identify a nonnatural cause for the personal loss and to seek redress, often within the legal system. For the pharmaceutical companies, the pressure is to identify drugs that not only are effective for the disorders under treatment but extraordinarily safe. To accomplish this task, companies are spending record amounts of money on research (Figure 5.3)—outspending, in the past few years, even the National Institutes of Health. The absolute amount

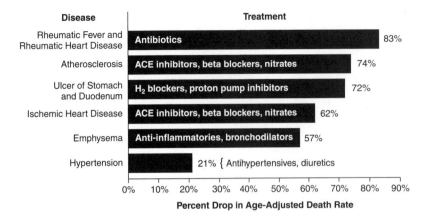

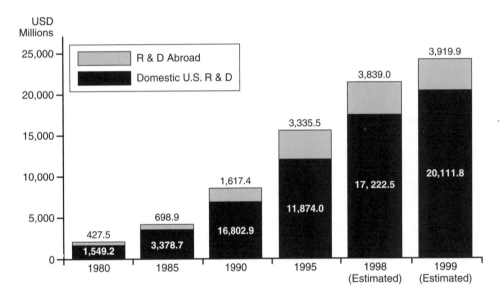

FIGURE 5.2. Some of the impacts of pharmaceutical agents on death rates in the United States. Vaccines have caused an even more impressive decline. (From Pharmaceutical Research and Manufacturers of America. *1999 Industry profile.* Washington, DC: Pharmaceutical Research and Manufacturers of America, 1999, with permission.)

FIGURE 5.3. The expenditures for research and development (R&D) by research-based pharmaceutical companies, including both U.S. and foreign company spending in the United States, and U.S. company spending abroad. (From Pharmaceutical Research and Manufacturers of America. *1999 Industry profile.* Washington, DC: Pharmaceutical Research and Manufacturers of America, 1999, with permission.)

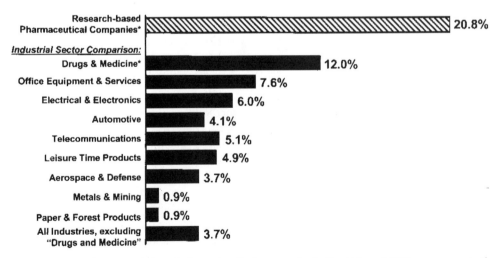

FIGURE 5.4. The research-based pharmaceutical companies in the U.S. and R&D as a percent of sales. About 80% of this R&D is devoted to new products; the other 20% is spent on improvements of existing products. (From Pharmaceutical Research and Manufacturers of America. *1999 Industry profile.* Washington, DC: Pharmaceutical Research and Manufacturers of America, 1999, with permission.)

Share of Prescription Units

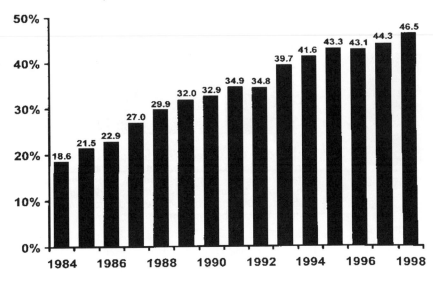

FIGURE 5.5. Generic drugs have dramatically increased their share of the market in the past few years. Although some large research and development (R&D)–oriented pharmaceutical companies operate generic subsidiaries, the generic business is primarily driven by volume and cost of goods. Virtually no R&D is sustained by this portion of the market. (From Pharmaceutical Research and Manufacturers of America. *1999 Industry profile.* Washington, DC: Pharmaceutical Research and Manufacturers of America, 1999, with permission.)

of research investment also is remarkable from the standpoint of research and development as a percentage of sales (Figure 5.4), with other industries averaging only 3.7%; by comparison, research-based pharmaceutical companies average over 20%. Considering the steady incursions of generic drugs in the marketplace (Figure 5.5)—generic companies perform virtually no research—the pressure is on big companies to maintain a flow of patented drugs in the marketplace to maintain the research momentum.

Challenges in Regulatory Aspects of Development

Not all of the challenges of developing a new drug are scientific. Many difficulties arise as a result of the regulation of the industry by various governmental bodies. The effect on drug development is, at first glance, more subtle than the scientific questions of safety and efficacy; the impact can be powerful and often is viewed negatively by the company.

Before discussing the regulatory aspects of drug development, it is important to recognize the remarkable contributions of governmental regulatory agencies—primarily the FDA in the United States—to the science of drug development, especially in the design of clinical studies. Before the thalidomide disaster in 1963, a drug merely needed to be proven safe to obtain a place in the market. Since then (in the United States), a drug must be proven *safe and effective.* The insistence of the FDA on *controlled* clinical studies (usually randomized and often blinded) has greatly advanced the science of clinical trials. The result has been a heightened standard for drug approval. This standard has not been achieved, however, without additional costs.

The cost is measured in both time and money. As the sophistication of the process increases, more time is required to take a molecule from discovery to the drug store. As can be seen in Figure 5.6, the time of development has greatly lengthened since the 1960s. Regulatory approval was an early culprit, but more recently, the need for larger

Development Time (Years)

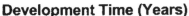

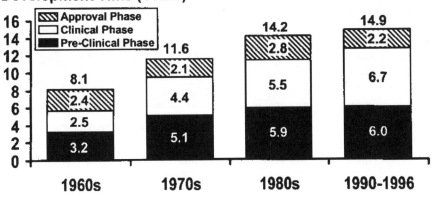

FIGURE 5.6. The time of development of a drug has almost doubled since the 1960s. The length of approval phase has actually decreased in recent years (in large part because of "user fees"), but the clinical and preclinical phases continue to lengthen. (From Pharmaceutical Research and Manufacturers of America. *1999 Industry profile.* Washington, DC: Pharmaceutical Research and Manufacturers of America, 1999, with permission.)

Number of Trials

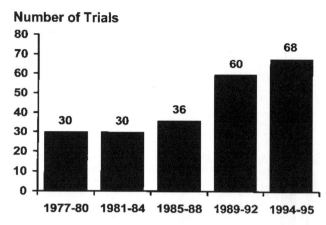

FIGURE 5.7. The increase in clinical trials per drug application, from 1977 to 1995. (From Pharmaceutical Research and Manufacturers of America. *1999 Industry profile*. Washington, DC: Pharmaceutical Research and Manufacturers of America, 1999, with permission.)

and more extensive clinical trials has caused the process to lengthen. This extension of time-to-market is costly not only because of the added studies conducted, but because it steals from the product's patent life.

Are more clinical trials actually being performed? As can be seen in Figure 5.7, the average number of clinical trials in each drug application has dramatically increased; this is mostly a response based on the *expectations* of the regulatory agencies. Whether this expectation is warranted is a matter of considerable debate. In any case, the most expensive aspect of drug development, the clinical trials process, has expanded greatly. This is further documented by the concomitant increase in the number of patients provided in each dossier (Figure 5.8).

Even the largest pharmaceutical companies have finite resources. When the cost of development of a drug increases, this means that fewer drugs can be pursued. Fur-

Share of GDP (%)

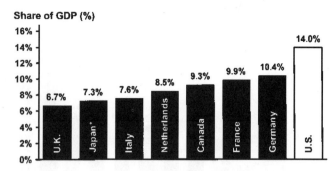

FIGURE 5.9. The United States outspends other developed countries on health care not only in absolute terms, but as a percentage of gross domestic product. (From Pharmaceutical Research and Manufacturers of America. *1999 Industry profile*. Washington, DC: Pharmaceutical Research and Manufacturers of America, 1999, with permission.)

ther, each individual drug, when it reaches the drug store, must now be more expensive—not only to cover the costs of its own development, but to fund future research.

Challenges in the Global Environment

The United States is not reluctant to invest in health care. Relative to other comparable countries, the United States devotes enormous resources, as shown in Figure 5.9. This is not to say that most of the costs are from drugs; clearly this is not the case, as is shown in Figure 5.10. The average person in the United States, as a matter of fact, spends on prescription drugs (Figure 5.11) somewhat less than on alcohol, but somewhat more than on tobacco!

The key to long-term success in pharmaceutical development lies in the ability of the companies to continue to be innovative to compete successfully in what has become an intensely competitive environment.

> The United States is, fortunately, in a position to benefit from this new international competition. We currently have the most highly developed biomedical research enterprise, many

Number of Patients

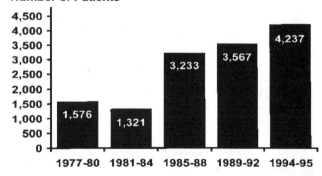

FIGURE 5.8. As expected from the increase in the number of clinical trials (Figure 5.7), the number of patients studied for each drug application has dramatically increased. (From Pharmaceutical Research and Manufacturers of America. *1999 Industry profile*. Washington, DC: Pharmaceutical Research and Manufacturers of America, 1999, with permission.)

Share of GDP (%)

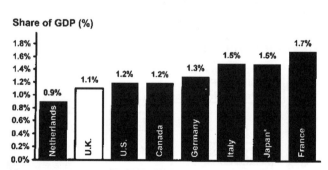

FIGURE 5.10. The United States is only average in the share of gross domestic product devoted to pharmaceuticals, compared with other developed countries. (From Pharmaceutical Research and Manufacturers of America. *1999 Industry profile*. Washington, DC: Pharmaceutical Research and Manufacturers of America, 1999, with permission.)

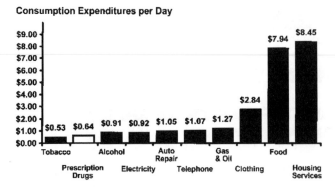

Consumption Expenditures per Day

FIGURE 5.11. Prescription drugs are relatively low on the scale of spending priorities in the United States. (From Pharmaceutical Research and Manufacturers of America. *1999 Industry profile.* Washington, DC: Pharmaceutical Research and Manufacturers of America, 1999, with permission.)

technological advantages, and a healthy biomedical industry. The opportunity is enormous if we can maintain an open trading system, free movement of capital and technology, and protection of intellectual property rights (5).

Further, "we must adopt policies that will help avoid the double-whammy of both paying for highly expensive health care and paying those costs in the form of profits to foreign companies" (5).

We are in the midst of one of the most exciting times in human history. The pace of development of new, more effective, drugs have never been faster. Whether the issue is approached from the viewpoint of the United States or a more global view is taken, one can only hope that the resources now devoted to finding new drugs—to combat both old and new diseases—will continue unabated.

REFERENCES

1. Stables JP, Kupferberg HJ. The NIH anticonvulsant drug development (ADD) program: preclinical anticonvulsant screening project. In: Avazini G, Regesta G, Tanganelli P, et al., eds. *Molecular and cellular targets for antiepileptic drugs.* London: John Libby, 1997.
2. Rundfeldt C, Netzer R. The novel anticonvulsant retigabine activates M-currents in Chinese hamster ovary-cells transfected with human KCNQ2/3 subunits. *Neurosci Lett* 2000;282:73–76.
3. Furst A, Fan AM. Principles and highlights of toxicology. In: Fan AM, Chang LW, eds. *Toxicology and risk assessment: principles, methods and applications.* New York: Marcel Dekker, 1996.
4. Pharmaceutical Research and Manufacturers of America. *1999 Industry profile.* Washington, DC: Pharmaceutical Research and Manufacturers of America, 1999.
5. Vaughn CC, Smith BRL, Porter RJ. The contributions of biomedical science and technology to U.S. economic competitiveness. In: Porter RJ, Malone TE, eds. *Biomedical research: collaboration and conflict of interest.* Baltimore: Johns Hopkins University Press, 1992.

Antiepileptic Drugs, 5th Edition. Edited by R.H. Levy, R.H. Mattson, B.S. Meldrum, and E. Perucca. Lippincott Williams & Wilkins, Philadelphia © 2002.

GENERAL PRINCIPLES

THE DEVELOPMENT OF ANTIEPILEPTIC DRUGS: REGULATORY PERSPECTIVE

RUSSELL KATZ*

REGULATORY BACKGROUND

In the United States, the legal bases for the use in people of drugs not approved for marketing (investigational drugs) and the standards for drug approval for marketing are contained in The Federal Food, Drug, and Cosmetic Act (the Act), a statute passed by Congress in 1938 and amended in 1962 and several times thereafter. To enact the provisions of the Act, the U.S. Food and Drug Administration (FDA), the governmental agency charged with regulating human research with investigational drugs and making decisions about drug approvability, has the authority to promulgate regulations that describe the various requirements of drug development and approval. These regulations, although not enacted by duly elected representatives (Congress), are the product of a detailed process of public notification and rule making, and have the force of law. Although the Act and regulations (and various documents written by the FDA and other organizations that provide nonbinding guidance to drug sponsors) together describe in detail all aspects of drug development and approval, this chapter focuses primarily on issues related to the requirements for assessing the effectiveness of proposed drug products, with particular emphasis on issues related to the demonstration of effectiveness for antiepileptic drugs (AEDs). A discussion of the many other issues involved in drug development in general can be found elsewhere (1).

The *sine qua non* for drug approval in the United States is a demonstration that the proposed drug product is effective; regardless of how safe a treatment may be, if it is not effective, it may not be approved. The standard applied by the FDA in determining effectiveness is defined in the Act as "substantial evidence" of effectiveness for the conditions described in approved product labeling. The Act defines substantial evidence as:

> ...evidence consisting of adequate and well-controlled investigations, including clinical investigations, by experts qualified by scientific training and experience to evaluate the effectiveness of the drug involved, on the basis of which it could be fairly and responsibly concluded by such experts that the drug will have the effect it purports or is represented to have under the conditions of use prescribed, recommended, or suggested in the labeling or proposed labeling thereof.

It is critical to recognize that the approval of a product is inherently linked to the labeling approved with it. That is, the labeling must accurately reflect what is known about the drug at the time of approval, and must include, among other things, a description of the patient population in whom the drug is considered to be effective, a description of the symptoms/signs benefited by the treatment, and a description of the effective dose(s) and of the risks associated with its use.

It also is critical to recognize that traditionally, the plural *investigations* has been interpreted to mean at least two such trials, thereby incorporating the well accepted scientific principle of independent replication or corroboration of experimental findings before they can be generally accepted. Typically, the FDA is expected to take an initial action on a new drug application within 10 months of its submission; for drugs that represent an advance over existing therapies, the initial action is supposed to occur within 6 months of the submission of the application.

In 1997, the Act was amended to include a new definition of substantial evidence, which permitted the FDA to make a finding of substantial evidence on the basis of a single adequate and well controlled clinical investigation and "confirmatory evidence." The relevant language in the amended Act is as follows:

> If the Secretary determines, based on relevant science, that data from one adequate and well-controlled clinical investigation and confirmatory evidence (obtained prior to or after such investigation) are sufficient to establish effectiveness, the Secretary may consider such data and evidence to constitute substantial evidence... .

Russell Katz, MD: Division of Neuropharmacological Drug Products Center for Drug Evaluation and Research, United States Food and Drug Administration, Washington, DC

*Dr. Katz is with the U.S. Food and Drug Administration (FDA). The views expressed in this chapter are his own and do not reflect an official statement from the FDA.

Although Congress gave no indication when this new standard should be used, or what it considered "confirmatory evidence," the FDA has produced a document that gives guidance on both of these points (2). In general, the FDA may rely on a single study to establish substantial evidence of effectiveness when that trial has demonstrated an important effect on mortality or irreversible morbidity or prevention of a disease with a potentially serious outcome, and where independent confirmation of the result would be difficult or impossible, for ethical or practical reasons. It is understood, therefore, that this new standard applies only in unusual circumstances; typically, drug approval still requires that substantial evidence consist of at least two, independent clinical trials demonstrating that the drug has the effect claimed for it in labeling.

Although the Act itself does not further describe the specific attributes of clinical investigations that the FDA may rely on as sources of evidence of effectiveness, these are described in detail in the regulations found at Title 21 of the Code of Federal Regulations, section 314.126 (21 CFR 314.126, "Adequate and well-controlled studies"). This section describes five specific trial designs (trials may incorporate aspects of several of these designs):

1. Placebo concurrent control. In this design, some patients are treated with investigational drug, whereas others are treated with placebo; treatment assignment invariably is random, and usually both patients and investigators are unaware of the treatment assignments (double-blind).
2. Dose-comparison concurrent control. In this design, patients are assigned to receive one of several doses of investigational drug; as in the placebo concurrent control, this design usually is random and double-blind.
3. No treatment concurrent control. In this design, some patients receive the investigational drug, whereas others receive no treatment; as in the other designs, treatment usually is randomly assigned.
4. Active treatment concurrent control. In this design, some patients are assigned (again, usually randomly) to the investigational drug, whereas others are assigned to treatment with a standard drug.
5. Historical control. In this design, all patients are treated with the investigational drug, and their responses are compared with "experience historically derived from the adequately documented natural history of the disease... ."

Although there are clinical circumstances in which each of these study designs is appropriate, because the natural history of most seizures in most patients with epilepsy is highly variable and unpredictable, well controlled studies of putative AEDs always must include a concurrent control, usually placebo or an "ersatz" placebo (see later).

The 1997 amended Act also introduced several additional provisions that have the potential to affect the development and approval of new treatments for epilepsy.

The Act, under its so-called Fast Track provisions, now provides for the approval of treatments for serious or life-threatening illnesses that demonstrate the "potential to address unmet medical needs" on the basis of substantial evidence of effectiveness on a surrogate marker that is reasonably likely to predict the clinical benefit of interest. Although this provision was first introduced into the Act in 1997, a similar provision has existed in the regulations since 1992. In those regulations, referred to as the Accelerated Approval regulations, the FDA for the first time codified its position that treatments for serious or life-threatening illnesses that provided meaningful benefits over existing treatments could be approved on the basis of an effect on a surrogate end point that "is reasonably likely, based on epidemiologic, therapeutic, pathophysiologic, or other evidence, to predict clinical benefit...."

A *validated* surrogate marker is a laboratory test or other measure that is not immediately linked to the patient's clinical symptoms or signs, but that is correlated with the patient's condition and its response to the applied treatment predicts the patient's clinical response on an appropriate outcome. For example, blood pressure is a validated surrogate marker for stroke, heart attack, and other serious outcomes because, in general, a hypertensive patient's blood pressure does not, in the short term, correlate with clinical symptoms (outside the far extremes of blood pressure, the patient is asymptomatic), but drug-induced decreases in elevated blood pressure have been shown to correlate with and predict decreasing rates of the long-term outcomes listed previously. An antihypertensive treatment therefore can be approved on the basis of its effect on blood pressure, not patient symptoms, because this effect has been shown to confer a clinical benefit in the future.

The law now, however, permits approval on the basis of a drug's effect on an unvalidated surrogate marker, one that can reasonably be *expected* (but not yet demonstrated) to predict the clinical outcome of interest (again, the regulations have permitted such approval since 1992). This new provision does require that an attempt be made to validate this surrogate after the drug is approved; if the surrogate is shown not to predict the clinical benefit of interest, it may be withdrawn from the market under expedited procedures.

The advantage of relying on an effect on a surrogate outcome as a basis for drug approval is that if the drug's desired effect is on a clinical outcome likely to occur far in the future after treatment initiation, the trials may be done in a reasonable length of time. In the example of the antihypertensive given previously, the clinical events of interest are expected to occur many years after treatment initiation. The reliance on a drug's effect on blood pressure to support approval permits the studies to be practically done. However, there are many potential pitfalls in relying on a drug's effect on an unvalidated surrogate marker as the basis for drug approval (3). Most critically, the fact that the drug has the desired effect on the surrogate may not mean that the drug will have the desired effect on the clinical outcome; indeed, the drug may have the expected effect on the surrogate, but an unexpected, deleterious effect on the clinical outcome of interest. Nonetheless, there are situations in which reliance on an unvalidated surrogate marker may be acceptable. To date, no AED has been approved on the basis of its effect on a surrogate marker; it is expected that an AED should produce a detectable beneficial effect on the clinical measure of interest (e.g., seizures) before it may be approved. Such effects are demonstrable in studies of reasonable duration, and therefore there is no need to rely on an indirect (surrogate) measure. However, there may be circumstances in which an effect on a surrogate marker may play an important part in the approval of AEDs in the future (see later).

The amended Act also offers an incentive to pharmaceutical sponsors to undertake studies in the pediatric population (defined as patients 16 years of age and younger), a segment of the population traditionally not included in studies performed to gain drug approval. Under this provision, sponsors can gain 6 months of additional marketing exclusivity for a drug (assuming that there is still a period of exclusivity attached to the product) if they perform studies in pediatric patients as requested by the FDA. This program is voluntary, but the prospect of 6 months of additional marketing has prompted many sponsors to conduct adequate studies in pediatric patients with seizures that presumably otherwise would not have been conducted.

However, because this provision is voluntary, and because the FDA had determined that studies in pediatric patients were vital for many drug products known to be used off-label in these patients, shortly after this amendment was instituted in 1997, the FDA adopted, in December 1998, regulations *requiring* that sponsors perform adequate trials in pediatric patients for those indications for which the drug is being developed in adults (21 CFR 314.55). Although the rule technically applies to all drugs, including drugs already approved, it has been applied primarily to drugs under development or for which new drug applications have been submitted since the rule went into effect in April 1999. Sponsors may submit an application with adult data only, but they must commit to performing the appropriate studies in pediatric patients for the same indications for which the drug is approved in adults in a specific time frame after initial approval; various penalties may be imposed if the studies are not completed in the appropriate time. Pediatric studies are required when gaining the appropriate claim in that population will provide a meaningful clinical benefit (defined as a significant improvement in the treatment, diagnosis, or prevention of a disease compared with other treatments approved for that indication in the relevant pediatric population, and the drug is in a drug class or indication for which there is a need for additional therapeutic options), or there would be substantial pediatric use for the indication and the absence of adequate pediatric labeling would pose a health risk. This requirement for pediatric studies may be waived if the treatment does not meet the criteria for meaningful benefit *and* substantial use, the sponsor demonstrates that the studies would be impossible or impractical to perform, the use would be unsafe in pediatric patients, or reasonable efforts to produce an appropriate dosage form (if necessary) have failed. Taken together, the 1997 provisions of the Act and the pediatric rule have had a profound effect on the number of adequate studies performed in pediatric patients, and in particular in pediatric patients with epilepsy.

EPILEPSY-SPECIFIC ISSUES

Until the early 1990s, the last new chemical entity approved in the United States for the treatment of epilepsy was valproic acid, approved in 1978 for the treatment of absence seizures and multiple seizure types that include absence seizures. In 1993, however, two new chemical entities were approved, felbamate and gabapentin, followed in 1994 by lamotrigine. Including these three, as of this writing, nine new chemical entities have been approved for the treatment of various seizure types, as well as various new dosage forms and routes of administration for several older AEDs (e.g., controlled-release forms of carbamazepine, injectable forms of valproic acid, rectally administered diazepam). In addition, many of the newer drugs initially approved for a specific indication (most new AEDs are initially approved for the treatment of partial seizures), as well as some of the older drugs, have subsequently been approved for additional seizure types and populations (e.g., primary generalized seizures, Lennox-Gastaut syndrome).

Starting with the newly approved drugs in the early 1990s, several issues have been considered important in the approval process.

Labeling

As noted earlier, the approval of a drug product in the United States is inextricably linked to the product labeling. Specifically, the labeling must accurately describe the population for whom the drug is useful as well as the effect seen for the drug in the trials that supported approval. Of course, in addition, the label must accurately reflect the known toxicities of the drug. Because of the requirement that the labeling accurately reflect the effects of the drug and the population in whom it has shown to be effective, the labeled indications for newly approved AEDs reflect a number of the specific conditions under which the drugs are studied. Specifically, drugs are approved as treatments for the specific seizure types found to be benefited by the treatment, for the specific population studied (adults, or, if studied in the pediatric population, the earliest age shown to be benefited is given), and the conditions of study (adjunctive therapy or monotherapy). Typically, AEDs are studied first in adults with partial seizures whose epilepsy is not adequately controlled and who already are being treated with several other AEDs. For this reason, a typical indication in product labeling for a newly approved AEDs might state that the drug is indicated as adjunctive therapy in adults with partial seizures.

This approach to labeling a newly approved AED is based on several considerations. First, when the new drug applications for the first three newly approved AEDs were presented to the FDA's Peripheral and Central Nervous Systems Drugs Advisory Committee (a group of non-FDA experts in various areas of neurology impaneled by the FDA and to whom the FDA presents selected issues and from whom the FDA solicits nonbinding advice), the Committee recommended this approach. Although the FDA was, and is, not obliged to take the Committee's advice, it was thought prudent to do so in this case. First, the FDA agreed that studying a drug solely under conditions in which the drug is given against a background of other AEDs could not support a conclusion that the drug would be effective when given alone. Although it may be generally considered that any AED that works when given in conjunction with other AEDs must be effective when given alone, there is little to no evidence from adequate controlled trials that establishes this for most AEDs. Even if one were to conclude (without evidence) that this must be true, the effective dose when the drug is given as monotherapy would not be known; this could be reliably known only if it was studied in an adequate trial. Even if a therapeutic plasma range were known for the drug under adjunctive conditions (although this is *not* known for any of the recently approved AEDs), establishing a dose of the drug that results in these plasma levels when the drug is given as monotherapy (e.g., from a pharmacokinetic study) still would not be adequate to establish that this plasma range confers seizure control when the drug is given alone. For these reasons, drugs studied only under adjunctive conditions are specifically and explicitly indicated as adjunctive treatment.

Similarly, drugs studied only in adults are not indicated as being effective in pediatric patients. The FDA has not been willing to extrapolate findings from adults to pediatric patients. At the moment, if a drug sponsor wishes to obtain approval for an indication in pediatric patients, they must perform an adequate study in the relevant subsegments of the pediatric population or submit other evidence that would convince the FDA that the drug's effect in adults implies that it also is effective in pediatric patients. Such an approach would need to establish that the disease (in this case, a particular seizure type) is the same in both populations, that the two populations are known to respond the same way to the applied treatment, and that there exists sufficient pharmacokinetic information in the relevant pediatric groups to support dosing recommendations. Although it may appear logical to assume, for example, that partial seizures in the adult are "the same" as partial seizures in pediatric patients, it is not immediately obvious that the pathophysiologic events leading to a partial seizure in the developed brain are identical to those causing a partial

seizure in the developing brain, even though the two events may appear phenomenologically similar. Further, given our lack of knowledge about (a) these pathophysiologic events, and (b) the complete mechanism of action of any AED, it is not obvious, in the absence of controlled trial data, how one could reasonably conclude that a drug will work the same way in the two populations. Finally, even if one were to conclude that these first two points could be assumed, one could not know what an effective dose would be in the pediatric patients without data from a controlled trial in pediatric patients. For these reasons, the FDA requires studies in pediatric patients to support a claim in this group.

Finally, the effects of a drug on a given seizure type are not ordinarily considered evidence of effectiveness for other seizure types. As with the aforementioned case with pediatric patients, given our lack of complete understanding about the biologic events underlying the cause of any specific seizure type and occurrence and our lack of detailed understanding of the mechanism of action of any of the available AEDs, one could not be certain of the effects of a drug on a seizure type not studied based on its effects on a different seizure type. Typically, therefore, for a sponsor to gain approval for a drug for a specific seizure type, the drug's effect on that seizure type must be documented in at least one adequate clinical trial. Specifically, if a drug is approved initially to treat, for example, partial seizures (on the basis of at least two clinical trials), it may be approved for another seizure type (e.g., primary generalized seizures) on the basis of a single additional, well controlled trial. This requirement for only a single trial in the latter seizure type is based on the view that adequate evidence already established the drug's effect as an AED; the FDA ordinarily considers this prior demonstration as "lending strength" to the finding from the single trial in the new seizure type, and concludes that substantial evidence of effectiveness has been presented for the new indication. There may, however, be instances in which the new seizure type is considered so fundamentally different from the previously approved seizure type that two trials may be required for approval of the former indication.

Clinical Trial Issues

Although theoretically any of the previously described study designs could be used to demonstrate an effect of a proposed AED, in practice only a relatively few are considered capable of yielding the valid evidence on which to base a finding of substantial evidence.

The overarching principle applied by the FDA in interpreting clinical trials with AEDs to date has been the principle that a (statistically significant) difference between the proposed treatment and the control treatment (which need not be placebo) must be demonstrated for the trial to be unambiguously interpretable. Such an outcome, in which a difference is seen between the proposed and control treatments, is the only outcome that can be interpreted without reliance on data external to the trial itself, making it the most powerful and reliable sort of evidence of effectiveness.

That this is so can be seen from an examination of the results of a trial in which no difference is seen between a proposed AED and an active control drug. This outcome is subject to two interpretive problems, only one of which can be potentially addressed without resort to information outside of the trial itself.

The problem with this outcome that is potentially addressable is that the new drug may, in fact, be worse than the old drug, but the study was not adequately powered (did not have enough patients) to detect this difference. This problem might be able to be addressed if sufficient numbers of patients were enrolled.

The more fundamental interpretive problem with such an outcome is that to support the conclusion that the new drug is effective, one must assume that the old (control) drug was effective, *in this specific trial* (4,5). Although this may seem to be a reasonable assumption if the old drug is approved, and therefore known to be effective, for the seizure type under study, it is not always true that drugs known to be effective are effective at all times in all patients, and, specifically, it is not known if it was effective in the particular trial performed. There are many examples of cases in which drugs known to be effective have been shown not to be distinguished from a placebo in a given clinical trial (4).

As noted, then, for an active controlled trial that does not demonstrate a difference between the treatment groups to be interpreted as demonstrating the effectiveness of the new drug, it must be concluded that the old drug was effective in that particular trial. However, as we have just seen, that may not always be true. The only way in which the effectiveness of the old (active control) drug in a particular trial can reasonably be assumed to be true is if it can be known with great certainty that the patients assigned to the active control would not have responded as they did had they been assigned to placebo. This, in turn, can be known reliably only if the natural history of the untreated condition is known with great precision, or if there is a robust database in which the active control has been shown repeatedly to be superior to placebo by a given amount (this is why active controlled trials that do not detect a difference between treatments often are referred to as a subset of historical controlled trials, the weakest source of evidence). Unfortunately, for most types of seizures, and for most, if not all, AEDs used as active controls, both types of information (natural history and response rates) are unavailable. Because this information is not available, active controlled trials of AEDs that do not demonstrate a difference between treatments are not interpretable, and are not relied on by the FDA as being capable of providing evidence of effectiveness.

On the other hand, an active controlled trial in which the new treatment is seen to be superior to the active control is easily interpreted as supporting effectiveness, assuming that the active control did not make the control patients worse than they would have been without treatment. Although

this assumption also may be untestable in a given trial, in most cases such an assumption is reasonable because it is quite rare that a drug known to be effective will make a separate cohort of patients worse than they would have been had they not been treated; the point is that it usually is unknown if an effective treatment *will be* effective at all times in all patient samples, or it is known that not infrequently many effective drugs are not effective in a given patient sample in a controlled trial. It is critical to point out, however, that such an outcome (in which patients assigned to the new drug perform better than those assigned to the old drug) ordinarily cannot support the conclusion that the new drug is superior to the old drug. For such a conclusion to be reached, one would need to be sure that the new drug was compared with the most effective dose of the old drug. Such a trial ordinarily would compare several doses of the new drug with the full range of available doses of the old drug, to ensure that the comparison was "fair"; such trials are difficult to do, and have rarely been done successfully.

Given, then, that a difference between treatments is necessary for a study to be accepted as contributing to a finding of substantial evidence of effectiveness, a number of clinical trial designs are considered acceptable by the FDA.

The most common study performed is the so-called placebo add-on design. In this study, patients on one to three concomitant AEDs are randomized to receive new drug or placebo added on to their current AED regimen. Such studies usually maintain patients on a dose of the experimental treatment thought to be therapeutic, or placebo, for 3 months, and the frequency of seizures is compared between the two groups. Again, this design is not capable of determining the superiority of the new drug to the concomitant AEDs being taken by the patients; it simply is capable of supporting the conclusion that the new drug, when added on to other AEDs, is superior to placebo added on to other AEDs; this is sufficient to establish that the drug has an antiseizure effect (when given as adjunctive therapy), and, if replicated, can support a finding of substantial evidence of effectiveness. In this study design, it is critical to ensure that the plasma levels of the concomitant AEDs are not systematically elevated in the drug-treated group compared with those in the placebo group (as might happen secondary to a pharmacokinetic interaction). If the plasma levels were significantly elevated, any effect seen might be due to the higher levels of the concomitant AEDs, and not to any intrinsic activity of the new drug.

Many other designs have contributed to a finding of substantial evidence of effectiveness, depending on the clinical condition under study. All are useful if, as noted, they can detect a favorable difference between the patients assigned to the investigational drug and those assigned to the control treatment.

A number of designs have been used to determine the effectiveness of an AED when used as monotherapy. Monotherapy studies pose a number of unique problems, mainly because some authors consider it unethical to treat patients with seizures with placebo alone (6). In some cases, however, patients have been randomized to receive different fixed doses of the experimental drug, with the goal of showing superiority of the high dose to the low dose. Such a study can be considered ethically acceptable if there is uncertainty about which dose (if any) of the drug is effective. For example, intravenous lorazepam was studied in patients with status epilepticus; in this study, patients were randomized to receive one of two doses. In this trial, the high dose was superior to the low dose, permitting a conclusion that the drug (at the high dose) was effective. Similarly, patients have been randomized to investigational drug or low-dose active control as monotherapy, and in these studies a finding of superiority of the investigational drug has supported a conclusion that the investigational drug is effective (but again, it does not support the conclusion that the investigational drug is superior to the active control). Some authors believe that this design is unethical because patients are randomized to a dose of the active control that is known not to be optimum, and that therefore the control patients are not being adequately treated; others feel that the design is ethical because they believe that the low dose of the active control is sufficient to prevent any serious seizure event (e.g., status), and it may, in any event, be effective (although such an outcome probably would make the study uninterpretable; see earlier).

A monotherapy design in which patients are treated with placebo alone has been used in patients with severe refractory epilepsy who are being evaluated for surgical treatment. In these patients, an attempt is made to remove all AEDs to evaluate further their potential for surgery. Given that these patients are having all of their medications removed for a period as part of their presurgical evaluation, investigators have randomized these patients to drug or placebo for brief periods (usually no more than 10 days) and assessed their response. Although this design is capable of detecting an antiseizure effect of some drugs (a therapeutic dose of drugs used in this paradigm must be able to be achieved quite rapidly), the study period is so brief that the FDA does not currently consider such a study as providing substantial evidence of effectiveness in monotherapy.

A placebo control–only design also has served as the basis for a finding of effectiveness in patients with a history of only a few seizures or in patients newly diagnosed with epilepsy. These patients would be expected to have few seizures, and would not be expected to suffer serious harm if not treated with active drug for a defined period. In addition, studies in patients not well controlled on several AEDs in which patients are randomly assigned to monotherapy with an investigational drug or placebo (or low-dose AED as a control) have been performed. In these studies, the usual primary measure of effectiveness is the time to meeting various exit criteria (several measures of increasing seizure activity). Some

find this design acceptable because it has the advantage of being interpretable, while protecting the patients' safety because they are withdrawn from the study when their seizures become worse (i.e., they meet exit criteria).

Another proposed monotherapy design involves treating patients with an investigational drug in open-label, uncontrolled conditions for a given duration (may be many months), and then randomly assigning them to continue on drug or placebo (randomized withdrawal design). This design has the additional advantage of permitting an assessment of long-term seizure control; if the drug is superior to placebo in the randomized phase, this implies that it had been effective during the open-label, uncontrolled, prerandomization phase.

However, as noted earlier, there is increasing concern among many (although certainly not all) investigators that the treatment of patients with seizures with placebo alone is unethical, and it is becoming increasingly difficult for sponsors to perform adequately designed monotherapy studies. The design of ethically acceptable but scientifically sound and interpretable monotherapy studies represents one of the great challenges for the future.

Finally, many investigators have expressed interest in developing trial designs that are capable of determining whether a proposed treatment can prevent or cure epilepsy. There are many unanswered questions about what features should be incorporated into such studies, including the population to be studied, the duration of such a study, and the appropriate outcome measures (e.g., it may be necessary for a sponsor to show not only that patients have no seizures, but that their electroencephalogram normalizes), including perhaps surrogate markers (e.g., imaging, structural, or functional). Although these are difficult questions, drugs developed to prevent or cure epilepsy, and the designs that would adequately demonstrate these effects, present perhaps the greatest and most exciting challenges for the future of the treatment of the patient with seizures.

REFERENCES

1. Katz R. The introduction of new drugs. In: Gennaro AR, ed. *Remington: the science and practice of pharmacy.* Easton, PA: Mack, 1995.
2. U.S. Department of Health and Human Services. *Guidance for industry: providing clinical evidence of effectiveness for human drug and biological products.* Washington, DC: U.S. Department of Health and Human Services, 1998.
3. Fleming TR, DeMets DL. Surrogate end points in clinical trials: are we being misled? *Ann Intern Med* 1996;125:605–613.
4. Temple RJ, Ellenberg SS. Placebo-controlled trials and active-control trials in the evaluation of new treatments. *Ann Intern Med* 2000;133:455–463.
5. Leber P. Hazards of inference: the active control investigation. *Epilepsia* 1989;30[Suppl 1]: S57–S63.
6. Chadwick D, Privitera M. Placebo-controlled studies in neurology: where do they stop? *Neurology* 1999;52:682–685.

GENERAL PRINCIPLES

ANTIEPILEPTIC DRUG MONOTHERAPY IN ADULTS: SELECTION AND USE IN NEW-ONSET EPILEPSY

RICHARD H. MATTSON

The new onset of epileptic seizures usually leads to initiation of antiepileptic drug (AED) treatment to prevent recurrence. Although this chapter is directed at treatment of adults, a number of basic principles involved in this process are common to all patients. These principles include how to select, how to initiate, and how to maintain AED treatment.

Before beginning treatment, it is necessary to decide whether to treat at all or withhold therapy. After a single (first) seizure, there is uncertainty that any further seizures will occur. The probabilities vary with many factors and range from 20% to 70% (1). Ultimately, the patient, family, and physician need to balance the relative risk to that individual of another seizure against the potential for harm occurring as a consequence of AED treatment. Finally, if treatment has been associated with a remission of seizures, a decision must be made as to when and if it is advisable to discontinue treatment and, if so, how it should be done. The issues are very similar to those surrounding initiation of therapy and depend on the risks and benefits of a recurrent seizure compared with the adverse effects of AED therapy.

If more than two unprovoked seizures have occurred, the probabilities of recurrence exceed 70% (2), and most often treatment is recommended. The selection of an initial AED from among the more than a dozen widely available requires a careful review of all the properties of the various drugs and the individual needs of the patient. After selection has been made, the treatment, start-up, and maintenance must be planned and implemented.

SEIZURE TYPE AND EPILEPSY SYNDROME

When first seen, the patient with adult-onset epilepsy presents with a history of some type of seizure (3). This is most commonly of tonic-clonic type with or without partial seizures or, less frequently, absence and myoclonic seizures. After evaluation is complete, a diagnosis of an epilepsy type or syndrome is made whenever possible (4). Localization-related (partial) epilepsy is the most common type and is of symptomatic or cryptogenic etiology. Less often, generalized idiopathic epilepsy appears in adult life. When possible, treatment is based on epilepsy syndrome because seizure types in a particular syndrome are likely to respond to the same AED. For example, valproate (VPA) is effective for tonic-clonic, absence, and myoclonic seizures often occurring in juvenile myoclonic epilepsy, whereas carbamazepine (CBZ) is especially effective for partial and tonic-clonic seizures characteristic of localization-related epilepsy. However, the epilepsy syndrome frequently is not identifiable, particularly at onset, so clinical trials often do not clearly distinguish the type. In addition, efficacy trials use seizure control as a primary outcome. For this reason, the focus of AED selection often emphasizes seizure rather than epilepsy type.

SELECTION CRITERIA

Selection of a drug for epilepsy treatment depends on multiple characteristics (Table 7.1).

A drug, of course, must be effective in preventing recurrent seizures. Total control is the usual goal, but may not be possible with monotherapy or even combined drug treatment. Efficacy may be limited to a specific seizure type for some compounds, whereas others have a broad spectrum of activity. The degree of efficacy or potency is important, but

Richard H. Mattson, MD: Professor of Neurology and Director of Medical Studies, Department of Neurology, Yale University School of Medicine and Veterans Administration, West Haven, Connecticut

TABLE 7.1. SELECTION CRITERIA

- Efficacy
- Safety
- Tolerability
- Pharmacokinetic properties
- Formulations
- Expense

some patients have easily controlled tonic-clonic seizures and the most potent drug may not be necessary, especially if the drug with greatest potency has poorer tolerability (5–7). For patients not fully controlled, measures such as reduction in number or rate of attacks or change in severity of seizures are important outcomes (8–10).

Adverse effects usually are divided into those of tolerability and safety. The latter is of particular importance. Serious medical hazard usually leads to avoidance or discontinuation of AEDs. Occasionally, a drug with a risk of systemic side effects of potentially life-threatening type may be justifiable for severe refractory epilepsy. Thus, a place exists for the use of felbamate (FLB) in selected patients (11).

Although safety is of greatest concern, tolerability is a more common problem in AED use. Some drugs, such as the barbiturates, produce sedation or some cognitive difficulty at high dose that compromises the quality of life. Virtually all AEDs can produce unwanted, annoying, and sometimes almost incapacitating side effects. These usually are correctable by reduction of dose, but this may then allow recurrence of seizures.

Pharmacokinetic properties include absorption, distribution to different body parts, biotransformation, and elimination. These determine how much and how often an AED must be given to maintain the most desirable pharmacodynamic effects. Hepatic metabolism is a major mode of clearance of all the older and a number of the newer AEDs. Many drugs share the same biotransforming enzyme

systems, resulting in frequent interactions that can make management more complex.

Formulations of some drugs have rapid absorption, with peak blood levels often producing transient side effects. This can be avoided by using more delayed- or extended-release formulations. At times, sprinkle, rectal, or parenteral formulations are needed or desirable, and are not available for all products.

Finally, expense is an issue. Some of the population have insurance or other sources of economic support for the cost of AEDs, but this is not true for many individuals. Although national health plans provide medication in some countries, in others the cost of the newer AEDs runs approximately three or more times that of the older, established compounds. In the United States, for example, cost for each of the new AEDs may range from $3,000 to $6,000 per year, compared with $100 to $1,500 for older AEDs.

LIFE-TABLE ANALYSIS

The relative advantages of each AED are based on the criteria described previously. A single outcome measure that allows comparison is the life-table analysis. The length of time a patient continues on drug is an indication of acceptable efficacy, safety, and tolerability. A large, blinded, randomized trial has been conducted comparing CBZ, phenobarbital (PB), phenytoin (PHT), or primidone (PRM) monotherapy in treatment of partial epilepsy in adults (12). Life-table analysis of patients with partial and tonic-clonic seizures revealed an outcome significantly less successful for PRM The primary reason was poor tolerability during initiation of therapy. For patients with partial seizures, CBZ and PHT were significantly more successful than either PB or PRM, in this case owing to differences in efficacy and tolerability (Figure 7.1). Later trials comparing CBZ and

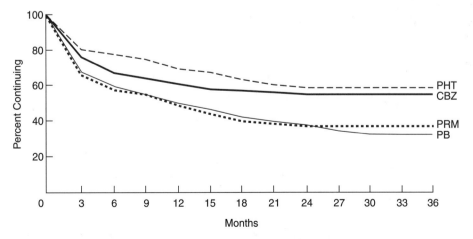

FIGURE 7.1. Partial seizure group remaining in study. Carbamazepine (CBZ) and phenytoin (PHT) were more successful than phenobarbital (PB) or primidone (PRM).

VPA failed to detect a difference in retention for tonic-clonic, partial, or all seizures combined (13–15).

The first active-control monotherapy trial of the new AEDs showed that FLB was more successful than low-dose VPA (16). Brodie and colleagues (17) compared CBZ with lamotrigine (LTG) as monotherapy in patients with new-onset epilepsy and overall found fewer withdrawals from the study in patients on LTG because of better tolerability (Figure 7.2). Steiner and coinvestigators (18) found equal retention in a similar trial comparing LTG and PHT. More recently, three independent clinical monotherapy trials in patients with partial epilepsy compared oxcarbazepine (OXC) with CBZ, PHT, or VPA, and in each case equal or superior retention was achieved with OXC (19–21). No efficacy differences were found in these trials, but OXC was better tolerated. In a somewhat more unusual design, topiramate (TPM) was compared in patients selected for treatment with CBZ or VPA according to the decision by the physician as to the optimal drug for therapy. Then the patient was randomized to high- versus low-dose TPM (200 or 100 mg) or continued on the original AED. Retention was not significantly different between CBZ, VPA, and either dose of TPM (22). In another large, double-blind study, patients with new-onset epilepsy were randomized to gabapentin (GBP) or LTG, and no differences in retention were found between the two drugs (23). Two studies indicate outcome for vigabatrin (VGB) therapy is comparable with CBZ in terms of retention (24,25). VGB showed better tolerability but less efficacy against seizures. Another

trial showed two doses of GBP (900 and 1,200 mg/day) were more successful than a low dose (300 mg/day) and produced results equivalent to those obtained in an unblinded comparison group treated with 600 mg CBZ (26).

It is evident that most studies of new AEDs have involved CBZ, although some have compared a study drug or drugs with PHT or VPA, and in these trials no significant differences have been detected. Only one trial has compared success between two or more of the new AEDs (23). LTG has shown somewhat better retention than CBZ in an elderly population of patients with new-onset epilepsy (27). The other new AEDs, levetiracetam (LEV), tiagabine (TGB), and zonisamide (ZNS), have not been sufficiently tested in randomized monotherapy studies of new-onset adult epilepsy to evaluate outcome. However, add-on trials have clearly demonstrated efficacy for each drug.

In summary, comparatively few differences are found in overall retention among either new or older AEDs in comparative trials using life-table analyses. Overall, 60% to 80% of patients with new-onset epilepsy remain on the drug to which they were randomized. Success is less if an intent-to-treat analysis is used and includes patients leaving the study for apparent non–study-related reasons. Outcome is somewhat better in studies including generalized epilepsy, in contrast to those limiting intake to partial epilepsy (12–15). The close similarity in success for the AEDs using life-table analyses makes it necessary to turn to alternative criteria for making treatment selection.

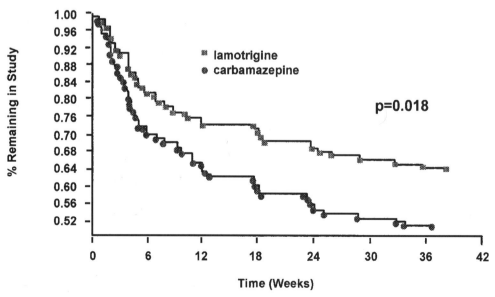

FIGURE 7.2. Continuation on carbamazepine (CBZ) or lamotrigine (LTG) monotherapy after double-blind randomization in adults with new-onset epilepsy. (From Brodie MJ, Richens A, Yeun AW. Double-blind comparison of lamotrigine and carbamazepine in newly diagnosed epilepsy. *Lancet* 1995;345:476–479, with permission.)

EFFICACY

Comparisons of efficacy are difficult because different outcome measures are used in clinical trials and results are not always comparable (10) (Table 7.2). For initial treatment, the most important goal is complete seizure control for a period of time (e.g., 6, 12, 24 months). Another frequently used measure is time to first (or *n*th) seizure. Time and percentage of patients entering remission provide similar information expressed in a different way. Because complete control is not possible for many patients, other measures of efficacy have been used. The number of seizures that occur in a test period can be compared between a study drug and another, or with placebo. Often this number is compared with a lead-in baseline test period. The reduction (or increase) in seizures is a measure of efficacy of the treatment. When the observation period is not the same for all subjects, the seizure number per period of time (week, month) can be used. The change in seizures commonly is expressed as a reduction relative to a baseline number. Outcome most often is expressed as the percentage of patients achieving a 50% or greater reduction. This outcome measure is used most often for studies involving patients with difficult-to-control epilepsy rather than new or early-onset disease, in which case total control often is achieved. Seizure severity may change even for a specific seizure type. For example, a tonic-clonic seizure may be less severe if unaccompanied by tongue biting, incontinence, or postictal confusion, or preceded by a lengthy aura. Several instruments have been developed to express the severity in numeric terms (8,9).

Compounding the problem of assessing efficacy of AEDs is the limitation of many studies in defining the inclusion and analysis of specific seizure types (3) or the epilepsy classification (4).

Tonic-Clonic Seizures

Evidence based on prospective, randomized trials suggests little, if any, difference in efficacy for treatment of tonic-clonic seizures. Most studies indicate tonic-clonic seizures are more fully controlled than those of partial type (5–7,12–14). Although modest differences are found in different studies, most standard and older AEDs successfully control approximately 60% of patients for a year of follow-up from the beginning of what should be adequate dosing. Because some patients enter remission after one or more seizures while on therapy, approximately 70% to 80% will come under control (14,15).

Some studies (28–32) suggest a higher percentage of patients with tonic-clonic seizures associated with idiopathic generalized epilepsy syndromes can be well controlled than those with secondarily generalized tonic-clonic seizures associated with localization-related epilepsy. Prospective, blinded large trials have not been conducted to address this issue. Retrospective analysis of the study of PHT compared to VPA revealed those patients with probable idiopathic generalized epilepsy had better control with VPA therapy (31). Because accurate diagnosis often is difficult, many trials do not restrict entry to a single epilepsy type (12,13,15,20,21).

In most studies, the trial design does not possess enough power to test for differences between drugs for tonic-clonic seizures. The problem arises in part from the fact that these seizures occur relatively infrequently compared with partial seizures. Consequently, a long duration of study is required to detect outcomes. In addition, tonic-clonic seizures are successfully controlled in a high percentage of cases, so detection of a significant difference becomes more difficult. Despite these limitations, all the older standard AEDs except ethosuximide (ESM) appear to be effective. Based on consensus evidence and nonrandomized trials, VPA is thought to be somewhat more effective than CBZ, PB, or PHT (33).

Partial Seizures

All the available AEDs except ESM are believed to be effective for partial seizures, although less so than for tonic-clonic seizures. The older multicenter studies (12–15) reveal better control of tonic-clonic than partial seizures over time. Some studies suggest that in more difficult control problems, CBZ and perhaps PHT are slightly more effective than the barbiturates or VPA. In the first Department of Veterans Affairs Cooperative (VA COOP) Study (12), CBZ provided better complete control of partial seizures than the barbiturates (PB and PRM). In the second VA COOP study (13), CBZ was more effective than VPA using time to first seizure (Figure 7.3), seizure score or seizure rate, but no difference was found for complete control for 1 year of treatment. Other investigators have not found a difference in efficacy between these two drugs. The apparent difference in efficacy may be explained by several factors. The VA patient population represented a more difficult-to-control group because only approximately half had never been previously treated. The numbers of subjects in the VA trial were very large, allowing detection of small differences. Finally, outcome measures were different in the various studies.

TABLE 7.2. EFFICACY END POINTS

- Complete seizure control
- Time to first (*n*th) seizure
- Number (%) entering remission
- Seizure number (rate)
- Seizure severity score
- Surrogate markers (electroencephalogram)

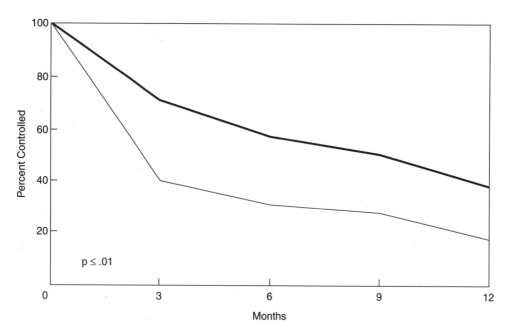

FIGURE 7.3. Time to first seizure, carbamazepine (CBZ) (top line) versus valproate (VPA), Department of Veterans Affairs Cooperative Study #264. (From Mattson RH, Cramer JA, Collins JF, et al. A comparison of valproate with carbamazepine for the treatment of complex partial seizures and secondarily generalized tonic/clonic seizures in adults. *N Engl J Med* 1992;327:765–771, with permission.) Difference *p* < .05.

Mixed Partial and Tonic-Clonic Seizures

Patients with partial (localization-related) epilepsies often experience both partial as well as generalized seizures, so it is appropriate to combine all groups together in assessing the outcome of treatment. The results parallel the findings for specific seizure types, with success being intermediate between patients with only partial or only tonic-clonic seizures because tonic-clonic seizures are more easily controlled than those of partial type. In the VA COOP Studies, approximately 40% to 50% could be completely controlled after treatment with one of the standard older AEDs (5,10,11). The study of Heller et al. also noted better control of tonic clonic than partial seizures (14).

Absence Seizures

Although absence seizures almost always have their onset before adult life, occasionally they are not recognized or are misdiagnosed earlier. Many early open studies established efficacy initially with use of trimethadione and other diones, and later with ESM and related analogs (34). VPA was found to have comparable efficacy with ESM in controlled trials (35). VPA also caused a dramatic decrease in the surrogate end point of spike–wave discharges on the electroencephalogram (36). Increasing evidence has indicated that LTG (37–40) is effective as both add-on therapy and monotherapy. TPM, ZNS, and perhaps LEV also may be effective (41,42). Controlled, comparative trials have not established the relative efficacy of these newer AEDs.

For treatment of absence seizures, only ESM and VPA possess known long-term efficacy. Benzodiazepines are very useful acutely, but tolerance develops over time. Absence seizures have been worsened or unmasked especially with the use of CBZ (43,44), but PHT also has been found to have an adverse effect at times. Recent reports indicate that AEDs that increase brain γ-aminobutyric acid (GABA; i.e., GBP, TGB and VGB) also may have an aggravating effect (44).

Myoclonic Seizures

No controlled trials have been done to compare the relative efficacy of the available AEDs in treatment of myoclonic seizures, but extensive experience has shown VPA to be highly effective (45–50). The benzodiazepines, including clonazepam, diazepam, and nitrazepam, are all effective and used especially for resistant seizures. Tolerance commonly develops after some months, limiting their value. Increasing evidence indicates TPM and ZNS are effective as well. LTG has been reported both to help and to aggravate myoclonic seizures (38,51,52)

Tonic and Atonic Seizures

Tonic or atonic seizures do not commonly arise in adulthood and usually are found in patients with refractory, extratemporal partial epilepsy in adults or in secondary generalized epilepsies with onset in childhood. Most AEDs have some effect in lessening severity. Empirical trial often is needed to find the most helpful drug. This is a condition that may well justify the use of FLB (9,53).

ADVERSE EFFECTS

Safety

Safety problems are infrequent, but may occur with use of all the AEDs, with the possible exception of GBP. Idiosyncratic hypersensitivity reactions with rash are seen in 5% to 10% after start-up, and usually occur within the first 6 months of therapy (12–15.). Rarely, these proceed to more serious toxicity, including Stevens-Johnson syndrome, epidermal toxic necrolysis, hepatitis, or aplastic anemia. Only VPA among the older drugs does not cause these hypersensitivity reactions. Among the new AEDs, LTG has been associated most frequently with idiosyncratic hypersensitivity reactions that sometimes have progressed to Stevens-Johnson syndrome or toxic epidermal necrolysis syndrome. Slow titration of the dose, especially when coadministered with VPA, minimizes the risk (54). In monotherapy trials, using a gradual increase in dosage, the frequency of rash was comparable with that with CBZ (17,23,27). OXC and ZNS also have been found to cause rash on occasion, but GBP, LEV, TGB, and TPM have an incidence comparable with placebo in clinical trials, a considerable safety advantage for these drugs.

Although CBZ was associated with aplastic anemia early after its introduction, this problem has proven to be very rare. On the other hand, CBZ commonly is associated with clinically unimportant leukopenia (12), hyponatremia, and, rarely, cardiac arrhythmias (13,55,56). All the older AEDs have been associated with rare idiosyncratic hepatitis, vasculitis, and multiorgan failure. These immunologically mediated problems are not seen with VPA use, but rare metabolic hepatic failure, pancreatitis, and thrombocytopenia all have been reported. PHT also can cause neuropathy and cerebellar degeneration.

All the older AEDs have been associated with some degree of decreased bone calcium and pathologic fractures. Although thought to be due in part to enzyme induction, the same changes are associated with use of VPA, a nonenzyme inducer (57).

The barbiturates also can produce chronic connective tissue disorders such as Dupuytren's contracture (58).

FLB has caused clinically significant aplastic anemia and hepatic failure, markedly limiting use of the drug (11). VGB can cause retinal damage and concentric visual field loss (59). Although it is available in most developed countries except the United States, future use of VGB likely will be reserved for those whose poorly controlled seizures justify the risk.

Tolerability

All AEDs can produce somnolence and mental slowing if dosage is too high or increased too rapidly. LTG and FLB

TABLE 7.3 ADVERSE EVENTS (% PATIENTS)

Week	CBZ	PB	PHT	PRM
Dizziness				
1	11	3	10	13
12	3	2	3	0
GI				
1	12	2	9	18
12	5	2	3	4

Veterans Administration cooperative study. (From Steiner TJ, Dellaportas CI, Findley LJ, et al. lamotrigine monotherapy in newly diagnosed untreated epilepsy: a double-blind, randomized comparison with phenytoin. *Epilepsia* 1999;40:601–607, with permission.) N= 240.

are least likely to have this effect in long-term use. CBZ most often produces visual disturbance or dizziness; PHT, ataxia and mental slowing or sedation; PB, sedation and affective/behavioral/cognitive change; and VPA, tremor and, at times, sedation. PRM causes dizziness and somnolence. All these older AEDs, including ESM, can cause gastrointestinal side effects, especially at start-up. PB is least likely of the older drugs to cause dizziness or gastrointestinal complaints (12,60) (Table 7.3).

Many of the new AEDs show superior tolerability in terms of central nervous system complaints (61–66). LTG, GBP, OXC, and VGB were better tolerated than CBZ in comparative testing (17,19,24,26,27). FLB, TPM, and ZNS sometimes are associated with gastrointestinal symptoms and, not infrequently, weight loss. This may be considered either a negative or positive effect, depending on the individual. TPM and, to some degree, TGB and ZNS appear to produce sedation and cognitive difficulties if given too rapidly. In addition to these complaints, FLB and, occasionally, LTG have been associated with headache and insomnia.

A major problem with many AEDs is an unwanted effect on cognition, mood, or behavior. Among the older AEDs, neuropsychological testing has consistently revealed deficits associated with use of PB (67,68). No consistent differences have been found among the other AEDs when comparable doses have been given (67). In VA COOP Study #264, a behavioral toxicity battery showed no differences from baseline to a retest after 6 months of treatment with CBZ or VPA, and no differences were found between the two drugs. The only AED effect detected was a failure to find a practice effect that was observed in a control group (69).

PHARMACOKINETICS

All of the older drugs are cleared at least partly by hepatic metabolism followed by renal elimination of inactive metabolites. As a consequence, drug interactions are complex and can result in changes in blood levels. PHT, PB, and PRM induce clearance of CBZ and VPA, whereas many drugs inhibit metabolism of CBZ and cause levels to rise, leading to side effects. Except for VPA, these AEDs may induce the clearance of other drugs, such as warfarin sodium, cyclosporine, and oral contraceptives, leading to less-than-expected effectiveness of the drugs and potential serious clinical outcomes. Knowledge and anticipation of these problems can obviate them, but for the occasional or new prescriber of AEDs, the subtleties of patient care with the older AEDs can make management difficult and, at times, dangerous.

The rate of clearance affects frequency of dosing. Most of the older drugs can be administered in twice-daily divided doses when used as monotherapy. CBZ and VPA may have shorter half-lives and if control requires high doses, variation between peak and trough levels can lead to insufficient control or transient excess dose side effects. To maintain reasonably constant blood/brain levels, three or four times daily regimens may be required; these often lead to decreased compliance and suboptimal clinical effect (70).

Most of the new AEDs have pharmacokinetic properties that make management easier (71). GBP, LEV, and VGB are renally eliminated. Although LTG, TPM, and ZNS undergo conjugation in the liver and their clearance can be increased or decreased by other drugs, they are not enzyme inducers and do not effect clearance of other compounds, with the exception of some lowering of sex hormone levels by TPM. OXC and TGB are primarily metabolized by the liver, but have minimal effects on the metabolism of other drugs, again with the exception of some decrease in sex hormone levels associated with OXC use. Both are, to some extent, inducible by drugs such as PHT and PB. Protein binding is not clinically significant for any of the new AEDs except TGB. The half-life of many of the new AEDs is sufficiently long to allow twice-daily dosing, with the exception of GBP, TGB, and VGB. Although these AEDs have half-lives of approximately 6 hours, they have a mechanism of GABA action that may cause a prolonged effect beyond what might be expected from blood level concentrations (72). GBP also has limited absorption because of saturable active L-amino transport. To achieve maximal levels for each dose, divided administration is advised.

FORMULATIONS

Most patients are able to take the AEDs orally, in pill or capsule form. However, some cause gastrointestinal irritation and some individuals, especially children or the mentally handicapped, will not or cannot take the pills. At times, chewable, liquid, or sprinkle formulations are desirable. For drugs with a short half-life or rapid absorption causing blood level peaks and poor tolerability, a delayed-release product can allow prolonged absorption, leading to more constant concentrations, improving efficacy as well as tolerability. When oral intake is not possible, a parenteral formulation allows administration of the drug if rapid clinical effect is required.

CBZ is available in regular tablets, chewable tablets [Tegretol 100 mg (Novartis, Summit, NJ)], and slow-release [Tegretol-XR, Retard, or Carbatrol (Athena Neurosciences, South San Francisco, CA)], but no parenteral formulation. After autoinduction and especially if coadministered with enzyme-inducing drugs like PB or PHT, peak-and-trough effects may occur unless multiple daily doses are administered. In these cases, the slow-release formulations are particularly useful clinically.

The other older standard AEDs (PB, PHT, VPA) have an extensive variety of formulations compared with the newer AEDs. PB has a slow clearance, so the amount given daily is only approximately 10% of total body stores. The rate of absorption is not important because peak effects are minimal. It is available in tablets as well as an elixir for oral administration. It also is available in a liquid in propylene glycol solution or as the sodium salt soluble in water. Both are suitable for parenteral administration. PHT is available as a tablet, a suspension, a delayed preparation (Dilantin; Pfizer, NY), and parenteral formulations. PHT is highly insoluble and is dissolved in propylene glycol at a pH of 11. The solution is highly irritating to tissue and must be given carefully and slowly by vein. A water-soluble prodrug, fosphenytoin (Cerebyx; Pfizer, NY), can safely be given intravenously (i.v.) or by intramuscular injection. VPA is available as a syrup, sprinkles, capsules, and delayed-absorption or extended-release tablets. A water-soluble parenteral formulation [Depacon (Abbott Laboratories, Abbott Park, IL), Epilim; Sanofi, NY] is very well tolerated when given i.v. at rapid rates.

The new AEDs have a limited number of formulations, although LTG and TPM are available as chewable tablets and sprinkles. No parenteral formulations have yet been marketed for these products, although many are water soluble and should not pose major difficulties for the development of parenteral formulations. The monohydroxy metabolite of OXC (MHD), has the potential for parenteral administration.

SPECIFIC OLDER ANTIEPILEPTIC DRUG PROFILES

Most of these older AEDs (Table 7.4) have been available for 40 years or more, in contrast to the newer AEDs, which have been extensively used for less than a decade. As a consequence, much more information has accumulated about optimal selection and use of these older drugs. These were reviewed in detail in the last edition of this book (73). We have a better awareness of their adverse effects, especially those that do not become evident until after long-term use. Examples include recognition of neuropathy with use of PHT, connective tissue disorders with use of the barbiturates, and teratogenesis with almost all the older AEDs. Even new AEDs may have such adverse effects not recognized in

TABLE 7.4. CONSIDERATIONS IN SELECTING OLDER STANDARD ANTIEPILEPTIC DRUGS

Drug	Advantages	Disadvantages	Comment
Carbamazepine	Very effective for partial and tonic-clonic seizures Minimal long-term sedative, cognitive, behavioral adverse effects	More frequent transient side effects during initiation of treatment; rash; complex pharmacokinetics; no parenteral formulation Leukopenia, hyponatremia	A drug of first choice for partial epilepsies
Ethosuximide	Very effective for treatment of absence seizures	Effective only for absence seizures Frequent gastrointestinal side effects	A drug of first choice for treatment of absence seizures
Phenobarbital	Very effective for tonic-clonic and effective for partial seizures Available from multiple routes of administration Inexpensive	Adverse sedative, cognitive, effective, behavioral effects; rash; chronic connective tissue effects; complex pharmacokinetics	No longer drug of first choice, but effective, relatively safe and very inexpensive
Phenytoin	Very effective for partial and tonic-clonic seizures Parenteral formulation available	Cosmetic side effects; pharmacokinetics are complex; rash; chronic neuropathy, cerebellar ataxia Saturation kinetics	A drug of first choice for partial epilepsies potent enzyme inducer; excellent for rapid initiation of treatment
Primidone	Very effective for tonic-clonic seizures; effective for partial seizures	Side effects common during initiation of therapy; other adverse effects same as phenobarbital	Not a drug of first choice, but when used alone is effective and minimally toxic; metabolized to phenobarbital
Valproate	Broad-spectrum efficacy for all seizure types; Intravenous formulation available	Weight gain; teratogenicity, tremor, alopecia; rare pancreatitis, hepatitis, bleeding disorder	First choice for idiopathic epilepsy; an alternative drug of first choice for partial epilepsy; excellent for rapid parenteral therapy

early use. VGB has proven to cause retinal dysfunction, but this was not recognized for a decade and a half despite special scrutiny of visual function in these patients (57).

Carbamazepine

CBZ was developed by Geigy Ltd. in the 1950s along with a number of related tricyclic compounds and first reported to be of use in both epilepsy and trigeminal neuralgia in the 1960s (56). Its use especially in the localization-related (partial) epilepsies with tonic-clonic and partial seizures has grown steadily over the years, to the point where it is widely regarded as one of, if not the drug of choice for these epilepsy types (33).

CBZ has been studied extensively for efficacy in a variety of designs, and no other AED has ever been known to possess greater efficacy. Some studies have found CBZ to have greater efficacy in treatment of partial (and sometimes tonic-clonic) seizures than the barbiturates, GBP, VPA, and VGB (10,11,22–24). No efficacy differences have been found between CBZ and PHT despite many comparative trials. In any given patient, however, one may prove more effective than the other. The efficacy of CBZ compared with LTG or TPM has not been defined because the trials were not designed with sufficient numbers of patients with partial seizures to detect differences that might be clinically significant. In contrast to efficacy for partial and secondarily generalized seizures, considerable observational reports

indicate CBZ does not help and may worsen or unmask absence and myoclonic seizures (43,44,51).

CBZ causes safety problems similar to those with other older AEDs. The most common problem is a hypersensitivity rash that occurs in approximately 10% of patients. The onset usually occurs within the first days or weeks of initiation of treatment. The rash may be mild and subside spontaneously or with lowering or temporarily discontinuing the drug. Rarely, this progresses to Stevens-Johnson syndrome or toxic epidermal necrolysis with multisystem involvement and serious morbidity as well as death. A more widely perceived risk of toxicity is the occurrence of agranulocytosis or aplastic anemia. This complication is quite rare and is estimated to occur only in 1 person in 100,000 or 200,000 people exposed to the drug. On the other hand, leukopenia of mild degree is a common accompaniment but of no clinical significance (except as a source of anxiety for the treating physician). Hyponatremia, usually of modest degree, also may occur. This rarely is of clinical importance unless some other factor leads to sodium loss such as use of some diuretics, low-sodium diet, or hemodilution from excessive solute-free fluid administration. Infrequently, cardiac arrhythmias have been reported during use of CBZ (13,57). Some gastrointestinal distress may occur at drug initiation but is not usually a persistent or significant safety problem.

Central nervous system adverse effects are dose and blood level related. In addition, they are especially prominent during initiation before tolerance and autoinduction have developed. Dizziness, blurred vision, and diplopia are most frequent, although as levels increase sedation can be a complaint. The problems may occur intermittently during peak concentrations of drug, but can be minimized by use of more frequent dosing of smaller quantities or use of slow-release formulations. Cognitive effects are minimal in most individuals, including both volunteer subjects and patients. In contrast to some AEDs that may aggravate depression, CBZ often is used in treatment of mood disorders. In long-term use, CBZ usually is free of adverse effects at doses that produce control in most patients.

The pharmacokinetic properties of CBZ are somewhat complex. Metabolized to an active metabolite, the 10,11-epoxide, CBZ is primarily oxidized by the hepatic cytochrome P450 (CYP) 3a isoenzyme system and undergoes autoinduction. As a consequence, blood concentrations decrease over days or weeks at a constant dose. CBZ can induce the metabolism and increase the clearance of a number of drugs as well as sex hormones, decreasing the amount available for efficacy. The metabolism of CBZ also is inducible by PHT and the barbiturates in particular. The resulting increased clearance my decrease the half-life to as short as 6 hours, necessitating frequent dosing to avoid wide swings in blood/brain concentrations and consequent loss in efficacy or excess effects. When used as monotherapy, the half-life of CBZ is closer to 9 to 12 hours, which often allows twice-daily or at most three-times–daily dosing. Inhibition by other medications can cause clearance to slow, levels to rise, and adverse effects to appear. Commonly used medications such as the macrolide antibiotics are just one example (56). CBZ is available in a variety of oral formulations, including slow-release capsules, but owing to marked insolubility is not available for parenteral use. CBZ is among the least expensive AEDs.

In summary, after almost four decades of use, CBZ has become the gold standard for treatment of partial and secondarily generalized tonic-clonic seizures on the basis of unexcelled efficacy, long-term safety, and modest cost. With more experience, some newer AEDs may become preferable because of better tolerability, safety, and pharmacokinetic properties.

Ethosuximide

ESM is an older standard AED with limited use in adults. It was introduced in the 1950s for the treatment of absence and similar seizures. It was safer than and largely replaced the diones, which had more adverse effects. No efficacy was found for treatment of tonic-clonic or partial seizures, limiting its use to add-on or joint therapy unless the patient had only childhood absence epilepsy. It has remained a drug of choice for this syndrome (34). When VPA became widely available in the 1970s and demonstrated efficacy for broad-spectrum seizure control as well as equal efficacy in treatment of absence seizures, the indication for ESM use

declined. However, it was found that some patients who did not respond to either AED had a better response to the combination. Some patients who had absence in addition to tonic-clonic seizures but had intolerable or toxic adverse effects from VPA could be treated with ESM and another AED in combination. ESM is available only in oral formulation and is not a primary drug choice for absence status epilepticus. A variety of adverse effects have been reported with use of ESM. Because the drug often has been combined with other drugs such as PB or PHT, it sometimes is difficult clearly to define the effect of ESM alone. Safety issues include the rare reports of Stevens-Johnson syndrome, aplastic anemia, and hepatic and renal failure. However, consistent reports suggest the most common problems associated with use of ESM are nausea, abdominal pain, and, at times, weight loss.

In summary, ESM has a small but valuable role as a first-line AED for absence seizures. It is very rare for these to appear in new-onset adult epilepsy in the absence of other seizure types, in which case VPA or even LTG or TPM are more likely choices.

Phenobarbital

PB, the oldest AED in general use, remains the most widely administered AED in the world. Introduced into use by Hauptman in 1912, PB was one of a group of barbiturates synthesized and studied by Bayer, the German chemical/pharmaceutical company, in the 1800s. Although used initially as a sedative, its dramatic effectiveness in epilepsy treatment became evident. Widespread use occurred only gradually, in part as a consequence of issues such as World War I.

Although current seizure terminology was not used in early reports, efficacy for treatment for partial and tonic-clonic seizures seemed well established. In one of the only "placebo"-controlled monotherapy trials in epilepsy, Sommerfeld-Ziskin and Ziskin (74) followed epilepsy patients after randomization to PB or placebo (diet) and found a marked decrease of seizures in the PB group after a year or more of follow-up. More recently, controlled studies of PB compared with other AEDs fail to reveal significant differences in efficacy except for the VA COOP Study #118, which indicated CBZ was somewhat more effective in preventing partial seizures (12). PB is not considered helpful in treating absence seizures, although animal models would have predicted broad-spectrum efficacy. PB has compared less favorably than most AEDs because of the occurrence of adverse effects. Safety issues are similar to those with many older AEDs, with rash appearing in 5% to 10% of patients and, rarely, much more serious problems, including Stevens-Johnson syndrome, aplastic anemia, and hepatitis. Chronic use also has been associated with connective tissue disorders, including Dupuytren's contracture, frozen shoulder, and other related conditions (59). The most common

problems associated with use of PB are those related to the central nervous system. Not surprisingly, in view of the fact that PB was first developed as a sedative, sleepiness is a common problem, especially at high doses. This is by no means invariable, and some patients tolerate quite high blood levels without complaint. Cognitive compromise not only has been a subjective complaint, but neuropsychological test batteries have consistently demonstrated some compromises compared with control subjects or patients on other standard AEDs (67,68). Behavior problems may be caused or aggravated especially in children with mental handicaps. The slow clearance and long half-life make once-daily dosing appropriate.

In summary, PB has proven to be as effective in controlling tonic-clonic seizures as any other AED, can be taken once daily, is available in parenteral formulations, and is very inexpensive. A greater prevalence of chronic adverse effects, especially of the psychological type, compared with many other AEDs has made PB a second-line AED choice except when cost is a primary consideration.

Phenytoin

PHT was studied by Tracy Putnam in an effort to find a chemical compound possessing an antiepileptic action with efficacy comparable with or better than that of PB, but without the sedative properties. In pioneering work using a cat electroshock model he had developed, he screened a number of hydantoins supplied by Parke-Davis. Diphenylhydantoin (PHT) was found to have the desired characteristics, and together with Houston Merritt, Putnam tested the drug in patients with epilepsy with considerable success. Introduced in 1938, PHT continues to be widely used and remains the most frequently prescribed AED in the United States. Clinical comparative trials have shown PHT treatment of patients with partial and tonic-clonic seizures to have equally successful retention compared with other AEDs (12,14,28–31,33). No study has found any other AED to have greater efficacy than PHT in treatment of partial and tonic-clonic seizures. In the VA COOP study #118, a significantly greater number of patients taking PHT entered into complete control at 1 year of follow-up compared with those on PB or PRM (75). On the other hand, PHT has no efficacy in control of absence, myoclonic, or atonic seizures and at times may aggravate these attacks (44,51).

Serious adverse effects are comparable with those of the other older AEDs. Rash occurs in approximately 5% to 10% of patients exposed to the drug. Rare occurrences of Stevens-Johnson syndrome, toxic epidermal necrolysis, hepatic failure, and aplastic anemia have all been reported, albeit rarely. Sedation can be experienced, especially as the dose rises. Mild mental slowing also may be noted, although carefully conducted neuropsychological test batteries do not reveal significant differences between PHT, CBZ, and VPA if doses and blood levels are in the usual range for treatment (67). Com-

monly, incoordination and ataxia appear as blood levels rise. Nystagmus often but not always parallels these side effects. Mental slowing and stupor appear with increasing overdose. Long-term side effects include hirsutism, which may constitute a cosmetic problem in children or women, particularly when affecting the face. Gingival hyperplasia is especially a problem in children or in adults with poor dental hygiene. Although the problem is much less evident in adults, it may occur in some patients despite scrupulous dental care. More important is the occasional development of peripheral neuropathy or cerebellar degeneration in some patients after long-term PHT therapy.

The pharmacokinetics of PHT are complex. Clearance occurs by oxidation to an inactive dihydroxy metabolite before renal excretion. The drug is metabolized primarily by the CYP4 hepatic isoenzyme system. This enzyme is saturable, resulting in rate-limiting clearance and an increasing half-life as blood concentration rises. This change at times may lead to unexpected increases or decreases in blood and brain levels with associated changes in clinical effect unless dosage is closely managed. On the other hand, the relatively long half-life makes once- or twice-daily dosing practical and enhances compliance. PHT is a potent inducer of hepatic enzymes and increases clearance of many AEDs, hormones, and medications administered for other medical problems. Awareness is necessary and appropriate increases in other medications need to be considered if PHT is coadministered.

PHT is available in an extensive number of formulations, facilitating use when rapid parenteral administration is indicated or when oral administration by tablet or capsule is not possible. It is well tolerated and is especially suitable when rapid start of treatment is indicated.

In summary, PHT is one of the oldest available AEDs and is unsurpassed in efficacy for controlling partial and tonic-clonic seizures. It also is available in many formulations and is useful for rapid loading of drug when prompt control of seizures is indicated. Its long half-life allows infrequent administration, and it is quite inexpensive. It is well tolerated at usual doses for most patients. Unfortunately, balancing these advantages are a number of undesirable characteristics. The pharmacokinetics are complex and can make dosing difficult. Adverse effects of a cosmetic type can be a problem for some patients. Of more concern is the development of long-term complications such as neuropathy or cerebellar degeneration. The introduction of many new AEDs with fewer adverse effects and more favorable pharmacokinetic properties suggests that, increasingly, PHT will be selected as one of a few drugs suitable for rapid start-up and for patients with difficult-to-control seizures.

Primidone

PRM was introduced in 1954 and in open trials was found to improve seizure control especially for patients with partial epilepsy. PRM also was used for treatment of juvenile myoclonic epilepsy with good success, particularly before the introduction of VPA (50).

Biotransformation of PRM to PB made it unclear if PRM was more than a prodrug. Considerable evidence from animal studies as well as patient trials has accumulated to indicate that when PRM is used as monotherapy, insufficient PB is found in the blood to account for all the clinical effect. PRM is primarily metabolized to PB and is cleared in approximately 8 to 12 hours, making twice-daily or three-times–daily dosing advisable to avoid peak effects. The metabolically derived PB has the same pharmacokinetic properties as PB that is used as monotherapy.

Although its adverse effects are similar to those of PB, PRM is associated with frequent dizziness, sedation, and gastrointestinal disturbance unless initiation and titration are carried out at very low doses (25 to 50 mg/day) and increased only as tolerated. The difficulty with start-up resulted in poorer retention in the VA COOP Study (12). However, once past that period, PRM was comparable in retention with CBZ, PB, and PHT (12). By some measures, both CBZ and PHT showed somewhat greater efficacy than PRM or PB (12,75).

In summary, PRM therapy is difficult to initiate and shares the long-term adverse effects of PB. It no longer is considered a first-line treatment for epilepsy, but for patients who have been successfully treated with this AED, it is reasonable to continue unless chronic adverse effects become evident. It is a first-line drug for tremor, so for patients with seizures and tremor it can treat both problems.

Valproate

VPA, the newest of the older drugs, was one of the first, if not the first, AED synthesized. Valproic acid, an oily compound, was used as a solvent, and it was in this context that Meurier et al. discovered its antiepileptic property serendipitously in 1963. Use soon spread to other countries from France, and its value for treatment of a wide variety of seizure types and epilepsy syndromes soon was evident. In contrast to CBZ, PB, and PHT, the primary AEDs available at the time, VPA was highly effective against absence and myoclonic seizures as well as tonic-clonic seizures. Indeed, efficacy against most seizure types made VPA the first true broad-spectrum agent. Despite extensive experience and a consensus that VPA is in general the drug of choice for treatment of the generalized epilepsies, the only controlled, comparative clinical trials were conducted for absence seizures decades ago. In those studies, VPA and ESM were equally effective. More recent trials have found VPA to be comparably effective in preventing partial and secondarily generalized tonic-clonic seizures (13–15). CBZ is somewhat more effective for partial seizure control using some outcome measures, but as with most of the AEDs, the differences in efficacy for treatment of partial (localization-related) epilepsies are modest (13). VPA is especially useful in patients with coexistent migraine headache or bipolar disease.

Serious toxicity is relatively uncommon. VPA is much less likely to cause hypersensitivity rash and related problems such as Stevens-Johnson syndrome than other AEDs having an aromatic ring structure (i.e., CBZ, PB, PRM, LTG, and PHT). Other systemic toxicities can be important. Hepatic failure with potentially fatal outcome has occurred primarily in children younger than 2 years of age and taking coadministered enzyme-inducing AEDs. For adolescent patients or in adults on monotherapy, the risk is very low. Bleeding disorders occur very infrequently and are due to disturbance of several factors. A somewhat dose-related decreased platelet count usually is not of clinical importance. Rare but potentially very serious pancreatitis also has been associated with VPA. Thinning of the hair, especially at high dosage, can occur but is transient. Gastrointestinal side effects were quite common at start-up, especially with the valproic acid formulation. Delayed- or slow-release formulations are much better tolerated. The most common adverse effect is weight gain, which is reported in some series to occur in approximately half the patients (13). This adverse effect is initially primarily a cosmetic issue, but over long term might predispose the patient to the many medical comorbidities of overweight (diabetes mellitus, hypertension, elevated lipids, and arteriosclerosis). However, such a risk is conceptual and no data are available to confirm it. An association between polycystic ovary syndrome and VPA use has been reported, but the frequency is debated. Another issue of importance to women of childbearing years is the teratogenic potential of VPA. Like most other older AEDs, VPA is associated with approximately a doubling in the incidence of congenital malformations, but VPA also is specifically associated with a 1% to 2% incidence of spina bifida, a particular concern to women of childbearing age.

Neurologic adverse effects are minimal at usual dosages. As dose and blood levels increase, an action tremor commonly appears, along with some sedation, but these are reversible. Neuropsychological testing reveals minimal compromise, and results are similar to those obtained with use of CBZ (67–69).

The pharmacokinetics of VPA are somewhat complex The drug is metabolized by oxidation and may produce active metabolites. If used together with an enzyme-inducing drug such as PHT, the clearance is increased and the half-life may be only 6 to 8 hours. This may lead to use of multiple doses daily unless delayed- or slow-release formulations are used. The absence of enzyme-inducing properties makes VPA easier to use with other inducible drugs or hormones than CBZ, PB, or PHT. VPA is available in virtually every desired formulation, including a water-soluble form for rapid parenteral administration.

In summary, despite a number of adverse effects, VPA was the first truly broad-spectrum AED that had efficacy for all the major seizure types. It remains the first drug for consideration in treatment of the idiopathic generalized epilepsies and associated absence, myoclonic, and tonic-clonic seizures, and is a reasonable alternative for all adult-onset epilepsies. Compared with the newer AEDs, it is relatively inexpensive. It is very well tolerated parenterally and is very suitable for patients requiring rapid initiation of treatment.

THE NEW ANTIEPILEPTIC DRUGS

Limitations in Information about New Antiepileptic Drugs

Our knowledge of AEDs when they initially are made available for marketing usually is quite limited, especially since the introduction of PHT. Government regulations and economic considerations have significantly influenced the type of trials and consequently the information available when compounds are released for clinical use. The trial designs have significant limitations in providing knowledge of when and how to treat epilepsy with new drugs (Table 7.5).

Formal evaluation of the new AEDs often has been done only in placebo-controlled studies, in which the drugs were used as add-on therapy in patients with partial seizures, with or without secondarily generalized tonic-clonic seizures, refractory to optimal standard care. Some drugs have been investigated in other refractory epilepsy types such as Lennox-Gastaut syndrome, and some have been used as acute treatment against placebo in a medication withdrawal epilepsy surgery evaluation protocol. Some of the studies used a dose-ranging protocol to identify an optimally safe and effective dose. In some monotherapy studies, one group of patients is treated with one dose that is too low to expect optimal effect. Such designs provide evidence of efficacy for regulatory purposes and licensing, but do not provide clinically useful information to indicate how a new drug compares with one already in use. Knowledge about the long-term efficacy and safety of these new drugs also is limited because the blinded, controlled treatment phase in most trials lasts only 3 to 4 months.

TABLE 7.5. LIMITATIONS OF PHASE II AND III CLINICAL TRIALS

- Focus on patients with refractory epilepsy
- Add-on design confounds identification of therapeutic and adverse effects attributable to new antiepileptic drug
- Most studies are of partial seizures
- Little or no data on:
  1. Efficacy/safety in other seizure/epilepsy types
  2. Efficacy/safety as monotherapy
  3. Long-term efficacy/safety
  4. Optimal doses
  5. Rare adverse events

The rationale for evaluating the new AEDs in various selected populations of patients with epilepsy is to allow therapeutic benefits to be readily detected and quantified in a short period. Sufficient power for statistical analysis is critical for government approval and licensing. Furthermore, the use of investigational drugs is more justifiable in patients whose seizures are poorly controlled and for whom the risk-to-benefit ratio of undefined potential toxicity is acceptable. Consequently, the efficacy studies usually indicate a modest degree of usefulness in very selected seizure and epilepsy types, and may give a limited view of the spectrum of efficacy of a new AED. For example, LTG seemed to have limited efficacy in early trials in which it was compared with placebo as an add-on therapy for patients with uncontrolled partial seizures. However, despite its modest efficacy as add-on therapy, LTG later was found to be as effective as CBZ or PHT in monotherapy trials involving patients with new-onset epilepsy (17,18).

The limited nature of the premarketing clinical trials also makes it difficult to assess the spectrum of efficacy of a new AED. For reasons previously stated, these studies primarily enroll patients with refractory partial seizures. Few trials are conducted in patients who have idiopathic generalized epilepsy with tonic-clonic, absence, or myoclonic seizures, because these individuals' seizures are more easily controlled with standard AEDs such as VPA and ESM. Based on data submitted to the U.S. Food and Drug Administration (FDA), LTG and TPM initially were approved in the United States only as adjunct therapy for partial seizures. Yet, increasing experience suggests that these drugs are effective for multiple seizure and epilepsy types (37–42). The dissociation between approved indication and common usage was most apparent for VPA. Although widely given for almost all seizure and epilepsy types, VPA was FDA approved only for the treatment of absence seizures for 20 years.

Because the premarketing clinical trials usually are conducted in patients with highly resistant seizures who are receiving combinations of AEDs, the true efficacy of the investigational drug alone is difficult to determine. One reason for this is that the observed effects may be due to pharmacodynamic or pharmacokinetic drug–drug interactions (71). For example, blood levels of LTG vary depending on the drug(s) with which it is coadministered. CBZ and PHT enhance LTG clearance, whereas VPA has an inhibitory effect. Therefore, LTG blood levels may be severalfold higher in a patient concomitantly receiving VPA plus LTG than LTG plus PHT, even when the LTG dose is kept constant. As a result, the efficacy of LTG may appear to be quite different under these two circumstances.

The uncertainty over optimal doses of investigational drugs is based on the design of initial studies. This also confounds assessment of how these agents should be administered when they become commercially available. For example, long-term clinical experience indicates that doses of GBP and LTG used in early clinical trials were suboptimal. In contrast, the doses used for initial TPM testing were much higher than necessary and may have contributed to more frequent reporting of poor tolerability. In its early trials, TPM was administered at doses up to 1,000 mg/day, whereas later analyses suggest that many patients obtained a good response and experienced fewer side effects when treated with TPM at 400 mg/day. As monotherapy, TPM doses as low as 100 mg/day were as effective as usual doses of CBZ or VPA in patients with new-onset epilepsy (22).

Adverse effects and tolerability of new AEDs are equally difficult to assess on the basis of data provided by the pre-marketing trials. Adverse effects reported in those studies may be the result of the investigational drug being evaluated, but they more likely occurred as a consequence of polytherapy. For example, dizziness was reported by 38% of patients in the add-on trials combining LTG with CBZ or PHT, but by only 8% of patients in studies of LTG monotherapy. These data indicate that LTG is well tolerated as monotherapy, and most of its neurotoxic effects can be attributed to combination treatment.

The relatively small number of patients entered into early clinical trials also precludes detection of rare or uncommon toxicities. This problem is highlighted by the late recognition of the risk of aplastic anemia and hepatic failure associated with FLB use (11).

The AEDs described as "new" vary considerably, from those that have been extensively used worldwide for 10 years, such as OXC, to the very new AED, LEV, which had very limited exposure when first brought to market.

Each of the new AEDs has advantages and disadvantages, which are summarized in Table 7.6 and described in greater detail in the following sections. Information available concerning many of these drugs is much less extensive than that for the older standard agents. For some, such as GBP, LTG, OXC, and ZNS, however, considerable use has already occurred, and the characteristics of these drugs are increasingly well known. For LEV, TGB, and, to some degree, TPM, knowledge about efficacy and adverse effects, as well as optimal usage, still is rapidly evolving (61–66).

INDIVIDUAL DRUG PROFILES

Felbamate

FLB (Felbatol; Wallace Laboratories, Cranbury, NJ) was marketed in 1994 after add-on studies and clinical trials investigating its use as monotherapy. These studies revealed

TABLE 7.6. CONSIDERATIONS IN SELECTION OF NEW ANTIEPILEPTIC DRUGS

Drug (Brand Name)	Advantages	Disadvantages	Comment
Felbamate (Felbatol)	Broad spectrum of efficacy, including Lennox-Gastaut syndrome; alerting	Rare fatal aplastic anemia and hepatitis; headache; insomnia; weight loss; drug interactions	Use limited owing to risks; inhibits metabolism of PB, PHT, and VPA: induces metabolism of CBZ
Gabapentin (Neurontin)	Effective in partial and tonic-clonic seizures; well tolerated and very safe; no known interactions	Limited absorption; short half-life; moderately limited spectrum of efficacy	Mechanism of action unknown but may enhance GABA synthesis and calcium channel function
Lamotrigine (Lamictal)	Broad spectrum of efficacy; sense of well-being; may be effective in Lennox-Gastaut syndrome	Hypersensitivity reactions occasionally severe; metabolism inducible by CBZ, PB, and PH, and inhibited by VPA	Extensive experience; excellent overall efficacy/tolerability, but requires slow dose titration
Levetiracetam (Keppra)	Effective for partial seizures; possible broad spectrum; well tolerated; no interactions	Long-term safety unknown	Delayed action in animal models, suggesting unique mechanism of action
Oxcarbazepine (Trileptal)	Very effective for partial and tonic-clonic seizures; extensive experience	Rash, hyponatremia	Pharmacodynamics similar to CBZ, but better pharmacokinetics
Tiagabine (Gabatril)	Effective in partial and tonic-clonic seizures	Undergoes hepatic metabolism; short half-life; affected by enzyme induction	Unique mechanism of action; blocks GABA reuptake
Topiramate (Topamax)	Very effective in partial and tonic-clonic seizures; may have broad spectrum of efficacy; weight loss	Possible cognitive or behavioral problems on initiation; risk of renal calculi; paresthesias; weight loss	Unique compound related to sugars; renal elimination; long half-life
Vigabatrin (Sabril)	Quite effective in partial and tonic-clonic seizures; infantile spasms; long duration of action; well tolerated	Visual field loss; may not be marketed in the USA; uncommon psychiatric symptoms (psychoses); weight gain	Unique mechanism of action; irreversibly inhibits GABA transaminase; serum levels not closely related to efficacy
Zonisamide (Zonegran)	Effective for partial and tonic-clonic seizures; perhaps broad spectrum	Renal calculi; sedation; dizziness	Related to sulfa drugs

CBZ, carbamazepine; PB, phenobarbital; PHT, phenytoin; VPA, valproate; GABA, γ-aminobutyric acid.

that FLB had some efficacy in patients with partial seizures, although its potency seemed to be modest. Investigation in one controlled monotherapy trial in patients with partial-onset seizures randomized patients to FLB or low-dose VPA (76). The study design allowed demonstration of efficacy in the investigational agent without exposing control patients to unacceptable risks—that is, low-dose VPA was expected to prevent convulsive seizures and status epilepticus, but to be insufficient for controlling partial seizures. Using this "pseudoplacebo:" design, the investigators demonstrated a significant difference in efficacy. The superiority of FLB over VPA was not proven because VPA was administered in a suboptimal dose.

In a second monotherapy trial, patients who had stopped taking AEDs for presurgical recording of seizures were randomized to FLB or placebo in addition to the anti-convulsant regimen at the end of the surgical evaluation (77). In this setting, placebo treatment was thought to be justifiable because AED therapy already was discontinued for an appropriate medical reason, and an additional seizure might provide even more useful information for a decision about possible surgical treatment. In this trial, FLB again demonstrated monotherapy efficacy in seizure control, albeit for a short period, compared with placebo. These new monotherapy clinical trial decisions have been used in testing subsequent new AEDs. The efficacy of FLB also has been demonstrated in the refractory population of patients with Lennox-Gastaut syndrome. As a result, FLB has been approved for use either as adjunct therapy or monotherapy in both adults with partial epilepsy and children with Lennox-Gastaut syndrome.

Unfortunately, FLB was associated with frequent adverse effects during its clinical evaluation, especially in patients to whom it was administered as adjunctive therapy and the dosage rapidly escalated. FLB has complex pharmacokinetic interactions with other agents. It decreases CBZ and increases PHT and VPA levels, which confounded assessment of its specific pharmacodynamic effects. Headache occasionally was reported by FLB-treated patients, and led some patients to discontinue treatment. Gastrointestinal distress also was reported, and weight loss was relatively common. However, because many patients had gained weight during prior CBZ or VPA therapy, this "adverse effect" was, at times, a welcome benefit. Similarly, insomnia (or alerting) associated with FLB proved to be of considerable value to the families of many infants and children previously treated with multiple sedating AEDs for epilepsy syndromes, such as Lennox-Gastaut syndrome. Even when seizure improvement was modest, the overall alerting effect was a significant positive benefit.

Of greatest importance in FLB's safety profile was the later realization of the risk of serious idiosyncratic reactions. Aplastic anemia and liver failure developed in some patients, and approximately one-third of these individuals died. Eventually, the probability of these serious events was estimated to be 1:2,000 to 1:5,000 exposed to FLB (11). Consequently, the manufacturer and the FDA advised that the drug be used only when the benefit warranted the significant risk. Clearly, selected patients fulfill these criteria, although FLB should be used only after treatment with the standard and other new AEDs has failed. It can be argued that a trial and failure with FLB should be considered before surgery, which itself carries a 1% to 3% risk of catastrophic outcome.

FLB should be used as monotherapy whenever possible because of the complex pharmacokinetic interactions and adverse effects encountered when it is coadministered with other AEDs. It should be continued only when a significant clinical benefit is achieved. Monitoring of blood cell counts and liver function tests is advised, although there is no proof that early recognition of aplastic anemia or hepatic failure, followed by discontinuation of FLB, prevents a catastrophic outcome.

In summary, FLB is an effective broad-spectrum AED whose potential toxicity limits use to those patients failing other drugs.

Gabapentin

Many placebo-controlled trials showed modest efficacy in treatment of partial and tonic-clonic seizures when GBP (Neurontin; Pfizer, NY) was used as an add-on to standard AED therapy (63,64). The dosage evaluated ranged from 600 to 1,800 mg/day, and these studies showed a dose–response pattern for seizure control. Based on the testing of the lower doses, the predicted effectiveness of GBP is probably less than subsequently demonstrated in studies in which doses up to 4,800 mg/day were found to be safe and effective. Open-label experience from extensive studies and other clinical trials established the long-term efficacy and safety of GBP in patients with refractory epilepsy, and indicated that such patients may benefit from and tolerate GBP doses higher than those used in the controlled clinical investigations.

GBP has been tested as monotherapy in a surgical evaluation model, in which patients were given GBP 300 or 3,600 mg/day after their third seizure. The higher dose was significantly more effective than the lower dose, providing protection against a subsequent seizure during an 8-day follow-up (78). A crossover study of monotherapy in incompletely controlled patients with partial seizures showed that in approximately 20% of patients, intractable seizures could be successfully managed with GBP monotherapy (600, 1,200, or 2,400 mg/day). However, the seizure exacerbation led many patients in this refractory epilepsy study to discontinue study participation, and no dose–response effect was identified among those who continued monotherapy (79).

A European dose-ranging GBP monotherapy trial of patients with new-onset epilepsy, however, demonstrated superior efficacy among patients who received GBP 900 or 1,200 mg/day, compared with 300 mg/day. It was found that the overall success rate, measured by retention in the study, by both higher doses was comparable with that achieved in an unblinded parallel group that received CBZ 600 mg/day. In this study, CBZ treatment failed primarily because of adverse effects, whereas GBP provided less seizure control but better tolerability (26).

A large, multicenter, double-blind monotherapy trial of patients with new-onset epilepsy compared GBP with LTG, and no differences in retention or seizure control could be detected over a 24-week period of observation (23)

On the other hand, GBP has been evaluated for the treatment of refractory generalized seizures in a double-blind, parallel-control trial using 1,200 mg/day and there was no benefit compared with placebo for the treatment of generalized tonic-clonic seizures, myoclonic seizures, or absence seizures (80). Anecdotal reports have suggested that, occasionally, absence seizures may increase with the use of GBP (44).

The side effect profile of GBP is very favorable. No serious systemic safety problems have arisen despite a very large patient exposure both for epilepsy and pain therapy. Indeed, it would appear that GBP is one of the safest drugs used in the entire field of medicine. However, experience based on extensive use has been available for less than a decade, and some chronic problems might eventually become evident. Other systemic adverse effects are uncommon. Gastrointestinal symptoms and weight gain occasionally are reported. Hypersensitivity reaction rash is very unusual, and seems to occur no more frequently than with the use of placebo.

Central nervous system tolerability also is excellent in most adults. Fatigue, dizziness, and ataxia, side effects commonly associated with start-up of most AEDs, have been reported early in drug administration, and seemed to be dose related. However, the frequency and severity of these complaints are relatively low. Approximately 9% of patients who received GBP in a controlled monotherapy trial withdrew because of drug-related adverse effects, a low number, not much greater than might be expected from placebo (23).

Cognitive/neuropsychological batteries have detected no impairment of performance with GBP use, whereas some psychological test results and quality-of-life measures improved after patients were crossed over from other AEDs to GBP monotherapy.

GBP also has a favorable pharmacokinetic profile. It is completely eliminated renally, and does not undergo hepatic metabolism. Consequently, in contrast to the older AEDs, there are no drug interactions to consider in patients receiving GBP. The elimination half-life of GBP is approximately 6 hours, which suggests that multiple dosing is advisable. However, there is some evidence that a more prolonged effect may occur, perhaps because of increased brain levels of GABA (72). Therefore, the duration of GBP's anti-

convulsant activity may be more prolonged than might be expected based on the blood concentrations.

GBP is absorbed into the systemic circulation and enters the central nervous system by active L-amino transport. This system is saturable, and may limit the amount of drug entering the circulation from the gastrointestinal tract or the brain from the blood in any given period. The renal elimination of GBP results in higher blood concentrations and slower elimination in patients with decreased renal function. Changes in elimination are directly related to creatinine clearance. Changes in dosage can be modified according to this expected clearance, but clinical response probably is more important. Blood level determination also may be of assistance.

In summary, GBP has been shown to be an effective AED for control of partial and secondarily generalized tonic-clonic seizures and has outstanding safety. The degree of efficacy has been difficult to assess. Add-on and initial monotherapy trials often used low dosages and were conducted in refractory patients. The small improvement in control suggested modest efficacy. However, in subsequent open trials, much higher dosages were well tolerated, and these should be considered before GBP therapy is considered a failure. Although the outcomes from available monotherapy trials do not allow comparison of efficacy with older drugs like CBZ or PHT, it may be argued that its favorable side effect profile and pharmacokinetic properties make it a treatment of first choice with selected patients having partial or tonic-clonic seizures, reserving more traditional but less well tolerated drugs such as CBZ, PHT, and VPA for patients in whom GBP monotherapy fails.

Lamotrigine

LTG (Lamictal; Glazo Smith Kline, Research Triangle, NC) was one of a number of antifolate compounds developed by Wellcome, Ltd. that proved to possess broad-spectrum anticonvulsant properties in animal models and was subsequently brought to clinical trials. Dose-related efficacy has been found in multiple studies in which LTG was given as an add-on with other AEDs in patients with refractory partial epilepsy. Approximately 20% more patients receiving LTG 400 mg/day, compared with placebo, experienced a ≥50% reduction in seizures. Although these results suggest modest efficacy, it must be remembered that the drug was tested in a group of patients with refractory seizures. The trials often were conducted as add-on therapy to enzyme-inducing AEDs, so the effective blood levels of LTG were considerably less than had it been given as monotherapy.

Clinical trial experience also suggests that, like VPA, LTG has a broad spectrum of antiepileptic efficacy. In monotherapy studies, enrolling patients with new-onset epilepsy of all types, LTG was found to be as effective as CBZ or PHT and better tolerated (15,16). In an active-control study, patients with partial seizures previously treated with CBZ or PHT were crossed to either LTG therapy (250mg twice daily) or low-dose VPA (500mg twice daily) (81). Significantly more patients were successfully maintained on LTG than VPA monotherapy. LTG also has efficacy in the treatment of absence and myoclonic seizures, as well as multiple seizures associated with the Lennox-Gastaut syndrome (37–40).

Systemic events have been infrequent in patients receiving LTG, except for idiosyncratic rash. Some gastrointestinal complaints may be reported on start-up, but otherwise the drug is well tolerated. Hypersensitivity reactions have occurred in approximately 10% of patients, but the incidence can be much higher. The probability of rash or more serious reactions such as Stevens-Johnson syndrome seems to be related to the rate of administration and corresponding blood levels (54). Therefore, the dose of LTG should be titrated slowly. This is particularly important when it is coadministered with VPA, which inhibits LTG clearance and causes a rapid increase in LTG blood concentrations. The usual adult dosage is 150 to 600 mg/day.

LTG's adverse effect profile was particularly difficult to assess in the premarketing clinical trials. Among patients with partial seizures who received LTG as add-on therapy to CBZ, neurotoxic side effects, including dizziness, diplopia, and ataxia, were common and often limited LTG use unless the CBZ dose was reduced. In marked contrast, however, the use of LTG monotherapy was only infrequently associated with neurologic side effects, thus confirming that the events that occurred in the add-on trials were attributable to the combination of drugs, rather than to LTG alone. LTG seems to have no adverse effects on cognition, and may have positive effects on mood and behavior (82).

LTG is metabolized in the liver, by glucuronidation, before renal elimination (71). Its half-life is approximately 24 hours when it is used as monotherapy or together with noninteracting drugs. Metabolism is induced by CBZ, PHT, and the barbiturates, and the half-life of LTG is reduced to approximately 12 hours when it is administered concomitantly with these enzyme inducers. As noted previously, VPA inhibits the metabolism of LTG, resulting in a doubling or tripling of the half-life. Although the metabolism of LTG is affected by other older AEDs, it is not an enzyme inducer and is minimally protein bound. Consequently, coadministered drugs are not affected by its use.

The long half-life allows once- or twice-daily dosing, which enhances compliance (70).

In summary, LTG has demonstrated good efficacy as a broad-spectrum AED, possesses favorable pharmacokinetic properties as monotherapy, has excellent long-term tolerability, is relatively nonsedating, and is antidepressant. The only important limitation is a hypersensitivity reaction that is comparable to that seen with the older AEDs (i.e., CBZ, PB, PHT), but can be serious. This adverse effect notwithstanding, LTG has evolved to be a first-line choice for epilepsy therapy.

Levetiracetam

LEV (Keppra; UCB Pharmaceuticals, New Smyrna, GA) is one of the newest AEDs, so less is known about its efficacy and adverse effects. In experimental animal models, LEV has demonstrated unique properties. It has no effect on acute seizures produced by Metrazol or electroshock, but is highly effective against genetic animal or kindled models of epilepsy. These experimental studies failed to reveal mechanisms of action similar to those of other AEDs (83).

Efficacy has been demonstrated in add-on trials of partial and secondarily generalized seizures. A combination of three multicenter, double-blind, placebo-controlled, parallel-group studies proved LEV at 1,000, 2,000, or 3,000 mg/day to be statistically significantly better than placebo for all seizures combined, as well as subgroups of simple, complex, or secondarily generalized tonic-clonic seizures (84). The spectrum of activity has not been fully explored, but spike–wave patterns were significantly suppressed in genetic mouse models and photic sensitivity in a small open clinical epilepsy trial. These results suggest efficacy against generalized seizures such as absence and myoclonic seizures (42).

Pharmacokinetic studies indicate fairly prompt and complete absorption and distribution. Elimination is renal. Interaction studies have shown no effect on the metabolism of other compounds, nor the converse.

Adverse effects have been few in current clinical trials and no safety problems have arisen, although numbers of patients exposed to LEV remain relatively small, so rare idiosyncratic reactions can easily go undetected at this phase in evaluation (85). Dosage has ranged widely from 600 to 4,800 mg/day and more, if needed and tolerated.

At present, the drug is available only for oral administration.

In summary, LEV's clinical spectrum, extent of efficacy, optimal dosing, and so forth, have yet to be well defined. However, the safety and pharmacokinetic properties of LEV are especially promising.

Oxcarbazepine

OXC (Trileptal; Novartis) is a tricyclic AED closely related to CBZ and developed in the 1960s by Geigy Limited. Although a new drug to the United States and a number of other countries, it has been widely used in parts of Europe since its introduction in Denmark in the early 1990s. It is marketed extensively throughout the world, and considerable information is available concerning its indications and safety.

OXC has been studied in comparative active-control clinical trials and demonstrated efficacy equal to the standard drugs CBZ, PHT, and VPA (17–19) in new-onset epilepsy. When administered in usual and tolerated dosages, effects are the same as those of CBZ. Occasionally, patients have responded better to OXC on an individual basis. OXC also has been used successfully as monotherapy for the treatment of uncontrolled partial and secondarily generalized tonic-clonic seizures (86–88). In a high-dosage (2,400 mg/day) versus low-dosage (300 mg/day) OXC trial, the high dosage was markedly more effective in preventing exit from the study than the low dosage ("pseudoplacebo"). These studies clearly established monotherapy efficacy for regulatory purposes. OXC is not effective against absence or myoclonic seizures, and like its close relative CBZ, it may at times cause aggravation of these seizure types. The usual adult dosages are 900 to 2,400 mg/day.

The adverse effects of OXC are very similar to those of CBZ. Visual disturbance and occasional sedation or gastrointestinal complaints may accompany high doses, but OXC is less likely to cause these symptoms with acute start-up. Idiosyncratic rash and related problems are comparable with those with CBZ, and a cross-sensitivity reaction occurs in approximately 25% of patients who have rash from earlier administration of CBZ (89). Hyponatremia is seen as well, although rarely of clinically significant degree. On the other hand, leukopenia, often associated with CBZ therapy, is not noted as commonly with OXC.

Although the clinical profile of efficacy and adverse effects is quite similar for OXC and CBZ, the pharmacokinetics are importantly distinctive. OXC is reduced, converting the keto to a hydroxyl group, producing monohydroxy OXC (MHD). This is the pharmacologically active metabolite. Although OXC has minimal effects on metabolism of other AEDs, it does sometimes cause elevation of PHT levels when given in high doses. Some reduction in oral contraceptive effects also has been reported. Unlike CBZ, there is no autoinduction.

OXC is available orally, in tablet form. A parenteral formulation of the water-soluble metabolite, MHD, which is the pharmacologically active metabolite, is undergoing development. This would provide a much-needed parenteral formulation for this important family of AEDs.

In summary, OXC, although closely related to CBZ, has several distinct advantages. It is equally as effective as CBZ and other standard AEDs in the treatment of partial and secondarily generalized seizures and overall is better tolerated, with fewer adverse effects. OXC's pharmacokinetics are more favorable, with fewer interactions than the standard AEDs. Clearly, this should be a drug of first choice for monotherapy and treatment of localization-related epilepsy, although like all the new AEDs, it is considerably more expensive than the older drugs.

Tiagabine

TGB (Gabaitril; Sanofi, France) was specifically designed and synthesized to inhibit GABA reuptake and prevent seizures, unlike most AEDs, which were discovered by serendipity. Compared with some of the more extensively used new AEDs such as GBP, LTG, and VGB, TGB has

been evaluated in relatively few studies. In add-on, placebo-controlled studies, TGB was associated with statistically significant efficacy (90,91). The results of a monotherapy trial suggested effectiveness by some measures, but no significant difference was found between low- and high-dose TGB, probably because efficacy was present at the low dose (92). Insufficient clinical information is available to predict the spectrum of efficacy for TGB. The usual dosage is 24 to 56 mg/day.

TGB usually is well tolerated. Treatment initiation and high dosages (>56 mg/day) occasionally elicit the usual AED-related central nervous system complaints of sedation, dizziness, tremor, and, less often, confusion. TGB also has been associated with some other cognitive complaints, although neuropsychological batteries conducted in some TGB clinical trials have failed to link its use to any significant disturbances (93). No serious safety problems have arisen.

TGB's pharmacologic properties are less favorable than most of the other new AEDs. TGB is metabolized in the liver and has a half-life of approximately 6 hours, although its clearance is even more rapid when it is administered with enzyme-inducing drugs. Nevertheless, TGB has been effective in clinical trials when administered in a twice-daily or three-times–daily regimen. TGB also is highly protein bound, although the clinical significance of any drug displacement is minimal in the absence of a meaningful blood level monitoring technique.

In summary, the role of TGB as an AED is still uncertain, but its use in its approved indication as adjunctive treatment seems to be appropriate. TGB is safe, reasonably well tolerated, and easy to administer as an adjunct; therefore, it may be an appropriate therapeutic selection in patients whose seizures do not respond adequately to standard AEDs.

Topiramate

TPM (Topamaz; Ortho-McNeil Pharmaceutical, Raritan, NJ), originally developed by Johnson and Johnson as an oral hypoglycemic, proved instead to be an effective AED. Clinical trials using TPM as an add-on drug for the treatment of partial and secondarily generalized tonic-clonic seizures revealed a ≥50% reduction in seizures in 40% to 50% of patients receiving TPM 200 to 400 mg/day. Little increased benefit was observed in doses up to 1,000 mg/day. A monotherapy study of crossover to 1,000 or 100 mg/day of TPM in patients with refractory partial seizure demonstrated a statistically significant advantage for the higher dose and also established efficacy as monotherapy (94). In newly diagnosed patients with epilepsy, both 100 and 200 mg/day dosages of TPM achieved success comparable with CBZ or VPA, and the 100 mg/day group experienced the best tolerability (22).

TPM also has been tested in patients with other seizure types, and preliminary evidence suggests its efficacy for treating generalized seizures, and that it may have a broad spectrum of efficacy similar to FLB and LTG (41,95). However, there is too little information to define clearly the spectrum and potency of TPM in clinical use compared with other AEDs.

TPM has especially favorable pharmacokinetic characteristics. It is well absorbed, water soluble, not significantly protein bound, eliminated primarily by the kidneys, and has a half-life of approximately 24 hours. When given with enzyme-inducing drugs such as CBZ, PHT, or barbiturates, oxidation and glucuronidation of TPM are enhanced, and clearance is approximately 40% more rapid than when it is administered as monotherapy or coadministered with non–enzyme-inducing drugs (71).

Although trials indicated considerable potency of TPM, they also revealed multiple side effects. Some of the reported adverse events were characteristic of other AEDs, such as fatigue, gastrointestinal upset, and dizziness, and many of those were mild and self-limiting. However, a subpopulation of approximately 15% of patients experienced psychological disturbances, including impaired thinking or irritability. The exact terms for this thinking disturbance are not always easy to translate from the standardized form and terminology used. Neuropsychological testing indicates modest but clear verbal memory difficulties in some patients (96). Nonetheless, these complaints caused some TPM-treated patients to withdraw from clinical trials. Although neurologic, and especially psychological, adverse effects seemed to be relatively prominent in the TPM clinical trials, many patients received high doses (800 or 1,000 mg/day) that now are recognized to contribute to side effects without increased efficacy, and dose escalation was too rapid to allow tolerance to develop.

However, other systemic side effects were infrequent. The incidence of idiosyncratic rash was no greater than that among placebo-treated patients, and in contrast to the experience with GBP, VGB, CBZ, and VPA, weight gain was not a problem, and some patients even lost weight. Renal calculi developed in approximately 1% to 3% of patients, but most of the stones passed without adverse sequelae. This side effect emphasizes the need for adequate fluid intake by patients receiving TPM. Paresthesias are a common side effect (25% to 33% of patients on monotherapy), usually affecting the arms, but are not usually a cause for discontinuing drug. Some reports indicate TPM may cause acute-angle glaucoma, but the frequency of this problem is unclear (97).

In summary, TPM seems to be a potent and generally safe new AED for the treatment of partial and secondarily generalized seizures. Some meta-analyses of add-on trials suggest it is the most potent of the new AEDs (63). Increasing evidence indicates TPM has broad-spectrum efficacy. The fact that adverse effects occurred more frequently with TPM than with other AEDs in initial trials may, in part, be attributable to very high doses given too quickly. Weight loss may be an advantage.

Vigabatrin

In placebo-controlled clinical trials, VGB (Sabril; Bridgewater, NJ) has demonstrated clear efficacy in the treatment of partial and secondarily generalized seizures, in which 40% to 50% of patients experienced a ≥50% reduction in seizures. In a monotherapy study, comparable success rates were achieved in patients treated with VGB and CBZ; VGB was better tolerated but less effective in controlling partial seizures (24,25). Uncontrolled trials suggest that absence and myoclonic seizures are not helped by VGB, and may even increase (44).

Safety has developed as a serious concern. Visual field defects have developed in approximately 30% of patients treated with VGB. Others report the problem less frequently, but it often is asymptomatic and not readily detected (57,98). Otherwise, VGB has a favorable profile. Its use has been associated with some sedation and weight gain, but serious systemic toxicity has not been reported (63–66). Information in the European literature indicates that in a small percentage of VGB-treated patients psychoses develop, particularly depression, which resolved with drug discontinuation.

The pharmacodynamic properties of VGB are especially favorable. Because of the irreversible inhibition of GABA transaminase, the effect of VGB on brain GABA levels persists long after the drug has been eliminated from the body. Although VGB is renally excreted, with a half-life of approximately 6 hours, GABA levels in the brain remain increased for ≥24 to 48 hours (72). Therefore, twice-daily and probably even once-daily administration is a reasonable treatment schedule. VGB has no known interactions with other drugs, except for slight lowering of PHT levels.

In summary, VGB is an effective drug for the treatment of partial and secondarily generalized seizures and shows promise in infantile spasms. The occurrence of visual compromise will probably limit use to those whose epilepsy severity justifies the risk.

Zonisamide

ZNS (Zonegran; Elan Pharmaceuticals) is a sulfa compound that was first developed by Dainippon Pharmaceutical Corporation in Japan and studied initially through license to Parke-Davis. Although the drug appeared promising, the occurrence of renal calculi led to discontinuation of trials in the United States, but they were continued in Japan and the drug was marketed and used extensively both there and in a number of other countries. The drug has been found to be statistically significantly more effective than placebo in add-on trials for partial and secondarily generalized tonic-clonic seizures. The number of patients achieving 50% or greater reduction in seizures averaged approximately 33% or a little more on dosages of 400 to 800 mg/day (65,66,99). This would place it at an intermediate level of efficacy, between GBP/LTG and VGB/TPM. Randomized, controlled monotherapy trials have not been reported despite extensive use in open trials. Some evidence of broad-spectrum efficacy is seen both in animal models and in limited trials, which have included the generalized epilepsies, with absence and myoclonic seizures. Specifically, Baltic myoclonic epilepsy has been aided by ZNS therapy (100,101).

Serious adverse effects have been infrequent. Approximately 3% of patients have had renal calculi, but these almost always have passed without invasive intervention (100). Other safety issues have been very uncommon. Some cross-reactivity has been seen in individuals allergic to sulfa drugs. Some somnolence, dizziness, and mental slowing can be seen during start-up, depending on rate of escalation and total dose. These are minimized with slow administration and limiting the dosage to necessary amounts to achieve control.

ZNS is renally excreted after conjugation, and has a half-life of 2 to 3 days as monotherapy, or 1 to 1.5 days for patients on enzyme-inducing drugs. ZNS is available in tablet form, with no parenteral formulation being available.

In summary, ZNS, like OXC, is a new compound to the U.S. market. However, extensive experience throughout the world over the past decade has allowed awareness of efficacy and adverse effects, although further trials of monotherapy and other epilepsy types are indicated (Table 7.6). It appears to have broad-spectrum AED potential.

ANTIEPILEPTIC DRUG SELECTION AND MANAGEMENT

When a decision has been made to initiate AED therapy for prevention of recurrent seizures, selection must be made from the many drugs available. *No one drug of choice can be defined for any seizure or epilepsy type.* Most adult-onset epilepsy is symptomatic or cryptogenic (etiology not determined) of partial (localization-related) type with partial or tonic-clonic seizures. The patient, family, and significant others, with advice and recommendations from the physician and other professionals, must decide which constellation of drug characteristics (as summarized in Tables 7.1 and 7.2) is most appropriate for each individual patient. However, CBZ has been tested against other drugs most often, has proven as effective as any other, and was somewhat more potent for treating partial seizures than some AEDs (i.e., GBP, PB, VGB, VPA). PHT has equal efficacy to CBZ but may have cumulative chronic adverse effects, as do PB and VPA. On the basis of systematic review, the Scottish Intercollegiate Guidelines Network (SIGN) considered CBZ the best selection overall (33). These guidelines were developed before the comparative trials of the newer AEDs in which both LTG and OXC were found to have better tolerability than the older drugs. One study also

indicated TPM compared favorably with CBZ and VPA. Another trial has shown GBP and LTG to be comparatively successful as monotherapy. Consequently, many reasonable options now exist.

The idiopathic generalized epilepsies with tonic-clonic, myoclonic, or absence seizures most often arise in childhood or early adolescence, but both juvenile myoclonic epilepsy and grand mal on awakening may first come to attention in adult life. For many years, VPA has been the consensus drug of choice and was recommended in the SIGN Guidelines, although no randomized, comparative trials with level I evidence have been conducted (33). The introduction of LTG and TPM with broad-spectrum antiseizure properties now offers reasonable alternatives to VPA when anticipated adverse effects of VPA are undesirable. LEV and ZNS also show potential, but evidence is insufficient to make definite recommendations.

Treatment Initiation

Other factors may dictate the most appropriate AED to use in therapy. Patients presenting with serial seizures often need prompt termination of attacks. Although this may be done with a benzodiazepine, some longer-acting AED therapy is required. This is easily accomplished with the use of parenteral PHT, VPA, or PB. For patients needing to achieve control quickly but not requiring parenteral administration, PB, PHT, GBP, or VPA can be brought to effective concentrations within a day or two with oral loading. In contrast, CBZ, LTG, TGB, TPM, and ZNS are associated with poor tolerability or increased risk of idiosyncratic rash with rapid titration. OXC and LEV appear to be intermediate in tolerability for rapid initiation.

Regardless of the adverse effects at initiation, many subside in time despite increasing dose and blood levels (Figure 7.4). The patient should be encouraged to allow some time for his or her body to adjust to the drug and not abandon treatment with the onset of side effects of nonserious type.

As a consequence of these issues of tolerability, specific rates of administration are recommended for each drug. Some general principles of starting treatment and rate of administration are shown in Table 7.7. The rate should be modified on an individual basis. If tolerance is poor, the dosage should be withheld or reduced for several days or weeks. If tolerance is good, more rapid escalation provides quicker protection against recurrent seizures. After increasing the dosage to what might be recommended for an individual's age and weight, further changes can be made on the basis of clinical response. These changes should take into account the pharmacokinetic properties of the drug (102,103). On maintenance dosages of PHT, a steady state would not be reached for approximately 7 to 10 days and, for PB, for several weeks. In general, the clinician can assume a steady state will be reached no sooner than five half-lives of the drug. For CBZ, the blood levels achieved by

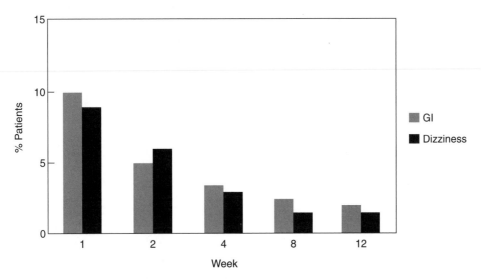

FIGURE 7.4. Functional tolerance to early side effects. Adverse events versus time on antiepileptic drug therapy, Department of Veterans Affairs Cooperative Study, 118. (From Mattson RH, Cramer JA, Collins JF. Early tolerance to antiepileptic drug side effects: a controlled trial of 247 patients. In: Koella WP, et al, eds. *Tolerance to beneficial and/or adverse effects of antiepileptic drugs*. New York: Raven Press, 1986:149–156, with permission.)

the first week decrease on a steady dose owing to autoinduction. The dosage subsequently is increased as needed to obtain seizure control. If CBZ is discontinued for any reason, deinduction occurs within a few days and restarting at the prior dosage results in much higher blood levels, often causing adverse effects. These metabolic changes may be especially important when CBZ is discontinued and then restarted in a presurgical/diagnostic epilepsy monitoring unit evaluation or if a patient is unable to take oral medication for whatever reason (104).

If rash appears, the drug should be withheld. Approximately half the instances of rash clear spontaneously and do not recur. A small percentage, however, may progress to multisystem involvement, including Stevens-Johnson syndrome, and treatment in someone who has had rash must be monitored closely, with prompt cessation of drug with any worsening. For patients with prior exposure to an AED that caused a rash, there is increased likelihood of cross-reactivity with older AEDs and probably LTG (82). Criteria for drug selection in these individuals should include a low risk of hypersensitivity. Such drugs include GBP, LEV, TGB, TPM, and VPA.

TABLE 7.7. INITIATION OF TREATMENT

- Discuss plan with patient and family
- Use a "test" dose at bedtime
- If side effects, delay next dose
- If side effects recur, reduce dose
- Increase dose as tolerated

When one of the older AEDs is selected, a decision also may need to be made whether to prescribe a generic or brand-name, originator product (105,106). With new-onset epilepsy, control often is achieved without using high doses of medication (4,5,10–13). Because the outcome is a clinical one, aided by AED blood levels, a properly manufactured generic should suffice in most cases. In fact, VA COOP Study #118 used generic PHT in the trial without difficulty. However, in a number of circumstances a generic product (or variable suppliers of the product) is not recommended. When seizures are more difficult to control, dosages need to be increased near or to the point of poor tolerability. In such situations, small fluctuations in bioavailability may be clinically quite important. CBZ and PHT are two AEDs that may have little room for variability. Small changes in AED levels may lead to side effects or loss of control. For products that have a short half-life, such as CBZ or VPA, extended-release formulations may prevent peak/trough effects that also can lead to adverse effects or breakthrough seizures. Valproic acid often causes more gastrointestinal side effects than a brand-name delayed-absorption VPA formulation. Other brand-name products may be important for some patients. Thus, a sprinkle, chewable, or liquid form is useful for those who cannot or will not swallow a tablet or capsule. Brand-name fosphenytoin is a much better tolerated parenteral formulation than generic PHT.

Older versus New Antiepileptic Drugs

When selecting an AED for initiating therapy (or as alternative therapy), it is unclear what place the new AEDs should occupy. No evidence exists that the newer compounds possess greater efficacy than the older ones, but pharmacokinetic properties are improved and, in some, tolerability and safety appear to be better. On the other hand, they usually are much more expensive. Consequently, unless there is a particular reason to select one of the newer drugs for starting therapy, CBZ, PB, PHT, and VPA are most appropriate for partial and secondarily generalized seizures associated with symptomatic epilepsy. ESM is indicated for pure absence seizures, and VPA for seizures of tonic-clonic, absence, and myoclonic type found in the idiopathic generalized epilepsies. When adverse effects or pharmacokinetic characteristics of the older drugs are undesirable for an individual patient, it is reasonable to select one of the newer AEDs.

Maintenance

Any problem after initiation of therapy is reason to schedule a visit, urgently if some systemic problem is suspected. Minor issues such as dose changes often can be dealt with by telephone (but documentation of the discussion should be made in the records). If logistically possible, a return visit within a few weeks or a month may be useful even if no problems have arisen. This presents further opportunity to provide patient education (preferably with a significant other as well) so the patient can knowledgeably collaborate in management of what quite possibly will be a long-term condition. Although much information may have been discussed at an initial visit, many facts may not have been heard, were misinterpreted, or were subsequently contradicted by readings or comments from family and friends.

Antiepileptic Drug Monitoring

Monitoring the concentration of AEDs in the blood has proven to be a valuable supplement to patient care, especially for compounds with complex pharmacokinetic properties like CBZ or PHT. There are specific times and situations when determination of blood levels is most useful (Table 7.8). On the other hand, routine monitoring was not found to yield better outcomes in patients whose physicians had such information compared with patients managed only by clinical response (107). Experience and open studies have indicated that there are blood AED concentrations most often associated with control and freedom from

TABLE 7.8. BLOOD ANTIEPILEPTIC DRUG MONITORING

- After starting drug at steady state
- When adding or subtracting an interacting drug
- When side effects are occurring
- When seizures break through
- Periodically to assess compliance

adverse effects, but these are based on population statistics, and do not apply to each individual patient. Consequently, most guidelines suggest concentrations of AEDs for effectiveness and freedom from side effects, yet many individuals obtain good control on low, or even "subtherapeutic" concentrations, and others may require and tolerate levels much higher. This principle applies to most, if not all, AEDs, and emphasizes that clinical outcome is the primary measure determining drug dosage. The desirable levels of drug with use of the new AEDs are not established, but there is no reason to believe they will not be as useful as has been proven true for the older drugs (108–110). The initial target concentrations of 2 to 5 μg/mL for drugs like GBP, LTG, and TPM probably were too low, and clinical experience suggests that maximal control while maintaining reasonable tolerability may not be realized until concentrations are in the 10- to 20-μg/mL range.

Safety Monitoring

In addition to obtaining blood AED levels, some testing for safety monitoring may be advisable. Initial evaluation of the cause of the epilepsy often will have included complete blood counts, liver function tests, blood urea nitrogen, and serum glucose and electrolytes. These values can serve as a baseline before initiating treatment. The utility of repeating these determinations on any regular basis is controversial (111). If the safety risks are relatively high, as with use of FLB, the manufacturer recommends regular monitoring. For rare idiosyncratic aplastic anemia, hepatitis, nephritis, or pancreatitis, it is unlikely regular testing is cost effective or clinically helpful. Rather, history and physical examination should provide evidence of systemic adverse effects to be further investigated with blood testing (112).

Compliance

Optimal drug selection, fine tuning of dosing based on pharmacokinetic properties, avoidance of adverse effects, and selection of the most suitable formulation all are of no value in seizure control if the patient does not take the medication as prescribed. The reasons for failure to take the AED are multiple and include denial of illness, insufficient education by medical personnel, subtle or expected adverse effects, complexity of regimen, and simple forgetfulness (112). Using electronic monitoring methods, Cramer et al. (70) found compliance fell off considerably with three- or four-times–daily prescribing, and whenever possible twice- or once-daily administration should be used. For drugs with a rapid absorption and short half-life, a slow-release formulation may allow such dosing and avoid peak/trough effects while enhancing compliance. Containers holding doses for each day or week as well as fitting intake to a fixed daily activity (e.g., meals, washing) also may be useful. Asking the patient when he or she takes the medication may reveal vagueness warranting further education. AED blood levels at clinic visits that are in the target range and refilling prescriptions at appropriate times are some indication of compliance, but do not mean medication is taken as prescribed. Patients may skip and later double-up on doses, a practice that may lead either to seizures or adverse effects despite the appearance of compliance. If breakthrough seizures occur, obtaining blood AED levels as soon as possible helps to determine if the drug or the patient has failed to maintain seizure control and possibly avert unnecessarily changing to another AED.

REFERENCES

1. Berg AT, Shinnar S. The risk of seizure recurrence following a first unprovoked seizure: a quantitative review. *Neurology* 1991; 41:965–972.
2. Hauser WA, Rich SS, Lee JR, et al. Risk of recurrent seizures after two unprovoked seizures. *N Engl J Med* 1998;338:429–434.
3. Commission on Classification and Terminology of the International League Against Epilepsy. Proposal for revised clinical and electroencephalographic classification of epileptic seizures. *Epilepsia* 1981;22:489–501.
4. Commission on Classification and Terminology of the International League Against Epilepsy. Proposal for revised classification of epilepsies and epileptic syndromes. *Epilepsia* 1989;30: 389–399.
5. Elwes R, Johnson AL, Shorvon SD, et al. The prognosis for seizure control in newly controlled epilepsy. *N Engl J Med* 1984;311:944–947.
6. Kwan P, Brodie MJ. Effectiveness of the first antiepileptic drug. *Epilepsia* 2001;42:1255–1261.
7. Mattson RH, Cramer JA, Collins JF, and the Department of Veterans Affairs Epilepsy Cooperative Studies No. 118 and No. 264 Groups. Prognosis for total control of complex partial and secondarily generalized tonic-clonic seizures. *Neurology* 1996; 47:68–76.
8. Cramer JA, Mattson RH. Quantitative approaches to seizure severity. In: Meinardi H, Cramer JA, Baker GA, et al., eds. New York: Plenum Press, 55–71.
9. Baker GA, Camfield C, Camfield P, et al. ILAE Commission report: Commission on Outcome Measures in Epilepsy 1994–1997. *Epilepsia* 1998;39:213–231.
10. Mattson RH. Monotherapy trials: endpoints. *Epilepsy Res* 2001; 45:1109–1117.
11. Pellock JM, Brodie MJ. Felbamate: 1997 update. *Epilepsia* 1997;38:1261–1264.
12. Mattson RH, et al. Comparison of carbamazepine, phenobarbital, phenytoin, and primidone in partial and secondarily generalized tonic/clonic seizures. *N Engl J Med* 1985;313:145–151.
13. Mattson RH, Cramer JA, Collins JF, et al. A comparison of valproate with carbamazepine for the treatment of complex partial seizures and secondarily generalized tonic/clonic seizures in adults. *N Engl J Med* 1992;327:765–771
14. Heller AJ, Chesterman P, Elwes RD, et al. Phenobarbitone, phenytoin, carbamazepine or sodium valproate for newly diagnosed adult epilepsy: a randomized comparative monotherapy trial. *J Neurol Neurosurg Psychiatry* 1995;58:44–50.
15. Richens A, Davidson DL, Cartlidge NE, et al. A multicentre comparative trial of sodium valproate and carbamazepine in adult onset epilepsy. *J Neurol Neurosurg Psychiatry* 1994;57: 682–687.
16. Sachdeo R, Kramer PLD, Rosenberg A, et al. Felbamate monotherapy for partial onset seizures. *Ann Neurol* 1992;32: 386–392.
17. Brodie MJ, Richens A, Yeun AW. Double-blind comparison of lamotrigine and carbamazepine in newly diagnosed epilepsy. *Lancet* 1995;345:476–479.
18. Steiner TJ, Dellaportas CI, Findley LJ, et al. lamotrigine monotherapy in newly diagnosed untreated epilepsy: a double-blind, randomized comparison with phenytoin. *Epilepsia* 1999; 40:601–607.
19. Dam M, Ekberg R, Loyning Y, et al. A double-blind study comparing oxcarbazepine and carbamazepine in patients with newly diagnosed, previously untreated epilepsy. *Epilepsy Res* 1989;3:70–76.
20. Christe W, Gunter K, Vigonius U, et al. A double-blind controlled clinical trial: oxcarbazepine versus sodium valproate in adults with newly diagnosed epilepsy. *Epilepsy Res* 1997;26: 451–460.
21. Bill PA, Vigonius U, Pohlmann H, et al. A double-blind controlled clinical trial of oxcarbazepine versus phenytoin in adults with previously untreated epilepsy. *Epilepsy Res* 1997;27:195–204.
22. Privitera MD, Brodie MJ, Mattson RH, et al. Topiramate, carbamazepine and valproate monotherapy: a double-blind comparison in the spectrum of newly diagnosed epilepsy (*in press*).
23. Brodie MJ, Chadwick DW, Anhut H, et al., and the Gabapentin Study Group 945-212. Gabapentin versus lamotrigine: a double-blind comparison in newly diagnosed epilepsy. *Epilepsia* (*in press*).
24. Kalvianien R, Aikia M, Saukkonen AM, et al. Vigabatrin vs carbamazepine monotherapy in patients with newly diagnosed epilepsy. *Arch Neurol* 1995;52:989–996.
25. Chadwick DW, and the Vigabatrin European Monotherapy Study Group. Safety and efficacy of vigabatrin and carbamazepine in newly diagnosed epilepsy: a multicentre, randomized double-blind study. *Lancet* 1999;354:13–19.
26. Chadwick DW, Anhut H, Greiner MJ, et al. A double-blind trial of gabapentin monotherapy for newly diagnosed partial seizures. *Neurology* 1998;51:1282–1288.
27. Brodie MJ, Overstall PW, Giorgi L, et al. Multicentre, double-blind, randomized comparison between lamotrigine and carbamazepine in elderly patients with newly diagnosed epilepsy. *Epilepsy Res* 1999;37:81–87.
28. Callaghan N, Kenny RA, O'Neill B, et al. A prospective study between carbamazepine, phenytoin and sodium valproate as monotherapy in previously untreated and recently diagnosed patients with epilepsy. *J Neurol Neurosurg Psychiatry* 1985;48: 639–644.
29. Turnbull DM, Rawlins MD, Weightman D, et al. A comparison of phenytoin and valproate in previously untreated adult epileptic patients. *J Neurol Neurosurg Psychiatry* 1982;45:55–59.
30. Ramsay RE, Wilder BJ, Berger JR, et al. A double-blind study comparing carbamazepine with phenytoin as initial seizure therapy in adults. *Neurology* 1983;33:904–910.
31. Wilder BJ, Ramsay E, Murphy JV, et al. Comparison of valproic acid and phenytoin in newly diagnosed tonic-clonic seizures. *Neurology* 1983;33:1474–1476.
32. Mattson RH, Cramer JA. Crossover from polytherapy to monotherapy in primary generalized epilepsy. *Am J Med* 1988; 84:23–28.
33. Scottish Intercollegiate Guidelines Network (SIGN). *Diagnosis and management of epilepsy in adults*. Edinburgh: SIGN, 1997.
34. Sherwin AL. ESM: clinical use. In: Levy RH, Mattson RH, Meldrum BS, eds. *Antiepileptic drugs*, 4th ed. New York: Raven Press, 1995:667–673.
35. Sato S, White BG, Penry JK, et al. Valproic versus ESM in the treatment of absence seizures. *Neurology* 1982;32:157–153.

36. Villareal HJ, Wilder BJ, Willmore LJ, et al. Effect of valproic acid on spike-wave discharges in patients with absence seizures. *Neurology* 1978;28:886–891.

37. Buoni S, Grosso S, Fois A. Lamotrigine in typical absence epilepsy. *Brain Dev* 1999;21:303–306.

38. Gericke CA, Picard F, de Saint-Martin A, et al. Efficacy of lamotrigine in idiopathic generalized epilepsy syndromes: a video-EEG-controlled, open study. *Epileptic Disord* 1999;1:159–165.

39. Frank LM, Enlow T, Holmes GL, et al. Lamictal (lamotrigine) monotherapy for typical absences in children. *Epilepsia* 2000; 41:357–359.

40. Panayiotopoulos CP. Treatment of typical absence seizures and related epileptic syndromes. *Paediatr Drugs* 2001;3:379–403.

41. Wheless JW. Use of topiramate in childhood generalized seizure disorders. *J Child Neurol* 2000;15[Suppl 1]:S7–S13.

42. French JA. The role of the new antiepileptic drugs. *Am J Manag Care* 2001;7[Suppl]:S209–S214.

43. Shields WD, Saslow E. Myoclonic, atonic and absence seizures following institution of carbamazepine therapy in children. *Neurology* 1983;33:1487–1489.

44. Perucca E, Gram L, Avanzini G, et al. Antiepileptic drugs as a cause of worsening seizures. *Epilepsia* 1998;39:5–17.

45. Convanis A, Gupta AK, Jeavons PM. Sodium valproate: monotherapy and polytherapy. *Epilepsia* 1982;23:693–720.

46. Delgado-Escueta AV, Enrile-Bascal F. Juvenile myoclonic epilepsy of Janz. *Neurology* 1984;34:285–294.

47. Bourgeois B, Beaumanoir A, Blasjev B, et al. Monotherapy with valproate in primary generalized epilepsies. *Epilepsia* 1987;28 [Suppl 2]:S8–S11.

48. Penry JK, Dean JC, Riela AR. Juvenile myoclonic epilepsy: long term response to therapy. *Epilepsia* 1989;30[Suppl 14]: 519–523.

49. Panayiotopoulos CP, Obeid T, Tahan AR. Juvenile myoclonic epilepsy: a 5-year prospective study. *Epilepsia* 1994;35: 285–296.

50. Janz D, Durner M. Juvenile myoclonic epilepsy. In: Engel J, Pedley TA, eds. *A textbook of epilepsy*. Philadelphia: Lippincott–Raven, 1997:2389–2400.

51. Genton P, Gelisse P, Thomas MD, et al. Do carbamazepine and phenytoin aggravate juvenile myoclonic epilepsy? *Neurology* 2000;55:1106–1109.

52. Biraben A, Allain H, Scarabin JM, et al. Exacerbation of juvenile myoclonic epilepsy with lamotrigine. *Neurology* 2000;55: 1758.

53. The Felbamate Study Group in Lennox-Gastaut Syndrome. Efficacy of felbamate in childhood epileptic encephalopathy (Lennox-Gastaut syndrome). *N Engl J Med* 1993;328:29–33.

54. Messenheimer J, Mullens EL, Giorgi I, et al. Safety review of adult clinical trial experience with lamotrigine. *Drug Saf* 1998; 18:281–296.

55. Kenneback G, Bergfeldt L, Vallin H, et al. Electrophysiologic effects and clinical hazards of carbamazepine treatment for neurologic disorders in patients with abnormalities of the cardiac conduction system. *Am Heart J* 1991;121:1421–1429.

56. Mattson RH. Carbamazepine. In: Engel J, Pedley TA, eds. *A textbook of epilepsy*. Philadelphia: Lippincott–Raven, 1997.

57. Sato Y, Kondo I, Ishida S, et al. Decreased bone mass and increased bone turnover with valproate therapy in adults with epilepsy. *Neurology* 2001;57:445–449.

58. Mattson RH, Cramer JA, McCutchen CM, and the VA Cooperative Epilepsy Study Group. Barbiturate related connective tissue disorders *Arch Intern Med* 1989;149:911–914.

59. Eke T, Talbot JF, Lawden MC. Severe persistent visual field constriction associated with vigabatrin. *BMJ* 1997;314:180–181.

60. Mattson RH, Cramer JA, Collins JF. Early tolerance to antiepileptic drug side effects: a controlled trial of 247 patients. In: Koella WP, et al., eds. *Tolerance to beneficial andor adverse effects of antiepileptic drugs*. New York: Raven Press, 1986:149–156.

61. Bialer M, et al. Progress report on new antiepileptic drugs: a summary of the Fourth Eilat Conference (EILAT IV). *Epilepsy Res* 1999;34:1–41.

62. Bialer M, Johannessen SI, Kupferberg HJ, et al. Progress report on new antiepileptic drugs: a summary of the Fifth Eilat Conference (EILAT V). *Epilepsy Res* 2001;43:11–58.

63. Marson AG, et al. New antiepileptic drugs: a systematic review of their efficacy and tolerability. *BMJ* 1996;313:1169–1174.

64. Cramer JA, et al. New antiepileptic drugs: comparison of key clinical trials. *Epilepsia* 1999;40:590–600.

65. Marson AG, Hutton JL, Leach JP, et al. Levetiracetam, oxcarbazepine, remacemide and zonisamide for drug resistant localization-related epilepsy: a systematic review. *Epilepsy Res* 2001; 46:259–270.

66. Cramer JA, Ben-Menachem EB, French J. Review of treatment options for refractory epilepsy and vagal nerve stimulation. *Epilepsy Res* 2001;47:17–25.

67. Meador KJ, Loring DW, Hun K, et al. Comparative cognitive effects of anticonvulsants. *Neurology* 1990;40:391–394.

68. Vining EPG, Mellits FD, Dorsen MM, et al. Psychologic and behavioral effects of antiepileptic drugs in children: a double-blind comparison between phenobarbital and valproic acid. *Pediatrics* 1987;80[Suppl 1]:165–174.

69. Prevey ML, Delaney RC, Cramer JA, et al. The effect of valproate on cognitive functioning: a comparison with carbamazepine. *Arch Neurol* 1996;53:1008–1016.

70. Cramer JA, Mattson RH, et al. How often is medication taken as prescribed? A novel assessment technique. *JAMA* 1989;261: 3273–3277.

71. Perucca E. The clinical pharmacokinetics of the new antiepileptic drugs. *Epilepsia* 1999;40[Suppl 9]:S7–S13.

72. Kocsis JD, Mattson RH. GABA levels in the brain: a target for new antiepileptic drugs. *Neuroscientist* 1996;2:326–334.

73. Mattson RH. Selection of antiepileptic drug therapy. In: Levy RH, Mattson RH, Meldrum B, eds. *Antiepileptic drugs*, 4th ed. New York: Raven Press, 1995:123–135.

74. Sommerfeld-Ziskin E, Ziskin E. Effect of phenobarbital on the mentality of epileptic patients. *Arch Neurol Psychiatry* 1940;43: 70–79.

75. Mattson RH, Cramer JA, and the VA Cooperative Study Group. Seizure remission after active epilepsy. *Epilepsia* 1990; 31:648(abstr).

76. Faught E, Sachdeo RC, Remler MP, et al. Felbamate monotherapy for partial onset seizures: an active control trial. *Neurology* 1993;41:1785–1789.

77. Bourgeois B, Leppik IE, Sackellares JC, et al. Felbamate: a double-blind controlled trial in patients undergoing presurgical evaluation in partial seizures. *Neurology* 1993;43:693–696.

78. Bergey GK, Morris HH, Rosenfeld W, et al., and the U.S. Gabapentin Study Group 88/89. Gabapentin monotherapy: I. an 8-day, double-blind, dose-controlled, multicenter study in hospitalized patients with refractory complex partial and secondarily generalized seizures. *Neurology* 1997;49:739–745.

79. Beydoun A, Fischer J, Labar DR, et al., and the U.S. Gabapentin Study Group 82/83. Gabapentin monotherapy: II. a 26-week, double-blind, dose-controlled, multicenter study of conversion from polytherapy in outpatients with refractory complex partial or secondarily generalized seizures. *Neurology* 1997;49:746–752.

80. Chadwick DW, Liederman DB, Sauerman W, et al. Gabapentin in generalized seizures. *Epilepsy Res* 1996;25:191–197.

81. Gillam F, Vasquez B, Sackellares JC, et al. An active-control trial of lamotrigine monotherapy for partial seizures. *Neurology* 1998;51:1018–1025.

82. Edwards KR, Sackellares JC, Vuong A, et al. Lamotrigine monotherapy improves depressive symptoms in epilepsy: a double-blind comparison with valproate. *Epilepsy Behav* 2001;2: 28–36.

83. Klitgard H, Matagne A, Gobert J, et al. Evidence for a unique profile of levetiracetam in rodent models of seizures and epilepsy. *Eur J Pharmacol* 1998;353:191–206.

84. Privitera M. Efficacy of levetiracetam: a review of three pivotal trials. *Epilepsia* 2001;42[Suppl 4]:S31–S35.

85. French J, Edrich P, Cramer JA. A systematic review of the safety profile of levetiracetam: a new antiepileptic drug. *Epilepsy Res* 2001;47:77–90.

86. Beydoun A, Sachdeo RC, Rosenfeld WE, et al. Oxcarbazepine monotherapy of partial-onset seizures: a multicenter, double-blind, clinical trial. *Neurology* 2000;54:2245–2251.

87. Sachdeo R, Beydoun A, Schacter S, et al. Oxcarbazepine (Trileptal) as monotherapy in patients with partial seizures. *Neurology* 2001;57:864–871.

88. Schachter SC, Vasquez B, Fisher RS, et al. Oxcarbazepine: a double-blind, randomized, placebo-control, monotherapy trial for partial seizures. *Neurology* 1999;52:732–737.

89. Beran RG. Cross-reactive skin eruptions with both carbamazepine and oxcarbazepine. *Epilepsia* 1993;34:163–165.

90. Kalviainen R, Brodie MJ, Duncan J, et al. A double-blind, placebo-controlled trial of TGB given three-times daily as add-on therapy for refractory partial seizures: Northern European TGB Study Group. *Epilepsy Res* 1998;30:31–40.

91. Uthman BM, Rowan AJ, Ahmann PA, et al. TGB for complex partial seizures: a randomized, add-on, dose-response trial. *Arch Neurol* 1998;55:56–62.

92. Schacter SC. TGB monotherapy in the treatment of partial epilepsy. *Epilepsia* 1995;36[Suppl 6]:S2–S6.

93. Dodrill CB, Arnett JL, Sommerville KW, et al. Cognitive and quality of life effects of differing dosages of TGB in epilepsy. *Neurology* 1997;48:1025–1031.

94. Sachdeo RC, Reife RA, Lim P, et al. Topiramate monotherapy for partial onset seizures. *Epilepsia* 1997;38:294–300.

95. Biton V, et al. A randomized, placebo-controlled study of topiramate in primary generalized tonic-clonic seizures. *Neurology* 1999;52:1330–1337.

96. Aldenkamp AP, Baker G, Mulder OG. et al. A multicenter clinical study to evaluate the effect on cognitive function of topiramate compared with valproate as add-on therapy to carbamazepine in patients with partial-onset seizures. *Epilepsia* 2000; 41:1167–1178.

97. Banta JT, Hoffman K, Budenz DL, et al. Presumed topiramate-induced bilateral acute angle-closure glaucoma. *Am J Ophthalmol* 2001;132:112–114.

98. Krauss GI, Johnson MA, Miller NR. Vigabatrin associated retinal cone system dysfunction: electroretinogram and ophthalmologic findings. *Neurology* 1998;50:614–618.

99. Faught E, Ayala R, Montouris GG, et al. Randomized controlled trial of zonisamide for the treatment of refractory partial-onset seizures. *Neurology* 2001;57:1774–1779.

100. Henry TR, Leppik IE, Gumnit RJ, et al. Progressive myoclonic epilepsies treated with zonisamide. *Neurology* 1988;38: 928–931.

101. Kyllerman M, Ben-Menachem E. Zonisamide for progressive myoclonus epilepsy. *Epilepsy Res* 1998;29:109–114.

102. Perucca E, Dulac O, Shorvon S, et al. Harnessing the clinical potential of antiepileptic drug therapy: dosage optimization. *CNS Drugs* 2001;15:609–621.

103. Porter RJ. How to use antiepileptic drugs. In: Levy RH, Mattson RH, Meldrum BS, eds. *Antiepieptic drugs*, 4th ed. New York: Raven Press, 1995:137–148.

104. Spencer SS, Packey DJ. Antiepileptic drug management before and after epilepsy surgery. In: Levy RH, Mattson RH, Meldrum BS, eds. *Antiepileptic drugs*, 4th ed. New York: Raven Press, 1995:189–200.

105. Crawford P, Hall WW, Chapell B, et al. Generic prescribing for epilepsy: is it safe? *Seizure* 1996;5:1–5.

106. Nuwer MR, Browne, TR, Dodson WE, et al. Generic substitutions for antiepileptic drugs. *Neurology* 1990;40:1647–1651.

107. Jannuzzi G, Cian P, Fattore C, et al. A multicenter randomized controlled trial on the clinical impact of therapeutic monitoring in patients with newly diagnosed epilepsy: the Italian TDM Study Group in Epilepsy. *Epilepsia* 2000;41:222–230.

108. Perucca E. Is there a role for therapeutic drug monitoring of new anticonvulsants? *Clin Pharmacokinet* 2000;38:191–204.

109. Tomson T, Johannessen SI. Therapeutic monitoring of the new antiepileptic drugs. *Eur J Clin Pharmacol* 2000;55:697–705.

110. Mattson RH. Antiepileptic drug monitoring: a reappraisal. *Epilepsia* 1995;36[Suppl 5]:S22–S29.

111. Pellock JM, Willmore LJ. A rational guide to routine blood monitoring in patients receiving antiepileptic drugs. *Neurology* 1991;41:961–964.

112. Cramer JA, Mattson R. Compliance with antiepileptic drug therapy. In: Levy RH, Mattson RH, Meldrum BS, eds. *Antiepileptic drugs*, 4th ed. New York: Raven Press, 1995: 149–159.

8

GENERAL PRINCIPLES

COMBINATION THERAPY AND DRUG INTERACTIONS

EMILIO PERUCCA
RENÉ H. LEVY

Up to the early 1970s, the use of combination therapy was standard practice among neurologists treating people with epilepsy: for example, a survey conducted in four European countries in 1975 showed that each patient received an average of 3.2 drugs, of which more than two-thirds were anticonvulsants (1). This practice was based on the never-proven assumption that the simultaneous prescription of two or more antiepileptic drugs (AEDs) ensured synergistic therapeutic activity while protecting against the risk of excessive toxicity. Phenobarbital and phenytoin were by far the most commonly coprescribed drugs, to the extent that many AED preparations available on the market at the time contained fixed-ratio combinations of these agents (2). There were other reasons for prescribing more than one drug at the same time. Because of the lack of broad-spectrum agents, patients with multiple seizure types often required combination therapy to obtain complete control of their seizures, the best example being the use of ethosuximide and phenobarbital to suppress absence and tonic-clonic seizures, respectively. It was also not uncommon to prescribe additional central nervous system (CNS) medications, such as bromide, atropine, caffeine, and amphetamine, in an attempt to potentiate antiepileptic efficacy or to counteract the sedative effects of first-line AEDs (2).

Unfortunately, the goal of seizure freedom with little or no toxicity was seldom achieved with these therapies. Some patients failed to achieve seizure control when excessively low dosages were prescribed, and the subsequent attempt to use higher dosages of multiple medications often resulted in unacceptable toxicity. In a comprehensive review from those times, Reynolds (3) was alarmed by the frequency and severity of side effects of AED therapy and identified poly-

therapy and use of high dosages as the main factors responsible for iatrogenic disease in patients with chronic epilepsy. This realization paved the way to a series of investigations in which the advantages of monotherapy became all too evident. It was fortunate that this development coincided with the availability of novel information on the importance of pharmacokinetic principles and on value of serum AED level monitoring, which allowed the use of individual anticonvulsants in a more efficient way.

In a landmark study, Shorvon and coworkers (4) assessed prospectively the value of phenytoin and carbamazepine monotherapy, assisted by serum level monitoring, in 51 patients with newly diagnosed partial or generalized tonic-clonic seizures. After a follow-up of 28 months (for phenytoin) or 12 months (for carbamazepine), 76% to 88% of these patients had their seizures completely controlled, a finding leading to the conclusion that "polypharmacy is largely, and possibly totally, unnecessary in newly diagnosed adult epileptics." Many subsequent studies have confirmed that monotherapy is effective and well tolerated both in adults and in children. Although response rates vary greatly in relation to seizure type and syndromic form, between 50% and 90% of patients with newly diagnosed epilepsy can have their seizures fully controlled using one appropriate drug at individualized dosages (6–13). Other studies have shown that, even in patients with chronic refractory epilepsy, reduction of polypharmacy often can be achieved successfully without deterioration in seizure control, and with appreciable benefit in terms of a lessened burden of side effects (14).

Based on the foregoing evidence, no physician currently will question the principle that the treatment of epilepsy should be optimally started with a single drug (15,16). Realization of the many advantages of monotherapy (Table 8.1), however, should not lead one to consider combination therapy as an evil to be avoided at all costs. Indeed, it has been convincingly shown that not all patients can be successfully managed with monotherapy, and in some situa-

Emilio Perucca, MD, PhD: Department of Internal Medicine and Therapeutics, Clinical Pharmacology Unit, University of Pavia, Pavia, Italy

René H. Levy, PhD: Professor and Chair, Department of Pharmaceutics; and Professor of Neurological Surgery, University of Washington School of Pharmacy and Medicine, Seattle, Washington

TABLE 8.1. ADVANTAGES OF MONOTHERAPY

- Effective seizure control in most patients
- Minimization of side effects
- Easier clinical management (response easily correlated to the prescribed drug)
- Avoidance of adverse drug interactions
- Simpler treatment schedule (better compliance)
- Lower treatment cost

tions the simultaneous use of more than one drug is necessary to obtain the best clinical response (17,18).

The present chapter provides a critical overview of the current role of combination therapy in the treatment of epilepsy. An attempt is made to identify situations in which multiple drug therapy is indicated and to provide information about specific drug combinations that may be particularly useful, as well as combinations that should be preferably avoided. Finally, brief consideration is given to the potential implications of combining AED therapy with other medications that a patient may require for unrelated medical conditions, such as hypertension, infection, or the need for contraception. Because the use of multiple drug therapy involves the possibility of pharmacokinetic and pharmacodynamic interactions, the basic principles underlying the mechanisms, prediction, and management of such interactions are briefly discussed.

WHEN SHOULD COMBINATION ANTIEPILEPTIC DRUG THERAPY BE USED?

As discussed earlier, there is consensus that combination AED therapy should be reserved for those patients whose seizures cannot successfully be controlled with a single drug. However, this statement fails to identify the precise moment at which combination therapy should actually be introduced in the treatment algorithm. Should AED combinations be used in patients who fail to respond to maximally tolerated doses of one initially prescribed AED, or should these combinations be reserved for those patients whose seizures persist despite sequential use of two or more AEDs, each given as monotherapy? There seems to be considerable variation in the attitude of prescribing physicians toward these strategies. For example, in a survey in 14 Mediterranean countries, the proportion of neurologists opting for combination therapy (instead of using alternative monotherapy) when initial monotherapy had failed ranged from 23% in France to 67% in Syria: in many countries, including Turkey, Greece, and Italy, physicians were almost equally divided in their attitude toward early introduction of polypharmacy (19).

A review of evidence from prospective studies provides valuable clues regarding when combination drug therapy should be preferentially tried. In what is perhaps the most frequently quoted abstract in the history of epileptology, Hakkarainen (20) randomized a total of 100 patients with newly diagnosed convulsive seizures to either carbamazepine or phenytoin and found that, after 1 year, 50 patients continued to have seizures while they were receiving the allocated treatment. When these patients were switched to monotherapy with the alternative drug, 17 (34%) became seizure free. Of the 33 patients who were refractory to *both* phenytoin and carbamazepine as monotherapy, only five (15%) had their seizures controlled when the two drugs were tried together. These results clearly indicate that a substantial proportion of patients refractory to an initial drug can have their seizures controlled by switching to alternative monotherapy, and only a few patients do well with combination therapy. Although the design of this study may be criticized on the grounds that carbamazepine and phenytoin, sharing a similar mechanism of action and CNS side effect profiles, may not be ideal drugs to combine, other studies support the conclusion that alternative monotherapy has significant merits in patients refractory to a single drug. In a randomized comparison of vigabatrin and carbamazepine in patients with newly diagnosed partial epilepsy, 11 of 25 (44%) patients who failed to respond to initial monotherapy had their seizures fully controlled when they were switched to monotherapy with the alternative drug (21). Only five of the 14 patients refractory to two sequential monotherapies had their seizures controlled by the same two drugs in combination. In a larger, single-center observational study, 67 of 248 patients (27%) refractory to initial monotherapy were rendered seizure free with a second or third drug used as monotherapy, and only 12 had their seizures controlled by combination therapy (13). An interim analysis of an ongoing randomizing study comparing add-on therapy with alternative monotherapy also failed to show major outcome differences between these two strategies (22). In other studies in which patients refractory to initial treatment were switched to combination therapy (18,23–26), response rates are generally comparable to those described for patients managed with alternative monotherapy, but the burden of side effects tends to be greater in patients receiving more than one drug (6). Thus, it is clear that alternative monotherapy is associated with a significant probability of therapeutic success when the initially prescribed AED has failed, and therefore it should be the preferred strategy in these patients. Although it could be argued that the early addition (rather than the substitution) of a second drug will allow more rapid achievement of seizure control in the small subgroup of patients who do require combination therapy, such a policy would expose to a high risk of adverse effects many patients whose seizures could be managed with a single drug.

Based on the evidence discussed earlier, it appears reasonable to restrict the use of combination therapy to those patients in whom sequential therapies with *at least* two appropriate AEDs, each prescribed at the maximally tolerated dosage (25), have failed. The value of adding a second and, sometimes, even a third drug in patients with long-standing refractory epilepsy is documented by many placebo-controlled add-on trials of newer AEDs (27–30), even though one cannot exclude that, at least in some of these patients, an improvement in seizure frequency could have been obtained by simply increasing the doses of baseline medication. In general, between 20% and 50% of patients with refractory partial epilepsies or symptomatic generalized epilepsies are expected to benefit from AED combinations (18,29), although the actual proportion of those who will be free of seizures will be considerably smaller, typically less than 20%. Earlier, more aggressive use of combination therapy may be justified in occasional cases, for example, in patients with notoriously refractory epilepsy syndromes.

Although the benefit of combination therapy in a subgroup of patients with difficult-to-treat epilepsies cannot be questioned, one should be cautious about the risk of overtreatment (16,31). Use of more than one drug, especially when high doses are administered, leads to a greater burden in terms of side effects (32), and it is important to evaluate in the individual patient whether the price paid in terms of greater toxicity is justified by the improvement in seizure control. In patients with chronic epilepsy, seizure frequency fluctuates over time, and it is not uncommon for a second AED to be added during a period of spontaneous exacerbation: under these conditions, the subsequent improvement in seizure frequency may be related to spontaneous amelioration (the so-called *regression to the mean*), rather than to the effect of the added drug (33). Because of this situation, the need for maintaining combination therapy should be reassessed at regular intervals, and monotherapy should be reinstituted whenever appropriate. Moreover, in some patients, the addition of a second drug may cause a paradoxical increase in seizure frequency as a manifestation of drug toxicity (23,34): failure to recognize this may lead to a vicious circle whereby a further increase in AED load produces even less seizure control.

ARE SOME ANTIEPILEPTIC DRUG COMBINATIONS BETTER THAN OTHERS?

From a theoretical standpoint, combining two drugs may lead to additive, supraadditive (synergistic), or infraadditive effects. An AED combination would be desirable if it produces supraadditive antiepileptic efficacy in the presence of simply additive toxicity or additive efficacy in the presence of infraadditive toxicity. In a series of careful studies, Bourgeois and coworkers (35–39) looked at pharmacodynamic effects of various combinations of conventional AEDs in animal models and failed to provide evidence of definitely

favorable interactions, except for valproate-ethosuximide (38) and, possibly, valproate-carbamazepine (39) combinations, which were associated with additive anticonvulsant activity and infraadditive toxicity. Results of studies of some of the newer AEDs suggest supraadditive anticonvulsant effects with some combinations (40,41), but the clinical relevance of these findings is difficult to assess, partly because we lack reliable models for predicting human neurotoxicity. Animal studies may be useful to generate hypotheses, but the ultimate demonstration of the usefulness of specific combinations can come only from the clinic.

Although it has been proposed that combining AEDs with different mechanisms of action should be therapeutically beneficial (42), in practice, our knowledge of the mechanisms of action of the various drugs, most of which have more than one primary action, is too incomplete to allow a rational application of this approach (27). Thus, AEDs are usually combined mainly on empirical grounds, by taking into consideration several general rules (Table 8.2). Clinical experience does suggest that some AED combinations may have a superior therapeutic index compared with others, the evidence being particularly convincing for valproate combined with ethosuximide in patients with refractory absence seizures (43) and for valproate combined with lamotrigine in patients with various refractory seizure

TABLE 8.2. CRITERIA FOR SELECTION OF ANTIEPILEPTIC DRUG COMBINATIONS

- Use AED combinations only when monotherapy with at least two appropriate drugs at maximally tolerated dosages failed to control seizures.
- Try to avoid combination of AEDs with closely overlapping side effect profiles. By converse, exploit potential antagonism for certain undesired effects (e.g., an AED that has caused weight gain may be combined usefully with an AED known to cause weight loss).
- Consider AED combinations for which there is clinical evidence of a favorable therapeutic index (e.g., valproate and ethosuximide, or valproate and lamotrigine).
- If a patient has multiple seizure types, use AEDs whose combined efficacy spectrum will provide protection against all seizures.
- Be aware of potentially adverse AED interactions, and adjust dosage if appropriate. Monitoring serum AED concentrations may be indicated.
- Observe carefully clinical response and individualize dosage as appropriate. If long-term response is unsatisfactory, reinstitute monotherapy or switch to an alternative combination.
- Remember that in many patients responding well to polytherapy, in may be possible to discontinue gradually the initial drug and reinstitute monotherapy.

AED, antiepileptic drug.
Modified from Genton P, Roger J. Antiepileptic drug monotherapy versus polytherapy: A historical perspective. *Epilepsia* 1997;38 (suppl. 5):S2–S5, with permission.

TABLE 8.3. SOME ANTIEPILEPTIC DRUGS COMBINATIONS CLAIMED TO BE PARTICULARLY ADVANTAGEOUS

Combination	Seizure Type	Level of Evidence	Reference
Valproate–carbamazepine	Partial	Extensive clinical experience but few controlled studies	Brodie and Mumford (42) Harden et al. (50) Walker and Koon (59)
Valproate–ethosuximide	Absence	Well documented	Rowan et al. (43)
Valproate–lamotrigine	Various	Well documented	Brodie et al. (44), Ferrie et al. (46) Panayiotopulos et al. (45), Pisani et al. (47)
Carbamazepine–vigabatrin	Partial	Speculative	Brodie and Mumford (42)
Lamotrigine–vigabatrin	Partial	Controversial	Stolarek et al. (51)
Tiagabine–vigabatrin	Partial	Anecdotal	Leach and Brodie (52)
Gabapentin–lamotrigine	Partial	Anecdotal	Pisani et al. (53)
Lamotrigine–topiramate	Partial	Anecdotal	Stephens et al. (54)

types (44–47). With these combinations, pharmacodynamic mechanisms of interaction are assumed to be at play, although pharmacokinetic changes may simultaneous occur. In a trial that clearly illustrates the complexities of these interactions, Pisani and coworkers (47) evaluated prospectively 13 patients with refractory complex partial seizures who had failed to respond to maximally tolerated dosages of either valproate or lamotrigine given separately. When the two drugs were given together, four patients became seizure free, and an additional four patients experienced seizure reductions of 62% to 78%. Although the addition of valproate to lamotrigine initially produced an increase in serum lamotrigine levels, the appearance of side effects, especially tremor, required a reduction in dose of both medications, and seizure control was finally achieved at serum drug concentrations that were lower than those achieved before combination therapy was instituted. Potential advantages have been claimed for other combinations (Table 8.3), but the evidence is mostly anecdotal, and interindividual variation can be considerable.

COMBINATION THERAPY AND DRUG INTERACTIONS

As discussed earlier, concomitant use of medications leads to the possible occurrence of drug interactions. Traditionally, these are classified into two groups: (a) pharmacokinetic interactions, which involve a change in the absorption, distribution, or elimination of the affected drug; and (b) pharmacodynamic interactions, which are thought to result in a change in pharmacologic response at the site of action. Interaction may occur between or among two or more AEDs, when they are used in combination therapy, or between AEDs and other drugs used for unrelated conditions. The following sections provide a brief overview on some important issues related to the mechanisms and management of drug interaction in patients with epilepsy.

PHARMACODYNAMIC INTERACTIONS

Unlike pharmacokinetic interactions, which usually involve an easily measured change in the blood concentration of the affected drug, pharmacodynamic interactions manifest themselves by a change in pharmacologic response that may be difficult to characterize objectively. This situation explains why these interactions have been investigated incompletely, even though their clinical relevance is probably considerable. As mentioned earlier, two drugs may interact pharmacodynamically, leading to additive, supraadditive, or infraadditive effects, at the level of both therapeutic response and toxicity (38,39).

Pharmacodynamic AED interactions may be adverse, neutral, or beneficial. Possibly favorable interactions are described earlier in the discussion of the preferential use of certain AED combinations. Adverse pharmacodynamic interactions, possibly explained by additive neurotoxicity (48), most often involve the appearance of CNS side effects in patients receiving polytherapy, even when the doses and blood levels of individual AEDs are in the low range. Just as some combinations seem to produce better therapeutic effects than others (43–47,49–54), evidence also indicates that certain specific combinations may be more likely to cause tolerability problems. For example, several studies have documented that the addition of lamotrigine to carbamazepine often results in symptoms suggestive of carbamazepine toxicity: this was initially explained as the possible result of a rise in serum carbamazepine-10,11-epoxide levels, but more recent studies indicate that the levels of this metabolite are unaffected by lamotrigine, and an adverse pharmacodynamic interaction is responsible for these manifestations (55).

PHARMACOKINETIC INTERACTIONS

Knowledge of the mechanisms underlying pharmacokinetic drug interactions expanded in the 1990s, and consequently it has become possible to develop a rational approach to their prediction. These interactions have been traditionally divided in three categories: interactions based on absorption, those based on distribution, and those based on elimination or metabolism. For AEDs, little information exists on interactions occurring within the lumen of the gastrointestinal tract. At the level of distribution, there is a significant body of literature on protein binding displacement, probably because of a lingering misconception that increases in the unbound fraction of a drug would result in increases in its unbound concentration and possibly enhanced toxicity. Eventually, it became apparent that AEDs have low extraction ratios, and thus changes in unbound fraction do not affect unbound concentrations. At the level of metabolism, significant qualitative predictions of changes in concentration of an AED became possible with a knowledge of the hepatic (and intestinal, if appropriate) enzymes responsible for its metabolic clearance (56). To characterize the effects of an AED on other drugs, it is necessary to define its inhibition and induction spectra.

ANTIEPILEPTIC DRUGS AS SUBSTRATES

Except for gabapentin, levetiracetam, and vigabatrin commonly used AEDs are metabolized by microsomal enzymes such as cytochromes P450 and glucuronyl transferases. Carbamazepine is a substrate for cytochromes CYP3A4 and some CYP2C isoforms, and this information is sufficient to explain increases in carbamazepine levels associated with coadministration of macrolide antibiotics (e.g., triacetyl oleandomycin, erythromycin, clarithromycin, roxithromycin, josamycin, azithromycin, flurithromycin, ponsinocycin, and spiramycin), diltiazem, verapamil, ketoconazole, danazol, propoxyphene, fluoxetine, fluvoxamine, and viloxazine (57). Induction of those isoforms (CYP3A4 and possibly CYP2Cs) explains the decreases in carbamazepine levels caused by phenytoin, phenobarbital, primidone, felbamate, and rifampicin.

Most of the fate of phenytoin is controlled by two enzymes, CYP2C9 and CYP2C19, and most of the drugs that elevate phenytoin levels are known inhibitors of one or both enzymes: amiodarone, phenylbutazone, miconazole, and sulfonamides inhibit CYP2C9, and cimetidine, felbamate, fluoxetine, omeprazole, ticlopidine, viloxazine, oxcarbazepine and topiramate inhibit CYP2C19, whereas fluconazole inhibits both enzymes (58). CYP3A4 contributes to the elimination of tiagabine and zonisamide (59,60), and induction of this isozyme explains the increase in the clearance of these drugs in patients receiving concomitant treatment with phenytoin, carbamazepine, phenobarbital and primidone. Although only a small fraction of the dose of topiramate is eliminated by oxidative metabolism in healthy subjects, induction of metabolism explains why the total clearance of topiramate is increased twofold when this drug is coadministered with phenytoin (61).

A glucuronosyltransferase, UGT1A4, plays an important role in the metabolism of lamotrigine, and most of a lamotrigine dose is recovered in urine in the form of a 5-*N*-glucuronide and a 2-*N*-glucuronide. This enzyme is inhibited by valproate, and it is induced (possibly with other glucuronosyltransferases) by phenytoin and carbamazepine. Coadministration of valproate is associated with appreciable elevations in lamotrigine levels, and, conversely, coadministration of inducers such as phenytoin, carbamazepine, or phenobarbital results in decreases in lamotrigine concentrations (62). Both types of interactions usually require dosage modifications.

Similarly, a significant portion of valproate clearance is controlled by glucuronidation, and this explains the decreases in valproate levels associated with phenytoin, carbamazepine, and phenobarbital (63). Oxcarbazepine is essentially a prodrug for the active 10-hydroxy metabolite resulting from reduction by a cytosolic enzyme. This metabolite is primarily glucuronidated, and its levels are also reduced in the presence of enzyme inducers (64).

ANTIEPILEPTIC DRUGS AS INHIBITORS

Some evidence indicates that oxcarbazepine topiramate, felbamate, valproate, and carbamazepine behave as weak inhibitors of the metabolism of phenytoin through the enzyme CYP2C19. This inhibition results in relatively small increases in phenytoin levels with appreciable intersubject variability.

Valproate is also a mild inhibitor of microsomal epoxide hydrolase, and its coadministration with carbamazepine is associated with elevations in carbamazepine-10,11-epoxide (65). The interaction of valproate with phenobarbital is associated with elevations in phenobarbital levels, probably caused by inhibition of uridine diphosphate glucosyltransferase (66). As mentioned earlier, another valproate inhibition interaction that requires attention is based on inhibition of UGT1A4 (and possibly other glucuronyl transferases), resulting in elevations in lamotrigine levels that usually require dosage adjustments (62).

ANTIEPILEPTIC DRUGS AS INDUCERS

In the field of drug interactions, phenobarbital, phenytoin, and carbamazepine rank among the most potent inducers of drug metabolism. They affect the disposition of many drugs, principally those that are substrates of CYP3A4 and CYP2C enzymes, as well as drugs metabolized by glucuronidation. The administration of phenobarbital, phenytoin, and carbamazepine is usually associated with decreases in levels of carbamazepine (heteroinduction and autoinduction) and other CYP3A4 substrates such as cyclosporine, oral contraceptives and corticosteroids. Oxcarbazepine, topiramate, and felbamate have a narrower spectrum of enzyme inducing activity, but they have also been found to reduce the blood levels of steroid oral contraceptives. As indicated earlier, the two AEDs that are eliminated principally by conjugation, valproate and lamotrigine, are induced by phenobarbital, phenytoin, and carbamazepine.

ROLES OF TRANSPORTERS

In the last few years, evidence has accumulated that transporters play a critical role in the disposition of some drugs and are involved in drug interactions. For example, P-glycoprotein, which had been initially characterized for its role in multidrug resistance in cancer chemotherapy, has been recognized to interact with many drugs (67). It functions as an efflux pump located in several tissues (intestinal wall, liver and biliary system, blood–brain barrier, kidney, and placenta). Digoxin is a substrate for P-glycoprotein, and inhibition of this pump by ketoconazole or quinidine is the probable mechanism for digoxin toxicity associated with these drug combinations. The roles of transporters in the disposition of AEDs is just emerging.

REFERENCES

1. Guelen PJM, Van der Klejin E, Woudstra U. Statistical analysis of pharmacokinetic parameters in epileptic patients chronically treated with antiepileptic drugs. In: Schneider H, Janz D, Gardner-Thorpe C, et al., eds. *Clinical pharmacology of antiepileptic drugs.* Berlin: Springer-Verlag, 1975:2–10.
2. Genton P, Roger J. Antiepileptic drug monotherapy versus polytherapy: a historical perspective. *Epilepsia* 1997;38[Suppl 5]:S2–S5.
3. Reynolds EH. Chronic antiepileptic toxicity: a review. *Epilepsia* 1975;16:319–352.
4. Shorvon SD, Chadwick D, Galbraith AW, et al. One drug for epilepsy. *BMJ* 1978;1:474–476.
5. Covanis A, Gupta AK, Jeavons PM. Sodium valproate: monotherapy and polytherapy. *Epilepsia* 1982;23:693–720.
6. Mattson RH, Cramer JA, Collins JF, et al. Comparison of carbamazepine, phenobarbital, phenytoin, and primidone in partial and secondarily generalized tonic-clonic seizures. *N Engl J Med* 1985;313:145–151.
7. Dulac O, Stern D, Rey E, et al. Sodium valproate monotherapy in childhood epilepsy. *Brain Dev* 1986;8:47–52.
8. Mattson RH, Cramer JA, Collins JF, et al. A comparison of valproate with carbamazepine for the treatment of complex partial seizures and secondarily generalized tonic-clonic seizures. *N Engl J Med* 1992;327:765–771.
9. De Silva M, MacArdle B, McGowan M, et al. Randomised comparative monotherapy trial of phenobarbitone, phenytoin, carbamazepine, or sodium valproate for newly diagnosed childhood epilepsy. *Lancet* 1996;347:709–713.
10. Heller AJ, Chesterman P, Elwes RDC, et al. Phenobarbitone, phenytoin, carbamazepine, or sodium valproate for newly diagnosed adult epilepsy: a randomised comparative monotherapy trial. *J Neurol Neurosurg Psychiatry* 1995;58:44–50.
11. Richens A, Davidson DLW, Cartlidge NEF, et al. A multicentre trial of sodium valproate and carbamazepine in adult-onset epilepsy. *J Neurol Neurosurg Psychiatry* 1994;57:682–687.
12. Verity CM, Hosking G, Easter DJ (on behalf of The Pediatric EPITEG Collaborative Group). A multicentre comparative trial of sodium valproate and carbamazepine in paediatric epilepsy. *Dev Med Child Neurol* 1995;37:977–108.
13. Kwan P, Brodie MJ. Early identification of refractory epilepsy. *N Engl J Med* 2000;342:314–319.
14. Shorvon S, Reynolds EH. Reduction in polypharmacy for epilepsy. *BMJ* 1979;2:1023–1025
15. Beghi E, Perucca E. The management of epilepsy in the 1990s: acquisitions, uncertainties and perspectives for future research. *Drugs* 1995;49:680–694.
16. Perucca E. Pharmacologic advantages of antiepileptic drug monotherapy. *Epilepsia* 1997;38[Suppl 5]:S6–S8.
17. Schmidt D, Gram L. Monotherapy versus polytherapy in epilepsy: a reappraisal. *CNS Drugs* 1995;3:194–208.
18. Krämer G. The limitations of antiepileptic drug monotherapy. *Epilepsia* 1997;38[Suppl 5]:S9–S13.
19. Baldy-Moulinier M, Covanis A, D'Urso S, et al. Therapeutic strategies against epilepsy in Mediterranean countries: a report from an international collaborative survey. *Seizure* 1998;7:513–520.
20. Hakkarainen H. Carbamazepine vs diphenylhydantoin vs their combination in adult epilepsy. *Neurology* 1980;30:354.
21. Tanganelli P, Regesta G. Vigabatrin vs carbamazepine monotherapy in newly diagnosed focal epilepsy: a randomized response conditional cross-over study. *Epilepsy Res* 1996;25:257–262.
22. Gatti G, for Biomed Add-on Study of Epilepsy (BASE). Randomized controlled study of alternative monotherapy versus add-on therapy in patients with refractory partial epilepsy: preliminary results. In: Velo G, Perucca E, eds. Abstracts of the VII World Conference on Clinical Pharmacology and Therapeutics and 4th Congress of the European Association for Clinical Pharmacology and Therapeutics, Florence, 15–20 July 2000. *Br J Clin Pharmacol* 2000: 180.
23. Schmidt D. Two antiepileptic drugs for intractable epilepsy with complex partial seizures. *J Neurol Neurosurg Psychiatry* 1982;45:1119–1124.
24. Smith DB, Mattson RH, Cramer JA, et al. Results of a nationwide Veterans Administration Cooperative Study comparing the efficacy and toxicity of carbamazepine, phenobarbital, phenytoin, and primidone. *Epilepsia* 1987;28[Suppl 3]:S50–S58.
25. Dean JC, Penry JK. Carbamazepine/valproate therapy in 100 patients with partial seizures failing carbamazepine monotherapy: long-term follow-up. *Epilepsia* 1988;29:687.
26. Perucca E. Pharmacoresistance in epilepsy: how should it be defined? *CNS Drugs* 1998;10:171–179.
27. Perucca E. The new generation of antiepileptic drugs: advantages and disadvantages. *Br J Clin Pharmacol* 1996;42:531–543.
28. Cramer JA, Fisher R, Ben-Menachem E, et al. New antiepileptic drugs: comparison of key clinical trials. *Epilepsia* 1999;40:590–600.
29. Gatti G, Bonomi I, Jannuzzi G, et al. The new antiepileptic drugs: pharmacological and clinical aspects. *Curr Pharmacol Design* 2000;6:839–860.
30. Marson AG, Kadir ZA, Chadwick DW. New antiepileptic drugs: a systematic review of their efficacy and tolerability. *BMJ* 1996;313:1169–1179.
31. Perucca E. Pharmacological principles as a basis for polytherapy. *Acta Neurol Scand Suppl* 1995;162:31–34.
32. Lammers MW, Hekster YA, Keyser A, et al. Monotherapy or polytherapy for epilepsy revisited: a quantitative assessment. *Epilepsia* 1995;36:440–446.
33. Spilker B, Segretti A. Validation of the phenomenon of regression of seizure frequency in epilepsy. *Epilepsia* 1984;25:443–449.
34. Perucca E, Gram L, Avanzini G, et al. Antiepileptic drugs as a cause of worsening of seizures. *Epilepsia* 1998;39:5–17.
35. Bourgeois BF, Dodson WE, Ferrendelli JA. Primidone, pheno-

barbital, and PEMA. II. Seizure protection, neurotoxicity, and therapeutic index of varying combinations in mice. *Neurology* 1983;33:291–295.

36. Bourgeois BF. Antiepileptic drug combinations and experimental background: the case of phenobarbital and phenytoin. *Naunyn Schmiedebergs Arch Pharmacol* 1986:333:406–411.

37. Bourgeois BF, Wad N. Combined administration of carbamazepine and phenobarbital: effect on anticonvulsant activity and neurotoxicity. *Epilepsia* 1988;29:482–487.

38. Bourgeois BF. Anticonvulsant potency and neurotoxicity of valproate alone and in combination with carbamazepine or phenobarbital. *Clin Neuropharmacol* 1988;11:348–359.

39. Bourgeois BF. Combination of valproate and ethosuximide: antiepileptic and neurotoxic interaction. *J Pharmacol Exp Ther* 1988;247:1128–1132.

40. Gordon R, Gels M, Wichmann J, et al. Interaction of felbamate with several other antiepileptic drugs against seizures induced by maximal electroshock in mice. *Epilepsia* 1993;34:367–371.

41. Swiader M, Kotowski J, Gasior M, et al. Interaction of topiramate with conventional antiepileptic drugs in mice. *Enr J Pharmacol* 2000.

42. Brodie MJ, Mumford JP, for the 012 Study Group. Double-blind substitution of vigabatrin and valproate in carbamazepine-resistant partial epilepsy. *Epilepsy Res* 1999;40:199–205.

43. Rowan AJ, Meijer JWA, de Beer-Pawlikowski N, et al. Valproate-ethosuximide combination therapy for refractory absence seizures. *Arch Neurol* 1983;40:797–802.

44. Brodie MJ, Yuen AC, and 105 Study Group. Lamotrigine substitution study: evidence for synergism with sodium valproate. *Epilepsy Res* 1997;26:423–432.

45. Panayiotopoulos CP, Ferrie CD, Knott C, et al. Interaction of lamotrigine with sodium valproate. *Lancet* 1993;341:445.

46. Ferrie CD, Panayiotopoulos CP. Therapeutic interaction of lamotrigine and sodium valproate in intractable myoclonic epilepsy. *Seizure* 1994;344:1375–1376.

47. Pisani F, Oteri G, Russo R, et al. The efficacy of valproate-lamotrigine comedication in refractory complex partial seizures: evidence for a pharmacodynamic interaction. *Epilepsia* 1999;40:1141–1146.

48. Deckers CLP, Hekster YA, Keyser A, et al. Reappraisal of polytherapy in epilepsy: a critical review of drug load and adverse effects. *Epilepsia* 1997;38:570–575.

49. Walker JE, Koon P. Carbamazepine vs valproate vs combined therapy for refractory partial complex seizures with secondary generalization. *Epilepsia* 1988;29:693.

50. Harden CL, Zisfein J, Atos-Radzion CE, et al. Combination valproate-carbamazepine therapy in partial epilepsies resistant to carbamazepine monotherapy. *J Epilepsy* 1993;6:91–94.

51. Stolarek I, Blacklaw J, Forrest G, et al. Vigabatrin and lamotrigin in regractory epilepsy. *J Neurol Neurosurg Psychiatry* 1994;57:921–924.

52. Leach JP, Brodie MJ. Synergism with GABAergic drugs in refractory epilepsy. *Lancet* 1994;343:1650.

53. Pisani F, Oteri G, Antonino F, et al. Complete seizure control following gabapentin-lamotrigine comedication. *Epilepsia* 40[Suppl 2]:253–254.

54. Stephens LJ, Sills GJ, Brodie MJ. Lamiotrigine and topiramate may be a useful combination. *Lancet* 1998;351:958–959.

55. Besag FMC, Berry DJ, Pool F, et al. Carbamazepine toxicity with lamotrigine: pharmacokinetic or pharmacodynamic interaction? *Epilepsia* 1998;39:183–187.

56. Levy RH, Thummel KE, Unadkat JD. Absorption, distribution, and elimination of antiepileptic drugs. In: Levy RH, Mattson RH, Meldrum BS, eds. *Antiepileptic drugs*, 4th ed. New York: Raven Press, 1995:13–30.

57. Levy RH, Wurden CJ. Carbamazepine: interactions with other drugs. In: Levy RH, Mattson RH, Meldrum BS, eds. *Antiepileptic drugs*, 4th ed. New York: Raven Press, 1995:543–554.

58. Levy RH, Bajpai M. Phenytoin: interactions with other drugs. II. Mechanistic aspects. In: Levy RH, Mattson RH, Meldrum BS, eds. *Antiepileptic drugs*, 4th ed. New York: Raven Press, 1995:329–338.

59. Bopp BA, Nequist GE, Rodrigues AD. Role of cytochrome P-450 3A subfamily in the metabolism of [C14]-tiagabine by human heptaic microsomes. *Epilepsia* 1995;36[Suppl 3]:159.

60. Nakasa H, Ohmari S, Kitada M. Formation of a 2-suphamoylacetylphenol from zonisamide under aerobic conditions in rat liver microsomes. *Xenobiotica* 1996;26:495–501.

61. Gisclon LG, Curtin CR, Kramaer LD. Steady-state (SS) pharmacokinetics (PK) of phenytoin (Dilantin) and topiramate (Topamax) in epileptic patients on monotherapyand during combination therapy. *Epilepsia* 1994;35[Suppl 8]:54.

62. Yuen AW, Land G, Weatherley BC, et al. Sodium valproate acutely inhibits lamotrigine metabolism. *Br J Clin Pharmacol* 1992;33:511–513.

63. Levy RH, Rettenmeier AW, Anderson GD, et al. Effects of polytherapy with phenytoin, carbamazepine, and stiripentol on formation of 4-ene-valproate, a hepatotoxic metabolite of valproic acid. *Clin Pharmacol Ther* 1999;48:225–235.

64. Tartara A, Galimberti CA, Manni R, et al. The pharmacokinetics of oxcarbazepine and its active metabolite 10-hydroxy-carbamazepine in healthy subjects and in epileptic patients. *Br J Clin Pharmacol* 1993;36:366–368.

65. Kerr BM, Levy RH. Carbamazepine: carbamazepine epoxide. In: Levy RH, Mattson RH, Meldrum BS, eds, *Antiepileptic drugs*, 4th ed. New York: Raven Press, 1995:529–542.

66. Kutt H. Phenobarbital: interactions with other drugs. In: Levy RH, Mattson RH, Meldrum BS, eds. *Antiepileptic drugs*, 4th ed. New York: Raven Press, 1995:389–400.

67. Silvermann JA. P-Glycoprotein. In: Levy RH, Thummel KE, Trager WE, et al., eds. *Metabolic drug interactions*. Philadelphia: Lippincott Williams & Wilkins, 2000:135–144.

GENERAL PRINCIPLES

LABORATORY MONITORING OF ANTIEPILEPTIC DRUGS

SVEIN I. JOHANNESSEN
TORBJÖRN TOMSON

Because drug action depends on drug disposition, knowledge of the fundamental pharmacokinetic properties of a given drug is important for optimal treatment. Drug treatment of epilepsy was one of the first areas to benefit from clinical pharmacokinetic studies. In the past, the most effective individual dosage was established by trial and error. The development of technology for quantifying drug concentrations in biologic fluids has, however, made it possible to study the relationship among drug dosage, drug concentration in body fluids, and pharmacologic effect and thereby provides new insight into drug therapy (1,2). It was soon recognized that the desired therapeutic effect of many antiepileptic drugs (AEDs) was achieved within specific ranges of serum levels for each drug: lower concentrations gave an unsatisfactory effect, and higher concentrations gave undesirable side effects. Therapeutic drug level monitoring has since become established for many drugs to optimize drug therapy regimens for individual patients.

Mainly because of indiscriminate overuse and misuse, therapeutic drug monitoring has attracted criticism (3,4), and its value in the treatment of epilepsy has sometimes been questioned. However, although randomized clinical trials have failed to demonstrate an impact of drug monitoring on the overall outcome of epilepsy treatment (5), better understanding of the relationship between pharmacokinetics and pharmacodynamics is likely to result in improved drug effectiveness and safety (6). Numerous reports have been published on the kinetics of AEDs and on the rational use of drug monitoring (6–16).

Svein I. Johannessen, PhD: Director of Research, The National Center for Epilepsy, Sandvika, Norway

Torbjörn Tomson, MD, PhD: Department of Neurology, Karolinska Hospital, Stockholm, Sweden

WHY DETERMINE SERUM ANTIEPILEPTIC DRUG LEVELS?

The role of therapeutic drug monitoring in the treatment of epilepsy reflects epilepsy-related factors as well as properties of the various AEDs. Because treatment is prophylactic and seizures occur at irregular intervals and sometimes have serious consequences, it may be difficult to find the optimal dose on clinical grounds alone. Occasionally, signs of toxicity may be insidious and difficult to interpret, in particular among patients with epilepsy who have associated mental handicaps. The chronic, sometimes lifelong treatment also makes it particularly important to monitor therapy to reduce the risk of long-term adverse effects. These arguments for therapeutic monitoring in epilepsy are valid irrespective of the type of AED. However, the usefulness of drug monitoring also depends on the pharmacologic properties of the drug to be monitored. Therapeutic monitoring is likely to be particularly useful if there is a pronounced interindividual variability in pharmacokinetics, if the kinetics in the individual patient may be altered by drug interactions, concurrent disease, or other conditions, if there is an established correlation between the drug concentration and its therapeutic and toxic effects, and if the therapeutic range is narrow.

The use of drug assays in therapy control rests on the assumption that the relationship between the serum concentration of the active drug and its effects is better than that between dose and effect. Some pharmacologic requirements need to be fulfilled in part or in full to obtain a meaningful relationship between the serum concentration of a drug and its effect. The drug should have a reversible action, and development of tolerance should not occur at receptor sites. It should act by itself and not through metabolites (unless these are measured), and the level of unbound drug at the site of sampling should ideally be equal to the unbound concentration at receptor sites. Hence, although the epilepsy-related rationale for drug monitoring is similar for all AEDs, the usefulness of this monitoring varies among AEDs, depending on their pharmacological properties.

THERAPEUTIC RANGE OF SERUM LEVELS

Most of the older AEDs have a more or less well-defined therapeutic range of serum levels (Table 9.1). This range must not be strictly interpreted, because many of the underlying studies are based on patients with severe epilepsy treated with several AEDs; controlled studies in patients using one drug only for newly diagnosed or moderate epilepsy are scarce. However, most patients are optimally treated with a drug when its steady-state serum levels are maintained within that range (17–19).

In mild epilepsy, seizure control is often attained at levels lower than the usually recommended range (20–22). In fact, investigators have suggested that the lower limit of the therapeutic range should be disregarded, and any concentration up to the toxic limit should be considered potentially therapeutic (6). The dose should thus not be increased just to reach the defined therapeutic serum levels in patients who become seizure free with low drug levels. Conversely, some patients with more severe epilepsy need "supratherapeutic" levels to achieve optimal effects. It is also possible that the optimal serum levels differ according to seizure type. Thus, the dose should be titrated to the "optimal serum level" for the individual patient.

The therapeutic ranges for phenytoin, phenobarbital, carbamazepine, ethosuximide, valproate, and clonazepam are reasonably well recognized (20,23–32) (Table 9.1). Further studies are necessary to determine the place of serum concentration monitoring for clobazam and for the newer AEDs (Table 9.1). In patients treated with clobazam, the serum levels are in the order of 0.1 to 1.0 μmol/L for the parent drug and 1 to 10 μmol/L for the metabolite, desmethylclobazam (33,34).

A retrospective analysis of patients treated with felbamate reveals that serum concentrations between 210 and 462 μmol/L are associated with optimal seizure control (35). Another study, however, suggests that adverse effects are more frequent in patients with felbamate concentrations >231 μmol/L than with lower concentrations (36).

Wide ranges of gabapentin plasma concentrations have been reported to be associated with seizure control. Therapeutic effects of gabapentin were evident in refractory patients with partial seizures only at serum concentrations >12 μmol/L (37). In another study (38), using high-dose gabapentin in patients with refractory partial seizures, plasma concentrations among responders ranged from 34 to 122 μmol/L.

For lamotrigine, a target range of 4 to 16 μmol/L was suggested early (39), but this range is probably too low because many patients benefit from and tolerate considerably higher concentrations. Morris et al. (40) proposed a target range of 12 to 55 μmol/L based on their own experience and on an open trial of patients with intractable

TABLE 9.1. PHARMACOKINETIC VARIABLES FOR MAJOR ANTIEPILEPTIC DRUGS

Drug	Elimination Half-life (h)	Time to Steady-state (days)	Therapeutic Range (μmol/L)	Comment on Value of Therapeutic Range
Older AEDs				
Carbamazepine	8–20	4–7	15–45	Of value
Clobazam	≈18	4–7	NE	Probably limited use
Clonazepam	20–60	5–10	60–220 nmol/L	Probably limited use
Ethosuximide	40–60	5–10	300–600	Of value
Phenobarbital	50–160	10–35	50–130	Of value
Phenytoin	7–60[a]	4–8	40–80	Necessary
Primidone	4–12	1–3	25–50	Monitor phenobarbital
Valproic acid (sodium valproate)	11–20	2–4	300–600	Of value
Newer AEDs[c]				
Felbamate	14–22	3–5	200–400	Potentially of value
Gabapentin	5–7	2	40–120	Probably limited use
Lamotrigine	8–33	3–15	10–60	Potentially of value
Levetiracetam	6–8	2	?	Probably limited use
Oxcarbazepine[b]	8–15	2–3	50–140	Potentially of value
Tiagabine	7–9	2	?	Potentially of value
Vigabatrin	5–7	1–2	?	Of little value
Topiramate	20–30	4–6	10–60	Potentially of value
Zonisamide	50–70	5–12	35–200	Potentially of value

AED, antiepileptic drug; NE, not established.
[a]Concentration dependent.
[b]Monohydroxy derivative.
[c]Therapeutic ranges (μmol/L) are tentative and given in round numbers because of lack of precise documentation.

seizures (41). Most studies have shown a wide range in plasma concentrations associated with seizure control and a considerable overlap in plasma concentrations of responders and nonresponders, as well as between patients with and without side effects (42–44).

For levetiracetam, the role of therapeutic drug monitoring has not yet been established.

The target range of serum levels for the active metabolite of oxcarbazepine has not yet been well defined. Friis et al. (45) found a mean trough level of approximately 80 µmol/L in their retrospective analysis of 947 patients, but the range in serum concentrations was wide (12 to 160 µmol/L), and the relation to effects and toxicity not analyzed in detail. Similarly, Van Parys and Meinardi (46) reported concentrations ranging from 12 to 128 µmol/L (mean, 70) in seizure-free adult patients. Neither the mean concentration nor the range differed from those in nonresponders. Borusiak et al. (47) reported somewhat higher concentrations in children, 60 to 220 µmol/L (mean, 120). Side effects were more frequent at plasma concentrations of 140 to 160 µmol/L. A population pharmacokinetic-pharmacodynamic assessment was made based on samples from 513 patients participating in three double-blind trials of oxcarbazepine (48). Generally, safety and efficacy responses could adequately be explained by oxcarbazepine dose alone, and plasma concentrations of the metabolite provided limited additional information.

Information on concentration-effect relations with tiagabine is scarce. However, a more pronounced reduction in seizures was observed at trough plasma concentrations >106 µmol/L in a preliminary analysis of data from a clinical trial of patients with complex partial seizures given three different dosages of tiagabine (49).

In contrast to most other AEDs, monitoring of serum levels of vigabatrin is not suitable as a guide to therapy. The mechanism of action of vigabatrin is irreversible inhibition of γ-aminobutyric acid (GABA)-transferase, the enzyme responsible for the catabolism of GABA. Because of the long-lasting inhibition, the antiepileptic effect of vigabatrin long outlasts its presence in serum.

Seizure control has been associated with topiramate serum levels between 10 and 16 µmol/L (50,51). A preliminary report based on topiramate as add-on therapy with other AEDs in patients with refractory epilepsy suggests that levels >12 µmol/L are necessary for effectiveness (52). In monotherapy, patients with topiramate concentrations >30 µmol/L have had a better response than those with lower levels (53).

In add-on studies of zonisamide, favorable clinical responses have been observed at serum levels of 94 to 141 µmol/L (54) and at 33 to 188 µmol/L in children (55). There was, however, a considerable overlap between serum concentrations of responders and nonresponders as well as between serum levels associated with seizure control and those related to side effects (56).

Although clearly further studies are needed, tentative serum concentration ranges for the newer AEDs are given in Table 9.1. As indicated earlier, seizure control is generally reported at a wide range of serum concentrations, and there is a significant overlap with concentrations observed in nonresponders and with patients reporting side effects (6,15). It is clear that the optimal concentration is individual, and this may vary considerably among patients, as indeed is also the case for the older AEDs.

Relationship between Dose and Serum Drug Level

Bioavailability

The bioavailability of a drug varies not only with the mode of administration but also between individuals and drugs. Usually, AEDs are given orally, but some can also be given intravenously, intramuscularly, and rectally. After oral administration, maximal serum levels of most AEDs are attained within 2 to 8 hours of the dose intake (6,9). The rate and extent of absorption can be influenced by several factors, as discussed in the following sections.

Biopharmaceutical Formulation.
The rate and extent of absorption are affected by the biopharmaceutical formulation and by differences between nongeneric and generic preparations. The changeover to a preparation with better bioavailability can give serum levels that are too high, with a subsequent risk of drug intoxication. Conversely, a preparation with poor bioavailability can lead to subtherapeutic serum levels and increased seizure frequency (57,58).

Preparation Form.
AEDs are marketed in solutions, syrups, standard tablets, enteric-coated tablets, slow-release tablets, capsules, and suppositories. Standard tablets are absorbed faster than enteric-coated tablets and slow-release (retard) tablets (59).

Gastrointestinal Content.
The degree of absorption of some drugs can be greater when they are taken under fasting conditions, and for other drugs, the converse is true.

Protein Binding and Distribution

On entering the circulation, most AEDs are partly bound to serum proteins and establish an equilibrium between free and bound fractions (6,9,60,61). Only a free drug dissolved in plasma can cross biologic membranes and can interact with specific brain receptors. There is then a dynamic equilibrium between AED molecules in the plasma and in cerebral extracellular fluid. Therefore, the drug concentration in the plasma is assumed to be a measure of drug concentration in the brain and thus provides a measure of antiepileptic effect because AEDs clearly exert their antiepileptic actions within the brain (62,63). Protein binding differs for each drug, but normally it is quite constant for one AED in the same patient. A reduction in binding can have clinical consequences with highly protein-bound drugs such as phenytoin, valproate, and tiagabine.

Factors Determining the Steady-State Concentration in Serum

The relationship between clinical effect and serum drug levels is evaluated during steady-state conditions. The time lapse before steady-state serum drug levels are attained after initiation of therapy depends on the biologic half-life of the drug (6,9) (Table 9.1). Theoretically, 97% of the final steady-state serum drug level is achieved five half-lives after the initiation of drug therapy. Five times the drug half-life is thus taken as a time interval necessary to achieve steady state. The same rule applies when dosage adjustments are made. Usually, more time is needed because the maintenance dose is often increased gradually. Therefore, the first blood sample related to steady-state concentrations should be drawn about 1 to 2 weeks after initiation of treatment, except for phenobarbital, for which a 3- to 4-week period is recommended because of the longer half-life of this drug. Because carbamazepine increases its own metabolism (autoinduction), the serum drug level may decrease somewhat in the initial dosage period. The time needed before the patient is adjusted to the optimal serum AED level regarding clinical efficacy may, of course, be considerably longer. Generally, the dose should be gradually increased with sufficient time to evaluate the clinical effect to limit adverse reactions.

The rate of elimination of a drug varies from one person to another. Besides genetic factors and interactions resulting from comedication, the rate of elimination depends on age and sex. Fertile women often have faster drug metabolism rates than do men. The rate of metabolism decreases with increasing age for both sexes. When related to age, children tend to require higher drug doses (in milligrams per kilogram) than adults to obtain comparable serum levels. Both renal and liver disease may markedly influence drug protein binding and elimination and can be of clinical importance. Under these conditions, it is therefore especially important that the dose of AED is increased slowly until seizure control is achieved, and the serum concentration is followed and carefully evaluated to avoid intoxications.

Drug Interactions

When a patient is treated with more than one drug, there is often a risk of drug interactions that may result in altered therapeutic outcome. Drug interactions may alter absorption, protein binding, receptor action, metabolism, and excretion of any therapeutic agent (15,51,64,65). The most commonly encountered drug interactions are changes in the rates of biotransformation as a consequence of enzyme induction or inhibition. Interactions between and among AEDs and between these and other drug classes are common. Thus, lower serum AED levels may result in loss in efficacy, and higher levels may result in increased adverse effects.

In long-term treatment of patients with epilepsy, it is important to be aware of the possibility of such drug interactions. Although some drug interactions are not clinically significant, others may cause a marked change in the clinical status of the patient. Change in drug levels in patients treated with the same drugs and dosage varies, and reliable predictions are very difficult to make. Thus, a drug interaction observed in one patient may not be observed in another. When one uses drug combinations that can lead to clinically significant interactions, it is therefore important to be observant for loss of efficacy or clinical signs of intoxication, and it is also necessary to monitor the drug levels 2 to 4 weeks after the addition or withdrawal of a drug. For instance, if an intoxication occurs and the interfering secondary drug cannot be withdrawn, the dose of the primary drug should be reduced, based on appropriate serum drug level monitoring.

WHAT TO MEASURE?

Total Serum Drug Levels Versus Free (i.e., Unbound) Serum Drug Levels

Because it is generally assumed that free (i.,e., unbound) drug in plasma is the therapeutically active fraction, the most meaningful way of evaluating clinically significant drug concentrations would be to measure the free drug concentration. However, current analytic methods for quantitation of these drugs measure the total concentration. The drug assays do not distinguish between protein-bound and free drug. Consequently, both fractions are measured and are expressed as a total drug concentration, which routinely is much easier to measure.

An important condition for using the total serum drug concentration as a guideline for the therapeutic or toxic effect is that the protein binding of a certain drug must be constant for the individual patient and the same for all patients. The protein binding differs for each drug depending on its physical and chemical properties, as well as on the physical characteristics of the serum protein. A drug may be either tightly or loosely bound, depending on its affinity for serum proteins. Displacement of a drug from its binding site may result in clinical toxicity because of increased concentration of unbound drug, even though the total level is unchanged.

Normally, the degree of binding is quite constant (9,66). A reduction in binding can take place under special conditions such as uremia (endogenous displacers). This can be of clinical importance for drugs that are highly bound, such as phenytoin. Newborns with hypoalbuminemia and especially those with hyperbilirubinemia have a reduced drug binding capacity that gives a greater free, and thus therapeutically active, drug fraction in serum. Under these circumstances, a drug with reduced binding capacity and consequently elevated free fraction may be clinically effective or toxic at lower total serum drug levels than would be expected. It is therefore important to consider these aspects when the dosage is determined. Several techniques are available for measurement of the protein binding and the free serum drug levels, including ultrafiltration and equilibrium dialysis (67).

At present, the value of routine monitoring of free drug levels is doubtful. More studies of the relationship between free drug levels and clinical effect are required to evaluate this approach. Therefore, free drug level measurements should be restricted to problem cases. It is of importance in patients who clinically fail to respond to AED therapy because of altered protein binding as a consequence of drug interactions or in special physiologic or pathologic states such as pregnancy, hypoalbuminemia, or hepatic or renal failure (68–71).

Drug Levels in Other Body Fluids

The free drug level can also be derived from the drug concentration in cerebrospinal fluid, saliva, or tears (60,72–77). Access to cerebrospinal fluid samples is, of course, limited, and studies of the concentration of AEDs in tears have been scarce until recently. Saliva, however, can be an alternative medium to serum for carbamazepine, phenytoin, primidone, and ethosuximide because the concentration in saliva reflects the concentration of free drug in serum. This is not the case for phenobarbital and valproate, owing to the physicochemical properties of these substances (72). However, the concentration of a drug in saliva can be influenced by the sampling conditions and by the contamination of mucus and of unswallowed residual drug and food. Under well-controlled sampling conditions, saliva measurements can be useful for determination of the concentration of free drug, especially when a change in the protein binding is suspected.

Because saliva can be collected by noninvasive techniques, this approach is helpful when multiple serial samples are needed, particularly in children. However, further clinical studies with sensitive analytic methods are needed to evaluate the use of saliva and tears as assay mediums. This is also the case for routine measurements of unbound drug concentration in serum.

Preliminary studies in patients and in healthy persons indicate that valproate concentrations in subcutaneous tissue sampled by microdialysis may reflect unbound serum concentrations (78). Further studies are needed to explore

whether this may become a useful method when serial sampling of unbound drug concentrations is required and to ascertain whether the technique could be applied to other AEDs.

Serum Levels of Drug Metabolites

The evaluation of therapeutic drug monitoring will be further refined when the active metabolites of AEDs also can be taken into account. So far, the role of metabolites is not clarified to that extent. One exception is the role of phenobarbital derived from primidone. Primidone is rapidly converted to phenylethylmalonamide and is more slowly converted to phenobarbital. Most physicians routinely prefer to measure and use the concentration of derived phenobarbital during primidone therapy and both primidone and phenobarbital in certain cases only. Routine determination of phenylethylmalonamide is then unnecessary.

Carbamazepine is also a drug with antiepileptic effects resulting from metabolites, the main metabolite being carbamazepine-10,11-epoxide (79). The epoxide levels may range from 10% to 50% of the serum levels of the parent compound. However, there is no constant relationship between the concentration of the epoxide and carbamazepine, and the ratio varies during the day in the individual patient and with comedication (60,80). One should measure both carbamazepine and the epoxide in clinical trials, but at present measuring the metabolite is not indicated for routine monitoring. Oxcarbazepine is the keto derivative of carbamazepine and is rapidly and almost completely metabolized to 10,11-dihydro-10-hydroxycarbazepine, and therefore, the serum level of this metabolite is measured.

WHEN SHOULD SERUM ANTIEPILEPTIC DRUG LEVELS BE MEASURED?

The importance of serum drug level monitoring in patients receiving long-term treatment has been emphasized. The clinical conditions for monitoring and determining when the serum drug level ideally should be measured will vary, depending on the pharmacological properties of the AED, but some general guidelines can be issued.

Initiation of Drug Therapy, Dose Adjustment, and Other Medication

Two to 3 weeks after initiation of drug therapy, when steady-state conditions are attained, the serum drug level should be measured and correlated with the clinical effect to see whether the dose is optimal. This is particularly relevant for AEDs with a narrow and well-defined target range. However, a drug level for most AEDs at this point may also be of value as reference for future situations with therapeutic failure. Dosage adjustment is a further indication for monitoring, in particular of AEDs with dose-dependent kinetics, and it is mandatory after dosage adjustments of phenytoin. The addition of comedication that may cause interactions also prompts monitoring of serum drug levels.

Therapy Failure, Intoxication, and Noncompliance

Inadequate serum drug levels can result from an insufficient dose prescribed (physician), from too low a dose taken (patient compliance) (81), or from a high rate of metabolism (genetic variability or induction). Correspondingly, a high concentration can be caused by too high a dose prescribed or taken or by a low rate of metabolism. Drug compliance is often poor in the treatment of patients with epilepsy.

At high serum drug concentrations, it may be necessary to withdraw the drug for several days. When serum drug concentrations have returned to an appropriate level, therapy can be reinstated at a lower dose.

Other Illnesses

Monitoring is essential in patients with other illnesses and treatment that can influence the disposition of the drug, the water balance, and thus the serum concentration and the seizure control (82). For instance, infections and long-lasting diarrhea may have such an influence.

Monitoring is important in patients with liver and renal dysfunction (83). In patients with severe hepatic disease, drug kinetics may be significantly altered (84–86). The serum protein binding may be reduced as reported for phenytoin, carbamazepine, and valproate. The same also applies to the capacity of the drug-metabolizing enzymes in the liver. However, the net effect of the total drug clearance may vary considerably, and monitoring of serum levels, together with close clinical observation of the patient, is important.

The clinical picture in renal disease may also vary, and the effect on drug disposition of AEDs may be different in individual patients (84,87). The unbound fraction (not the free concentration) of phenytoin and valproate is increased, but it is rarely necessary to reduce daily doses because of the concomitant increase in total drug clearance. Accordingly, a therapeutic effect may be observed at lower total drug levels than usual. The risk of adverse effects caused by drug interactions is considerably increased in patients with renal or liver disease.

Pregnancy

During pregnancy, it is especially important to maintain good seizure control without side effects to avoid harm to the mother and fetus from the seizures and the drugs. Any major changes in AED therapy should be made before the patient conceives. Women considering pregnancy should be placed on the simplest feasible medication regimen. Levels should be closely monitored to determine the lowest dose that will achieve comfortable serum drug levels to keep the risk of drug-induced abnormalities in the child as low as possible.

During pregnancy, several pharmacokinetic parameters of most AEDs are changed significantly, resulting in decreased steady-state serum levels, but the free (i.e., unbound) drug level may be unchanged. Total serum AED levels and, for some AEDs, if possible, free levels, should be measured at regular intervals throughout pregnancy. If an AED dose is increased during pregnancy, the dose should be returned to prepregnancy levels during the first weeks of the puerperium, to avoid toxicity. Drug levels must be checked periodically for at least the first 2 months after delivery (88,89).

Routine Control

Routine control of the serum AED levels is useful because this gives the best basis for comparison if the clinical situation should change. In adults with well-controlled seizures, the serum drug levels may be routinely checked once a year in connection with a medical checkup. Children should be evaluated more frequently during growth when altered drug disposition can be expected. Frequent monitoring is essential at the earliest onset of puberty because metabolic patterns undergo rapid changes at this time. Seizure control can easily worsen because of increasing weight and altered drug disposition.

Sampling Conditions

Whenever possible, the blood sampling time for individual patients should be standardized to ensure comparable conditions. Ideally, the samples should be taken during drug fasting in the morning; in outpatients, the morning dose can be postponed a couple of hours to ensure this condition. For determination of valproate and other AEDs with a short half-life, it is mandatory that the sample be taken during drug fasting in the morning because these drugs have great variations in the serum level between dose intakes. When toxic symptoms of drug are suspected during the day, it is best to draw the sample at the time of maximal serum drug level or at the time when the toxic symptoms are most pronounced. However, one has to keep in mind that the therapeutic ranges are based on trough levels. The following patient data are necessary for a meaningful evaluation of drug levels: age, weight, sex, diagnosis, indications for analysis, clinical conditions of relevance, all drugs in use with total daily doses, and sampling time in relation to the last drug intake.

ASSAY METHODS

Numerous methods are available for the determination of serum AED levels, including various gas chromatographic, liquid chromatographic, and immunoassay procedures (2,90). Analytically, it is easier to determine the level of a single drug than that of a mixture of drugs. Because patients often are treated with more than one drug, it is necessary to use selective methods for drug measurement.

An immunoassay for specific measurement of a single drug is often preferred. These assays have several advantages over other currently used methods because they are precise, reproducible, and rapid for determination of drugs in microsamples. However, they are not as suitable for drug screening as are certain chromatographic methods.

QUALITY CONTROL

Active participation in both internal and external quality control schemes to ensure reliable results is necessary for any laboratory engaged in the routine determination of AEDs. Optimal analytic quality is important for effective therapy; otherwise, the patient can easily be mistreated, and the analytic technique, as well as the laboratory, can become discredited. International cooperation on voluntary quality control schemes of AEDs has improved the analytic performance of many laboratories engaged in therapeutic drug monitoring (91,92).

PITFALLS IN THERAPEUTIC ANTIEPILEPTIC DRUG MONITORING

No strict correlation exists between efficacy and toxicity of AEDs and their serum level for an individual patient. The degree of seizure control and toxicity varies widely among patients with the same serum drug levels. No therapeutic or optimum range is applicable to all patients. The optimum serum drug level depends partly on the severity of the epilepsy and partly on the pharmacodynamic response to a drug. Therefore, drug monitoring is not a substitute for clinical judgment. It is the patient who is being treated, not the serum drug level (3,93–96).

A serum level judged on a single sample may be misleading for drugs with wide diurnal serum level fluctuations as with carbamazepine and valproate, especially if slow-release tablets are not used. Therefore, the blood sampling time must be standardized whenever possible. If peak-related side effects are suspected, a kinetic profile with several measurements in the same day will provide more information than a single trough level.

One has to keep in mind the analytic problems in determination of AEDs. Accuracy may be a problem in many laboratories in spite of quality control programs. If unexpected values are reported, repeated measurements should be carried out before taking clinical action.

CONCLUDING REMARKS

In the future, more emphasis should be placed on rational and cost-effective therapeutic monitoring (97,98). Methods that produce rapid results are of greater relevance and lead to more efficient patient care than assays that involve time lapses of hours or days before the clinician can take action.

For the older AEDs, the therapeutic range and the place of serum drug level monitoring were established long after the introduction of the drugs. Many newer AEDs have been marketed in recent years, and others are in clinical trials (99). The role of therapeutic monitoring of these drugs and of possible comedication needs further investigations. Development and testing of newer AEDs should include an evaluation of therapeutic drug monitoring as early as possible in specifically designed clinical studies, preferably using monotherapy.

REFERENCES

1. Johannessen SI, Morselli PL, Pippenger CE, et al., eds. *Antiepileptic therapy: advances in drug monitoring.* New York: Raven Press, 1980.
2. Pippenger CE, Penry JK, Kutt H, eds. *Antiepileptic drugs: quantitative analysis and interpretation.* New York: Reven Press, 1978.
3. Chadwick D. Overuse of monitoring of blood concentrations of antiepileptic drugs. *BMJ* 1987;294:723–724.
4. Schoenenberger RA, Tanasijevic MJ, Jha A, et al. Appropriateness of antiepileptic drug level monitoring. *JAMA* 1995;274: 1622–1626.
5. Iannuzzi G, Cian P, Fattore C, et al. A multicentre randomized controlled trial on the clinical impact of therapeutic drug monitoring in patients with newly diagnosed epilepsy. *Epilepsia* 2000; 41:222–230.
6. Perucca E. Is there a role for therapeutic drug monitoring of the new anticonvulsants? *Clin Pharmacokinet* 2000;38:191–204.
7. Commission on Antiepileptic Drugs. Guidelines for therapeutic monitoring on antiepileptic drugs. *Epilepsia* 1993;34:585–587.
8. Levy RH, Pitlick WH, Eichelbaum M, et al., eds. *Metabolism of antiepileptic drugs.* New York: Raven Press, 1984.
9. Morselli PL, Franco-Morselli R. Clinical pharmacokinetics of antiepileptic drugs in adults. *Pharmacol Ther* 1980;10:65–101.
10. Schmidt D, Jacob R. Clinical and laboratory monitoring of antiepileptic medication. In: Wyllie E, ed. *The treatment of epilepsy: principles and practice.* Philadelphia: Lea & Febiger, 1993:798–809.
11. Johannessen SI. Plasma drug concentration monitoring of anticonvulsants: practical guidelines. *CNS Drugs* 1997;7:349–365.
12. Eadie MJ. Therapeutic drug monitoring: antiepileptic drugs. *Br J Clin Pharmacol* 1998;46:185–193.
13. Brodie MJ. Routine measurement of new antiepileptic drug concentrations: a critique and a prediction. In: French J, Leppik I, Dichter MA, eds. Antiepileptic drug development. *Adv Neurol* 1998;76:223.

14. Patsalos PN. New antiepileptic drugs. *Ann Clin Biochem* 1999; 36:10–19.

15. Tomson T, Johannessen SI. Therapeutic monitoring of the new antiepileptic drugs. *Eur J Clin Pharmacol* 2000;55:697–705.

16. Glauser TA, Pippenger CE. Controversies in blood-level monitoring: re-examining its role in the treatment of epilepsy. *Epilepsia* 2000;41[Suppl 8]:S6–S15.

17. Schmidt D, Einicke I, Haenel F. The influence of seizure type on the efficacy of plasma concentrations of phenytoin, phenobarbital, and carbamazepine. *Arch Neurol* 1986;43:263–265.

18. Turnbull DM, Rawlins MD, Weightman D, et al. "Therapeutic" serum concentration of phenytoin: the influence of seizure type. *J Neurol Neurosurg Psychiatry* 1984;47:231–234.

19. Vaida FJE, Aicardi J. Reassessment of the concept of a therapeutic range of anticonvulsant plasma levels. *Dev Med Child Neurol* 1983;25:660–671.

20. Lund L. Anticonvulsant effect of diphenylhydantoin relative to plasma levels. *Arch Neurol* 1974;31:289–294.

21. Shorvon SD, Galbraith AW, Laundy M, et al., eds. *Antiepileptic therapy: advances in drug monitoring.* New York: Raven Press, 1980:213–220.

22. Strandjord RE, Johannessen SI. Carbamazepine as the only drug in patients with epilepsy: serum levels and clinical effect. In: Johannessen SI, Morselli PL, Pippenger CE, et al., eds. *Antiepileptic therapy: advances in drug monitoring.* New York: Raven Press, 1980:229–235.

23. Baruzzi A, Bordo B, Bossi L, et al. Plasma levels of di–propylacetate and clonazepam in epileptic patients. *Int J Clin Pharmacol* 1977;15:403–408.

24. Cereghino JJ. Serum carbamazepine concentration and clinical control. *Adv Neurol* 1975;11:309–329.

25. Eichelbaum M, Bertilsson L, Lund L, et al. Plasma levels of carbamazepine and carbamazepine 10,11-epoxide during treatment of epilepsy. *Eur J Clin Pharmacol* 1976;9:417–421.

26. Gram L, Flachs H, Würtz-Jørgensen A, et al. Sodium valproate, serum level and clinical effect in epilepsy: a controlled study. *Epilepsia* 1979;20:303–312.

27. Henriksen O, Johannessen SI. Clinical observations of sodium valproate in children: an evaluation of therapeutic serum levels. In: Johannessen SI. Morselli PL, Pippenger CE, et al., eds. *Antiepileptic therapy: advances in drug monitoring.* New York: Raven Press, 1980:253–261.

28. Monaco F, Riccio A, Benna P, et al. Further observations on carbamazepine plasma levels in epileptic patients: relationships with therapeutic and side effects. *Neurology* 1976;26:936–943.

29. Penry JK, Porter RJ, Dreifuss FE. Ethosuximide: relation of plasma levels to clinical control. In: Woodbury DM, Penry JK, Schmidt RP, eds. *Antiepileptic drugs.* New York: Raven Press, 1972:431–441.

30. Schottelius DD, Fincham RW. Clinical application of serum primidone levels. In: Pippenger CE, Penry JK, Kutt H, eds. *Antiepileptic drugs: quantitative analysis and interpretation.* New York: Raven Press, 1978:273–282.

31. Sjö O, Hvidberg EF, Naestoft J, et al. Pharmacokinetics and side-effects of clonazepam and its 7-amino-metabolite in man. *Eur J Clin Pharmacol* 1975;8:249–254.

32. Sundqvist A, Tomson T, Lundkvist B. Valproic acid in patients with juvenile myoclonic epilepsy on monotherapy: a dose-effect study. *Ther Drug Monit* 1998;20:149–157.

33. Streete JM, Berry DJ, Newbery JE. The analysis of clobazam and its metabolite desmethylclobazam by high-performance liquid chromatography. *Ther Drug Monit* 1991;13:339–344.

34. Wang J, Hug D, Gautschi K, et al. Clobazam for treatment of epilepsy. *J Epilepsy* 1993;6:180–184.

35. Troupin AS, Montouris G, Hussein G. Felbamate: therapeutic range and other kinetic information. *J Epilepsy* 1997;10:26–31.

36. Harden CL, Trifiletti T, Kutt H. Felbamate levels in patients with epilepsy. *Epilepsia* 1996;37:280–283.

37. Sivenius J, Kälviäinen R, Ylinen A, et al. Double blind study of gabapentin in the treatment of partial seizures. *Epilepsia* 1991; 32:539–542.

38. Wilson EA, Sills GJ, Forrest G, et al. High dose gabapentin in refractory partial epilepsy: clinical observations in 50 patients. *Epilepsy Res* 1998;29:161–166.

39. Brodie MJ, Richens A, Yuen AWC. Double-blind comparison of lamotrigine and carbamazepine in newly diagnosed epilepsy. *Lancet* 1995;345:476–479.

40. Morris RG, Black AB, Harris AL, et al. Lamotrigine and therapeutic drug monitoring: retrospective survey following the introduction of a routine service. *Br J Clin Pharmacol* 1998;46: 547–551.

41. Schapel G, Black A, Lam E, et al. Combination vigabatrin and lamotrigine therapy for intractable epilepsy. *Seizure* 1996:5: 51–56.

42. Bartoli A, Guerrini R, Belmonte A, et al. The influence of dosage, age and comedication on steady-state plasma lamotrigine concentrations in epileptic children: a prospective study with preliminary assessment of correlations with clinical response. *Ther Drug Monit* 1997:19:252–260.

43. Kilpatric ES, Forrest G, Brodie M. Concentration-effect and concentration-toxicity relations with lamotrigine: a prospective study. *Epilepsia* 1996;37:534–538.

44. Eriksson A-S, Nergårdh A, Hoppu K. The efficacy of lamotrigine in children and adolescents with refractory generalized epilepsy: a randomized, double-blind, cross-over study. *Epilepsia* 1998;39:495–501.

45. Friis ML, Kristensen O, Boas J, et al. Therapeutic experiences with 947 epileptic out-patients in oxcarbazepine treatment. *Acta Neurol Scand* 1993;87:224–227.

46. Van Parys JAP, Meinardi H. Survey of 260 patients treated with oxcarbazepine (Trileptal) on a named-patient basis. *Epilepsy Res* 1994;19:79–85.

47. Borusiak P, Korn-Merker E, Holert N, et al. Oxcarbazepine in treatment of childhood epilepsy: a survey of 46 children and adolescents. *J Epilepsy* 1998;11:355–360.

48. Nedelman JR, Gasparini M, Hossain M, et al. Oxcarbazepine: analysis of concentration-efficacy/safety relationships. *Neurology* 1999;52[Suppl 2]:A524–A525.

49. Rowan AJ, Gustavson L, Shu V, et al. Dose concentration relationship in a multicentre tiagabine (Gabitril) trial. *Epilepsia* 1997;38[Suppl 3]:40.

50. Reife RA, Pledger G, Doose D, et al. Topiramate PK/PD analysis. *Epilepsia* 1995;36[Suppl 3]:S152.

51. Perruca E, Bialer M. The clinical pharmacokinetics of the newer antiepileptic drugs: focus on topiramate, zonisamide and tiagabine. *Clin Pharmacokinet* 1996;31:29–46.

52. Penovich PE, Schroeder-Gustafson M, Gates JR, et al. Clinical experience with topiramate: correlation of serum levels with efficacy and adverse events. *Epilepsia* 1997;38[Suppl 8]:181.

53. Twyman RE, Ben-Menachem E, Veloso F, et al. Plasma topiramate (TPM) concentrations vs therapeutic response during monotherapy. *Epilepsia* 1999;40[Suppl 7]:111–112.

54. Wilensky AJ, Friel PN, Ojemann LM, et al. Zonisamide in epilepsy: a pilot study. *Epilepsia* 1985;26:212–220.

55. Mimaki T, Mino M, Sugimoto T, et al. Antiepileptic effect and serum levels of zonisamide in epileptic patients with refractory seizures. In: Sunshine I, ed. *Recent developments in therapeutic drug monitoring and clinical toxicology.* Marcel Dekker, New York, 1992:437–442.

56. Mimaki T. Clinical pharmacology and therapeutic drug monitoring of zonisamide. *Ther Drug Monit* 1998;20:593–597.

57. Lund L. Clinical significance of generic inequivalence of two dif-

ferent pharmaceutical formulations of phenytoin. *Eur J Clin Pharmacol* 1974;7:119–124.

58. Peterson H de Coudres. Brand-name antiepileptic drugs versus generics. In: Resor SR Jr, Kutt H, eds. *The medical treatment of epilepsy.* New York: Marcel Dekker, 1992:493–495.
59. Johannessen SI, Henriksen O. Comparison of the serum concentration profiles of Tegretol and two new slow-release preparations. In: Wolf P, Dam M, Janz D, et al., eds. *Advances in epileptology: XVth epilepsy international symposium.* New York: Raven Press, 1987:421–424.
60. Johannessen SI, Gerna M, Bakke J, et al. CSF concentrations and serum protein binding of carbamazepine and carbamazepine-10,11-epoxide in epileptic patients. *Br J Clin Pharmacol* 1976;3: 575–582.
61. Johannessen SI, Strandjord RE. Absorption and protein binding in serum of several anti-epileptic drugs. In: Schneider H, Janz D, Gardner-Thorpe C, et al., eds. *Clinical pharmacology of antiepileptic drugs.* New York: Springer-Verlag, 1975:262–273.
62. Morselli PL, Baruzzi A, Gerna M, et al. Carbamazepine and carbamazepine-10,11-epoxide concentrations in human brain. *Br J Clin Pharmacol* 1977;4:535–540.
63. Sherwin AL, Eisen AA, Sokolowski CD. Anticonvulsant drugs in human epileptogenic brain: correlation of phenobarbital and diphenylhydantoin levels with plasma. *Arch Neurol* 1973;29:73–77.
64. Kutt H. Pharmacokinetic interactions with antiepileptic medication. In: Wyllie E, ed. The treatment of epilepsy. Principles and practice. Philadelphia: Lea & Febiger, 1993;775-784.
65. Pitlick WH, ed. Antiepileptic drug interactions. New York: Demos Publications, 1989.
66. Johannessen SI. Antiepileptic drugs: pharmacokinetic and clinical aspects. *Ther Drug Monit* 1981;3:17-37.
67. Pacifici GM, Viani A. Methods of determining plasma and tissue binding of drug: pharmacokinetic consequences. *Clin Pharmacokinet* 1992;23:449–468.
68. Baird-Lambert J, Manglick MP, Wall M, et al. Identifying patients who might benefit from free phenytoin monitoring. *Ther Drug Monit* 1987;9:134–138.
69. Lenn NJ, Robertson M. Clinical utility of unbound antiepileptic drug blood levels in the management of epilepsy. *Neurology* 1992;42:988–990.
70. Levy RH, Schmidt D. Utility of free level monitoring of antiepileptic drugs. *Epilepsia* 1985;25:199–205.
71. Svensson CK, Woodruff MN, Baxter JG, et al. Free drug concentration monitoring in clinical practice: rationale and current status. *Clin Pharmacokinet* 1986;11:450–469.
72. Blom GF, Guelen PJM. The distribution of anti-epileptic drugs between serum, saliva and cerebrospinal fluid. In: Gardner-Thorpe C, Janz D, Meinardi H, et al., eds. *Antiepileptic drug monitoring.* Tunbridge Wells, UK: Pitman Medical, 1977:287–297.
73. Drobitch RK, Svensson CK. Therapeutic drug monitoring in saliva: an update. *Clin Pharmacokinet* 1992;23:365–379.
74. Johannessen SI, Henriksen O. Serum levels of di-*n*-propylacetate in epileptic patients. *Pharm Weekbl [Sci]* 1977;112:287–289.
75. Johannessen SI, Strandjord RE. Concentration of carbamazepine (Tegretol) in serum and cerebrospinal fluid in patients with epilepsy. *Epilepsia* 1973;14:373–379.
76. Monaco F, Piredda S, Mastropaolo C, et al. Diphenylhydantoin and primidone in tears. *Epilepsia* 1981;22:185–188.
77. Schmidt D, Kupferberg HJ. Diphenylhydantoin, phenobarbital, and primidone in saliva, plasma, and cerebrospinal fluid. *Epilepsia* 1975;16:735–741.
78. Lindberger M, Tomson T, Ståhle L. Validation of microdialysis

sampling for subcutaneous extracellular valproic acid in humans. *Ther Drug Monitor* 1998;20:358–362.

79. Tomson T, Almqvist O, Nilsson BY, et al. Carbamazepine-epoxide in epilepsy: a pilot study. *Arch Neurol* 1990;47:888–892.
80. Johannessen SI, Baruzzi A, Gomeni R, et al. Further observations on carbamazepine and carbamazepine-10,11-epoxide kinetics in epileptic patients. In: Gardner-Thorpe C, Janz D, Meinardi H, et al., eds. *Antiepileptic drug monitoring.* Tunbridge Wells, UK: Pitman Medical, 1977:110–127.
81. Leppik IE. Compliance in the treatment of epilepsy. In: Wyllie E, ed. *The treatment of epilepsy: principles and practice.* Philadelphia: Lea & Febiger, 1993:810–816.
82. Kutt H. Effect of acute and chronic diseases on the disposition of antiepileptic drugs. In: Morselli PL, Pippenger CE, Penry JK, eds. *Antiepileptic drug therapy in pediatrics.* New York: Raven Press, 1983:293–302.
83. Asconapé JJ, Penry JK. Use of antiepileptic drugs in the presence of liver and kidney diseases: a review. *Epilepsia* 1982;23[Suppl 1]:S65–S79.
84. Hooper WD, Bochner F, Eadie MJ, et al. Plasma protein binding of diphenylhydantoin: effects of sex hormones, renal and hepatic diseases. *Clin Pharmacol Ther* 1974; 15:276–282.
85. Hooper WD, Dubetz DK, Bochner F, et al. Plasma protein binding of carbamazepine. *Clin Pharmacol Ther* 1975;17:433–440.
86. Klotz U, Rapp T, Müller WA. Disposition of valproic acid in patients with liver disease. *Eur J Clin Pharmacol* 1978;13:55–60.
87. Gugler R, Müller G. Plasma protein binding of valproic acid in healthy subjects and in patients with renal disease. *Br J Clin Pharmacol* 1978;5:441–446.
88. Tomson T, Gram L, Sillanpää M, et al. Recommendation for the management and care of pregnant women with epilepsy. In: Tomson T, Gram L, Sillanpää M, et al., eds. *Epilepsy and pregnancy.* Petersfield, XX: Wrightson Biomedical Publishing, 1997:201–208.
89. Johannessen SI. Pharmacokinetics of valproate in pregnancy: mother, foetus, newborn. *Pharm Weekbl [Sci]* 1992;14:114–117.
90. Meijer JWA. Knowledge, attitude, and practice in antiepileptic drug monitoring. *Acta Neurol Scand Suppl* 1991;83:134.
91. Pippenger CE, Penry JK, White BG, et al. Interlaboratory variability in determination of plasma antiepileptic drug concentrations. *Arch Neurol* 1976;33:351–355.
92. Wilson JF, Tsanaclis LM, Perrett JE, et al. Performance of techniques for measurement of therapeutic drugs in serum: a comparison based on external quality assessment data. *Ther Drug Monit* 1992;14:98–106.
93. Beardsley RS, Freeman JM, Appel FA. Anticonvulsant serum levels are useful only if the physician appropriately uses them: an assessment of the impact of providing serum level data to the physicians. *Epilepsia* 1983;24:330–335.
94. Dodson EW. Level off. *Neurology* 1989;39:1009–1010.
95. Pena AIA, Lope ES. Can a single measurement of carbamazepine suffice for therapeutic monitoring? *Clin Chem* 1987;33:812–813.
96. Woo E, Chan YM, Yu YL, et al. If a well-stabilized epileptic patient has a subtherapeutic antiepileptic drug level, should the dose be increased? A randomized prospective study. *Epilepsia* 1988;29:129–139.
97. Pippenger CE. The cost-effectiveness of therapeutic drug monitoring. *Ther Drug Monit* 1990;12:418.
98. Vozeh S. Cost-effectiveness of therapeutic drug monitoring. *Clin Pharmacokinet* 1987;13:131–140.
99. Bialer M, Johannessen SI, Levy RH, et al. Progress report on new antiepileptic drugs: a summary of the Fifth Eilat Conference. *Epilepsy Res* 2001;43:11–58.

GENERAL PRINCIPLES

SAFETY MONITORING OF ANTIEPILEPTIC DRUGS

L. JAMES WILLMORE

Treatment of patients with epilepsy that is guided by the goals of complete seizure control without intolerable drug side effects is commonly compromised when control cannot be achieved because titration is limited by secondary drug toxicity (1,2). Good patient management requires establishment of a therapeutic alliance with active patient involvement. Toxic effects of drugs serve as one end point, independent of blood level monitoring, to allow clinical titration to efficacy. Although adverse effects from dose-related central nervous system toxicity of antiepileptic drugs (AEDs) are components of the pharmacologic effects of drugs, it is the unpredictable and dangerous idiosyncratic side effects that are of concern in monitoring patients during long-term treatment.

Idiosyncratic effects of drugs are rare but may be life-threatening. Physicians use scheduled monitoring laboratory studies in the hope of protecting patients against such serious problems, with the expectation of detecting dangerous reactions in time to intervene. Some physicians use regularly scheduled monitoring of drug blood levels along with a program of accumulating hematologic data, routine serum chemistry studies, and urinalysis (3). Pharmaceutical companies and published regulatory materials appear to require this monitoring strategy by incorporating standard recommendations for drug use as published in the *Physicians' Desk Reference* (4) in the United States and the *Compendium of Pharmaceuticals and Specialties* (5) in Canada. Although these reference sources appear to define the medicolegal *standard of practice* for many clinicians, in fact, these documents preserve observations about a specific and well-defined group of patients under close scrutiny during drug trials. Some

reports in these documents are amended when data show that specific warnings are needed to protect patients. Contrary to clinical practice, and these publications, scientific criteria based on accumulated evidence fail to support routine monitoring because such archival data rarely predict the occurrence of serious drug reactions. Although habits and practice vary both within the United States and in other countries, routine studies should be obtained at baseline, before starting treatment with a new drug, by measuring biochemical function and structural circulating elements in the blood (6) (Table 10.1).

All the established AEDs and some of the newer drugs (7–9) have caused serious idiosyncratic drug reactions that do not depend on drug dose and are unpredictable in their occurrence. All organs have been affected, but skin involvement tends to be the most common (Table 10.2). Established AEDs, used in millions of patients, are known to cause agranulocytosis, aplastic anemia, blistering skin rash, hepatic necrosis, allergic dermatitis, serum sickness, and pancreatitis. Newly available drugs used in many fewer patients throughout the world have caused allergic dermatitis and serious skin reactions (Table 10.2). Other than with felbamate (FBM), additional numerous serious reactions have yet to be reported with any credibility with these newer medications.

L. James Willmore, MD: Associate Dean and Professor, Department of Pharmacology and Physiology, Saint Louis University School of Medicine; and Attending Neurologist, Department of Neurology, Saint Louis University Hospital, Saint Louis, Missouri

TABLE 10.1. BASELINE SCREENING STUDIES BEFORE BEGINNING ANTIEPILEPTIC DRUG TREATMENT

Complete blood count with differential and platelets
Glucose, blood urea nitrogen, electrolytes, calcium, phosphorus, magnesium, creatinine, urate, serum iron, cholesterol, bilirubin, alkaline phosphatase, aspartate aminotransferase, alanine aminotransferase, total protein, albumin globulin, prothrombin time, partial thromboplastin time

TABLE 10.2. IDIOSYNCRATIC REACTIONS TO ANTIEPILEPTIC DRUGS

Reaction	CBZ	ETH	FBM	GBP	LEV[a]	LTG	PB	PHT	TPM	TGB	OXC	VPA
Agranulocytosis	X	X	X				X	X				X
Stevens-Johnson syndrome	X	X				X	X	X				X
Aplastic anemia	X	X	X					X				X
Hepatic failure	X	X					X	X				X
Allergic dermatitis	X	X	X	X		X	X	X	X	X	X	X
Serum sickness	X	X					X	X				X
Pancreatitis	X							X				X

CBZ, carbamazepine; ETH, ethosuximide; FBM, felbamate; GBP, gabapentin; LEV, levetiracetam; LTG, lamotrigine; PB, phenobarbital; PHT, phenytoin; TPM, topiramate; TGB, tiagabine; OXC, oxcarbazepine; VPA, valproic acid.
[a]Too few patient exposures for LEV.

MANAGEMENT PLANNING

After a drug is selected for use, the physician must review the relative benefits and risks with the patient and must document, in the patient's record, that this discussion took place. This process of review and information forms the basis for informal informed consent. The patient should be taught the criteria for success and should be reminded about the necessary process of trial and error in drug selection and about the methods for changing drugs. Because common dose-related side effects are used to aid in management, but interfere with treatment, this process should be one of negotiation. The patient must know the nature of the side effects, what must be tolerated, and how the physician will use these side effects in the titration process. Serious, life-threatening, idiosyncratic effects of a selected drug must be reviewed in clear terms, but within the context of rarity. Although the patient must participate in this therapeutic alliance and be ready to communicate should symptoms develop, the physician must identify patients who are without advocates or whose ability to communicate is impaired. These special patients may need the design of a monitoring strategy, a plan not needed by most patients with epilepsy. A program of screening may be useful in some high-risk patients (1).

CLINICAL MONITORING

Clinical monitoring is useful, especially when viewed within the context of the incidence of serious adverse reactions. Although routine monitoring of hepatic function revealed elevation of values in 5% to 15% of patients treated with carbamazepine (CBZ), fewer than 20 patients with significant hepatic complications were reported in the United States from 1978 to 1989 (10). Fewer cases of pancreatitis were reported. Transient leukopenia occurs in up to 12% of adults and children treated with CBZ (11,12). Aplastic anemia or agranulocytosis, unrelated to the afore-mentioned benign leukopenia, occurs in two per 575,000, with a mortality rate of approximately one in 575,000 treated patients per year (10). Only four of the 65 cases of agranulocytosis or aplastic anemia occurred in children.

Of patients developing exfoliative dermatitis alone or as part of systemic hypersensitivity, blood test abnormalities were not found until patients developed clinical symptoms. Presymptomatic blood studies fail to predict disease development. Test abnormalities such as benign leukopenia or transient hepatic enzyme elevations do not predict the occurrence of life-threatening reactions. A genetic abnormality in arene oxide metabolism may occur in those patients at higher risk of some types of adverse responses, such as hepatitis (13). A screening test for such defects is not available. The data show that routine monitoring, as practiced commonly, does not allow anticipation of life-threatening effects associated with CBZ treatment. Findings for phenytoin (PHT) and phenobarbital (PB) are similar (1).

Assessment of patients developing hepatotoxicity from treatment with valproate (VPA) suggests that the highest risk is in children <2 years old who are being treated with several AEDs. Most fatalities occurred in the first 6 months of treatment, but some patients developed hepatotoxicity up to 2 years after VPA initiation. Children <2 years of age who were receiving polytherapy had a one in 500 to 800 chance of developing fatal VPA hepatotoxicity. Negative predictors were documented. Patients at negligible risk were those >10 years old who were treated with VPA alone and who were free of indication of underlying metabolic or neurologic disorders. Children at intermediate risk were those between age 2 and 10 years and who were receiving monotherapy and all patients requiring polytherapy. The risk of fatal VPA hepatotoxicity continues to decline with increasing age, even in polytherapy, after the first decade of life (14).

Additional risk characteristics include patients with presumed metabolic disorders or with severe epilepsy complicating mental retardation and organic brain disease

(15,16,17,18). Although this pattern of incidence provides useful clinical guidelines, most clinicians consider them too restrictive or insufficiently detailed to allow identification of patients at highest risk (19). This lack of more specific guidelines to identify patients at highest risk for development of VPA hepatotoxicity has caused the use of that drug to be restricted in patients with intractable epilepsy. Further complicating management strategies, routine laboratory monitoring does not predict the development of fulminant and irreversible hepatic failure (20). Some patients progressing to fatal hepatotoxicity never develop abnormalities of specific hepatic function tests. Conversely, abnormalities of serum ammonia, carnitine, fibrinogen, and hepatic function tests have been reported to occur without the presence of clinically significant hepatotoxicity. Drug interactions should be considered as well (21,22). Reporting clinical symptoms and identification of patients at greatest risk of fatal hepatotoxicity are more reliable means for monitoring. Vomiting is the most frequently reported initial symptom in fatal cases (15,16). Combined symptoms of nausea, vomiting, and anorexia occurred in 82% of patients with reported VPA-associated hepatotoxicity, whereas lethargy, drowsiness, and come were reported in 40% (23,24). Although some patients may have reversal of hepatotoxicity by early drug discontinuation, fatalities still result after such prompt action (25). No biochemical markers have been identified to differentiate those patients who survive from those with a fatal outcome (25).

Whether children or adults, most patients reported with fatal hepatotoxicity had neurologic abnormalities, including mental retardation, encephalopathy, and decline of neurologic function. In patients >21 years old, two of four had degenerative disease of the nervous system. One report stated that nine of 16 patients with hepatic fatalities were neurologically abnormal (26). In one series, all patients in the 11- to 20-year age group were neurologically abnormal. In one review, only seven of 26 adults reported with fatal hepatic failure related to VPA were considered to be neurologically normal (27).

The specific biochemical disorders associated with VPA hepatotoxicity include urea cycle defects, organic acidurias, multiple carboxylase deficiency, mitochondrial or respiratory chain dysfunction, cytochrome aa_3 deficiency in muscle, pyruvate carboxylase deficiency, and hepatic pyruvate dehydrogenase complex deficiency (brain) (19,28,29). Clinical disorders associated with VPA toxicity include GM_1 gangliosidosis type 2, spinocerebellar degeneration, Friedreich's ataxia, Lafora's body disease, Alper's disease, and MERRF (myoclonic epilepsy with ragged red fiber myopathy) syndrome (23). Patients with such disorders must be identified because of their higher risk of VPA hepatotoxicity.

High-risk patients usually are identified by clinical assessment. Medical history, health status at the initiation of AED treatment, and both patient and physician awareness of clinically important symptoms and signs are more likely to suggest the need for further evaluation.

LIMITATIONS OF ROUTINE LABORATORY MONITORING

Two prospective studies evaluated the efficacy of routine blood and urine screening in patients being treated on a long-term basis with AEDs. Camfield et al. (30) performed blood and urine testing in 199 children to evaluate liver, blood, and renal function at initiation of therapy and at 1,3, and 6 months. These investigators repeated the screening studies every 6 months. There were no serious clinical reactions in these patients treated with PB, PHT, CBZ, or VPA. Studies were repeated in 6% because of abnormal but clinically insignificant results, and in two children therapy was discontinued unnecessarily. These investigators concluded that routine monitoring provided no useful information and sometimes led to unnecessary responses. A second study of 662 adults treated with CBZ, PHT, PB, or primidone failed to detect significant laboratory abnormalities during 6 months of monitoring (31). The authors concluded that routine screening was not cost effective or of significant value for asymptomatic patients. Treatment of 480 patients with either CBZ or VPA in a double-blind, controlled trial also demonstrated a lack of usefulness of routine laboratory monitoring (32).

LABORATORY ABNORMALITIES

Laboratory standards vary. Certain changes are expected and acceptable for patients undergoing long-term AED therapy. In asymptomatic patients, few significant abnormalities occur at three times the upper limit of normal for hepatic functions tests. Leukocyte counts as low as 2×10^9/L are frequently insignificant and do not, in and of themselves, predict bone marrow suppression. Such changes occur in at least 10% of patients treated with CBZ or PHT, are usually transient, and do not predict the occurrence of aplastic anemia or agranulocytosis. Platelet counts >100,000 also are usually asymptomatic and do not predict the development of thrombocytopenia.

Regular monitoring of hematology, chemistry, and other routine studies may be most helpful only if the patient is immediately presymptomatic and presenting with abnormal symptoms and signs (33). Thus, regularly scheduled laboratory monitoring for all patients treated with AEDs both is wasteful and does not lead to the desired result of identifying patients at risk of development of life-threatening adverse drug reactions. Camfield et al. (33) estimated that if every patient with epilepsy in North America were tested three times each year for complete blood count, serum amino aspartate, and transaminase levels, the cost would be more than $400,000,000 annually. A modification of recommendations regarding routine monitoring has been suggested by the Canadian Association for Child Neurology (33).

Although obtaining routine, scheduled screening studies is the habit of most clinicians, the key to treatment monitoring is patient and parent education and counseling. All concerned about a patient must be aware of potential complications and the symptoms that may herald the occurrence of an adverse event. Furthermore, physicians must be willing to evaluate patients on an urgent basis when changes suggesting the development of significant adverse drug reactions are reported. Such symptoms include bruising, bleeding, rash, abdominal pain, vomiting, jaundice, lethargy, coma, and deterioration in seizure control. Exacerbation of seizures or marked shortening of the seizure-free interval is a cause both for review of treatment and survey for the presence of adverse drug effects. The development of any of these possibly ominous symptoms is the best indication for repeating laboratory evaluations.

Although the data suggest that routine, scheduled monitoring is neither cost effective nor helpful, the physician must obtain baseline studies before initiation of an AED. Baseline studies are listed in Table 10.1. Review and retention of such pretreatment data in the medical record may identify patients with heretofore unidentified illness and may allow comparison should symptoms develop and laboratory studies need to be repeated.

AT-RISK PROFILES

Because prediction of the occurrence of serious adverse effects is not possible by routine laboratory monitoring, one useful strategy may be to identify high-risk patients. Glauser (7) has attempted to construct "at risk" clinical profiles for some of the AEDs. Profiles rely on reports of patients who developed idiopathic drug reactions and then constructing a profile based on common occurrences among such cohorts. Drugs allowing profiling include FBM, lamotrigine (LMT), and VPA. VPA has a risk profile for hepatotoxicity that is too nonspecific to be of much practical help. Patients at risk of developing hepatic

failure during treatment with VPA include those <2 years old who are being treated with several AEDs and who have a known metabolic disease associated with developmental delay (10–12). Patients fitting the at-risk profile need detailed laboratory screening for the presence of metabolic disorders. Studies suggested (6) include serum lactate, serum pyruvate, serum carnitine, urinary organic acids, and routine hematologic and chemical screening. Prothrombin time and partial thromboplastin time along with arterial blood gases and ammonia are useful as well (Table 10.3).

NEW DRUGS: MONITORING STRATEGIES

As new drugs are developed and are added to the regimen available for treating patients with epilepsy, physicians have an obligation to review source documents about those medications and to devise a strategy for treatment and monitoring. Drug development is performed by treating selected patients. Age ranges are defined, epilepsy syndromes and seizure types are identified, and patients with associated illness or need for concomitant medications are excluded. Studies are performed exposing limited numbers of patients to a drug for a finite period. During such studies, patients undergo intense scrutiny to identify treatment-related symptoms or adverse effects of a drug. These restrictions in study design may fail to uncover drug interactions or the occurrence of serious adverse effects of a drug.

Because data are limited, initiation of treatment with a newly available drug requires special caution. Although the process of informed consent remains informal, patients should be given as much information as possible. Industry-produced materials may prove useful, but the physician should also provide copies of package inserts coupled with material they prepare describing how the drug is to be used and any monitoring strategy planned. Although the guiding principle of monitoring of patients who are treated with established drugs is parsimony in terms of obtaining routine chemical and hematologic studies, based on the knowledge that such monitoring is ineffective in detecting the occurrence of serious adverse events, such is not the case with a newly introduced drug. As with the established drugs, baseline data should be obtained. Communication is still key; the patient must be prepared to contact the physician, and the physician must facilitate that communication. Chemical and hematologic monitoring with use of a new drug may be recommended in the materials a company develops in concert with regulatory functions of the Food and Drug Administration in the United States. Although recommendations may seem excessively conservative, it may be wise to follow those guidelines until a larger experience is obtained and data become available. This admonition is best illustrated by the experience reported in the communications about FBM.

TABLE 10.3. ASSESSMENT FOR HIGH-RISK PATIENTS TREATED WITH VALPROATE

At risk:
  Younger than 2 years of age
  Treated with multiple drugs
  Known metabolic disease
  Delayed development
Specific screening studies:
  Serum lactate and pyruvate
  Plasma carnitine
  Urinary metabolic screen with organic acids
  Ammonia and arterial blood gases

From DeVries SI. Haematological aspects during treatment with anticonvulsant drugs. *Epilepsia.* 1965;7:1–15, with permission.

TABLE 10.4. GUIDELINES FOR USE OF FELBAMATE

Risk factors
  Nonspecific
    Caucasian
    Adult
    Female
  Suggestive
    Prior cytopenia
    Allergy to another antiepileptic drug
    Prior immune disorder
Laboratory screening
  New antiepileptic drug panel
Atopaldehyde studies

Specific Drugs

Felbamate

Serious idiosyncratic reactions to FBM, including aplastic anemia, occur with an incidence of approximately one per 4,000 to 8,000, as compared with an incidence of 2 to 2.5 per million persons in the general population (7,34–37). The rate of death resulting from aplastic anemia from FBM is more than 20 times the rate associated with CBZ (7,35,36). Some features related to patients developing aplastic anemia during FBM treatment include the occurrence of an immunologic disorder, such as lupus erythematosus, a condition found in 33% of affected patients (7,35,36), a history of cytopenia, occurring in 42% of patients, and a history of an allergic reaction or toxic reaction to another AED, observed in 52% of patients (7,35,36).

Clinical risk profiles for FBM suggest a screening strategy. Although some features, such as being a white woman, are not specific, the occurrence a prior AED allergic reaction, cytopenia, a history of an immune disorder, especially lupus erythematosus, and less than 1 year of treatment are more worrisome. Screening studies to measure the excretion of atopaldehyde and the ratio of monocarbamate metabolites may offer a method for screening of patients treated with FBM. Table 10.4 lists screening guidelines for patients to be treated with FBM.

Hepatotoxic effects of FBM seem less clearly associated with risk factors. Of the 18 reported patients, an estimated incidence for all patients was 1 per 18,500 to 25,000, a pattern similar to that found during treatment with VPA. However, detailed review suggested that only seven of these 18 patients actually suffered hepatic injury from FBM, numbers that are more than likely too few to construct a risk profile (7). Because atopaldehyde, an electrophylic and cytotoxic substance, can be formed from the monocarbamate metabolite of FBM, a measure of the ratio of excreted mercapturic acid to carbamoyl derivatives indirectly reflects the ability of a patient's liver to conjugate glutathione to the atopaldehyde (38–40). Kits for evaluating patients are available from the manufacturer of FBM and should be used when treating patients with that drug.

Lamotrigine

LMT is known to cause serious dermatologic reactions (41). Although erythematous rash with a morbilliform pattern or urticaria and patterns with a maculopapular component are most common (34,41–45), some patients can develop erythema mulitforme and blistering reactions such as the Stevens-Johnson syndrome or toxic epidermal necrolysis. Simple rashes require careful assessment to ensure that a hypersensitivity syndrome is not developing. Sensitivity reactions include fever, lymphadenopathy, elevated liver enzymes, and altered numbers of circulating cellular elements of blood (41).

In drug trials in the United States, rash was observed in about 10% of patients, with 3.8% having to discontinue and 0.3% hospitalized (41). Most serious rashes developed within 6 weeks of beginning treatment with LMT. In children treated in drug trials, rash was observed in 12.9%, with serious rash in 1.1% with half of those with Stevens-Johnson syndrome (41). More than 80% of patients with complete data developing serious rash were being treated with VPA or had been given doses at a rate higher than recommended (41). Overall, children treated with LMT have a threefold increased risk of developing serious rash compared with adults. Apparently, when specific treatment

TABLE 10.5. SUGGESTED GUIDELINES FOR USE OF LAMOTRIGINE

Provide information for patients and parents about rash		
Weeks 1 and 2	**Weeks 3 and 4**	**To Achieve Maintenance**
For adult patients receiving inducing drugs such as phenytoin, carbamazepine, or barbiturates (but not valproate):		
50 mg/day	100 mg/day (in divided doses)	Add 50–100 mg every 1–2 wk to 200–400 mg/day
For patients treated with valproate		
25 mg every other day	25 mg/day	Add 25–50 mg every 1–2 wk to 100–200 mg/day

guidelines are followed, the incidence of serious rash may possibly be reduced (41,45,46). Table 10.5 lists the suggested treatment plan for LMT use.

RECOMMENDATIONS FOR MANAGEMENT

1. Baseline laboratory studies should be obtained before initiation of treatment with an AED. Data are unavailable about the yield of such testing, but baseline studies provide a benchmark and could identify patients with special risk factors that could influence drug selection.
2. Blood and urine monitoring in otherwise healthy and asymptomatic patients treated with most AEDs is not necessary. FBM is the exception.
3. High-risk patients must be identified at the beginning of treatment. These patients include those with biochemical disorders, altered systemic health, neurodegenerative disease, or a history of significant adverse drug reactions. Monitoring must be designed to the specific clinical situation.
4. Patients without an advocate and those who are unable to communicate require a different strategy. Although data are unavailable, blood monitoring should be obtained for patients with multiple handicaps who are institutionalized. Monitoring should include basic hematology and chemistry tests, with additional studies based on the patient's clinical situation.
5. When treating a patient with a newly available drug, one should provide detailed information to the patient or the caregiver. One should follow recommended guidelines for blood monitoring until the numbers of patients treated in this country increase and data become available.

REFERENCES

1. Schmidt D. *Adverse effects of antiepileptic drugs.* New York: Raven Press, 1982.
2. Pellock JM. Efficacy and adverse effects of antiepileptic drugs. *Pediatr Clin North Am* 1989;36:435–448.
3. DeVries SI. Haematological aspects during treatment with anticonvulsant drugs. *Epilepsia* 1965;7:1–15.
4. *Physicians' desk reference,* 54th ed. Oradell, NJ: Medical Economics, 1999.
5. Krogh CME. *Compendium of pharmaceuticals and specialities,* 34th ed. Ottawa: Canadian Pharmaceutical Association, 1999.
6. Pellock JM, Willmore LJ. A rational guide to routine blood monitoring in patients receiving antiepileptic drugs. *Neurology* 1991; 41:961–964.
7. Glauser TA. Idiosyncratic reactions: new methods of identifying high-risk patients. *Epilepsia* 2000;41:S16–S29.
8. Park BK, Pirmohamed M, Kitteringham NR. Idiosyncratic drug reactions: a mechanistic evaluation of risk factors. *Br J Clin Pharmacol* 1992;34:377–395.
9. Pirmohamed M, Kitteringham NR, Park BK. The role of active metabolites in drug toxicity. *Drug Saf* 1994;11:114–144.
10. Seetharam MN, Pellock JM. Risk-benefit assessment of carbamazepine in children. *Drug Saf* 1991;6:148–158.
11. Pellock JM. Carbamazepine side effects in children and adults. *Epilepsia* 1987;28:S64–S70.
12. Hart RG, Easton JD. Carbamazepine and hematological monitoring. *Ann Neurol* 1982;11:309–312.
13. Spielberg SP, Gordon GB, Blake DA, et al. Predisposition to phenytoin hepatotoxicity assessed *in vitro.* N Engl J Med 1981;305:722–727.
14. Bryant AE III, Dreifuss FE. Valproic acid hepatic fatalities. III. U.S. experience since 1986. *Neurology* 1996;46:465–469.
15. Dreifuss FE, Santilli N, Langer DH, et al. Valproic acid hepatic fatalities: a retrospective review. *Neurology* 1987;37:379–385.
16. Dreifuss FE, Langer DH, Moline KA, et al. Valproic acid hepatic fatalities. II. US experience since 1984. *Neurology* 1989;39: 201–207.
17. Willmore LJ. Clinical manifestations of valproate hepatotoxicity. In: Levy RH, Penry JK, eds. *Idiosyncratic reactions to valporate: clinical risk patterns and mechanisms of toxicity.* New York: Raven Press, 1991:3–7.
18. Willmore LJ. Clinical risk patterns: summary and recommendations. In: Levy RH, Penry JK, eds. *Idiosyncratic reactions to valproate: clinical risk patterns and mechanisms of toxicity.* New York: Raven Press, 1991:163–165.
19. Willmore LJ, Triggs WJ, Pellock JM. Valproate toxicity: risk-screening strategies. *J Child Neurol* 1991;6:3–6.
20. Willmore LJ, Wilder BJ, Bruni J, et al. Effect of valproic acid on hepatic function. *Neurology* 1978;28:961–964.
21. Kifune A, Kubota F, Shibata N, et al. Valproic acid-induced hyperammonemic encephalopathy with triphasic waves. *Epilepsia* 2000;41:909–912.
22. Hamer HM, Knake S, Schomburg U, et al. Valproate-induced hyperammonemic encephalopathy in the presence of topiramate. *Neurology* 2000;54:230–232.
23. van Egmond H, Degomme P, de Simpel H, et al. A suspected case of late-onset sodium valproate-induced hepatic failure. *Neuropediatrics* 1987;18:96–98.
24. Kuhara T, Inoue Y, Matsumoto M, et al. Markedly increased ω-oxidation of valproate in fulminant hepatic failure. *Epilepsia* 1990;31:214–217.
25. Konig SA, Siemes H, Blaker F, et al. Severe hepatotoxicity during valproate therapy: an update and report of eight new fatalities. *Epilepsia* 1994;35:1005–1015.
26. Scheffner D, Konig St, Rauterberg-Ruland I, et al. Fatal liver failure in 16 children with valproate therappy. *Epilepsia* 1988;29: 530–542.
27. Konig SA, Schenk M, Sick C, et al. Fatal liver failure associate with valproate therapy in a patient with Friedreich's disease: review of valproate hepatotoxicity in adults. *Epilepsia* 1999;40: 1036–1040.
28. Jellinger K, Seitelberger F. Spongy encephalopathies in infancy: spongy degeneration of CNS and progressive infantile poliodystrophy. In: Goldensohn ES, Appel SA, eds. *Scientific approaches to clinical neurology.* Philadelphia: Lea & Febiger, 1977:363.
29. Prick M, Gabreels F, Renier W, et al. Pyruvate dehydrogenase deficiency restricted to brain. *Neurology* 1981;31:398–404.
30. Camfield C, Camfield P, Smith E, et al. Asymptomatic children with epilepsy: little benefit from screening for anticonvulsant-induced liver, blood or renal damage. *Neurology* 1986;36: 838–841.
31. Mattson RH, Cramer JA, Collins JF, et al. Comparison of carbamazepine, phenobarbital, phenytoin, and primidone in partial and secondarily generalized tonic-clonic seizures. *N Engl J Med* 1985;313:145–151.
32. Mattson RH, Cramer JA, Collins JF, et al. A comparison of valproate with carbamazepine for the treatment of complex partial

seizures and secondarily generalized tonic-clonic seizures in adults. *N Engl J Med* 1992;327:765–771.

33. Camfield P, Camfield C, Dooley J, et al. Routine screening of blood and urine for severe reactions to anticonvulsant drugs in asymptomatic patients is of doubtful value. *Can Med Assoc J* 1989;140:1303–1305.

34. Pellock JM. Managing pediatric epilepsy syndromes with new antiepileptic drugs. *Pediatrics* 1999;104:1106–1116.

35. Pellock JM. Felbamate. *Epilepsia* 1999;40:S57–S62.

36. Pellock JM, Brodie MJ. Felbamate: 1997 update. *Epilepsia* 1997; 38:1261–1264.

37. Patton W, Duffull S. Idiosyncratic drug-induced haematological abnormalities: incidence, pathogenesis, management and avoidance. *Drug Saf* 1994;11:445–462.

38. Kapetanovic IM, Torchin CD, Thompson CD, et al. Potentially reactive cyclic carbamate metabolite of the antiepileptic drug felbamate produced by human liver tissue *in vitro. Drug Metab Dispos* 1998;26:1089–1095.

39. Thompson CD, Gulden PH, Macdonald TL. Identificaiton of modified atropaldehyde mercapturic acids in rat and human urine after felbamate admistration. *Chem Res Toxicol* 1997;10: 457–462.

40. Thompson CD, Barthen MD, Hooper DW. Quantification in patient uring samples of felbamate and three metabolites: acid carbamate and two mercapturic acids. *Epilepsia* 1999;40:769–776.

41. Guberman AH, Besag FMC, Brodie MJ, et al. Lamotrigine-associated rash: risk/benefit consideratins in adults and children. *Epilepsia* 1999;40:985–991.

42. Schlienger RG, Shapiro LE, Shear NH. Lamotrigine-induced severe cutaneous adverse reactions. *Epilepsia* 1998;39:S22–S26.

43. Pellock JM. Overview of lamotrigine and the new antiepileptic drugs: the challenge. *J Child Neurol* 1997;12:S48–S52.

44. Willmore LJ, Messenheimer JA. Adult experience with lamotrigine. *J Child Neurol* 1997;12:S16–S18.

45. Messenheimer JA, Mullens EJ, Giorgi L, et al. Safety review of adult clinical trial experience with lamotrigine. *Drug Saf* 1998; 18:281–296.

46. Motte J, Trevathan E, Arvidsson JFV, et al. Lamotrigine for generalized seizures associated with the Lennox-Gastaut syndrome. *N Engl J Med* 1994;337:1807–1812.

GENERAL PRINCIPLES

USE OF ANTIEPILEPTIC DRUGS IN CHILDREN

OLIVIER DULAC

Managing epilepsy in the neonate and child requires an understanding of the unique biochemical and pharmacologic characteristics of this age range. Accurate classification of seizures and identification of epilepsy syndromes, coupled with a thorough neurologic assessment to define etiology, and a comprehensive assessment of the patient's health and social situation are essential to good treatment. Effective management also requires communication with the patient's parents, to ensure that they understand the goals of the treatment, which depend of the type of epilepsy and its prognosis, the side effects of medications, the diagnostic process, and treatment monitoring strategies. Parents need to have realistic expectations regarding seizure control, and they must understand the need to try drugs in sequence. After each prescription is written, a leaflet giving the main characteristics of the drug prescribed, focusing on the usual dose administered, the first signs of potential side effects, and the concurrent medications that are contraindicated or need special attention, should be given to the parents and read to them. The child's parents also need to know from the onset of treatment what the criteria for cessation of treatment will be. "Treatment for life" does not exist, despite frequent claims to the contrary, including those made by the medical profession.

CHARACTERISTICS OF EPILEPSY IN NEONATES AND CHILDREN

The first peak of incidence of epilepsy is in the first decade of life (1). In one cohort, the incidence was 120 per 100,000 in the first year of life (2), decreasing to 40 per 100,000 for the remainder of the first decade. The most common identifiable cause is either prenatal or a consequence of acute circulatory failure (3). However, for more than three-fourths of children with epilepsy, the cause cannot be determined. Seizures are more likely to be occasional and the result of acute brain damage in the newborn than in the infant and in the infant than in the child.

The type of seizures observed in adults may also occur in children. Partial seizures may be observed from the very first months of life (1,4). Some types of seizures are specific to the newborn period and infancy. For example, clusters of spasms are rarely observed after 1 year of age (5), although they may occur later (6), even without the expected hypsarrhythmic electroencephalographic (EEG) pattern (7). Many children have several types of seizures; one epidemiologic study reported more than 1.6 seizure types per patient <10 years old (1). Seizures are not the only expression of epilepsy in children, however. Motor and cognitive functions may be affected, and some patients with a form of epilepsy that produces speech disorders, the Landau-Kleffner syndrome, never have seizures.

Some types of epilepsy are age specific. The combination of specific seizure types, cognitive and motor characteristics, and EEG patterns, beginning within a specific age range, serves to define epilepsy syndromes that are age related and depend partly on particular stages of brain cortical maturation. This concept is of critical importance because the cause is unknown in most children (8).

Intractability of epilepsy is correlated with educational difficulties. More than 60% of patients with seizures persisting for >2 years after onset fail in school, compared with a 25% rate of failure among those patients with rapid seizure control (9).

EFFECTS OF ANTIEPILEPTIC DRUGS ON THE CLINICAL PATTERN

The selection of an antiepileptic drug (AED) for a specific patient is usually based on clinical observation, because controlled data do not apply to individual patients. Carbamazepine (CBZ) is often considered more effective to treat

Olivier Dulac, MD: Professor, Department of Pediatric Neurology, University of René Descartes, Paris, France

partial seizures than generalized seizures, whereas the reverse is true for valproate (VPA) (10–12). However, one randomized trial in children with newly diagnosed partial or generalized Torric-Clount seizures failed to disclose any difference in efficacy of both compounds, whatever the seizure type, partial or generalized (13).

AEDs may modify the clinical pattern of seizures by (a) controlling the type of seizures experienced by the patient or (b) changing the type of seizures. For example, in a given patient, a drug may result in control of secondarily generalized seizures, including epileptic spasms, whereas simple or complex partial seizures remain unaffected (14). This response may be clinically relevant because generalized seizures are more incapacitating than partial seizures from the cognitive point of view (15). An additional seizure pattern may emerge as a result of adverse effects of the AEDs, and it may worsen of the patient's condition, as may occur in the case of (a) tonic status epilepticus in patients with Lennox-Gastaut syndrome who are treated with benzodiazepines (16) or (b) myoclonic status in patients with myoclonic epilepsy who are treated with CBZ or vigabatrin (VGB) (14). Thus, the choice of a drug must be governed not only by seizure types but also by the identification of any specific epilepsy syndrome. Although this may be difficult at onset of the seizure disorder, when the diagnosis remains uncertain, it soon becomes feasible because, in one epidemiologic study of prevalence, proper syndromic diagnosis could be established in >90% of cases with established epilepsy (17).

ANTIEPILEPTIC DRUG EFFICACY IN EPILEPSY SYNDROMES

The occurrence of seizures requires identification of other potentially related clinical characteristics to define the epilepsy syndrome. A specific seizure type may be associated with several epilepsy syndromes, each having a different response to AED treatment. For example, simple partial seizures appear to respond differently to treatment, depending on whether the seizures are the result of a brain lesion or of a condition such as benign partial epilepsy with centrotemporal spikes (BPECTS). Although preliminary observations suggest that CBZ is more effective than VPA in patients with symptomatic partial epilepsy, both drugs are associated with the same rate of efficacy in patients with BPECTS (10). An AED may improve seizure control in some epilepsy syndromes, whereas it may worsen seizure control in others. Some specific responses to drugs may be expected with some of the epilepsy syndromes (18–20). For example, CBZ may worsen continuous spike waves in slow-wave sleep (21). Table 11.1 shows those drugs that are more likely to be dangerous in specific epilepsy syndromes.

The diagnosis of a specific epilepsy syndrome is challenging. Although the patient may have specific seizures

TABLE 11.1. POTENTIAL AGGRAVATION IN VARIOUS EPILEPSY SYNDROMES

	PB	CBZ	VGB	PHT	LTG
Idiopathic generalized epilepsy		+	+		
Absences	+	+	+	+	
Dravet's syndrome	+	+	+		+
Epileptogenic encephalopathies					
Continuous spike-waves in sleep	+	+	+	+	
Infantile spasms	+	+		+	
Lennox-Gastaut syndrome	+	+	+		

PB, phenobarbital; CBZ, carbamazepine; VGB, vigabatrin; PHT, phenytoin; LTG, lamotrigine.

from the onset, the characteristic EEG pattern necessary to establish the diagnosis may not be observed for some time, and early diagnosis may not be possible. A patient with seizures that are typical of those observed in BPECTS may not have centrotemporal spikes on a given EEG. Patients with myoclonic-astatic epilepsy (22) are commonly thought to have Lennox-Gastaut syndrome. In severe myoclonic epilepsy of infancy (Dravet's syndrome) (23,24), the observation of myoclonic jerks and spike-wave discharges on the EEG will be delayed for several years. Alternating unilateral seizures may, at the onset, be thought to result from focal epilepsy. However, patients with focal epilepsy may have generalized seizures when the condition starts during the first year of life, with focal seizures appearing later (25).

An epileptic syndrome may have a clinical pattern evolving through several stages, each with a different response to AEDs. Both VPA and the benzodiazepines are effective at the onset of Dravet's syndrome. By the age of 3 to 4 years, phenytoin (PHT) and VGB may have become effective, possibly because episodes of status epilepticus have produced additional epileptogenic brain injury (23). Accumulating evidence indicated that some disorders currently considered specific epilepsy syndromes are, in fact, heterogeneous. A syndrome with different causes may have different responses to treatment. This is best illustrated by infantile spasms that have a better response to VGB than to steroids when the spasms are caused by tuberous sclerosis (26), but they may fail to respond to VGB monotherapy when they are cryptogenic with negative neuroradiology but psychomotor delay before the first spasms (27). Thus, an etiologic diagnosis, in addition to identification of the syndrome, is required whenever possible before any treatment decision is made.

Precise identification of the epilepsy syndrome is often difficult during the first weeks or months of the disease. Thus, it is often wise to administer a compound that has a relatively large spectrum of activity and that is not known to cause syndrome specific worsening, particularly VPA.

Before marketing new compounds for epilepsy, some data should be available regarding not only efficacy but also potential harm in the various specific syndromes of childhood epilepsy. Regarding efficacy, controlled trials need only small numbers of patients when they select patients with one given epilepsy syndrome and eventually one type of origin. Thus, it was possible to demonstrate the efficacy of VGB in infantile spasms, whatever the cause (28), with <50 patients and in those with epilepsy resulting from tuberous sclerosis with only 22 patients (29). It was also possible to show the efficacy of stiripentol combined with clobazam and VPA in Dravet's syndrome with only 41 patients (30).

TOLERABILITY OF DRUG THERAPY

Several of the AEDs have age-specific adverse effects, particularly in patients with associated metabolic abnormalities. Acute hepatic failure is 30 to 100 times more frequent in infants than in adults (31–39). Infants <2 years of age are in the most vulnerable group for the occurrence of inborn errors of metabolism, which predispose to VPA hepatotoxicity, and these infants are in the age group of patients in need of VPA therapy (31–33,39–41). VPA is more likely to be used in polytherapy in infants than in adults. For example, acetylsalicylic acid often used to be administered for fever in infants, and the combination of this drug with VPA in the presence of fever seems to be particularly strongly associated with drug-induced Reye-like hepatic failure (34,42). Drug interactions between macrolides and CBZ have been most commonly reported in children (35,43). Ethosuximide may cause hallucinations in adolescents (36,44). Whether this effect of ethosuximide is the result of age-related specific effects of AEDs or, alternatively, a specific age-related characteristic of the epilepsy for which this drug is administered remains unclear because treatment of absence epilepsy with high doses of ethosuximide is required in adolescents. Skin rash associated with lamotrigine (LTG) is more common when the drug is used in combination with VPA (37,45). This type of drug combination is effective in patients with generalized epilepsy, a common type of epilepsy in childhood (38,46). Thus, the cause of epilepsy may contribute to the occurrence of side effects of AEDs in children.

ANTIEPILEPTIC DRUGS AND COGNITIVE FUNCTIONS IN PEDIATRIC PATIENTS

Behavior and cognitive functions are affected by preexisting brain injury coupled with psychological isolation (31,32,39,40). Seizures, frequent spike-wave activity, and AED effects may all exacerbate these problems, and distinguishing the leading cause of cognitive disorder is often challenging. Half the children exhibit fluctuations of cognitive functions and behavior over periods of a few months (33,41). However, some epilepsy syndromes in infants and children are associated with marked mental deterioration within a few weeks. This finding applies particularly to patients with generalized paroxysmal activity, whether primarily or secondarily generalized, with the epilepsy syndromes unclassified as either partial or generalized. In partial epilepsy, the type of cognitive deficit depends of the topography of the epileptogenic focus (34,42).

Toxic circulating levels of AEDs may alter intellectual functioning. Cognitive disorders are easily overlooked, as shown in studies of school-age children treated with phenobarbital (PB) (35,36,43,44) or CBZ (37,45). PB-induced depression may be overlooked (38,46). These complications of treatment are of particular concern because children are rapidly developing cognitive functions. Cognitive impairment caused by drugs may abate within a few weeks after beginning treatment. Polypharmacy and underlying poor neuropsychological functioning increase the risk of developing behavioral side effects. In addition, the use of several drugs may alter a patient's ability to develop tolerance to cognitive alterations when compared with the use of monotherapy. Observational data and standardized tests are not available regarding cognitive test performance in children <6 years of age who are treated with AEDs.

PHARMACOKINETICS

The effect of a drug on a target organ is determined by the drug concentration at the site of action. Both seizure control and toxic effects depend on the quantity of circulating free drug not bound by plasma proteins that is in equilibrium with brain water. Commonly available methods for monitoring serum levels of AEDs measure total drug levels. Although monitoring total plasma levels provides useful information in most instances, this may not be the case for highly protein-bound drugs when the ratio of unbound to free drug is altered. PHT, VPA, and CBZ are highly bound to proteins. Any changes that alter protein binding could influence the relationship between total drug concentration and clinical effect.

In neonates and very young children, albumin, globulins, and circulating glycoproteins are reduced in concentration (47), thus limiting the capacity for protein binding by AEDs. Further, high levels of free fatty acids and bilirubin are capable of displacing some AEDs from protein binding sites (48,49).

In the newborn, permeability of the blood–brain barrier to small molecules is increased, resulting in increased extracellular volume. Because cerebrospinal fluid production is diminished, the sink effect is reduced, with increasing drug concentrations in brain extracellular fluids (50). The factors causing variable rates in central nervous system concentration include the negative log of dissociation constant of a drug, cerebral blood flow, and acid-base equilibrium (51).

Gastrointestinal System

AED absorption is delayed in the newborn. This pattern is caused by several factors, including achlorhydria. Stomach acid secretion increases during the first 20 to 30 months of life. Absorption also is affected by erratic and prolonged gastric emptying, a pattern that persists until 6 to 8 months of age (52). The principal factor affecting drug absorption is immaturity of the intestinal mucosa (53). These changes cause variable bioavailability of PHT (54,55). In contrast to the situation in neonates and very young children, drug absorption may be more rapid in children than in adults. This change causes a higher peak concentration of drug, with a subsequent increase of dose-related adverse effects (56). For example, CBZ syrup causes somnolence within 1 hour of dosing; this drug formulation should be given in divided doses throughout the day (57).

Conversely, age has little effect on rectal absorption of the AEDs (58,59). It is the formulation that may affect rectal bioavailability and absorption velocity. Liquid formulations are more rapidly absorbed than suppositories. This is particularly relevant for diazepam when one is treating a patient with a prolonged seizure or status epilepticus.

Parenteral Routes of Administration

The intramuscular route of administration is not reliable, particularly in acute conditions in which the patient's cardiovascular function is altered. As for the intravenous route, most formulations are developed for adults, and concentrations are too high for proper administration in small children. Thus, the drug needs to be diluted, with a risk of error.

Changes in Body Composition

The distribution in the body depends of the size of the various compartments, the relative liposolubility and hydrosolubility of the compound, and its binding to plasma proteins. In the first year of life, the extracellular water represents a higher proportion of body weight than in adults. Until puberty, the lipidic compartment comprises a bigger proportion of body weight than in the adult. Drug binding to plasma proteins is weaker in the first year of life than later in life because the concentrations of albumin and α_1-glycoprotein are low.

The bigger volume of distribution of drugs in the newborn explains the need for an increased loading dose, compared with adults, to reach the same blood level. It also explains in part the longer half-life.

Hepatic Function

Clearance of an AED from the plasma is influenced by the capacity of the liver to metabolize the drug. Because drug clearance determines steady-state drug concentrations, any age-related alteration in clearance by the liver will affect observed serum drug concentrations. One key variable is the rate of elimination of an active metabolite as compared with the elimination of the parent drug. This relationship can cause symptoms of toxicity because a metabolite may not be eliminated rapidly, whereas the serum level of the parent drug appears unchanged.

Some, but not all, metabolic pathways are reduced in the newborn, with reduced plasma clearance. The requested dose per body weight is therefore lower than in adults to reach the same plasma level. Drug metabolism may be modified in favor of the most mature pathway (60). For example, diazepam, which in adults is desmethylated by cytochrome CYP2C into nordiazepam and then is hydroxylated by cytochrome CYP3A into oxazepam before glycuronic acid conjugation and urine elimination, accumulates in the newborn as nonglucuronated oxazepam and nordiazepam because of the immaturity of glucuroconjugation.

The rate of metabolism by liver microsomes is influenced by drug exposure (61). PB (62), PHT (63), and CBZ (80) induce hepatic metabolism. Conjugation with glucuronic acid is significantly reduced until 18 to 24 months of age. Inefficient oxidative plasma clearance endures until the second or third week of life. After that time, there is a gradual increase in the rate of drug metabolism, which, over a period of weeks to months, reaches rates considerably higher than those in adults (56). For this reason, the dosage requirements in milligrams per kilogram for most AEDs are higher in children than in adults.

Renal Function

Filtration reaches the adult rate at the end of the first month of life and tubular function within the second month. This feature may be relevant for drugs that are mainly eliminated by the kidney, such as VGB, gabapentin, and primidone.

SPECIFIC DRUGS

Phenytoin

Data regarding bioavailability of PHT in the newborn are conflicting, with poor absorption reported by some authors (55), but not confirmed by others (64). This point is important when one is attempting oral treatment after intravenous administration for status epilepticus, however, because impaired bioavailability interferes with the switch to oral treatment. The drug's half-life is longer in the neonate (15 to 105 hours) and shorter in infants (2 to 7 hours) than it is in adults (24 to 48 hours). Nonlinear pharmacokinetics causes the therapeutic index to be narrow, because mild alteration in the dose may produce major changes in the blood level with a high risk of intoxication or loss of efficacy. Therefore, at onset of treatment, monitoring of plasma level is critical to prevent side effects and to determine the rate of dosage increase. In addition, the plasma level of the drug should be monitored until the proper steady state has been reached.

A review of the charts of 80 infants aged up to 20 months who were receiving PHT showed that, if properly monitored, this compound is very efficient when it is administered intravenously for status epilepticus. However, when the drug was given orally, it was difficult to determine the appropriate dose and to maintain the patient at a given plasma level for a clinically relevant period (65). Fewer than 10% of patients in this series benefited from the drug given orally. Thus, in practice, oral administration of PHT is not recommended in infancy.

A model for loading of patients with status epilepticus has been developed (66), and the plasma level is correlated with efficacy and side effects, including a paradoxical increase in seizure frequency with high blood levels. Dilantin (the trade name for the parenteral formulation of PHT) must be diluted in a large amount of physiologic saline to avoid precipitation in the tube. When the drug is given orally by gastric tube to children who cannot swallow tablets because they are unconscious, bioavailability may be poor, and blood levels should therefore be monitored (67).

The newborn babies of mothers treated with PHT are prone to develop neonatal hemorrhage that should systematically be prevented with vitamin K_1, given to the mother during the last month of pregnancy and to the baby at birth. Many children, particularly those with mental disability, have problems with gingival hypertrophy and hypertrichosis.

Fosphenytoin

Fosphenytoin is the phosphatase ester of PHT; thus, it is a prodrug of PHT that is changed into PHT by esterases. It is soluble in water, and its pH is lower than that of PHT, features that permit both intravenous and intramuscular administration in the adult. Unfortunately, very few data are available on children, and they mostly concern children between 5 and 18 years of age, with findings similar to those in adults. Very few data are available on children <5 years old (68). Only four infants have been reported, and PHT blood levels between 10 and 20 µg/kg could not be reached in these patients (69).

Valproate

Age-related changes in pharmacokinetics of VPA should be anticipated because of the high percentage of drug that is protein bound and its metabolic route of elimination (70). Dehydrogenation of VPA results in the formulation of 2-ene, 3-ene and 4-ene VPA compounds. The 4-ene metabolites are highest in infants and decline with age. The 2-ene

compound has antiepileptic potency (71). VPA binds to albumin at high- and low-affinity sites. This binding is saturable, and thus the free fraction increases with dose.

VPA interferes with the metabolism of several AEDs, including LTG, CBZ, PB, PHT, and felbamate (FBM), as well as with drugs other than AEDs, and so the dose of the concomitant medication needs to be reduced. The drug's half-life is 60 to 100 hours in newborns and 10 to 15 hours in children.

VPA-associated hepatic failure is of major concern when one is selecting this drug for infants and young children. It appears to be age related, with a higher risk in infants treated with polytherapy (39). The hepatic failure occurs within the first 6 months of VPA treatment, and it begins with vomiting, increased seizures, and drowsiness. At this stage, cessation of treatment after measuring prothrombin and transaminase levels may prevent a fatal outcome (72). The risk of hepatotoxicity may be influenced by the need to use the drug in a group of patients who may be either (a) selectively vulnerable because of underlying disease or (b) at risk because of unidentified metabolic abnormality (41). One specific disorder, the hepatocerebral syndrome of Alper, produces intractable epilepsy and hepatic failure, occasionally causing attribution of hepatic failure to VPA. Monitoring strategies in children, including regular or scheduled measurement of blood chemistry studies, fail to detect hepatic dysfunction, and thus communication with parents or caregivers regarding the clinical state of the patient is the best defense against abnormalities in hepatic function (70).

Pancreatitis also has a peak of incidence in association with VPA therapy in childhood (73). Stomach ache, nausea, and anorexia are frequent in patients taking the solution or syrup formulations, unfortunately the only two available for infants and young children.

Dose escalation should be progressive, over 10 to 14 days, to prevent the occurrence of confusion and drowsiness. The parenteral administration of VPA is useful when oral administration is not possible because of gastrointestinal disorders or surgical intervention. However, this drug has not been studied extensively for use in status epilepticus.

Carbamazepine

CBZ is insoluble in aqueous solution, and it behaves as a neutral lipophilic substance (74). It is biotransformed into CBZ-10,11-epoxide (75–77). The epoxide is formed at the 10,11 double bond on the azepine ring, catalyzed by the hepatic monoxygenases (78). The epoxide is then hydrated by the microsomal epoxide hydrolase (79). Because of solubility problems, gastrointestinal absorption of CBZ is both slow and unpredictable (80). Bioavailability is variable and unpredictable in neonates and infants (81). The elimination half-life varies greatly with age (80,82,83). After establishment of autoinduction, it is <10 hours in children and even shorter in infants. To overcome excessive fluctuation in plasma levels, a controlled-release formulation has been developed. Unfortunately, this formulation is not suitable for infants and young children, the age group for which it would be the most useful because it is the age at which the half-life is the shortest and peak-related side effects are the most prominent.

CBZ has problematic drug interactions with other AEDs and with various other medications as well. Enzyme inducers cause a fall in blood CBZ levels. Inhibition of the activity of epoxide hydroxylase, as occurs with VPA concomitant medication, increases the concentration of the epoxide (84). Both CBZ and the epoxide have antiepileptic properties (85,86). However, compounds such as stiripentol that inhibit the transformation of CBZ into the epoxide at the cytochrome P450 level permit better tolerability of high levels of CBZ with better antiepileptic effect (87).

CBZ is bound to albumin at 65% to 85%. CBZ-10,11-epoxide is also protein bound, but by a lesser percentage (88). The starting dose is 5 mg/kg, going to 10 to 20 mg/kg by 2- to 3-mg/kg increments every week. Infants require up to 30 mg/kg (37,89).

Diplopia is a common concentration-dependent side effect. Treatment with CBZ may be associated with transient somnolence after use of the syrup. This effect is the result of the combination of rapid absorption and short half-life that requires higher doses by body weight in infants than in adults. Nystagmus, vertigo, headache, and ataxia may occur (90,68). These side effects disappear when the dose is reduced, and they tend to decrease after 2 to 3 weeks of treatment, probably as a result of autoinduction. The most severe reactions are hematopoietic, hepatic, renal, and skin reactions (90). The incidence of a rash may be up to 10% (10), but it may be reduced by slow titration when starting the drug. However, Lyell's syndrome does occur, and the outcome is very severe. Hyponatremia is rarely, if ever, a problem in children. CBZ toxicity resulting from an interaction with the macrolide antibiotics, including josamycin, needs to be anticipated because use of this class of antibiotics in children is so common, particularly in school-age children.

In the newborn born of a mother treated with CBZ, there is a risk of vitamin K deficiency requiring vitamin K supplementation. The risk of seizure exacerbation is probably the most difficult problem to handle in infants and children. Myoclonus in patients with idiopathic generalized epilepsy (91), absence and atonic seizures (92) in children, infantile spasms (93,94), and spike activity, particularly during sleep (21), may all be accentuated or triggered by CBZ.

Oxcarbazepine

Oxcarbazepine (OXC) is a derivative of CBZ that has similar efficacy but better tolerability, particularly in children.

Its hepatic metabolism converts it into the monohydroxy derivative of OXC. The metabolic interactions of OXC are very limited. The drug's half-life is in the adult range in children ≤5 years of age, but it is significantly lower in younger children and infants (unpublished data). The incidence of skin rash is four times lower than with CBZ. Hyponatremia may be an issue in children (95). No effect on growth has been observed (96). No soluble formulation is currently available.

Like CBZ, the drug has been shown to be effective in partial epilepsy in children (97–100). Its efficacy was similar to that of PHT in a controlled study (101). As with CBZ, there is a risk of increased seizures, particularly myoclonic and absence seizures, infantile spasms, and conditions characterized by major spike-wave activity, although the effect in partial epilepsy is similar to that in patients with mental retardation (102).

Felbamate

FBM has a complex hepatic metabolism, with clinically relevant metabolic interactions with CBZ, VPA, PB, and PHT. Inducing compounds reduce FBM's half-life by 30%, whereas FBM reduces the clearance of PB, PHT, and VPA but increases the clearance of CBZ. CBZ E levels are increased by FBM.

Bone marrow failure and hepatic failure are the major concerns. Thirty-four patients with FBM-associated aplastic anemia have been reported, with 13 known fatalities. No case of bone marrow failure has been observed in children <13 years of age, but exposure in the lower age groups has been limited. Hepatic failure is lethal in one-third of cases, the overall risk is similar to that associated with VPA, and children <5 years of age have been affected (103). The identification of a reactive metabolite, atropaldehyde, and human leukocyte antigen studies suggest that high-risk patients may be identified. One should monitor transaminases and blood cell counts, every 2 weeks at onset and for several months, then less often. A few cases of anaphylactic reactions and other idiosyncratic reactions including Stevens-Johnson syndrome have been recorded.

FBM has been shown to be effective in double-blind studies both in pediatric partial epilepsy and in adults and children with Lennox-Gastaut syndrome. The combination with VPA may be particularly useful, with a mean decrease in seizure frequency of 60% and a 40% decrease in the frequency of drop attacks in one series when VPA was added to FBM (104). Improved behavior has also been reported, as a result of reduced seizure frequency (105). The main indication is therefore for children with Lennox-Gastaut syndrome, provided they respond clearly within the first 2 or 3 months of treatment. A few clinical observations have mentioned an effect in infantile spasms (106), but if this is the case, the effect is mild.

Lamotrigine

LTG is metabolized by the liver. Its half-life is decreased by enzyme-inducing concomitant medication and is increased by VPA. These interactions are clinically relevant, for example, with a risk of the loss of antiepileptic activity if VPA is removed without modifying the LTG dose. The incidence of the major side effect, skin rash, is increased by the combination with VPA and with rapid titration. Titration must be particularly slow in combination with VPA, starting with a maximum of 0.2 mg/kg for the first 2 weeks, then 0.5 mg/kg for the next 2 weeks, then 2 mg/kg for another 2 weeks before the usual dose of 2 to 5 mg/kg can be reached. Conversely, the combination with VPA may be more effective in some patients than LTG monotherapy. The reason for this enhanced effect is not restricted to metabolic interactions with raised plasma LTG levels, but it may include a pharmacodynamic effect, yet to be elucidated (46). Tolerance is good, with headache and nausea occurring mainly if titration is too rapid. A combination with CBZ is reported to be poorly tolerated, even with moderate doses and blood levels of CBZ, and it results in side effects usually encountered in patients receiving high doses of CBZ (107). Again, a pharmacodynamic phenomenon may be the cause.

Generalized epilepsies, namely, Lennox-Gastaut syndrome and absence epilepsies, are the best indications for this drug (45), although some patients with infantile spasms may occasionally benefit, at the point at which the condition has become Lennox-Gastaut syndrome (108). Efficacy has also been demonstrated in a double-blind study of children with partial epilepsy (109). The combination with VPA may be useful in this setting. Moreover, a double-blind study has shown the efficacy of this drug in Lennox-Gastaut syndrome (110). In this case, a paradoxical increase in seizure frequency with high doses of LTG has occasionally been observed (not published). Regarding myoclonic astatic-epilepsy starting after the age of 2 years, with major slow spike-wave activity, several clinical observations suggest good efficacy of LTG if it is given early in the course of the disorder. Conversely, LTG has worsened >80% of patients with severe myoclonic epilepsy in infancy, a disorder that is characterized by recurrent convulsive seizures beginning in the middle of the first year of life and often triggered by fever (19). This finding may seem paradoxical because this generalized epilepsy shares a major myoclonic component with myoclonic-astatic epilepsy.

Improved cognitive function has been claimed in patients with Lennox-Gastaut syndrome, but it remains difficult to determine whether the improvement is indeed the result of some psychotropic effect independent of the control of seizures. Patients with infantile and juvenile ceroid lipofuscinosis have been shown to benefit from this compound, in nonblinded conditions (111).

Vigabatrin

VGB is an irreversible inhibitor of γ-aminobutyric acid (GABA) transaminase. It increases the concentration of GABA in the synapse, and this is the supposed mode of the antiepileptic action. The drug is not metabolized by the liver, but it is excreted by the kidneys, and the dose should be reduced when the patient has low creatinine clearance (112). Titration can be rapid, with good tolerability.

Side effects are mild in infant and children. Hyperactivity may occur, especially in children who have a history of hyperactivity or mental retardation, and it disappears when the dose is reduced (113). Increased body weight occurs rarely, but the weight gain in these patients may be very marked. The most impressive side effect, visual field defects, was discovered almost 10 years after the drug reached the market, with several hundred thousand patient-years of treatment completed. One-third of the patients have the defect on visual field testing, but only a few patients have a clinical complain that leads to the investigation (114).

The drug is particularly effective in infantile spasms, especially in patients with tuberous sclerosis and focal cortical dysplasia (in preparation). Efficacy in infantile spasms has been established in one double-blind placebo-controlled study (115), as well as in two randomized studies comparing the compound to either adrenocorticotropic hormone or hydrocortisone (29,116). The latter study exclusively included patients with tuberous sclerosis. In this particular disease, cessation of spasms may be followed by the occurrence of focal seizures. In these cases, however, major improvement of cognitive function has been reported, despite the persistent focal seizures, and patients reach a cognitive level similar to that of patients who experienced only focal seizures starting in the same age range (15). For all these studies, VGB was administered as the first-line drug. The number of patients included in each study was very small, and freedom from seizures was the end point, thus demonstrating high specificity of this compound in this type of epilepsy. In infants with spasms, the drug is currently used as first-line therapy in most European countries (27,117,118). At a dose of 100 to 150 mg/kg, the drug is active in >65% of patients with cryptogenic cases and >55% of patients with symptomatic cases, with one-third of the latter experiencing relapse, whereas this is very uncommon in cryptogenic cases. One major issue is the appropriate duration of treatment in responders, a duration that probably depends on the cause of the seizures: 6 to 12 months in patients with cryptogenic cases, but longer in tuberous sclerosis, in which the risk of recurrence is higher. The addition of steroids in nonresponders raises the proportion of responders to nearly 100% of patients with cryptogenic cases. In older patients, however, who have not received the drug within the first 2 to 3 years of the disease, VGB is much less effective. Increased seizures have even been reported in patients who have developed the patterns of Lennox-Gastaut syndrome (14). In patients with tuberous sclerosis, this contrast is even more striking. Patients >4 years old who have persistent infantile spasms may note a worsening of their condition with the occurrence of major hyperactivity, after the introduction of VGB.

The administration of VGB is more troublesome in patients with partial epilepsy, given the lack of valuable data regarding retinal function in this age range. Nevertheless, the drug has been shown to be effective in a randomized double-blind withdrawal trial (119). Patients with severe partial epilepsy not responsive to other drugs usually effective and patients for whom a rapid decline in cognitive function related to frequent seizures requires a compound with a possibly rapid titration should be tried on VGB at the dose of 40 to 80 mg/kg (120). Indeed, within a few days, too short a period for retinal toxicity to appear, the eventual benefit can be observed, or the drug can be discontinued. Finally, absence seizures and myoclonic epilepsy may be worsened by VGB (14).

Topiramate

Topiramate (TPM) is poorly protein bound; it is moderately metabolized (30%) in monotherapy but metabolized more thoroughly in polytherapy with enzyme-inducing compounds (50%). The kidney mainly excretes it. Thus, the dose needs to be reduced when renal clearance is <60 mL/min/1.73 m^2. The clearance of TPM is higher in children than in adults, and, consequently, plasma TPM concentrations in children are about 30% lower than those found in adults receiving comparable dosages (120). Kidney stones occur rarely, if at all, in children. Poor appetite and weight loss are frequent. Modified mood with some kind of depression with hallucinations may occur, especially at the onset of treatment, when the dose titration is too rapid. Cognitive dulling was observed in 41% of patients in one series, and 31% stopped treatment because of drug intolerance (121). The incidence reaches 54% in mentally handicapped children (122). Factors that increase the risk of behavior disorders are mainly a history of such disorders and LTG concomitant medication (123). Ataxia and coordination disorders may also occur. With high doses, speech difficulties may affect the child; this is quite specific to TPM (124). Case reports mention central hyperventilation related to the administration of TPM because of its inhibitory action on carbonic anhydrase (125). TPM may inhibit the metabolism of PHT.

TPM has been shown to be effective as add-on drug in refractory partial epilepsy in children from the age of 4 years (126): given a mean 10 mg/kg at maintenance, 14% children became seizure free, and 57% had a >50% decrease in seizure frequency. In generalized tonic-clonic seizures, TPM was also effective, with 44% of children aged 3 to 16 years having a >75% decrease in seizure frequency when they received 1 to 16 mg/kg (mean, 7 mg/kg), but no clue was

given regarding the syndromic form in these patients (127). Patients with Lennox-Gastaut syndrome experienced a moderate effect; a double-blind study showed a 14% decrease in seizure frequency (128), and in open follow-up with 10 mg/kg, 15% became free of drop attacks, and 55% had a >50% decrease in drop attacks (97). However, the clinical relevance of incomplete responses in patients with daily seizures remains to be established. Fewer than a dozen patients with infantile spasms who had not received VGB were given TPM in very high doses (mean, 29 mg/kg, ≤50 mg/kg), and four of 11 became seizure free (97). TPM was claimed to be effective in five children with Angelman's syndrome (129). One case with dramatic improvement of progressive myoclonic epilepsy is on record (122). In practice, the initial dose should be no more than 0.5 to 1 mg/kg/day for 2 weeks, followed by increases every other week, usually up to 5 mg/kg.

Gabapentin

Gabapentin is readily absorbed, and it is neither protein bound or metabolized by the liver. Thus, it has no significant metabolic interactions. Excretion is mainly through the kidney. Hyperactivity may be an issue, mainly for patients who have mental retardation or a history of hyperactivity (130).

This drug has an effect on partial epilepsy in children, but the only study performed failed to demonstrate any effect in the newborn (although these patients had very severe cases). The efficacy in childhood partial epilepsy is very mild; in a double-blind placebo-controlled trial, no difference in the number of responders could be identified, and only three patients became seizure free compared to one in the placebo group (115). In one series, only three of 52 children with uncontrolled partial seizures benefited in the long term (131). A controlled study failed to demonstrate an effect in childhood absence epilepsy (132).

Ethosuximide

In children, ethosuximide has a long half-life of 30 hours, and this permits a single daily dose at night. Bone marrow toxicity, which is very rare, cannot be predicted by hematologic monitoring. Ethosuximide is indicated in absence seizures and myoclonus, and some patients with epileptic encephalopathy and continuous spike waves in sleep may benefit.

Phenobarbital and Primidone

PB causes insidious cognitive and behavioral effects (133). Vining et al. (35) compared results of cognitive tests in 28 children with febrile seizures who were treated with PB with results in control subjects who were treated with VPA. PB caused significant difficulties in full-scale and performance intelligence quotient, contraction praxis, attention, mood, and the ability to finish a task. Farwell et al. (36) performed serial assessments of cognitive performances of children treated prophylactically for febrile seizures with PB. These investigators found cognitive decline in patients receiving PB. Hyperactivity in response to PB administration may be insignificant, or it may occur in as many as 42% of patients. Occasionally, dose reduction of PB may result in improvement of hyperactivity or disordered sleep that was not identified as being caused by PB. PB-induced hyperactivity does not appear to correlate with PB blood levels (35). Rash complicates PB treatment in 1% to 3% of patients; exfoliative dermatitis may occur rarely. Rickets has occurred among disabled children with pigmented skin who are treated with multiple AEDs. Dependency to PB may develop; withdrawal symptoms of anxiety, somnolence, tremor, and convulsions with possible seizure exacerbation may occur. Attacks of acute intermittent porphyria may be precipitated by administration of drugs causing enzyme induction, including PB. Primidone is poorly tolerated in children because of associated somnolence and drug-induced hyperactivity.

Benzodiazepines

Diazepam is an important drug for the treatment of convulsive status epilepticus. The drug is highly protein bound; the metabolite desmethyldiazepam is also active. In the newborn, it has slow catabolism, with a half-life ranging from 40 to 400 hours. Therefore, the drug and its active metabolites accumulate, producing hypotonia and breathing difficulties. The drug is absorbed rectally in infants and children (58,59), more rapidly as a solution than as a suppository. Rectal administration of the solution is useful for infants and children experiencing convulsive status epilepticus because parents administer the drug rectally. However, intravenous administration reaches blood levels sufficient to stop status epilepticus more rapidly, and it is preferred whenever possible.

Clonazepam is useful intravenously for the treatment of status epilepticus. Clonazepam produces hypotonia, somnolence, and ataxia. For the oral treatment of epilepsy in infants and children, it should therefore not be the benzodiazepine of first choice.

Clobazam is certainly the benzodiazepine of choice for the oral treatment of chronic epilepsy in infants and children. It is relatively well tolerated, and the usual side effects encountered with the other compounds of the group, namely, somnolence, hypotonia, and ataxia, are much less frequent with clobazam, although some children become irritable and aggressive. Absorption is rapid and reaches maximum concentration within 2 hours. Protein binding is 85%, and there is complete metabolic transformation through cytochrome P450 into desmethylclobazam, which

is active and has a longer half-life (50 hours) than clobazam (20 hours). The steady state is reached within 10 days.

Lorazepam is commonly used in infants and children for the treatment of status epilepticus. It may be more efficient than diazepam, particularly by rectal administration (134).

Tiagabine

Tiagabine (TGB) is an inhibitor of GABA reuptake. Therefore, it increases the concentration of GABA in the synaptic cleft. Few data are available in children. The pharmacokinetics of TGB after a single 0.1 mg/kg dose was studied in 25 children receiving concomitant medication (135). Areas under the curve were significantly higher (.002), and clearance values were significantly lower ($p > .02$) in children comedicated with VPA compared with children taking enzyme inducers such as CBZ and PHT. Moreover, the half-life of TGB was twice as long in patients taking VPA compared with patients receiving enzyme inducers. When adjusted for body surface, kinetic parameters in children were similar to those found in historical adult controls receiving comparable comedication. However, when adjusted for body weight, clearance values were higher in children than in adults.

Ascending doses of TGB (0.25 to 1.5 mg/kg/day) were added to previous medication in 52 children >2 years old (136). The median reduction in seizure frequency for patients with partial seizures was 33%, whereas there was no change for those with generalized seizures. A single patient with pharmacoresistant epilepsy and multifocal spikes experienced total seizure control (137). In 14 patients with both seizures and spastic tetraplegia, TGB was given at the starting dose of 0.1 to 0.2 mg/kg/day and was increased to 1.1 mg/kg (138). Half of the patients experienced improved tone, strength, coordination, range of motion, and relaxation of extremities, with less ataxia and wobbling.

The main *side effects* of TGB affect the *central nervous system*: asthenia, nervousness, dizziness, and somnolence. Like other GABAergic drugs, TGB has the potential to worsen myoclonus and absence seizures. In addition, it may precipitate *nonconvulsive status epilepticus*. Two patients experienced status epilepticus in one series (136). One 12-year-old child with perisylvian microgyria developed frontal lobe status after 1 week of total seizure control, at the dose of 1 mg/kg, with disappearance of status epilepticus after the dose was decreased by 25% (139).

In view of the evidence reviewed earlier, the use of TGB in children should be restricted to resistant partial epilepsy, and consideration should be given to the risk of nonconvulsive status epilepticus.

Zonisamide

Some authors believe that zonisamide (ZNS), added to clonazepam and VPA or a barbiturate, can reduce the cascade of myoclonia in progressive myoclonus epilepsies for ≥2 years, but relapse may occur thereafter (140). Of 11 patients with infantile spasms resistant to vitamin B$_6$ who were receiving ZNS, four responded with cessation of spasms and hypsarrhythmia, at 4 to 5 mg/kg/day, but half had a relapse (141). At 4 to 20 mg/kg, ZNS was effective in both patients with cryptogenic cases and in 28% of the symptomatic cases, but again, half the patients had a relapse (142). Kishi et al. (143) found that ZNS is useful for patients with atypical infantile spasms, when steroids cannot be administered. One patient with epileptogenic encephalopathy had an excellent response to ZNS (144). The effect of ZNS add-on therapy was weaker in patients with intellectual disability (41% of patients experiencing a >50% seizure decrease) than in those without intellectual disability (67% responder rate; $p < .0l$); in monotherapy, tolerability was also poorer in patients with intellectual disability (145).

In two children aged 1 and 3 years, ZNS induced *behavior disorders* at plasma ZNS levels within or even lower than the therapeutic range (146). One 2-year-old child exhibited fever and *oligohidrosis* resulting from abnormal perspiration, with acute chorea, tremor, and cogwheel hypertonia that disappeared within 2 weeks of cessation of the drug (147). Acetylcholine stimulation testing may be helpful in predicting this complication, with a sensitivity of 1 and a false-positive rate of 0.67 (148). Three patients were reported with *urinary lithiasis;* alkaline urine and hypercalciuria seem to be predisposing factors (149).

The indications of ZNS are still to be identified on the basis of controlled trials, particularly for infantile spasms, in which a comparison should be done with VGB. Parents should be aware of the risk of perspiration abnormalities and nephrolithiasis.

CONCLUSION

In addition to proper pediatric formulation, four sets of pediatric data should be collected early in the development of new compounds, to optimize the benefit:risk ratio as soon as possible: pharmacokinetics, tolerability, pediatric syndrome-specific potential of worsening, and, eventually, efficacy in pediatric-specific epilepsy syndromes. Whether duplicating in children the efficacy controlled studies already performed in adults for types of epilepsy observed in both adults and children are clinically relevant and ethically sound remains to be established.

REFERENCES

1. Hauser WA. Seizure disorders: the changes with age. *Epilepsia* 1992;33[Suppl 4]:S6–S14.
2. Luna D, Chiron C, Pajot N, et al. *Epidémiologie des épilepsies de l'enfant dans le département de l'Oise (France).* London: John Libbey Eurotext, 1988.
3. Nelson KB, Ellenberg JH. Predisposing and causative factors in childhood epilepsy. *Epilepsia* 1987;28[Suppl 1]:S16–S24.
4. Duchowny MS. Complex partial seizures in infancy. *Arch Neurol* 1987;44.
5. Jeavons PM, Bower BD, Dimitrakoudi M. Long-term prognosis of 150 cases of "West syndrome." *Epilepsia* 1973;14:153–164.
6. Bednarek N, Motte J, Soufflet C, et al. Evidence of late-onset infantile spasms. *Epilepsia* 1998;39:55–60.
7. Gobbi G, Bruno L, Pini A, et al. Periodic spasms: an unclassified type of epileptic seizure in childhood. *Dev Med Child Neurol* 1987;29:766–775.
8. Roger J, Bureau M, Dravet C, et al. *Epileptic syndromes in infancy, childhood, and adolescence.* London: John Libbey, 1992.
9. Desguerre I, Chiron C, Loiseau J, et al. Epidemiology of idiopathic generalized epilepsies. In: Malafosse A, Genton P, Hirsch E, et al., eds. *Idiopathic generalized epilepsies: clinical experimental and genetic aspects.* London: John Libbey, 1994:19–25.
10. Chaigne D, Dulac O. Carbamazepine versus valproate in partial epilepsies of childhood. *Adv Epilepsy* 1989;17:198–200.
11. Dulac O, Bouguerra L, Rey E, et al. Monothérapie par la carbamazepine dans les épilepsies de l'enfant. *Arch Fr Pediatr* 1983;40:415–419.
12. Dulac O, Steru D, Rey E, et al. Sodium valproate monotherapy in childhood epilepsy. *Brain Dev* 1986;8:47–52.
13. Verity CM, Hosking G, Easter DJ. A multicentre comparative trial of sodium valproate and carbamazepine in paediatric epilepsy: the Paediatric EPITEG Collaborative Group. *Dev Med Child Neurol* 1995;37:97–108.
14. Lortie A, Chiron C, Mumford J, et al. The potential for increasing seizure frequency, relapse and appearance of new seizure types with vigabatrin. *Neurology* 1993;43[Suppl 5]:S24–S27.
15. Jambaqué I, Chiron C, Dumas C, et al. Mental and behavioural outcome of infantile epilepsy treated by vigabatrin in tuberous sclerosis patients. *Epilepsy Res* 2000;38:151–160.
16. Tassinari CA, Dravet C, Roger J, et al. Tonic status epilepticus precipitated by intravenous benzodiazepine in five patients with Lennox-Gastaut. *Epilepsia* 1972;13:421–435.
17. Berg AT, Shinnar S, Levy SR, et al. How well can epilepsy syndromes be identified at diagnosis? A reassessment 2 years after initial diagnosis. *Epilepsia* 2000;41:1335–1341.
18. Perucca E, Gram L, Avanzini G, et al. Antiepileptic drugs as a cause of worsening seizures. *Epilepsia* 1998;39:5–17.
19. Guerrini R, Dravet C, Genton P, et al. Lamotrigine and seizure aggravation in severe myoclonic epilepsy. *Epilepsia* 1998;39:508–512.
20. Uldall P, Bulteau C, Pedersen SA, et al. Tiagabine adjunctive therapy in children with refractory epilepsy: a single-blind dose escalating study. *Epilepsy Res* 2000;42:159–168.
21. Marescaux C, Hirsch E, Finck S, et al. Landau-Kleffner syndrome: a pharmacological study of five cases. *Epilepsia* 1990;31:768–777.
22. Doose H. Myoclonic astatic epilepsy of early childhood. In: Roger J, et al., eds. *Epileptic syndromes in infancy, childhood and adolescence.* London: John Libbey Eurotext, 1992:103–114.
23. Dravet C, Bureau M, Guerrini R, et al. Severe myoclonic epilepsy in infants. In: Roger J, et al., eds. *Epileptic syndromes in infancy, childhood, and adolescence.* London: John Libbey Eurotext, 1992:75–88.
24. Sarisjulis N, Gamboni B, Plouin P, et al. Diagnosing idiopathic/cryptogenic epilepsy syndromes in infancy. *Arch Dis Child* 2000;82:226–230.
25. Luna D, Dulac O, Plouin P. Ictal characteristics of cryptogenic partial epilepsies in infancy. *Epilepsia* 1989;30:827–832.

26. Chiron C, Dulac O, Beaumont D, et al. Therapeutic trials of vigabatrin in refractory infantile spasms. *J Child Neurol* 1991; 6[Suppl 2]:S52–S59.

27. Villeneuve N, Soufflet C, Plouin P, et al. Traitement des spasmes infantiles par le vigabatrin en monothérapie de première intention: è propos de 70 nourrissons. *Arch Pediatr* 1998;5:731–738.

28. Appleton RE, Peters AC, Mumford JP, et al. Randomised, placebo-controlled study of vigabatrin as first-line treatment of infantile spasms. *Epilepsia* 1999;40:1627–1633.

29. Chiron C, Dumas C, Jambaqué I, et al. Randomized trial comparing vigabatrin and hydrocortisone in infantile spasms due to tuberous sclerosis. *Epilepsy Res* 1997;26:389–395.

30. Chiron C, Marchand MC, Tran A, et al. Stiripentol in severe myoclonic epilepsy in infancy: a randomised placebo-controlled syndrome-dedicated trial. STICLO study group. *Lancet* 2000; 356:1638–1642.

31. Freeman JM, Jacobs J, Vining E, et al. Epilepsy in the inner city schools: a school based program that makes a *difference*. *Epilepsia* 1984;25:438–442.

32. Stores G. School children with epilepsy at risk for learning and behavior problems. *Dev Med Child Neurol* 1978;20:502–508.

33. Bourgeois BFD, Prensky AL, Palkes HS, et al. Intelligence in epilepsy: a prospective study in children. *Ann Neurol* 1983;14: 438–444.

34. Bulteau C, Jambaqué I, Viguier D, et al. Epileptic syndromes, cognitive assessment and school placement: a study of 251 children. *Dev Med Child Neurol* 2000;42:319–327.

35. Vining EPG, Mellitis ED, Dorsen MM, et al. Psychologic and behavioral effects of antiepileptic drugs in children: a double-blind comparison between phenobarbital and valproic acid. *Pediatrics* 1987;80:165–174.

36. Farwell JR, Lee YJ, Hirtz DG, et al. Phenobarbital for febrile seizures: effects on intelligence and on seizure recurrence. *N Engl J Med* 1990,322:364–369.

37. O'Dougherty M, Wright FS, Cox S, et al. Carbamazepine plasma concentration: relationship to cognitive impairment. *Arch Neurol* 1987;44:863–867.

38. Brent DA, Crumrine PK, Varma RR, et al. Phenobarbital treatment and major depressive disorder in children with epilepsy. *Pediatrics* 1987;80:909–917.

39. Dreifuss FE, Langer DH. Hepatic considerations in the use of antiepileptic drugs. *Epilepsia* 1987;28[Suppl 2]:S23–S29.

40. Egger J, Harding BN, Boyd SG, et al. Progressive neuronal degeneration in childhood liver disease. *Clin Pediatr* 1987; 26:167–173.

41. Willmore LJ, Triggs WJ, Pellock JM. Valproate toxicity: risk-screening strategies. *J Child Neurol* 1991;6:3-6.

42. Dreifuss FE, Langer DH, Moline KA, et al. Valproic acid hepatic fatalities. II. US experience since 1984. *Neurology* 1989; 39:201–207.

43. Mesdjian E, Dravet C, Cenraud B, et al. Carbamazepine intoxication due to triacetyloleandomycin administration in epileptic patients. *Epilepsia* 1980;21:489–496.

44. Roger J, Grangeon H, Guey J, et al. Psychiatric and psychological complications of ethosuximide treatment in epilepsies. *Encephale* 1968;57:407–438.

45. Schlumberger E, Chavez F, Palacios L, et al. Lamotrigine in the treatment of 120 children with epilepsy. *Epilepsia* 1994;35: 359–367.

46. Pisani F, Oteri G, Russo MF, et al. The efficacy of valproate-lamotrigine comedication in refractory complex partial seizures: evidence for a pharmacodynamic interaction. *Epilepsia* 1999; 40:1141–1146.

47. Pacifici GM, Taddeuci-Brunelli G, Rane A. Clonazepam serum protein binding during development. *Clin Pharmacol Ther* 1984;35:354–359.

48. Kurz H, Mauser-Granshorn A, Suckel HH. Differences in the binding of drugs to plasma proteins from newborn and adult man. *Eur J Clin Pharmacol* 1977;11:463–467.

49. Kurz H, Michels H, Suckel HH. Differences in the binding of drugs to plasma proteins from the newborn and adult man. *Eur J Clin Pliarmacol* 1977; 11:469–472.

50. White HS, Kemp JW, Woodbury DM. Effects of central nervous system maturation on drug metabolism. In: Morselli PL, et al., eds. *Antiepileptic drug therapy in pediatrics.* New York: Raven Press, 1983:13–35.

51. Morselli PL. Development and physiological variables important for drug kinetics. In: Morselli PL, et al., eds. *Antiepiletpic drug therapy in pediatrics.* New York: Raven Press, 1983:1–12.

52. Cavell B. Gastric emptying in preterm infants. *Acta Paediatr Scand* 1979;68:725–730.

53. Heiman G. Enteral absorption and bioavailability in children in relation to age. *Eur J Clin Pharmacol* 1980;18:43–50.

54. Jalling B, Boreus LO, Rane A, et al. Plasma concentration of diphenylhydantoin in young infants. *Pharmacol Clin* 1970;2: 200–202.

55. Painter MJ, Pippenger C, McDonald H, et al. Phenobarbital and diphenylhydantoin levels in neonates with seizures. *J Pediatr* 1978;92:315–319.

56. Morselli PL, Franco-Morselli R, Bossi L. Clinical pharmacokinetics in newborns and infants: age related differences and therapeutic implications. *Clin Pharmacokinet* 1980;5:485–527.

57. Hoppner RJ, Kuger A, Meijer JNA, et al. Correlation between daily fluctuations of carbamazepine serum levels and intermittent side-effects. *Epilepsia* 1980;21:341–350.

58. Dulac O, Aicardi J, Rey E, et al. Blood levels of diazepam after single rectal administration in infants and children. *J Pediatr* 1978;93:1039–1041.

59. Knudsen FV. Plasma diazepam in infants after rectal administration in solution and by suppositories. *Acta Paediatr Scand* 1977;67:699–704.

60. Morselli PL, Principi N, Togoni G, et al. Diazepam elimination in premature and full term infants and children. *J Perinat Med* 1973;1:133–141.

61. Aranda JV, MacLeod SM, Renton KW, et al. Hepatic microsomal drug oxidation and electron transport in newborn infants. *J Pediatr* 1974;85:534–542.

62. Boreus LO, Jalling B, Kallberg N. Clinical pharmacology of phenobarbital in the neonatal period. In: Morselli PL, et al., eds. *Basic and therapeutic aspects of perinatal pharmacology.* New York: Raven Press, 1975:331–340.

63. Loughnan PM, Greenwald A, Purton WN, et al. Pharmacokinetics observations of phenytoin disposition in the newborn and young infant. *Arch Dis Child* 1977; 52:302–309.

64. Wisner KL, Perel JM. Serum levels of valproate and carbamazepine in breastfeeding mother-infant pairs. *J Clin Psychopharmacol* 1998;18:167–169.

65. Sicca F, Contaldo A, Rey E, et al. Phenytoin administration in the newborn and infant. *Brain Dev* 2000;22:35–40.

66. Richard MO, Chiron C, D'Athis P, et al. Phenytoin monitoring in status epilepticus in infants and children. *Epilepsia* 1993;34: 144–150.

67. Bauer LA. Interference of oral phenytoin absorption by continuous nasogastric feeding. *Neurology* 1982;32:570–572.

68. Pellock JM. *Fosphenytoin use in children.* Neurology 1996;46 [Suppl 1]:S14–S16.

69. Takeoka M, Krishnamoorthy KS, Soman TB, et al. Fosphenytoin in infants. J Child Neurol 1998;13:537–540.

70. Pellock JM, Willmore LJ. A rational guide to routine blood monitoring in patients receiving antiepileptic drugs. *Neurology* 1991;41:961–964.

71. Loscher W, Nau H. Pharmacological evaluation of various

metabolites and analogues of valproic acid. anticonvulsant and toxic potencies in mice. *Neuropharmacology* 1985;24:427–435.

72. König SA, Siemes H, Blaker F, et al. Severe hepatotoxicity during valproate therapy: an update and report of eight new fatalities. *Epilepsia* 1994;35:1005–1015.

73. Asconape JJ, Penry JK, Dreifuss FE, et al. Valproate-associated pancreatitis. *Epilepsia* 1993;34:177–183.

74. Leppik IE. Metabolism of antiepileptic medication: newborn to elderly. *Epilepsia* 1992;33[Suppl 4]:S32–S40.

75. Patsalos PN, Stephenson TJ, Krishna S, et al. Side-effects induced by carbamazepine-10,11-epoxide. *Lancet* 1985;2:496.

76. Schoeman JF, Elyas, AA, Brett EM, et al. Correlation between plasma carbamazepine-10,11-epoxide concentration and drug side effects in children with epilepsy. *Dev Med Child Neurol* 1984;26:756–764.

77. Schoeman JF, Elyas AD, Brett EM, et al. Altered ratio of carbamazepine-10,11-epoxide in plasma of children: evidence of anticonvulsant drug interaction. *Dev Med Child Neurol* 1984; 26:749–755.

78. Riley RJ, Kitteringham NR, Park BK. Structural requirements for bioactivation of anticonvulsants to cytotoxic metabolites *in vitro*. *Br J Clin Pharmacol* 1989;28:482–487.

79. Bender AD, Post A, Meier JP, et al. Plasma protein binding of drugs as a function of age in adult human subjects. *J Pharm Sci* 1975;64:1711–1713.

80. Morselli PL, Bossi L. Carbamazepine absorption, distribution and excretion. In: Woodbury DM, et al., eds. *Antiepileptic drugs*. New York: Raven Press, 1982:465–482.

81. Rey E, D'athis P, De Lauture D, et al. Pharmacokinetics of carbamazepine in the neonate and in the child. *Int J Clin Pharmacol Biopharm* 1979;17:90–96.

82. Hockings N, Pail A, Moody APJ, et al. The effects of age on carbamazepine pharmacokinetics and adverse effects. *Br J Clin Pharmacol* 1986;22:725–728.

83. Battino D, Bossi L, Croci D, et al. Carbamazepine plasma levels in children and adults: influence of age, dose and associated therapy. *Ther Drug Monit* 1980;2:315–322.

84. Mc Lachlan M. Anatomic structural and vascular changes in the ageing kidney. In: Nunez JFM, et al., eds. *Renal function and diseases in the elderly*. London: Butterworth, 1987:3–26.

85. Albright PS, Bruni J. Effects of carbamazepine and its epoxide metabolites on amygdala-kindled seizures in rats. *Neurology* 1984;34:1383–1386.

86. Bourgeois OFD, Wad N. Individual and combined antiepileptic and neurotoxic activity of carbamazepine and carbamazepine-10,11-epoxide in mice. *J Pharmacol Exp Ther* 1984; 231:411–415.

87. Perez J, Chiron C, Musial C, et al. Stiripentol: efficacy and tolerability in children with epilepsy. *Epilepsia* 1999;40:1618–1626.

88. Cloyd JC, Lackner TE, Leppik, IE. Antiepileptics in the elderly: pharmacoepidemiology and pharmacokinetics. *Arch Fam Med* 1994;3:589–598.

89. Porter RJ. How to initiate and maintain carbamazepine therapy in children and adults. *Epilepsia* 1987;28:S59–S63.

90. Pellock JM. Carbamazepine side effects in children and adults. *Epilepsia* 1987;28:S64–S70.

91. Snead OC, Hosey LC. Exacerbation of seizures in children by carbamazepine. *N Engl J Med* 1985;313;916–922.

92. Shields WD, Saslow E. Myoclonic, atonic and absence seizures following the institution of carbamazepine therapy in children. *Neurology* 1983;33:1487–1489.

93. Talwar D, Arora MS, Sher PK. EEG changes and seizure exacerbation in young children treated with carbamazepine. *Epilepsia* 1994;35:1154–1159.

94. Martinovitch Z, Plouin P, Chiron C, et al. Infantile spasms exacerbation with carbamazepine treatment.

95. Borusiak P, Korn-Merker E, Holert N, et al. Hyponatremia induced by oxcarbazepine in children. *Epilepsy Res* 1998;30: 241–246.

96. Rattya J, Vainionpaa L, Knip M, et al. The effects of valproate, carbamazepine, and oxcarbazepine on growth and sexual maturation in girls with epilepsy. *Pediatrics* 1999;103:588–593.

97. Glauser TA, Clark PO, McGee K. Long term response to topiramate in patients with West syndrome. *Epilepsia* 2000;41 [Suppl 1]:S91–S94.

98. Glauser TA, Levisohn PM, Ritter F, et al. Topiramate in Lennox-Gastaut syndrome: open-label treatment of patients completing a randomized controlled trial. Topiramate YL study group. *Epilepsia* 2000;41[Suppl 1]:S86–S90.

99. Glauser TA, Nigro M, Sachdeo R, et al. Adjunctive therapy with oxcarbazepine in children with partial seizures: the Oxcarbazepine Pediatric Study Group. *Neurology* 2000;54: 2237–2244.

100. Gaily E, Granström ML, Liukkonen E. Oxcarbazepine in the treatment of early childhood epilepsy. *J Child Neurol* 1997;12: 496–498.

101. Guerreiro MM, Vigonius U, Pohlmann H, et al. A double blind controlled clinical trial of oxcarbazepine versus phenytoin in children and adolescents with epilepsy. *Epilepsy Res* 1997;27: 205–213.

102. Gaily E, Granström ML, Liukkonen E. Oxcarbazepine in the treatment of epilepsy in children and adolescents with intellectual disability. *J Intellect Disabil Res* 1998;42[Suppl 1]:41–45.

103. Pellock JM. Felbamate. *Epilepsia* 1999;40[Suppl 5]:S57–S62.

104. Siegel H, Kelley K, Stertz B, et al. The efficacy of felbamate as add-on therapy to valproic acid in the Lennox-Gastaut syndrome. *Epilepsy Res* 1999;34:91–97.

105. Gay PE, Mecham GF, Coskey JS, et al. Behavioral effects of felbamate in childhood epileptic encephalopathy (Lennox-Gastaut syndrome). *Psychol Rep* 1995;77:1208–1210.

106. Hurst DL, Rolan TD. The use of felbamate to treat infantile spasms. *J Child Neurol* 1995;10:134–136.

107. Besag F, Wallace SJ, Dulac O, et al. Lamotrigine for the treatment of epilepsy in childhood. *J Pediatr* 1995;127:991–997.

108. Veggiotti P, Cieuta C, Rey E, et al. Lamotrigine in infantile spasms. *Lancet* 1994;344:1375–1376.

109. Duchowny M, Pellock JM, Graf WD, et al. A placebo-controlled trial of lamotrigine add-on therapy for partial seizures in children: Lamictal Pediatric Partial Seizure Study Group. *Neurology* 1999;53:1724–1731.

110. Motte J, Trevathan E, Arvidsson JF, et al. Lamotrigine for generalized seizures associated with the Lennox-Gastaut syndrome: Lamictal Lennox-Gastaut Study Group. *N Engl J Med* 1997; 337:1807–1812.

111. Aberg LE, Bäckman M, Kirveskari E, et al. Epilepsy and antiepileptic drug therapy in juvenile neuronal ceroid lipofuscinosis. *Epilepsia* 2000;41:1296–1302.

112. Jacqz-Aigrain E, Guillonneau M, Rey E, et al. Pharmacokinetics of the S(+) and R(−) enantiomers of vigabatrin during chronic dosing in a patient with renal failure. *Br J Clin Pharmacol* 1997;44:183–185.

113. Luna D, Dulac O, Pajot N, et al. Vigabatrin in the treatment of childhood epilepsies: a single-blind placebo-controlled study. *Epilepsia* 1989;30:430–437.

114. Gross-Tsur V, Banin E, Shahar E, et al. Visual impairment in children with epilepsy treated with vigabatrin. *Ann Neurol* 2000;48:60–64.

115. Appleton R, Fichtner K, LaMoreaux L, et al. Gabapentin as add-on therapy in children with refractory partial seizures: a 12-week, multicentre, double-blind, placebo-controlled study. Gabapentin Paediatric Study Group. *Epilepsia* 1999;40: 1147–1154.

116. Vigevano F, Cilio MR. Vigabatrin versus ACTH as first-line treatment for infantile spasms: a randomized, prospective study. *Epilepsia* 1997;38:1270–1274.

117. Aicardi J, Mumford JP, Dumas C, et al. Vigabatrin as initial therapy for infantile spasms: a European retrospective survey. Sabril IS Investigator and Peer Review Groups. *Epilepsia* 1996;37:638–642.

118. Granström ML, Gaily E, Liukkonen E. Treatment of infantile spasms: results of a population-based study with vigabatrin as the first drug for spasms. *Epilepsia* 1999;40:950–957.

119. Chiron C, Dulac O, Gram L. Vigabatrin withdrawal randomized study in children. *Epilepsy Res* 1996;25:209–215.

120. Jambaqué I, Chiron C, Kaminska A, et al. Transient motor aphasia and recurrent partial seizures in a child: language recovery upon seizure control. *J Child Neurol* 1998;13:296–300.

121. Dooley JM, Camfield PR, Smith E, et al. Topiramate in intractable childhood onset epilepsy—a cautionary note. *Can J Neurol Sci* 1999;26:271–273.

122. Uldall P, Buchholt JM. Clinical experiences with topiramate in children with intractable epilepsy. *Eur J Paediatr Neurol* 1999;3:105–111.

123. Gerber PE, Hamiwka L, Connolly MB, et al. Factors associated with behavioral and cognitive abnormalities in children receiving topiramate. *Pediatr Neurol* 2000;22:200–203.

124. Aldenkamp AP, Baker G, Mulder OG, et al. A multicenter, randomized clinical study to evaluate the effect on cognitive function of topiramate compared with valproate as add-on therapy to carbamazepine in patients with partial-onset seizures. *Epilepsia* 2000;41:1167–1178.

124. Laskey AL, Korn DE, Mootjani BI, et al. Central hyperventilation related to administration of Topiramate. *Pediatr Neurol* 2000;22:305–308.

125. Ritter F, Glauser TA, Elterman RD, et al. Effectiveness, tolerability and safety of topiramate in children with partial onset seizures: Topiramate YP study group. *Epilepsia* 2000;41[Suppl 1]:S82–S85.

126. Montouris GD, Biton V, Rosenfeld WE. Nonfocal generalized tonic-clonic seizures: response during long-term topiramate treatment. Topiramate YTC/YTCE study group. *Epilepsia* 2000;41[Suppl 1]:S77–S81.

127. Sachdeo RC, Glauser TA, Ritter F, et al. A double-blind, randomized trial of topiramate in Lennox-Gastaut syndrome: Topiramate YL Study Group. *Neurology* 1999;52:1882–1887.

128. Franz DN, Glauser TA, Tudor C, et al. Topiramate therapy of epilepsy associated with Angelman's syndrome. *Neurology* 2000;54:1185–1188.

129. Mikati MA, Choueri R, Khurana DS, et al. Gabapentin in the treatment of refractory partial epilepsy in children with intellectual disability. : *J Intellect Disabil Res* 1998;42[Suppl 1]:57–62.

130. Korn-Merker E, Borusiak P, Boenigk HE. Gabapentin in childhood epilepsy: a prospective evaluation of efficacy and safety. *Epilepsy Res* 2000;38:27–32.

131. Trudeau V, Myers S, LaMoreaux L, et al. Gabapentin in naive childhood absence epilepsy: results from two double-blind, placebo-controlled, multicenter studies. *J Child Neurol* 1996; 11:470–475.

132. Camfield CS, Chaplin S, Doyle AB, et al. Side effects of phenobarbital in toddlers: behavioral and cognitive aspects. *J Pediatr* 1979;95:361–365.

133. Appleton R, Sweeney A, Choonara I, et al. Lorazepam versus diazepam in the acute treatment of epileptic seizures and status epilepticus. *Dev Med Child Neurol* 1995;37:682–688.

134. Reference to come.

135. Gustavson LE, Boellner SW, Granneman GR, et al. A single-dose study to define tiagabine pharmacokinetics in pediatric patients with complex partial seizures. *Neurology* 1997;48:1032–1037.

136. Uldall P, Bulteau C, Pedersen SA, et al. Tiagabine adjunctive therapy in children with refractory epilepsy: a single-blind dose escalating study. *Epilepsy Res* 2000;42:159–168.

137. Akman CI, Schubert R. The role of tiagabine in the treatment of intractable epilepsy of childhood with multifocal independent spikes: a case report. *Clin Electroencephalogr* 2000;31:207–210.

138. Holden KR, Titus MO. The effect of tiagabine on spasticity in children with intractable epilepsy: a pilot study. *Pediatr Neurol* 1999;21:728–730.

139. Piccinelli P, Borgatti R, Perucca E, et al. Frontal nonconvulsive status epilepticus associated with high-dose tiagabine therapy in a child with familial bilateral perisylvian polymicrogyria. *Epilepsia* 2000;41:1485–1488.

140. Wallace SJ. Myoclonus and epilepsy in childhood: a review of treatment with valproate, ethosuximide, lamotrigine and zonisamide. *Epilepsy Res* 1998;29:147–154.

141. Suzuki Y, Nagai T, Ono I, et al. Zonisamide monotherapy in newly diagnosed infantile spasms. *Epilepsia* 1997;38:1035–1038.

142. Yanai S, Hanai T, Narazaki O. Treatment of infantile spasms with zonisamide. *Brain Dev* 1999;21:157–161.

143. Kishi T, Nejihashi Y, Kajiyama M, et al. Successful zonisamide treatment for infants with hypsarrhythmia. *Pediatr Neurol* 2000;23:274–277.

144. Ohno M, Shimotsuji Y, Abe J, et al. Zonisamide treatment of early infantile epileptic encephalopathy. *Pediatr Neurol* 2000;23:341–344.

145. Iinuma K, Minami T, Cho K, et al. Long-term effects of zonisamide in the treatment of epilepsy in children with intellectual disability. *J Intellect Disabil Res* 1998;42[Suppl 1]:68–73.

146. Kimura S. Zonisamide-induced behavior disorder in two children. *Epilepsia* 1994;35:403–405.

147. Shimizu T, Yamashita Y, Satoi M, et al. Heat stroke–like episode in a child caused by zonisamide. *Brain Dev* 1997;19:366–368.

148. Okumura A, Ishihara N, Kato T, et al. Predictive value of acetylcholine stimulation testing for oligohidrosis caused by zonisamide. *Pediatr Neurol* 2000;23:59–61.

149. Kubota M, Nishi-Nagase M, Sakakihara Y, et al. Zonisamide-induced urinary lithiasis in patients with intractable epilepsy. *Brain Dev* 2000;22:230–233.

GENERAL PRINCIPLES

ANTIEPILEPTIC DRUG USE IN WOMEN

MARTHA J. MORRELL

Women and men with epilepsy share many of the same burdens—the unpredictability of seizures, the need to take daily medications for years or even a lifetime, the social stigma, and the psychological consequences arising from societal misunderstanding. In addition, women with epilepsy must be concerned about the potential effect of reproductive sex steroid hormones on the seizure threshold, about the impact of epilepsy and antiepileptic drugs (AEDs) on reproductive physiology, and about the risks to pregnancy and the fetus from maternal seizures and AEDs. Other considerations include the potential of gender to alter AED pharmacokinetics and pharmacodynamics. As health care providers gain greater sophistication in the treatment of epilepsy and as new therapies become available, gender emerges as a significant consideration in designing the optimal treatment for the whole patient.

HORMONES AND SEIZURES

Steroid hormones modulate brain excitability. This alters the epilepsy phenotype at puberty, over the menstrual cycle, and at menopause. Physiologic changes in steroid hormones are also likely to influence efficacy of AEDs. As such, ovarian steroids may be considered pharmacoactive compounds that alter the seizure threshold—estrogens acting as proconvulsants and progesterones as anticonvulsants (1).

Steroid Hormone Effects on Neuronal Excitability

The effects of hormones on neuronal excitability are best understood for estrogen and progesterone, the principal ovarian steroid hormones (2–4). In all experimental models

Martha J. Morrell, MD: Professor of Clinical Neurology, Department of Neurology, Columbia University, College of Physicians and Surgeons; and Director, Columbia Comprehensive Epilepsy Center, New York, New York

of epilepsy seizure susceptibility alters with fluctuations of these hormones similar to physiologic changes over a reproductive cycle (5,6).

Estrogen has a seizure-activating effect in experimental models of epilepsy and in the human cerebral cortex. Estrogen lowers the electroshock seizure threshold (7–9), creates new cortical seizure foci when applied topically (10), activates preexisting cortical epileptogenic foci (11), and increases the severity of chemically induced seizures (12). Intravenous estrogen activates electroencephalographic epileptiform activity in some women with partial epilepsy (13).

In contrast to estrogen, progesterone exerts a seizure-protective effect in experimental models of epilepsy. High doses of progesterone and its reduced metabolite pregnenolone induce sedation and anesthesia in rats and in humans. Spontaneous interictal spikes produced by cortical application of penicillin are reduced by progesterone (14). Progesterone also suppresses kindling (15), heightens the seizure threshold to chemical convulsants (16,17), elevates the electroshock seizure threshold (8,18), attenuates ethanol withdrawal convulsions (17), and suppresses focal seizures (19) in animal models of epilepsy.

Steroid hormones modulate cortical excitability by several distinct mechanisms of action (3). In the classic model, the steroid hormone binds to an intracellular receptor (intracytoplasmic for glucocorticoids, intranuclear for estrogen and progesterone). Binding transforms the receptor to an active form that binds to DNA and leads to gene activation and protein synthesis, a process requiring 30 minutes to several hours. Many neuroactive effects of steroids are evident in seconds to minutes, a finding suggesting that some actions are mediated by mechanisms other than the classic model, probably at the level of the neuronal membrane. Sex steroid hormones exert immediate, short-duration effects on neuronal membrane excitability by altering γ-aminobutyric acid (GABA)–mediated inhibition and glutamate-mediated excitation (20) (Table 12.1).

TABLE 12.1. MEMBRANE AND GENOMIC EFFECTS OF OVARIAN STEROIDS ON NEURONAL EXCITABILITY[a]

	GABA$_A$ Receptor	NMDA Receptor in Hippocampus	GABA Concentration	GABA$_A$ Receptor Number
Estrogen	Reduces Cl influx	Activates	Decreases	Reduces number
Progesterone	Increases Cl influx	Inhibits	Increases	Increases number

GABA, γ-aminobutyric acid; NMDA, *N*-methyl-D-aspartate.
[a]Effects of estrogen and progesterone on neuronal excitability are mediated by altering the resting membrane potential. Estrogen reduces inhibition and increases excitation. Progesterone increases inhibition and reduces excitation.

A sex steroid hormone recognition site is present on a recombinantly expressed GABA$_A$ receptor complex derived from human complementary DNA (cDNA) (21). Neurosteroids, such as the ovarian steroids, act at two sites on the GABA$_A$ receptor complex: directly on the chloride channel and at a distinct site that mediates the action of GABA and benzodiazepines (22–25).

Estrogen reduces the effectiveness of GABA-mediated neuronal inhibition by reducing chloride conductance through the GABA$_A$ receptor complex. Excitatory neurotransmission is modulated by estrogen through agonist binding sites on the *N*-methyl-D-aspartate (NMDA) receptor complex in the CA-1 region of the hippocampus (26).

Progesterone and progesterone metabolites function as allosteric receptor antagonists or inverse agonists at the GABA$_A$ receptor complex (27–29), thus potentiating GABA-induced chloride conductance by increasing the frequency (benzodiazepine-like effects) and duration (barbiturate-like effect) of channel opening (24,30,31). In addition, progesterone may alter the potency of AEDs. Benzodiazepine binding to the GABA$_A$ receptor complex increases by >50% in the presence of pregnenolone, the major reduced metabolite of progesterone (32).

Genomic effects of ovarian steroids alter excitability with a longer latency and for a longer duration. Estrogen increases neuronal excitability by inhibiting GABA synthesis in the arcuate nucleus, in the ventromedial nucleus of the hypothalamus, and in the centromedial group of the amygdala (33), probably through regulation of messenger RNA (mRNA) encoding for glutamic acid decarboxylase, the rate-limiting enzyme for GABA synthesis (34,35). Estrogen affects mRNA encoding for GABA$_A$ receptor subunits (36). Progesterone also modulates GABA amino decarboxylase (34), alters expression of mRNA encoding for GABA$_A$ receptor subunits (34,36), and reduces glutamate activity (37–39).

Neuronal morphology is altered with physiologic changes in estrogen. Estrogen exposure profoundly alters the morphology of CA-1 hippocampal neurons taken from ovariectomized animals, by increasing dendritic spines and excitatory synaptic connections within 12 to 24 hours of exposure (40,41). Conversely, when estrogen levels fall, these changes reverse within a similar period.

The sensitivity of neurons to the modulating effects of individual steroid hormones may be dynamic, changing after puberty and in response to fluctuations in basal levels of steroid hormones over a reproductive cycle (16,42). The pubertal surge in estrogen appears to have a neuronal priming effect. In contrast to the situation in postpubertal rats, estrogen does not alter the rate of amygdala kindling in prepubertal male and female rats. Rats castrated prepubertally have higher seizure thresholds to minimal and maximal electroshock than do animals castrated after puberty (8). Several experimental models of epilepsy in rodents suggest that the sensitivity of the GABA$_A$ receptor complex to neurosteroids varies to maintain homeostatic regulation of brain excitability (6,24,43). In rodents, the threshold dose for seizure onset induced by chemical convulsants (biculline, picrotoxin, pentylenetetrazol, and strychnine) changes over the estrus cycle. Female rats in estrus (equivalent to the premenstrual phase in humans) are more sensitive to chemical convulsants than are females in diestrus and males, whereas infusion of progesterone increases the seizure threshold more for females in diestrus (equivalent to human low-progesterone follicular phase) (43). Estrogens also exert differential effects on neuronal excitability, depending on cycling status. Enhanced neuronal excitability occurs when female rats in low-estrogen states are given estrogen, but not when estrogen is given during a high-estrogen state (diestrus) (44).

Catamenial Seizures

Women with epilepsy frequently display menstrual cycle-associated seizure patterns. The debate in the literature about whether catamenial (menstrual-associated) seizure patterns exist can be explained by the difference in seizure patterns across ovulatory and anovulatory menstrual cycles. Authors who have not differentiated ovulatory and anovulatory menstrual cycles (45) have not detected catamenial patterns. Authors who have identified cycles as ovulatory or anovulatory find distinct and reproducible seizure patterns in ovulatory cycles (46,47), with seizures more likely to occur in the perimenstrual and ovulatory phases, times when estrogen levels are relatively high and progesterone is relatively low.

The endocrine profile differs in ovulatory and anovulatory cycles. The hypothalamic trophic hormone gonadotropin-releasing hormone stimulates release of the pituitary gonadotropin, luteinizing hormone (LH), and follicle-stimulating hormone (FSH). FSH stimulates formation of an ovarian follicle. Estrogen is the predominant ovarian sex hormone during the follicular phase (first half) of the menstrual cycle. A midcycle LH surge triggers ovulation and transforms the follicle into the corpus luteum, which secretes progesterone throughout the second, or luteal, phase of the cycle. If fertilization does not occur, the follicle involutes, and progesterone secretion stops. The uterine lining is then shed, to complete a cycle of about 28 days in length. During anovulatory cycles, estrogen levels remain high throughout the cycle, and progesterone remains low.

Hormone-mediated seizure patterns differ across ovulatory and anovulatory cycles. Catamenial seizure patterns may not be evident over all cycles in an individual woman because of the high likelihood of anovulatory cycles in women with epilepsy. During ovulatory cycles, most seizures arise about 3 days before the onset of menstrual flow and persist for a total of 6 days. These seizures may be triggered by the perimenstrual progesterone withdrawal. For women with catamenial seizure patterns, more than three-fourths of all seizures arise in this 6-day window of time (47). Seizures occurring at ovulation may be triggered by the estrogen surge. In contrast to the perimenstrual and ovulatory seizure preponderance over ovulatory cycles, seizures are more dispersed and are often more frequent during an anovulatory cycle, probably because of the relative high and persistent concentration of estrogen unopposed by the luteal surge in progesterone.

Other mechanisms may also contribute to perimenstrual seizure exacerbation. Perimenstrual reductions in serum concentrations of AEDs have been described, perhaps related to increased volume of distribution or increased metabolism (48).

Treatment of Hormonally Sensitive Seizures

The most effective treatment for any type of seizure is usually one of the first-line AEDs used in monotherapy. Women whose seizures display a catamenial association may also respond to adjunctive therapy with a carbonic anhydrase inhibitor or with hormonal therapy.

Acetazolamide (Diamox) is a weak carbonic anhydrase inhibitor with mild diuretic actions. Oral acetazolamide may be helpful as adjunctive therapy for catamenial seizures, although this is not a labeled indication in the United States. One small trial described a ≥50% reduction in seizures in 45% of women taking acetazolamide either intermittently or continuously for catamenial seizures. Fifteen percent of the women reported loss of efficacy over 6 to 24 months (49).

The anticonvulsant properties of acetazolamide may be related to its ability to cause a mild, transient metabolic acidosis. Because tolerance to the anticonvulsant properties of the drug may develop, intermittent therapy may be preferable. In women with catamenial seizures and predictable menstrual cycles, acetazolamide may be used for 10 to 14 days, surrounding the time of seizure vulnerability. The usual dosage is 250 to 1,000 mg in two divided doses. Side effects include gastrointestinal disturbance, sedation, headache, and hypersensitivity reactions, particularly in those sensitive to sulfonamides. Bone marrow depression and renal colic arise rarely, as do electrolyte disturbances such as hypokalemia and hyperglycemia in patients with diabetes mellitus. Acetazolamide has teratogenic and embryocidal effects in rats and mice. This appears to be a species-specific effect; nevertheless, acetazolamide should not be used in pregnant women.

Several small studies have evaluated the effectiveness of progesterones and antiestrogens as AEDs. Synthetic oral progestins have not been helpful (50), although parenteral medroxyprogesterone (Depo-provera) reduces the seizure frequency in some women when it is given in large enough doses to cause amenorrhea (50,51). This can be given as medroxyprogesterone, 120 to 150 mg intramuscularly every 6 to 12 weeks (52). Adverse effects include hot flashes, irregular vaginal breakthrough bleeding, breast tenderness, and a 6- to 12-month delay before the return of menstrual cycles. Natural progesterone is available as extract of soy in suppository and lozenge form. The progesterone may be given over the initial luteal phase of the cycle as 100 to 200 mg three to four times a day, with an average dose of 600 mg to achieve a serum level of 5 to 25 ng/mL (52,53). Natural progesterone comes as 200-mg lozenges and can be given as one-half to one lozenge three times daily on days 14 to 25, one-fourth to one-half lozenge three times daily on days 26 and 27, and one-fourth lozenge three times daily on day 28. Another alternative is prometrium, 100 mg capsules, using a similar dosage schedule. A progesterone topical cream may be helpful for women with ovulatory seizures. This can be used several days before ovulation is anticipated. Reversible side effects include asthenia, emotional depression, breast tenderness, and acne. Progesterone therapy may be most advantageous in women who have inadequate luteal phase cycles, as determined by serum progesterone levels of <5 ng/mL during the midluteal phase (53). Progesterone therapy should be avoided during or in anticipation of pregnancy, and in the absence of scrupulous contraception.

Antiestrogens, such as clomifene, are typically used to treat infertility and as cancer chemotherapeutic agents. Clomifene has been reported to reduce seizures in women with intractable partial epilepsy, but it is associated with potentially significant side effects such as hot flashes, polycystic ovaries, and unplanned pregnancy (52). Many antiestrogens are under development. Some may eventually have a role in the treatment of hormone-sensitive seizures.

Menopause, Epilepsy, and Antiepileptic Drugs

Women with epilepsy may find that seizures improve after menopause, especially if seizures displayed catamenial patterns. However, the perimenopause may be a time of seizure exacerbation. About 2 to 3 years before ovulation stops, cycles become irregular, and there are fluctuations in concentrations of gonadal steroids. This is a time when seizure patterns may change and seizure frequency may worsen (54). One survey suggests that postmenopausal estrogen replacement may exacerbate seizures in some women with epilepsy (55).

EFFICACY AND TOLERABILITY OF ANTIEPILEPTIC DRUGS IN WOMEN

AED pharmacokinetics and pharmacodynamics may differ in men and women. Women have smaller body size, higher body fat, lower body water, and less muscle mass. Contraceptive sex steroid hormones and hormone replacement therapy, as well as endogenous ovarian steroid hormones, may also alter AED pharmacology and efficacy.

Since 1993, the U.S. Food and Drug Administration (FDA) and the Department of Health and Human Services (DHHS) have mandated that clinical evaluation of new drugs include study and evaluation of gender differences (56). An efficacy analysis by gender is available for most of the newly marketed AEDs, but not for the older AEDs. Gabapentin, felbamate, lamotrigine, tiagabine, and topiramate were as effective and well tolerated in women as in men during premarketing trials (57). Zonisamide showed equal efficacy by gender but was better tolerated in women (58).

DRUG INTERACTIONS

Hormonal contraception may be ineffective in women receiving hepatic cytochrome P450 enzyme–inducing AEDs, with a failure rate exceeding 6% per year (59–61). A United States–based national survey found that most neurologists and obstetricians were not aware of this significant potential interaction (62). Another survey of more than 3,500 health care providers, including pediatricians, general practitioners, and family practice physicians, confirmed this knowledge deficit (63). Most oral contraceptives contain only sufficient hormone to inhibit ovulation, and even subtle increases in metabolism may lead to contraceptive failure. Some AEDs promote metabolism of contraceptive steroids and also increase production of sex hormone binding globulin, a protein that avidly binds steroid hormones and renders them biologically inactive (64).

Ethinylestradiol and mestranol, a prodrug converted to active ethinylestradiol, are synthetic estrogens contained within oral contraceptives at a usual dose of 35 μg of ethinylestradiol. Ethinylestradiol undergoes significant first-pass metabolism with individual bioavailablity ranging from 10% to 75 %. First-pass metabolism occurs by sulfation in the gut, followed by glucuronidation or hydroxylation in the liver. Hydroxylation is catalyzed by the cytochrome CYP3A4. Synthetic progestins contained in oral contraceptives are levonorgestrel, norethindrome, norethisterone, desogestrel, norgestimate, and gestodene. Bioavailablity is ≤80%, and there is no significant first-pass effect. CYP3A4 also appears to be involved in progesterone metabolism.

Phenytoin (PHT), phenobarbital (PB), and carbamazepine (CBZ) are broad-spectrum inducers of hepatic cytochrome P450 enzymes. Enzyme induction increases metabolism of the estrogenic, and probably progestational, component and also increases steroid hormone protein binding, thus reducing the hormone concentration. PHT and CBZ each reduce the concentration of 50 μg of ethinylestradiol by about 50%, and they reduce the concentration of levonorgestrel by about 30% (65). Sodium valproate (VPA) did not change concentrations of ethinylestradiol or levonorgestrel in six women with epilepsy (66).

Felbamate, oxcarbazepine, and topiramate are weak inducers of CYP3A4 only. The effects of felbamate on an oral contraceptive containing 30 μg ethinylestradiol and 75 mg gestodene were assessed in a randomized double-blind, placebo-controlled study of healthy premenopausal female volunteers. Felbamate was associated with a 42% decrease in gestodene and had a minor effect on ethinylestradiol (67). The effects of oxcarbazepine on oral contraceptives containing 50 μg of ethinylestradiol and 250 μg of levonorgestrel were assessed in healthy women volunteers. Oxcarbazepine was associated with a reduction of 47% in plasma concentrations of both hormones (68). Healthy women volunteers receiving topiramate and oral contraceptives containing norethindrone, 1 mg, and ethinylestradiol, 35 μg, had an 18% to 30% reduction in concentration of ethinylestradiol, with no change in the progesterone norethindrone (69). Table 12.2 provides a list of AEDs categorized by their effect on cytochrome P450 enzymes.

To provide acceptable contraceptive efficacy, women taking cytochrome P450–inducing AEDs must receive at least 50 μg of the estrogen component (70,71). Long-term progesterone-only contraceptive systems such as subdermal levonorgestrel are also prone to failure because of increased steroid metabolism (72,73). Intramuscular medroxyprogesterone has not been evaluated for efficacy in women taking cytochrome P450–inducing AEDs. For women taking these enzyme-inducing AEDs in whom pregnancy is contraindicated, use of a barrier contraceptive should be advised.

TABLE 12.2.   CATEGORIZATION OF ANTIEPILEPTIC DRUGS BY EFFECTS ON CYTOCHROME P450 LIVER ENZYMES[a]

Drugs That Induce Cytochrome P450 Enzymes and May Adversely Interact with Hormonal Contraception	Drugs That Inhibit or Have No Effect on Cytochrome P450 Enzymes and Do Not Adversely Interact with Hormonal Contraception
Carbamazepine	Gabapentin
Felbamate	Lamotrigine
Oxcarbazepine	Levetiracetam
Phenobarbital	Tiagabine
Phenytoin	Valproate
Primidone	Zonisamide
Topiramate	

[a]Drugs that induce this enzyme system may decrease the concentration of biologically active hormone and therefore reduce efficacy of hormonally based contraception. Drugs that inhibit or have no effect on this enzyme system do not affect the efficacy of hormonal contraception.

ANTIEPILEPTIC DRUG EFFECTS ON REPRODUCTIVE HORMONES AND HEALTH

Fertility

Women with epilepsy are less likely to have children than are other women. Although studies of incident population of persons with seizures or epilepsy do not show a fertility deficit (74,75), all studies of prevalent populations report lower birth rates. Birth rates are reduced by one-third to as much as two-thirds compared with nonepileptic women (76–80). Social factors may contribute to lower birth rates. Women with epilepsy are less likely to marry. Moreover, women with epilepsy may voluntarily choose not to have children. This choice may come about from concern about parenting or concern about transmission of epilepsy, or it may be based on advice provided by family, friends, and health care providers. More important than social pressures is the reproductive dysfunction associated with epilepsy and with AEDs (81).

Hypothalamic-Pituitary Hormone Abnormalities

Disruption of the hypothalamic-pituitary axis is one mechanism for infertility in women with epilepsy (82). The hypothalamic-pituitary axis supports the female reproductive cycle. Hypothalamic gonadotropin-releasing hormone regulates the release of pituitary FSH and LH according to an ultradian cycle of about 28 days (the menstrual cycle) and observing a circadian cycle in addition. Disruption of either of these cycles can lead to ovulatory failure.

Seizures alter hypothalamic hormone release, which then disrupts gonadotropin hormone, and pituitary hormone release (83). In humans, high-frequency epileptic discharges in the hippocampus are associated with a surge in pituitary prolactin (84,85). About 20 minutes after a seizure involving mesial temporal lobe structures (all generalized tonic-clonic and most complex partial seizures),

prolactin levels increase by three to five times baseline and remain elevated for 2 hours (86,87). Ictal elevations in LH are also observed.

In addition to ictal perturbations of LH, interictal abnormalities are also described. Elevations in circadian pulsatile secretions of LH in women with generalized epilepsy (88) and reductions in circadian pulsatile LH release in women with temporal lobe epilepsy (89) suggest that epilepsy syndromes may differentially alter LH release. Disturbances in LH release in either direction are associated with anovulatory cycles (Morrell et al., 2002, *in press*).

Sex Steroid Hormones

Sex steroid hormone concentrations are altered in women receiving AEDs that change the activity of cytochrome P450 liver enzymes. AEDs that induce the hepatic microsomal enzyme system (the cytochrome P450 system) increase metabolism of gonadal and adrenal steroid hormones and induce the synthesis of sex hormone binding globulin, a binding protein for steroid hormones. Increased protein binding decreases the free, biologically active fraction of hormone. Women taking the enzyme-inducing AEDs PHT, CBZ, and PB have significant reductions in estradiol and in gonadal and adrenal androgens, and they have significant elevations in sex hormone binding globulin compared with women without epilepsy who are not taking AEDs (90–95; Morrell et al., 2002, *in press*). Women taking VPA (which does not induce liver cytochrome enzymes) have higher gonadal and adrenal androgen levels (96). Women with epilepsy who are receiving gabapentin or lamotrigine in monotherapy had no differences in gonadal steroids compared with nonepileptic controls (Morrell et al., 2001).

Polycystic Ovaries

Approximately 30% of women with epilepsy have polycystic-appearing ovaries, compared with about 15% of reproductive-age women without epilepsy (97). Whether these women have polycystic ovary syndrome is not known (98). Polycystic ovary syndrome is characterized by obesity, acne and hirsutism, elevated LH, elevated androgens, abnormal lipid profile, chronic anovulation, and polycystic ovaries. All these features need not be present. An abnormality in the insulin receptor causing insulin resistance is the basis for this gynecologic syndrome (99). Health consequences of polycystic ovary syndrome include infertility, dyslipidemia, glucose intolerance and diabetes, and endometrial cancer (100).

Women with epilepsy who are taking AEDs may develop some of these features, including anovulatory cycles, menstrual cycle length abnormalities, abnormal LH:FSH ratio, obesity, and polycystic ovaries (96). Twenty-five to 40% of menstrual cycles in women with epilepsy are anovulatory (in contrast to about 10% of cycles in women without epilepsy). Abnormally long or short menstrual cycles (less than 23 days or more than 35 days), significant cycle variability, and midcycle bleeding are signs of ovulatory dysfunction in women with epilepsy. VPA is especially closely associated with polycystic ovaries, hyperandrogenism, and hyperinsulinemia. In part, this may be related to VPA-induced weight gain and obesity (94,101). Whereas 25% to 30% of women with epilepsy who are taking AEDs other than VPA have polycystic-appearing ovaries, this number may be as high as 60% for women receiving VPA (96) (Morrell et al., 2002, *in press*).

Isojarvi et al. (96) found the prevalence of polycystic ovaries to be highest in women receiving VPA before the age of 20 years. In contrast to a rate of 32% in women receiving VPA after age 20 years and a rate of 18% in women receiving AEDs other than VPA after the age of 20, 60% of women receiving VPA before they were 20 years old and 25% of women receiving other AEDs before age 20 had polycystic-appearing ovaries. Elevations in insulin were reported in the women in this study who were receiving VPA. In addition, VPA-associated elevations in androgens were found in about 20% of these reproductive-age women (96). Androgen elevations have also been reported in prepubertal girls (102).

VPA-associated polycystic ovaries, hyperandrogenism, and hyperinsulinemia appear to be reversible. Sixteen women who had these features when they took VPA were changed to lamotrigine (94). The polycystic-appearing ovaries resolved within 1 year in most of these patients. Testosterone and insulin concentrations normalized within several months. A cross-sectional observational study of 93 women with epilepsy also found an association between current use of VPA and higher prevalence of polycystic ovaries. However, women with epilepsy who were receiving VPA for ≥3 years in the past were no more likely to have polycystic-appearing ovaries than were women who had never taken VPA (Morrell et al., 2002, *in press*).

Sexual Dysfunction

Sexual dysfunction affects 30% to 40% of persons with epilepsy. Women with epilepsy may have diminished sexual interest and desire (103,104). More than one-third report dyspareunia, vaginismus, and lack of vaginal lubrication, symptoms of a disorder of sexual arousal (105). Direct measurement of genital blood flow showed a diminished genital blood flow response in persons with localization related epilepsy of temporal lobe origin in response to erotic visual stimuli (106).

AEDs may contribute to sexual dysfunction by direct cortical effects or secondarily through alterations in the hormones supporting sexual behavior. Occasional or chronic impotence occurred in 12% of men beginning treatment of epilepsy with a single drug, and it was most likely to be associated with barbiturate use (107). Decreased libido or impotence occurred in 22% of men receiving primidone. AEDs also reduce the biologically active fraction of steroid hormones by increasing steroid hormone protein binding and metabolism (108–110). Reductions in androgens by enzyme-inducing AEDs may impair erectile function in men (111) and may reduce sexual desire in men and in women. Reductions in estrogen contribute to the physiologic arousal dysfunction experienced by women with epilepsy.

Detecting Reproductive Dysfunction in the Woman with Epilepsy

Until the relationship of epilepsy, AEDs, and these reproductive endocrine and ovarian abnormalities is better understood, clinicians must be alert to signs of reproductive dysfunction. These signs are listed in Table 12.3. Keeping a diary with length of the menstrual cycle and the timing and duration of menstrual flow is the most sensitive indicator for most reproductive cycle disorders. Women with menstrual dysfunction should be referred for gynecologic evaluation and care. A suggested evaluation is provided in Table 12.4.

TABLE 12.3. SYMPTOMS AND SIGNS OF REPRODUCTIVE DYSFUNCTION

- Weight gain of more than 10% or body mass index of more than 27 kg/m²
- Hirsutism (increased body and facial hair and scalp hair loss)
- Acne
- Menstrual cycle shorter than 23 days or longer than 35 days
- Menstrual cycle with more than 5 days' variability from cycle to cycle
- Midcycle menstrual bleeding
- History of difficulty conceiving or first trimester miscarriage
- Disorder of sexual desire or sexual arousal

TABLE 12.4. EVALUATION STRATEGY FOR WOMEN WITH EPILEPSY AND REPRODUCTIVE DYSFUNCTION

- Physical, gynecologic, and neurologic examinations
- Complete blood count, liver function tests, fasting glucose, and lipid panel
- Thyroid function tests
- Pituitary hormones
  - Luteinizing hormone and follicle-stimulating hormone
  - Prolactin
- Gonadal and adrenal steroids
  - Estradiol, progesterone, testosterone, dihydroepiandrostenedione (DHEA)
- Transvaginal ovarian ultrasound

EFFECTS OF ANTIEPILEPTIC DRUGS ON BONE HEALTH

AEDs may alter bone mineral metabolism and may compromise bone health, especially in women who have smaller bone mass. Women using the established AEDs are at higher risk of bone disorders such as osteopenia, osteomalacia, and fractures (112–114). A prospective study evaluating the risk of hip fractures in women >65 years of age found that women taking AEDs were twice as likely to have a hip fracture (115).

Bone biochemical abnormalities described in people with epilepsy include hypocalcemia, hypophosphatemia, elevated serum alkaline phosphatase, elevated parathyroid hormone (PTH), and reduced levels of vitamin D and its active metabolites (116–118). The most severe bone and biochemical abnormalities are found in patients taking AED polytherapy (116,117) and in patients who have taken AEDs for a longer period (112).

AEDs may alter bone mineral metabolism by inducing vitamin D metabolism (61,117). Decreased Vitamin D leads to decreased intestinal calcium absorption, hypocalcemia and a compensatory increase in circulating PTH, resulting in increased mobilization of bone calcium stores. Because VPA does not induce the hepatic cytochrome P450 enzyme system, this mechanism does not explain the reduction in bone density associated with the drug (114). AEDs may also interfere directly with intestinal calcium absorption and could directly affect bone cell function, possibly through inhibition of cellular responses to PTH (113,118). Research is currently under way to define effects of individual AEDs on bone metabolism. In the meantime, women with epilepsy should receive adequate daily calcium and vitamin D and should engage regularly in gravity-resisting exercise.

ANTIEPILEPTIC DRUGS AND LIPID METABOLISM

Increased total cholesterol and low-density lipoproteins (LDLs) are associated with cardiovascular disease in women as well as men. Changes in lipid metabolism and body weight associated with use of some AEDs may create a long-term adverse health effect. Some AEDs are associated with abnormalities in cholesterol and lipid profiles (119–122). CBZ, PB and PHT increase high density lipoproteins. CBZ has cholesterol lowering effects, and PB and PHT may exert a similar cholesterol lowering action. Counteracting these favorable lipid trends, elevations in low density lipoproteins are reported with CBZ and PB. VPA increases low- and high-density lipoproteins and leads to an unfavorable lipid profile. VPA-associated obesity and increases in insulin may account for VPA-associated dyslipidemia (94). Until the nature and mechanisms of AED-associated alterations in lipid metabolism are better understood, clinicians should monitor cholesterol and lipid profiles in women and men receiving AEDs.

PRINCIPLES OF ANTIEPILEPTIC DRUGS USE IN PREGNANCY

Approximately 1% of all pregnancies are in women with epilepsy. The number of women with epilepsy who become pregnant has grown over the years, as marriage rates have increased for women with epilepsy (123), as parenting has become more socially supported, and as the medical management of pregnancy in women with epilepsy has improved. Pregnancy outcome can be maximized if the health care provider is alert to the following concerns: the importance of maintaining seizure control during pregnancy, the potential for fetal loss, and the risk of AED-associated teratogenicity and neurodevelopmental delay. Counseling and relatively minor treatment modifications can reduce the risk of an adverse pregnancy outcome.

Seizure frequency may change during pregnancy. Approximately 35% of pregnant women with epilepsy experience an increase in seizure frequency, 55% have no change, and 10% have a decrease in seizure frequency (124,125). The factors that are believed to alter seizure frequency include changes in sex hormones, in AED metabolism, in sleep schedules, and in medication compliance.

AED concentrations may change during pregnancy. Physiologic changes during pregnancy that can alter AED pharmacokinetics and total AED concentrations include decreased gastric tone and motility, nausea and vomiting, which arise in 40% of women during the first trimester, an increase in plasma volume of 40% to 50%, and an increase in renal clearance. The pharmacokinetics of some AEDs is more profoundly affected than is that of others, probably because of the pregnancy-related differential effects on cytochrome P450 enzymes. Two cytochrome P450 enzymes, CYP2C9 and CYP2C19, are induced to a greater extent than is CYP3A4. This could account for the greater reduction in PHT compared with CBZ, which is principally metabolized by CYP3A4, and VPA, which is predominantly eliminated by glucuronidation and β-oxidation (64,126). Although the total concentration falls for many AEDs, there tends to be an increase in the percentage of unbound or free drug because of a reduction in albumin and, thus, in protein binding (127). Therefore, it is necessary to follow the non–protein-bound drug concentration, especially for AEDs that are highly protein bound, such as CBZ, PHT, and VPA. Dose adjustments should aim to maintain a stable non–protein-bound fraction. The concentration of AED in fetal serum is proportional to the free (non–protein-bound) maternal concentration (128).

Women with epilepsy are at greater risk of fetal loss. Early or late miscarriage and preterm delivery are three to five times more likely than in women without epilepsy. The reasons for fetal loss are not entirely understood, but they are more likely to be related to maternal seizures than to fetal exposure to AEDs (129,130). Fetal heart rate decelerations indicate fetal distress and are reported with maternal seizures (131). These observations underscore the importance of seizure control during pregnancy.

The first reports of birth defects associated with fetal exposure to AEDs came from small, retrospective case series that described drug-specific syndromes after exposure to trimethadione, PHT, PB, CBZ, VPA, and benzodiazepines. However, the features of these syndromes were more similar than dissimilar, with typical features being cleft lip and palate, cardiac septal defects, urogenital defects, and dysmorphisms of the face and digits. The effects of individual AEDs were further obscured in the early studies because women were likely to be receiving AED polypharmacy.

The older AEDs (benzodiazepines, PHT, CBZ, PB, and VPA) are associated with a higher risk of fetal major malformations, including cleft lip and palate and cardiac defects (atrial septal defect, tetralogy of Fallot, ventricular septal defect, coarctation of the aorta, patent ductus arteriosus, and pulmonary stenosis) (132–134). The incidence of these major malformations in infants born to mothers

with epilepsy taking any one of these AEDs is 4% to 6 %, compared with 2% to 4% for the general population. Neural tube defects (spina bifida and anencephaly) occur in 0.5% to 1% of infants exposed to CBZ (135) and in 1% to 2% of infants exposed to VPA during the first month of gestation (136). Risks of malformations are highest in fetuses exposed to multiple AEDs and those exposed to higher doses.

Minor congenital anomalies associated with AED exposure include facial dysmorphism and digital anomalies, which arise in 6% to 20 % of infants exposed to antiepileptic drugs *in utero* (137). This represents a twofold increase over the general population. However, these anomalies are usually subtle and are often outgrown.

Concerns are mounting that exposure to AEDs *in utero* may confer a long-lasting neurodevelopmental or neurocognitive deficit (138,139). Fetal head growth retardation has been associated with maternal use of AEDs (140). Although prospective trials are lacking, retrospective studies show that children exposed *in utero* to VPA in monotherapy or polytherapy are more likely to require special educational resources (141). Prospective studies are under way to define more clearly the neurodevelopmental risks of AED exposure to the developing brain.

As outlined in Table 12.5, several large, observational studies confirm that fetuses exposed to AEDs *in utero* are at risk of morphologic abnormalities: 193 pregnancies from 145 women with epilepsy were compared with 24,094 pregnancies in women without epilepsy. Children born to women with epilepsy who took AEDs during pregnancy had low birth weight, decreased body length, and decreased head circumference (142). Another prospective multicenter study also found reduced birth weight and body length in children born to mothers with epilepsy who were taking AEDs (143). A prospective study of 983 babies born to women with epilepsy in Japan, Italy, and Canada found a 7% rate of malformations for exposed children compared

TABLE 12.5. SUMMARY OF LARGEST STUDIES USING CONTROL GROUPS AND EVALUATING MAJOR CONGENITAL MALFORMATIONS IN CHILDREN EXPOSED TO ANTIEPILEPTIC DRUGS IN UTERO

| | | No. of Malformations and Rate | | |
	Data Collection Period	Children of Women with Epilepsy on AEDs	Control Subjects	Additional Findings
Netherlands (188,189)	1972–1992	52 (3.7%)	29 (1.5%)	Additional risk with polytherapy
Japan, Italy, Canada (144)	1978–1991	80 (9.0%)	3 (3.1%)	Valproate dose correlated with malformations
United Kingdom (190)	1988–1993	10 (3.4%)	6 (1%)	No cases of spina bifida
Iceland (74)	1972–1990	13 (5.9%)		
Denmark (142)	1989–1994	4 (4.6%)	280 (1%)	
United States (146)	1986–1993	18 (5.7%)	9 (1.8%)	Major malformations, microcephaly, growth retardation, midface hypoplasia or hypoplasia of fingers in 20.6% of AED-exposed infants vs. 8.5% of control subjects

AED, antiepileptic drug.

with a 3.1% rate for children not exposed to an AED *in utero* (144). There was no difference in incidence of malformation by exposure to any one AED.

The risk of teratogenicity is partly related to the extent of fetal exposure to the AED (145). The risk is highest in fetuses exposed to higher dosages and to AED polytherapy. Holmes et al. (146) assessed women with a history of seizures on and off AEDs delivering at one of five maternity hospitals in the Boston area. Identified mother-infant pairs were compared with control pairs of nonepileptic mothers and infants. Considering major malformations alone, 4.5% of women with epilepsy who were taking a single AED gave birth to a child with a major malformation, whereas 8.6% of women who were taking two or more AEDs had a child with a major malformation. No women with a history of seizures who were not taking an AED gave birth to a child with a major malformation. Major malformations were detected in 1.8% of infants born to controls. When major malformations, growth retardation, microcephaly, hypoplasia of the midface, and hypoplasia of the fingers were considered, 20.6% of the infants born to mothers with epilepsy who were taking AEDs had one or more of these birth defects, in contrast to 28% of the infants born to mothers who were taking two or more AEDs, 6.1% of the infants born to mothers with a history of seizures but who were not taking AEDs, and 8.5% of controls.

This study confirms observations made in the 1990s. AEDs increase the risk of major malformations and anomalies, and the risk increases with exposure to multiple AEDs. There is no study yet that provides the answer to the question "Which drug is best to use in pregnancy?" The design of the Holmes study was not able to capture the difference in incident versus prevalent epilepsy, nor was it able to assess the effects of ethnicity and preventive health behaviors such as folic acid supplementation.

Several mechanisms have been postulated to explain the teratogenicity of AEDs. Some AEDs may be teratogenic because of free radical (arene oxide) intermediates (147,148). CBZ, PB, and PHT are metabolized by cytochrome P450 enzyme–dependent oxidative intermediates, which are further metabolized by hydroxylation by epoxide hydrolase to nonreactive dihydrodiols. PB, PHT, and CBZ induce formation of the epoxide intermediate, and VPA inhibits epoxide hydrolase (149,150). Therefore, polytherapy with an enzyme-inducing AED and VPA would promote epoxide formation and would inhibit epoxide breakdown. These unstable intermediates bind with RNA and disrupt DNA synthesis and organogenesis. Higher concentrations of oxide metabolites are associated with a greater risk of fetal malformations, and susceptibility to oxidative-related teratogenicity may be genetically determined (151–153). Another putative mechanism for AED-related teratogenicity is alteration in endogenous retinoid concentrations (154).

Some AEDs may cause a deficiency of folic acid (155). PB, PHT, and CBZ are associated with folate malabsorp-tion, whereas VPA inhibits methionine synthetase, an enzyme promoting the conversion of homocysteine to methionine, a step requiring folic acid as a cofactor (156). Elevation of homocysteine has been associated with higher risk of neural tube defects (157). Administration of folic acid helps to overcome the enzyme inhibition and reduce homocysteine levels.

Folic acid supplementation at conception and through pregnancy reduces the risk of giving birth to a child with neural tube defects in women without epilepsy (158–165). The Medical Research Council (166) vitamin study conclusively demonstrated that folic acid supplementation of 4 mg/day reduces the recurrence risk of neural tube defects in women who had previously given birth to a child with a neural tube defect. The Czech Cooperative Vitamin Study found that first occurrence rates of neural tube defects were significantly reduced by periconceptional supplementation of folic acid, 0.4 mg/day (167). The U.S. Centers for Disease Control and Prevention recommends that all women of childbearing potential receive routine supplementation of folic acid of at least 0.4 mg/day (168).

The protective effect of folic acid in pregnant women without epilepsy has led to the recommendation that folic acid be provided to women with epilepsy, although there are no studies as yet conclusively demonstrating the relevance of this mechanism in AED-mediated teratogenicity. In fact, folic acid supplementation does not necessarily protect against nonneural tube defects. In the Czech study, the rate of cleft lip and palate was not reduced in women receiving periconceptional folic acid (167). How relevant these observations are to women with epilepsy is not yet established. One study associated lower serum levels of folic acid with a higher risk of malformations in children of mothers taking AEDs during pregnancy (169). However, in a more recent study, folic acid supplementation provided to women receiving folic acid antagonists during pregnancy (including AEDs) did not reduce the risk of nonneural tube defects such as cleft lip or palate and cardiovascular and urinary tract malformations (170). One report of a child born with a neural tube defect to a mother taking VPA, 2,000 mg/day, and folic acid suggests that folic acid is not absolutely protective against this malformation (171). However, an ongoing assessment of pregnancy outcomes in children born to mothers with epilepsy reports a reduction in children born with major malformations, coincident with more widespread folic acid supplementation (172).

The malformations associated with AEDs are all generated in the first trimester of pregnancy, and neural tube defects are formed by day 28 after conception. Most women cannot know whether they are pregnant until a menstrual cycle is missed (day 15). In the United States, more than 50% of pregnancies are unplanned (173), and more than 40% of women with planned pregnancies do not consult a health care provider before pregnancy. Therefore, interventions must be designed to maximize fetal outcome

TABLE 12.6. TERATOGENICITY ANTIEPILEPTIC DRUGS: ANIMAL REPRODUCTIVE TOXICOLOGY

AED	IUGR	Skeletal[a]	Orofacial Clefts	Cardiovascular	Urogenital	NTDs
Carbamazepine	+		+		+	+
Felbamate	+					
Gabapentin	+	+				
Lamotrigine	+	+				
Levetiracetam	+	+				
Oxcarbazepine[b]	+	+				
Phenobarbital	+	+	+	+	+	
Phenytoin	+	+	+		+	
Tiagabine	+					
Topiramate	+	+[c]				
Valproic acid		+		+		+
Zonisamide	+	+		+		

AED, antiepileptic drug; IUGR, intrauterine growth retardation; NTDs, neural tube defects.
[a]Delayed ossification.
[b]Teratogenic at maternal toxic dose.
[c]Limb agenesis at high dose in rodents.

before conception. Many professional societies, including the American Academy of Neurology (70), the American College of Obstetric and Gynecologic Physicians (174), and the Canadian Society of Medical Geneticists (175) recommend that all women of childbearing age taking AEDs receive supplemental folic acid supplementation at 0.4 to 5.0 mg/day.

Since 1993, some new AEDs have been introduced. There is little information regarding effects of some of these drugs on the developing human fetus. Animal reproductive toxicology studies for AEDs provide some useful information but may not be specifically predictive of the human experience. Data from the FDA on fetal outcome in animals exposed to the AEDs is presented in Table 12.6.

The U.S. Institute of Medicine has advocated for inclusion of pregnant and lactating women in clinical drug trials

(176). However, the DHHS still places severe restrictions on participation in drug trials for pregnant and lactating women (177). Therefore, prospective, widely inclusive registries are the best means for obtaining information on pregnancy outcome after AED exposure. Information about pregnancy outcomes for fetuses exposed to the newer AEDs is provided in Table 12.7.

Prospective registries have been established to learn more about pregnancy and fetal outcome in women using AEDs, as discussed later. A registry should be contacted regarding any woman who becomes pregnant while taking AEDs.

Management of epilepsy in reproductive-age women should focus on maintaining effective control of seizures while minimizing fetal AED exposure (70,174,178). This applies to dosage and to the number of AEDs. Medication reduction or substitution should take place before concep-

TABLE 12.7. HUMAN PREGNANCY EXPERIENCE WITH THE NEWER ANTIEPILEPTIC DRUGS

Antiepileptic Drug	Premarketing and Postmarketing Experience
Felbamate[a]	10 pregnancies: 1 SAb, 2 Tab, 7 normal outcomes
Gabapentin[b]	16 pregnancies: 5 Tab, 3 births with defects on polytherapy
Levetiracetam	No information available
Lamotrigine[b]	289 pregnancy reports with 293 outcomes (2 sets if twins, 1 set of triplets): 12 SAb (no defects), 27 TAb (2 with defects, both polytherapy); 242 normal outcomes 13 births with defects: 10 polytherapy, 3 monotherapy
Oxcarbazepine[c]	12 pregnancies: 3 SAb, 9 normal outcomes
Tiagabine[a]	23 pregnancies: 4 SAb, 8 TAb, 1 birth with defects on polytherapy
Topiramate[a]	8 pregnancies: 5 TAb, 3 normal outcomes
Zonisamide[b]	Premarketing: 9 pregnancies: 3 SAb, 3 TAb, 1 birth with hypospadias on polytherapy 26 births in Japan: 2 births with defects on polytherapy (1 anencephaly, 1 atrial septal defect)

SAb, spontaneous abortion; TAb, therapeutic abortion.
[a]Premarketing data.
[b]Premarketing and postmarketing data.
[c]Named patient distribution.

tion. Altering medication during pregnancy increases the risk of breakthrough seizures and exposes the fetus to an additional AED. The recommended management during pregnancy is AED monotherapy at the lowest effective dose. The best drug to choose is the drug most likely to be effective and well tolerated for that woman's seizure type. At this time, there is not sufficient information to identify any particular AED as the drug of choice during pregnancy. In addition, if there is a family history of neural tube defects, an agent other than CBZ or VPA may be considered. The FDA use in pregnancy categories for the marketed AEDs are provided in Table 12.8.

Once a patient is pregnant, prenatal diagnostic testing includes a maternal serum α-fetoprotein and a level II (anatomic) ultrasound at 14 to 18 weeks. This strategy identifies >95% of infants with neural tube defects. In some instances, amniocentesis may be indicated.

AEDs have also been associated with an increased risk of early fetal hemorrhage. This may result from an AED-related vitamin K deficiency with a reduction in vitamin K–dependent clotting factors (179). Vitamin K deficiency in the newborn is suspected because of reports of PIVKAs (proteins induced by vitamin K absence) detected in umbilical cord blood of neonates born to women taking CBZ, PB, and PHT (180). This abnormality is corrected by maternal supplementation with oral vitamin K (181). Therefore, the American Academy of Neurology (70) recommends that vitamin K supple-

TABLE 12.8. U.S. FOOD AND DRUG ADMINISTRATION–ASSIGNED PREGNANCY CATEGORIES FOR ANTIEPILEPTIC DRUGS

Category C: Either studies in animals have revealed adverse effects on the fetus (teratogenic or embryocidal effects, or others) and there are no controlled studies in women, or studies in women and animals are not available. Drugs should be given only if the potential benefits justify the potential risk to the fetus.
 Felbamate
 Gabapentin
 Lamotrigine
 Levetiracetam
 Oxcarbazepine
 Tiagabine
 Topiramate
 Zonisamide
Category D: There is positive evidence of human fetal risk, but the benefits from use in pregnant women may be acceptable despite the risk (e.g., if the drug is needed in a life-threatening situation or for a serious disease for which safer drugs cannot be used or are ineffective).
 Carbamazepine
 Phenobarbital
 Phenytoin
 Primidone
 Valproic acid, Divalproce sodium

mentation be provided (vitamin K_1 at 10 mg/ day) over the last month of gestation.

ANTIEPILEPTIC DRUG PREGNANCY REGISTRIES

Information about the teratogenic potential of an AED is obtained in animals as part of preclinical development. These animal studies do not necessarily predict the human response, although the animal studies did indicate the teratogenic potential of the older AEDs.

Information about the frequency and specific type of teratogenic risk of a pharmaceutical compound is difficult to acquire in humans. Pregnant women are excluded from investigational drug trials, even many phase IV trials. Therefore, information about reproductive toxicology is obtained from preclinical animal studies, from unintended pregnancies occurring during human premarketing trials, and from spontaneous postmarketing reports. Governmental efforts in the United States include the FDA MedWatch effort and the human birth defects surveillance program of the Centers for Disease Control and Prevention. Individual pharmaceutical companies collect reports of adverse fetal outcomes, and some have sponsored drug specific registries. The scientific community has, until recently, relied on retrospective (and usually small) series evaluating fetal outcome after gestational AED exposure.

More than 2,000 prospective pregnancies are needed to detect a drug effect that occurs in 4% to 8% of exposed fetuses. To detect both the frequency and the type of birth defects associated with exposure to an agent, data must be acquired on all pregnancy exposures, and the number of normal as well as abnormal outcomes must be determined. Retrospective registries do not supply the numerator needed to determine incidence.

A review of the literature on AED-associated teratogenesis underscores the importance of obtaining prospective information on human pregnancies. The time and duration of gestational exposure to the AED were often unknown, nor were other risks for adverse fetal outcome assessed, such as tobacco and alcohol use during pregnancy. Ultimately, it is difficult to associate a pharmaceutical agent with adverse fetal outcome without considering the independent and interactive effects of other variables contributing to fetal outcome, such as genetics and environmental factors.

The ideal pregnancy registry is prospective and population based, uses predefined methods of data collection, contains data on timing of AED exposure and a detailed treatment schedule, uses standard definitions for pregnancy outcome, malformations, and anomalies, and includes prolonged follow-up after birth. Registries must include a large number of patients to evaluate less frequent exposures and ideally compares treated and untreated women with epilepsy and nonepileptic controls. Variables collected should include family history of birth defects, classification of maternal epilepsy, exposure to other pharmaceutical compounds, high-risk behavior, and maternal age. At this time, the European Registry comes closest to this ideal and has been very successful in recruiting subjects.

BREAST-FEEDING

Breast-feeding is strongly recommended by most health organizations to promote maternal-child bonding and to reduce the risk of infection and immunologic disorders later in the child's life (182,183). AEDs cross into breast milk to variable extents. Passage is by simple diffusion, and the ratio is determined by the drug's molecular weight, the negative log of the dissociation constant, lipophilicity, and the extent of protein binding. Protein binding is the most important variable in determining the concentration of AED in breast milk in relation to the maternal serum concentration (184,185). For PHT, CBZ, VPA, and TGB, the concentration in breast milk is negligible because of their high protein binding. Ethosuximide, PB, and PRM result in measurable concentrations. Lamotrigine reaches approximately 30% of the maternal serum concentration (186). AED protein binding and concentrations in breast milk are listed in Table 12.9.

For most women, the best advice is seriously to consider breast-feeding. Once started, the infant can be observed for proper weight gain and sleep cycles. The mother must also be advised that AED metabolism and clearance will remain elevated as long as breast-feeding continues. When breast-feeding stops, the mother may experience an increase in serum AED concentrations requiring a dosage adjustment.

CONCLUSION

As multiple AEDs become available, selection of a treatment regimen considers medication effectiveness, which is a combination of efficacy and tolerability. Epilepsy phenotype may vary according to cycles of ovarian steroid hormones. Although the efficacy of marketed AEDs appears to be equivalent across gender, tolerability may differ. AED-related bone loss may affect men and women equally, but women, because of their lower bone mass, may be at greater risk of symptomatic bone disease. Lipid abnormalities related to VPA may be more profound in women than in men because women appear to be more susceptible to VPA-associated weight gain. Women may also suffer more significant consequences of AED-related alterations in steroid hormones, manifesting as failure of hormonal contraceptive or as ovulatory dysfunction. Women face the fear of AED-related birth defects. The teratogenic potential of AEDs will be better defined as global registries develop to record pregnancy outcomes after AED exposure.

Reproductive and metabolic health may be compromised in persons with epilepsy, and women appear to be at particular risk. Because the health care provider appreciates these risks, early diagnosis and intervention in patients with dyslipidemia, bone disease, and reproductive health dysfunction is possible, and interventions to maximize metabolic and reproductive health can be instituted. Interventions include changing to an alternative AED or implementing symptomatic treatment. More recent assessments of care delivered to women with epilepsy demonstrate that health care practices are often not in accordance with recommended best practice (63,187). Appreciating gender differences in epilepsy presentation and treatment response is essential to ensure the best care for the woman with epilepsy.

TABLE 12.9. ANTIEPILEPTIC DRUG PROTEIN BINDING, PASSAGE INTO MILK, AND ACCUMULATION IN INFANTS

Antiepileptic Drug	Percentage Protein Bound	Milk:Plasma Ratio	Concentrations in Infants
Carbamazepine	75	0.17–0.69	Not therapeutic
Carbamazepine–epoxide	60	0.3–0.5	
Ethosuximide	0	0.77–1.0	Therapeutic
Felbamate	25	Not known	Not known
Gabapentin	0	0.73	Not known
Lamotrigine	55	0.47–0.77	Therapeutic
Levetiracetam	<10	Not known	Not known
Oxcarbazepine	60	0.5	Not known
Oxcarbazepine–MHD	40		
Phenytoin	90	0.06–0.69	Not therapeutic
Primidone	0	0.4–0.96	Therapeutic
Tiagabine	96	Not known	Not known
Topiramate	15	Not known	Not known
Valproate	90	0.01–0.1	Not therapeutic
Vigabatrin	0	0.04–0.22	Not known
Zonisamide	40	Not known	Not known

MHD, monohydroxy derivative.

REFERENCES

1. Morrell MJ. Catamenial epilepsy and issues of fertility, sexuality and reproduction. In: Wyllie E, ed. *The treatment of epilepsy: principles and practice*, 3rd ed. Baltimore: Lippincott Williams & Wilkins, 2001:671–680.
2. Pfaff DW, McEwen BS. Actions of estrogens and progestins on nerve cells. *Science* 1983;219:808–814.
3. McEwen BS. Multiple ovarian hormone effects on brain structure and function. *J Gend Specif Med* 1998;1:33–41.
4. Woolley CS, Schwartzkroin PA. Hormonal effects on the brain. *Epilepsia* 1998;39[Suppl 8]:S2–S8.
5. Thomas J, McLean JH. Castration alters susceptibility of male rats to specific seizures. *Physiol Behav* 1991;49:1177–1179.
6. Finn DA, Gee KW. The estrous cycle, sensitivity to convulsants and the anticonvulsant effect of a neuroactive steroid. *J Pharmacol Exp Ther* 1994;271:164–170.
7. Wooley DE, Timiras PS. Estrous and circadian periodicity and electroshock convulsions in rats. *Am J Physiol* 1962;202:379–382.
8. Wooley DE, Timiras PS. The gonad-brain relationship: effects of female sex hormones and electroshock convulsions in the rat. *Endocrinology* 1962;70:196–209.
9. Stitt SL, Kinnard WJ. The effect of certain progestins and estrogens on the threshold of electrically induced seizure patterns. *Neurology* 1968;18:213–216.
10. Marcus EM, Watson CW, Goldman PL. Effects of steroids on cerebral electrical activity: epileptogenic effects of conjugated estrogens and related compounds in the cat and rabbit. *Arch Neurol* 1966;15:521–532.
11. Logothetis J, Harner R. Electrocortical activation by estrogens. *Arch Neurol* 1960;3:290–297.
12. Hom AC, Buterbaugh GG. Estrogen alters the acquisition of seizures kindled by repeated amygdala stimulation or pentylentetrazol administration in ovariectomized female rats. *Epilepsia* 1986;27:103–108.
13. Logothetis J, Harner R, Morrell F, et al. The role of estrogens in catamenial exacerbation of epilepsy. *Neurology* 1959;9:352–360.
14. Landgren S, Backstrom T, Kalistratov G. The effect of progesterone on the spontaneous interictal spike evoked by the application of penicillin to the cat's cerebral cortex. *J Neurol Sci* 1976;36:119–133.
15. Holmes GL, Kloczko N, Weber DA, et al. Anticonvulsant effect of hormones on seizures in animals. In: Porter RJ, Mattson RH, Ward AM Jr, et al., eds. *Advances in epileptology: XVth Epilepsy International Symposium*. New York: Raven Press, 1984:265–268.
16. Wilson MA. Influences of gender, gonadectomy, and estrous cycle on GABA/BZ receptors and benzodiazepine response in rats. *Brain Res Bull* 1992;29:165–172.
17. Finn DA, Roberts AJ, Crabbe JC. Neuroactive steroid sensitivity in withdrawal seizure-prone and -resistant mice. *Alcohol Clin Exp Res* 1995;19:410–415.
18. Spiegel E, Wycis H. Anticonvulsant effects of steroids. *J Lab Clin Med* 1945;30:947–953.
19. Tauboll E, Lindstrom S. The effect of progesterone and its metabolite 5-alpha-pregnan-3-alpha-ol-20-one on focal epileptic seizures in the cat's visual cortex *in vivo*. *Epilepsy Res* 1993;14:17–30.
20. Brann DW, Hendry LB, Mahesh VB. Emerging diversities in the mechanism of action of steroid hormones. *J Steroid Biochem Mol Biol* 1995;52:113–133.
21. Lan NC, Chen JS, Belelli D, et al. A steroid recognition site is functionally coupled to an expressed GABA$_A$-benzodiazepine receptor. *Eur J Pharmacol* 1990;188:403–406.
22. Belelli D, Lan NC, Gee KW. Anticonvulsant steroids and the GABA/benzodiazepine receptor-chloride ionophore complex. *Neurosci Biobehav Rev* 1990;14:315–322.
23. Majewska MD. Neurosteroids: endogenous bimodal modulators of the GABA-A receptor: mechanism of action and physiological significance. *Prog Neurobiol* 1992;38:379–395.
24. Finn DA, Gee KW. The influence of estrous cycle on neurosteroid potency at the gamma-aminobutyric acid. *J Pharmacol Exp Ther* 1993;265:1374–1379.
25. Costa E, Auta J, Guidotti A, et al. The pharmacology of neurosteroidogenesis. *J Steroid Mol Biol* 1994;49:385–389.
26. Weiland NG. Estradiol selectively regulates agonist binding sites on the *N*-methyl-D-aspartate receptor complex in the CA-1 region of the hippocampus. *Endocrinology* 1992;131:662–668.
27. Harrison NL, Majewska MD, Harrington JW, et al. Structure-activity relationships for steroid interaction with the gamma-aminobutyric acid-A receptor complex. *J Pharmacol Exp Ther* 1987;241:346–353.
28. Gee KW, Bolger MB, Brinton RE, et al. Steroid modulation of the chloride ionophore in rat brain: structure-activity requirements, regional dependence and mechanism of action. *J Pharmacol Exp Ther* 1988;246:803–812.
29. Steiger A, Trachsel L, Guldner J, et al. Neurosteroid pregnenolone induces sleep-EEG changes in man compatible with inverse agonist GABA$_A$-receptor modulation. *Brain Res* 1993;615:267–274.
30. Majewska MD, Harrison NL, Schwartz RD, et al. Steroid hormone metabolites are barbiturate-like modulators of the GABA receptor. *Science* 1986;232:1004–1007.
31. Morrow L, Pace JR, Purdy RH, et al. Characterization of steroid interactions with gamma-aminobutyric acid receptor-gated chloride ion channels: evidence for multiple steroid recognition sites. *Mol Pharmacol* 1989;37:263–70.
32. McAuley JW, Kroboth PD, Stiff DD, et al. Modulation of [^{3}H]flunitrazepam binding by natural and synthetic progestational agents. *Pharmacol Biochem Behav* 1993;45:77–83S.
33. Wallis CJ, Luttge WG. Influence of estrogen and progesterone on glutamic acid decarboxylase activity in discrete regions of rat brain. *J Neurochem* 1980;34:609–613.
34. Weiland NG. Glutamic acid decarboxylase messenger ribonucleic acid is regulated by estradiol and progesterone in the hippocampus. *Endocrinology* 1992;131:2697–2702.
35. McCarthy MM, Kaufman LC, Brooks PJ, et al. Estrogen modulation of mRNA for two forms of glutamic acid decarboxylase (GAD) in rat brain. *Neuroscience* 1993;19:1191.
36. Peterson SL, Reeves A, Keller M, et al. Effects of estradiol (E$_2$) and progesterone (P$_4$) on expression of mRNAS encoding GABA$_A$ receptor subunits. *Neuroscience* 1993;19:1191.
37. Smith SS, Waterhouse BD, Chapin JK, et al. Progesterone alters GABA and glutamate responsiveness: a possible mechanism for its anxiolytic action. *Brain Res* 1987;400:353–359.
38. Smith SS, Waterhouse BD, Woodward DJ. Locally applied progesterone metabolites alter neuronal responsiveness in the cerebellum. *Brain Res Bull* 1987;18:739–747.
39. Weiland NG, Orchinik M, Brooks PJ, et al. Allopregnanolone mimics the action of progesterone on glutamate decarboxylase gene expression in the hippocampus. *Neuroscience* 1993;19:1191.
40. Woolley CS, Wenzel HJ, Schwartzkroin PA. Estradiol increases the frequency of multiple synapse boutons in the hippocampal CA-1 region of the adult female rat. *J Comp Neurol* 1996;373:108–117.
41. Woolley CS, Weiland NG, McEwen BS, et al. Estradiol increases the sensitivity of hippocampal CA-1 pyramidal cells to NMDA receptor-mediated synaptic input with correlation with dendritic spine density. *J Neurosci* 1997;17:1848–1859.

42. Kawakami M, Sawyer CH. Neuroendocrine correlates of changes in brain activity thresholds by sex steroids and pituitary hormones. *Horm Brain Thresh* 1959;65:652–668.

43. Finn DA, Ostrom R, Gee KW. Estrus cycle and sensitivity to convulsants and the anticonvulsant effect of 3α-hydroxy-5α-pregnan-20–one(3α,5α-P). *Neuroscience* 1993;19:1539.

44. Teyler TJ, Vardaris RM, Lewis D, et al. Gonadal steroids: effects on excitability of hippocampal pyramidal cells. *Science* 1980; 209:1017–1029.

45. Duncan S, Read CL, Brodie MJ. How common is catamenial epilepsy? *Epilepsia* 1993;34:827–831.

46. McAuley JW, Moore JL, Long, et al. Characterizing cyclical seizures in an outpatient epilepsy clinic. *Epilepsia* 1996;37 [Suppl 5]:94.

47. Herzog AG, Klein P, Ransil BJ. Three patterns of catamenial epilepsy. *Epilepsia* 1997;38:1082–1088.

48. Bäckstrom T, Jorpes P. Serum phenytoin, phenobarbital, carbamazepine, albumin;and plasma estradiol, progesterone concentration during the menstrual cycle in women with epilepsy. *Acta Neurol Scand* 1979;59:63–71.

49. Lim LL, Foldvary N, Mascha E, et al. Acetazolamide in women with catamenial epilepsy. *Epilepsia* 2001;42:746–749.

50. Mattson RH, Cramer JA, Caldwell BV, et al. Treatment of seizures with medroxyprogesterone acetate: preliminary report. *Neurology* 1984;34:1255–1258.

51. Zimmerman AW, Holden KR, Reiter EO, et al. Medroxyprogesterone acetate in the treatment of seizures associated with menstruation. *J Pediatr* 1973;83:959–63.

52. Herzog AG. Reproductive endocrine considerations and hormonal therapy for women with epilepsy. *Epilepsia* 1991;32 [Suppl 6]:527–533.

53. Herzog AG. Progesterone therapy in women with complex partial and secondary generalized seizures. *Neurology* 1995;45: 1660–1662.

54. Abbasi F, Krumholz A, Kittner SJ, et al. Effects of menopause on seizures in women with epilepsy. *Epilepsia* 1999;40: 205–210.

55. Harden CL, Pulver MC, Ravdin L, et al. The effect of menopause and perimenopause on the course of epilepsy. *Epilepsia* 1999;40:1402–1407.

56. Food and Drug Administration, US Department of Health and Human Services. Guidelines for the study of and evaluation of gender differences in the clinical evaluation of drugs. *Fed Reg* 1993;58:39406–39416.

57. Morrell MJ. The new antiepileptic drugs and women: efficacy, reproductive health, pregnancy, and fetal outcome. *Epilepsia* 1996;37[Suppl 6]:S34–S44.

58. Yerby M, Morrell MJ. Efficacy, safety and tolerability of zonisamide in women: sexual dysfunction and hormonal abnormalities in women with epilepsy. *Epilepsia* 2000;41[Suppl 7]: 199.

59. Coulam CB, Annegers JF. Do oral anticonvulsants reduce the efficacy of oral contraceptives? *Epilepsia* 1979;20:519–526.

60. Mattson RH, Cramer JA, Darney PD, et al. Use of oral contraceptives by women with epilepsy. *JAMA* 1986;256:238–240.

61. Perrucca E. Clinical implications of hepatic microsomal enzyme induction by antiepileptic drugs. *Pharmacol Ther* 1987;33: 139–144.

62. Krauss GL, Brandt J, Campbell M, et al. Antiepileptic medication and oral contraceptive interactions: a national survey of neurologists and obstetricians. *Neurology* 1996;46:1534–1539.

63. Morrell MJ, Sarto GE, Osborne Shafer P, et al. Health issues for women with epilepsy: a descriptive survey to assess knowledge and awareness among healthcare providers. *J Womens Health Gend Based Med* 2000;9:959–965..

64. McAuley JW, Anderson GD. Treatment of epilepsy in women of reproductive age: pharmacokinetic considerations. *Clin Pharmacokinet. In press.*

65. Crawford P, Chadwick DJ, Martin C, et al. The interaction of phenytoin and carbamazepine with combined oral contraceptive steroids. *Br J Clin Pharmacol* 1990;30:892–896.

66. Crawford P, Chadwick D, Cleland P, et al. The lack of effect of sodium valproate on the pharmacokinetics of oral contraceptive steroids. *Contraception* 1986;33:23–29.

67. Saano V, Glue P, Banfield CR, et al. Effects of felbamate on the pharmacokinetics of a low-dose combination oral contraceptive. *Clin Pharmacol Ther* 1995;58:523–531.

68. Fattore C, Cipolla G, Gatti G, et al. Induction of ethinylestradiol and levonorgestrel metabolism by oxcarbazepine in healthy women. *Epilepsia* 1999;40:783–787.

69. Rosenfeld WE, Doose DR, Walker SA, et al. Effect of topiramate on the pharmacokientics of an oral contraceptive containing norethindrone and ethinyl estradiol in patients with epilepsy. *Epilepsia* 1997;38:317–323.

70. American Academy of Neurology, Quality Standards Subcommittee. Practice Parameter: management issues for women with epilepsy. *Neurology* 1998;51:944–948.

71. Zahn CA, Morrell MJ, Collins SD, et al. Management issues for women with epilepsy: a review of the literature. American Academy of Neurology Practice Guidelines. *Neurology* 1998;51: 949–956.

72. Haukkamaa M. Contraception by Norplant subdermal capsules is not reliable in epileptic patients on anticonvulsant treatment. *Contraception* 1986;33:559–565.

73. Odlind V, Olsson SE. Enhanced metabolism of levonorgestrel during phenytoin treatment in a woman with Norplant implants. *Contraception* 1986;33:257–261.

74. Olafsson E, Hallgrimsson JT, Hauser WA, et al. Pregnancies of women with epilepsy: a population-based study in Iceland. *Epilepsia* 1998;39:887–892.

75. Olafsson E, Hauser WA, Gudmundsson G. Fertility in patients with epilepsy: a population- based study. *Epilepsia* 1998;51: 71–73.

76. Dansky LV, Andermann E, Andermann F. Marriage and fertility in epileptic patients. *Epilepsia* 1980;21:261–271.

77. Webber MP, Hauser WA, Ottman R, et al. Fertility in persons with epilepsy: 1935–1974. *Epilepsia* 1986;27:746–752.

78. Schupf N, Ottman R. Likelihood of pregnancy in individuals with idiopathic/cryptogenic epilepsy: social and biologic influence. *Epilepsia* 1994;35:750–756.

79. Schupf N, Ottman R. Reproduction among individuals with idiopathic/cryptogenic epilepsy: risk factors for reduced fertility in marraige. *Epilepsia* 1996;37:833–840.

80. Wallace H, Shorvon S, Tallis R. Age-specific incidence and prevalence rates of treated epilepsy in an unselected population of 2,052,922 and age-specific fertility rates of women with epilepsy. *Lancet* 1998;352:1970–1973.

81. Herzog AG, Seibel MM, Schomer DL, et al. Reproductive endocrine disorders in women with partial seizures of temporal lobe origin. *Arch Neurol* 1986;43:341–346.

82. Franceschi M, Perego L, Cavagnini F, et al. Effects of long-term antiepileptic therapy in the hypothalamic-pituitary axis in man. *Epilepsia* 1984;25:46–52.

83. Meo R, Bilo L, Nappi C, et al. Derangement of the hypothalamic GnRH pulse generator in women with epilepsy. *Seizure* 1993;2:241–252.

84. Dana-Haeri J, Trimble MR, Oxley J. Prolactin and gonadotrophin changes following generalized and partial seizures. *J Neurol Neurosurg Psychiatry* 1983;46:331–335.

85. Sperling MR, Pritchard PB, Engel J, et al. Prolactin in partial epilepsy: an indicator of limbic seizures. *Ann Neurol* 1986; 20:716–722.

86. Pritchard PB, Wannamaker BB, Sagel J, et al. Endocrine function following complex partial seizures. *Ann Neurol* 1983;14: 27–32.

87. Pritchard PB. The effect of seizures on hormones. *Epilepsia* 1991;32[Suppl 6]:S46–S50.

88. Bilo L, Meo R, Valentino R, et al. Abnormal pattern of luteinizing hormone pulsatility in women with epilepsy. *Fertil Steril* 1991;55:705–711.

89. Drislane FW, Coleman AE, Schomer DL, et al. Altered pulsatile secretion of luteinizing hormone in women with epilepsy. *Neurology* 1994;44:306–310.

90. Levesque LA, Herzog AG, Seibel MM. The effect of phenytoin and carbamazepine on serum dehydroepiandrosterone sulfate in men and women who have partial seizures with temporal lobe involvement. *J Clin Endocrinol Metab* 1986;63:243–245.

91. Macphee GJ, Larkin JG, Butler E, et al. Circulating hormones and pituitary responsiveness in young epileptic men receiving long-term antiepileptic medication. *Epilepsia* 1988;29:468–475.

92. Isojarvi JIT, Parakinen AJ, Ylipalosaari PJ, et al. Serum hormones in male epileptic patients receiving anticonvulsant medication. *Arch Neurol* 1990;47:670–676.

93. Isojarvi JIT, Parakinen AJ, Rautio A, et al. Serum sex hormone levels after replacing carbamazepine with oxcarbazepine. *Eur J Clin Pharmacol* 1995;47:461–464.

94. Isojarvi JIT, Rattya J, Myllyla VV, et al. Valproate, lamotrigine, and insulin-mediated risks in women with epilepsy. *Ann Neurol* 1998;43:446–451.

95. Stoffel-Wagner B, Bauer J, Flugel D, et al. Serum sex hormones are altered in patients with chronic temporal lobe epilepsy receiving anticonvulsant medication. *Epilepsia* 1998;39:1164–1673.

96. Isojarvi JIT, Laatikainen TJ, Pakarinen AJ, et al. Polycystic ovaries and hyperandrogenism in women taking valproate for epilepsy. *N Engl J Med* 1993;329:1383–1388.

97. Clayton RN, Ogden V, Hodgkinson J, et al. How common are polycystic ovaries in normal women and what is their significance for the fertility of the population? *Clin Endocrinol.* 1992; 37:127–34.

98. Polson DW, Wadsworth J, Adams J, et al. Polycystic ovaries: a common finding in normal women. *Lancet* 1988;1(8590): 870–872.

99. Ben-Shlomo I, Franks S, Adashi EY. The polycystic ovary syndrome: nature or nurture? *Fertil Steril* 1995;63:953–954.

100. Lobo RA. A disorder without identity: "HCA," "PCO," "PCOD," "PCOS," "SLS." What are we to call it?! *Fertil Steril* 1995;63:1158–1160.

101. Biton V, Mirza W, Montouris G, et al. Weight change associated with valproate and lamotrigine monotherapy in patients with epilepsy. *Neurology* 2001;56:172–177.

102. Vainionpaa LK, Rattya J, Knip M, et al. Valproate-induced hyperandrogenism during pubertal maturation in girls with epilepsy. *Ann Neurol* 1999;45:444–450.

103. Morrell MJ. Sexual dysfunction in epilepsy. *Epilepsia* 1991;32 [Suppl 5]:S38–S45.

104. Morrell MJ. Sexuality in epilepsy. In: Engel J, Pedley TA, eds. *Epilepsy: a comprehensive textbook.* New York: Lippincott–Raven, 1997:2021–2026.

105. Morrell MJ, Guldner GT. Self-reported sexual function and sexual arousability in women with epilepsy. *Epilepsia* 1996;37: 1204–1210.

106. Morrell MJ, Sperling MR, Stecker M, et al. Sexual dysfunction in partial epilepsy: a deficit in physiological sexual arousal. *Neurology* 1994;44:243–247.

107. Mattson RH, Cramer JA, Collins JF, et al. Comparison of carbamazepine, phenobarbital, phenytoin, and primidone in partial and secondarily generalized tonic-clonic seizures. *N Engl J Med* 1985;313:145–151.

108. Dana-Haeri J, Oxley J. Reduction of free testosterone by antiepileptic drugs. *BMJ* 1982;284:85–6.

109. Luhdorf K. Endocrine function and antiepileptic treatment. *Acta Neurol Scand Suppl* 1983;67:15–19.

110. Beastall GH, Cowan RA, Gray JMB, et al. Hormone binding globulins and anticonvulsant therapy. *Scott Med J* 1985;30: 101–105.

111. Fenwick PBC, Mercer C, Grant R, et al. Nocturnal penile tumescence and serum testosterone levels. *Arch Sex Behav* 1986; 15:13–21.

112. Chang S, Ahn C. Effects of antiepileptic drug therapy on bone mineral density in ambulatory epileptic children. *Brain Dev* 1994;16:382–385.

113. Valimaki M, Tiihonen M, Laitinen K, et al. Bone mineral density measured by dual-energy x-ray absorptiometry and novel markers of bone formation and resorption in patients on antiepileptic drugs. *J Bone Miner Res* 1994;9:631–637.

114. Sheth R, Wesolowski C, Jacob J, et al. Effect of carbamazepine and valproate on bone mineral density. *J Pediatr* 1996;127: 256–262.

115. Cummings LN, Giudice L, Morrell MJ. Ovulatory function in epilepsy. *Epilepsia* 1995;36:355–359.

116. Bogliun G, Beghi E, Crespi V, et al. Anticonvulsant drugs and bone metabolism. *Acta Neurol Scand* 1986;74:284–288.

117. Gough H, Goggin T, Bissessar A, et al. A comparative study of the relative influence of different anticonvulsant drugs, UV exposure and diet on vitamin D and calcium metabolism in outpatients with epilepsy. *Q J Med* 1986;230:569–577.

118. Marcus R. Secondary forms of osteoparosis. In: Coe F, Favus M, ed. *Disorders of bone and mineral metabolism.* New York: Raven Press, 1992, 889–904.

119. Louma PV, Sotaniemi EA, Peklonen RO, et al. Plasma high density lipoprotein cholesterol and hepatic cytochrome P450 concnetrations in epileptics undergoing anticonvulsant treatment. *Scand J Clin Lab Invest* 1980;40:163–167.

120. Calandre EP, Rodriguez-Lopez C, Blazquez A, et al. Serum lipids, lipoproteins and apolipoproteins A and B in epileptic patients treated with valproic acid, carbamazepine or phenobarbital. *Acta Neurol Scand* 1991;83:250–253.

121. Eiris JM, Lojo S Del Rio MC, et al. Effects of long term treatment with antiepileptic drugs on serum lipid levels in children treated with anticonvulsants. *Neurology* 1995;45:1155–1157.

122. Verrotti A, Domizio S, Angelozzi B, et al. Changes in serum lipids and lipoproteins in epileptic children treated with anticonvulsants. *J Paediatr Child Health* 1997;33:242–245.

123. Fisher RS, Vickrey BG, Gibson P, et al. The impact of epilepsy from the patient's perspective. I. Descriptions and subjective perceptions. *Epilepsy Res* 2000;41:39–51.

124. Schmidt D, Beck-Mannagetta G, Janz D, et al. The effect of pregnancy on the course of epilepsy: a prospective study. In: Janz D, Dam M, Richens A, eds. *Epilepsy, pregnancy and the child.* New York: Raven Press, 1982:39–49.

125. Hauser WA, Hesdorffer DC. Risk factors. In: Hauser WA, Hesdorffer DC, eds. *Epilepsy: frequency, causes and consequences.* New York: Demos, 1990:53–100.

126. Tomson T, Lindbom U, Ekqvist B, et al. Disposition of carbamazepine and phenytoin in pregnancy. *Epilepsia* 1994;35:131–135.

127. Yerby MS, Friel PN, McCormick K. Pharmacokinetics of anticonvulsants in pregnancy: alterations in plasma protein binding. *Epilepsy Res* 1990;5:223–228.

128. Takeda A, Okada H, Tanaka H, et al. Protein binding of four antiepileptic drugs in maternal and umbilical cord serum. *Epilepsy Res* 1992;13:147–151.

129. Steegers-Teunissen RPM, Renier WO, et al. Factors influencing the risk of abnormal pregnancy outcome in epileptic women: a multicentre prospective study. *Epilepsy Res* 1994;18:261–269.

130. Schupf N., Ottman R. Reproduction among individuals with idiopathic/cryptogenic epilepsy: risk factors for spontaneous abortion. *Epilepsia* 1997;38:824–829.

131. Teramo K, Hiilesmaa V, Brady A, et al. Fetal heart rate during a maternal grand mal epileptic seizure. *J Perinat Med* 1979;7:3.

132. Annegers JF, Hauser WA, Elveback LR, et al. Congenital malformations and seizure disorders in the offspring of parents with epilepsy. *Int J Epidemiol* 1978;7:241–247.

133. Friis ML. Facial clefts and congenital heart defects in children of parents with epilepsy: genetic and environmental etiologic factors. *Acta Neurol Scand* 1989:79:433–459.

134. Koch S, Loesche G, Jager-Roman E, et al. Major birth malformations and antiepileptic drugs. *Neurology* 1992;42[Suppl 5]:83–88.

135. Rosa FW. Spina bifida in infants of women treated with carbamazepine during pregnancy. *N Engl J Med* 1991;324:674–677.

136. Omtzigt JGC, Los FJ, Grobee DE, et al. The risk of spina bifida aperta after first-trimester exposure to valproate in a prenatal cohort. *Neurology* 1992;42[Suppl 5]:119–125.

137. Gaily E, Granstrom M L. Minor anomalies in children of mothers with epilepsy. *Neurology* 1992;42[Suppl 5]:128–131.

138. Gaily E, Kantola-Sorsa E, Granstrom ML. Intelligence of children of epileptic mothers. *J Pediatr* 1988;113:677–684.

139. Koch S, Titze K, Zimmerman RB, et al. Long-term neuropsychological consequences of maternal epilepsy and anticonvulsant treatment during pregnancy for school-age children and adolescents. *Epilepsia* 1999;40:1237–1243.

140. Hiilesmaa VK, Teramo K, Granstrom ML, et al. Fetal head growth retardation associated with maternal antiepileptic drugs. *Lancet* 1981;2:165–167.

141. Adab N, Jacoby A, Smith D, et al. Additional educational needs in children born to mothers with epilepsy. *J Neurol Neurosurg Psychiatry* 2001;70:15–21.

142. Hvas CL, Henriksen TB, Ostergaard JR, et al. Epilepsy and pregnancy: effect of antiepileptic drugs and lifestyle on birthweight. *Br J Obstet Gynecol* 2000;107:896–902.

143. Battino D, Kaneko S, Andermann E, et al. Intrauterine growth in the offspring of epileptic women: a prospective multicenter study. *Epilepsy Res* 1999;36:53–60.

144. Kaneko S, Battino D, Andermann E, et al. Congenital malformations due to antiepileptic drugs. *Epilepsy Res* 1999;33:145–158.

145. Kaneko S, Otani K, Fukushima Y, et al. Teratogenecity of antiepilepsy drugs: analysis of possible risk factors. *Epilepsia* 1988;29:459–467.

146. Holmes LB, Harvey EA, Coull BA, et al. The teratogenicity of anticonvulsant drugs. *N Engl J Med* 2001;344:1132–1138.

147. Finnell RH, Buehler BA, Kerr BM, et al. Clinical and experimental studies linking oxidative metabolism to phenytoin-induced teratogenesis. *Neurology* 1992;42:25–31.

148. Miranda AF, Wiley MJ, Wells PG. Evidence for embryonic peroxidase-catalyzed bioactivation and glutathione-dependent cytoprotection in phenytoin teratogenicity: modulation by eicosatetraynoic acid and buthione sulfoximine in murine embryo culture. *Toxicol Appl Pharmacol* 1994;124:230–241.

149. Kerr BM, Levy RH Inhibition of epoxide hydrolase by anticonvulsants and risk of teratogenicity. *Lancet* 1989;1:610–611.

150. Wegner C, Nau H. Alteration of embryonic folate metabolism by valproic acid during organogenesis: implications for mechanism of teratogenesis. *Neurology* 1992;42[Suppl 5]:17.

151. Strickler SM, Dansky LV, Miller MA, et al. Genetic predisposition to phenytoin-induced birth defects. *Lancet* 1985;2:746–749.

152. Buehler BA, Delimont D, Van Waes M, et al. Prenatal prediction of risk of the fetal hydantoin syndrome. *N Engl J Med* 1990;322:1567–1572.

153. Finnell RH. Genetic differences in susceptibility to anticonvulsant drug induced developmental defects. *Pharmacol Toxicol* 1991;69:223–227.

154. Nau H, Tzimas G, Mondry M, et al. Antiepileptic drugs alter endogenous retinoid concentration: a possible mechanism of teratogenesis of anticonvulsant therapy. *Life Sci* 1995;57:53–60.

155. Tomson T, Lindbom U, Sundqvist A, et al. Red cell folate levels in pregnant epileptic women. *Eur J Clin Pharmacol* 1995;48:305–308.

156. Steegers-Theunissen RPM, Boers GHJ, Trijbels FJM, et al. Neural-tube defects and derangement of homocysteine metabolism. *N Engl J Med* 1991;324:199–200.

157. Mills JL, McPartlin JM, Kirke PN, et al. Homocysteine metabolism in pregnancies complicated by neural tube defects. *Lancet* 1995;345:149–151.

158. Laurence KM, James N, Miller MH, et al. Double-blind, randomized controlled trial of folate treatment before conception to prevent the recurrence of neural-tube defects. *BMJ* 1981;282:1509–1511.

159. Dansky L, Andermann E, Roseblatt D, et al. Anticonvulsants, folate levels and and pregnancy outcome. *Ann Neurol* 1987;21:176–182.

160. Yates JRW, Ferguson-Smith MA, Shenkin A, et al. Is disordered folate metabolism the basis for the genetic predisposition to neural tube defects? *Clin Genet* 1987;31:279–287.

161. Milunsky A, Jick H, Jick SS, et al. Multivitamin/folic acid supplementation in early pregnancy reduces the prevalence of neural tube defects. *JAMA* 1988;262:2847–2852.

162. Mulinare J, Corder JF, Erickson JD, et al. Periconceptional use of multivitamins and the occurrence of neural tube defects. *JAMA* 1988;260:3141–3145.

163. Werler MM, Shapiro S, Mitchell AA. Periconceptional folic acid exposure and risk of occurrent neural tube defects. *JAMA* 1993;269:1257–1261.

164. Daly LE, Kirke PN, Molloy A, et al. Folate levels and neural tube defects: implications for treatment. *JAMA* 1995;274:1698.

165. Gordon N. Folate metabolism and neural tube defects. *Brain Dev* 1995;17:307–311.

166. Medical Research Council Vitamin Research Group. Prevention of neural tube defects: results of the Medical Research Council Vitamin Study. *Lancet* 1991;338:131–137.

167. Czeizel AE, Dudas I. Prevention of the first occurrence of neural tube defects by periconceptional vitamin suplementation. *N Engl J Med* 1992;327:1832–1835.

168. Centers for Disease Control. Recommendations for the use of folic acid to reduce the number of cases of spina bifida and other neural tube defects. *MMWR Morb Mortal Wkly Rep* 1992;41:1–7.

169. Ogawa Y, Kaneko S, Otani K, et al. Serum folic acid levels in epileptic mothers and their relationship to congenital malformations. *Epilepsy Res* 1991;8:75–78.

170. Hernandez-Diaz S, Werler MM, Walker AM, et al. Folic acid antagonists during pregnancy and the risk of birth defects. *N Engl J Med* 2000;343:1608–1614.

171. Craig J, Morrison P, Morrow J, et al. Failure of periconceptional folic acid to prevent a neural tube defect in the offspring of a mother taking sodium valproate. *Seizure* 1999;8:253–254.

172. Oguni M, Dansky L, Andermann E, et al. Improved pregnancy outcome in epileptic women in the last decade: relationship to maternal anticonvulsant therapy. *Brain Dev* 1992;14:371–380.

173. Grimes DA. Unplanned pregnancies in the U.S. *Obstet Gynecol* 1986;67:438–442.

174. American College of Obstetric and Gynecologic Physicians Educational Bulletin. Seizure disorders in pregnancy. *X* 1996;231:1–13.

175. Van Allen M, Fraser FC, Dallaire L, et al. Recommendations on the use of folic acid supplementation to prevent the recurrence of neural tube defects. *Can Med Assoc J* 1993;149:1239–1243.

176. Institute of Medicine. *Women and health research: ethical and legal issues of including women in clinical studies.* Washington, DC: National Academy Press, 1994:1–25.

177. Department of Health and Human Services (DHHS). Additional DHHS protections pertaining to research, development and related activities involving fetuses, pregnant women and human in vitro fertilization. Title 45, Code of Federal Regulations. Part 46, subpart B, March 15, 1994.

178. Commission on Genetics, Pregnancy, and the Child, International League Against Epilepsy. Guidelines for the care of women of childbearing age with epilepsy. *Epilepsia* 1993;34:588–589.

179. Thorp JA, Gaston L, Caspers DR, et al. Current concepts and controversies in the use of vitamin K. *Drugs* 1995;49:376–387.

180. Cornelissen M, Steegers-Theunissen R, Kollee L, et al. Increased incidence of neonatal vitamin K deficiency resulting from maternal anticonvulsant therapy. *Am J Obstet Gynecol* 1993;168:923–928.

181. Cornelissen M, Steegers-Theunissen R, Kollee L, et al. Supplementation of vitamin K in pregnant women receiving anticonvulsant therapy prevents neonatal vitamin K deficiency. *Am J Obstet Gynecol* 1993;168:884–888.

182. American Academy of Pediatrics. The transfer of drugs and other chemicals into human milk. *Pediatrics* 1994;93:137–150.

183. Ito S. Drug therapy for breast-feeding women. *N Engl J Med* 2000;343:118–126.

184. Bar-Oz B, Nulman I, Koren G, et al. Anticonvulsants and breast-feeding: a critical review. *Pediatr Drugs* 2000;2:113–126.

185. Hagg S, Spigset O. Anticonvulsant use during lactation. *Drug Saf* 2000;22:425–440.

186. Ohman I, Vitols S, Tomson T. Lamotrigine in pregnancy: pharmacokinetics during delivery, in the neonate and during lactation. *Epilepsia* 2000;41:709–713.

187. Seale C, Morrell MJ, Nelson L, et al. Analysis of the prenatal and gestational care given to women with epilepsy. *Neurology* 1998;51:1039–1045.

188. Samren E, vanDuijn C, Koch S, et al. Maternal use of antiepileptic drugs and the risk of major congenital malformation: a joint European prospective study of human teratogenesis associated with maternal epilepsy. *Epilepsia* 1997;38:981–990.

189. Samren EB, van Duijn CM, Christiaens GC, et al. Antiepileptic drug regimens and major congenital abnormalities in the offspring. *Ann Neurol* 1999;46:739–746.

190. Canger R, Battino D, Canevini MP, et al. Malformations in offspring of women with epilepsy: a prospective study. *Epilepsia* 1999;4:1231–1236.

GENERAL PRINCIPLES

EPILEPSY IN THE ELDERLY

ILO E. LEPPIK
JAMES C. CLOYD

The elderly comprise the most rapidly growing segment of the population, and onset of epilepsy is higher in this age group than in any other. The incidence of a first seizure is 52 to 59 per 100,000 in persons 40 to 59 years of age, but it rises to 127 per 100,000 in those ≥60 years old (1). Among persons ≥65 years, the active epilepsy prevalence rate is approximately 1.5%, about twice the rate of younger adults. In 1995, approximately 2.3 million residents of the United States had been diagnosed with epilepsy: 1.4 million were adults aged 15 to 64 years, 300,000 were children aged ≥14 years, and 550,000 were persons >65 years of age. Approximately 181,000 persons developed epilepsy in 1995, and approximately 68,000 of these were >65 years old (2). As the elderly population continues to grow steadily, increasing numbers of older persons are likely to require accurate diagnosis and effective treatment. The foregoing data are based mostly on a community-based population. The prevalence of epilepsy and antiepileptic drug (AED) use is much higher in nursing homes. In a review of 45,405 people ≥65 years old who were living throughout the United States in long-term care facilities serviced by Pharmacy Corporation of America, at least one AED was taken by 4,573 (10.1%) of the residents (3). Later studies have confirmed that the prevalence of AED use in the nursing home population varies between 10% and 11% (4–6). Approximately 1.5 million elderly people reside in nursing homes; thus, as many as 150,000 elderly nursing home patients may be taking AEDs.

In the elderly, the most common identifiable cause of epilepsy is stroke, which accounts for 30% to 40% of all cases (7). Brain tumor, head injury, and Alzheimer's disease are other major causes. However, in many patients, the precise cause cannot be identified. Assessment of AED treatment efficacy and toxicity in elderly patients is challenging because seizures are sometimes difficult to observe, signs and symptoms of toxicity can be attributed to other causes (e.g., Alzheimer's disease, stroke) or to comedications, and the patient may not be able to self-report problems accurately.

ANTIEPILEPTIC DRUG USE IN THE ELDERLY

In addition to their use in epilepsy, AEDs are prescribed for various other disorders, including neuralgias, aggressive behavior disorders, essential tremor, and restless legs syndrome, conditions prevalent in the elderly. Treatment of older patients with AEDs, as with many other medications, is complicated by increased sensitivity to drug effects, narrow therapeutic ranges, complex pharmacokinetics, and the increased likelihood of drug interactions because of multiple drug therapy (8–11). Elderly persons also have a high probability of concomitant disorders. Use of antipsychotic therapy may also increase seizures (12,13). As a cause of adverse reactions in the elderly, AEDs rank fifth among all drug categories (14). Nonetheless, the frequent use of AEDs by nursing home residents and the growing number of elderly persons in the general population suggest that hundreds of thousands of older persons are being treated with these medications.

Phenytoin (PHT) is the most commonly used AED in nursing homes. In a 1995 study of 21,551 nursing home residents in 24 states on one day in the spring of 1995, 10.5% had an AED order (4). Of these patients, 9.2% had a seizure or epilepsy indication recorded. Of the AEDs, 6.2% of these patients were taking PHT, 1.8% used carbamazepine, 0.9% used valproic acid, 1.7% used phenobarbital, and all other AEDs combined, 1.2% (Table 13.1). The diagnosis of epilepsy is generally made only after a person has had two or more seizures. However, many physicians may begin treatment with AEDs after a single seizure in elderly patients because the risks of a second seizure are perceived to be high. Treatment in the elderly carries more risks

Ilo E. Leppik, MD: Director of Research, MINCEP Epilepsy Care, Minneapolis, Minnesota

James C. Cloyd, PharmD: Professor and Director, Epilepsy Research and Education Program, College of Pharmacy, University of Minnesota, Minneapolis, Minnesota

TABLE 13.1. MOST COMMONLY USED ANTIEPILEPTIC DRUGS IN A NURSING HOME POPULATION (N = 21,551)

Antiepileptic Drug	No. of Residents (%)
Phenytoin	1,344 (6.2)
Carbamazepine	397 (1.8)
Valproic acid	198 (0.9)
Phenobarbital	375 (1.2)
All others	268 (1.2)

Cloyd JC, Lackner TE, Leppik IE. Antiepileptics in the elderly. Pharmacoepidemiology and pharmacokinetics. *Archives of Fam Med* 1994;3(7):589–598, with permission.

than in younger persons because elderly persons may experience more side effects, they have a greater risk of drug interactions, and they may be less able to afford the costs of medications. Thus, both the benefits and risks of treatment may be greater in the elderly.

At the present time, data are limited regarding the clinical use of AEDs in the elderly. The paucity of information makes it difficult to recommend specific AEDs with any confidence that the outcomes will be optimal. Nevertheless, decisions need to be made, and indeed they are being made. Many of the recommendations will be modified as new knowledge is obtained, and at the present time, the "comfort level" with some drugs may play a larger role than actual experience or data.

Elderly persons differ in many respects from younger adults, and simply using information applicable to the younger age group will not lead to the best outcome (Table 13.2). Elderly persons represent a much more heterogeneous population, but they may, for purposes of simplification, be considered to consist of the elderly healthy (EH), except for epilepsy, and the elderly with multiple medical problems (EMMP). A drug choice optimal for one group

TABLE 13.2. PHARMACOKINETICS OF ANTIEPILEPTIC DRUGS IN ELDERLY AND YOUNGER ADULTS

Drug	Protein Binding (%)		Half-life (h)	
	60+ Yr	<60 Yr	60+ Yr	<60 Yr
Carbamazepine	NA	75–85	NA	12–24
Felbamate	NA	25–35	NA	13–23
Gabapentin	NA	<10	NA	5–8
Lamotrigine	NA	55	31	29
Levetiracetam	<10%	<10%	NA	8–10
Oxcarbazepine	Low	Low	NA	8–10
Phenobarbital	NA	45–50	NA	75–126
Phenytoin	80–93	87–93	40–60	20–40
Valproic Acid	87–95	90–95	11–17	9–18
Zonisamide	Low	Low	NA	24–60

NA, reliable data not available.
Compiled from refs. 1,3,5,21–23,29,36,37,45,48–53,58,63.

TABLE 13.3. CHOOSING ANTIEPILEPTIC DRUGS FOR THE ELDERLY HEALTH AND THE ELDERLY WITH MULTIPLE MEDICAL PROBLEMS

Antiepileptic Drug	Healthy Elderly	Elderly with Multiple Medical Problems
Carbamazepine	Good	Avoid patients with cardiac and renal disease
Felbamate	Too risky for routine use	Use caution
Gabapentin	Good	Very good
Lamotrigine	Good	Good
Levetiracetam	Good	Very good
Oxcarbazepine	Good	Avoid patients receiving diuretics
Phenytoin	Good	Good, avoid using with protein-bound drugs
Phenobarbital	Too sedating	Too sedating
Valproate	Good	Avoid in patients with Parkinson's disease
Tiagabine	Good	Good
Topiramate	Good	Good, but check cognition
Zonisamide	Good	Good

Table based on author's personal opinion and experience.

may not be appropriate for the others. Even the EH will have a decline in functioning of the various organ systems, leading to lower hepatic and renal clearance of AEDs and a possible increase in sensitivity of the central nervous system (CNS) to side effects. In addition, the cost of AEDs is an important factor for many patients. These issues are greatly complicated for the EMMP population. In addition, the state of health many change rapidly, so a choice appropriate for one period may not be acceptable later. Each available drug is discussed in terms of the benefits and risks for the EH and EMMP populations (Table 13.3).

Effect of Advancing Age on Pharmacodynamics and Pharmacokinetics

Age-related changes in physiology result in clinically significant alterations in both drug response and drug disposition. Changes in receptor number and sensitivity, alterations in cellular biochemistry, and the nature of the disorder can affect both pharmacologic and toxicologic effects (15–17). Elderly patients taking carbamazepine or valproic acid for epilepsy realize optimal seizure control, but they are also more likely to experience adverse events, at lower plasma concentrations than younger patients (18). Castleden et al. (19) have shown that elderly persons exhibit greater cognitive impairment after a dose of nitrazepam than do younger patients, although plasma concentrations are similar.

Age-related changes in physiology can alter all aspects of pharmacokinetics: absorption, distribution, metabolism, and elimination. Advanced age is associated with increased gastric pH, diminished gastrointestinal fluids, and slower intestinal transit, and reduced absorptive area. Each of these changes can affect either or both the rate and extent of absorption. Age-related reduction in intestinal and hepatic blood flow, intestinal drug transport and metabolism, and hepatic metabolism can also affect the systemic bioavailability of some drugs. Gastric pH and intestinal transit time may exhibit intrapatient day-to-day variability, whereas other processes tend to decline slowly. Age-related alterations in absorption are most likely to affect slowly absorbed AEDs, particularly those administered as solid dosage forms, extended release formulations, or drugs absorbed by active transport (gabapentin). Depending on the process or processes affected, alterations in gastrointestinal physiology can either increase or decrease bioavailability, resulting in loss of seizure control or onset of side effects.

Total serum drug concentration reflects both drug bound to serum proteins and unbound drug. For most drugs, unbound concentration in serum is in direct equilibrium with the concentration at the site of action. Because drug concentration at the site of action determines the magnitude of both desired and toxic responses, unbound drug in serum provides the best correlation with drug response (20). Total serum drug concentration is useful for monitoring therapy when the drug is not highly protein bound (less than 75%) or when the ratio of unbound to total drug concentration remains relatively stable. This is not the case for highly bound AEDs such as carbamazepine, PHT, tiagabine, and valproic acid; these drugs frequently undergo age-related alterations in protein binding.

Older persons experience a gradual reduction in serum albumin and increased α_1-acid glycoprotein (AAG) concentrations (20–22). By age 65 years, many persons have low normal albumin concentrations or are frankly hypoalbuminemic (23). Albumin concentration may be further reduced by conditions such as malnutrition, renal insufficiency, and rheumatoid arthritis. As serum albumin levels decline, the likelihood increases that drug binding will decrease. This has the effect of lowering the total serum drug concentration while unbound serum drug concentration remains unchanged. The concentration of AAG, a reactant serum protein, increases with age; further elevations occur during pathophysiologic stress such as stroke, heart failure, trauma, infection, myocardial infarction, surgery, and chronic obstructive pulmonary disease (22). Administration of enzyme-inducing AEDs also increases AAG (24). When the concentration of AAG rises, the binding of weakly alkaline and neutral drugs such as carbamazepine (and its epoxide metabolite) to AAG can increase, thereby causing higher total serum drug and metabolite concentrations.

Thus, measurements of total concentrations of highly bound AEDs in the elderly are misleading. For example, an elderly person with a low serum albumin level could have a PHT free fraction of 20% on the basis of reduced binding,

rather than the usual 10% seen in younger adults. In such a patient, a total PHT level of 20 mg/L with a 20% free fraction corresponds to an unbound concentration of 4.0 mg/L; the same 4.0 mg/L of unbound concentration in a younger person with normal binding and clearance would be associated with a total drug level of 40 mg/L. Not recognizing this situation may lead to inappropriate clinical decisions.

The age-related physiologic changes having the greatest effect on pharmacokinetics are reduction in liver mass resulting in decreased drug metabolizing capacity and diminished kidney function (25–28). Hepatic drug metabolism declines approximately 10% per decade beginning at age 40 years (27,28). A decrease in drug-metabolizing capacity results in a slower unbound clearance that, in turn, will cause an increase in unbound and, if there is no change in protein binding, total drug concentrations. Studies to date have included an insufficient number of people >85 years of age to know whether the decrease in drug metabolism continues in the oldest old. The effect of advancing age on enzyme induction has not been well characterized.

Renal function, as measured by glomerular filtration rate, also decreases by approximately 10% with each decade of age, beginning at age 40 years (26). Creatinine clearance is a reliable marker of glomerular filtration and correlates well with unbound renal clearance of drugs eliminated by the kidneys. Elderly persons eliminate renally cleared drugs and active metabolites more slowly than do younger adults.

The total clearance of the major AEDs, which are predominately eliminated by the liver, is influenced by both the extent of protein binding and the intrinsic metabolizing capacity (intrinsic clearance) of unbound drug. Because total clearance determines steady-state total drug concentration, age-related alterations in protein binding or intrinsic clearance can affect serum drug concentrations. Age-related reductions in intrinsic clearance cause a rise in both unbound and, if there is no simultaneous decrease in protein binding, serum drug concentrations.

If an elderly patient has a decrease in both hepatic drug metabolizing capacity and protein binding, the effect on total and unbound drug will depend on the relative magnitude of change for each parameter. If the decrease in protein binding is greater than the reduction in unbound clearance, total drug concentration can remain unchanged or can even decline in the presence of rising unbound drug concentration. Measurement of unbound concentration in elderly patients is essential when altered protein binding is suspected or when response (either therapeutic or toxic) does not correlate with total drug concentration.

Despite the effects of age-related physiologic changes on pharmacodynamics and drug disposition and the widespread use of AEDs in the elderly, few studies on AED pharmacokinetics, drug interaction, efficacy, or safety in the elderly have been published (28–31). The available reports generally involve single-dose evaluations in small samples of

TABLE 13.4. ROUTES OF ANTIEPILEPTIC DRUG ELIMINATION IN THE ELDERLY

Drug	Metabolism/Route of Elimination	Comments
Carbamazepine	Hepatic	Protein binding decreased with reduced serum albumin.
		Estimated dosage requirements 40% less than for younger adults.
Felbamate	Hepatic	Many drug interactions.
Gabapentin	Renal	Elimination correlates with creatinine clearance. Dosage may need to be 30%–50% less than for younger adults.
Lamotrigine	Hepatic–glucuronide conjugation	Effect of advancing age on conjugation reactions are not well understood; doses may need to be altered.
Phenobarbital	Hepatic and renal	
Phenytoin	Hepatic	Protein binding decreased with reduced serum albumin. Initial dosage 2–3 mg/kg. Subsequent increases should be small (<10% of dose).
Primidone	Hepatic	Half-life and clearance similar to younger adults. Dosage may not need to be adjusted (45).
Topiramate	Hepatic and renal	Dosage may need to be reduced in elderly patients with diminished renal function.
Valproic acid	Hepatic	Protein binding decreased with reduced serum albumin. Dosage may need to be 30%–40% less than for younger adults.

NA, information not available for elderly patients.

the young old, that is, persons 65 to 74 years old. The absence of data on AED pharmacokinetics in the oldest old increases the possibility of therapeutic failure and adverse reactions in this population (32). (A summary of available pharmacokinetic information in the elderly is presented in Table 13.4.)

Older patients appear to be more sensitive to the CNS and systemic adverse effects of AEDs, especially cognition (33,34). In one study, PHT was the only drug among several factors that was associated with a significant increase in nonvertebral fractures among community-dwelling elderly women (34). This study also found that both elderly men and women taking moderate doses of benzodiazepines, including clonazepam, had a greater likelihood of hip fractures (34). These reports indicate that elderly persons, as a group, are more sensitive to both the pharmacodynamic effects and the toxic effects of AEDs, although there is substantial intrapatient variability.

Phenytoin

PHT is poorly soluble and slowly absorbed, reaching peak concentrations after a single dose ranging from 6 to 18 hours. Age-related alterations in gastrointestinal function could have an impact on PHT absorption. Preliminary results from our studies indicate that oral PHT bioavailability in elderly patients ranges from 40% to 100%. Other investigators have observed fluctuations ranging from 50%

to 150% in PHT concentrations among 15 frail nursing home patients while receiving maintenance therapy with the same daily dose and formulations. These reports suggest that the elderly may be susceptible to intrapatient alterations in PHT bioavailability resulting in clinical significant changes in drug concentration.

Studies in elderly patients have shown decreases in PHT binding to albumin and increases in the free fraction (35,36). The binding of PHT to serum proteins correlates with the albumin concentration, which is typically low normal to subnormal in the elderly. As the drug concentration rises and the albumin concentration falls, PHT binding is likely to decrease.

PHT elimination in the elderly is reduced. One study compared the pharmacokinetics of PHT at steady state after oral administration in 34 elderly (60 to 79 years), 32 middle-aged (40 to 59 years), and 26 younger adults (20 to 39 years) with epilepsy. All subjects had normal albumin concentrations and liver function and received no other medications, including other AEDs known to alter hepatic metabolism. The maximum rate of metabolism (V_{max}) declined gradually with age; the elderly group had a mean V_{max} that was 20% smaller than in the younger adults (37). Other smaller studies have also shown that PHT metabolism is reduced in the elderly (25,38–41). The smaller V_{max} means that PHT metabolism becomes saturated at lower concentrations than in younger patients. Thus, smaller maintenance doses of PHT are needed to attain desired unbound serum concentrations, and relatively small changes in dose (≤10%) are recommended when making dosing adjustments. Thus, in the elderly, a daily dose of 3 mg/kg appears to be appropriate, rather than the 5 mg/kg per day used in younger adults (42). This 3 mg/kg dose is only 160 mg/day for a 52-kg woman or 200 mg/day for a 66-kg man. The reduced elimination also results in extended half-lives. Most elderly patients with total PHT concentrations ≥10 mg/L have PHT half-lives of >40 hours. Personal observation (Cloyd and Leppik) would indicate that elderly patients can be safely given PHT doses once a day with minimal fluctuation in drug concentrations and improved compliance.

One nursing home survey revealed that residents were taking PHT doses similar to those used in younger adults (3). Thus, there is a great potential for inadvertent overdose in the nursing home population. Because of protein binding, the total levels in these persons may appear to be normal, but measurement of the unbound level may be necessary to detect overdoses (43,44). In patients with both reduced metabolism and binding to serum albumin, unbound PHT concentration increases while the total drug concentration decreases. In such cases, the total drug concentration does not correlate with response. Patients may achieve seizure control with what is thought to be subtherapeutic concentrations, or they may experience toxicity when total serum concentrations are in the therapeutic range. Measurement of unbound PHT concentrations is necessary for elderly patients who have the following: (a) decreased serum albumin concentration or total PHT concentrations that are near the upper boundary of the therapeutic range; (b) total concentrations that decline over time; (c) a low total concentration relative to the daily dose; or (d) total concentrations that do not correlate with clinical response. A range of 5 to 15 mg/L may be more appropriate as a therapeutic range for the elderly (42).

PHT is effective for localization-related epilepsies, and thus it has an efficacy profile appropriate for the elderly. However, no studies regarding the effectiveness of PHT in the elderly have been published. Some evidence from the Veterans Administration cooperative study would suggest it is equally effective as carbamazepine, phenobarbital, and primidone, but the number of subjects in that study was small. PHT has drug-drug interactions, and it needs to be used cautiously in EMMP patients receiving other medications.

PHT does have some effects on cognitive functioning, especially at higher levels (33). It is not known whether the elderly will be more sensitive to this problem. In addition, PHT may cause imbalance and ataxia. It is likely that EMMP patients, especially those with CNS disorders, may be more sensitive to these effects. One study investigated the risk factors for nonvertebral fractures in elderly, community-dwelling elderly women. Among the various lifestyle, demographic, and health factors that contributed

to an increase risk, PHT, despite relatively low usage, was the only drug with a significant effect (34). PHT also is known to be a mild blocker of cardiac conduction, and it should be used cautiously in persons with cardiac conduction defects, especially heart blocks. Treatment with antineoplastic drugs may decrease PHT concentrations (45). Drug interactions with PHT are a major problem in treating the elderly (8,9).

Carbamazepine

Young adults typically require 10 to 20 mg/kg/day taken in three or four divided doses to attain serum carbamazepine concentrations within the usual therapeutic range (46). Carbamazepine doses were much lower in one nursing home study, whereas trough serum carbamazepine concentrations remained within the usual therapeutic range (5). One study evaluated carbamazepine clearance in seven elderly (mean age, 82.3 years) using daily dose and trough serum concentrations. Clearance was 40% lower than in a group of younger patients 41.0±19.6 versus 71.4±35.8 mL/hr/kg, respectively (3). This decrease is the same magnitude as seen with PHT and valproic acid in elderly patients. The smaller clearance results in a prolonged elimination half-life. These changes in carbamazepine pharmacokinetics require lower doses and less frequent dosing in elderly patients.

Carbamazepine is effective for localization-related epilepsies, and thus it has an efficacy profile appropriate for the elderly. However, no studies regarding the ability of carbamazepine in the elderly have been published. Some evidence from the VAH cooperative study would suggest that it is equally effective as PHT, phenobarbital, and primidone, but the number of subjects in the study was small. There seems to be a reduction of the drug's clearance with advancing age, so doses will need to be lower in both EH and EMMP patients. What is not known is whether its metabolism will be autoinducible to the same extent that it is in younger populations. Thus, one will need to monitor drug levels after initiation of treatment and adjust doses accordingly.

Carbamazepine has some significant drug-drug and drug-food interactions with medications that inhibit the cytochrome P450 enzyme, CYP3A4, responsible for carbamazepine metabolism. Among the inhibitors are erythromycin, fluoxetine, ketoconazole, propoxyphene (Darvon), and grapefruit juice. EH patients will need to be cautioned about the use of these medications. Many other drug interactions occur, so carbamazepine is one AED that must be used cautiously in EMMP patients receiving other medications.

Carbamazepine at higher levels does have some effects on cognitive functioning. It is not known whether the elderly will be more sensitive to this problem. In addition, carbamazepine may cause imbalance and ataxia. It is likely that EMMP patients, especially those with CNS disorders, may be more sensitive to these effects.

One of the major concerns with carbamazepine is its effect on sodium levels. Hyponatremia is a well-known phenomenon with carbamazepine use, and it may cause significant problems in younger adults, especially in the presence of polydipsia. Although little is known about carbamazepine and sodium balance in the elderly, this could well be a major issue, especially if patients are receiving diuretics or are on salt-restricted diets. This issue needs to be investigated further. Carbamazepine also is known to affect cardiac rhythms, and it should be used cautiously, if at all, in persons with rhythm disturbances.

One of the pharmacokinetic problems of carbamazepine is its short half-life, associated with the possible need to take the drug multiple times a day. In the elderly, however, the drug's half-life may be longer. In any case, the new slow-release formulations (Carbatrol and Tegretol XR) have overcome these limitations. Carbamazepine is a moderately priced drug, and it should not present a significant cost issue, especially if lower doses are needed.

Phenobarbital

Phenobarbital is effective for localization-related epilepsies, and thus it has an efficacy profile appropriate for the elderly (47). However, the VAH cooperative study demonstrated that phenobarbital and primidone have effects on cognitive functioning, most prominent at higher levels (48). The elderly will be more sensitive to this problem. Thus, although phenobarbital is the least expensive of all the AEDs, its effects on cognition and mood make this an undesirable drug for the elderly, both the EH, who are trying to maintain independent living conditions, and EMMP patients, who may have underlying intellectual deficits.

Valproic Acid

Only a few small studies have compared the pharmacokinetics of valproic acid in young and old patients (30,49,50). In a study of steady-state valproate pharmacokinetics in six young adult and six elderly volunteers (66 to 72 years), the average unbound fraction of valproate was 10.7% in the elderly compared with 6.4% in younger subjects. In elderly subjects, mean unbound concentration was 57% higher and unbound clearance was 65% lower than in younger adults (49). In another study comparing single-dose intravenous valproate pharmacokinetics in seven young adult volunteers and in six residents of long-term care units (75 to 87 years), total clearance was similar in the two groups. Serum elimination half-life was twice as long in the elderly as in the younger subjects, 14.9 versus 7.2 hours (50). Valproic acid, like PHT, is associated with reduced protein binding and unbound clearance in the elderly. As a result, the desired clinical response may be

achieved with a lower dose than usual. Because the serum elimination half-life is prolonged, the dosing interval can be extended. If the albumin concentration has fallen or if the patient's clinical response does not correlate with total drug concentration, measurement of unbound drug should be considered.

Felbamate

Felbamate is effective for localization-related epilepsies, and it appears to have a broader spectrum of effectiveness than some of the other AEDs. Thus, it has an efficacy profile that may be very appropriate for the elderly. Felbamate is primarily metabolized by the liver and is known to have certain drug-drug interactions, both inhibitory and inductive (51). Thus, it does not appear to be a drug that will be easy to use in EMMP patients. Because of its association with aplastic anemia and hepatic failure, felbamate has a higher risk profile than the other AEDs and may have limited use in the elderly.

Gabapentin

Gabapentin is effective for localization-related epilepsies, and thus it has an efficacy profile appropriate for the elderly. Gabapentin is not metabolized by the liver, but rather it is renally excreted (52). Creatinine clearance is reduced with advancing age, so doses will need to be lower in both EH and EMMP patients. Thus, one will need to monitor drug levels after initiation of treatment and adjust doses accordingly. Because gabapentin has no drug-drug interactions, it may be especially useful in EMMP patients. Gabapentin may have some cognitive side effects, especially at higher levels, and the elderly may be more sensitive to this problem.

One of the problems with gabapentin is its short half-life, associated with the possible need to take the drug multiple times a day. In the elderly, however, the drug's half-life may be longer. Gabapentin is a high-priced drug, and it may present a significant cost issue, especially if higher doses are needed. A study comparing carbamazepine with gabapentin and lamotrigine is in progress, and more information regarding the various safety and efficacy issues will be available when the VAH study is completed.

Lamotrigine

Because lamotrigine is effective for localization-related epilepsies, it has an efficacy profile appropriate for the elderly. One study comparing it with carbamazepine was favorable (53). Lamotrigine is primarily metabolized by the liver by glucuronidation (54). It is not known whether there is a reduction of its glucuronidation with advancing age. Thus, one will need to monitor drug levels after initiation of treatment and adjust doses accordingly.

Lamotrigine elimination is reduced by drugs such as valproic acid, which block glucuronidation. Thus, some caution may need to be observed in EMMP patients who are taking other drugs.

Tiagabine

Tiagabine is effective for localization-related epilepsies and has an efficacy profile appropriate for the elderly. It is primarily metabolized by the liver. There may be a reduction of its clearance with advancing age, but this may be overshadowed by the susceptibility to increased metabolizing by inducing drugs. Experience with this drug in elderly is limited.

Topiramate

Topiramate has an efficacy profile appropriate for the elderly. Topiramate is both metabolized by the liver and excreted unchanged in the urine. There may be a reduction of its clearance with advancing age, so levels will need to be monitored. Topiramate does have some effects on cognitive functioning, especially word finding. The elderly may be more sensitive to this problem.

Benzodiazepines

Benzodiazepines used for the treatment of epilepsy include diazepam, lorazepam, clorazepate, and clonazepam. Diazepam and lorazepam are administered intravenously for the acute treatment of status epilepticus, and clorazepate and clonazepam are given orally as maintenance therapy.

Diazepam is highly protein bound (>99%) and undergoes oxidative metabolism to form an active metabolite, desmethyldiazepam. Protein binding declines with age, resulting in an increased free fraction and a greater distribution volume of diazepam and desmethyldiazepam. Unbound clearance is reduced, thus prolonging the serum elimination half-life of the drug and its metabolite. Lorazepam is less highly bound (90%) and is metabolized by conjugation to lorazepam glucuronide. The free fraction of lorazepam rises with age, and the volume of distribution is increased, but less than with diazepam. The elimination half-life of lorazepam is similar in the young and the elderly. Direct comparisons of the pharmacokinetics of clonazepam and clorazepate in the young and the elderly have not been published.

Elderly persons tend to be more sensitive to drugs that act on the CNS. Among such drugs, the benzodiazepines have undergone the most extensive pharmacodynamic investigation. In a study of diazepam sedation, this side effect was increased in the elderly, although unbound drug concentrations did not differ from those in younger subjects (55). The increased sensitivity of the elderly to such drugs is apparently independent of drug concentration, either in the serum or at the site of action.

Drug Interactions

Drug interactions involving AEDs pose a major problem because epilepsy in the elderly is often accompanied by other disorders. In one survey, half the patients in long-term care facilities were taking five or more other maintenance medications in addition to an AED (3) (Table 13.5). Many of these comedications have clinically significant pharmacodynamic or pharmacokinetic interactions with AEDs. For example, CNS depressants such as psychotropics can exaggerate the side effects of several AEDs. Pharmacokinetic interactions between AEDs and comedications can also occur by altering the absorption, hepatic metabolism, or protein binding of either drug. Pharmacokinetic drug interactions can be multidimensional: valproic acid competes with PHT for plasma protein binding site, whereas PHT induces valproate metabolism and valproate inhibits PHT metabolism. Additionally, some drug interactions alter the concentrations of active AED metabolites. For example, valproate inhibits carbamazepine epoxide conversion to its inactive metabolite and results in an increase in carbamazepine epoxide, whereas carbamazepine itself may remain unchanged.

PHT absorption may be significantly reduced by certain antacids. The calcium cations often used in antacids may interact with PHT and may form insoluble complexes (56, 57). Aluminum or magnesium hydroxide may decrease gabapentin absorption. There do not appear to be clinically significant interactions affecting the bioavailability of other AEDs.

Protein binding interactions that displace AEDs generally do not alter unbound drug concentrations. Hence, dosage adjustments may not be needed, but this should be verified by measuring unbound levels.

The most clinically significant drug interactions involving AEDs are those that affect metabolism (58). Medications that inhibit hepatic enzymes responsible for drug metabolism decrease the clearance of affected drugs and result in a rise in serum concentrations. Drugs that induce hepatic enzymes increase the clearance of affected drugs and produce a decrease in serum concentration. Discontinuation of an inhibitor or inducer produces the opposite effect.

TABLE 13.5. FREQUENCY OF USE OF COMEDICATIONS WITH POTENTIAL PHARMACOKINETIC OR PHARMACODYNAMIC INTERACTIONS WITH THE ANTIEPILEPTIC DRUGS IN 4,291 RESIDENTS OF NURSING HOMES

Drug Category	Percentage Use with Antiepileptic Drugs
Antidepressants	18.9
Antipsychotics	12.7
Benzodiazepines	22.4
Thyroid supplements	14.0
Antacids	8.0
Calcium channel blockers	6.9
Warfarin	5.9
Cimetidine	2.5

TABLE 13.6. ISOENZYME-MEDIATED ANTIEPILEPTIC DRUG METABOLISM AND ISOENZYME-SPECIFIC DRUG INTERACTIONS

Drug Category	CYP 1A2	CYP 2C9	CYP 2C19	CYP 3A4	UGTs[a]
Antiepileptic drug	CBZ (minor)	PHT PB VPA (minor)	PHT DZP	CBZ Midazolam Tiagabine Zonisamide	VPA LTG Lorazepam MHD
Inducers	Omeprazole Cigarette smoking Charbroiled meats	CBZ OXC PB PHT Rifampin St. John's wort	CBZ PB PHT Rifampin	CBZ OXC MHD[b] St. John's wort	CBZ LTG PB PHT Rifampin
Inhibitors	Ciprofloxacin Enoxacin Fl:uroxamine	Cimetidine Fluconazole Sertraline Paroxetine VPA OXC Isoniazid (?)	Cimetidine Omeprazole Felbamate Topiramate	Cimetidine Ketoconazole Itraconazole Fluconazole Erythromycin Clarithromycin Fluoxetine Grapefruit	VPA

CPY, cytochrome P 450; UGT, glucuronosyltransferases; CBZ, carbamazepine; PHT, phenytoin; PB, phenobarbital; VPA, valproate; LTG, lamotrigine; MHD, monohydroxy derivative of OXC.
[a]VPA glucuronidation is catalyzed by UGT 1A9 and UGT 2B7; LTG by UGT 1A3 and UGT 1A4; and lorazepam by UGT 2B7. The isoenzymes responsible for 10-OH-CBZ glucuronidation have not been identified.
[b]Variable effect on CYP 3A substrates.

An important consideration when managing therapy in the elderly is the effect of frequent changes in drugs and doses. A drug interaction reference should be checked to determine whether a specific interaction occurs (57). A list of the clinically important interactions listed by AED and the affected isoenzyme is presented in Table 13.6.

Alternate Routes of Administration

Some elderly patients may be unable or unwilling to take oral medications because of oroesophageal conditions, other physical disabilities, or altered mental status. Elderly patients also have an increased risk of seizure emergencies such as status epilepticus that require acute management. These circumstances necessitate the use of alternative routes of administration. The most commonly used method when providing maintenance therapy is a feeding gastrostomy or nasogastric tube. Carbamazepine, felbamate, PHT, phenobarbital, primidone, and valproic acid have liquid formulations that may be given through feeding tubes. Solutions such as valproic acid syrup should be well absorbed, although this has not been substantiated, and some patients experience nausea or vomiting (59). Absorption of suspensions, the contents of capsules, and crushed tablets may be more problematic. The bioavailability of PHT suspension through a gastrostomy or nasogastric tube may be reduced when the drug is coadministered with enteral feedings (60). Therefore, administration of suspension should be sepa-

rated from enteral feedings by several hours, and the tube should be thoroughly flushed after a dose. The bioavailability of carbamazepine suspension through nasogastric or gastric tubes is not known. In some patients, divalproex sodium and carbamazepine sprinkle particles adhere to the end of tubes and can cause gastric fluid to leak externally around gastric tubes (21).

Rectal administration is a viable option for some, but not all, AEDs. For short-term use (days), preparation of solutions or suspension using available commercial products are preferred, and there is some information about bioavailability and safety. When rectal administration extends over weeks or longer, suppositories should be considered because of ease of administration and patient comfort. Valproic acid syrup, carbamazepine suspension, and suspensions of crushed lamotrigine or topiramate tablets can be administered rectally to adults on a temporary basis. Bioavailability varies from 50% for lamotrigine to 80% to 100% for the other drugs, but the rate of absorption is slow for carbamazepine (61). Diazepam is absorbed very well rectally. The elderly are likely to absorb rectally administered AEDs to the same extent as younger adults, although such studies have not been done. PHT, regardless of formulation, is poorly absorbed rectally (62). Intramuscular administration of PHT sodium and valproate sodium should be avoided because both are associated with tissue injury (63).

A water-soluble PHT prodrug, fosphenytoin, may be administered intravenously or intramuscularly either as maintenance therapy when the oral route is not available or to treat seizure emergencies. The bioavailability of intramuscular fosphenytoin approaches 100% in younger adults, and preliminary results from our group indicate that it is also rapidly and completely absorbed in elderly patients. This finding suggests that intramuscular fosphenytoin may be useful in treating seizure emergencies when intravenous therapy is not possible. Injectable forms of PHT sodium and fosphenytoin may be given intravenously, but both require monitoring of blood pressure and of heart rate and rhythms, especially in the elderly. Valproate sodium injectable may be given as a rapid intravenous infusion without altering blood pressure or cardiac function (63,64).

Seizure emergencies in the elderly can be treated with rectal diazepam. The risk of respiratory depression is low, although extra caution should be exercised in elderly patients taking multiple CNS depressants or with pulmonary disease. Intranasal administration of midazolam injectable has been reported in children and younger adults and may be an option in elderly patients. The same precautions apply to intranasal midazolam as with rectal diazepam.

CONCLUSION

The use of AEDs in the elderly poses many issues not yet thoroughly studied. Consequently, many of the remarks in this chapter are subject to change as new data become available. Nevertheless, certain conclusions can be drawn. Elderly patients must have AED concentrations monitored more closely, and unbound levels are needed for some drugs. One must be particularly cautious in using dose recommendations developed for younger adults. Because of drug interactions, one must be familiar with routes of elimination of the AEDs and the influences of other drugs. PHT is the most commonly used AED in the elderly in the United States, but it has significant drawbacks. Similarly, carbamazepine may have the side effect of hyponatremia. The newer AEDs may have a more prominent role in the elderly, but more studies are needed.

ACKNOWLEDGMENT

Preparation of this chapter was supported in part by National Institutes of Health–National Institute of Neurological diseases and Stroke grant no. P50 NS16308.

REFERENCES

1. Hauser WA. Epidemiology of seizures in the elderly. In: Rowan AJ, Ramsay RE, eds. *Seizures and epilepsy in the elderly.* Boston: Butterworth-Heinemann, 1997:7–20.

2. Epilepsy Foundation of America. *Epilepsy: a report to the nation.* Landover, MD: Epilepsy Foundation of America 1999.

3. Cloyd JC, Lackner TE, Leppik IE. Antiepileptics in the elderly: pharmacoepidemiology and pharmacokinetics. *Arch Fam Med* 1994;3:589–598.

4. Garrard, J, Cloyd JC, Gross C, et al. Factors associated with antiepileptic drug use among nursing home elderly. *J Geriatr Med Sci* 2000;55:384–392.

5. Lackner TE, Cloyd JC, Thomas LW, et al. Antiepileptic drug use in nursing home residents: effect of age, gender, and comedication on patterns of use. *Epilepsia* 1998;39:1083–1087.

6. Schachter SS, Cramer GW, Thompson GD, et al. An evaluation of antiepileptic drug therapy in nursing facilities. *J Am Geriatr Soc* 1998;46:1137–1141.

7. Hauser WA, Hesdorffer DC, eds. *Epilepsy: frequency, causes and consequences.* New York: Demos, 1990:1–51.

8. Nation RL, Evans AM, Milne RW. Pharmacokinetic drug interactions with phenytoin. I and II. *Clin Pharmacokinet* 1990;18:37–60, 131–150.

9. Neef C, de Voogd-van den Straaten I. An interaction between cytostatic and anticonvulsant drugs. *Clin Pharmacol Ther* 1988;43:372–375.

10. Sirven JI. Acute and chronic seizures in patients older than 60 years. *Mayo Clin Proc* 2001;76:175–183.

11. Stephen LJ, Brodie MJ. Epilepsy in elderly people. *Lancet* 2000;355:1441–1446.

12. Cold JA, Wells BG, Froemming JH. Seizure activity associated with antipsychotic therapy. *DCIP* 1991;24:601–606.

13. Itil TM, Soldatos C. Epileptogenic side effects of psychotropic drugs: practical recommendations. *JAMA* 1980;244:1460–1463.

14. Moor SA, Teal TW, eds. Adverse drug reaction surveillance in the geriatric population: a preliminary review. In: *Proceedings of the Drug Information Association Workshop on Geriatric Drug Use: clinical and social perspectives.* Washington, DC: Pergamon Press, 1985.

15. Roberts J, Tumer N. Pharmacodynamic basis for altered drug action in the elderly. *Clin Geriatr Med* 1988;4:127–49.

16. Sherwin AL, Loynd JS, Bock GW, et al. Effects of age, sex, obesity, and pregnancy on plasma diephenythydantoin levels. *Epilepsia* 1974;15:507–521.

17. Vestal RE, Gurwitz JH. Geriatric pharmacology. In: Carruthers SG, Hoffman BB, Melmon KL, et al., eds. *Clinical pharmacology: basic principles in therapeutics,* 4th ed. New York: McGraw-Hill, 2000:1151–1177.

18. Ramsay RE, Rowan AJ, Slater JD, et al. Effect of age on epilepsy and its treatment: results of the VA Cooperative Study. *Epilepsia* 1994;35[Suppl 8]:91.

19. Castleden CM, George CF, Marcer D, et al. Increased sensitivity to nitrazepam in old age. *BMJ* 1977;1:10–12.

20. Wallace SM, Verbeeck RK. Plasma protein binding of drugs in the elderly. *Clin Pharmacokinet* 1987;12:41–72.

21. Cloyd JC, Kriel RL. Bioavailability of rectally administered valproic acid syrup. *Neurology* 1981;31:1348–1352.

22. Verbeeck RK, Cardinal JA, Wallace SM. Effect of age and sex on the plasma binding of acidic and basic drugs. *Eur J Clin Pharmacol* 1984;27:91–97.

23. Greenblatt DJ. Reduced serum albumin concentrations in the elderly: a report from the Boston Collaborative Drug Surveillance Program. *J Am Geriatr Soc* 1979;27:20–22.

24. Tiula E, Neuvonen PJ. Antiepileptic drugs and alpha-1 acid glycoprotein. *N Engl J Med* 1982;307:1148.

25. Bach B, Hansen JM, Kampmann JP, et al. Disposition of antipyrine and phenytoin correlated with age and liver volume in man. *Clin Pharmacokinet* 1981;6:389–396.

26. Rowe JW, Andres R, Tobin JD, et al. The effect of age on creatinine clearance in men: a cross-sectional and longitudinal study. *J Gerontol* 1976;31:155–163.

27. Woodhouse KW, Wynne HA. Age-related changes in liver size and hepatic blood flow: the influence on drug metabolism in the elderly. *Clin Pharmacokinet* 1988;15:287–294.

28. Wynne HA, Cope LH, Mutch E, et al. The effect of age on liver volume and apparent liver blood flow in healthy man. *Hepatology* 1989;9:297–301.

29. Faught E. Epidemiology and drug treatment of epilepsy in elderly people. *Drugs Aging* 1999;15:255–269.

30. Perucca E, Grimaldi R, Gatti G, et al. Pharmacokinetics of valproic acid in the elderly. *Br J Clin Pharmacol* 1984;17:665–669.

31. Willmore LJ. Choice and use of newer anticonvulsant drugs in older patients. *Drugs Aging* 1999;17:441–452.

32. Faich GA, Dreis M, Tomita D. National adverse drug reaction surveillance 1986. *Arch Intern Med* 1988;148:785–787.

33. Read CL, Stephen LJ, Stolarek IH, et al. Cognitive effects of anticonvulsant monotherapy in elderly patients: a placebo-controlled study. *Seizure* 1998;7:159–162.

34. Bohannon AD, Hanlon JT, Landerman R, et al. Association of race and other potential risk factors in community-dwelling elderly women. *Am J Epidemiol* 1999;149:1002–1009.

35. Patterson M, Hazelwood R, Smithhurst B, et al. Plasma protein binding of phenytoin in the aged: *in-vivo* studies. *Br J Clin Pharmacol* 1982;13:423–425.

36. Umstead GS, Morales M, McKercher Pl. Comparison of total, free, and salivary phenytoin concentrations in geriatric patients. *Clin Pharm* 1986;5:59–62.

37. Bauer LA, Blouin RA. Age and phenytoin kinetics in adult epileptics. *Clin Pharmacol Ther* 1982;31:301–304.

38. Hayes MJ, Langman MJS, Short AH. Changes in drug metabolism with increasing age. II. Phenytoin clearance and protein binding. *Br J Clin Pharmacol* 1975;2:73–79.

39. Houghton GW, Richens A, Leighton M. Effects of age, height, weight and sex on serum phenytoin concentrations in epileptic patients. *Br J Clin Pharmacol* 975;2:251–256.

40. Lambie DC, Caird FL. Phenytoin dosage in the elderly age. *Ageing* 1977;6:133–137.

41. Troupin AS, Johannessen SI. Epilepsy in the elderly: a pharmacologic perspective. In: Smith DB, ed. *Epilepsy: current approaches to diagnosis and treatment.* New York: Raven Press, 1990: 141–153.

42. Leppik IE. *Contemporary diagnosis and management of the patient with epilepsy,* 5th ed. New Town, PA: Handbooks in Health Care, 2000:159.

43. Drinka PJ, Miller J, Voeks SK, et al. Phenytoin binding in a nursing home. *J Geriatr Drug Ther* 1988;3:73–82.

44. Edwards GB, Culberton VL, Anresen GB, et al. Free phenytoin concentrations in geriatrics. *J Geriatr Drug Ther* 1988;3:97–102.

45. Bollini P, Riva R, Albani F, et al. Decreased phenytoin levels during antineoplastic therapy: a case report. *Epilepsia* 1983;24: 75–78.

46. Morselli PL. Carbamazepine: absorption, distribution and excretion. In: Levy RH, Mattson RM, Dreifuss FE, et al., eds. *Antiepileptic drugs,* 3rd ed. New York: Raven Press, 1989:473–490.

47. Eadie MJ, Lander CM, Hooper WD, et al. Factors influencing plasma phenobarbitone levels in epileptic patients. *Br J Clin Pharmacol* 1977;4:41–47.

48. Mattson R, et al. Comparison of carbamazepine, phenobarbital, phenytoin, and primidone in partial and secondarily generalized tonic-clonic seizures. *N Engl J Med* 1985;313:145–151.

49. Bauer LA, Davis R, Wilensky A, et al. Valproic acid clearance: unbound fraction and diurnal variation in young and elderly adults. *Clin Pharmacol Ther* 1985;37:697–700.

50. Bryson SM, Verma N, Scott PJW, et al. Pharmacokinetics of valproic acid in young and elderly subjects. *Br J Clin Pharmacol* 1983;16:104–105.

51. Graves NM. Felbamate. *Ann Pharmacother* 1993;27:1073–1081.

52. Richens A. Clinical pharmacokinetics of gabapentin. In: Chadwick D, ed. *New trends in epilepsy management: the role of gabapentin.* London: Royal Society of Medicine Services, 1993:41–46.

53. Brodie MJ, Overstall PW, Giorgi L. Multicentre, double-blind, randomised comparison between lamotrigine and carbamazepine in elderly patients with newly diagnosed epilepsy: the UK Lamotrigine Elderly Study Group. *Epilepsy Res* 1999;37:81–87.

54. Peck AW. Clinical pharmacology of lamotrigine. *Epilepsia* 1991;32[Suppl 2]:S9–S12.

55. Cook PJ, Flanagan R, James IM. Diazepam tolerance: effect of age, regular sedation and alcohol. *BMJ* 1984;289:351–353.

56. Cacek AT. Review of alterations in oral phenytoin bioavailability associated with formulation, antacids, and food. *Ther Drug Monit* 1986;8:166–171.

57. Hansten PD, Horn JR, eds. *Drug interactions: a clinical perspective and analysis of current developments.* Vancouver, WA: Applied Therapeutics, 1993:331–371.

58. Cusack BJ. Drug metabolism in the elderly. *J Clin Pharmacol* 1988;28:571–576.

59. Jones-Saete C, Kriel RL, Cloyd JC. External leakage from feeding gastrostomies in patients receiving valproate sprinkle. *Epilepsia* 1992;33:692–695.

60. Haley CJ, Nelson J: Phenytoin-enteral feeding interaction. *Ann Pharmacother* 1989;23:796–798.

61. Graves NM, Kriel RL, Jones-Saete C, et al. Relative bioavailability of rectally administered carbamazepine suspension in humans. *Epilepsia* 1985;26:429–433.

62. Fuerst RH, Graves NM, Kriel RL, et al. Absorption and safety of rectally administered phenytoin. *Eur J Drug Metab Pharmacokinet* 1988;13:257–260.

63. Devinsky O, Leppik IE, Willmore LJ, et al. Safety of intravenous valproate. *Ann Neurol* 1995;38:670–674.

64. Dreifuss FE, Rosman NP, Cloyd JC, et al. A comparison of rectal diazepam gel and placebo for acute repetitive seizures. *N Engl J Med* 1998;338:1869–1875.

65. Bachman KA, Belloto RJ. Differential kinetics of phenytoin in elderly patients. *Drugs Aging* 1999;15:235–250.

66. Bender AD, Post A, Meier JP, et al. Plasma protein binding of drugs as a function of age in adult human subjects. *J Pharm Sci* 1975;64:1711–1713.

67. Bernus I, Dickinson RG, Hooper WD, et al. Anticonvulsant therapy in aged patients: clinical pharmacokinetic considerations. *Drugs Aging* 1997;10:278–289.

68. Dawling S, Crome P. Clinical pharmacokinetic considerations in the elderly: an update. *Clin Pharmacokinet* 1989;17:236–263.

69. Sandor P, Sellers EM, Dumbrell M, et al. Effect of short- and long-term alcohol use on phenytoin kinetics in chronic alcoholics. *Clin Pharmacol Ther* 1981;30:390–397.

GENERAL PRINCIPLES

TREATMENT OF STATUS EPILEPTICUS

BRIAN K. ALLDREDGE

Generalized convulsive status epilepticus is the most life-threatening manifestation of an acute seizure episode. It is precipitated by a wide range of medical and neurologic conditions and represents the failure of normal neuronal mechanisms that limit typical convulsive seizures (1).

Population-based studies indicate that 102,000 to 152,000 cases of status epilepticus occur in the United States each year. The annual incidence is 41 to 61 per 100,000 persons and is highest during the first year of life and after the age of 60 years. The overall 30-day mortality rate after status epilepticus is 22%, with an estimated 22,200 to 42,000 deaths each year in the United States. The mortality rate in children is 3%, and is significantly lower than the 26% mortality rate in adults (2).

Historically, most clinical studies have defined status epilepticus as 30 minutes of either continuous seizures or repeated seizures without full recovery of consciousness. However, it is widely acknowledged that aggressive treatment should begin much earlier. Most secondarily generalized seizures in adults end within 2 minutes of onset (3), and in children seizures that last longer than 5 minutes are unlikely to stop spontaneously (4). Recently, an operational definition of status epilepticus as "≥5 minutes of (a) continuous seizures or (b) two or more discrete seizures between which there is incomplete recovery of consciousness" has been proposed (1,5), and has been used in one prospective study of out-of-hospital treatment (6).

Patient outcome after an episode of status epilepticus is affected by the interaction between several factors, including (a) age of the patient, (b) the etiology of acute seizures, (c) prolonged duration of seizures, and (d) concomitant physiologic disturbances (5,7).

This chapter focuses on the drug treatment of generalized convulsive status epilepticus in both hospital and non-hospital settings. Detailed discussions of the causes, clinical features, pathophysiology, and general medical management of status epilepticus are available in other reviews (5,8,9) and in a definitive text by Shorvon (10).

PRINCIPLES OF DRUG TREATMENT

The primary goal of drug treatment for status epilepticus is rapid cessation of seizures. Termination of the somatic manifestations of seizures alone is not sufficient; effective therapy must terminate both clinical and electrical seizure activity. In choosing drugs to treat status epilepticus, factors that should be considered include (a) the latency from beginning drug administration to the onset of clinical efficacy, (b) the duration of the clinical antiseizure effect, and (c) the effect of treatment on consciousness and cardiorespiratory function. Intravenous drug administration is preferred when treatment is administered by medical personnel and adequate support measures are available to manage the medical complications from ongoing seizures and their treatment.

A variety of pharmacokinetic and pharmacodynamic factors influence the clinical utility of drugs used for status epilepticus. The entry of most drugs and xenobiotics into the brain is limited by endothelial tight junctions that constitute the blood–brain barrier. Most drugs that have a rapid onset of clinical antiseizure effect are highly lipophilic compounds that reach peak brain concentrations quickly after intravenous administration. Carrier-mediated transport mechanisms also may play a role in enhancing the efficiency of brain entry, particularly for hydrophilic compounds (11). For highly lipophilic drugs such as benzodiazepines, the duration of antiseizure effect is largely affected by the rate and extent of drug movement out of brain tissue. These agents redistribute into other peripheral compartments (primarily lipoid tissues), resulting in a decline in brain and blood concentrations that is largely independent of drug elimination by the processes of metabolism and excretion. The biphasic decline in plasma drug concentration versus time for these drugs can be described by a *two-compartment model* (Figure 14.1). The first phase primarily represents *distribution* of drug from the *central compartment* (blood

Brian K. Alldredge, PharmD: Professor, Department of Clinical Pharmacy and Neurology, University of California, San Francisco, San Francisco, California

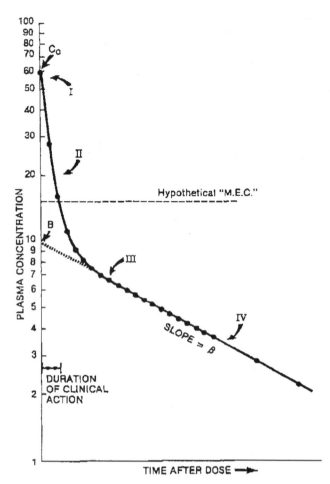

FIGURE 14.1. Simulated plasma drug concentration versus time relationships (semilogarithmic) from a two-compartment pharmacokinetic model after intravenous administration. Co is the peak concentration in plasma (or in the "central compartment"). B is the zero-order intercept of the elimination phase of the plasma concentration curve when extrapolated back to time zero. For highly lipophilic drugs, the initial phase primarily represents the distribution of drug from brain and blood to various body tissues. Note that this initial decline in plasma concentration may be sufficient to terminate clinical activity if the plasma level falls below some minimum effective concentration (MEC). The second phase represents elimination by metabolism or excretion. (Reprinted from Greenblatt DJ, Shader RI. *Pharmacokinetics in clinical practice.* Philadelphia: WB Saunders, 1985, with permission.)

and brain for many lipophilic drugs) to various tissues representing a *peripheral compartment*. The second phase represents drug *elimination* by metabolism and excretion.

Once the diagnosis of status epilepticus is established, appropriate antiepileptic drug treatment should begin immediately. Both experimental and clinical evidence support this approach. Meldrum and Brierley demonstrated that irreversible brain injury was more likely in freely convulsing baboons when seizures lasted longer than 80 minutes (12). Physiologic complications from prolonged seizures (e.g., hyperthermia and hypotension) potentiated

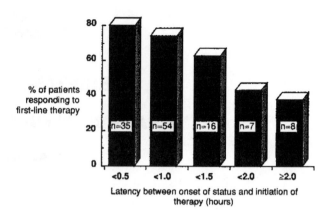

FIGURE 14.2. Relationship between duration of status epilepticus before administration of antiepileptic drugs and response to first-line therapy (usually, diazepam followed by phenytoin). Numbers in the bars refer to the total number of patients in each duration group. (Reprinted from Lowenstein DH, Alldredge BK. Status epilepticus at an urban public hospital in the 1980s. *Neurology* 1993;43:483–488, with permission.)

this damage (12). Numerous clinical reports also support a correlation between increased duration of status epilepticus and neurologic sequelae in patients (7,13–15). Another advantage of early intervention is that status epilepticus is more likely to respond to drug treatment when therapy is initiated as soon as possible. In the lithium–pilocarpine model of status epilepticus in rats, Walton and Treiman found that diazepam was progressively less effective in terminating seizures as the duration of seizures lengthened (16). Clinical evidence in support of this observation was found in a study in which the response of status epilepticus to initial treatment (usually diazepam followed by phenytoin) declined from 80% in those patients whose treatment began within 30 minutes of the onset of seizures, to less than 40% when treatment was initiated 2 hours or longer after seizures began (14) (Figure 14.2).

ANTIEPILEPTIC DRUG THERAPIES

Benzodiazepines

Benzodiazepines are widely preferred as initial antiepileptic drug therapy for status epilepticus because they are potent and have a rapid onset of effect. The most commonly used agents are lorazepam and diazepam (5,9,17). Clonazepam also is effective as initial therapy, although this author knows of no prospective, controlled comparisons with other benzodiazepines. The intravenous preparation of clonazepam is not available for use in the United States. Midazolam has been used as initial therapy for status epilepticus (18); however, the primary utility of this agent is related to its rapid absorption after nonintravenous routes of administration (see section on Out-of-Hospital Treatment). The antiseizure effect of these agents is related to allosteric interaction with the benzodiazepine binding site on the γ-

TABLE 14.1. PHARMACOKINETIC FEATURES OF BENZODIAZEPINES USED FOR STATUS EPILEPTICUS

	Lorazepam	Diazepam	Midazolam	Clonazepam
Protein binding (%)	90	97	96	86
Distribution half-life (hr)	2–3	0.3	0.06	0.5
Primary elimination route	glucuronidation	demethylation oxidation	oxidation	nitro reduction acetylation
Elimination half-life (hr)	8–25	28–54	2–4	20–60
Active metabolites	none	N-desmethyldiazepam oxazepam	α-hydroxy-midazolam	none

hr, hour.

aminobutyric acid, subtype A (GABA$_A$) receptor, resulting in enhanced GABA-mediated neuronal inhibition. Pharmacokinetic features of benzodiazepines that are relevant to their use in status epilepticus are summarized in Table 14.1. The primary adverse effects of intravenous benzodiazepines are respiratory depression (3% to 11% of patients) and impaired consciousness (20% to 60%) (6,19,20). Hypotension and cardiac dysrhythmias are uncommon.

Lorazepam has a longer distribution half-life than other benzodiazepines, indicating a slower rate of egress from blood and brain to peripheral tissues. It is this property that is likely responsible for the prolonged duration of action of lorazepam (12 to 24 hours) (5). Although lorazepam is less lipophilic than diazepam and has been shown to reach peak brain and cerebrospinal fluid concentrations more slowly than diazepam in animals (21,22), randomized, comparative studies show the two drugs to have a similar onset of clinical antiseizure effect (6,20). Two prospective, double-blind studies have compared lorazepam 4 mg and diazepam 10 mg (both administered intravenously) as initial in-hospital treatment of status epilepticus in adults. In both studies, if the first injection was not effective, a repeat dose was given. Status epilepticus was terminated in 89% to 91% of patients given lorazepam and 76% to 84% of patients given diazepam. These differences were not statistically significant (20,23). Because lorazepam has a longer duration of action than diazepam and the two agents do not differ with regard to onset of effect and efficacy in status epilepticus, recent treatment paradigms recommend lorazepam over diazepam as initial treatment (5,17).

As discussed, diazepam is highly effective for termination of status epilepticus. However, its utility is limited by a short duration of antiseizure effect. This is related to the short residence time of the drug in brain tissue (24,25). Ramsay and colleagues studied the concentrations of diazepam in brain and plasma after intravenous administration to cats (26). As shown in Figure 14.3, peak brain and plasma concentrations of diazepam were attained within 1 minute. Thereafter, brain and plasma concentrations declined in parallel. At 45 minutes postinjection, plasma diazepam levels had declined to less than 200 ng/mL, a concentration that has been associated with clinical efficacy in status epilepticus (26). This observation is consistent with

clinical reports. Peak plasma concentrations of diazepam decline by 50% within 20 minutes of intravenous administration in humans (27). Also, as much as 47% to 50% of patients treated with intravenous diazepam experience early breakthrough seizures after initial cessation of status epilepticus (28,29).

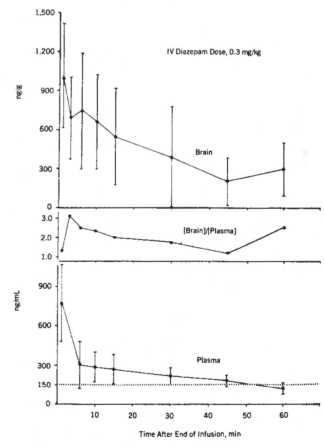

FIGURE 14.3. Brain concentrations (*upper panel*), plasma concentrations (*lower panel*), and brain/plasma concentration ratios (*middle panel*) of diazepam after intravenous administration to cats. Concentration values are means and standard deviations. (Reprinted from Ramsay RE, Hammond EJ, Perchalski RJ, et al. Brain uptake of phenytoin, phenobarbital, and diazepam. *Arch Neurol* 1979;36:535–539, with permission.)

Phenytoin and Fosphenytoin

Phenytoin is effective for the termination of status epilepticus, but its utility as initial therapy is limited by the slow rate of drug administration and the attendant delay in attaining maximal antiseizure effect. For this reason, phenytoin most often is administered after a benzodiazepine. In this regard, phenytoin is useful for maintenance of a long-lasting antiseizure effect, and it may effectively terminate status epilepticus when a benzodiazepine fails.

The usual intravenous loading dose of phenytoin is 20 mg/kg. This dosage should be reduced in the elderly (to 15 mg/kg) and in patients who have a baseline phenytoin level of 10 mg/L or more (5,9). If the initial loading dose of phenytoin is ineffective, an additional 5 to 10 mg/kg may be given. Phenytoin should be administered at a maximal rate of 50 mg/min. Peak brain concentrations are attained at the end of an intravenous infusion (30). Thus, a delay in maximal antiseizure effect of approximately 30 minutes can be expected when intravenous phenytoin is administered to an adult of average size. In a randomized comparison of four treatment regimens, Treiman and colleagues found that phenytoin 18 mg/kg was less effective than lorazepam 0.1 mg/kg as initial therapy for patients with overt (clinically evident) generalized convulsive status epilepticus (43.6% and 64.9% response rates, respectively; *p* = .002). Efficacy was initially assessed 20 minutes after beginning the drug infusions (31). The slower administration rate for phenytoin (mean infusion time, 33 minutes) may account for the inferior response rate.

Hypotension is a common adverse effect during intravenous infusion of phenytoin. The risk is highest in elderly patients and in those with preexisting cardiac disease, and when administration rates exceed 50 mg/min (32). Cardiac arrhythmias also may occur. Under these circumstances, slowing or stopping the infusion is recommended. Phenytoin is less likely to depress consciousness than benzodiazepines or phenobarbital.

Fosphenytoin is a phosphate ester prodrug of phenytoin with several potential advantages. Unlike parenteral phenytoin solution, fosphenytoin is water soluble (and compatible with all common intravenous solutions) and does not require a propylene glycol diluent or adjustment to alkaline pH. For these reasons, fosphenytoin causes fewer local injection site reactions and it can be administered at a faster rate than intravenous phenytoin. Conversion to phenytoin occurs with a half-life of 15 minutes and is catalyzed by nonspecific phosphatases that are ubiquitous in blood and body tissues. At recommended infusion rates, both phenytoin and fosphenytoin yield therapeutic unbound phenytoin concentrations (1 mg/mL) in blood within 10 minutes after beginning the infusion (33). Thus, the lag time in fosphenytoin conversion to phenytoin is overcome by a more rapid administration rate. In an open-label study, fosphenytoin was safe and well tolerated in the treatment of status epilepticus (34). Walton and colleagues compared fosphenytoin and phenytoin administered to nonconvulsing rats and found lower initial brain concentrations of phenytoin immediately after the end of the fosphenytoin infusion (35). The significance of this finding in humans is unknown because no studies have been conducted to compare the two drugs. Doses of fosphenytoin are expressed in terms of the milligrams of phenytoin that are yielded after cleavage of the phosphate ester bond. Thus, administering a dose of 1,000 mg phenytoin equivalents (PE) of fosphenytoin is equivalent to administration of 1,000 mg of phenytoin. The recommended dose of fosphenytoin for status epilepticus is 20 mg/kg PE and the maximal infusion rate is 150 mg/min PE. If ineffective, a supplemental dose of 5 to 10 mg/kg PE fosphenytoin may be given.

Phenobarbital

Phenobarbital has been shown to be effective as initial therapy for status epilepticus in two randomized trials. Shaner and colleagues compared phenobarbital (infusion rate, 100 mg/min) with simultaneous treatment with diazepam and phenytoin (infusion rates, 2 mg/min and 50 mg/min, respectively), and found phenobarbital-treated patients to have a shorter latency from initiation of treatment to cessation of seizures (36). In the randomized, blinded trial of Treiman et al., phenobarbital (100 mg/min) stopped overt status epilepticus in 58.2% of patients. In this study, phenobarbital was equivalent to other treatments (lorazepam, phenytoin alone, or diazepam followed by phenytoin) with regard to efficacy and safety end points (31). Loading doses of phenobarbital can cause significant depression of consciousness. Also, hypotension and respiratory depression are more common when phenobarbital is combined with a benzodiazepine (37). For these reasons, phenobarbital most often is reserved for patients who fail to respond to a benzodiazepine and phenytoin. In this setting, the recommended dose of phenobarbital is 20 mg/kg, and support measures for respiration and blood pressure should be readily available (9).

Valproate

Experience with intravenous valproate for the treatment of status epilepticus has increased despite lack of formal approval by the U.S. Food and Drug Administration and recommendation only for slow intravenous administration (20 mg/min). Loading doses of 21 to 28 mg/kg valproate given intravenously result in a mean postinfusion serum concentration of 133 mg/L (range, 64 to 204 mg/L) (38). Infusion rates of 200 mg/min in adults and 3 mg/kg/min in children are safe and well tolerated (39,40).

Open-label experience has shown valproate to be effective in both adults and children with various types of status epilepticus (i.e., generalized convulsive, partial, and generalized nonconvulsive status epilepticus) (41–44). The circumstances of valproate use vary widely in these reports from administration as initial therapy (43) to treatment after the failure of benzodiazepines, phenytoin, and barbiturates (44). In addition, a variety of dosing regimens were used and widely variable response rates (30–83%) are reported. No controlled clinical trials have compared valproate with other therapies for status epilepticus. Thus, the preferred place of valproate in an overall approach to management is unknown. Based on available evidence, the recommended loading dose of valproate for status epilepticus in adults and children is 20 to 25 mg/kg (diluted 1:1 with D_5W) administered at 3 to 6 mg/kg/min (up to 200 mg/min).

Apparent advantages of intravenous valproate include minimal effects on level of consciousness and cardiorespiratory function. Hypotension has been reported with intravenous valproate in the treatment of status epilepticus (45), but it appears to be uncommon. Sinha and Naritoku reported the successful administration of intravenous loading doses of valproate to 13 adult (primarily elderly) patients with medically refractory status epilepticus and cardiovascular instability. Most patients required vasopressive agents for blood pressure support before treatment with valproate. No significant changes in blood pressure, pulse, or vasopressor use were reported with valproate infusion rates of 6 to 100 mg/min (46).

Other Therapies

Alternative therapies that have been used for in-hospital management of status epilepticus include lidocaine, paraldehyde, and chlormethiazole. Although effective, these agents have not been shown to be more efficacious or safer than the treatments discussed previously. In small case series, intravenous lidocaine 1 to 3 mg/kg (usually followed by a maintenance infusion) has been effective for terminating status epilepticus refractory to other agents (47). Some authors suggest that lidocaine may have a unique role in the treatment of status epilepticus in neonates and in patients with respiratory disease (48–50). Chlormethiazole is used in the United Kingdom, Europe, and Australia, but is not approved in the United States. The recommended dose in adults is 320 to 820 mg (40 to 100 mL of a 0.8% solution) given at a rate of 5 to 15 mL/min, followed by a continuous infusion of 0.5 to 1 mL/min titrated upward according to response (10). A continuous infusion is necessary because of the short distribution half-life. Chlormethiazole causes sedation and respiratory depression that is potentiated by benzodiazepines and barbiturates. Paraldehyde can be given by rectal and intramuscular routes for the treatment of status epilepticus. Historically, the drug has been useful for the treatment of acute alcohol-related seizures and for patients in whom intravenous access is not feasible. Its use is limited by foul odor, lack of widespread availability, and require-

ments for light-protected storage and use with glass syringes (10).

Refractory Status Epilepticus

Status epilepticus fails to respond to standard treatment with benzodiazepines, phenytoin, and barbiturates in 10% to 15% of patients (14). These patients are at increased risk for permanent neurologic damage and death from prolonged electrical seizure activity and from severe physiologic complications associated with both seizures and intensive drug therapies (51). Mortality rates for refractory status epilepticus range from 32% to 77% (52). Definitive therapy with high-dose midazolam, barbiturates (usually pentobarbital), or propofol usually is necessary. These therapies also should be considered for patients at earlier stages of treatment if status epilepticus has been ongoing for 60 to 90 minutes or longer. Patients should be managed in an intensive care unit during treatment because ventilatory assistance and hemodynamic support usually are required.

The optimal treatment for refractory status epilepticus has not been defined. The number of patients who have been treated with midazolam, pentobarbital, and propofol in this setting is relatively small, and no randomized, controlled comparisons of treatments have been conducted. In adults, midazolam usually is administered as a single dose of 0.2 mg/kg by slow intravenous injection, followed by a continuous infusion of 0.075 to 10 µg/kg/min (53). Midazolam is highly effective for initial control of refractory status epilepticus; however, tachyphylaxis and breakthrough seizures are detected in approximately 50% of patients during continuous electroencephalographic (EEG) monitoring (54). Escalation of the midazolam infusion rate often is necessary. With prolonged, high-dose therapy, the half-life of midazolam is significantly prolonged owing to accumulation in peripheral tissues. This may lead to unexpected delays in the return of consciousness and spontaneous respiration during gradual withdrawal of midazolam (55).

The recommended dose of propofol is 1 to 2 mg/kg, followed by a maintenance infusion of 2 to 10 mg/kg/hr. Rates of successful treatment with propofol are similar to those with high-dose midazolam (52,56). However, in one retrospective comparison, the overall mortality rate was higher in propofol-treated patients (8 of 14 patients; 57%) than in those who received midazolam (1 of 6 patients; 17%) (52). Another retrospective study of propofol for refractory status epilepticus reported a higher mortality rate with this agent (7 of 8 patients; 88%) compared with patients treated with pentobarbital (4 of 8 patients; 50%) (56). In neither study was the mortality rate with propofol significantly higher than with the comparison treatment.

Pentobarbital is highly effective for control of refractory status epilepticus. However, myocardial depression, hypotension, and delayed postinfusion respiratory recovery are limitations (51,57,58). Nonetheless, there is no clear evidence for significant differences between pentobarbital and other therapies with regard to overall mortality. The recommended dose of pentobarbital is 10 to 15 mg/kg administered intravenously over 1 hour, followed by a continuous infusion of 0.5 to 1 mg/kg/hr.

For all of the aforementioned therapies, dosages should be adjusted to suppression of all electrographic seizures. Intravenous fluids and vasopressive agents may be required to treat hypotension. Once seizures have been controlled for 12 to 24 hours, therapy should be gradually weaned. Continuous EEG monitoring is required during high-dose treatment and while therapy is gradually withdrawn.

OUT-OF-HOSPITAL TREATMENT

Traditionally, status epilepticus has been managed in hospitals and emergency departments using drugs administered by the intravenous route. However, status epilepticus often occurs outside of the hospital. In a review of 804 paramedic encounters for seizures over a 3-month period in San Francisco, 117 (14%) were for multiple seizures or status epilepticus (59). Given the demonstrated value of early intervention in seizure emergencies, there is interest in developing and evaluating out-of-hospital therapies to stop status epilepticus or to prevent the evolution of acute seizure events into a more prolonged seizure state.

Prehospital Therapy

Recently, many emergency medical services (EMS) systems have adopted the practice of paramedic administration of benzodiazepines for out-of-hospital status epilepticus. Diazepam is the drug of choice in most EMS systems, and patients usually are transported to an emergency department for further evaluation and treatment. Despite the intuitive appeal of this approach, the equipment and consultant resources available to paramedics in the field differ significantly from those in hospitals. This may affect the management of status epilepticus, related physiologic complications, and adverse effects from medical treatment in a way that alters the balance between efficacy and safety (60,61).

The value of paramedic treatment for out-of-hospital status epilepticus was studied in a randomized, double-blind clinical trial (6). Adults with repeated or continuous seizures for more than 5 minutes were treated with either lorazepam 2 mg, diazepam 5 mg, or placebo by slow intravenous injection. An identical dose was given if seizures persisted. Patients received active antiepileptic drug therapy at the discretion of the treating physician when they arrived at a hospital. The primary outcome variable was termination of status epilepticus by the time the patient arrived at an emergency department. Response rates were 59.1% for lorazepam, 42.6% for diazepam, and 21.1% for placebo.

With adjustment for covariates (cause of status epilepticus, time interval from status epilepticus onset to study treatment, and time interval from treatment to emergency department arrival), lorazepam and diazepam were more effective than placebo. The trend favoring lorazepam over diazepam did not reach statistical significance. Out-of-hospital respiratory or circulatory complications occurred in 10.6% of lorazepam-treated patients, 10.3% in the diazepam group, and 22.5% in the placebo group ($p = .08$). The rates of cardiorespiratory complications that persisted to the time of emergency department arrival were approximately 50% of those in the field, suggesting that paramedics effectively managed these conditions. The three treatment groups did not differ with regard to neurologic outcome or mortality rates. A practical issue regarding the use of lorazepam in this setting is that the drug is heat labile and requires frequent restocking or refrigerated storage on ambulances in warm climates (62).

Despite the demonstrated value of paramedic drug treatment with benzodiazepines for out-of-hospital status epilepticus, many patients in the aforementioned trial did not respond to treatment. Intensive medical care was required in 73% of patients who continued in status epilepticus until emergency department arrival, and in 32% of those whose seizures ended. Thus, further study is required to identify more effective drugs or treatment regimens for this condition. Experience with the management of children with out-of-hospital status epilepticus is limited. Paramedic administration of intravenous or rectal diazepam significantly shortens the total duration of status epilepticus (63). However, one small case series of children treated with intravenous diazepam by paramedics found an unacceptably high rate of respiratory depression and intubation-related complications (64).

Alternate Routes of Drug Administration

Drugs and drug products available for administration by nonintravenous routes also are available for the out-of-hospital management of patients with seizure emergencies. Benzodiazepine antiseizure agents are most useful in this regard because they are potent, can be administered in small volumes, and are rapidly absorbed when the appropriate drug/route combination is chosen. Agents that are effective after transmucosal administration can be given by family members and caregivers after these individuals are properly trained. These therapies also may be considered by medical and paramedical personnel as treatment options for patients in whom venous access is unavailable. Throughout the following discussion, it should be kept in mind that none of these treatments is approved for the treatment of status epilepticus and that most published experience is in patients with prolonged or repetitive seizures who have not met defined criteria for status epilepticus.

Rectal Administration

Diazepam is rapidly and reliably absorbed after rectal administration. Bioavailability is 80% to 100% and peak drug concentration are attained within 30 minutes of rectal administration of the parenteral solution to children (65–67). A gel formulation of diazepam (Diastat) also is available for rectal use, and it has the advantages of improved retention characteristics and availability in pre-measured doses in an applicator with a flexible plastic tip. Rectal diazepam has been reported to be effective for acute repetitive seizures, prolonged seizures, and status epilepticus (68–71). Clinical effect is evident approximately 15 minutes after administration. The recommended dose of diazepam for rectal administration is 0.5 mg/kg for children younger than 6 years of age, 0.3 mg/kg for children 6 to 12 years of age, and 0.2 mg/kg for patients 12 years of age or older. Somnolence, ataxia, and incoordination occur occasionally after treatment. Respiratory depression is rare even when recommended doses are exceeded (67,72). Lorazepam and midazolam are not recommended for rectal administration because of unreliable absorption (73,74).

Intranasal Administration

Intranasal administration of midazolam for acute seizures has gained popularity, particularly for children. The nasal mucosa is highly vascularized, which aids in drug absorption. However, the volume of drug that can be administered without being swallowed is small, approximately 0.5 mL per nostril. Peak concentrations of midazolam occur within 12 minutes after administration to children, and the estimated bioavailability is 55% (75). Oral bioavailability is 15% to 27%; therefore, drug that is swallowed will likely contribute little to the clinical effect (73). When administered to 20 children with prolonged generalized seizures, intranasal midazolam was effective in all patients within 5 minutes (76). Adolescents and adults have been effectively treated despite the large volume of medication required (77). A recent randomized comparison of intravenous diazepam and intranasal midazolam for prolonged febrile seizures in children demonstrated potential advantages for midazolam. The mean time from arrival at the hospital to cessation of seizures was shorter in patients treated with midazolam (6.1 minutes; 95% confidence interval, 6.3 to 6.7 minutes) than in patients treated with intravenous diazepam (8.0 minutes; 95% confidence interval, 7.9 to 8.3 minutes) (78). The recommended dose of intranasal midazolam is 0.2 mg/kg, with half the dose administered in each nostril. The parenteral solution should be used, but it can cause local irritation and tastes bitter (75).

Buccal Administration

In healthy volunteers, midazolam is 75% bioavailable after buccal administration, and peak plasma concentrations occur within 30 minutes (79). The pharmacodynamic effect of midazolam appears even more quickly. Scott and colleagues reported changes in the 8- to 30-Hz frequencies on the EEG within 5 to 10 minutes after buccal administration of midazolam to nonepileptic subjects (80). The clinical efficacy of buccal administration of the parenteral midazolam solution also has been demonstrated. In a non-blinded, randomized comparison in 42 patients, buccal midazolam stopped prolonged seizures in 75% of episodes, compared with a 59% response with rectal diazepam (*p* = .16) (81). The recommended dose of buccal midazolam is 0.2 mg/kg. Treatment is administered by parting the lips of the patient and squirting the solution between the cheek and gingiva. This route is advantageous over intranasal administration because the volume of drug need not be restricted. However, studies comparing the two routes have not been conducted. Both intranasal and buccal administration have advantages over rectal treatment with regard to ease of access and greater social acceptability.

Intramuscular Administration

Of the benzodiazepines available for intramuscular administration, midazolam is absorbed most rapidly. Peak plasma concentrations occur within 30 minutes and bioavailability is 90% (82). Suppression of interictal spikes in people with epilepsy is evident within 5 minutes of intramuscular administration (83).

In open-label use, intramuscular midazolam is effective for terminating status epilepticus in adults and children (84–86). Chamberlain and colleagues randomly assigned children with status epilepticus to intramuscular midazolam or intravenous diazepam and found both treatments to be equally effective for terminating seizures within 10 minutes of administration (overall, 92% response) (86). When the two treatments were compared with regard to time from patient arrival in the emergency department to cessation of seizures, midazolam was superior to diazepam (7.8 versus 11.2 minutes, respectively; *p* = .047) (86). Respiratory depression after intramuscular midazolam is rare, but has been reported (87). The recommended dose of intramuscular midazolam is 0.2 mg/kg.

SUMMARY

Status epilepticus is a neurologic emergency that requires prompt recognition and aggressive drug treatment. An organized, systematic approach to drug selection and administration results in more rapid control of seizures (88). Figure 14.4 gives a recommended approach to drug treatment. A comparable sequence of treatment and dosages may be used for status epilepticus in children. However, drug administration rates should be appropriately

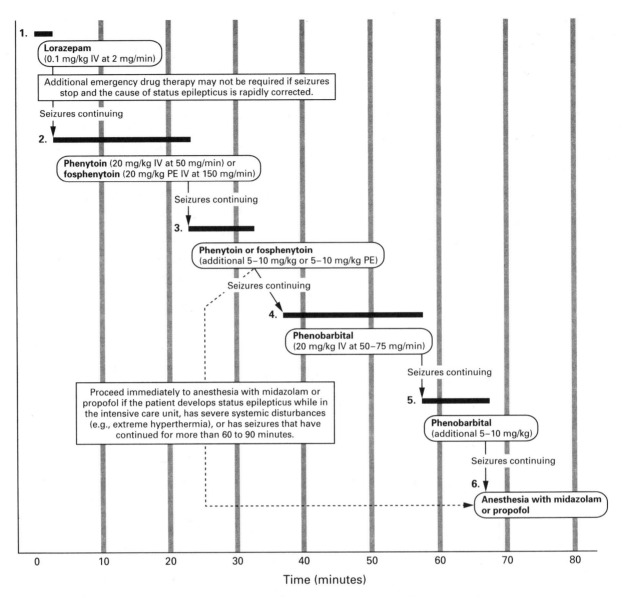

FIGURE 14.4. Antiepileptic drug therapy for status epilepticus in adults. Horizontal bars indicate approximate duration of drug infusions. Doses (mg/kg) are appropriate for children; however, infusion rates should be adjusted as follows: lorazepam 0.5 to 2 mg/min; phenytoin 1 mg/kg/min; fosphenytoin 3 mg/kg/min; phenobarbital 2 mg/kg/min. The maximal infusion rates recommended in adults should not be exceeded (89). (Reprinted from Lowenstein DH, Alldredge BK. Status epilepticus. *N Engl J Med* 1998;338:970–976, with permission.)

adjusted (89). When status epilepticus occurs outside of the hospital, several treatment options are available. Paramedic administration of intravenous lorazepam and diazepam has been shown to be safe and effective in adults. For out-of-hospital status epilepticus, this treatment approach is preferred. When emergency medical services are not available, transmucosal drug administration may be considered. Rectal diazepam, buccal midazolam, and intranasal midazolam have been reported to be effective in a variety of acute seizure conditions. However, experience with these therapies for the treatment of status epilepticus is limited.

REFERENCES

1. Lowenstein DH, Bleck T, Macdonald RL. It's time to revise the definition of status epilepticus. *Epilepsia* 1999;40:120–122.
2. DeLorenzo RJ, Hauser WA, Towne AR, et al. A prospective, population-based epidemiologic study of status epilepticus in Richmond, Virginia. *Neurology* 1996;46:1029–1035.
3. Theodore WH, Porter RJ, Albert P, et al. The secondarily generalized tonic-clonic seizure: a videotape analysis. *Neurology* 1994; 44:1403–1407.
4. Shinnar S, Berg AT, Moshe SL, et al. How long do new-onset seizures in children last? *Ann Neurol* 2001;49:659–664.

5. Lowenstein DH, Alldredge BK. Status epilepticus. *N Engl J Med* 1998;338:970–976.
6. Alldredge BK, Gelb AM, Isaacs SM, et al. A comparison of lorazepam, diazepam, and placebo for the treatment of out-of-hospital status epilepticus. *N Engl J Med* 2001;345:631–637.
7. Towne AR, Pellock JM, Ko D, et al. Determinants of mortality in status epilepticus. *Epilepsia* 1994;35:27–34.
8. Treiman DM. Therapy of status epilepticus in adults and children. *Curr Opin Neurol* 2001;14:203–210.
9. Working Group on Status Epilepticus. Treatment of convulsive status epilepticus: recommendations of the Epilepsy Foundation of America's Working Group on Status Epilepticus. *JAMA* 1993; 270:854–859.
10. Shorvon S. *Status epilepticus: its clinical features and treatment in children and adults.* Cambridge: Cambridge University Press, 1994.
11. Naora K, Shen DD. Mechanism of valproic acid uptake by isolated rat brain microvessels. *Epilepsy Res* 1995;22:97–106.
12. Meldrum BS, Brierley JB. Prolonged epileptic seizures in primates. *Arch Neurol* 1973;28:10–17.
13. Rowan AJ, Scott DF. Major status epilepticus: a series of 42 patients. *Acta Neurol Scand* 1970;46:573–584.
14. Lowenstein DH, Alldredge BK. Status epilepticus at an urban public hospital in the 1980s. *Neurology* 1993;43:483–488.
15. Aminoff MJ, Simon RP. Status epilepticus: causes, clinical features and consequences in 98 patients. *Am J Med* 1980;1980: 657–666.
16. Walton NY, Treiman DM. Response of status epilepticus induced by lithium and pilocarpine to treatment with diazepam. *Exp Neurol* 1988:267–275.
17. Walker MC. The epidemiology and management of status epilepticus. *Curr Opin Neurol* 1998;11:149–154.
18. Galvin GM, Jelineck GA. Midazolam: an effective intravenous agent for seizure control. *Arch Emerg Med* 1987;4:169–172.
19. George KA, Dundee JW. Relative amnestic actions of diazepam, flunitrazepam and lorazepam in man. *Br J Clin Pharmacol* 1977; 4:45–50.
20. Leppik IE, Derivan AT, Homan RW, et al. Double-blind study of lorazepam in status epilepticus. *JAMA* 1983;249:1452–1454.
21. Arendt RM, Greenblatt DJ, deJong RH, et al. In vitro correlates of benzodiazepine cerebrospinal fluid uptake, pharmacodynamic action and peripheral distribution. *J Pharmacol Exp Ther* 1983; 227:98–106.
22. Walton NY, Treiman DM. Lorazepam treatment of experimental status epilepticus in the rat: relevance to clinical practice. *Neurology* 1990;40:990–994.
23. Andermann F, Cendes F, Reiher J, et al. A prospective double-blind study of the effects of intravenously administered lorazepam and diazepam in the treatment of status epilepticus. *Epilepsia* 1992;33[Suppl 2]:3.
24. Greenblatt DJ, Divoll M. Diazepam versus lorazepam: relationship of drug distribution to duration of clinical action. In: Delgado-Escueta AV, Wasterlain CG, Treiman DM, et al., eds. *Status epilepticus: mechanisms of brain damage and treatment,* vol 34. New York: Raven Press, 1983:487–491.
25. Browne TR. The pharmacokinetics of agents used to treat status epilepticus. *Neurology* 1990;40[Suppl 2]:28–32.
26. Ramsay RE, Hammond EJ, Perchalski RJ, et al. Brain uptake of phenytoin, phenobarbital, and diazepam. *Arch Neurol* 1979;36: 535–539.
27. Booker HE, Celesia CG. Serum concentrations of diazepam with epilepsy. *Arch Neurol* 1973;29:191–194.
28. Naquet CF, Tutton JC, Smith BH. First attempt at treatment of experimental status epilepticus in animals and spontaneous status epilepticus in man with diazepam (Valium). *Electroencephalogr Clin Neurophysiol* 1965;18:427.
29. Bell DS. Dangers of treatment of status epilepticus with diazepam. *BMJ* 1969;1:159–161.
30. Wilder BJ, Ramsay RE, Willmore LJ, et al. Efficacy of intravenous phenytoin in the treatment of status epilepticus: kinetics of central nervous system penetration. *Ann Neurol* 1977;1: 511–518.
31. Treiman DM, Meyers PD, Walton NY, et al. A comparison of four treatments for generalized convulsive status epilepticus. *N Engl J Med* 1998;339:792–798.
32. Cranford RE, Leppik IE, Patrick B, et al. Intravenous phenytoin: clinical and pharmacokinetic aspects. *Neurology* 1978;28: 874–880.
33. Kugler AR, Knapp LE, Eldon MA. Attainment of therapeutic phenytoin concentrations following administration of loading doses of fosphenytoin: a metaanalysis. *Neurology* 1996;46 [Suppl]:A176.
34. Fischer JH, Allen FH, Runge J, et al. Fosphenytoin (Cerebyx) in status epilepticus: safety, tolerance, and pharmacokinetics. *Epilepsia* 1996;37[Suppl 5]:202.
35. Walton NY, Uthman BM, El Yafi K, et al. Phenytoin penetration into brain after administration of phenytoin or fosphenytoin. *Epilepsia* 1999;40:153–156.
36. Shaner DM, McCurdy SA, Herring MO, et al. Treatment of status epilepticus: a prospective comparison of diazepam and phenytoin versus phenobarbital and optional phenytoin. *Neurology* 1988;38:202–207.
37. Goldberg MA, McIntyre HB. Barbiturates in the treatment of status epilepticus. In: Delgado-Escueta AV, Wasterlain CG, Treiman DM, et al., eds. *Status epilepticus: mechanisms of brain damage and treatment.* New York: Raven Press, 1983:499–503.
38. Venkataraman V, Wheless JW. Safety of rapid intravenous infusion of valproate loading doses in epilepsy patients. *Epilepsy Res* 1999;35:147–153.
39. Yu KTT, Mills SM, Thompson NM. Safety and efficacy of intravenous valproate loading in pediatric status epilepticus and acute repetitive seizures. *Epilepsia* 2001;42[Suppl 7]:188–189.
40. Limdi N, Faught E. The safety of rapid valproic acid infusion. *Epilepsia* 2000;41:1342–1345.
41. Price DJ. Intravenous valproate: experience in neurosurgery. In: Chadwick D, ed. *Fourth international symposium on sodium valproate and epilepsy.* Jersey, UK: Royal Society of Medicine Services, 1989:197–203.
42. Naritoku DK, Sinha S. Outcome of status epilepticus treated with intravenous valproate. *Neurology* 2001;56[Suppl 3]: A235–A236.
43. Giroud M, Gras D, Escousse A, et al. Use of injectible valproic acid in status epilepticus: a pilot study. *Drug Invest* 1993;5: 154–159.
44. Uberall MA, Trollmann R, Wunsiedler U, et al. Intravenous valproate in pediatric epilepsy patients with refractory status epilepticus. *Neurology* 2000;54:2188–2189.
45. White JR, Santos CS. Intravenous valproate associated with significant hypotension in the treatment of status epilepticus. *J Child Neurol* 1999;14:822–823.
46. Sinha S, Naritoku DK. Intravenous valproate is well tolerated in unstable patients with status epilepticus. *Neurology* 2000;55: 722–724.
47. Walker IA, Slovis CM. Lidocaine in the treatment of status epilepticus. *Acad Emerg Med* 1997;4:918–922.
48. Pascual J, Cuidad J, Berciano J. Role of lidocaine (lignocaine) in managing status epilepticus. *J Neurol Neurosurg Psychiatry* 1992; 55:49–51.
49. Hellstrom-Westas L, Westgren U, Rosén I, et al. Lidocaine for treatment of severe seizures in newborn infants: I. clinical effects and cerebral activity monitoring. *Acta Paediatr Scand* 1988; 77:79–84.

50. Hellstrom-Westas L, Svenningsen NW, Westgren U, et al. Lidocaine for treatment of severe seizures in newborn infants: II. blood concentrations of lidocaine and metabolites during intravenous infusion. *Acta Paediatr Scand* 1992;81:35–39.
51. Bleck TP. Advances in the management of refractory status epilepticus. *Crit Care Med* 1993;21:955–957.
52. Prasad A, Worrall BB, Bertram EH, et al. Propofol and midazolam in the treatment of refractory status epilepticus. *Epilepsia* 2001;42:380–386.
53. Parent JP, Lowenstein DH. Treatment of refractory generalized status epilepticus with continuous infusion of midazolam. *Neurology* 1994;44:1837–1840.
54. Claassen J, Hirsch LJ, Emerson RG, et al. Continuous EEG monitoring and midazolam infusion for refractory nonconvulsive status epilepticus. *Neurology* 2001;57:1036–1042.
55. Naritoku DK, Sinha S. Prolongation of midazolam half-life after sustained infusion for status epilepticus. *Neurology* 2000;54:1366–1368.
56. Stecker MM, Kramer TH, Raps EC, et al. Treatment of refractory status epilepticus with propofol: clinical and pharmacokinetic findings. *Epilepsia* 1998;39:18–26.
57. Yaffe K, Lowenstein DH. Prognostic factors of pentobarbital therapy for refractory generalized status epilepticus. *Neurology* 1993;43:895–900.
58. Osorio I, Reed RC. Treatment of refractory generalized tonic-clonic status epilepticus with pentobarbital anesthesia after high-dose phenytoin. *Epilepsia* 1989;30:464–471.
59. Alldredge BK, Corry MD, Allen F, et al. Identification and management of out-of-hospital seizures by paramedics. *Epilepsia* 1998;39[Suppl 6]:70.
60. Lowenstein DH, Alldredge BK, Allen F, et al. The prehospital treatment of status epilepticus (PHTSE) study: design and methodology. *Control Clin Trials* 2001;22:290–309.
61. Valenzuela TD, Copass MK. Clinical research on out-of-hospital emergency care. *N Engl J Med* 2001;345:689–690.
62. Gottwald MD, Akers LC, Liu P-K, et al. Prehospital stability of diazepam and lorazepam. *Am J Emerg Med* 1999;17:333–337.
63. Alldredge BK, Wall DB, Ferriero DM. Effect of prehospital treatment on the outcome of status epilepticus in children. *Pediatr Neurol* 1995;12:213–216.
64. Shaner SA, Shanahan RJ. Intravenous diazepam administration by paramedics in the treatment of status epilepticus in children. *Ann Neurol* 1989;26:472–473.
65. Moolenaar F, Bakker S, Visser J, et al. Biopharmaceutics of rectal administration of drugs in man: IX. comparative biopharmaceutics of diazepam after single rectal, oral, intramuscular and intravenous administration in man. *Int J Pharmaceut* 1980;5:127–137.
66. Dulac O, Aicardi J, Rey E, et al. Blood levels of diazepam after single rectal administration in infants and children. *J Pediatr* 1978;93:109–141.
67. Knudsen FU. Plasma diazepam in infants after rectal administration in solution and by suppository. *Acta Paediatr Scand* 1977;66:563–567.
68. Dreifuss FE, Rosman NP, Cloyd JC, et al. A comparison of rectal diazepam gel and placebo for acute repetitive seizures. *N Engl J Med* 1998;338:1869–1875.
69. Hoppu K, Santavuori P. Diazepam rectal solution for home treatment of acute seizures in children. *Acta Paediatr Scand* 1981;70:369–372.
70. Lombroso CT. Intermittent home treatment of status and clusters of seizures. *Epilepsia* 1989;30[Suppl 2]:S11–S14.
71. Kriel RL, Cloyd JC, Hadsall RS, et al. Home use of rectal diazepam for cluster and prolonged seizures: efficacy, adverse reactions, quality of life, and cost analysis. *Pediatr Neurol* 1991;7:13–17.
72. Brown L, Bergen DC, Kotagal P, et al. Safety of Diastat when given at larger-than-recommended doses for acute repetitive seizures. *Neurology* 2001;56:1112.
73. Payne K, Mattheyse FJ, Liebenberg D, et al. The pharmacokinetics of midazolam in paediatric patients. *Eur J Clin Pharmacol* 1989;37:267–272.
74. Dooley JM, Tibbles JAR, Rumney PG, et al. Rectal lorazepam in the treatment of acute seizures in childhood. *Ann Neurol* 1985;18:412–413.
75. Rey E, Delaunay L, Pons G, et al. Pharmacokinetics of midazolam in children: comparative study of intranasal and intravenous administration. *Eur J Clin Pharmacol* 1991;41:355–357.
76. Lahat E, Goldman M, Barr J, et al. Intranasal midazolam for childhood seizures. *Lancet* 1998;352:620.
77. Scheepers M, Scheepers B, Clarke M, et al. Is intranasal midazolam an effective rescue medication in adolescents and adults with severe epilepsy? *Seizure* 2000;9:417–422.
78. Lahat E, Goldman M, Barr J, et al. Comparison of intranasal midazolam with intravenous diazepam for treating febrile seizures in children: prospective randomised study. *BMJ* 2000;321:83–86.
79. Schwagmeier R, Alincic S, Striebel HW. Midazolam pharmacokinetics following intravenous and buccal administration. *Br J Clin Pharmacol* 1998;46:203–206.
80. Scott RC, Besag FMC, Boyd SG, et al. Buccal absorption of midazolam: pharmacokinetics and EEG pharmacodynamics. *Epilepsia* 1998;39:290–294.
81. Scott RC, Besage FMC, Neville BGR. Buccal midazolam and rectal diazepam for treatment of prolonged seizures in childhood and adolescence: a randomized trial. *Lancet* 1999;353:623–626.
82. Bell DM, Richards G, Dhillon S, et al. A comparative pharmacokinetic study of intravenous and intramuscular midazolam in patients with epilepsy. *Epilepsy Res* 1991;10:183–190.
83. Jawad S, Oxley J, Wilson J, et al. A pharmacodynamic evaluation of midazolam as an antiepileptic compound. *J Neurol Neurosurg Psychiatry* 1986;49:1050–1054.
84. Mayhue FE. IM midazolam for status epilepticus in the emergency department. *Ann Emerg Med* 1988;17:643–645.
85. Egli M, Albani C. Relief of status epilepticus after i.m. administration of the new short-acting benzodiazepine midazolam (Dormicum). In: *12th World Congress of Neurology, Kyoto, Japan, September 20–25, 1981*. Amsterdam: Excerpta Medica, 1981, 44.
86. Chamberlain JM, Altieri MA, Futterman C, et al. A prospective, randomized study comparing intramuscular midazolam with intravenous diazepam for the treatment of seizures in children. *Pediatr Emerg Care* 1997;13:92–94.
87. Taylor JW, Simon KB. Possible intramuscular midazolam-associated cardiorespiratory arrest and death. *DICP Ann Pharmacother* 1990;24:695–697.
88. Gilbert KL. Evaluation of an algorithm for treatment of status epilepticus in adult patients undergoing video/EEG monitoring. *J Neurosci Nurs* 2000;32:101–107.
89. Hanhan UA, Fiallos MR, Orlowski JP. Status epilepticus. *Pediatr Clin North Am* 2001;48:683–694.

GENERAL PRINCIPLES

PREVENTION OF EPILEPTOGENESIS

ASLA PITKÄNEN

GENERAL PRINCIPLES OF EPILEPTOGENESIS

Epileptogenesis refers to the dynamic processes underlying the appearance and natural history of epilepsy (1). It is part of the "epileptic process" that can be divided into three phases: initial brain damaging insult → latency phase or epileptogenesis (no seizures) → appearance of spontaneous seizures (newly diagnosed epilepsy) (Figure 15.1). Various brain insults, including head trauma, stroke, encephalitis, or status epilepticus (SE) can cause neuronal damage and can initiate epileptogenesis (2). After a latency period that may last from weeks to months to years, spontaneous recurrent seizures begin, and the diagnosis of epilepsy is made. Finally, as experimental and human data show, neurobiologic changes as well as clinical symptoms can continue to be altered even after the spontaneous seizures have become recurrent.

In humans, epileptogenesis and the progressive aspects of epilepsy are best understood in patients with seizure onset in the temporal lobe. Moreover, most of the animal models of epileptogenesis mimic the generation of symptomatic temporal lobe epilepsy (TLE) in mature brain. Finally, experimental and clinical attempts to prevent epileptogenesis have focused on preventing symptomatic epilepsy with focal onset of seizures. Therefore, this chapter reviews the currently available strategies aimed at preventing epileptogenesis triggered by brain damage and the development of symptomatic TLE.

NEUROBIOLOGIC BASIS OF EPILEPTOGENESIS

Understanding neurobiologic changes underlying epileptogenesis at the molecular level is key to designing rational therapies to prevent epileptogenesis in patients who are at risk. The dearth of human samples emphasizes the importance of using adequate animal models in such studies. Kin-

Asla Pitkänen, MD, PhD: Professor of Neurobiology, A.I. Virtanen Institute, University of Kuopio, Kuopio, Finland

dling is perhaps the most often used model of epileptogenesis (3). *Kindling* refers to a phenomenon in which an initially subconvulsive stimulus eventually evokes seizures when it is administered repeatedly. Unlike in the genesis of symptomatic TLE in humans, however, in kindling, the following pertain: (a) the electrical stimulus is applied to a

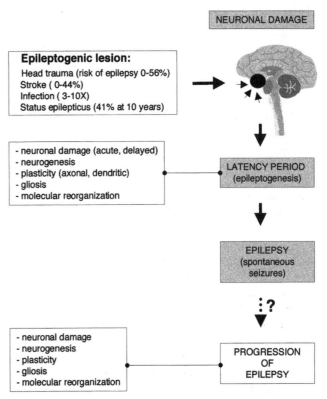

FIGURE 15.1. The epileptic process leading to the development of human symptomatic temporal lobe epilepsy includes three phases: brain injury (trauma, stroke, infection, status epilepticus) → latency period (epileptogenesis) → spontaneous seizures (epilepsy). Available data suggest that several parallel pathologic processes occur during epileptogenesis. These processes include neuronal damage (acute and delayed), plasticity (axonal and dendritic), gliosis, neurogenesis, and molecular reorganization. Some data suggest that remodeling of neuronal circuits continues after the spontaneous seizures begin (see text).

structurally *intact brain;* (b) the "epileptogenic phase" (development of kindling) includes *evoked seizures* that result in neuronal damage, axonal plasticity, and memory impairment; and finally, (c) the development of *spontaneous seizures is rare.* With these caveats in mind, kindling may actually model the progression of cryptogenic TLE better than the epileptogenesis preceding the occurrence of spontaneous seizures.

Experimental available data are from models in which epileptogenesis results in the occurrence of spontaneous seizures triggered by inducing SE either chemically, with kainic acid, pilocarpine, or lithium-pilocarpine, or electrically, by stimulating the amygdala, hippocampus, perforant pathway, or angular bundle. Data obtained from these models indicate that several neurobiologic events can progress in a parallel and serial manner during epileptogenesis. These events include neuronal damage, gliosis, axonal and dendritic plasticity, changes in the extracellular matrix, and molecular reorganization (Figure 15.1). The following discussion summarizes the major aspects of the reorganization of neuronal circuits occurring during epileptogenesis (4).

Neuronal Loss

In experimental models, SE that lasts for 30 to 40 minutes is long enough to induce neuronal loss and epileptogenesis. In addition to acute necrotic neuronal damage in various brain areas, SE induces delayed programmed cell death that can continue for several days or even weeks. Based on experimental data, activation of caspases by both intrinsic (mitochondrial origin) and extrinsic (death receptor–mediated) pathways is involved in programmed cell death.

Histologic findings, magnetic resonance (MR) imaging volumetry data, and MR spectroscopy data indicate that SE may also damage various regions of the human brain, including the hippocampus, amygdala, medial temporal cortex, striatum, thalamus, and cerebellum. An elevation in serum neuron-specific enolase (a marker of brain injury) after convulsive or nonconvulsive SE is another indicator favoring the idea that SE may cause structural damage to the human brain. In primates, an 82-minute duration of SE is enough to induce histologic damage, SE lasting 1.5 hours is sufficient to elevate serum neuron specific enolase, and SE lasting 45 to 72 minutes is enough to reduce hippocampal volume. Further, serial MR volumetry imaging studies of the hippocampus demonstrated that, after prolonged focal febrile seizures as well as after SE associated with encephalitis, the progression of hippocampal volume loss can continue for several months or years. Whether a direct relationship exists between the hippocampal damage and the development of TLE remains to be shown. It has been demonstrated, however, that the risk of later epileptogenesis is higher in individuals with SE associated with structural damage than in subjects without such damage (5). Taken together, these data provide a testable hypothesis

that neuroprotective treatment started during or after SE and targeted to alleviate delayed or programmed cell death will prevent epileptogenesis.

Axonal Plasticity

The best understood form of axonal plasticity in TLE is mossy fiber sprouting. Mossy fibers are granule cell axons that normally innervate hilar cells and the apical dendrites of CA3 pyramidal cells. Probably because of the death of their normal target neurons in the hilus and CA3 during the epileptic process, mossy fibers sprout and innervate postsynaptic targets in abnormal locations, including the granule cell dendrites in the inner molecular layer of the dentate gyrus and basal dendrites of CA3 pyramidal cells in the hippocampus proper. Through these contacts, granule cells form excitatory circuitries with adjacent granule cells in the epileptic brain.

The contribution of mossy fiber sprouting to the circuitry that generates spontaneous seizures as an end result of epileptogenesis has been questioned by several investigators (4). For example, axonal remodeling also occurs in the CA1 field of the hippocampus proper in experimental animals, as well as in the CA1 and the entorhinal cortex in humans. Otherwise, prevention of mossy fiber sprouting by cycloheximide, a protein synthesis inhibitor, does not prevent the development of epilepsy despite the prevention of mossy fiber sprouting. Further, the density of sprouting is not associated with the latency to the appearance of the spontaneous seizures or their frequency. In addition to the sprouting of excitatory axons, there are reports that the inhibitory axons may also sprout.

Assuming that the sprouting of excitatory axons and the formation of new synapses with other excitatory neurons are responsible for decreasing the seizure threshold and the development of spontaneous seizures, prevention or guidance of axonal sprouting forms an appealing target for the design of new antiepileptogenic compounds. In fact, previous attempts to prevent or delay epileptogenesis in kindling or spontaneous seizure models have revealed an association between the delay in epileptogenesis and the reduction in mossy fiber sprouting (see later). Whether a functional causality exists between the two phenomena remains to be shown. There is, however, also the possibility that manipulation of the naturally occurring plastic response compromises normal recovery (6).

Dendritic Plasticity

In addition to neuronal output regions (axons), neuronal input regions (dendrites) undergo morphologic plasticity in epilepsy. These include changes in spine number and morphology as well as in dendritic branching. According to observations in the rat pilocarpine model, plastic changes in spine morphology and density are dynamic (7). The density of spines in granule cells decreased by 95% within 2 weeks of the onset of SE. Some recovery occurs by the time spontaneous seizures appear.

Neurogenesis

The infragranular region in the adult dentate gyrus contains progenitor cells that may differentiate into neurons after single seizures or SE in rat models of TLE (8). Some of the newly formed neurons in the dentate gyrus have the immunochemical phenotype of granule cells, and they project to the CA3 subfield of the hippocampus. In contrast, investigators have described that some newly formed neurons along the hilar-CA3 border have the immunohistochemical phenotype and intrinsic electrophysiologic properties of granule cells, but they are synchronized with spontaneous rhythmic bursts of CA3 pyramidal cells of the hippocampus proper, and consequently they may contribute to the abnormal hyperexcitability in the epileptic hippocampus (9). Whether manipulation of the rate of neurogenesis modifies epileptogenesis remains to be investigated.

Gliosis

After neuronal damage by SE, the number and morphology of astrocytes expressing glial fibrillary acidic protein increase dramatically and chronically (10). Regulation of the extracellular microenvironment, in particular, buffering of extracellular potassium ion increases and clearance of glutamate by astrocytes, is critical for the control of neuronal excitability. Astrocytes can regulate synaptogenesis and neurite outgrowth as well as long-distance signaling through glial networks. The association of these astrocytic functions with epileptogenesis remains to be explored.

Activation of microglia occurs after various brain insults, such as SE or stroke, which are associated with epilepsy later in life. The proposed functions of microglial cells include the release of cytokines, proteases, reactive oxygen species, and nitrogen intermediates. Therefore, these cells are proposed to have a significant role in cell death processes after brain injury that can precipitate epileptogenesis. Manipulation of microglial function provides another route by which the severity of overall neuronal damage can be affected after brain-damaging insults such as stroke or SE that are associated with an enhanced risk of epilepsy later in life.

Molecular Reorganization

In situ hybridization, immunohistochemical tests, and high-output molecular screening techniques have demonstrated changes in the expression of many genes after SE and during epileptogenesis. For example, Nedivi and colleagues (11) estimated that 500 to 1,000 genes become expressed after kainate-induced SE. More recently, we analyzed hippocampal tissue in rats using complementary DNA arrays containing more than 5,000 genes. Tissue samples were collected 2 weeks after the onset of SE in animals that were monitored with videoelectroencephalography to confirm the induction of the epileptogenic phase. Our data indicate upregulation of 88 genes and downregulation of 32 genes. Of these, 27 have been previously described to be expressed in brain, seven have been shown to have role in epilepsy or seizures, and 16 are expressed in other pathologic conditions of the brain (12). It remains to be seen whether these data will guide us to an understanding of the molecular basis of previously described neurobiologic changes, such as neuronal damage, plasticity, gliosis, or neurogenesis occurring during epileptogenesis.

EFFECT OF CURRENTLY AVAILABLE ANTIEPILEPTIC DRUGS ON EPILEPTOGENESIS

Neuronal loss appears to be a common factor that precedes the appearance of spontaneous seizures after SE both in experimental models and humans. Therefore, we hypothesize that a compound would be antiepileptogenic in the following circumstances: (a) if it alleviates neuronal damage caused by brain insults that are associated with an increased risk of epilepsy later in life, even when its administration starts during or after the beginning of the insult (e.g., during ischemia or SE); (b) if the compound delays or suppresses the development of kindling; and finally, (c) if the compound prevents (or at least delays) the development of epilepsy in models, in which spontaneous seizures develop after brain damage (e.g., SE). Table 15.1 summarizes the neuroprotective and antiepileptogenic effects of currently available antiepileptic drugs (AEDs).

Neuroprotection after Brain Damaging Insults

Neuroprotective effects of most of the currently used AEDs have been tested in ischemia models. Both sodium channel blockers (carbamazepine, phenytoin, lamotrigine) and compounds enhancing γ-aminobutyric acid (GABA)ergic neurotransmission (clonazepam, tiagabine, topiramate, vigabatrin) alleviate ischemia-induced neuronal damage in rats when treatment is started during ischemia or soon after the beginning of reperfusion (Table 15.1). Surprisingly, fewer data are available regarding the neuroprotective effects of compounds used to treat SE or of AEDs on SE-induced damage (Table 15.1). Thus far, most of the compounds enhancing GABAergic transmission have a mild neuroprotective effect. In addition, treatment afterward with lamotrigine and valproate alleviates SE-induced neuronal loss.

TABLE 15.1. NEUROPROTECTIVE AND ANTIEPILEPTOGENIC EFFECTS OF DRUGS USED TO TREAT STATUS EPILEPTICUS OR SEIZURES IN HUMANS

Drug	Brain Damage Associated with an Increased Risk of Epilepsy		Epileptogenesis		Epilepsy
	Ischemia-induced Damage (Posttreatment)	SE-induced Damage (Posttreatment)	Development of Kindling (Pretreatment)	Development of Spontaneous Seizures (Posttreatment)	Seizure-induced Damage (Pretreatment)
SE medication					
Diazepam	↓ (34,35,36,68)	↓ (37)	↓ (38)	ND	↓ (39,67)
Enflurane	ND	ND	ND	ND	ND
Etomidate	ND	↓ (40)	ND	ND	ND
Halothane	ND	↓ (41)	ND	ND	ND
Isoflurane	ND	±0 (42)	ND	ND	ND
Lorazepam	ND	ND	ND	ND	ND
Midazolam	ND	ND	ND	ND	ND
Pentobarbitone	ND	ND	ND	ND	↓ (43)
Propofol	↓ (44)	↓ (45)	ND	ND	ND
Thiopentol	ND	ND	ND	ND	ND
Antiepileptic drug					
Carbamazepine	↓ (46)	ND	±0 or ↑ (38,47,48)	ND	±0 or ↓ (49,50,51)
Clobazam	ND	ND	↓ (38)	ND	ND
Clonazepam	↓ (52)	ND	↓ (38)	ND	ND
Ethosuximide	ND	ND	↓ (38)	ND	ND
Felbamate	↓ (53,54,55)	ND	ND	ND	ND
Gabapentin	ND	ND	ND	ND	ND
Lamotrigine	↓ (46,56,57,58)	↓ (59)	±0 or ↓ (60,61)	ND	↓ (59,62)
Levetiracetam	ND	ND	↓ (13)	ND	ND
Oxcarbazepine	ND	ND	±0 or ↑ (38,48)	ND	ND
Phenobarbital	ND	±0 or ↓ (63,64)	↑ (38,47)	±0 (16,63)	±0 or ↓ (63,65,67)
Phenytoin	±0 or ↓ (46,66)	ND	±0 or ↑ (38)	ND	±0 (67)
Primidone	ND	ND	ND	ND	ND
Tiagabine	↓ (68,69,70,71)	ND	↓ (72,73)	ND	↓ (74)
Topiramate	↓ (75,76)	↓ (77)	↓ (78)	ND	ND
Valproate	ND	↓ (16)	↓ (38,47)	↓ (?) (16)	±0 (67)
Vigabatrin	↓ (79)	±0 or ↓ (14,80,81)	↓ (82)	±0 (14,15)	↓ (51,83)
Zonisamide	ND	ND	ND	ND	ND

±0, no effect found; ↑, enhanced rate of kindling or more severe damage; ↓, decreased rate of kindling or less severe damage; ND, data not available; SE, status epilepticus.
Reference reporting the effect is indicated as a number in parenthesis. In all studies included in the Table, neuroprotective effect was assessed by using histologic techniques. Only data obtained in *in vivo* animal models are included in the table.

Delay of Kindling

Studies investigating the effects of AEDs on the development of kindling indicate that most of the sodium channel blockers do not delay the development of kindling, whereas all compounds enhancing GABAergic transmission do have such an effect (Table 15.1). However, when stimulation is reapplied after the drug washes out, the rats typically become kindled. This finding makes it difficult to assess whether AEDs have any direct effects on neurobiologic alterations leading to epileptogenesis or whether the delay of kindling is just associated with the suppression of afterdischarges. Levetiracetam, a newer compound with unknown mechanisms, also delays the development of kindling (13). Unlike any other compound, levetiracetam, used during the induction of kindling, shortens the dura-

tion of afterdischarges from 62 to 41 seconds and the duration of seizures from 53 to 34 seconds after kindling has been established following a washout period (13). Whether this finding predicts a disease-modifying effect of levetiracetam in experimental models with spontaneous seizures and in humans remains to be investigated.

Prevention of the Development of Spontaneous Seizures

Next one can hypothesize that compounds that alleviate neuronal damage caused by epileptogenic brain insults and also delay the development of kindling are the best candidate AEDs for the prevention of epileptogenesis and the development of spontaneous seizures after SE. These compounds include clonazepam, phenobarbital, valproate, lamotrigine, tiagabine, topiramate, and vigabatrin (Table 15.1). So far, phenobarbital, valproate, and vigabatrin have been tested. In one study, vigabatrin treatment (75 mg/kg/day) that was started 2 days after SE induced by amygdala stimulation in adult rats and was continued for 10 weeks had no clear antiepileptogenic effects. Moreover, seizure frequency and duration did not differ from those noted in vehicle-treated rats, a finding suggesting that vigabatrin administration during epileptogenesis has no disease-modifying effects (14). André, Marescaux, and Nehlig and coworkers did not demonstrate any antiepileptogenic effects of vigabatrin treatment (250 mg/kg/day) that was started after pilocarpine administration in the lithium-pilocarpine model (15). Bolanos et al. (16) investigated the antiepileptogenic effect of phenobarbital (70 mg/kg/day) and valproate (1200 mg/kg/day) in a kainic acid model in 35-day-old rats. Phenobarbital-treated rats developed spontaneous seizures like the vehicle-treated animals. The valproate-treated group, however, had no spontaneous seizures. In this study, only behaviorally generalized seizures were recorded, a practice that compromised the interpretation of the data because partial or subclinical electrographic seizures may have remained undetected.

Clinical trials aimed at preventing epileptogenesis in humans have tested the efficacy of prophylactic treatment with carbamazepine, phenytoin, and valproate in patients with head trauma (17) or valproate in patients with newly diagnosed tumors (18). As these studies demonstrate, there have been no beneficial effects. It is uncertain whether the lack of an effect in humans could have been predicted by preclinical animal studies because the compounds studied in spontaneous seizure models do not include, for example, phenytoin. Moreover, in experimental studies, epileptogenesis was induced by SE, whereas in human studies, the antiepileptogenic effect was assessed after head trauma.

AEDs have been designed to prevent the initiation and spread of spontaneous seizures; that is, they are expected to work on the neuronal circuits that have already undergone modifications, rather than on the networks in which the modifications preceding seizure occurrence are still ongoing. The difference in the molecular mechanisms of epileptogenesis and ictogenesis (seizure initiation) is probably a critical factor underlying the lack of an association between antiepileptic efficacy and antiepileptogenic effects.

OTHER APPROACHES USED TO PREVENT EPILEPTOGENESIS OR TO MODIFY THE SEVERITY OF DEVELOPING EPILEPSY

In addition to AEDs, several other treatment strategies have been attempted to prevent epileptogenesis in experimental models. In a kindling model, pretreatment with the *N*-methyl-D-aspartic acid (NMDA) antagonist MK-801 (19),

enhancement of noradrenergic transmission with intraperitoneal injection of epinephrine bitartrate (20), pretreatment with intraperitoneal injection of the immunosuppressant calcineurin inhibitors cyclosporine or FK506 (21), intrahippocampal injection of brain-derived neurotrophic factor (22) or blockade of receptor function with TrkB receptor bodies (23), intracerebroventricular infusion of nerve growth factor antibodies (24), and intrahippocampal administration of peptides blocking the nerve growth factor receptor (25) prevent or delay kindling and associated plastic changes in the mossy fiber pathway.

Contrary to the idea of using compounds that suppress neuronal activity (e.g., AEDs), several studies indicate that the stimulation of neuronal activity using sensory stimuli, environmental enrichment, or electrically generated stimuli reduces neuronal damage and epileptogenesis in spontaneous seizure models and also delays the development of kindling (26). Finally, experiments using gene therapy to increase the expression of proteins restoring energy metabolism or blocking programmed cell death (27), as well as vaccination against NMDA-type glutamate receptors (28) to protect brain from stroke or SE-induced injury, provide novel ideas to be tested in experimental antiepileptogenesis trials.

Even though no treatments convincingly prevent or reduce the risk of epileptogenesis after brain injury, some treatments do have disease-modifying effects. For example, a ketogenic diet (29) and intraventricular administration of basic fibroblast growth factor (30), started during or after kainate-induced SE, reduced the frequency and duration of spontaneous seizures, even though these regimens did not prevent the development of epilepsy in all animals. Moreover, mice chronically treated with an L-type calcium channel blocker (nicarpidine) starting at the time of pilocarpine-induced SE had milder cognitive deterioration than did vehicle-treated controls (31).

The conspicuous heterogeneity of approaches that have been tested to prevent epileptogenesis in experimental models is indicative of the lack of understanding of the underlying mechanisms of the disease. Breakthroughs in our understanding of the molecular mechanisms of epileptogenesis are necessary for rational systematic attempts to prevent epilepsy after brain injury in the future.

DO NEUROBIOLOGIC ALTERATIONS UNDERLYING EPILEPTOGENESIS CONTINUE AFTER THE BEGINNING OF SPONTANEOUS SEIZURES?

Data from experimental and human studies suggest that the different categories of neurobiologic alterations occurring during SE-induced epileptogenesis can be induced by brief seizures that typically last for less than 2 minutes (4). Using stereologic cell counting methods, silver staining techniques, markers of apoptosis, or immunohistochemical staining of subpopulations of neurons, several laboratories have reported that even a few brief seizures can induce neuronal damage in the amygdala and the hilus of the dentate gyrus in the kindling model of TLE in rat. The severity of damage correlates with the number of seizures the animal has experienced. In humans, histologic analyses, MR imaging volumetry, and MR spectroscopy, as well as serum neuron-specific enolase studies, suggest that recurrent seizures induce progressive damage. Further, programmed cell death contributes to seizure-induced damage in rats and probably also in humans (32). In all these studies, only a subpopulation of patients with drug-refractory seizures had progressive damage. Whether this is related to the genotype of the patient or to other factors remains to be explored.

In addition to neuronal damage, the density of mossy fiber sprouting increases according to the number of seizures in the kindling model. Similarly, data provide evidence that sprouting may be an ongoing phenomenon in the human dentate gyrus (33) and the entorhinal cortex (4). Whether ongoing axonal remodeling is related to the progressive neuronal loss or seizure-induced stimulation of axonal plasticity remains to be determined. Brief kindled seizures in adult rats may induce differentiation of progenitor cells into neurons in the infragranular region of the dentate gyrus. One sees increased astrocytosis and activated microglia in samples taken from kindled animals or in patients operated on for drug-refractory TLE. Finally, seizures induce alterations in the expression of certain molecular markers.

Taken together, extensive evidence favors the idea that molecular, cellular, and network reorganization continues after the diagnosis of epilepsy, particularly in patients who are not free of seizures. More data are, however, needed to link each of these alterations with the progression in the frequency or type of seizures, as well as with the progression of other symptoms, such as memory impairment in individual patients. If there is a connection, therapeutic prevention of such modifications in patients who are not seizure free would require consideration.

Another question is whether there is any evidence that ongoing treatments have any neuroprotective or disease-modifying effects in patients who continue to have seizures. Previous studies of the neuroprotective effects of AEDs indicate that pretreatment with phenobarbital, tiagabine, lamotrigine, and vigabatrin alleviates SE-induced neuronal damage, even though these drugs do not completely suppress seizure activity (Table 15.1). Conversely, compounds delaying the development of kindling could also have a disease-modifying effect if they would shorten the seizure duration (Table 15.1). As my colleagues and I have demonstrated, carbamazepine and valproate shorten the duration of spontaneous seizures in an amygdala stimulation model in rat (unpublished). Whether long-term use will provide neuroprotective or seizure-shortening effects that will trans-

late into a functional benefit for drug-refractory patients with epilepsy remains to be studied.

FUTURE PERSPECTIVES

Prevention of epileptogenesis is a major challenge for specialists in epilepsy. More data are needed to fill in the lacunae of our current knowledge about the natural course of epileptogenesis in humans and about markers that can be used to identify those who are at highest risk. Development of new experimental models that better mimic human epileptogenesis after experimental stroke, head trauma, or encephalitis or meningitis will provide tools to answer certain questions, such as the following: How similar are the molecular mechanisms of epileptogenesis after various brain insults? Preclinical testing using these models may also better predict the antiepileptogenic efficacy of new treatments in seizures of different origins. Appreciation that epileptogenesis and ictogenesis have very different neurobiologic bases will undoubtedly guide researchers toward the discovery of compounds that more selectively target epileptogenic, rather than ictogenic, mechanisms. Considering that different molecular pathways are activated in parallel during epileptogenesis, it remains to be seen whether future antiepileptogenic treatment will consist of monotherapy or polytherapy.

Neuroprotection appears to be a critical component related to epileptogenesis. Whether alleviation of neuronal loss after brain-damaging insults will result in a delay or prevention of epileptogenesis remains a testable hypothesis. Otherwise, continuous remodeling of neuronal circuitries in established epilepsy, at least in some drug-refractory patients, will challenge the future treatment of epilepsy to include not only the antiepileptic effect but also features such as neuroprotection.

REFERENCES

1. Engel J Jr. *Seizures and epilepsy.* Philadelphia: FA Davis, 1989: 221–239.
2. Hauser WA. Incidence and prevalence. In: *Epilepsy: a comprehensive textbook.* Philadelphia: Lippincott–Raven, 1997:47–57.
3. Goddard GV, McIntyre DC, Leech CK. A permanent change in brain function resulting from daily electrical stimulation. *Exp Neurol* 1969;25:295–330.
4. Pitkänen A, Salmenperä T, Partanen K et al. Seizure-induced damage to the medial temporal lobe: association with impairment in emotional behavior and memory performance. In: Sillanpää M, Gram L, Johannessen SI, et al., eds. *Epilepsy and mental retardation.* Petersfield, UK: Wrightson Biomedical Publishing, 1999:147–163.
5. Hesdorffer DC, Logroscino G, Cascino G, et al. Risk of unprovoked seizure after acute symptomatic seizure: effect of status epilepticus. *Ann Neurol* 1998;44:908—912.
6. Hernandez TD. Preventing post-traumatic epilepsy after brain injury: weighting costs and benefits of anticonvulsant prophylaxis. *Trends Pharmacol Sci* 1997;18:59–62.
7. Isokawa M. Remodelling dendritic spines of dentate granule cells

in temporal lobe epilepsy patients and the rat pilocarpine model. *Epilepsia* 2000;41[Suppl 6]:S14–S17.

8. Parent JM, Yy TW, Leibowitz RT, et al. Dentate granule cell neurogenesis is increased by seizures and contributes to aberrant network reorganization in the adult rat hippocampus. *J Neurosci* 1997;17:3727–3738.

9. Scharfman HE, Goodman JH, Sollas AL. Granule-like neurons at the hilar/CA3 border after status epilepticus and their synchrony with area CA3 pyramidal cells: functional implications of seizure-induced neurogenesis. *J Neurosci* 2000;20: 6144–6158.

10. Heinemann U, Gabriel S, Schuchmann S, et al. Contribution of astrocytes to seizure activity. *Adv Neurol* 1999;79:583–590.

11. Nedivi E, Hevroni D, Naot D, et al. Numerous candidate plasticity-related genes revealed by differential cDNA cloning. *Nature* 1993;363:718–722.

12. Lukasiuk K, Pitkänen A. Analysis of changes in gene expression during the period of epileptogenesis in the rat model of temporal lobe epilepsy using high density cDNA arrays. *Eur J Neurosci* 2000;12 [Suppl 11];209(abst).

13. Löscher W, Hönack D, Rundfeldt C. Antiepileptogenic effects of the novel anticonvulsant levetiracetam (ucb L059) in the kindling model of temporal lobe epilepsy. *J Pharmacol Exp Ther* 1998;284:474–479.

14. Halonen T, Nissinen J, Pitkänen A. Chronic elevation of brain GABA levels beginning two days after status epilepticus does not prevent epileptogenesis in rats. *Neuropharmacology* 2001;

15. André V, Ferrandon A, Marescaux C, Nehlig A. Vigabatrin protects against hippocampal damage but is not antiepileptogenic in the lithium-pilocarpine model of temporal lobe epilepsy. *Epilepsy Res* 2001;47:99–117.

16. Bolanos AR, Sarkisian M, Yang Y, et al. Comparison of valproate and phenobarbital treatment after status epilepticus in rats. *Neurology* 1998;51:41–48.

17. Temkin NR, Dikmen SS, Winn HR. Clinical trials for seizure prevention. *Adv Neurol* 1998;76:179–188.

18. Glantz MJ, Cole BF, Friedberg MH, et al. A randomized, blinded, placebo-controlled trial of divalproex sodium prophylaxis in adults with newly diagnosed brain tumors. *Neurology* 1996;46:985–991.

19. Sutula T, Koch J, Golarai G, et al. NMDA receptor dependence of kindling and mossy fiber sprouting: evidence that the NMDA receptor regulates patterning of hippocampal circuits in the adult brain. *J Neurosci* 1996;16:7398–7406.

20. Welsh KA, Gold PE. Epinephrine proactive retardation of amygdala-kindled epileptogenesis. *Behav Neurosci* 1986;100:236–245.

21. Moya LJMP, Matsui H, de Barros GAM, et al. Immunosuppressants and calcineurin inhibitors, cyclosporin A and FK506, reversibly inhibit epileptogenesis in amygdaloid kindled rat. *Brain Res* 1994;648:337–341.

22. Osehobo P, Adams B, Sazgar M, et al. Brain-derived neurotrophic factor infusion delays amygdala and perforant path kindling without affecting paired-pulse measures of neuronal inhibition in adult rats. *Neuroscience* 1999;92:1367–1375.

23. Binder DK, Routbort MJ, Ryan TE, et al. Selective inhibition of kindling development by intraventricular administration of trkB receptor body. *J Neurosci* 1999;19:1424–1436.

24. Van der Zee CEEM, Rashid K, Le K, et al. Intraventricular administration of antibodies to nerve growth factor retards kindling and blocks mossy fiber sprouting in adult rats. *J Neurosci* 1995;15:5613–5323.

25. Rashid K, Van der Zee EEM, Ross GM, et al. A nerve growth factor peptide retards seizure development and inhibits neuronal sprouting in a rat model of epilepsy. *Proc Natl Acad Sci USA* 1995;92:9495–9499.

26. Kelly ME, McIntyre DC. Hippocampal kindling protects several structures from the neuronal damage resulting from kainic acid-induced status epilepticus. *Brain Res* 1994:634:245–256.

27. McLaughlin J, Roozendaal B, Dumas T, et al. Sparing of neuronal function postseizure with gene therapy. *Proc Natl Acad Sci USA* 2000;97:12804–12809.

28. During MJ, Symes CW, Lawlor PA, et al. An oral vaccine against NMDAR1 with efficacy in experimental stroke and epilepsy. *Science* 2000;287:1453–1460.

29. Muller-Schwarze AB, Tandon P, Liu Z, et al. Ketogenic diet reduces spontaneous seizures and mossy fiber sprouting in the kainic acid model. *Neuroreport* 1999;10:1517–1522.

30. Liu Z, Holmes GL. Basic fibroblast growth factor is highly neuroprotective against seizure-induced long-term behavioral deficits. *Neuroscience* 1997;76:1129–1138.

31. Ikegaya Y, Nishiyama N, Matsuki N. L-type Ca^{2+}-channel blocker inhibits mossy fiber sprouting and cognitive deficits following pilocarpine seizures in immature mice. *Neuroscience* 2000; 98:647–659.

32. Henshall DC, Clark RSB, Adelson PD, et al. Alterations in bcl-2 and caspase gene family protein expression in human temporal lobe epilepsy. *Neurology* 2000;55:250–257.

33. Proper EA, Oestreicher AB, Jansen GH, et al. Immunohistochemical characterization of mossy fiber sprouting in the hippocampus of patients with pharmaco-resistant temporal lobe epilepsy. *Brain* 2000;123:19–30.

34. Schwartz RD, Huff RA, Yu X, et al. Postischemic diazepam is neuroprotective in the gerbil hippocampus. *Brain Res* 1994;647: 153–160.

35. Schwartz RD, Yu X, Katzman MR, et al. Diazepam, given postischemia, protects selectively vulnerable neurons in the rat hippocampus and striatum. *J Neurosci* 1995;15:529–539.

36. Voll CL, Auer RN. Postischemic seizures and necrotizing ischemic brain damage: neuroprotective effects of postischemic diazepam and insulin. *Neurology* 1991;41:423–428.

37. Ben-Ari Y, Tremblay E, Ottersen OP, et al. The role of epileptic activity in hippocampal and "remote" cerebral lesions induced by kainic acid. *Brain Res* 1980;191:79–97.

38. Schmutz M, Klebs K, Baltzer V. Inhibition or enhancement kindling evolution by antiepileptics. *J Neural Transm* 1988;72: 245–257.

39. Ben-Ari Y, Tremblay E, Ottersen OP, et al. Evidence suggesting secondary epileptogenic lesions after kainic acid: pretreatment with diazepam reduces distant but not local brain damage. *Brain Res* 1979;165:362–365.

40. Lee J, Kim D, Hong H, et al. Protective effect of etomidate on kainic acid–induced neurotoxicity in rat hippocampus. *Neurosci Lett* 2000;286:179–182.

41. Walker MC, Perry H, Scaravilli PN, et al. Halothane as a neuroprotectant during constants stimulation of the perforant path. *Epilepsia* 1999;40:359–364.

42. Kawaguchi M, Kimbro JR, Drummond JC, et al. Isoflurane delays but does not prevent cerebral infarction in rats subjected to focal ischemia. *Anesthesiology* 2000;92:1335–1342.

43. Lee MG, Chou JY, Lee KH, et al. MK-801 augments pilocarpine-induced electrographic seizure but protects against brain damage in rats. *Prog Neuropsychopharmacol Biol Psychiatry* 1997; 21:331–344.

44. Young Y, Menon DK, Tisavipat N, et al. Propofol neuroprotection in a rat model of ischemia reperfusion injury. *Eur J Anaesthesiol* 1997;14:320–326.

45. Ahuja S, Germano IM. Anticonvulsant and neonatal protective effects of propofol on experimental status epilepticus. *J Epilepsy* 1998;11:168–176.

46. Rataud J, Debarnot F, Mary V, et al. Comparative study of voltage-sensitive sodium channel blockers in focal ischemia and electric convulsions in rodents. *Neurosci Lett* 1994;172:19–23.

47. Silver JM, Shin C, McNamara JO. Antiepileptogenic effects of conventional anticonvulsants in the kindling model of epilepsy. *Ann Neurol* 1991;29:356–363.

48. Weiss SRB, Post RM. Carbamazepine and carbamazepine-10,11-epoxide inhibit amygdala-kindled seizures in the rat but do not block their development. *Clin Neuropharmacol* 1987;10:272–279.

49. Lahtinen H, Ylinen A, Lukkarinen U, et al. Failure of carbamazepine to prevent behavioural and histopathological sequels of experimentally induced status epilepticus. *Eur J Pharmacol* 1996;297:213–218.

50. Vezzani A, Wu HQ, Angelico P, et al. Quinolinic acid-induced seizures, but not nerve cell death, are associated with extracellular Ca^{2+} decrease assessed in the hippocampus by brain dialysis. *Brain Res* 1988;454:289–297.

51. Pitkänen A, Tuunanen J, Halonen T. Vigabatrin and carbamazepine have different efficacies in the prevention of status epilepticus induced neuronal damage in the hippocampus and amygdala. *Epilepsy Res* 1996;24:29–45.

52. Marciani MG, Santone G, Sancesario G, et al. Protective effects of clonazepam on ischemic brain damage induced by 10-minute bilateral carotid occlusion in Mongolian gerbils. *Funct Neurol* 1993;8:114–119.

53. Wasterlain CG, Adams LM, Schwartz PH, et al. Posthypoxic treatment with felbamate is neuroprotective in a rat model of hypoxia-ischemia. *Neurology* 1993;43:2303–2310.

54. Bertorelli R, Smirne S, Adami M, et al. Neuroprotective effects of felbamate on global ischemia in Mongolian gerbils. *Pharmacol Res* 1996;34:59—64.

55. Wasterlain CG, Adams LM, Wichmann JK, et al. Felbamate protects CA1 neurons from apoptosis in a gerbil model of global ischemia. *Stroke* 1996;27:1236–1240.

56. Shuaib AS, Mahmood RH, Wishart T, et al. Neuroprotective effects of lamotrigine in global ischemia in gerbils: a histological, *in vivo* microdialysis and behavioral study. *Brain Res* 1995;702:199–206.

57. Crumrine RC, Bergstrand K, Cooper AT, et al. Lamotrigine protects hippocampal CA1 neurons from ischemic damage after cardiac arrest. *Stroke* 1997;28:2230–2237.

58. Smith SE, Meldrum BS. Cerebroprotective effect of lamotrigine after focal ischemia in rats. *Stroke* 1995;26:117–122.

59. Halaney T, Nissinen J, Pitkänen A. Effect of lamotrigine treatment on status epilepticus-induced neuronal damage and memory impairment in rats. *Epilepy Res* 2001;46:205–223.

60. O'Donnell RA, Miller AA. The effect of lamotrigine upon development of cortical kindled seizures in the rat. *Neuropharmacology* 1991;30:253–258.

61. Stratton SC, Large CH, Cox B, Davies G, Hagan RM. Antiepileptogenic-like effects of lamotrigine in a rat amygdala model. *Epilepsy Res* 2002, in press.

62. Maj R, Fariello RG, Ukmar G, et al. PNU-151774E protects against kainate-induced status epilepticus and hippocampal lesions in the rat. *Eur J Pharmacol* 1998;359:27–32.

63. Mikati MA, Holmes GL, Chronopoulos, A et al. Phenobarbital modifies seizure-related brain injury in the developing brain. *Ann Neurol* 1994;36:425–433.

64. Sutula T, Cavazos J, Golarai G. Alteration of long-lasting structural and functional effects of kainic acid in the hippocampus by brief treatment with phenobarbital. *J Neurosci* 1992;12:4173–4187.

65. Ault B, Gruenthal M, Amstrong DR, et al. Efficacy of baclofen and phenobarbital against the kainic acid limbic seizure-brain damage syndrome. *J Pharmacol Exp Ther* 1986;239:612–617.

66. Hayakawa T, Hamada Y, Maihara T, et al. Phenytoin reduces neonatal hypoxic-ischemic brain damage in rats. *Life Sci* 1994;54:387–392.

67. Fuller TA, Olney JW. Only certain anticonvulsants protect against kainate neurotoxicity. *Neurobehav Toxicol Teratol* 1981;3:355–361.

68. Johansen FF, Diemer DH. Enhancement of GABA neurotransmission after cerebral ischemia in the rat reduces loss of hippocampal CA1 pyramidal cells. *Acta Neurol Scand* 1991;84:1–6.

69. Inglefield JR, Perry JM, Schwartz RD. Postischemic inhibition of GABA reuptake by tiagabine slows neuronal death in the gerbil hippocampus. *Hippocampus* 1995;5:460–468.

70. Chen Xu W, Yi Y, Qiu L, et al. Neuroprotective activity of tiagabine in a focal embolic model of cerebral ischemia. *Brain Res* 2000;874:75–77.

71. Yang Y, Li Q, Wang CX, et al. Dose-dependent neuroprotection with tiagabine in a focal cerebral ischemia model in rat. *NeuroReport* 2000;11:2307–2311.

72. Dalby NO, Nielsen EB. Tiagabine exerts an anti-epileptogenic effect in amygdala kindling epileptogenesis in the rat. *Neurosci Lett* 1997;229:135–137.

73. Morimoto K, Sato H, Yamamoto Y, et al. Antiepileptic effects of tiagabine, a selective GABA uptake inhibitor, in the rat kindling model of temporal lobe epilepsy. *Epilepsia* 1997;38:966–974.

74. Halonen T, Nissinen J, Jansen JA, et al. Tiagabine prevents seizures, neuronal damage and memory impairment in experimental status epilepticus. *Eur J Pharmacol* 1996;299:69–81.

75. Lee SR, Kim SP, Kim JE. Protective effect of topiramate against hippocampal neuronal damage after global ischemia in the gerbils. *Neurosci Lett* 2000;281:183–186.

76. Yang YY, Shuaib A, Li Q, et al. Neuroprotection by delayed administration of topiramate in a rat model of middle cerebral artery embolization. *Brain Res* 1998;804:169–176.

77. Niebauer M, Gruenthal M. Topiramate reduces neuronal injury after experimental status epilepticus. *Brain Res* 1999;837:263–269.

78. Amano K, Hamada K, Yagi K, et al. Antiepileptic effects of topiramate on amygdaloid kindling in rats. *Epilepsy Res* 1998:31:123–128.

79. Shuaib A, Murabit MA, Kanthan R, et al. The neuroprotective effects of gamma-vinyl GABA in transient global ischemia: a morphological study with early and delayed evaluations. *Neurosci Lett* 1996;204:1–4.

80. Pitkänen A, Jolkkonen E, Nissinen J, et al. Effect of vigabatrin treatment on status epilepticus -induced neuronal damage and mossy fiber sprouting in the rat hippocampus. *Epilepsy Res* 1999;33:67–85.

81. Jolkkonen J, Halonen T, Jolkkonen E, et al. Seizure-induced damage to the hippocampus is prevented by modulation of the GABAergic system. *Neuroreport* 1996;7:2031–2035.

82. Shin C, Rigsbee LC, McNamara JO. Anti-seizure and antiepileptogenic effect of (γ-vinyl (γ-aminobutyric acid in amygdaloid kindling. *Brain Res* 1986;398:370–374.

83. Ylinen AMA, Miettinen R, Pitkänen A, et al. Enhanced GABAergic inhibition preserves hippocampal structure and function in a model of epilepsy. *Proc Natl Acad Sci USA* 1991:88:7650–7653.

BENZODIAZEPINES

BENZODIAZEPINES

MECHANISMS OF ACTION

ROBERT L. MACDONALD

Benzodiazepines (BDZs) are used as anticonvulsant drugs primarily to treat status epilepticus and to terminate serial seizures, but they are also used clinically for antianxiety, as muscle relaxants, and for their hypnotic activity. The primary target of BDZs is a receptor for the neutral amino acid γ-aminobutyric acid (GABA). GABA, the major inhibitory neurotransmitter in the central nervous system, is released from GABAergic neurons and binds to both GABA$_A$ receptors (GABARs) and GABA$_B$ receptors. The GABAR is a macromolecular protein that forms a chloride ion–selective channel and contains binding sites for GABA, anticonvulsant BDZs and barbiturates, anesthetic steroids, and the convulsant β-carbolines and picrotoxin (26,47,49) (Figure 16.1; Table 16.1). The GABA$_B$ receptor does not form an ion channel but is coupled by guanosine triphosphate binding proteins to calcium or potassium ion channels. BDZs enhance GABAR-mediated inhibition but do not alter GABA$_B$ receptor-mediated inhibition.

BENZODIAZEPINES ENHANCE GABAERGIC INHIBITION BY BINDING TO BENZODIAZEPINE RECEPTORS

An effect of BDZs on GABAergic inhibition was initially suggested by finding that diazepam enhanced presynaptic inhibition in the cat spinal cord (70), and it was further supported by the finding that diazepam had a GABA-mimetic action on cerebellar cyclic guanosine monophosphate content (21,22). The first direct demonstration that BDZs enhance postsynaptic GABA responses was made using vertebrate spinal cord neurons in cell culture (20,44). Based on the direct effect of diazepam and chlordiazepoxide on GABA responses, it was suggested that BDZs interact directly with a postsynaptic GABA receptor to enhance GABA receptor current by an allosteric mechanism.

The basis for the interaction of BDZs with GABARs was established when a BDZ binding site on the GABAR (the BDZ receptor) was discovered and was characterized (54,81) (Figure 16.1). The BDZ receptor represented the site for BDZs to enhance GABAR current allosterically. The demonstration of high-affinity BDZ binding to mammalian brain fractions and the reciprocal interaction of GABA and BDZ binding were consistent with the physiologic demonstration that BDZs were acting by direct modulation of GABAR function (31,44,81,84).

However, the nature of the BDZ receptor was shown to be more complex by the discovery of compounds that bound to the BDZ receptor but had unexpected actions (10,11). The ethyl ester of β-carboline-3-carboxylate was isolated from human urine and rat brain and was shown to displace [^{3}H]diazepam potently from BDZ receptors. However, this and related β-carbolines were shown to reduce GABAR current and to be convulsant and anxiogenic despite their binding to the BDZ receptor. Thus, these compounds were described as *inverse agonists*. In addition, an imidazobenzodiazepine, flumazenil, was shown to bind to BDZ receptors but to have little intrinsic activity and thus appeared to be a BDZ receptor antagonist. Furthermore, compounds with partial agonist or partial antagonist activities were described (11). Thus, the BDZ receptor can effectively increase (BDZ agonist action) or decrease (BDZ inverse agonist action) postsynaptic GABAergic inhibition, depending on the nature of the BDZ receptor ligand (9).

In addition to binding BDZ receptor ligands with positive and negative efficacy, the BDZ receptor was shown to exist in multiple forms. Triazolopyridazines such as CL 218,872 were shown to displace [^{3}H]flunitrazepam more potently from cerebellar than from hippocampal membranes, a finding suggesting the existence of BZ1 (CL 218,872–sensitive) and BZ2 (CL 218,872–insensitive) receptors (39). Both BZ1 and BZ2 receptors were coupled to the GABA binding site, thus suggesting GABAR heterogeneity.

Robert L. Macdonald, MD, PhD: Professor and Chairman, Department of Neurology, Vanderbilt University, Nashville, Tennessee

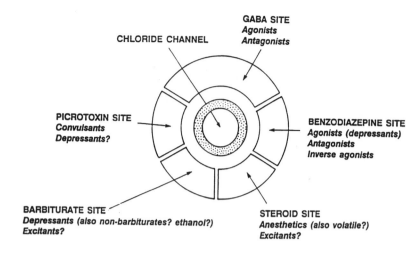

FIGURE 16.1. Schematic "donut" model of the GABA_A receptor-chloride ion channel complex. Each of the sections represents a distinct functional binding domain for the drug class indicated, as well as the chloride channel itself in the middle. No implications about the protein subunit structure are made in this model. (From Olsen RW, Sapp DM, Bureau MH, et al. Allosteric actions of CNS depressants including anesthetics on subtypes of the inhibitory GABA_A receptor-chloride channel complex. In: Rubin E, Miller KW, Roth SH, eds. Molecular and cellular mechanisms of alcohol and anesthetics. *Ann NY Acad Sci* 1991;625:145–154, with permission.)

MOLECULAR BIOLOGY OF GABA RECEPTORS

Our understanding of the molecular biology of GABARs evolved rapidly in the 1990s. The molecular structure of the GABAR was determined by photoaffinity labeling the GABAR with the BDZ [³H]flunitrazepam (54,75). Initially, a single 51-kd polypeptide was specifically labeled in crude brain homogenates. Subsequently, additional 53-, 55-, and 59-kd BDZ binding polypeptides were obtained and were shown to vary among brain regions, during development, in one-dimensional peptide mapping of proteolytic fragments, and in binding specificity (73), consistent with the presence of a family of gene products. This conclusion was subsequently confirmed by molecular cloning.

The GABAR was then purified (76), and it was demonstrated that the purified receptor bound BDZs and muscimol and was composed of two subunits, an α subunit and a β subunit (78). Photoaffinity labeling demonstrated that α subunits were labeled with BDZs and β subunits were

labeled with GABA agonists (18,37,38). Immunolabeling, immunoprecipitation, and Western blot analysis of GABA and BDZ binding sites demonstrated conservation of GABARs within different brain regions and across species (32,52). Subsequently, microheterogeneity of both subunits was observed by protein staining, photoaffinity labeling, and immunoblotting (15,16,30,57). What originally appeared to be two polypeptide bands actually contained more than a dozen polypeptides of similar size.

Purification of bovine GABAR α and β subunits allowed Barnard and colleagues to clone the complementary DNA (cDNA) sequences (71). Several important features were initially identified in these two subunits but were later found in all subsequent GABAR subunits (Figure 16.2). First, both subunit proteins were homologous to each other, having approximately 35% amino acid identity, and they had conserved hydropathy profiles, a finding suggesting a conserved transmembrane topology and common evolution. This general structure was similar to the four-transmembrane domain model of the nicotinic cholinergic receptor (nAchR) (58), a finding suggesting that these receptors (and later glycine and serotonin receptors) formed a supergene family of ligand-gated ion channels. Second, there existed a β-structural loop formed from the disulfide linkage of two cysteine residues that were 14 amino acids apart in the *N*-terminal segment of the proteins. Third, numerous sites for *N*- and *O*-linked glycosylation were identified in the *N*-terminal segment of the proteins. Finally, there was a high concentration of Thr and Ser residues in the second transmembrane region (TM2) that, again based on analogy to nAchRs, was believed to line the ion channel pore. However, a major difference between the two subunits was the proposed intracellular loop located between TM3 and TM4, the region most dissimilar between the two subunits. Moreover, a consensus phosphorylation sequence for cyclic adenosine monophosphate–dependent protein kinase was located within this loop of the β, but not the α, subunit.

TABLE 16.1. γ-AMINOBUTYRIC ACID A RECEPTOR PHARMACOLOGY

Selective agonists	Muscimol, GABA
Competitive antagonist	Bicuculline
Noncompetitive TBPS antagonists	Picrotoxin, PTZ
Channel blocker	Penicillin
BDZ receptor agonists	Diazepam, clonazepam
BDZ receptor inverse agonists	DMCM, βCCM
BDZ receptor antagonist	Flumazenil
Barbiturate receptor agonists	Pentobarbital, phenobarbital
Steroid receptor agonist	Alphaxalone
Channel selectivity	Cl–
Subunits	α, β, γ, δ, ε, π, θ, ρ

GABA, γ-aminobutyric acid; BDZ, benzodiazepine; CCM, DMCM, ; PTZ, ; TBPS, .

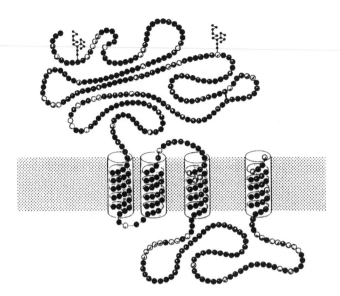

FIGURE 16.2. Generic GABA_A receptor protein subunit sequence and topologic structure. The *N*-terminal half of the polypeptide is suggested to be extracellular, with probable sites for asparagine glycosylation (polymeric *black circles* at positions 10 and 110) and the conserved cystine bridge at positions 138 to 152. Four putative membrane-spanning domains are shown as α-helical cylinders within the cell membrane *(stippled)*, with the C-terminal at the extracellular end of the fourth membrane-spanning region. A large putative intracellular loop is present between the third and fourth membrane-spanning regions. (Modified from Olsen RW, Tobin AJ. Molecular biology of GABA_A receptors. *FASEB J* 1990;4:1469–1480, with permission.)

After the identification of the first two GABAR subunit cDNAs, it was discovered that mammals had multiple families of subunits (α,β,γ,δ,ε,π,θ, and ρ) and multiple subunit subtypes including α (1–6), β (1–3), γ (1–3), and ρ (1—3) (4,23,24,34,36,40,42,43,60,72), which all share similar structural features and basic functional properties (Table 16.2). Within a family, the amino acid similarity ranges from 70% to 80%, and between families, it ranges from 30% to 40%. Further GABAR subunit diversity has been shown to result from alternative splicing of subunit mes-

senger RNA (mRNA) transcripts. Two forms of the γ2 subtype, a short form (γ2S, the original clone) and a long form (γ2L), were cloned (81). The γ2L variant differed from the γ2S variant by differential splicing and insertion of eight amino acids into the intracellular loop between TM3 and TM4. Interestingly, this insert contained a consensus phosphorylation sequence for protein kinase C.

MOLECULAR STRUCTURE OF GABA RECEPTORS

The current understanding of the molecular structure of the GABAR–ion channel complex is that it is heteropentameric glycoprotein (approximately 275 kd), composed of multiple combinations of polypeptide subunits. The subunits form a quasisymmetric structure around the ion channel, with each subunit contributing to the wall of the channel (50). The model is based heavily on analogy with the nAchR.

The existence of 19 or so subunit subtypes leads to several questions about the molecular structure of GABARs. It is not known how many oligomeric GABAR isoforms exist in nature, and the subunit composition of each GABAR isoform is unclear. It is likely that different combinations of subunit subtypes form different GABAR isoforms in different neuronal populations. Thus, it was not surprising to discover differential regional expression in the central nervous system and spinal cord of various subunit subtype mRNAs (41). Localization of the GABAR gene products, including mRNA by *in situ* hybridization and polypeptides by immunocytochemistry, is giving a picture of where each is found and their possible overlap or coexistence in the same cells. The distribution of mRNAs in the central nervous system determined by *in situ* hybridization is very different for each subunit subtype. Some subtype mRNAs are only expressed in specific cell types; for example α6 mRNA is demonstrated only in cerebellar granule cells (18). Other subtypes, such as for the β2 subtype, have a more ubiqui-

TABLE 16.2. γ-AMINOBUTYRIC ACID A RECEPTOR SUBUNIT BIOCHEMISTRY

Subunits	α	β	γ	δ	ρ
No. of subtypes	6	4	4	1	2
No. of splice variants	0	1	1	0	0
Size range (kd)	48–64	51	48	48	52
Percentage AA homology, intrafamily	70–80	70–80	70–80	NA	70–80
Percentage AA homology, interfamily	30–40	30–40	30–40	30–40	30–40
Consensus sequence sites for phosphorylation	α4, α6: PKA PKC	β1–β4: PKA PKC	γ1, γ3: PTK γ2S/L: PTK PKC	?	ρ1, ρ2: PKC

AA, ?; NA, not available; PKA, protein kinase A; PKC, protein kinase C; PTK, .

tous distribution, whereas various α,β, and γ subtypes and the one δ subtype show very different regional as well as developmental distributions (51,59,65,72). Thus, differential expression and assembly of various GABAR subtypes could produce a multitude of receptor isoforms. However, the specific subunit composition, stoichiometry, and number of different GABAR isoforms are unknown.

BENZODIAZEPINE REGULATION OF RECOMBINANT GABA RECEPTORS

After cloning of GABAR subunits, GABAR expression in *Xenopus* oocytes or mammalian cell lines was performed to determine whether functional GABAR channel assembly occurred and to determine the pharmacologic properties of expressed GABARs (5,6,62,63,64,76,82). Coexpression of α1, β1, and γ2 subtypes in *Xenopus* oocytes produced GABARs with reproducible BDZ pharmacology. GABAR responses were potentiated by diazepam and were inhibited by inverse agonist β-carbolines, and these effects were blocked by the BDZ receptor antagonist flumazenil. Complete BDZ receptor pharmacology was also demonstrated by binding assays to human embryonic kidney (HEK) 293 cell membranes after transient coexpression of the three GABAR subunits. An appropriate rank order of potency of several BDZ receptor ligands was demonstrated.

The molecular basis for BI and BZII binding sites was determined using transient expression of αxβ12S (x = 1, 2, or 3) subunit combinations in HEK 293 cells (63). The combination of α1β1γ2S GABAR subtypes produced BZI binding sites, and either α2β1γ2S or α3β1γ2S GABAR subtype combination produced BZII binding sites. These receptor isoforms were differentiated based on binding of the BZI selective compounds, zolpidem and CL 218,872. BDZ receptor pharmacology was not altered by substituting any other β subtype. Seeburg and colleagues further studied the effect of expressing α4, α5, and α6 subtypes with β1 and γ2S subtypes. Expression of the α5 subtype with β1 and γ2S subtypes also created BZII BDZ binding sites, although they had even lower affinity for zolpidem than either α2 or α3 subtype–containing receptors (60). Expression of the α6 subtype with β1 and γ2S subtypes produced a receptor isoform that did not bind the prototypical BDZs, diazepam and flunitrazepam, or β-carbolines, but it did bind the inverse agonist imidazobenzodiazepine Ro 15-4513 and flumazenil (74). Binding of GABA agonists was not impaired. A similar BDZ receptor profile was discovered for the α4 subtype expressed with β1 and γ2S subtypes (82). Thus, BDZ pharmacology of recombinant GABARs appears to depend on the α subtype. The original BZI and BZII classification was altered to include the increased BDZ receptor heterogeneity and contains BZI

(α1), BZIIA (α2 and α3), BZIIB (α5), and BZIII (α4 and α6) receptors (27).

FUNCTIONAL DOMAINS FOR BENZODIAZEPINE ACTION

A single amino acid was identified as the covalent attachment site for photoaffinity labeling with [³H] flunitrazepam, H102 in bovine α1 (H101 in rat, also present in α2, α3, α5) (28,79,80). Replacement of the H in the α1 subtype with R as in the α6 subtype reduced BDZ binding, whereas replacement of R100 in the α6 subtype with H as in the α1 subtype resulted in BDZ binding (87). A mouse knock-in for point mutation H101R in the α1 subtype lost sensitivity to the sedative-hypnotic action of BDZs, but not the anxolytic or motor-impairing effects, which must be mediated by α2, α3, α5 subtypes (67). Comparison of other amino acids with histidine at this position revealed that α1 H101 is critical for BDZ binding and efficacy (29). Additional studies revealed that the α4 subtype, also producing GABARs with low affinity for BDZ agonists, has R, not H, in the corresponding position 101. Mutagenesis also implicated P161 and I211 in the BDZ binding site on α6 (88). In addition, the variable selectivity of α subunits for BDZs allowed determination of a residue involved in this specificity: residue α1G200 = α3E225 was shown to be responsible for differences in α1 versus α2/3 subtypes in affinity for CL 218,872 and other ligands (61), a finding suggesting that these residues may participate in the BDZ binding pocket.

The γ subunit is required for benzodiazepine binding by GABARs, and γ2T142 was shown to affect BDZ binding (53). Other residues in the γ2 subtype (F77, T55, M57) have been implicated in BDZ binding (12,13). Chimeras between γ2 and α1 subtypes showed that γ2 K41-W82 and γ2 R114-D161 are needed for BDZ binding in HEK cells, but the chimera of *N*-terminal 1-161γ2 with the rest of the α1 subtype sequence (expressed with the β2 subtype) gave poor BDZ enhancement of GABAR currents in oocytes and poor GABA enhancement of BDZ binding in HEK cells (7). Residues found in β subunits to affect GABA binding (1) were mutagenized in the α1 subtype (α1Y159, Y161, T206, Y209) and were found to affect BDZ binding (2,14,89). The latter are situated near the already mentioned G200 residue (69). This correspondence of domains for BDZ binding pockets with those for GABA binding in the same pentamer was noted (12,77,79) as a possible evolutionary modification of an agonist site into one for an exogenous allosteric modulator. A sequence homology surrounding the residues in the α1 subtype implicated in binding muscimol and flunitrazepam (79) suggested the structural connection, as well as a functional correlate: in whatever manner GABA binding on β/α subunits is conformationally coupled to channel opening, BDZ binding on α/γ subunits may also promote that physical change.

REGULATION OF GABA RECEPTOR CHANNELS BY BENZODIAZEPINE RECEPTOR LIGANDS

Development of the single-channel recording technique has permitted direct study of native GABAR channels on neurons and recombinant GABARs expressed in mammalian cells (8,33,48). When GABA is applied to outside-out patches obtained from mouse spinal cord neurons in cell culture, the GABAR channel opens and closes rapidly, so relatively square current pulses are recorded (Figure 16.3). The GABAR channel opens to multiple conductance levels. A 27- to 30-ps conductance level is the predominant or main conductance level (Figure 16.3C, *double asterisks)* and conductance levels of 17 to 19 ps and 11 to 12 ps occur less frequently (Figure 16.3C, *single asterisk)*. Although the GABAR channel opens to multiple conductance levels, current through the main conductance level is responsible for >95% of the current through the channel.

The equilibrium single-channel gating properties of the main conductance level of the GABAR in murine spinal cord neurons in culture have been characterized (48,68,85). The GABAR opens in bursts of openings interrupted by brief closures (Figure 16.3). The GABAR has been shown to open into three different open states with mean durations of 0.5, 2.5, and 7.3 milliseconds. Increasing GABA concentration produces GABAR single-channel currents that increase in dura-

tion. The studies suggest that the receptor has two binding sites for GABA molecules, and the singly bound receptor opens primarily to the brief 0.5-millisecond state, whereas the doubly bound receptor opens primarily to the longer 2.5- and 7.3-millisecond states. The mean open channel duration increases with GABA concentration because more doubly bound receptor is formed. The GABAR has been shown also to enter into multiple closed states including two brief closed states with mean durations of 0.2 and 2.8 milliseconds and at least three closed states with longer mean durations.

BDZs enhance GABAR current (20,44,45) by binding to the BDZ receptor on GABARs (55,56,83,86). The β-carboline, methyl 6,7-dimethoxy-4-ethyl-β-carboline-3-carboxylate (DMCM), reduces GABA-mediated inhibition also by interacting with the BDZ receptor. To enhance GABAR current, a drug may increase channel conductance, increase channel open and burst frequencies, or increase channel open and burst durations. Conversely, to reduce GABAR current, a drug may decrease channel conductance, decrease channel open and burst frequencies, or decrease channel open and burst durations. By determining the drug-induced alterations produced in the open, closed, and burst properties of GABAR single-channel currents, the mechanisms of action of the BDZs and β-carbolines on GABAR channels were determined. At clinically relevant concentrations (<100 nmol/L), single-channel recordings demonstrated diazepam increased receptor opening frequency without altering mean open time or conductance (66,86) (Figure 16.4). These results contrast with the

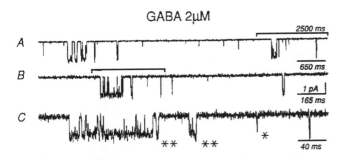

GABA 2μM

FIGURE 16.3. Single-channel currents are shown at increasing time resolution *(a–c)* for GABA (2 μmol/L). GABA-evoked bursting single-channel inward (downgoing) currents with at least two current amplitudes when outside-out patches are voltage clamped at −75 mV. The larger 2.04-pA (27-picosecond) channel *(double asterisks)* occurred more frequently compared with a smaller 1.48-pA (20-picosecond) channel *(single asterisk).* The portion outlined for each tracing is presented expanded in time in the tracing beneath it. Attenuated brief channel openings seen at lower temporal resolution may be seen at true amplitudes at higher temporal resolution. Time calibration for each trace is shown on the *right* below the trace. Current calibration applies throughout. (Modified from Twyman RE, Macdonald RL. Neurosteroid regulation of GABA$_A$ receptor single channel kinetic properties. *J Physiol (Lond)* 1992;456:215–245, with permission.)

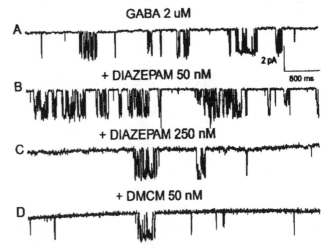

GABA 2 uM

FIGURE 16.4. A: GABA opened chloride channels resulting in single and bursting inward currents. **B,C:** GABA (2 μm) with diazepam (50 nm) resulted in increased opening frequency. **D:** GABA with DMCM (50 nm) resulted in decreased opening frequency. Data were obtained from different excised outside-out patches. Time and current calibration bars are applicable to all traces shown. (From Rogers CJ, Twyman RE, Macdonald RL. Benzodiazepine and β-carboline regulation of single GABA$_A$ receptor channels of mouse spinal neurones in culture. *J Physiol (Lond)* 1994;475:69–82, with permission.)

increase in burst duration with little effect on burst frequency seen in the presence of phenobarbital (86). For diazepam, these results could be explained by an increased affinity of the GABAR at one, but not both, of the GABA binding sites. Another explanation is that BDZs could reduce the rate of entry into a desensitized state without altering the gating of the bound GABAR channel.

Reduction of GABAR currents by an inverse agonist for the BDZ receptor is produced by a mechanism opposite to the action of BDZ receptor agonists. The inverse agonist β-carboline, DMCM, did not alter GABAR conductance or average open and burst durations (66), but it did reduce open and burst frequencies. These results suggest that modulation of GABAR single-channel kinetics by DMCM could be explained by a reduction of the affinity of GABA binding at the first, but not second, GABA binding site. Again, an alternative interpretation is that β-carbolines increase the rate of entry into a desensitized state without altering the gating of the bound GABAR.

OTHER ACTIONS OF BENZODIAZEPINES

Although the primary action of anticonvulsant BDZs is to enhance GABAergic inhibition by binding to the BDZ receptor on GABARs, other actions of BDZs have been described. BDZs have been demonstrated to modify sodium channel function in a manner similar to that of the anticonvulsants phenytoin, carbamazepine, and sodium valproate (46). Diazepam has been shown to block trains of action potential in rat diaphragm muscle fibers and to decrease peak inward sodium current of frog myelinated nerve fibers. This effect on the sodium channel produces a voltage-dependent block of high-frequency repetitive firing of cultured mammalian neurons (50). The effect of diazepam to limit repetitive firing occurred at diazepam concentrations achieved in the treatment of status epilepticus and was not blocked by the BDZ receptor antagonist flumazenil. Thus, the effects of BDZs on sodium channels are not mediated through the BDZ receptor, but instead represent direct effects of BDZs on sodium channels.

BDZs have also been demonstrated to reduce voltage-dependent calcium currents (69). Diazepam and the convulsant Ro-54864 reduced the duration of voltage-dependent calcium currents in mouse neurons in cell culture. However, the effect was produced at supertherapeutic concentrations of diazepam not likely achieved in ambulatory patients. Similarly, diazepam reduced the calcium conductance in identified leech neurons (35) and guinea pig myenteric neurons (19) at supertherapeutic concentrations. Thus, although BDZs decrease voltage-dependent calcium currents in neurons, the effect is unlikely to be clinically relevant because of the high concentrations of BDZs that are required.

There have been additional reports of BDZ interactions with other channels and neurotransmitter receptors. BDZs

were reported to enhance calcium-mediated potassium conductance (17), and they reduced the effect of excitatory amino acids (3,25). However, these observations have not been substantiated, and it is generally accepted that BDZs do not have significant interactions with excitatory amino acid receptors or potassium channels.

CONCLUSION

It is firmly established that BDZs have primary action as anticonvulsants by interacting with GABARs at the BDZ binding site and allosterically modifying GABAR current to enhance inhibition. However, the great advances made in understanding the molecular biology of the GABAR demonstrate that there are multiple GABAR isoforms with differential sensitivity to BDZ receptor ligands. Thus, BDZ receptor ligands targeted to BZI, BZII, or BZIII receptors have different clinical actions. Studies are currently under way to determine specific GABAR isoforms in the central nervous system. Once this is accomplished, then specific anticonvulsant drugs will be developed that will target those specific GABAR isoforms. It is certainly possible that in the future there will be BDZ receptor ligands with selective anxiolytic or anticonvulsant actions without undesired side effects.

Although BDZs have their primary action to enhance GABAR current, a significant interaction of BDZs with sodium channels has been reported. This interaction occurs only at concentrations of BDZs that are achieved in the treatment of status epilepticus. The effects of BDZs at these high concentrations are similar to those of phenytoin, carbamazepine, and sodium valproate, findings suggesting that BDZs may recruit a second mechanism of action when these drugs are given in high doses to patients with status epilepticus.

REFERENCES

1. Amin J, Weiss DS. GABA$_A$ receptor needs two homologous domains of the β-subunit for activation by GABA but not by pentobarbital. *Nature* 1993;366:565–569.
2. Amin J, Brooks-Kayal A, Weiss DS. Two tyrosine residues on the α subunit are crucial for benzodiazepine binding and allosteric modulation of GABA$_A$ receptors. *Mol Pharmacol* 1997;51:833–841.
3. Assumpção JA, Bernardi N, Brown J, et al. Selective antagonism by benzodiazepines of neuronal responses to excitatory amino acids in the cerebral cortex. *Br J Pharmacol* 1979;67:563–568.
4. Bateson AL, Lasham A, Darlison MG. γ-Aminobutyric acid A receptor heterogeneity is increased by alternative splicing of a novel β-subunit gene transcript. *J Neurochem* 1991;56:1437–1440.
5. Benke D, Mertens S, Trzeciak A, et al. GABA$_A$ receptors display association of γ2-subunit with α1- and β2/β3-subunits. *J Biol Chem* 1991;266:4478–4483.
6. Blair LA, Levitan ES, Marshall J, et al. Single subunits of the GABA$_A$ receptor form ion channels with properties of the native receptor. *Science* 1988;242:577–579.
7. Boileau AJ, Kucken AM, Evers A, et al. Molecular dissection of benzodiazepine binding and allosteric coupling using chimeric GABA$_A$ receptor subunits. *Mol Pharmacol* 1998;53:295–303.

8. Bormann J, Hamill OP, Sakmann B. Mechanism of anion permeation through channels gated by glycine and γ-aminobutyric acid in mouse cultured spinal neurones. *J Physiol (Lond)* 1987; 385:243–286.

9. Braestrup C, Nielsen M, Honoré T, et al. Benzodiazepine receptor ligands with positive and negative efficacy. *Neuropharmacology* 1983;22:1451–1457.

10. Braestrup C, Nielsen M, Olsen CE. Urinary and brain β-carboline-3-carboxylates as potent inhibitors of brain benzodiazepine receptors. *Proc Natl Acad Sci USA* 1980;77:2288–2292.

11. Braestrup C, Schmiechen R, Neef G, et al. Interaction of convulsive ligands with benzodiazepine receptors. *Science* 1982;216: 1241–1243.

12. Buhr A, Baur R, Malherbe P, et al. Point mutations of the α1β2γ2 GABA$_A$ receptor affecting modulation of the channel by ligands of the benzodiazepine binding site. *Mol Pharmacol* 1996; 49:1080–1084.

13. Buhr A, Baur R, Sigel E. Subtle changes in residue 77 of the γ subunit of α1β2γ2 GABA$_A$ receptors drastically alter the affinity for ligands of the benzodiazepine binding site. *J Biol Chem* 1997; 272:11799–11804.

14. Buhr A, Schaerer MT, Baur R, et al. Residues at positions 206 and 209 of the α1 subunit of GABA$_A$ receptors influence affinities for benzodiazepine binding site ligands. *Mol Pharmacol* 1997;52:676–682.

15. Bureau MH, Olsen RW. Multiple distinct subunits of the γ-aminobutyric acid-A receptor protein show different ligand-binding affinities. *Mol Pharmacol* 1990;37:497–502.

16. Bureau MH, Olsen RW. GABA$_A$ receptor subtypes: ligand binding heterogeneity demonstrated by photoaffinity labeling and autoradiography. *J Neurochem* 1993;61:1479–1491.

17. Carlen PL, Gurevich N, Polc P. Low-dose benzodiazepine neuronal inhibition: enchanced Ca^{2+}-mediated K$^+$-conductance. *Brain Res* 1983;271:358–364.

18. Casalotti SO, Stephenson FA, Barnard EA. Separate subunits for agonist and benzodiazepine binding in the gamma amnobutyric acid A receptor oligomer. *J Biol Chem* 1986;261:15013–15016.

19. Cherubini E, North RA. Benzodiazepines both enhance γ-aminobutyrate responses and decrease calcium action potentials in guinea-pig myenteric neurones. *Neuroscience* 1985;14:309–315.

20. Choi DW, Farb DH, Fischbach GD. Chlordiazepoxide selectively augments GABA action in spinal cord cell cultures. *Nature* 1977;269:342–344.

21. Costa E, Guidotti A, Mao CC. Evidence for involvement of GABA in the action of benzodiazepines: studies on rat cerebellum. *Adv Biochem Psychopharmacol* 1975;XX: 113–130.

22. Costa E, Guidotti A, Mao CC, et al. New concepts on the mechanism of action of benzodiazepines. *Life Sci* 1975;17:167–185.

23. Cutting GR, Curristin S, Zoghbi H, et al. Identification of a putative gamma-aminobutyric acid (GABA) receptor subunit ρ2 cDNA and colocalization of the genes encoding ρ2 (GABRR2) and ρ1 (GABRR1) to human chromosome 6q14-q21 and mouse chromosome-4. *Genomics* 1992;12:801–806.

24. Cutting GR, Lu L, O'Hara BF, et al. Cloning of the gamma-aminobutyric acid (GABA) rho1 cDNA: a GABA receptor subunit highly expressed in the retina. *Proc Natl Acad Sci USA* 1991; 88:2673–2677.

25. DeBonnel G, DeMontigny C. Benzodiazepines selectively antagonize kainate-induced activation in the rat hippocampus. *Eur J Pharmacol* 1983;93:45–54.

26. DeLorey TM, Olsen RW. γ-Aminobutyric acid A receptor structure and function. *J Biol Chem* 1992;267:16747–16750.

27. Doble A, Martin IL. Multiple benzodiazepine receptors: no reason for anxiety. *Trends Pharmacol Sci* 1992;13:76–81.

28. Duncalfe LL, Carpenter MR, Smillie LB, et al. The major site of photoaffinity labeling of the γ-aminobutyric acid type A receptor

by [^{3}H] flunitrazepam is histidine 102 of the α subunit. *J Biol Chem* 1996;271:9209–9214.

29. Dunn SMJ, Davies M, Munton AL, et al. Mutagenesis of the rat α1 subunit of the GABA$_A$ receptor reveals the importance of residue 101 in determining the allosteric effects of benzodiazepine site ligands. *Mol Pharmacol* 1999;56:768–774.

30. Fuchs K, Adamiker D, Sieghart W. Identification of α2- and α3-subunits of the GABA$_A$-benzodiazepine receptor complex purified from the brains of young rats. *FEBS Lett* 1990;261:52–54.

31. Gavish M, Snyder SH. Benzodiazepine recognition sites on GABA receptors. *Nature* 1980;287:651–652.

32. Häring P, Stähli C, Schoch P, et al. Monoclonal antibodies reveal structural homogeneity of γ-aminobutyric acid/benzodiazepine receptors in different brain areas. *Proc Natl Acad Sci USA* 1985; 82:4837–4841.

33. Hamill OP, Bormann J, Sakmann B. Activation of multiple-conductance state chloride channels in spinal neurones by glycine and GABA. *Nature* 1983;305:805–808.

34. Herb A, Wisden W, Luddens H, et al. The third gamma-subunit of the γ-aminobutyric acid type-A receptor family. *Proc Natl Acad Sci USA* 1992;89:1433–1437.

35. Johansen J, Taft WC, Yang J, et al. Inhibition of Ca^{2+} conductance in identified leech neurons by benzodiazepines. *Proc Natl Acad Sci USA* 1985;82:3935–3939.

36. Kato K. Novel GABA$_A$ receptor α subunit is expressed only in cerebellar granule cells. *J Mol Biol* 1990;214:619–624.

37. Kirkness EF, Turner AJ. The γ-aminobutyrate/benzodiazepine receptor from pig brain: purification and characterization of the receptor complex from cerebral cortex and cerebellum. *Biochem J* 1986;233:265–270.

38. Kirkness EF, Turner AJ. Antibodies directed against a nonapeptide sequence of the γ-aminobutyrate (GABA)/benzodiazepine receptor α-subunit. *Biochem J* 1988;256:2291–294.

39. Klepner CA, Lippa AS, Benson DI, et al. Resolution of two biochemically and pharmacologically distinct benzodiazepine receptors. *Pharmacol Biochem Rev* 1979;11:457–462.

40. Knoflach F, Rhyner T, Villa M, et al. The β-subunit of the GABA$_A$ receptor confers sensitivity to benzodiazepine receptor ligands. *FEBS Lett* 1991;293:191–194.

41. Laurie DJ, Seeburg PH, Wisden W. The distribution of 13-GABA$_A$ receptor subunit messenger RNAs in the rat brain. II. Olfactory bulb and cerebellum. *J Neurosci* 1991;12:1063–1076.

42. Levitan ES, Schofield PR, Burt DR, et al. Structural and functional basis for GABA$_A$ receptor heterogeneity. *Nature* 1988;335:76–79.

43. Luddens H, Pritchett DB, Kohler M, et al. Cerebellar GABA$_A$ receptor selective for a behavioural alcohol antagonist. *Nature* 1990;346:648–651.

44. Macdonald RL, Barker JL. Benzodiazepines specifically modulate GABA-mediated postsynaptic inhibition in cultured mammalian neurones. *Nature* 1978;271:563–564.

45. Macdonald RL, Barker JL. Enhancement of GABA-mediated postsynaptic inhibition in cultured mammalian spinal cord neurons: a common mode of anti-convulsant action. *Brain Res* 1979; 167:323–336.

46. Macdonald RL, Kelly RM. Drug mechanisms of action of currently prescribed and newly developed antiepileptic drugs. *Epilepsia* 1994;35:S41–S50.

47. Macdonald RL, Olsen R. GABA$_A$ receptor channels. *Annu Rev Neurosci* 1994;17:569–602.

48. Macdonald RL, Rogers CJ, Twyman RE. Kinetic properties of the GABA$_A$ receptor main-conductance state of mouse spinal cord neurons in culture. *J Physiol (Lond)* 1989;410:479–499.

49. Macdonald RL, Twyman RE. Kinetic properties and regulation of GABA$_A$ receptor channels. In: Narahashi T, ed. *Ion Channels*, vol 4. New York: Plenum Press, 1992:315–343.

50. McLean MJ, Macdonald RL. Benzodiazepines, but not beta car-

bolines, limit high frequency repetitive firing of action potentials of spinal cord neurons in cell culture. *J Pharmacol Exp Ther* 1988;244:789–795.

51. MacLennan AJ, Brecha N, Khrestchatisky M, et al. Independent cellular and ontogenetic expression of mRNAs encoding three α polypeptides of the rat GABA$_A$ receptor. *Neuroscience* 1991;43: 69–380.

52. Mamalaki C, Stephenson FA, Barnard EA. The GABA$_A$ benzodiazepine receptor is a heterotetramer of homologous and subunits. *EMBO J* 1987;6:561–565.

53. Mihic SJ, Whiting PJ, Klein RL, et al. A single amino acid of the human GABA$_A$ receptor γ2 subunit determines benzodiazepine efficacy. *J Biol Chem* 1994;269:32768–32783.

54. Möhler H, Battersby MK, Richards JG. Benzodiazepine receptors protein identified and visualized in brain tissue by a photoaffinity lable. *Proc Natl Acad Sci USA* 1980;11:1660–1670.

55. Olsen RW. GABA-benzodiazepine-barbiturate receptor interactions. *J Neurochem* 1981;37:1–13.

56. Olsen RW. The γ-aminobutyric acid/benzodiazepine/barbiturate receptor chloride ion channel complex of mammalian brain. In: Edelman GM, Gall WE, Cowan WM, eds. *Synaptic function.* New York: Neuroscience Research Foundation/Wiley, 1987:257–271.

57. Park D, DeBlas AL. Peptide subunits of γ-aminobutyric acid A/benzodiazepine receptors from bovine cerebral cortex. *J Neurochem* 1991;56:1972–1979.

58. Popot JL, Changeux JP. Nicotinic receptor of acetylcholine: structure of an oligomeric integral membrane protein. *Physiol Rev* 1984;64:1162–1239.

59. Poulter MO, Barker JL, O'Carroll AM, et al. Differential and transient expression of GABA$_A$ receptor-subunit mRNAs in the developing rat CNS. *J Neurosci* 1992;12:2888–2900.

60. Pritchett DB, Seeburg PH. Gamma-aminobutyric acid A receptor α5-subunit creates novel type II benzodiazepine receptor pharmacology. *J Neurochem* 1990;54:1802–1804.

61. Pritchett DB, Seeburg PH. γ-Aminobutyric acid type A receptor point mutation increases the affinity of compounds for the benzodiazepine site. *Proc Natl Acad Sci USA* 1991;88:1421–1425.

62. Pritchett DB, Sontheimer H, Gorman CM, et al. Transient expression shows ligand gating and allosteric potentiation of GABA$_A$ receptor subunits. *Science* 1988;242:1306–1308.

63. Pritchett DB, Sontheimer H, Shivers BD, et al. Importance of a novel GABA$_A$ receptor subunit for benzodiazepine pharmacology. *Nature* 1989;338:582–585.

64. Puia G, Vicini S, Seeburg PH, et al. Influence of recombinant γ-aminobutyric acidA receptor subunit compositions on the action of allosteric modulators of γ-aminobutyric acid-gated Cl- currents. *Mol Pharmacol* 1991;39:691–696.

65. Richards JG, Schoch P, Haefely W. Benzodiazepine receptors: new vistas. *Semin Neurosci* 1991;3:191–203.

66. Rogers CJ, Twyman RE, Macdonald RL. Benzodiazepine and β-carboline regulation of single GABA$_A$ receptor channels of mouse spinal neurones in culture. *J Physiol* 1994;475:69–82.

67. Rudolph U, Crestani F, Benke D, et al. Benzodiazepine actions medated by specific GABA$_A$ receptor subtypes. *Nature* 1999;401: 796–800.

68. Sakmann B, Hamill OP, Bormann J. Patch-clamp measurements if elementary chloride currents activated by the putative inhibitory transmitters GABA and glycine in mammalian spinal neurons. *J Neural Transm Suppl* 1983;18:83–95.

69. Schaerer MT, Buhr A, Baur R, et al. Amino acid residue 200 on the α1 subunit of GABA$_A$ receptors affects the interaction with selected benzodiazepine binding site ligands. *Eur J Pharmacol* 1998;354:283–287.

70. Schmidt RF, Vogel ME, Zimmerman M. Die Wirkung von Diazepam and die Präsynaptische Hemmung und andere Rückenmarksreflexe. *Naunyn Schmiedebergs Arch Exp Pathol Pharmakol* 1967;258:69–82.

71. Schofield PR, Darlison MG, Fujita N, et al. Sequence and functional expression of the GABA$_A$ receptor shows a ligand-gated receptor superfamily. *Nature* 1987;328:221–227.

72. Shivers BD, Killisch I, Sprengel R, et al. Two novel GABA$_A$ receptor subunits exist in distinct neuronal subpopulations. *Neuron* 1989;3:327–337.

73. Sieghart W, Drexler G. Irreversible binding of [^{3}H]flunitrazepam to different proteins in various brain regions. *J Neurochem* 1983;-41:47–55.

74. Sieghart W, Eichinger A, Richards JG, et al. Photoaffinity labelling of benzodiazepine receptor proteins with the partial inverse agonist [^{3}H]Ro15-4513: a biochemical and autoradiographic study. *J Neurochem* 1987;48:46–52.

75. Sieghart W, Karobath M. Molecular heterogeneity of benzodiazepine receptors. *Nature* 1980;286:285–287.

76. Sigel E, Barnard EA. A γ-aminobutyric acid/benzodiazepine receptor complex from bovine cerebral cortex: improved purification with preservation of regulatory sites and their interactions. *J Biol Chem* 1984;259:7219–7223.

77. Sigel E, Buhr A. The benzodiazepine binding site of GABA$_A$ receptors. *Trends Pharmacol Sci* 1997;18:425–429.

78. Sigel E, Stephenson FA, Mamalaki C, et al. A γ-aminobutyric acid/benzodiazepine receptor complex of bovine cerebral cortex: purification and partial characterization. *J Biol Chem* 1983;258:6965–6971.

79. Smith GB, Olsen RW. Functional domains of GABA$_A$ receptors. *Trends Pharmacol Sci* 1995;16:162–168.

80. Smith GB, Olsen RW. Deduction of amino acid residues in the GABA$_A$ receptor α subunits photoaffinity labeled with the benzodiazepine flunitrazepam. *Neuropharmacology* 2000;39:55–64.

81. Squires RF, Braestrup C. Benzodiazepine receptors in rat brain. *Nature* 1977;266:732–734.

82. Stephenson FA, Duggan MJ, Pollard S. The γ2 subunit is an integral component of the γ-aminobutyric acidA receptor but the α1 polypeptide is the principal site of the agonist benzodiazepine photoaffinity labeling reaction. *J Biol Chem* 1990;265:21160–21165.

83. Study RE, Barker JL. Diazepam and (±) pentobarbital: fluctuation analysis reveals different mechanisms for potentiation of γ-aminobutyric acid responses in cultured central neurons. *Proc Natl Acad Sci USA* 1981;78:7180–7184.

84. Tallman JF, Paul SM, Skolnick P, et al. Receptors for the age of anxiety: pharmacology of the benzodiazepines. *Science* 1980;207: 274–281.

85. Twyman RE, Macdonald RL. Neurosteroid regulation of GABA$_A$ receptor single channel kinetic properties. *J Physiol (Lond)* 1992; 456:215–245.

86. Twyman RE, Rogers CJ, Macdonald RL. Differential mechanisms for enhancement of GABA by diazepam and phenobarbital: a single channel study. *Ann Neurol* 1989;25:213–220.

87. Wieland HA, Lüddens H, Seeburg PH. A single histidine in GABA$_A$ receptors is essential for benzodiazepine agonist binding. *J Biol Chem* 1992;267:1426–1429.

88. Wieland HA, Lüddens H. Four amino acid exchanges convert a diazepam-insensitive inverse agonist-preferring GABA$_A$ receptor into a diazepam-preferring GABA$_A$ receptor. *J Med Chem* 1994; 37:4576–4580.

89. Wingrove PB, Thompson SA, Wafford KA, et al. Key amino acids in the γ subunit of the GABA$_A$ receptor that determine ligand binding and modulation at the benzodiazepine site. *Mol Pharmacol* 1997;52:874–881.

Antiepileptic Drugs, 5th Edition. Edited by R.H. Levy, R.H. Mattson, B.S. Meldrum, and E. Perucca. Lippincott Williams & Wilkins, Philadelphia © 2002.

BENZODIAZEPINES

CHEMISTRY, BIOTRANSFORMATION, AND PHARMACOKINETICS

GAIL D. ANDERSON
JOHN W. MILLER

CLOBAZAM

Chemistry and Metabolic Scheme

Clobazam (7-chloro-1-methyl-5-phenyl-1,5-benzodiazepine-2,4-dione) is a benzodiazepine in which the imine group in the fourth and fifth position of the diazepine ring is substituted by an amide (Figure 17.1). It has a molecular weight of 301 and is a crystalline powder, which is relatively insoluble in water. Clobazam has marked antiepileptic properties (1), and it is said to be less sedating than other commonly used benzodiazepines (2,3). The primary metabolite of clobazam, *N*-desmethylclobazam, contributes significantly to the pharmacologic effect of clobazam, because it has higher serum levels than clobazam after administration (4).

Absorption

Bioavailability. Clobazam is rapidly and completely absorbed (5); food has variable effects on this process (6). After a single 10-mg oral dose, a peak concentration of 164 to 325 ng/mL is reached in 0.5 to 2 hours (7) in healthy volunteers and in patients with epilepsy. After a 30-mg oral dose (8), peak levels of clobazam are reached in 1 to 3 hours, with a delayed peak of *N*-desmethylclobazam. Diurnal variation in absorption has been suggested (9).

Routes of Administration and Formulations. Clobazam is not available for intravenous (i.v.) or intramuscular (i.m.) injection. Rectal solutions are initially absorbed more rapidly than capsules or suppositories, but they reach similar peaks of 200 to 400 ng/mL after doses of 30 mg (10). *N*-desmethylclobazam peaks in about 24 hours, with similar peak concentrations, time to peak, and area under the curve for oral capsules, rectal solution, and rectal suppositories (10). However, there is less variability in levels with rectal administration.

Distribution

Clobazam is highly lipophilic and is rapidly distributed in fat and in the brain, before being redistributed widely (11,12). It has a large volume of distribution (VD), measured at 81±20 L in healthy subjects after a single oral 20-mg dose (13).

Plasma Protein Binding. Clobazam is about 85% protein bound (4). Hepatic disease decreases protein binding and approximately doubles VD relative to healthy subjects (13). A strong correlation exists between salivary and plasma concentrations of clobazam within a wide range of concentrations (14).

Cerebrospinal Fluid, Brain, and Other Tissues. In preclinical studies, ^{14}C-clobazam was found to distribute evenly in the brain and body tissues in rats and dogs without evidence of accumulation (12). However, at autopsy of a 6-year-old child who had received clobazam on a long-term basis, *N*-desmethylclobazam levels exceeded clobazam levels by 15-fold or more, and liver and brain levels exceeded those in serum (15).

Transplacental Passage. Clobazam does cross the human placenta, and a neonatal withdrawal syndrome has been observed with prenatal exposure (16).

Breast Milk. The ratio of milk to plasma for clobazam plus *N*-desmethylclobazam after 2 days of treatment is 0.13:0.36, with a maximal dose of 0.038 to 0.05 mg/kg/day to the child (17). It is suggested that the infant be monitored for signs of sedation. Based on the high protein bind-

Gail D. Anderson, PhD: Professor, Department of Pharmacy, University of Washington, Seattle, Washington

John W. Miller, MD, PhD: Professor, Department of Neurology, University of Washington; and Director, Regional Epilepsy Center, Harborview Medical Center, Seattle, Washington

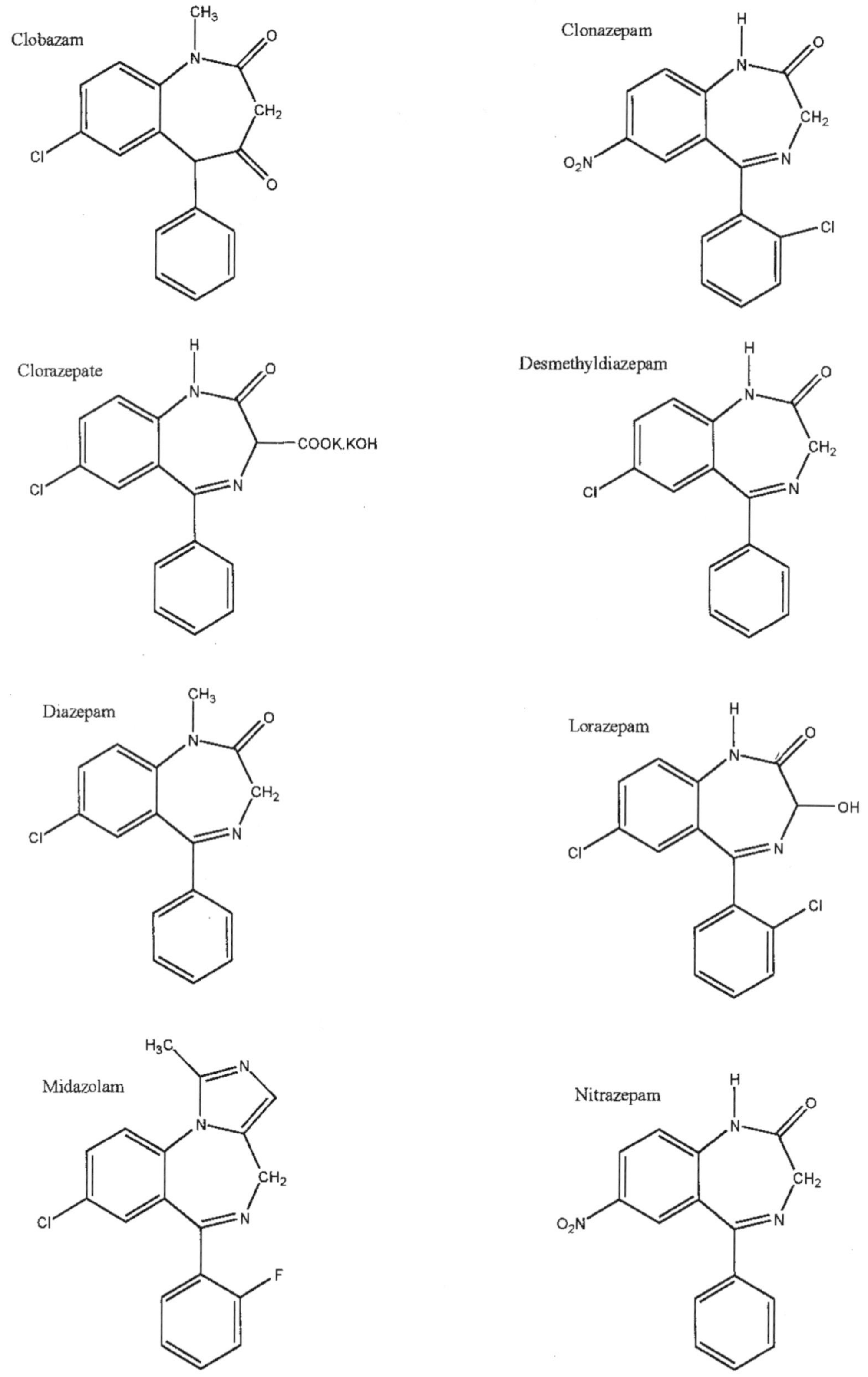

FIGURE 17.1. Chemical structure of the benzodiazepines.

ing of clobazam, infant exposure should be minimal, and breast-feeding is safe.

Routes Of Elimination

Although eight metabolites of clobazam exist in humans, the active metabolite *N*-desmethylclobazam is the most important (12).

Biotransformation. The main pathway is demethylation to *N*-desmethylclobazam, but hydroxylation also occurs. Unlike the 1,4-benzodiazepines, this hydroxylation occurs not at the 3 position of the heterocyclic ring, but at the 4 position before it is conjugated (12). This process leads to the formation of the other metabolites, 4-hydroxyclobazam and 4-hydroxydesmethylclobazam (18).

Renal Excretion. Renal excretion of unmetabolized clobazam is not significant (19).

Clearance and Half-Life

Healthy Subjects. The elimination half-life ($t\frac{1}{2}$) of clobazam ranges from 10 to 30 hours, whereas that of *N*-desmethylcobazam is 36 to 46 hours, thus accounting for its important contribution to the biologic action of clobazam (12).

Comedicated Epileptic Patients. The pharmacokinetics of a 30-mg oral clobazam dose was compared between patients receiving long-term antiepileptic drug therapy and control subjects (8). Although absorption was similar, clobazam was more rapidly and completely metabolized in the comedicated patients, presumably because of induction of hepatic metabolism (Table 17.1). As a result of this, *N*-desmethylclobazam levels were higher in the patients. Because it has been shown that *N*-desmethylclobazam is an effective antiepileptic agent when it is directly administered (20,21), this metabolite appears to be primarily responsible for the antiepileptic effects of clobazam in comedicated patients. Another study also found increased *N*-desmethylclobazam:clobazam ratios in patients comedicated with carbamazepine, phenytoin, or phenobarbital (22,23).

Elderly Patients. Study of the elimination of a single clobazam dose (24) revealed a statistically significant doubling of the $t\frac{1}{2}$ in elderly men (47.7 versus 16.6 hours), with trend toward a higher $t\frac{1}{2}$ in elderly women (48.6 versus 30.7 hours). The clearance is reduced (24).

Other Concurrent Conditions. Hepatic disease may alter both protein binding and clobazam elimination, with a potentially profound effect on clobazam levels (4).

Relationship between Serum Concentration and Dose and Effect

Because of the active metabolite *N*-desmethylcobazam, no clear correlation exists between clobazam levels and effect (25–27). Studies relating *N*-desmethylcobazam levels to psychometrically measured effects have not been performed, but this metabolite has effects on γ-aminobutyric acid–mediated chloride currents in cultured neurons that are identical to those of a similar range of clobazam concentrations (28).

CLONAZEPAM

Chemistry and Metabolic Scheme

Clonazepam [5-(2-chlorophenol)-1,3-dihydro-7-nitro-2H-1,4 benzodiazepin-2-one] is a light yellow crystalline powder with a molecular weight of 315.7 and negative log of dissociation constant (pK_a) of 1.5 and 10.5 (Figure 17.1) (29).

TABLE 17.1. CLOBAZAM PHARMACOKINETICS. VALUES REPORTED AS MEAN ±STANDARD DEVIATION OR RANGE IN DIFFERENT POPULATION

Population	T_{max} (h)	F	V (L/kg)	Fraction Bound (%)	Half-life (h)	Clearance (mL/min/kg)	References
Children	—	—	194	—	16 *N*-desmethylclobazam: 15	—	225
Adults: monotherapy	1.3–1.7	0.87	0.87–1.83	82–90	16.6–48.6 *N*-desmethylclobazam: 36–46	0.36–0.63	5–7,12,24
Elderly	Male, 1.6 Female, 1.5	—	Male, 1.4 Female, 1.83	Male, 86.5–90.4 Female, 85.0–89.2	Male, 47.7 Female, 48.6	Male, 0.36 Female, 0.48	24
Hepatic cirrhosis	2.5	—	178	—	51	—	13
Acute hepatitis	3.0	—	173	—	47	—	13

T_{max}, time of peak concentration; F, bioavailability; V, volume of distribution.

Absorption

Bioavailability. After oral administration, the bioavailability of clonazepam was >80% in seven of eight healthy subjects (30). The time of peak plasma concentrations ranged from 1 to 4 hours (30,31). After rectal administration in adult patients (32) and six children (33), clonazepam was well absorbed and resulted in peak concentrations in 10 to 30 minutes but with substantial interindividual variation. Absorption of clonazepam after intranasal and buccal administration was compared with an i.v. bolus in seven healthy subjects (34). The bioavailability of both formulations was approximately 40%. The time to peak ranged from 15 to 30 minutes for the intranasal formulation and from 30 to 90 minutes for the buccal administration. The rate and extent of absorption of clonazepam were decreased in patients with higher than normal gastric pH who were treated with ranitidine compared with absorption in patients with a normal gastric pH who were treated with caffeine (35).

Routes of Administration and Formulations. Clonazepam is available for oral administration as tablets and drops and as a parenteral formulation for i.v. administration.

Distribution

After i.v. administration, the distribution of clonazepam is described by a two-compartment model with a distribution $t\frac{1}{2}$ ranging from 0.7 to 3.4 hours (30). The VD ranges from 1.5 to 4.4 L/kg in healthy adults (30). In neonates, the apparent VD was similar to adults and ranged from 1.8 to 4.4 L/kg with a distribution $t\frac{1}{2}$ of 0.1 to 2.1 hours (36).

Plasma Protein Binding. Clonazepam protein binding is 86% in healthy subjects and is slightly decreased in patients with liver cirrhosis or reduced renal function and before hemodialysis in patients with chronic uremia (37).

Cerebrospinal Fluid, Brain, and Other Tissues. Studies in rodents have demonstrated that brain and plasma concentrations are proportional to dose with brain concentrations approximately three to four times higher than plasma (38).

Transplacental Passage. Two case reports have described placental transfer of clonazepam. In a woman treated with clonazepam for 1 week before delivery, the umbilical arterial and venous plasma levels were approximately equal to the maternal plasma concentration at delivery (39). In another case report of a woman treated with clonazepam throughout her pregnancy, clonazepam concentrations in the umbilical cord blood were 60% of the maternal serum concentration at delivery. The infant suffered neonatal apnea within a few hours of birth, possibly because of clonazepam-induced respiratory depression (40).

Breast Milk. After 12 days of breast-feeding, the infant described earlier had a serum clonazepam concentration of only 1 ng/mL, which could still be from the initial interuterine dose and not from breast milk specifically. Based on the high protein binding of clonazepam, infant exposure should be minimal, and breast-feeding should be safe.

Routes of Elimination

Biotransformation. Clonazepam is extensively metabolized by reduction of the nitro group at the 7 position to form 7-amino-clonazepam and hydroxylated to form 3-hydroxyclonazepam (41); 7-amino-clonazepam is sequentially metabolized by acetylation to form 7-acetamido-clonazepam. Plasma concentrations of 7-amino-clonazepam are approximately equal to and tend to parallel those of clonazepam during long-term administration (42).

Genetics and Isozymes. The initial reduction to 7-amino-clonazepam is catalyzed by the cytochrome CYP3A4 (43), and the subsequent acetylation occurs through *N*-acetyltransferase, which is polymorphically distributed (44). However, because the metabolite is not active, the genetic polymorphism is not clinically significant. The isozyme responsible for hydroxylation has not been identified.

Renal Excretion. Less than 1% of the dose of clonazepam is excreted unchanged in the urine (31,42). In one study, urinary recovery of clonazepam and of its primary metabolites accounted for 41% to 61% after a single oral dose, and fecal recovery ranged from 8% to 31% (41). In this study, approximately 40% to 50% of the recovered dose consisted of 7-amino-clonazepam and 7-acetamido-clonazepam, with approximately 30% excreted as hydroxylated metabolites.

Clearance and Half-Life

Healthy Subjects. The reported $t\frac{1}{2}$ and clearance of clonazepam range from 17 to 56 hours and 94 to 125 mL/hr/kg, respectively (30,31).

Comedicated Epileptic Patients. Coadministration of clonazepam with drugs that induce or inhibit CYP3A4 will alter clonazepam plasma clearance. Phenobarbital and phenytoin significantly increase the clearance of clonazepam by 19% to 24% and 46% to 58%, respectively, with resulting decreases in clonazepam $t\frac{1}{2}$ (45). Clonazepam plasma concentrations decreased by 19% to 37% over 5 to 15 days after administration of carbamazepine (46). Coadministration of clonazepam with fluoxetine (47) or sertraline (48) did not alter clonazepam clearance in healthy subjects.

Children. In a group of 18 neonates, the $t\frac{1}{2}$ ranged from 22 to 81 hours, with a prolonged $t\frac{1}{2}$ of 140 hours reported in one neonate (36) (Table 17.2). The corresponding clearance

TABLE 17.2. CLONAZEPAM PHARMACOKINETICS

Population	T_{max} (h)	F	V (L/kg)	Fraction Bound (%)	Half-life (h)	Clearance (mL/hr/kg)	References
Neonates	—	—	1.8–4.4	—	22–81	25–150	36
Children	2–3	—	2.1 ± 0.6	—	28 ± 4.6	53 ± 24	49,50
Adults:	1–4	>0.8	1.5–4.4	86	17–56	94–125	30,31
Monotherapy							
Polytherapy with inducers	—	—	2.3–7.7	87	12–46	96–208	45,46

T_{max}, time of peak concentration; F, bioavailability; V, volume of distribution.
Values reported as mean ± standard deviation or range in different populations.

ranged from 25 to 150 mL/hr/kg. In a study of nine children ages 2 to 18 years, the oral clearance of clonazepam showed a ninefold variation and ranged from 7 to 64 mL/hr/kg, with a mean of 25 mL/hr/kg (49). In another study of four children ages 7 to 12 years, the oral clearance of clonazepam was 37 to 89 mL/hr/kg. The t½ ranged from 22 to 33 hours (50).

Relationship between Serum Concentration and Dose

In children receiving clonazepam monotherapy, maintenance doses of clonazepam ranging from 0.028 to 0.11 mg/kg resulted in plasma concentrations of 13 to 72 ng/mL, with an excellent linear correlation between dose and serum concentration (50). In children receiving concurrent carbamazepine monotherapy, clonazepam doses of 0.03 to 0.18 mg/kg resulted in plasma concentrations of 13.8 to 67.9 ng/mL (51). A linear correlation between dose and serum concentrations has been demonstrated in adults, with doses of 1.2 to 2.9 mg/day dose resulting in serum concentrations of 4 to 36 ng/mL (52).

Relationship between Serum Concentration and Effect

In general, a clear relationship between serum concentration and effect has not been established. In children with absence seizures, efficacy was found with concentrations between 13 and 72 ng/mL (50). In patients with various epilepsy types, a clonazepam dose of 6 mg/day resulted in plasma concentrations of 25 to 30 ng/mL. On discontinuation of clonazepam in 14 patients, four patients who developed withdrawal symptoms had significantly higher 7-amino-clonazepam plasma concentrations than those without withdrawal symptoms but with similar clonazepam plasma concentrations (42). The significance of this observation is unknown.

CLORAZEPATE

Chemistry and Metabolic Scheme: Clorazepate dipotassium (7-chloro-1,3-dihydro-2-oxo-5-phenyl-1H-1,4-ben-zodiazepine-3-carboxylic acid, monopotassium salt, monopotassium hydroxide) is a prodrug that is rapidly and completely decarboxylated to form desmethyldiazepam (DMD) (Figure 17.1). DMD is a major metabolite of other benzodiazepines including diazepam, chlordiazepoxide, and prazepam. Chemically, clorazepate is an off-white to pale yellow, fine, crystalline powder with a molecular weight of 408.93. It is soluble in water (100 and 200 mg/mL), ethanol (0.6 mg/mL), and isopropanol (0.7 mg/mL) and in organic solvents (<0.5 mg/mL) (53). At pH levels of <4, >90% of clorazepate is converted to DMD within 10 minutes (54).

Absorption

Bioavailability. After oral administration, clorazepate is converted rapidly and completely in the stomach to DMD, and therefore the pharmacokinetics properties of clorazepate are described in terms of DMD. After oral administration of clorazepate, peak concentrations of DMD occur within 0.5 to 2 hours. The slow-release formulation, designed for once-daily administration, peaks in approximately 12 hours (55). Bioavailability of DMD after an oral or i.m. dose of clorazepate is approximately 90% to 100% (56,57). After either i.v. or i.m. administration, clorazepate decarboxylation to DMD is slower, with a chlorazepate elimination t½ of 2.3 to 2.4 hours (57). Because low gastric pH is required to convert clorazepate to DMD, any condition or medication that increases pH could alter the therapeutic efficacy of clorazepate. Administration of clorazepate with sodium bicarbonate at doses that increased the gastric pH to greater than 6 resulted in an increase in the time to peak serum concentrations and a decrease in the maximum serum concentration of DMD (58). However, studies in patients with a Billroth gastrectomy and impaired or absent gastric acid secretion did not demonstrate altered conversion of clorazepate to DMD (59). In some studies, coadministration with magnesia and alumina antacid suspension (60,61) reduced but did not significantly alter single-dose or steady-state DMD serum concentrations. Administration of clorazepate in patients after abdominal radiation resulted in a significantly decreased area under the concentration time curve for DMD compared with control subjects (62).

Routes of Administration and Formulations. Clorazepate is available as oral tablets, as capsules, as a slow-release preparation, and in some countries as a parenteral formulation that can be administered by i.v. or i.m. routes.

Distribution

After absorption, DMD distributes into the body in two phases, which can be characterized by a two-compartment model. The distribution $t\frac{1}{2}$ ranges from 0.7 to 2.2 hours. The VD ranges from 1 to 1.8 L/kg and is increased in obesity (56,63,64). Increasing age, female sex (65), and obesity (63) are associated with increased VD.

Plasma Protein Binding. DMD is highly protein bound predominately to albumin (96% to 98%), and the extent of binding is decreased with decreasing albumin plasma concentrations (65,66).

Cerebrospinal Fluid, Brain, and Other Tissues. Cerebrospinal fluid (CSF) concentrations of DMD correlate with its unbound serum concentrations and are approximately 4% of plasma concentrations (66). DMD rapidly crosses the blood–brain barrier. After long-term use of diazepam, DMD accumulates in the CSF (67). On autopsy in patients who had been treated with clorazepate or diazepam, DMD was concentrated in the adrenal gland, liver, and heart; intermediate concentrations were found in kidney, brain, and lung, and low concentrations were noted in skeletal muscle and fat (68).

Transplacental Passage. In a study evaluating i.m. clorazepate in pregnant women during the first stage of labor, clorazepate crossed the placental barrier slowly (68), in contrast to DMD, which was transported rapidly across the placenta to the fetus. DMD showed excess accumulation in heart and lungs of the fetus when diazepam was administered (69).

Breast Milk. DMD enters breast milk and reaches a concentration of 15% to 50% of the maternal plasma concentrations. However, the serum concentrations in the newborn are minimal.

Routes of Elimination

As stated earlier, clorazepate is a prodrug, which is rapidly converted to DMD in the stomach and is designed to produce therapeutic plasma concentrations of DMD.

Biotransformation. DMD is excreted unchanged (5% to 9% of the dose), it undergoes sequential metabolism to a glucuronide conjugate (25%), or it is hydroxylated to oxazepam, a reaction catalyzed by CYP2C19 and CYP3A4 (50%) (70). (Temazepam is demethylated to oxazepam, which is eliminated unchanged, and as a glucuronide conjugate.)

Genetics. See the later discussion of diazepam regarding CYP2C19 genetic polymorphism.

Biliary and Renal Excretion. After oral administration, <1% of the dose is recovered in the urine as unchanged clorazepate. When given by either i.v. or i.m. routes, approximately 7% is recovered as unchanged clorazepate. Between 15% and 20% of the dose is recovered in the feces because of biliary secretion (53,71).

Clearance and Half-life

Healthy Subjects. The $t\frac{1}{2}$ of DMD ranges from 55 to 100 hours, and clearance ranges from 0.18 to 0.27 mL/min/kg (56,61,65,72). In spite of the long $t\frac{1}{2}$, clorazepate is given in divided doses or as a slow-release formulation because of its rapid absorption, resulting in relatively high peak concentrations that have been associated with toxicity (Table 17.3). The $t\frac{1}{2}$ of DMD is prolonged in obese patients as a result of increased VD.

TABLE 17.3. DMD PHARMACOKINETICS AFTER ADMINISTRATION OF CLORAZEPATE

Population	T_{max} (h)	F	V (L/kg)	Fraction Bound (%)	Half-life (h)	Clearance (mL/min/kg)	References
Neonates					73–138	—	73
Adults: Monotherapy	p.o.: 0.5–2	1.0	0.7–2.2	96–98	40–130	0.18–0.27	56,61, 65,72
	i.m.: 2.7–11	0.91					
Polytherapy with inducers	p.o.: 0.5–1.5	—	1.63 ± 0.24	—	40.8 ± 9.96	0.47 ± 0.8	64
Elderly:							
Male	p.o.: 0.5–4.0	—	0.8–1.6	—	50–219	0.06–0.23	65
Female	0.5–4.0		0.9–2.5		48–116	0.12–0.41	
Obesity	p.o.: 0.5–2.5	—	1.0–2.5	—	64–369	0.05–0.23	63
Pregnancy	i.m.: 11 ± 2.2	—	3.1 ± 0.96	—	180 ± 100	0.37 ± 0.3	74

T_{max}, time of peak concentration; F, bioavailability; V, volume of distribution; p.o., oral; i.m., intramuscular.
Values reported as mean ± standard deviation or range in different populations.

Comedicated Epileptic Patients. The $t\frac{1}{2}$ of DMD is reduced in patients who are comedicated with enzyme inducers, presumably because of increased clearance (64). Cimetidine increases the $t\frac{1}{2}$ of DMD by decreasing the clearance in both young and elderly subjects (72).

Children. Neonates have a prolonged $t\frac{1}{2}$ (73).

Elderly Patients. The $t\frac{1}{2}$ of DMD is increased and the clearance reduced in elderly men, but not in elderly women (65, 72).

Other Concurrent Conditions. The $t\frac{1}{2}$ of DMD was prolonged in pregnant women because of an increased VD; however, there was no significant difference in clearance (74). The $t\frac{1}{2}$ was increased and the clearance was decreased in patients with liver disease (75). Smoking decreases the $t\frac{1}{2}$ and increases the clearance of DMD (76). Genetic variability in CYP2C19 is responsible for significant intersubject variability in clearance.

Relationship Between Serum Concentration and Dose and Serum Concentration and Effect. After administration of clorazepate either by the oral or i.m. route, there is a two- to threefold range in DMD peak concentrations and area under the concentration time curve. Clorazepate is a prodrug and is inactive. The effect of clorazepate is the result of its active metabolites, DMD, temazepam, and oxazepam.

DIAZEPAM

Chemistry and Metabolic Scheme

Diazepam (7-chloro-1,3-dihyro-1-methyl-5-phenyl-2H-1, 4 benzodiazepin-2-one) is a yellowish crystalline substance with a molecular weight of 284.8 and a melting point of 125° to 126°C (Figure 17.1). The pKa of diazepam is 3.4. Diazepam is soluble in chloroform, ethanol, dioxane, and dilute hydrochloric acid, but it is not soluble in water (77).

ABSORPTION

Bioavailability. On oral administration, 5-, 10-, or 20-mg doses of diazepam are rapidly and completely absorbed, with peak concentrations occurring within 30 to 90 minutes (78,79). Slow-release oral capsules peak in 3.8 hours; i.m. administration results in poor and irregular absorption, with plasma levels only approximately 60% of those obtained after oral administration (80,81). Rectal administration of a 0.5 to 1.0 mg/kg diazepam solution results in peak concentrations within 60 minutes (82,83). A rectal gel formulation is rapidly and completely absorbed within 30 to 60 minutes after rectal administration with an estimated

absolute bioavailability of 90% (84). Diazepam rectal suppositories exhibit slow and variable absorption and are not suitable for the treatment of acute seizures (82,85).

Routes of Administration and Formulations. Diazepam is administered by oral, i.v., i.m., and rectal routes and is available as an oral solution, tablets, a sustained-release capsule, a rectal suppository and gel, and a parenteral formulation.

Distribution

After i.v. administration, diazepam distributes into the body in two phases, which can be characterized by a two-compartment mathematical model. Diazepam distributes quickly into lipoid tissues and rapidly crosses the blood–brain barrier (86). The VD ranges from 1 to 2 L/kg (87). Female patients have a larger VD (1.87 L/kg) than male patients (1.34 L/kg) (88). Elderly persons have a larger VD (1.4 L/kg) than young persons (0.88 L/kg) (89). There is no significant difference in the VD in neonates, infants, or children (87).

Plasma Protein Binding. Diazepam is highly protein bound, and binding is significantly related to albumin, α_1-acid glycoprotein, and free fatty acid concentrations (90). Protein binding ranges from 97% to 99% (75,86). Protein binding is decreased in patients with reduced liver cirrhosis (75), in acute and chronic renal failure (91–93), in the elderly (93), and in the fetus and newborn (69). By the end of the first week, protein binding reaches adult levels, paralleled by changes in free fatty acid concentration (94,95).

Cerebrospinal Fluid, Brain, and other Tissues. The CSF concentrations of diazepam and DMD correlate with unbound concentrations (2% and 4% of plasma concentrations, respectively) (66). After an i.v. dose of diazepam, the time of onset in patients with status epilepticus ranges from immediate effect to 10 minutes (median, 2 minutes), a finding suggesting a rapid distribution into brain (96). Animal studies have demonstrated that brain concentrations of diazepam are obtained rapidly after i.v. administration and then decline in parallel to changes in plasma concentrations (97). Diazepam was concentrated in the adrenal gland, liver and heart, and kidney with lower concentrations in lung, fat, and brain at autopsy in patients who had been treated with diazepam (98).

Transplacental Passage. Both diazepam and DMD distribute across the placenta. DMD accumulates in fetal heart and lung (69).

Breast Milk. Because of the extensive protein binding of diazepam and DMD, the ratio of milk to plasma is low, ranging from 0.1 to 0.5, so the infant receives <5% of the therapeutic pediatric dose (99). However, during prolonged treatment with diazepam, the infant should be observed for signs of excess sedation.

Routes of Elimination

Biotransformation. Diazepam is extensively metabolized to several active metabolites including DMD, temazepam, and oxazepam (100). DMD is formed by a demethylation reaction catalyzed by CYP2C19 (major) and CY3A4 (70). DMD accumulates in blood to concentrations severalfold higher than diazepam. DMD is hydroxylated to oxazepam, a reaction catalyzed by CYP2C19, which is either excreted unchanged or undergoes sequential metabolism to a glucuronide conjugate. Diazepam is also hydroxylated to temazepam, a reaction catalyzed by CYP3A4 (70). Temazepam is demethylated to oxazepam or is excreted unchanged.

Genetics. Diazepam and DMD pharmacokinetics has been studied in subjects phenotyped for the CYP2C19 polymorphism. In a study in groups of poor and extensive metabolizers of CYP2C19, (101) the mean $t\frac{1}{2}$ of DMD was significantly longer in poor metabolizers of CYP2C19 (161 hours) than extensive metabolizers (116 hours). The mean $t\frac{1}{2}$ of diazepam was approximately the same in the Chinese extensive metabolizers of CYP2C19 (85 hours) and poor metabolizers (88 hours) but twice that of whites, who were extensive metabolizers (40.8 hours). A study in Korean patients (102) found the $t\frac{1}{2}$ of both diazepam (59.7 versus 91.0 hours) and DMD (95.9 versus 213.1 hours) to be sig-

nificantly shorter in extensive metabolizers of CYP2C19 compared with poor metabolizers. Similar results were found in a group of white patients who were poor and extensive CYP2C19 metabolizers (103).

Biliary and Renal Excretion. Diazepam is not excreted into the bile in significant amounts (75). Only a small percentage (2% to 3%) of diazepam is excreted unchanged in the urine (89).

Clearance and Half-Life

Healthy Subjects. The $t\frac{1}{2}$ of diazepam is approximately 1 to 2 days and is independent of dose (Table 17.4). DMD has a significantly longer $t\frac{1}{2}$ of 3 to 4 days and will accumulate, reaching two to five times higher concentrations at steady state than diazepam. Mean plasma clearance ranges from 14 to 35 mL/min in extensive metabolizers of CYP2C19 and from 9 to 12 mL/min in poor metabolizers of CYP2C19.

Comedicated Epileptic Patients. Patients comedicated with hepatic enzyme-inducing drugs (carbamazepine, phenytoin, phenobarbital, primidone) have a decreased $t\frac{1}{2}$ of diazepam and DMD (104).

Children. Neonates and infants have decreased hydroxylation and glucuronidation capacity, which may result in a decreased clearance of diazepam (105).

Elderly Patients. There is no age-related difference in diazepam clearance after single or multiple doses (89).

TABLE 17.4. DIAZEPAM AND DMD PHARMACOKINETICS AFTER DIAZEPAM ADMINISTRATION

Population	T$_{max}$ (h)	F	V (L/kg)	Fraction Bound (%)	Half-life (h)	Clearance (mL/min)	References
Neonates/infants	—	—	1.3 ± 0.2	Neonate: 84	Newborns: D: 31 ± 2 Infants: 10 ± 2	—	226
Children	p.o.: 30–90 i.m.: 30–60 Rectal gel: 10–30	—	2.6 ± 0.5	—	D: 17 ± 3 DMD:	—	100
Adults: Monotherapy	p.o.: 30–90 i.m.: 30–60 Rectal gel: 10–30	1.0	0.95–2.0	D: 96–99 DMD: 97	D: 28–54	D: 15–35 DMD 7.4–11.3	78,79
Polytherapy with inducers	—	—	 DMD: 1.6	—	D: 36 ± 5	D: 18.7 ± 2.3 DMD: 35.8 ± 7.4	104
Elderly	—	1.0	0.8–2.2	94.2 ± 0.38	D: 80–100 DM: 151 ± 60	D: 10–32 DM: 4.3 ± 1.5	89
Hepatic disease	—	—	0.6–1.7	95.3 ± 1.8	D: 59–116 h DMD: 108 ± 40	D: 8–24 DM: 4.6	75,104
Renal disease	—	—	—	92.0 ± 7.7	—	D: 28 ± 10	91–93
Pregnancy	—	—	—	—	D: 65 ± 29	—	69

T$_{max}$, time of peak concentration; F, bioavailability; DMD, desmethyldiazepam; V, volume of distribution; D, diazepam; p.o., oral; i.m., intramuscular.
Values reported as mean ± standard deviation or range in different populations.

Other Concurrent Diseases. Clearance is decreased, and $t\frac{1}{2}$ of DMD is significantly increased in patients with acute viral hepatitis and alcoholic cirrhosis when diazepam is administered (75,104).

Relationship between Serum Concentration and Dose

Diazepam plasma concentrations vary up to 10-fold after a single oral dose, threefold after multiple oral doses, and severalfold after i.v., i.m., and rectal administration (77,87).

Relationship between Serum Concentration and Effect

After multiple doses of diazepam, the pharmacologic effect of diazepam results from a combination of the effects of diazepam, DMD, temazepam, and oxazepam. In contrast, after a single dose of diazepam, metabolite accumulation does not occur to the extent of providing an initial effect; however, the prolonged $t\frac{1}{2}$ of DMD contributes to the duration of effect (77,87).

LORAZEPAM

Chemistry and Metabolic Scheme

Lorazepam (7-chloro-5(2-chlorophenyl)-1,3-dihydro-3-dihyroxy-2H-1,4-benzodiazepine-2-one) is a white, odorless, crystalline powder with a molecular weight of 321.16 and a melting point of approximately 168 °C (Figure 17.1). It has pK_a values of 1.3 and 11.5 and is virtually insoluble in water and undissociated at physiologic pH (106).

Absorption

Bioavailability. After oral administration in six healthy subjects, the bioavailability of lorazepam was >90%, with the time of peak concentrations within 1 to 2 hours (107,108). After i.m. administration of lorazepam, peak concentrations occur with 1 to 2 hours, and bioavailability is >90%. Sublingual administration of lorazepam resulted in a time lapse before absorption of approximately 23 minutes in nine of 10 subjects. The mean absorption $t\frac{1}{2}$ was 29 minutes, and bioavailability was 98% (108).

Routes of Administration and Formulations. Lorazepam is available as oral and sublingual tablets and as a parenteral solution for i.v. and i.m. administration.

Distribution

After both i.v. and i.m. administration, the distribution of lorazepam is described by a two-compartment model with a distribution $t\frac{1}{2}$ ranging from 1 to 30 minutes (107,108).

The VD ranges from 0.85 to 1.5 L/kg in healthy subjects (108,109). In critically ill neonates, the VD is approximately the same as in adults. In a study of 15 healthy elderly subjects, the VD was slightly less (0.99 L/kg) compared with young subjects (1.1 L/kg) (110). The VD in obese patients is significantly larger than in normal-weight controls. When normalized for body weight, there is no significant difference (111). In patients with liver cirrhosis, the VD was significantly increased compared with healthy subjects because of decreased protein binding (112).

Plasma Protein Binding. Lorazepam is approximately 93% protein bound to albumin, and binding is independent of concentration (113) and sex (114). Protein binding is decreased in the elderly (88%) (114) and in patients with concurrent liver disease (87%) (112).

Cerebrospinal Fluid, Brain, and other Tissues. Approximately 10% to 15% of the corresponding plasma concentration of lorazepam is found in the CSF; that this is approximately equal to the unbound fraction suggests that passage into the CSF is passive (115). Transport of lorazepam into CSF has been investigated in rodent (116) and mammalian models (117). In rats, lorazepam accumulates in brain tissue to concentrations approximately 40 times unbound concentrations in the serum, a finding suggesting that lorazepam is bound to receptors in the brain (116). In a study comparing i.v. lorazepam with diazepam in healthy subjects, the electroencephalographic effect did not reach maximum until 30 minutes after infusions of either low or high doses of lorazepam compared with 2.5 minutes with diazepam (118). In a follow-up study, the $t\frac{1}{2}$ for equilibration between plasma and the brain was 0.15 hour (119).

Transplacental Passage. Lorazepam distributes readily into the placenta (120–122). Single i.v. doses of lorazepam during labor result in approximately equal plasma concentrations in the infant at birth (121). A large study of 53 neonates born to 51 mothers receiving lorazepam demonstrated that umbilical cord blood concentrations were slightly lower than maternal plasma concentrations at time of delivery. Three-fourths of the infants requiring ventilation at birth had cord lorazepam concentrations >45 ng/mL (122).

Breast Milk. Because of its high protein binding, transfer of lorazepam into breast milk is minimal, and breast-feeding should be safe.

Routes of Elimination

Biotransformation. Lorazepam is extensively metabolized by the liver to a glucuronide conjugate at the 3-hydroxy position, a reaction catalyzed by uridine diphosphate glucuronosyltranferase. Minor metabolism also includes a 2-quinazoline carboxylic acid and hydroxylorazepam (123). Plasma concentrations of lorazepam glucuronide are twice as high as those of lorazepam (124). The glucuronide metabolite is inactive and does not contribute to the pharmacologic effect of lorazepam (123).

Biliary and Renal Excretion. Less than 1% of lorazepam is excreted unchanged by the kidneys (107,124). Approximately 75% of the lorazepam dose is recovered as lorazepam glucuronide, with 13% recovered as minor metabolites (123). After administration of ^{14}C-lorazepam to healthy subjects, 88% of the dose was recovered, with 78% as lorazepam glucuronide, and fecal recovery accounted for only 7% (124). Lorazepam undergoes significant enterohepatic recirculation. When enterohepatic recirculation was interrupted by administration of neomycin and cholestyramine, lorazepam oral and systemic clearance increased by 34% and 24%, respectively (125).

Clearance and Half-Life

Healthy Subjects. The clearance and t$\frac{1}{2}$ of lorazepam have been determined in numerous studies with various dosage forms. The ranges of clearances and t$\frac{1}{2}$ are 0.91 to 1.75 mL/min/kg and 17 to 56 hours, respectively (107–109, 112,118,222). A slight decrease in clearance with a 3-mg i.v. dose (1.88±0.23 mL/min/kg) compared with a 1.6-mg i.v. dose (2.08±0.22 mL/min/kg) has been reported (118). In contrast, pharmacokinetic studies of three patients who took overdoses of lorazepam found that the t$\frac{1}{2}$ of lorazepam was approximately the same as was found with therapeutic doses, a finding suggesting non–dose-dependent elimination (126).

Comedicated Epileptic Patients. Even though lorazepam is commonly used in patients who are also receiving other enzyme-inducing antiepileptic drugs, there are no pharmacokinetic studies in this patient population (Table 17.5). Based on the hepatic induction profile of carbamazepine, phenytoin, and phenobarbital, lorazepam clearance should be significantly increased and t$\frac{1}{2}$ decreased with concurrent use of hepatic enzyme inducers. Valproate decreases the clearance of lorazepam by approximately 40% (127).

Children. Neonates receiving lorazepam by maternal transmission at birth cleared lorazepam slowly. Full-term infants continued to excrete lorazepam for at least 8 days, and preterm infants excreted the drug for at least 11 days (122). The clearance was approximately 25% of that found in adults, with a resulting prolonged t$\frac{1}{2}$ in critically ill neonates receiving i.v. lorazepam (128). In a study designed to evaluate the effects of cystic fibrosis, the control group consisted of children and adolescents ages 7 to 19 years. There was no significant difference in the pharmacokinetics of lorazepam compared with adult values taken from the literature (129). There is no information on the pharmacokinetics of lorazepam in infants and children ages 1 to 7 years. Because glucuronidation reaches adult levels by ages 2 to 3 years (130), after the age of 3 years, clearance corrected for body weight should be approximately the same as for adults. In infants and children <3 years old, doses should be reduced because of a decreased glucuronidation capacity and presumably decreased clearance.

Elderly Patients. Lorazepam clearance was slightly reduced by 22% in a group of 15 elderly healthy subjects compared with young subjects. There was no difference in t$\frac{1}{2}$ (110).

Obesity. In one study, the clearance of lorazepam was increased in obesity; however, as with the VD, when normalized for body weight, no significant difference was noted (111). Therefore, there was no resulting difference in t$\frac{1}{2}$.

TABLE 17.5. LORAZEPAM PHARMACOKINETICS

Population	T$_{max}$ (h)	F	V (L/kg)	Fraction Bound (%)	Half-life (h)	Clearance (ml/min/kg)	References
Neonates	—	—	0.76 ± 0.37	—	40.2 ± 16.5	0.232 ± 0.11	128
Children	—	—	0.8 ± 0.06	—	7.7–17.3	0.8 ± 0.08	129
Adults: Monotherapy 107–109,112,118,227	p.o.: 2.4 ± 0.3	0.99 ± 0.06	0.85–1.5	93.2 ± 1.8	7–26	0.91–1.76	
	i.m.: 1.2 ± 0.3	0.96 ± 0.04					
	s.l.: 2.3 ± 0.7	0.94 ± 0.07					
Elderly	i.m.: 1.03 ± 0.16 p.o.: 0.95 ± 0.19	—	0.99 ± 0.03	87–89	15.9 ± 1.1	0.77 ± 0.06	110,114
Obesity	—	—	1.25 ± .10	89.1 ± 0.4	16.5 ± 1.7	0.98 ± 0.12	111
Hepatic cirrhosis	—	—	2.01 ± 0.82	88.6 ± 2.5	41.2 ± 24.5	0.81 ± 0.48	112
Acute hepatitis	—	—	1.52 ± 0.64	91.0 ± 1.9	28.3 ± 8.9	0.74 ± 0.34	112
Cystic fibrosis	—	—	1.5 ± 0.1	—	6.9–17.3	1.8 ± 0.2	129

T$_{max}$, time of peak concentration; F, bioavailability; V, volume of distribution; p.o., oral; i.m., intramuscular; s.l., subcutaneous.
Values reported as mean ± standard deviation or range in different populations.

Other Concurrent Conditions. There is no significant difference in the pharmacokinetics of lorazepam in patients with acute hepatitis (112). In contrast, liver cirrhosis is associated with an increase in the VD of lorazepam resulting in a doubling of the mean $t_{1/2}$. Because of the lack of renal excretion of unchanged drug, the clearance of lorazepam is unaffected by renal impairment. Only 8% of lorazepam is removed by 6 hours of hemodialysis (131). There was no difference in the pharmacokinetics of lorazepam between patients with well-controlled insulin-dependent diabetes mellitus and healthy controls (132). In a group of patients with cystic fibrosis, the clearance of lorazepam was approximately double, and $t_{1/2}$ was 50% compared with an age-matched control population (129). Lorazepam clearance was decreased by 37%, and $t_{1/2}$ was increased in a group of tetraplegic patients compared with healthy subjects. The clearance in paraplegic patients was decreased, although not to the same extent as in the tetraplegic patients (133).

Relationship between Serum Concentration and Dose

The relationship between dose and serum concentration for all routes of lorazepam administration is linear. Oral doses of 2 or 4 mg of lorazepam result in peak plasma concentrations of 23 to 36 μg/mL or 39 to 68 μg/mL, respectively (107,108). For multiple doses, plasma clearance varies twofold, which will result in a corresponding twofold variation in steady-state plasma concentrations.

Relationship between Serum Concentration and Effect

A study in patients with intractable partial complex seizures suggested a narrow therapeutic range of 20 to 30 ng/mL for seizure control, with side effects occurring at concentrations >33 ng/mL (134). Lorazepam plasma concentrations of 30 to 100 ng/mL resulted in good seizure control in a group of patients with status epilepticus (135). A pharmacokinetic-pharmacodynamic study of the amnesic effects of lorazepam found a 50% effective concentration of 12 to 15 ng/mL (136).

MIDAZOLAM

Chemistry and Metabolic Scheme

Midazolam (8-chloro-6-(2-fluorophenyl)-1-methyl-4H-imidazo[1,5-a][1,4]benzodiazepine) is an imidazobenzodiazepine that readily forms soluble salts (pK$_a$ 6.15) because of the nitrogen in position 2 or the imidazole ring (137,138). It has a molecular weight of 362 (Figure 17.1) (137).

Absorption

Bioavailability. Midazolam is administered parenterally as a salt in an acidic aqueous solution. However, at physiologic pH, it is highly lipophilic. As a result, it has very rapid onset and a short duration of action after single i.v. or i.m. doses. Peak sedation is achieved within 3 minutes in healthy adults after i.v. infusion (138). Midazolam is compatible with 5% dextrose in water, normal saline, and lactated Ringer's solution.

Routes of Administration and Formulations. Midazolam is commonly used as a midazolam hydrochloride solution at acidic pH (3.3 to 3.5). Midazolam can be administered intermittently or continuously by the i.v. or i.m. route. Because parenteral formulations do not require propylene glycol or other lipoidal substituents, local irritation from injections are minimal. After i.m. injection, peak levels are reached in 20 to 30 minutes, with 91% bioavailability for midazolam hydrochloride (138). The parenteral formulation has been administered by the oral, rectal, buccal, (139,140) and intranasal (141,142) routes; an oral tablet is available in Europe, and an oral syrup is available in the United States. Testing of the oral midazolam syrup indicates that when 1 mg/kg is administered as an oral syrup (143), adequate sedation is produced within 30 minutes. However, because midazolam is rapidly cleared by the liver, only about half of an orally administered dose reaches the systemic circulation as unchanged drug (144). In children, oral bioavailability is as low as 27% because of first-pass hepatic metabolism (145).

Distribution

After i.v. administration, midazolam has a rapid phase of disappearance because of distribution, with a $t_{1/2}$ of 6 to 15 minutes (144), followed by slower disappearance resulting from biotransformation. In healthy subjects, the VD is 1 to 2.5 L/kg (146–152), and it increases with obesity (153) and in the elderly (154,155).

Plasma Protein Binding. The plasma binding of midazolam is 97% (137).

Cerebrospinal Fluid, Brain, and other Tissues. In experimental animals, midazolam has been shown to equilibrate between plasma and CSF within a few minutes of i.v. administration and then to enter cerebral tissue rapidly (117).

Routes of Elimination

Midazolam is rapidly eliminated by hepatic and intestinal metabolism, a reaction catalyzed entirely by CYP3A4, with a hepatic extraction ratio of 0.3 (156).

Biotransformation. Metabolism occurs by oxidation of the imidazole ring, predominately to 1-hydroxymidazolam (75%), with small amounts of 4-hydroxymidazolam (3%) and 1,4-dihydroxymidazolam (1%) (157–161). This is followed by glucuronidation. The main metabolite, 1-hydroxymidazolam, has about 10% of the biologic activity of midazolam and an elimination $t\frac{1}{2}$ of 1 hour (146,161).

Genetics. Midazolam metabolism entirely depends on CYP3A, and its hepatic clearance has been used as a phenotyping probe for this cytochrome P450 enzyme subfamily (156,162). A higher proportion of isoform CYP3A5 favors production of 1-hydroxymidazolam, whereas 1,4-hydroxyl production is favored when more CYP3A4 is present (163–165). Although considerable individual variation in these isoforms exist, clinically significant differences have not been found between African-American and European-American populations (166).

Renal Excretion. Approximately 45% to 57% of midazolam is renally excreted as glucuronide conjugates, with only 0.03% of midazolam excreted unchanged (137).

Clearance and Half-Life

Healthy Subjects. The $t\frac{1}{2}$ of midazolam ranges from 1.5 to 4 hours, and clearance ranges from 0.24 to 0.53 L/min (146,148,149).

Comedicated Epileptic Patients. Midazolam metabolism is decreased by drugs that inhibit the activity of CYP3A4, such as erythromycin, clarithromycin, ketoconazole, dilti-azem, verapamil, and cimetidine (149,167,168) (Table 17.6). Long-term administration of agents such as carbamazepine, phenytoin, and barbiturates, which induce hepatic metabolism, decrease midazolam bioavailability appreciably.

Children. In neonates, the $t\frac{1}{2}$ of midazolam is prolonged, with a decreased clearance compared with adults (169,170). The $t\frac{1}{2}$ of midazolam is somewhat shorter in children, and the clearance is somewhat higher (137,145,171,172).

Elderly Patients. In these patients, the midazolam VD may be increased, and the $t\frac{1}{2}$ may be prolonged (154, 155).

Other Concurrent Conditions. The clearance of midazolam is reduced in patients with hepatic disease (173), congestive heart failure (174), and decreased cardiac output or hepatic blood flow (175). Renal failure increases the free fraction of midazolam because of reduced plasma protein binding; one study found that it did not significantly affect midazolam elimination (176), although another found prolongation of the $t\frac{1}{2}$ to 13 hours in patients with renal failure who were in an intensive care unit (177).

Relationship between Serum Concentration and Dose and Effect

A good relationship has been found between midazolam plasma or serum concentration and psychometrically measured effects after oral (149,178), i.m. (179), and i.v. (149,178–180) administration. Subjective effects occur at a threshold of levels of 30 to 100 ng/mL (149,178,179).

TABLE 17.6. MIDAZOLAM PHARMACOKINETICS

Population	T_{max} (h)	F	V (L/kg)	Fraction Bound (%)	Half-life (h)	Clearance (mL/min/kg)	References
Neonates	—	—	—	—	6.52–12	3.9–6.85	169,170
Children	—	—	—	—	0.78–2.4	6.4–15.4	145,171,172
Adults: monotherapy	i.m.: 0.24–0.51 p.o.: 0.5–0.97	i.v., i.m.: 1.0 p.o.: 0.40	0.7–1.7	96	1.36–4	6.4–11.1	144, 147–149, 151,161,179
Elderly	Male, 0.71–0.85 Female, 0.54–0.74	—	Male, 119–139 Female, 113–137	—	Male p.o.: 3.43–5.35 i.v.: 4.2–7.0 Female p.o.: 2.65–4.55 i.v.: 3.2–4.8	Male, 296–382 Female, 383–481	153
Obesity	0.77–1.01	—	284–338	—	i.v. 7.56–9.24 p.o.: 5.09–6.79	434–510 mL/min	153
Chronic renal failure	—	—	3.48–4.1	—	3.83–5.33	9.85–12.95	176

T_{max}, time of peak concentration; F, bioavailability; V, volume of distribution; i.m., intramuscular; i.v., intravenous; p.o., oral.
Values reported as mean or range in different populations.

NITRAZEPAM

Chemistry and Metabolic Scheme

Nitrazepam (1,3-dihydro-7-nitro-5-phenyl-2H-1,4-benzo-diazepine-2-one) is a benzodiazepine derivative (Figure 17.1) that is used as a sedative-hypnotic agent (181,182) and to treat selected forms of epilepsy in some countries (183–186). It is a yellow, odorless, tasteless crystalline powder, which is insoluble in water, but soluble in chloroform, ethanol, ether, and diluted inorganic acids. It has a molecular weight of 281.3 and a melting point of 226° to 229°C. It has pK_a values of 3.2 and 10.8 (187).

Absorption

Bioavailability. Mean peak plasma concentrations of 35 to 47 ng/mL are reportedly achieved after an oral dose of 5 mg of nitrazepam, and levels of 83 to 164 ng/mL occur after 10-mg doses both in healthy young and elderly patients of both sexes. Peak levels are usually achieved in less than an hour (188–194). Rectal administration leads to similar peak levels in approximately 18 minutes (191).

Routes of Administration and Formulations. Nitrazepam is administered by oral, i.v., i.m., and rectal routes. Oral bioavailability is reportedly total with oral administration (191), but it is only 80% when the drug is given rectally. There is some evidence that peak level times vary among different oral preparation brands (189).

Distribution

The distribution of nitrazepam can be explained in a two-compartment open model either after i.v. administration or after the peak concentration has been reached (187–189, 191,195,196). The initial rapid decline of concentration resulting from redistribution has a $t\frac{1}{2}$ of 17 minutes. The mean VD in young healthy subjects is 2.0 L/kg (191,196) after i.v. administration and 2.4 L/kg after oral administration (197). One study (198) found no gender differences; another (194) found a larger VD in women (2.56 versus 1.82 L/kg). Elderly subjects have a somewhat larger VD than young subjects (194,197,199), although this difference is small at steady state (199).

Plasma Protein Binding. Nitrazepam is highly protein bound, with an 85.8% to 86.8% bound fraction (184). Protein binding is decreased in patients with hepatic cirrhosis (81.1% versus 86.2% in healthy controls) (199), but VD is unaffected. Similarly, binding is also decreased in patients with chronic renal insufficiency (83.2% versus 85%) (200). Protein binding in healthy elderly patients is similar to that in young subjects (194,201).

Cerebrospinal Fluid, Brain, and Other Tissues. Evidence suggests that equilibration between plasma and CSF concentrations occurs slowly (202), because after a 5-mg oral dose, the percentage ratio of CSF to plasma concentrations increases from 8% at 2 hours to 15.6% at 36 hours. Animal studies have found a brain to plasma concentration ratio of 60% at 15 to 30 minutes after i.v. administration (203), but brain concentrations are lower in younger rats (204). Excretion of nitrazepam into saliva is variable and does not reliably reflect free plasma concentration (197, 205,206). On postmortem examination of patients who had taken nitrazepam on a long-term basis, similar concentrations of nitrazepam were present in peripheral blood and in the liver, but nitrazepam was concentrated in the vitreous humor and bile (207). Significant redistribution did not occur after death (207).

Transplacental Passage. Nitrazepam does cross the human placenta, with lower concentrations than plasma early on, but with equilibrium with maternal tissues in late pregnancy (208).

Breast Milk. Nitrazepam is excreted into breast milk only in low concentrations (184,209,210). However, sedation has nonetheless been reported in nursing infants of mothers who take nitrazepam (211).

Routes of Elimination

Nitrazepam elimination is primarily urinary and is independent of dose and administration route (184,187).

Biotransformation. Nitrazepam undergoes nitroreduction, which is mediated not only by hepatic enzymes but also by intestinal microflora (212). Subsequent acetylation to 7-aminonitrazepam and the hydroxylation of a small fraction of this metabolite occur in the liver (184,213,214). A secondary metabolic route to benzophenones also exists (187).

Genetics. The acetylation of 7-aminonitrazepam is genetically polymorphic, but this is not clinically significant because 7-aminonitrazepam is not pharmacologically active (215,216).

Biliary and Renal Excretion. About half of a single oral dose of nitrazepam is excreted in the urine within a week (184,217). Most of this is in the form of the metabolites 7-acetamidonitrazepam and 7-aminonitrazepam, with less than 1% unchanged. Nitrazepam and its metabolites are found in bile at five to 12 times plasma concentrations (36,207), and 8% to 20% of nitrazepam doses are excreted in the feces (217).

TABLE 17.7. NITRAZEPAM PHARMACOKINETICS

Population	T$_{max}$ (h)	F	V (L/kg)	Fraction Bound (%)	Half-life (h)	Clearance (mL/min/kg)	References
Neonates	—	—		85–88	—	—	197
Adults: monotherapy	1.35–2.47	0.54–0.93	2.5–2.9	85–88	21–40	1.51–1.91	184,188,195,197,228,229
Elderly	4–8	—	3.1–6.5	—	24.2–56.6	—	220,228
Obesity	—	—	2.45–2.79	79.9–80.7	31.3–35.7	—	193
Hepatic Cirrhosis	—	—	2.17	81.1	30.5	59 mL/min	199
Chronic renal failure	—	—	3.84–4.48	83.2	20.4–42.6	1.9–6.5	200

T$_{max}$, time of peak concentration; F, bioavailability; V, volume of distribution.
Values reported as range in different populations.

Clearance and Half-Life

Healthy Subjects. The t$\frac{1}{2}$ of nitrazepam ranges from 18 to 31 hours (184,188,189,191,192,194,195,199,218,219), with similar results after single oral or i.v. doses or with long-term treatment for 14 to 24 days (184,220).

Comedicated Epileptic Patients. The only clinically significant interaction that has been reported for nitrazepam is potentiation of its effect by coadministration of sodium valproate (221) (Table 17.7.). However, induction of the hepatic microsomal enzyme system by rifampin does increase nitrazepam clearance significantly (222), a finding suggesting that, as with other benzodiazepines, nitrazepam pharmacokinetics may be influenced by hepatic enzyme-inducing antiepileptic drugs.

Elderly Patients. Somewhat increased mean t$\frac{1}{2}$ of 38 to 40 hours have been reported in the elderly (199,220).

Other Concurrent Conditions. The t$\frac{1}{2}$ is also prolonged in obesity because of the increased VD (191). The clearance of nitrazepam is unaffected by chronic renal or hepatic disease (199,200).

Relationship between Serum Concentration and Dose and Effect

Long-term daily nitrazepam doses of 170 to 390 µg/kg have been found to lead to plasma concentrations of 40 to 180 ng/mL in children with epilepsy (220). The peak sedative effects of a single oral dose of 5 mg have been seen about 2 hours before peak plasma concentrations have been reached (223). Moreover, a lack of correlation between the residual effects of nitrazepam and plasma levels has been described (205,218,224).

REFERENCES

1. Gastaut H, Low M. Antiepileptic properties of clobazam, a 1,5 benzodiazepine in man. *Epilepsia* 1979;20:437–446.

2. Feely M. Fortnightly review: drug treatment of epilepsy. *BMJ* 1999;318:106–109.

3. Schmidt D, Bourgeois B. A risk-benefit assessment of therapies for Lennox-Gastaut syndrome. *Drug Saf* 2000;22:467–477.

4. Shorvon SD. Benzodiazepines: clobazam. In: Levy RH, Mattson RH, Meldrum BS, eds. *Antiepileptic drugs,* 4th ed. New York: Raven Press, 1995:763–777.

5. Rupp W, Badian M, Christ O, et al. Pharmacokinetics of single and multiple doses of clobazam in humans. *Br J Clin Pharmacol* 1979;7:51S–57S.

6. Divoll M, Greenblatt D, Ciraulo D, et al. Clobazam kinetics: intrasubject variability and effect of food on absorption. *J Clin Pharmacol* 1982;22:69–73.

7. Tedeschi G, Riva R, Baruzzi A. Clobazam plasma concentrations: pharmacokinetic study in healthy volunteers and data in epileptic patients. *Br J Clin Pharmacol* 1981;11:619–621.

8. Jawad S, Richenbs A, Oxley J. Single dose pharmacokinetic study of clobazam in normal volunteers and epileptic patients. *Br J Clin Pharmacol* 1984;18:873–877.

9. Guentert TW. Time-dependence in benzodiazepinepharmacokinetics: mechanisms and clinical significance. *Clin Pharmacokinet* 1984;9:203–210.

10. Davies IB, McEwen J, Pidgen AW, et al. Comparison of N-desmethylclobazam and N-desmethyldiazepam: two active benzodiazepine metabolites. In: Hindmarch I, Stonier PD, Trimble MR, eds. *Clobazam: psychopharmacology and clinical applications.* International Congress and Symposium Series no. 74. London: Royal Society of Medicine, 1985:11–16.

11. Aucamp AK. Aspects of the pharmacokinetics and pharmacodynamics of benzodiazepines with particular reference to clobazam. *Drug Dev Res Suppl* 1982;1:117–126.

12. Volz M, Christ O, Kellner H-M, et al. Kinetics and metabolism of clobazam in animals and man. *Br J Clin Pharmacol* 1979;7 [Suppl 1]:41S–50S.

13. Monjanel-Mouterde S, Antoni M, Bun H, et al. Pharmacokinetics of a single oral dose of clobazam in patients with liver disease. *Pharmacol Toxicol* 1994;74:345–350.

14. Gorodischer R, Burtin P, Verjee Z, et al. Is saliva suitable for therapeutic monitoring of anticonvulsants in children? An evaluation in the routine clinical setting. *Ther Drug Monit* 1997;19:637–642.

15. Fraser AD, Isner AF, Heifetz SA. Tissue distribution of ethosuximide and clobazam in a seizure related fatality. *J Forensic Sci* 1988;33:1058–1063.

16. McElhatton PR. The effects of benzodiazepines use during pregnancy and lactation. *Reproductive Toxicol* 1994;8:461–475.

17. Bar-Oz B, Nulman I, Koren G, et al. Anticonvulsants and breast-feeding: a critical review. *Pediatr Drugs* 2000;2:113–126.

18. Hanks GWBJCP. Clobazam: pharmacological and therapeutic profile. *Br J Clin Pharmacol* 1979;7:151S–155S.

19. Bernus I, Dickinson RG, Hooper WD, et al. Anticonvulsant therapy in aged patients. *Drugs Aging* 1997;10:278–289.
20. Callaghan N, Gogin T. Clobazam as adjunctive treatment in drug resistant epilepsy: report on an open prospective study. *Ir Med J* 1984;77:240–244.
21. Dailley C, Freely M, Gent JP, et al. A preliminary evaluation of *N*-desmethylclobazam in epilepsy. *Br J Pharmacol* 1986;89:705.
22. Sennoune S, Mesdjian E, Bonneton J, et al. Interactions between clobazam and standard antiepileptic drugs in patients with epilepsy. *Ther Drug Monit* 1982;14:269–274.
23. Theis JGW, Koren G, Daneman R, et al. Interactions of clobazam with conventional antiepileptics in children. *J Child Neurol* 1997;12:208–213.
24. Greenblatt DJ, Divoll M, Surrendra KP, et al. Clobazam kinetics in the elderly. *Br J Clin Pharmacol* 1981;12:631–636.
25. Dulac O, Figueroa D, Rey E, et al. Monothérapie par le clobazam dans les épilepsies de l'enfant. *Presse Med* 1983;12: 1067–1069.
26. Schmidt D, Rhode M, Wolf P, et al. Tolerance to the antiepileptic effect of clobazam. In: Grey H-H, Froscher W, Koella WP, et al., eds. *Tolerance to beneficial and adverse effects of antiepileptic drugs.* New York: Raven Press, 1986:109–118.
27. Shimizu H, Abe J, Futagi Y, et al. Antiepileptic effects of clobazam in children. *Brain Dev* 1982;4:57–62.
28. Nakamura F, Suzuki S, Nishimura S, et al. Effects of clobazam and its active metabolite on GABA-activated currents in rat cerebral neurons in culture. *Epilepsia* 1996;37:728–735.
29. Sato S, Malow BA. Clonazepam. In: Levy RH, Mattson RH, Meldrum BS, eds. *Antiepileptic drugs,* 4th ed. New York: Raven Press, 1995:725–734.
30. Berlin A, Dahlstrom H. Pharmacokinetics of the anticonvulsant drug clonazepam evaluated from single oral and intravenous doses and repeated oral administration. *Eur J Clin Pharmacol* 1975;9:155–159.
31. Kaplan SA, Alexander K, Jack ML, et al. Pharmacokinetic profiles of clonazepam in dog and humans and of flunitrazepam in dog. *J Pharm Sci* 1974;63:527–532.
32. Klosterskov Jensen P, Abild K, Nohr Poulsen M. Serum concentration of clonazepam after rectal administration. *Acta Neurol Scand* 1983;68:417–420.
33. Rylance GW, Poulton J, Cherry RC, et al. Plasma concentrations of clonazepam after single rectal administration. *Arch Dis Child* 1986;61:186–188.
34. Schols-Hendriks MW, Lohman JJ, Janknegt R, et al. Absorption of clonazepam after intranasal and buccal administration. *Br J Clin Pharmacol* 1995;39:449–451.
35. Meyer MC, Straughn AB. Biopharmaceutical factors in seizure control and drug toxicity. *Am J Hosp Pharm* 1993;50[Suppl 5]: S17–S22.
36. Andre M, Boutroy MJ, Dubruc C, et al. Clonazepam pharmacokinetics and therapeutic efficacy in neonatal seizures. *Eur J Clin Pharmacol* 1986;30:585–589.
37. Pacifici GM, Viani A, Rizzo G, et al. Plasma protein binding of clonazepam in hepatic and renal insufficiency and after hemodialysis. *Ther Drug Monit* 1987;9:369–373.
38. Greenblatt DJ, Miller LG, Shader RI. Clonazepam pharmacokinetics, brain uptake, and receptor interactions. *J Clin Psychiatry* 1987;48[Suppl]:4–11.
39. de Groot G, Maes RAA, Thiery M. Placental transfer of clonazepam: a case study. *IRCS Med Sci* 1977;5:589.
40. Fisher JB, Edgren BE, Mammel MC, et al. Neonatal apnea associated with maternal clonazepam: a case report. *Obstet Gynecol* 1985;66[Suppl]:34S–35S.
41. Eschenhof VE. Untersuchungen uber das Schicksal des antikonvulsivums Clonazepam im Organismus der Ratte, des Hundes und des Menschen. *Arzneimittelforschung* 1973;23:390–400.
42. Sjo O, Hvidberg EF, Naestoft J, et al. Pharmacokinetics and side-effects of clonazepam and its 7-amino-metabolite in man. *Eur J Clin Pharmacol* 1975;8:249–254.
43. Seree EJ, Pisano PJ, Placidi M, et al. Identification of the human and animal hepatic cytochrome P450 involved in clonazepam metabolism. *Fundam Clin Pharmacol* 1993;7:69–75.
44. Miller ME, Garland WA, Min BH, et al. Clonazepam acetylation in fast and slow acetylators. *Clin Pharmacol Ther* 1981;30: 343–347.
45. Khoo KC, Mendels J, Rothbart M, et al. Influence of phenytoin and phenobarbital on the disposition of a single oral dose of clonazepam. *Clin Pharmacol Ther* 1980;28:368–375.
46. Lai AA, Levy RH, Cutler RE. Time-course of interaction between carbamazepine and clonazepam in normal man. *Clin Pharmacol Ther* 1978;24:316–323.
47. Greenblatt DJ, Preskorn SH, Cotreau MM, et al. Fluoxetine impairs clearance of alprazolam but not clonazepam. *Clin Pharmacol Ther* 1992;52:479–486.
48. Bonate PL, Kroboth PD, Smith RB, et al. Clonazepam and sertraline: absence of drug interaction in a multiple-dose study. *J Clin Psychopharmacol* 2000;20:19–27.
49. Walson PD, Edge JH. Clonazepam disposition in pediatric patients. *Ther Drug Monit* 1996;18:1–5.
50. Dreifuss FE, Penry JK, Rose SW, et al. Serum clonazepam concentrations in children with absence seizures. *Neurology* 1975; 25:255–258.
51. Hosoda N, Miura H, Takanashi S, et al. The long-term effectiveness of clonazepam therapy in the control of partial seizures in children difficult to control with carbamazepine monotherapy. *Jpn J Psychiatry Neurol* 1991;45:471–473.
52. Labbate LA, Pollack MH, Otto MW, et al. The relationship of alprazolam and clonazepam dose to steady-state concentration in plasma. *J Clin Psychopharmacol* 1994;14:274–276.
53. Wilensky AJ. Benzodiazepines: chlorazepate. In: Levy RH, Mattson RH, Meldrum BS, eds. *Antiepileptic drugs,* 4th ed. New York: Raven Press, 1995:751–762.
54. Abruzzo CW, Brooks MA, Cotler S, et al. Differential pulse polarographic assay procedure and *in vitro* biopharmaceutical properties of dipotassium chlorazepate. *J Pharmacokinet Biopharm* 1976;4:29–41.
55. Carrigan PJ, Chao GC, Barker WM, et al. Steady-state bioavailability of two clorazepate dipotassium dosage forms. *J Clin Pharmacol* 1977;17:18–28.
56. Greenblatt DJ, Divoll MK, Soong MH, et al. Desmethyldiazepam pharmacokinetics: studies following intravenous and oral desmethyldiazepam, oral clorazepate, and intravenous diazepam. *J Clin Pharmacol* 1988;28:853–859.
57. Bertler A, Lindgren S, Magnusson JO, et al. Pharmacokinetics of chlorazepate after intravenous and intramuscular administration. *Psychopharmacology (Berl)* 1983;80:236–239.
58. Abruzzo CW, Macasieb T, Weinfeld R, et al. Changes in the oral absorption characteristics in man of dipotassium clorazepate at normal and elevated gastric pH. *J Pharmacokinet Biopharm* 1977;5:377–390.
59. Ochs HR, Greenblatt DJ, Allen MD, et al. Effect of age and Billroth gastrectomy on absorption of desmethyldiazepam from clorazepate. *Clin Pharmacol Ther* 1979;26:449–456.
60. Chun AH, Carrigan PJ, Hoffman DJ, et al. Effect of antacids on absorption of clorazepate. *Clin Pharmacol Ther* 1977;22: 329–335.
61. Shader RI, Ciraulo DA, Greenblatt DJ, et al. Steady-state plasma desmethyldiazepam during long-term clorazepate use: effects of antacids. *Clin Pharmacol Ther* 1982;31:180–183.
62. Sokol GH, Greenblatt DJ, Lloyd BL, et al. Effect of abdominal radiation therapy on drug absorption in humans. *J Clin Pharmacol* 1978;18:388–396.

63. Abernethy DR, Greenblatt DJ, Divoll M, et al. Prolongation of drug half-life due to obesity: studies of desmethyldiazepam (clorazepate). *J Pharm Sci* 1982;71:942–944.

64. Wilensky AJ, Levy RH, Troupin AS, et al. Clorazepate kinetics in treated epileptics. *Clin Pharmacol Ther* 1978;24:22–30.

65. Shader RI, Greenblatt DJ, Ciraulo DA, et al. Effect of age and sex on disposition of desmethyldiazepam formed from its precursor clorazepate. *Psychopharmacology (Berl)* 1981;75:193–197.

66. Kanto J, Kangas L, Siirtola T. Cerebrospinal fluid of diazepam and its metabolites in man. *Acta Pharmacol Toxicol* 1975;36:328–334.

67. Handel J. Cummulation in cerebrospinal fluid of the *N*-desmehtylmetabolite after long-term treatment with diazepam in man. *Acta Pharmacol Toxicol* 1975;37:17–22.

68. Rey E, Pons G, Richard MO, et al. Pharmacokinetics of the individual enantiomers of vigabatrin (gamma-vinyl GABA) in epileptic children. *Br J Clin Pharmacol* 1990;30:253–257.

69. Mandelli M, Morselli PL, Nordio S, et al. Placental transfer of diazepam and its disposition in the newborn. *Clin Pharmacol Ther* 1975;17:564–572.

70. Andersson T, Miners JO, Veronese ME, et al. Diazepam metabolism by human liver microsomes is mediated by both S-mephenytoin hydroxylase and CYP3A isoforms. *Br J Clin Pharmacol* 1994;38:131–137.

71. Staak M, Moosmayer A, Besserer K, et al. Pharmakokinetische untrersuchungen nach oraler und parenteraler applikation von Dikaium: Chlorazepat. *Arzneimittelforschung* 1982;32:272–275.

72. Divoll M, Greenblatt DJ, Abernethy DR, et al. Cimetidine impairs clearance of antipyrine and desmethyldiazepam in the elderly. *J Am Geriatr Soc* 1982;30:684–689.

73. Rey E, Giraux P, d'Athis P, et al. Pharmacokinetics of the placental transfer and distribution of clorazepate and its metabolite nordiazepam in the feto-placental unit and in the neonate. *Eur J Clin Pharmacol* 1979;17:181–185.

74. Rey E, d'Athis P, Giraux P, et al. Pharmacokinetics of clorazepate in pregnant and non-pregnant women. *Eur J Clin Pharmacol* 1979;17:175–180.

75. Klotz U, Avant GR, Hoyumpa A, et al. The effects of age and liver disease on the disposition and elimination of diazepam in adult man. *J Clin Invest* 1975;55:347–359.

76. Norman TR, Fulton A, Burrows GD, et al. Pharmacokinetics of *N*-desmethyldiazepam after a single oral dose of clorazepate: the effect of smoking. *Eur J Clin Pharmacol* 1981;21:229–233.

77. Schmidt D. Benzodiazepines: diazepam. In: Levy RH, Mattson RH, Meldrum BS, eds. *Antiepileptic drugs,* 4th ed. New York: Raven Press, 1995:705–724.

78. Kaplan SA, Jack ML, Alexander K, et al. Pharmacokinetic profile of diazepam in man following single intravenous and oral and chronic oral administration. *J Pharm Sci* 1973;62:1789–1796.

79. Garattini S, Marcucci F, Morselli PL, et al. The significance of measuring blood levels of benzodiazepines. In: Davies DS, Prichard BNC, eds. *Biological effects of drugs in relation to their plasma concentrations.* London: MacMillan, 1973:211–225.

80. Gamble JAS, Dundee JW, Assaf RAE. Plasma diazepam levels after single dose oral an dintramuscular administration. *Anaesthesia* 1975;30:164–169.

81. Hillestad L, Hansen T, Melson H, et al. Diazepam metabolism in normal man. I. Serum concentrations and clinical effects after intravenous, intramuscular, and oral administration. *Clin Pharmacol Ther* 1974;16:479–484.

82. Knudsen FU. Plasma-diazepam in infants after rectal administration in solution and by suppository. *Acta Paediatr Scand* 1979;66:563–567.

83. Meberg A, Langslet A, Bredesen JE, et al. Plasma concentration of diazepam and *N*-desmethyldiazepam in children after a single rectal or intramuscular dose of diazepam. *Eur J Clin Pharmacol* 1978;14:272–276.

84. Cloyd JC, Lalonde RL, Beniak TE, et al. A single-blind, crossover comparison of the pharmacokinetics and cognitive effects of a new diazepam rectal gel with intravenous diazepam. *Epilepsia* 1998;39:520–526.

85. Schwartz DE, Vecchi M, Ronco A, et al. Blood levels after administration of 7-chloror-1,3 dihydro-1-methyl-5-phenyl-2H-1,4-benzodiazepine-2–one (diazepam) in various forms. *Arzneimittelforschung* 1966;16:1109–1110.

86. Van Der Kleijn E, Van Rossum JM, Muskens ETJM, et al. Pharmacokinetics of diazepam in dogs, mice and humans. *Acta Pharmacol Toxicol* 1971;29[Suppl 3]:109–127.

87. Mandelli M, Tognoni G, Garattini S. Clinical pharmacokinetics of diazepam. *Clin Pharmacokinet* 1978;3:72–91.

88. Ochs HR, Greenblatt DJ, Divoll M, et al. Diazepam kinetics in relation to age and sex. *Pharmacology* 1981;23:24–30.

89. Herman RJ, Wilkinson GR. Disposition of diazepam in young and elderly subjects after acute and chronic dosing. *Br J Clin Pharmacol* 1996;42:147–155.

90. Routledge P, Stargel W, Kitchell B, et al. Sex-related differences in the plasma protein binding of lignocaine and diazepam. *Br J Clin Pharmacol* 1981;11:245–250.

91. Tiula E, Haapanen EJ, Neuvonen PJ. Factors affecting serum protein binding of phenytoin, diazepam and propranolol in acute renal disease. *Int J Clin Pharmacol Ther Toxicol* 1987;25:469–475.

92. Kangas L, Kanto J, Forsstrom J, et al. The protein binding of diazepam and *N*-demethyldiazepam in patients with poor renal function. *Clin Nephrol* 1975;5:114–118.

93. Viani A, Rizzo G, Carrai M, et al. The effect of ageing on plasma albumin and plasma protein binding of diazepam, salicylic acid and digotoxin in healthy subjects and patients with renal impairment. *Br J Clin Pharmacol* 1992;33:299–304.

94. Kuhnz W, Nau H. Differences in *in vitro* binding of diazepam and desmethyldiazepam to maternal and fetal plasma proteins at birth: relation to free fatty acid concentration and other parameters. *Clin Pharmacol Ther* 1983;34:220–226.

95. Nau H, Luck W, Kuhnz W. Decreased serum protein binding of diazepam and its major metabolite during the first postnatal week relate to increased free fatty acid levels. *Br J Clin Pharmacol* 1984;17:92–98.

96. Leppik IE, Derivan AT, Homan RW, et al. Double-blind study of lorazepam and diazepam in status piilepticus. *JAMA* 1983;249:1452–1454.

97. Ramsay RE, Hammond EJ, Perchalski RJ, et al. Brain uptake of phenytoin, phenobarbital and diazepam. *Arch Neurol* 1979;36:535–539.

98. Friedman H, Ochs HR, Greenblatt DJ, et al. Tissue distribution of diazepam and its metabolite desmethyldiazepam: a human autopsy study. *J Clin Pharmacol* 1985;25:613–615.

99. Hagg S, Spigset O. Anticonvulsant use during lactation. *Drug Saf* 2000;22:425–440.

100. Kanto J, Sellman R, Haataja M, et al. Plasma and urine concentrations of diazepam and its metabolites in children, adults and in diazepam-intoxicated patients. *Int J Clin Pharmacol* 1978;16:258–264.

101. Zhang Y, Reviriego J, Lou Y-Q, et al. Diazepam metabolism in native Chinese poor and extensive hydroylators of S-mephenytoin: interethnic differences in comparison with white subjects. *Clin Pharmacol Ther* 1990;48:496–502.

102. Sohn D-R, Kusaka M, Ishizaki T, et al. Incidence of S-mephenytoin hydroxylation deficiency in a Korean population and the interphenotypic differences in diazepam pharmacogenetics. *Clin Pharmacol Ther* 1992;52:160–169.

103. Bertilsson L, Henthorn TK, Sanz E, et al. Importance of genetic factors in the regulation of diazepam metabolism: relationship to S-mephenytoin, but no desbrisoquin hydroxylation pathways. *Clin Pharmacol Ther* 1989;45:348–355.

104. Hepner GW, Vesell ES, Lipton A, et al. Disposition of aminopyrine, antipyrine, diazepam, and indocyanine green in patients with liver disease or on anticonvulsant drug therapy: diazepam breath test and correlations in drug elimination. *J Lab Clin Med* 1977;90:440–456.

105. Morselli PL, Principi N, Tognoni G, et al. Diazepam elimination in premature and full term infants, and children. *J Perinat Med* 1973;1:133–141.

106. Horman RW, Treiman DM. Lorazepam. In: Levy RH, Mattson RH, Meldrum BS, eds. *Antiepileptic drugs,* 4th ed. New York: Raven Press, 1995:779–790.

107. Greenblatt DJ, Shader RI, Franke K, et al. Pharmacokinetics and bioavailability of intravenous, intramuscular, and oral lorazepam in humans. *J Pharm Sci* 1979;68:57–63.

108. Greenblatt DJ, Divoll M, Harmatz JS, et al. Pharmacokinetic comparison of sublingual lorazepam with intravenous, intramuscular, and oral lorazepam. *J Pharm Sci* 1982;71:248–252.

109. Greenblatt DJ, Joyce TH, Comer WH, et al. Clinical pharmacokinetics of lorazepam. II. Intramuscular injection. *Clin Pharmacol Ther* 1977;21:222–230.

110. Greenblatt DJ, Allen MD, Locniskar A, et al. Lorazepam kinetics in the elderly. *Clin Pharmacol Ther* 1979;26:103–113.

111. Abernethy DR, Greenblatt DJ, Divoll M, et al. Enhanced glucuronide conjugation of drugs in obesity: studies of lorazepam, oxazepam and acetaminophen. *J Lab Clin Med* 1983;101:873–880.

112. Kraus JW, Desmond PV, Marshall JP, et al. Effect of aging and liver disease on disposition of lorazepam. *Clin Pharmacol Ther* 1978;24:411–419.

113. Moschitto LJ, Greenblatt DJ. Concentration-independent plasma protein binding of benzodiazepines. *J Pharm Pharmacol* 1983;35:179–180.

114. Divoll M, Greenblatt DJ. Effect of age and sex on lorazepam protein binding. *J Pharm Pharmacol* 1982;34:122–123.

115. Ochs HR, Busse J, Greenblatt DJ, et al. Entry of lorazepam into the cerebrospinal fluid. *Br J Clin Pharmacol* 1980;10:405–406.

116. Walton NY, Treiman DM. Lorazepam treatment of experimental status epilepticus in the rat: relevance to clinical practice. *Neurology* 1990;40:990–994.

117. Arendt RM, Greenblatt DJ, de Jong RH, et al. *In vitro* correlates of benzodiazepine cerebrospinal fluid uptake, pharmacodynamic action and peripheral distribution. *J Pharmacol Exp Ther* 1983;227:98–106.

118. Greenblatt DJ, Ehrenberg BL, Gunderman J, et al. Kinetic and dynamic study of intravenous lorazepam: comparison with intravenous diazepam. *J Pharmacol Exp Ther* 1989;250:134–140.

119. Greenblatt DJ, von Moltke LL, Ehrenberg BL, et al. Kinetics and dynamics of lorazepam during and after continuous intravenous infusion. *Crit Care Med* 2000;28:2750–2757.

120. Kanto J, Aaltonen L, Liukko P, et al. Tranfer of lorazepam and its conjugate across the human placenta. *Acta Pharmacol Exp Toxicol* 1980;47:130–134.

121. McBride RJ, Dundee JW, Moore J, et al. A study of the plasma concentrations of lorazepam in mother and neonate. *Br J Anaesth* 1979;51:971–977.

122. Whitelaw AGL, Cummings AJ, McFadyen IR. Effect of maternal lorazepam on the neonate. *BMJ* 1981;282:1106–1108.

123. Elliott HW. Metabolism of lorazepam. *Br J Anaesth* 1976;48:1017–1023.

124. Greenblatt DJ, Schillings RT, Kyriakopoulos AA, et al. Clinical pharmacokinetics of lorazepam: absorption and distribution of oral ^{14}C-lorazepam. *Clin Pharmacol Ther* 1976;20:329–341.

125. Herman RJ, Duc Van J, Szakacs CBN. Disposition of lorazepam in human beings: enterohepatic recirculation and first-pass effect. *Clin Pharmacol Ther* 1989;46:18–25.

126. Divoll M, Greenblatt DJ, Lacasse Y, et al. Pharmacokinetic study of lorazepam overdose. *Am J Psychiatry* 1980;137:1414–1415.

127. Anderson GD, Gidal BE, Kantor ED, et al. Lorazepam-valproate interaction: studies in normal subjects and isolated perfused rat liver. *Epilepsia* 1994;35:221–225.

128. McDermott CA, Kowalczyk AL, Schnitzler ER, et al. Pharmacokinetics of lorazepam in critically ill neonates with seizures. *J Pediatr* 1992;120:479–483.

129. Kearns GL, Mallory GB, Crom WR, et al. Enhanced hepatic drug clearance in patients with cystic fibrosis. *J Pediatr* 1990;117:972–979.

130. Dutton GJ. Developmental aspects of drug conjugation with special reference to glucuronidation. *Annu Rev Pharmacol Toxicol* 1978;18:17–35.

131. Morrison G, Chiang ST, Koepke HH, et al. Effect of renal impairment and hemodialysis on lorazepam kinetics. *Clin Pharmacol Ther* 1984;35:646–652.

132. Herman RJ, Chaudhary A, Szakacs CB, et al. Disposition of lorazepam in diabetes: differences between patients treated with beef/pork and human insulins. *Eur J Clin Pharmacol* 1995;48:253–258.

133. Segal JL, Brunnenmann SR, Eltorai IM, et al. Decreased systemic clearance of lorazepam in humans with spinal cord injury. *J Clin Pharmacol* 1991;31:651–656.

134. Walker JE, Homan RW, Crawford IL. Lorazepam: a controlled trial in patients with intractable partial complex seizures. *Epilepsia* 1984;25:464–466.

135. Walker JE, Horman RW, Vasko MR, et al. Lorazepam in status epilepticus. *Ann Neurol* 1979;6:207–213.

136. Blin O, Jacquet A, Callamand S, et al. Pharmacokinetic-pharmacodynamic analysis of mnesic effects of lorazepam in healthy volunteers. *Br J Clin Pharmacol* 1999;48:510–512.

137. Blumer JL. Clinical pharmacology of midazolam in infants and children. *Clin Pharmacokinet* 1998;35:37–37.

138. Kanto JH. Midazolam: the first water-soluble benzodiazepine. Pharmacology, pharmacokinetics and efficacy in insomnia and anesthesia. *Pharmacotherapy* 1985;5:138–154.

139. Scott RC, Besag FMC, Boyd SG, et al. Buccal absorption of midazolam: pharmacokinetics and EEG pharmacodynamics. *Epilepsia* 1998;39:290–294.

140. Scott RC, Besag FMC, Neville BGR. Buccal midazolam and rectal diazepam for treatment of prolonged seizures in childhood and adolescence: a randomised trial. *Lancet* 1999;353:623–626.

141. Koren G. Intranasal midazolam for febrile seizures: a step forward in treating a common and distressing condition. *BMJ* 2000;321:64–65.

142. Lahat E, Goldran M, Barr J, et al. Intranasal midazolam for childhood seizures. *Lancet* 1998;352:620.

143. Marshall J, Rodarte A, Blumer J, et al. Pediatric pharmacodynamics of midazolam oral syrup. *J Clin Pharmacol* 2000;40:578–589.

144. Reves JG. Benzodiazepines. In: Prys-Roberts C, Hug CCJ, eds. *Pharmacokinetics of anesthesia.* Oxford: Blackwell Scientific Publications, 1984:157–186.

145. Payne K, Matteyse FJ, Liebenberg D, et al. The pharmacokinetics of midazolam in paediatric patients. *Eur J Clin Pharmacol* 1989;37:267–272.

146. Ziegler WH, Schalch E, Leishman B, et al. Comparison of the effects of intravenously administered midazolam, triazolam and their hydroxy metabolites. *Br J Clin Pharmacol* 1983;16:63S–69S.

147. Klotz U, Ziegler G. Physiologic and temporal variation in hepatic elimination of midazolam. *Clin Pharmacol Ther* 1982; 32:107–112.

148. Smith MT, Eadie MJ, Brophy TO. The pharmacokinetics of midazolam in man. *Eur J Clin Pharmacol* 1981;19:271–278.

149. Allonen H, Ziegler G, Klotz U. Midazolam kinetics. *Clin Pharmacol Ther* 1981;30:653–661.

150. Greenblatt DJ, Locniskar A, Ochs HR, et al. Automated gas chromatography for studies of midazolam pharmacokinetics. *Anesthesiology* 1981;55:176–179.

151. Heizmann P, Eckert M, Ziegler QH. Pharmacokinetics and bioavailability of midazolam in man. *Br J Clin Pharmacol* 1983; 16:43S–49S.

152. Kanto J, Sjovall S, Erkkola R, et al. Placental transfer and maternal midazolam kinetics. *Clin Pharmacol Ther* 1983;33: 786–791.

153. Greenblatt DJ, Abernethy DR, Locniskar A, et al. Effect of age, gender, and obesity on midazolam kinetics. *Anesthesiology* 1984; 61:27–35.

154. Harper KW, Collier PS, Dundee JW, et al. Age and nature of operation influence the pharmacokinetics of midazolam. *Br J Anaesth* 1985;57:866–871.

155. Kanto J, Aaltonen L, Himberg JJ, et al. Midazolam as an intravenous induction agent in the elderly: a clinical and pharmacokinetic study. *Anesth Analg* 1986;65:15–20.

156. Thummel KE, Shen DD, Podoll TD, et al. Use of midazolam a human cytochrome P450 3A probe. I. *In vitro–in vivo* correlations in liver transplant patients. *J Pharmacol Exp Ther* 1994; 271:549–556.

157. Gerecke M. Chemical structure and properties of midazolam compared with other benzodiazepines. *Br J Clin Pharmacol* 1983;16:11S–16S.

158. Heizmann P, Ziegler WH. Excretion and metabolism of ^{14}C-midazolam in humans following oral dosing. *Arzneimittelforschung* 1981;31:2220–2223.

159. Arndt RM, Greenblatt DJ, Garland WA. Quantitation by gas chromatography of the 1- and 4-hyroxy metabolites of midazolam in human plasma. *Pharmacology* 1984;29:158–164.

160. Rubio F, Miwa BJ, Garland WA. Determination of midazolam and two metabolites of midazolam in human plasma by gas chromatography-negative chemical-ionization mass spectrometry. *J Chromatogr* 1982;233:157–165.

161. Amrein R, Hetzel W, Bonetti EP, et al. Clinical pharmacology of dormicum (midazolam) and anexate (fluemazenil). *Resuscitation* 1988;16:S5–S27.

162. Kronbarch T, Mathys D, Ulmeno M, et al. Oxidation of midazolam and triazolam by human liver cytochrome P450IIIA4. *Mol Pharmacol* 1989;36:89–96.

163. Gorski JC, Hall SD, Jones DR, et al. Regioselective biotransformation of midazolam by members of the human cytochrome P450 (CYP3A) subfamily. *Biochem Pharmacol* 1994;47: 1643–1653.

164. Haehner BD, Gorski JC, Vandenbranden M, et al. Bimodal distribution of renal cytochrome P450 3A activity in humans. *Mol Pharmacol* 1996;50:52–59.

165. Paulussen A, Kavrijsen K, Bohets H, et al. Two linked mutations in transcripional regulatory elements of the CYP3A5 gene constitute the major genetic determinant of polymorphic activity in humans. *Pharmacogenetics* 2000;10:415–424.

166. Wandel C, Witte JS, Hall JM, et al. CYP3A activity in African American and European American men: population differences and functional effect of the CYP3A4*1B5′-promoter region polymorphisms. *Clin Pharmacol Ther* 2000;68:82–91.

167. Olkkola KT, Aranko K, Luurila H, et al. A potential hazardous interaction between erythromycin and midazolam. *Clin Pharmacol Ther* 1993;53:298–305.

168. Backman JT, Olkkola KT, Aranko K, et al. Dose of midazolam should be reduced during diltiazem and verapamil treatments. *Br J Clin Pharmacol* 1994;37:221–225.

169. Jacqz-Aigrain E, Wood C, Robieux I. Pharmacokinetics of midazolam in critically ill neonates. *Eur J Clin Pharmacol* 1990; 39:191–192.

170. Jacqz-Aigrain E, Daoud P, Zburtin P, et al. Pharmacokinetics of midazolam during continuous infusion in critically ill neonates. *Eur J Clin Pharmacol* 1992;42:329–332.

171. Jones RD, Visram AR, Chan MM, et al. A comparison of three induction agents in paediatric anaesthesia: cardiovascular effects an recovery. *Anaesth Intensive Care*;22:545–555.

172. Reves JG, Glass PS, Lubarsky DA. Nonbarbiturate intravenous anesthetics. In: Miller RD, editor. *Anesthesia,* 4th ed. New York: Churchill Livingstone, 1994:247–289.

173. Pentikainen PJ, Valisalmi L, Himberg JJ, et al. Pharmacokinetics of midazolam following intravenous and oral administration in patients with chronic liver disease and in healthy subjects. *J Clin Pharmacol* 1989;29:272–277.

174. Patel IH, Soni PP, Fukuda EK, et al. The pharmacokinetics of midazolam in patients with congestive heart failure. *Br J Clin Pharmacol* 1990;29:565–569.

175. Trouvin JH, Farinotti R, Haberer JP, et al. Pharmacokinetics of midazolam in anaesthetised cirrhotic patients. *Br J Anaesth* 1988;60:762–767.

176. Vinik HR, Reves JG, Greenblatt DJ, et al. The pharmacokinetics of midazolam in chronic renal failure patients. *Anesthesiology* 1983;59:390–394.

177. Driessen JJ, Vree TB. Pharmacokinetics of benzodiazepines used for ICU sedation. In: Vincent JL, ed. *Update in intensive care and emergency medicine,* vol 81. Berlin: Springer-Verlag, 1989:586–595.

178. Crevoisier CH, Ziegler WH, Eckert M, et al. Relationship between plasma concentration and effect of midazolam after oral and intravenous administration. *Br J Clin Pharmacol* 1983; 16:51S–61S.

179. Crevoisier CH, Eckert M, Heizmann P, et al. Relation between the clinical effect and the pharmacokinetics of midazolam following i.m. and i.v. administration. *Arzneimittelforschung* 1981; 31:2211–2215.

180. Kanto J, Aaltonen L, Erkkola R, et al. Pharmacokinetics and sedative effect of midazolam in connection with caesarean section performed under epidural analgesia. *Acta Anaesthesiol Scand* 1984;28:116–118.

181. Janknegt R, van der Kuy A, Declerck G, et al. Hypnotics: drug selection by means of the system of objectified judgement analysis (SOJA) method. *Pharmacoeconomics* 1996;10: 152–163.

182. Uchiumi M, Sugiyama T, Suzuki M, et al. Effects of a single dose of zolpidem, triazolam and nitrazepam on daytime sleepiness. *Jpn J Neuropsycholopharmacol* 1994;16:45–56.

183. Sternbach LH, Fryer RI, Keller O, et al. Quinazolines and 1-4 benzodiazepines. X. Nitro-substituted 5-phenyl-1,4-benzodiazepine derivatives. *J Med Pharm Chem* 1963;6:261–265.

184. Rieder J, Wendt G. Pharmacoketics and metabolism of the hypnotic nitrazepam. In: Garattini S, Mussini E, Randall L, eds. *The benzodiazepines.* New York: Raven Press, 1973:999–127.

185. Sawada H, Hara A. Novel metabolite of nitrazepam in the rabbit urine. *Experientia* 1976;32:987–988.

186. Yanagi Y, Haga F, Endo M, et al. Comparative study of azepam and its desmethyl derivative (nitrazepam) in rats. *Xenobiotica* 1975;5:245–257.

187. Baruzzi A, Michelucci R, Tassinari CA. Benzodiazepines: nitrazepam. In: Levy RH, Mattson RH, Meldrum BS, eds. *Antiepileptic drugs,* 4th ed. New York: Raven Press, 1995: 735–749.

188. Breimer DD, Bracht H, De Boer AG. Plasma level profile of nitrazepam (Modagon) following oral administration. *Br J Clin Pharmacol* 1977;4:709–711.

189. De Boer AG, Rost-Kaiser J, Bracht H, et al. Assay of underivatized nitrazepam and clonazepam in plasma by capillary gas chromatography applied to pharmaokinetic and bioavailability studies in humans. *J Chromatogr* 1978;145:105–114.

190. Holm V, Melander A, Wahlin-Boll E. Influence of food and of age on nitrazepam kinetics. *Drug Nutr Interact* 1982;1:307–311.

191. Jochemsen R, Hogendoorn JJH, Dingemanse J, et al. Pharmacokinetics and bioavailability of intravenous, oral, and rectal nitrazepam in humans. *J Pharmacokinet Biopharm* 1982;10:231–245.

192. Jochemsen R, Van der Graaff M, Boeijinga JK, et al. Influence of sex, menstral cycle and oral contraception on the disposition of nitrazepam. *Br J Clin Pharmacol* 1982;13:319–324.

193. Abernethy DR, Greenblatt DJ, Locniskar A, et al. Obesity effects on nitrazepam disposition. *Br J Clin Pharmacol* 1986;22:551–557.

194. Greenblatt DJ, Abernethy DR, Locniskar A, et al. Age, sex and nitrazepam kinetics: relation to antipyrine disposition. *Clin Pharmacol Ther* 1985;38:697–703.

195. Kangas L, Allonen H, Lammintausta R, et al. Pharmacokinetics of nitrazepam in saliva and serum after a single oral dose. *Acta Pharmacol Toxicol* 1979;45:20–24.

196. Rieder J. Plasma levels and derived pharmacokinetic characteristics of unchanged nitrazepam in man. *Arzneimittelforschung* 1973;23:212–218.

197. Kangas L, Allonene H, Lammintausta R, et al. Pharmacokinetics of nitrazepam in human plasma and saliva. *Acta Pharmacol Toxicol* 1977;41:56.

198. Jochemsen R, van der Graaff M, Boeijinga JK, et al. Influence of sex, menstrual cycle and oral contraception on the disposition of nitrazepam. *Br J Clin Pharmacol* 1982;13:319–324.

199. Jochemsen R, Van Beusekom BR, Spoelstra P, et al. Effect of age and liver cirrhosis on the pharmacokinetics of nitrazepam. *Br J Clin Pharmacol* 1983;15:295–302.

200. Ochs HR, Oberem U, Greenblatt DJ. Nitrazepam clearance unimpaired in patients with renal insufficiency. *J Clin Psycholopharmacol* 1992;12:183–185.

201. Ho PC, Triggs EJ, Heazlewood V, et al. Determination of nitrazepam and temazepam in plasma by high-performance liquid chromatography. *Ther Drug Monit* 1983;5:303–307.

202. Kangas L, Kanto J, Siirtola T, et al. Cerebrospinal fluid concentrations of nitrazepam in man. *Acta Pharmacol Toxicol* 1977;41:65–73.

203. Tanayama S, Momose S, Kanai Y. Comparative studies on the metabolic disposition of 8–chloro-6-phenyl-4H-S-triazolo[4,3-a][1,4] benzodiazepine (D-40TA) and nitrazepam after single and repeated administration in rats. *Xenobiotica* 1974;4:229–236.

204. Hewick DS, Shaw V. Tissue distribution of radioactivity after injection of C14-nitrazepam in young and old rats. *J Pharm Pharmacol* 1978;30:318–319.

205. Hart BJ, Wilting J, de Gier JJ. Complications in correlation studies between serum, free serum and saliva concentrations of nitrazepam. *Methods Find Exp Clin Pharmacol* 1987;9:127–131.

206. Hart BJ, Wilting J, de Gier JJ. The stability of benzodiazepines in saliva. *Methods Find Exp Clin Pharmacol* 1988;10:21–26.

207. Robertson MD, Drummer OH. Postmortem distribution and redistribution of nitrobenzodiazepines in man. *J Forensic Sci* 1998;43:9–13.

208. Kangas L, Kanto J, Erkkola R. Transfer of nitrazepam across the human placenta. *Eur J Clin Pharmacol* 1977;12:355–357.

209. Matheson I, Lunde PK, Bredesen JE. Midazolam and nitrazepam in the maternity ward: milk concentrations and clinical effects. *Br J Clin Pharmacol* 1990;30:787–793.

210. McElhatton PR. The effects of benzodiazepine use during pregnancy and lactation. *Reprod Toxicol* 1994;8:461–475.

211. Speight ANP. Floppy infant syndrome and maternal diazepam and/or nitrazepam. *Lancet* 1977;2:878.

212. Hewick DS, Shaw V. The importance of the intestinal microflora in nitrazepam metabolism in the rat. *Br J Pharmacol* 1978;62:427.

213. Bartosek I, Kvetina J, Guaitani A, et al. Comparative study of nitrazepam metabolism in perfused isolated liver laboratory animals. *Eur J Pharmacol* 1970;11:378–382.

214. Bartosek I, Musini E, Saronio C, et al. Studies on nitrazepam reduction *in vitro*. *Eur J Pharmacol* 1970;11:249–253.

215. Karim AKMB, Price Evans DA. Polymorphic acetylation of nitrazepam. *J Med Genet* 1976;13:17–19.

216. Eze LC. High incidence of the slow nitrazepam acetylator phenotype in a Nigerian population. *Biochem Genet* 1987;25:225–229.

217. Kangas L. Urinary elimination of nitazepam and its main metabolites. *Acta Pharmacol Toxicol* 1979;45:16–19.

218. Kangas L, Kanto J, Syvalahti E. Plasma nitrazepam concentrations after an acute intake and their correlation to sedation and serum growth hormone levels. *Acta Pharmacol Toxicol* 1977;41:65–73.

219. Moller Jesen K. Determination of nitrazepam in serum by gas-liquid chromatography. *J Chromatogr* 1975;111:389–396.

220. Kangas L, Lisalo E, Kanto J, et al. Human pharmacokinetics of nitrazepam: effect of age and diseases. *Eur J Clin Pharmacol* 1979;15:163–170.

221. Jeavons PM. Choice of drug therapy in epilepsy. *Practitioner* 1977;219:542–556.

222. Brockmeyer NH, Mertins L, Klimek K, et al. Comparative effects of rifampin and/or probenecid on the pharmacokinetics of temazepam and nitrazepam. *Int J Clin Pharmacol Ther Toxicol* 1990;28:387–393.

223. Grundstrom R, Holmberg G, Hansen T. Degree of sedation obtained with various doses of diazepam and nitrazepam. *Acta Pharmacol Toxicol* 1978;43:13–18.

224. Hojer J, Baehrendtz S, Magnusson A, et al. A placebo-controlled trial of flumzenil given by continuous infusion in severe benzodiazepine overdosage. *Acta Anaesthesiol Scand* 1991;35:584–590.

225. Bun H, Monjanel-Mouterde S, Noel F, et al. Effects of age and antiepileptic drugs on plasma levels and kinetics of clobazam and *N*-desmethylclobazam. *Pharmacol Toxicol* 1990;67:136–140.

226. Kanto J, Erkkola R, Sellman R. Distribution and metabolism of diazepam in early and late human pregnacy: postnatal metabolism of diazepam. *Acta Pharmacol Toxicol* 1974;35[Suppl 36].

227. Caille G, Spenard J, Lacasse Y, et al. Pharmacokinetics of two lorazepam formulation, oral and sublingual after multiple doses. *Biopharm Drug Disp* 1983;4:31–42.

228. Castleden CM, George CF, Marcer D, et al. Increased sensitivity to nitrazepam in old age. *BMJ* 1977;1:10–12.

229. Iisalo E, Kangas L, Ruikka I. Pharmacokinetics of nitrazepam in young volunteers and aged patients. *Br J Clin Pharmacol* 1977;4:646.

BENZODIAZEPINES

CLINICAL EFFICACY AND USE IN EPILEPSY

DIETER SCHMIDT

Although the general use of benzodiazepines is increasingly out of favor, mainly because of the development of tolerance, dependence, and withdrawal in this class of drugs, their value for the treatment of epilepsy remains largely unchallenged. Benzodiazepines including diazepam, clonazepam, and lorazepam remain drugs of first choice for the treatment of early status epilepticus (1). In addition, the rectal administration of diazepam has become very useful for the acute treatment of ongoing seizures and serial seizures and for the prevention of febrile seizures (2). Benzodiazepines such as clobazam or clonazepam are very valuable for adjunctive therapy in some patients with refractory epilepsy. The mechanism of action, the chemistry, the biotransformation and pharmacokinetics, and the adverse effects of benzodiazepines are discussed in Chapters 16, 17, and 19, as well as in the literature (3–5). This chapter deals with the clinical efficacy and the use of clobazam, clonazepam, diazepam, lorazepam, midazolam, and nitrazepam in the short-term and long-term treatment of epilepsy.

CLOBAZAM

Clobazam has a 1,5 substitution instead of the usual 1,4-diazepine structure. The structure results in a reduction of the sedative effects when compared with diazepam in animal studies, without losing its anticonvulsant effect (5). Although it is not promoted commercially, clobazam continues to be widely used by many specialists for epilepsy, for at least two reasons. First, clobazam tablets and capsules are rapidly and highly effective as adjunctive therapy for partial and generalized seizures, for intermittent therapy, and for controlling nonconvulsive status epilepticus. Second, clobazam is better tolerated than other benzodiazepines. These features have made clobazam an excellent second-line therapy in some patients with resistant epilepsy. The main disadvantage is the development of tolerance in as many as

Dieter Schmidt, MD: Head, Epilepsy Research Group Section, Berlin, Germany

50% of patients within weeks or months. Clobazam has been marketed in Europe since the 1970s and in Canada since 1988, but it is not available in the United States.

Clinical Efficacy

In nine placebo-controlled add-on trials in refractory epilepsy, clobazam was shown to be very effective as an adjunctive drug, leading to a mean reduction of seizures by 30% in patients with partial seizures unresponsive to other antiepileptic drugs (5). In several studies, a 50% reduction was seen in as many as half of the patients studied (6,7). This finding compares favorably with many of the currently available antiepileptic drugs. In addition, numerous open, single-arm studies were undertaken in patients with secondarily generalized seizures, Lennox-Gastaut syndrome, startle epilepsy, nonconvulsive status epilepticus, electrical status during slow-wave sleep, reflex epilepsies, alcohol withdrawal seizures, and benign childhood partial epilepsies (5). More recently, clobazam was tested in a large double-blind trial as first-line monotherapy in children with newly diagnosed partial epilepsy, and the drug was reported to be similar, in efficacy and tolerability, to monotherapy with phenytoin or carbamazepine (8,9).

Clobazam has a mild anxiolytic effect that is useful for many patients with chronic partial epilepsy. As discussed earlier, the development of tolerance is a clinical problem, and efforts to limit tolerance by drug holidays, treatment on alternate days starting with a low dose, or overcoming loss of efficacy with a higher dose have largely been unsuccessful. In view of the development of tolerance in many patients, it is not surprising that no clear relationship has been found between the serum concentration of clobazam or of the main metabolite and seizure control, and an optimum range of serum concentrations in chronic epilepsy has not been established.

Clinical Use

Clobazam should be considered as adjunctive therapy whenever treatment with a single first-line antiepileptic drug has not led to sufficient seizure control (Table 18.1).

TABLE 18.1. CLINICAL USE OF BENZODIAZEPINES IN EPILEPSY

Drug	Clinical Use	Main Advantages	Main Disadvantages
Clobazam	First-line adjunctive therapy for refractory partial and generalized seizures, intermittent therapy, nonconvulsive status epilepticus	Highly effective, better tolerated than other benzodiazepines, rapid onset of action	Tolerance in 50%, withdrawal problems
Clonazepam	Second-line adjunctive therapy in partial and generalized seizures (especially absence and myoclonic seizures), Lennox-Gastaut syndrome, and the premonitory stage of status epilepticus and early status epilepticus Second-line therapy for established status epilepticus	Useful second-line adjunctive drug	Strong sedation, hypersalivation in some patients, tolerance
Diazepam	First-line treatment for the premonitory and early stages of status epilepticus (i.v., bolus, or rectal solution). Second-line for established status epilepticus (i.v. infusion) Nonconvulsive status epilepticus Intermittent prophylaxis of febrile seizures, and home treatment of acute repetitive seizures (rectal solution or gel)	Highly effective, rapid onset of action, several methods of administration	Sedation, tolerance, withdrawal problems
Lorazepam	First-line treatment for the early stage of status epilepticus (i.v. bolus) and for treatment of exit-of-hospital status epilepticus	Longer duration of action than diazepam, can be repeated often, rate of injection less critical	Sedation, frequent and rapid development of tolerance
Midazolam	Second-line treatment for the early stages of) status epilepticus (i.m, i.v. bolus, rectal solution	Effective, rapid onset of action, can be given i.m.	Respiratory depression, sedation
Nitrazepam	Second- to third-line adjunctive therapy in partial and generalized seizures (especially myoclonic seizures and infantile spasms)	Last resort for severe childhood epilepsies	Severe sedation and muscular hypotonia in some patients

i.v., intravenous; i.m., intramuscular.
Common practice use is given, individual preference may vary, and the list of clinical use is not exhaustive (see text).

Although antiepileptic drug choice is to an extent arbitrary, given the lack of pragmatic large-scale trials to establish preference, clobazam is a valuable add-on drug because it is widely effective. In my practice, I use it primarily for patients with partial seizures, in whom it is rapidly effective; one knows, usually within 2 to 3 weeks of prescribing a 10-mg tablet or capsule at night, whether it will work. Clobazam is also a useful adjunctive drug for some patients with other seizures, such as patients with Lennox-Gastaut syndrome or reflex epilepsies. Clobazam can also be used for a short course of maintenance treatment after intravenous (i.v.) benzodiazepines in myoclonic status epilepticus, complex partial status epilepticus, and atypical absence status epilepticus. Furthermore, because of its high efficacy and modest side effects, clobazam is ideal for bridging a short period of increased seizure susceptibility (e.g., during examinations, overnight travel, attending a party, switching antiepileptic drugs). In the patient with catamenial epilepsy, it may be useful. In tonic status epilepticus, seizures may be worsened, and clobazam should be used with care.

Clobazam is usually administered orally at a dose of 10 to 20 mg/day, preferably taken at night or in a twice-daily regimen. The only available preparation is a 10-mg tablet or capsule. Higher doses should be generally avoided because the efficacy does not increase, and side effects become more common. If tolerance develops, the drug is slowly withdrawn at a rate of 10 mg per month. Although clobazam is a very well tolerated benzodiazepine at the recommended dosage, general precautions for the use of benzodiazepines apply.

CLONAZEPAM

Clonazepam is one of the oldest benzodiazepines available and is a potent anticonvulsant. Nevertheless, it has largely fallen out of favor for use in chronic epilepsy, mainly because of the development of tolerance, withdrawal symptoms, sedation, and bronchial hypersecretion (4). Clonazepam is still used as a second-line drug in the treatment of status epilepticus, both convulsive and nonconvulsive. In recent years, however, it has largely been superseded by the other benzodiazepines diazepam, midazolam, and lorazepam. Clonazepam was introduced in Europe in the 1970s and is marketed worldwide.

Clinical Efficacy

Clonazepam was introduced before controlled trials became mandatory for evaluation of efficacy and tolerability of antiepileptic drugs. It was studied in the 1970s and 1980s in a few, often small controlled clinical trials as adjunctive therapy in patients with partial and generalized seizures unresponsive to standard treatment (4). Clonazepam is a potent antiepileptic drug for adjunctive therapy of generalized absence and myoclonic seizures and also for partial seizures. However, because of sedation, problems during withdrawal, and hypersalivation, it is increasingly used as a second-line adjunctive drug only when better-tolerated adjunctive antiepileptic drugs have not been helpful. It has been evaluated in single-arm studies in partial and generalized epilepsy, and the effects have generally been modest. It has been used in benign rolandic epilepsy and also in epilepsia partialis continua. In the generalized epilepsies, the effectiveness of this drug is similar to that of ethosuximide for absence seizures (4,10), and it can be useful in myoclonic seizures, such as in juvenile myoclonic epilepsy and in Lennox-Gastaut syndrome. Clonazepam is also useful for bridge therapy while antiepileptic drugs are being changed or withdrawn (11). It is still used widely in the treatment of various forms of status epilepticus (Table 18.2). Its indications are the same as for diazepam, and its effectiveness is similar (1). Clonazepam can be given i.v. or as an oral and rectal solution. A few drops of the solution are swallowed as a last resort by some patients to control incipient seizures at home or when these patients are out of the house. Tolerance to the anticonvulsant effects (and the sedative and motor side effects) may occur within days in some patients, whereas in others tolerance to the anticonvulsant effect is seen after weeks and months. The mechanism underlying the development of tolerance remains elusive, and various maneuvers (as described earlier, in the section on clobazam) to overcome or to avoid tolerance are largely ineffective. Clonazepam may impair swallowing of saliva through muscle hypotonia and, as a consequence, may lead to pneumonia in some patients and also to drooling. Withdrawal of clonazepam may present also a problem, despite its long half-life, and it should be done cautiously. My experience is to do this in outpatients at a rate not faster than 0.25 mg per month. Withdrawal symptoms, which may be seen in as many as 50% of patients, include rebound seizures, anxiety, tremor, insomnia, and, in some patients, psychotic episodes. In view of the development of tolerance, it is not surprising that no clear relationship has

been found between the serum concentration of clonazepam and seizure control, and an optimum range of serum concentrations in chronic epilepsy has not been established.

Clinical Use

Clonazepam is still used as an adjunctive drug in patients with a wide range of partial and generalized seizures who do not respond to standard treatment and better-tolerated adjunctive therapy (Table 18.1). It is used especially for the long-term treatment of myoclonic seizures and as a short course of maintenance therapy in myoclonic status epilepticus, as well as in atypical absence status epilepticus. Tonic status epilepticus can be worsened by clonazepam. Clonazepam is more widely used in children than in adults. Clonazepam is available as 0.5- and 2-mg tablets and as an oral solution. The initial oral dose is usually 0.25 mg, which is increased gradually to 0.5 mg and, if necessary, <4.0 mg/day, given at night or in twice-daily regimens. In children, the usual maintenance dose is between 1 and 3 mg/day (13).

Clonazepam is also a second-line drug for treatment of convulsive or nonconvulsive status epilepticus, but it has been superseded in many centers by diazepam, midazolam, and lorazepam. As an i.v. bolus, clonazepam is used in early status epilepticus, whereas for established status epilepticus, a short i.v. infusion may be used (1). Clonazepam has a similar onset of action but a longer duration of action and a lower rate of early relapse than diazepam. The drug accumulates during prolonged infusion, leading to hypotension, sedation, and, finally, respiratory arrest. Too rapid an infusion may lead to severe hypotension and syncope, and continuous infusion should be avoided if possible.

The usual preparation for emergency treatment is a 1-mL ampule containing 1 mg clonazepam. For treatment of early status epilepticus, clonazepam is usually given as a 1-mg bolus injection over 1 minute in adults, whereas 0.25 to 0.5 mg may be used in children. This dose can be repeated three times over a period of 3 hours, and clonazepam can also be given very slowly in dextrose (5%) or 0.9% sodium chloride solution (1 to 2 mg in 250 mL). Reduction of epileptiform electroencephalographic activity and a parallel decrease of seizures were seen in children after a single intramuscular (i.m.) injection of 0.02 mg/kg body weight/day (12), a finding suggesting that much lower doses may be useful, at least in some children.

DIAZEPAM

Diazepam is the most widely used benzodiazepine in epilepsy and is a drug of first choice for the treatment of the premonitory stages of status epilepticus, for early status epilepticus, for serial seizures, for prolonged seizures, and

TABLE 18.2. COMPARATIVE EFFICACY OF DIAZEPAM AND CLONAZEPAM IN VARIOUS TYPES OF STATUS EPILEPTICUS

	Diazepam	Clonazepam
Tonic-clonic status epilepticus	177/224 (79%)	21/24 (88%)
Absence status epilepticus	44/72 (61%)	56/67 (84%)
Partial status epilepticus	59/67 (88%)	35/40 (88%)

[a]Some patients had multiple injections or infusions, and most had additional therapy (1).

for the prophylaxis of febrile seizures. The usefulness of diazepam in treatment of status with its well-proven efficacy and rapid onset of action is, however, limited by frequent seizure relapse after initial control by bolus injection and by the unwelcome accumulation after repeated injection or continuous infusion with a risk of sudden respiratory depression, sedation, and hypotension (1,13). The rectal administration of diazepam solutions or gel is convenient, safe, and effective. Use of suppositories, i.m. administration, or long-term oral administration of diazepam is not recommended for treatment of epilepsy because of limited efficacy, poor tolerability, and general risks of this class of drugs. Diazepam was introduced in Europe in the 1970s and is marketed worldwide.

Clinical Efficacy

A single i.v. bolus of diazepam at a dose of 5 to 10 mg at a rate of 1 to 5 mg/min has been reported to stop initial seizure activity in 88% of patients with various seizure types in status epilepticus (2) (Table 18.2). In one study, i.v. diazepam, given as a bolus of 2 mg/min, stopped convulsions in 32% of patients after 3 minutes, in 68% of patients after 5 minutes, and in 80% of patients after 10 minutes (14). When bolus injections failed, a symptomatic cause was often found, such as acute infectious encephalopathies, several cerebral anoxia, and acute cerebral infarction. Seizures were controlled in 76% of the episodes treated with 10 mg diazepam i.v. and in 89% treated with 4 mg lorazepam i.v. in a double-blind study of status epilepticus (15). Both drugs were injected over a period of 2 minutes. Adverse effects occurred in 12.5%, including respiratory depression and sedation. A prospective comparison of i.v. diazepam plus phenytoin versus i.v. phenobarbital in the treatment of status epilepticus found both regimens similarly effective and comparable in safety (16). However, the combination of diazepam with phenobarbital is not recommended (see the later discussion on clinical use). In a large double-blind study of a total of 384 patients with convulsive status epilepticus, i.v. diazepam (0.15 mg/kg body weight) followed by i.v. phenytoin (18 mg/kg) was less effective and less easy to use than i.v. lorazepam and was as efficacious as phenobarbital (17).

The main disadvantages of diazepam (when given alone) are seizure relapse after i.v. injection and accumulation after prolonged infusion (Table 18.1). Seizure relapse is common and limits the usefulness of diazepam in status epilepticus. Only 50% of patients are seizure free 2 hours after a single injection (18): the relapse is caused by diazepam's rapid redistribution, resulting in an abrupt fall of its concentration in the brain, with a significant loss of anticonvulsant effect. Additional treatment is necessary, and numerous proposals have been made including the use of i.v. phenytoin, phenobarbital, lidocaine, and clonazepam (1), as well as a constant infusion of diazepam.

Continuous Infusion

The use of continuous diazepam infusion in patients with refractory status epilepticus was shown to be effective in 12 of 18 patients after failure of a bolus injection of 20 mg diazepam and an i.v. loading of 15 mg/kg phenytoin in the opposite arm (14). When seizures persisted, a continuous infusion of diazepam 4 to 8 mg/hr with 50 mg of diazepam in 500 mL dextrose/water was given for 3 hours. When diazepam is used as an infusion, a maximum of 20 mg should be dissolved and thoroughly mixed in a minimum of 250 mL of solvent. This solution will not precipitate in a 5% to 10% glucose solution or in a 0.9% saline solution. The infusion should be given immediately after mixing, and a large-caliber vein should be used. Significantly, compared with i.v. bolus injection, diazepam by continuous infusion may result in a lower incidence of respiratory depression and hypotension. Early clinical observations in adult patients with refractory status epilepticus reported control of seizures without side effects with continuous diazepam infusions ranging from 10 to 48 mg/day for 12 to 24 hours (18) to 75 to 100 mg/day and 140 to 200 mg /day for 2 to 7 days in adults and 3 to 4 mg /kg/day for 21 hours to 8 days in infants (2,19). Current recommendations for diazepam i.v. infusion for treatment of convulsive status epilepticus are 2 to 3 mg/kg/day in adults and 0.3 to 1.0 mg/kg/day in children (13). However, development of tolerance was noted with infusions lasting longer than 1 day (2). In view of the development of tolerance, it is not surprising that no clear relationship has been found between the serum concentration of diazepam or of its main metabolite and seizure control.

Although limited published data indicate that continuous i.v. infusions of diazepam are safe and effective, critics point out that diazepam accumulates on repeated injections or during continuous infusion, and this accumulation carries a high risk of causing sudden respiratory depression, sedation, and hypotension (1,13). Continuous electroencephalographic monitoring has been recommended to evaluate clinical effectiveness.

Rectal Solution or Gel

Although i.v. administration is the preferred immediate treatment, venous access is often difficult to achieve, and medical personnel may not be immediately available at the site of the emergency. In contrast, the rectal solution or gel of diazepam can immediately be given by parents at home or at any site, and it can be administered by paramedical personnel either for prehospital treatment or in the emergency room. In fact, visits to the emergency room may be reduced, and quality of life may improve.

The rectal solution of diazepam has been effectively used in children for the emergency treatment of ongoing seizures at home (20,21). An initial dose of 0.5 mg/kg was employed with a maximum of 20 mg per single dose. The convulsions were stopped within 15 minutes in 80% of the episodes. (20). Side effects occurred in four of 17 children and included temporary respiration difficulties in one patient aged 16 years who was receiving concomitant phenobarbital treatment and who had received 0.5 mg/kg of rectal diazepam. Urticaria and pruritus occurred in two children, and dizziness was noted in one 13-year-old patient.

Improvement in the quality of life was seen in 58% of patients after rectal administration of 0.3 to 0.5 mg/kg injectable solution in one study (21). Emergency room visits decreased, and cost savings were noted. The authors of this report concluded that rectal diazepam appears to be a practical method for the effective treatment of severe seizures at home (20,21). Home use of rectal diazepam solution (0.5 mg/kg) led to prompt cessation of seizures in 15 of 17 families, whereas in two, rectal diazepam was unsuccessful, and hospital treatment was needed (22). Rectal diazepam solution, in a dosage ranging from 0.4 to 1.2 mg/kg, has also been successful in the treatment of convulsions in the children's emergency room. In 71% of 55 children, convulsions ceased within 5 minutes, and in a further 7%, convulsions stopped within 5 to 10 minutes. In 16%, rectal diazepam was ineffective, but there was a rapid response to i.v. diazepam. Convulsions lasting more than 15 minutes could be controlled in only 46% in comparison with 81% for shorter convulsions. Four children had transient respiratory depression (23). In a prospective study, 44 children aged 6 months to 5 years were treated with a rectal solution of diazepam during 59 generalized seizures in a hospital. Diazepam i.v. solution was administered rectally with a disposable plastic syringe and a 6-cm-long plastic tube with a blunt tip. Children aged <3 years received 0.5 to 0.9 mg/kg per dose, whereas children >3 years old were given a dose of 0.6 to 0.8 mg/kg. Rectal diazepam was effective in 80% of the episodes. In 10%, rectal diazepam failed, although i.v. diazepam was effective, and in 10%, treatment with diazepam failed after rectal and i.v. administration. No significant respiration depression or other serious side effects were observed (24). The rapid and reliable anticonvulsant effect of diazepam given rectally makes this regimen a valuable alternative when i.v. administration is not feasible.

Rectal administration is also effective for the prevention of recurrent febrile convulsions. When diazepam solution (in a dose of 5 mg in children aged <3 years and 7.5 mg in those >3 years old) was administered rectally whenever the children's temperature was 38.5°C or more, recurrence rate was 12% compared with 39% for the randomized control group, who received diazepam rectally only for the acute treatment of an ongoing seizure. The risk of subsequent epilepsy was not lowered, however (25). No significant side effects were observed in this study. In another study conducted in Denmark, rectal diazepam (5 mg in children aged <3 years and 7.5 mg in those >3 years old) was given at home every 12 hours in children with previous febrile seizures whenever the children's temperature was 38.5° C or higher. Twenty-three of 89 children had a recurrence within 1 year, and 69 had side effects, none of which was serious. A control group receiving valproic acid suppositories showed a similar recurrence rate of 14 of 80 children. The recurrence rates with both treatments were low compared with figures for untreated controls in Denmark (32%), a finding suggesting that intermittent treatment was effective (26). Successful treatment of febrile seizures at home with rectal diazepam solution in a dose of 5 mg (children weighing <12 kg) or 10 mg (children weighing <12 kg) has been confirmed in a large study in Italy (27).

A single rectal administration of diazepam (20 to 30 mg) has also been used successfully to prevent serial seizures in adult patients with drug-resistant epilepsy who are prone to serial seizures. The onset of effect was noted approximately 10 minutes after drug administration, and the effective dose was 0.50 mg/kg (28,29). Preliminary data indicate that rapid achievement of diazepam serum concentrations of 500 to 700 ng/mL are needed for single-dose seizure control, and concentrations of >150 to 200 ng/mL are necessary for maintenance of seizure control (2).

A rectal diazepam gel became available in the United States in 1998. In several placebo-controlled trials, single and repeated rectal diazepam gel application in a dose of 0.2 to 0.5 mg/kg acutely reduced seizures in children, adolescents, and adults with episodes or clusters of repetitive seizures in a nonmedical or home setting (30–34). Somnolence was the only remarkable side effect, and respiratory depression was not seen (35). Local tolerability was good. Children received one dose at the onset of acute repetitive seizures and a second dose 4 hours later. Adults received three doses: one dose at seizure onset, and two more doses 4 and 12 hours after onset. Treatment was administered by a caregiver, such as a parent, who had received special training.

Oral Treatment

A single 20-mg oral dose of diazepam significantly reduced the incidence of serial seizures at plasma concentrations of 273±190 (SD) ng/mL (2). Oral intermittent diazepam given as prophylaxis of recurrent febrile seizures showed no difference to placebo (36–38). After excluding many protocol violators, however, and analyzing children actually receiving diazepam, investigators found a statistically significant reduction in the risk of febrile seizures (39). Oral diazepam is rarely used and is not recommended for the long-term treatment of epilepsy (2,13). Controlled trials showed that diazepam is less effective than phenytoin or phenobarbital for the treatment of generalized tonic-clonic seizures and is about as effective as pheneturide, a now obsolete agent, for the treatment of partial seizures (2). Sharing the fate of oral diazepam, clorazepate, a prodrug that is converted to the active antiepileptic drug *N*-desmethyldiazepam, is only rarely used for the treatment of epilepsy (40).

Clinical Use

Diazepam is a drug of first choice to treat the premonitory stage of status epilepticus and early status epilepticus, serial seizures, and ongoing acute seizures (Table 18.2). Diazepam, i.v. at a dose of 10 to 20 mg, given at a rate of 1 to 5 mg/min, is an effective and safe first-line emergency treatment of the premonitory stage of status epilepticus and early status epilepticus in adults. In children, the dose is 0.25 to 0.5 mg/kg at a rate of 1 to 5 mg/min. Administration can be repeated once after 15 minutes if status epilepticus continues. When diazepam is injected slowly, side effects are rare in patients without risk factors. Resuscitation because of respiratory or cardiovascular depression is rarely necessary, but it should be available when risk factors are present. These factors include the following: rapid bolus injection; pretreatment with sedative drugs (e.g., phenobarbital); advanced heart, lung, or liver disease; and status epilepticus secondary to acute brain disease. If seizures continue after 30 minutes, infusion of diazepam is a second-line option in established status epilepticus. Alternative and preferred options include i.v. infusion of phenobarbital, phenytoin, or fosphenytoin (1,2,13). If diazepam infusion is used, preliminary experience suggests that an initial loading dose of 20 mg should be administered to control the seizures temporarily in an adult patient in an intensive care unit, followed by a continuous i.v. infusion of diazepam 2 mg/kg/day. The rate of infusion should be determined clinically; monitoring of plasma diazepam and *N*-desmethyl-diazepam concentrations may be useful to detect accumulation, and close supervision of safety and tolerability (e.g., sudden respiratory depression and hypotension) and intensive videoelectroencephalographic monitory are strongly recommended. As pointed out earlier, accumulation may occur and may lead to sudden respiratory depression. If diazepam or alternative regimens including phenytoin or phenobarbital are not effective and status epilepticus continues for 1 hour, general anesthesia and muscle relaxants should be given (1).

When the i.v. route cannot be accessed without delay, the rectal administration of diazepam solution is the procedure of choice. Rectal diazepam is effective and safe for the immediate home treatment of prolonged seizures and serial seizures and for the initial treatment of status epilepticus. Furthermore, rectal diazepam is effective and safe for intermittent prophylaxis of febrile seizures and serial seizures.

Diazepam suppositories and i.m. and oral diazepam are not suited for emergency treatment. Oral diazepam may be clinically useful after i.v. use for a short course of maintenance therapy of myoclonic status epilepticus and complex partial status epilepticus. Diazepam can worsen tonic status epilepticus and should be used with caution. The possible teratogenic effect and the development of sedation and possibly a withdrawal syndrome in the neonate suggest a critical benefit: risk evaluation before diazepam is used during pregnancy. Although nursing is not generally discouraged, it may result in neonatal plasma concentrations in the range of 30% to 75% of the serum concentration of nursing mothers. Long-term diazepam exposure is fraught with the risk of overdose, dependence, and withdrawal, as well as poor efficacy because of the development of tolerance. Therefore, long-term use of this drug is neither safe nor effective for the treatment of chronic epilepsy, nor is it recommended for the prophylaxis of febrile seizures. The recommended rectal dose is 10 to 30 mg in adults, 0.5 to 0.75 mg/kg in children aged 2 to 5 years, 0.3 mg/kg in children aged 6 to 10 years, and 0.2 mg/kg in children aged <12 years. The administration can be repeated. If the rectal administration is not retained because of mucosal irritation, the dose should be repeated immediately. Training of relatives or nonmedical persons is recommended. One should keep the tube pressed together during extraction; resucking of the drug back into the tube is avoided.

The usual dosage of an i.v. bolus injection of undiluted drug is 10 to 20 mg in adults and 0.25 to 0.5 mg/kg in children at a rate of 1 to 5 mg/min. The bolus can be repeated at intervals of at least 15 minutes. If seizures persist in a patient with refractory status epilepticus in an intensive care unit, a continuous i.v. infusion of diazepam 2 mg/kg/day is one option. The rate of infusion should be clinical, and close supervision of safety and tolerability is strongly recommended.

LORAZEPAM

Lorazepam is considered by many physicians the preferred drug for the treatment of the early stage of status epilepticus. It has a longer duration of action and a smaller risk of respiratory depression and hypotension than diazepam (1). It has also been used for refractory status epilepticus.

Clinical Efficacy

Lorazepam was compared with diazepam for the treatment of status epilepticus, serial seizures, and ongoing acute seizures (3). Seizures were controlled in 76% of the episodes treated with 10 mg diazepam i.v. and in 89% of those treated with 4 mg lorazepam i.v. in a double-blind study of status epilepticus (15). The efficacy of lorazepam (4 to 10 mg i.v.) and of clonazepam (1 mg i.v.) was comparable in an early series of 64 patients with status epilepticus (41). Lorazepam was more effective than diazepam in patients with other epileptic seizures excluding generalized tonic-clonic seizures. Twelve percent of these seizure types were not controlled by lorazepam, and 32% of the episodes were not controlled by diazepam. In a large double-blind study of a total of 384 patients with convulsive status epilepticus, lorazepam (in an i.v. dose of 0.1 mg/kg and a maximal rate of administration of 2 mg/min) was more effective than phenytoin and was as efficacious as and easier to use than phenobarbital or a combination of diazepam and phenytoin (17). More clinical experience is needed to determine whether lorazepam can replace diazepam or phenytoin in the treatment of status epilepticus, but results from these studies (17,41) indicate that lorazepam is at least as effective as diazepam or the combination of diazepam and phenytoin in the initial treatment of status epilepticus. In a open, randomized study in children, lorazepam and diazepam were similarly effective in stopping acute seizures, but lorazepam caused respiratory depression less often, and no patient receiving lorazepam required admission to the intensive care unit for either respiratory depression or persisting status epilepticus (42), a finding confirming earlier observations that the rate of endotracheal intubation may be lower when lorazepam rather than diazepam is used for treatment of status epilepticus in children (43). Lorazepam, in high doses ranging up to 9 mg/hr, has also been used as an alternative to pentobarbital for treatment of refractory status epilepticus (44). There is large clinical experience with lorazepam in newborns, children, and adults. In a short-term placebo-controlled trial, 1 mg twice daily of oral lorazepam was effective as adjunctive therapy for partial seizures unresponsive to standard antiepileptic drugs (45).

In a recent comparison of 2 mg i.v. lorazepam, 5 mg i.v. diazepam and placebo for the treatment of out-of-hospital treatment of status epilepticus, both drugs were safe and more effective than placebo when administered by paramedics in adults with prolonged or repetitive generalize convulsive seizures (45a). An identical second injection was given if needed. Status epilepticus had been terminated in more patients treated with lorazepam (59.1%) or diazepam (42.6%) than patients given placebo (21.1%). The odds ratio for termination of status epilepticus at arrival was 1.9 (95% confidence interval, 0.8 to 4.4) in the lorazepam group as compared to the diazepam group. The rates of respiratory or circulatory complications after the study treatment had been administered were 10.6% for the lorazepam group, 10.3% for the diazepam group, and 22.5% for the placebo group. The authors concluded that lorazepam was likely to be a better therapy than diazepam for paramedic treatment of out-of-hospital status epilepticus in adults.

Clinical Use

An i.v. bolus of lorazepam is primarily used for the early treatment of status epilepticus as an alternative to diazepam (Table 18.1). During subsequent management, additional antiepileptic drugs are necessary because tolerance may develop within 24 hours The clearance of lorazepam is largely unaffected by mild to moderate renal and liver disease. Lorazepam is rarely used for oral treatment in epilepsy. The usual dosage of lorazepam in adults is an i.v. bolus of 0.07 mg/kg, usually 4 mg, repeated after 10 minutes if nec-

essary; in children, a bolus of 0.1 mg/kg is recommended. The rate of injection should not exceed 1 mg/min.

MIDAZOLAM

Midazolam, as an i.v. bolus or as an i.m. or rectal solution, has been used as an alternative to diazepam or lorazepam for the treatment of the premonitory stage of status epilepticus and of early status epilepticus. It is more water soluble than diazepam and is rapidly absorbed after i.m., nasal, and buccal administration (46,47). Midazolam can be used when i.v. administration is inconvenient or is not possible.

Clinical Efficacy

Comparisons of buccal and i.m. midazolam with rectal diazepam have shown similar efficacy and onset of action (47). Midazolam i.m. is as effective as i.v. diazepam in stopping ongoing seizures, but it may have a faster onset of action (48). There is limited clinical experience with the use of midazolam in the treatment of status epilepticus in children and adults both for initial treatment and for infusion in refractory status. Cardiovascular depression, hypotension, and apnea have been reported requiring intubation for artificial respiration (49).

Clinical Use

Like diazepam, midazolam is short acting, and additional antiepileptic drugs are necessary in the management of status epilepticus to prevent relapse of seizures (Table 18.1). As with diazepam, the half-life of midazolam is prolonged in severe hepatic disease, and a 50% lower dose should be given. The usual dosage for i.m. injection is 5 to 10 mg in adults and 0.15 to 0.3 mg/kg in children; this can be repeated once. The i.v. bolus is 0.1 to 0.3 mg/kg, at a rate not exceeding 2 mg/min, which can also be repeated once. For buccal instillation, 10 mg can be given by catheter and syringe in children and adults.

NITRAZEPAM

Nitrazepam is largely confined to second-line or third-line treatment of severe childhood epilepsies, mainly West's syndrome (Table 18.1). Although quite effective, it is rarely used nowadays because of severe, and in some patients intolerable, drowsiness, ataxia, increase in bronchial secretions, hypersalivation (from nitrazepam-induced hypotonia of the muscles involved in the swallowing of saliva), and aspiration pneumonia in some patients (50). Nitrazepam has largely been superseded in the treatment of infantile spasms (West's syndrome) by vigabatrin, valproate, steroids, or adrenocorticotropic hormone.

Clinical Efficacy and Use

Nitrazepam was introduced to the market at a time when controlled trials were not generally required for evaluation of efficacy. Nitrazepam seems to be effective for infantile spasms, in which it is associated with a response of 52% to 68% and fewer side effects compared with high-dose adrenocorticotropic hormone. The drug is also used as adjunctive therapy in the severe symptomatic generalized epilepsies such as Lennox-Gastaut syndrome and in severe myoclonic epilepsies. The unfavorable side effect profile precludes the wide use of nitrazepam, except for patients in whom standard therapy and better-tolerated second-line drugs have been ineffective. Apart from the dose-related side effects discussed earlier, leukopenia may occur, and sudden withdrawal may result in rebound seizures and delirium tremens. The usual dosage is <1 mg/kg/day in children and <0.5 mg/kg/day in adults. In most patients, the dose is between 1.25 and 10 mg/day.

REFERENCES

1. Shorvon S. *Status epilepticus.* Cambridge: Cambridge University Press, 1994:199.
2. Schmidt D. Benzodiazepines: diazepam. In: Levy RH, Mattson RH, Meldrum BS, eds. *Antiepileptic drugs,* 4th ed. New York: Raven Press, 1995:705–724.
3. Homan RW, Treiman DW. Benzodiazepines: lorazepam. In: Levy RH, Mattson RH, Meldrum BS, eds. *Antiepileptic drugs,* 4th ed. New York: Raven Press, 1995:779–790.
4. Sato S, Malow BA. Benzodiazepines: clonazepam. In: Levy RH, Mattson RH, Meldrum BS, eds. *Antiepileptic drugs,* 4th ed. New York: Raven Press, 1995:725–734.
5. Shorvon SD. Benzodiazepines: clobazam. In: Levy RH, Mattson RH, Meldrum BS, eds. *Antiepileptic drugs,* 4th ed. New York: Raven Press, 1995:763–777.
6. Keene DL, Whiting S, Humphreys P. Clobazam as an add-on drug in the treatment of refractory epilepsy of childhood. *Can J Neurol Sci* 1990;17:317–319.
7. Schmidt D, Rohde M, Wolf P, et al. Clobazam for refractory focal epilepsy: a controlled trial. *Arch Neurol* 1986;43:824–826.
8. Anonymous. Clobazam has equivalent efficacy to carbamazepine and phenytoin as monotherapy for childhood epilepsy: Canadian Study Group for Childhood Epilepsy . *Epilepsia* 1998;39: 952–959.
9. Bawden HN, Camfield CS, Camfield PR, et al. The cognitive and behavioural effects of clobazam and standard monotherapy are comparable. *Epilepsy Res* 1999;33:133–143.
10. Dreifuss FE, Penry JK, Rose SW, et al. Serum clonazepam concentrations in children with absence seizures. *Neurology* 1975;23:255–258.
11. Sanders PT, Kopczynski AM, Lesser RP, et al. Effectiveness of clonazepam bridge therapy for reducing seizures and side effects during initiation of chronic anticonvulsants. *Epilepsia* 1998;39 [Suppl 6]:51.
12. Dahlin M, Knutsson E, Amark P, et al. Reduction of epileptiform activity in response to low-dose clonazepam in children with epilepsy: a randomized double-blind study. *Epilepsia* 2000;41: 308–315.
13. Shorvon S. *Handbook of epilepsy treatment.* Oxford: Blackwell Science, 2000:1–248.
14. Delgado-Escueta AV, Enrile-Bascal F. Combination therapy for status epilepticus: intravenous diazepam and phenytoin. *Adv Neurol* 1983;34:477–485.
15. Leppik IE, Derivan AT, Homan RW, et al. Double-blind study of lorazepam and diazepam in status epilepticus. *JAMA* 1983;249: 1452–1454.
16. Shaner DM, McCurdy SA, Herring MO, et al. Treatment of status epilepticus: a prospective comparison of diazepam and phenytoin versus phenobarbital and optional phenytoin. *Neurology* 1988;38:202–207.
17. Treiman DM, Meyers PD, Walton NY, et al. A comparison of four treatments for generalized convulsive status epilepticus. *N Engl J Med* 1998;792–798.
18. Schwab RS. Intravenous diazepam in the treatment of prolonged seizure activity. *N Engl J Med* 1967;276:779–784.
19. Thong YH, Abramson DC. Continuos infusion of diazepam in infants with severe recurrent convulsions. *Med Ann DC* 1974;43: 63–65.
20. Hoppu K, Santavuori P. Diazepam rectal solution for home treatment of acute seizures in children. *Acta Paediatr Scand* 1981;70: 369–372.
21. Kriel RL, Cloyd JC, Hadsall RS, et al. Home use of rectal diazepam for cluster and prolonged seizures: efficacy, adverse reactions, quality of life, and cost analysis. *Pediatr Neurol* 1991;7:13–17.
22. Camfield CS, Camfield PR, Smith E, et al. Home use of rectal diazepam to prevent status epilepticus in children with convulsive disorders. *J Child Neurol* 1989;4:125–126.
23. Sykes RM, Okonofua JA. Rectal diazepam solution in the treatment of convulsions in the children's emergency room. *Ann Trop Paediatr* 1988;8:259–261.
24. Knudsen FU. Rectal administration of diazepam in solution in the acute treatment of convulsions in infants and children. *Arch Dis Child* 1979;54:855–857.
25. Knudsen FU. Effective short-term diazepam prophylaxis in febrile convulsions. *J Pediatr* 1985;106:487–490.
26. Daugbjerg P, Brems M, Mai J, et al. Intermittent prophylaxis in febrile convulsions: diazepam or valproic acid? *Acta Neurol Scand* 1990;82:17–20.
27. Ventura A, Basso T, Bortolan G, et al. Home treatment of seizures as a strategy for the long-term management of febrile convulsions in children. *Helv Paediatr Acta* 1982;37:581–587.
28. Milligan NM, Dhillon S, Griffiths A, et al. A clinical trial of single dose rectal and oral administration of diazepam for the prevention of serial seizures in adult epileptic patients. *J Neurol Neurosurg Psychiatry* 1984;47:235–240.
29. Remy C, Jourdi N, Villemain D, et al. Intrarectal diazepam in epileptic adults. *Epilepsia* 1992;33:353–358.
30. Cereghino JJ, Mitchell WG, Murphy J, et al. Treating repetitive seizures with a rectal diazepam formulation: a randomized study. The North American Diastat Study Group. *Neurology* 1998;51: 1274–1282.
31. Dreifuss FE, Rosman NP, Cloyd JC, et al. A comparison of rectal diazepam gel and placebo for acute repetitive seizures. *N Engl J Med* 1998;338:1869–1875.
32. Kriel RL, Cloyd JC, Pellock JM, et al. Rectal diazepam gel for treatment of acute repetitive seizures: the North American Diastat Study Group. *Pediatr Neurol* 1999;20:282–288.
33. Mitchell WG, Shellenberger K, Groves L, et al. Rectal diazepam gel (Diastat) for the acute repetitive seizures: results of a double-blind, placebo-controlled study in children and adults with epilepsy. *Epilepsia* 1996;37[Suppl 5]:154.
34. Pellock JM, Mitchell WG, Cloyd JC. Diastat (diazepam rectal gel) in the treatment of acute repetitive seizures in adults. *Epilepsia* 1998;39[Suppl 6]:126–127.
35. Shellenberger K, Groves L, Franklin J, et al. Diastat (diazepam

rectal gel) therapy of acute epileptic seizures does not compromise respiratory function. *Epilepsia* 1997;38[Suppl 8]:57–58.

36. Uhari M, Rantala H, Vainionpaa L, et al. Effect of acetaminophen and of low intermittent doses of diazepam on prevention of recurrences of febrile seizures. *J Pediatr* 1995;126:991–995.

37. Autret E, Billard C, Bertrand P, et al. Double-blind, randomized trial of diazepam versus placebo for prevention of recurrence of febrile seizures. *J Pediatr* 1990;117:490–494.

38. Rantala H, Tarkka R, Uhari, M. A meta-analytic review of the preventive treatment of recurrences of febrile seizures. *J Pediatr* 1997;131:922–925.

39. Rosman NP, Colton T, Labazzo J, et al. A controlled trial of diazepam administered during febrile illnesses to prevent recurrence of febrile seizures. *N Engl J Med* 1993;329:79–84.

40. Wilensky AJ. Benzodiazepines: clorazepate. In: Levy RH, Mattson RH, Meldrum BS, eds. *Antiepileptic drugs,* 4th ed. New York: Raven Press, 1995:751–762.

41. Sorel L, Mechler L, Harmant J. Comparative trial of intravenous lorazepam and clonazepam in status epilepticus. *Clin Ther* 1981; 4:326–336.

42. Appleton R, Sweeney A, Choonara I, et al. Lorazepam versus diazepam in the acute treatment of epileptic seizures and status epilepticus. *Dev Med Child Neurol* 1995;37:682–688.

43. Chiulli DA, Terndrup TE, Kanter RK. The influence of diazepam or lorazepam on the frequency of endotracheal intubation in childhood status epilepticus. *J Emerg Med* 1991;9:13–17.

44. Labar DR, Ali A, Root J. High-dose intravenous lorazepam for the treatment of refractory status epilepticus. *Neurology* 1994;44: 1400–1402.

45. Walker JE, Homan RW, Crawford IL. Lorazepam: a controlled trial in patients with intractable complex partial seizures. *Epilepsia* 1984;25:464–466.

45a. Allredge BK, Gelb AM, Marshall Isaacs S, et al. A comparison of lorazepam, diazepam, and placebo for the treatment of out-of-hospital status epilepticus. *N Engl J Med* 2001;345:631–637.

46. Jawad S, Richens A, Oxley J. Pharmacodynamic and clinical evaluation of midazolam in epilepsy. *Acta Neurol Scand* 1984;70:219.

47. Scott RC, Besag FMC, Neville BGR. Buccal midazolam and rectal diazepam for treatment of prolonged seizures in childhood and adolescence: a randomised trial. *Lancet* 1999;353: 623–626.

48. Chamberlain JM, Altieri MA, Futterman H, et al. A prospective, randomized study comparing intramuscular midazolam with intravenous diazepam for the treatment of seizures in children. *Pediatr Emerg Care* 1997;13:92–94.

49. Bebin M, Beck TP. New anticonvulsant drugs: focus on flunarizine, fosphenytoin, midazolam and stiripentol. *Drugs* 1994;48: 153–171.

50. Baruzzi A, Michelucci R, Tassinari CA. Benzodiazepines: nitrazepam. In: Levy RH, Mattson RH, Meldrum BS, eds. *Antiepileptic drugs,* 4th ed. New York: Raven Press, 1995: 735–749.

BENZODIAZEPINES

ADVERSE EFFECTS

ROBERTO MICHELUCCI
CARLO ALBERTO TASSINARI

The benzodiazepines (BZDs) represent a large and popular class of drugs with similar mechanisms of action, clinical indications, and efficacy and toxicity profiles. Although all the BZDs have anticonvulsant activity in a variety of animal models, only a few have been developed for the management of epilepsy. Some of these, such as diazepam (DZP) and lorazepam (LZP), are mainly used for epilepsy emergencies (e.g., status epilepticus) whereas other compounds, such as clonazepam (CZP) and clobazam (CLB), are usually employed for long-term treatment. Depending on the route of administration—oral, rectal, intravenous (i.v.), or intramuscular (i.m.)—and the clinical application (acute or chronic), the spectrum of adverse effects and toxicity issues vary widely. Therefore, in the present chapter, the adverse effects of BZDs are reviewed separately according to the route of administration and clinical application. A section concerning the manifestations and management of overdose follows.

ADVERSE EFFECTS OF BENZODIAZEPINES IN THE MAINTENANCE TREATMENT OF EPILEPSY

CZP, CLB, and, to a lesser extent, DZP, LZP, nitrazepam (NZP), and clorazepate (CLP) may be administered orally as add-on drugs in epileptic patients refractory to previous medications. The fact that the BZDs are mostly used as adjunctive therapy may lead to an overestimation of their potential of toxicity, resulting from pharmacokinetic and pharmacodynamic interactions. The adverse effects of BZDs as long-term therapy include dose-related toxicity, hypersensitivity reactions, paradoxical effects, withdrawal effects, side effects from drug interactions, teratogenicity, and effects on neonates.

Roberto Michelucci, MD, PhD: Deputy Chief, Department of Neurological Sciences, Bellaria Hospital, Bologna, Italy

Carlo Alberto Tassinari, MD: Neurological Chief, Department of Neurological Sciences, University of Bologna, Bologna, Italy

Dose-Related Toxicity

Common dose-related effects involve the central nervous system (CNS), occur mostly at the beginning of treatment, and disappear with dose reduction. They also tend to lessen with the duration of treatment because of the development of tolerance.

For most BZDs, there seems to be some correlation between plasma drug concentrations after a single dose and CNS-related effects (1–5). At about 200 ng/mL of DZP, subjects tended to become slightly tired and drowsy (2). After i.m. administration of 10 mg of DZP, coordinative and reactive skills were impaired for as long as 5 hours at plasma concentrations exceeding 180 ng/mL (3). Using a sensitive neurophysiologic test, Bittencourt et al. (6) demonstrated a clear correlation between NZP and DZP concentrations and their effect on the peak velocity of saccadic eye movements (which is a measure of brainstem reticular formation function). With prolonged treatment, however, the relationship between plasma concentration and the effect of BZD drugs tends to become blurred because of the development of tolerance. Although dose dependency of side effects during maintenance treatment has been advocated for most BZDs, no relationship was found between the adverse effects and the plasma concentration of CZP (7,8). With DZP, disturbing side effects such as marked drowsiness, vertigo, ataxia, and impaired performance were associated with plasma concentrations >900 to 1,000 ng/mL (4). However, interindividual variability in response at any given concentration is considerable, and measurement of drug levels has no important role in optimizing BZD treatment.

Sedation or Drowsiness. This symptom is the most frequent complaint and is reported to occur in 10% to 85% (median, 62%) of patients receiving CZP (9) and in >40% of those taking DZP and NZP (10). Conversely, CLB has been associated with less sedative effects. In a review of 70 double-blind clinical trials comparing the effects of DZP, CLB, and placebo for anxiety and other psychiatric indications, Koeppen (11) found that the incidence of sedation was 26% with CLB, 46% with DZP, and 10% with placebo. These results were obtained, however, with high doses of CLB (>30 mg a day) and DZP (>15 mg/day). When adverse reactions to CLB were analyzed in epileptic patients, drowsiness was found to occur less frequently, probably because of lower doses employed (12). In a double-blind placebo controlled study of 10 healthy volunteers, CLB (20 to 30 mg/day) had fewer side effects than LZP (2 to 3 mg/day) (13). In healthy volunteers, CLB (10 and 20 mg) was also significantly less sedative than CZP (0.5 and 1.5 mg), although neither drug affected the ventilatory response to carbon dioxide (14).

Ataxia. Incoordination or ataxia is probably the second most common side effect of long-term BZD use. It is sometimes associated with dizziness and dysarthria. NZP, DZP, and CZP are more frequently observed to cause incoordination or ataxia, but this adverse effect has been reported for all the marketed BZDs, including CLB and CLP. Ataxia was found in 7% to 43% of patients treated with CZP (9) and in 5% to 50% of patients taking DZP and NZP as long-term therapy for seizure control (10). Ataxia was also mentioned in four of 23 open-label studies of CLB in epilepsy reviewed by Koeppen (12).

Behavioral Abnormalities. Significant behavioral and personality changes such as hyperactivity, restlessness, short attention span, irritability, and aggression may occur during long-term therapy with BZDs. Children are particularly likely to experience alterations in behavior and emotional state, but the elderly may be also susceptible. Behavioral effects have been reported in 2% to 51% (median, 12%) of patients taking CZP (9). NZP has been shown to induce symptoms of CNS stimulation, such as nightmares, insomnia, and agitation (15,16). Adverse personality changes, especially irritability, can occur during CLP therapy, particularly in association with primidone (17). Although CLB seems to induce behavioral effects less commonly (18), increased irritability, depression, and disinhibition may occur with CLB in chronically institutionalized patients (19). Sheth et al. (20) described seven developmentally disabled children treated with CLB for refractory epilepsy who developed a severe behavior disorder (aggressive agitation, self-injurious behavior, insomnia, incessant motor activity) 10 to 55 days after initiation of drug therapy. These disturbances resolved promptly on drug discontinuation.

Cognitive and Psychomotor Impairment. Several studies demonstrated that the administration of BZDs may impair human performances and psychomotor skills, mostly after single doses or short-term administration (21,24,25). When BZDs are administered repeatedly, these effects tend to be less prominent. Although some reviews state that no clear differentiation existed between the types of performances affected by the BZDs (22), other reviews have indicated that the performances to which mental speed is essen-

tial may be particularly affected (23). Of particular interest are the data concerning the residual effects of NZP on skills related to driving or other daily activities (21). Although some studies failed to detect negative effects of CLB on psychomotor performance (26), CLB may cause a slight impairment in some cognitive tests, mainly on retrieval processes and mental rapidity (27).

Studies of presurgical patients strongly suggest that BZDs can impair recall of events that follow the administration of these drugs. Studies in normal volunteers have also demonstrated clearly detrimental effects of BZDs on the ability to recall stimuli presented after drug administration. In clinical practice, anterograde amnesia has been reported with LZP at usual doses (28).

Other Clinically Relevant Side Effects. Muscle weakness, fatigue, and hypotonia are sometimes reported during BZD treatment; CZP, CLB, and NZP are particularly prone to cause this effect (9,16,18). BZDs should not be given to myasthenic patients. Visual disturbances, including nystagmus, blurred vision, and diplopia, may occur with any BZD, but they are not common (10). Although BZDs apparently have varying effects on appetite and weight, increased appetite and weight gain are more frequently reported (10). A significant weight gain was observed in nine of 81 patients taking CZP for more than 2 weeks (29), and it was also mentioned in five of 23 open studies with CLB reviewed by Koeppen (12). Acute psychotic reactions have been reported with BZD treatment but are exceptionally rare (9,10).

Hypersecretion and Drooling. Increased salivation and hypersecretion of the tracheobronchial tree have been noted with all the BZDs in children, but these findings are absent or negligible in adults (10). CZP and NZP are particularly prone to induce these effects (7,9,30,31). Although these symptoms are usually attributed to salivary and bronchial hypersecretion (7,31), Wyllie et al. (32) performed manometric examinations in two children with NZP-induced drooling and aspiration and demonstrated a delay of the cricopharyngeal relaxation during swallowing. These investigators suggested that NZP-induced drooling and aspiration may be caused by impaired swallowing.

Nitrazepam-Induced Death in Children. In 1987, Murphy et al. (33) observed an association between NZP and death in children with epilepsy who were receiving NZP at dosages ranging from 0.9 to 2.5 mg/kg/day. Consequently, a dosage of NZP <0.8 mg/kg/day was recommended in children (33). In a prospective study of esophageal manometry in 14 children receiving NZP for myoclonic epilepsy, Lim et al. (34) demonstrated swallowing incoordination with delayed cricopharyngeal relaxation in four of 14 patients. One of these patients developed respiratory distress and bronchospasm, which improved dramatically together with normalization of manometric findings after NZP was discontinued. In light of these results, a disturbance of swallowing was postulated as a possible cause of unexplained sudden death in children, and esophageal manometry was suggested as a helpful technique for defining patients at risk of sudden death (34). Rintahaka et al. (35) reported 21 deaths in 302 children who entered into a NZP study for intractable epilepsy. NZP therapy (at dosages ranging from 0.15 to 2.55 mg/kg/day) was associated with a statistically increased risk of mortality in young children (<3.4 years) with refractory epilepsy. Dysphagia, recurrent respiratory tract infections, gastroesophageal reflux, and aspiration apparently increased the likelihood of death in patients taking NZP. It is not known whether the risk of increased mortality in young children with intractable epilepsy is a NZP-specific problem or is common to other BZDs.

Hypersensitivity Reactions

BZDs rarely produce allergic reactions (10), and these drugs are commonly recommended in the management of seizures in patients with hypersensitivity reactions to antiepileptic drugs (36).

Rashes have been attributed to BZDs by several authors (31,37–39). Leukopenia has been reported to be caused by DZP (40), CZP (41), and NZP (42), and it is apparently reversible. Thrombocytopenic purpura has been described in association with CZP (43), whereas systemic lupus erythematosus has been associated with CLB (44). Hepatic necrosis has been associated with CLP (45) and DZP (46). Esophageal burn was reported in one patient taking CLP (47), and allergic intestinal nephritis occurred in one patient receiving oral DZP (48).

Paradoxical Effects

Long-term oral treatment with BZDs, particularly NZP and CZP, has been reported to cause a paradoxical increase in seizure frequency (42,49,50) or the appearance of new seizure types (51,52). Peterson (42) reported that six of 108 epileptic patients treated with oral NZP had an exacerbation of seizures. Similarly, increased frequency and severity of grand mal seizures were observed in 14 patients after NZP oral administration (50). In a survey of a large patient population treated with various oral BZDs, Alvarez et al. (53) reported that 5.8% of patients may have suffered from seizure aggravation. Worsening of seizures appeared to be more common in patients treated with CZP and particularly concerned tonic seizures and absences. In a retrospective study analyzing approximately 2,500 phases of add-on therapy in a total of 1,006 patients suffering from focal epilepsy, CLB and CZP were found to increase seizure frequency in 2% of cases (54). Oral BZDs, particularly CZP, have been correlated with precipitation of tonic-like microseizures in infants with West's syndrome (51,52).

Withdrawal Effects

In persons who do not have epilepsy, abrupt withdrawal of BZDs has been associated with convulsions, worsening of insomnia, psychosis, and delirium tremens (10,55–57). Particular attention has been devoted to the occurrence of *de novo* nonconvulsive status epilepticus after BZD withdrawal in nonepileptic patients (58–60). The clinical picture consists of acute mental confusion with an electroencephalographic (EEG) correlate of diffuse spike-and-wave discharges occurring in middle-aged or elderly patients with a history of long-term BZD use. These episodes may be misdiagnosed as acute BZD intoxication, and the diagnosis may be difficult if the EEG is delayed or is not performed; however, treatment with the specific BZD antagonist flumazenil aggravates the confusional state, whereas DZP administration leads to rapid recovery (58–60). Instances of grand mal seizures or convulsive status epilepticus have been also reported, usually after LZP has been discontinued (61).

In epileptic patients, abrupt withdrawal of BZDs commonly produces an increase of seizure frequency and severity, sometimes leading to convulsive status epilepticus. A "negative myoclonus" state has been reported after discontinuation of CLB (62). Although slow tapering is associated with a lower risk of precipitation of seizures, no optimal rate of withdrawal has been calculated for any BZD. Safe discontinuation rates for CZP were estimated to be <0.04 mg/kg/day (63) and 0.2 mg/day (64). Paradoxically, discontinuation of a BZD may result in amelioration of seizure activity in some patients (65).

Side Effects as a Result of Interaction with Other Drugs

BZDs may interact with other drugs, usually through pharmacodynamic mechanisms. It is well known that BZDs potentiate the action of CNS depressant drugs, such as ethanol or barbiturates, and BZDs may produce CNS depression and respiratory irregularities when they are given in association with amphetamines and methylphenidate (66). Feldman (17) reported the deleterious effects on behavior of the combination of CLP and primidone. The ability of BZDs to interact with other drugs through pharmacokinetic mechanisms is minimal. However, an increase in phenytoin levels, sometimes leading to intoxication, has been reported after CZP (67) or CLB (68) introduction. CLB may also induce an increase in the levels of carbamazepine (69) and carbamazepine-10,11-epoxide (70). A case of carbamazepine intoxication with negative myoclonus after addition of CLB has been reported (71). Cocks et al. (72) found that CLB may elevate valproate levels, and these investigators suggested that a combination of valproate and CLB, particularly at high doses, should be avoided because toxicity may be common. Conversely, valproate may induce a clinically significant potentiation of the effects of NZP (73), LZP (74), and DZP (75).

Teratogenicity and Effects on Postnatal Development

The possible teratogenic effects of BZDs are difficult to assess but appear to be mild. No definite causal relationship has been established, even though an association between first trimester intake of BZDs and oral clefts (especially cleft palate) was found in some retrospective studies (76,77), but not in others (78,79). Oral clefts have been reported with DZP, NZP, oxazepam, and chlordiazepoxide assessed as a group (77), as well as in individual case reports. The actual risk of having a child with cleft lip and cleft palate has been estimated to be 0.4% with DZP (80). Multiple limb anomalies were reported in a newborn child whose mother had taken CLP during the first trimester (81). Intake of BZDs in early pregnancy, as verified by case records and controls (82) and detection of high serum levels (83), has also been associated with an increased risk of CNS malformations and dysmorphism. An amplifying action of BZDs on valproate teratogenicity has been suggested (84).

Newborns, especially premature newborns, exposed to BZDs *in utero* during the late third trimester or at the time of delivery may present with the floppy infant syndrome consisting of floppy movement, poor sucking, hypotonia, hypothermia, poor reflexes, low Apgar scores, and apnea (66,85,86). A BZD withdrawal syndrome has also been observed in neonates (86).

ADVERSE EFFECTS OF BENZODIAZEPINES GIVEN AS ACUTE THERAPY IN EPILEPSY

BZDs play a prominent role in the emergency management of epilepsy. DZP, CZP, LZP, and midazolam (MDL) are commonly given i.v. for the treatment of status epilepticus (10,87,88); however, alternative routes of administration are feasible for the management of ongoing or serial seizures at home or when i.v. injection is inconvenient because of thrombophlebitis or technical difficulties during status epilepticus. These alternative routes include rectal (for DZP, MDL, LZP, CZP) or i.m. (for MDL) administration. Nasal administration of MDL for the treatment of acute seizures has also been described (89).

Intravenous Administration

Adverse effects of i.v. BZDs include systemic and CNS toxicity, local tissue irritation, and paradoxical effects.

Systemic and Central Nervous System Toxicity

Acute adverse effects consist mostly of hypotension and CNS-related events, specifically respiratory depression and profound sedation.

Diazepam. Browne and Penry (10) reviewed 401 patients with status epilepticus who were treated with DZP and found 16 cases of severe respiratory depression, along with 10 of marked hypotension. In a consecutive series of 33 patients, respiratory depression occurred in only one patient who received 25 mg, and there was mild to moderate respiratory depression in three other patients at doses of 10 mg (90). In another series of 98 patients, apnea appeared after i.v. injection of 5 and 10 mg in two patients with aminophylline-induced and lidocaine-induced seizures (91). Mild to severe hypotension and temporary respiratory depression were reported in 5.2% of 246 patients receiving multiple therapy (92). One of these patients died. Appleton et al. (93) reported a 15% incidence of respiratory depression in 53 patients treated with i.v. DZP, with half of these patients requiring repeated multiple doses. Overall, a review of the pertinent literature demonstrates that respiratory depression and hypotension occur more frequently when DZP is used in combination with other agents, such as barbiturates (94), lidocaine and epinephrine (95), methaqualone (96), chlordiazepoxide, and amobarbital (97). Additional risk factors include severe brain damage as a cause of status epilepticus (98), older age (99), and decompensated liver disease (100). Although the literature is reassuring about the risks, the rate of bolus injection is a critical factor. It has been claimed that the rate of bolus injection should not exceed 2 to 5 mg/min, to avoid serious respiratory depression (101). The propylene glycol solvent may contribute to the cardiorespiratory effects attributed to DZP (66).

Clonazepam. The acute side effect profile of i.v. CZP is similar to that of DZP. As with DZP, the risk of respiratory depression and hypotension is greatest after acute brain injury, in patients who have already received barbiturates, and in the elderly (98). CZP sedates and depresses levels of consciousness and is more potent than DZP in this regard (92).

Lorazepam. Like DZP and CZP, LZP has the potential for producing respiratory depression and hypotension, but prior medication with other antiepileptic drugs does not seem to increase the risk or severity of adverse reactions (102). Moreover, the risk of respiratory depression seems to be greater after the first injection of LZP than on subsequent injections (103). The incidence of respiratory depression with LZP therapy in status epilepticus ranges between 3% (93) and 10% (90), a rate substantially similar to that reported with DZP, although some studies suggested a lower risk with LZP (93). In the Veterans Administration comparative study of four treatments for generalized convulsive status epilepticus, LZP (0.1 mg/kg) was found to have the same incidence of adverse reactions as DZP (0.15 mg/kg) and phenytoin (18 mg/kg) (104).

Midazolam. In early studies of preoperative anesthetic practice, apnea was reported in 10% to 77% of patients who received i.v. MDL (0.2 to 0.36 mg/kg) (105). In status epilepticus, the i.v. dose used is lower than that previously used for anesthesia, and apnea has not been reported but is a potential risk. Toxicity is more likely to occur in elderly patients (88).

Local Tissue Irritation

Venous thrombosis, phlebitis, and pain may occur at the site of infusion of DZP or CZP. Thrombophlebitis occurred in 3.5% of >1,500 i.v. injections given during gastroscopy and may have been the result of drug precipitation caused by rapid injection (106,107). However, in a review provoked by a startling article about the loss of a limb after i.v. DZP administration, no significant local vascular complications were found among 15,813 injections (108). Overall, the dangers of local complications of i.v. BZDs appear to be negligible.

Paradoxical Effects

Paradoxical effects, such as the induction of tonic status epilepticus, have been described with the i.v. use of DZP, CZP, NTZ, and LZP, especially in children prone to this seizure type (109–111) (Figure 19.1). Tassinari et al. (109) gave the first account of this complication: in five children with Lennox-Gastaut syndrome, the i.v. injection of DZP (10 mg) triggered very frequent tonic seizures, amounting to tonic status, in 5 seconds to 11 minutes. The sleep-inducing properties of BZDs did not seem to be a critical factor in the appearance of tonic seizures in these patients.

Rectal Administration

Numerous studies have stressed the good safety profile of rectally administered BZDs, usually DZP (112–114).

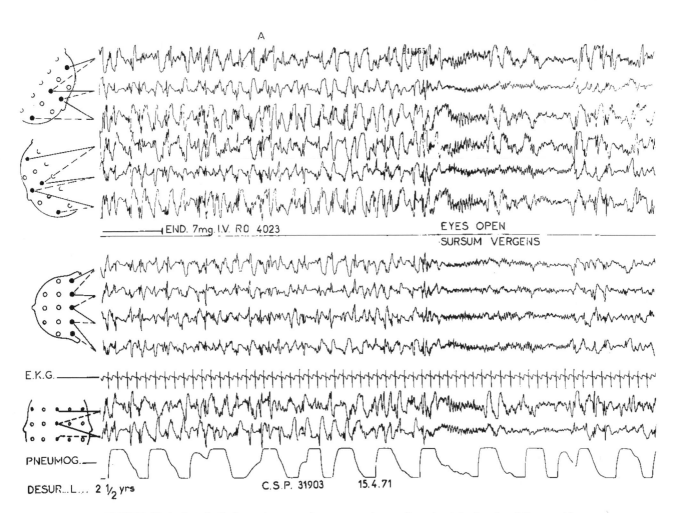

FIGURE. 19.1. Paradoxical reaction to an intravenous benzodiazepine injection in a 2.5-year-old child with Lennox-Gastaut syndrome. The patient has "atypical absence status" with diffuse slow spike-and-wave (SW) discharges. A few seconds after receiving a 7-mg injection of clonazepam (Ro-4023), the patient had a tonic seizure, characterized by initial flattening of the tracing and a progressively increasing-amplitude diffuse polyspike discharge. The child opened the eyes, and the eyeballs rose upward. Additional tonic seizures, with the same electroclinical manifestations, occurred over the next few minutes, with persistence of diffuse slow SW discharges between the seizures. (Courtesy of Drs. C.H. Dravet and J. Roger, Centre St. Paul, University of Marseille, France, *unpublished data*, 1971.)

Overall, these studies have shown that the rectal administration of DZP induces sedation in 17% to 33% of patients, with no respiratory depression. At variance with these favorable results, a 9% incidence of respiratory depression, after the use of rectal DZP as monotherapy, was observed in a prospective study including 97 children with 130 episodes of acute seizures (115). Moreover, Brodtkorb et al. (116) emphasized the risks of long-term or excessive administration of rectal DZP, which may cause a cyclic reappearance of seizures or the combination of toxic and withdrawal effects in some patients.

Intramuscular Administration

MDL is the only BZD used in acute epilepsy that can be given with benefit by i.m. injection. Reports of respiratory depression after i.m. MDL injection for status epilepticus have not been published. There is, however, one report of a patient who developed apnea 20 minutes after receiving 10 mg i.m. MDL (88). Ghilain et al. (117) reported one patient with bradycardia, and three patients with a slight decrease in blood pressure, among 14 patients treated with i.m. MDL.

MANIFESTATIONS AND MANAGEMENT OF OVERDOSE

An extensive survey of hospital admissions for drug overdose in the United States showed that 13% involved BZD ingestion, usually in combination with other drugs (e.g., barbiturates, sedative-hypnotics, ethanol, or miscellaneous drug combinations) (118).

Signs of BZD overdose vary with the particular drug, the doses taken, and the age of the patient. Generally, when BZDs are taken at relatively low doses, patients are somewhat somnolent and exhibit ataxia (119). At higher doses, patients are often comatose and areflexic; when awake, these patients exhibit nystagmus, ataxia, dysarthria, and occasionally hypotension (120). Both very young and very old patients may develop these manifestations at lower doses (21). Respiratory depression, which is an infrequent sign in patients with exclusive BZD overdosage, has been reported with higher frequency in cases of multiple drug ingestion, sometimes leading to death (21). By contrast, death after the ingestion of BZDs alone is exceedingly rare (121). Out of 102 patients with NZP overdoses, only six were deeply comatose, and these patients recovered uneventfully in 12 hours (122). Nonetheless, death has been reported after an overdose with an undetermined amount of NZP (123). After massive DZP overdoses, patients with plasma concentrations <20,000 ng/mL DZP and 5,000 ng/mL *N*-desmethyldiazepam have survived (66). Levels of *N*-desmethyldiazepam of 10,000 ng/mL have been observed in patients who ingested large amounts

of CLP but who remained conscious with ataxia (124). Rapid clinical recovery from BZD overdose does not result from rapid elimination of metabolites—which have a long half-life—but is more likely to be related to the development of tolerance to the depressant effects of the drug (66).

A few case studies provide suggestive evidence that the effects of high doses of LZP may differ from those of other BZDs. Overdose with LZP has resulted in hallucinations (125), delirium (126), and transient global amnesia (127). Bullous skin lesions have been reported in patients with coma induced by DZP (128) and NZP (129). Exocrine sweat gland necrosis may also occur after DZP overdose (128). Comatose patients with NZP (130) or LZP (131) intoxication may show the peculiar EEG pattern of *alpha coma*. A case of nonfatal cardiac arrest was reported after DZP overdose (70 mg) in a 2-year-old child (132).

Treatment of BZD overdose consists of general supportive care, close observation, and, in most serious cases, admission to intensive care units. Apart from standard intensive care treatment, the BZD receptor antagonist flumazenil is usually given by i.v. repeated single injections or continuous infusion (133) to reverse BZD-induced CNS depression. Activated charcoal (134), exchange transfusion (135), and physostigmine (136) have been also employed in DZP intoxication. In an early study (137), the sedative effects of LZP were reversed with an infusion of 1 mg/kg of aminophylline.

CONCLUSION

BZDs are widely used for the treatment of epileptic disorders. When administered orally as long-term therapy, BZDs produce dose-related CNS effects, particularly sedation, ataxia, and behavioral and cognitive changes. Many of these effects, which occur in 20% to 60% of patients, tend to decrease over a few weeks because of the development of tolerance. Less frequent, but clinically significant, side effects include fatigue, blurred vision, and memory disturbances. Drooling can be caused by impaired swallowing or hypersecretion in NZP-treated children; moreover, impaired swallowing has been claimed to be responsible for the increased risk of death among young children given NZP for intractable epilepsy. Abrupt BZD withdrawal has been associated with a risk of seizures, psychosis, and status epilepticus, both in epileptic and nonepileptic patients. When administered i.v. for the acute management of status epilepticus, BZDs may cause respiratory depression and hypotension. These events are more frequent when BZDs are used in combination with other sedative agents or in patients with severe brain damage, old age, and liver impairment. Additional effects include damage at the site of injection (which is negligible for LZP and MDL) and paradoxical induction of tonic status epilepticus in patients with Lennox-Gastaut syndrome. BZDs are relatively safe in overdose, and fatalities are exceedingly rare. Signs of acute intoxication range from somnolence and ataxia to areflexic coma. Hallucinations, delirium, and transient global amnesia have been reported with LZP. Apart from supportive treatment, the BZD receptor antagonist flumazenil can be given by i.v. injection to reverse BZD-induced CNS depression.

REFERENCES

1. Hillestad L, Hansen T, Melsom H, et al. Diazepam metabolism in normal man: serum concentrations and clinical effects after intravenous, intramuscular, and oral administration. *Clin Pharmacol Ther* 1974;16:479–484.

2. Korttila K, Linnoila M. Absorption and sedative effects of diazepam after oral administration and intramuscular administration into the vastus lateralis muscle and the deltoid muscle. *Br J Anaesth* 1975;47:857–862.

3. Korttila K, Linnoila M. Psychomotor skills related to driving after intramuscular administration of diazepam and meperidine. *Anesthesiology* 1975;42:685–691.

4. Morselli PL. Psychotropic drugs-benzodiazepines. In: Morselli PL, ed. *Drug disposition during development.* New York: Spectrum Publications, 1977:449–459.

5. Kanto J. Plasma concentrations of diazepam and its metabolites after peroral, intramuscular and rectal administration. *Int J Clin Pharmacol* 1975;12:427–432.

6. Bittencourt PRM, Wade P, Smith AT, et al. The relationship between peak velocity of saccadic eye movements and serum benzodiazepine concentration. *Br J Clin Pharmacol* 1981;12:523–533.

7. Baruzzi A, Bordo B, Bossi L, et al. Plasma levels of di-*n*-propylacetate and clonazepam in epilepsy patients. *Int J Clin Pharmacol Biopharm* 1977;15:403–408.

8. Sjo O, Hvidber EF, Naestoft J, et al. Pharmacokinetics and side effects of clonazepam and its 7-amino-metabolite in man. *Eur J Clin Pharmacol* 1975;8:249–254.

9. Dreifuss FE, Sato S. Clonazepam. In: Woodbury DM, Penry JK, Pippenger CE, eds. *Antiepileptic drugs,* 2 nd ed. New York: Raven Press, 1982:737–752.

10. Browne IR, Penry JK. Benzodiazepines in the treatment of epilepsy. *Epilepsia* 1973;14:277–310.

11. Koeppen D. Clinical experience with clobazam (1968–1981). In: Hindmarch I, Stonier PD, eds. *Clobazam.* London: Royal Society of Medicine, 1981:193–198.

12. Koeppen D. A review of clobazam studies in epilepsy. In: Hindmarch I, Stonier PD, Trimble MR,eds. *Clobazam: human psychopharmacology and clinical applications.* London: Royal Society of Medicine, 1985:207–215.

13. Saletu B, Grunberger J, Berner P, et al. On differences between 1,5 and 1,4 benzodiazepines: pharmaco-EEG and psychometric studies with clobazam and lorazepam. In: Hindmarch I, Stonier PD, Trimble MR, eds. *Clobazam:human psychopharmacology and clinical applications.* London: Royal Society of Medicine, 1985:23–46.

14. Wildin JD, Pleuvry BJ, Mawer GE, et al. Respiratory and sedative effects of clobazam and clonazepam in volunteers. *Br J Clin Pharmacol* 1990;29:169–177.

15. Girdwood RH. Nitrazepam nightmares. *BMJ* 1973;1:353.

16. Baruzzi A, Michelucci R, Tassinari CA. Nitrazepam. In: Levy RH, Mattson RH, Meldrum BS, eds. *Antiepileptic drugs,* 4th ed. New York: Raven Press,1995:735–749.

17. Feldman RG. Clorazepate in temporal lobe epilepsy. *JAMA* 1976;236:2603.

18. Shorvon SD. Clobazam. In: Levy RH, Mattson RH, Meldrum BS, eds. *Antiepileptic drugs,* 4th ed. New York: Raven Press, 1995:763–777.

19. Allen J, Oxley J, Robertson M, et al. Clobazam as adjunctive treatment in refractory epilepsy. *BMJ* 1983;286:1246–1247.

20. Sheth RD, Goulden KJ, Ronen GM. Aggression in children treated with clobazam for epilepsy. *Clin Neuropharmacol* 1994; 17:332–337.

21. Woods JH, Katz JC, Winger G. Abuse liability of benzodiazepines. *Pharmacol Rev* 1987;39:251–413.

22. McNair DM. Antianxiety drugs and human performance. *Arch Gen Psychiatry* 1973,29:611–617.

23. Wittenborn JR. Effects of benzodiazepines on psychomotor performance. *Br J Clin Pharmacol* 1979;7: 61S-76S.

24. Lahtinen U, Lahtinen A, Pekkola P. The effect of nitrazepam on manual skill, grip strength, and reaction time with special reference to subjective evaluation of effects on sleep. *Acta Pharmacol Toxicol* 1978;42:130–134.

25. Moodley P, Golombok S, Lader M. Effects of clorazepate dipotassium and placebo on psychomotor skills. *Percept Mot Skills* 1985;61:1121–1122.

26. Hindmarch I, Gudgeon AC. The effects of clobazam and lorazepam on aspects of psychomotor performance and car handling ability. *Br J Clin Pharmacol* 1980;10:145–150.

27. Cull CA, Trimble MR. Anticonvulsant benzodiazepines and performance. In: Hindmarch I, Stonier PD, Trimble MR, eds. *Clobazam: human psychopharmacology and clinical applications.* London: Royal Society of Medicine, 1985:23–46.

28. Scharf MB, Khosla N, Lysaght R, et al.. Anterograde amnesia with oral lorazepam. *J Clin Psychiatry* 1983;44:362–364.

29. Hanson RA, Menkes JH. A new anticonvulsant in the management of minor motor seizures. *Dev Med Child Neurol* 1972; 14:3–14.

30. Pinder RM, Brogden RN, Speight TM, et al. Clonazepam (Rivotril-Roche): an independent report. *Curr Ther Res* 1977;18: 25–32.

31. Millichap JG, Ortiz WR. Nitrazepam in myoclonic epilepsies. *Am J Dis Child* 1966;112:242–248.

32. Wyllie E, Wyllie R, Cruse RP, et al. The mechanism of nitrazepam-induced drooling and aspiration. *N Engl J Med* 1986;314: 35–38.

33. Murphy JV, Sawasky F, Marquardt KM, et al. Deaths in young children receiving nitrazepam. *J Pediatr* 1987;111:145–147.

34. Lim HCN, Nigro MA, Beirwaltes P, et al. Nitrazepam-induced cricopharyngeal dysphagia, abnormal esophageal peristalsis and associated bronchospasm:probable cause of nitrazepam related sudden death. *Brain Dev* 1992;14:309–314.

35. Rintahaka PJ, Nakagawa JA, Shewmon DA, et al. Incidence of death in patients with intractable epilepsy during nitrazepam treatment. *Epilepsia* 1999;40:492–496.

36. Griebel ML. Acute management of hypersensitivity reactions and seizures. *Epilepsia* 1998;39[Suppl 7]:S17–S21.

37. Markham CH. The treatment of myoclonic seizures of infancy and childhood with LA-1. *Pediatrics* 1964;34:511–518.

38. Greenblatt DJ, Allen MD. Toxicity of nitrazepam in the elderly: a report from the Boston Collaborative Drug Surveillance Program. *Br J Clin Pharmacol* 1978;5:407–413.

39. Arndt KA, Jick H. Rates of cutaneous reactions to drugs: a report from the Boston Collaborative Drug Surveillance Program. *Drug Intell Clin Pharmacol* 1976;9:648–654.

40. Haerten K, Pöttgen W. Leukopenie nach Banzodiazepin-Derivaten. *Med Welt* 1975;26:1712–1714.

41. Bittner-Manicka M, Wasilewski R. Preliminary clinical evaluation of Rivotril in epilepsy. *Neurol Neurochirur Pol* 1976;26:519–525.

42. Peterson WG. Clinical study of Mogadon, a new anticonvulsant. *Neurology* 1967;17:878–880.

43. Veall RM, Hogarth HC. Thrombocytopenia during treatment with clonazepam. *BMJ* 1975;4:462.

44. Caramaschi P, Biasi D, Carletto A, et al. Clobazam-induced systemic lupus erythematosus. *Clin Rheumatol* 1995;14:116.

45. Parker JL. Potassium clorazepate (Tranxene)–induced jaundice. *Postgrad Med J* 1979;55:908–910.

46. Cunningham ML. Acute hepatic necrosis following treatment with amitriptyline and diazepam. *Br J Psychiatry* 1965;111:1107–1109.

47. Maroy B, Moullot PH. Esophageal burn due to clorazepate dipotassium (Tranxene). *Gastrointest Endosc* 1986;32:240.

48. Sadjadi SA, McLaughlin K, Shah RM. Allergic interstitial nephritis due to diazepam. *Arch Intern Med* 1987;147:579.

49. Browne TR. Clonazepam. *N Engl J Med* 1978;299:812–816.

50. Gibbs FA, Anderson EM. Treatment of hypsarrhythmia and infantile spasms with a Librium analogue. *Neurology* 1965;1115:1173–1176.

51. Ohtahara S, Ohtsuka Y, Miyaka S, et al. Induced-microseizures: clinical and electroencephalographic study. *Tenkan* Kenkyu 1983;1:51–60.

52. Otani K, Tagawa T, Futagi Y, et al. Induced microseizures in West syndrome. *Brain Dev* 1991;13:196–199.

53. Alvarez N, Hartford E, Doubt C. Epileptic seizures induced by clonazepam. *Clin Electroencephalogr* 1981;12:57–65.

54. Elger CE, Bauer J, Schermann J, et al. Aggravation of focal epileptic seizures by antiepileptic drugs. *Epilepsia* 1998;39 [Suppl 3]:S15–S18.

55. Darcy L. Delirium tremens following withdrawal of nitrazepam. *Med J Aust* 1972;2:450.

56. Preskorn SH, Denner LJ. Benzodiazepines and withdrawal psychosis. *JAMA* 1977;237:36–38.

57. Martinez-Cano H, Vela-Bueno A, de Iuta M, et al. Benzodiazepine withdrawal syndrome seizures. *Pharmacopsychiatry* 1995;28:257–262.

58. Thomas P, Lebrun C, Chatel M. *De novo* absence status epilepticus as a benzodiazepine withdrawal syndrome. *Epilepsia* 1993;34:355–358.

59. Primavera A, Cocito L. Acute confusion in a chronic benzodiazepine patient. *Gen Hosp Psychiatry* 1995;17:456–462.

60. Kanemoto K, Miyamoto T, Abe R. Ictal catatonia as a manifestation of *de novo* absence status epilepticus following benzodiazepine withdrawal. *Seizure* 1999;8:364–366.

61. Gatzonis SD, Angelopoulos EK, Daskalopoulou EG, et al. Convulsive status epilepticus following abrupt high-dose benzodiazepine discontinuation. *Drug Alcohol Depend* 2000;59:95–97.

62. Gambardella A, Aguglia U, Oliveri RL, et al. Negative myoclonic status due to antiepileptic drug tapering: report of three cases. *Epilepsia* 1997;38:819–823.

63. Sugai K. Seizures with clonazepam: discontinuation and suggestions for safe discontinuation rates in children. *Epilepsia* 1993;34:1089–1097.

64. Chataway J, Fowler A, Thompson PJ, et al. Discontinuation of clonazepam in patients with active epilepsy. *Seizure* 1993;2:295–300.

65. Borusiak P, Bettendorf U, Karenfort M, et al. Seizure-inducing paradoxical reaction to antiepileptic drugs. *Brain Dev* 2000;22:243–245.

66. Schmidt D. Diazepam. In: Levy RH, Mattson RH, Meldrum BS, eds. *Antiepileptic drugs,* 4th ed. New York: Raven Press, 1995:705–724.

67. Huang CY, Mc Lead JG, Sampson D, et al. Clonazepam in the treatment of epilepsy. *Med J Aust* 1974;2:5–8.

68. Zifkin B, Sherwin A, Andermann F. Phenytoin toxicity due to interaction with clobazam. *Neurology* 1991;41: 313–314.

69. Wolf P. Clobazam in drug-resistant patients with complex focal seizures-report of an open study. In: Hindmarch I, Stonier PD, Trimble MR, eds. *Clobazam: human psychopharmacology and clinical applications.* London: Royal Society of Medicine, 1985:167–171.

70. Munoz JJ, De-Salamanca RE, Diaz-Obregon C, et al. The effect of clobazam on steady state plasma concentrations of carbamazepine and its metabolites. *Br J Clin Pharmacol* 1990;29:763–765.

71. Genton P, Nguyen VH, Mesdjian E. Carbamazepine intoxication with negative myoclonus after the addition of clobazam. *Epilepsia* 1998;39:1115–1118.

72. Cocks A, Critchley EMR, Hayward HW, et al. The effect of clobazam on the blood levels of sodium valproate. In: Hindmarch I, Stonier PD, Trimble MR, eds. *Clobazam: human psychopharmacology and applications.* London: Royal Society of Medicine, 1985:155–157.

73. Jeavons PM. Choice of drug therapy in epilepsy. *Practitioner* 1977;219:542–556.

74. Anderson GD, Gidal BE, Kantor ED, et al. Lorazepam-valproate interaction: studies in normal subjects and isolated perfused rat liver. *Epilepsia* 1994;35:221–225.

75. Dhillon S, Richens A. Valproic acid and diazepam interaction *in vivo. Br J Clin Pharmacol* 1982;13:553–560.

76. Aarskog D. Association between maternal intake of diazepam and oral clefts. *Lancet* 1975;2:921.

77. Saxen I, Saxen L. Association between maternal intake of diazepam and oral clefts. *Lancet* 1975;2:498.

78. Czeizel A. Diazepam, phenytoin, and aetiology of cleft lip and or cleft palate. *Lancet* 1976;1:810.

79. McElhatton PR. The effects of benzodiazepine use during pregnancy and lactation. *Reprod Toxicol* 1994;8:461–475.

80. Safra MJ, Oakley GP Jr. Valium: an oral cleft teratogen? Cleft Palate J 1976;13:198–200.

81. Patel DA, Patel AR. Clorazepate and congenital malformations. *JAMA* 1980;224:135–136.

82. Milkovich L, Van den Berg BJ. Effects of prenatal meprobamate and chlordiazepoxide hydrochloride in human embryonic and foetal development. *N Engl J Med* 1974;291:1268–1271.

83. Laegreid L, Olegard R, Conradi N, et al. Congenital malformations and maternal consumption of benzodiazepines: a case-control study. *Dev Med Child Neurol* 1990;132:432–441.

84. Laegreid L, Kyllerman M, Hedner T, et al. Benzodiazepine amplification of valproate teratogenic effects in children of mothers with absence epilepsy. *Neuropediatrics* 1993;24:88–92.

85. Gillberg C. "Floppy infant syndrome" and maternal diazepam. *Lancet* 1977;2:244.

86. Weber LWD. Benzodiazepines in pregnancy: academical debate or teratogenic risk? *Biol Res Preg* 1985;6:151–167.

87. Tassinari CA, Michelucci R. The use of diazepam and clonazepam in epilepsy. *Epilepsia* 1998;39[Suppl 1]:S7–S14.

88. Shorvon SD. The use of clobazam, midazolam, and nitrazepam in epilepsy. *Epilepsia* 1998;39[Suppl 1]:S15–S23.

89. Jeanuet PY, Roulet E, Maeder IM, et al. Home and hospital treatment of acute seizures in children with nasal midazolam. *Eur J Paediatr Neurol* 1999;3:73–77.

90. Leppik IE, Derivan AT, Homan RW, et al. Double-blind study of lorazepam and diazepam in status epilepticus. *JAMA* 1983;249:1452–1454.

91. Aminoff MJ, Simon RP. Status epilepticus: causes, clinical features and consequences in 98 patients. *Am J Med* 1980;69:657–666.

92. Schmidt D. How to use benzodiazepines. In: Morselli PL, Pippenger CR, Penry JK, eds. *Antiepileptic drug therapy in pediatry.* New York: Raven Press, 1983:269–278.

93. Appleton R, Sweeney A, Choonara I, et al. Lorazepam versus diazepam in the acute treatment of epileptic seizures and status epilepticus. *Dev Med Child Neurol* 1995;37:682–688.

94. Schwab RS. Intravenous diazepam in the treatment of prolonged seizure activity. *N Engl J Med* 1967;276:779–784.

95. Sherman PM. Cardiac arrest with diazepam. *J Oral Surg* 1974; 32:567.

96. Doughty A. Unexpected danger of diazepam. *BMJ* 1970;2:239.

97. Greenblatt DJ, Koch-Weser J. Adverse reactions to intravenous diazepam: a report from the Boston Collaborative Drug Surveillance Program. *Am J Med Sci* 1973;266:261–266.

98. Tassinari CA, Daniele O, Michelucci R, et al. Benzodiazepines: efficacy in status epilepticus. In: Delgado-Escueta AV, Wasterlain CG, Treiman DM, Porter RJ, eds. *Status epilepticus.* New York: Raven Press, 1983:465–475.

99. Reidenberg MM, Levy M, Warner H, et al. Relationship between diazepam dose, plasma level, age, and central nervous system depression. *Clin Pharmacol Ther* 1978;23:371–374.

100. Greenblatt DJ, Koch-Weser J. Clinical toxicity of chlordiazepoxide and diazepam in relation to serum albumin concentration: a report from the Boston Collaborative Drug Surveillance Program. *Eur J Clin Pharmacol* 1974;7:259–262.

101. Shorvon S. *Status epilepticus: its clinical features and treatment in children and adults.* Cambridge: Cambridge University Press, 1994:209.

102. Mitchell WG, Crawford TO. Lorazepam is the treatment of choice for status epilepticus. *J Epilepsy* 1990;3:7–10.

103. Crawford TO, Mitchell WG, Snodgrass SR. Lorazepam in childhood status epilepticus and serial seizures: effectiveness and tachyphylaxis. *Neurology* 1987;37:190–195.

104. Treiman DM, Meyers PD, Walton NY, et al. A comparison of four treatments for generalized convulsive status epilepticus. *N Engl J Med* 1998;339:792–798.

105. Dundee JW, Halliday NJ, Harper KW, et al. Midazolam: a review of its pharmacological properties and therapeutic use. *Drugs* 1984;28:519–543.

106. Langdon DE, Harlan JR, Bailey RL. Thrombophlebitis with diazepam used intravenously. *JAMA* 1973;223:184–185.

107. Jusko WJ, Gretsch M, Gassett R. Precipitation of diazepam from intravenous preparations. *JAMA* 1973;225:176.

108. Tassinari CA, Roger J, Dravet C, et al. Comments on a startling article: loss of a limb following intravenous diazepam. *Pediatrics* 1975;6:898–899.

109. Tassinari CA, Dravet C, Roger J, et al. Tonic status epilepticus precipitated by intravenous benzodiazepines in five patients with Lennox-Gastaut syndrome. *Epilepsia* 1972;13:421–435.

110. Bittencourt PR, Richens A. Anticonvulsant-induced status epilepticus in Lennox-Gastaut syndrome. *Epilepsia* 1981;22: 129–134.

111. Martin D. Intravenous nitrazepam in the treatment of epilepsy. *Neuropaediatrie* 1970;2:27–37.

112. Cereghino JJ, Mitchell WG, Murphy J, et al. Treating repetitive seizures with a rectal diazepam formulation: a randomized study. *Neurology* 1998;51:1274–1282.

113. Dreifuss FE, Rosman NP, Cloyd JC, et al. A comparison of rectal diazepam gel and placebo for acute repetitive seizures. *N Engl J Med* 1998;338:1869–1875.

114. Mitchell WG, Conry JA, Crumrine PK, et al. An open-label study of repeated use of diazepam rectal gel (Diastat) for episodes of acute breakthrough seizures and clusters: safety, efficacy and tolerance. *Epilepsia* 1999;40:1610–1617.

115. Norris E, Marzouk O, Nunn A, et al. Respiratory depression in children receiving diazepam for acute seizures: a prospective study. *Dev Med Child Neurol* 1999;41:340–343.

116. Brodtkorb E, Aamo T, Henriksen O, et al. Rectal diazepam: pitfalls of excessive use in refractory epilepsy. *Epilepsy Res* 1999;35: 123–133.

117. Ghilain S, Van Rijkevorsel-Harmant K, Harmant J, et al. Midazolam in the treatment of epileptic seizures. *J Neurol Neurosurg Psychiatry* 1988;51:732.

118. Greenblatt DJ, Allen MD, Noel BJ, et al. Acute overdosage with benzodiazepine derivatives. *Clin Pharmacol Ther* 1977;21: 497–514.

119. Bardhan KD. Cerebellar syndrome after nitrazepam overdosage. *Lancet* 1969;1:1319–1320.

120. Greenblatt DJ, Woo E, Allen MD, et al. Rapid recovery from massive diazepam overdose. *JAMA* 1978;240:1872–1874.

121. Davis JM, Bartlett E, Termini BA. Overdosage of psychotropic drugs: a review. I. Major and minor tranquilizers. *Dis Nerv Syst* 1968;29:157–164.

122. Matthew H, Roscoe P, Wright N. Acute poisoning: a comparison of hypnotic drugs. *Practitioner* 1972;208:254–258.

123. Giusti GV, Chiarotti M. Lethal nitrazepam intoxications: report of two cases. *Z Rechtsmed* 1979;84:75–78.

124. Wilensky AJ. Clorazepate. In: Levy RH, Mattson RH, Meldrum BS, eds. *Antiepileptic drugs,* 4th ed. New York: Raven Press, 1995:751–762.

125. Vand den Beerg AA. Hallucinations after oral lorazepam in children. *Anaesthesia* 1986;41:330–331.

126. Blitt CD, Petty WC. Reversal of lorazepam delirium by physostigmine. *Anesth Analg* 1975;54:607–608.

127. Sandy KR. Transient global amnesia induced by lorazepam. *Clin Neuropharmacol* 1985;8:297–298.

128. Varma A-J, Fisher BK, Sarin MK. Diazepam-induced coma with bullae and eccrine sweat gland necrosis. *Arch Intern Med* 1977;137:1207–1210.

129. Ridley CM. Bullous lesions in nitrazepam overdosage. *BMJ* 1971;3:28.

130. Carrol WM, Mastaglia FL. Alpha and beta coma in drug intoxication uncomplicated by cerebral hypoxia. *Electroencephalogr Clin Neurophysiol* 1979;46:95–105.

131. Guterman B, Sebastian P, Sodha N. Recovery from alpha coma after lorazepam overdose. *Clin Electroencephalogr* 1981;12: 205–208.

132. Berger R, Green G, Melnick A. Cardiac arrest caused by oral diazepam intoxication. *Clin Pediatr* 1975;14:842–844.

133. Löscher W, Schmidt D. New drugs for the treatment of epilepsy. *Curr Opin Invest Drugs* 1993;2:1067–1095.

134. Traeger S-M, Haug MT. Reduction of diazepam serum half life and reversal of coma by activated charcoal in a patient with severe liver disease. *J Toxicol Clin Toxicol* 1986;4:329–337.

135. Thearle MJ, Dunn PM, Hailey DM. Exchange transfusion for diazepam intoxication at birth followed by jejunal stenosis. *Proc R Soc Med* 1973;66:349–350.

136. Larson GF, Hurlbert BJ, Wingard DW. Physostigmine reversal of diazepam-induced depression. *Anesth Analg* 1977;56: 348–351.

137. Wangler MA, Kilpatrick DS. Aminophylline is an antagonist of lorazepam. *Anesth Analg* 1985;64:834–836.

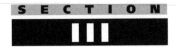

CARBAMAZEPINE

CARBAMAZEPINE

MECHANISMS OF ACTION

ROBERT L. MACDONALD

Carbamazepine (CBZ) is an iminostilbene and a structural congener of the tricyclic antidepressant drug imipramine (Figure 20.1). CBZ has been shown to be effective in the treatment of simple partial, complex partial, and generalized tonic-clonic seizures, but it is ineffective against generalized absence seizures (10,85,89,101). CBZ and the anticonvulsant drug phenytoin (Figure 20.1) have been shown to be effective in treatment of partial seizures and tonic-clonic seizures when they are used alone or as initial therapy (42,83), and both CBZ and phenytoin are drugs of first choice in the treatment of these seizure disorders (60). However, CBZ may be more effective in the treatment of complex partial seizures when complete seizure control is used as an end point (94). CBZ is an effective anticonvulsant drug in experimental animals (30,100), and it has an anticonvulsant profile that is similar to that of phenytoin (39,43). It is effective against maximal electroshock seizures at nontoxic doses but is not active against subcutaneous metrazol-induced seizures. CBZ may also be effective in the short-term and long-term treatment of manic-depressive illness (77), and it is the drug of choice for treatment of trigeminal neuralgia (6). CBZ is administered to adults in doses of 10 to 20 mg/kg/day to achieve total plasma concentrations of 4 to 12 μg/mL (16 to 48 μmol/L) (9, 46). The lower range of plasma concentrations are adequate to control seizures in patients with primary or secondarily generalized tonic-clonic seizures alone, but the higher plasma concentrations are required to treat seizures in patients with partial seizures with or without tonic-clonic seizures (87). CBZ is a lipid-soluble drug that is 65% to 80% bound to plasma proteins (38), and cerebrospinal fluid concentrations vary from 19% to 33% of total plasma concentrations (23). Assuming that 25% of total plasma CBZ is unbound, free plasma and cerebrospinal fluid concentrations are likely to be 1 to 3 μg/mL (4.2 to 12.6 μmol/L) (38).

ACTIONS ON EPILEPTIFORM DISCHARGES

The effect of CBZ has been studied in organized neuronal preparations such as the hippocampal slice. In this preparation, CBZ has been demonstrated to reduce spontaneous bursts recorded from the CA1 region of the rat hippocampal slice that were induced by low-calcium, high-magnesium solutions (29,36,72), low-calcium, low-magnesium solutions (20), and veratridine application (74). These effects were produced in the absence of synaptic transmission because the slices were bathed in a low-calcium solution or veratridine. These results were produced at CBZ concentrations that did not block single antidromically evoked action potentials. Because the effect on paroxysmal bursting in hippocampal pyramidal neurons was produced

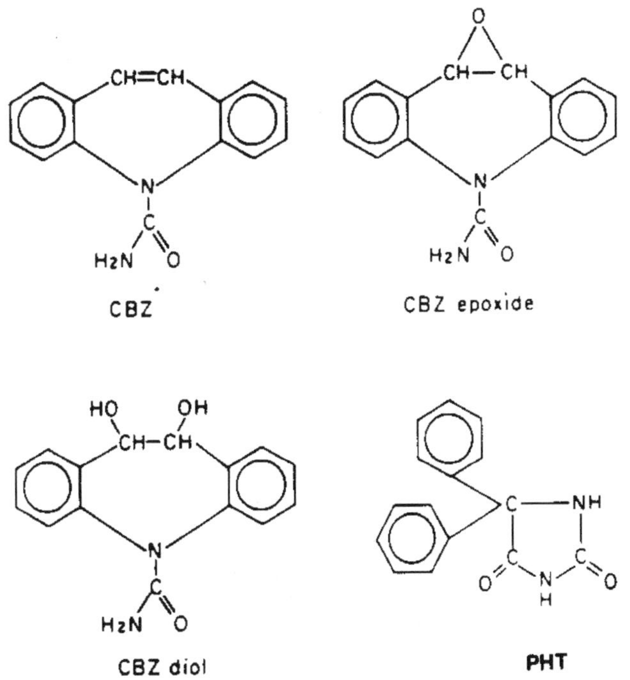

FIGURE 20.1. The structure of carbamazepine (CBZ), the CBZ metabolites, CBZ epoxide and CBZ diol, and phenytoin are presented.

Robert L. Macdonald, MD, PhD: Professor and Chair, Department of Neurology, Vanderbilt University, Nashville, Tennessee

when chemical synaptic transmission was blocked, the antiepileptic effect of CBZ was likely to reduce membrane excitability of pyramidal neurons directly.

The effects of CBZ on hippocampal epileptiform discharges have been shown to be age dependent. CBZ eliminated repetitive afterdischarges in immature rat CA3 hippocampal pyramidal neurons produced by penicillin without altering epileptiform bursts, a finding also suggesting an effect on neuronal excitability (96). Hippocampal slices exposed to the convulsant 4-aminopyridine generate several types of spontaneous discharges, two short-duration bursts and long polyspike bursts (7, 103). In hippocampal slices from adult rats, CBZ abolished long bursts without altering the short "interictal-like" bursts (7,106). Addition of 4-aminopyridine to hippocampal slices from immature animals produced ictal-like and interictal-like discharges, whereas in slices from mature animals, 4-aminopyridine produced only ictal-like activity (26). In immature slices, CBZ blocked ictal-like discharges at relatively low concentrations (50 µmol/L) and blocked interictal-like discharges only at higher concentrations (100 µmol/L). In contrast, CBZ did not block the interictal-like discharges in the adult slices even at the higher concentration. Thus, CBZ appears to have selective actions on convulsant-induced bursting, and the effect is different in developing and mature hippocampus.

MECHANISMS OF ACTION

Multiple mechanisms of action for CBZ have been proposed. However, these can be divided into two basic mechanisms of drug action: (a) an action of CBZ on neuronal sodium channels to reduce sustained, high-frequency repetitive firing of action potentials; and (b) actions of CBZ on synaptic transmission and neurotransmitter receptors including purine, monoamine, acetylcholine, and *N*-methyl-D-aspartate (NMDA) receptors. Although evidence has been reported supporting both these mechanisms, current experimental evidence suggests that the major mechanism of action of CBZ is to reduce the ability of neurons to fire at high frequency by enhancing sodium channel inactivation. This mechanism and the others are discussed later.

REDUCTION OF SUSTAINED HIGH-FREQUENCY REPETITIVE FIRING

In early studies, CBZ was shown to reduce the excitability of peripheral nerves (35,44). These original observations suggested that CBZ directly reduced the sodium conductance underlying the action potential because increased threshold, decreased conduction velocity, and decreased action potential height occurred. However, it is likely that the CBZ concentrations used in these experiments were

supratherapeutic. Schauf et al. (86) demonstrated directly that CBZ reduced sodium current in *Myxicola* giant axons. This effect was not specific for sodium currents because potassium currents were also reduced. The CBZ effect occurred only at very high CBZ concentrations (0.25 to 1.0 µm). Thus, early studies demonstrated that CBZ directly affected sodium channels, but only at supratherapeutic concentrations.

Early studies also suggested that CBZ may have some effect on spontaneous or evoked repetitive firing recorded from peripheral nerves. Honda and Allen (35) demonstrated that CBZ reduced spontaneous firing of action potentials recorded from peripheral nerves immersed in isotonic sodium oxalate or phosphate solutions. Hershkowitz and Raines (32) studied the effect of CBZ on muscle spindle discharges. These investigators correlated effects on spindle discharges with blood levels and demonstrated that CBZ depressed several aspects of muscle spindle discharges at concentrations that had little or no effect on nerve conduction velocity. These researchers demonstrated that CBZ depressed muscle spindle activity in a manner similar to that produced by local anesthetics. The sustained and prolonged repetitive firing of spontaneous activity and the static stretch response were sensitive to CBZ block, but the brief response to muscle stretch was spared. In addition, CBZ was demonstrated to reduce repetitive afterdischarges originating from small unmyelinated nerves in production of neuromuscular posttetanic potentiation in cat soleus neuromuscular preparations at CBZ concentrations similar to those suppressing spontaneous activity in static stretch responses of muscle spindles (33). This effect on posttetanic repetitive afterdischarges recorded from isolated ventral root filaments occurred at concentrations that did not affect conduction velocity of the motor nerves (33).

The effect of CBZ on repetitive firing was not limited to neuromuscular preparations. CBZ reduced high-frequency repetitive firing of action potentials recorded from mouse spinal cord (Figure 20.2), from neocortical and hippocampal pyramidal neurons grown in primary dissociated cell culture (52,61,64,65), and from hippocampal pyramidal neurons in the slice (36). When depolarized, spinal cord and cortical neurons sustain high-frequency repetitive discharges. In the presence of CBZ at therapeutic free serum concentrations (>1 µmol/L or 4.2 µg/mL), there was a concentration-dependent reduction in the number of action potentials evoked with 500-millisecond depolarizing pulses and in the percentage of neurons manifesting sustained repetitive firing. No effect was produced on single action potentials at concentrations of CBZ <10.6 µmol/L (2.5 µg/mL). In addition to CBZ, its active metabolite, CBZ epoxide (Figure 20.1), was also effective in producing limitation of high-frequency repetitive firing at concentrations comparable to those of CBZ (Figure 20.2). However, an inactive metabolite of CBZ, CBZ diol (Figure 20.1), did not affect high-frequency repetitive firing until concentra-

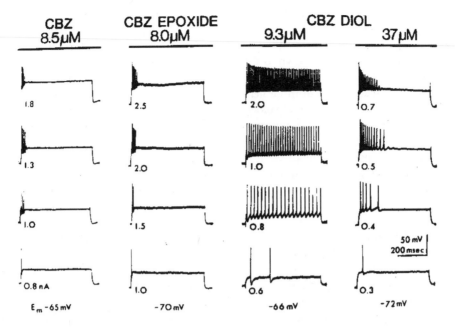

FIGURE 20.2. Carbamazepine (CBZ), CBZ epoxide, and CBZ diol reduced sustained high-frequency repetitive firing in spinal cord neurons. Each column shows recordings from a single spinal cord neuron bathed in a solution high in magnesium salt. Sustained high-frequency repetitive firing was limited by CBZ and CBZ epoxide at low, clinically relevant concentrations. CBZ diol had no effect at a clinically relevant concentration but did limit sustained repetitive firing at a high nontherapeutic concentration. (From McLean MJ, Macdonald RL. Carbamazepine and 10,11-epoxycarbamazepine produce use- and voltage-dependent limitation of rapidly firing action potentials of mouse central neurons in cell culture. *J Pharmacol Exp Ther* 1986;238:727–738, with permission.)

tions were an order of magnitude higher than those effective for CBZ (Figure 20.2). Thus, CBZ and its active metabolite limited sustained high-frequency repetitive firing of action potentials at therapeutic free serum concentrations that did not modify single action potentials.

The effect of CBZ on repetitive firing had three major properties. First, the effect was *voltage dependent*. The reduction of sustained repetitive firing by CBZ could be enhanced by evoking the action potentials from a reduced membrane potential and could be reversed by evoking the repetitive train after membrane hyperpolarization. Second, the effect was *use dependent* (14). When limitation of repetitive firing was produced, the first action potential in the action potential train was unaffected. However, with successive action potentials in the train there was a reduction in the maximal rate of rise of the action potentials and in the action potential heights until failure of firing occurred. Third, the effect was *time dependent*. After a train of action potentials was evoked to produce a reduction of firing in the presence of CBZ, subsequent action potentials evoked after the train were also reduced in amplitude and maximum rate of rise. This reduction in action potential properties lasted several hundred milliseconds after the initial conditioning train.

These results suggest that CBZ affects sodium channels. However, the effect is likely to be on the inactivation process of sodium channels. It has been proposed that CBZ binds to sodium channels only in the inactive state, and therefore it limits repetitive firing only when the membrane is depolarized, so a few of the channels are in the inactive state (64). Blockade of repetitive firing can be reversed by hyperpolarizing the membrane to remove all sodium channel inactivation. Furthermore, because inactivation is enhanced by CBZ, initial action potentials in the train are unaffected, but subsequent action potentials in the train are more strongly affected because of the prolonged inactivation of sodium channels opened during early action potentials in the train. Finally, recovery of sodium channels from inactivation is thought to be prolonged, and therefore the reduction in action potentials produced in a train persists for several hundred milliseconds. Thus, it has been proposed that CBZ limits high-frequency repetitive firing by binding to sodium channels in the inactive state and by slowing the rate of recovery of these channels from inactivation. In addition to CBZ, several other antiepileptic drugs that are effective against generalized tonic-clonic and partial seizures, including phenytoin (62) and valproic acid (63), block high-frequency repetitive firing (52,54,55), possibly by a similar mechanism.

The action of CBZ on inactivated sodium channels has been confirmed using voltage-clamp techniques. In studies of peripheral nerve and muscle (15,88), neuroblastoma cells in culture (49,115), human NT2-N cells in culture (98), acutely dissociated hippocampal neurons (45,98,104), and rat brain type IIA sodium channels stably expressed in Chinese hamster ovary cells (82), CBZ has been shown to slow the rate of recovery from inactivation and to shift the voltage dependency of steady-state inactivation to more negative voltages and thus to produce a frequency- and voltage-dependent block of sodium channels. The block appears to be selective for the inactive form of the closed channel. Thus, it is likely that CBZ binds preferentially to the inactive form of the sodium channel, an action consistent with the modulated receptor hypothesis of local anesthetic drug action proposed by Hille (34).

In addition to its effect on sodium action potentials and currents, CBZ has been demonstrated to reduce veratridine-stimulated calcium flux (17,24), as well as batrachotoxin-activated sodium influx in N18 neuroblastoma cells and rat brain synaptosomes (116). Veratridine and batrachotoxin both bind to voltage-dependent sodium channels. Therefore, the block of calcium or sodium transport activated by either veratridine or batrachotoxin suggests an action of CBZ on voltage-dependent sodium channels. Furthermore, CBZ inhibited binding of [³H]batrachotoxinin A 20-α-benzoate to sodium channels of rat brain synaptosomes (114). Batrachotoxin causes persistent activation, not block, of sodium channels by binding to high-affinity states of the channel. Thus, it appears that CBZ blocks high-frequency sustained repetitive firing of action potentials and spontaneous burst discharges, veratridine- and batrachotoxin-induced sodium flux, and [³H]batrachotoxinin binding by binding to sodium channels and enhancing voltage-dependent sodium channel inactivation.

SYNAPTIC ACTIONS

In spinal cord, CBZ did not alter monosynaptic reflex discharges at systemic doses that depressed polysynaptic discharges and posttetanic potentiation (39,44,99,100). However, the blood levels required to reduce posttetanic potentiation were supratherapeutic (39), and CBZ failed to alter posttetanic potentiation in the rat hippocampal slice (36). CBZ also reduced synaptic transmission in the spinal trigeminal nucleus of cats (6,25,31,84) and in the nucleus centrum medianum of the thalamus (31). Similarly, the extracellular excitatory postsynaptic potential field potential recorded in hippocampal CA1 apical dendrites and evoked by stratum radiatum stimulation was reduced by CBZ at moderate concentrations (10 to 100 μmol/L) (36). These studies suggest that CBZ may decrease excitatory synaptic transmission. However, these studies do not clarify whether the effect of CBZ is presynaptic or postsynaptic.

In addition to the effects on the process on synaptic transmission, CBZ has been reported to alter neurotransmitter levels, metabolism, and receptors. The primary neurotransmitter receptors studied have included adenosine, monoamine, acetylcholine, γ-aminobutyric acid (GABA), and glutamate receptors.

CBZ may modify excitatory amino acid receptor responses. CBZ did not modify postsynaptic responses to glutamate in a normal magnesium solution (64), and CBZ (400 μmol/L) failed to affect sodium-dependent or [³H]L-glutamate binding to hippocampal synaptic membranes (36). CBZ did not inhibit activation of non-NMDA receptors in cultured rat hippocampal neurons (3), and it attenuated α-amino-3-hydroxy-5-methyl-4-isoxazole propionate (AMPA) receptor-mediated depolarizations in the rat cortical wedge only at high, supratherapeutic concentrations (76). These data suggest that AMPA-like and kainatelike excitatory amino acid responses are not affected by CBZ.

In contrast, CBZ may alter NMDA receptor responses. CBZ reduced NMDA-activated currents in cultured spinal cord neurons in a concentration-dependent fashion, and it had minimal effects on NMDA-activated currents at relatively low concentrations (>10 μmol/L) (47). Consistent with an effect on NMDA receptors, CBZ reduced NMDA-induced elevation of intracellular calcium concentration in primary cultures of cerebellar granule neurons at a relatively low concentration (50 μmol/L) (8,37), and it reduced NMDA-induced depolarizations in cortical wedges prepared from genetically epilepsy-prone DBA/2 mice at therapeutic CBZ concentrations (1 to 10 μmol/L) (48). Maximal reduction of NMDA-induced depolarizations were produced at CBZ concentrations of 10 to 80 μmol/L, and at higher concentrations (100 to 200 μmol/L), CBZ paradoxically increased the depolarizations. The reduction of NMDA-induced depolarizations by CBZ was noncompetitive, with a reduction in the maximal depolarization but little effect on the half-maximal NMDA concentration. In contrast, the enhancement of the NMDA-induced depolarization at higher NMDA concentrations was "competitive," with a left shift in the concentration response curve and no alteration in the magnitude of the maximum depolarization. However, in the rat hippocampus, responses to NMDA (97) and NMDA-induced increases in the discharge rate of low-magnesium–induced field potentials (105) were not affected by CBZ, and CBZ did not displace [³H]MK801 to mouse cortical membranes at therapeutic concentrations (28). These data suggest that although CBZ may have anticonvulsant action, at least in part, by reduction of the NMDA receptor current, this mechanism of action remains unproven.

A role of CBZ in modifying adenosine receptor responses was suggested by the finding that CBZ inhibited adenosine-stimulated cyclic adenosine monophosphate accumulation in rat cortical slices (50), and CBZ modified the specific binding of adenosine agonists to rat brain membranes (58,90–92,108). CBZ specifically displaced the adenosine A1 agonist [³H]cyclohexyl adenosine (CHA) and antagonist [³H]diethylphenylxanthine binding (57,58,107, 108), and the inhibition of adenosine receptor binding by CBZ was competitive (58). CBZ was less potent in inhibiting the binding of the adenosine A2 agonist [³H]5′-*N*-ethylcarboxamidoadenosine (27,91), a finding suggesting that CBZ binds preferentially to A1 receptors. Consistent with these results, CBZ was shown to displace an A1 adenosine receptor ligand from human hippocampus (19). To determine whether CBZ is an agonist or antagonist at A1 adenosine receptors, the effects of the nucleotide guanosine triphosphate and temperature on CBZ binding have been studied. Guanosine triphosphate has been shown to reduce the affinity of agonists for receptors without altering the affinity of antagonists (16,75,102), and antagonist binding potency has been shown to increase at lower temperatures, whereas agonist binding potency increases at higher temperatures (51). Because the potency of CBZ to displace [³H]CHA is unaffected by guanosine triphosphate (91) and is increased at lower temperatures (57), it is likely that CBZ is an A1 adenosine receptor antagonist. The functional significance of CBZ antagonist action at A1 adenosine receptors, however, is unclear. In studies in hippocampal slice, CBZ did not appear to have an action mediated by adenosine receptors (72). The depressant effect of adenosine on the population spike recorded in CA1 was completely blocked by caffeine, but the depressant effect of CBZ was not modified by caffeine. Furthermore, a role for adenosine receptors in CBZ action could not be supported in the immature rat hippocampus *in vitro* (95). Despite a clear demonstration that CBZ is an antagonist at A1 adenosine receptors, it is unlikely that this interaction is responsible for the anticonvulsant properties of CBZ. No correlation has been found between the potency of a series of CBZ analogs as inhibitors of either agonist or antagonist binding and their ability to inhibit maximal electroshock seizures (58). Adenosine receptor agonists, not adenosine receptor antagonists, have anticonvulsant effects (1,2,21,22,56,119). Furthermore, in amygdala-kindled seizures in the rat, CBZ, but not CHA, was an anticonvulsant (111), and adenosine receptor antagonists did not block the anticonvulsant effect of CBZ (110). In the striatum, CBZ has been shown to modify extracellular dopamine levels (71). The effect of CBZ is consistent with A1 antagonist and A2 agonist activity. Thus, although it appears established that CBZ is an A1 adenosine receptor antagonist, it is unlikely that the anticonvulsant properties of CBZ are derived from actions at adenosine receptors.

Investigators have suggested that monoamines may be involved in the actions of CBZ. The threshold for inducing electroshock seizures was reduced after administration of drugs that deplete brain monoamines (4,11,40,41,81). In contrast, the threshold for inducing electroshock seizures was elevated by administration of monoamine precursors or inhibitors of monoamine catabolism (12,40,78). After an intraventricular injection of 6-hydroxydopamine (6-OHD),

which reduced forebrain catecholamines, CBZ was less effective in raising the electroconvulsive threshold current (80,81). Pretreatment with desipramine, which protected noradrenergic neurons from 6-OHD toxicity, blocked the 6-OHD effect on the CBZ anticonvulsant effect. CBZ, however, was shown to increase dopamine, its metabolites, and its precursors in the striatum and hippocampus at therapeutic plasma concentrations (69). Reduction of brain serotonin levels by destruction of raphe neurons did not alter the CBZ anticonvulsant effect (80). However, CBZ has been shown to increase extracellular serotinin levels (18,70). Both the uptake and release of [³H]norepinephrine from brain synaptosomes was inhibited by 100 μmol/L CBZ (79). These results suggest that norepinephrine may be involved in the action of CBZ. However, Westerink et al. (113) found no change in 3,4-dihydroxyphenyl acidic acid and homovanillic acid, the metabolites of dopamine, in corpus striatum, nucleus accumbens, and tuberculum olfactorium of the rat after CBZ treatment. CBZ did not alter extracellular norepinephrine levels in rat hippocampus (118). Furthermore, CBZ did not alter the firing rate of noradrenergic neurons in the locus ceruleus (73). With these conflicting studies, a role for CBZ on catecholamine metabolism remains uncertain.

An effect of CBZ on *cholinergic* responses in the brain has also been reported. CBZ was shown to produce an increase in striatal and hippocampal acetylcholine levels and a decrease in choline levels (13,66). Neither choline acetyltransferase nor cholinesterase activity was affected by CBZ. CBZ also increased release and synthesis (66).

Certain antiepileptic drugs have been demonstrated to enhance *GABAergic* synaptic transmission by enhancing the postsynaptic action of GABA at GABAA receptors (53,54). However, on spinal cord neurons in cell culture, no effect of CBZ was found on postsynaptic responses to iontophoretically applied GABA (64), and CBZ did not alter GABAergic inhibition in the hippocampal slice (36). Furthermore, CBZ did not alter the binding of the GABAA receptor agonist [³H]muscimol to rat brain synaptic membranes after either short-term or long-term treatment (67,68). These results suggest that CBZ does not modify GABAA receptor function.

CBZ has been shown to interact with peripheral benzodiazepine sites. Peripheral benzodiazepine binding sites were labeled with [³H]Ro 5-4864 (4′-cholorodiazepam), and CBZ produced a competitive displacement of the labeled ligand with a rather high dissociation constant of 45 μmol/L (58). Furthermore, Ro 5-4864 antagonized the anticonvulsant effect of CBZ, and the effect of Ro 5-4864 was reversed by PK-11195, a compound that displaced Ro 5-4864 binding to peripheral benzodiazepine sites (111). CBZ also upregulated the binding of [³H]PK-11195 to platelets after 4 weeks of treatment (112), and CBZ inhibited the binding of [³H]diazepam to cultured astrocytes but not to cultured neurons (5). In amygdala-kindled rats made tolerant to the anticonvulsant effect of CBZ, cross-tolerance was obtained with the anticonvulsant effects of PK-11195, but not to diazepam, a finding consistent with a CBZ interaction with peripheral, but not central, benzodiazepine receptors (109). However, no change in [³H]Ro 5-4864 binding was obtained in rat brain after long-term CBZ treatment (59), and Ro 5-4864 is a convulsant compound that antagonizes GABA$_A$ receptor responses by binding to the TBPS site on the GABA$_A$ receptor (93). Although the available evidence supports an interaction of CBZ with peripheral benzodiazepine sites, it is unclear whether this interaction occurs at a clinically relevant concentration and how CBZ would produce an anticonvulsant action by binding to this site. On balance, it appears unlikely that CBZ exerts it anticonvulsant action by interacting with peripheral benzodiazepine sites.

CONCLUSION

CBZ and its active metabolite CBZ epoxide both limit sustained high-frequency repetitive firing of sodium-dependent action potentials. It is likely that they do so by binding to the inactive form of sodium channels, thereby producing use- and voltage-dependent block of sodium channels. Thus, CBZ is more effective in reducing high-frequency repetitive firing when neurons are depolarized because more channels are in the inactive state. Under normal physiologic conditions, it is likely that vertebrate myelinated and unmyelinated axons have a large negative membrane potential, and therefore, propagated action potentials are relatively resistant to the action of CBZ. In contrast, the cell body of neurons is subject to synaptic depolarization and inward currents that produce burst firing. This is particularly true in neurons undergoing epileptic discharge. CBZ is therefore effective in limiting high-frequency action potentials generated in bursting neurons.

In addition to altering neuronal excitability, CBZ may alter the process of synaptic transmission by affecting presynaptic sodium channels. It has been demonstrated that [³H]BTX-B binding sites are not restricted to cell bodies and axons but are present in synaptic zones with a heterogeneous distribution in the nervous system (117). In the hippocampal slice, stimulation of stratum radiatum elicited extracellular field potentials recorded from the CA1 pyramidal cell layer. The field potentials consisted of a fiber spike, which reflects axonal propagation, and a population spike, which reflects effective synaptic transmission. Veratridine, which displaces [³H]BTX-B binding, produces a specific reduction in the synaptically evoked population spike without affecting the fiber spike. This effect of veratridine is antagonized by CBZ. It is likely therefore that CBZ blocks presynaptic sodium channels and the firing of action potentials; this would secondarily reduce voltage-dependent calcium entry and synaptic transmission.

Although the most likely mechanism of action of CBZ is to block high-frequency repetitive firing of action potentials

by interacting with sodium channels, additional actions of CBZ have been suggested. CBZ has been reported to block NMDA receptor currents at therapeutically relevant concentrations. Whereas this observation has not been fully characterized, it is possible that this action of CBZ may act in concert with the effect of CBZ on sodium channels to produce its anticonvulsant effect. At present, it is not possible to determine the relative contribution, if any, of blockade of NMDA currents to the anticonvulsant mechanism of CBZ.

In summary, CBZ is likely to act both presynaptically, to block release of neurotransmitter by blocking firing of action potentials, and postsynaptically, by blocking the development of high-frequency repetitive discharge initiated at cell bodies and possibly by blocking NMDA receptor currents. These combined presynaptic and postsynaptic effects are likely to form the basis of the anticonvulsant actions of CBZ.

REFERENCES

1. Albertson TE, Joy RM, Stark LG. Caffeine modification of kindled amygdaloid seizures. *Pharmacol Biochem Behav* 1983;19:339–343.
2. Albertson TE, Stark LG, Joy RM, et al. Aminophylline and kindled seizures. *Exp Neurol* 1983;81:703–713.
3. Ambrósio AF, Silva AP, Malva JO, et al. Carbamazepine inhibits L-type Ca²⁺ channels in cultured rat hippocampal neurons stimulated with glutamate receptor agaonist. *Neuropharmacology* 1999;38:1349–1359.
4. Azzaro AJ, Wenger GR, Craig CR, et al. Reserpine-induced alterations in brain amines and their relationship to changes in the incidence of minimal electro-shock seizures in mice. *J Pharmacol Exp Ther* 1972;180:558–568.
5. Bender AS, Hertz L. Evidence for involvement of the astrocytic benzodiazepine receptor in the mechanism of action of convulsant and anticonvulsant drugs. *Life Sci* 1988;43:477–484.
6. Blom S. Tic douloureau treated with a new anticonvulsant: experiences with.G32883. *Arch Neurol* 1963;2:357–366.
7. Brückner C, Heinemann U. Effects of standard anticonvulsant drugs on different patterns of epileptiform discharges induced by 4-aminopyridine in combined entorhinal cortex-hippocampal slices. *Brain Res* 2000;859:15–20.
8. Cai Z, McCaslin PP. Amitriptyline, desipramine, cyproheptadine and carbamazepine, in concentrations used therapeutically, reduce kainate- and N-methyl-D-aspartate-induced intracellular Ca²⁺ levels in neuronal culture. *Eur J Pharmacol* 1992;219:53–57.
9. Cereghino JJ. Carbamazepine: relation of plasma concentration to seizure control. In: Woodbury DM, Penry JK, Pippenger CE, eds. *Antiepileptic drugs.* New York: Raven Press, 1982:507–519.
10. Cereghino JJ, Brock JT, Van Meter JC, et al. Carbamazepine for epilepsy: a controlled prospective evaluation. *Neurology* 1974;24:401–410.
11. Chen G, Ensor CR, Bohner B. A facilitation action of reserpine on the central nervous system. *Proc Soc Exp Biol Med* 1954;86:507–510.
12. Chen G, Ensor CR, Bohner B. Studies of drug effects on electrically induced extensor seizures and clinical implications. *Arch Int Pharmacodyn Ther* 1968;172:183–218.
13. Consolo S, Bianchi S, Ladinski H. Effect of carbamazepine on cholinergic parameters in rat brain areas. *Neuropharmacology* 1976;15:653.

14. Courtney KR. Mechanism of frequency-dependent inhibition of sodium currents in myelinated nerve by the lidocaine derivative GEA 968. *J Pharmacol Exp Ther* 1975;195:225–236.

15. Courtney KR, Etter EG. Modulated anticonvulsant block of sodium channels in nerve and muscle. *Eur J Pharmacol* 1983; 88:1–9.

16. Creese I, Usdin TB, Snyder SH. Dopamine receptor binding regulated by guanine nucleotides. *Mol Pharmacol* 1979;16: 69–76.

17. Crowder JM, Bradford HF. Common anticonvulsants inhibit Ca^{2+} uptake and amino acid neurotransmitter release *in vitro*. *Epilepsia* 1987;28:378–382.

18. Dailey JW, Reith MEA, Yan Q-S, et al. Carbamazepine increases extracellular serotonin concentration: lack of antagonism by tetrodotoxin or zero Ca^{2+}. *Eur J Pharmacol* 1997;328: 153–162.

19. Deckert J, Berger W, Kleopa K, et al. Adenosine A1 receptors in human hippocampus: inhibition of [^{3}H]8–cyclopentyl-1,3 dipropylxanthine binding by antagonist drugs. *Neurosci Lett* 1993;150:191–194.

20. Dost R, Rundfeldt C. The anticonvulsant retigabine potently suppresses epileptiform discharges in the low Ca^{++} and low Mg^{++} model in the hippocampal slice preparation. *Epilepsy Res* 2000;38:53–66.

21. Dunwiddie TV, Fredholm BB. Adenosine A1 receptors inhibit adenylate cyclase activity and neurotransmitter release and hyperpolarize pyramidal neurons in rat hippocampus. *J Pharmacol Exp Ther* 1989;249:31–37.

22. Dunwiddie TV, Worth T. Sedative and anticonvulsant effects of adenosine analogs in mouse and rat. *J Pharmacol Exp Ther* 1982;220:70–76.

23. Eadie MJ, Tyrer JH. Carbamazepine. In: *Anticonvulsant therapy*. Edinburgh: Churchill Livingstone, 1980:132–161.

24. Ferrendelli JA, Daniels-McQueen S. Comparative actions of phenytoin and other anticonvulsant drugs on potassium- and veratridine-stimulated calcium uptake in synaptosomes. *J Pharmacol Exp Ther* 1982;220:29–34.

25. Fromm GH, Killian JM. Effect of some anticonvulsant drugs on the spinal trigeminal nucleus. *Neurology* 1967;17:275–280.

26. Fueta Y, Avoli M. Effects of antiepileptic drugs on 4-aminopyridine-induced epileptiform activity in young and adult rat hippocampus. *Epilepsy Res* 1992;12:207–215.

27. Fujiwara Y, Sato M, Otsuki S. Interaction of carbamazepine and other drugs with adenosine (A1 and A2) receptors. *Psychopharmacology* 1986;90:332–335.

28. Grant KA, Snell LD, Rogawski MA, et al. Comparison of the effects of the uncompetitive *N*-methyl-D-aspartate antagonist (±)-5-aminocarbonyl-10,11-dihydro-5H-dibenzo[a,d]cyclohepten-5,10-imine (ADCI) with its structural analogs dizocilpine (MK-801) and carbamazepine on ethanol withdrawal seizures. *J Pharmacol Exp Ther* 1992;260:1017–1022.

29. Heinemann U, Feranceschetti S, Hamon B, et al. Effects of anticonvulsants on spontaneous epileptiform activity which develops in the absence of chemical synaptic transmission in hippocampal slices. *Brain Res* 1985;325:349–353.

30. Hernandez-Peon R. Anticonvulsant action of G32883. *Third Proc Int Neuropsychopharmacologicum* 1964;3:303–311.

31. Hernandez-Peon R. Central action of G32883 upon transmission of trigeminal pain impulses. *Med Pharmacol Exp (Basel)* 1965;12:73–80.

32. Hershkowitz N, Raines A. Effects of carbamazepine on muscle spindle discharges. *J Pharmacol Exp Ther* 1978;204:581–591.

33. Hershkowitz N, Dretchen KL, Raines A. Carbamazepine suppression of post-tetanic potentiation at the neuromuscular junction. *J Pharmacol Exp Ther* 1978;207:810–816.

34. Hille B. Local anesthetics: hydrophilic and hydrophobic pathways for the drug-receptor reaction. *J Gen Physiol* 1977;69: 497–515.

35. Honda H, Allen M. The effect of an iminostilbene derivative (G32883) on peripheral nerve. *J Med Assoc Ga* 1973;62:38–42.

36. Hood TW, Siegfried J, Haas HL. Analysis of carbamazepine actions in hippocampal slices of the rat. *Cell Mol Neurobiol* 1983;3:213–222.

37. Hough CJ, Irwin RP, Gao X-M, et al. Carbamezepine inhibition of *N*-methyl-D-aspartate–evoked calcium influx in rat cerebellar granule cells. *J Pharmacol Exp Ther* 1996;276: 143–149.

38. Johannessen SI, Gerna M, Bakke J, et al. CSF concentrations and serum protein binding of carbamazepine and carbamazepine 10,11-epoxide in epileptic patients. *Br J Clin Pharmacol* 1976;3:575–582.

39. Julien RM, Hollister RP. Carbamazepine: mechanism of action. *Adv Neurol* 1975;11:263–277.

40. Kilian M, Frey HH. Central monoamines and convulsive thresholds in mice and rats. *Neuropharmacology* 1973;12: 681–692.

41. Koe BK, Weissman A. The pharmacology of para-chlorophenylalanine, a selective depletor of serotonin stores. *Adv Pharmacol* 1968;6B:29–47.

42. Kosteljanetz M, Christiansen J, Dam AM, et al. Carbamazepine vs phenytoin. *Arch Neurol* 1979;36:22–24.

43. Krall RL, Penry JK, White BG, et al. Antiepileptic drug development. II. Anticonvulsant drug screening. *Epilepsia* 1978;19: 409–428.

44. Krupp P. The effect of Tegretol on some elementary neuronal mechanisms. *Headache* 1969;9:42–46.

45. Kuo C-C, Chen R-S, Chen R-C. Carbamazepine inhibition of neuronal Na^{+} currents: quantitative distinction from phenytoin and possible therapeutic implications. *Mol Pharmacol* 1997;51: 1077–1083.

46. Kutt H. Clinical pharmacology of carbamazepine. In: Pippenger CE, Penry JK, Kutt H, eds. *Antiepileptic drugs: quantitative analysis and interpretation*. New York: Raven Press, 1978: 307–314.

47. Lampe H, Bigalke H. Carbamazepine blocks NMDA-activated currents in cultured spinal cord neurons. *Neuroreport* 1990;1: 8–10.

48. Lancaster JM, Davies JA. Carbamazepine inhibits NMDA-induced depolarizations in cortical wedges prepared from DBA/2 mice. *Experientia* 1992;48:751–753.

49. Lang DG, Wang CM, Cooper BR. Lamotrigine, phenytoin and carbamazepine interactions on the sodium current present in AN4TG1 mouse neuroblastoma cells. *J Pharmacol Exp Ther* 1993;266:829–835.

50. Lewin E, Bleck B. Cyclic AMP accumulation in cerebral cortical slices: effect of carbamazepine, phenobarbital, and phenytoin. *Epilepsia* 1977;18:237–242.

51. Loshe MJ, Lenschow V, Schwabe J. Two affinity states for Rz adenosine receptors in brain membranes, analysis of guanine nucleotide and temperature, effects on radioligand binding. *Mol Pharmacol* 26:1–9.

52. Macdonald RL. Mechanisms of anticonvulsant drug action. In: Meldrum BS, Pedley TA, eds. *Recent advances in epilepsy*. New York: Churchill Livingstone, 1983:1–23.

53. Macdonald RL. Seizure disorders and epilepsy. In: Johnston MV, Macdonald RL, Young AB, eds. *Principles of drug therapy in neurology*. Philadelphia: FA Davis, 1992:87–117.

54. Macdonald RL, McLean MJ. Anticonvulsant drugs: mechanisms of action. *Adv Neurol* 1986;44:713–735.

55. Macdonald RL, McLean MJ, Skerritt JH. Anticonvulsant drug mechanisms of action. *Fed Proc* 1985;44:2634–2639.

56. Maitre M, Chesielski L, Lehmann A, et al. Protective effect of

adenosine and nicotinamide against audiogenic seizure. *Biochem Pharmacol* 1974;23:2807–2816.

57. Marangos PJ, Patel J, Smith KD, et al. Adenosine antagonist properties of carbamazepine. *Epilepsia* 1987;28:387–394.

58. Marangos PJ, Post RM, Patel J, et al. Specific and potent interactions of carbamazepine with brain adenosine receptors. *Eur J Pharmacol* 1983;93:175–182.

59. Marangos PJ, Weiss SRB, Montgomery P, et al. Chronic carbamazepine treatment increases brain adenosine receptors. *Epilepsia* 1985;26:493–498.

60. Mattson RH, Cramer JA, Collins JF, et al. Comparison of carbamazepine, phenobarbital, phenytoin, and primidone in partial and secondarily generalized tonic-clonic seizures. *N Engl J Med* 1985;313:145–151.

61. McLean MJ, Macdonald RL. Selective effects of anticonvulsant drugs on high frequency repetitive firing of action potentials in mouse spinal cord neurons in cell culture. *Neurology* 1983;33:213.

62. McLean MJ, Macdonald RL. Multiple actions of phenytoin on mouse spinal cord neurons in cell culture. *J Pharmacol Exp Ther* 1983;227:779–789.

63. McLean MJ, Macdonald RL. Sodium valproate, but not ethosuximide, produces use- and voltage-dependent limitation of high frequency repetative firing of action potentials of mouse central neurons in cell culture. *J Pharmacol Exp Ther* 1986;237:1001–1011.

64. McLean MJ, Macdonald RL. Carbamazepine and 10,11-epoxycarbamazepine produce use- and voltage-dependent limitation of rapidly firing action potentials of mouse central neurons in cell culture. *J Pharmacol Exp Ther* 1986;238:727–738.

65. McLean MJ, Taylor CP, Macdonald RL. Phenytoin and carbamazepine limit sustained high frequency repetitive firing of action potentials of hippocampal neurons in cell culture and tissue slices. *Soc Neurosci Abstr* 1984;10:873.

66. Mizuno K, Okada M, Murakami T, et al. Effects of carbamazepine on acetylcholine release and metabolism. *Epilepsy Res* 2000;40:187–195.

67. Motohashi N. GABA receptor alterations after chronic lithium administration: comparison with carbamazepine and sodium valproate. *Prog Neuropsychopharmacol Biol Psychiatry* 1992;16:571–579.

68. Motohashi N, Ikawa K, Kariya T. GABA_B receptors are up-regulated by chronic treatment with lithium or carbamazepine: GABA hypothesis of affective disorders? *Eur J Pharmacol* 1989;166:95–99.

69. Okada M, Hirano T, Mizuno K, et al. Biphasic effects of carbamazepine on the dopaminergic system in rat striatum and hippocampus. *Epilepsy Res* 1997;28:143–153.

70. Okada M, Hirano T, Mizuno K, et al. Effects of carbamazepine on hippocampal serotonergic system. *Epilepsy Res* 1997;31:187–198.

71. Okada M, Kiryu K, Kawata Y, et al. Determination of the effects of caffeine and carbamazepine on striatal dopamine release by *in vivo* microdialysis. *Eur J Pharmacol* 1997;321:181–188.

72. Olpe HR, Baudry M, Jones RSG. Electrophysiological and neurochemical investigations on the action of carbamazepine on the rat hippocampus. *Eur J Pharmacol* 1985;110:71–80.

73. Olpe HR, Jones RSG. The action of anticonvulsant drugs on the firing of locus coeruleus neurons: selective activating effect of carbamazepine. *Eur J Pharmacol* 1983;91:107.

74. Otoom SA, Alkadhi KA. Action of carbamazepine on epileptiform activity of the verartidine model in CA1 neurons. *Brain Res* 2000;885:289–294.

75. Peroutka SJ, Lebovitz RM, Snyder SH. Serotonin receptor binding sites affected differentially by guanine nucleotides. *Mol Pharmacol* 1979;16:700–708.

76. Phillips I, Martin KF, Thompson KS, et al. Weak blockade of AMPA receptor-mediated depolarisations in the rat corticial wedge by phenytoin but not lamotrigine or carbamazepine. *Eur J Pharmacol* 1997;337:189–195.

77. Post RM, Uhde TW, Wolff EA. Profile of clinical efficacy and side effects of carbamazepine in psychiatric illness: relationship to blood and CSF levels of carbamazepine and its -10,11–epoxide metabolite. *Acta Psychiatr Scand* 1984;69:104–120.

78. Prockop DJ, Shore PA, Brodie BB. An anticonvulsant effect of monoamine oxidase inhibitors. *Experientia* 1959;15:145–147.

79. Purdy RE, Julien RM, Fairhurst AS, et al. Effect of carbamazepine on the *in vitro* uptake and release of norepinephrine in adrenergic nerves of rabbit aorta and in whole brain synaptosomes. *Epilepsia* 1977;18:251.

80. Quattrone A, Crunelli V, Samanin R. Seizure susceptibility and anticonvulsant activity of carbamazepine, diphenylhydantoin and phenobarbital in rats with selective depletions of brain monoamines. *Neuropharmacology* 1978;17:643–647.

81. Quattrone A, Samanin R. Decreased anticonvulsant activity of carbamazepine in 6-hydroxydopamine–treated rats. *Eur J Pharmacol* 1977;41:333–336.

82. Ragsdale DS, Scheuer T, Catterall WC. Frequency and voltage-dependent inhibition of type IIA Na⁺ channels, expressed in a mammalian cell line, by local anesthetic, antiarrhythmic, and antitconvulsant drugs. *Mol Pharmacol* 1991;40:756–765.

83. Ramsay RE, Wilder B, Berger J, et al. A double-blind study comparing carbamazepine with phenytoin as initial seizure therapy in adults. *Neurology* 1983;33:904–910.

84. Rasmussen P, Rushede J. Facial pain treated with carbamazepine (Tegretol). *Acta Neurol Scand* 1970;46:385–408.

85. Rodin EA, Rim CS, Rennick PM. The effects of carbamazepine on patients with psychomotor epilepsy: results of a double blind study. *Epilepsia* 1974;15:547–561.

86. Schauf CL, Floyd AD, Marder J. Effects of carbamazepine in the ionic conductances of myxicola giant axons. *J Pharmacol Exp Ther* 1974;189:538–543.

87. Schmidt D, Einicke I, Haenel F. The influence of seizure type on the efficacy of plasma concentrations of phenytoin, phenobarbital, and carbamazepine. *Arch Neurol* 1986;43:263–265.

88. Schwarz JR, Grigat G. Phenytoin and carbamazepine: potential- and frequency-dependent block of Na currents in mammalian myelinated nerve fibers. *Epilepsia* 1989;30:286–294.

89. Simonsen J, Zander Olsen P, Kuhl V, et al. A comparative controlled study between carbamazepine and diphenylhydantoin in psychomotor epilepsy. *Epilepsia* 1976;17:169–176.

90. Skerritt JH, Davies LP, Johnston GAR. A purinergic component in the anticonvulsant action of carbamazepine? *Eur J Pharmacol* 1982;82:195–197.

91. Skerritt JH, Davies LP, Johnston GAR. Interactions of the anticonvulsant carbamazepine with adenosine receptors. I. Neurochemical studies. *Epilepsia* 1983;24:643–642.

92. Skerritt JH, Johnston GAR, Chen Chow S. Interactions of the anticonvulsant carbamazepine with adenosine receptors. II. Pharmacological studies. *Epilepsia* 1983;24:643–650.

93. Skerritt JH, Werz MA, McLean MJ, et al. Diazepam and its anomalous *p*-chloro-derivative Ro 5-4864: comparative effects on mouse neurons in cell culture. *Brain Res* 1984;3l0:99–l05.

94. Smith DB, Mattson RH, Cramer JA, et al. Veterans Administration Epilepsy Cooperative Study Group: results of a nationwide Veterans Administration cooperative study comparing the efficacy and toxicity of carbamazepine, phenobarbitol, phenytoin, and primidone. *Epilepsia* 1987;28:S50–S558.

95. Smith KL, Swann JW. Does carbamazepine act via an adenosine receptor? *Epilepsia* 1985;26:524.

96. Smith KL, Swann JW. Carbamazepine suppresses synchronized

afterdischarging in disinhibited immature rat hippocampus *in vitro. Brain Res* 1987;400:371–376.

97. Stone TW. Interactions of carbamazepine, chlormethiazole and pentobarbitone with adenosine on hippocampal slices. *Gen Pharmacol* 1988;19:67–72.

98. Sun L, Lin SS. The anticonvulsant SGB-017 (ADCI) blocks voltage-gated sodium channels in rat and human neurons: comparison with carbamazepine. *Epilepsia* 2000;41:263–270.

99. Theobald W, Krupp P, Levin P. Neuropharmacologic aspects of the therapeutic action of carbamazepine in trigeminal neuralgia. In: Hassler R, Walker AE, eds. *Trigeminal neuralgia: pathogenesis and pathophysiology.* Stuttgart: Thieme, 1970:107–115.

100. Theobald W, Kunz HA. Zur pharmacologie des Antiepileptikums 5-carbmyl-5H-dibenzo b,f azepin. *Arzneimittelforschung* 1963;13:122–125.

101. Troupin A, Ojemann LM, Halpern L, et al. Carbamazepine: a double-blind comparison with phenytoin. *Neurology* 1977;27:511–519.

102. U'Pritchard DC, Snyder SH. Guanyl nucleotide influences on [³H]ligand binding to alpha-noradrenergic receptors in calf brain membranes. *J Biol Chem* 1978;253:3444–3452.

103. Voskuyl RA, Albus H. Spontaneous epileptiform discharges in hippocampal slices induced by 4-aminopyridine. *Brain Res* 1985;34:54–66.

104. Vreugdenhil M, Wadman WJ. Modulation of sodium currents in rat CA1 neurons by carbamazepine after kindling epileptogenesis. *Epilepsia* 1999;40:1512–1522.

105. Walden J, Grunze H, Bingmann D, et al. Calcium antagonistic effects of carbamazepine as a mechanism of action in neuropsychiatric disorders: studies in calcium dependent model epilepsies. *Eur Neuropsychopharmacol* 1992;2:455–462.

106. Watts AE, Jefferys JGR. Effects of carbamazepine and baclofen on 4-aminopyridine-induced epileptic activity in rat hippocampal slices. *Br J Pharmacol* 1993;108:819–823.

107. Weir RL, Anderson SM, Daly JW. Inhibition of N6-[³H]cyclohexyladenosine binding by carbamazepine. *Epilepsia* 1990;31:503–512.

108. Weir RL, Padgett W, Daly JW, et al. Interaction of anticonvulsant drugs with adenosine receptors in the central nervous system. *Epilepsia* 1984;25:492–498.

109. Weiss SRB, Post RM. Contingent tolerance to carbamazepine: a peripheral-type benzodiazepine mechanism. *Eur J Pharmacol* 1991;193:159–163.

110. Weiss SRB, Post RM, Marangos PJ, et al. Adenosine antagonists, lack of effect on the inhibition of kindled seizures in rats by carbamazepine. *Neuropharmacology* 1985;24:535–638.

111. Weiss SRB, Post RM, Patel J, et al. Differential mediation of the anticonvulsant effects of carbamazepine and diazepam. *Life Sci* 1985;36:2413–2419.

112. Weizman A, Tanne Z, Karp L, et al. Carbamzepine up-regulates the binding of [³H]PK 11195 to platelets of epileptic patients. *Eur J Pharmacol* 1987;141:471–474.

113. Westerink BH., Lejeune B, Korf J, et al. On the significance of regional dopamine metabolism in the rat brain for the classification of centrally acting drugs. *Eur J Pharmacol* 1977;42:179–190.

114. Willow M, Caterall WA. Inhibition of binding of [³H]batrachotoxin A 20—benzoate to sodium channels by the anticonvulsant drugs diphenylhydantoin and carbamazepine. *Mol Pharmacol* 1982;22:627–635.

115. Willow M, Gonoi T, Catterall WA. Voltage clamp analysis of the inhibitory actions of diphenylhydantoin and carbamazepine on voltage-sensitive sodium channels in neuroblastoma cells. *Mol Pharmacol* 1985;27:549–558.

116. Willow M, Kuenzel EA, Caterall WA. Inhibition of voltage-sensitive sodium channels in neuroblastoma cells and synaptosomes by the anticonvulsant drugs diphenylhydantoin and carbamazepine. *Mol Pharmacol* 1984;25:228–234.

117. Worley PF, Baraban JM. Site of anticonvulsant action on sodium channels: autoradiographic and electrophysiological studies in rat brain. *Neurobiology* 1987;84:3051–3055.

118. Yan QS, Jobe PC, Dailey JW. Evidence that a serotonergic mechanism is involved in the anticonvulsant effect of fluoxetine in genetically epilepsy-prone rats. *Eur J Pharmacol* 1994;252:105–112.

119. Zwillich CW, Sutton FD, Neff TA, et al. Theophylline-induced seizures in adults. *Ann Intern Med* 1975;82:784–787.

Antiepileptic Drugs, 5th Edition. Edited by R.H. Levy, R.H. Mattson, B.S. Meldrum, and E. Perucca. Lippincott Williams & Wilkins, Philadelphia © 2002.

CARBAMAZEPINE

CHEMISTRY, BIOTRANSFORMATION, AND PHARMACOKINETICS

EDOARDO SPINA

Carbamazepine (CBZ) is an iminodibenzyl derivative with anticonvulsant properties that is structurally related to the tricyclic antidepressants. It is one of the most commonly prescribed drugs for epilepsy, but it also is used in the treatment of other neurologic conditions, such as chronic pain syndromes and trigeminal neuralgia, as well as in a variety of psychiatric disorders (1,2).

CHEMISTRY AND METABOLIC SCHEME

The chemical name of CBZ is 5H-dibenz[b,f]azepine-5-carboxamide or 5-carbamoil-5H-dibenz[b,f]azepine. It is a white or yellowish-white, crystalline, almost odorless powder, tasteless or with a slightly bitter taste. CBZ has a molecular weight of 236.3 and a melting point between 189°C and 193°C. Unlike tricyclic antidepressants, which are basic substances, CBZ is a neutral compound because its carbamoyl side chain is part of a nonionized urea moiety (3). CBZ is a highly lipophilic agent, as indicated by a partition coefficient of (P) 58 in the system n-octanol/aqueous buffer pH = 7.4, which is soluble in various organic solvents, such as alcohol and acetone, but practically insoluble in water. CBZ is prepared by chemical synthesis and exists in several crystal modifications, with the α and β forms being of primary interest. Solid dosage formulations usually contain the β-modification, whereas in aqueous syrup formulations CBZ is present as the dihydrate. Crystalline CBZ is chemically stable under normal storage conditions at room temperature.

CBZ is extensively metabolized in the body, and several metabolites are formed by parallel or sequential reactions catalyzed by different enzymes (Figure 21.1). The pharmacokinetic parameters of CBZ are summarized in Table 21.1.

Edoardo Spina, MD, PhD: Associate Professor, Section of Pharmacology, Department of Clinical and Experimental Medicine and Pharmacology, University of Messina, Policlinico Universitario, Messina, Italy

ABSORPTION

Absorption of CBZ from the gastrointestinal tract is rather slow and extremely variable (4). Single-dose studies have shown that peak plasma CBZ concentrations usually occur between 4 and 8 hours after oral administration of regular tablets, but peaks as late as 24 hours have been reported, depending on the formulation (4–9). After reaching a maximum, plasma concentrations typically plateau for 10 to 30 hours before declining (5,7). Peak plasma CBZ concentrations are reached more rapidly (within an average of 3 hours) in patients on long-term treatment owing to the autoinduction process (see section on Biotransformation) (4). The delayed and irregular absorption of CBZ from conventional tablets probably is related to its very slow dissolution in the gastrointestinal fluid or to its anticholinergic properties, which may modify the gastrointestinal transit time (4,5). Earlier kinetic studies found evidence of dose-independent absorption of CBZ in the range of 50 to 600 mg (5,7,8). More recent investigations, however, indicate that the rate and extent of CBZ absorption appear to be dose dependent and that the time to reach maximal concentration is prolonged when the dose is increased (4,10). It has been suggested that CBZ undergoes a simultaneous first-order and zero-order absorption, with approximately 35% of the available dose absorbed at a zero-order rate (11). Oral solutions of CBZ are absorbed more rapidly and produce higher peaks than tablets (12,13). On the other hand, controlled-release formulations ensure a smoother absorption profile and allow less frequent administration (14).

Bioavailability

Because of the lack of an injectable formulation, the absolute bioavailability of CBZ in humans has not been determined. However, based on the recovery of radiolabeled CBZ in urine and feces after single-dose administration of ^{14}C-CBZ in a gelatin capsule, the oral bioavailability has

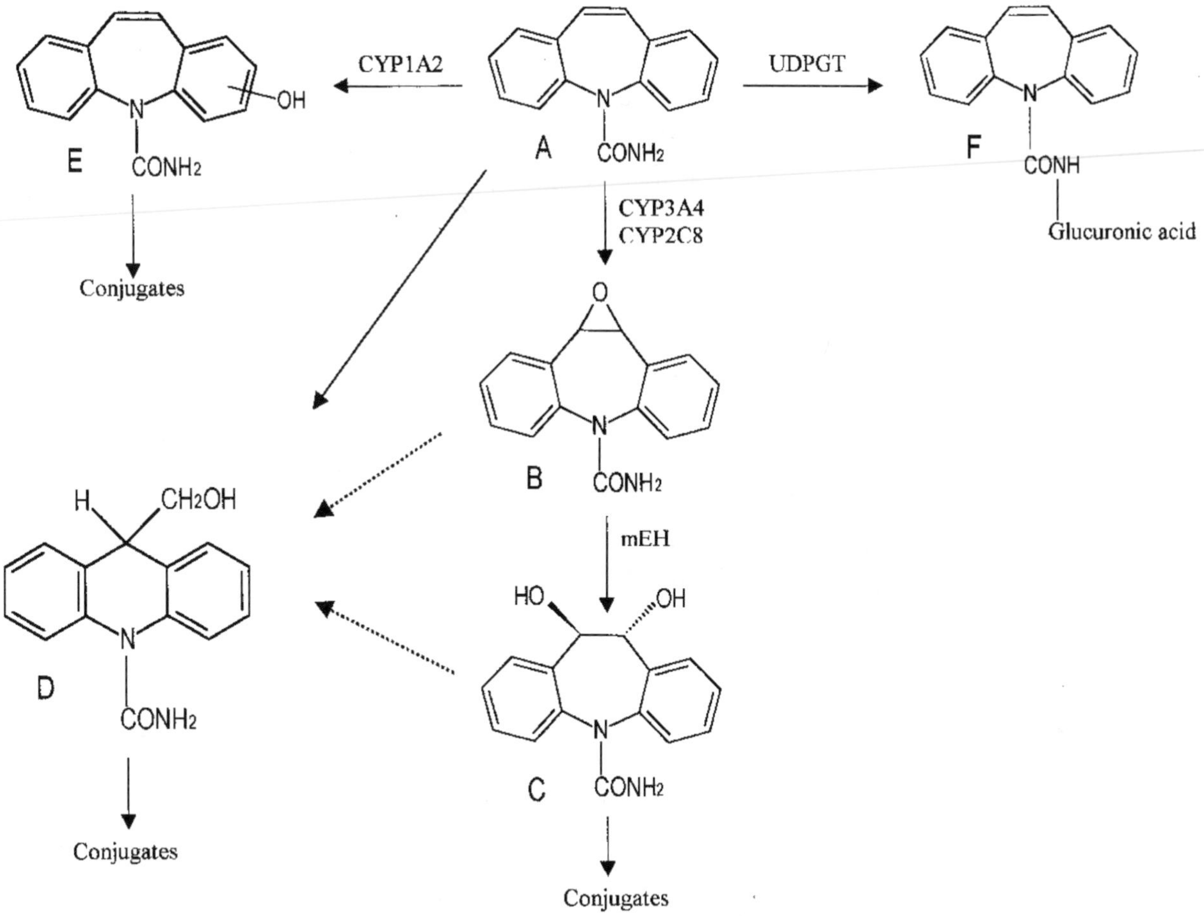

FIGURE 21.1. Biotransformation of carbamazepine in humans, and the enzymes catalyzing the major metabolic reactions. A, carbamazepine; B, carbamazepine-10,11-epoxide; C, *trans*-10,11-dihydroxy-10,11-dihydrocarbamazepine; D, 9-hydroxymethyl-10-carbamoyl acridan; E, 1-, 2-, 3-, and 4-hydroxycarbamazepine; F, carbamazepine *N*-glucuronide; CYP, cytochrome P450; mEH, microsomal epoxide hydrolase; UDPGT, uridine diphosphate glucuronosyltransferase.

TABLE 21.1. PHARMACOKINETIC PARAMETERS OF CARBAMAZEPINE

	Mean ± SD	Range
T_{max} (h)	—	2–24[a]
Bioavailability (%)	—	75–85[b]
Volume of distribution (L/kg)	1.20 ± 0.45	0.88–1.86[c]
	1.07 ± 0.22	0.79–1.40[d]
Protein binding (%)	72.1 ± 1.2	70.2–74.0[d]
Half-life (h)	35.6 ± 15.3	18.5–54.7[c]
	35.9 ± 8.3	23.9–46.4[d]
	35.3 ± 10.0	26.0–52.9[e]
Total clearance (L/h)	1.82 ± 1.19	1.06–3.59[c]
	1.52 ± 0.21	1.14–1.60[d]
Urinary excretion (% of the dose)		
Unchanged CBZ	—	0.5–1[f]
CBZ epoxide	—	1–2
trans-CBZ-diol	—	20–60
9-HM-10-CA	—	5–11
Hydroxy-CBZ	—	5–10

SD, standard deviation; T_{max}, time to maximum effectAQ2; CBZ, carbamazepine.
[a]Ref. 9.
[b]Ref. 15.
[c]Ref. 6.
[d]Ref. 7.
[e]Ref. 5.
[f]Refs. 60, 62, 84.

been estimated to range from 75% to 85% (15). In a pharmacokinetic study with a parenteral formulation for experimental use, comparison of the oral and intravenous routes of CBZ administration in two healthy subjects showed complete bioavailability of the oral dose (16). Data from different studies indicate that the oral bioavailability of CBZ is similar whether given as conventional tablets, solutions, suspensions, syrups, or newly developed chewable or sustained-release formulations (12–14,17–21). The relative bioavailability of a rectally administered suspension of CBZ was found to be similar to that of an orally administered tablet (22,23). However, in a study of children with epilepsy, the relative bioavailability of a suppository for rectal administration was found to be 80% compared with slow-release tablets (24). The bioavailability of CBZ was slightly, but not significantly, increased when tablets were taken with meals, probably because of enhanced solubilization of the drug by the bile secreted after food ingestion (5).

Formulations and Routes of Administration

For human use, CBZ is commercially available for oral and rectal administration (1). Oral preparations consist of various solid dosage forms, including controlled-release formulations, and a syrup. The marketed formulations include tablets of 100, 200, or 400 mg, chewable tablets of 100 or 200 mg, controlled-release tablets of 100, 200, or 400 mg, and a suspension of 100 mg/5 mL. Solid-dose preparations with modified-release characteristics have been developed to reduce peak-related toxic effects and to decrease clinically troublesome fluctuations in plasma CBZ concentrations during the dosage interval (14). In addition, sustained-release formulations may be administered only once or twice daily, compared with three or four daily doses of conventional formulations, thus improving patient compliance. CBZ also is supplied as suppositories of 125 or 250 mg for rectal administration. Because of the low solubility of CBZ in water, no parenteral preparation has been marketed, although an injectable formulation has been used in a pharmacokinetic study in humans (16) and in animal models (25).

The major metabolite of CBZ, carbamazepine-10,11-epoxide (CBZ epoxide), has been directly administered orally to humans in the form of a suspension, a solution, and an enteric-coated tablet (26–28). Because it is unstable in an acid environment, it is advisable to coadminister the suspension or solution formulations with antacids.

DISTRIBUTION

CBZ is a neutral and fairly lipophilic compound that easily crosses the blood–brain barrier and other biologic membranes of the body and rapidly distributes to various organs and tissues, without any preferential affinity for specific

regions. After administration of single oral doses to healthy volunteers and patients, the apparent volume of distribution of CBZ has been found to range between 0.79 and 1.86 L/kg (6,7). These values have been calculated assuming complete bioavailability of the drug, and the real volumes therefore might be slightly lower and less variable. The apparent volume of distribution of CBZ epoxide, calculated after direct administration to healthy subjects, was found to range between 0.59 and 1.57 L/kg (26,28).

Plasma Protein Binding

Both CBZ and its major metabolite are bound to plasma proteins, primarily to albumin and, to a lesser extent, to α_1-acid glycoprotein. The plasma protein binding of CBZ ranges between 70% and 80%, as determined *in vitro* by equilibrium dialysis and ultrafiltration and *in vivo* by estimating the concentration of the drug simultaneously in plasma and in cerebrospinal fluid or saliva (7,29–31). The protein binding is independent of total plasma concentrations over the therapeutic range, but may be reduced at supratherapeutic levels (29). Plasma protein binding of CBZ epoxide has been reported to range between 50% and 60%, and the epoxide metabolite seems not to bind to α_1-acid glycoprotein (31,32).

Protein binding of CBZ appears to be slightly lower in newborns and children than in adults, with a free fraction of 30% to 35% for parent drug and 55% to 60% for the epoxide metabolite (33–36). One study has reported an elevation of free CBZ concentrations in plasma of elderly patients, probably due to an age-related decrease in levels of nonglycated albumin, which appears to be the major ligand of CBZ in serum (37). No significant modifications in CBZ protein binding have been observed during pregnancy (34,38). However, the unbound fractions of CBZ and CBZ epoxide have been reported to increase slightly throughout pregnancy from 21% to 27% for parent drug and from 42% to 52% for the metabolite (39). Patients with hepatic diseases were found to have slightly lower plasma protein binding compared with normal subjects, whereas there were no significant differences in binding capacity between patients with renal disease and healthy individuals (29). The free CBZ fraction was reported to be moderately decreased in patients with disease states associated with an increased α_1-acid glycoprotein concentration, such as inflammation, myocardial infarction, cancer, and trauma (40). Unlike phenytoin and valproic acid, the plasma protein binding of CBZ shows very little interindividual variation, suggesting that there is no need to monitor free rather than total plasma concentrations (41).

Cerebrospinal Fluid, Brain, Saliva, and Other Tissues

Both CBZ and CBZ epoxide readily pass into the central nervous system, and their concentrations in cerebrospinal fluid reflect the free fraction of the drug. The cerebrospinal fluid concentrations of CBZ have been reported to range from 17% to 31% of the total plasma concentrations, whereas those of CBZ epoxide were found to be approximately 45% to 55% of the corresponding total plasma levels (30,42,43). In patients undergoing brain surgery for tumor removal, the ratio between brain and plasma concentrations ranged from 0.8 to 1.6 for CBZ and from 0.5 to 1.5 for CBZ epoxide (44,45). The postmortem concentrations of CBZ and its epoxide metabolite in frontal cortex were approximately 1.4 and 1.1 times higher, respectively, than those simultaneously present in serum (46).

Salivary concentrations of CBZ and CBZ epoxide in humans are similar to the unbound concentrations in plasma, and have been reported to range from 20% to 30% of plasma concentrations for parent drug and from 30% and 40% for the metabolite (31,47,48). Determination of salivary CBZ concentrations may represent a useful and easy tool for measuring unbound drug (47). CBZ concentrations in tears also reflect the free fraction of the drug in plasma (49). On the other hand, CBZ appears to have a limited penetration into red blood cells, as indicated by erythrocyte-to-plasma ratios of 0.14 to 0.38 (29,50).

Transplacental Passage

CBZ penetrates the placenta extensively and rapidly and distributes to different tissues and organs of the fetus homogeneously (51). Fetal plasma concentrations of CBZ, determined in human umbilical cord, were found to range between 50% and 80% of maternal levels (51–53). There is *in vitro* evidence that human fetal liver during weeks 15 to 21 of gestation is able to metabolize CBZ to its 10,11-epoxide (54). Accordingly, CBZ epoxide also has been detected in fetal tissues and amniotic fluid (51). Concentrations of CBZ and its epoxide metabolite in amniotic fluid were found to be 2 to 2.5 times higher than corresponding free concentrations in maternal serum (55). Such a difference might be related to a higher presence of maternal proteins.

Breast Milk

Both CBZ and the epoxide metabolite are transferred to breast milk (51). Concentrations of CBZ in breast milk have been reported to be approximately 30% to 40% of those in maternal plasma, whereas the corresponding value for CBZ epoxide was approximately 50% (56,57). The possible daily amount of CBZ transferred to the newborn during breast-feeding has been estimated to range between 2 and 5 mg (57). The effect of such a dose on the newborn has yet to be evaluated.

ROUTES OF ELIMINATION

CBZ is eliminated by biotransformation followed by urinary and biliary excretion of the parent drug and the formed metabolites. After administration of a single oral dose of ^{14}C-labeled CBZ, 72% of the radioactivity was excreted in the urine, and the remaining 28% was recovered in feces (15).

Biotransformation

CBZ is extensively metabolized in the body, with less than 2% of an oral dose excreted unchanged in urine (3,15). Biotransformation of CBZ appears to occur mainly in the liver, although animal studies suggest that the lung also contributes, approximately by 5%, to the total body clearance of the drug (58). Several metabolites are formed by parallel or consecutive reactions, as indicated in Figure 21.1. The major pathways of CBZ biotransformation include the epoxide-diol pathway, aromatic hydroxylation, and conjugation reactions. It has been estimated that metabolites from these three major routes account for 80% to 90% of total urinary radioactivity (3,15)

The epoxide-diol pathway is quantitatively the most important in CBZ biotransformation and it consists of an initial oxidation of the 10,11 double bond of the seven-membered azepine ring followed by a hydrolysis reaction. CBZ is first oxidized to the chemically stable CBZ epoxide, which is pharmacologically active. Except for a small amount excreted as such in urine (~1% of the dose), this primary metabolite is extensively hydrolyzed (hydrated) to *trans*-10,11-dihydroxy-10,11-dihydrocarbamazepine (*trans*-CBZ-diol). The diol, which is present in human plasma mainly as its S,S-enantiomer (59), is then excreted into the urine, where it accounts for approximately 35% of a carbamazepine dose, partly as unconjugated and partly as its mono-O-glucuronide (60). A minor metabolite of the epoxide-diol pathway is 9-hydroxymethyl-10-carbamoyl acridan (9-HM-10-CA), which is almost completely conjugated with glucuronic acid before excretion in urine (61). However, this metabolite appears to be formed mainly from CBZ itself and only in small part through the epoxide-diol pathway (62).

An additional, but quantitatively less important, pathway of CBZ metabolism is represented by hydroxylation at different positions of the six-membered aromatic rings, with the formation of four possible phenolic products, 1-, 2-, 3-, and 4-hydroxycarbamazepine (3). Animal studies indicate that reactive arene oxides are intermediates of these reactions (63). Two other metabolites of this pathway carry a hydroxyl group in position 2 and a methoxy group in position 1 or 3. These phenolic metabolites are then conjugated with glucuronic acid and, to a lesser extent, with sulfuric acid and excreted in urine. Only traces of these metabolites are excreted unconjugated.

Conjugation reactions usually are regarded as the third most important route of CBZ biotransformation (3). The drug may be directly conjugated with glucuronic acid. Glucuronidation occurs at the amino group of the carbamoyl side chain. Unlike most other glucuronides, this *N*-glucuronide conjugate cannot be hydrolyzed with β-glucuronidase. Glucuronidation also occurs as a secondary metabolic process, and almost all CBZ metabolites carrying free hydroxyl groups are converted to their *O*-glucuronides. These conjugated metabolites are susceptible to cleavage with β-glucuronidase. As an additional secondary conjugation process, CBZ and its phenolic metabolites can be conjugated with sulfuric acid.

With regard to the pharmacologic activity of CBZ metabolites, it is well established that CBZ epoxide has anticonvulsant effects in animal models of epilepsy and might therefore contribute to the clinical effects of CBZ in humans (64). Conversely, *trans*-CBZ-diol is devoid of anticonvulsant activity, whereas 9-HM-10-CA and 2- and 3-hydroxy-CBZ have shown only little or no activity in animal tests (3).

It is well documented that CBZ induces its own metabolism during long-term therapy (autoinduction) (6,62,65). Combination therapy with other anticonvulsants (e.g., phenytoin or phenobarbital) further induces CBZ metabolism (heteroinduction) (62,66,67). The autoinduction process involves the epoxide-diol pathway, and it has been demonstrated that both the CBZ epoxidation and the subsequent epoxide hydrolysis are induced, although the latter reaction to a lesser extent (60,62). There is conflicting evidence concerning the susceptibility to autoinduction of the formation of 9-HM-10-CA and aromatic hydroxylation (62,68). On the other hand, glucuronidation of diol, phenolic, or acridan metabolites appears not to be autoinducible (68). The course of the autoinduction process appears to be complex, discontinuous, and prolonged (69). There is evidence that it may start within 24 hours of first exposure to CBZ (70) and seems to be complete during the first 3 to 5 weeks of treatment (71). According to further studies (72,73), the process of autoinduction is complete within 1 week of starting CBZ therapy or dose change, and it appears to be dose dependent.

There has been a recent increase in knowledge of the specific enzymes involved in the major pathways of CBZ biotransformation, particularly cytochrome P450 (CYP) isoenzymes. Studies with purified or cloned CYP enzymes have demonstrated that the epoxidation of CBZ is mediated by CYP3A4 and CYP2C8, with CYP3A4 playing the most important role (74). These isoforms are induced by repeated administration of CBZ (75,76) and by phenobarbital (77). The subsequent hydrolysis of the epoxide to form *trans*-diol is catalyzed by a microsomal epoxide hydrolase, which is responsible for the inactivation of epoxides derived from the oxidative metabolism of xenobiotics (78). This enzyme also may be induced by repeated doses of CBZ (60,62,75) and by phenobarbital (79), although to a lesser extent than the CYP isoforms responsible for the formation of CBZ epoxide. The CYP1A2 isoform appears to be the major enzyme responsible for the aromatic hydroxylation of

CBZ (80). Direct *N*-glucuronidation of CBZ as well as glucuronidation of its metabolites are catalyzed by microsomal uridine diphosphate glucuronosyltransferase (UDPGT) (3). The specific UDPGT isoform responsible for these reactions is yet unidentified.

With regard to the genetic aspects of CBZ metabolism, of the different CYP isoenzymes involved in its oxidative reactions—namely, CYP1A2, CYP2C8, and CYP3A4—only the CYP2C8 isoform is polymorphically expressed (81). Wide interindividual variability has been reported in the expression of CYP1A2 and CYP3A4 in humans, but to date no specific polymorphisms have been identified (3). Microsomal epoxide hydrolase is universally expressed, with no evidence for enzyme-deficient phenotypes (82). Polymorphisms have been described for the UDPGT variant catalyzing glucuronidation of bilirubin, but it is not known if it is involved in CBZ glucuronidation (3).

Biliary and Renal Excretion

As previously stated, approximately 28% of an oral dose of ¹⁴C-labeled CBZ was found in the feces, suggesting both incomplete absorption and a nonnegligible biliary excretion of unidentified metabolites (15). In this respect, only 1% of a single 400-mg oral dose of CBZ was eliminated by bile within 72 hours, indicating no significant enterohepatic circulation (83). However, these results do not exclude the possibility of a more consistent biliary excretion of conjugated metabolites.

CBZ is eliminated in the urine mainly as metabolites, and elimination is faster in patients receiving other antiepileptic drugs. In epileptic patients stabilized on CBZ treatment, 20% to 60% of the daily dose is excreted as the *trans*-CBZ-diol, 5% to 11% as 9-HM-10-CA, 5% to 10% as phenolic metabolites, 1% to 2% as CBZ epoxide, and 0.5% as unchanged CBZ (60,62,84).

CLEARANCE AND HALF-LIFE

The elimination of CBZ is well described by a one-compartment open model and follows an apparent first-order process, as demonstrated by the log-linear terminal phase of the typical plasma concentration–time curve after a single dose to a normal subject (6,8). However, because of the autoinduction process, the plasma elimination of CBZ is considerably more rapid during maintenance therapy than after single-dose administration to healthy volunteers, leading to a condition defined as time-dependent kinetics (69,85). In this situation, clearance values increase and half-lives decrease with time, with the result that steady-state CBZ levels are lower than those predicted from single-dose kinetic studies. As a consequence, higher doses are needed to maintain the same plasma concentrations. Therefore, the values of the elimination parameters of CBZ depend on whether the drug has been studied after administration of its first dose or after there has been time for autoinduction to occur. The apparent plasma half-life and total-body clearance usually exhibit large interindividual differences, not only in relation to various pathophysiologic factors and coadministration of other drugs, but because the autoinduction process reaches different levels in different individuals.

Healthy Subjects

In healthy subjects, after administration of a single dose of CBZ, the plasma half-life has been reported to range from 18 to 55 hours and the corresponding clearance values from 0.013 to 0.061 L/hr/kg or from 1.14 to 1.80 L/hr (5–7). In a study of epileptic patients, the plasma half-life of CBZ declined from 35.6 ± 15.3 hours after the initial single dose to 20.9 ± 5.0 hours after repeated administration (6).

The renal clearance values for CBZ epoxide and *trans*-CBZ-diol in epileptic patients are (mean ± standard deviation) 9.7 ± 3.9 and 70.9 ± 13.9 mL/min, respectively (60). After massive CBZ overdosage, renal clearances of CBZ and CBZ epoxide were low (1 and 8 mL/min, respectively) and flow dependent, whereas renal clearance of *trans*-CBZ-diol was approximately 160 to 350 mL/min and independent of the urine flow (86).

After direct administration of CBZ epoxide to healthy volunteers, the half-life of the epoxide metabolite was found to range from 5 to 11 hours, and corresponding clearance values ranged from 0.063 to 0.136 L/hr/kg (26,28).

Comedicated Epileptic Patients

The elimination of CBZ is increased in patients receiving enzyme-inducing anticonvulsants (62,66,67). Eichelbaum et al. (85) studied CBZ kinetics in three groups of subjects: (a) healthy volunteers, (b) epileptic patients on CBZ monotherapy, and (c) epileptic patients comedicated with other anticonvulsants. The plasma clearances were 0.020 ± 0.003, 0.055 ± 0.007 and 0.113 ± 0.033 L/hr/kg in the three groups, respectively, and the corresponding half-life values were 26.2 ± 6.1, 12.3 ± 0.8, and 8.2 ± 3.3 hours. The increased clearance in the patients was due mainly to an induction of the epoxide-diol pathway, as reflected by an increased urinary excretion of the *trans*-CBZ-diol metabolite. The effect of other drugs on CBZ elimination is discussed in Chapter 23.

Children

The clearance of CBZ appears to be age dependent, with the highest disposition rate during infancy and early childhood (87,88). A within-subject study, conducted over several years, indicated that the major modifications in clearance occur between 9 and 13 years of age and that adult values are reached at 15 to 17 years of age (89). The apparent plasma half-life of CBZ is shorter in children than in adults and has been reported to range from 3 to 32 hours (65,90). In a study of children 10 to 13 years of age, the half-life of CBZ declined from 25 to 32 hours after the first single dose, to 18 to 22 hours after 4 to 6 days of treatment, and to 10 to 14 hours after 4 weeks of therapy (65). In the same children, the mean first dose clearance was 0.028 ± 0.031 L/hr/kg, which doubled to 0.056 ± 0.011 L/hr/kg after 17 to 32 days of treatment. Because of the increased clearance, children need relatively larger total daily doses of CBZ, on a milligram per kilogram basis, than adults (88,91).

Elderly

The pharmacokinetics of a single 400-mg oral dose of CBZ were compared in a group of six young healthy volunteers aged between 20 and 25 years and in a group of five elderly volunteers aged between 66 and 84 years. No age-dependent modifications in elimination parameters were detected (92). However, an age-related decrease in the apparent oral clearance of CBZ was reported in a more recent population pharmacokinetic analysis (93).

Pregnancy

Data on the elimination of CBZ during pregnancy are conflicting. Some studies found no significant changes in the total plasma concentrations and in the intrinsic clearance of CBZ during pregnancy (38,94). The observation of an increased CBZ epoxide/CBZ ratio, associated with a decrease in levels of *trans*-CBZ-diol, was explained as the result of inhibition of the epoxide hydrolase rather than increased epoxidation (38). Other studies reported a decrease in total plasma concentrations of CBZ, whereas unbound concentrations remained constant (39,95). An increase in total plasma clearance of CBZ, largely dependent on an increased epoxide formation, has been documented during pregnancy in women comedicated with an anticonvulsant (96)

Other Possible Determinants of Intersubject Variability

There are no specific studies available on the effect of liver, renal, or cardiac diseases on the elimination parameters of CBZ (2,4). Moreover, no significant interethnic differences in CBZ kinetics and metabolism are to be expected, based on observations in Asian or African patients compared with whites (4).

RELATIONSHIP BETWEEN SERUM CONCENTRATION AND DOSE

Most studies have reported a poor or weak correlation between the dose and plasma concentration of either CBZ or CBZ epoxide (30,42,97,98). In this respect, plasma levels of the metabolite were found to correlate more closely with CBZ dose than levels of the parent drug (60,99). In patients taking the same daily dose, there is a threefold to eightfold interindividual variability in steady-state plasma concentrations of CBZ and its epoxide metabolite, largely dependent on the different factors affecting the elimination of CBZ (30,42,60,97–100). When CBZ is used as monotherapy, the plasma CBZ epoxide concentrations usually are 10% to 50% of those of the parent drug, without a clear relationship between concentrations of both compounds (99,101). Apparently, the ratio of CBZ epoxide to CBZ in plasma shows wide interindividual and intraindividual variability according to a number of factors, including age, physiologic status, concurrent drug therapy, dose regimens, and dosage schedule (30,36,42,60,91,98,99, 102). Furthermore, it has been clearly documented that steady-state plasma concentrations of both CBZ and CBZ epoxide oscillate markedly during the dosing intervals. Fluctuations of 40% to 150% for CBZ and 40% to 500% for the epoxide have been described (103–105). The magnitude of these interdosage fluctuations is influenced both by the absorption characteristics of the CBZ dosage form in use and by its elimination half-life. To minimize drug fluctuations, slow-release formulations have been commercialized (14).

In individual patients receiving CBZ monotherapy, it has been shown that steady-state plasma CBZ concentrations increase linearly with the dose over the range from 200 to 1,300 mg/day (106). However, at high doses, plasma levels of CBZ were found to increase less than proportionately in relation to the magnitude of drug dosage increases (68,107–109). Such a curvilinear relationship between dose and plasma CBZ concentration is due mainly to ongoing dose-dependent autoinduction of its metabolism (72,73); alternatively, the nonlinearity may be explained by a dose dependency in the absorption of CBZ (10).

RELATIONSHIP BETWEEN SERUM CONCENTRATION AND EFFECT

Several studies have investigated the relationship between plasma CBZ concentrations and clinical effects in epilepsy. The therapeutic range of plasma concentrations of CBZ for treating epilepsy has been estimated at 4 to 12 μg/mL or 17 to 51 μmol/L (110), although different intervals have been proposed, such as 4 to 8 μg/mL (111), 4 to 10 μg/mL (97), 6 to 10 μg/mL (112), 6 to 12 μg/mL (113), or 8 to 12 μg/mL (114). The lower limit of the therapeutic range is not clearly defined, and good seizure control has been observed over a wide range of plasma concentrations. Although earlier studies (112,114), conducted mostly in patients with intractable seizures, indicated that an effective response could not be achieved at concentrations lower

than 4 to 6 μg/mL, other investigations in a broader range of epileptic patients showed that lower levels also could be effective. In this respect, Callaghan et al. (100) reported plasma CBZ concentrations from 1.2 to 8.0 μg/mL in 10 of 13 patients with complete seizure control. Shorvon et al. (111) treated 25 newly diagnosed patients with generalized tonic-clonic or partial seizures with CBZ as monotherapy, using a target concentration range of 4 to 8 μg/mL. Five patients achieved good control of seizures in spite of plasma CBZ concentrations less than 4 μg/mL. Seizures were completely controlled in 17 patients with levels within the targeted range, although they remained uncontrolled in 3 patients despite serum concentrations of 4 to 8 μg/mL. The upper limit of the therapeutic range also is poorly defined. However, although side effects have been reported to occur over a wide range of CBZ concentrations (100,114), they are more likely to appear at concentrations exceeding 10 to 12 μg/mL (110). In massive CBZ poisoning, plasma concentrations above 40 μg/mL have been associated with an increased risk of coma, seizures, respiratory failure, and cardiac conduction defects (115). During recovery from CBZ overdosage, plasma CBZ concentrations above 25 μg/mL were associated with coma and seizures, levels in the range 15 to 25 μg/mL with combativeness, hallucinations, and choreiform movements, and levels of 11 to 15 μg/mL with ataxia and drowsiness (116).

Some methodologic shortcomings may explain the discrepancies among studies (101,117). In particular, when trying to establish a therapeutic range, correlations should be studied at different dosages in the same patients or by randomization of groups of subjects to predefined dosages or plasma concentrations. It is remarkable that such data are available in only one study (111).

The concentration–response relationship for CBZ may be complicated by pharmacokinetic factors, such as the autoinduction of CBZ metabolism, the presence of an active metabolite, and variability in plasma protein binding. As previously stated, CBZ undergoes autoinduction of metabolism with a decrease in the plasma level–dose relationship and in half-life values during maintenance therapy, with a further decrease in the presence of concomitant antiepileptic drugs. Consequently, considerable interdosage fluctuations may occur in relation to the dosing interval. Therefore, collection of samples should be standardized with respect to time of dosing. A correlation between interdosage fluctuations in plasma CBZ concentrations and occurrence of intermittent side effects has been described (103,118,119). No conclusive evidence is available regarding the contribution of the active metabolite CBZ epoxide to the overall therapeutic and toxic effects (117). It is likely that, under usual conditions, CBZ epoxide does not contribute appreciably to clinical effects. However, in situations associated with abnormally elevated CBZ epoxide concentrations, such as in patients treated with inhibitors of epoxide hydrolase (Chapter 23), development of CBZ toxicity may be attributable almost completely to markedly increased concentrations of CBZ epoxide in plasma. Another factor that may complicate the concentration–response relationship for CBZ is represented by differences in plasma protein binding. However, in the case of CBZ, the extent of drug binding is relatively modest (70% to 80%) and shows limited interindividual variability, so that monitoring free instead of total plasma CBZ concentrations has not proved advantageous (41).

Pharmacodynamic factors also may contribute to explain the variability in the CBZ level–response relationship. In particular, the therapeutic response of individual patients to a given plasma CBZ concentration appears to be considerably conditioned by the type and severity of epilepsy (120). In addition, the possibility of pharmacodynamic interactions with other anticonvulsants needs to be considered. When CBZ is coadministered with enzyme-inducing anticonvulsants, therapeutic and toxic effects usually occur at low plasma drug concentrations (121,122).

A limited number of studies have investigated the relationship between plasma CBZ levels and clinical response in clinical indications other than epilepsy. In a controlled study of patients with trigeminal neuralgia, optimal pain control was achieved at the concentration range of 5.7 to 10.1 µg/mL (106). In another investigation, involving patients with neuralgic pain, plasma CBZ concentrations in the range 2 to 7 µg/mL were found to be associated with a 25% to 75% reduction in pain in 50% of patients (123). On the other hand, no correlation between plasma concentration of CBZ and clinical effects was found in 18 affectively ill patients treated with CBZ as monotherapy (43).

CONVERSION

Conversion factor:

$$CF = \frac{1,000}{\text{mol. wt. CBZ}} = \frac{1,000}{236.3}$$

Conversion:

$$(\text{µg/mL}) \times 4.23 = \text{µmol/L}$$
$$(\text{µmol/L}) \div 4.23 = \text{µg/mL}$$

REFERENCES

1. Anonymous. Carbamazepine. In: Dollery C, ed. *Therapeutic drugs*, 2nd ed. London: Churchill Livingstone, 1999:C44–C48.
2. Dickinson RG, Eadie MJ, Vajda FJE. Carbamazepine. In: Eadie MJ, Vajda FJE, eds. *Antiepileptic drugs: pharmacology and therapeutics: handbook of experimental pharmacology*, vol 138. Berlin: Springer-Verlag, 1999:271–317.
3. Faigle JW, Feldmann KF. Carbamazepine: chemistry and biotransformation. In: Levy RH, Mattson RH, Meldrum BS, eds. *Antiepileptic drugs*, 4th ed. New York: Raven Press, 1995:499–513.
4. Morselli PL. Carbamazepine: absorption, distribution, and excretion. In: Levy RH, Mattson RH, Meldrum BS, eds. *Antiepileptic drugs*, 4th ed. New York: Raven Press, 1995:515–528.
5. Levy RH, Pitlick WH, Troupin AS, et al. Pharmacokinetics of carbamazepine in normal man. *Clin Pharmacol Ther* 1975;17:657–668.
6. Eichelbaum M, Ekbom K, Bertilsson L, et al. Plasma kinetics of carbamazepine and its epoxide in man after single and multiple doses. *Eur J Clin Pharmacol* 1975;8:337–341.
7. Rawlins MD, Collste P, Bertilsson L, et al. Distribution and elimination kinetics of carbamazepine in man. *Eur J Clin Pharmacol* 1975;8:91–96.
8. Gerardin AP, Abadie FV, Campestrini JA, et al. Pharmacokinetics of carbamazepine in normal humans after single and repeated oral doses. *J Pharmacokinet Biopharm* 1976;4:521–535.
9. Popovic J, Mikov M, Jakovljevic V. Pharmacokinetics of carbamazepine derived from a new tablet formulation. *Eur J Drug Metab Pharmacokinet* 1995;20:297–300.
10. Kumps AH. Dose-dependency of the ratio between carbamazepine serum levels and dosage in patients with epilepsy. *Ther Drug Monit* 1981;3:271–274.
11. Riad LE, Chan KKW, Wagner WE, et al. Simultaneous first- and zero-order absorption of carbamazepine tablets in humans. *J Pharm Sci* 1986;75:897–900.
12. Wada JA, Troupin AS, Friel P, et al. Pharmacokinetic comparison of tablet and suspension dosage forms of carbamazepine. *Epilepsia* 1978;19:251–255.
13. Bloomer D, Dupuis LL, MacGregor D, et al. Palatability and relative bioavailability of an extemporaneous carbamazepine oral suspension. *Clin Pharm* 1987;6:646–649.
14. Bialer M. Pharmacokinetic evaluation of sustained release formulations of antiepileptic drugs. *Clin Pharmacokinet* 1992;22:11–21.
15. Faigle JW, Feldmann KF. Pharmacokinetic data of carbamazepine and its major metabolites in man. In: Schneider H, Janz D, Gardner-Thorpe C, et al., eds. *Clinical pharmacology of antiepileptic drugs*. Berlin: Springer-Verlag, 1975:159–165.
16. Gerardin A, Dubois JP, Moppert J, et al. Absolute bioavailability of carbamazepine after oral administration of a 2% syrup. *Epilepsia* 1990;31:334–338.
17. Neuvonen PJ. Bioavailability and central side effects of different carbamazepine tablets. *Int J Clin Pharmacol Ther Toxicol* 1985;23:226–232.
18. Chan KK, Sawchuk RJ, Thompson TA, et al. Bioequivalence of carbamazepine chewable and conventional tablets: single-dose and steady-state studies. *J Pharm Sci* 1985;74:866–870.
19. Patsalos PN. A comparative pharmacokinetic study of conventional and chewable carbamazepine in epileptic patients. *Br J Clin Pharmacol* 1990;29:574–577.
20. Thakker KM, Mangat S, Garnett WR, et al. Comparative bioavailability and steady state fluctuations of Tegretol commercial and carbamazepine OROS tablets in adult and pediatric epileptic patients. *Biopharm Drug Dispos* 1992;13:559–569.
21. Reunanen M, Heinonen EH, Nyman L, et al. Comparative bioavailability of carbamazepine from two slow-release preparations. *Epilepsy Res* 1992;11:61–66.
22. Graves NM, Kriel RL, Jones-Saete C, et al. Relative bioavailability of rectally administered carbamazepine suspension in humans. *Epilepsia* 1985;26:429–433.
23. Neuvonen PJ, Tokola O. Bioavailability of rectally administered carbamazepine mixture. *Br J Clin Pharmacol* 1987;24:839–841.
24. Arvidsson J, Nilsson HL, Sandstedt P, et al. Replacing carbamazepine slow-release tablets with carbamazepine suppositories: a pharmacokinetic and clinical study in children with epilepsy. *J Child Neurol* 1995;10:114–117.

25. Loscher W, Honack D. Intravenous carbamazepine: comparison of different parenteral formulations in a mouse model of convulsive status epilepticus. *Epilepsia* 1997;38:106–113.

26. Tomson T, Tybring G, Bertilsson L. Single-dose kinetics and metabolism of carbamazepine-10,11-epoxide. *Clin Pharmacol Ther* 1983;33:58–65.

27. Sumi M, Watari N, Umezawa O, et al. Pharmacokinetic study of carbamazepine and its epoxide metabolite in humans. *J Pharmacobiodyn* 1987;10:652–661.

28. Spina E, Tomson T, Svensson J-O, et al. Single-dose kinetics of an enteric-coated formulation of carbamazepine-10,11-epoxide, an active metabolite of carbamazepine. *Ther Drug Monit* 1988; 10:382–385.

29. Hooper WD, Dubetz DK, Bochner F, et al. Plasma protein binding of carbamazepine. *Clin Pharmacol Ther* 1975;17: 433–440.

30. Johannessen SI, Gerna M, Bakke J, et al. CSF concentrations and serum protein binding of carbamazepine and carbamazepine-10,11-epoxide in epileptic patients. *Br J Clin Pharmacol* 1976;3:575–582.

31. MacKichan JJ, Duffner PK, Cohen ME. Salivary concentrations and plasma protein binding of carbamazepine and carbamazepine-10,11-epoxide in epileptic patients. *Br J Clin Pharmacol* 1981;12:31–37.

32. MacKichan JJ, Zola EM. Determinants of carbamazepine and carbamazepine-10,11-epoxide binding to serum protein, albumin and alpha 1-acid glycoprotein. *Br J Clin Pharmacol* 1984; 18:487–493.

33. Pynnonen S, Sillanpaa M, Frey H, et al. Carbamazepine and its 10,11-epoxide in children and adults with epilepsy. *Eur J Clin Pharmacol* 1977;11:129–133.

34. Kuhnz W, Steldinger R, Nau H. Protein binding of carbamazepine and its epoxide in maternal and fetal plasma at delivery: comparison to other anticonvulsants. *Dev Pharmacol Ther* 1984;7:61–72.

35. Groce JB III, Casto DT, Gal P. Carbamazepine and carbamazepine-epoxide serum protein binding in newborn infants. *Ther Drug Monit* 1985;7:274–276.

36. Riva R, Contin M, Albani F, et al. Free and total serum concentrations of carbamazepine and carbamazepine-10,11-epoxide in infancy and childhood. *Epilepsia* 1986;26:320–322.

37. Koyama H, Sugioka N, Uno A, et al. Age-related alteration of carbamazepine-serum protein binding in man. *J Pharm Pharmacol* 1999;51:1009–1014.

38. Yerby MS, Friel PN, Miller DQ. Carbamazepine protein binding and disposition in pregnancy. *Ther Drug Monit* 1985;7: 269–273.

39. Yerby MS, Friel PN, McCormick K, et al. Pharmacokinetics of anticonvulsants in pregnancy: alterations in plasma protein binding. *Epilepsy Res* 1990;5:223–228.

40. Baruzzi A, Contin M, Perucca E, et al. Altered serum protein binding of carbamazepine in disease states associated with an increased α_1-acid glycoprotein concentration. *Eur J Clin Pharmacol* 1986;31:85–89.

41. Perucca E. Free level monitoring of antiepileptic drugs: clinical usefulness and case studies. *Clin Pharmacokinet* 1984;9[Suppl 1]:71–78.

42. Eichelbaum M, Bertilsson L, Lund L, et al. Plasma levels of carbamazepine and carbamazepine-10,11-epoxide during treatment of epilepsy. *Eur J Clin Pharmacol* 1976;9:417–421.

43. Post RM, Uhde TW, Ballenger JC, et al. Carbamazepine and its -10,11-epoxide metabolite in plasma and CSF: relationship to antidepressant response. *Arch Gen Psychiatry* 1983;40:673–676.

44. Morselli PL, Baruzzi A, Gerna M, et al. Carbamazepine and carbamazepine-10,11-epoxide concentration in human brain. *Br J Clin Pharmacol* 1977;4:535–540.

45. Friis ML, Christiansen J, Hvidberg EF. Brain concentration of carbamazepine and carbamazepine-10,11-epoxide in epileptic patients. *Eur J Clin Pharmacol* 1978;14:47–51.

46. Rambeck B, Schnabel R, May T, et al. Postmortem concentrations of phenobarbital, carbamazepine and its metabolite carbamazepine-10,11-epoxide in different region of the brain and in the serum: analysis of autoptic specimens from 51 epileptic patients. *Ther Drug Monit* 1993;15:91–98.

47. Chambers RE, Homeida M, Hunter KR, et al. Salivary carbamazepine concentrations. *Lancet* 1977;1:656–657.

48. Westenberg HGM, van der Kleijn E, Oei TT, et al. Kinetics of carbamazepine and carbamazepine and carbamazepine-epoxide, determined by use of plasma and saliva. *Clin Pharmacol Ther* 1978;23:320–328.

49. Monaco F, Mutani R, Mastropaolo C, et al. Tears as the best practical indicator of unbound fraction of an anticonvulsant drug. *Epilepsia* 1979;20:705–710.

50. Pynnonen S, Yrjana T. The significance of the simultaneous determination of carbamazepine and its 10,11-epoxide from plasma and human erythrocytes. *Int J Clin Pharmacol* 1977; 15:222–226.

51. Pynnonen S, Kanto J, Sillanpaa M, et al. Carbamazepine: placental transport, tissue concentrations in foetus and newborn and level in milk. *Acta Pharmacol Toxicol* 1977;41:244–253.

52. Meyer FP, Quednow B, Potrafki A, et al. Pharmacokinetics of anticonvulsants in the perinatal period. *Zentralbl Gynakol* 1988; 110:1195–1205.

53. Takeda A, Okada H, Tanaka H, et al. Protein binding of four antiepileptic drugs in maternal and umbilical cord serum. *Epilepsy Res* 1992;13:147–151.

54. Piafsky KM, Rane A. Formation of carbamazepine epoxide in human fetal liver. *Drug Metab Dispos* 1978;6:502–503.

55. Omtzigt JG, Los FJ, Meijer JWA, et al. The 10,11-epoxide–10,11-diol pathway of carbamazepine in early pregnancy in maternal serum, urine, and amniotic fluid: effect of dose, comedication, and relation to outcome of pregnancy. *Ther Drug Monit* 1993;15:1–10.

56. Kuhnz W, Jager-Roman E, Rating D, et al. Carbamazepine and carbamazepine-10,11-epoxide during pregnancy and postnatal period in epileptic mothers and their nursed infants: pharmacokinetic and clinical effects. *Pediatr Pharmacol* 1983;3:199–208.

57. Froescher W, Eichelbaum M, Niesen M, et al. Carbamazepine levels in breast milk. *Ther Drug Monit* 1984;6:266–271.

58. Wedlund PL, Chang SL, Levy RH. Steady-state determination of the contribution of lung metabolism to the total body clearance of drugs: application to carbamazepine. *J Pharm Sci* 1983; 72:860–862.

59. Eto S, Tanaka N, Noda H, et al. Chiral separation of 10,11-dihydro-10,11-trans-dihydrocarbamazepine, a metabolite with two asymmetric carbons, in human serum. *J Chromatogr B Biomed Appl* 1996;677:325–330.

60. Bourgeois BFD, Wad N. Carbamazepine-10,11-diol steady-state serum levels and renal excretion during carbamazepine therapy in adults and children. *Ther Drug Monit* 1984;6:259–265.

61. Eto S, Tanaka N, Noda H, et al. 9-Hydroxymethyl-10-carbamoylacridan in human serum is one of the major metabolites of carbamazepine. *Biol Pharm Bull* 1995;18:926–928.

62. Eichelbaum M, Tomson T, Tybring G, et al. Carbamazepine metabolism in man: induction and pharmacogenetic aspects. *Clin Pharmacokinet* 1985;10:80–90.

63. Madden S, Maggs JL, Park BK. Bioactivation of carbamazepine in the rat in vivo: evidence for the formation of reactive arene oxide(s). *Drug Metab Dispos* 1996;24:469–479.

64. Kerr BM, Levy RH. Carbamazepine: carbamazepine epoxide. In: Levy RH, Mattson RH, Meldrum BS, eds. *Antiepileptic drugs*, 4th ed. New York: Raven Press, 1995:529–541.

65. Bertilsson L, Hojer B, Tybring G, et al. Autoinduction of carbamazepine metabolism in children examined by a stable isotope technique. *Clin Pharmacol Ther* 1980;27:83–88.

66. Christiansen J, Dam M. Influence of phenobarbital and diphenylhydantoin on plasma carbamazepine levels in patients with epilepsy. *Acta Neurol Scand* 1973;49:543–546.

67. Eichelbaum M, Kothe KW, Hoffmann F, et al. Kinetics and metabolism of carbamazepine during combined antiepileptic drug therapy. *Clin Pharmacol Ther* 1979;26: 366-371.

68. Bernus I, Dickinson RG, Hooper WD, et al. Dose-dependent metabolism of carbamazepine in humans. *Epilepsy Res* 1996; 24:163–172.

69. McNamara PJ, Coburn WA, Gibaldi M. Time course of carbamazepine self-induction. *J Pharmacokinet Biopharm* 1979;7: 63–68.

70. Bernus I, Dickinson RG, Hooper WD, et al. Early stage autoinduction of carbamazepine metabolism in humans. *Eur J Clin Pharmacol* 1994;47:355–360.

71. Bertilsson L, Tomson T, Tybring G. Pharmacokinetics: time-dependent changes: autoinduction of carbamazepine epoxidation. *J Clin Pharmacol* 1986;26:459–462.

72. Mikati MA, Browne TR, Collins JF. Time course of carbamazepine autoinduction. *Neurology* 1989;39:592–594.

73. Kudriakova TB, Sirota LA, Ruzova GI, et al. Autoinduction and steady-state pharmacokinetics of carbamazepine and its major metabolites. *Br J Clin Pharmacol* 1992;33:611–615.

74. Kerr BM, Thummel KE, Wurden CJ, et al. Human liver carbamazepine metabolism: role of CYP3A4 and CYP2C8 in 10,11-epoxide formation. *Biochem Pharmacol* 1994;47:1969–1979.

75. Tybring G, von Bahr C, Bertilsson L, et al. Metabolism of carbamazepine and its epoxide metabolite in human and rat liver in vitro. *Drug Metab Dispos Biol Fate Chem* 1981;9:561–564.

76. Regnaud L, Sirois G, Chakrabati S. Effect of four-day treatment with carbamazepine at different dose levels on microsomal enzyme induction, drug metabolism and drug toxicity. *Pharmacol Toxicol* 1988;62:3–6.

77. Wagner J, Schmid K. Induction of microsomal enzymes in rat liver by oxcarbazepine, 10,11-dihydro-10-hydroxy-carbamazepine and carbamazepine. *Xenobiotica* 1987;17:951–956.

78. Kitteringham NR, Davis C, Howard N, et al. Interindividual and interspecies variation in hepatic microsomal epoxide hydrolase activity: studies with cis-stilbene, carbamazepine-10,11-epoxide and naphthalene. *J Pharmacol Exp Ther* 1996;278: 1018–1027.

79. Spina E, Martines C, Fazio A, et al. Effect of phenobarbital on the pharmacokinetics of carbamazepine-10,11-epoxide, an active metabolite of carbamazepine. *Ther Drug Monit* 1991;13: 109–112.

80. Johnson CM, Thummel KE, Kroetz DL, et al. Metabolism of CBZ by cytochrome P450 isoforms 3A4, 2C8 and 1A2. *Pharm Res* 1992;9:s-301.

81. Rettie AE, Koop DR, Haining RL. CYP2C. In: Levy RH, Thummel KE, Trager WF, et al., eds. *Metabolic drug interactions*. Philadelphia: Lippincott Williams & Wilkins, 2000: 75–86.

82. Kroetz DL, Kerr BM, McFarland LV, et al. Measurement of *in vivo* microsomal epoxide hydrolase activity in white subjects. *Clin Pharmacol Ther* 1993;53:306–315.

83. Terhaag B, Richter K, Diettrich H. Concentration behavior of carbamazepine in bile and plasma of man. *Int J Clin Pharmacol Biopharm* 1978;16:607–609.

84. Eichelbaum M, Kothe KW, Hoffmann F, et al. Use of stable labelled carbamazepine to study its kinetics during chronic carbamazepine treatment. *Eur J Clin Pharmacol* 1982;23: 241–244.

85. Suzuki K, Kaneko S, Sato T. Time-dependency of serum carbamazepine concentration. *Folia Psychiatr Neurol Jpn* 1978;32: 199–209.

86. Vree TB, Janssen TH, Hekster YA, et al. Clinical pharmacokinetics of carbamazepine and its epoxy and hydroxy metabolites in humans after an overdose. *Ther Drug Monit* 1986;8: 297–304.

87. Battino D, Bossi L, Croci D, et al. Carbamazepine plasma levels in children and adults: influence of age and associated therapy. *Ther Drug Monit* 1980;2:315–322.

88. Leppick IE. Metabolism of antiepileptic medication: newborn to elderly. *Epilepsia* 1992;33[Suppl 4]:32–40.

89. Albani F, Riva R, Contin M, et al. A within-subject analysis of carbamazepine disposition related to development in children with epilepsy. *Ther Drug Monit* 1992;14:457–460.

90. Rey E, d'Athis P, de Lauture D, et al. Pharmacokinetics of carbamazepine in the neonate and in the child. *Int J Clin Pharmacol Biopharm* 1979;17:90–96.

91. Rylance GW, Edwards C, Gard PR. Carbamazepine-10,11-epoxide in children. *Br J Clin Pharmacol* 1984;18:935–939.

92. Hockings N, Pall A, Moody J, et al. The effects of age on carbamazepine pharmacokinetics and adverse effects. *Br J Clin Pharmacol* 1986;22:725–728.

93. Graves NM, Brundage RC, Wen Y, et al. Population pharmacokinetics of carbamazepine in adults with epilepsy. *Pharmacotherapy* 1998;18:273–281.

94. Tomson T, Lindbom U, Ekqvist B, et al. Disposition of carbamazepine and phenytoin in pregnancy. *Epilepsia* 1994;35: 131–135.

95. Battino D, Binelli S, Bossi L, et al. Plasma concentrations of carbamazepine and carbamazepine-10,11-epoxide during pregnancy and after delivery. *Clin Pharmacokinet* 1985;10:279–284.

96. Bernus I, Hooper WD, Dickinson RG, et al. Metabolism of carbamazepine and co-administered anticonvulsants during pregnancy. *Epilepsy Res* 1995;21:65–75.

97. Monaco F, Riccio A, Benna P, et al. Further observations on carbamazepine plasma levels in epileptic patients: relationship with therapeutic and side effects. *Neurology* 1976;26:936–943.

98. Rapeport WG. Factors influencing the relationship between carbamazepine plasma concentration and its clinical effects in patients with epilepsy. *Clin Neuropharmacol* 1985;8:141–149.

99. McKauge L, Tyrer JH, Eadie MJ. Factors influencing simultaneous concentrations of carbamazepine and its epoxide in plasma. *Ther Drug Monit* 1981;3:63–70.

100. Callaghan N, O'Callaghan M, Duggan B, et al. Carbamazepine as a single dose in the treatment of epilepsy: a prospective study of serum levels and seizure control. *J Neurol Neurosurg Psychiatry* 1978;11:309–329.

101. Bertilsson L, Tomson T. Clinical pharmacokinetics and pharmacological effects of carbamazepine and carbamazepine-10, 11-epoxide: an update. *Clin Pharmacokinet* 1986;11:177–198.

102. Brodie MJ, Forrest G, Rapeport WG. Carbamazepine-10,11-epoxide concentrations in epileptics on carbamazepine alone and in combination with other anticonvulsants. *Br J Clin Pharmacol* 1983;16:747–750.

103. Tomson T. Interdosage fluctuations in plasma carbamazepine concentration determine intermittent side effects. *Arch Neurol* 1984;41:830–834.

104. Elyas AA, Patsalos PN, Agbato OA, et al. Factors influencing simultaneous concentrations of total and free carbamazepine and carbamazepine-10,11-epoxide in serum of children with epilepsy. *Ther Drug Monit* 1986;8:288–292.

105. Macphee GJ, Butler E, Brodie MJ. Intradose and circadian variation in circulating carbamazepine and its epoxide in epileptic patients: a consequence of autoinduction of metabolism. *Epilepsia* 1987;28:286–294.

106. Tomson T, Tybring G, Bertilsson L, et al. Carbamazepine ther-

apy in trigeminal neuralgia: clinical effects in relation to plasma concentration. *Arch Neurol* 1980;37:699–703.

107. Cotter LM, Eadie MJ, Hooper WD, et al. The pharmacokinetics of carbamazepine. *Eur J Clin Pharmacol* 1977;12:451–456.

108. Perucca E, Bittencourt P, Richens A. Effect of dose increments on serum carbamazepine concentration in epileptic patients. *Clin Pharmacokinet* 1980;5:576–582.

109. Tomson T, Svensson JO, Hilton-Brown P. Relationship between intraindividual dose to plasma concentration of carbamazepine: indication of dose-dependent induction of metabolism. *Ther Drug Monit* 1989;11:533–539.

110. Johannessen SI. Laboratory monitoring of antiepileptic drugs. In: Levy RH, Mattson RH, Meldrum BS, eds. *Antiepileptic drugs*, 4th ed. New York: Raven Press, 1995:179–188.

111. Shorwon SD, Chadwick D, Galbraith AW, et al. One drug for epilepsy. *BMJ* 1978;1:474–476.

112. Simonsen N, Olsen IZ, Kuhl V, et al. A comparative controlled study between carbamazepine and diphenylhydantoin in psychomotor epilepsy. *Epilepsia* 1976;17:169–176.

113. Porter RJ, Theodore WH. Nonsedative regimens in the treatment of epilepsy. *Arch Intern Med* 1983;143:945–947.

114. Troupin A, Moretti-Ojemann L, Halpern L, et al. Carbamazepine: a double-blind comparison with phenytoin. *Neurology* 1977;27:511–519.

115. Hojer J, Malmlund HO, Berg A. Clinical features of 28 consecutive cases of laboratory confirmed massive poisoning with carbamazepine alone. *J Toxicol Clin Toxicol* 1993;31:449–458.

116. Weaver DF, Camfield P, Fraser A. Massive carbamazepine overdose : clinical and pharmacologic observations in five episodes. *Neurology* 1988;38:755–759.

117. Bialer M, Levy RH, Perucca E. Does carbamazepine have a narrow therapeutic plasma concentration range? *Ther Drug Monit* 1998;20:56–59.

118. Hoppener RJ, Kuyer A, Meijer JWA, et al. Correlation between daily fluctuations of carbamazepine serum levels and intermittent side effects. *Epilepsia* 1980;2:341–350.

119. Riva R, Albani F, Ambrosetto G, et al. Diurnal fluctuations in free and total steady-state plasma levels of carbamazepine and correlation with intermittent side effects. *Epilepsia* 1984;25:476–481.

120. Schmidt D, Einicke I, Haenel F. The influence of seizure type on the efficacy of plasma concentrations of phenytoin, phenobarbital, and carbamazepine. *Arch Neurol* 1986;43:263–265.

121. Kutt H, Solomon G, Wasterlain C, et al. Carbamazepine in difficult to control epileptic outpatients. *Acta Neurol Scand Suppl* 1975;60:27–32.

122. Riva R, Contin M, Albani F, et al. Lateral gaze nystagmus in carbamazepine-treated epileptic patients: correlation with total and free plasma concentrations of parent drug and its 10,11 epoxide metabolite. *Ther Drug Monit* 1985;7:277–282.

123. Moosa RS, McFayden ML, Miller R, et al. Carbamazepine and its metabolites in neuralgias: concentration–effect relations. *Eur J Clin Pharmacol* 1993;45:297–301.

CARBAMAZEPINE

INTERACTIONS WITH OTHER DRUGS

COLLEEN J. WURDEN
RENÉ H. LEVY

Carbamazepine (CBZ) is associated with clinically relevant drug interactions with a variety of other therapeutic agents. CBZ is almost completely cleared by metabolism, with less than 5% of a dose excreted unchanged in urine (1). The main pathway of metabolism is conversion to the active 10,11-epoxide (CBZE). Cytochrome P450 (CYP) 3A4 (CYP3A4) has been identified as the primary isoform that catalyzes the oxidation to the epoxide, whereas CYP2C8 is a minor contributor to this pathway in human liver (2). CYP3A4 also is constitutively expressed in the human intestine. Microsomes prepared from intestinal tissue can catalyze the epoxidation of CBZ, although the *in vivo* contribution of the intestine to the total clearance of CBZ probably is small (3). The epoxide subsequently is hydrated to a *trans*-dihydrodiol by microsomal epoxide hydrolase (4). In patients receiving CBZ chronically, 30% to 50% of a dose is excreted as the diol in urine (5). Because 90% of CBZ epoxide is converted to CBZ diol (6), it can be concluded that 30% to 50% of a dose of CBZ goes through the epoxidation pathway and a significant fraction of the primary metabolism is mediated by CYP3A4.

Several other characteristics of CBZ increase its susceptibility to interactions with other drugs. CBZ has a narrow therapeutic range, and, in an effort to maintain seizure control with a single anticonvulsant agent, plasma CBZ concentrations often are maximized to the upper limit of tolerance. Also, CBZ is a low-clearance drug, and thus sensitive to enzyme induction or enzyme inhibition, especially because a large number of drugs inhibit or induce CYP3A4.

Because CBZ is an inducer of CYP3A4 and other metabolic enzymes, another type of drug interaction resulting in subtherapeutic plasma concentrations of other agents can occur. Last, because CBZE can contribute to both thera-

peutic effect and toxicity, its interactions must be taken into consideration (7).

EFFECTS OF OTHER DRUGS ON CARBAMAZEPINE

Inhibition of Carbamazepine Metabolism

Inhibition of CBZ metabolism can occur when a coadministered drug competes with CBZ for binding to metabolic enzymes. Inhibitory drug interactions occur when the coadministered drug binds to CYP3A4 and reaches concentrations at the site of the enzyme that are high enough relative to the K_i (affinity of the inhibitor for binding to the enzyme) to inhibit a significant fraction of the CYP3A4 population. Inhibition of isoforms other than CYP3A4 has not been implicated in drug interactions resulting in decreased clearance of CBZ. Conversion to CBZE accounts for 30% to 50% of total CBZ clearance (5); thus, inhibition of this pathway can result in 1.5- to 2-fold increases in steady-state plasma levels of CBZ. Because CBZE is pharmacologically active, interactions leading to changes in the plasma concentration of this metabolite (e.g., due to inhibition of epoxide hydrolase) also can be clinically relevant, and they also are described in this section.

The binding affinity (K_m) of CBZ to CYP3A4 determined in expressed CYP3A4 is 442 μmol/L (10-fold higher than therapeutic concentrations). Therefore, CBZ concentrations *in vivo* are far below those required to cause significant inhibition of CYP3A4 (2). Accordingly, there have been no reported interactions with CBZ resulting in decreased clearance of another CYP3A4-metabolized drug.

Anticonvulsants

Lamotrigine

Although lamotrigine has been reported occasionally to increase the plasma concentration of CBZE, possibly by inhibiting epoxide hydrolase, most studies found no changes in plasma CBZ or CBZE concentration after addition of

Colleen J. Wurden, MD: Department of Pharmaceutics, University of Washington School of Pharmacy and Medicine, Seattle, Washington

René H. Levy, PhD: Professor and Chair, Department of Pharmaceutics, Professor of Neurophysical Surgery, University of Washington School of Pharmacy and Medicine, Seattle, Washington

lamotrigine (8), and one study in healthy volunteers showed no effect of lamotrigine on the kinetic parameters of orally administered CBZE (9). Based on these findings, lamotrigine's ability to potentiate the adverse effects of CBZ probably can be attributed to a pharmacodynamic interaction (10).

Remacemide

Remacemide (300 mg twice daily) increased plasma CBZ concentrations by 20% to 30% without consistent changes in the concentrations of CBZE, suggesting concomitant inhibition of the epoxidation pathway (11). In addition, the areas under the under the plasma concentration versus time curves (AUCs) of remacemide and its active metabolite were 60% and 30%, respectively, in patients who received CBZ compared with values observed in healthy volunteers treated only with remacemide, suggesting that CBZ induces the clearance of remacemide (11).

Stiripentol

Stiripentol is a broad-spectrum inhibitor of oxidative metabolic enzymes, including CYP3A4 (12). The formation clearance of CBZ to CBZE was inhibited by stiripentol in seven epileptic patients by 50% (0.212 to 0.091 mL/min/kg) (13). In agreement, in human liver microsomal incubations with therapeutic concentrations of CBZ (14 μg/mL) and stiripentol (7 μg/mL), stiripentol inhibited CBZE formation velocity by 40% to 50%. Additional studies in our laboratory found that stiripentol also inhibited the metabolism of CBZ to two minor metabolites, 2-OH-CBZ and 3-OH-CBZ, that account for approximately 20% of CBZ clearance *in vivo* and appear to be formed by multiple CYP isoforms in microsomal incubations (unpublished results).

Valproic Acid

Administration of the anticonvulsant valproic acid is widely reported to increase the ratio of CBZE to CBZ. Also, valproic acid coadministration increased the CBZE half-life and decreased CBZE clearance in six patients (14). Although in theory, increased CBZE plasma concentrations could contribute to symptoms of CBZ toxicity, this has not been clearly demonstrated, and the interaction may be clinically insignificant (15,16).

Valpromide

Valpromide, the amide derivative of valproic acid, is used in many countries as an antiepileptic and as a mood-stabilizing agent. Compared with valproic acid, valpromide is a much more potent inhibitor of epoxide hydrolase, and by this mechanism it can lead to a very marked increase in plasma CBZE concentration (16). The interaction is clinically relevant because it often results in signs of CBZ intoxication.

Vigabatrin

Vigabatrin is a newer anticonvulsant that is not metabolized by liver enzymes; however, addition of vigabatrin to CBZ monotherapy causes elevated CBZ plasma levels. In most studies, vigabatrin has not been found to affect plasma CBZ levels (17). In a recent investigation in 66 epileptic patients, however, mean CBZ concentrations were increased by an average of 14% (9.41 versus 11.31 μg/mL, $p < .001$) after the addition of vigabatrin (average dose, 31.1 mg/kg/day; average CBZ dose, 16.7 mg/kg/day) (18).

Antidepressants

Fluoxetine

The addition of fluoxetine to maintenance regimens of CBZ in patients and healthy volunteers resulted in increased plasma CBZ concentrations in some but not all studies (19–22). There are two case reports describing patients who received CBZ chronically. The addition of fluoxetine to their drug regimens resulted in CBZ plasma level increases of 33% to 63% (22). Fluoxetine was reported significantly to decrease both oral and intrinsic clearance of CBZ in a clinical study with six patients (21). Conversely, at least one clinical trial with CBZ and fluoxetine in eight subjects found that steady-state plasma concentrations of CBZ and CBZE were not affected by coadministration of fluoxetine (23). In human liver microsomes, we found that fluoxetine could mildly inhibit conversion of CBZ to CBZE only at concentrations 25 times therapeutic (unpublished results). Fluoxetine also was a weak inhibitor of the CYP3A4 probe activity, 10-hydroxylation of (R)-warfarin. Gidal et al. obtained results similar to ours in human liver microsomes (20). *In vitro* kinetic studies determined the K_i for fluoxetine inhibition of the CYP3A4-mediated 1'-hydroxylation of midazolam to be 65.7 μmol/L (100-fold higher than therapeutic), which also suggests that fluoxetine is not a reversible CYP3A4 inhibitor at clinical concentrations (24).

Other research indicates that fluoxetine coadministration has the potential to decrease the clearance of alprazolam, a compound that is metabolized by CYP3A4 (25–27). The impairment was attributed mainly to inhibition of alprazolam clearance by norfluoxetine, a primary circulating metabolite of fluoxetine, because the decrease in alprazolam clearance persisted for 12 days after discontinuation of fluoxetine, when norfluoxetine still was detectable in plasma but fluoxetine was not (27). Norfluoxetine appears to be a more potent inhibitor of CYP3A4 than fluoxetine and is known to accumulate in the plasma after multiple dosing of fluoxetine. In human liver microsomes, the K_i for inhibition of conversion of midazolam to 1'-hydroxymidazolam by norfluoxetine was 19.1 μmol/L (24). Because this metabolite has a lower K_i for CYP3A4 than its parent, we investigated the possibility that inhibition of CBZ metabolism was the result of inhibition by this metabolite. *In vitro*, norfluoxetine demonstrated an ability to inhibit the CYP3A4-mediated epoxidation of CBZ and 10-hydroxylation of (R)-warfarin only at norfluoxetine concentrations that were 25 times higher than expected in plasma *in vivo* (unpublished results). Also, norfluoxetine did not significantly inhibit formation of either of the phenolic metabolites of CBZ. Our *in vitro* results suggest that fluoxetine and its metabolite, norfluoxetine, are not potent reversible inhibitors of CBZ metabolism. In agreement with these results, concurrent fluoxetine administration did not result in decreased clearance of the CYP3A4 substrates, cyclosporine, triazolam, and terfenadine (28–30). Recently, however, fluoxetine was shown to bind irreversibly to and inactivate CYP3A4 *in vitro* at rates sufficient to affect *in vivo* concentrations of CYP3A4, resulting in inhibition of clearance (31).

Fluvoxamine

Fluvoxamine is a moderate inhibitor of CYP3A4 and inhibited the *in vitro* metabolism of alprazolam, terfenadine, and triazolam, which are metabolized predominantly by CYP3A4 (32–34). In addition, fluvoxamine decreased the clearance of alprazolam by 55% in 10 healthy men (35). Interactions between CBZ and fluvoxamine have been suggested in case reports (36,37). Addition of fluvoxamine 600 mg/day to the regimen of a patient previously maintained on CBZ increased plasma concentrations of CBZ from 7.3 to 12.4 μg/mL (38). However, no interaction was observed in a controlled study of fluvoxamine addition to steady-state CBZ therapy in seven subjects (23).

Viloxazine

Viloxazine has been suggested to be less epileptogenic than conventional antidepressants and therefore can be used in depressed epileptic patients. Viloxazine was added to the therapeutic regimen of six epileptic patients with symptoms of depression, and plasma levels of CBZ increased 55%, from 7.5 ± 3.2 to 11.6 ± 4.8 μg/mL (39). CBZ epoxide levels also increased from 0.76 ± 0.32 to 0.88 ± 0.40 μg/mL. These results suggest that viloxazine is an inhibitor of oxidative metabolism to the epoxide, as well as inhibiting epoxide clearance to the *trans*-diol. However, further work to determine the effect of viloxazine on CBZE clearance after administration of CBZE demonstrated no decrease in clearance to the *trans*-diol metabolite (40).

Nefazodone

The steady-state AUC of CBZ increased from 60.77 ± 8.44 to 74.98 ± 12.88 μg/hr/mL ($p < .001$) in 12 subjects after the addition of nefazodone (200 mg/day for 5 days). Also, during the combined administration period, the steady-state AUC of nefazodone decreased from 7,326 ± 3,768 to 542 ± 191 ng /hr/mL, suggesting that CBZ induces the clearance of nefazodone (41).

Other Psychoactive Agents

Loxapine

Elevation of the CBZE:CBZ ratio in plasma, possibly related to inhibition of epoxide hydrolase, has been reported in patients receiving CBZ and the antipsychotic loxapine; however, no adverse effects were noted (42).

Valnoctamide

Valnoctamide, a valproic acid derivative used in some countries as an over-the-counter tranquilizer, has been shown to inhibit epoxide hydrolase both *in vitro* and *in vivo*, and by this mechanism to increase the plasma concentration of CBZE in CBZ-treated patients (43). The interaction can result in clinical signs of CBZ intoxication.

Calcium Channel Blockers

Diltiazem

Coadministration of CBZ and diltiazem has been reported to increase CBZ plasma concentrations up to 50% (44–47). Two diltiazem metabolites (*N*-desmethyl-diltiazem and *N,N*-didesmethyl-diltiazem) are more potent inhibitors (11 and 200 times, respectively) of CYP3A4-mediated testosterone-6-β-hydroxylation than diltiazem, suggesting that these metabolites are most likely the major contributors to this interaction (48).

Verapamil

Verapamil (120 mg three times a day) was given as adjunctive therapy to six patients with refractory partial epilepsy receiving CBZ. Within a few days, symptoms of CBZ neurotoxicity developed in all six patients. There was a mean rise of 46% in total and 33% in free plasma CBZ concentrations in five of these patients (49). Verapamil is extensively metabolized in the liver by several CYP isoenzymes, including CYP3A4, CYP2C8, and CYP1A2, to several metabolites (50,51). However, the *in vitro* K_i values determined for the inhibition of CYP3A4 by verapamil are significantly higher than levels attained therapeutically. In addition, K_m values determined for verapamil metabolism by CYP3A4 and CYP2C8 also are significantly higher than therapeutic verapamil plasma concentrations, suggesting that simple competitive inhibition by verapamil *in vivo* is unlikely (50). *In vitro*, inhibition of CBZ metabolism was found to be minor at therapeutic concentrations of verapamil (unpublished results from our laboratory). One metabolite of verapamil, norverapamil, accumulates *in vivo* at plasma levels comparable with the parent drug, and could contribute to inhibition of CBZ metabolism (52). In addition, verapamil concentrations at the active site of the enzyme may be significantly higher than measured in plasma because mouse liver concentrations are 1,000-fold higher than mouse plasma concentrations (53).

Macrolide Antibiotics

For the purposes of drug interactions, macrolide antibiotics can be classified into three groups (54). The first includes troleandomycin and erythromycin, which are metabolized by CYP3A4 to nitrosoalkanes that form stable complexes with the heme of CYP and render it inactive (55). CBZ interactions with erythromycin and troleandomycin have been reported on multiple occasions since the late 1970s (56). Mesdjian et al. described 17 patients on CBZ who became intoxicated within 24 to 48 hours after receiving troleandomycin (8 to 33 mg/kg/day) (57). Symptoms of toxicity disappeared 2 to 3 days after troleandomycin was withdrawn. Erythromycin interaction reports typically note a twofold to fourfold increase in serum CBZ concentrations within 24 to 72 hours after the addition of erythromycin.

Josamycin, flurithromycin, roxithromycin, clarithromycin, miocamycin, and midecamycin comprise the second group, which form complexes to a lesser extent, are less potent inhibitors, and sometimes cause drug interactions. Slight but statistically significant decreases in plasma clearance of CBZ were reported after single or multiple doses of josamycin in healthy volunteers and in patients with epilepsy, although none of the subjects had symptoms of CBZ toxicity (58,59). In normal volunteers, coadministration of flurithromycin (500 mg three times daily for 10 days) resulted in a slight but statistically significant increase in CBZ AUC and a 25% decrease in the AUC of the CBZE metabolite, suggesting inhibition of this pathway of CBZ clearance (60). Coadministration of roxithromycin did not affect the clearance of CBZ (61). Administration of clarithromycin (500 mg/day) to a patient maintained on CBZ resulted in increased plasma concentration of CBZ and decreased plasma concentration of CBZE, indicating inhibition of the epoxide pathway of CBZ elimination (62). Miocamycin caused a 13% increase in the CBZ AUC and a 26% decrease in the AUC of CBZE (63).

Members of the third group—spiramycin, rokitamycin, dirithromycin, and azithromycin—do not inactivate CYP and do not appear to modify the clearance of other compounds cleared by CYP3A4 (54,64).

Isoniazid

Addition of the antitubercular agent isoniazid to the therapeutic regimen of 13 patients receiving CBZ resulted in elevated plasma CBZ concentrations and signs of CBZ toxicity in 10 of those patients (65). In one patient, CBZ clearance decreased 45% when isoniazid (300 mg for 3 days) was coadministered (66). Another patient demonstrated elevated CBZ serum levels and symptoms of CBZ toxicity 5 days after the addition of isoniazid to his regimen (67). *In vitro* experiments demonstrated that isoniazid is a potent inhibitor of CBZ epoxidation and of CYP3A4-mediated (R)-10-warfarin hydroxylation at a therapeutically relevant concentration (unpublished results). These findings suggest that isoniazid is a CYP3A4 inhibitor. In support of this hypothesis, the involvement of CYP3A4 in the metabolism of vincristine is well established, and isoniazid is suspected of inhibiting vincristine clearance in at least one published case report (68).

Antifungals

Ketoconazole

Ketoconazole is a potent CYP3A4 inhibitor that causes clinically significant drug interactions with CYP3A4 substrates such as cyclosporine, tacrolimus, triazolam, midazolam, alprazolam, and terfenadine (69). In one study, addition of ketoconazole (200 mg/day orally for 10 days) to eight patients stabilized on CBZ resulted in a 29% increase in mean plasma CBZ levels (70). This effect was less pronounced than expected based on ketoconazole interactions reported with other CYP3A4 substrates.

Fluconazole

There is at least one report of a patient who experienced CBZ toxicity after the addition of fluconazole to his drug regimen. Plasma CBZ levels increased from 11.1 to 24.5 µg/mL after taking 150 mg of fluconazole for 3 days. CBZ plasma levels returned to normal after discontinuation of fluconazole (71). This, in relation to the finding with ketoconazole, contradicts the rank order of inhibition potencies found with other CYP3A4 substrates (69).

Ritonavir

Ritonavir, an antiretroviral agent, has been reported to be a potent mechanism-based inhibitor of CYP3A4, and there are at least two case reports of elevated CBZ plasma levels after comedication with ritonavir (72). A patient receiving CBZ (350 mg/day for 8 years) and zonisamide (140 mg/day) had a CBZ plasma concentration of 9.5 µg/mL before receiving ritonavir. Twelve hours after a single 200-mg dose of ritonavir, the serum CBZ concentration was increased markedly to 17.8 µg/mL (73). Another patient became toxic on CBZ when his antiviral drug regimen was changed from stavudine (40 mg twice daily), lamivudine (150 mg twice daily), and indinavir (800 mg three times daily) to lamivudine (150 mg twice daily), didanosine (400 mg/day), ritonavir (600 mg twice daily), and saquinavir (400 mg twice daily). At the time of the antiviral drug change, CBZ plasma concentrations were 6.5 µg/mL. The patient developed dizziness and a progressive gait disorder that initially was attributed to left hemiparesis. CBZ plasma levels were checked 2 months later and found to be 18 µg/mL; after CBZ therapy was discontinued, the gait disorder disappeared (74).

Metronidazole

Metronidazole has been reported to increase plasma CBZ levels, possible by inhibiting its metabolism (75).

Propoxyphene

CBZ toxicity resulting from the coadministration of CBZ and propoxyphene has been the subject of a multitude of case reports in the literature (76–78). Also, in two clinical trials, propoxyphene (65 mg three times per day for 3 to 7 days) added to drug regimens of patients stabilized on CBZ resulted in increased plasma levels of CBZ by 45% to 77% (79,80). In a population kinetics study, the doses of CBZ and propoxyphene were found to be lower among patients who used a combination of the two drugs than among those who used only one. However, the mean level of CBZ in the serum was significantly higher and the serum CBZE level was significantly lower among the patients who used the combination of CBZ and propoxyphene, indicating an inhibition of the metabolism of CBZ (81). Propoxyphene (65 mg/day) was found to inhibit the clearance of alprazolam (a drug that appears to be metabolized exclusively by CYP3A4) by 40% (1.3 to 0.8 mL/min/kg) in eight patients, further suggesting that propoxyphene is an inhibitor of CYP3A4 metabolism (82).

In human liver microsomes, concentration-dependent inhibition of CBZ-10,11-epoxidation by propoxyphene was observed, although inhibition was mild. Formation of the 10-hydroxylated metabolite of (R)-warfarin, a probe of CYP3A4 activity, paralleled the findings with CBZ, suggesting that propoxyphene is a weak inhibitor of CBZ metabolism by CYP3A4 (unpublished data from our laboratory).

The inhibition noted clinically may result from contribution of the propoxyphene metabolite, norpropoxyphene, which has been shown to inhibit microsomal oxidative metabolism and to accumulate in the plasma at levels up to 13 times those of its parent compound (83,84). Alternatively, tissue distribution studies in the rat demonstrated that propoxyphene distributed into tissues at concentrations that were 10 to 20 times greater than in blood (85). Highest concentrations were observed in liver. These results, in conjunction with our *in vitro* study results, suggest that the observed clinical drug interaction may be the result of inhibition of the CYP3A4-mediated metabolism of CBZ by propoxyphene or its metabolite. In addition, the *N*-dealkylation of propoxyphene has been suggested to result in irreversible inhibition of CYP3A4 (31).

Cimetidine

Although CBZ intoxication has been reported after addition of cimetidine, the interaction is not identified consistently and probably is of limited clinical relevance (8). Any increase in CBZ concentration appears to be relatively small and may be transient. This was demonstrated in a study of eight subjects who received CBZ (300 mg twice daily) for 42 days (days 1 to 42) and cimetidine (400 mg three times a day) for 7 days (days 29 to 35). CBZ plasma concentrations increased 17% after 2 days of cimetidine treatment but returned to the precimetidine level by the seventh day of cimetidine administration (86).

Danazol

Danazol, a synthetic estrogen used in the management of endometriosis, inhibits the epoxide-*trans*-diol elimination of CBZ, resulting in 50% to 100% increases in steady-state plasma CBZ levels. A study of one patient maintained on CBZ (600 mg/day for 5 years) demonstrated an increase in CBZ plasma steady-state concentrations (41.6 to 68.4 μmol/L) after 33 days of danazol comedication (600 mg/day) (87). Another patient's previously stable CBZ plasma level increased from 38 to 76 μmol/L after beginning danazol administration (88). A study of six women with epilepsy and fibrocystic breast disease reported a 91% mean increase in CBZ concentration (from 7.55 to 14.45 μg/mL) after danazol was added (89).

Nicotinamide

Nicotinamide caused elevation of CBZ levels in two patients, with high correlations between CBZ clearance and nicotinamide doses (90).

Induction of Carbamazepine Metabolism

Metabolism of CBZ *in vivo* is induced by some other anticonvulsants, resulting in decreased plasma concentrations of CBZ. *In vitro* evidence obtained from incubation of CBZ in human liver microsomes demonstrated that CBZE formation velocity in livers obtained from donors who received CYP enzyme-inducing agents (e.g., rifampin, dexamethasone, and phenytoin) was 1.9-fold higher than that in livers from uninduced donors (2). Because most CBZE formation is mediated by CYP3A4, induction of CYP3A4 by these agents is suggested.

Phenytoin, Phenobarbital, and Primidone

Several studies have consistently demonstrated that CBZ metabolism is highly inducible by other antiepileptic drugs, including phenytoin, phenobarbital, and primidone (8). In patients receiving multiple drugs, the inducing effects of multiple anticonvulsants can be additive in terms of reducing CBZ concentrations (91). Christiansen and Dam (92,93) showed in 123 patients that the slope of the relationship between plasma level and dose of CBZ is reduced separately by phenytoin, phenobarbital, and the combination of phenytoin and phenobarbital. Schneider (94) reported similar findings in 184 patients receiving 8 different combinations of CBZ and other drugs. This study showed that primidone also has a significant effect in decreasing the slope of the relationship between plasma CBZ level and dose, presumably as a consequence of enzyme induction. In 142 patients, Johannessen and Strandjord (95) also found that phenytoin or phenobarbital, or a combination of both, could reduce the plasma level-to-dose ratio of CBZ. They emphasized the need to monitor CBZ levels during polytherapy to achieve the proper dosage increments. Rane et al. (96) compared the mean CBZ levels in children on monotherapy and polytherapy and found that the ratio of plasma level to dose was lower in the group on polytherapy, but the concentration of CBZE metabolite was significantly higher.

Several other studies have found that the ratio of CBZE to CBZ steady-state plasma levels was higher in patients taking CBZ with other antiepileptic drugs than in those taking CBZ only (93,94,96–98). There is some evidence that epoxide hydrolase also is subject to induction by pretreatment with inducing agents such as phenytoin and phenobarbital (99,100).

Korczyn et al. studied the plasma levels of CBZ and the epoxide and dihydrodiol metabolites in two groups of patients (monotherapy versus polytherapy) and concluded that other anticonvulsant agents induce the epoxidation of CBZ as well as the conversion of the epoxide to the dihydrodiol (101). Induction of CBZE clearance by phenobarbital was demonstrated in six epileptic patients stabilized on phenobarbital and in six drug-free, healthy volunteers (7). The plasma clearance of a single dose of CBZ epoxide was significantly higher in the patient group than in the control (220.2 ± 63.5 versus 112.5 ± 46). Because CBZ epoxide is almost completely converted to *trans*-CBZ diol by microsomal epoxide hydrolase, it appears that phenobarbital induces this enzyme (4,5). The clinical significance of these interactions has not been shown.

Coadministration of CBZ and phenytoin appears to result in a simultaneous dual effect, inhibition or induction of phenytoin metabolism by CBZ (see page 253, under "Phenytoin") and induction of CBZ metabolism by phenytoin. The mean serum concentration of CBZ was 59% lower in patients receiving CBZ in combination with phenytoin, compared with patients receiving only CBZ (102). Conversely, reduction of phenytoin dosage resulted in increased CBZ concentrations (103). In another study that examined serum concentrations of CBZ and its major metabolites, CBZE and CBZ-diol, phenytoin comedication decreased CBZ serum levels and increased the concentrations of both CBZE and CBZ-diol (104). These results suggest that phenytoin is an inducer of CYP3A4 and CBZ epoxidation.

Felbamate

Felbamate has been identified as an inducer of CYP3A4 (105). Several studies show a decrease in serum concentrations of CBZ with felbamate comedication. Addition of felbamate to 22 patients on stable CBZ monotherapy resulted in a decrease of 10% to 42% in CBZ levels (106). A double-blind, crossover, placebo-controlled study of 32 patients stabilized on CBZ and phenytoin demonstrated that felbamate decreased mean CBZ concentrations (7.5 to 6.1 µg/mL) and increased CBZE concentrations (1.8 to 2.4

µg/mL) (107,108). Because of the increase in plasma CBZE levels and a concomitant pharmacodynamic interaction, felbamate often potentiates the adverse effects of CBZ.

Oxcarbazepine

Oxcarbazepine has been found to produce a modest reduction in the plasma levels of CBZ at steady state (109).

St. John's Wort

St. John's Wort, a herbal medicine used as an antidepressant and for other indications, is an inducer of CYP3A4. At a dosage of 900 mg/day, St. John's Wort has been found to reduce plasma CBZ levels after a single dose of CBZ (110), but in a separate study, steady-state plasma CBZ levels were not affected by St. John's wort given at the same dosage (111).

Plasma Protein Binding Interactions

CBZ is only 75% bound in human plasma, and interactions resulting from displacement of CBZ by other drugs or from displacement of coadministered drugs by CBZ are likely to be free from clinical consequences. The influence of several drugs on the plasma binding of CBZ at a concentration of 5 µg/mL was studied by ultrafiltration. It was found that phenobarbital, phenytoin, and nortriptyline had no effect on the protein binding of CBZ, whereas ethosuximide showed a very slight increase in the percentage of CBZ bound to protein (112). Valproic acid was found to cause a 25% increase in the free fraction of CBZ (23.5% to 29.5%), although wide fluctuations in the CBZ dose-to-plasma level relationship are likely to obscure any clinical effect (113,114).

EFFECT OF CARBAMAZEPINE ON OTHER DRUGS: INDUCTION

The number of drug interaction reports resulting from CYP induction by CBZ has been increasing. CBZ autoinduces its own metabolism through the CYP3A4-mediated pathway during long-term administration (115–117). In humans, the induction half-life of CYP3A4 appears to be approximately 4 days, and therefore a period of 3 to 4 weeks of CBZ administration is required to achieve steady state (118). The increased clearance is associated with a shortened half-life and a reduction in the total serum CBZ concentration at steady state compared with single dose. One study in four patients found that the average steady-state concentration of CBZ was reduced by 50% after 3 weeks of drug administration (115). Induction of CYP3A4 by CBZ has been confirmed in human hepatocyte cultures (119). This inductive effect on CYP3A4 also decreases the plasma concentrations of other coadministered drugs that are CYP3A4 substrates. It is likely, however, that CBZ induces other CYP isoforms because *in vivo*, CBZ appears to increase the metabolic clearances of olanzapine, bupropion, the active (S) enantiomer of warfarin, and phenytoin, which appear to be substrates of CYP1A2, CYP2B6, CYP2C9, and CYP2C9/CYP2C19, respectively. The hypothesis of induction of CYP1A2 is supported by another study that found that CBZ treatment increased the percentage of labeled caffeine exhaled as carbon dioxide, a method used to assess CYP1A2 activity *in vivo* (120).

Anticonvulsants

Benzodiazepines

Alprazolam

CBZ (300 mg/day for 10 days) significantly decreased the plasma concentration of a single oral dose of alprazolam by increasing the oral clearance (0.90 versus 2.13 mL/min/kg) and shortening the elimination half-life (17.1 versus 7.7 hours) (121) (121a). Alprazolam is cleared primarily by CYP3A4, and the induction of this enzyme by CBZ is the likely cause for the increased clearance of this drug.

Clobazam

Clobazam is a benzodiazepine used as adjuvant therapy for intractable seizures. A pharmacokinetic study in healthy volunteers found that CBZ (200 mg twice daily for 2 weeks) decreased clobazam plasma steady-state concentrations by 61% and increased concentrations of its major metabolite, *N*-desmethylclobazam, by 44% (122). The results of a study in epileptic children also showed that CBZ decreased clobazam serum concentrations and increased the concentrations of *N*-desmethylclobazam.

Clonazepam

Clonazepam plasma concentrations may be reduced by CBZ (123). CBZ (200 mg/day) decreased clonazepam steady-state concentrations by 19% to 37% after a 5- to 15-day administration period (118).

Clorazepate

Enzyme-inducing anticonvulsants reduce the plasma levels of the active metabolite of clorazepate, *N*-desmethyldiazepam (124).

Diazepam

Enzyme-inducing anticonvulsants, including CBZ, have been found to cause a reduction in the plasma concentration of diazepam and concomitantly to increase the plasma levels of its active metabolite, *N*-desmethyldiazepam (125).

Midazolam

The AUC of an oral 15-mg dose of midazolam in patients on chronic CBZ therapy was reduced to 5.7% of the AUC in noninduced control subjects (126). This dramatic effect was attributed to the significant first-pass metabolism of midazolam and the induction of both intestinal and hepatic CY3A4 by CBZ. Because after intravenous (i.v.) administration, midazolam clearance depends more on liver blood flow than on microsomal enzyme activity, the reduction of plasma midazolam levels in patients treated with CBZ would be expected to be far less significant when midazolam is given i.v., such as in the treatment of status epilepticus.

Ethosuximide

When CBZ (200 mg/day) was added to the regimen of healthy subjects receiving 250 mg/day of ethosuximide, ethosuximide clearance increased significantly after 10 days of CBZ therapy, with a synchronous decrease in ethosuximide half-life from 54 to 45 hours (127).

Felbamate

Felbamate clearance is increased significantly by enzyme-inducing anticonvulsants, including CBZ (128).

Lamotrigine

CBZ also is an inducer of uridine diphosphate-glucuronosyl transferase, and this appears to be the basis for increased rate of lamotrigine clearance when these drugs are used together. The half-life of lamotrigine is reduced from 24 to 15 hours in patients receiving enzyme-inducing anticonvulsants, including CBZ (129).

Phenobarbital and Primidone

Phenobarbital is a product of primidone metabolism, and serum phenobarbital concentrations increased significantly when CBZ was added to the regimen of four patients receiving primidone (130). The increase in phenobarbital levels appears to be due to increased conversion from primidone rather than inhibition of phenobarbital clearance, because one study demonstrated no change in phenobarbital clearance in 25 patients taking both phenobarbital and CBZ (131).

Phenytoin

The effect of CBZ on phenytoin pharmacokinetics appears to be variable. CBZ has been reported to shorten phenytoin half-life and reduce phenytoin plasma concentrations at steady state (132–136). However, there also have been reports of CBZ causing prolonged phenytoin half-life and increased plasma phenytoin concentrations (137–139). In particular, one study found that CBZ caused an increase in steady-state phenytoin concentrations in half of the patients studied and no change in the remainder (138). These data suggest that CBZ may both induce and inhibit the enzymes responsible for phenytoin biotransformation, and that the prevailing effect may vary from patient to patient.

Phenytoin is metabolized predominantly by CYP2C9 (140) and to a smaller extent by CYP2C19 (141). Induction of CYP2C9 is suggested as the cause of decreased anticoagulation reported in patients stabilized on warfarin and then prescribed CBZ (142). Inducibility of CYP2C19 by rifampicin has been demonstrated, but there are no reports regarding inducibility of CYP2C19 by CBZ (143). *In vitro*, CBZ has been shown to inhibit the CYP2C19-mediated 4′-hydroxylation of (S)-mephenytoin, with a K_i value of 35 μmol/L (therapeutic range of CBZ is 25 to 50 μmol/L) (unpublished data from our laboratory). The available evidence suggests that the effect of CBZ on phenytoin pharmacokinetics could be the result of a balance between induction of CYP2C9 and inhibition of CYP2C19.

Tiagabine

Tiagabine is extensively metabolized in the liver, largely by CYP3A4, with less than 1% excreted unchanged (129). The monotherapy half-life of tiagabine is 5 to 8 hours and is shortened to 2 to 3 hours when coadministered with CYP3A4 inducers, including CBZ. Tiagabine does not alter the clearance of CBZ.

Topiramate

Topiramate metabolic clearance is increased by concomitant CBZ administration, whereas CBZ clearance is unchanged (144). When patients were changed from CBZ plus topiramate to topiramate monotherapy, topiramate clearance was reduced by approximately 50%, suggesting that an adjustment in topiramate dosage may be required when CBZ is discontinued (145).

Valproic Acid*

Several studies indicate that CBZ increases the plasma clearance of valproic acid, probably through induction of the metabolic processes responsible for valproic acid elimination. Six healthy subjects received 250 mg of valproic acid twice daily for 4 weeks; a very small dose of CBZ (200 mg once daily) was added after 4 days of valproic acid therapy (146). A significant decrease in steady-state blood valproic acid levels was apparent after 2 weeks of CBZ therapy.

The effects of CBZ on specific metabolic pathways of valproic acid were examined in epileptic patients (147). The formation of Δ^4-valproate (hepatotoxic metabolite of valproic acid) was increased by 105% in the presence of CBZ. The clearances by several other pathways, ω and ω-1 oxi-

dation (both CYP mediated) as well as glucuronidation, also were increased.

Zonisamide

Zonisamide is metabolized partly by CYP3A4 (148). The plasma half-life of zonisamide is reduced from 60 hours in healthy subjects to 36.4 hours in patients receiving CBZ (149,150). In another study, CBZ was found to decrease the zonisamide steady-state plasma concentration-to-dose ratio, indicating that zonisamide clearance is increased by CBZ coadministration (151).

Antidepressants

Tricyclic Antidepressants

In addition to CYP2D6 (a noninducible enzyme) and CYP1A2, CYP3A4 is partially responsible for a minor fraction of demethylation of the tertiary amine tricyclic antidepressants (amitriptyline, clomipramine, and imipramine), and CBZ may induce the metabolism of these drugs (152). One study found that children receiving CBZ required higher doses of imipramine than control subjects (153). Despite the higher imipramine dosages, the CBZ group had lower plasma concentrations of imipramine and its active metabolite, desipramine. CBZ has been associated with a decrease in amitriptyline serum levels (42%) and in the levels of its active metabolite, nortriptyline (40%) (154). Because the metabolites of imipramine and amitriptyline are active, induction of metabolite clearances may play a role in the diminished effects of these drugs.

The clearance of nortriptyline appeared to be increased by the addition of CBZ in a 73-year-old woman (155). Average serum concentrations decreased from 355 ± 49 nmol/L (13 samples over 2 years) to 140 and 134 nmol/L (at two separate measurements) 9 weeks after beginning CBZ (600 mg/day). The main metabolic pathway of nortriptyline is mediated by CYP2D6 (high affinity) and CYP3A4 (low affinity) (156).

Bupropion

Patients with mood disorders received a single oral dose of bupropion (150 mg) while receiving placebo (n = 17) or chronic blind CBZ (n = 12). The AUC of bupropion was 90% lower in patients receiving CBZ, suggesting that CBZ induces the clearance of bupropion (157). Bupropion undergoes extensive biotransformation primarily to hydroxybupropion by CYP2B6 (158,159).

Other Antidepressants

The metabolism of many other antidepressants, including mianserin (160) and nefazodone (41), is accelerated by concomitant treatment with enzyme-inducing anticonvulsants.

*Type your question here, and then click Search.

Antipsychotic Drugs

Clozapine

Clozapine is an atypical antipsychotic drug that is used mainly for the treatment of refractory schizophrenia. Clozapine is eliminated by oxidation in the liver, predominantly by CYP1A2. CBZ was found to decrease the plasma levels of clozapine by 47% in a study of 12 patients (161). Another study compared patients receiving clozapine alone with those also receiving CBZ, and found that patients on CBZ had a mean 50% lower concentration-to-dose ratio than the monotherapy group ($p < .001$), indicating that CBZ is an inducer of the metabolism of clozapine (162).

Haloperidol

Comedication with CBZ and haloperidol is associated with lower haloperidol plasma levels and worse clinical outcome than haloperidol alone (163). In a study of 231 schizophrenic patients, patients who received CBZ and haloperidol concomitantly had a mean haloperidol concentration-to-dose ratio that was 37% less than that of subjects who received haloperidol alone (164). Several other studies found that haloperidol plasma levels are reduced by more than 50% after the addition of CBZ (165).

Olanzapine

Olanzapine is an antipsychotic agent cleared mainly by CYP1A2. Olanzapine clearance was compared before and after a 2-week treatment with CBZ (200 mg twice daily) in 12 healthy volunteers. The olanzapine AUC was significantly decreased after the addition of CBZ (336 ± 103 hr·mg/L versus 223 ± 59 hr·mg/L, $p < .001$), suggesting that CBZ is an inducer of CYP1A2 (166).

Risperidone

Risperidone is an antipsychotic agent cleared mainly by CYP2D6, although CYP3A4 is a contributor. In five patients assessed with and without CBZ comedication, dose-normalized plasma risperidone and 9-hydroxyrisperidone levels were significantly lower when the patients received combination therapy, suggesting that CBZ can induce the clearance of this drug (167). This interaction seems to have considerable clinical significance, particularly in patients with deficient CYP2D6 activity (168).

Steroids

Oral Contraceptives

Breakthrough bleeding and contraceptive failure have been reported in women taking oral contraceptives (169,170). In a pharmacokinetic study of four women who received a single dose of oral contraceptive containing ethinyl estradiol (50 µg) and levonorgestrel (250 µg) before and 8 to 12 weeks after beginning therapy with CBZ (171), the AUCs of ethinyl estradiol and levonorgestrel were decreased by 40% when CBZ was added, suggesting that CBZ induced the metabolism of both hormone components of the oral contraceptive preparation. CYP3A4 is the major enzyme responsible for the 2-hydroxylation of ethinyl estradiol (172,173).

Other Steroids

Enzyme-inducing anticonvulsants, including CBZ, have been found to increase the metabolic clearance of prednisolone, methylprednisolone, dexamethasone, and many other steroids (8). These interactions can result in inadequate response when these steroids are used therapeutically or diagnostically.

Cyclosporine

CBZ has been reported to induce the metabolism of the immunosuppressive drug, cyclosporine, which is metabolized by CYP3A4 (174–176). Cyclosporine pharmacokinetics were studied in three pediatric renal transplant recipients receiving CBZ doses of 16.4 to 20.8 mg/kg/day and compared with control patients. Steady-state trough concentrations of cyclosporine were significantly lower in the CBZ group (57 ± 14 ng/mL versus 162 ± 22 ng/mL), even though the CBZ patients received higher cyclosporine doses (16.2 ± 8.8 mg/kg/day versus 10.8 ± 5.2 mg/kg/day) (177).

Oral Anticoagulants

Patients stabilized on warfarin exhibit increased prothrombin times after the addition of CBZ to their drug regimens, suggesting that CBZ induces warfarin metabolism (142). Also, a patient maintained on CBZ and warfarin discontinued her CBZ without consulting her physician and suffered excessive hyperprothrombinemia and hemorrhage (178). Up to twofold reductions in warfarin dosage have been required when CBZ therapy was discontinued (179). Warfarin is an enantiomeric compound, with the clearance of the more active (S)-warfarin mediated by CYP2C9 and the less active (R)-warfarin by CYP3A4 (180,181). Although it is likely that induction of CYP3A4 increases the biotransformation of the (R) enantiomer, the degree of the clinical interaction between CBZ and warfarin suggests that CYP2C9 also is induced by CBZ. The metabolism of other coumarin anticoagulants also has been found to be stimulated to a clinically important extent by CBZ (182).

Dihydropyridine Calcium Antagonists

Nimodipine is a calcium channel blocking agent administered as a racemic mixture to prevent cerebral vasospasm in patients with subarachnoid hemorrhage, and to improve cerebral function in elderly patients. In epileptic patients taking CBZ, there was a sevenfold decrease in the AUC of nimodipine (183). The plasma levels of other dihydropyridine calcium antagonists, including nisoldipine, nifedipine and felodipine, are markedly reduced by enzyme-inducing anticonvulsants (8).

Chemotherapeutic Agents

Doxycycline

In five patients on long-term CBZ therapy, the half-life of doxycycline (8.4 hours) was significantly shorter than the mean half-life of 15.1 hours in nine control patients (184).

Indinavir

CBZ is prescribed for treatment of seizures or postherpetic neuralgia in human immunodeficiency virus–infected patients. In one case report, the plasma concentration of the antiretroviral drug indinavir (800 mg every 8 hours) was decreased up to 16 times after the addition of CBZ (200 mg/day) (185).

Itraconazole

Plasma concentrations of the antifungal itraconazole are markedly reduced by concomitant administration of CBZ. Induction of itraconazole metabolism is of clinical relevance in systemic mycoses because treatment failures have occurred in patients receiving CBZ and itraconazole. Bonay et al. described a patient who had undetectable plasma itraconazole concentrations during coadministration with CBZ (186). Three weeks after withdrawal of CBZ, plasma itraconazole concentrations increased and reached the therapeutic range without modification of the antifungal dosage (186).

Vincristine

The antineoplastic agent, vincristine, is at least partially metabolized by CYP3A4. One clinical study found vincristine clearance was 63% higher in a patient group receiving CBZ (eight patients) or phenytoin (one patient) compared with a control patient group, suggesting that CBZ is an inducer of vincristine clearance (187).

Fentanyl

The primary route of fentanyl clearance is *N*-dealkylation to norfentanyl, and this step is catalyzed predominantly by CYP3A4 (188). The effect of chronic anticonvulsant therapy on the minimum dose of fentanyl required during cranial surgery was studied in four groups of patients receiving either no anticonvulsants; CBZ alone; CBZ with either valproic acid or phenytoin; and CBZ, valproic acid, and either phenytoin or primidone. The patients receiving any of the anticonvulsant therapies required significantly more fentanyl during anesthesia (189).

Neuromuscular Blocking Agents

Patients receiving CBZ have been found to exhibit a reduced sensitivity to some neuromuscular blocking agents. Both enzyme induction and pharmacodynamic factors may be involved in these interactions (8).

Other Drugs

Because CYP3A4 and other enzymes that are induced by CBZ metabolize a large number of drugs, the clearance of many other compounds is likely to be increased in patients taking CBZ. In particular, because the enzyme-inducing spectrum of CBZ is similar to that of phenytoin and phenobarbital, it is likely that many of the interactions mediated by enzyme induction with the latter drugs (Chapters 53 and 60) also are seen with CBZ.

CONCLUSIONS

Identification of CYP3A4 as the primary catalytic enzyme for the main clearance pathway of CBZ allows an understanding of the effects of several drugs on plasma CBZ concentrations. Drugs that inhibit CYP3A4 increase plasma CBZ. CYP3A4 is inducible, and this explains the decreases in CBZ levels during coadministration of CYP3A4 inducers. Also, CBZ appears to induce CYP3A4, CYP2C9, CYP2C19, and CYP1A2, resulting in decreased plasma concentrations of substrates of these isoforms when they are prescribed with CBZ.

ACKNOWLEDGMENT

Work on this chapter was supported in part by National Institutes of Health grant P01 GM 32165.

REFERENCES

1. Lertratanangkoon K, Horning MG. Metabolism of carbamazepine. *Drug Metab Dispos* 1982;10:1–10.
2. Kerr BM, Thummel KE, Wurden CJ, et al. Human liver carbamazepine metabolism: role of CYP3A4 and CYP2C8 in 10,11-epoxide formation. *Biochem Pharmacol* 1994;47:1969–1979.
3. Kerr BM, Sanins SM, Thummel KE, et al. Metabolism of carbamazepine by hepatic and intestinal P450 3A4. *Pharm Res* 1991;8:S239.
4. Bertilsson L, Tomson T. Clinical pharmacokinetics and phar-

macological effects of carbamazepine and carbamazepine-10,11-epoxide: an update. *Clin Pharmacokinet* 1986;11:177–198.

5. Eichelbaum M, Tomson T, Tybring G, et al. Carbamazepine metabolism in man: induction and pharmacogenetic aspects. *Clin Pharmacokinet* 1985;10:80–90.

6. Bertilsson L, Tomson T. Kinetics and metabolism of carbamzepine-10,11-epoxide in man. In: Levy RH, Pitlick WH, Eichelbaum M, et al., eds. *Metabolism of antiepileptic drugs.* New York: Raven Press, 1982:19–26.

7. Spina E, Martines C, Fazio A, et al. Effect of phenobarbital on the pharmacokinetics of carbamazepine-10,11-epoxide, an active metabolite of carbamazepine. *Ther Drug Monit* 1991;13:109–112.

8. Spina E, Pisani F, Perucca E. Clinically significant pharmacokinetic drug interactions with carbamazepine: an update. *Clin Pharmacokinet* 1996;31:198–214.

9. Pisani F, Xiao B, Fazio A, et al. Single-dose pharmacokinetics of carbamazepine-10,11-epoxide in patients on lamotrigine monotherapy. *Epilepsy Res* 1994;19:245–248.

10. Besag FM, Berry DJ, Pool F, et al. Carbamazepine toxicity with lamotrigine: pharmacokinetic or pharmacodynamic interaction? *Epilepsia* 1998;39:183–187.

11. Leach JP, Blacklaw J, Jamieson V, et al. Mutual interaction between remacemide hydrochloride and carbamazepine: two drugs with active metabolites. *Epilepsia* 1996;37:1100–1106.

12. Tran A, Rey E, Pons G, et al. Influence of stiripentol on cytochrome P450-mediated metabolic pathways in humans: in vitro and in vivo comparison and calculation of in vivo inhibition constants. *Clin Pharmacol Ther* 1997;62:490–504.

13. Kerr BM, Martinez-Lage JM, Viteri C, et al. Carbamazepine dose requirements during stiripentol therapy: influence of cytochrome P-450 inhibition by stiripentol. *Epilepsia* 1991;32:267–274.

14. Pisani F, Caputo M, Fazio A, et al. Interaction of carbamazepine-10,11-epoxide, an active metabolite of carbamazepine, with valproate: a pharmacokinetic study. *Epilepsia* 1990;31:339–342.

15. McKee PJ, Blacklaw J, Butler E, et al. Variability and clinical relevance of the interaction between sodium valproate and carbamazepine in epileptic patients. *Epilepsy Res* 1992;11:193–198.

16. Pisani F, Fazio A, Oteri G, et al. Sodium valproate and valpromide: differential interactions with carbamazepine in epileptic patients. *Epilepsia* 1986;27:548–552.

17. Grant SM, Heel RC. Vigabatrin: a review of its pharmacodynamic and pharmacokinetic properties and therapeutic potential in patients with epilepsy and disorders of motor control. *Drugs* 1991;41:889–926.

18. Jedrzejczak J, Dlawichowska E, Owczarek K, et al. Effect of vigabatrin addition on carbamazepine blood serum levels in patients with epilepsy. *Epilepsy Res* 2000;39:115–120.

19. Gernaat HB, Van de Woude J, Touw DJ. Fluoxetine and parkinsonism in patients taking carbamazepine. *Am J Psychiatry* 1991;148:1604–1605.

20. Gidal BE, Anderson GD, Seaton TL, et al. Evaluation of the effect of fluoxetine on the formation of carbamazepine epoxide. *Ther Drug Monit* 1993;15:405–409.

21. Grimsley SR, Jann MW, Carter JG, et al. Increased carbamazepine plasma concentrations after fluoxetine coadministration. *Clin Pharmacol Ther* 1991;50:10–5.

22. Pearson HJ. Interaction of fluoxetine with carbamazepine [Letter; comment]. *J Clin Psychiatry* 1990;51:126.

23. Spina E, Avenoso A, Pollicino AM, et al. Carbamazepine coadministration with fluoxetine or fluvoxamine. *Ther Drug Monit* 1993;15:247–250.

24. Ring BJ, Binkley SN, Roskos L, et al. Effect of fluoxetine, norfluoxetine, sertraline and desmethyl sertraline on human CYP3A catalyzed 1′-hydroxy midazolam formation in vitro. *J Pharmacol Exp Ther* 1995;275:1131–1135.

25. von Moltke LL, Greenblatt DJ, Cotreau-Bibbo MM, et al. Inhibitors of alprazolam metabolism in vitro: effect of serotonin- reuptake-inhibitor antidepressants, ketoconazole and quinidine. *Br J Clin Pharmacol* 1994;38:23–31.

26. Lasher TA, Fleishaker JC, Steenwyk RC, et al. Pharmacokinetic pharmacodynamic evaluation of the combined administration of alprazolam and fluoxetine. *Psychopharmacology* 1991;104:323–327.

27. Greenblatt DJ, Preskorn SH, Cotreau MM, et al. Fluoxetine impairs clearance of alprazolam but not of clonazepam. *Clin Pharmacol Ther* 1992;52:479–486.

28. Bergstrom RF, Goldberg MJ, Cerimele BJ, et al. Assessment of the potential for a pharmacokinetic interaction between fluoxetine and terfenadine. *Clin Pharmacol Ther* 1997;62:643–651.

29. Strouse TB, Fairbanks LA, Skotzko CE, et al. Fluoxetine and cyclosporine in organ transplantation: failure to detect significant drug interactions or adverse clinical events in depressed organ recipients. *Psychosomatics* 1996;37:23–30.

30. Wright CE, Lasher-Sisson TA, Steenwyk RC, et al. A pharmacokinetic evaluation of the combined administration of triazolam and fluoxetine. *Pharmacotherapy* 1992;12:103–106.

31. Mayhew BS, Jones DR, Hall SD. An in vitro model for predicting in vivo inhibition of cytochrome P450 3A4 by metabolic intermediate complex formation. *Drug Metab Dispos* 2000;28:1031–1037.

32. von Moltke LL, Greenblatt DJ, Court MH, et al. Inhibition of alprazolam and desipramine hydroxylation in vitro by paroxetine and fluvoxamine: comparison with other selective serotonin reuptake inhibitor antidepressants. *J Clin Psychopharmacol* 1995;15:125–131.

33. von Moltke LL, Greenblatt DJ, Duan SX, et al. Inhibition of terfenadine metabolism in vitro by azole antifungal agents and by selective serotonin reuptake inhibitor antidepressants: relation to pharmacokinetic interactions in vivo [See comments]. *J Clin Psychopharmacol* 1996;16:104–112.

34. von Moltke LL, Greenblatt DJ, Harmatz JS, et al. Triazolam biotransformation by human liver microsomes in vitro: effects of metabolic inhibitors and clinical confirmation of a predicted interaction with ketoconazole. *J Pharmacol Exp Ther* 1996;276:370–379.

35. Fleishaker JC, Hulst LK. A pharmacokinetic and pharmacodynamic evaluation of the combined administration of alprazolam and fluvoxamine. *Eur J Clin Pharmacol* 1994;46:35–39.

36. Fritze J, Unsorg B, Lanczik M. Interaction between carbamazepine and fluvoxamine. *Acta Psychiatr Scand* 1991;84:583–584.

37. Martinelli V, Bochetta A, Palmas AM, et al. An interaction between carbamazepine and fluvoxamine. *Br J Clin Pharmacol* 1993;36:615–616.

38. Bonnet P, Vandel S, Nezelof S, et al. Carbamazepine, fluvoxamine: is there a pharmacokinetic interaction? [Letter]. *Therapie* 1992;47:165.

39. Pisani F, Fazio A, Oteri G, et al. Carbamazepine-viloxazine interaction in patients with epilepsy. *J Neurol Neurosurg Psychiatry* 1986;49:1142–1145.

40. Perucca E, Pisani F, Spina E, et al. Effects of valpromide and viloxazine on the elimination of carbamazepine-10,11-epoxide, an active metabolite of carbamazepine. *Pharmacol Res* 1989;21:111–112.

41. Laroudie C, Salazar DE, Cosson JP, et al. Carbamazepine-nefazodone interaction in healthy subjects. *J Clin Psychopharmacol* 2000;20:46–53.

42. Collins DM, Gidal BE, Pitterle ME. Potential interaction between carbamazepine and loxapine: case report and retrospective review. *Ann Pharmacother* 1993;27:1180–1187.

43. Pisani F, Haj-Yehia A, Fazio A, et al. Pharmacokinetics of valnoctamide in epileptic patients and its interaction with carbamazepine: in vitro/in vivo correlation. *Epilepsia* 1993;34: 954–959.

44. Brodie MJ, MacPhee GJ. Carbamazepine neurotoxicity precipitated by diltiazem. *BMJ* 1986;292:1170–1171.

45. Bahls FH, Ozuna J, Ritchie DE. Interactions between calcium channel blockers and the anticonvulsants carbamazepine and phenytoin. *Neurology* 1991;41:740–742.

46. Maoz E, Grossman E, Thaler M, et al. Carbamazepine neurotoxic reaction after administration of diltiazem. *Arch Intern Med* 1992;152:2503–2504.

47. Eimer M, Carter BL. Elevated serum carbamazepine concentrations following diltiazem initiation. *Drug Intell Clin Pharm* 1987;21:340–342.

48. Sutton D, Butler AM, Nadin L, et al. Role of CYP3A4 in human hepatic diltiazem N-demethylation: inhibition of CYP3A4 activity by oxidized diltiazem metabolites. *J Pharmacol Exp Ther* 1997;282:294–300.

49. Macphee GJ, McInnes GT, Thompson GG, et al. Verapamil potentiates carbamazepine neurotoxicity: a clinically important inhibitory interaction. *Lancet* 1986;1:700–703.

50. Tracy TS, Korzekwa KR, Gonzalez FJ, et al. Cytochrome P450 isoforms involved in metabolism of the enantiomers of verapamil and norverapamil. *Br J Clin Pharmacol* 1999;47:545–552.

51. Kroemer HK, Gautier JC, Beaune P, et al. Identification of P450 enzymes involved in metabolism of verapamil in humans. *Naunyn Schmiedebergs Arch Pharmacol* 1993;348:332–337.

52. Woodcock BG, Hopf R, Kaltenbach M. Verapamil and norverapamil plasma concentrations during long-term therapy in patients with hypertrophic obstructive cardiomyopathy. *J Cardiovasc Pharmacol* 1980;2:17–23.

53. Sekerci S, Tulunay M. Interactions of calcium channel blockers with non-depolarising muscle relaxants in vitro. *Anaesthesia* 1996;51:140–144.

54. Periti P, Mazzei T, Mini E, et al. Pharmacokinetic drug interactions of macrolides. *Clin Pharmacokinet* 1992;23:106–131.

55. Pessayre D, Larrey D, Funck-Brentano C, et al. Drug interactions and hepatitis produced by some macrolide antibiotics. *J Antimicrob Chemother* 1985;16[Suppl A]:181–194.

56. Babany G, Larrey D, Pessayre D. Macrolide antibiotics as inducers and inhibitors of cytochrome P450 in experimental animals and man. *Prog Drug Metab* 1988;11:61–98.

57. Mesdjian E, Dravet C, Cenraud B, et al. Carbamazepine intoxication due to triacetyloleandomycin administration in epileptic patients. *Epilepsia* 1980;21:489–496.

58. Albin H, Vincon G, Pehourcq F, et al. Influence of josamycin treatment on carbamazepine kinetics [in French]. *Therapie* 1982;37:151–156.

59. Vincon G, Albin H, Demotes-Mainard F, et al. Effects of josamycin on carbamazepine kinetics. *Eur J Clin Pharmacol* 1987;32:321–323.

60. Barzaghi N, Gatti G, Crema F, et al. Effect of flurithromycin, a new macrolide antibiotic, on carbamazepine disposition in normal subjects. *Int J Clin Pharmacol Res* 1988;8:101–105.

61. Saint-Salvi B, Tremblay D, Surjus A, et al. A study of the interaction of roxithromycin with theophylline and carbamazepine. *J Antimicrob Chemother* 1987;20[Suppl B]:121–129.

62. Albani F, Riva R, Baruzzi A. Clarithromycin-carbamazepine interaction: a case report. *Epilepsia* 1993;34:161–162.

63. Couet W, Istin B, Ingrand I, et al. Effect of ponsinomycin on single-dose kinetics and metabolism of carbamazepine. *Ther Drug Monit* 1990;12:144–149.

64. Principi N, Esposito S. Comparative tolerability of erythromycin and newer macrolide antibacterials in paediatric patients. *Drug Saf* 1999;20:25–41.

65. Valsalan VC, Cooper GL. Carbamazepine intoxication caused by interaction with isoniazid. *BMJ* 1982;285:261–262.

66. Wright JM, Stokes EF, Sweeney VP. Isoniazid-induced carbamazepine toxicity and vice versa: a double drug interaction. *N Engl J Med* 1982;307:1325–1327.

67. Block SH. Carbamazepine-isoniazid interaction. *Pediatrics* 1982;69:494–495.

68. Carrion C, Espinosa E, Herrero A, et al. Possible vincristine-isoniazid interaction. *Ann Pharmacother* 1995;29:201.

69. Venkatakrishnan K, von Moltke LL, Greenblatt DJ. Effects of the antifungal agents on oxidative drug metabolism: clinical relevance. *Clin Pharmacokinet* 2000;38:111–180.

70. Spina E, Arena D, Scordo MG, et al. Elevation of plasma carbamazepine concentrations by ketoconazole in patients with epilepsy. *Ther Drug Monit* 1997;19:535–538.

71. Nair DR, Morris HH. Potential fluconazole-induced carbamazepine toxicity. *Ann Pharmacother* 1999;33:790–792.

72. von Moltke LL, Durol AL, Duan SX, et al. Potent mechanism-based inhibition of human CYP3A in vitro by amprenavir and ritonavir: comparison with ketoconazole. *Eur J Clin Pharmacol* 2000;56:259–261.

73. Kato Y, Fujii T, Mizoguchi N, et al. Potential interaction between ritonavir and carbamazepine. *Pharmacotherapy* 2000; 20:851–854.

74. Garcia BA, Latorre IA, Porta EJ, et al. Protease inhibitor-induced carbamazepine toxicity. *Clin Neuropharmacol* 2000 Jul-Aug;23(4):216–218.

75. Patterson BD. Possible interaction between metronidazole and carbamazepine. *Ann Pharmacother* 1994;28:1303–1304.

76. Kubacka RT, Ferrante JA. Carbamazepine-propoxyphene interaction. *Clin Pharm* 1983;2:104.

77. Oles KS, Mirza W, Penry JK. Catastrophic neurologic signs due to drug interaction: Tegretol and Darvon. *Surg Neurol* 1989;32: 144–151.

78. Yu YL, Huang CY, Chin D, et al. Interaction between carbamazepine and dextropropoxyphene. *Postgrad Med J* 1986;62: 231–233.

79. Dam M, Christensen J. Interaction of propoxyphene with carbamazepine. *Lancet* 1977;2:509.

80. Hansen BS, Dam M, Brandt J, et al. Influence of dextropropoxyphene on steady state serum levels and protein binding of three anti-epileptic drugs in man. *Acta Neurol Scand* 1980; 61:357–367.

81. Bergendal L, Friberg A, Schaffrath AM, et al. The clinical relevance of the interaction between carbamazepine and dextropropoxyphene in elderly patients in Gothenburg, Sweden. *Eur J Clin Pharmacol* 1997;53:203–206.

82. Abernethy DR, Greenblatt DJ, Morse DS, et al. Interaction of propoxyphene with diazepam, alprazolam and lorazepam. *Br J Clin Pharmacol* 1985;19:51–57.

83. Peterson GR, Hostetler RM, Lehman T, et al. Acute inhibition of oxidative drug metabolism by propoxyphene (Darvon). *Biochem Pharmacol* 1979;28:1783–1789.

84. Inturrisi CE, Colburn WA, Verebey K, et al. Propoxyphene and norpropoxyphene kinetics after single and repeated doses of propoxyphene. *Clin Pharmacol Ther* 1982;31:157–167.

85. Emmerson JL, Welles JS, Anderson RC. Studies on the tissue distribution of d-propoxyphene. *Toxicol Appl Pharmacol* 1967; 11:482–488.

86. Dalton MJ, Powell JR, Messenheimer JA Jr, et al. Cimetidine and carbamazepine: a complex drug interaction. *Epilepsia* 1986; 27:553–558.

87. Kramer G, Theisohn M, von Unruh GE, et al. Carbamazepine-

danazol drug interaction: its mechanism examined by a stable isotope technique. *Ther Drug Monit* 1986;8:387–392.

88. Hayden M, Buchanan N. Danazol-carbamazepine interaction [Letter]. *Med J Aust* 1991;155:851.

89. Zielinski JJ, Lichten EM, Haidukewych D. Clinically significant danazol-carbamazepine interaction. *Ther Drug Monit* 1987;9:24–27.

90. Bourgeois BF, Dodson WE, Ferrendelli JA. Interactions between primidone, carbamazepine, and nicotinamide. *Neurology* 1982;32:1122–1126.

91. Tomson T, Spina E, Wedlund JE. Minor additive inducing effects of phenobarbital on carbamazepine clearance in patients on combined carbamazepine-phenytoin therapy. *Ther Drug Monit* 1987;9:117–119.

92. Christiansen J, Dam M. Influence of phenobarbital and diphenylhydantoin on plasma carbamazepine levels in patients with epilepsy. *Acta Neurol Scand* 1973;49:543–546.

93. Christiansen J, Dam M. Drug interaction in epileptic patients. In: Schneider H, Janz D, Gardner-Thorpe C, et al., eds. *Clinical pharmacology of anti-epileptic drugs*. Berlin: Springer-Verlag, 1975:197–200.

94. Schneider H. Carbamazepine: the influence of other antiepileptic drugs on its serum level. In: Schneider H, Janz D, Gardner-Thorpe C, et al., eds. *Clinical pharmacology of anti-epileptic drugs*. Berlin: Springer-Verlag, 1975:186–196.

95. Johannessen SI, Strandjord RE. Concentration of carbamazepine (Tegretol) in serum and in cerebrospinal fluid in patients with epilepsy. *Epilepsia* 1973;14:373–379.

96. Rane A, Hojer B, Wilson JT. Kinetics of carbamazepine and its 10,11-epoxide metabolite in children. *Clin Pharmacol Ther* 1976;19:276–283.

97. Dam M, Jensen A, Christiansen J. Plasma level and effect of carbamazepine in grand mal and psychomotor epilepsy. *Acta Neurol Scand Suppl* 1975;60:33–38.

98. Westenberg HG, van der Kleijn E, Oei TT, et al. Kinetics of carbamazepine and carbamazepine-epoxide, determined by use of plasma and saliva. *Clin Pharmacol Ther* 1978;23:320–328.

99. Rane A, Peng D. Phenytoin enhances epoxide metabolism in human fetal liver cultures. *Drug Metab Dispos* 1985;13:382–385.

100. Tybring G, von Bahr C, Bertilsson L, et al. Metabolism of carbamazepine and its epoxide metabolite in human and rat liver in vitro. *Drug Metab Dispos* 1981;9:561–564.

101. Korczyn AD, Ben-Zvi A, Kaplanski J, et al. Plasma levels of carbamazepine and metabolites: effect of enzyme inducers. In: Meinardi H, Rowan AJ, eds. *Advances in epileptology*. Amsterdam: Swets & Zeitlinger, 1978:278–279.

102. Rambeck B, May T, Juergens U. Serum concentrations of carbamazepine and its epoxide and diol metabolites in epileptic patients: the influence of dose and comedication. *Ther Drug Monit* 1987;9:298–303.

103. Chapron DJ, LaPierre BA, Abou-Elkair M. Unmasking the significant enzyme-inducing effects of phenytoin on serum carbamazepine concentrations during phenytoin withdrawal. *Ann Pharmacother* 1993;27:708–711.

104. Liu H, Delgado MR. Interactions of phenobarbital and phenytoin with carbamazepine and its metabolites' concentrations, concentration ratios, and level/dose ratios in epileptic children. *Epilepsia* 1995;36:249–254.

105. Glue P, Banfield CR, Perhach JL, et al. Pharmacokinetic interactions with felbamate. In vitro-in vivo correlation. *Clin Pharmacokinet* 1997;33:214–224.

106. Albani F, Theodore WH, Washington P, et al. Effect of felbamate on plasma levels of carbamazepine and its metabolites. *Epilepsia* 1991;32:130–132.

107. Wagner ML, Graves NM, Marienau K, et al. Discontinuation

of phenytoin and carbamazepine in patients receiving felbamate. *Epilepsia* 1991;32:398–406.

108. Wagner ML, Remmel RP, Graves NM, et al. Effect of felbamate on carbamazepine and its major metabolites. *Clin Pharmacol Ther* 1993;53:536–543.

109. Barcs G, Walker EB, Elger CE, et al. Oxcarbazepine placebo-controlled, dose ranging trial in refractory partial epilepsy. *Epilepsia* 2000;41:1597–1607.

110. Burstein AH, Alfaro RM, Piscitelli SC, et al. Effect of St. John's wort on carbamazepine single dose pharmacokinetics in healthy volunteers. *J Clin Pharmacol* 2000;68:605–612.

111. Burstein AH, Horton RL, Dunn T, et al. Lack of effect of St. John's wort on carbamazepine pharmacokinetics in healthy volunteers. *Clin Pharmacol Ther* 2000;68:605–612.

112. Rawlins MD, Collste P, Bertilsson L, et al. Distribution and elimination kinetics of carbamazepine in man. *Eur J Clin Pharmacol* 1975;8:91–96.

113. Mattson GF, Mattson RH, Cramer JA. Interaction between valproic acid and carbamazepine: an in vitro study of protein binding. *Ther Drug Monit* 1982;4:181–184.

114. Bourgeois BF. Pharmacologic interactions between valproate and other drugs. *Am J Med* 1988;84:29–33.

115. Eichelbaum M, Ekbom K, Bertilsson L, et al. Plasma kinetics of carbamazepine and its epoxide metabolite in man after single and multiple doses. *Eur J Clin Pharmacol* 1975;8:337–341.

116. Bertilsson L, Hojer B, Tybring G, et al. Autoinduction of carbamazepine metabolism in children examined by a stable isotope technique. *Clin Pharmacol Ther* 1980;27:83–88.

117. Pitlick WH, Levy RH, Tropin AS, et al. Pharmacokinetic model to describe self-induced decreases in steady-state concentrations of carbamazepine. *J Pharm Sci* 1976;65:462–463.

118. Lai AA, Levy RH, Cutler RE. Time-course of interaction between carbamazepine and clonazepam in normal man. *Clin Pharmacol Ther* 1978;24:316–323.

119. Pichard L, Fabre I, Fabre G, et al. Cyclosporin A drug interactions: screening for inducers and inhibitors of cytochrome P-450 (cyclosporin A oxidase) in primary cultures of human hepatocytes and in liver microsomes. *Drug Metab Dispos* 1990;18:595–606.

120. Parker AC, Pritchard P, Preston T, et al. Induction of CYP1A2 activity by carbamazepine in children using the caffeine breath test. *Br J Clin Pharmacol* 1998;45:176–178.

121. Yuan R, Flockhart DA, Balian JD. Pharmacokinetic and pharmacodynamic consequences of metabolism-based drug interactions with alprazolam, midazolam, and triazolam. *J Clin Pharmacol* 1999;39:1109–1125.

121a. Furukori H, Otani K, Yasui N, et al. Effect of carbamazepine on the single oral dose pharmacokinetics of alprazolam. *Neuropsychopharmacology* 1998;18:364–369.

122. Levy RH, Lane EA, Guyot M, et al. Analysis of parent drug-metabolite relationship in the presence of an inducer: application to the carbamazepine-clobazam interaction in normal man. *Drug Metab Dispos* 1983;11:286–292.

123. Murphy K, Delanty N. Primary generalized epilepsies. *Curr Treat Options Neurol* 2000;2:527–542.

124. Wilensky AJ, Ojemann LM, Temkin NR, et al. Clorazepate kinetics in treated epileptics. *Clin Pharmacol Ther* 1978;24:22–30.

125. Dhillon S, Richens A. Pharmacokinetics of diazepam in epileptic patients and normal volunteers following intravenous administration. *Br J Clin Pharmacol* 1981;12:841–844.

126. Backman JT, Olkkola KT, Ojala M, et al. Concentrations and effects of oral midazolam are greatly reduced in patients treated with carbamazepine or phenytoin. *Epilepsia* 1996;37:253–257.

127. Warren JW Jr, Benmaman JD, Wannamaker BB, et al. Kinetics

of a carbamazepine-ethosuximide interaction. *Clin Pharmacol Ther* 1980;28:646–651.

128. Palmer KJ, McTavish D. Felbamate: a review of its pharmacodynamic and pharmacokinetic properties, and therapeutic potential in the management of epilepsy. *Drugs* 1993;45:1041–1065.

129. Benedetti MS. Enzyme induction and inhibition by new antiepileptic drugs: a review of human studies. *Fundam Clin Pharmacol* 2000;14:301–319.

130. Callaghan N, Feely M, Duggan F, et al. The effect of anticonvulsant drugs which induce liver microsomal enzymes on derived and ingested phenobarbitone levels. *Acta Neurol Scand* 1977;56:1–6.

131. Eadie MJ, Lander CM, Hooper WD, et al. Factors influencing plasma phenobarbitone levels in epileptic patients. *Br J Clin Pharmacol* 1977;4:541–547.

132. Hansen JM, Siersboek-Nielsen K, Skovsted L. Carbamazepine-induced acceleration of diphenylhydantoin and warfarin metabolism in man. *Clin Pharmacol Ther* 1971;12:539–543.

133. Cereghino JJ, Meter JC, Brock JT, et al. Preliminary observations of serum carbamazepine concentration in epileptic patients. *Neurology* 1973;23:357–366.

134. Hooper WD, Dubetz DK, Eadie MJ, et al. Preliminary observations on the clinical pharmacology of carbamazepine ("Tegretol"). *Proc Aust Assoc Neurol* 1974;11:189–198.

135. Lai ML, Lin TS, Huang JD. Effect of single- and multiple-dose carbamazepine on the pharmacokinetics of diphenylhydantoin. *Eur J Clin Pharmacol* 1992;43:201–203.

136. Windorfer A, Sauer W. Drug interactions during anticonvulsant therapy in childhood: diphenylhydantoin, primidone, phenobarbitone, clonazepam, nitrazepam, carbamazepine and dipropylacetate. *Neuropadiatrie* 1977;8:29–41.

137. Browne TR, Szabo GK, Evans JE, et al. Carbamazepine increases phenytoin serum concentration and reduces phenytoin clearance. *Neurology* 1988;38:1146–1150.

138. Zielinski JJ, Haidukewych D, Leheta BJ. Carbamazepine-phenytoin interaction: elevation of plasma phenytoin concentrations due to carbamazepine comedication. *Ther Drug Monit* 1985;7:51–53.

139. Zielinski JJ, Haidukewych D. Dual effects of carbamazepine-phenytoin interaction. *Ther Drug Monit* 1987;9:21–23.

140. Veronese ME, Mackenzie PI, Doecke CJ, et al. Tolbutamide and phenytoin hydroxylations by cDNA-expressed human liver cytochrome P4502C9 [published erratum appears in *Biochem Biophys Res Commun* 1991;180:1527]. *Biochem Biophys Res Commun* 1991;175:1112–1118.

141. Bajpai M, Roskos LK, Shen DD, et al. Roles of cytochrome P4502C9 and cytochrome P4502C19 in the stereoselective metabolism of phenytoin to its major metabolite. *Drug Metab Dispos* 1996;24:1401–1403.

142. Schlienger R, Kurmann M, Drewe J, et al. Inhibition of phenprocoumon anticoagulation by carbamazepine. *Eur Neuropsychopharmacol* 2000;10:219–221.

143. Zhou HH, Anthony LB, Wood AJ, et al. Induction of polymorphic 4'-hydroxylation of S-mephenytoin by rifampicin. *Br J Clin Pharmacol* 1990;30:471–475.

144. Sachdeo RC, Sachdeo SK, Walker SA, et al. Steady-state pharmacokinetics of topiramate and carbamazepine in patients with epilepsy during monotherapy and concomitant therapy. *Epilepsia* 1996;37:774–780.

145. Bourgeois BF. Drug interaction profile of topiramate. *Epilepsia* 1996;37[Suppl 2]:S14–S17.

146. Bowdle TA, Levy RH, Cutler RE. Effects of carbamazepine on valproic acid kinetics in normal subjects. *Clin Pharmacol Ther* 1979;26:629–634.

147. Levy RH, Morselli PL, Bianchetti G, et al. Interaction between valproic acid and carbamazepine in epileptic patients. In: Levy RH, Pitlick WH, Eichelbaum M, et al., eds. *Metabolism of antiepileptic drugs.* New York: Raven Press, 1982:45–51.

148. Nakasa H, Nakamura H, Ono S, et al. Prediction of drug-drug interactions of zonisamide metabolism in humans from in vitro data. *Eur J Clin Pharmacol* 1998;54:177–183.

149. Ito T, Yamaguchi T, Miyazaki H, et al. Pharmacokinetic studies of AD-810, a new antiepileptic compound: phase I trials. *Arzneimittelforschung* 1982;32:1581–1586.

150. Ojemann LM, Shastri RA, Wilensky AJ, et al. Comparative pharmacokinetics of zonisamide (CI-912) in epileptic patients on carbamazepine or phenytoin monotherapy. *Ther Drug Monit* 1986;8:293–296.

151. Shinoda M, Akita M, Hasegawa M, et al. The necessity of adjusting the dosage of zonisamide when coadministered with other anti-epileptic drugs. *Biol Pharm Bull* 1996;19:1090–1092.

152. Chiba K, Kobayashi K. Antidepressants. In: Levy RH, Thummel KE, Trager WF, et al., eds. *Metabolic drug interactions.* Philadelphia: Lippincott Williams & Wilkins, 2000:233–244.

153. Brown CS, Wells BG, Cold JA, et al. Possible influence of carbamazepine on plasma imipramine concentrations in children with attention deficit hyperactivity disorder. *J Clin Psychopharmacol* 1990;10:359–362.

154. Leinonen E, Lillsunde P, Laukkanen V, et al. Effects of carbamazepine on serum antidepressant concentrations in psychiatric patients. *J Clin Psychopharmacol* 1991;11:313–318.

155. Brosen K, Kragh-Sorensen P. Concomitant intake of nortriptyline and carbamazepine. *Ther Drug Monit* 1993;15:258–260.

156. Venkatakrishnan K, von Moltke LL, Greenblatt DJ. Nortriptyline E-10-hydroxylation in vitro is mediated by human CYP2D6 (high affinity) and CYP3A4 (low affinity): implications for interactions with enzyme-inducing drugs. *J Clin Pharmacol* 1999;39:567–577.

157. Ketter TA, Jenkins JB, Schroeder DH, et al. Carbamazepine but not valproate induces bupropion metabolism. *J Clin Psychopharmacol* 1995;15:327–333.

158. Hesse LM, Venkatakrishnan K, Court MH, et al. CYP2B6 mediates the in vitro hydroxylation of bupropion: potential drug interactions with other antidepressants. *Drug Metab Dispos* 2000;28:1176–1183.

159. Faucette SR, Hawke RL, Lecluyse EL, et al. Validation of bupropion hydroxylation as a selective marker of human cytochrome P450 2B6 catalytic activity. *Drug Metab Dispos* 2000;28:1222–1230.

160. Nawishi S, Hathaway N, Turner P. Interaction of anticonvulsant drugs with mianserin and nomifensine. *Lancet* 1981;2:870–871.

161. Tiihonen J, Vartiainen H, Hakola P. Carbamazepine-induced changes in plasma levels of neuroleptics. *Pharmacopsychiatry* 1995;28:26–28.

162. Jerling M, Lindstrom L, Bondesson U, et al. Fluvoxamine inhibition and carbamazepine induction of the metabolism of clozapine: evidence from a therapeutic drug monitoring service. *Ther Drug Monit* 1994;16:368–374.

163. Hesslinger B, Normann C, Langosch JM, et al. Effects of carbamazepine and valproate on haloperidol plasma levels and on psychopathologic outcome in schizophrenic patients. *J Clin Psychopharmacol* 1999;19:310–315.

164. Hirokane G, Someya T, Takahashi S, et al. Interindividual variation of plasma haloperidol concentrations and the impact of concomitant medications: the analysis of therapeutic drug monitoring data. *Ther Drug Monit* 1999;21:82–86.

165. Levy RH, Kerr BM. Clinical pharmacokinetics of carbamazepine. *J Clin Psychiatry* 1988;49[Suppl]:58–62.

166. Lucas RA, Gilfillan DJ, Bergstrom RF. A pharmacokinetic interaction between carbamazepine and olanzapine: observa-

tions on possible mechanism. *Eur J Clin Pharmacol* 1998;54: 639–643.

167. Spina E, Avenoso A, Facciola G, et al. Plasma concentrations of risperidone and 9-hydroxyrisperidone: effect of comedication with carbamazepine or valproate. *Ther Drug Monit* 2000;22: 481–485.

168. Spina E, Scordo MG, Avenoso A, et al. Adverse drug interaction between risperidone and carbamazepine in a patient with chronic schizophrenia and deficient CYP2D6 activity. *J Clin Psychopharmacol* 2001;21:108–109.

169. Back DJ, Orme ML. Pharmacokinetic drug interactions with oral contraceptives. *Clin Pharmacokinet* 1990;18:472–484.

170. Rapport DJ, Calabrese JR. Interactions between carbamazepine and birth control pills. *Psychosomatics* 1989;30:462–464.

171. Crawford P, Chadwick DJ, Martin C, et al. The interaction of phenytoin and carbamazepine with combined oral contraceptive steroids. *Br J Clin Pharmacol* 1990;30:892–896.

172. Guengerich FP. Oxidation of 17 alpha-ethynylestradiol by human liver cytochrome P-450. *Mol Pharmacol* 1988;33: 500–508.

173. Kerlan V, Dreano Y, Bercovici JP, et al. Nature of cytochromes P450 involved in the 2-/4-hydroxylations of estradiol in human liver microsomes. *Biochem Pharmacol* 1992;44:1745–1756.

174. Alvarez JS, Del Castillo JAS, Ortiz MJA. Effect of carbamazepine on cyclosporin blood level. *Nephron* 1991;58:235–236.

175. Yee GC, McGuire TR. Pharmacokinetic drug interactions with cyclosporin: part I. *Clin Pharmacokinet* 1990;19:319–332.

176. Combalbert J, Fabre I, Fabre G, et al. Metabolism of cyclosporin A: IV. purification and identification of the rifampicin-inducible human liver cytochrome P-450 (cyclosporin A oxidase) as a product of P450IIIA gene subfamily. *Drug Metab Dispos* 1989;17:197–207.

177. Cooney GF, Mochon M, Kaiser B, et al. Effects of carbamazepine on cyclosporine metabolism in pediatric renal transplant recipients. *Pharmacotherapy* 1995;15:353–356.

178. Denbow CE, Fraser HS. Clinically significant hemorrhage due to warfarin-carbamazepine interaction. *South Med J* 1990;83:981.

179. Cropp JS, Bussey HI. A review of enzyme induction of warfarin metabolism with recommendations for patient management. *Pharmacotherapy* 1997;17:917–928.

180. Kunze KL, Wienkers LC, Thummel KE, et al. Warfarin-fluconazole: I. inhibition of the human cytochrome P450-dependent metabolism of warfarin by fluconazole: in vitro studies. *Drug Metab Dispos* 1996;24:414–421.

181. Rettie AE, Korzekwa KR, Kunze KL, et al. Hydroxylation of warfarin by human cDNA-expressed cytochrome P-450: a role for P-4502C9 in the etiology of (S)-warfarin-drug interactions. *Chem Res Toxicol* 1992;5:54–59.

182. Schlienger R, Kurmann M, Drewe J, et al. Inhibition of phenprocoumon anticoagulation by carbamazepine. *Eur Neuropsychopharmacol* 200;10:219–221.

183. Tartara A, Galimberti CA, Manni R, et al. Differential effects of valproic acid and enzyme-inducing anticonvulsants on nimodipine pharmacokinetics in epileptic patients. *Br J Clin Pharmacol* 1991;32:335–340.

184. Penttila O, Neuvonen PJ, Aho K, et al. Interaction between doxycycline and some antiepileptic drugs. *BMJ* 1974;2: 470–472.

185. Hugen PW, Burger DM, Brinkman K, et al. Carbamazepine—indinavir interaction causes antiretroviral therapy failure. *Ann Pharmacother* 2000;34:465–470.

186. Bonay M, Jonville-Bera AP, Diot P, et al. Possible interaction between phenobarbital, carbamazepine and itraconazole. *Drug Saf* 1993;9:309–311.

187. Villikka K, Kivisto KT, Maenpaa H, et al. Cytochrome P450-inducing antiepileptics increase the clearance of vincristine in patients with brain tumors. *Clin Pharmacol Ther* 1999;66: 589–593.

188. Feierman DE, Lasker JM. Metabolism of fentanyl, a synthetic opioid analgesic, by human liver microsomes: role of CYP3A4. *Drug Metab Dispos* 1996;24:932–939.

189. Tempelhoff R, Modica PA, Spitznagel EL. Anticonvulsant therapy increases fentanyl requirements during anaesthesia for craniotomy. *Can J Anaesth* 1990;37:327–332.

23

CARBAMAZEPINE

CLINICAL EFFICACY AND USE IN EPILEPSY

PIERRE LOISEAU

The efficacy of carbamazepine (CBZ) in patients with epilepsy was first demonstrated in the early 1960s and the drug was licensed in Europe soon after its discovery. The threat of serious adverse reactions (hematopoietic disturbances) delayed its use in North America. It was later demonstrated that the risk had been exaggerated. Along with valproic acid (VPA), CBZ belongs to the second generation of anticonvulsants, considered as having less neurotoxicity than older drugs such as phenytoin (PHT), phenobarbital (PB), and primidone (PRM), and it has been increasingly prescribed as a first-line drug. With the introduction of many new antiepileptic drugs (AEDs) in the 1990s, the question now is its place in a wider armamentarium of antiepileptic medication.

SPECTRUM OF EFFICACY

Evidence supporting the efficacy of CBZ as an anticonvulsant is derived from a host of studies with various designs. Some of these studies are summarized here.

Randomized, Controlled Trials

CBZ effectivness has been compared with that of a placebo or of active drugs, either alone or as an add-on medication.

Carbamazepine versus Placebo

CBZ or placebo was added for 3-week periods to baseline therapy of PB and PHT in 37 hospitalized adult patients with intractable psychomotor epilepsy. Secondarily generalized seizures were reduced by 55% and psychomotor seizures by 83% when the patients were on CBZ (1). Twenty-three difficult-to-control outpatients of all ages with grand mal or psychomotor seizures received CBZ and placebo for 3 months

each. The preexisting medication was unchanged, but the CBZ dosage was increased, according to tolerance, up to 1,200 mg; complete control was not achieved in any, but ≥50% improvement occurred in 12 patients (2).

Carbamazepine versus Phenytoin

CBZ and PHT were compared in 24 adult epileptic patients with behavior disorders. They received the two drugs as sole medication, each for a 6- month period; no significant difference was found between the two drugs with regard to efficacy, but CBZ, compared with PHT, reduced significantly the severity of personality disorders (3). Thirty-eight patients (>12 years of age) with psychomotor seizures (31 previously treated) received CBZ or PHT as sole medication, each for 16 weeks. The effect of both drugs was the same, but some patients, however, responded better either to CBZ or to PHT (4). CBZ and PHT as sole drug were given to 47 adult outpatients with moderately severe seizure disorders (5). This double-blind study confirmed the conclusions of a pilot study (6): Both drugs were approximately equally effective, but significantly fewer patients experienced side effects while on CBZ. Efficacy of CBZ and PHT was compared in adult patients with partial (n = 10), primary generalized (n = 4), undetermined (n = 4), or secondarily generalized epilepsy (n = 1). Each treatment period lasted 10 weeks, and all medication except PB or PRM was discontinued gradually while CBZ or PHT was increased to a dose of approximately 15 mg/kg for CBZ and 6 mg/kg for PHT; the dose subsequently was adjusted on the basis of plasma levels. No statistically significant differences were found between CBZ and PHT with regard to seizure control (7). Hakkarainen (8) reported a 3-year study of 100 consecutive adults with newly diagnosed epilepsy in which half the patients were randomly allocated to CBZ or to PHT treatment. After the first year, complete control of seizures was achieved in 50 patients (26 on CBZ and 24 on PHT). For nonresponders, the treatment was changed from CBZ to PHT or vice-versa for the second year; complete

---

Pierre Loiseau, MD: Honorary Professor, Department of Neurology, Bordeaux Medical University, Bordeaux, France

control of seizures was achieved in another eight patients on CBZ and in nine on PHT. For the remaining 33 nonresponders, combined CBZ and PHT treatment was used for the third year, and 5 (15%) of these patients became totally seizure free. New referrals were randomly assigned to receive as initial therapy either CBZ plus placebo or PHT plus placebo, and increases in dosage were made until plasma concentrations were adequate or seizure control was attained. Complete control was achieved in 85% of the 70 who completed the 2-year study, without difference between the two drugs (9). A randomized, double-blind study substituted PHT monotherapy with CBZ or oxcarbazepine in adult outpatients with unsatisfactory seizure control of partial or generalized tonic-clonic seizures (GTCS) or with unwanted side effects; seven (39%) of the patients in CBZ group became seizure free or showed >50% reduction in seizure frequency during the maintenance phase (1 year) compared with the seizure control on PHT therapy (10). In a randomized, double-blind study in young children, CBZ and PHT were equally effective (11).

Carbamazepine versus Phenobarbital

Behavioral and anticonvulsant effects of CBZ versus PB were evaluated in 21 adult patients; after 2 months on the original double-blind prescription, a crossover was made to the other compound for an additional 4-month period. Although no significant difference in efficacy during the final months of each drug treatment phase was found, significant behavioral improvement was noted when on CBZ (12). Children with untreated, newly diagnosed partial seizures received either CBZ (n = 15) or PB (n = 18) for 12 months; if necessary, the dose was gradually increased to the maximum amount tolerated or until the serum level was 10 to 12 mg/L for CBZ and 32 to 40 mg/L for PB. There was a statistically nonsignificant trend toward better seizure control with CBZ (13).

Carbamazepine versus Primidone

Patients with either predominantly psychomotor seizures (n = 31) or GTCS only (n = 14) were initially stabilized on therapeutic doses of PHT and either CBZ or PRM, while all other medications were progressively withdrawn; after 3 months of treatment, their drugs were switched for a second 3-month period. Both drugs had a similar efficacy in partial as well as generalized seizures (14).

Carbamazepine versus Clonazepam

Thirty-six previously untreated patients, 6 to 72 years of age, with newly diagnosed complex partial seizures were randomly allocated to 6-month treatment with either CBZ or clonazepam; 10 of 19 patients on CBZ and 8 of 17 on clonazepam became seizure free (15).

Carbamazepine versus Valproic Acid

In a small study, 25 adult patients (18 untreated, 7 uncontrolled when on PB or PHT) were randomly divided into two treatment groups with VPA (n = 15) or CBZ (n = 10). After 3 months of treatment, any patient who had a seizure while on the first drug was changed to the other drug; no significant difference in seizure control was noted (16). Mattson et al. (17) conducted a multicenter, randomized, double-blind, parallel trial comparing CBZ with VPA in the treatment of 480 adults with complex partial seizures (206 patients) or secondarily GTCS (274 patients). The medication was prescribed initially at dosages adjusted to achieve serum levels in the middle of the therapeutic range. Dosages later were decreased if side effects required change or increased if control was inadequate. Patients were followed 1 to 5 years. For secondarily GTCS, significant differences were not detected between CBZ and VPA, even if a trend favored CBZ. For patients with GTCS only, a retrospective analysis revealed CBZ to be significantly more effective than VPA (18). For complex partial seizures, CBZ was significantly more effective than VPA by a number of outcome measures, but not for total seizure control. In a smaller study, either CBZ or VPA as sole medication was given in 33 previously untreated or insufficiently treated patients, aged 10 to 70 years, who had experienced at least 2 complex partial seizures; complete control during the 24-week maintenance period was achieved in 64% of the patients in both groups (19). The Adult EPITEG Collaborative Group compared CBZ and VPA in adult patients with newly diagnosed partial and secondarily or primarily GTCS. By the end of the 3-year trial period, 80% of the patients available for assessment had achieved 12 months' remission and 60% had achieved 24 months' remission, with a similar proportion in each treatment group (20).

Carbamazepine versus Oxcarbazepine

The Scandinavian Oxcarbazepine Study Group (21) randomly allocated adult patients with previously untreated epilepsy (primarily GTCS or partial seizures with or without secondary generalization) to treatment with either CBZ (n = 82) or oxcarbazepine (n = 83). During the 48-week treatment period, somewhat more patients obtained seizure control (60% versus 52%) or >50% reduction in seizure frequency (81.4% versus 80.2%) with CBZ, a statistically nonsignificant difference.

Carbamazepine versus Vigabatrin

The efficacy and safety of CBZ and vigabatrin (VGB) monotherapy in patients with partial seizures were compared in two randomized, controlled, response-conditional, crossover, open-label trials. In the first trial (22), after 1 year 26 of 50 (52%) patients in the CBZ group and 16 of 50

(32%) in the VGB group were seizure free. In the second study (23), complete control of seizures was obtained in 20 of 39 (51.3%) patients treated with CBZ, and in 17 of 37 (45.9%) patients treated with VGB, a statistically nonsignificant difference. The combination of the two drugs suppressed the seizures in 5 of 14 resistant cases. Although both agents had a similar efficacy in partial seizures without secondary generalization, CBZ was superior to VGB in patients with secondarily generalized seizures (five of seven and two of six patients treated, respectively).

Carbamazepine versus Lamotrigine

Adults with newly diagnosed, untreated epilepsy were randomized to CBZ (n = 129) or lamotrigine (LTG; n = 131) as sole drugs for a treatment duration of 48 weeks; seizures were partial with or without secondary generalization in 73 patients for each group, and primarily GTCS in 62 patients in the CBZ group and 60 in the LTG group. No difference was found between the two drugs at the time of first seizure or in the proportion of patients remaining seizure free in the last 24 weeks of the trial (38% for CBZ and 39% for LTG); no difference according to seizure type was noted (24). Another trial compared CBZ and LTG as monotherapy in the same category of patients; there was no significant differences between three treatment groups with respect to the number of patients who completed the 24-week treatment seizure free, although the higher LTG dose (200 mg/day) possibly was most effective, with 60.4% seizure-free patients compared with 51.3% (LTG 100 mg/day) and 54.7% (CBZ 600 mg/day) (25).

Carbamazepine versus Phenytoin versus Phenobarbital

Efficacy and tolerance of CBZ were evaluated in a prospective, double-blind study in 45 drug-resistant adult patients; during each of the three 21-day treatment periods, one-third of the patients were assigned to receive PHT (300 mg/day), PB (300 mg/day), or CBZ (1,200 mg/day). CBZ was equal in efficacy to PHT or PB (26). Polymedicated patients with frequent complex partial seizures received CBZ, PHT, or PB in a prospective, double-blind, crossover study; CBZ and PB were more active than PHT, with improvement in 67%, 61%, and 33% of the patients, respectively (27).

Carbamazepine versus Phenytoin versus Valproic Acid

Efficacy of CBZ, PHT, and VPA was compared in 181 new referrals with epilepsy (5 to 69 years of age) over a 14- to 24-month follow-up period (28). One of the three drugs was given initially to all patients on a randomized basis. If the patient failed to respond to the first drug or experienced side effects, a second drug was randomly allocated as single treatment, and, if necessary, a third single drug was prescribed. Patients with GTCS became seizure free in 73% of cases on PHT, 39% on CBZ, and 59% on VPA; a >50% improvement was noted in 8%, 36%, and 19% of cases, respectively. Patients with partial seizures became seizure free in 57% of cases on PHT, 33% on CBZ, and 44% on VPA, and a >50% improvement was noted in 19%, 39%, and 33% of cases, respectively.

Carbamazepine versus Phenytoin versus Phenobarbital versus Primidone

CBZ efficacy was found equivalent to that of PB, PHT, or PRM in 45 mentally subnormal adult inpatients with GTCS (29). In a large, double-blind trial, 622 adult patients were randomly assigned to monotherapy with CBZ, PB, PHT, or PRM and were followed for 2 years or until the drug failed to control seizures or caused unacceptable side effects. Patients had previously been untreated (58%) or undertreated and had simple or complex partial seizures (265 patients) or secondarily GTCS (357 patients) as their predominant seizure type. Overall treatment success was highest with CBZ or PHT, intermediate with PB, and lowest with PRM. Differences in failure rates were explained mostly by the fact that PRM and PB caused more toxic effects. Seizure control was only 39% at 12 months for all patients and all seizure types, and was similar among the drugs tested. CBZ provided significantly better control of partial seizures (30) compared with the barbiturates.

Carbamazepine versus Phenytoin versus Phenobarbital versus Sodium Valproate

In 243 previously untreated adult epileptic patients, no significant differences between the four drugs were found for either measure of efficacy, with 27% remaining seizure free and 75% entering 1 year of remission by 3 years of follow-up (31). Seizure type (partial versus generalized seizures) had no influence on the comparative efficacy.

OTHER STUDIES

CBZ was discovered long before the Good Clinical Practice Guidelines were formulated, and the drug was licensed, at least in Europe, on the basis of open studies that contemporary health authorities considered sufficient for approval. The results of the first administration of CBZ to humans were simultaneously reported by Bonduelle and colleagues and by Lorgé at the Third International Congress of Neuropsychopharmacology (Munich, 1962). The first retrospective or prospective series studies, in which CBZ was prescribed as an add-on medication, date back to the early 1960s.

Polytherapy

Some of these studies are summarized as examples.

Lorgé added CBZ to the therapeutic regimen of 132 adult patients with different types of epileptic seizures, most of whom had been uncontrolled for many years; the follow-up period ranged from 3 months to 3 years. Twenty-five percent of patients became seizure free and a further 37% had a >50% reduction in seizure frequency; the author concluded that CBZ was an effective antiepileptic agent in all seizure types except absence seizures and was particularly effective in grand mal and psychomotor seizures, and he called attention to its psychotropic effect and its lack of serious side effects (32). Bonduelle et al. prescribed CBZ as add-on therapy in 100 patients of all ages (26 <16 years of age) with PB-resistant seizures. After 1 year, 26 were seizure free, 25 experienced infrequent seizures, and 18 had a >50% reduction in seizure frequency; mood and behavior were considered as improved in almost half the patients (33). Gamstorp (34) gave CBZ to 58 children, 55 of whom had difficult-to-treat partial or generalized seizures. CBZ sometimes was added to the drugs given previously and sometimes replaced one or two of these drugs. Twenty-two patients became seizure free and eight were considerably improved. In three patients, CBZ seemed to increase the number of attacks and cause a deterioration in behavior, with improvement when the drug was stopped. The 24 improved patients remained under observation (35). Of the 19 controlled patients, 13 remained entirely seizure free, 8 for more than 8 years. Of the six patients who relapsed, five had mild and infrequent attacks and only one had a severe relapse 6 months after the initial response. In 1975, Gamstorp (36) reviewed the records of 43 patients with psychomotor epilepsy treated with CBZ at a dose of 20 mg/kg/day. Twenty-three of the 38 children who tried CBZ and tolerated it became seizure free, and 6 were considerably improved. Huf and Schain reported the long-term use of CBZ over a 5-year period; at the time of evaluation, 50 (82%) of 61 children with drug-resistant epilepsy were regarded by their parents as having improved seizure control: 13 were seizure free, and 37 had ≥50% reduction in seizure frequency; no patients were believed to be aggravated (37). Many other studies were conducted with a roughly similar methodology and similar results (38,39).

Some of these studies raised suspicions over the development of tolerance (36). Parsonage reported a retrospective open study of 100 adult patients with refractory complex partial seizures; at the time of review, 11 patients were fully controlled, 22 had a reduction of seizure frequency >50%, 20 had a reduction <50%, 30 were unchanged, and in 15 the seizures showed an increased frequency (however, the drug was withdrawn on this account only in 4 of them) (38). Good control of seizures had been maintained in a number of patients for as long as 12 years, and development of tolerance is not mentionned (38).

Monotherapy

The King's College Hospital group undertook a prospective study of 25 outpatients with GTCS or partial seizures who were treated initially with CBZ and followed for a mean of 1 year. At the end of the period of observation, 21 of 25 (84%) were completely controlled (40). In a prospective study, CBZ was prescribed as a single drug to 11 previously untreated patients and 17 pharmacoresistant patients with either partial or generalized seizures. Ten new referrals and one patient with chronic epilepsy became seizure free, and a >50% reduction in seizure frequency occurred in one new referral and nine refractory patients; the mean follow-up period was 14 months (range, 7 to 32 months) (41). During a 5-year period, CBZ monotherapy was started in 286 patients with various seizure types; CBZ was the drug of first choice in 64%. Of the 253 patients treated for over 3 months at the time of evaluation, 141 were seizure free, and a satisfactory therapeutic effect (no seizure or a reduction in seizure frequency ≥75%) was achieved in a total of 188 patients (74%). In 31 patients (12%), there was an increase in seizure frequency compared with the period immediately before CBZ monotherapy (42). Sixty-eight children with various epilepsy types received CBZ as sole drug for a mean period of 10 months; CBZ was the first therapy in 13 children, whereas in others PB or VPA had been unsuccessful. The seizures disappeared in 43% of cases (43). In another study, polytherapy was replaced by CBZ monotherapy in 43 adult outpatients with chronic epilepsy of various types. Reduction of polytherapy and maintenance of monotherapy was successful in 31 (72%) of the patients; in the monotherapy group, a reduction of >50% in seizure frequency was observed in 25% of the patients with a mean follow-up period of 2 years (44).

Psychotropic Effects of Carbamazepine in Patients with Epilepsy

Reports on psychotropic effects in patients with epilepsy when treated with CBZ have been conflicting, with regard both to their reality and to their mechanisms when their existence was admitted. The first investigators noticed in their patients a frequent and sometimes dramatic improvement in mood and behavior (32,33,45,46). A survey of 40 published reports, concerning approximately 2,500 patients, allowed Dalby (47) to state that a beneficial psychotropic effect was present in 50% of patients. On the other hand, a few studies did not demonstrate any clear-cut change (1,2,29). The question of a psychotropic effect of CBZ treatment therefore was addressed by means of objective neuropsychological testing or rating scales (1,3,12,13,26,48–50). A review was published in 1985 (51).

Changes observed may be summarized as follows : (a) better alertness, with better attention and concentration;

(b) better mood, with reduction of depression and anxiety; and (c) better behavior, with less irritability and aggressiveness. Three nonexclusive factors might be responsible for these changes, which could be classified into two separate categories, intellectual and affective functioning, but in reality encompass a broad range of interrelated functions (52):

1. A direct psychotropic effect of CBZ. Two series of arguments favor a direct action on mood. A correlation between higher levels of CBZ and reduced levels of anxiety and depression was found (49,53). Many investigators have noticed that patients with a past history of emotional or behavioral disturbances were more likely to improve when on CBZ than those without such a history (47). Gamstorp (34) noted that "CBZ did not seem to cause any change in the behavior of patients who had seem mentally normal before the trial." More direct evidence in support of the psychotropic effects of CBZ derives from its efficacy in patients who have neither seizure disorders nor epileptiform EEG patterns (39,51) (Chapter 26).
2. A reduction in or control of seizures (26). According to some authorities, this factor may play a role, but is not indispensable. However, one may assume that it is important when CBZ is effective, dramatically reducing the number of seizures and, hence, improving the patient's quality of life (54) and improving cognition, because both epileptic seizures and interictal epileptiform discharges may cause cognitive disturbances and structural brain damage.
3. Substitution of CBZ for sedative AEDs. The cognitive effects of AEDs have been widely investigated during the past 30 years (55). Double-blind studies compared the behavior and the neuropsychological performances of patients on CBZ or on other drugs. Patients on CBZ were better, but reanalyses of the early studies have shown that the differential cognitive effects of AEDs are subtle (56). These studies do not demonstrate a psychotropic effect of CBZ, but only that, to some extent, CBZ is less neurotoxic than PHT, PB, and PRM. They do not prove that CBZ has no negative effect. Performances were improved after its withdrawal (57,58).

In summary, CBZ has been prescribed as an add-on drug in patients with refractory epilepsy and as one-drug treatment in untreated patients or in previously treated chronic patients, children as well as adults. The overall efficacy results, as measured by control of seizures, ranked CBZ as one of the most effective AEDs. In monotherapy studies, complete control often was achieved, and a reduction of seizure frequency by at least 75% was obtained in 60% to 90% of patients. Reports mainly based on clinical observation suggested additional beneficial psychotropic effects.

MODE OF USE

Indications

Adults

CBZ is effective against the entire range of partial seizures (i.e., simple and complex seizures) with or without secondary generalization (59). In terms of epilepsies and epileptic syndromes, it is a drug of first choice in cryptogenic as well as in symptomatic localization-related epilepsies. CBZ efficacy against GTCS also is well documented. In terms of epileptic syndromes, it can be prescribed in idiopathic generalized epilepsies with GTCS, excepting juvenile myoclonic epilepsy, and in epilepsies without unequivocal generalized or focal seizures.

Children

"Carbamazepine is effective in children when it is administered in the appropriate situation" (60). CBZ is a first-line drug for any patient with partial seizures and secondarily generalized seizures. In terms of epileptic syndromes, its efficiency is documented in cryptogenic and symptomatic localization-related epilepsies, and in idiopathic benign epilepsies of childhood (61). CBZ use in generalized epilepsies is more controversial. Undoubtedly, children with GTCS due to idiopathic epilepsies have been included in some studies, with excellent result. However, there have been reports of children whose seizures were made worse by CBZ (see section on Contraindications).

Dosing Recommendations

CBZ therapy must begin gradually; a full therapeutic dosage may not be achieved for many days or even weeks (59).

Starting Dosage

An evening dosage of 100 mg (half a 200-mg scored tablet) is recommended in adults and children older than 12 years of age; in younger children, a lower dosage is used, depending on the patient's weight (scored chewable tablet or suspension).

Titration Rate

The procedure of rapidly achieving a therapeutic concentration by use of loading doses is not possible with CBZ because of the transient side effects that would occur during initiation of therapy (62). Dizziness, unsteadiness, blurred vision or double vision, sedation, nausea, and vomiting have been noted by early investigators and were well documented in controlled studies in adults, for example with a dosage regimen of 400 mg on the first day, 800 mg on the second day, and 1,200 mg on the third day (26). The side effects peaked on the third day. Even if they are mild and transient, they can lead to patients stopping the medication. Furthermore, a rapid titration substantially increases the risk of skin rash and hypersensitivity syndrome. The most convincing report was published in the 1980s (63). Patients undergoing craniotomy for a variety of neurosurgical conditions associated with a high risk of epilepsy received CBZ 200 mg for three oral doses at 8-hour intervals in the 24 hours preceding surgery, and 200 mg three times daily as a maintenance dose thereafter. In 8 of 48 (16.6%) patients, exanthematous skin eruptions developed, a much higher incidence than usual. Therefore, the initial dosage must be increased slowly to the full therapeutic dosage over a variable period. When the clinical situation allows it, a weekly interval is preferred (59). In case of frequent seizures, the interval should be shorter (e.g., every second day), with a slower increase if side effects appear. In general, dosage is increased until seizures cease or dose-related side effects occur. In case of side effects, the total daily dose is reduced by 100 or 200 mg.

Initial Target Maintenance Dosage

Because both low doses and low plasma concentrations may give complete seizure control in many patients, at least in patients with newly diagnosed epilepsy, it is important not to hurry and to make individual adjustments based on clinical grounds. Patients with newly diagnosed epilepsy were controlled with a mean CBZ dose of 7.5 mg/day, whereas patients with chronic epilepsy were controlled only with a mean CBZ dose of 10.3 mg/kg (64). In general, there is little correlation between dosage and therapeutic efficacy (26,62,64,65). Doses giving control ranged from 600 to 1,600 mg in adults (38) (i.e., 3 to 15.9 mg/kg) (64).

CBZ induces its own metabolism during prolonged administration, which results in increased clearance (Chapter 21). Thus, sequential increases in dosage may be necessary over the first few weeks of treatment (9).

Optimal Range of Maintenance Dosages

The mean effective dosage is probably 20 mg/kg in children younger than 5 years of age and 10 mg/kg in other patients. However, there is no one dosage of CBZ appropriate for all patients.

Three reasons may explain persisting seizures: poor compliance, an inadequate dosing regimen, and a truly CBZ-resistant epilepsy. Plasma level determinations allow easy detection of poorly compliant patients. Because of a poor correlation between dosage and efficacy, it was recommended that CBZ dosage be adjusted by plasma level monitoring. It was assumed that the serum CBZ level was posi-

tively correlated with the degree of seizure control (66). Optimum seizure control was reported to occur with CBZ plasma concentration in the range of 5 to 10 mg/L (67). Other authorities stated that such a wide range of serum levels was associated with seizure control that it was not possible to define a therapeutic range for CBZ (41,64). The relation of plasma levels to drug efficacy and toxicity is inexact. When large groups of patients are considered, it is not uncommon to find that uncontrolled patients have higher plasma levels than controlled patients. Plasma level monitoring is a useful tool for the clinician, but has no definitive value. In uncontrolled patients, it is necessary to push the drug to the maximum clinically tolerated dose, regardless of its plasma level.

Dosage Intervals

The plasma concentration of carbamazepine is characterized by rapid absorbtion and a relatively short elimination half-life, which may lead to considerable fluctuation of the level between doses. Interdosage fluctuations in CBZ plasma concentrations with high peak levels are considered to be responsible for transient side effects occurring 2 to 4 hours after drug intake (i.e., peak-related side effects) (68–70). In patients receiving comedication with enzyme inducers, such as PHT, PB, and PRM, the CBZ elimination half-life is rather short, ranging from 5.6 to 16 hours (mean, 8.2 hours). For these reasons, some epileptologists concluded that CBZ should be administered no fewer than four or five times a day. Such frequent dosing would be very uncomfortable for most outpatients and would lead to poor compliance. Even a thrice-daily administration, as recommended (71), probably is unnecessary for many patients. Two or three doses provide approximately the same amount of CBZ available in circulation, with a mean fluctuation of 57% ± 20% and 56% ± 29%, respectively (72). A twice-a-day schedule would be as effective (6,59). However, when high doses of CBZ are necessary, acute toxicity could be avoided by splitting the dosage into a thrice-daily pattern.

Extended-Release Carbamazepine

Because detrimental consequences might result from large plasma drug level fluctuations, with either breakthrough seizures at the trough level times or intermittent peak-related side effects, new CBZ formulations were developed in the late 1980s. They have prolonged absorption (slow-release, extended-release, controlled-release) characteristics (CBZ-CR). They give higher minimum serum levels (C_{min}) and lower maximum serum levels (C_{max}). In adults, the mean daily fluctuation was 30% ± 10% with CBZ-CR twice-daily administration, whereas it was 61% ± 17% with CBZ thrice daily (72). In children, the interdose variation in CBZ plasma concentration was 21% for the patients receiving CBZ-CR and 41% for the patients receiving comparable doses of the standard CBZ preparation (73). A once-daily evening dose of CBZ-CR was considered to give therapeutically efficient 24-hour levels (74). In a multicenter, double-blind, crossover trial of CBZ versus CBZ-CR in 30 patients, fluctuations of CBZ and CBZ-epoxide levels at steady state were significantly lower for CBZ-CR, leading to a significant decrease in intermittent side effects (75). In adult patients, fewer cognitive side effects of CBZ were observed when fluctuations in the serum concentration were smoothed by slow-release absorption (76). More recently, a randomized, double-blind, two-way, crossover study compared the pharmacokinetics of twice-daily CBZ-CR and four-times-daily immediate-release CBZ in 24 adult patients with epilepsy. No differences were found for area under the curve, C_{max}, and C_{min} (77). Patients who had been on high-dosage conventional CBZ reported significant reductions in side effects with CBZ-CR, and several patients were noted to have improved seizure control because higher doses were possible with fewer side effects (78). Similar advantages occur with use of other delayed-release formulations (Tegretol XR and Carbatrol).

Generics

Controversy over generic drugs has existed for decades, and therapeutic equivalence and bioequivalence are issues with generic drugs (79). A variety of case reports and uncontrolled studies reported differences between generic and brand products, and among generics. These differences could result in loss of seizure control or in development of toxic effects. Such a loss of control in patients switched from Tegretol to a generic CBZ product, with subsequent recovery of control on switching back to Tegretol, was reported (80).

Current Role in Epilepsy Management

Monotherapy is the rule in untreated patients (81), and may be possible in certain patients previously treated with unsatisfactory results, but not in all of them (82). The advantages of a single-drug treatment are well established (83). CBZ currently is the most frequently prescribed first-line drug for the treatment of partial tonic-clonic seizures and GTCS in both adults and children. Conversely, it is ineffective against some particular types of generalized seizures (see later). Patients remaining uncontrolled at the maximum tolerable dose of CBZ should be given another treatment, which may be alternative monotherapy. However, certain patients whose seizures are not controlled with a single drug benefit from drug combination (84). After failure of monotherapies, bitherapies must be considered, despite pharmacokinetic and pharmacodynamic problems of interactions, because of solutions to these problems

(85,86). Several reports are in favor of the efficacy of bitherapy in the 20% to 30% of patients who are not controlled with one drug only. Addition of VPA in 100 CBZ-resistant patients resulted in 17% seizure free, and improvement was noted in 39% (87). Confirmation was given in a smaller study (88). The aim of a randomized, double-blind study in patients with partial seizures uncontrolled on CBZ monotherapy was to see how many did better on bitherapy (89). Approximately 10% of the 215 adult patients remained seizure free during the final 3-month treatment period. This study suggests that when a Na^+ blocking agent, such as CBZ, fails, adding a γ-aminobutyric acid agonist-drug, such as VPA or VGB, may be successful. However, some drug-resistant patients do benefit from PHT/CBZ combination therapy without a significant increase in drug toxicity (8,90).

CBZ withdrawal, for failure as well as for success, always should be progressive to prevent withdrawal seizures.

Use in Special Populations

Infants and Children

Because children metabolize CBZ faster than adults, larger doses can be recommended in children (60). The younger the patient, the higher the CBZ clearance rate, and hence the higher the dosage required. This statement is true mainly for infants (91). However, even in children, twice-daily administration is feasible (36,43,92).

Women of Childbearing Potential

CBZ decreases the efficacy of contraceptive pills by induction of cytochrome P450 isoenzyme 3A (CYP3A)–mediated metabolism of oral contraceptive corticosteroids (Chapter 22). Epidemiologic data suggest that there may be an association between the use of CBZ during pregnancy and fetal malformations (93). Breast-feeding usually is not contraindicated (94).

The Elderly

No systematic studies in geriatric patients have been conducted, but in daily practice as well as in clinical studies, elderly patients were prescribed CBZ without harm. Nonspecific problems include (a) a possible increased sensitivity to the effects of medication owing to age-dependent changes in pharmacokinetics and pharmacodynamics; and (b) frequent comedication, with risks of meaninful drug interactions (Chapters 13 and 22).

Comedicated Patients

Patients being treated for epilepsy can be at risk when they are prescribed other drugs for concomitant diseases (95) because of drug–drug interactions (Chapter 22). Clinically,

CBZ metabolism induction by other drugs is less important than its inhibition by CYP3A4 inhibitors. Toxic symptoms and signs may develop in the patient in a few days. The combination of CBZ and VPA must be prescribed with caution. By inhibiting epoxide hydrolase, VPA increases CBZ-epoxide levels (96). This may result in side effects. Another inconvenience of an increase in CBZ-epoxide is the increase in formation of arene oxides with probable teratogenicity, which means that the combination of CBZ and VPA must be avoided in pregnancy. The combination also must be avoided in infants because CBZ increases the formation of delta-4 VPA, a probably hepatotoxic metabolite (97).

Precautions

CBZ should be prescribed with caution in patients with a history of cardiac, hepatic, or renal damage and adverse hematologic reactions to other drugs.

CBZ adverse effects are discussed fully in Chapter 26. In patient management, the skin, the central nervous system, and the blood must be checked for evidence of toxicity. Rashes occur in approximately 5% to 10% of patients. They appear in most cases within the first few months after initiation of therapy. They usually are transient, but can precede a Stevens-Johnson syndrome. Our personal policy is to stop the therapy. It is important to determine if neurotoxicity is peak dependent or dose dependent. When it is peak dependent, subdividing the daily dosage is sufficient. When it is dose dependent, the daily dosage must be decreased. A wide range of serum levels was associated with these side effects (28). However, concentrations greater than 12 mg/L usually have been associated with toxic signs (2,66).

Because of very rare aplastic anemias and rather common benign leukopenias, hematologic monitoring has been recommended. It no longer is requested by many European neurologists (42). Porter (59) suggested checking the white blood cell count weekly for 1 month and biweekly for 6 additional weeks after initiation of therapy.

Routine laboratory monitoring may be helpful for early detection of chronic adverse reactions, but severe adverse reactions can occur despite careful surveillance (98).

Contraindications

CBZ should not be used in patients with known sensitivity to any of the tricyclic antidepressants, and its use with monoamine oxidase inhibitors is not recommended.

In the 1990s, there was a growing awareness that AEDs can worsen epileptic conditions by aggravating preexisting seizures or by triggering new seizure types (99,100). To date, exacerbation of seizures and worsening of electroencephalographic (EEG) recordings by CBZ has been reported in a number of case reports, and there is accumu-lating evidence that CBZ is relatively contraindicated in certain types of seizures and specific epilepsy syndromes. An increase of GTCS and absences and precipitation of atonic and myoclonic seizures in children have been reported (101–107). It has been well known since the early 1970s that CBZ is not indicated in the treatment of typical absence seizures. Nonetheless, of 18 consecutive referrals of children with resistant typical absences only, 8 were erroneously treated with CBZ either as sole drug or as an add-on. Frequency of absence seizures increased in four children, and in two of these myoclonic jerks developed that resolved on withdrawal of CBZ (108). CBZ-related aggravation is not limited to children. In adult patients, CBZ therapy resulted in exacerbation or *de novo* appearance of absence or myoclonic seizures (109–113).

In summary, exacerbation of seizures can result from CBZ therapy. At particularly high risk are children with symptomatic or cryptogenic generalized or multifocal severe epilepsy, characterized by mixed seizure types, and generalized, synchronous, spike–wave discharges. Patients with any of the idiopathic epilepsies also are at risk for CBZ-associated seizures, whatever their age, particularly when they experience absence seizures or myoclonic jerks. An EEG might help screen higher-risk patients, and serial EEGs are recommended when starting CBZ therapy in patients at risk: Seizure exacerbation almost invariably is accompanied by the development of generalized epileptiform discharges.

SUMMARY

Many studies have demonstrated CBZ efficacy against cryptogenic and symptomatic localization-related epilepsies, undetermined epilepsies, and some seizure types in a number of forms of idiopathic generalized epilepsies. Its efficacy in symptomatic generalized epilepsy is controversial, and it may worsen absence and myoclonic seizures. It is effective as single-drug treatment and in combination therapy. However, monotherapy always is preferable. In previously untreated patients, a moderate dosage often is sufficient. In seizures that are difficult to control, CBZ must be pushed to the maximally tolerated dose. Plasma level monitoring is more useful in polytherapy than in monotherapy. Dose choice is determined on a clinical and not a laboratory basis. CBZ was shown to be as effective as other AEDs, with less long-term side effects than PB, PRM, or PHT. It is a drug of choice because of either a direct psychotropic effect or indirect beneficial effects resulting from a lack of neurotoxicity.

REFERENCES

1. Rodin EA, Rim CS, Rennick PM. Effect of carbamazepine on patients with psychomotor epilepsy: result of a double-blind study. *Epilepsia* 1974;15:547–561.

2. Kutt H, Solomon G, Wasterlain C, et al. Carbamazepine in difficult to control epileptic out-patients. *Acta Neurol Scand Suppl* 1975;60:27–32.

3. Rajotte P, Jilek W, Jilek L, et al. Propriétés antiépileptiques et psychotropes de la carbamazépine (Tégrétol). *Union Med Can* 1967;96:1200–1206.

4. Simonsen N, Olsen IZ, Kuhl V, et al. A comparative controlled study between carbamazepine and diphenylhydantoin in psychomotor epilepsy. *Epilepsia* 1976;17:169–176.

5. Troupin AS, Ojeman LM, Halpern L, et al. Carbamazepine: a double-blind comparison with phenytoin. *Neurology* 1977;27:511–519.

6. Troupin AS, Green JR, Levy R. Carbamazepine as an anticonvulsant: a pilot study. *Neurology* 1974;24:863–869.

7. Kosteljanetz M, Christiansen J, Mouritzen Dam A, et al. Carbamazepine vs. phenytoin: a controlled trial in focal motor and generalized epilepsy. *Arch Neurol* 1979;36:22–24.

8. Hakkarainen H. Carbamazepine and diphenylhydantoin as monotherapy or in combination in the treatment of adult epilepsy. *Neurology* 1980;30:354.

9. Ramsay RE., Wilder BJ, Berger JR, et al. A double-blind study comparing carbamazepine with phenytoin as initial therapy in adults. *Neurology* 1983;33:904–910.

10. Reinikainen K, Keränen T, Hallikaien E, et al. Substitution of diphenylhydantoin by oxcarbazepine or carbamazepine: double-blind study. *Acta Neurol Scand Suppl* 1984;98:89–90.

11. Stein J. Carbamazepine versus phenytoin in young epileptic children. *Drug Ther* 1989;19:76–77.

12. Marjerrisson G, Jedlicki SM, Keogh RET, et al. Carbamazepine: behavioral, anticonvulsant and EEG effects in chronically-hospitalized epileptics. *Dis Nerv Syst* 1968;29:133–136.

13. Mitchell WG, Chavez JM. Carbamazepine versus phenobarbital for partial seizures in children. *Epilepsia* 1987;28:56–60.

14. Rodin EA, Rim CS, Rennick PM. A comparison of the effectiveness of primidone versus carbamazepine in epileptic out-patients. *J Nerv Ment Dis* 1976;163:41–46.

15. Mikkelsen B, Berggreen P, Joensen P, et al. Clonazepam (Rivotril) and carbamazepine (Tegretol) in psychomotor epilepsy: a randomized multicenter trial. *Epilepsia* 1981;22:415–420.

16. Shakir RA. Sodium valproate, phenytoin and carbamazepine as sole anticonvulsants. In: Parsonage MJ, Cadwell DS, eds. *The place of sodium valproate in the treatment of epilepsy.* London: Royal Society of Medecine International Congress and Symposium Series, 1980:7–16.

17. Mattson RH, Cramer JA, Collins JF. A comparison of valproate with carbamazepine for the treatment of complex partial seizures and secondarily generalized tonic-clonic seizures. *N Engl J Med* 1992;327:765–771.

18. Mattson RH. Carbamazepine. In: Engel J, Pedley T, eds. *Epilepsy: a comprehensive textbook.* Philadelphia: Lippincott-Raven, 1997:1491–1502.

19. So EL, Lai CW, Pellock J, et al. Safety and efficacy of valproate and carbamazepine in the treatment of complex partial seizures. *J Epilepsy* 1992;5:149–152.

20. Richens A, Davidson DLW, Cartlidge NEF, et al. A multicentre comparative trial of sodium valproate and carbamazepine in adult onset epilepsy. *J Neurol Neurosurg Psychiatry* 1994;57:682–687.

21. Dam M, Ekberg R, Loyning Y, et al. A double-blind study comparing oxcarbazepine and carbamazepine in patients with newly diagnosed, previously untreated epilepsy. *Epilepsy Res* 1989;3:70–76.

22. Kälviäinen R, Mervaala E, Sivenius J, et al. Vigabatrin: clinical use. In: Levy RH, Mattson RH, Meldrum BS, eds. *Antiepileptic drugs,* 4th ed. New York: Raven Press, 1995:925–930.

23. Tanganelli P, Regesta G. Vigabatrin vs. carbamazepine monotherapy in newly diagnosed focal epilepsy: a randomized response conditional cross-over study. *Epilepsy Res* 1996;25:257–262.

24. Brodie MJ, Richens A, Yuen AWC. Double-blind comparison of lamotrigine and carbamazepine in newly diagnosed epilepsy. *Lancet* 1995;345:476–479.

25. Reunanen M, Dam M, Yuen AWC. A randomised open multicentre comparative trial of lamotrigine and carbamazepine as monotherapy in patients with newly diagnosed or recurrent epilepsy. *Epilepsy Res* 1996;23:149–155.

26. Cereghino JJ, Brock JT, Van Meter JC, et al. Carbamazepine for epilepsy: a controlled prospective evaluation. *Neurology* 1974;24:401–410.

27. Benassi E, Loeb C, Desio G, et al. Carbamazepine, diphenylhydantoin, phenobarbital: a prospective trial in 18 temporal lobe epilepsy. In: Johannessen SI, Morselli PL, Pippenger CE, et al., eds. *Antiepileptic therapy: advances in drug monitoring.* New York: Raven Press, 1980:195–202.

28. Callaghan N, Kenny RA, O'Neill B, et al. A prospective study between carbamazepine, phenytoin and sodium valproate as monotherapy in previously untreated and recently diagnosed patients with epilepsy. *J Neurol Neurosurg Psychiatry* 1985;41:639–644.

29. Bird CAK, Griffin BP, Milkazevska JM, et al. Tegretol (carbamazepine): a controlled trial of a new anticonvulsant. *Br J Psychiatry* 1966;112:737–742.

30. Mattson RH, Cramer JA, Collins JF, et al. Comparison of carbamazepine, phenobarbital, phenytoin, and primidone in partial and secondarily generalized tonic-clonic seizures. *N Engl J Med* 1985;313:145–151.

31. Heller AJ, Chesterman P, Elwes RDC, et al. Phenobarbitone, phenytoin, carbamazepine, or sodium valproate for newly diagnosed adult epilepsy: a randomized comparative monotherapy trial. *J Neurol Neurosurg Psychiatry* 1995;58:44–50.

32. Lorgé M. Klinische Erfahrungen mit einen neuen Antiepilepticum, Tegretol (G 32.883), mit besonderer Wirkung auf die epileptische Wesenveränderung. *Schweiz Med Wochenschr* 1963;93:1042–1058.

33. Bonduelle M, Bouygues P, Sallou C, et al. Expérimentation clinique de l'anti-épileptique G. 32.883 (Tégrétol): résultats portant sur 100 cas observés en trois ans. *Rev Neurol (Paris)* 1964;110:209–215.

34. Gamstorp I. A clinical trial of Tegretol in children with severe epilepsy. *Dev Med Child Neurol* 1966;8:296–300.

35. Gamstorp I. Long-term follow-up of children with severe epilepsy treated with carbamazepine (Tegretol®, Geigy). *Acta Paediatr Scand Suppl* 1970;206:96–97.

36. Gamstorp I. Treatment with carbamazepine: children. *Adv Neurol* 1975;11:237–248.

37. Huf R, Schain RJ. Long-term experiences with carbamazepine (Tegretol) in children with seizures. *J Pediatr* 1980;97:310–312.

38. Parsonage M. Treatment with carbamazepine: adults. *Adv Neurol* 1975;11:221–234.

39. Sillanpää M. Carbamazepine: pharmacology and clinical use. *Acta Neurol Scand Suppl* 1981;88:1–202.

40. Shorvon SD, Chadwick D, Galbraith AW, et al. One drug for epilepsy. *BMJ* 1978;1:474–476.

41. Callaghan N, O'Callaghan M, Duggan B, et al. Carbamazepine as a single drug in the treatment of epilepsy: a prospective study of serum levels and seizure control. *J Neurol Neurosurg Psychiatry* 1978;41:907–912.

42. Klee JG, Andersen EB, Philbert A. Carbamazepine (Tegretol) monotherapy in epilepsy: a retrospective study in out-patients. In: Dam M, Gram L, Penry JK, eds. *Advances in epileptology:*

XIIth Epilepsy International Symposium. New York: Raven Press, 1981:509–514.

43. Dulac O, Bouguerra L, Rey E, et al. Monothérapie par la carbamazépine dans les épilepsies de l'enfant. *Arch Fr Pediatr* 1983; 40:415–419.

44. Keränen T, Reinikainen K, Riekkinen PJ. Carbamazepine monotherapy versus polytherapy in chronic epilepsies. *Acta Neurol Scand Suppl* 1984;98:87–88.

45. Jongmans JWM. Report on the antiepileptic effect of Tegretol. *Epilepsia* 1964;5:74–82.

46. Arieff AJ, Mier M. Anticonvulsant and psychotropic action of Tegretol. *Neurology* 1966;16:107–110.

47. Dalby MA. Behavioral effects of carbamazepine. *Adv Neurol* 1975;11:331–341.

48. Thompson PJ, Trimble MR. Anticonvulsant drugs and cognitive functions. *Epilepsia* 1982;23:531–544.

49. Andrewes DB, Bullen JG, Tomlinson L, et al. A comparative study of the cognitive effects of phenytoin and carbamazepine in new referrals with epilepsy. *Epilepsia* 1986;22:128–134.

50. Smith B, Mattson RH, Cramer JA, et al. Results of a nationwide Veterans Administration cooperative study comparing the efficacy and toxicity of carbamazepine, phenobarbital, phenytoin and primidone. *Epilepsia* 1987;28[Suppl 3]:550–558.

51. Evans RW, Gualteri CT. Carbamazepine: a neuropsychological and psychiatric profile. *Clin Neuropharmacol* 1985;8:221–241.

52. Devinsky O. Cognitive and behavioral effects of antiepileptic drugs. *Epilepsia* 1995;36[Suppl 2]:S46–S65.

53. Macphee GJA, MacPhail EM, Butler E, et al. Controlled evaluation of a supplementary dose of carbamazepine on psychomotor function in epileptic patients. *Eur J Clin Pharmacol* 1986;31:195–199.

54. Aldenkamp AP, Alpherts WCJ, Sandstedt P, et al. Antiepileptic drug-related cognitive complaints in seizure-free children with epilepsy before and after drug discontinuation. *Epilepsia* 1998; 39:1070–1074.

55. Vermeulen J, Aldenkamp AP. Cognitive side-effects of chronic antiepileptic drug treatment: a review of 25 years of research. *Epilepsy Res* 1995;22:65–95.

56. Kälviäinen R, Äikiä M, Riekkinen PJ Sr. Cognitive adverse effects of antiepileptic drugs: incidence, mechanisms and therapeutic implications. *CNS Drugs* 1996;5:358–368.

57. Gallassi R, Moreale A, Loruso S, et al. Carbamazepine and phenytoin: comparison of cognitive effects in epileptic patients during monotherapy and withdrawal. *Arch Neurol* 1988;45: 892–894.

58. Duncan JS, Shorvon SD, Trimble MR. Effects of removal of phenytoin, carbamazepine, and valproate on cognitive function. *Epilepsia* 1990;31:584–591.

59. Porter RJ. How to initiate and maintain carbamazepine therapy in children and adults. *Epilepsia* 1987;28[Suppl 3]:S59–S63.

60. Dodson WE. Carbamazepine efficacy and utilization in children. *Epilepsia* 1987;28[Suppl 3]:S17–S24.

61. Lerman P, Kivity-Ephraim S. Carbamazepine sole anticonvulsant for focal epilepsy of childhood. *Epilepsia* 1974;15:229–234.

62. Cereghino JJ. Serum carbamazepine concentration and clinical control. *Adv Neurol* 1975;11:309–330.

63. Chadwick D, Shaw MDM, Foy P, et al. Serum anticonvulsant concentrations and the risk of drug induced skin eruptions. *J Neurol Neurosurg Psychiatry* 1984;47:642–644.

64. Strandjord RE, Johannessen SI. Single-drug therapy with carbamazepine in patients with epilepsy: serum levels and clinical effect. *Epilepsia* 1980;21:655–662.

65. Theodore WH, Narang PK, Holmes MD, et al. Carbamazepine and its epoxide: relation of plasma levels to toxicity and seizure control. *Ann Neurol* 1989;25:194–196.

66. Schneider H. Carbamazepine: an attempt to correlate serum levels with antiepileptic and side effects. In: Schneider H, Janz D, Gardner-Thorpe C, et al., eds. *Clinical pharmacology of antiepileptic drugs.* Berlin: Springer-Verlag, 1975:151–158.

67. Bertilsson L. Clinical pharmacokinetics of carbamazepine. *Clin Pharmacokinet* 1978;3:128–143.

68. Höppener RJ, Kuyer A, Meijer JWA. Correlations between daily fluctuations of carbamazepine serum levels and intermittent side-effects. *Epilepsia* 1980;21:341–350.

69. Riva R, Albani F, Ambrosetto G, et al. Diurnal fluctuations of free and total steady-state plasma levels of carbamazepine and correlation with intermittent side-effects. *Epilepsia* 1984;25:476–481.

70. Tomson T. Interdosage fluctuations in plasma carbamazepine concentration determine intermittent side-effects. *Arch Neurol* 1984;41:830–833.

71. Henriksen O, Johannessen SI, Munthe-Kaas AW. How to use carbamazepine. In: Morselli PL, Pippenger CE, Penry JK, eds. *Antiepileptic drugs in pediatrics.* New York: Raven Press, 1983: 227–243.

72. Johannessen SI, Henriksen O. Comparison of the serum concentration profiles of Tegretol and two new slow-release preparations. *Adv Epileptol* 1987;16:421–423.

73. Ryan SW, Forsythe I, Hartley R, et al. Slow release carbamazepine in treatment of poorly controlled seizures. *Arch Dis Child* 1990;65:930–935.

74. Stefan H, Schäfer H, Kreiten K, et al. Once daily evening dose of carbamazepine sustained release: profiles of 24-hour plasma levels. *Adv Epileptol* 1987;16:425–426.

75. Canger R, Belvedre D, Cornaggia CM, et al. Studio clinico-farmacocinetico della CBZ convenzionale versus la CBZ a rilasco controllato (CR): trial multicentrico in doppio cieco, cross-over. *Boll Lega Ital Epil* 1987;58/59:309–311.

76. Aldenkamp AP, Alpherts WCJ, Moerland MC, et al. Controlled release carbamazepine: cognitive side effects in patients with epilepsy. *Epilepsia* 1987;28:507–514.

77. Garnett WR, Levy B, McLean AM, et al. Pharmacokinetic evaluation of twice-daily extended-release carbamazepine (CBZ) and four-time-daily immediate-release CBZ in patients with epilepsy. *Epilepsia* 1998;39:274–279.

78. Tikku D, Sachdeo RC, Kaufman KR. Open-label prospective clinical evaluation of Tegretol XR in patients with epilepsy. *Epilepsia* 1999;40[Suppl 7]:68–69.

79. Bialer M, Yacobi A, Moros D, et al. Criteria to assess in vivo performance and bioequivalence of generic controlled-release formulations of carbamazepine. *Epilepsia* 1998;39:513–517.

80. Sachdeo RC, Belendiuk G. Generic versus branded carbamazepine. *Lancet* 1987;1:1432.

81. Reynolds EH, Shorvon SD. Monotherapy or polytherapy for epilepsy? *Epilepsia* 1981;22:1–10.

82. Perucca E. Pharmacological principles as a basis for polytherapy. *Acta Neurol Scand Suppl* 1995;162:31–34.

83. Perucca E. Pharmacologic advantages of antiepileptic drug monotherapy. *Epilepsia* 1997;38[Suppl 5]:S6–S8.

84. Schmidt D, Gram L. Monotherapy versus polytherapy in epilepsy. In: Mallarkey G, Palmer, KJ, eds. *Issues in epilepsy.* Auckland, New Zealand: Adis, 1999:67–81.

85. Deckers CLP, Hekster YA, Keyser A, et al. Reappraisal of polytherapy in epilepsy: a critical review of drug load and adverse effects. *Epilepsia* 1997;38:570–575.

86. Ferrendelli JA. Pharmacology of antiepileptic drug polypharmacy. *Epilepsia* 1999;40[Suppl 5]:S81–S83.

87. Dean JC, Penry JK. Carbamazepine/valproate therapy in 100 patients with partial seizures failing carbamazepine monotherapy: long-term follow-up. *Epilepsia* 1988;29:687.

88. Walker JE, Koon R. Carbamazepine versus valproate versus

combined therapy for refractory partial complex seizures with secondary generalization. *Epilepsia* 1988;29:693.

89. Brodie MJ, Mumford JP, 012 Study Group. Double-blind substitution of vigabatrin and valproate in carbamazepine-resistant partial epilepsy. *Epilepsy Res* 1999;34:199–205.

90. Lorenzo NY, Bromfield EB, Theodore WH. Phenytoin and carbamazepine: combination versus single-drug therapy for intractable partial seizures. *Ann Neurol* 1988;24:136.

91. Morselli PL. Carbamazepine: absorption, distribution and excretion. *Adv Neurol* 1975;11:279–293.

92. Jeavons PM. Monotherapy with sodium valproate and carbamazepine. In: Clifford Rose F, ed. *Research progress in epilepsy.* Bath, UK: Pitman, 1983:406–412.

93. Samren E, Lindhout D. Major malformations associated with maternal use of anti-epileptic drugs. In: Tomson T, Gram L, Sillanpää M., et al., eds. *Epilepsy and pregnancy.* Chichester, UK: Wrightson Biomedical, 1997:43–61.

94. Yerby MS. Problems and management of the pregnant woman with epilepsy. *Epilepsia* 1987;28[Suppl 3]:S29–S38.

95. Loiseau P. Treatment of concomitant illnesses in patients receiving anticonvulsants: drug interactions of clinical significance. *Drug Saf* 1998;19:495–510.

96. Levy RH, Moreland TA, Morselli PL, et al. Carbamazepine/valproic acid interaction in man and in rhesus monkey. *Epilepsia* 1984;25:338–345.

97. Levy RH, Rettenmeier AWA, Anderson GD, et al. Effects of polytherapy with phenytoin, carbamazepine, and stiripentol on formation of 4-ene valproate, a hepatotoxic metabolite of valproic acid. *Clin Pharmacol Ther* 1990;48:225–235.

98. Wyllie E, Wyllie R. Routine laboratory monitoring for serious adverse effects of antiepileptic medications: the controversy. *Epilepsia* 1991;32[Suppl 5]:S74–S79.

99. Perucca E, Gram L, Avanzini G, et al. Antiepileptic drugs as a cause of worsening of seizures. *Epilepsia* 1998;39:5–17.

100. Guerrini R, Belmonte A, Genton P. Antiepileptic drug-induced worsening of seizures in children. *Epilepsia* 1998;39[Suppl 3]:S2–S10.

101. Shields WP, Saslow E. Myoclonic, atonic and absence seizures following institution of carbamazepine therapy in children. *Neurology* 1983;33:1487–1489.

102. Johnsen SD, Tarby TJ, Sidell AD. Carbamazepine-induced seizures. *Ann Neurol* 1984;16:392–393.

103. Hurst DL. Carbamazepine-induced absences and minor motor seizures. *Neurology* 1985;35[Suppl 1]:286.

104. Snead OC, Hosey LC. Exacerbation of seizures in children by carbamazepine. *N Engl J Med* 1985;313:916–921.

105. Lerman P. Seizures induced or aggravated by anticonvulsants. *Epilepsia* 1986;27:706–710.

106. Caraballo R, Fontana E, Michelizza B, et al. Carbamazepina, assence atipiche, crisi atoniche e stato di PO continua del sonno (POCS). *Boll Lega Ital Epil* 1989;66/67:379–381.

107. Dhuna A, Pascual-Leone A, Talwar D. Exacerbation of partial seizures and onset of nonepileptic myoclonus with carbamazepine. *Epilepsia* 1991;32:275–278.

108. Parker APJ, Agathonikou A, Robinson RO, et al. Inappropriate use of carbamazepine and vigabatrin in typical absence seizures. *Dev Med Child Neurol* 1998;40:517–519.

109. Sachdeo RC, Chokroverty S. Enhancement of absences with carbamazepine. *Epilepsia* 1985;26:534.

110. So EL, Ruggles KH, Cascino GD, et al. Seizure exacerbation and status epilepticus related to carbamazepine 10,11-epoxide. *Ann Neurol* 1994;35:743–746.

111. Liporace JD, Sperling MR, Dichter MA. Absence seizures and carbamazepine in adults. *Epilepsia* 1994;35:1026–1028.

112. Talwar D, Arora MS, Sher PK. EEG changes and seizure exacerbation in young children treated with carbamazepine. *Epilepsia* 1994;35:1154–1159.

113. Sözüer DT, Atakli D, Atay T, et al. Evaluation of various antiepileptic drugs in juvenile myoclonic epilepsy. *Epilepsia* 1996;37[Suppl 4]:S77.

CARBAMAZEPINE

CLINICAL EFFICACY AND USE IN OTHER NEUROLOGIC DISORDERS

ETTORE BEGHI

Carbamazepine (CBZ) has been one of the most extensively investigated antiepileptic drugs for the treatment of neurological disorders other than epilepsy. CBZ exerts a use-dependent inhibition of sodium channels and reduces the frequency of sustained repetitive firing of action potentials in neurons. CBZ also may inhibit the release of somatostatin and have some calcium antagonistic effects (1,2). These mechanisms of action may explain the efficacy of CBZ in conditions like neuropathic pain and pain syndromes, hemifacial spasm, restless legs syndrome (RLS), or myotonia. The analgesic effects of CBZ are correlated with the plasma levels of the drug (3). However, most of the evidence on the use of CBZ in these disorders comes from nonrandomized studies or from small randomized trials. This prevents solid conclusions on the clinical efficacy of this drug in many of these conditions.

NEUROPATHIC PAIN

Neuropathic pain is a spectrum of neuralgic pain syndromes that includes trigeminal neuralgia and neuralgias affecting other cranial or peripheral nerves (glossopharyngeal, superior laryngeal, postherpetic), diabetic neuropathy, thalamic syndrome, phantom limb pain, tabetic pain, cancer pain, and others.

Trigeminal and Other Chronic Neuralgias

CBZ has been extensively investigated for the treatment of trigeminal neuralgia, a paroxysmal form of facial pain commonly affecting the second and third division of the trigeminal nerve. The results of randomized clinical trials on the use of CBZ in patients with trigeminal or other neuralgias are illustrated in Table 24.1 (4–11). The daily dose ranged from 100 to 2,400 mg. The drug was manifestly superior to placebo and was more effective or better tolerated than

other active comparators (tizanidine, tocainide, pimozide). Pain relief was obtained in up to 84% of cases and persisted after prolonged treatment in up to 80% (8,12). In a systematic review of three placebo-controlled studies (13), the odds ratio (OR) for efficacy of CBZ was 4.9 [95% confidence interval (CI), 3.4 to 6.9]; however, patients on active treatment had more adverse events (OR, 3.7; 95% CI, 2.2 to 6.2) and were more frequently withdrawn from treatment (OR, 6.2; 95% CI, 1.2 to 31.7). The number-needed-to-treat for effectiveness of CBZ compared with placebo was 2.6 (95% CI, 2.0 to 3.4), and that for adverse events was 3.7 (95% CI, 2.4 to 7.8) (14).

The efficacy of CBZ in neuropathic pain other than trigeminal neuralgia is supported by less consistent findings (Table 24.2). The drug has been compared with placebo, prednisolone, nortriptyline–fluphenazine, or transcutaneous electrical nerve stimulation (TENS) for the management of pain in patients with diabetes (15,16), stroke (17), herpes zoster (18,19), and Guillain-Barré syndrome (20). CBZ 150 to 1,000 mg/day was better than placebo and TENS, similar to nortriptyline–fluphenazine, and less effective than prednisolone and amitriptyline. Nonrandomized studies (mostly case reports and case series) reported CBZ being effective in glossopharyngeal neuralgia, phantom limb pain, multiple sclerosis, thalamic syndrome, and miscellaneous neuralgias (2).

Based on the results of the randomized clinical trials, CBZ can still be considered as a first-line drug for the treatment of trigeminal neuralgia. The starting dose may be 100 to 200 mg. In most cases, the daily dose should be increased gradually until pain relief is achieved, up to 1,000 to 1,200 mg. In this population of predominantly elderly patients, adverse effects may appear if dosing is not very low and gradual . Occasionally, further dose increments may be suggested. The daily dose of 2,400 mg should never be exceeded. Given the spontaneous remission of pain and the toxic effects of long-term treatment with CBZ, treatment withdrawal should be recommended after 2 to 3 months in patients with pain relief. In patients not responding to CBZ, phenytoin, gabapentin, lamotrigine, or topiramate

Ettore Beghi, MD: Chief, Neurophysiology Unit, "San Gerardo" Hospital, Monza, Italy; and Head, Neurological Disorders Laboratory, Institute for Pharmacological Research "Mario Negri," Milan, Italy

TABLE 24.1. RANDOMIZED CLINICAL TRIALS OF CARBAMAZEPINE FOR TRIGEMINAL AND OTHER CRANIAL NEURALGIAS

Ref.	No. Treated (age, yr) [Disease]	Treatment Duration [Double-Blind Period]	Daily Dose, mg [Comparator]	Significant Results [No. Improved]	Adverse Events[a] [No. Withdrawals]
4	9 (37–76) [Trigeminal]	3 days	600 [PLC]	CBZ preferred by 8/9; CBZ and PLC equally effective in 1/9	(11 taking CBZ in open trial also assessed) CBZ 14/20; PLC 3/9 [CBZ1/20; PLC 0/9]
5	77 (20–84) [Trigeminal]	4 wk (two 2-wk periods)	400–800 [PLC]	Reduction of pain severity to 57% with CBZ and 15% with PLC (32% difference) No. paroxysms reduced by 68% (PLC 26%). Effect of triggers reduced by 68% (PLC 40%) [CBZ 144/268; PLC 35/190]	CBZ 38/77; PLC 20/77 [CBZ 1/77; PLC 0/77]
6	42 (36–83) [Trigeminal 30; postherpetic 6; tabetic 2; atypical facial pain 4]	10 days	400–1,000 [PLC]	[Mild improvement to complete recovery with CBZ in 100% with trigeminal neuralgia, postherpetic and tabetic pain; PLC response minimal or absent in all patients]	(Only trigeminal neuralgia) CBZ 23/36 [CBZ 3/30]
7	37 (?) [Trigeminal]	2 wk	100–2,400 [PLC]	[CBZ 15/20; PLC 6/24]	Drowsiness: CBZ 10/37 Ataxia: CBZ 7/37 [CBZ 2/37; PLC 0/24]
8	71 (30–80+) [Trigeminal typical 40; atypical 16; other facial pain 15]	One or two 5-day periods	400–600 [PLC]	[Typical trigeminal: CBZ 33/40; PLC 8/40; atypical: CBZ 13/15; PLC 1/15; other facial pain: CBZ 8/15; PLC 2/15]	(Including long-term assessment) CBZ 9/71 [CBZ 4/71; PLC 0/71]
9	12 (47–72) [Trigeminal]	3 wk	900 [TZN 18]	[CBZ 4/6; TZN 1/5]	[TZN 3/6; CBZ 0/6]
10	12 (41–78) [Trigeminal]	2 wk	Max. tolerated dose [TCN 60/kg]	[12/12 on both drugs]	TCN 3/12; [TCN 1/12; CBZ 0/12]
11	48 (48–68) [Trigeminal]	8 wk	300–1,200 [PMZ 4–12; PLC]	Arbitrary symptom score reduced by 78% with PMZ and 50% with CBZ [PMZ 18/48; CBZ 27/48]	PMZ 40/48 CBZ 21/48

CBZ, carbamazepine; PLC, placebo; PMZ, pimozide; TCN, tocainide; TZN, tizanidine.
[a] No. with any event or, if unavailable, with most common events.

TABLE 24.2. RANDOMIZED CLINICAL TRIALS OF CARBAMAZEPINE FOR NEUROPATHIC PAIN OTHER THAN TRIGEMINAL NEURALGIA

Ref.	No. Treated (age, yr) [Disease]	Treatment Duration [Double-Blind Period]	Daily Dose, mg [Comparator]	Significant Results [No. Improved]	Adverse Events[a] [No. Withdrawals]
15	30 (21–81) [Diabetic neuropathy]	2 wk	Up to 600 [PLC]	[CBZ 28/30; PLC 19/30]	Somnolence: CBZ 16/30 Dizziness: CBZ 12/30 [CBZ 2/30; PLC 0/30]
16	16 (?) [Diabetic neuropathy]	4 wk	600 [FPZ/NTP 1.5/30]	Visual analogue scale no difference between treatments	CBZ 3/16; FPZ 8/16 [CBZ 2?]
17	15 (53–74) [Stroke]	4 wk	Up to 800 [AMT up to 75; PLC]	Mean pain intensity at week 4 (10-step verbal scale): CBZ 4.2; AMT 4.2; PLC 5.3 [CBZ 5/14; AMT 10/15; PLC 1/15]	CBZ 13/14; AMT 14/15; PLC 7/15 [CBZ 1/14; AMT 0/15; PLC 0/15]
18	29 (NR) [Postherpetic neuralgia]	8 wk	150–1,000+ CLP 10–75 [TNS]	Mean improvement (pain difference) with CBZ+CLP: 43.1 points [CBZ+CLP 11/12 TNS 2/4]	[CBZ 3/16; TCN 2/13]
19	40 (50–86) [Acute herpes zoster]	4 wk	400 [PDN 40 for 10 days, then tapered]	Healing faster with PDN Neuralgia: CBZ 13/20; PDN 3/20	None
20	12 (22–54) [Guillain-Barré syndrome]	7 days	300 [PLC]	Pain score (range 0–5): CBZ 1.7; PLC 3.1 Sedation score (range 0–6): CBZ 2.3; PLC 4.2 Pethidine requirement: CBZ 1.7 mg/kg/day; PLC 3.7 mg/kg/day	None significant

ADL, activities of daily living; AMT, amitriptyline; ASP, aspirin; CBZ, carbamazepine; CLP, clonazepam; FPZ, fluphenazine; NR, not reported; NTP, nortriptyline; PDN, prednisolone; PLC, placebo; TNS, transcutaneous electrical nerve stimulation. [a] No. with any event or, if unavailable, with most common events.

could be attempted as monotherapy or in combination. Patients with intractable pain may require either percutaneous thermocoagulation of the trigeminal ganglion or direct exploration of the trigeminal root.

The use of CBZ also can be considered for the treatment of glossopharyngeal neuralgia, based on common pathophysiologic mechanisms. Less consistent findings support the use of the drug in other chronic pain syndromes, for which no definite guidelines can be proposed. Because the risk of adverse treatment events and drug withdrawal is high with CBZ, the drug should be used only with constant reference to its risk–benefit profile.

MIGRAINE AND TENSION-TYPE HEADACHE

The frequency of migraine and tension-type headache and their ill-defined pathogenic mechanisms, spectrum of severity, and variable response to treatment prompted the investigation of some anticonvulsant drugs, including valproic acid, clonazepam, lamotrigine, and CBZ.

There is only one double-blind, crossover, placebo-controlled study assessing the efficacy of CBZ in the treatment of migraine (21). In this study, 48 patients aged 14 to 60 years were treated with CBZ 600 mg/day or equivalent placebo for 6 weeks. CBZ was better than placebo in reducing the number of attacks and increasing the number of responders. Adverse events were most common in patients given active treatment (CBZ, 30/45; placebo, 11/48), but only one case on CBZ needed to withdraw from treatment. Despite these encouraging findings, evidence is insufficient to support the use of CBZ in migraine, tension-type, or other chronic headache syndromes.

RESTLESS LEGS SYNDROME AND OTHER SLEEP DISORDERS

RLS is a common sensorimotor disorder with an estimated prevalence of 1% to 5%, characterized by unpleasant sensation in the legs occurring predominantly during sleep (22). This syndrome may cluster in families and be secondary to other clinical conditions, like anemia, pregnancy, or peripheral neuropathies. The effects of CBZ in patients with RLS have been tested in two randomized clinical trials. In a small, placebo-controlled, crossover study in six patients, CBZ up to 600 mg/day reduced the number of attacks in three cases (placebo, 0) (23). The apparent efficacy in RLS was confirmed in a larger, double-blind, placebo-controlled study involving 174 patients. In this study, CBZ up to 300 mg/day was significantly more effective than placebo (24). The median daily dose of CBZ was 236 mg and the median drug plasma concentration was 12 μmol/L. Thirty-four patients receiving CBZ experienced unwanted effects (six withdrawals). However, in this trial, even placebo showed a

significant therapeutic effect, which indicates the need of placebo-controlled studies to confirm the efficacy of any treatment of this disorder. The treatment of RLS usually is symptomatic and is causal only in the secondary forms. The treatments of choice include dopaminergic drugs and benzodiazepines. CBZ 200 to 300 mg/day can be used as a second-choice drug for idiopathic or cryptogenic RLS.

Nocturnal paroxysmal dystonia and episodic nocturnal wandering are complex motor attacks occurring during sleep and characterized by sudden arousal followed by dystonic posturing and semipurposeful activity (25). The attacks may remit with CBZ, given at very low dosages in open trials, and recur after treatment withdrawal.

MYOTONIA

Myotonia is a clinical manifestation of different muscle disorders characterized by altered muscle membrane physiology. CBZ (600 and 800 mg/day) has been compared with phenytoin (200 and 300 mg/day) and placebo for the treatment of myotonia in six patients with myotonic dystrophy (26). In this double-blind, crossover study, each treatment was given for 15 days. CBZ was similar to phenytoin (but better than placebo) in decreasing the time of myotonic afterdischarges and improving myotonic symptoms, with no dose differences.

Because there are no standard reference treatments, CBZ might be indicated as a therapeutic option for myotonia. The risk–benefit profile of the drug and the availability of alternative drugs [phenytoin (Chapter 61), diazepam] must be considered when starting treatment of patients with myotonia. Additional randomized trials are needed to assess the efficacy of CBZ and other drugs in the treatment of myotonia.

DEMENTIA

The use of CBZ has been considered for the symptomatic treatment of agitation and aggressiveness in patients with dementia. Although the rationale for the effects of CBZ in agitation of patients with dementia is unknown, its use has been advocated on the basis of its apparent efficacy on agitation, aggression, irritability, and impulsivity in several clinical disorders, despite the negative results of a small controlled study (27). In a multicenter, double-blind, placebo-controlled, 6-week study of 51 patients with Alzheimer's disease or vascular dementia and agitation living in nursing homes, CBZ was started at 100 mg/day and given at a modal daily dose of 300 mg (mean serum concentration of 5.3 μg/mL) (28). Active treatment was better than placebo in reducing agitation and aggression, as indicated by the significant reduction of the scores of the Brief Psychiatric Rating Scale (CBZ, 7.7 points; placebo, 0.9 points) and by the improvement of the Clinical Global Impression rating (CBZ, 77%; placebo, 21%). Agitation and hostility were the most affected behavioral abnormalities. Extra time required to attend to behavioral problems was significantly lower with CBZ. However, adverse events (mostly drowsiness, disorientation, and ataxia) were more common with active treatment (59% versus 29%), and dropouts were reported only with CBZ (four cases). Subsequent withdrawal of CBZ showed reversion to baseline state in patients previously showing improved behavior, compared with no change in patients stopping placebo (29). On this basis, chronic CBZ use at low to average daily doses might be considered an alternative option for the treatment of agitation and aggressiveness in patients with dementia.

ATTENTION-DEFICIT/HYPERACTIVITY DISORDER

Attention-deficit/hyperactivity disorder (ADHD) is a rather common clinical condition that is present in approximately 3% of school-age children and adolescents (30). Despite several psychopharmacologic options, there are many nonresponders in whom the persisting behavioral symptoms may affect academic and social functioning. CBZ has been repeatedly assessed as a treatment option in children and adolescents with ADHD, and a meta-analysis has been performed of the international reports concerning the efficacy of the drug in this study population (31). Seven open studies (189 patients; CBZ daily dose, 100 to 800 mg) and three double-blind, placebo-controlled studies (57 patients; CBZ daily dose, 200 to 600 mg) reported CBZ being effective in ADHD, with significant changes from baseline in impulsivity, distractibility, and motor overactivity. The meta-analysis of the three controlled studies showed CBZ being significantly superior ($p = .018$) to placebo, with 71% of patients experiencing substantial improvement (placebo, 26%). Sedation (7% to 13%), rash (5%), and ataxia (2%) were the most common adverse events, which were reported as mild and transient. Based on this meta-analysis, CBZ 200 to 600 mg/day can be considered safe and effective for children with ADHD.

OTHER CONDITIONS

Hemifacial spasm is a chronic movement disorder of the face characterized by twitching, tonic spasm, and synkinesis of the muscles innervated by the facial nerve. The recommended treatment of hemifacial spasm is the local injection of type A botulinum toxin. Pharmacotherapy of hemifacial spasm includes membrane-stabilizing anticonvulsants like CBZ and phenytoin; however, the efficacy of these drugs is sustained only by small open trials with inadequate follow-up.

CBZ (400 and 600 mg/day) was effective in reducing cerebellar tremor in a small, single-blind, placebo-controlled trial (32). By contrast, CBZ seems ineffective in the treatment of tinnitus (33,34) and stuttering (35).

REFERENCES

1. Waterhouse E, DeLorenzo RJ. Mechanisms of action of antiepileptic drugs: An overview. In: Shorvon S, Dreifuss F, Fish D, et al., eds. *The treatment of epilepsy.* Oxford: Blackwell Science, 1996:123–137.
2. Swerdlow M. Anticonvulsant drugs and chronic pain. *Clin Neuropharmacol* 1984;7:51–82.
3. Tomson T, Ekbom K. Trigeminal neuralgia: time course of pain in relation to carbamazepine dosing. *Cephalalgia* 1981;1:91–97.
4. Rockliff BW, Davis EH. Controlled sequential trials of carbamazepine in trigeminal neuralgia. *Arch Neurol* 1966;15:129–136.
5. Campbell FG, Graham JG, Zilkha KJ. Clinical trial of carbamazepine (Tegretol) in trigeminal neuralgia. *J Neurol Neurosurg Psychiatry* 1966;29:265–167.
6. Killian JM, Fromm GH. Carbamazepine in the treatment of neuralgia. *Arch Neurol* 1968;19:129–136.
7. Nicol CF. A four year double blind study of Tegretol in facial pain. *Headache* 1969;9:54–57.
8. Rasmussen P, Riishede J. Facial pain treated with carbamazepine (Tegretol). *Acta Neurol Scand* 1970;46:385–408.
9. Viming ST, Lyberg T, Lataste X. Tizanidine in the management of trigeminal neuralgia. *Cephalalgia* 1986;6:181–182.
10. Lindstrom P, Lindblom U. The analgesic effect of tocainide in trigeminal neuralgia. *Pain* 1987;28:45–50.
11. Lechin F, van der Dijs B, Lechin ME, et al. Pimozide therapy for trigeminal neuralgia. *Arch Neurol* 1989;46:960–963.
12. Carnaille H, De Coster J, Tyberghein J, et al. Etude statistique de près de 700 cas de facialgies traiteès par le Tégrétol. *Acta Neurol Belg* 1966;66:175–196.
13. McQuay H, Carroll D, Jadad AR, et al. Anticonvulsant drugs for management of pain: a systematic review. *BMJ* 1995;311:1047–1052.
14. Wiffen P, Collins S, McQuay H, et al. Anticonvulsant drugs for acute and chronic pain. In: *Cochrane database of systematic reviews.* 2000:CD00133.
15. Rull JA, Quibrera R, Gonzales-Millan. Symptomatic treatment of peripheral diabetic neuropathy with carbamazepine (Tegretol): Double blind crossover trial. *Diabetologia* 1969;5:215–218.
16. Gomez-Perez FJ, Choza R, Rios JM, et al. Nortriptyline-fluphenazine vs carbamazepine in the symptomatic treatment of diabetic neuropathy. *Arch Med Res* 1996;27:525–529.
17. Leijon G, Boivie J. Central post-stroke pain: A controlled trial of amitriptyline and carbamazepine. *Pain* 1989;36:27–36.
18. Gerson GR. Studies on the concomitant use of carbamazepine and clomipramine for the relief of post-herpetic neuralgia. *Postgrad Med J* 1977;53[Suppl 4]:104–109.
19. Keczkes K, Basheer AM. Do corticosteroids prevent post-herpetic neuralgia? *Br J Dermatol* 1980;102:551–555.
20. Tripathi M, Kaushik S. Carbamazepine for pain management in Guillain-Barre syndrome patients in the intensive care unit. *Crit Care Med* 2000;28:655–658.
21. Rompel H, Bauermeister PW. Aetiology of migraine and prevention with carbamazepine (Tegretol): Results of a double-blind, cross-over study. *S Afr Med J* 1970;44:75–80.
22. Wetter TC, Pollmacher T. Restless legs and periodic leg movements in sleep syndromes. *J Neurol* 1997;244[Suppl 1]:S37–S45.
23. Lundvall O, Abom PE, Holm R. Carbamazepine in restless legs: A controlled pilot study. *Eur J Clin Pharmacol* 1983;25:323–324.

24. Telstad W, Sorensen O, Larsen S, et al. Treatment of the restless legs syndrome with carbamazepine: A double blind study. *BMJ* 1984;288:444–446.

25. Montagna P. Nocturnal paroxysmal dystonia and nocturnal wandering. *Neurology* 1992;42[Suppl 6]:61–67.

26. Sechi GP, Traccis S, Durelli L, et al. Carbamazepine versus diphenylhydantoin in the treatment of myotonia. *Eur Neurol* 1983;22:113–118.

27. Chambers CA, Bain J, Rosbottom R, et al. Carbamazepine in senile dementia and overactivity: A placebo controlled double blind trial. *IRCS Med Sci* 1982;10:505–506.

28. Tariot PN, Erb R, Podgorski CA, et al. Efficacy and tolerability of carbamazepine for agitation and aggression in dementia. *Am J Psychiatry* 1998;155:54–61.

29. Tariot PN, Jakimovich L, Erb R, et al. Withdrawal from controlled carbamazepine therapy followed by further carbamazepine treatment in patients with dementia. *J Clin Psychiatry* 1999;60:684–689.

30. Safer DJ, Krager JM. A survey of medication treatment for hyperactive/inattentive students. *JAMA* 1988;260:2256–2258.

31. Silva RR, Munoz DM, Alpert M. Carbamazepine use in children and adolescents with features of attention-deficit hyperactivity disorder: A meta-analysis. *J Am Acad Child Adolesc Psychiatry* 1996;35:352–358.

32. Sechi GP, Zuddas M, Piredda M, et al. Treatment of cerebellar tremors with carbamazepine: A controlled trial with long-term follow-up. *Neurology* 1989;39:1113–1115.

33. Hulshof JH, Vermeij P. The value of carbamazepine in the treatment of tinnitus. *J Otorhino Laryngol Relat Spec* 1985;47:262–266.

34. Yang DJ. Tinnitus treated with combined traditional Chinese medicine and Western medicine. *Chung Hsi I Chieh Ho Tsa Chih [Chin J Mod Dev Trad Med]* 1989;9:259–260, 270–271.

35. Harvey JE, Culatta R, Halikas JA, et al. The effects of carbamazepine on stuttering. *J Nerv Ment Dis* 1992;180:451–457.

SUGGESTED READING

Beghi E. The use of anticonvulsants in neurological conditions other than epilepsy: A review of the evidence from randomized controlled trials. *CNS Drugs* 1999;11:61–82.

CARBAMAZEPINE

CLINICAL EFFICACY AND USE IN PSYCHIATRIC DISORDERS

MICHAEL R. TRIMBLE

The use of antiepileptic drugs in the management of patients with psychiatric problems but who do not have epilepsy has a long history. In fact, going back to the nineteenth and early twentieth centuries, much more phenobarbital and bromides were prescribed to patients with psychiatric conditions, mainly in the neurotic spectrum, than were ever prescribed for epilepsy. This trend continued in the mid-twentieth century, the nonepileptic indications for phenytoin being broad and encompassing a number of conditions that today would be categorized as anxiety related. In the same vein, drugs such as the benzodiazepines are known to have powerful anxiolytic effects, as well as being anticonvulsants.

Thus, the profile of the antiepileptic drugs is intimately biologically entwined with the underlying neurobiology of psychiatric disorders. This is further reinforced by the fact that benzodiazepine inverse agonists can precipitate not only anxiety and panic attacks, but seizures. There also is an interesting literature on the development of psychiatric syndromes in epileptic patients who have their antiepileptic drugs stopped (e.g., for surgery) and, either with or without the development of withdrawal seizures, can develop a variety of psychopathologic symptoms.

The history of the introduction of carbamazepine for use in psychiatry goes back to the 1970s, shortly after the drug was introduced in the management of epilepsy. In these times (indeed, as of today) in Japan, most patients with epilepsy were treated by psychiatrists. Psychiatrists were thus using the newly discovered anticonvulsant properties of carbamazepine in patients with epilepsy, but at the same time noticed an effect of the drug on mood. These same psychiatrists therefore used carbamazepine in the management of patients with affective disturbances and noted an effect on bipolar disorders. These observations were taken up widely thereafter, both in Europe and the United States,

and there now is a considerable body of evidence showing that carbamazepine has an effect on mood regulation.

This review is divided into three sections, the first dealing with the clinical evidence in epilepsy, the second in patients without epilepsy, and the third with some underlying theoretical principles.

CARBAMAZEPINE AS A MOOD-STABILIZING AGENT: STUDIES IN EPILEPSY

Ever since its introduction into the clinical management of epilepsy, carbamazepine has been reported to possess psychotropic properties (1). In an extensive review, Dalby reported that 90% of the published reports of carbamazepine in epilepsy mentioned its psychotropic effects, and that in 40 reports of over 2,000 patients, such effects were seen in approximately 50% of patients. The psychotropic effect was described as follows:

> The psychotropic action [of carbamazepine] is uniformly described as an increase in psychic tempo in patients with the so-called epileptic personality. The slowness, sluggishness and stickiness of the perseverations and the apathy and lack of initiative of the patients with longstanding severe epilepsy, usually uncontrolled on large doses of phenobarbital, phenytoin and primidone, diminishes and a quickening of thought and action occurs. The affective changes, such as irritability, aggressive tendencies, impulsivity, dysphoric episodes, and states of depression and anxiety are reduced or abolished giving way to an elevation of mood (1).

A number of controlled investigations in epileptic patients are available. Some of these directly assess affective symptoms; others are of patients with less well defined behavior problems, in some studies patients with learning disability being included. Rajotte et al. (2) noted a significant improvement in behavior with carbamazepine compared with placebo on behavior rating scales in a double-blind, crossover trial. Similar results were obtained by Marjerrison et al. (3) and Cereghino (4). Rodin et al. (5)

Michael R. Trimble, MD: Professor of Behavioral Neurology, Department of Neurology, Institute of Neurology, London, United Kingdom

stabilized 45 patients on phenytoin and either primidone or carbamazepine. After 3 months, those on carbamazepine were changed to primidone, and vice versa. Patients were assessed using the Minnesota Multiphasic Personality Inventory (MMPI). Patients scored higher on the psychopathic deviate scale of the MMPI and became more depressed when on primidone, whereas on carbamazepine they became less depressed. In a similarly designed study, Dodrill and Troupin (6) compared carbamazepine with phenytoin over a 4-month period using a double-blind, crossover design, with patients randomly assigned to the drug of study. On the MMPI, every clinical scale favored the carbamazepine treatment period, the results being statistically significant for the F scale, which relates to feelings, attitudes, and emotions. Interestingly, in the aforementioned studies, the psychotropic effects of carbamazepine appeared dissociated from its effect on seizures.

Several studies were carried out evaluating changes of behavior in patients with epilepsy using serum level monitoring of the antiepileptic drugs. In one study of children with epilepsy, Trimble and Corbett (7) analyzed correlations between behavior deviance scores for conduct disorder and serum levels of antiepileptic drugs. The higher deviance scores were associated with higher levels of some anticonvulsants (particularly phenobarbital), whereas for carbamazepine the correlation was negative. A significant difference between the correlations for phenobarbital and carbamazepine was noted.

There are three studies in adult patients showing a similar relationship between serum levels of carbamazepine and scores on behavior rating scales. Rodin and Schmaltz (8) gave the Bear-Fedio Personality Inventory, a scale specifically constructed to assess interictal behavior changes in epilepsy, to 148 patients with epilepsy. They noted significant associations between rating scale scores and carbamazepine, but not for other anticonvulsants. Specifically, they reported that carbamazepine levels were significantly inversely correlated with the total score of psychopathology, and subscores of elation, philosophical interests, a sense of personal destiny, altered sexuality, and hypergraphia.

Andrewes et al. (9) administered to 42 newly referred patients with epilepsy the Mood Adjective Check List and followed the progress of patients receiving monotherapy either with phenytoin or carbamazepine. Again, significant associations were noted between mood scores and serum levels of carbamazepine—the higher the level of carbamazepine, the lower the ratings for anxiety, fatigue, and depression

Robertson et al. (10) provided further data on this relationship. They used the Research Diagnostic Criteria for Major Affective Disorder in patients with epilepsy, and measured serum levels of anticonvulsant drugs. Patients on phenobarbital were more likely to report higher depression scores, whereas patients on carbamazepine rated themselves as less depressed and had lower anxiety scores, and a nega-

tive correlation was found between trait anxiety and serum carbamazepine levels.

The association of phenobarbital with affective disorder, and the contrast with carbamazepine, also were seen in the studies of Brent and colleagues (11,12). An overrepresentation of patients with epilepsy was noted in a consecutive series of suicide attempters seen at a children's hospital. They noted that of 131 consecutive suicide attempts made by 126 children seen over a period of 5 years, 9 had epilepsy. This was over 15 times the expected frequency. The attempters with epilepsy made more medically serious attempts, showed more premeditation, and had a higher frequency of suicidal attempts both before and after the index event than did nonepileptic children. Eight of these nine children were on phenobarbital.

The authors then carried out a comparative study of affective disorder in 15 children with epilepsy treated with phenobarbital compared with 24 treated with carbamazepine. The groups were similar over a wide range of demographic and seizure-related variables, but patients on phenobarbital showed a much higher frequency of major affective disorder (40% versus 4%) and of suicidal ideation (47% versus 4%). Depression was particularly noted in those children who had a family history of major affective disorder among first-degree relatives. The contribution of the antiepileptic drugs, however, was supported by the fact that the diagnosis of major depressive disorder was made within 12 months of the initiation of the medication in 33% of the phenobarbital group, and in none of the carbamazepine group. Sixteen patients in the carbamazepine group had been treated previously with phenobarbital. Eight reported having an affective disorder on the phenobarbital, and all eight lost their affective symptoms when switched to carbamazepine.

Other studies have examined the behavioral toxicity profile of antiepileptic drugs, including carbamazepine, looking at the effect of the drugs on mood. Thompson and Trimble (13) followed a group of 20 patients who underwent a reduction in the number of anticonvulsants they were prescribed, and 15 patients who underwent a similar reduction, but who had one of their medications substituted for carbamazepine. There was no consistency in either group regarding which antiepileptic drug was withdrawn. They also had 10 patients who did not undergo any anticonvulsant drug changes. The profile of their mood was studied on three occasions, at baseline, at 3 months, and then at 6 months; in addition to the ratings of mood, a number of cognitive tasks were performed. The overall findings suggested that the drug changes made in both groups of patients resulted in improvements of performance on psychological tests, and that these were not simply the result of practice. Patients changing to carbamazepine, either alone or in combination with existing medication, displayed more widespread improvements in test performance, particularly with regard to measures of memory, than those that did not have the carbamazepine substitution. Interestingly, these patients were also shown to improve in mood. When patients with initial high rating scales scores for mood disorder were examined, a significant antidepressant affect was noted on switching to carbamazepine.

These studies of people with epilepsy often are difficult to interpret because of the methodologic issues concerned. Thus, patients have epilepsy, and any change of seizure frequency may be expected to alter patients' mood. Further, patients often are on polytherapy, and any reduction of polytherapy toward monotherapy may bring about improvements in mood that perhaps are secondary to resolution of drug side effects or improvement of cognitive function. Third, the monitoring of patients in terms of their mood often has been based on purely clinical grounds and the rating scales used (with few exceptions) have been validated in patients with psychiatric illness, and therefore may not necessarily be of value in patients with epilepsy.

Nevertheless, there is an interesting trend that runs through the literature on carbamazepine since its introduction, namely, that it does appear to have a positive effect on behavior in patients with epilepsy. The most commonly reported behaviors that seem to be improved when the drug is prescribed lie along an affective spectrum, but include improvements in aggressive and irritable behaviors; carbamazepine also has some relationship to elation (8), suggesting possible control of hypomania and mania.

CARBAMAZEPINE AND AFFECTIVE DISORDERS IN NONEPILEPTIC PATIENTS

The terminology used in the following studies varies, particularly since the introduction of the third and fourth editions of the *Diagnostic and Statistical Manual of Mental Disorders* (DSM-III and DSM-IV), the latter being the standardized statistical and classification manual used by most psychiatrists. The early studies were carried out using basic clinical descriptions.

In the diagnostic manuals, under the affective disorders, several conditions are described. The syndromes most treated with carbamazepine have been bipolar disorders, either for the acute treatment of mania *per se*, or for the longer-term prophylaxis of bipolar affective disorders.

Thus, DSM-IV (14) distinguishes mood episodes (manic or hypomanic episodes) from mood disorders. Among the mood disorders, a distinction is made between bipolar 1 disorders (mania with or without evidence of a previous depressive episode) and bipolar 2 disorders, which essentially are recurrent major depressive episodes with hypomanic episodes. Until the introduction of carbamazepine for the management of bipolar disorders, the mainstay of treatment was lithium. Lithium was shown not only to have an effect on acute mania, but to prevent the recurrence of episodes of affective disorder in patients with bipolar disorder. However, lithium has many disadvantages. Not only does it have significant side effects, some of which may be profound (e.g., renal problems or hypothyroidism), it is associated with cognitive obtunding, and many patients find it difficult to take. Further, serum level monitoring is carried out because it is quite easy to induce lithium toxicity, which, if unrecognized, can lead to permanent neurologic impairment.

Lithium, in contrast to carbamazepine, is not anticonvulsant (if anything, in overdose it is convulsant) and clearly has a limited spectrum of clinical activity in the sense that it is not used as widely as carbamazepine in neurologic syndromes, such as for paroxysmal pains. However, some of the early studies in psychiatric patients suggested that patients responding to lithium may have a clinical profile different from those responding to carbamazepine.

Carbamazepine in Acute Mania

Many of the observations have been anecdotal, but over time at least 12 double-blind studies have been carried out comparing the effects of carbamazepine in acute mania with placebo, lithium, or neuroleptic medication. These studies reveal that it is equivalent to lithium over a period of up to 8 weeks and that the time course of the antimanic effect is, if anything, a little slower than with neuroleptics, but equivalent to lithium. These studies have been reviewed in detail by others (15,16).

More recent studies include those of Okuma et al. (17), who compared carbamazepine and lithium in a double-blind trial for 4 weeks. Carbamazepine was noted to be equivalent to lithium in outcome. Small et al. (18) compared carbamazepine with lithium in a double-blind trial that lasted 8 weeks, and again found no difference between the two drugs. Review of some of the clinical data suggested that patients who responded best to carbamazepine were those who were more manic at onset, were more dysphoric, and had a history of rapid cycling in the year before admission. Interestingly, these variables were said to be associated with a poorer response to lithium.

On account of these studies, and clinical impressions, carbamazepine now finds a role in the clinical management of patients with acute mania. There are several advantages to this drug over the use of neuroleptics, not the least being that if patients are kept on a drug prophylactically, the possibility of the later development of extrapyramidal disorders with neuroleptic drugs is avoided. This is particularly relevant for patients who are refractory to lithium and require an alternative to it.

The dose of carbamazepine used in acute mania is somewhat higher initially than in epilepsy because it is important to bring the symptoms under rapid control. This increases the possibility of provoking central nervous system (CNS) side effects. However, in mania, dosages often can be increased quite rapidly (by 200 mg/day) and tolerated until clinical responses are observed. Dosages up to 1,800 mg/day often are used. There is no relationship between the serum levels of carbamazepine and the antimanic effect; the mean levels of carbamazepine in those treated successfully often are below the upper limits of tolerance. In clinical practice, there are some patients who are treated on a combination of lithium and carbamazepine, which may tend toward greater CNS toxicity. Patients with underlying neurologic disease (secondary manias) are particularly susceptible to these problems.

Carbamazepine as Prophylaxis in Bipolar Disorder

There are at least 14 controlled (or partially controlled) studies of the use of carbamazepine in the prophylaxis of bipolar disorder, and these have been reviewed by Post and colleagues (19). In addition, there have been many uncontrolled studies. Most studies have been in comparison with lithium, although some have used placebo. Another clinical design has been to switch patients from lithium to carbamazepine if they have not responded to lithium.

In reviewing the literature on the use of carbamazepine in psychiatric disorders generally, there have been over 500 reports involving more than 2,000 patients, and most have had bipolar affective disorder. With regard to long-term prophylaxis, Post et al. summarized the 14 controlled or partially controlled studies in this area. Essentially, of 629 patients prescribed carbamazepine, a good response was noted in 390 (62%). Most of these studies were double-blind, and several of them randomized.

The early studies came from Japan (20,21). Since then, studies have been undertaken by Post and colleagues and by several groups in Europe (22–25). These studies demonstrated an equivalence between carbamazepine and lithium for prophylaxis, and certain patients appeared to respond preferentially. Patients who are referred to as *rapid cyclers*, namely, patients with an unstable bipolar disorder with rapid fluctuations (more than four episodes a year), are known to respond poorly to lithium and seem to do better on carbamazepine, or on a combination of carbamazepine and lithium, than on lithium alone. Indeed, there are several reports of lithium nonresponders gaining additional clinical improvement with carbamazepine added to the regime (26).

Serum Levels and Side Effects

The doses of carbamazepine given in prophylaxis of affective disorder are similar to those prescribed for epilepsy, but no study has shown any dose–effect relationship, or indeed serum level–effect relationship. In general, patients are started on 200 mg and titrated slowly. Mean serum levels, where they have been assessed, are within the therapeutic range for epilepsy. Unwanted side effects typical for carbamazepine are seen in a rather higher percentage of patients without epilepsy, and occur in up to a third. Although these are mainly gastrointestinal and neurologic, a rash has been reported in up to 15% of psychiatric patients (27). Thyroid function often is minimally affected, with a lowered plasma level of thyroxine and raised thyroid-stimulating hormone, but hypothyroidism itself is rare (28). However, thyroid function should be monitored, especially when carbamazepine is combined with lithium.

Hyponatremic syndromes are seen and may pose a particular problem in psychotic patients, who may become polydipsic, exacerbating the problems with sodium levels. Interestingly, this effect on sodium is the opposite to that of lithium, which tends to lead to sodium retention.

No clinical information has been gathered on the distinction between slow-release and conventional carbamazepine prescriptions in the treatment of affective disorders, although patients with psychiatric problems, and especially patients with mood disorders, can be remarkably noncompliant with medication and may be prone to abuse their prescriptions. Obviously, the use of slow-release preparations, given on a twice-daily basis, is a clinical advantage when using carbamazepine with psychiatric disorders.

THE USE OF CARBAMAZEPINE IN OTHER PSYCHIATRIC DISORDERS

In addition to its use in bipolar affective disorder and mania, carbamazepine has been used in several other psychiatric conditions, although controlled clinical information is sparse. In uncontrolled studies, moderate or marked clinical effects were reported when carbamazepine was added to existing therapy in 61% of 182 patients with schizoaffective or schizophrenic disorders (29). The carbamazepine usually is given in addition to a neuroleptic drug, and the initial hope was that carbamazepine would either replace the neuroleptic or would lead to a decrease of neuroleptic use, and hence to a diminution of the possible long-term side effects of the traditional antipsychotic drugs. In addition to the clinical reports, there are double-blind case studies and some clinical crossover studies comparing carbamazepine with placebo, which was added to existing neuroleptic treatments. These studies suggest responses in approximately 50% of schizophrenic patients. Although there are some reports of improvement in core schizophrenic symptoms (hallucinations and delusions), the main effects appear to be on other aspects of behavior, particularly the affective symptoms, aggressive disorders, and excitability.

Schizoaffective disorder also has been studied. Greil et al. gave 90 patients with schizoaffective disorder either lithium or carbamazepine, and although no significant difference was noted on treatment outcome, there were fewer side effects with carbamazepine (30). Patients with schizodepressive syndromes appeared to respond better than patients with schizomanic presentations.

One problem that arises in treating schizophrenic patients with carbamazepine is lowering of the serum levels of any prescribed neuroleptic drugs, particularly haloperidol, due to the liver enzyme induction by carbamazepine. Reports of deterioration of the psychotic state after the administration of carbamazepine may reflect this pharmacokinetic interaction rather than a pharmacodynamic effect. Several investigators have noted exacerbations of psychosis on withdrawal of carbamazepine, which may reflect the therapeutic benefit of this drug, and is in keeping with the carbamazepine withdrawal syndromes reported in epileptic patients (31).

Carbamazepine and Aggressive Disorders

In some of the studies quoted previously, one of the behavioral syndromes that seems to respond to carbamazepine is dysphoric, aggressive behavior. A behavioral syndrome that most often is reported to respond to carbamazepine is episodic dyscontrol. This disorder has an interesting history, with earlier clinical descriptions coming from Munro et al. (32). They examined patients who previously had been investigated by Robert Heath. He monitored the activity of neurons in the limbic system using implanted electrodes, and demonstrated that patterns of sudden onset of aggression correlated with aberrant electrical activity in these areas, particularly in the hippocampus. These episodes tended to occur in patients with probable neurologic diatheses, but similar changes were reported in patients with and without epilepsy. These patients were differentiated from patients with life-long impulsive aggression, usually associated with personality disorders. In episodic dyscontrol, the episodes of aggression seemed to be uncharacteristic; they were of rapid onset after trivial provocation and they subsided rapidly, with the patients often feeling remorse afterward. Electroencephalographic (EEG) abnormalities often were noted on surface electrodes, and a history of brain trauma sometimes was present.

This disorder, referred to earlier as *episodic dyscontrol*, reemerges in DSM-IV as *intermittent explosive disorder*. Over time, it has been thought to be related to epilepsy, although the clinical and neurophysiologic evidence does not support that. Nonetheless, early trials of anticonvulsants suggested they may be of value in the treatment of episodic dyscontrol, although no double-blind, controlled studies exist.

Typical of the case reports is that of Stone et al. (33) of a man in whom explosive, aggressive feelings with suicidal ideas and explosive anger suddenly developed. An EEG was carried out that showed bursts of 6-per-second spike-and-wave complexes during hyperventilation, and bursts of 6- and 12-per-second rhythmic sharp waves in the mid-temporal areas. On carbamazepine his symptoms evaporated.

Other situations where carbamazepine has been used are in the management of aggressive disorders associated with the borderline personality disorder, and for the management of drug withdrawal syndromes.

With regard to the former, Cowdry and Gardner (34) compared four psychotropic agents in patients with borderline personality disorders and monitored their behavior, particularly aggressive behavior. The drugs used were alprazolam, carbamazepine, trifluoperazine, and tranylcypromine. In terms of the overall clinical effects, the most interesting finding was that patients given alprazolam showed a deterioration of their aggressive behavior, and those on carbamazepine showed a highly statistically significant improvement.

In alcoholism, the main benefit of carbamazepine in withdrawal states is that it is both psychotropic and anticonvulsant, and may therefore prevent the onset of withdrawal seizures as well as preventing craving (35). A further advantage of carbamazepine over the use of benzodiazepines is that there is less likely to be a withdrawal syndrome on stopping the drug, and much less abuse potential.

Although in some of the aforementioned studies, the presence of EEG abnormalities in patients may suggest a superior response to an anticonvulsant drug such as carbamazepine, the data do not really confirm that.

THEORETICAL BASIS FOR THE USE OF ANTIEPILEPTIC DRUGS IN PSYCHIATRIC DISORDERS

There are clear overlaps in the basic neurochemistry of epilepsy and a number of psychiatric syndromes, in particular revolving around neurotransmitters such as γ-aminobutyric acid (GABA), glutamate, and serotonin. Low levels of serotonin and low serotonin turnover rates lend to depressive, aggressive, and impulsive behavior, and also are proconvulsant (36). GABA agonism is clearly anticonvulsant, but may be associated with the development of psychiatric syndromes, particularly in epilepsy (37). Dopamine is known to be both anticonvulsant and propsychotic, and there is good evidence for an involvement of dopamine in both mood disorders and psychoses.

Carbamazepine is structurally related to the tricyclic antidepressants, and its mode of action is different from some other anticonvulsants such as phenytoin and phenobarbital. Its biochemical actions, apart from its effect at sodium channels, include partial agonism at adenosine receptors, an increase in the firing rate of the locus ceruleus, and a decrease in dopamine turnover (38). Furthermore, it increases the turnover of serotonin, which may imply some influence over affective tone.

In animal models, carbamazepine has been shown to be more effective than other standard antiepileptics in inhibiting the seizures developed from amygdylar kindling (39), suggesting some limbic system selectivity for the drug. Indeed, it is the model of kindling that has been most put forward to explain the association between severe psychiatric disorders and epilepsy, as well as the effect of anticonvulsant agents on these syndromes. This has been reviewed on many occasions (38). In summary, the suggestion is that a kindling-like process (probably more a sensitization) leads to the development of recurrent manic depressive episodes, which are seen (as with some seizure disorders) to recur more frequently and at shorter intervals as time progresses. The episodes become triggered by less meaningful environmental events, and eventually take on a spontaneity. Such models also have been used to explain the development of other psychopathologic processes such as the addictive behaviors and the symptoms of both alcohol withdrawal and cocaine abuse (40).

Although there is no evidence that kindling *per se* (which is an animal model for the development of seizures) occurs in patients with psychiatric disorders, the concept of sensitization, the CNS mechanisms that may underlie this, and the effect of certain drugs such as the antiepileptics on biochemical processes related to sensitization and kindling, are being actively explored.

CONCLUSION

In this chapter, the evidence for the use of carbamazepine in nonepileptic psychiatric disorders is reviewed. Much of the evidence stems from studies conducted over a decade ago, and, since the value of its use in bipolar disorder was noted by the Japanese in the 1960s, carbamazepine has found widespread use in psychiatric settings. It is now approved in over 100 countries for use in affective disorders, and in the United States is the only drug approved by the Food and Drug Administration for the long-term prophylaxis of bipolar disorder, apart from lithium.

It also has found use in a spectrum of other clinical problems. It has been used mainly in bipolar affective disorders, but also has been prescribed for conditions as diverse as the aggressive, dysphoric, and excited behavior of schizophrenia, through episodic dyscontrol, through effects on craving and management of alcohol withdrawal. In the latter conditions, few or no clinical trials have been carried out, and none now are likely to be performed. In spite of this, its use, particularly for the management of aggressive disorders, seems well established, and indeed in a number of countries it remains one of the first-line drugs for treatment of alcohol withdrawal. Its use in bipolar disorder still is being explored because it has become clear that, as with lithium, there are a number of patients who simply do not respond to the drug, either because of side effects, or because it is ineffective. Nonetheless, the introduction of the use of carbamazepine into clinical practice for the management of psychiatric disorders has led to a considerable interest in the use of other anticonvulsant drugs in psychiatry. A number of these are being investigated, either in acute mania or more for the treatment of chronic bipolar disorder. Although the term *antiepileptic* has been used throughout this chapter for this group of drugs, the fact that carbamazepine is used widely outside epilepsy (and is used in other neurologic conditions) emphasizes the value of retaining the term *anticonvulsant*.

REFERENCES

1. Dalby MA. Behavioural effects of carbamazepine. *Adv Neurol* 1975;332–334.
2. Rajotte P, Jilekl Peralrs A, et al. Proprietes antiepiletiques et psychotropes de la carbamazepine (Tegretol). *Union Med Can* 1967;96:1200–1206.
3. Marjerrison G, Jedlicki SM, Keogh RP, et al. Carbamazepine: behavioural, anticonvulsant and EEG effects in chronically hospitalised epileptics. *Dis Nerv Syst* 1968;29:133–136.
4. Cereghino JJ. Carbamazepine: relation of plasma concentration to seizure control. In: Woodbury DM, Penry JK, Pippenger PE, eds. *Antiepileptic drugs.* New York: Raven Press, 1982:507–519.
5. Rodin EA, Choon SR, Kitano H, et al. A comparison of the effectiveness of primidone versus carbamazepine in epileptic outpatients. *J Nerv Ment Dis* 1976;163:41–46.
6. Dodrill CB, Troupin AS. Psychotropic effects of carbamazepine in epilepsy: a double-blind comparison with phenytoin. *Neurology* 1977;27:1023–1208.
7. Trimble M , Corbett J. Behavioural and cognitive disturbances in epileptic children. *J Ir Med Assoc* 1980;73[Suppl]:21–28.
8. Rodin EA, Schmaltz S. The Bear-Fedio Personality Inventory and temporal lobe epilepsy. *Neurology* 1984;34:591–596.
9. Andrewes DG, Tomlinson L, Elwes RDC, et al. A comparative study of the cognitive effects of phenytoin and carbamazepine in new referrals with epilepsy. *Epilepsia* 1986;27:128–134.
10. Robertson MM, Trimble MR, Townsend HRA. The phenomenology of depression in epilepsy. *Epilepsia* 1987;28:364–372.
11. Brent DA. Overrepresentation of epileptics in a consecutive series of suicide attempters seen at a children's hospital. *J Am Acad Child Psychiatry* 1986;25:242–246
12. Brent DA, Krumrine PK, Varma RR, et al. Phenobarbital treatment and major depressive disorder in children with epilepsy. *Pediatrics* 1987;80:909–917.
13. Thompson PJ, Trimble MR. Anticonvulsive drugs and cognitive functions. *Epilepsia* 1982;23:531–545.
14. American Psychiatric Association. *Diagnostic and statistical manual of mental disorders,* 4th ed. Washington, DC: American Psychiatric Press, 1994.
15. Post RM. Effectiveness of carbamazepine in the treatment of bipolar affective disorders. In: McElroy S, Pope HG, eds. The use of anticonvulsants in psychiatric disorders: recent advances. Clifton, NJ: Oxford Health Care, 1988:1–23.
16. Dunn RT, Frye MS, Kimbrell TA, et al. The efficacy and use of anticonvulsants in mood disorders. *Clin Neuropharmacol* 1998; 21:215–235.
17. Okuma T, Yamashita I, Takahashi R, et al. Comparison of the antimanic efficacy of carbamazepine and lithium carbonate by double blind controlled study. *Pharmacopsychiatry* 1990;23: 143–150.
18. Small JG, Klapper MH, Milstein V, et al. Carbamazepine compared with lithium in the treatment of mania. *Arch Gen Psychiatry* 1991;48:81–89.

19. Post RM, Denicoff D, Frye MA, et al. Re-evaluation of carbamazepine prophylaxis in bipolar disorder. *Br J Psychiatry* 1997; 170:202–204.

20. Okuma T, Kishimoto A, Inoue K. Anti-manic and prophylactic effects of carbamazepine (Tegretol) on manic depressive psychosis. *Seishin Igaku* 1975;17:617–630.

21. Kishimoto A, Ogura C, Hazama H. Long-term prophylactic effects of carbamazepine in affective disorder. *Br J Psychiatry* 1983;143:327–331.

22. Watkins S, Callender K, Thomas DR, et al. The effect of carbamazepine and lithium on remission from affective illness. *Br J Psychiatry* 1987;150:180–182.

23. Lusznat RM, Murphy DP, Nunn CMH. Carbamazepine vs lithium in the treatment and prophylaxis of mania. *Br J Psychiatry* 1988;153:198–204.

24. Froscher W, Stoll KD. Carbamazepine in manic syndromes. A controlled double-blind study. *Nervenarzt* 1985;56:43–47.

25. Silverstone T, Coxhead N, Cookson J. Carbamazepine vs lithium in bipolar disorder. In: *8th World Congress in Psychiatry, Athens 1989*. International Congress Series. Amsterdam: Excerpta Medica, 1989(abstr 1205).

26. Nolen WA. Carbamazepine, a possible adjunct or alternative to lithium in bipolar disorders. *Acta Psychiatr Scand* 1983;67:218–225.

27. Elphick M, Lyons, F, Cowen P. Low tolerability of carbamazepine in psychiatric patients may restrict its clinical usefulness. *J Psychopharmacol* 1988;2:1–4.

28. Roy-Byrne PP, Joffe RT, Uhde TW, et al. Carbamazepine and thyroid function in affectively ill patients. *Arch Gen Psychiatry* 1984;41:1150–1153.

29. Post RM. Anticonvulsants as adjuncts to neuroleptics in the treatment of schizo-affective and schizophrenic patients. In: Post RM, Trimble MR, Pippenger CE, eds. *Clinical use of anticonvulsants in psychiatric disorders*. New York: Demos Press, 1989: 153–164.

30. Greil W, Ludwig-Mayerhofer W, Erazo N, et al. Lithium versus carbamazepine in the maintenance treatment of schizoaffective disorder: a randomised study. *Eur Arch Psychiatry Clin Neurosci* 1997;247:42–50.

31. Ketter TA, Post RM, Theodore WH. Positive and negative psychiatric effects of antiepileptic drugs in patients with seizure disorders. *Neurology* 1999;53[Suppl 2]:s53–s57.

32. Munro RR. Episodic behaviour disorders and limbic ictus. In: Doane BK, Livingston KE, eds. *The limbic system*. New York: Raven Press, 1986:251–266.

33. Stone JL, McDaniel KD, Hughes JR, et al. Episodic dyscontrol disorder and paroxysmal EEG abnormalities: successful treatment with carbamazepine. *Biol Psychiatry* 1986;21:208–212.

34. Cowdry RW, Gardner DL. Pharmacotherapy of borderline personality disorder: alprazolam, carbamazepine, trifluoperazine and tranylcypromine. *Arch Gen Psychiatry* 1988;45:111–119.

35. Mayo-Smith MF. Pharmacological management of alcohol withdrawal. *JAMA* 1997;278:144–151.

36. Trimble MR. *Biological psychiatry*, 2nd ed. Chichester, UK: John Wiley & Sons, 1997.

37. Trimble MR. Anticonvulsant-induced psychiatric disorders. *Drug Safe* 1996;15:159–166.

38. Post RM, Weiss SRB. Kindling and manic-depressive illness. In: Bolwig T, Trimble MR, eds. *The clinical relevance of kindling*. Chichester, UK: John Wiley & Sons, 1989.

39. Albright PS, Burnham WI. Development of a new pharmacological seizure model. *Epilepsia* 1980;21:681–689.

40. Ballenger JC, Post RM. Addictive behaviour in kindling. In: Bolwig TG, Trimble MR, eds. *The clinical relevance of kindling*. Chichester, UK: John Wiley & Sons, 1989:231–258.

CARBAMAZEPINE

ADVERSE EFFECTS

GREGORY L. HOLMES

Carbamazepine (CBZ) is one of the major antiepileptic drugs (AEDs) used in the treatment of epilepsy in children and adults. One of the advantages of CBZ is the excellent side effect profile; CBZ rarely produces adverse cosmetic effects such as gingival hypertrophy, does not interfere significantly with cognitive function, attention, or behavior, and rarely is associated with life-threatening events.

However, as with all currently available AEDs, CBZ is associated with some adverse events. Most of the side effects are mild and dose related, although severe idiosyncratic adverse events can occur. Although a large number of idiosyncratic adverse effects have been attributed to CBZ therapy, it often is very difficult, in the myriad of anecdotal cases reported, to establish CBZ as conclusively responsible for the side effects. In the case of most severe adverse side effects, the patient is taken off the medication, and if the adverse event subsides, the clinician concludes that CBZ is the culprit. Unless a rechallenge with CBZ is attempted, it is very difficult to prove decisively that CBZ is the responsible agent for the adverse event. However, because with some adverse events rechallenge would be considered dangerous, the relationship between CBZ and the adverse event may remain cloudy.

INCIDENCE OF SIDE EFFECTS

All AEDs have side effects; in a study of 355 primarily adult patients receiving chronic AED therapy, 42% had 1 or more adverse reactions during the study period (1). When the individual AEDs were compared in patients on monotherapy, 15.5% of patients receiving CBZ had side effects at the first visit. This percentage should be compared with a 31% overall rate of side effects with AEDs. Many CBZ-related side effects improve with time; only 7% of patients had side effects at the time of their last visit.

Gregory L. Holmes, MD: Professor of Neurology, Department of Neurology, Harvard Medical School; and Director, Center for Research in Pediatric Epilepsy, Children's Hospital, Boston, Massachusetts

When questioned about possible side effects, many patients note some; however, in most cases these are mild and not of sufficient magnitude to warrant discontinuation of the drug. In a study evaluating side effects of AEDs in children, Herranz et al. (2) found that 43% of 35 children taking CBZ had side effects at some point; however, in only 3% did the side effects lead to withdrawal of the drug. CBZ was the best tolerated of the AEDs evaluated. Pellock (3) found that 70% of children treated with CBZ as monotherapy or as combination therapy had side effects. However, other authors have found a lower rate of side effects in children (4,5). Okuno et al. (4) found that only 20 of 90 (22%) children treated with CBZ had side effects, most of which were mild and transient.

NEUROLOGIC ADVERSE EFFECTS

As with most AEDs, most of the side effects with CBZ involve the central nervous system. Nausea, headache, dizziness, incoordination, vertigo, tiredness, and diplopia are the most frequent symptoms (6–12). Nystagmus, tremor, and ataxia may be detected with a neurologic examination. These side effects usually are dose related and reversible, and they appear to be more common in the elderly (13). There are significantly fewer side effects when the patient is on monotherapy than when he or she is on polytherapy (11).

Neurologic side effects in children are similar to those in adults (2,5). In a study of 35 children receiving CBZ monotherapy, the most common side effect, drowsiness, occurred in 11% (2). Drowsiness also was the most common side effect, present in 43% of the patients, in a review by Pellock (3). Other commonly reported neurologic side effects in the Pellock series included incoordination in 20% and vertigo in 6%. Although diplopia was reported in only one child by Herranz et al. (2), this side effect likely goes unrecognized in nonverbal children. Other authors have reported a high incidence of this side effect in both children and adults (7,11). It is known that CBZ prolongs the duration of saccadic eye movements (14).

A high incidence of drowsiness and other adverse effects occurs when the drug is first started, especially if therapy is initiated at full dosage (10,15). Although tolerance to some of the side effects occurs rapidly (16), when possible, the dosage should be slowly increased because the rate of change of CBZ escalation is an important determinant of cognitive and motor dysfunction (17).

The short half-life of CBZ results in considerable fluctuation of CBZ levels, even when the drug is given multiple times daily. Many of the neurologic adverse effects occur at peak plasma levels of the drug (18–20). When peak blood CBZ levels are below 8 µg/mL, neurologic side effects are unusual, whereas levels greater than 12 µg/mL are associated with a higher risk of adverse effects (21). Some authors have reported that the unbound CBZ levels correlate better with neurotoxicity than total CBZ levels in serum (21,22). Because side effects of CBZ tend to occur at the time of a rapid peak concentration, use of sustained- or controlled-release CBZ can significantly reduce the incidence of side effects (16,23–25).

CBZ is metabolized through oxidation to the active metabolite carbamazepine-10,11-epoxide (CBZ epoxide) (26). The epoxide has been implicated as the responsible agent for side effects (11,27), with several studies demonstrating a correlation between plasma CBZ epoxide concentration and side effects (11,27,28). However, Tomson et al. (29) crossed patients over from CBZ to CBZ epoxide. Despite high epoxide levels, no patients reported increased side effects. In fact, the authors noted a trend toward improvement when patients were switched to the epoxide therapy. Likewise, Theodore et al. (30) did not find epoxide levels to correlate with side effects. Riva et al. (22) found that the correlation of epoxide levels with the presence of nystagmus was no better than that with CBZ serum levels alone.

In most patients, neurologic side effects are easily managed (3). Because some side effects occur at peak concentrations, reduction of peak levels and associated toxicity may be achieved by giving the same daily dosage at more frequent intervals (29). Tomson (29) found that CBZ levels were 79% ± 29% higher than trough levels on a twice-daily dosage schedule and 40% ± 13% higher during four-times-daily administration. The appearance and intensity of side effects were related to the fluctuations in CBZ levels and were thus substantially reduced during the four-times-daily regimen.

Controlled-release CBZ reduces fluctuations in CBZ levels (24,31,32). Although the controlled-release preparation is likely to reduce some of the side effects seen at peak concentration (25), many patients tolerate the daily fluctuations of CBZ well. For example, Pieters et al. (24) did not find that changing from conventional CBZ to controlled-release CBZ altered attention or vigilance in children.

Movement Disorders

Abnormal involuntary movements occasionally have been reported in connection with CBZ treatment (33–36).

These movements have included tics (37,38), asterixis (39), and dystonia (34,40). Movement disorders typically develop in patients on AED polytherapy (34,35), in patients with brain damage (34), or in patients with toxic plasma levels of CBZ (33).

Peripheral Nerves and Muscle

Rarely, AEDs may lead to electromyographic signs of peripheral neuropathy (41). Lühdorf et al. (42) performed electromyography and nerve conduction velocity studies in 12 patients before and 3 months after CBZ treatment. No interval changes were noted. Likewise, Danner et al. (43) found no changes in nerve conduction velocity or the electromyogram in patients receiving CBZ. CBZ does not appear to cause a myopathy or result in weakness (14).

Exacerbation of Seizures

CBZ has been increasingly recognized to exacerbate or precipitate seizures in some patients. Initially described by Snead and Hosey in 1985 (44), the observation that CBZ can precipitate a new type of seizure or increase seizure frequency has been noted by other authors (45–47). Snead and Hosey (44) described 15 children with seizures in whom one or more seizure type was exacerbated during treatment with CBZ. The most common seizure type exacerbated was generalized atypical absences (11 patients). Four patients had an increase in generalized tonic-clonic or tonic seizures. The authors reported that a bilaterally synchronous spike-and-wave discharge of 2.5 to 3 cycles per second was predictive of increased atypical absence seizures with CBZ, whereas generalized bursts of spikes and slow waves of 1 to 2 cycles per second placed the patient at risk for increased tonic-clonic seizures. CBZ also may exacerbate epileptiform activity on the electroencephalogram (EEG) (48).

HYPERSENSITIVITY REACTIONS
Skin Rash

The incidence of rash with CBZ varies from 2% to 17% in various series (3,8,12,21,49,50). In most patients the rash is mild and not associated with any other systemic signs. The rash may disappear even when the drug is continued. A variety of cutaneous manifestations may be seen, of which the maculopapular, morbilliform, and urticarial types are the most common. If the rash persists, it is recommended that the drug be discontinued because serious and potentially life-threatening skin reactions (i.e., exfoliative dermatitis, Steven-Johnson syndrome, and Lyell's syndrome), although rare, do occur (3,50,51). CBZ-induced hair loss has been reported (52).

Murphy et al. (53) treated 20 patients with CBZ drug rashes with prednisone and antihistamines. Sixteen patients were able to continue CBZ, whereas four had to discontinue the drug.

Other Allergic Reactions

In addition to the rashes seen with CBZ, more extensive hypersensitivity reactions with systemic signs such as fever, skin rashes, hepatosplenomegaly, and lymphadenopathy occasionally may occur (54–58). A variety of various other organ systems may be involved, and vasculitis (55,59), myocarditis (60), interstitial pneumonia (61–65), membranous glomerulopathy (66), pseudolymphoma (58,67), and tubulointerstitial nephritis (68) have been implicated in these CBZ-induced hypersensitivity reactions.

The exact etiology of these multiorgan hypersensitivity reactions is unknown. There is some evidence that they may be type III or IV hypersensitivity reactions (51). Deposition of immune complexes, with CBZ or its metabolites acting as the antigenic stimulus, may be responsible for the multiorgan involvement (54,59). Although corticosteroids and immunosuppressive therapy may be needed (60), discontinuation of CBZ typically causes the symptoms to disappear.

The diagnosis of drug hypersensitivity to CBZ can be established by either *in vivo* reexposure or *in vivo* stimulation tests (51). These tests should be performed if there is any doubt about the diagnosis, or if continued treatment with CBZ is crucial.

SYSTEMIC LUPUS ERYTHEMATOSUS

Systemic lupus erythematosus (SLE) may be induced by CBZ (69–72). As with other rare side effects, it often is difficult to form a definite connection between CBZ and the development of SLE. In contrast with many other skin reactions, the symptoms of SLE usually appear 6 to 12 months after the initiation of CBZ therapy (69,71). Discontinuation of the drug may lead to a gradual improvement and eventual disappearance of the symptoms (72). A positive antinuclear factor titer may persist after the drug is discontinued and clinical symptoms resolve (69,71).

HEPATIC AND GASTROINTESTINAL SIDE EFFECTS

Hepatic enzyme induction is a well known effect of treatment with CBZ, and asymptomatic elevation of liver enzymes commonly is observed during the course of CBZ therapy, occurring in 5% to 10% of patients (3). In one series comprising more than 200 children, 6% had elevation of liver enzymes (3). The modest rise in liver enzymes was of no clinical significance (3). Studies comparing phenobarbital, phenytoin, and CBZ indicate similar enzyme-inducing potentials of these drugs, as measured by antipyrine clearance and urinary excretion of D-glucaric acid (73,74).

Although rare, more severe CBZ-associated hepatotoxicity has been reported (56,75–83). CBZ-induced hepatotoxicity appears to have two different forms (79,80). The first is a hypersensitivity-induced granulomatous hepatitis with cholestasis (78,79,84). Levy et al. (78) reported three patients with CBZ-induced granulomatous hepatitis. All patients had onset of symptoms approximately 3 to 4 weeks after starting the drug, fever and laboratory evidence of hepatic dysfunction, and granulomatous infiltration on biopsy. All patients improved after discontinuation of the drug. Furthermore, in one patient fever and rash developed on rechallenge with one dose of CBZ. Mitchell et al. (84) described an additional two patients in whom hepatitis developed within 1 month of starting CBZ. Symptoms and signs resolved after discontinuation of the drug.

The second form of hepatotoxicity is a direct toxic effect of CBZ (or its metabolites) on the liver that results in acute hepatitis and hepatocellular necrosis without significant cholestasis (79,80). The hepatitis due to CBZ exposure also is a hypersensitivity reaction, presumably mediated by an immunologic mechanism and typically occurring in the setting of a generalized hypersensitivity response (75).

Most patients who experience hepatic dysfunction have taken CBZ for less than 1 month and have associated fever or rash (78,84). Rechallenge with the drug has resulted in recurrence of the symptoms (78,85). Even with discontinuation of the drug, fatalities can occur (75,86). It has been suggested that the CBZ epoxide metabolite may be the hepatotoxic substance because there has been no correlation between toxicity and CBZ serum concentrations (80,81). Acute hepatitis appears to be rare in children (81,87).

Common gastrointestinal side effects of CBZ consist of vomiting, nausea, and diarrhea (2,88,89). Herranz et al. (2), in a study of 35 children treated with CBZ monotherapy, found that 14% had gastrointestinal disturbances. Pellock (3), in a review of adverse effects in 220 children treated with CBZ as monotherapy or polytherapy, reported that 9% had gastrointestinal side effects. Although pancreatitis has developed in a few patients treated with CBZ (90,91), it is not currently possible to definitively determine a causal link.

Additional gastrointestinal adverse effects reported with CBZ include acute cholangitis (92), eosinophilic colitis (88), constipation (93), and inhibition of intestinal folic acid absorption (94).

HEMATOLOGIC TOXICITY

Hematologic abnormalities are probably the most feared idiosyncratic reactions associated with CBZ. The package insert for Tegretol (Novartis Pharmaceutical Inc., Summit,

NJ) contains a warning regarding bone marrow suppression. Fortunately, recent studies demonstrate that severe idiosyncratic hematologic toxicities, such as aplastic anemia, megaloblastic anemia, agranulocytosis, or thrombocytopenia, are rare among patients taking CBZ (3,95,96).

Transient leukopenia commonly occurs in approximately 10% to 20% of patients treated with CBZ (6,51, 97,98), whereas persistent leukopenia has been reported in approximately 2% of patients treated with CBZ (95). Livingston et al. (7) reported moderate leukopenia [3,000 to 3,500 white blood cells (WBCs)/mm^3] in 9 of 225 patients and marked leukopenia (2,000 to 3,000 WBCs/mm^3) in 4 of 225 patients, usually within the first 3 months of treatment. Despite continuation of CBZ, cell counts returned to normal and in no case did isolated leukopenia precede more widespread marrow suppression.

Some authors have reported that younger patients have a lower prevalence of transient or persistent leukopenia than do older patients (10,15,99). However, in a study of 200 children taking CBZ, leukopenia, defined as a WBC count of less than 4,000/mm^3, occurred in 17% of patients younger than 12 years of age and in 8% of children 12 to 17 years of age (100). In a study of 220 children receiving CBZ therapy, Pellock (3) found that 28 (13%) had leukopenia with WBC counts below 4,000/mm^3, but only 5 (2%) had counts below 3,000/mm^3. None of the leukopenias progressed, and all of the patients remained on CBZ. Most of the children had low WBC counts before starting CBZ, viral infections, or both.

Leukopenia does not appear to be dose related. Transient leukopenia is more common in patients with low WBC counts before treatment (98). The proportion of T lymphocytes and B lymphocytes apparently is not altered by CBZ (97).

In rare cases, CBZ may cause serious hematologic toxicity (i.e., aplastic anemia, persistent leukopenia, and thrombocytopenia). Although CBZ-associated aplastic anemia is rare, the mortality rate is high (50,95,96,101). Hart and Easton (95), based on evidence available in 1982, estimated the prevalence of aplastic anemia to be <1/50,000. Pellock (3) estimated the risk to be smaller: 5.1 per million for aplastic anemia, 1.4 for agranulocytosis, and 2.2 for deaths associated with these events. A precise estimation of the risk for development of aplastic anemia during CBZ treatment is difficult because patients often are on other medications or have other risk factors for aplastic anemia. Neither the duration of treatment nor the age of the patient appear to be major factors in the development of aplastic anemia. It is uncertain whether aplastic anemia is dose related.

Rarely, isolated thrombocytopenia can occur during treatment with CBZ (9,102–104). As with the WBC count, there may be a transient decrease in the platelet count at the beginning of CBZ therapy (9,95).

There is a debate as to how frequent complete blood cell counts should be obtained in patients on CBZ (21). Dodson (21) recommends that the WBC count be measured at 6 weeks, 3 months, and 6 months. If the leukocyte count is consistently above 3,500/mm^3 and the granulocyte count is above 1,200/mm^3, Dodson recommends that the frequency of measurements can be reduced. If the neutrophil count is below 1,200/mm^3, the frequency of the observations should be increased. If the neutrophil count is below 900/mm^3, it is recommended that the CBZ dosage be reduced. However, other clinicians do not perform routing hematologic monitoring, obtaining studies only when the patient has symptoms of a blood dyscrasia. It does not appear that routine monitoring of the complete blood cell and platelet counts allows early detection and discontinuation of drug before the process becomes irreversible (12,21,105).

If both anemia and neutropenia occur, obtaining a reticulocyte count, serum iron concentration, and iron-binding capacity provides an indirect indication of hematopoietic activity (21). The combination of a normal or elevated reticulocyte count with a normal or low iron level is reassuring that the bone marrow is active. A low reticulocyte count with an increased serum iron concentration indicates that hematopoietic activity is reduced. In this case, CBZ should be stopped.

ENDOCRINOLOGIC EFFECTS

Antidiuretic Hormone and Water Retention

Hyponatremia and water retention are well known side effects of CBZ (106–111). The risk increases with age and with serum level of the drug (112–115). Hyponatremia secondary to CBZ is more common among the elderly (46,116), and is quite unusual in children (113,117). Hyponatremia appears to be related to serum drug level: patients whose CBZ levels are ≥6 µg/mL have a 3.5-fold greater prevalence than do those with lower levels (113). Hyponatremia is more frequent in patients on monotherapy, suggesting that other AEDs may prevent the antidiuresis induced by CBZ (114).

There may be several mechanisms by which CBZ has an antidiuretic effect. CBZ has been reported to have both a direct antidiuretic hormone (ADH) effect or ADH-promoting activity and ADH-releasing effect (51,118,119). Evidence favoring a renal effect of CBZ arises from the finding that the antidiuretic effect may be reversed by demeclocycline, a drug used to treat the syndrome of inappropriate ADH through a nephrogenic, dose-dependent inhibition of ADH-sensitive adenylate cyclase activity (119,120).

Evidence supporting a direct hypothalamic effect comes from studies demonstrating that hyponatremia may be normalized by concomitant treatment with phenytoin (115), an AED known to alter water balance by inhibiting ADH release (121). Some investigators have observed increased arginine vasopressin levels (a measure of ADH activity) during CBZ treatment (118,122), suggesting a hypothalamic effect. However, Stephens et al. (123), in a study of normal volunteers, measured ADH by radioimmunoassay and demonstrated a decrease, not an increase, in ADH levels.

Because several of the symptoms of hyponatremia—dizziness, headache, drowsiness, and nausea—may mimic side effects of CBZ, hyponatremia should be considered when these symptoms occur (51,109). Excessive intake of fluids should be discouraged in patients on CBZ. Finally, caution is in order when elderly patients on a low-salt diet are treated with CBZ.

Thyroid Hormones

Thyroid function test results frequently are abnormal in patients taking AEDs, including CBZ (124–133). In one of the largest studies, Isojärvi et al. (128) measured circulating thyroid hormones, as well as the pituitary function, in 63 male patients with epilepsy receiving either CBZ, phenytoin, or valproate as monotherapy or a combination of CBZ plus phenytoin or CBZ plus valproate. Patients on CBZ, phenytoin, CBZ plus phenytoin, and CBZ plus valproate had lower levels of circulating thyroxine (T_4) and free thyroxine (FT_4) than control patients. Serum T_4 and FT_4 concentrations were unaffected by valproate monotherapy. Triiodothyronine (T_3) levels were normal in all groups studied. Despite low T_4 and FT_4 serum levels, the serum thyrotropin [thyroid-stimulating hormone (TSH)] concentration was slightly elevated only in patients treated with a combination of CBZ plus valproate. The TSH responses to thyrotropin-releasing hormone (TRH) after 20 minutes were slightly lower in the patient group receiving phenytoin monotherapy than in the untreated patients, whereas other TRH responses to TSH were unchanged in the other patient groups.

The decrease in serum T_4 usually is small to moderate. Rootwelt et al. (131) found that in patients starting on CBZ, serum levels of T_4 fell to a stable 70% of the basal level after 1 to 2 weeks, whereas T_3 decreased transitorily to 85% of the basal level. TSH showed a complementary, but somewhat delayed transitory increase.

CBZ activates liver microsomal enzymes, thereby increasing peripheral metabolism of thyroid hormones (134). A CBZ-induced conversion and metabolism of T_4 to T_3 and of T_3 itself could explain the changes in thyroid hormone levels during CBZ therapy. In addition, thyroid hormones and CBZ bind competitively to thyroxine-binding globulin (131). Competitive binding to TBG by CBZ results in a reduction of protein-bound T_4 and an increase in FT_4 (124).

Despite changes in serum levels of T_4, patients usually remain clinically euthyroid (131). This observation could be explained by an increased peripheral use of, or sensitivity to, T_4. Overt hypothyroidism has been described in only two patients, one treated with CBZ monotherapy and one receiving a combination of CBZ and phenytoin (134). The significance, if any, of low serum T_4 and FT_4 levels in asymptomatic patients is uncertain. In patients with normal TRH levels and no clinical signs of hypothyroidism replacement, therapy does not appear to be indicated.

Because of the increased peripheral metabolism of thyroid hormones with CBZ, treating T_4-supplemented hypothyroid patients with CBZ may require an increase in the dose of T_4 to maintain the euthyroid state (135).

Adrenal Cortical Function

CBZ can cause an increase in free cortisol levels (136). In spite of this, cushingoid symptoms have not been observed during treatment with the drug. The significance, if any, of this observation therefore is unclear.

Sex Hormones

The effect of CBZ and other AEDs on sex hormones has been of considerable interest to many investigators because reproductive dysfunction and hyposexuality frequently are reported in patients with epilepsy (137–139). As noted by Herzog and Levesque (140) and Isojärvi (141), the cause of these complaints likely is multifactorial, with psychosocial, AED, seizure-related, and hormonal factors. A number of investigators have measured sex hormones in patients on AEDs to determine if changes in sexual function are related to hormonal changes.

Testosterone exists in the serum in three forms: free, albumin bound, and sex hormone–binding globulin (SHBG) bound (140). The SHBG-bound fraction is not biologically active, whereas the free testosterone and albumin-bound testosterone are available to tissues. Because of CBZ-induced hepatic synthesis of SHBG, serum levels of SHBG increase during therapy with CBZ treatment (128,142). However, serum total testosterone concentration does not change or increase, the free androgen index (one indicator of the non–SHBG-bound portion of testosterone) decreases, and the serum free testosterone level remains unchanged or decreases (128,142–144). The low free testosterone found in some patients may be secondary to increased metabolism (145).

The significance of changes in hormonal levels with CBZ is uncertain. Although Leiderman et al. (146) did not find a correlation between sexual desire and total serum testosterone concentration in men with temporal lobe epilepsy, Toone et al. (147) found that hyposexuality correlated with lower levels of free, rather than of total, testosterone. Isojärvi et al. (128) did not find serum free testosterone levels or the free androgen index to correlate with sexual dysfunction in their patients. In contrast, Herzog et al. (140,148), found that patients with reproductive or sexual dysfunction had a higher likelihood of abnormally low non–SHBG-bound testosterone than did men with epilepsy without sexual dysfunction.

Because AEDs affect the levels of other hormones, including estradiol, gonadotropin, and thyroid hormone, the relationship between AEDs and sexual function is complex. Seizures *per se*, particularly those involving the limbic system, can lead to reproductive dysfunction and hyposexuality, making the assessment of the hormonal status in patients with epilepsy even more complicated (140).

Reports concerning the serum levels of prolactin (PRL) and gonadotropin in patients with epilepsy receiving AEDs are controversial: Some authors have reported elevated levels of these hormones, whereas others have observed unaltered levels (142). Franceschi et al. (149) reported elevated PRL levels in patients with epilepsy receiving CBZ as single-drug therapy. They found no alteration in the basal levels of gonadotropin. Dana-Haeri et al. (150) did not find any changes in basal PRL or follicle-stimulating hormone (FSH) levels in male patients with epilepsy treated with CBZ, but found a significant rise in the mean basal level of luteinizing hormone (LH). Bonuccelli et al. (151) studied the spontaneous secretion of PRL in a small group of male patients with epilepsy receiving CBZ and found no change in PRL. Furthermore, 21-day treatment with CBZ did not cause any change in LH levels in healthy volunteers (145). Isojärvi et al. (142) found no difference in the mean gonadotropin or PRL levels in CBZ-treated patients and control subjects. It is not clear whether alteration of sex hormones plays a role in impotence among men with epilepsy.

To study the effects of CBZ on pituitary responsiveness, Isojärvi et al. (152) studied the effects of LH-releasing hormone, TRH, and metoclopramide on FSH, LH, and PRL in patients taking CBZ. The mean basal concentration of serum LH was significantly lower in the CBZ-treated female patients than in untreated women. In addition, the mean basal concentration of PRL was lower and the response of PRL to TRH was higher in male patients treated with CBZ. These results demonstrate that CBZ has an effect on pituitary responsiveness. The clinical relevance of these findings is not clear.

Effect of Carbamazepine on Oral Contraceptives

Because of the liver enzyme–inducing potential of CBZ, the drug may augment the degradation of estrogen and progesterone. Consequently, the effect of oral contraceptives may be impaired (153). Breakthrough bleeding and a number of unintended pregnancies have occurred in patients treated with CBZ.

BONE METABOLISM

Although biochemical changes in the metabolism of vitamin D are observed during treatment with CBZ (154), whether clinically apparent osteomalacia develops during treatment with the drug is controversial (155–157). In a study of 21 patients with epilepsy receiving CBZ as the only AED, hypocalcemia was detected in 3, hypophosphatemia in 1, and elevated serum alkaline phosphatase in 4 patients (155). Serum 25-hydroxyvitamin D values were significantly lower in the patients than in the control subjects. Although there was no difference in bone mineral density between the patients and control subjects, an increased amount of trabecular resorption surfaces was found in patients treated with CBZ, leading the authors to conclude that CBZ therapy may lead to vitamin D deficiency and osteomalacic skeletal changes. O'Hare et al. (154) also reported hypocalcemia in 10% of patients on CBZ monotherapy. Serum calcium was significantly lower and alkaline phosphatase significantly higher in patients than in matched control subjects. None of the patients was symptomatic. The authors postulated that calcium abnormalities were secondary to induction of hepatic microsomal enzymes.

CARDIOVASCULAR TOXICITY

Although rare, CBZ has been implicated in a number of cardiovascular abnormalities, including congestive heart failure (158), aggravation of the sick sinus syndrome (159), hypertension (6), and conduction defects resulting in bradycardia or Stokes-Adams attacks (107,160–164). Cardiac side effects, which seem to be especially likely to develop in older patients (in whom the incidence of conduction disturbances is highest), may develop after years of CBZ therapy. Rechallenge with CBZ after insertion of a pacemaker has supported a causal relationship between the CBZ and conduction disturbances (162). The conduction defect may be dose related.

Kasarskis et al. (165), in a review of 40 previous cases of CBZ-induced cardiac dysfunction, suggested that two distinct forms of CBZ-associated cardiac dysfunction occur. In the first form, sinus tachycardia occurs in the setting of a massive CBZ overdose. The 14 patients with this form were characterized by a young age (mean, 25.2 ± 12.6 years; range, 1.5 to 55 years), markedly elevated serum CBZ levels (mean, 227 μmol/L; range, 97.4 to 1,012 μmol/L), the absence of preexisting cardiac dysfunction, and an equal sex distribution. The second group consisted almost exclusively of elderly women who had potentially life-threatening bradyarrhythmias or atrioventricular conduction delay, associated with either therapeutic or modestly elevated serum CBZ levels. The mean age in the second group was 65.0 ± 18.4 years (range, 10 to 87 years). In the 26 patients with the second form, cardiac dysfunction appeared without warning during routine clinical management of either seizures or trigeminal neuralgia.

In healthy, young individuals, the risk of CBZ-induced cardiac dysfunction appears low (166). Patients with underlying cardiac disease may be at higher risk for conduction defects. Although heart block rarely is reported in children, patients with tuberous sclerosis and cardiac rhabdomyoma may be at increased risk for conduction block (167). Durelli et al. (45) found that in a patient with a myotonic cardiomyopathy, CBZ treatment resulted in a grade 1 heart block that appeared to increase in severity with increasing dosage of the drug.

These clinical observations are supported by experimental work with dogs (168). Parenteral CBZ results in a prolongation of atrioventricular conduction and a decreased rate of phase 4 depolarization of autonomic fibers. It appears that CBZ at low or therapeutic doses can worsen a preexisting atrioventricular block, and that the drug at higher levels can induce conduction delays *de novo* in otherwise normal elderly people (> 65 years) (165).

RENAL ADVERSE EFFECTS

Isolated renal side effects of CBZ therapy are rare. Cases of acute renal failure due to presumed CBZ-induced acute interstitial nephritis (68,169), and a case of membranous glomerulopathy presumably caused by a type III allergic reaction to CBZ (66) have been reported. CBZ also has been implicated in urinary retention (170).

HEME BIOSYNTHESIS

Several studies indicate that CBZ may influence heme biosynthesis (171,172), and reports of CBZ-induced attacks of nonhereditary porphyria exist (173,174). Conversely, CBZ is recommended by some authors for use in patients with acute intermittent porphyria (175,176).

IMMUNOGLOBULIN FUNCTION

Levels of the immunoglobulin G (IgG) subclass IgG_2 have been reported to be decreased in patients on CBZ (177). The significance, if any, of altered concentrations of IgG subclasses with CBZ is likely to be slight. There are no significant differences in concentrations of serum (178,179) or nasal immunoglobulins (178) or in frequency of respiratory tract infections between patients receiving CBZ and control subjects (178). These findings are in contrast to phenytoin, in which reduced concentrations of serum and nasal IgA have been reported (180).

RETINAL ABNORMALITIES

A reversible retinopathy possibly secondary to CBZ was reported in two adult patients treated with CBZ for more than 7 years (181). Both patients had sudden reduction of visual acuity without other side effects. Lesions in the retinal epithelium were noted in both patients. Discontinuation of the drug led to improvement in visual function and in the morphologic changes. The tricyclic psychotropic drugs are known to have toxic effects on the retinal pigment epithelium. Because CBZ is chemically similar to the tricyclics, it is possible that the development of retinal lesions in these two patients is not coincidental. Color vision can be affected by AEDs. López et al. (182) found that color visual perception was impaired in 82% (30 of 37) of patients taking either CBZ, phenytoin, or valproate. In the CBZ group, abnormalities in the blue-yellow axis occurred in 66.7% (8 of 12) of the patients. None of these patients complained of disturbances in color vision.

NEUROPSYCHOLOGICAL EFFECTS

CBZ may cause a variety of psychic disturbances, including asthenia, restlessness, insomnia, agitation, and anxiety (50). In addition, CBZ has been implicated in sporadic cases of psychosis (50). Overall, the incidence of psychiatric symptoms with CBZ is low and appears to be lower than with some of the other AEDs (183)

Two patients in whom signs of an encephalopathic process developed while on CBZ have been reported (184,185). The first patient (184) presented with confusion, spasticity, hyperreflexia, bilateral extensor plantar responses, and ataxia, whereas the second (185) became mute and manifested a spastic quadriparesis. Both patients improved dramatically when CBZ was discontinued.

In unpublished cases, the author has cared for three children with partial seizures in whom expressive aphasia developed over several months while on CBZ. EEGs showed bilateral frontotemporal lobe spikes that markedly increased during sleep. After withdrawal of CBZ, speech returned to baseline status and the number of epileptiform discharges during both the awake and sleep states decreased. It is suspected that CBZ, by increasing the epileptiform discharges, caused the aphasia.

COGNITIVE FUNCTION

The risks of cognitive impairment with nontoxic chronic CBZ appear low (16,23,186–188). Cognitive improvement may occur when patients are switched from barbiturates or polytherapy to CBZ (10). Most studies examining cognitive effects have used the immediate-release preparations of CBZ. It is likely that both children and adults will perform better with the sustained-release preparations.

Aman et al. (189) evaluated 50 children with well controlled seizures receiving CBZ monotherapy with a battery of cognitive and motor tasks. Testing was performed both after CBZ was administered, presumably at a time of peak concentration, and before CBZ administration, when CBZ concentrations were at trough levels. During testing at peak concentration, response time varied as a function of the test; response time was increased for matching familiar figures and for auditory–visual integration, but decreased for short-term memory tasks. In addition, at peak concentrations the children had fewer extraneous movements while seated; that is, they were less restless, had an improved attention span, and had steadier motor movements. Of note was the finding that concentration of CBZ in the saliva did not correlate with any variables measured.

O'Dougherty et al. (190) studied the relationship between serum CBZ concentrations and cognitive performance in 11 children with partial seizures. Neuropsychological tests demonstrated a mild beneficial effect of CBZ on eye–hand coordination and, with low serum levels, better rapid processing of items in memory. No changes in simple reaction time, sustained attention, behavioral adjustment, or motor performance with the preferred hand were observed at low or moderate CBZ levels. Efficiency of learning new information and memory scanning rate showed a level-dependent relationship with CBZ. Poor performances were significantly associated with higher plasma CBZ levels. As discussed by Trimble (191), the relationship between performance on cognitive tasks and serum levels of CBZ in children appears to vary as a function of the task.

As do children, adults function quite well when serum CBZ levels are within the therapeutic range (187). In a study of 22 adults (mean age, 36 years) studied with a battery of neuropsychological measures involving motor speed, reaction time, attention, and memory, there was no consistent relationship between results on the test battery and serum concentration of CBZ (192). Further support for the lack of significant cognitive impairment with CBZ comes from a large study on the effects of withdrawal of AEDs on cognitive function in children. Aldenkamp et al. (23) found that the impact of AED treatment on cognitive functions appears to be limited in magnitude.

OVERDOSAGE

Massive CBZ overdoses have been well described by numerous authors (79,193–205). Although CBZ overdosage is serious, death rarely occurs with a CBZ overdose (206,207). Fisher and Cysyk (207) reviewed 23 cases of CBZ overdosage reported in the literature. Only two deaths were recorded. The highest serum level report was 65 mg/L (200). A patient who consumed 400 tablets of 200 mg CBZ survived after hemoperfusion (201).

Overdoses of CBZ have been associated with symptoms resembling the central anticholinergic syndrome caused by tricyclic antidepressants (205,207). The most prevalent symptoms of CBZ overdosage are nystagmus, mydriasis, ophthalmoplegia, cerebellar and extrapyramidal signs, and impairment of consciousness progressing to a comatose state, possibly accompanied by seizures, myoclonus, and respiratory depression (208). Cardiac symptoms consist of tachycardia, arrhythmia, conduction disturbances, and low blood pressure. Gastrointestinal and anticholinergic symptoms also may supervene. Coma may develop at serum CBZ levels as low as 80 μmol/L (209,210). Life-threatening cardiac events are rare with CBZ overdose, although cardiorespiratory problems can occur with serum CBZ levels exceeding 35 μg/mL (208).

Weaver et al. (211) described four stages in CBZ overdosage: I—coma, seizures [CBZ levels >25 μg/mol (105 μmol/L)]; II—combativeness, hallucinations, choreiform movements [15 to 25 μg/mL (65 to 105 μmol/L)]; III—drowsiness, ataxia [11 to 15 μg/mL (45 to 65 μmol/L)]; and IV—potentially catastrophic relapse [11 μg/mL (45 μmol/L)].

During CBZ intoxication, there is a prolongation of the CBZ half-life and elevation of the CBZ epoxide/CBZ ratio (211). The concentration of CBZ epoxide may exceed that of the parent compound (195,211). It has been suggested that the evolution of the intoxication correlates more closely with the course of the CBZ epoxide level than with the concentration of CBZ itself, which declines rapidly (79,211).

Because of the anticholinergic-like action of the drug, delayed gastric emptying often is present, leading to impaired absorption of the drug. In addition, when ingested in large quantities, the drug may form a concretion. For that reason, gastric emptying may continue for as long as 12 hours or more in asymptomatic patients and up to 60 hours in symptomatic patients (208). Activated charcoal, metoclopramide, which enhances gut motility, and vigorous cathartics also have been recommended (204,208,212). Relapses can occur owing to delayed absorption of CBZ from the intestine (196,205,211). Because of the high degree of protein binding of CBZ, forced diuresis, peritoneal dialysis, and hemodialysis are not recommended (201,208). Charcoal hemoperfusion, a technique in which blood is pumped through a column containing activated carbon granules coated with acrylic hydrogen polymer, has been used successfully to treat patients with overdosage (194,195,198,199). Charcoal hemoperfusion is associated with thrombocytopenia, coagulopathy, hypothermia, and hypocalcemia. Recently, high-efficiency dialysis, which uses a highly permeable membrane and a high dialysate flow, has been used safely for a patient with a CBZ overdosage (193). This technique appears effective and safe.

CONCLUSION

It is quite likely that CBZ will remain one of the major AEDs as we enter the twenty-first century. The drug will likely remain popular not only because of its efficacy in controlling a variety of seizures but because of its excellent safety profile. Although CBZ may cause a number of side effects, most are mild and easily managed. Fortunately, severe adverse reactions are rather infrequent.

ACKNOWLEDGMENTS

This work was supported in part by the National Institute of Neurological and Communicative Disorders (NS27984). The author acknowledges the contribution of Drs. Lennart Gram and Peder Klosterskov Jensen, who wrote the chapter on carbamazepine toxicity in the third edition of this book. Their contribution greatly aided the author in the preparation of this review.

REFERENCES

1. Collaborative Group for Epidemiology of Epilepsy. Adverse reactions to antiepileptic drugs: a follow-up study of 355 patients with chronic antiepileptic drug treatment. *Epilepsia* 1988;29:787–793.
2. Herranz JL, Armijo JA, Artega R. Clinical side effects of phenobarbital, primidone, phenytoin, carbamazepine, and valproate during monotherapy in children. *Epilepsia* 1988;29:794–804.
3. Pellock JM. Carbamazepine side effects in children and adults. *Epilepsia* 1987;28[Suppl 3]:S64–S70.
4. Okuno T, Ito M, Nakano S, et al. Carbamazepine therapy and long-term prognosis in epilepsy of childhood. *Epilepsia* 1989; 30:57–61.
5. Pellock JM, McIntyre HB, Rivera VM. Carbamazepine: a retrospective usage survey of prescribing and monitoring habits. *J Epilepsy* 1989;2:169–173.
6. Killian JM, Fromm GH. Carbamazepine in treatment of neuralgia: use and side effects. *Arch Neurol* 1968;19:129–136.
7. Livingston S, Villamater C, Sakata Y, et al. Use of carbamazepine in epilepsy: results in 87 patients. *JAMA* 1967;200: 204–208.
8. Redpath TH, Gayford JJ. The side effects of carbamazepine therapy. *Oral Surg* 1968;26:299–303.
9. Rodin EA, Rim CS, Rennick PM. The effects of carbamazepine on patients with psychomotor epilepsy: results of a double-blind study. *Epilepsia* 1974;15:547–561.
10. Schain RJ, Ward JW, Guthrie D. Carbamazepine as an anticonvulsant in children. *Neurology* 1977;27:476–480.
11. Schoeman JF, Elyas AA, Brett EM, et al. Correlation between plasma carbamazepine-10,11-epoxide concentration and drug side effects in children with epilepsy. *Dev Med Child Neurol* 1984;26:756–764.
12. Mattson RH. Carbamazepine. In: Engel J Jr, Pedley TA, eds. *Epilepsy: a comprehensive textbook.* Philadelphia: Lippincott-Raven, 1997:1491–1502.
13. Reynolds EH. Neurotoxicity of carbamazepine. *Adv Neurol* 1975;11:345–353.
14. Noachtar S, von Maydell B, Fuhry L, et al. Gabapentin and carbamazepine affect eye movements and posture control differently: a placebo-controlled investigation of acute CNS side effects in healthy volunteers. *Epilepsy Res* 1998;31:47–57.
15. Davis EH. Clinical trials of Tegretol in trigeminal neuralgia. *Headache* 1969;9:77–82.
16. van der Meyden CH, Bartel PR, Sommers DK, et al. Effect of acute doses of controlled-release carbamazepine on clinical, psychomotor, electrophysiological, and cognitive parameters of brain function. *Epilepsia* 1992;33:335–342.
17. Delcker A, Wilhelm H, Timmann D, et al. Side effects from increased doses of carbamazepine on neuropsychological and posturographic parameters of humans. *Eur Neuropsychopharmacol* 1997;7:213–218.
18. Höppener RJ, Kuyer A, Meijer JWA, et al. Correlation between daily fluctuations of carbamazepine serum levels of intermittent side effects. *Epilepsia* 1980;21:341–350.
19. Keranen T, Silvenius J. Side effects of carbamazepine, valproate and clonazepam during long-term treatment of epilepsy. *Acta Neurol Scand Suppl* 1983;97:69–80.
20. Tedeschi G, Casucci G, Allocca S, et al. Neuroocular side effects of carbamazepine and phenobarbital in epileptic patients as measured by saccadic eye movements analysis. *Epilepsia* 1989; 30:62–66.
21. Dodson WE. Carbamazepine and oxcarbazepine. In: Dodson WE, Pellock JM, eds. *Pediatric epilepsy: diagnosis and therapy.* New York: Demos, 1993:303–314.
22. Riva R, Contin M, Albani F, et al. Lateral gaze nystagmus in carbamazepine-treated epileptic patients: correlation with total and free plasma concentrations of parent drug and its 10,11 epoxide metabolite. *Ther Drug Monit* 1985;7:277–282.
23. Aldenkamp AP, Alpherts WCJ, Moerland MD, et al. Controlled-release carbamazepine: cognitive side effects in patients with epilepsy. *Epilepsia* 1987;28:507–514.
24. Pieters MSM, Jennekens-Schinkel A, Stijnen T, et al. Carbamazepine (CBZ) controlled release compared with conventional CBZ: a controlled study of attention and vigilance in children with epilepsy. *Epilepsia* 1992;33:1137–1144.
25. Mirza WU, Rak IW, Thadani VM, et al. Six-month evaluation of Carbatrol (extended-release carbamazepine) in complex partial seizures. *Neurology* 2000;51:1727–1729.
26. Strandjord RE, Johannessen SI. Single-drug therapy with carbamazepine in patients with epilepsy: serum levels and clinical effects. *Epilepsia* 1980;21:655–662.
27. Meijer JWA, Binnie CD, Debets RMC, et al. Possible hazard of valpromide-carbamazepine combination therapy in epilepsy. *Lancet* 1984;1:802.
28. Patsalos PN, Stephenson TJ, Krishna S, et al. M. Side-effects induced by carbamazepine-10,11-epoxide. *Lancet* 1985;8:496.
29. Tomson T. Interdosage fluctuations in plasma carbamazepine concentration determine intermittent side effects. *Arch Neurol* 1984;41:830–834.
30. Theodore WH, Narang PK, Holmes MD, et al. Carbamazepine and its epoxide: relation of plasma levels to toxicity and seizure control. *Ann Neurol* 1989;25:194–196.
31. Steven RE, Limsakun T, Evans G, et al. Controlled, multidose, pharmacokinetic evaluation of two extended-release carbamazepine formulations (Carbatrol and Tegretol-XR). *J Pharm Sci* 1998;87:1531–1534.
32. Garnett WR, Levy B, McLean AM, et al. Pharmacokinetic evaluation of twice-daily extended-release carbamazepine (CBZ) and four-times-daily immediate-release CBZ in patients with epilepsy. *Epilepsia* 1998;39:274–279.
33. Bradbury AJ, Bentick B, Todd PJ. Dystonia associated with carbamazepine toxicity. *Postgrad Med J* 1982;58:525–526.

34. Crosley CJ, Swender PT. Dystonia associated with carbamazepine administration: experience in brain-damaged children. *Pediatrics* 1979;63:612–615.

35. Jacome D. Carbamazepine induced dystonia. *JAMA* 1979;241: 2263.

36. Wendland KL. Myoclonus following doses of carbamazepine. *Nervenarzt* 1968;39:231–233.

37. Neglia JP, Glaze DG, Zion TE. Tics and vocalizations in children treated with carbamazepine. *Pediatrics* 1984;73:841–844.

38. Robertson PL, Garofalo EA, Silverstein FS, et al. Carbamazepine-induced tics. *Epilepsia* 1993;34:965–968.

39. Ambrosetto G, Riva R, Baruzzi A. Hyperammonemia in asterixis induced by carbamazepine: two case reports. *Acta Neurol Scand* 1984;69:186–189.

40. Bimpong-Bita K, Froescher W. Carbamazepine-induced choreoathetoid dyskinesias. *J Neurol Neurosurg Psychiatry* 1982; 45:560.

41. Geraldini W, Faedda MT, Sideri G. Anticonvulsant therapy and its possible consequence on the peripheral nervous system: a neurographic study. *Epilepsia* 1984;25:502–505.

42. Lühdorf K, Nielsen CJ, Oerbæk K, et al. Motor and sensory conduction velocities and electromyographic findings in man before and after carbamazepine treatment. *Acta Neurol Scand* 1983;67:103–107.

43. Danner R, Lang H, Yale C. Prospective neurometric studies during the beginning of carbamazepine and phenytoin therapy. *Acta Neurol Scand* 1984;69:207–217.

44. Snead OC, Hosey LC. Exacerbation of seizures in children by carbamazepine. *N Engl J Med* 1985;313:916–921.

45. Dhuna A, Pascual-Leone A, Talwar D. Exacerbation of partial seizures and onset of nonepileptic myoclonus with carbamazepine. *Epilepsia* 1991;32:275–278.

46. Radó JP, Juhos E, Sawinsky I. Dose-response relations in drug-induced inappropriate secretion of ADH: effects of clofibrate and carbamazepine. *Int J Clin Pharmacol* 1975;12:315–319.

47. Genton P. When antiepileptic drugs aggravate epilepsy. *Brain Dev* 2000;22:75–80.

48. Sachdeo R, Chokroverty S. Increasing epileptiform activities in the EEG in presence of decreasing clinical seizures after carbamazepine. *Epilepsia* 1985;26:522.

49. Chadwick D, Shaw MDM, Foy P, et al. Serum anticonvulsant concentrations and the risk of drug induced skin eruptions. *J Neurol Neurosurg Psychiatry* 1984;47:642–644.

50. Sillanpää M. Carbamazepine: pharmacology and clinical uses. *Acta Neurol Scand Suppl* 1981;88:1–202.

51. Gram L, Jensen PK. Carbamazepine: toxicity. In: Levy R, Mattson R, Meldrum B, et al., eds. *Antiepileptic drugs*, 3rd ed. New York: Raven Press, 1989:555–565.

52. Shuper A, Stahl BA, Weitz R. Carbamazepine-induced hair loss. *Drug Intell Clin Pharm* 1985;19:924.

53. Murphy JM, Mashman J, Miller JD, et al. Suppression of carbamazepine-induced rash with prednisone. *Neurology* 1991;41: 144–145.

54. Lewis IJ, Rosenbloom L. Glandular fever-like syndrome, pulmonary eosinophilia and asthma associated with carbamazepine. *Postgrad Med J* 1982;58:100–101.

55. Mullick FG, McAllister HA, Wagner BM, et al. Drug related vasculitis: clinicopathologic correlations in 30 patients. *Hum Pathol* 1979;10:313–325.

56. Ponte CD. Carbamazepine-induced thrombocytopenia, rash, and hepatic dysfunction. *Drug Intell Clin Pharm* 1983;17: 642–644.

57. Stewart CR, Vengrow MI, Riley TL. Double quotidian fever caused by carbamazepine. *N Engl J Med* 1980;302:1262.

58. Yates P, Stockdill G, McIntyre M. Hypersensitivity to carbamazepine presenting as pseudolymphoma. *J Clin Pathol* 1986; 39:1224–1228.

59. Harats N, Shalit M. Carbamazepine induced vasculitis. *J Neurol Neurosurg Psychiatry* 1987;50:1241–1243.

60. Taliercio CP, Olney BA, Lie JT. Myocarditis related to drug hypersensitivity. *Mayo Clin Proc* 1985;60:463–468.

61. De Swert LF, Ceuppens JL, Teuwen D, et al. Acute interstitial pneumonitis and carbamazepine therapy. *Acta Paediatr Scand* 1984;73:285–288.

62. Lee T, Cochrane GM. Pulmonary eosinophilia and asthma associated with carbamazepine. *BMJ* 1981;282:440.

63. Schmidt M, Brugger E. Case of carbamazepine-induced interstitial pneumonia. *Med Klin* 1980;75:29–31.

64. Stephan WC, Parks RD, Tempest B. Acute hypersensitivity pneumonitis associated with carbamazepine therapy. *Chest* 1978;74:463–464.

65. Taylor MW, Smith CC, Hern JE. An unexpected reaction to carbamazepine. *Practitioner* 1981;225:219–220.

66. Hordon LD, Turney JH. Membranous glomerulopathy associated with carbamazepine. *BMJ* 1987;294:375.

67. Shuttleworth D, Graham-Brown RAC, Williams AJ, et al. Pseudo-lymphoma associated with carbamazepine. *Clin Exp Dermatol* 1984;9:421–423.

68. Hogg RJ, Sawyer M, Hecox K, et al. Carbamazepine-induced acute tubulointerstitial nephritis. *J Pediatr* 1981;98:830–832.

69. Bateman DE. Carbamazepine induced systemic lupus erythematosus: case report. *BMJ* 1985;291:632–633.

70. Di Giorgio CM, Rabinowicz AL, Olivas R. Carbamazepine-induced antinuclear antibodies and systemic lupus erythematous-like syndrome. *Epilepsia* 1991;32:128–129.

71. McNicholl B. Carbamazepine induced systemic lupus erythematosus. *BMJ* 1985; 291:1126.

72. Toepfer M, Sitter T, Lochmüller H, et al. Drug-induced systemic lupus erythematosus after 8 years of treatment with carbamazepine. *Eur J Clin Pharmacol* 1998;54:193–194.

73. Perucca E, Hedges A, Makki KA, et al. A comparative study of the relative enzyme inducing properties of anticonvulsant drugs in epileptic patients. *Br J Clin Pharmacol* 1984;18:401–410.

74. Shaw PN, Houston JB, Rowland M, et al. Antipyrine metabolite kinetics in healthy human volunteers during multiple dosing of phenytoin and carbamazepine. *Br J Clin Pharmacol* 1985; 20:611–618.

75. Gram L, Bentsen KD. Hepatic toxicity of antiepileptic drugs: a review. *Acta Neurol Scand Suppl* 1983;97:81–90.

76. Hopen G, Nesthus I, Laerum OD. Fatal carbamazepine-associated hepatitis: report of two cases. *Acta Med Scand* 1981;210: 333–335.

77. Levander HG. Granulomatous hepatitis in a patient receiving carbamazepine. *Acta Med Scand* 1980;208:333–335.

78. Levy M, Goodman MW, Van Dyne BJ, et al. Granulomatous hepatitis secondary to carbamazepine. *Ann Intern Med* 1981;95: 64–65.

79. Luke DR, Rocci ML, Schaible DH, et al. Acute hepatotoxicity after excessively high doses of carbamazepine on two occasions. *Pharmacotherapy* 1986;6:108–111.

80. Soffer EE, Taylor RJ, Bertram PD, et al. Carbamazepine-induced liver injury. *South Med J* 1983;76:681–683.

81. Zucker P, Daum F, Cohen MI. Fatal carbamazepine hepatitis. *J Pediatr* 1977;91:667–668.

82. Haase MR. Carbamazepine-induced hepatorenal failure in a child. *Pharmacotherapy* 2000;19:667–671.

83. Morales-Diaz M, Pinilla-Roa E, Ruiz I. Suspected carbamazepine-induced hepatotoxicity. *Pharmacotherapy* 1999;19: 252–255.

84. Mitchell MC, Boitnott JK, Arregui A, et al. Granulomatous

hepatitis associated with carbamazepine therapy. *Am J Med* 1981;71:733–735.

85. Ramsay ID. Carbamazepine-induced jaundice. *BMJ* 1967;4: 155.

86. Horowitz S, Patwarden R, Marcus, E. Carbamazepine hepatotoxicity. *Epilepsia* 1986;27:592.

87. Galeone D, Lamontanara G, Torelli D. Acute hepatitis in a patient treated with carbamazepine. *J Neurol* 1985;232: 301–303.

88. Anttila V-J, Valtonen M. Carbamazepine-induced eosinophilic colitis. *Epilepsia* 1992;33:119–121.

89. Iyer V, Holmes JW, Richardson RL. Intractable diarrhea from carbamazepine. *Epilepsia* 1992;33:185–187.

90. Soman M, Swenson CA possible case of carbamazepine-induced pancreatitis. *Drug Intell Clin Pharm* 1985;19:925–927.

91. Tsao CY, Wright FS. Acute chemical pancreatitis associated with carbamazepine intoxication. *Epilepsia* 1993;34:174–176.

92. Larrey D, Hadengue A, Pessayre D, et al. Carbamazepine-induced acute cholangitis. *Dig Dis Sci* 1987;32:554–557.

93. Ettinger AB, Shinnar S, Sinnett MJ, et al. Carbamazepine-induced constipation. *J Epilepsy* 1992;5:191–193.

94. Hendel J, Dam M, Gram L, et al. The effects of carbamazepine and valproate on folate metabolism in man. *Acta Neurol Scand* 1984;69:226–231.

95. Hart RB, Easton JD. Carbamazepine and hematological monitoring. *Ann Neurol* 1982;11:309–312.

96. Pisciotta AV. Hematological toxicity of carbamazepine. *Adv Neurol* 1975;11:355–368.

97. Gilhus NE, Matre R. Carbamazepine effects on mononuclear blood cells in epileptic patients. *Acta Neurol Scand* 1986;74: 181–185.

98. Killian JM. Tegretol in trigeminal neuralgia with special references to hematopoietic side effects. *Headache* 1969;9:58–63.

99. Huf R, Schain RJ. Long-term experience with carbamazepine (Tegretol) in children with seizures. *J Pediatr* 1980;97:310–312.

100. Silverstein FS, Boxer L, Johnston MV. Hematological monitoring during therapy with carbamazepine in children. *Ann Neurol* 1983;13:685–686.

101. Franceschi M, Ciboddo G, Truci G, et al. Fatal aplastic anemia in a patient treated with carbamazepine. *Epilepsia* 1988;29: 582–583.

102. Baciewicz G, Yerevanian BI. Thrombocytopenia associated with carbamazepine: case report and review. *J Clin Psychiatry* 1984; 45:315–316.

103. Pearce J, Ron MA. Thrombocytopenia after carbamazepine. *Lancet* 1968;2:223.

104. Rutman JY. Effects of carbamazepine on blood elements. *Ann Neurol* 1978;3:373.

105. Pellock JM, Willmore LJ. A rational guide to blood monitoring in patients receiving antiepileptic drugs. *Neurology* 1991;41: 961–964.

106. Appleby L. Rapid development of hyponatremia during low-dose carbamazepine therapy. *J Neurol Neurosurgery Psychiatry* 1984;47:1138.

107. Byrne E, Wong CH, Chambers DG, et al. Carbamazepine therapy complicated by nodal bradycardia and water intoxication. *Aust N Z J Med* 1979;9:295–296.

108. Meinders AE, Cejka V, Roberston GL. The antidiuretic action of carbamazepine in man. *Clin Sci Mol Med* 1974;47:289–299.

109. Perucca E, Richens A. Water intoxication produced by carbamazepine and its reversal by phenytoin. *Br J Clin Pharmacol* 1980;9:302P–304P.

110. Stephens WP, Coe JY, Baylis PH. Plasma arginine vasopressin concentrations and antidiuretic action of carbamazepine. *BMJ* 1978;1:1445–1447.

111. Carville S, Clarke D, Cassidy G. The management of epilepsy in a hospital for people with a learning disability. *Seizure* 1999; 8:175–180.

112. Kalff R, Houtkooper HA, Meyer JWA, et al. Carbamazepine and sodium levels. *Epilepsia* 1984;25:390–397.

113. Lahr MB. Hyponatremia during carbamazepine therapy. *Clin Pharmacol Ther* 1985;37:693–696.

114. Perucca E, Garratt A, Hebdige S, et al. Water intoxication in epileptic patients receiving carbamazepine. *J Neurol Neurosurg Psychiatry* 1978;41:713–718.

115. Sordillo P, Sagransky DM, Mercado R, et al. Carbamazepine-induced syndrome of inappropriate antidiuretic hormone secretion: reversal by concomitant phenytoin therapy. *Arch Intern Med* 1978;138:299–301.

116. Koivikko MJ, Valikangas SL. Hyponatremia during carbamazepine therapy in children. *Neuropediatrics* 1983;14:93–96.

117. Helin I, Nilsson KO, Bjerre I, et al. Serum sodium and osmolality during carbamazepine treatment in children. *BMJ* 1977; 2:558.

118. Ashton MG, Ball SG, Thomas TH, et al. Water intoxication associated with carbamazepine treatment. *BMJ* 1977;1: 1134–1135.

119. Ringel RA, Brick JF. Perspective on carbamazepine-induced water intoxication: reversal by demeclocycline. *Neurology* 1986;36:1506–1507.

120. Ballardie FW, Mucklow JC. Partial reversal of carbamazepine-induced water intolerance by demeclocycline. *Br J Clin Pharmacol* 1984;17:763–765.

121. Fichman MP, Kleeman CR, Bethune JE. Inhibition of antidiuretic hormone secretion by diphenylhydantoin. *Arch Neurol* 1970;22:45–53.

122. Smith NJ, Espir MLE, Baylis PH. Raised plasma arginine vasopressin concentration in carbamazepine-induced water intoxication. *BMJ* 1977;2:804.

123. Stephens WP, Espir MLE, Tattersall RB, et al. Water intoxication due to carbamazepine. *BMJ* 1977;1:754–755.

124. Bentsen KD, Gram L, Veje A. Serum thyroid hormones and blood folic acid during monotherapy with carbamazepine and valproate: a controlled study. *Acta Neurol Scand* 1983;67: 235–241.

125. Connacher AA, Borsey DQ, Browning MC, et al. The effective evaluation of thyroid status in patients on phenytoin, carbamazepine or sodium valproate attending an epilepsy clinic. *Postgrad Med J* 1987;63:841–845.

126. Ericsson UB, Bjerre I, Forsgren M, et al. Thyroglobulin and thyroid hormones in patients on long-term treatment with phenytoin, carbamazepine, and valproic acid. *Epilepsia* 1985;26:594–596.

127. Isojärvi JIT, Pakarinen AJ, Myllylä VV. Thyroid function in epileptic patients treated with carbamazepine. *Arch Neurol* 1989;46:1175–1178.

128. Isojärvi JIT, Pakarinen AJ, Ylipalosaari PJ, et al. Serum hormones in male epileptic patients receiving anticonvulsant medication. *Arch Neurol* 1990;47:670–676.

129. Kaneko S, Otani K, Fukushima Y, et al. Effect of antiepileptic drugs on hGH, TSH, and thyroid hormone concentrations during pregnancy. *Int J Biol Res Pregnancy* 1982;3:148–151.

130. Liewendahl K, Majuri H, Helenius T. Thyroid function tests in patients on long-term treatment with various anticonvulsant drugs. *Clin Endocrinol* 1978;8:185–191.

131. Rootwelt K, Ganes T, Johannessen SI. Effect of carbamazepine, phenytoin and phenobarbitone on serum levels of thyroid hormones and thyrotropin in humans. *Scand J Clin Lab Invest* 1978;38:731–736.

132. Strandjord RE, Aanderud S, Myking OL, et al. Influence of car-

bamazepine on serum thyroid and triiodothyronine in patients with epilepsy. *Acta Neurol Scand* 1981;63:111–121.

133. Yeo PP, Bates D, Howe JG, et al. Anticonvulsants and thyroid function. *BMJ* 1978;1:1581–1583.

134. Aanderud S, Myking OL, Strandjord RE. The influence of carbamazepine on thyroid hormones and thyroxine-binding globulin in hypothyroid patients substituted with thyroxine. *Clin Endocrinol* 1981;15:247–252.

135. De Luca F, Arrigo T, Pandullo E, et al. Changes in thyroid function tests induced by 2 month carbamazepine treatment in L-thyroxine-substituted hypothyroid children. *Eur J Pediatr* 1986;145:77–79.

136. Lühdorf K. Endocrine functions and anti-epileptic treatment. *Acta Neurol Scand Suppl* 1983;94:15–19.

137. Cramer JA, Jones EE. Reproductive function in epilepsy. *Epilepsia* 1991;32[Suppl 6]:S19–S26.

138. Herzog AG. Reproductive endocrine considerations and hormonal therapy for women with epilepsy. *Epilepsia* 1991;32 [Suppl 6]:S27–S33.

139. Morrell MJ. Sexual dysfunction in epilepsy. *Epilepsia* 1991;32 [Suppl 6]:S38–S45.

140. Herzog AG, Levesque LA. Testosterone, free testosterone, non-sex hormone-binding globulin-bound testosterone, and free androgen index: which testosterone measurement is most relevant to reproductive and sexual function in men with epilepsy? *Arch Neurol* 1992;49:133–134.

141. Isojärvi JI, Parkarinen AJ, Ulipalosaari PJ, et al. Serum hormones in male epileptic patients receiving anticonvulsant medications. *Arch Neurol* 1990;47:670–676.

142. Isojärvi JI, Pakarinen AJ, Myllylä VV. Effects of carbamazepine therapy on serum sex hormone levels in male patients with epilepsy. *Epilepsia* 1988;29:781–786.

143. Dana-Haeri J, Oxley J, Richens A. Reduction of free testosterone by antiepileptic drugs. *BMJ* 1982;284:85–86.

144. Isojärvi JI, Pakarinen AJ, Myllylä VV. Effects of carbamazepine on the hypothalamic-pituitary-gonadal axis in male patients with epilepsy: a prospective study. *Epilepsia* 1989;30:446–452.

145. Connell JMC, Rapeport WG, Beastall GH, et al. Changes in circulating androgens during short term carbamazepine therapy. *Br J Clin Pharmacol* 1984;17:347–351.

146. Leiderman DB, Csernansky JG, Moses JA Jr. Neuroendocrinology and limbic epilepsy: relationship to psychopathology, seizure variables, and neuropsychological function. *Epilepsia* 1990;31:270–274.

147. Toone BK, Wheeler H, Nanjee M, et al. Sex hormones, sexual activity and plasma anticonvulsant levels in male epileptics. *J Neurol Neurosurg Psychiatry* 1983;46:824–826.

148. Herzog AG, Drislane FW, Schomer DL, et al. Abnormal pulsatile secretion of luteinizing hormone in men with epilepsy: relationship to laterality and nature of paroxysmal discharges. *Neurology* 1990;40:1557–1561.

149. Franceschi M, Perego L, Cavagnini F, et al. Effects of long-term antiepileptic therapy on the hypothalamic-pituitary axis in man. *Epilepsia* 1984;25:46–52.

150. Dana-Haeri J, Oxley J, Richens A. Pituitary responsiveness to gonadotrophin-releasing and thyrotrophin-releasing hormones in epileptic patients receiving carbamazepine or phenytoin. *Clin Endocrinol* 1984;20:163–168.

151. Bonuccelli U, Murialdo G, Martino E, et al. Effects of carbamazepine on prolactin secretion in normal subjects and in epileptic subjects. *Clin Neuropharmacol* 1985;8:165–174.

152. Isojärvi JIT, Myllylä VV, Pakarinen AJ. Effects of carbamazepine on pituitary responsiveness to luteinizing hormone-releasing hormone, thyrotropin-releasing hormone, and metoclopramide epileptic patients. *Epilepsia* 1989;30:50–56.

153. Coulam CB, Annegers JF. Do anticonvulsants reduce the efficacy of oral contraceptives? *Epilepsia* 1979;20:519–526.

154. O'Hare JA, Duggan B, O'Driscoll B, et al. Biochemical evidence for osteomalacia with carbamazepine therapy. *Acta Neurol Scand* 1980;62:282–286.

155. Hoikka V, Alhava EM, Karjalainen P, et al. Carbamazepine and bone mineral metabolism. *Acta Neurol Scand* 1984;69:77–80.

156. Tjellesen L, Nilas L, Christiansen C. Does carbamazepine cause disturbances in calcium metabolism in epileptic patients? *Acta Neurol Scand* 1983;68:13–19.

157. Tjellesen L, Gotfredsen A, Christiansen C. Effect of vitamin D2 and D3 on bone-mineral content in carbamazepine-treated epileptic patients. *Acta Neurol Scand* 1983;68:424–428.

158. Terrence CF, Fromm G. Congestive heart failure during carbamazepine therapy. *Ann Neurol* 1980;8:200–201.

159. Hewetson KA, Ritch AES, Watson RDS. Sick sinus syndrome aggravated by carbamazepine therapy for epilepsy. *Postgrad Med J* 1986;62:497–498.

160. Beermann B, Edhag O, Vallin H. Advanced heart block aggravated by carbamazepine. *Br Heart J* 1975;37:668–671.

161. Benassi E, Bo G-P, Cocito L, et al. Carbamazepine and cardiac conduction disturbances. *Ann Neurol* 1987;22:280–281.

162. Boesen F, Anderson EB, Jensen EK, et al. Cardiac conduction disturbances during carbamazepine therapy. *Acta Neurol Scand* 1983;68:49–52.

163. Hamilton DV. Carbamazepine and heart block. *Lancet* 1978; 1:1365.

164. Herzberg L. Carbamazepine and bradycardia. *Lancet* 1978;1: 1097–1098.

165. Kasarskis EJ, Kuo C-S, Berger R, et al. Carbamazepine-induced cardiac dysfunction: characterization of two distinct clinical syndromes. *Arch Intern Med* 1992;152:186–191.

166. Puletti M, Iani C, Curione M, et al. Carbamazepine and the heart. *Ann Neurol* 1991;29:575–576.

167. Weig SG, Pollack P. Carbamazepine-induced heart block in a child with tuberous sclerosis and cardiac rhabdomyoma: implications for evaluation and follow-up. *Ann Neurol* 1993;34:617–619.

168. Steiner C, Wit AL, Weiss MP, et al. The antiarrhythmic actions of carbamazepine (Tegretol). *J Pharmacol Exp Ther* 1970;173: 323–335.

169. Hegbrant J, Kurkus J, Öqvist B. Carbamazepine-related acute renal failure. *Neurology* 1993;43:446–447.

170. Steiner I, Birmanns B. Carbamazepine-induced urinary retention in long-standing diabetes mellitus. *Neurology* 1993;43: 1855–1856.

171. Moore MR, McGuire G, Brodie MJ, et al. Carbamazepine and haem biosynthesis. *Lancet* 1983;2:846.

172. Rapeport WG, Connell JC, Thompson GG, et al. Effect of carbamazepine on haem biosynthesis in man. *Eur J Clin Invest* 1984;14:107–110.

173. Rideout JM, Wright DJ, Lim CK, et al. Carbamazepine-induced non-hereditary acute porphyria. *Lancet* 1983;2:464.

174. Yeung Laiwah AAC, Rapeport WG, Thompson GG, et al. Carbamazepine-induced non-hereditary acute porphyria. *Lancet* 1983;1:790–792.

175. Lai C-W. Carbamazepine in seizure management in acute intermittent porphyria. *Neurology* 1981;31:232.

176. Bonkowsky HL. Carbamazepine in seizure management in acute intermittent porphyria. *Neurology* 1981;31:1579–1580.

177. Gilhus NE, Lea T. Carbamazepine: effect on IgG subclasses in epileptic patients. *Epilepsia* 1988;29:317–320.

178. Gilhus NE, Strandjord RE, Aarli J. Respiratory disease in patients with epilepsy on single-drug therapy with carbamazepine and phenobarbital. *Eur Neurol* 1982;21:284–288.

179. Pacifici R, Paris L, Di Carlo S, et al. Immunologic aspects of

carbamazepine treatment in epileptic patients. *Epilepsia* 1991;
32:122–127.

180. Gilhus NE, Aarli J. Respiratory disease and nasal immunoglob-ulin concentrations in phenytoin-treated epileptic patients. *Acta Neurol Scand* 1981;63:34–43.

181. Nielsen NV, Syversen K. Possible retinotoxic effect of carba-mazepine. *Acta Ophthalmol* 1986;64:287–290.

182. López L, Thomson A, Rabinowicz AL. Assessment of colour vision in epileptic patients exposed to single-drug therapy. *Eur Neurol* 1999;41:201–205.

183. Chadwick D. Safety and efficacy of vigabatrin and carba-mazepine in newly diagnosed epilepsy: a multicentre ran-domised double-blind study. *Lancet* 1999;354:13–19.

184. Smith CR. Encephalomyelopathy as an idiosyncratic reaction to carbamazepine: a case report. *Neurology* 1991;41:760761.

185. Stommel EW. Carbamazepine encephalopathy. *Neurology* 1992;
42:705.

186. Dodrill CB, Troupin AS. Neuropsychological effects of carba-mazepine and phenytoin: a reanalysis. *Neurology* 1991;41:
141–143.

187. Meador KJ, Loring DW, Huh K, et al. Comparative cognitive effects of anticonvulsants. *Neurology* 1990;40:391–394.

188. Troupin A, Ojemann LM, Halpern L, et al. Carbamazepine: a double-blind comparison with phenytoin. *Neurology* 1977;27:
511–519.

189. Aman MG, Werry JS, Paxton JW, et al. W. Effects of carba-mazepine on psychomotor performance in children as a func-tion of drug concentration, seizure type, and time of medica-tion. *Epilepsia* 1990;31:51–60.

190. O'Dougherty W, Wright FS, Cox S, et al. Carbamazepine plasma concentration: relationship to cognitive impairment. *Arch Neurol* 1987;44:863–867.

191. Trimble MR. Antiepileptic drugs, cognitive function, and behavior in children: evidence from recent studies. *Epilepsia* 1990;31[Suppl 4]:S30–S34.

192. Reinvang I, Bjarveit S, Johannessen S, et al. Cognitive function and time-of-day variation in serum carbamazepine concentra-tion in epileptic patients treated with monotherapy. *Epilepsia* 1991;32:116–121.

193. Schuerer DJE, Brophy PD, Maxvold NJ, et al. High-efficiency dialysis for carbamazepine overdose. *Clin Tox* 2000;38:321–323.

194. Chan KM, Aguanno JJ, Janssen R, et al. Charcoal hemoperfu-sion for treatment of carbamazepine poisoning. *Clin Chem* 1981;27:1300–1302.

195. de Groot G, van Heijst AN, Maes RA. Charcoal hemoperfusion

in treatment of two cases of acute carbamazepine poisoning. *J Toxicol Clin Toxicol* 1984;22:349–362.

196. de Zeeuw RA, Westenberg HGM, van der Kleijn E, et al. An unusual case of carbamazepine poisoning with a near-fatal relapse after two days. *Clin Tox* 1979;14:263–269.

197. Denning DW, Matheson L, Bryson SM, et al. Death due to car-bamazepine self-poisoning: remedies reviewed. *Hum Toxicol* 1985;4:255–260.

198. Gay N, Byra W, Eisinger R. Carbamazepine poisoning: treat-ment by hemoperfusion. *Nephron* 1981;27:202–203.

199. Leslie PJ, Heyworth R, Prescott LF. Cardiac complications of carbamazepine intoxication: treatment by haemoperfusion. *BMJ* 1983;286:1018.

200. May D. Acute carbamazepine intoxication: clinical spectrum and management. *South Med J* 1984;77:24–26.

201. Nilsson C, Sterner G, Idvall J. Charcoal hemoperfusion for treatment of serious carbamazepine poisoning. *Acta Med Scand* 1984;216:137–140.

202. O'Neal W Jr, Whitten KM, Baumann RJ, et al. Lack of serious toxicity following carbamazepine overdosage. *Clin Pharmacol* 1984;3:545–547.

203. Rockoff S, Baselt R. Severe carbamazepine poisoning. *Clin Tox* 1981;18:935–939.

204. Sethna M, Solomon G, Cedarbaum J, et al. Successful treat-ment of massive carbamazepine overdose. *Epilepsia* 1989;30:
71–73.

205. Sullivan JB, Rumack BH, Peterson RG. Acute carbamazepine toxicity resulting from over-dose. *Neurology* 1981;31:621–624.

206. Berry DJ, Wiseman HM, Volans GN. A survey of non-barbitu-rate anticonvulsant drug overdosage reported to the poisons information service (UK). *Hum Toxicol* 1983;2:357–360.

207. Fisher RS, Cysyk B. A fatal overdose of carbamazepine: case report and review of literature. *J Toxicol Clin Toxicol* 1988;26:
477–486.

208. Mack RB. Julius seizure: carbamazepine (Tegretol) poisoning. *N C Med J* 1985;46:41–42.

209. Lehrman SN, Bauman ML. Carbamazepine overdose. *Am J Dis Child* 1981;135:768–769.

210. Tartara A, Manni R, Maurelli M, et al. Carbamazepine poison-ing: a case report. *Ital J Neurol Sci* 1986;7:165–166.

211. Weaver DF, Camfield P, Fraser A. Massive carbamazepine over-dose: clinical and pharmacologic observations in five episodes. *Neurology* 1988;38:755–759.

212. Boldy DA, Heath A, Ruddock S, et al. Activated charcoal for carbamazepine poisoning. *Lancet* 1987;1:1027.

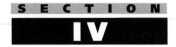

SECTION IV

FELBAMATE

FELBAMATE

JOHN M. PELLOCK
JAMES L. PERHACH
R. DUANE SOFIA

Felbamate (FBM), a dicarbamate compound related to meprobamate, was initially synthesized in the 1950s. Because it had no tranquilizing or sedative activity, FBM was not initially developed until 1986, when efficacy in a wide range of seizure models was reported (1). FBM was synthesized and developed by Wallace Laboratories (Cranbury, NJ) and became the first of the "new-generation" antiepileptic drugs (AEDs) approved for marketing in the United States in 1993. Its clinical success as a potent, broad-spectrum AED is well documented, but the appearance of life-threatening idiosyncratic reactions has markedly reduced its use to a third- or fourth-line agent for use in patients with refractory epilepsy.

The 1995 fourth edition of *Antiepileptic Drugs* dedicated six chapters to this novel AED (2–7), discussing modes of action, chemistry and biotransformation, pharmacokinetics, FBM drug interactions, clinical use, and toxicity. The current chapter summarizes those writings and offers updates, particularly regarding clinical use and toxicity.

ANTICONVULSANT ACTIVITY

The anticonvulsant effects of FBM were evaluated by Swinyard et al. (1) against maximal electroshock seizure (MES) and subcutaneous Metrazol (s.c.MET) tests, where the drug was administered to mice and rats by the oral route (Table 27.1). FBM protected mice against MES with a resultant median effective dose (ED_{50}) of 81 mg/kg. The oral ED_{50} in the MES tests in rats was 48 mg/kg. FBM also was effec-

John M. Pellock, MD: Chairman, Division of Child Neurology, Professor of Neurology, Pediatrics, Pharmacy, and Pharmaceutics, Medical College of Virginia; Hospitals and Physicians, Virginia Commonwealth University Health Care Systems, Richmond, Virginia

James L. Perhach, PhD, FCP: Senior Director, Clinical Pharmacology, Perdue Pharma L.P., Princeton, New Jersey

R. Duane Sofia, PhD: Vice President, Department of Preclinical Research, Wallace Laboratories, Cranbury, New Jersey

tive against chemically induced convulsions. The oral ED_{50}s in the s.c.MET test were 548 and 238 mg/kg in mice and rats, respectively (2).

FBM demonstrated a high degree of safety in mice and rats as measured by neurotoxicity and calculated protective indices (PI). The median toxic dose (TD_{50}) in mice from the rotorod test was 1,545 mg/kg (Table 27.1) after oral dosing. In the rat, the oral TD_{50} was estimated at >3,000 mg/kg (Table 27.1). Compared with phenytoin (PHT), carbamazepine (CBZ), phenobarbital, and valproic acid (VPA), FBM demonstrated the lowest potential for neurotoxicity (i.e., the highest TD_{50} value). Thus, protective indices (TD_{50}/ED_{50}) for FBM after oral administration to mice and rats provide for a significantly large margin of safety or, in other words, a very wide therapeutic window (2).

The anticonvulsant effects of FBM were further substantiated in kindling models of epilepsy using cornea- and amygdala-kindled rats (8). In pentylenetetrazol-kindled rats, FBM significantly reduced the intensity of behavioral seizures, and seizure frequency was reduced in monkeys made chronically epileptic by injections of aluminum hydroxide (9). There was a marked increase in seizure rate when FBM was withdrawn. Yamaguchi and Rogawski (10) also have shown that FBM was effective in protecting mice against 4-aminopyridine–induced seizures, using lethality as the end point. These findings are consistent with the ability of FBM to inhibit seizure spread. FBM also was effective in two models of status epilepticus in the rat (11).

Interactions, Safety, and Neuroprotection

The ability of FBM to enhance the anticonvulsant activities of PHT, VPA, CBZ, phenobarbital, and diazepam, and, conversely, the effects of these drugs on the anticonvulsant action of FBM, were evaluated in mice. Initial experiments showed that FBM enhanced the protective effects of diazepam, PHT, VPA, and CBZ in the MES test. Based on early data (2), it is apparent that a positive interaction often

TABLE 27.1. PROFILE OF ANTICONVULSANT ACTIVITY OF ORALLY ADMINISTERED FELBAMATE AND PROTOTYPICAL ANTIEPILEPTIC DRUGS IN MICE AND RATS[a]

| | Mice | | | | | Rats | | | | |
| | | MES | | s.c. MET | | | MET | | s.c. MET | |
Substance	TD_{50}[b] (mgkg)	ED_{50} (mgkg)	PI[c]	ED_{50} (mgkg)	PI[c]	TD_{50} (mgkg)	ED_{50} (mgkg)	PI[c]	ED_{50} (mgkg)	PI[c]
Felbamate	1,545.0 (1,299.1–1,986.9)	81.1 (72.0–92.8)	19.1	548.2 (433.7–750.7)	2.8	>3,000.0	47.8 (41.0–57.3)	>63	238.1 (132.1–549.3)	>12
Phenytoin	86.7 (80.4–96.1)	9.0 (7.40–10.6)	10.0	No protection	NE	>3,000.0	29.8 (21.9–38.9)	>100	No protection	NE
Carbamazepine	217.2 (131.5–270.1)	15.4 (12.4–17.3)	14.0	48.1 (40.8–57.4)	4.5	813.1 (488.8–1,233.9)	8.5 (3.4–10.5)	95.7	No protection	NE
Phenobarbital	96.8 (79.9–115.0)	20.1 (14.8–31.6)	4.8	12.6 (8.0–19.1)	7.7	61.1 (43.7–95.9)	9.1 (7.6–11.9)	6.7	11.5 (7.7–15.0)	5.3
Valproic acid	1,264.4 (800.0–2,250.0)	664.8 (605.3–718.0)	1.9	388.3 (348.9–438.6)	3.3	280.2 (191.3–352.8)	489.5 (351.1–728.4)	0.6	179.6 (146.7–210.4)	1.6

MES, maximal electroshock seizure test; s.c. MET, subcutaneous Metrazol seizure threshold; TD_{50}, median toxic dose; ED_{50}, median effective dose; NE, not evaluable.
[a]Values in parentheses are 95% confidence limits.
[b]Toxic dose (rotorod performance).
[c]Protective index (TD_{50}/ED_{50}).
From Swinyard EA, Sofia RD, Kupferberg HJ. Comparative anticonvulsant activity and neurotoxicity of felbamate and four prototype antiepileptic drugs in mice and rats. *Epilepsia* 1986;27:27–34, with permission.

occurs between FBM and standard AEDs in laboratory animal seizure models. The results of the safety pharmacology studies with FBM clearly point to its excellent safety profile in various body systems (2).

The neuroprotective effect of FBM was shown *in vitro* by inhibition of hypoxic injury in a hippocampal slice (12) and *in vivo* by Wasterlain et al. in a neonatal rat model (13). Moreover, posthypoxic treatment with FBM in this same model produced both dose-dependent and time-dependent neuroprotective effects (14). A neuroprotective effect of FBM also was observed after kainic acid–induced status epilepticus (15) and suggested that FBM had no adverse effects on learning and memory.

Mechanism of Action

Although the precise mechanism of action for the anticonvulsant and neuroprotective effects of FBM has not been fully elucidated, several hypotheses have been proposed and tested to suggest four potential mechanisms, all antiexcitatory (2,16).

FBM interferes with voltage-gated sodium channels, resulting in the blockade of sustained, repetitive neuronal firing and prevention of seizure spread (8). It indirectly antagonizes *N*-methyl-D-aspartate (NMDA) by interfering with the binding of glycine to strychnine-insensitive glycine receptors (17). Because glycine acts as an obligatory coagonist for glutamate acting at the NMDA receptor subtype, glycine blockage therefore may lead to a reduction of NMDA receptor–modulated cationic conductance. FBM has no direct NMDA receptor blocking action (2). A third mechanism involves non-NMDA excitatory amino acid receptors. FBM protects against seizures induced by quisqualate and kainate (8) and those induced by α-amino-3-hydroxy-5-methyl-4-

isoxazole propionic acid (AMPA), the natural agonist for these receptor subtypes (18). FBM also inhibits voltage-activated calcium currents at clinically relevant concentrations (19). This may inhibit release of excitatory neurotransmitters and also explain FBM's antiabsence effect.

FBM probably does not substantially affect inhibitory neurotransmission (16). It does not bind to γ-aminobutyric acid (GABA), benzodiazepine, or picrotoxin sites on the GABA$_A$–chloride ionophore complex, and does not affect chloride influx, with or without the presence of GABA (20). Although GABA-potentiating action has been suggested (21), millimolar concentrations are required, whereas the antiexcitatory mechanisms require only the micromolar concentrations of FBM readily achievable in the brain with clinical doses (2).

CHEMISTRY

Felbamate (Felbatol; Wallace Laboratories) is the generic name for 2-phenyl-1,3-propanediol dicarbamate, with the empiric formula $C_{11}H_{14}N_2O_4$ and a molecular weight of 238.24 (the conversion factor from concentration to molarity is 1,000/238.24 = 4.20) (3) (Figure 27.1).

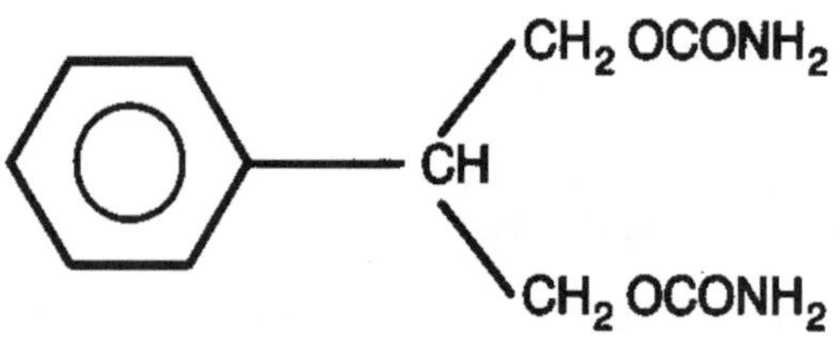

FIGURE 27.1. Felbamate structure.

A molecule of FBM is composed of a phenyl ring attached to the middle carbon of the 1,3-propanediol chain. The two hydrogens of the aliphatic primary hydroxyl groups are replaced by a carbamyl group, $CONH_2$. This leads to a symmetric, achiral, nonionic substance with medium lipophilicity and a high degree of hydrophobicity.

PHYSICOCHEMICAL PROPERTIES

The melting point determined for various commercial-scale lots of drug by differential scanning calorimetry ranged 149.5°C to 150.8°C; FBM reference standard of 99.9% purity had a melting point of 150.3°C to 151.2°C. The solubility of FBM is very low in water and relatively low in common organic solvents. The drug has good solubility only in solvents with strong hydrogen bonding capability to break up the intermolecular hydrogen bonds of FBM in its crystal lattice, such as dimethylsulfoxide or dimethylacetamide. The partition coefficients reveal medium lipophilicity of FBM. This important property allows the drug to cross cell membranes easily and manifests itself in the drug's distribution throughout tissues and organs.

Chemical stability studies of aqueous FBM solutions at acidic to neutral pH indicate that it is relatively stable. In the presence of 0.4 N hydrochloric acid at 40°C, only 1.3% of FBM was hydrolyzed after 24 hours. However, at alkaline pH, the carbamate groups underwent hydrolysis. Treatment with 0.01 N sodium hydroxide for 24 hours at 40°C hydrolyzed 28.9% of the drug; among the hydrolysis products, 19% consisted of the monocarbamate (MCF) and 1.8% of the 2-phenyl-1,3-propanediol. FBM solutions also exhibited considerable stability to oxygenation; bubbling of oxygen through a solution at 40°C for 24 hours led to a loss of 2.4%. When kept at 37°C for 24 hours in human plasma or simulated gastric and intestinal fluid, no significant change could be detected.

BIOTRANSFORMATION

Structurally, FBM is a relatively simple molecule and as such it undergoes only a few enzymatic biotransformation reactions (i.e., hydroxylations of the aromatic phenyl ring or the aliphatic C-2 on the propanediol chain or hydrolysis of the carbamate groups). These primary hydroxy metabolites then are conjugated in secondary biotransformation steps (phase II reactions with glucuronic acid) or, in the case of the primary alcohol hydroxy groups, oxidized further. The conjugation of FBM itself also is possible because a *N*-glucuronide conjugate of meprobamate has been reported (22). Because the solubility of FBM in aqueous biologic fluids is very low, the aforementioned metabolic reactions would permit the drug to be eliminated in the form of more water-soluble products. Pharmacokinetic studies in animals

(23) and humans (24) have indicated that, indeed, the main route of excretion for both FBM and its metabolites is the urine; much less is excreted in the feces.

However, in none of the species studied so far is FBM completely metabolized; a significant amount of drug is excreted unchanged, pointing to a low first-pass effect. The structures of the identified and hypothesized metabolites of FBM are shown in Figure 27.2.

Animal Metabolites

The biotransformation of FBM in rats, rabbits, and dogs has been studied with [^{14}C]FBM as tracer (25). Three metabolites were isolated from rat or dog urine and the isolated compounds positively identified by their high-performance liquid chromatography (HPLC) retention times and mass spectra in the EI and CI mode compared with synthetic reference standards of the metabolites (26). In addition to their identification, ^{14}C HPLC profiles of the metabolites and unchanged drug were obtained for urine and bile of the three species and for plasma of dogs and rats and feces of dogs. Because a pharmacokinetic study with [^{14}C]FBM in these species (27) showed that up to one-third of the ^{14}C in plasma is accounted for by metabolites, ^{14}C metabolic profiling in dog and rabbit plasma also was performed. Approximately 6% or less of the ^{14}C was in the form of the *para*-hydroxyfelbamate (pOHF) and 2-hydroxyfelbamate (2OHF) metabolites, but the low concentration of ^{14}C in the plasma samples precluded a more accurate balance for metabolites. The amount of unchanged drug in plasma varied from 72% to 100%. The major portion of the urinary ^{14}C was accounted for by the unchanged drug and the pOHF, 2OHF, and MCF metabolites; the remaining ^{14}C was in the form of polar, water-soluble compounds, including conjugates. Because urine is the major route of ^{14}C excretion, the urinary ^{14}C metabolic profiles represent a good overall picture of FBM biotransformation. The rat appears to have the most active metabolism of FBM, in which the formation of the pOHF metabolite predominates. In the rabbit and dog, less of the dose is metabolized and the two hydroxy metabolites are formed in approximately equal amounts, with small amounts of the hydrolysis product MCF also present.

The amount of ^{14}C excreted in feces was smaller than in urine. The ^{14}C in dog feces was composed of the two hydroxy metabolites with a pOHF/2OHF ratio of approximately 1.4, accounting for 60% to 70% of the ^{14}C; that accounted for by unchanged drug varied from 15% to 29%. This indicates that some biliary excretion of the metabolites in free or conjugated form must occur. Studies in bile duct–cannulated rats or dogs dosed with [^{14}C]FBM confirmed the existence of hepatobiliary recirculation of FBM and its metabolites. After enzyme hydrolysis with glucuronidase/sulfatase, up to half of the ^{14}C in the bile of rats collected at 2 hours was pOHF and only 3% was 2OHF. In

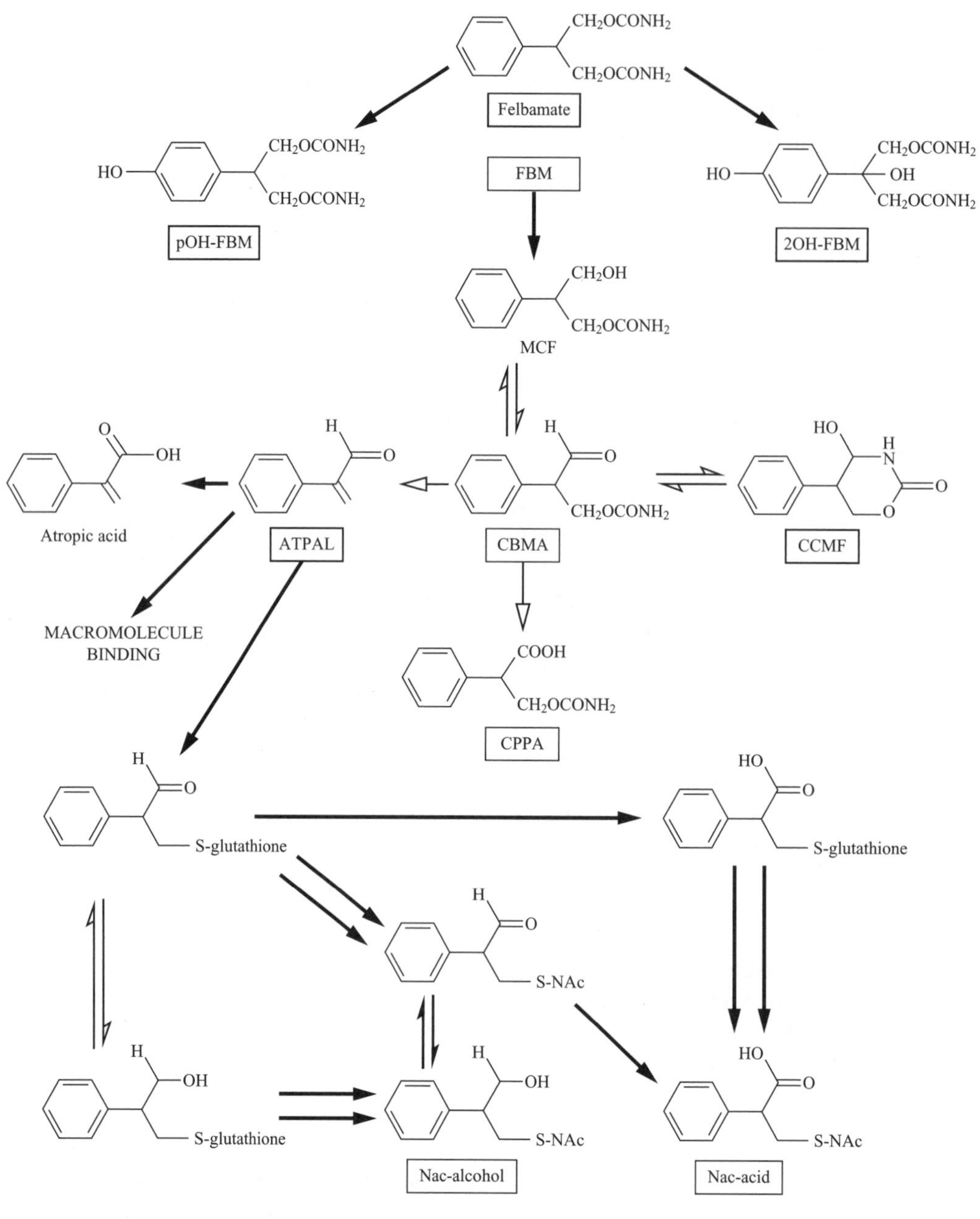

FIGURE 27.2. Metabolic pathway.

dog bile collected at 48 hours, 40% was pOHF and 25% 2OHF, and in rabbit bile at 72 hours, 24% was pOHF and 11% was 2OHF. In all the bile samples, unchanged FBM accounted for less than 10% of the biliary ^{14}C.

The sum of all conjugated ^{14}C metabolites in animal urine was estimated based on the solvent-extractable ^{14}C before and after enzymatic hydrolysis with β-glucuronidase/sulfatase. It ranged from 20% to 35% in rat urine, 20% to 30% in rabbit urine, and 10% to 20% in dog urine. The amounts of conjugated metabolites in native bile were estimated at 50% for the rat, 15% for the rabbit, and 70% for the dog. No conjugates were observed in dog feces.

There is no indication of a significant degree of extrahepatic biotransformation of FBM, but more detailed studies of metabolism in animal tissues have not been carried out. Cornford et al. (28) could not detect FBM metabolites in the brain tissue of mice at 5 minutes after an intracarotid injection of 4 mg/kg [^{14}C]FBM. A tissue distribution study in rats dosed with 100 mg/kg [^{14}C]FBM demonstrated extensive distribution of ^{14}C to all tissues (29). In a separate study, the concentration of FBM and its metabolites was determined in rat brain and cerebrospinal fluid (CSF) (AD) and heart tissue (Wallace Laboratories, unpublished data). In rats after a single oral dose of 500 mg/kg, only the 2OHF metabolite was present in measurable concentrations in plasma [maximal concentration (C_{max}) 7.8 μg/mL], brain and CSF (C_{max} 2.7 μg/g), and heart tissue (C_{max} 6.6 μg/g). The presence of the metabolites at these low concentrations is of limited importance because the anticonvulsant activity of the metabolites in the rat model is much lower than that of FBM.

Human Metabolites

The biotransformation of FBM in male volunteers dosed with a single dose of 100 or 1,000 mg [14C]FBM has been studied by 14C metabolic profiling in plasma and urine using HPLC ultraviolet and 14C monitoring (30). In plasma samples from both groups, FBM accounted for most of the 14C, but actual metabolite concentrations were too low to be accurately determined. The highest urinary 14C excretion rates were observed during the 4- to 8- and 8- to 1-hour periods. Approximately 50% of the urinary 14C was unchanged drug; the sum of the two hydroxy metabolites accounted for another 10% to 15%, with the pOHF/2OHF ratio in hydrolyzed urine equal to 1.8. The MCF metabolite amount varied from 0.7% to 2.7%, and the remaining 14C was in the form of polar unidentified components. Hydrolysis of the urine with β-glucuronidase/sulfatase caused a decrease in this polar fraction by 16%; this amount probably represents glucuronides or sulfate esters of the three metabolites and the *N*-glucuronide of FBM. The polar fraction of the urinary 14C remaining after enzyme hydrolysis of the conjugates (25.8% of 14C) has been examined in attempts to identify additional metabolites (31). Mass spectrometry analysis and HPLC comparison with a synthetic reference positively identified the major component of the polar fraction as 3-carbamolyoxy-2-phenylpropionic acid (CPPA) in the free form (Figure 27.3 for structure). This metabolite, accounting for approximately 12% of the urinary 14C in a 4- to 8-hour urine sample, is most likely formed by the oxidation of the MCF metabolites. The percentage indicates that enzyme hydrolysis of FBM to MCF is a major biotransformation pathway in humans. The presence of CPPA in dog urine also has been confirmed.

Further research has led to a hypothesis that the FBM metabolite, monocarbamate alcohol, undergoes stepwise oxidation to acid carbamate through an aldehyde intermediate, aldehyde carbamate, and that this aldehyde either is in a dynamic equilibrium with cyclic carbamate or is nonenzymatically converted to atropaldehyde (32). The conjugation and elimination of atropaldehyde would appear to be routine in patients with adequate stores of glutathione (33). This hypothesis further suggested that atropaldehyde might be biologically reactive and could contribute to the toxicity seen in some patients treated with FBM (Figure 27.2).

Evidence to support the formation of the cyclic carbamate intermediate metabolite, 4-hydroxy-5-phenyl tetrahydro-1,3-oxazin-2-one, from MCF and its metabolism to CPPA has been demonstrated *in vitro* using human liver S9 fractions and microsomes (34)

Sex and Age Differences in Biotransformation

Age but not sex has a significant effect on the pharmacokinetics of FBM in rats (29) and dogs (35,36). To explain those differences in the 14C metabolic profile in urine and feces of 5-week-old and adult dogs has been determined by HPLC (35). Although no qualitative differences in the 14C profiles were apparent, the amount of FBM metabolized in the very young dogs was approximately twice that in adults. The increase was distributed evenly between the two hydroxy metabolites and the polar fraction, and the pOHF/2OHF ratio did not change much.

In a tissue distribution study in adult and neonatal Sprague-Dawley rats dosed with 500 mg/kg [14C]FBM, a more dramatic difference in kinetics and biotransformation was observed (29). Large quantitative differences in plasma 14C profiles were apparent. The plasma concentrations of 2OHF in neonatal rats at peak time were 10-fold higher than in adults, but the pOHF metabolite concentrations were only slightly lower. Brain concentrations of 2OHF in the study showed the same trend: In adults the C_{max} at 12 hours was 2.7 μg/g, in neonates at 16 hours it was 54.4 μg/g.

Species Differences in Biotransformation

Based on urinary 14C metabolic profiles of enzyme hydrolyzed urine, no large differences in FBM metabolism between species have been observed. The urine is the major excretion route in all species.

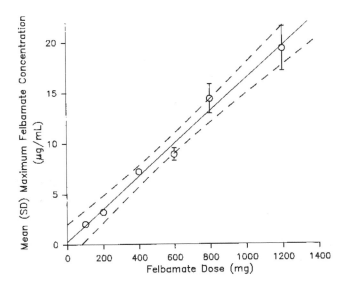

FIGURE 27.3. Felbamate concentration versus dose.

With regard to phase II metabolic reactions, there appears to be a species difference in the extent of conjugation for each of the three metabolites. This is based on the indirect estimation of the amount of conjugates in the urine before and after hydrolysis with β-glucuronidase/sulfatase (Wallace Laboratories, unpublished data). Approximately 40% of the amount of the pOHF metabolite is conjugated in the rat, 30% in the dog, and 35% in the rabbit. In the case of the 2OHF metabolite, 20% is conjugated in the rat and rabbit and 50% in the dog. The relatively small amounts of the MCF metabolite in urine appear to be approximately 75% in conjugated form in both rabbit and dog urine. The existence of the *N*-glucuronide of FBM in animal urine is not supported by data; however, in human urine the difference in the amount of FBM before and after enzymatic hydrolysis does indicate the presence of the *N*-glucuronide.

Induction of the Rat Hepatic Cytochrome P450 System

FBM was found to be a mild rat hepatic cytochrome P450 (CYP) inducer. In male Sprague-Dawley rats dosed daily with 1,000 mg/kg FBM for 5 days, the total CYP isozyme content was increased twofold compared with untreated animals. The drug was found to be approximately 25 times less potent than the standard inducing agent, sodium phenobarbital (37). The capacity of FBM for autoinduction of metabolism in the rat was demonstrated by *in vitro* incubations with rat hepatic microsomes from animals pretreated with FBM (38) in which, similar to microsomes in phenobarbital-pretreated rats (see section on *in vitro* biotransformation), the amount of drug metabolized doubled from 10% to approximately 20% to 25%, with the increase exclusively in the amount of the 2OHF metabolite.

CONVERSION

Conversion factor:

$$CF = \frac{1,000}{\text{mol. wt.}} = \frac{1,000}{238.24} = 4.20$$

Conversion:

$$(\mu g/mL) \times 4.20 = \mu mol/L$$
$$(\mu mol/L) \div 4.20 = \mu g/mL$$

ABSORPTION, DISTRIBUTION, AND EXCRETION

Absorption

FBM is well absorbed after oral administration. This assessment of absorption was obtained from an open-label, parallel study using a single dose of [^{14}C]FBM administered orally to six healthy male subjects (30). Three subjects ingested approximately 100 mg and the other three ingested 1,000 mg of FBM labeled with approximately 80 to 85 μCi of ^{14}C. After oral administration of 100 or 1,000 mg [^{14}C] FBM, over 90% of each ^{14}C dose was recovered in the urine, with less than 5% in the feces. Plasma FBM concentrations paralleled and were only slightly less than the ^{14}C-labeled concentrations. For both ^{14}C and FBM, plasma concentrations increased proportionately with the dose.

Single-Dose Studies

In one study, single oral doses of 100, 200, 400, 600, or 800 mg of FBM or placebo were administered to five different groups of male subjects under double-blind conditions (39). In another study, single doses of 1,200 mg of FBM were administered to eight male subjects (40). Plasma samples were assayed for FBM by a specific HPLC method (41).

Based on $AUC_{0\to\infty}$ (area under the plasma concentration–time curve) and C_{max} data, plasma FBM concentrations increased proportionally after administration of single doses of 100 to 1,200 mg (Figure 27.3). No evidence of nonlinearity was detected over the dose range studied. The mean ± standard deviation (SD) apparent clearance after a single 1,200 mg dose of FBM as a solution was 25.8 ± 2.9 (mL/hr)/kg.

The absorption of the commercial FBM suspension and tablets has been determined to be bioequivalent to the FBM capsules used in the clinical development of FBM. The absorption rate is similar for all formulations tested, although more rapid for the solution and capsules. The extent of absorption was the same for all dosage forms. The tablet and suspension are absorbed with peak times of 2 to 6 hours.

Multiple-Dose Studies

The steady-state pharmacokinetics and dose proportionality of FBM after oral administration of 400, 800, 1,200, 2,400, and 3,600 mg/day were evaluated in healthy men (400, 800, and 1,200 mg/day) and in newly diagnosed or untreated subjects with epilepsy (42,43). Ten otherwise healthy female subjects with epilepsy participated in the latter study. After 2 weeks at each dosage level, plasma samples were obtained and assayed (41). FBM C_{max}, C_{min} (trough), and AUCτ were proportional to dose. Multiple daily doses of 1,200, 2,400, and 3,600 mg/day gave C_{min} values of 30 ± 5, 55 ± 8, and 83 ± 21 μg/mL, respectively. In a separate dose proportionality study, subjects who had received other AEDs chronically and then converted to 3,600 mg/day of FBM were shown to tolerate doses of FBM up to 6,000 mg/day (44). After 3,600, 4,200, 4,800, 5,400, and 6,000 mg/day of FBM, mean steady-state C_{min} (trough) FBM concentrations of 87.5, 100.0, 118.6, 122.3, and 134.3 μg/mL, respectively, were observed. Proportional increases in AUCτ also were observed. Time to C_{max} did not differ. Food, antacids, and sex of the patient do not effect the pharmacokinetics of FBM (45,46).

Effects of Age

FBM gave dose-proportional steady-state plasma concentrations of 17, 32, and 49 μg/mL in children 4 to 12 years of age at doses of 15, 30, and 45 mg/kg/day, respectively (47). The plasma concentration of FBM in children (≤12 years of age) receiving 45 mg/kg/day is less than the FBM plasma concentration in adults receiving a comparable FBM dosage.

Effect of Renal Impairment

Subjects with four levels of renal dysfunction [creatinine clearance >80 mL/min (normal), >30 to 80, >10 to 30, or 5 to 10 mL/min] were administered a single oral dose of 1,200 mg FBM. Compared with control subjects, apparent total-body clearance, renal clearance, and urinary excretion of FBM were decreased, and half-life, C_{max}, and AUC values were increased in subjects with renal dysfunction. Renal clearance of FBM accounted for approximately 30% of apparent total body clearance in the control group and from 9% to 22% in the patients with renal failure. Renal clearance of FBM was significantly correlated with creatinine clearance ($R^2 = 0.75$; $p < .001$). These data suggest that initial dosage and titration of FBM may require adjustment in patients with renal dysfunction (48).

Distribution

Protein Binding

FBM is the predominant plasma species after oral administration. Binding of FBM to human plasma protein was independent of FBM concentrations between 10 and 310 μg/mL. Binding ranged from 22% to 25%, was mostly to albumin, depended on albumin concentration, and did not alter the protein binding of other AEDs (49).

Tissue Distribution

After administration of a single 100 mg/kg dose of [^{14}C] FBM (~50 μCi) to male rats, peak concentrations were reached and maintained from 2 to 4 hours. Tissue concentrations at 2, 4, 8, 24, and 48 hours after dosing indicated a broad dispersal of FBM across major organs, including liver, kidney, heart, lung, spleen, muscle, gonads, eyes, and brain. Peak brain concentration was observed at 4 hours, but was nearly at maximum at 2 hours. No accumulation of ^{14}C occurred in any of the individual tissues, based on peak

^{14}C levels at 48 hours. Disappearance of FBM from the brain paralleled that from the plasma (50). Similar uniform distribution was observed in pregnant female rats and fetal tissue. Autoradiographic analyses of frozen brain sections of rats suggested that FBM distributes relatively uniformly throughout the brain (51).

Cornford et al. have shown that FBM extraction in a single transcapillary passage was 5% to 20%, and drug uptake in rat brain was not concentration dependent (51). FBM is moderately lipophilic, and lipid-mediated blood–brain barrier penetration of FBM is similar to that of PHT and phenobarbital. Plasma protein does not affect FBM's entry into the brain. Erythrocyte-borne FBM also may supply the brain.

Although no systemic evaluation has been conducted, brain FBM concentrations in humans have been reported to be approximately 0.6 to 0.7 those of plasma. These data are somewhat confounded by the absence of precise plasma collection methods and the presence of other AEDs (52). The distribution ratio of [^{14}C] FBM between red blood cells and plasma or saline was found to be 0.97 to 0.99 (40). Comparable results were observed with dog whole blood and red blood cell suspensions in saline. The distribution and binding to red blood cells was reversible. FBM has been detected in human milk. No data on FBM's presence in saliva or tears are available.

Volume of Distribution

Preclinical data indicated that FBM is relatively uniformly distributed in the body tissues. Data from humans indicate that the apparent volume of distribution is 756 ± 82 mL/kg after a 1,200-mg dose in adults. The volume of distribution in monkeys after intravenous administration of 25 mg/kg was 930 mL/kg.

Elimination and Excretion

After oral administration, FBM concentrations parallel and are only slightly less than those of radioactivity. Approximately 40% to 50% of the absorbed dose (1,000 mg of [^{14}C]FBM) appears unchanged in unhydrolyzed urine, and an additional 52% to 58% is present as metabolites and conjugates (53). Similar profiles of elimination have been observed in rats, rabbits, and dogs (13). In hydrolyzed human urine, approximately 8% to 14% is present as pOHF, 4% to 6% as 2OHF, and 1% to 4% as FBM monocarbamate. None of these has significant anticonvulsant activity. These same metabolites were seen in urine from laboratory animals receiving FBM (35).

Clearance

The clearance of FBM from plasma is independent of the dose of FBM. The mean ± SD apparent clearances for healthy volunteers were 36.9 ± 17.7, 38.2 ± 16.8, and 27.6 ± 6.9 (mL/hr)/kg for FBM doses of 400, 800, and 1,200 mg/day. For subjects with newly diagnosed epilepsy, it ranged from 26.8 ± 4.0 to 30.1 ± 7.8 (mL/hr)/kg for FBM doses of 1,200 to 3,600 mg/day (48). For subjects with epilepsy converted from other AEDs, FBM's clearance ranged from 31.7 ± 9.2 to 32.1 ± 6.8 (mL/hr)/kg after administration of 4,200 to 6,000 mg/day (44).

Half-Life

Mean terminal elimination half-lives for radioactivity and FBM ranged from 16 to 22 hours regardless of dose (53). Comparable half-lives were observed for healthy male subjects receiving a 1,200-mg dose of FBM (39). Early reports of a shorter half-life are related to the fact that these subjects were not receiving FBM monotherapy and samples were not collected for a sufficient time (54).

INTERACTIONS WITH OTHER DRUGS

Prediction of Interactions Based on *In Vitro* Studies

In vitro studies show that FBM is a substrate for CYP3A4 and CYP2E1. Compounds that induce CYP3A4 (e.g., CBZ, PHT, and phenobarbital) increase FBM clearance. However, the CYP3A4 inhibitors gestodene, ethinyl estradiol, and erythromycin have little or no effect on FBM trough plasma concentrations, consistent with the fact that the pathway is relatively minor for FBM under normal (noninduced) conditions.

FBM has been shown *in vitro* to inhibit CYP2C19, which would account for its effect on PHT clearance, and it has been postulated that this could be the mechanism underlying the reduced clearance of phenobarbital by FBM.

Although not yet examined *in vitro*, FBM appears to induce the activity of CYP3A4, which would account for its reducing plasma concentrations of CBZ or the progestin gestodene (55).

Effect of Felbamate on Other Antiepileptic Drugs

Phenytoin

During a late phase I trial (54) and subsequent clinical trials, investigators (56–59) identified an interaction on coadministration of FBM and PHT that resulted in an increase in PHT concentrations, necessitating a decrease in PHT dose.

Further clarification of the effects of FBM on the pharmacokinetics of PHT was sought by Sachdeo et al. (60) in an open-label, rising FBM dose (1,200, 1,800, 2,400, 3,600 mg/day) study in 10 patients with epilepsy (5 men, 5 women, 19 to 50 years of age). Patients were established on

PHT monotherapy (200 to 500 mg/day) for a minimum of 2 weeks. Only one PHT dosage adjustment of approximately 20% was permitted during the study. This occurred after the development of signs and symptoms associated with PHT toxicity. Patients then were grouped according to when the dose of PHT was reduced, as well as how many FBM dose increments they completed.

FBM caused an increase in the steady-state plasma concentrations of PHT that was observed at a dose as low as 1,200 mg/day of FBM. Overall (10 patients), the mean steady-state trough plasma concentration of PHT increased from a baseline value of 17 ± 5 μg/mL to 21 ± 5 μg/mL after 1,200 mg/day of FBM, a mean increase of 24%. In six patients whose FBM dose was further increased to 1,800 mg/day, an additional increase in PHT trough concentrations of approximately 20% was observed. Three patients completed the study at 3,600 mg/day of FBM with one PHT dosage reduction before the increase in FBM dose to 2,400 mg/day. Their trough PHT concentration increased from 17 ± 2.9 μg/mL at baseline to 24 ± 3.7 μg/mL when the FBM dose was increased from 1,200 to 1,800 mg/day. The concentration fell to 22.7 ± 4.5 μg/mL when the PHT dose was reduced by 20% and 2,400 mg/day of FBM was administered. The trough concentration increased to 26.4 ± 4.1 μg/mL when the FBM dose was increased to 3,600 mg/day. PHT maximal plasma concentrations and AUCs exhibited parallel increases. Based on these observations, the following dosage recommendations have been formulated: On initiation of therapy with FBM at 1,200 mg/day, an initial PHT dose reduction of approximately 20% is suggested. Subsequent reductions in the PHT dose on implementation of further increases in the FBM dose should be individualized and based on clinical signs, symptoms, and plasma PHT concentrations.

The plasma protein binding of PHT was virtually unchanged (>91%) after FBM administration. The increases in PHT concentrations depended on FBM concentration and dose, suggesting that FBM inhibited PHT metabolism. (The mechanism of this interaction is discussed in the chapter on mechanistic aspects of PHT interactions.)

Valproic Acid

The effects of coadministration of FBM on the disposition of VPA were studied in a randomized, three-period, crossover study in patients with epilepsy previously stabilized on VPA monotherapy (9.5 to 26.2 mg/kg/day) (61). A baseline period, when only VPA was administered, was followed by a two-period crossover, during which patients randomly received a daily dose of either 1,200 or 2,400 mg FBM for a period of 2 weeks.

Nausea and headache were the most common adverse events reported. Coadministration of 1,200 and 2,400 mg/day of FBM increased the mean (± SD) AUC for VPA from a baseline value of 802 ± 174 to 1,025 ± 207 and to

1,236 ± 290 µg/hr/mL, respectively (increases of 28% and 54%). Increases of a similar magnitude were observed for the average maximum and trough steady-state concentrations. Increasing the FBM dose from 1,200 to 2,400 mg/day also resulted in a proportional increase in the value of the aforementioned parameters. The apparent total-body clearance of VPA decreased from 0.175 mL/min/kg at baseline to 0.138 (−21%) and 0.115 mL/min/kg (−34%) at respective doses of 1,200 and 2,400 mg/day of FBM.

FBM did not influence the protein binding of VPA. Thus, the data suggest that the decrease in total-body clearance can be attributed to a decrease in metabolic clearance of VPA through the inhibition of β-oxidation (62).

Carbamazepine

A decrease in the steady-state plasma concentration of CBZ, ranging between 20% and 25%, has been observed in a number of clinical trials after introduction of FBM. However, in several of the trials CBZ and PHT were coadministered, and a possible role for PHT cannot be excluded. To elucidate the mechanism of the interaction, the pharmacokinetics of CBZ in nine patients with epilepsy were determined during CBZ monotherapy (≥800 mg/day) and, after coadministration of FBM, up to a maximum daily dose of 3,000 mg (62).

Subsequent to coadministration of FBM, the apparent total-body clearance increased from a mean (± SD) of 229.4 ± 68.7 to 324.3 ± 109.2 mL/hr/kg, a mean increase of 41%. Correspondingly, CBZ plasma concentration decreased from 7.46 ± 1.65 µg/mL to 5.14 ± 1.14 µg/mL (−31%). In contrast, the mean plasma concentration of CBZ 10,11-epoxide increased from 0.99 ± 0.26 µg/mL to 1.56 ± 0.42 µg/mL (57%). No significant change (7%) in CBZ diol concentration was observed.

The increase in steady-state CBZ 10,11-epoxide concentration can be explained either by induction of CBZ metabolism to the epoxide or by inhibition of epoxide hydrolysis to the diol. The relative contribution of each mechanism can be assessed by evaluating the metabolite-to-parent ratio. The epoxide-to-CBZ ratio increased by 138%. Most of this increase was due to an increase in the formation clearance of CBZ 10,11-epoxide.

The plasma protein binding of CBZ, CBZ 10,11-epoxide, and CBZ diol was unchanged (63) during coadministration with FBM at a daily dose of 3,000 mg, thus excluding a protein binding interaction.

Effect of Other Antiepileptic Drugs on Felbamate

Phenytoin

The consequence of a controlled discontinuation of PHT in four patients treated with FBM, PHT, and CBZ was an increase in FBM plasma concentrations. The corresponding mean decrease in the apparent total-body clearance of FBM

was 21% (64). This observation was confirmed in a study of patients with epilepsy who were coadministered PHT and FBM (60). In this study, PHT (200 to 500 mg/day) caused an approximate doubling of the apparent total-body clearance of FBM (53 to 61 mL/hr/kg). Interestingly, in spite of the increase in clearance, the pharmacokinetics of FBM were still linear over the dose range 400 to 1,200 mg administered three times daily.

Carbamazepine

Patients who had successfully completed a gradual decrease in PHT dose experienced further increases in FBM plasma concentrations as their CBZ dose was decreased (64). A further mean reduction of 16.5% in apparent total-body clearance was reported. These data suggest that CBZ induced the clearance of FBM. In an open-label study with nine patients on CBZ monotherapy (≥800 mg/day) (62), the mean apparent clearance of FBM was approximately 40% greater than that observed in normal volunteers (26 mL/hr/kg). The mean half-life (14.6 hours) in patients coadministered CBZ was shorter (54) than in normal volunteers (20 hours).

Valproic Acid

VPA appears to have minimal effects on FBM steady-state plasma concentrations. An assessment of the effect of VPA on the pharmacokinetics of FBM was obtained from an open-label study in which patients on VPA monotherapy (9.2 to 26.2 mg/kg/day) were coadministered FBM 1,200 or 2,400 mg/day in a randomized, crossover fashion (65). No dose-dependent changes in clearance were observed. FBM clearance values after multiple-dose treatment at 1,200 or 2,400 mg/day were 25.9 and 27.6 mL/hr/kg, respectively, and terminal elimination half-life values were 22.2 and 21.7 hours, respectively. These values were the same as those reported in normal volunteers. AUC and trough plasma concentration increased linearly when the dose of FBM increased from 1,200 to 2,400 mg/day.

Gabapentin

Gabapentin has been reported to reduce the clearance of FBM and increase its serum concentration. The reported clearance of FBM decreased from 0.67 to 0.42 mL/kg/day with an accompanying increase in half-life to 35 hours (146% of baseline) (66).

Other Pharmacokinetic Interactions

No clinically relevant pharmacokinetic interactions were noted between FBM and lamotrigine, clonazepam, vigabatrin, or the active monohydroxy metabolite of oxcarbazepine. Information on the mechanisms underlying FBM's drug–drug interaction profile permits predictions to

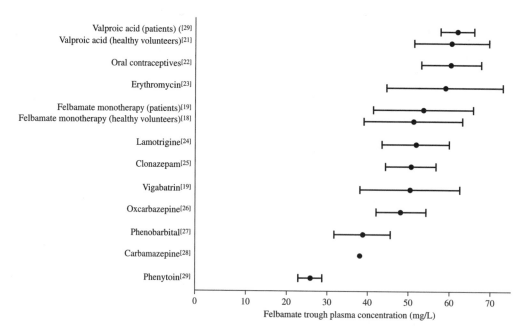

FIGURE 27.4. Effects of other drugs.

be made concerning the likelihood of interactions with other compounds.

A summary of the effects of other drugs on FBM trough concentrations is depicted in Figure 27.4.

CLINICAL USE

FBM was the first of a new generation of AEDs to be approved in the United States after a gap of nearly 15 years. The experience with FBM has provided many lessons. The Central Nervous System Advisory Committee of the U.S. Food and Drug Administration (FDA) recommended FBM for approval in December 1992. FBM was marketed in the United States on July 30, 1993 for monotherapy and adjunctive treatment of partial seizures with or without generalization, in adults, and as adjunctive therapy for partial and generalized seizures associated with Lennox-Gastaut syndrome, in children. The clinical development program used novel study designs (67). These included the relatively acute administration of FBM after withdrawal from other AEDs in patients undergoing presurgical evaluations, and trials allowing FBM monotherapy. Before its launch, approximately 4,000 patients were exposed with FBM, with >900 receiving the drug for ≥6 months, and >500 treated for at least 1 year (6,68,69).

Efficacy

Localization-Related Epilepsies

Five studies evaluated the effect of FBM in patients with localization-related epilepsy (6); three studies used double-

blind, placebo-controlled, add-on designs. Theodore et al. (70) used a three-period crossover study of FBM designed to estimate the importance of carryover effects, in 28 patients at a single center who had at least two complex partial seizures a week while taking CBZ (Figure 27.5). The decreases in seizure frequency compared with placebo—14%overall, 27% for partial seizures, and 12% for generalized tonic-clonic seizures—were not significant. FBM reduced CBZ levels by 24%. The maximum dose of FBM, 50 mg/kg, or 3,000 mg/day, was well tolerated. Mean FBM levels were 39 ± 11.5 mg/L. The only adverse effects occurring significantly more frequently with FBM than with placebo were nausea, diplopia, and blurred vision.

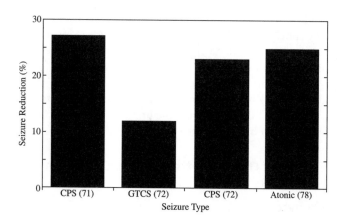

FIGURE 27.5. Percentage reduction of seizures in patients treated with felbamate compared with placebo in three double-blind, add-on trials of complex partial seizures (CPS), secondarily generalized tonic-clonic seizures, (GTCS), and atonic seizures. Numbers in parentheses are reference numbers.

Leppik et al. (71) reported a two-center study of FBM in 56 patients taking PHT and CBZ. Seizure frequency was 4.2% lower with FBM than during baseline and 23.4% lower than with placebo. The mean FBM dose was 2300 mg/day, and the mean plasma FBM level 32.5 mg/L. Although an unblinded monitor adjusted doses during the study to keep PHT and CBZ levels within each patient's baseline range, CBZ levels were 19% lower. Headache, dizziness, blurred vision, ataxia, nausea, and vomiting were reported more frequently when patients were taking FBM than when they were taking placebo.

In a multicenter study of 64 patients (72) who were being monitored for possible epilepsy surgery, the time to fourth seizure was significantly longer with 3,600 mg/day FBM (mean plasma FBM level, 65.1 mg/L) than with placebo. Forty-six percent of patients on FBM, compared with 88% on placebo, reached the fourth seizure end point (Figure 27.5). Patient were maintained on at least one other drug during the study. Headache, insomnia, and gastrointestinal disturbances were more common with FBM.

Two studies using an identical design compared FBM 3,600 mg/day with VPA 15 mg/kg/day (mean daily doses, 1,082 and 1,225 mg, respectively). The low doses of VPA were intended to protect patients from dangerous seizure exacerbation, but be less effective than FBM, in an attempt to test monotherapy efficacy versus an "active control" (73). Sachdeo et al. (74) randomized 44 patients (mean plasma FBM levels, 78.4 mg/L) and Faught et al. (75) randomized 111 patients (mean plasma FBM levels, 65 ± 23 mg/L) who had uncontrolled partial seizures during a 56-day baseline period, with other AEDs discontinued. During the 112-day trials, patients on VPA were significantly more likely to drop out owing to increased seizure frequency or severity: 40% on FBM versus 78% on VPA in one (75), and 18% versus 91% in the other study (74) (Figure 27.6). Combined data from the two studies showed that 29% of the

patients on FBM, compared with 11% on low-dose VPA, had a reduction in seizure frequency of 50% or greater (76).

Generalized Epilepsies

In one study (77), FBM (45 mg/kg or 3,600 mg/day) or placebo was administered for 70 days to 73 patients with Lennox-Gastaut syndrome, aged 4 to 36 years (mean, 13 years), who had a history of multiple seizure types (including at least 90 atonic or atypical absence seizures a month), were taking up to two AEDs, had a slow spike-and-wave pattern on the electroencephalogram (EEG), and had no evidence of progressive neurologic disease. The main outcome variable was seizure count, as recorded in 4-hour periods of video-EEG monitoring, which did not have a statistically significant effect. When seizure counts by the parents or guardians were compared, FBM reduced seizure frequency by 19% compared with baseline, whereas the reduction was 7% for placebo (p = .01). Atonic seizure frequency was reduced by 34% with FBM and by 9% with placebo (p = .002). The effect of FBM on atonic seizures appeared to be greater at a dose of 45 mg/kg/day (mean plasma FBM level, 43.8 mg/L) than at a dose of 15 mg/kg/day. Subsequent data analysis (78–81) showed that 47% of patients had a reduction of 57% in atonic seizures. Of interest is the seeming correlation of efficacy with rising serum levels. Doses of 5,000 to 6,000 mg/day have been administered to adults and those greater than 60 to 90 mg/kg/day to children (78–80). Anorexia, vomiting, and sleepiness occurred more frequently with FBM than with placebo. Global evaluation scores on a seven-point scale, from ratings by parents or guardians, were significantly better with FBM than with placebo. A subsequent follow-on, open-label study demonstrated that after 12 months, improvement on FBM was sustained. Also, a ≥50% reduction in seizure frequency was observed in 62% of children who initially received placebo after FBM was added (81).

Reports in small patient groups suggest that FBM may be effective in absence (82) or juvenile myoclonic epilepsy (83) and infantile spasms (71) when other drugs have failed.

Toxicity

Clinical Trials

More than 1,600 subjects were enrolled in the FBM clinical trials (7). The average age of the patients studied was 30 years. The patients in the Lennox-Gastaut trials included children as young as 4 years of age (77,81).

In all the clinical trials, the overall mean duration of exposure to FBM was 372 days. A total of 910 patients received FBM as monotherapy. For patients receiving adjunctive therapy, the mean duration of treatment was 347 days. The mean duration of treatment was 286 days for the monotherapy group. For patients receiving both adjunctive

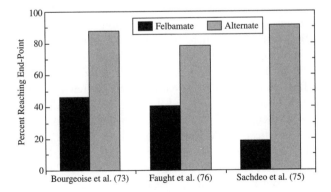

FIGURE 27.6. Percentage of patients taking felbamate compared with placebo (73) or low doses of valproic acid (75,76) who reached a defined seizure frequency or severity end point. Patients on felbamate were more likely to complete the trial in each study. Numbers in parentheses are reference numbers.

therapy and monotherapy, the mean duration was 383 days. In the children who received FBM, the overall duration of exposure was 293 days. Seventy-six children received FBM as monotherapy for a mean of 268 days, and 306 received FBM as adjunctive therapy for a mean of 274 days. Children who received both adjunctive therapy and monotherapy were treated for a mean of 383 days (7).

Most clinical trials with FBM followed the current recommended dosage schedule. Children were started on 15 mg/kg/day, increased at 7-day intervals to 30 mg/kg/day, and finally 45 mg/kg/day, or 3,000 mg. Adults began at 1,200 mg/day in three or four divided doses, and were increased every 7 days to 2,400 mg, and finally to 3,600 mg a day. The FBM dosage could be increased more quickly (6 to 7 days) when it was used as monotherapy (74,75). The presurgical study rapidly titrated FBM successfully up to 3,600 mg over a 3-day period without significant side effects (72).

Reports of overdosage with FBM have been limited. There is one report of attempted suicide by a subject who ingested 12,000 mg of FBM in a 12-hour period. Mild gastric distress and resting heart rate of 100 beats/min were the only problems reported. Overall, there have been no serious adverse effects from overdosages of FBM. If overdosages do occur, general supportive measures are recommended. It is not known if FBM is dialyzable (7).

On the basis of more recent clinical experience, it appears that a slower increase of FBM dosage, similar to that recommended outside the United States, may alleviate the most common adverse effects. In clinical practice, many of the adverse effects seem to be associated with rapid increases of the drug to target doses, and the adverse effects are exacerbated when FBM is used as adjunctive therapy (69).

Experimental Toxicology

Acute FBM toxicity evaluated in the mouse and rat indicated central nervous system stimulation, including hypoactivity, decreased muscle tone, ptosis, ataxia, loss of righting reflex, prostration, tremor, labored breathing, and death. The oral median lethal dose (LD_{50}) for rats and mice was >5,000 mg/kg. The intraperitoneal LD_{50} ranged from 475 to 2,233 mg/kg in the mouse and from 1,625 to 4,500 mg/kg in the rat (7).

In subchronic toxicity studies, body weight or body weight gain was significantly reduced in a dose-dependent manner in animals receiving FBM. Food consumption also was reduced. In both the 13-week and 1-year toxicity studies in dogs (up to 1,000 mg/kg and at 300 mg/kg, respectively), limb rigidity, seizures, ataxia, emesis, and salivation were noted; these symptoms typically were observed within the first 2 weeks of dosing. There were no consistent drug-related changes in clinical chemistry or hematologic parameters in any of the studies. Morphologic changes in the liver indicative of enzyme induction (i.e., increase in cytoplasmic vol-

ume, cytoplasmic vesiculation, and hepatic cell parenchyma) and the presence of intracytoplasmic myelin figures were observed in the high-dose FBM groups in both the subchronic and chronic toxicity study in the rat and the subchronic toxicity study in mice, but not in either dog study.

Carcinogenicity studies revealed that the oral administration of FBM did not increase the incidence of malignant or nonmalignant neoplasms or affect the longevity of either mice or rats. FBM showed no *in vitro* mutagenic effects. In addition, FBM in doses up to 2,000 mg/kg did not significantly increase the number of chromosomal aberrations per cell or the proportion of aberrant metaphases in rat bone marrow cells (7). In reproductive toxicity studies, FBM was nonteratogenic in the rat or rabbit because there were no visceral or skeletal variations or malformations observed in fetuses. In the rat, fetal exposure to drug and metabolites readily occurred because unrestricted placental transfer of [^{14}C] FBM was apparent from the maternal–fetal blood flow ^{14}C ratio.

Adverse Effects

During premarketing studies, the most common adverse reactions in adults receiving FBM monotherapy were anorexia, vomiting, insomnia, nausea, and headache. Similar symptoms were seen when FBM was used as adjunctive therapy, along with dizziness and somnolence. Adverse effects (5% incidence) were much higher when FBM was used as adjunctive therapy (G) (Table 27.2). Nausea, anorexia, and dizziness were reported in more than 5% of adult patients who received FBM as adjunctive therapy. Nausea was the only adverse effect that had a probable or definite relationship in more than 11% of adults on adjunctive therapy with FBM. The most common reasons for stopping FBM during adjunctive therapy were nausea, vomiting, anorexia, and insomnia. Most subjects did not require changes in FBM dosage. Almost all of the adverse effects resolved during the course of the studies, and were most likely the result of interactions between FBM and the standard AEDs. Whereas FBM interacts with CBZ by reducing the average plasma CBZ concentration by approximately 20%, there was an increase in the CBZ epoxide concentration of approximately 50%, and it is likely that many of the adverse effects were associated with the CBZ epoxide levels. FBM can increase PHT levels by approximately 20%. Thus, when FBM was introduced, PHT levels rose if the appropriate dosage reduction was not made, causing dose-related adverse effects. FBM also increased both the free and total plasma VPA levels. Because of the interactions of FBM, appropriate reductions in the doses of CBZ, PHT, and VPA may avoid many of the adverse effects.

In FBM monotherapy trials, nausea was the only problem that had a probable or definite relationship in more than 10% of adults on FBM monotherapy. Gastrointestinal complaints were the most common adverse effects and included nausea followed by anorexia, vomiting and dyspepsia, abdominal pain, diarrhea, and constipation. Neurologic symptoms reported included headache, the most common problem, dizziness, somnolence, and tremor. General physical complaints included fatigue and weight loss as the most common, followed by reports of injury and influenza-like symptoms. Insomnia was by far the most common psychological adverse effect, followed by nervousness and depression. There also were reports of diplopia and abnormal vision, as well as upper respiratory tract infections such as pharyngitis. Rash was uncommon, but rarely reported were leukopenia, thrombocytopenia, agranulocytosis, and Stevens-Johnson syndrome, usually when FBM was taken with other drugs (67,85).

The initial long-term safety data on FBM use in adults indicated that the most commonly occurring adverse effects were similar to those seen in earlier studies. There was no increase in the number of adverse effects reported in patients treated for 6 months or longer.

The issue of anorexia and weight loss was addressed in patients receiving FBM monotherapy for partial seizures (75). The reported incidence of weight loss and anorexia secondary to FBM ranges from 2% to 10% (7). The patients had a mean weight loss of 3 pounds from the baseline to the last trial visit, but the weight decrease was considered an adverse effect in only two of the patients.

The overall dropout rate from the clinical trials because of adverse effects or intercurrent illness in adult patients receiving FBM was 12%. The problems necessitating FBM discontinuation were gastrointestinal, 4.3%; psychological, 2.2%; whole-body, 1.7%; neurological, 1.5%; and dermatologic, 1.5% (7). More recently, seemingly rare urolithiasis during normal therapy and massive crystalluria and acute renal failure with FBM overdose have been reported (86,87).

Children

The adverse effects of FBM in children were much more common with adjunctive therapy than with monotherapy (7) (Table 27.2). A variety of symptoms occurred with FBM use as adjunctive therapy; anorexia was the most common gastrointestinal symptom, followed by vomiting, diarrhea, nausea, abdominal pain, and constipation. Similar symptoms were reported in patients receiving FBM monotherapy. Neurologic symptoms consisted of headache, somnolence, and dizziness. Adverse effects were far fewer in the FBM monotherapy group. Insomnia and nervousness were the most frequent psychological complaints. A few patients reported rash.

In children, only somnolence and anorexia (both 5.8%) and insomnia (5.5%) were considered probably or definitely related to FBM use (7). These adverse effects were reported in patients receiving FBM as adjunctive therapy. Less than 1% of patients receiving FBM adjunctive therapy had severe adverse effects. FBM was infrequently discontin-

ued for the following reasons: gastrointestinal, neurologic, dermatologic, psychological, or whole-body complaints. The only specific problem in children that required withdrawal of FBM was rash.

The long-term adverse effects of FBM use in children were somnolence, anorexia, vomiting, and insomnia. The incidence of weight loss as an adverse effect was 2% in children receiving FBM as adjunctive therapy and 3% in children receiving FBM as monotherapy. The weight reduction was 3% to 5% of the patient's pretreatment body weight and was approximately 0.6 to 4 pounds. The weight loss appears to reach a plateau as FBM therapy is continued. Although weight loss usually is seen as a beneficial side effect, some multihandicapped children with feeding or weight gain difficulties have been removed from FBM because of the severity of this associated symptom.

Overall, the dropout rate from the clinical trials because of adverse effects in pediatric patients was approximately 10%, and the most common reasons for discontinuation of FBM were gastrointestinal and neurologic complaints.

CLINICAL LABORATORY VALUES IN ADULTS AND CHILDREN

The clinical laboratory testing done in the clinical trials of FBM in both adults and children indicated that monitoring of clinical laboratory values was not necessary for the safe use of FBM. Monitoring concurrent AED and FBM levels may be helpful, along with careful clinical assessment, to help manage adverse effects. The subsequent identification of idiosyncratic reactions has put a new light on this recommendation (69).

Several articles have discussed the relative risks of FBM-associated aplastic anemia or hepatic failure and its subsequent use in patients (69,90,91). The following sections present the hypothetical mechanism through which FBM may produce toxicity, an estimate of risks involved for patients, and recommendation for clinical use.

Hypothesis

Research efforts attempting to understand the unexpected occurrence of aplastic anemia and liver toxicity after use of FBM have focused on its metabolism. It has been hypothesized that FBM toxicity results from FBM bioactivation to a highly reactive α,β-unsaturated aldehyde, 2-phenylpropenal, whose chemical structure and reactivity are similar to known chemical alkylators such as the cyclophosphamide metabolite, acrolein, and lipid peroxidation products, such as 4-hydroxynonenal. These efforts strongly support the hypothesis that 2-phenylpropenal may be the reactive metabolite mediating FBM toxicity (93–100). Thompson et al. (94) propose that in most patients undergoing FBM therapy, 2-phenylpropenal probably is detoxified by glutathione in the liver and undergoes further processing in the kidneys to the corresponding mercapturates (94). Excretion of mercapturates have been observed in the urine of all patients being treated with FBM (94,95). It is likely that a *small* number of patients receiving FBM therapy may become glutathione depleted, resulting in a compromised ability to detoxify 2-phenylpropanel, thereby increasing the risk for FBM toxicity.

Given the hypothesis that glutathione-depleted patients are at risk for FBM toxicity, a patient metabolite urinalysis assay was developed to monitor patients taking FBM for their epilepsy (95). The urine metabolite assay is based on our understanding of FBM metabolism. FBM is metabolized to an intermediate aldehyde carbamate metabolite that has two ultimate fates: oxidation to the corresponding acid carbamate, or β-elimination to form 2-phenylpropenal. The formation of 2-phenylpropenal can be measured by quantification of the corresponding mercapturates in patient urine. Given that the patient population metabolizes FBM in a regular manner, the ratio of acid carbamate to mercapturates in patient urine should produce a constant number. In fact, the results of the first 31 patients tested produced a constant ratio of 2.2 (95). Patients who then become glutathione depleted should excrete relatively fewer mercapturates, resulting in an increase in the ratio of acid carbamate to mercapturates.

The results from the first 31 patients were encouraging and supported the metabolite urine assay as a means to monitor patients at potential risk for FBM toxicity. More recently, Dieckhaus et al. (101) reported the use of single–time-point urine collection over 24-hour urine collection, demonstrating trends in the ratio of acid carbamate to mercapturates in 1,000 patients naive to FBM therapy. Evaluation of the first 1,000 patients revealed an outlier whose ratio was greater than 20 SD from the norm who presented with neutropenia. Taken together, the data suggest that FBM patient urine metabolite monitoring may be a useful means of predicting patients who may be at risk for FBM toxicity. Further work is underway to explore and validate this hypothesis.

Idiosyncratic Reactions

A single case of aplastic anemia associated with combination CBZ and FBM therapy was reported in February 1994. By mid-1994, a trickle of similar reports began to appear. On August 1, 1994, Carter Wallace, supported by the FDA, sent letters to nearly 250,000 physicians alerting them to this new risk associated with FBM treatment, and urgently recommended discontinuation of FBM in most patients, but in September 1994 the FDA Advisory Committee voted to allow FBM to remain on the market. By the autumn of 1994, cases of hepatic failure, including four deaths, also had been associated with FBM treatment (69).

Although physicians and patients were warned not to discontinue FBM abruptly, some individuals stopped tak-

ing it immediately and had serious exacerbations of their seizure disorder. Several incidences of status epilepticus resulted (69,88). Some patients chose to continue treatment with FBM because they had experienced a remarkable improvement in seizure control and often in their quality of life as well (68). FBM continues to be used in approximately 10,000 to 15,000 patients previously controlled on FBM or in those with refractory partial or generalized epilepsy, but it now is used as a third- or fourth-line AED.

Aplastic Anemia

Currently, approximately 36 cases of FBM-associated aplastic anemia have been reported. By 1999, 33 cases in the United States and a few additional cases internationally had been reported (91). Only one has been identified since 1999. The demographics of the patients reported to have aplastic anemia reveal that they were predominately female (67%), white (94%), adults (mean age, 42.5 years), receiving a mean FBM dose of 3,129 mg/day (range, 800 to 5400 mg/day), and the mean time to onset was 173 days (range, 23 to 339 days). The incidence of aplastic anemia attributed to FBM using all 33 reported cases was estimated at 300 per million patients treated.

Evaluation of the demographic characteristics and patient history revealed several features that appeared regularly and may profile the patient who is at risk. Aside from being predominantly female, 17 of the 33 patients (52%) had a prior history of anticonvulsant allergy or toxicity (especially rash), 14 had a history of prior cytopenia (42%), and 11 (33%) had evidence of immune disease (Table 27.3). Whether those patients with prior serious anticonvulsant allergy/toxicity, immune disorder, and prior history of cytopenia are truly at risk remains to be determined. It also is important to consider that four patients in whom aplastic anemia developed had none of the aforementioned risk factors (92).

On review of the first 31 reports received by the Slone Epidemiology Unit of Boston University using the International Agranulocytosis and Aplastic Anemia Study guide-

TABLE 27.3. PROFILE OF THE PATIENT AT RISK FOR FELBAMATE-RELATED APLASTIC ANEMIA

Potential Risk Factor	Percentage of Patients (n = 33)[a]
Age >17 yr	97
Female sex	67
Concomitant medications	79
Concomitant anticonvulsants	55
History significant for anticonvulsant toxicity/allergy	52
History of prior cytopenia	42
History of immune disease	33

[a]Analysis includes all reported cases to date, regardless of definitive diagnosis of aplastic anemia.

lines, only 23 cases (74%) met the criteria for aplastic anemia (92). FBM was judged to be the only plausible cause (unlikely confounding factors) in 3 cases (13%) and confounded but a likely possible cause in 11 cases; there was at least one other plausible cause in another 9 patients. In the worst-case scenario (using all 23 cases defined as aplastic anemia), the estimated incidence is 109 cases per million. In the best-case scenario (i.e., the 3 cases with unlikely confounding factors), the incidence is as low as 27 per million patients treated. This is opposed to an incidence of 2 to 2.5 per million in the general population. The overall risk for development of aplastic anemia when initiating FBM has been estimated at 1/3,000 to 1/5,000 cases per year, but one would have expected several more cases to have been identified subsequently (90,91). The risk of aplastic anemia with FBM may be 20 times that with CBZ therapy (91).

A review of the demographic profile of patients with reported aplastic anemia suggests that there may be a patient profile to aid in evaluating the individual patient at risk. Available data suggest the "at-risk" patient appears to be a middle-aged woman with a clinical history of a previous cytopenia (particularly thrombocytopenia), evidence of an underlying immunologic disorder (lupus, arthritis, or elevated antinuclear antibodies), and a significant history of prior anticonvulsant allergy. There has been only one pediatric patient diagnosed with aplastic anemia. However, this 13-year-old postpubertal girl with a history of mental retardation had a pre-FBM exposure diagnosis of systemic lupus erythematosus (91).

Hepatotoxicity

Eighteen cases of hepatic failure were reported in patients receiving FBM; evaluation indicated that 78% were female, 50% were 17 years of age or older, and the mean time to presentation was 217 days (range, 25 to 939 days). Of the patients, 16 were receiving other anticonvulsants. Using all reported cases of hepatic failure, the estimated incidence is 164 per million patients treated.

A further review suggested that only seven had a likely connection with FBM. Other cases were complicated by status epilepticus, viral hepatitis, shock liver, and paracetamol (acetaminophen) toxicity. The age range for those with a likely relationship to FBM was 5 to 56 years, and six of the seven patients were female. Using a numerator of 7, the incidence of hepatic failure would be approximately 64 per million patients treated. This incidence overlaps with the overall occurrence of VPA-associated hepatic failure, but for FBM there seems to be no clear age prediction, as seen with VPA (91).

Recommendations

A practice advisory was issued concerning "the use of FBM in the treatment of patients with intractable epilepsy" by the American Academy of Neurology, Subcommittee on Quality Standards in 1999 (91). They found sufficient evidence to recommend the use of FBM in several partial and generalized epilepsy syndromes, and balanced the severity of these conditions against the risk of life-threatening serious adverse effects (Table 27.4).

The clinical profile of patients at greatest risk and the proposed metabolic hypothesis presented previously may allow further delineation of patients at greatest risk.

FBM should be reserved for treatment of those adults and children with severe epilepsy refractory to other therapies, especially for patients with Lennox-Gastaut syndrome. Before beginning FBM treatment, a careful history concerning past indications of hematologic and hepatic toxicity, and of autoimmune disease, should be sought. Baseline routine hematologic and liver function tests should be performed, and patients and their families must be carefully informed of the potential risks; in the United States, written consent is recommended. Dose escalations should be made slowly, and dosages of comedication must be cor-

TABLE 27.4. THE USE OF FELBAMATE IN THE TREATMENT OF PATIENTS WITH INTRACTABLE EPILEPSY

A. Patients for whom risk/benefit ratio supports use because there is class I evidence for benefit
   1. Patients with Lennox-Gastaut syndrome older than age 4 yr unresponsive to primary AEDs
   2. Intractable partial seizures in patients older than 18 yr of age who have failed standard AEDs at therapeutic levels (monotherapy: data indicate a better risk/benefit ratio for felbamate used as monotherapy)
   3. Patients on felbamate >18 mo
B. Patients for whom the current risk/benefit assessment *does not support* the use of felbamate
   1. New-onset epilepsy in adults or children
   2. Patients who have experienced significant prior hematologic adverse events
   3. Patients in whom follow-up and compliance will not allow careful monitoring
   4. Patients unable to discuss risks/benefits (i.e., with mental retardation, developmental disability) and for whom no parent or legal guardian is available to provide consent.
C. Patients in whom risk/benefit ratio is unclear and based on case reports and expert opinion (class III) only, but under certain circumstances depending on the nature and severity of the patient's seizure disorder, felbamate use may be appropriate
   1. Children with intractable partial epilepsy
   2. Other generalized epilepsies unresponsive to primary agents
   3. Patients who experience unacceptable sedative or cognitive side effects with traditional AEDs
   4. Lennox-Gastaut syndrome in patients younger than 4 yr of age unresponsive to other AED

AED, antiepileptic drug.
From Kaufman DW, Kelly JP, Anderson T, et al. Evaluation of the case reports of aplastic anemia among patients treated with felbamate. *Epilepsia* 1997;38:1265–1269, with permission.

rected for known interactions where possible. A move to monotherapy should be a goal before FBM is added, using a clear, well-thought-out plan. There must be frequent and thorough clinical monitoring visits, and patients must be educated about symptoms that might herald either hematologic or hepatic toxicity. Urinary monitoring for FBM metabolites, as described earlier, may offer additional evidence of degree of risk, but is not established as a standard. If the desired clinical effect is not achieved at a reasonable dose in a timely manner, FBM should be discontinued.

CONCLUSION

FBM was introduced in the United States in 1993 as the first new AED after nearly 15 years. Efficacy was established for both partial and generalized epilepsy in adjunctive and monotherapy studies, after a number of preclinical studies suggesting a broad spectrum of activity. Its initial clinical toxicity profile suggested an acceptable risk as patients brightened and lost weight, rather than the contrary. The subsequent identification of life-threatening aplastic anemia and hepatotoxicity have relegated FBM to the status of a less preferred AED, but one that should be considered in the treatment of refractory epilepsy.

REFERENCES

1. Swinyard EA, Sofia RD, Kupferberg HJ. Comparative anticonvulsant activity and neurotoxicity of felbamate and four prototype antiepileptic drugs in mice and rats. *Epilepsia* 1986;27:27–34.
2. Sofia RD. Felbamate. In: Levy RH, Mattson RH, Meldrum BS, eds. *Antiepileptic drugs*, 4th ed. New York: Raven Press, 1995:791–797.
3. Kurcharczyk N. Felbamate: chemistry and biotransformation. In: Levy RH, Mattson RH, Meldrum BS, eds. *Antiepileptic drugs*, 4th ed. New York: Raven Press, 1995:799–806.
4. Perhach JL, Sumaker RC. Felbamate: absorption, distribution and excretion. In: Levy RH, Mattson RH, Meldrum BS, eds. *Antiepileptic drugs*, 4th ed. New York: Raven Press, 1995:807–812.
5. Banfield CR, Levy RH. Felbamate: interactions with other drugs. In: Levy RH, Mattson RH, Meldrum BS, eds. *Antiepileptic drugs*, 4th ed. New York: Raven Press, 1995:813–816.
6. Theodore WH, Jensen PK, Kwan RMF. Felbamate: clinical use. In: Levy RH, Mattson RH, Meldrum BS, eds. *Antiepileptic drugs*, 4th ed. New York: Raven Press, 1995:817–822.
7. Bebin EM, Sofia RD, Freifuss FE. Felbamate: toxicity. In: Levy RH, Mattson RH, Meldrum BS, eds. *Antiepileptic drugs*, 4th ed. New York: Raven Press, 1995:823–827.
8. White HS, Wolf HH, Swinyard EA, et al. A neuropharmacological evaluation of felbamate as a novel anticonvulsant. *Epilepsia* 1992;33:564–572.
9. Lockard JS, Levy RH, Moore DF. Drug alteration of seizure cyclicity. *Adv Epileptol* 1987;16:725–732.
10. Yamaguchi S, Rogawski MA. Effects of anticonvulsant drugs on 4-aminopyridine-induced seizures in mice. *Epilepsy Res* 1992;11:9–16.
11. Sofia RD, Gordon R, Gels M, et al. Effects of felbamate and other anticonvulsant drugs in two models of status epilepticus in the rat. *Res Commun Chem Pathol Pharmacol* 1993;79:335–341.
12. Wallis RA, Panizzon KL, Fairchild MD, et al. Protective effects of felbamate against hypoxia in the rat hippocampal slice. *Stroke* 1992;4:547–551.
13. Wasterlain CG, Adams LM, Hattori H, et al. Felbamate reduces hypoxic-ischemic brain damage *in vivo*. *Eur J Pharmacol* 1992;212:275–278.
14. Wasterlain CG, Adams LM, Schwartz PH, et al. Post-hypoxic treatment with felbamate is neuroprotective in a rat model of hypoxia-ischemia. *Neurology* 1994;43:2303–2310.
15. Chronopoulos A, Stafstrom C, Thurber S, et al. Neuroprotective effect of felbamate after kainic acid-induced status epilepticus. *Epilepsia* 1993;34:359–366.
16. Faught E. Felbamate. In: Wyllie E, ed. *The treatment of epilepsy: principles and practice*, 3rd ed. Philadelphia: Lippincott Williams & Wilkins, 2001.
17. McCabe RT, Wasterlan CG, Kucharczyk N, et al. Evidence for anticonvulsant and neuroprotectant action of felbamate mediated by strychnine-insensitive glycine receptors. *J Pharmacol Exp Ther* 1993;264:1248–1252.
18. DeSarro G, Ongini E, Bertorelli R, et al. Excitatory amino acid neurotransmission through both NMDA and non-NMDA receptors is involved in the anticonvulsant activity of felbamate in DBA/2 mice. *Eur J Pharmacol* 1993;262:11–19.
19. Stefani A, Spadoni F, Barnardi E. Voltage-activated calcium channels: targets of antiepileptic drug activity? *Epilepsia* 1997;38:959–965.
20. Ticku MK, Kamatchi GL, Sofia RD. Effect of anticonvulsant felbamate on $GABA_A$ receptor system. *Epilepsia* 1991;32:289–391.
21. Rho JM, Donevan SD, Rogawaki MA. Mechanism of action of the anticonvulsant felbamate: opposing effects on N-methyl-D-aspartate and gamma-aminobutyric acid receptors. *Ann Neurol* 1994;35:229–243.
22. Tsukamoto H, Yoshimura H, Tatsumi K. Metabolic fate of meprobamate (3): a new metabolic pathway of carbamate group—the formation of meprobamate N-glucuronide in animal body. *Chem Pharm Bull* 1963;11:421–426.
23. Berger FM, Ludwig BJ. United States Patent no. 2884444, 1959.
24. Choi YM, Kucharczyk N, Sofia RD. Synthesis of ^{14}C-labeled felbamate from phenylacetic-(methylene-^{14c}) acid. *Label Comp Radiopharm* 1986;23:545–552.
25. Yang JT, Morris M, Wong KK, et al. Felbamate metabolism in the rat, rabbit and dog. *Drug Metab Dispos* 1991;19:1126–1134.
26. Choi YM, Kucharczyk N, Sofia RD. Synthesis of 2-(4-hydroxyphenyl)-1,3-propanediol dicarbamate, 2-phenyl-2-hydroxy-1,3-propanediol dicarbamate, and 2-phenyl-1,3-propanediol monocarbamate. *Tetrahedron* 1986;42:6399–6404.
27. Adusumalli VE, Yang JT, Wong KK, et al. Felbamate pharmacokinetics in the rat, rabbit and dog. *Drug Metab Dispos* 1991;19:1116–1125.
28. Cornford EM, Young D, Paxton JW, et al. Blood-brain barrier penetration of felbamate. *Epilepsia* 1992;33:944–954.
29. Adusumalli VE, Wichmann JK, Kucharczyk N, et al. Distribution of the anticonvulsant felbamate to CSF and brain tissue of adult and neonatal rats. *Drug Metab Dispos* 1993;21:1079–1085.
30. Shumaker RC, Fantel C, Kelton E, et al. Evaluation of the elimination of [^{14}C] felbamate in healthy men. *Epilepsia* 1990;31:642.
31. Adusumalli VE, Choi YM, Romanyshyn LA, et al. Isolation and identification of 3-carbamoyloxy-2phenylopropionic acid as a

major human urinary metabolite of felbamate. *Drug Metab Dispos* 1993;21:710–716.

32. Thompson CD, Kinter MT, Macdonald TL. Synthesis and *in vitro* reactivity of 3-carbamoyl-2-phenylopropionaldehyde and 2-phenylopropenal: putative reactive metabolites of felbamate. *Chem Res Toxicol* 1996;9:1225–1229.

33. Thompson CD, Gulden P, Macdonald TL. Identification of modified atropaldehyde mercapturic acids in rat and human urine after felbamate administration. *Chem Res Toxicol* 1997;19:457–462.

34. Kapetanovic IM, Torchin CD, Thompson CD, et al. A potentially reactive cyclic carbamate metabolite of the antiepileptic drug felbamate produced by human liver tissue in vitro. *Drug Metab Dispos* 1998;28:1089–1095.

35. Yang JT, Morris M, Wong KK, et al. Felbamate metabolism in pediatric and adult beagle dogs. *Drug Metab Dispos* 1992;29:84–88.

36. Adusumalli VE, Gilchrist JR, Wichmann JK, et al. Pharmacokinetics of felbamate in pediatric and adult beagle dogs. *Epilepsia* 1992;33:955–960.

37. Segelman FH, Kelton E, Terzi RM, et al. The comparative potency of phenobarbital and five 1,3-propanediol dicarbamates for hepatic cytochrome P450 induction rats. *Res Commun Chem Pathol Pharmacol* 1985;48:467–470.

38. Adusumalli VE, Wong KK, Kucharczyk N, et al. Felbamate in vitro metabolism by rat liver microsomes. *Drug Metab Dispos* 1991;19:1135–1138.

39. Perhach JL, Weliky I, Newton JJ, et al. Felbamate. In: Meldrum BS, Porter RJ, eds. *New anticonvulsant drugs*. London: J Libbey, 1986:117–123.

40. Ward DL, Shumaker RC. Comparative bioavailability of felbamate in healthy men. *Epilepsia* 1990;31:642.

41. Romanyshyn LA, Wichmann JK, Kucharczyk N, et al. Simultaneous determination of felbamate and three metabolites in human plasma by high performance liquid chromatography. *Ther Drug Monit* 1994;16:83–89.

42. Ward DL, Weliky I, Shumaker RC, et al. Dose proportionality of Felbatol™ bid to healthy men. *Epilepsia* 1992;33(3):83.

43. Sachdeo RC, Narang-Sachdeo SK, Howard JR, et al. Steady-state pharmacokinetics and dose proportionality of felbamate after oral administration of 1200, 2400, and 3600 mg/day of felbamate. *Epilepsia* 1993;34(6):80.

44. Sachdeo S, Howard J, Dix R, et al. Tolerability and steady-state pharmacokinetics of felbamate following monotherapy over the oral dose range of 3600 to 6000 mg/day in subjects with epilepsy. *Neurology* 1994;44:296.

45. Gudipati RM, Raymond RH, Ward DL, et al. Effect of food on the absorption of felbamate in healthy male volunteers. *Neurology* 1992;42:332.

46. Sachdeo RC, Narang-Sachdeo SK, Howard JR, et al. Effect of antacid on the absorption of felbamate in subjects with epilepsy. *Epilepsia* 1993;34(6):79–80.

47. Ritter FJ, Leppik IE, Dreifuss FE, et al. Efficacy of felbamate in childhood epileptic encephalopathy (Lennox-Gastaut syndrome). *N Engl J Med* 1993;328:29–33.

48. Glue P, Sulowicz W, Colucci R, et al. Single dose pharmacokinetics of felbamate in patients with renal dysfunction. *Br J Clin Pharmacol* 1997;44:91–93.

49. Wagner ML, Graves NM, Leppik IE, et al. The effect of felbamate on valproate disposition. *Epilepsia* 1991;32(3):15.

50. Adusumalli VE, Wichmann JK, Kucharczyk N, et al. Distribution of the anticonvulsant felbamate to cerebrospinal fluid and brain tissue of adult and neonatal rats. *Drug Metab Dispos* 1993;21:1079–1085.

51. Cornford EM, Young D, Paxton JW, et al. Blood-brain barrier penetration of felbamate. *Epilepsia* 1992;33:944–954.

52. Adusumalli VE, et al. Drug concentrations in human brain tissue samples from epileptic patients treated with felbamate. *Drug Metab Dispos* 1994;22:168–170.

53. Shumaker RC, Fantel C, Kelton E, et al. Evaluation of the elimination of (^{14}C) felbamate in healthy men. *Epilepsia* 1990;31:642.

54. Wilensky AJ, Friel PN, Ojemann LM, et al. Pharmacokinetics of W-554 (ADD 03055) in epileptic patients. *Epilepsia* 1985;26:602–606.

55. Glue P, Banfield CR, Perhach JL, et al. Pharmacokinetic interactions with felbamate: *in vitro-in vivo* correlation. *Clin Pharmacokinet* 1997;33:214–223.

56. Fuerst RH, Graves NM, Leppik IE, et al. Felbamate increases phenytoin but decreases carbamazepine concentrations. *Epilepsia* 1988;29:488–491.

57. Fuerst RH, Graves NM, Leppik IE, et al. A preliminary report on alteration of carbamazepine and phenytoin metabolism by felbamate. *Drug Intell Clin Pharm* 1986;20:67.

58. Graves NM, Holmes GB, Fuerst RH, et al. Effect of felbamate on phenytoin and carbamazepine serum concentrations. *Epilepsia* 1987;30:225–229.

59. Holmes GB, Graves NM, Leppik IE, et al. Felbamate: bidirectional effects on phenytoin and carbamazepine serum concentrations. *Epilepsia* 1987;28:578.

60. Sachdeo R, Wagner M, Sachdeo S, et al. Steady-state pharmacokinetics of phenytoin when coadministered with Felbatol™ (felbamate) *Epilepsia* 1992;33(3):84.

61. Wagner M, Graves NM, Leppik IE, et al. The effect of felbamate on valproate disposition. *Epilepsia* 1991;32(3):15.

62. Howard JR, Dix RK, Shumaker RC, et al. Effect of felbamate on carbamazepine pharmacokinetics. *Epilepsia* 1992;33(3):84–85.

63. Albani F, Theodore WH, Washington P, et al. Effect of felbamate on plasma levels of carbamazepine and its metabolites. *Epilepsia* 1991;32:130–132.

64. Wagner M, Graves NM, Marineau K, et al. Discontinuation of phenytoin and carbamazepine in patients receiving felbamate. *Epilepsia* 1991;32:398–406.

65. Ward DL, Wagner ML, Perhach JL, et al. Felbamate steady-state pharmacokinetics during co-administration of valproate. *Epilepsia* 1991;32(3):8.

66. Troupin AS, Montouris G, Hussein G. Felbamate: therapeutic range and other kinetic information. *J Epilepsy* 1997;10:26–31.

67. Brodie MJ. Felbamate: a new antiepileptic drug. *Lancet* 1993;341:1445–1446.

68. Brodie MJ, Pellock JM. Taming the brain storms: felbamate updated. *Lancet* 1995;346:918–919.

69. Pellock JM, Brodie MJ. Felbamate: 1997 update. *Epilepsia* 1997;38:1261–1264.

70. Theodore WH, Raubertas R, Porter RJ, et al. Felbamate: a clinical trial for complex partial seizures. *Epilepsia* 1991;32:392–397.

71. Leppik IE, Dreifuss FE, Pledger GW, et al. Felbamate for partial seizures: results of a controlled clinical trial. *Neurology* 1991;41:1785–1789.

72. Bourgeois B, Leppik IE, Sackellares JC, et al. Felbamate: a double-blind controlled trial in patients undergoing presurgical evaluation of partial seizures. *Neurology* 1993;43:693–696.

73. Pledger GW, Kramer LD. Clinical trials of investigational antiepileptic drugs: monotherapy designs. *Epilepsia* 1991;32:716–721.

74. Sachdeo R, Kramer LD, Rosenberg A, et al. Felbamate monotherapy: controlled trial in patients with partial onset seizures. *Ann Neurol* 1992;32:386–392.

75. Faught E, Sachdeo RC, Remler MP, et al. Felbamate monotherapy for partial-onset seizures; an active control trial. *Neurology* 1993;43:688–692.

76. Jensen PK. Felbamate in the treatment of refractory partial onset seizures. *Epilepsia* 1993;34[Suppl 7]:S25–S29.

77. Felbamate Study Group in the Lennox-Gastaut Syndrome. Efficacy of felbamate in childhood epileptic encephalopathy (Lennox-Gastaut syndrome). *N Engl J Med* 1993;328:29–33.

78. Jensen PK. Felbamate in the treatment of Lennox-Gastaut syndrome. *Epilepsia* 1994;35[Suppl 5]:S54–S57.

79. Bourgeois BFD. Felbamate. *Semin Pediatr Neurol* 1997;4:3–8.

80. Pellock JM. Treatment of epilepsy in the new millennium. *Pharmacotherapy* 2000;20[Suppl]:1295–1385.

81. Dodson WE. Felbamate in the treatment of Lennox-Gastaut syndrome: results of a 12 month, open label study following a randomized clinical trial. *Epilepsia* 1993;34[Suppl 7]:S18–S24.

82. Devinsky O, Kothari M, Rubin R, et al. Felbamate for absence seizures. *Epilepsia* 1992;33[Suppl 3]:84.

83. Sachdeo RC, Murphy JV, Kamin M. Felbamate in juvenile myoclonic epilepsy. Epilepsia 1992;33[Suppl 3]:118.

84. Hurst DL, Rolan TD. The use of felbamate to treat infantile spasms. *J Child Neurol* 1995;10:134–136.

85. Abramowicz M, ed. Felbamate. *Med Lett Drugs Ther* 1993;35.

86. Sparagana SP, Stand WR, Adams RC. Felbamate urolithiasis. *Epilepsia* 2001;42:682–685.

87. Rengstorff DS, Milstone AP, Seger DL, et al. Felbamate overdose complicated by massive crystalluria and acute renal failure. *J Clin Toxicol* 2000;38:667–669.

88. Welty TE, Privitera M, Shukla R. Increased seizure frequency with felbamate withdrawal in adults. *Arch Neurol* 1998;55:641–645.

89. Siegel H, Kelley K, Stertz B, et al. The efficacy of felbamate as add-on therapy to valproic acid in the Lennox-Gastaut syndrome. *Epilepsy Res* 1999;34:91–97.

90. French J, Smith M, Faught E, et al. The use of felbamate in the treatment of patients with intractable epilepsy: practice advisory. *Neurology* 1999;52:1540–1545.

91. Pellock JM. Felbamate in epilepsy therapy: evaluating the risks. *Drug Saf* 1999;3:225–239.

92. Kaufman DW, Kelly JP, Anderson T, et al. Evaluation of the case reports of aplastic anemia among patients treated with felbamate. *Epilepsia* 1997;38:1265–1269.

93. Thompson CD, Kinter MT, Macdonald TL. Synthesis and *in vitro* reactivity of 3-carbamoyl-2-phenylpropionaldehyde and 2-phenylpropenal: putative reactive metabolites of felbamate. *Chem Res Toxicol* 1996;9:1225–1229.

94. Thompson CD, Gulden PH, Macdonald TL. Identification of modified atropaldehyde mercapturic acids in rat and human urine after felbamate administration. *Chem Res Toxicol* 1997;10:457–462.

95. Thompson, CD, Barthen MT, Hopper DW, et. al. Quantification in patient urine samples of felbamate and three metabolites: acid carbamate and two mercapturic acids. *Epilepsia* 1999;40:769–776.

96. Kapetanovic IM, Torchin CD, Thompson CD, et. al. A potentially reactive cyclic carbamate metabolite of the anti-epileptic drug felbamate produced by human liver tissue *in vitro. Drug Metab Dispos* 1998;26:1089–1095.

97. Thompson CD, Miller TA, Barthen MT, et al. The synthesis, in vitro reactivity, and evidence for formation in humans of 5-phenyl-1,3-oxazinane-2,4-dione, a metabolite of felbamate. *Drug Metab Dispos* 2000;28:434–439.

98. Dieckhaus CM, Miller TA, Sofia RD, et al. A mechanistic approach to understanding species differences in felbamate bioactivation: relevance to drug-induced idiosyncratic reactions. *Drug Metab Dispos* 2000;28:814–822.

99. Dieckhaus CM, Santos WL, Sofia RD, et al. The chemistry, toxicology and identification in rat and human urine of 4-hydroxy-5-phenyltetrahydro-1,3-oxazin-2-one: a reactive metabolite in felbamate bioactivation. *Chem Res Toxicol* 2001 (*in press*).

100. Dieckhaus CM, Roller SR, Santos, WL, et al. The role of glutathione S-transferases A1-1, M1-1 and P1-1 in the detoxification of 2-phenylpropenal, a reactive felbamate metabolite. *Chem Res Toxicol* 2001 (*in press*).

101. Dieckhaus CM, Roller SR, Johnson MA, et al. Felbamate metabolite patient urinalysis to monitor potential drug-induced idiosyncratic reactions. *Epilepsia* 2001 (*in press*).

GABAPENTIN

28

GABAPENTIN

MECHANISMS OF ACTION

CHARLES P. TAYLOR

Gabapentin (Neurontin or 1-[aminomethyl]cyclohexaneacetic acid) is a novel amino acid derived by addition of a cyclohexyl group to the chemical backbone of γ-aminobutyric acid (GABA) (74), the major rapid inhibitory neurotransmitter of mammalian brain (Figure 28.1A). X-ray crystallography and molecular modeling studies also indicate a structural similarity between gabapentin and L-leucine (Figure 28.1B). Gabapentin is an effective and safe anticonvulsant in extensive and well-controlled clinical trials (3,50). As a chemical derivative of GABA, gabapentin was expected originally to mimic the actions of GABA at inhibitory synaptic receptors in the brain and to mimic the action of baclofen or to prevent seizures by increasing rapid chloride-dependent inhibition. However, with one controversial exception, subsequent studies have shown that gabapentin is inactive at $GABA_A$ and $GABA_B$ receptors. In fact, many studies *in vivo* and *in vitro* have failed to pinpoint the mechanism of anticonvulsant action of gabapentin clearly.

Gabapentin interacts with a specific high-affinity binding site in mammalian brain membranes that is an auxiliary protein subunit of voltage-gated calcium channels. In addition, gabapentin reduces the release of several neurotransmitters in a manner that may be related to this high-affinity binding site. This chapter reviews the pharmacology of gabapentin.

The cellular mechanisms of anticonvulsant drugs are the subject of several reviews (70,91,96), and the pharmacology of gabapentin has been summarized in the literature (24,92). In addition to gabapentin, agents that have shown significant efficacy for treatment of refractory partial seizures in controlled clinical trials include sodium channel modulators (phenytoin, carbamazepine, zonisamide, and lamotrigine) and drugs that interact with GABA receptors or GABA metabolism or uptake (phenobarbital, vigabatrin, and the GABA-uptake blocker tiagabine; perhaps also valproic acid and felbamate). Of these clinically proven anti-

convulsants, only gabapentin and vigabatrin are amino acids, a feature suggesting that the mechanisms of both drugs may relate to the neurotransmitter or metabolic amino acids of the brain.

EFFECT OF GABAPENTIN ON EPILEPTIFORM DISCHARGES IN LABORATORY ANIMALS

Anticonvulsant Actions in Animal Models

To date, no published reports have shown that gabapentin alters seizurelike discharges *in vitro*, although one report indicates that gabapentin has an additive effect with vigabatrin to alter seizurelike discharges in rat hippocampal slices (46). Another unpublished study showed that gabapentin application, at 100 μmol/L for 60 minutes, did not inhibit stimulus-induced burst firing in hippocampal slices, a model of seizures in isolated hippocampal tissue (W. Wilson et al., *unpublished data,* methods of ref. 79). However, *in vivo,* gabapentin reduces the behavioral seizure score, and at higher dosages, it shortens the local afterdischarge duration in rats kindled by repeated electrical stimulation of the limbic system, a model of partial seizures (44,57,104). Furthermore, gabapentin treatment reduces the duration and development of maximal dentate activation (108), a model of epileptic seizures in anesthetized rats (85). In addition, systemic administration of gabapentin to rodents prevents seizures from a variety of different electrical and chemical stimuli (Table 28.1). Tonic extensor seizures from many different chemical agents are prevented, whereas threshold clonic seizures from several agents are not. In contrast to the prototype agents phenytoin and carbamazepine (39), clonic seizures from pentylenetetrazol are prevented by gabapentin. Gabapentin is active at low doses and thus prevents seizures from maximal electroshock in rats after doses equivalent to or lower than those of phenytoin or carbamazepine. With an intravenous dose of gabapentin (15 mg/kg) that prevents seizures from maximal electroshock in practically all rats, plasma gabapentin concentrations are approximately 5.0 μg/mL (30 μmol/L) at the time of peak anticonvulsant action (102).

Charles P. Taylor, PhD: Director, Department of CNS Pharmacology, Pfizer Global Research and Development, Ann Arbor, Michigan

A

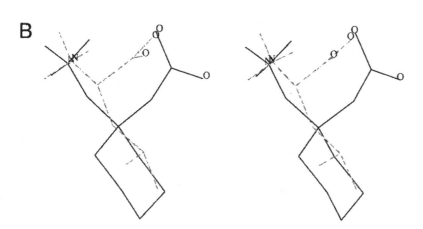

γ-aminobutyric acid (GABA)

gabapentin

(S)-3-isobutyl GABA

(R)-3-isobutyl GABA

B

FIGURE 28.1. A: Chemical structures of gabapentin in comparison with the inhibitory neurotransmitter γ-aminobutyric acid (GABA) and the enantiomers of 3-isobutyl GABA (pregabalin and R(–)-3-isobutyl GABA. Gabapentin and pregabalin cross the blood–brain barrier in animals and prevent seizures when these agents are given systemically, whereas GABA does not. Although the two-dimensional structures of gabapentin and GABA are similar, three-dimensional models show differences in the spacing of amino and carboxyl functional groups. **B:** Computer-generated molecular model of gabapentin superimposed on a similar model for L-leucine. This stereo pair may be viewed either with a stereo viewer or by slightly crossing the eyes to superimpose the two images. The carboxyl and amino moieties of the two molecules match closely in three-dimensional space, as do the lipophilic hydrocarbon moieties. These results suggest that gabapentin may be expected to mimic the actions of L-leucine and similar branched-chain neutral amino acids at a variety of biologic sites. The computer-modeled structure agrees with three-dimensional crystal structure of gabapentin (crystal coordinates deposited with the Cambridge structural database, Cambridge CB2 1E2, United Kingdom). (B, from E. Lunney, Pfizer Global R & D, *unpublished data* and Ibers JA. Gabapentin and gabapentin monohydrate. *Acta Crystallographica* 2001;57:641–643, with permission.

TABLE 28.1. ACTIVITY OF GABAPENTIN IN ANIMAL MODELS OF SEIZURES

Species	Convulsant Agent	Dose Route	ED$_{50}$ (mgkg)
Mouse	Tonic extensor seizures (maximal electroshock)	i.p.	78
Rat	Tonic extensor seizures (maximal electroshock)	i.v., p.o.	7.2, 9.1
Mouse	Tonic extensor seizure (thiosemicarbazide)	i.v., p.o.	6.3, 5.0[a]
Mouse	Tonic extensor seizure (3-mercaptopropionic acid)	p.o.	31[a]
Mouse	Tonic extensor seizure (strychnine)	p.o.	34[a]
Mouse	Tonic extensor seizure (pentylenetetrazole)	p.o.	52[a]
Mouse	Tonic extensor seizure (*N*-methyl-D-aspartate)	i.p.	>240[c]
Rat	Tonic extensor seizure (kainate)	i.p.	>300
Mouse	Threshold clonic seizure (pentylenetetrazole)	i.p.	47
Mouse	Threshold clonic seizure (bicuculline)	i.p.	>500
Mouse	Threshold clonic seizure (picrotoxin)	i.p.	>500
Mouse	Threshold clonic seizure (strychnine)	i.p.	>500
Rat	Behavioral seizure score (hippocampal kindled rats)	i.p.	30[b]
DBA/2J mouse	Tonic extensor seizure (audiogenic)	p.o.	2.5
Wistar rat (strain)	Absence seizures (electroencephalogram)	i.p.	Not effective (25–100 mg/kg)
Gerbil (genetic strain)	Tonic extensor seizure	p.o.	15
Baboon (genetic strain)	Photogenic myoclonus	i.v.	Not effective (1.0–240 mg/kg)

ED$_{50}$, median effective dose; i.p., intraperitoneal; i.v., intravenous; p.o., oral.
[a]From Bartoszyk et al. (1); others are unpublished data.
[b]Lowest effective dose.
[c]At this dose, seizures were significantly delayed but not prevented.

Gabapentin is active in several genetic models of seizures. However, unlike the anticonvulsants valproate, ethosuximide, and the benzodiazepines (53), gabapentin fails to prevent spike-and-wave events in the electroencephalogram of rats with genetic absence seizures. Gabapentin did not alter generalized seizure activity in *lethargic* mice (a second genetic model of absence) (34). In comparison with other antiepileptic drugs, the spectrum of anticonvulsant activity with gabapentin suggests efficacy for treatment of partial seizures and generalized tonic-clonic seizures but not for generalized absence. The profile of activity of gabapentin in animal models of seizure activity suggests that gabapentin may have a different pharmacologic mechanism than that of other antiepileptic drugs.

Another novel GABA derivative, S-(+)-3-isobutylGABA or pregabalin (94), has shown a profile of anticonvulsant activity very similar to that of gabapentin. The two enantiomers (optical isomers) of pregabalin differ greatly in their anticonvulsant potency and thus offer a tool with which to study various mechanisms that may be involved in the anticonvulsant action of pregabalin. The enantiomers of pregabalin are stereoselective for their inhibition of [3H]-gabapentin binding, a finding suggesting that anticonvulsant activity may relate to potency for displacing [3H]-gabapentin binding (94) (see also the later discussion of binding).

In contrast to most other anticonvulsants, the time of peak anticonvulsant action with gabapentin is delayed about 2 hours after intravenous administration, past the time of peak drug concentration in either the blood plasma or the brain interstitial space (102) (Figure 28.2). This delay suggests that anticonvulsant action may be caused by biochemical changes that require gabapentin to be present in brain for a substantial period. Alternatively, gabapentin may require prolonged binding to an extracellular receptor before its anticonvulsant action becomes significant. Existing data do not distinguish among these possibilities.

Other Pharmacologic Actions

Gabapentin is active in several animal models of spasticity (5). Spasticity was the initial therapeutic target of clinical studies with gabapentin, and subsequently, efficacy for treating spasticity has been demonstrated in clinical studies (13,26,66). In addition, studies have shown that gabapentin is active both in animal models of analgesia (1,21, 36,59,61,107) and in clinical trials for treatment of neuropathic pain (4,73). Similarly, gabapentin is active in animal models of anxiety (78), and it reduces anxiety scores in clinical studies (60). The cellular mechanisms of

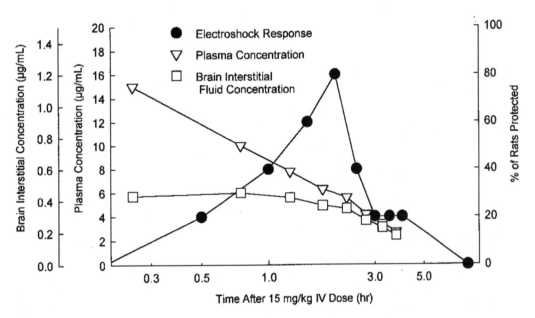

FIGURE 28.2. The anticonvulsant activity of gabapentin reaches a maximum approximately 3 hours after intravenous administration (electroshock response, *closed circles*). However, gabapentin concentrations in blood plasma *(open triangles)* and in brain interstitial space *(open squares)* peak soon after dosing and are declining at the time of maximal anticonvulsant action (concentrations may be converted to micromolar by multiplying by 5.8). These results indicate that the anticonvulsant mechanism of gabapentin requires significant time to be expressed and suggest that biochemical changes must take place before anticonvulsant effects are seen. (From Welty DF, Wang Y, Busch JA, et al. Pharmacokinetics and pharmacodynamics of CI-1008 (pregabalin) and gabapentin in rats using maximal electroshock. *Epilepsia* 1997;38:35–36, with permission.)

gabapentin for reducing spasticity, anxiety, and pain are not well understood, but they may overlap with mechanisms that are relevant for treatment of epilepsy (see later). Finally, high doses of gabapentin reduce neuronal pathology both *in vitro* (72) and in an animal model of amyotrophic lateral sclerosis (28). However, the mechanism of neuroprotective effects of gabapentin may differ from those for epilepsy and the other indications mentioned earlier (101). Furthermore, the proposed neuroprotective mechanism, that is, inhibition of branched-chain amino acid aminotransferase (BCAA-T) (35,41), probably occurs only at high concentrations of gabapentin that are not reached with clinical treatments.

Gabapentin, at 300 mg/kg, administered intravenously to mice, causes a 30% reduction in spontaneous locomotor activity and a slight reduction in behavioral responsiveness, but mice are still able to walk normally and to respond to sensory stimulation; no sleeping, catalepsy, or changes in pinnal or corneal reflexes are observed. At higher doses, gabapentin causes ptosis, exophthalmos, ataxia, muscle relaxation, and further slowing of behavioral responses. These results indicate that gabapentin has a weaker tendency for causing dose-related behavioral side effects than prototype anticonvulsants such as phenytoin or carbamazepine, which cause unresponsiveness and depress respiration at doses of $\geq$100 mg/kg when these agents are given intravenously to mice or rats (C. P. Taylor and M. G. Vartanian, *unpublished data*).

IN VITRO ACTIONS OF GABAPENTIN

Effects on GABA Receptors, GABA Turnover, and GABA Function

Despite previous findings that gabapentin is inactive as an agonist or antagonist at $GABA_B$ receptors, a recent study indicates that gabapentin is an agonist of one subtype of recombinant heterodimeric $GABA_B$ receptor, $GABA_B1a/2b$, a subtype thought to act mostly postsynaptically (55). Other recent results (39a,97a) indicate that gabapentin does not directly interact with $GABA_B$ receptor but may indirectly activate $GABA_A$ receptors by elevating extracellular GABA concentration. In addition, the actions of gabapentin on neurotransmitter release (D. Dooley et al., *personal communication*) and in an electrophysiologic model with anesthetized rats (84) are not reversed by antagonists of $GABA_B$ receptors. Therefore, it remains to be demonstrated whether a $GABA_B$ agonistlike action of gabapentin is relevant for anticonvulsant pharmacology.

Gabapentin increases the apparent rate of synthesis of GABA by up to twice control levels in several brain regions, a finding suggesting that altered GABA metabolism may underlie anticonvulsant action (43). However, the time course of changes in GABA synthesis induced by gabapentin does not correspond very well with the time course of anti-

convulsant effects, so the relevance of this effect remains unclear. Regardless of the mechanism responsible, gabapentin treatment in human patients causes a rapid and sustained elevation of whole-tissue GABA concentration in brain (63,64), and these changes in GABA concentration may lead to changes in GABA synaptic function. However, the pool of GABA measured in such studies is largely confined anatomically within GABAergic neurons of brain, and only a very small fraction of total GABA is free in extracellular space, where it is able to interact with neuronal GABA receptors. One analysis suggests that increased cellular concentration of GABA *in vitro* (106) can cause a steady inhibitory $GABA_A$-mediated current in cultured neurons. If such a mechanism also occurs *in vivo*, it would reduce brain excitability and thus could reduce or prevent seizure activity.

Gabapentin and pregabalin alter the inhibition of evoked potentials in hippocampus of anesthetized rats (86,108), a finding suggesting a change in GABA function in rat brain *in vivo*. This effect differs from that of baclofen (84), but the relevance and cellular mechanisms involved are not clear. Furthermore, gabapentin appears to *reduce* inhibition mediated by GABAergic interneurons in this *in vivo* model, and this is difficult to reconcile with an anticonvulsant effect. Despite this difficulty, these results suggest that gabapentin treatment alters the function of GABAergic inhibition in hippocampal neurons *in vivo*.

In vitro data with isolated optic nerve segments from neonatal rats suggest that gabapentin enhances the release of GABA from reversal of the GABA transporter (38). High-pressure liquid chromatography studies of optic nerve tissue (54) indicate that the effect of gabapentin in this system differs from that of vigabatrin, which increases GABA concentration in nerve segments (and brain tissues) by inhibiting GABA degradation. In this system, GABA can be released in a calcium-independent manner by application of the inhibitor and substrate of GABA transporters, nipecotic acid (56). The released GABA acts at $GABA_A$ receptors on axons and causes an easily measured depolarization. Preincubation of optic nerves with gabapentin (100 μmol/L for 1 hour) increases depolarizations from application of 1.0 mmol/L nipecotic acid. Nipecotic acid responses in optic nerve are not altered by acute application of gabapentin, and acute application causes no GABA agonistlike or antagonistlike effects. Furthermore, nipecotic acid responses both in control conditions and after enhancement by gabapentin are completely blocked by the $GABA_A$ antagonist bicuculline, a finding indicating that the effect is caused by changes in GABA release. Similar results with gabapentin have been obtained with field potential records and neuronal voltage-clamp records from the CA1 area of rat hippocampal slices (32,33,39a).

Previous studies have shown that increases in extracellular potassium or application of glutamate agonists release GABA from cultured brain cells both by calcium-dependent and calcium-independent mechanisms, the latter arising from alterations in the equilibrium of GABA transport (22,65). Some of the anticonvulsant effects of gabapentin therefore may arise from increased nonsynaptic GABA release during seizure activity, which has previously been hypothesized to be altered in epileptic brain tissues (17,22).

Gabapentin's prevention of seizures in rodents from administration of GABA antagonists or GABA synthesis inhibitors and findings of increased brain GABA concentrations in humans suggest that gabapentin may enhance GABA activity in brain by a novel means, in comparison with benzodiazepines, barbiturates, or GABA uptake inhibitors (52).

Recent findings (103a) indicate that application of gabapentin or pregabalin to rat neuronal cultures for two hours increases the fraction of GAT1 GABA transportor protein located at cell membranes.

Effects on Neurotransmitter Release

Gabapentin slightly reduces the release of several monoamine neurotransmitters from mammalian brain tissue slices *in vitro* (68,75), and this action has been reexamined with both gabapentin and pregabalin (15). This more recent study shows that the actions of gabapentin are most pronounced when slices are stimulated for many seconds by modest concentrations of potassium to evoke release (rather than by electrical stimulation or high potassium concentrations). Under these conditions, the release of preloaded norepinephrine is

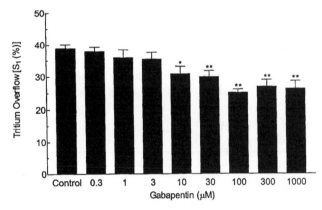

FIGURE 28.3. Gabapentin reduces the release of tritiated norepinephrine from rat neocortical brain slices *in vitro* (15). Tritium overflow (from [³H]norepinephrine that was preloaded into rat neocortex tissue) was evoked by a 120-second application of elevated potassium solution (25 mmol/L). Fractions (5 mL) were collected from superfusate samples (1 mL/min) and were analyzed for tritium. Each data point represents the mean from six or more replicate experiments. Significant differences from the control group were seen with 10 μmol/L and greater of gabapentin (*single asterisk* denotes *p < 0.05*; *double asterisks* denote *p < 0.01* by ANOVA). *Error bars* denote standard error of the mean. Gabapentin had a maximal inhibition of approximately 40% and an IC₅₀ for this effect of approximately 9 μmol/L. (From Dooley DJ, Donovan CM, Pugsley TA. Stimulus-dependent modulation of [³H]norepinephrine release from rat neocortical slices by gabapentin and pregabalin. *J Pharmacol Exp Ther* 2000; 296:1086–1098, with permission.)

reduced about 35% by 100 μmol/L gabapentin, and the half-maximal concentration is near 10 μmol/L (Figure 28.3). These studies also show that the effects of gabapentin and pregabalin are not additive, and so both compounds are likely to share a common cellular mechanism. The relevance of changes in monoamine release for anticonvulsant action is unclear, but changes in the release of other neurotransmitters could easily be relevant, and gabapentin also has been reported to reduce glutamate release from brain slices (16, 48). Although the molecular mechanism of reduced neurotransmitter release has not been clearly established, it is likely that changes in intracellular calcium are involved, because gabapentin also limits the increase in calcium fluorescence caused by potassium application to synaptosomes (21a,51, 97), and this could relate to binding of gabapentin to the α2δ auxiliary calcium channel protein (21). Furthermore, the actions of gabapentin on neurotransmitter release differ from those of the GABA_B agonist baclofen (68). This has been confirmed by findings that a selective GABA_B antagonist did not alter the effects of gabapentin on norepinephrine release *in vitro* (D. Dooley et al., *personal communication*). Despite all these effects of gabapentin on release of neurotransmitters in biochemical studies, the application of either gabapentin or pregabalin does not alter synaptic potentials in anesthetized rats evoked by single action potentials (86) and has only rather subtle inhibitory effects on synaptic currents in CA1 neurons (54a,97) or entorhinal neurons (21a) in tissue slices. The findings to date suggest that neurotransmitter release is modified by gabapentin only in a relatively subtle manner and particularly under conditions of prolonged depolarization or activation of cellular second messengers.

Effects on Cytosolic Enzymes of Brain Tissue

Gabapentin has been studied for effects on several enzymes that metabolize amino acids in rat brain tissues (25) (Figure 28.4). Several effects have been found, but they only occur with concentrations of gabapentin greater than those relevant for human therapy. Specifically, the activity of glutamic acid decarboxylase (GAD), BCAA-T, GABA transaminase (GABA-T), glutamate dehydrogenase (GDH), glutamine synthase, glutaminase, alanine aminotransferase, aspartate aminotransferase and γ-glutamyl transferase have been studied. These results are summarized in Table 28.2.

GAD is the primary synthetic enzyme for GABA, and it has been proposed that anticonvulsant actions of valproic acid may result from increased GAD activity (45). Studies with gabapentin and pregabalin show that they both enhance GAD activity in protein extracts partially purified from porcine brain (93). It is possible that the increased GABA turnover observed in rat brain after administration of gabapentin (43) results from activation of GAD. However, *in vitro* results need to be confirmed with purified isoenzymes of GAD. The high concentrations (and doses) of gabapentin

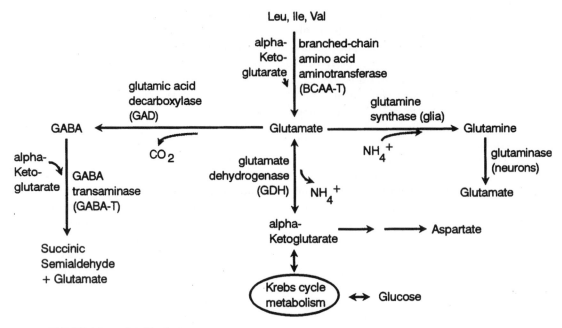

FIGURE 28.4. Simplified schematic diagram showing pathways of amino acid metabolism in the brain. *In vitro,* gabapentin interacts with branched-chain amino acid aminotransferase (BCAA-T), glutamic acid decarboxylase (GAD), glutamate dehydrogenase (GDH), and γ-aminobutyric acid transaminase (GABA-T), but not with glutaminase or glutamine synthase. It is unclear which of these interactions (if any) are necessary for anticonvulsant actions.

needed to enhance GAD activity suggest that this mechanism may not be relevant for anticonvulsant activity in humans.

BCAA-T of rat brain is the primary enzyme that metabolizes cytosolic L-leucine, L-isoleucine, or L-valine together with α-ketoglutarate to form glutamate; the other product of this reaction, α-ketoglutarate, is formed in glia and is exported to neurons (35,41). In a partially purified *in vitro* enzyme preparation, gabapentin inhibits BCAA-T activity (25). Gabapentin is a competitive inhibitor of BCAA-T metabolism of L-leucine, L-isoleucine, and L-valine, with

antagonist affinity constant (K_i) values of 300 to 1,300 μmol/L for gabapentin and Michaelis constant (K_m) values of 500 to 1,000 μmol/L for L-leucine, L-isoleucine, or L-valine (A. Goldlust et al., *personal communication*). In contrast, pregabalin is a weak noncompetitive inhibitor of BCAA-T, with K_i values about 20-fold higher. Relatively high concentrations of gabapentin decrease the *de novo* synthesis of glutamate in isolated retinal tissues (41) by this mechanism and this effect may also relate to changes in glutamine metabolism (6,41). BCAA-T inhibition by gabapentin may account for neuro-

TABLE 28.2. SUMMARY OF THE ACTIVITY OF GABAPENTIN AT ENZYMES OF RAT BRAIN INVOLVED IN GLUTAMATE AND GABA METABOLISM

Enzyme	Compound	Action (at 10.0 mmol/L)	Inhibition Type	K_i (Apparent)
GDH$_{synaptosomal}$	Gabapentin	Threefold enhancement	None	
GDH$_{synaptosomal}$	L-Leucine	Sixfold enhancement	None	
Glutamate decarboxylase (93)	Gabapentin	78% Enhancement (at 2.5 mmol/L)	None	
Branched-chain amino acid aminotransferase	Gabapentin	64% Inhibition	Competitive	0.8 mmol/L
GABA aminotransferase (rat brain)	Gabapentin	32% Inhibition	Mixed (competitive and noncompetitive)	23 mmol/L
Glutamine synthase	Gabapentin	No effect		
Glutaminase	Gabapentin	No effect		
Alanine aminotransferase (rat brain)	Gabapentin	No effect		
Aspartate aminotransferase (rat brain)	Gabapentin	No effect		
γ-glutamyltransferase (rat brain, substrate activity)	Gabapentin	<50% of glutamine		

K_i, antagonist affinity constant; GDH, glutamate dehydrogenase; GABA, γ-aminobutyric acid.
From refs. 25 and 93, with permission.

protective action of gabapentin (101), both in a transgenic model of amyotrophic lateral sclerosis (28) and in an *in vitro* model (72). However, it seems unlikely that BCAA-T inhibition accounts for the anticonvulsant action of gabapentin because of the high doses and concentrations required. In any case, activity at this enzyme suggests a biologic similarity between gabapentin and endogenous amino acids such as L-leucine (Figure 28.1B).

GABA-T is the primary degradative enzyme for the neurotransmitter GABA and converts it to succinic semialdehyde and glutamate. This enzyme is the primary target of the irreversible enzyme inhibitor and anticonvulsant agent vigabatrin (γ-vinyl GABA, (40,42)). Gabapentin inhibits GABA-T activity, but in contrast to vigabatrin, inhibition is very weak and completely reversible, with both competitive and noncompetitive components (apparent K_i near 25 mmol/L). The two enantiomers of pregabalin also inhibit GABA-T with K_i values of 6.6 and 64 mmol/L for pregabalin and the R enantiomer, respectively (A. Goldlust et al., *personal communication*). The concentrations of soluble GABA in the whole brain are in the range of 1,000 to 2,000 μmol/L (19) and are even higher within GABAergic neurons. In comparison, concentrations of gabapentin in brain tissues are probably too low to be significant on GABA-T. In addition, the spectrum of pharmacologic actions of gabapentin in animals is different from that of vigabatrin (58), a finding suggesting that GABA-T inhibition may not be significant with gabapentin.

GDH is found mostly in the mitochondria of rat brain neurons. It is responsible for the degradation of cytosolic glutamate under certain conditions and also for synthesis of glutamate under other conditions. L-leucine and its chemical analog 2-aminobicyclo[2.2.1] heptane-2-carboxylic acid (BCH) enhance the action of GDH when added at millimolar concentrations, and presumably as a result, they increase synaptosomal ammonia concentrations (18). Likewise, 10 mmol/L of gabapentin and pregabalin significantly increase GDH activity from rat brain (11,25). However, this effect occurs only at millimolar concentration and therefore is unlikely to be relevant for clinical treatment.

Effects on Neurotransmitter Receptors and Ion Channels

Radioligand Binding Studies

Gabapentin has been tested in a wide range of standardized radioligand binding assays and electrophysiologic responses *in vitro* and is remarkably silent in most tests (14). Gabapentin failed to displace radioligand binding at concentrations up to 100 μmol/L in standardized assays for GABA_A, GABA_B (including the subtypes GABA_B1a/2 and GABA_B1b/2) (39a,97a), benzodiazepine, glutamate, *N*-methyl-D-aspartic acid (NMDA), quisqualate, kainate, glycine, MK-801, and strychnine-insensitive glycine recep-

tors. In addition, gabapentin was inactive at the following: A1 and A2 adenosine receptors; α₁, α₂, and β-adrenergic receptors; D1 and D2 dopamine receptors; histamine H1 receptors; S1 and S2 serotonin receptors; M1, M2, and nicotinic acetylcholine receptors; δ, κ, and μ opiate receptors; leukotriene B₄, D₄, and thromboxane A₂ receptors; phorbol ester dibutyrate receptors; and binding sites on calcium channels labeled by nitrendipine and diltiazem and on sodium channels labeled by batrachotoxinin. These negative results suggest that gabapentin has a novel mechanism of action in comparison with many other drugs active in the central nervous system.

Gabapentin had little or no effect in several electrophysiologic tests with intracellular voltage records from cultured mouse spinal cord neurons *in vitro* (69) or in rat hippocampal slices *in vitro* (29). Furthermore, gabapentin did not alter responses to the application of GABA_A or GABA_B agonists in rat hippocampal slices or cultured neocortical neurons (39a,97a). Unlike GABA_A or GABA_B agonists or glutamate agonists, application of gabapentin (up to 500 μmol/L) did not alter resting neuronal membrane potential (69). Gabapentin had no effect on inhibitory responses of spinal cord neurons to GABA or glycine (69).

NMDA-Dependent Responses

Different studies have reported mixed results with gabapentin on responses dependent on NMDA receptors. When gabapentin was added to solutions bathing rat neocortical wedges (methods of ref. 30), it caused no responses and did not alter responses to the application of glutamate agonists NMDA, kainic acid, D,L-α-amino-3-hydroxy-5-methyl-isoxazole propionic acid (AMPA), or the NMDA antagonists 3-(2-carboxypiperazine-4-yl)propyl-1-phosphonic acid (CPP) or 7-chlorokynurenic acid with or without added glycine (L. Robichaud and P. Boxer, *personal communication*). Furthermore, the application of 100 μmol/L gabapentin did not change single-channel NMDA responses in outside-out patches with respect to the frequency of openings, mean open duration, burst duration, or mean number of openings per burst (69). In contrast to these negative results, another study (27) indicates that gabapentin enhances NMDA-induced currents in acutely isolated dorsal horn neurons, but only when the catalytic subunit of protein kinase C is applied intracellularly or when neurons are taken from acutely inflamed rats. Furthermore, the gabapentin effect reported by Gu and Huang (27) is accounted for by shifting the concentration–response curve so a lower concentration of the required coagonist, glycine, is required. Therefore, gabapentin is not expected to modulate NMDA receptors in saturating concentrations or very low concentrations of glycine. Enhancement of NMDA responses by gabapentin does not reconcile easily with an anticonvulsant effect. However, Gu and Huang (27) speculate that they recorded primarily from GABAergic interneurons, which may have increased excitability in response to gabapentin. These results, like those from neurotransmitter release studies (see earlier), suggest that gabapentin action in cellular systems may require altered states of cytosolic protein phosphorylation or sustained depolarization before they can be observed. Furthermore, the results of Gu and Huang raise the possibility that the effects of gabapentin may vary widely in different types of neurons (e.g., GABA neurons versus glutamate neurons).

Voltage-Gated Sodium Channels

Acute application of gabapentin had no effect on sustained repetitive firing of sodium-dependent action potentials of mouse spinal cord neurons or voltage-clamped calcium currents in dorsal root ganglion neurons (69). However, a different report indicates that gabapentin reduces sustained repetitive action potentials in cultured spinal cord cells when it is applied for longer periods (99). The modulation of action potentials by sustained gabapentin application probably occurs by a different mechanism from that of phenytoin, carbamazepine, or lamotrigine (67), because gabapentin and pregabalin do not interact with batrachotoxinin binding (105) even at high concentrations (*unpublished data*). Voltage-clamped sodium currents in a Chinese hamster ovary (CHO) cell line expressing sodium channel α subunits are not altered even by prolonged application of gabapentin (90), and sodium currents in acutely isolated neocortex neurons are not altered by gabapentin (81). Furthermore, gabapentin does not alter veratridine-induced cell death in cultured neocortical neurons (D. M. Rock, *personal communication*), whereas phenytoin, carbamazepine, and lamotrigine counteract veratridine. Therefore, the modulation of repetitive action potentials by gabapentin (99) appears to arise from a different molecular site of action than those of phenytoinlike anticonvulsants and needs further study.

Voltage-Gated Calcium Channels

The actions of gabapentin on voltage-clamped calcium currents also have been controversial. A study with acutely isolated rat neurons reported a small decrease in calcium currents (80), and this has been confirmed more recently by the same group (81). However, another published study with acutely isolated human neurons reported no effect of gabapentin (76), and a more recent study has not shown changes in calcium currents with gabapentin applied to neuronal pyramidal cell bodies (97). This latter report suggested that calcium influx in synaptosomes (isolated presynaptic endings) was indeed sensitive to gabapentin, and this has been shown independently using fluorescent tracer methods (21a,51), a finding suggesting that presynaptic calcium channels may be more sensitive to gabapentin than channels on cell bodies. Another a study reported inhibition of calcium

currents by gabapentin in cultured rat sensory neurons (89), but inhibition was only consistent and pronounced when neurons were previously exposed to an analog of cyclic adenosine monophosphate that activates protein kinase A. It is tempting to speculate that reduced calcium channel action is involved with the anticonvulsant action of gabapentin, particularly in light of high-affinity binding to the α2δ protein that interacts with calcium channels. However, it appears from the work published so far that gabapentin does not block calcium channels directly and completely (as do dihydropyridines or conotoxins). Furthermore, the reduced calcium channel function with gabapentin may not occur under all conditions, but may instead require the presence of presynaptic proteins (as in synaptosomes) or activation of specific cytosolic kinases. Additional work in this area is still needed to confirm the existing results with gabapentin and to clarify the conditions that are necessary for calcium channel modulation to occur.

EFFECTS OF GABAPENTIN ON MEMBRANE AMINO ACID TRANSPORT

Naturally occurring amino acids (and also gabapentin) are dually ionized at neutral pH. Because of this, they are not very soluble in lipids and have very little permeability to cell membranes by diffusion. To facilitate the transport of various amino acids across cell membranes, several families of specialized, membrane-bound proteins have evolved (12). Because gabapentin is an analog of a naturally occurring amino acid, it may be carried by one or more of the endogenous transport systems that are present in a variety of tissues. Initial studies of transport with gabapentin focused on transporters for glutamate and GABA that have specialized and highly selective transport mechanisms. Gabapentin and pregabalin at concentrations up to 1 mmol/L do not alter the uptake of [^{3}H]-GABA or [^{3}H]-D-aspartate into synaptosomes, cultured astrocytes, or CHO tumor cells. These results indicate that gabapentin is not a substrate or an inhibitor of either GABA or glutamate transporters (87).

System L Transport

Studies in humans and animals (82) and *in vitro* (83) show that gabapentin is transported across gut membranes into the bloodstream by a saturable mechanism similar to the large, neutral amino acid carrier (system L) of gut tissues. The transport of [^{3}H]-gabapentin and [^{3}H]-L-phenylalanine are mutually inhibitory, a finding indicating a common transport mechanism. These results and others published in the same report (82) indicate that one mechanism of gabapentin transit from gut to bloodstream is through a sodium-independent system L–like amino acid transporter.

The system L transporter and several other amino acid transporters have been characterized by radiotracer techniques in CHO tumor cells (87). System L actually represents a family of related sodium-independent transporters in various tissues that are relatively selective for neutral BCAAs and aromatic amino acids (12). Experiments with system L in CHO cells extend and confirm the notion that gabapentin competes with leucine for transport by system L.

The transport of [^{3}H]-gabapentin into CHO cells with different concentrations of substrate is shown in Figure 28.5A. Transport is mostly saturable, with Michaelis-Menten kinetics (K_m value of 35 µmol/L and V_{max} of 4.4 nmol/min/mg). These values of K_m and V_{max} are similar to those reported elsewhere for L-leucine. Uptake of gabapentin was inhibited more than 90% by L-leucine, L-valine, L-

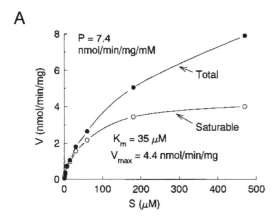

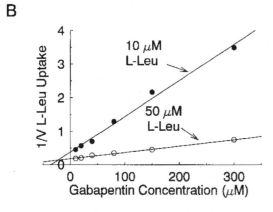

FIGURE 28.5. Tritiated gabapentin is transported into Chinese hamster ovary cells *in vitro* by system L. **A:** The initial rate of transport is saturable, with a K_m or half-maximum rate of transport at about 35 µmol/L. **B:** Inhibition of L-leucine transport by gabapentin is competitive with a K_i value of about 25 µmol/L, very similar to the K_m values for gabapentin transport (compare with A) and L-leucine transport (not shown). These data and others (see text) indicate that gabapentin and several other amino acids (L-leucine, L-isoleucine, L-valine, L-phenylalanine, and others) share a common transport mechanism, namely system L. (From T.-Z. Su and D. Oxender, Parke-Davis Research, *unpublished data*; also from Su TZ, Lunney E, Campbell G, et al. Transport of gabapentin, a gamma-amino acid drug, by system I alpha-amino acid transporters: a comparative study in astrocytes, synaptosomes, and CHO cells. *J Neurochem* 1995;64:2125–2131, with permission.)

isoleucine, L-phenylalanine, and the synthetic leucine analog BCH (2-aminobicyclo[2.2.1] heptane-2-carboxylic acid). The synthetic system A–specific amino acid analog MeAIB (methylaminoisobutyric acid) did not significantly inhibit gabapentin uptake. Thus, gabapentin behaves like a substrate of system L in CHO cells. A Dixon plot of the data with gabapentin inhibition of [^{3}H]-L-leucine uptake (Figure 28.5B) gives a K_i value similar to that for unlabeled L-leucine, consistent with competitive inhibition by a single transporter. Finally, both gabapentin and L-leucine facilitate the efflux of the other compound when they are added at the extracellular side of the membrane (this is called *transstimulation of efflux* and is a measure of heteroexchange). The heteroexchange of L-leucine and gabapentin confirms that a single transporter (system L) carries both amino acids.

System L transport also occurs in neuronal membranes and in astrocytes (6). In these systems, influx of [^{3}H]-gabapentin was more than 90% independent of sodium and was reciprocally inhibited by L-leucine, BCH, and unlabeled gabapentin. Thus, rat brain membranes have facilitated transport for gabapentin, a finding that may explain the accumulation of gabapentin in whole brain tissues (mostly representing cytosol) at higher concentrations than in the brain interstitial space (102).

Gabapentin is rapidly permeable to the blood–brain barrier (98,102) and is transported into brain tissues by a saturable mechanism accounted for by system L (47). In spite of the clear evidence that gabapentin is a transported by system L in various tissues, this appears not to account for anticonvulsant actions, because nonmetabolized substrates of system L transport such as BCH do not share the anticonvulsant properties of gabapentin in animal models.

TRITIATED GABAPENTIN BINDING

Studies with [^{3}H]-gabapentin reveal a specific binding site in brain (88). An elegant series of biochemical and molecular studies shows conclusively that the gabapentin binding site is identical with the $\alpha2\delta$ auxiliary protein subunit of voltage-gated calcium channels (23). A Scatchard analysis of specific binding activity shows a single site with apparent affinity constant or K_d of 38±2.8 nmol/L and density of binding sites or B_{max} of 4.6±0.4 pmol/mg protein (Figure 28.6A). [^{3}H]-Gabapentin binding is not altered by a wide variety of neuroactive substances including glutamate, GABA, NMDA, glycine, other anticonvulsants, or common neurotransmitters. In contrast, [^{3}H]-gabapentin binding is competitively blocked by low micromolar or high nanomolar concentrations of L-leucine, L-isoleucine, L-valine, and L-phenylalanine (7,95), but the significance of these findings remain unclear. However, the results with endogenous amino acids suggest that in brain tissues *in vivo*, the [^{3}H]-gabapentin binding site is saturated with endogenous BCAAs such as L-leucine.

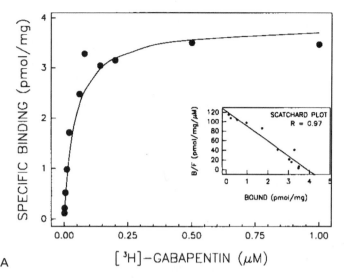
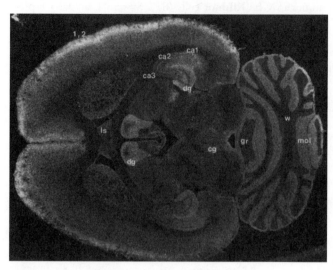

A   B

FIGURE 28.6. A: [3H]-Gabapentin binding to rat neocortex synaptic plasma membranes is saturable. Specific binding, defined by binding displaced by 100 μmol/L of (R,S)3-isobutyl γ-aminobutyric acid (GABA), was determined at increasing concentration of [3H]-gabapentin. Analysis of the Scatchard plot **(inset)** yielded a 50% saturation (K_d) value of 38 nmol/L and a maximum density of binding sites (B_{max}) of 4.6 pmol/mg protein. **B:** The autoradiographic localization of [3H]-gabapentin binding sites in a coronal section of rat brain tissue is shown. Highest densities of binding are seen in neocortex layers I and II *(1, 2)* and dendritic regions of hippocampus (CA1, CA2, and CA3 subfields and dentate gyrus or *dg*). The molecular layer of cerebellum *(mol)* also has a high density of binding, whereas the granule layer of cerebellum *(gr)*, lateral septum *(ls)*, and white matter *(w)* have low densities. [A, From Suman-Chauhan et al. (88); B, from Hill et al. (31), with permission.]

α2δ Protein has been cloned and functionally expressed at the cell membrane in a number of recombinant cell systems. α2δ Function is necessary for the high-level expression and function of the main ion-conducting calcium channel protein, α1. The function of α2δ proteins has been reviewed previously (20). Furthermore, four distinct α2δ–like proteins have been cloned and expressed in recombinant systems. Each of the four types function together with other calcium channel subunits (37). However, [3H]-gabapentin binds significantly only to the α2δ1 and α2δ2 isoforms, and not to α2δ3 or α2δ4 (49). The α2δ1 isoform is expressed widely in various tissues (e.g., brain, striate and cardiac muscle, glands), whereas expression of type 2 is somewhat more restricted to the central nervous system. It is not known which subtypes contribute most to the pharmacology of gabapentin for prevention of seizures. Mutagenesis studies of the α2δ1 protein have shown that binding of [3H]-gabapentin occurs to the extracellular portion of the protein, which binds gabapentin in the absence of the transmembrane domain (8), and requires several individual identified amino acid residues (100).

Autoradiographic studies (31) show that specific binding of gabapentin is highest in the superficial layers of neocortex and dendritic layers of hippocampus, with low levels of binding in white matter and brainstem (Figure 28.6B). Thus, gabapentin binding is densest in areas rich in synapses. [3H]-Gabapentin binding is displaced by unla-

beled gabapentin and by several structural analogs of gabapentin including pregabalin and additional gabapentin and pregabalin analogs (10,88). The two enantiomers of pregabalin have different potencies for binding at the gabapentin site, and the same stereospecificity for these enantiomers is seen in anticonvulsant studies with whole animals (94). Together, these findings indicate that the anticonvulsant actions of gabapentin and chemically similar compounds relate to binding at the [3H]-gabapentin site.

CONCLUSION

Gabapentin has significant anticonvulsant action in well-controlled clinical studies. The profile of anticonvulsant activity in a variety of animal models suggests that gabapentin differs pharmacologically from other anticonvulsants. Several *in vitro* actions of gabapentin are summarized in Table 28.3, along with information on concentration dependence that helps to assess the relevance for anticonvulsant or behavioral actions. Although numerous pharmacologic actions have been reported *in vitro*, it is not yet clear which actions are the most relevant for preventing seizures. The access of gabapentin from the gut to the brain depends on system L amino acid transport. Gabapentin is a potent ligand for displacement of [3H]-gabapentin binding

TABLE 28.3. SUMMARY OF IN VITRO ACTIONS OF GABAPENTIN.

Test System	Primary Observation	Concentration of Gabapentin	Direct Action?	Reference
[^{3}H]-Gabapentin binding to α2δ protein	Specific binding inhibited by gabapentin and derivatives, L-leucine	IC_{50} = 0.8 μmol/L	Yes, also occurs with binding to solubilized or recombinant protein	88
Action potential firing (cultured mouse spinal neurons)	Reduced action potential firing (prolonged treatment)	IC_{50} = 20 μmol/L for application times 60 min	Probably indirect, [voltage-clamped Na$^+$ currents not blocked (81)]	99
Monoamine neurotransmitter release (striatal or neocortical brain slices)	10%–40% Decrease in release of [^{3}H]-norepinephrine, [^{3}H]-dopamine, and [^{3}H]-serotonin	10–100 μmol/L (IC_{50} ~10 μmol)	Direct action on Ca^{2+} channels (?) or vesicle release machinery (?)	15, 68, 75
Ca^{2+} fluorescence and [^{3}H]-norepinephrine release in synaptosomes	Reduced release and fluorescence by 15%–30%	~10 μmol/L	Direct action on Ca^{2+} channels (?)	21a, 51, 97
[^{3}H]-Glutamate release in trigeminal nucleus slices	Reduced in tissue pretreated with substance P	~10 μmol/L	May be a direct action on Ca^{2+} channels or vesicle release machinery	48
Ca^{2+} channel function (voltage clamp) with cultured or acutely isolated neurons	~15%–50% decrease in current	1–100 μmol/L	Direct effect? may require activation of protein kinase A	2, 80, 81, 89
Reduced synaptic currents in voltage-clamped neuronal tissue slices	Up to 50% decrease in synaptic currents	10–100 μmol/L	Unknown, presynaptic (?)	54a, 62, 77 97
Enhanced reversal of GABA transport (rat optic nerve and hippocampal slices)	Increase in electrophysiologic response to 1 mmol/L nipecotic acid or increased GABA$_A$ current	100 μmol/L	Unknown	32, 33, 38
Enhanced GABA transporter activity in cultured neurons	100% increase in initial rate of GABA transport	EC_{50} approx. 20 μmol/L	Unknown	
Cell death from blockade of glutamate uptake (rat spinal cord cultures)	Reduced cell death of motor neurons	100 μmol/L	Blockade of BCAA-T and reduced glutamate synthesis (?)	41, 71, 101
NMDA response (voltage clamp with isolated spinal cord neurons)	25% Increase in NMDA current (shift in glycine dependence)	100 μmol/L	Probably indirect, requires protein kinase C catalytic subunit	27, 69
Glutamic acid decarboxylase enzyme activity	45% Enhanced V_{max}, no change in K_M (58)	1 mmol/L	Apparently; occurs in partially purified enzyme *in vitro*	93
BCAA-T enzyme activity	Competitive inhibition	K_i = 0.7 mmol/L, calculated inhibition *in vivo* ~10%	Apparently; occurs in partially purified enzyme *in vitro*	25, 35, 41
GABA transaminase enzyme activity	Mixed-type competitive and noncompetitive inhibition	K_i = 25 mmol/L, calculated inhibition *in vivo* <1%	Apparently; occurs in partially purified enzyme *in vitro*	25

GABA, γ-aminobutyric acid; BCAA-T, branched-chain amino acid aminotransferase; NMDA, *N*-methyl-D-aspartate; V_{max}, rate constant of enzyme activity; KM, affinity constant of enyme activity; Ki, affinity constant of inhibition.

to the α2δ protein, and this binding activity appears to correlate with anticonvulsant activity (9,10).

Gabapentin has a pronounced three-dimensional structural similarity to L-leucine (Figure 28.1), and gabapentin mimics the action of L-leucine at several sites, such as [^{3}H]-gabapentin binding, system L transport, BCAA-T enzyme, and GDH enzyme. In contrast to L-leucine, gabapentin does not appear to be metabolized by enzymes of brain cytosol. It seems unlikely that L-leucine–like actions are necessary for the anticonvulsant effects of gabapentin,

because other L-leucine analogs such as BCH do not share the anticonvulsant activity of gabapentin.

The findings of Kocsis et al. (38,54,32,33) suggest that gabapentin increases the nonsynaptic release of GABA from neuronal tissues, and the human studies of Petroff et al. (63, 64) indicate that gabapentin increases brain GABA concentrations. It is tempting to speculate that changes in GABA transporter function or GABA cellular concentration may be involved in the molecular basis of these effects. Numerous studies have addressed effects of gabapentin on sodium channels, calcium channels, and NMDA receptors. To date, these have not offered a single consistent view of gabapentin action. However, it is hoped that additional studies soon will give a more complete picture of the cellular and molecular basis of the anticonvulsant action of gabapentin. Such studies may also give insight into basic mechanisms involved in the disease of epilepsy and the onset of seizures.

ACKNOWLEDGMENTS

I wish to thank many colleagues and investigators who have studied gabapentin including Mark Vartanian, Barbra Stewart, Ti-Zhi Su, Arie Goldlust, Dale Oxender, David Rock, Greg Campbell, Mark Weber, Sean Donevan, David Hill, Jason Brown, Nick Gee, David Dooley, Susan Hutson, Kay LaNone, Kathy Sutton, Roland Jones, Sean Donevan, Jim Offord, Michael Quick, Jeff Kocsis, Leonard Meltzer, Beth Lunney, Sandy McKnight, Devin Welty, Janet Stringer, Ognen Petroff, Jeff Kocsis, and George Richerson.

REFERENCES

1. Abdi S, Lee DH, Chung JM. The anti-allodynic effects of amitriptyline, gabapentin, and lidocaine in a rat model of neuropathic pain. *Anesth Analg* 1998;87:1360–1366.
2. Alden KJ, Garcia J. Differential effect of gabapentin on neuronal and muscle calcium currents. *J Pharmacol Exp Ther* 2001; 297:727–735.
3. Andrews J, Chadwick D, Bates D. Gabapentin in partial epilepsy. *Lancet* 1990;335:1114–1117.
4. Backonja M, Beydoun A, Edwards KR, et al. Gabapentin for the symptomatic treatment of painful neuropathy in patients with diabetes mellitus. *JAMA* 1998;280:1831–1836.
5. Bartoszyk GD, Meyerson N, Reimann W, et al. Gabapentin. In: Meldrum BS, Porter RJ, eds. Curent Problems in Epilepsy, Vol 4, London, John Libbey, P., 1986; 147–163.
6. Brookes N. Interaction between the glutamine cycle and the uptake of large neutral amino acids in astrocytes. *J Neurochem* 1993;60:1923–1928.
7. Brown JP, Dissanayake VU, Briggs AR, et al. Isolation of the [³H]gabapentin-binding protein/alpha 2 delta Ca2⁺ channel subunit from porcine brain: development of a radioligand binding assay for alpha 2 delta subunits using [³H]leucine. *Anal Biochem* 1998;255:236–243.
8. Brown JP, Gee NS. Cloning and deletion mutagenesis of the alpha2 delta calcium channel subunit from porcine cerebral cortex: expression of a soluble form of the protein that retains [³H]gabapentin binding activity. *J Biol Chem* 1998;273: 25458–25465.
9. Bryans JS, Davies N, Gee NS, et al. Identification of novel ligands for the gabapentin binding site on the alpha2delta subunit of a calcium channel and their evaluation as anticonvulsant agents. *J Med Chem* 1998;41:1838–1845.
10. Bryans JS, Wustrow DJ. 3-substituted GABA analogs with central nervous system activity: a review. *Med Res Rev* 1999;19: 149–177.
11. Cho SW, Cho EH, Choi SY. Activation of two types of brain glutamate dehydrogenase isoproteins by gabapentin. *FEBS Lett* 1998;426:196–200.
12. Christensen HN. Role of amino acid transport and countertransport in nutrition and metabolism. *Pharmacol Rev* 1990;70:43–77.
13. Cutter NC, Scott DD, Johnson JC, et al. Gabapentin effect on spasticity in multiple sclerosis: a placebo-controlled, randomized trial. *Arch Phys Med Rehabil* 2000;81:164–169.
14. Diener HC, Hacke W, Hennerici M, et al. Lubeluzole in acute ischemic stroke: a double-blind, placebo-controlled phase II trial. *Stroke* 1996;27:76–81.
15. Dooley DJ, Donovan CM, Pugsley TA. Stumulus-dependent modulation of [³H]norepinephrine release from rat neocortical slices by gabapentin and pregabalin. *J Pharmacol Exp Ther* 2000;296:1086–1098.
16. Dooley DJ, Mieske CA, Borosky SA. Inhibition of K(+)-evoked glutamate release from rat neocortical and hippocampal slices by gabapentin. *Neurosci Lett* 2000;280:107–110.
17. During M, Ryder KM, Spencer DD. Hippocampal GABA transporter function in temporal-lobe epilepsy. *Nature* 1995; 376:174–177.
18. Ericinska M, Nelson D. Activation of glutamate dehydrogenase by leucine and its nonmetalizable analogue in rat brain synaptosomes. *J Neurochem* 1990;54:1335–1343.
19. Ericinska M, Nelson D, Wilson DF, et al. Neurotransmitter amino acids in the CNS. I. Regional changes in amino acid levels in rat brain during ischemia and reperfusion. *Brain Res* 1990;304:9–22.
20. Felix R. Voltage-dependent Ca2+ channel alpha2delta auxiliary subunit: structure, function and regulation. *Receptors Channels* 1999;6:351–362.
21. Field MJ, Oles RJ, Lewis AS, et al. Gabapentin (Neurontin) and S-(+)-3-isobutyl GABA represent a novel class of selective antihyperalgesic agents. *Br J Pharmacol* 1997;121:1513–1522.
21a. Fink K, dolley DJ, Meder WP, et al. Inhibition of neuronal Ca²⁺ influx by gabapentin and pregabalin in the human cortex. *Neuropharmacol* 2002;42:229–236.
22. Gaspary HL, Wang W, Richerson GB. Carrier-mediated GABA release activates GABA receptors on hippocampal neurons. *J Neurophysiol* 1998;80:270–281.
23. Gee NS, Brown JP, Dissanayake VU, et al. The novel anticonvulsant drug, gabapentin (Neurontin), binds to the alpha2delta subunit of a calcium channel. *J Biol Chem* 1996;271:5768–5776.
24. Goa KL, Sorkin EM. Gabapentin: a review of its pharmacological properties and clinical potential in epilepsy. *Drugs* 1993; 46:409–427.
25. Goldlust A, Su TZ, Welty DF, et al. Effects of anticonvulsant drug gabapentin on the enzymes in metabolic pathways of glutamate and GABA. *Epilepsy Res* 1995;22:1–11.
26. Gruenthal M, Mueller M, Olson WL, et al. Gabapentin for the treatment of spasticity in patients with spinal cord injury. *Spinal Cord* 1997;35:686–689.
27. Gu Y, Huang L-YM. Gabapentin actions on NMDA channels are PKC dependent. *Mol Pharmacol* 2001.
28. Gurney ME, Cutting FB, Zhai P, et al. Benefit of vitamin E, riluzole, and gabapentin in a transgenic model of familial amyotrophic lateral sclerosis. *Ann Neurol* 1996;39:147–157.
29. Haas HL, Wieser HG. Gabapentin: action on hippocampal slices of the rat and effects in human epilepticss. Paper presented at the Northern European Epilepsy Meeting, York, UK, 1986.
30. Harrison NL, Simmonds MA. Quantitative studies on some antagonists of *N*-methyl-D-aspartate in slices of rat cerebral cortex. *Br J Pharmacol* 1985;84:381–391.
31. Hill DR, Suman CN, Woodruff GN. Localization of [³H]gabapentin to a novel site in rat brain: autoradiographic studies. *Eur J Pharmacol* 1993;244:303–309.
32. Honmou O, Kocsis JD, Richerson GB. Gabapentin potentiates the conductance increase induced by nipecotic acid in CA1 pyramidal neurons *in vitro*. *Epilepsy Res* 1995;20:193–202.

33. Honmou O, Oyelese AA, Kocsis JD. The anticonvulsant gabapentin enhances promoted release of GABA in hippocampus: a field potential analysis. *Brain Res* 1995;692:273–277.

34. Hosford DA, Wang Y. Utility of the lethargic (lh/lh) mouse model of absence seizures in predicting the effects of lamotrigine, vigabatrin, tiagabine, gabapentin, and topiramate against human absence seizures. *Epilepsia* 1997;38:408–414.

35. Hutson SM, Berkich D, Drown P, et al. Role of branched-chain aminotransferase isoenzymes and gabapentin in neurotransmitter metabolism. *J Neurochem* 1998;71:863–874.

36. Jun JH, Yaksh TL. The effect of intrathecal gabapentin and 3-isobutyl gamma-aminobutyric acid on the hyperalgesia observed after thermal injury in the rat. *Anesth Analg* 1998;86:348–354.

37. Klugbauer N, Lacinova L, Marais E, et al. Molecular diversity of the dalcium channel alpha-2-delta subunit. *J Neurosci* 1999;19:684–691.

38. Kocsis JD, Honmou O. Gabapentin increases GABA-induced depolarization in rat neonatal optic nerve. *Neurosci Lett* 1994;169:181–184.

39. Krall RL, Penry JK, White BG, et al. Antiepileptic drug development. II. Anticonvulsant drug screening. *Epilepsia* 1978;19:409–428.

39a. Lanneau C, Green A, Hirst WD, et al. Gabapentin is not a GABA_B receptor agonist. *Neuropharmacol* 2001;41:965–975.

40. Larsson OM, et al. Differential effect of gamma-vinyl GABA and valproate on GABA-transaminase from cultured neurons and astrocytes. *Neuropharmacology* 1986;25:617–625.

41. Lieth E, LaNoue KF, Berkich D, et al. Nitrogen shuttling between neurons and glial cells during glutamate synthesis. *J Neurochem* 2001;76:1712–1723.

42. Lippert B, Metcalf BW, Jung MJ, et al. 4-Amino-hex-5-enoic acid, a selective catalytic inhibitor of 4-aminobutyric-acid aminotransferase in mammalian brain. *Eur J Biochem* 1977;74:441–445.

43. Loscher W, Honack D, Taylor CP. Gabapentin increases aminooxyacetic acid-induced GABA accumulation in several regions of rat brain. *Neurosci Lett* 1991;128:150–154.

44. Loscher W, Reissmuller E, Ebert U. Anticonvulsant efficacy of gabapentin and levetiracetam in phenytoin-resistant kindled rats. *Epilepsy Res* 2000;40:63–77.

45. Löscher W. Valproate enhances GABA turnover in the substantia nigra. *Brain Res* 1989;501:198–203.

46. Luecke A, Musshoff U, Koehling R, et al. Gabapentin potentiation of the antiepileptic efficacy of vigabatrin in an in vitro model of epilepsy. *Br J Pharmacol* 1998;124:370–376.

47. Luer MS, Hamani C, Dujovny M, et al. Saturable transport of gabapentin at the blood-brain barrier. *Neurol Res* 1999;21:559–562.

48. Maneuf YP, McKnight AT. Gabapentin inhibits substance P- and calcitonin gene-related peptide-facilitated K+-evoked release of [3H]-glutamate from rat caudal trigeminal nucleus slices. *Soc Neurosci Abstr* 2000;26:1931–1931.

49. Marais E, Klugbauer N, Hofmann F. Calcium channel alpha-2-delta subunits: structure and gabapentin binding. *Mol Pharmacol* 2001;59:1243–1248.

50. McLean MJ, Ramsey RE, Leppik I, et al. Gabapentin as add-on therapy in refractory partial epilepsy: a double-blind, placebo-controlled, parallel-group study. *Neurology* 1993;43:2292–2298.

51. Meder WP, Dooley DJ. Modulation of K+-induced synaptosomal calcium influx by gabapentin. *Brain Res* 2000;875:157–159.

52. Meldrum BS. GABAergic mechanisms in the pathogenesis and treatment of epilepsy. *Br J Clin Pharmacol* 1989;27:3S–11S.

53. Michelitti G, Vergnes M, Marescaux C, et al. Antiepileptic drug evaluation in a new animal model: spontaneous petit mal epilepsy in the rat. *Arzneimittelforshung* 1985;35:483–485.

54. Mirchandani GR, Agulian S, Abi-Saab W, et al. Vigabatrin increases total GABA levels in rat optic nerve while gabapentin and pregabalin do not. *Soc Neurosci Abstr* 1999;25:1868–1868.

54a. Misner DL, Kansagara AG, Bonhaus DW. Effects of gabapentin on hippocampal CA1 neurons. *Soc Neurosci Abstr* 2001;27:711.5.

55. Ng GYK, Bertrand S, Sullivan R, et al. Gamma-aminobutyric acid type B receptors with specific heterodimer composition and postsynaptic actions in hippocampal neurons are targets of anticonvulsant gabapentin action. *Mol Pharmacol* 2001;59:144–152.

56. Ochi S, Lim JY, Rand MN, et al. Transient presence of GABA in astrocytes of the developing optic nerve. *Glia* 1993;9:188–198.

57. Otsuki K, Morimoto K, Sato K, et al. Effects of lamotrigine and conventional antiepileptic drugs on amygdala- and hippocampal-kindled seizures in rats. *Epilepsy Res* 1998;31:101–112.

58. Palfreyman MG, Schechter PJ, Buckett WR, et al. The pharmacology of GABA-transaminase inhibitiors. *Biochem Pharmacol* 1981;30:817–824.

59. Pan H-L, Chen S-R, Eisenach JC. Gabapentin suppresses ectopic nerve discharges and reverses allodynia in neuropathic rats. *J Pharmacol Exp Ther* 1998;288:1026–1030.

60. Pande AC, Davidson JR, Jefferson JW, et al. Treatment of social phobia with gabapentin: a placebo-controlled study. *J Clin Psychopharmacol* 1999;19:341–348.

61. Partridge BJ, Chaplan SR, Sakamoto E, et al. Characterization of the effects of gabapentin and 3-isobutyl-gamma-aminobutyric acid on substance P–induced thermal hyperalgesia. *Anesthesiology* 1998;88:196–205.

62. Patel MK, Gonzalez MI, Bramwell S, et al. Gabapentin inhibits excitatory synaptic transmission in the hyperalgesic spinal cord. *Br J Pharmacol* 2000;130:1731–1734.

63. Petroff OA, Hyder F, Rothman DL, et al. Effects of gabapentin on brain GABA, homocarnosine, and pyrrolidinone in epilepsy patients. *Epilepsia* 2000;41:675–680.

64. Petroff OA, Rothman DL, Behar KL, et al. The effect of gabapentin on brain gamma-aminobutyric acid in patients with epilepsy. *Ann Neurol* 1996;39:95–99.

65. Pin JP, Bockaert J. Two distinct mechanisms, differentially affected by excitatory amino acids, trigger GABA release from fetal mouse striatal neurons in primary culture. *J Neurosci* 1989;9:648–656.

66. Priebe MM, Sherwood AM, Graves DE, et al. Effectiveness of gabapentin in controlling spasticity: a quantitative study. *Spinal Cord* 1997;35:171–175.

67. Ragsdale DS, Scheuer T, Catterall WA. Frequency and voltage-dependent inhibition of type IIA Na+ channels, expressed in a mammalian cell line, by local anesthetic, antiarrhythmic, and anticonvulsant drugs. *Mol Pharmacol* 1991;40:756–765.

68. Reimann W. Inhibition by GABA, baclofen and gabapentin of dopamine release from rabbit caudate nucleus: are there common or different sites of action? *Eur J Pharmacol* 1983;94:341–344.

69. Rock DM, Kelly KM, Macdonald RL. Gabapentin actions on ligand- and voltage-gated responses in cultured rodent neurons. *Epilepsy Res* 1993;16:89–98.

70. Rogawski MA, Porter RJ. Antiepileptic drugs: pharmacological mechanisms and clinical efficacy with consideration of promising developmental stage compounds. *Pharmacol Rev* 1990;42:223–286.

71. Rothstein JD, Kuncl RW. Neuroprotective strategies in a model of chronic glutamate-mediated motor neuron toxicity. *J Neurochem* 1995;65:643–651.

72. Rothstein JD. Therapeutic horizons of amyotrophic lateral sclerosis. *Curr Opinions Neurobiol* 1996;6:679–687.

73. Rowbotham MC, Harden N, Stacey B, et al. Gabapentin for

the treatment of postherpetic neuralgia: a randomized controlled trial. *JAMA* 1998;280:1837–1842.

74. Satzinger G. Antiepileptics from gamma-aminobutyric acid. *Arzneimittelforschung* 1994;44:261–266.

75. Schlicker E, Reimann W, Gothert M. Gabapentin decreases monoamine release without affecting acetylcholine release in the brain. *Arzheimittelforschung* 1985;35:1347–1349.

76. Schumacher TB, Beck H, Steinhauser C, et al. Effects of gabapentin, phenytoin and carbamazepine on calcium currents in hippocampal granule cells from patients with temporal lobe epilepsy. *Epilepsia* 1997.

77. Shimoyama M, Shimoyama N, Hori Y. Gabapentin affects glutamatergic excitatory neurotransmission in the rat dorsal horn. *Pain* 2000;85:405–414.

78. Singh L, Field MJ, Ferris P, et al. The antiepileptic agent gabapentin (Neurontin) possesses anxiolytic-like and antinociceptive actions that are reversed by D-serine. *Psychopharmacology (Berl)* 1996;127:1–10.

79. Stasheff SF, Bragdon AC, Wilson WA. Induction of epileptiform activity in hippocampal slices by trains of electrical stimuli. *Brain Res* 1985;344:296–301.

80. Stefani A, Spadoni F, Bernardi G. Gabapentin inhibits calcium currents in isolated rat brain neurons. *Neuropharmacology* 1998;37:83–91.

81. Stefani A, Spadoni F, Giacomini P, et al. The effects of gabapentin on different ligand- and voltage-gated currents in isolated cortical neurons. *Epilepsy Res* 2001;43:239–248.

82. Stewart BH, Kugler AR, Thompson PR, et al. A saturable transport mechanism in the intestinal absorption of gabapentin is the underlying cause of the lack of proportionality between increasing dose and drug levels in plasma. *Pharm Res* 1993;10:276–281.

83. Stewart BH, Reyner EL, Lu RH. Mechanism of gabapentin (Neurontin) transport across monolayers of human colon adenocarcinoma cells (CACO-2). *Amino Acids* 1993;5:204–204.

84. Stringer JL, Lorenzo N. The reduction in paired-pulse inhibition in the rat hippocampus by gabapentin is independent of GABA(B) receptor activation. *Epilepsy Res* 1999;33:93–97.

85. Stringer JL, Lothman EW. Maximal dentate activation: a tool to screen compounds for activity against limbic seizures. *Epilepsy Res* 1990;5:169–176.

86. Stringer JL, Taylor CP. The effects of gabapentin in the rat hippocampus are mimicked by two structural analogs, but not by nimodipine. *Epilepsy Res* 2000;41:155–162.

87. Su TZ, Lunney E, Campbell G, et al. Transport of gabapentin, a gamma-amino acid drug, by system l alpha-amino acid transporters: a comparative study in astrocytes, synaptosomes, and CHO cells. *J Neurochem* 1995;64:2125–2131.

88. Suman CN, Webdale L, Hill DR, et al. Characterisation of [³H]gabapentin binding to a novel site in rat brain: homogenate binding studies. *Eur J Pharmacol* 1993;244:293–301.

89. Sutton KG, Scott RH, Lee K, et al. Gabapentin inhibits high threshold calcium channel currents in cultured dorsal root ganglion neurones. *Soc Neurosci Abstr* 2000;26:234.4.

90. Taylor CP. The anticonvulsant lamotrigine blocks sodium currents from cloned alpha-subunits of rat brain Na⁺ channels in a voltage-dependent manner but gabapentin does not. *Soc Neurosci Abstr* 1993;23:1631.

91. Taylor CP. *Mechanisms of new antiepileptic drugs*, 3rd ed. Delgado-Escuelo AU, Wilson WA, Oslen RW, et al, eds. Philadelphia; Lippincott Williams & Wilkins, 1999:1011–1026.

92. Taylor CP, Gee NS, Su TZ, et al. A summary of mechanistic hypotheses of gabapentin pharmacology. *Epilepsy Res* 1998;29:233–249.

93. Taylor CP, Vartanian MG, Andruszkiewicz R, et al. 3-alkyl GABA and 3-alkylglutamic acid analogues: two new classes of anticonvulsant agents. *Epilepsy Res* 1992;11:103–110.

94. Taylor CP, Vartanian MG, Yuen PW, et al. Potent and stereospecific anticonvulsant activity of 3-isobutyl GABA relates to in vitro binding at a novel site labeled by tritiated gabapentin. *Epilepsy Res* 1993;14:11–15.

95. Thurlow RJ, Hill DR, Woodruff GN. Comparison of the uptake of [³H]-gabapentin with the uptake of L-[³H]-leucine into rat brain synaptosomes. *Br J Pharmacol* 1996;118:449–456.

96. Upton N. Mechanisms of action of new antiepileptic drugs: rational design and serendipitous findings. *Trends Pharmacol Sci* 1994;15:456–463.

97. vanHooft JA, Dougherty D, Endeman D, et al. Gabapentin inhibits presynaptic but not postsynaptic voltage-operated calcium channels in rat neocortex and hippocampus. *Soc Neurosci Abstr* 2000;26:662.7.

97a. Vartanian MG, Donovan DM, Weber ML, et al. Gabapentin does not interact with the GABA_B receptor. *Soc Neurosci Abstr* 2001;27:603.3.

98. Vollmer KO, vonHodenberg A, Koelle EU. Pharmacokinetics and metabolism of gabapentin in rat, dog and man. *Arzneimittelforschung* 1986;36:830–839.

99. Wamil AW, McLean MJ. Limitation by gabapentin of high frequency action potential firing by mouse central neurons in cell culture. *Epilepsy Res* 1994;17:1–11.

100. Wang M, Offord J, Oxender DL, et al. Structural requirement of the calcium-channel subunit alpha2delta for gabapentin binding. *Biochem J* 1999;342:313–320.

101. Welty DF, Schielke GP, Rothstein JD. Potential treatment of amyotrophic lateral sclerosis by the anticonvulsant gabapentin: a hypothesis. *Ann Pharmacother* 1995;29:1164–1167.

102. Welty DF, Schielke GP, Vartanian MG, et al. Gabapentin anticonvulsant action in rats: disequilibrium with peak drug concentrations in plasma and brain microdialysate. *Epilepsy Res* 1993;16:175–181.

103. Welty DF, Wang Y, Busch JA, et al. Pharmacokinetics and pharmacodynamics of CI-1008 (pregabalin) and gabapentin in rats using maximal electroshock. *Epilepsia* 1997; 35–36.

103a. Whitworth TL, Quick MW. Upregulation of γ–aminobutyric acid transporter expression: role of alkylated γ–aminobutyric acid derivatives. *Bioch Soc Trans* 2001;29:736–741.

104. Williamson J, Lothman EW, Taylor CP, et al. Comparison of S-(+)-3-isobutyl GABA and gabapentin against kindled hippocampal seizures. *Epilepsia* 1997;38:29–29.

105. Willow M, Catterall WA. Inhibition of the binding of [³H]batrachotoxinin A 20-α-benzoate to sodium channels by the anticonvulsant drugs diphenylhydantoin and carbamazepine. *Mol Pharmacol* 1982;22:627–635.

106. Wu Y, Wang W, Richerson GB. GABA transaminase inhibition induces spontaneous and enhances depolarization-evoked GABA efflux through reversal of the GABA transporter. *J Neurosci* 2001;21:2630–2639.

107. Xiao W-H, Bennett GJ. Gabapentin has an antinociceptive effect mediated via a spinal site of action in a rat model of painful peripheral neuropathy. *Analgesia* 1996;2:267–273.

108. Xiong Z-Q, Stringer JL. Effects of felbamate, gabapentin and lamotrigine on seizure parameters and excitability in the rat hippocampus. *Epilepsy Res* 1997;27:187–194.

GABAPENTIN

CHEMISTRY, BIOTRANSFORMATION, PHARMACOKINETICS, AND INTERACTIONS

FRANK J. E. VAJDA

OVERVIEW

Gabapentin (GBP), although designed as a γ-aminobutyric acid (GABA) analog, is not clearly GABAmimetic. First synthesized and tested in animals at Goedecke, in Freiburg, GBP has a simple pharmacokinetic profile, minimal propensity for drug interactions, and a lack of idiosyncratic reactions to date; thus, it is a valuable and safe drug (1,2). It was demonstrated early that GBP was not metabolized extensively either in rodents or in humans and that it penetrates the brain readily (3,4). GBP is 1-(aminomethyl)-cyclohexaneacetic acid. Absorption appears to be dependent on transport by the L-system amino acid transporter. Its elimination half-life is relatively short. It is cleared unchanged by the kidney (5). It is not protein bound, not metabolized, and has no significant drug–drug interactions (6). It is the first antiepileptic drug (AED) since bromide to be eliminated entirely by the kidney, a property shared with vigabatrin (7). It does not induce hepatic oxidation; thus, it may be a drug of choice in acute intermittent porphyria. In addition to its use in epilepsy, GBP has been evaluated in neuropsychiatric and pain disorders to define its psychoactive properties (8).

CHEMISTRY AND METABOLIC SCHEME

GBP is a conformationally restricted analog of GABA, not metabolically converted to GABA or its antagonists, nor is it an inhibitor of GABA uptake or degradation. It has higher lipid solubility than GABA (9). Structurally, GBP

incorporates GABA into a cyclohexane ring (Figure 29.1). A bitter-tasting crystalline substance with a molecular weight of 171.34, it is highly water soluble (octanol:aqueous pH 7.4 buffer partition coefficient log P = −1.10). It has two negative log of dissociation constant (pKa) values at 3.68 and 10.70 at 25°C and is a zwitterion at physiologic pH (5). Significantly, GBP resembles the bulky hydrophobic amino acids, L-leucine and L-phenylalanine, despite its not having a chiral carbon or an amino group α to the carboxyl group. GBP has a melting point of 165 to 167°C. As confirmed by x-ray structure analysis, the pseudoring configuration of the GABA molecule is integrated into a lipophilic cyclohexane system (10).

BIOAVAILABILITY

Accumulation after multiple dose administration is predictable from single dose data (11,12). After intravenous administration, the pharmacokinetics of GBP is best described by a three-compartment model (10), with half-life values for each phase being 0.1, 0.6, and 5.3 hours, respectively. The contribution of the terminal phase is 90% of the total area under the plasma concentration curve, which may be of significance in penetration of the

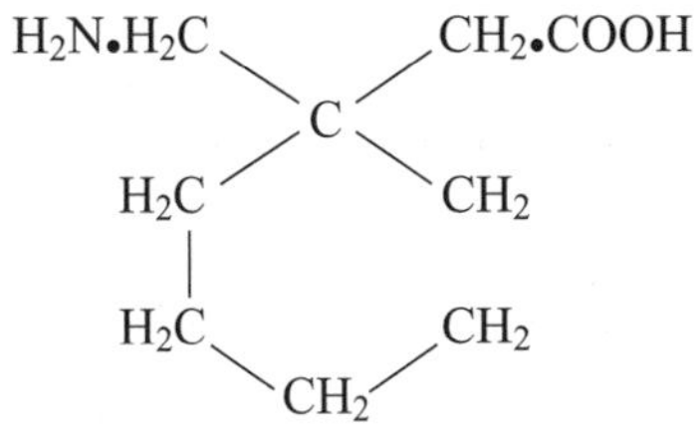

FIGURE 29.1. Formulas for gabapentin.

Frank J.E. Vajda, MD, FRACP: Professorial Fellow, Department of Medicine, University of Melbourne; and Director, Raoul Wallenberg Australian Centre for Clinical Neuropharmacology, St. Vincent's Hospital, Victoria, Australia

blood–brain barrier (13). Bioavailability of GBP is found to be 40% to 60% after oral administration of single 300- to 600-mg doses (10,14), and it is reported to be approximately 35% at a steady dosage of 1,500 mg three times daily. Time of maximum concentration is achieved in 2 to 3 hours. Maximum brain levels are expected after 1 hour after intravenous administration. Volume of distribution is calculated at steady state to be approximately 50 to 58 L (15). The only pharmacokinetic parameter significantly different between genders is maximum concentration, which is higher in women, likely the result of a smaller volume distribution.

FORMULATIONS

GBP formulations are available as 100-, 300-, 400-, and 800-mg capsules. A liquid syrup form of GBP has limited use in younger children (16). GBP is supplied only for administration orally.

PLASMA PROTEIN BINDING

The degree of protein binding is virtually nil for GBP (1,17).

CEREBROSPINAL FLUID, BRAIN, AND OTHER TISSUES

GBP levels in human brain are 80% of those in serum, a finding confirming animal distribution studies (18,19). Concentrations in human cerebrospinal fluid (CSF) are 5% to 35% of plasma levels, and tissue concentrations are approximately 80% of plasma levels (14,20). Ben Menachem and colleagues evaluated penetration of GBP into human CSF and its effects on free and total GABA, homovanillic acid, and 5-hydroxyindoleacetic acid. Five patients were given a single oral dose of GBP, 600 mg (four patients) and 1,200 mg (one patient). Plasma and CSF were collected for 72 hours. CSF:plasma GBP ratios were 0.1 after 6 hours. Free and total GABA concentrations were unchanged, but CSF 5-hydroxyindoleacetic acid and homovanillic acid concentrations increased at 24 and 72 hours (21). A study of simultaneous estimation of influx and efflux blood–brain barrier permeabilities of GBP used microdialysis. Rats were administered intravenous infusions of [^{14}C]GBP to achieve clinically relevant steady-state plasma concentrations. Total brain tissue GBP concentration was significantly higher at steady state than extracellular fluid concentration, owing to intracellular accumulation and tissue binding (22). A comparison of uptake of [^{3}H]GBP with uptake of L-[^{3}H]leucine into rat brain showed that GBP inhibits uptake of certain excitatory

amino acids in this synaptosomal preparation (23). Isolation and characterization of a [^{3}H]GBP binding protein from pig cerebral cortex membranes were reported. Purified L-type Ca^{2+} channel complexes were fractionated. [^{3}H]GBP binding activity closely followed elution of the $\alpha2\delta$ subunit (24). GBP was shown to bind most specifically in those areas of the brain where glutamate synapses are predominant (4). Binding of GBP at these sites is not altered by other AEDs, but it is consistently displaced stereospecifically by various other L-amino acids (15,19,20).

TRANSPORTERS

GBP is an artificial amino acid, and it was postulated that passage of GBP across cell membranes required facilitated transport by one of the saturable dose transport systems, ordinarily concerned with L-leucine and L-phenylalanine transport (4,25). The reason for the lack of proportionality after an oral dose was thought to be that GBP and the amino acids were mutually inhibitory and concentration dependent.

TRANSPLACENTAL PASSAGE AND BREAST MILK

No data are available on the transplacental passage of GBP in humans. It is not known whether the drug is safe in pregnancy, hence it is not used extensively. Data on breast milk have not been reported.

PHARMACOKINETICS IN ANIMALS

GBP is well absorbed in rats and dogs, with an elimination half-life of 2 to 3 hours and 3 to 4 hours, respectively. After intravenous administration, similar blood and brain concentrations were obtained in rats after a short distribution phase. More than 93% of [^{14}C]GBP was eliminated renally, as unchanged substance. Biotransformation to *N*-methyl GBP was found only in dogs (5,26). Pharmacokinetics was linear in the range of 400 to 500 mg/kg intravenously in rats, not sex dependent or changed on multiple dosage (3). Colonic GBP absorption in dogs was poor and consistent with membrane transport rate-limiting absorption of hydrophilic AEDs (27).

PHARMACOKINETICS IN HUMANS

Although oral absorption of GBP has been reported to saturate at doses >1,500 mg/day, other investigators report that high doses of GBP are absorbed and can be effective (28). Other reports suggest that bioavailability is 57% with a single dose of 300 mg and decreases to 35% with 1,600 mg three times daily (29). Data are conflicting on the effect of food on enhancement of absorption (1). High protein intake has been associated with increased GBP absorption. Both L-leucine and L-phenylalanine may compete with the intestinal transport of GBP. In 10 volunteers receiving a single dose of GBP 600 mg, after fasting and after a high-protein meal, maximum concentration was significantly increased and time to maximum concentration was significantly shorter after protein consumption (30). In another study after fasting or after a protein meal, pharmacokinetic parameters showed no statistically significant differences (31).

ELIMINATION

Renal clearance of GBP is linearly related to creatinine clearances (30,32). Because GBP elimination is affected by disease- and age-related decreases in renal function, dosage guidelines are based on renal function (33). In patients with renal impairment, peak plasma GBP levels are increased. After a single oral dose of GBP, elimination half-life increased to 16 hours in patients with a mean creatinine clearance of 41 mL/min and to 43 hours with a mean creatinine clearance of 13 mL/min. GBP is removed by hemodialysis.. A maintenance dose after dialysis should provide steady-state plasma concentrations comparable to those attained in the setting of normal renal function (34). A case of successful hemodialysis and hemoperfusion for treatment of valproate and GBP poisoning was reported (35). The elimination half-life of GBP in monotherapy is approximately 6 to 9 hours (11,22,36). Steady-state plasma concentrations of GBP can be reached within 1 to 2 days in patients with normal renal function (1,3,11,14).

BIOTRANSFORMATION AND EFFECTS ON LIVER ENZYMES

To investigate the influence of prolonged GBP administration on liver enzyme activity, a controlled trial of GBP was carried out using antipyrine clearance as a model for enzyme induction. None of the antipyrine parameters were affected by GBP administration (10). Because GBP is not metabolized in humans, neither isoenzymes nor genetic factors operating to give rise to metabolic differences among individuals are known or expected. In humans, no metabolites were found. (10,11).

CLEARANCE IN CHILDREN

Observations to date have not disclosed major differences in GBP kinetics between children and adults (1,39).

CLEARANCE IN ELDERLY PATIENTS

Old age is associated with decreased renal function; hence elimination of GBP by the kidney is impaired in elderly (33). GBP should be used cautiously and in reduced doses. GBP does not require routine laboratory monitoring, and because of lack of enzyme induction or alteration of metabolism of other drugs, it may represent an alternative to conventional drugs in the management of older patients (40). Morris recommends investigation of renal function parameters in patients who have experienced GBP toxicity at low blood levels. These patients include the elderly and those with known renal disease (16).

RELATIONSHIP BETWEEN SERUM CONCENTRATION AND DOSE

At doses of 4.8 g/day, bioavailability was estimated to be 35% (11). At doses of 300 to 600 mg three times daily, trough plasma concentrations were generally in the range of 1 to 10 μg/mL (10,15). After multiple oral doses of GBP, dose linearity was demonstrated (41). After a single dose of 300 mg (capsule), plasma concentrations of 2.7 μg/mL were obtained in 2 to 3 hours. After oral administration of 300 mg every 8 hours, peak plasma levels averaged 4 μg/mL. Because of individual variability in absorption and excretion of GBP, some patients do not develop significantly elevated plasma GBP levels until they are receiving high doses. A possible therapeutic range is of the order of 1 to 4 μg/mL. A value of 10 μg/mL without clinical toxicity may be grounds for discontinuation of the drug, if no therapeutic response has been achieved. Although in general four elimination half-lives are required to reach steady-state levels after starting treatment or after dose modification, there is suggestive evidence that the duration of action of GBP may be longer than predicted from its half-life, but multiple doses are still needed to maximize gastrointestinal absorption (1,42). In one major study, mean GBP levels in plasma were higher in responders than in nonresponders, and higher drug levels were related to increased efficacy of the drug (43). Improved seizure control tended to correlate with dose (44). Mattson suggests that for AEDs in which correlation between blood concentrations and clinical outcome is less clear, such as GBP, other indirect measures such as determination of serum GABA concentration or magnetic resonance spectroscopy may prove useful (45).

RELATIONSHIP BETWEEN SERUM CONCENTRATION AND EFFECT

Data are insufficient to recommend routine monitoring of GBP levels, although there is a possibility that measurement of plasma levels may be useful in high-dose treatment to

TABLE 29.1. GABAPENTIN PHARMACOKINETIC PARAMETERS

Pharmacokinetic Parameter	Values
Absorption	2–3 h (dose-dependent)
Oral bioavailability	<60% (35%–60%)
T_{max}	2–3 h
C_{max} after single dose of 300 mg	2.5–3.0 µg/mL
Metabolism	Nil
Plasma protein binding	Nil
V_d standardized for weight	0.65–1.4 L/kg
Half-life	6–7 h
Clearance	100–300 mL/min
Renal elimination	Proportional to creatinine clearance
Dose frequency	3 per day
Enzyme induction	Nil

T_{max}, time to maximum effect; C_{max}, maximum plasma concentration; V_d, volume of distribution; h, hours. From Perucca E. The clinical pharmacokinetics of the new antiepileptic drugs. *Epilepsia* 1999;40(suppl 9):S7–S13; Wong MO, Eldon MA, Keane WF, et al. Disposition of gabapentin in anuric subjects on hemodialysis. *J Clin Pharmacol* 1995;35:622–626; Gram L. Pharmacokinetics of new antiepileptic drugs. *Epilepsia* 1996;37 (suppl 6):S12–S16, with permission.

identify the level beyond which further dose increases fail to be absorbed (Table 29.1) (1,46–48).

DRUG INTERACTIONS

GBP neither induces nor inhibits hepatic microsomal enzymes, nor does it affect the plasma concentrations of most concurrently administered AEDs (11,15,46). Other AEDs have no effect on GBP pharmacokinetics (1). In animal studies, an augmentation of the antiepileptic effects of vigabatrin by GBP was demonstrated in guinea pig hippocampal slices. The combination of GBP and vigabatrin simultaneously decreased the repetition rate of epileptiform field potentials to a level significantly different from the effect by vigabatrin alone (49). In a study of 12 healthy women receiving 2.5 mg of norethisterone acetate and 30 µg ethinyl estradiol daily for three consecutive menstrual cycles, concurrent GBP administration did not alter the pharmacokinetics of either hormone. Thus, GBP is unlikely to cause contraceptive failure (50).

GBP may conceivably interact with drugs excreted predominantly by renal mechanisms. Most of the absorbed GBP, approximately 10% of lamotrigine, and 50% of absorbed felbamate are excreted unchanged in the urine; thus, a potential exists for GBP interaction with these drugs at a renal site (15). Interaction of GBP with felbamate has been reported. In a retrospective pharmacokinetic study of felbamate, 18 patients were taking felbamate and GBP simultaneously. Eleven patients were taking these two drugs alone. The mean half-life of felbamate in this cohort was

almost 50% higher than in patients receiving felbamate monotherapy, probably as a result of 37% lower clearance (51). Concomitant administration of GBP has not affected the plasma concentrations of carbamazepine or of its epoxide metabolite, phenobarbitone, phenytoin, or valproate. (32,37,52–54). These results are consistent with the effects of GBP observed in clinical studies (43,44) and other interaction studies related to the newer AEDs (36).

A case report indicated that GBP added to three AEDs (phenytoin, carbamazepine, and clobazam) caused a clinically significant rise in phenytoin plasma levels and signs of phenytoin toxicity. After cessation of GBP, levels of phenytoin returned to normal. Rechallenge with GBP caused further evidence of toxicity and a rise in phenytoin levels (55). Interactions of GBP have been reported with an antacid containing aluminum and magnesium hydroxide (56), which decreased the concentration of GBP by 15%; this interaction was not thought to be of clinical significance (15). Cimetidine also caused a similar effect, by a renal mechanism (11). The lack of clinically significant drug interactions is one of the drug's most favorable characteristics, contributing to its safety.

REFERENCES

1. Perucca E. The clinical pharmacokinetics of the new antiepileptic drugs. *Epilepsia* 1999;40[Suppl 9]:S7–S13.
2. McLean MJ. Management of convulsive disorders with the newer antiepileptic drugs: current review. In: Pollock JM, ed. *Broadening the spectrum of clinical uses of antiepileptic drugs.* London: Royal Society of Medicine, 2000:5–22.
3. Vollmer KO, von Hodenberg A, Kölle EU. Pharmacokinetics and metabolism of gabapentin in rat, dog and man. *Arzneimittelforschung* 1986; 36:830–839.
4. Taylor CP. Emerging perspectives on the mechanism of action of gabapentin. *Neurology* 1994;44[Suppl 5]:S10–S16.
5. Bartoszyk GD, Meyerson N, Reimann W, et al. Gabapentin. In: Meldrum BS, Porter RJ, eds. *New anticonvulsant drugs.* London: Libbey, 1986:147–164.
6. McLean MJ. Gabapentin in the management of convulsive disorders. *Epilepsia* 1999;40[Suppl 6]:S39–S50.
7. Bourgeois BF. New antiepileptic drugs. *Arch Neurol* 1998;55: 1181–1183.
8. Harden CL, Lazar LM, Pick LH, et al. A beneficial effect on mood in partial epilepsy patients treated with gabapentin. *Epilepsia* 1999;40:1129–1134.
9. Rogawski MA, Porter RJ. Antiepileptic drugs: pharmacological mechanisms and clinical efficacy with consideration of promising developmental stage compounds. *Pharmacol Rev* 1990;42: 223–286.
10. Schmidt B. Potential antiepileptic drugs. In: Levy RH, Dreifuss FE, Mattson RH, et al., eds. *Antiepileptic drugs,* 3rd ed. New York: Raven Press, 1989:925–935.
11. Richens A. Clinical pharmacokinetics of gabapentin. In: Chadwick D, ed. *New trends in epilepsy management: the role of gabapentin.* London: Royal Society of Medicine Services, 1993: 41–46.
12. Vollmer KO, Turck D, Bockbrader HN, et al. Summary of Neurontin (gabapentin) clinical pharmacokinetics. *Epilepsia* 1992;33 [Suppl 3]:77.

13. Vollmer KO, Anhut H, Thomann P, et al. Pharmacokinetic model of absolute bioavailability of the new anticonvulsant gabapentin. In: Manelis J, et al., eds. *Advances in epileptology.* New York: Raven Press, 1989:209–211.

14. McLean MJ. Gabapentin. *Epilepsia* 1995;36[Suppl 2]:S73–S85.

15. McLean MJ. Clinical pharmacokinetics of gabapentin. *Neurology* 1994;44[Suppl 5]:S17–S22.

16. Morris GL. Gabapentin. *Epilepsia* 1999;40[Suppl 5]:S63–S70.

17. Andrews CO, Fischer JH. Gabapentin: a new agent for the management of epilepsy. *Ann Pharmacother* 1994;28: 1188–1196.

18. Foot M, Wallace J. Gabapentin. In: Pisani F, Perucca E, Avanzani G, et al., eds. *New antiepileptic drugs.* Amsterdam: Elsevier, 1991: 109–114.

19. Ojemann LM, Friel PH, Ojemann GA. Gabapentin concentration in human brain. *Epilepsia* 1988;29:694.

20. Ben-Menachem E, Hedner T, Persson LI, et al. Seizure frequency and CSF gabapentin, GABA, and monoamine metabolite concentrations after 3 months treatment with 900 mg or 1,200 mg gabapentin daily in patients with intractable complex partial seizures. *Neurology* 1990;40[Suppl 1]:158.

21. Ben-Menachem E, Persson LI, Hedner T. Selected CSF biochemistry and gabapentin concentrations in the CSF and plasma in patients with partial seizures after a single oral dose of gabapentin. *Epilepsy Res* 1992;11:45–49.

22. Wang Y, Welty DF. The simultaneous estimation of the influx and efflux blood–brain barrier permeabilities of gabapentin using a microdialysis-pharmacokinetic approach. *Pharm Res* 1996;13: 398–403.

23. Thurlow RJ, Hill DR, Woodruff GN. Comparison of the autoradiographic binding distribution of [^{3}H]gabapentin with excitatory amino acid receptor and amino acid uptake site distributions in rat brain. *Br J Pharmacol* 1996;118:457–465.

24. Gee NS, Brown JP, Dissanayake VUK, et al. The novel anticonvulsant drug gabapentin (Neurontin) binds to the 2delta subunit of a Ca^{++} channel. *J Biol Chem* 1996;271:5768–5776.

25. Stewart BH, Kugler AR, Thompson PR, et al. A saturable transport mechanism in the intestinal absorption of gabapentin is the underlying cause of the lack of proportionality between increasing dose and drug levels in plasma. *Pharm Res* 1993;10:276–271.

26. von Hodenberg A, Vollmer KO. Metabolism of ^{14}C-gabapentin in rat, dog and man. *Naunyn Schmiedebergs Arch Pharmacol* 1983;324:R74.

27. Stevenson CM, Kim J, Fleisher D. Colonic absorption of antiepileptic agents. *Epilepsia* 1997;38:63–67.

28. Wilson EA, Forest G, Brodie MJ. High dose gabapentin is absorbed and can be effective. *Epilepsia* 1996; [Suppl 4]:127 (abst).

29. Leppik IE. Role of new and established antiepileptic drugs. *Epilepsia* 1998;39[Suppl 5]:S2–S6.

30. Gidal BE, Maly MM, Budde J, et al. Effect of high protein meal on gabapentin pharmacokinetics. *Epilepsy Res* 1996;23:71–76.

31. Benetello P, Furlanut M, Fortunato M, et al. Oral gabapentin disposition in patients with epilepsy after a high-protein meal. *Epilepsia* 1997;38:1140–1142.

32. Comstock TI, Sica DA, Bockbrader HN, et al. Gabapentin pharmacokinetics in subjects with various degrees of renal function. *J Clin Pharmacol* 1990;30:862.

33. Boyd RA, Türck D, Abel RB, et al. Effects of age and gender on single-dose pharmacokinetics of gabapentin. *Epilepsia* 1999;40: 474–479.

34. Haltenson CE, Keane WF, Turck D, et al. Disposition of gabapentin (GAB) in hemodialysis (HD) patients. *J Clin Pharmacol* 1992;32:751.

35. Fernandez MC, Walter FG, Kloster JC, et al. Hemodialysis and hemoperfusion for treatment of valproic acid and gabapentin poisoning. *Vet Hum Toxicol* 1996;38:438–443.

36. Anhut H, Leppik I, Schmidt, B, et al. Drug interaction study on the new anticonvulsant gabapentin with phenytoin in epileptic patients. *Naunyn Schmiedebergs Arch Pharmacol* 1988;337 [Suppl]:29.

37. Graves NM, Holmes GB, Leppik E, et al. Pharmacokinetics of gabapentin in patients treated with phenytoin. *Pharmacotherapy* 1989;9:196.

38. Johannessen SI. Pharmacokinetic and interaction profile of topiramate: review and comparison with other newer antiepileptic drugs. *Epilepsia* 1997; 38[Suppl 1]:S18–S23.

39. Khurana DS, Riviello J, Helmers S. Efficacy of gabapentin therapy in children with refractory partial seizures. *J Pediatr* 1996; 128:29–33.

40. Haider A, Tuchek JM, Haider S. Seizure control: how to use the new antiepileptic drugs in older patients. *Geriatrics* 1996;51: 42–45.

41. Turck D, Vollmer KO, Bockbrader HN, et al. Dose-linearity of new anticonvulsant gabapentin after multiple oral doses. *Eur J Clin Pharmacol* 1989;36:A310.

42. Leppik IE. Antiepileptic drugs in development: prospects for the near future. *Epilepsia* 1994;35[Suppl 4]:S29–S40.

43. UK Gabapentin Study Group. Gabapentin in partial epilepsy. *Lancet* 1990;335:1114–1117.

44. US Gabapentin Study Group No. 5. Gabapentin as add-on therapy in refractory partial epilepsy: a double-blind, placebo controlled, parallel-group study. *Neurology* 1993;43:2292–2298.

45. Mattson RH. Antiepileptic drug monitoring: a reappraisal. *Epilepsia* 1995;36[Suppl 5]:S22–S29.

46. Goa KL, Sorkin EM. Gabapentin: a review of its pharmacological properties and clinical potential in epilepsy. *Drugs* 1993; 46: 409–427.

47. Wong MO, Eldon MA, Keane WF, et al. Disposition of gabapentin in anuric subjects on hemodialysis. *J Clin Pharmacol* 1995;35:622–626.

48. Gram L. Pharmacokinetics of new antiepileptic drugs. *Epilepsia* 1996;37[Suppl 6]:S12–S16.

49. Lucke A, Musshoff U, Kohling R, et al. Gabapentin potentiation of antiepileptic efficacy of vigabatrin in an *in vitro* model of epilepsy. *Br J Pharmacol* 1998;124:370–376.

50. Eldon MA, Underwood BA, Randenitis EJ, et al. Gabapentin does not interact with a contraceptive regimen of norethindrone acetate and ethinyl estradiol. *Neurology* 1998;50:1146–1148.

51. Hussein G, Troupin AS, Montouris G. Gabapentin interaction with felbamate. *Neurology* 1996;47:1106–1107.

52. Graves NM, Leppik IE, Wagner ML, et al. Effect of gabapentin on carbamazepine levels. *Epilepsia* 1990;31:644–645.

53. Hooper WD, Kavanagh MC, Herkes GK, et al. Lack of pharmacokinetic interaction between phenobarbitone and gabapentin. *Br J Clin Pharmacol* 1991;31:171–174.

54. Radulovic LL, Wilder BJ, Leppik IE, et al. Lack of interaction of gabapentin with carbamazepine or valproate. *Epilepsia* 1994;35: 155–161.

55. Tyndel F. Interaction of gabapentin with other antiepileptics. *Lancet* 1994;343:1363–1364.

56. Busch JA, Radulovic LI, Bockbrader HN, et al. Effect of Maalox TC on single-dose pharmacokinetics of gabapentin capsules in healthy subjects. *Pharm Res* 1992;9[Suppl 10]:S315.

30

GABAPENTIN

CLINICAL USE

ANTHONY G. MARSON
DAVID W. CHADWICK

Gabapentin is one of the newer antiepileptic drugs, which was licensed for use in the United Kingdom and the United States in 1993. The previous chapters in this section outline our current knowledge of the mechanisms of action and the pharmacokinetic properties of gabapentin. In this chapter, we summarize our current knowledge about the clinical effects of gabapentin and hence the evidence that informs its clinical use. Given that randomized controlled trials are the most reliable method for assessing the effects of treatments (1,2), the focus of this chapter is on the results of randomized controlled trials.

At present, antiepileptic drugs are investigated first of all in drug-refractory populations (3), most of whom have localization-related (partial) epilepsy. Once an effect is demonstrated, the new drug may then be tested as monotherapy in a less refractory or drug-naive population. In this chapter, we follow the development of gabapentin and outline evidence about its effect as an add-on treatment before discussing evidence for its effect as monotherapy.

ADD-ON USE

Drug-Refractory Localization-Related Seizures

The effect of gabapentin on seizure frequency in patients with drug-resistant localization-related seizures was investigated in six randomized placebo controlled trials (4–9), one of which recruited children (4), with the remainder recruiting adults. For the trial recruiting children, 85% of the participants had localization-related seizures and 15% had generalized seizures, and the data from this trial are discussed

here. A systematic review and meta-analysis of these trials have been reported (10,11). The primary outcome of this systematic review was whether patients had a 50% or greater reduction in seizure frequency during the treatment phase of the trial compared with a prerandomization baseline phase. One of the six trials (5) did not have a baseline phase and could not contribute to the meta-analysis. The remaining trials recruited 750 adults and 247 children and had treatment phases ranging from 12 to 14 weeks (Table 30.1). In the adult trials overall, patients were allocated to doses of 600, 900, 1200 or 1,800 mg/day, whereas in the trial recruiting children, doses ranging from 600 to 1,800 mg/day were taken depending on weight.

Ignoring dose, the overall relative risk (95% confidence intervals) for a ≥50% reduction in seizure frequency was 1.81 (1.32 – 2.49), a finding indicating a statistically significant effect of gabapentin. Data from the adult studies were used in regression models for dose, and they showed increasing effect with increasing dose (Table 30.2). At 1,800 mg/day, 28.5% of patients had a ≥50% reduction in seizure frequency, a finding indicating that approximately seven patients would need to be treated to see one with a 50% response. Regression models show no plateau of effect at the doses tested, and it could be that higher doses would show a greater effect.

As a global outcome measure, this systematic review reported the proportion of patients who had treatment withdrawn during the course of the trial. The relative risk of treatment withdrawal for gabapentin compared with placebo was 1.04 (0.71 to 1.52), indicating no significant effect, although the confidence intervals are wide. This systematic review also reported side effects, and the following were significantly associated with gabapentin (relative risk 99% confidence intervals), dizziness 2.19 (1.24 to 3.89), fatigue 2.30 (1.11 to 4.75), somnolence 1.91 (1.20 to 3.05).

The effect of add-on gabapentin on cognition in patients with localization-related seizures was reported in one crossover trial (5). No effect on cognition was found, although the trial was small and lacked the power to detect

Anthony G. Marson, MD, MRCP: Lecturer in Neurology, Department of Neurological Science, University of Liverpool; and Senior Registrar, The Walton Centre for Neurology and Neurosurgery, Liverpool, United Kingdom

David W. Chadwick, MD: Professor of Neurology, Department of Neurological Science, University of Liverpool; and Consultant Neurologist, The Walton Centre for Neurology and Neurosurgery, Liverpool, United Kingdom

TABLE 30.1. TRIALS CONTRIBUTING TO THE METAANALYSIS

Trial	Doses Tested (mg/day) No. Randomized	Length of Treatment Period	Age Range, Yr, (% Male)	Number of Other AEDs Taken
Anhut, 1994	900 mg, 111	12 wk	12–67 (56)	≤2
	1,200 mg, 52			
Appleton, 1999	600–1,800 mg, 119	12 wk	3–12 (54)	≤3
Sivenius, 1991	900 mg, 18	12 wk	16–59 (47)	≤2
	1,200 mg, 9			
U.K. Gabapentin, 1990	1,200 mg, 61	14 wk	14–73 (39)	≤2
U.S. Gabapentin, 1993	600 mg, 53	12 wk	16–70 (66)	≤2
	1,200 mg, 101			
	1,800 mg, 54			

AED, antiepileptic drug.

potentially important effects because only 28 patients were randomized.

Generalized Seizures

The effect of gabapentin on drug-refractory generalized seizures was investigated in one randomized controlled trial (12). This trial had a treatment period of 14 weeks, and the published report gives data for 71 patients who were randomized to placebo and for 58 who were randomized to gabapentin. There was a nonsignificant trend in favor of gabapentin for the outcome ≥50% reduction in the frequency of generalized tonic clonic seizures, with 17.5% of the placebo group and 27.5% of the gabapentin group achieving this outcome. There was no clear trend for absence or myoclonic seizures.

Conclusion

There is clear evidence that gabapentin reduces seizure frequency and appears well tolerated when it is used as an add-on treatment for patients with localization-related seizures. The maximum dose tested was 1,800 mg, but given that no plateau of therapeutic effect was seen at doses tested, it is likely that higher doses would show a greater effect. There is insufficient evidence to support the use of gabapentin as an add-on treatment for patients with generalized seizures.

The evidence discussed so far was generated primarily by or in collaboration with the pharmaceutical industry, with the primary objective being to meet the requirements of regulatory authorities rather than to inform clinical practice. As a result, the evidence reviewed so far has certain important limitations, which need to be borne in mind when one tries to use this evidence to inform clinical practice.

First, these trials are all placebo-controlled trials. The clinician, however, has numerous drugs to choose from and needs to know how gabapentin compares with other drugs such as lamotrigine or topiramate rather than placebo. This issue will need to be addressed in head-to-head randomized controlled trials. Second, epilepsy is a chronic condition, and trials of 12 to 14 weeks' duration are too short to inform us of the longer-term effects of antiepileptic drugs. Third, outcomes such as percentage reduction in seizure frequency and ≥50% reduction in seizure frequency have little clinical meaning and are difficult to put into context at the bedside. In view of these and other difficulties, there is a clear need for more evidence about the effects of gabapentin add-on therapy from trials that both reflect and inform clinical practice.

TABLE 30.2. RESULTS OF REGRESSION MODELS FOR DOSE IN METAANALYSIS

Dose (mg/day)	Percent Responders (95% CI)	No. Needed to Treat (95% CI)
0 (placebo)	9.9 (7.2–13.5)	—
600	14.4 (12.0–17.3)	24.5 (15.5–31.4)
900	17.3 (14.6–20.3)	15.6 (9.3–20.5)
1,200	20.6 (21.5–36.7)	11.8 (5.6–17.5)
1,800	28.5 (21.5–36.7)	6.7 (3.0–10.5)

CI, confidence interval.

MONOTHERAPY

Localization-Related Seizures

Gabapentin was compared with carbamazepine in one randomized controlled trial that recruited patients with newly diagnosed localization-related seizures (13). This study was undertaken with the purpose of demonstrating an effect for the purpose of pursuing a possible monotherapy license. This trial had a treatment phase of 24 weeks' duration, with 74 patients allocated to 600 mg of carbamazepine per day and 72, 72, and 74 patients allocated to 300 mg, 600 mg, and 1,800 mg of gabapentin per day, respectively. Two main outcomes were reported, the first of which was "time to trial exit." Patients could exit the trial if they experience one tonic-clonic seizure, three simple or complex partial seizures, or status epilepticus or if they developed a new seizure type necessitating drug withdrawal. For this outcome, patients taking 900 and 1,800 mg gabapentin had significantly longer times to exit than patients taking 300 mg gabapentin. However, no difference was found between 900 or 1,800 mg of gabapentin and 600 mg of carbamazepine, although the trend was in favor of carbamazepine. The second outcome combined time to exit as stated earlier with time to treatment withdrawal resulting from adverse effects. For this outcome, no significant differences were found, although the trend was in favor of 900 mg of gabapentin. The authors reported the difference in the proportion of patients not exiting the trial for individual doses of gabapentin compared with carbamazepine. For this second outcome, there were estimated to be 9.6% more patients staying on 900 mg gabapentin than 600 mg of carbamazepine. The 95% confidence intervals were −6.5% to 26%. Although these confidence intervals do not indicate a significant difference, the lower confidence interval indicates that gabapentin is not more that 6.5% worse for this outcome, and this would be in keeping with the concept of noninferiority (14). This finding must be treated with caution, however, given that numerous comparisons have been made, and this observation could be a chance effect.

One randomized controlled trial was reported in which the effect of gabapentin monotherapy was investigated in a population with refractory localization-related seizures (15). In this trial, patients taking one or two antiepileptic drugs and experiencing a minimum of four seizures during an 8-week prospective baseline period were randomized to 600 mg (94 patients), 1,200 mg (90 patients), or 2,400 mg (91 patients) of gabapentin per day. There was no standard comparator (e.g., carbamazepine) in this trial, and the primary aim was to demonstrate an increase in effect with increasing dose of gabapentin monotherapy. The treatment period was of 26 weeks' duration. In the first 10 weeks, gabapentin was added, and an attempt was made to convert to gabapentin monotherapy. The primary outcome in this trial was time to exit, in which patients could exit the trial if they had status epilepticus or met certain criteria for worsening of seizure frequency or intensity. This trial found no difference among doses for this outcome, with median times to exit of 77, 81, and 75 days for 600, 1,200, and 2,400 mg/day, respectively. Because there was no standard comparator, this trial provides no evidence of how gabapentin monotherapy compares with a standard alternative. Given that no dose effect was found, this trial provides no evidence to support an effect of gabapentin monotherapy.

A third monotherapy study was reported (16), which used the "surgical paradigm." This trial recruited patients who had had their antiepileptic drugs withdrawn while they were undergoing seizure monitoring with a view to epilepsy surgery. Patients were allocated to 300 mg (42 patients) or 3,600 mg (40 patients) of gabapentin per day, with a treatment period of 8 days. The primary outcome was time to study exit measured in hours, in which exit criteria included a single tonic-clonic seizure, four simple or complex partial seizures, and status epilepticus. Time to exit was significantly longer (p = .001) for patients allocated to 3,600 mg gabapentin. Although this trial provides evidence of an effect of gabapentin monotherapy, it does not reflect and does little to inform clinical practice.

Generalized Seizures

The only reported trials of gabapentin monotherapy in patients with generalized seizures recruited children presenting with childhood absence epilepsy. Trudeau and colleagues (17) report combined data from two identical trials in which gabapentin monotherapy was compared with placebo. The trials had a treatment phase of 2 weeks' duration, and 15 patients were randomized to gabapentin and 18 to placebo. The primary outcome was the reduction in seizure frequency at the end of the treatment period compared with the prerandomization baseline period. Seizure frequency was assessed using ambulatory electroencephalographic monitoring, with patients monitored for 24 hour before randomization and at the end of the treatment period. No significant difference between gabapentin and placebo was found, and hence there is no evidence to support the use of gabapentin in the treatment of absence seizures.

CONCLUSION

There is no evidence from randomized controlled trials to support an effect of gabapentin in patients with generalized seizures. There is some evidence from two trials of an effect of gabapentin monotherapy against localization-related seizures; however, one of these trials does not inform clinical practice (16). In the second trial (13), some evidence of a dose effect for gabapentin was found, although compared with carbamazepine, no significant advantage was found for any of the doses of gabapentin tested. Confidence limits for 900 mg of gabapentin would be consistent with noninferiority. Given that this was not seen for 1,800 mg of gabapentin and that this observation could be a chance effect, this trial does not provide any strong evidence that would support the use of gabapentin monotherapy in patients with localization-related seizures. From the perspective of informing clinical practice, this trial has other limitations. In particular it is of relatively short duration (24 weeks), and the outcomes (time to exit) do not reflect outcomes of importance in every day practice, such as time to 12-month remission.

IMPLICATIONS FOR RESEARCH

Clearly, many questions relating to the clinical effects of gabapentin, both as monotherapy and as add-on therapy, remain unanswered. What evidence there is has been generated by or in collaboration with the pharmaceutical industry, with the primary aim of meeting the requirements of regulatory authorities, rather that to inform clinical practice. There is a clear need for further pragmatic randomized controlled trials of gabapentin as well as other newer antiepileptic drugs. Such trials should both reflect and inform clinical practice and should use outcomes of importance to both patients and clinicians. One such trial is under way in the United Kingdom (18) and compares monotherapy with gabapentin, lamotrigine, oxcarbazepine, topiramate, carbamazepine, and valproate.

REFERENCES

1. Cook DJ, Guyatt GH, Laupacis A, et al. Clinical recommendations using levels of evidence for antithrombotic agents. *Chest* 1995;104[Suppl 4]:227S–230S.
2. Sackett DL. Rules of evidence and clinical recommendations on use of antithrombotic agents. *Chest* 1986;89[Suppl 2]:2S–3S.
3. Commission on Antiepileptic Drugs of the International League Against Epilepsy. Guidelines for the clinical evaluation of antiepileptic drugs. *Epilepsia* 1989;30:400–408.
4. Appleton R, Fichtner K, LaMoreaux L, et al. Gabapentin as add-on therapy in children with refractory partial seizures: a 12-week, multicentre, double-blind, placebo-controlled study. Gabapentin Paediatric Study Group. *Epilepsia* 1999;40:1147–1154.
5. Leach JP, Girvan J, Paul A, et al. Gabapentin and cognition: a double blind, dose ranging, placebo controlled study in refractory epilepsy. *J Neurol Neurosurg Psychiatry* 1997;62:372–376.
6. Sivenius J, Kalviainen R, Ylinen A, et al. Double blind study of gabapentin in the treatment of partial seizures. *Epilepsia* 1991;32: 539–542.
7. Anhut H, Ashman P, Feuerstein TJ, et al. Gabapentin (Neurontin) as add-on therapy in patients with partial seizures: a double-blind, placebo-controlled study: the International Gabapentin Study Group. *Epilepsia* 1994;35:795–801.
8. UK Gabapentin Study Group. Gabapentin in partial epilepsy. *Lancet* 1990;335:1114–1117.
9. US Gabapentin Study Group No. 5. Gabapentin as add-on therapy in refractory partial epilepsy: a double-blind, placebo-controlled, parallel-group study. *Neurology* 1993;43:2292–2298.
10. Marson AG, Kadir ZA, Hutton JL, et al. Gabapentin for drug resistant partial epilepsy. In: *The Cochrane Library,* issue 3. Oxford: Update Software, 2000.
11. Marson AG, Kadir ZA, Hutton JL, et al. The new antiepileptic drugs: a systematic review of their efficacy and tolerability. *Epilepsia* 1997;38:859–880.
12. Chadwick D, Leiderman DB, Sauermann W, et al. Gabapentin in generalized seizures. *Epilepsy Res* 1996;25:191–197.
13. Chadwick DW, Anhut H, Greiner MJ, et al. A double-blind trial of gabapentin monotherapy for newly diagnosed partial seizures: International Gabapentin Monotherapy Study Group 945-77. *Neurology* 1998;51:1282–1288.
14. EMEA (Europan agency for the evaluation of medicinal products). Points to consider on switching between superiority and non-inferiority. *http:www.eudra.orghumandocspdfsewp048229en.pdf,* 2000.
15. Beydoun A, Fischer J, Labar DR, et al. Gabapentin monotherapy. II. A 26-week, double-blind, dose-controlled, multicenter study of conversion from polytherapy in outpatients with refractory complex partial or secondarily generalized seizures: the US Gabapentin Study Group 82/83. *Neurology* 1997;49:746–752.
16. Bergey GK, Morris HH, Rosenfeld W, et al. Gabapentin monotherapy. I. An 8-day, double-blind, dose-controlled, multicenter study in hospitalized patients with refractory complex partial or secondarily generalized seizures: the US Gabapentin Study Group 88/89. *Neurology* 1997;49:739–745.
17. Trudeau V, Myers S, LaMoreaux L, et al. Gabapentin in naive childhood absence epilepsy: results from two double-blind, placebo-controlled, multicenter studies. *J Child Neurol* 1996;11:470–475.
18. SANAD. http://www.liv.ac.uk/neuroscience/sanad.

GABAPENTIN

CLINICAL EFFICACY AND USE IN OTHER NEUROLOGICAL DISORDERS

BERND SCHMIDT

Gabapentin (GBP) is the first of the newer antiepileptic drugs (AEDs) that expanded its use, shortly after it was labeled and marketed for partial seizures with or without secondary generalization, into a broad range of neurologic and psychiatric indications. Now, most prescriptions for GBP worldwide are for conditions other than epilepsy. Following the lead of GBP, for most of the newer AEDs, marketing approval for additional indications, particularly for pain syndromes, bipolar disorder, and migraine, is sought early after the drug is first launched as an AED, or development programs for those other indications are pursued at the same time. In the future, it may be that the development of a drug as an AED may become only a sideline of other neuropsychiatric indications targeted first, because of the much larger market share and attractiveness of other central nervous system indications, compared with epilepsy, provided the mechanism of action of novel molecules suggests true broad-spectrum central nervous system activity.

On October 23, 2000, gabapentin (Neurontin) was approved by the German regulatory authorities for "neuropathic pain in adults," particularly diabetic polyneuropathy and postherpetic neuralgia, following the lead of Austria, Switzerland, the United Kingdom, Ireland, Italy, Brazil, Chile, Columbia, Ecuador, Peru, Venezuela, Mexico, the Philippines, and Singapore. The drug's package insert recommends the following GBP dosage regimen: initial dose of three times 300 mg from day 1, or a titration to 900 mg/day within 3 days, followed by an increase to 1,800 mg/day within a week, not too exceed a maximum daily dose of 3,600 mg.

NEUROPATHIC PAIN SYNDROMES

For neurologic disorders other than epilepsy, GBP's efficacy has been documented best by controlled randomized clinical trials of symptomatic treatment for neuropathic pain syndromes associated with diabetes and for postherpetic neuralgia. Based on these data, marketing approval for the indication of neuropathic pain was granted in some countries. In a double-blind trial, 165 patients with chronic painful diabetic neuropathies (diabetes type 1 and 2) were randomly assigned to receive ≤3,600 mg/day GBP or placebo for 8 weeks. At the 8-week study end point, for the intent-to-treat population, there was a significantly different ($p = .001$) mean daily pain score, used as a primary outcome variable, in favor of GBP over placebo. Consistent with the primary measure were significant improvements on total pain, mean sleep interference, and visual analogue scale (VAS) and present pain intensity (PPI) scores of the Short-Form McGill Pain Questionnaire. All other comedications that could have influenced pain or pain perception were excluded; antidiabetic medication had to be kept constant, and during the trial, hemoglobin A_1C values remained unchanged in both groups. An interesting feature of the trial results is that the mean curves for the GBP and placebo group were already significantly separate in the first week for the parameter sleep interference and in the second treatment week for all pain rating scales, a finding suggesting that the doses used during the initial 4-week titration period may be effective (900 to 1,800 mg/day).

Overall, 67% of the patients taking GBP made it through the forced titration ≤3,600 mg/day, and 6% withdrew because of adverse events. Dizziness (23%) and somnolence (22%) were the two adverse events occurring significantly more frequently than with placebo (1).

In a study with a very similar design, GBP was investigated in postherpetic neuralgia in a much older and comorbid patient population than the patients in the previously mentioned study, who had diabetic neuropathy. In the postherpetic neuralgia trial, 229 patients, whose mean age was 73 years and who had a median history of postherpetic pain for 28 years, were randomized to receive either ≤3,600 mg/day GBP or placebo for 8 weeks. Two-

Bernd Schmidt, MD, PhD: Head, Department of Neurology and Psychiatric Clinic, Wittnau, Germany

thirds of these patients were not taking any concomitant pain medication, and one-third received tricyclic antidepressants, opioids, or both, in stable doses throughout the study. After the first 4 weeks of forced GBP titration, 83% of the patients reached doses of ≥2,400 mg/day, and 65% received stable doses of 3,600 mg/day. The average daily pain score, the primary efficacy parameter, for the GBP-treated group was significantly reduced (*p* = .001) compared with the placebo-treated group from week 2 until the end of study week 8, without signs of tolerance. Significant differences in favor of the GBP-treated group were also achieved for secondary parameters such as daily sleep rating scores, total pain, or the Short-Form McGill Pain Questionnaire. Dizziness led to withdrawal in 5% and somnolence in 4% of the patients. In addition, somnolence was the most common adverse event (27%), followed by dizziness (23%). Serious adverse events were not reported in this older group of patients with herpetic neuralgia (2). Neither placebo-controlled study has any available data on long-term results .

A third randomized controlled trial compared two active regimens for diabetic peripheral neuropathy—GBP, 900 to 1,800 mg/day, versus amitriptyline hydrochloride (AMI), 25 to 75 mg/day—in a double-blind 6-week crossover design, with an intermediate 1-week washout. Only 25 patients were enrolled, 19 of whom completed both arms of the crossover trial and were evaluated. Both drugs (mean achieved doses: GBP, 1,565 mg/day; AMI, 59 mg/day) provided significant pain relief from 2 weeks onward, compared with baseline pain diary scores. However, at the end of treatment, there was no statistical difference in pain intensity scores between GBP and AMI. The authors agree that, to avoid a type II error, approximately 260 patients per paired crossover period would have been needed to draw valid conclusions on comparative efficacy. In the GBP-treated group, sedation and dizziness were the most frequent adverse events, and, as expected, in the AMI group, dry mouth and weight gain were the most common (3).

In an attempt to compare efficacy between studies and therapeutic regimens for treatment of diabetic neuropathic pain and postherpetic pain, numbers needed to treat (NNTs) were calculated for patients achieving >50% pain relief. In painful diabetic neuropathy, the NNT for use of all types of tricyclic antidepressants was 3.0 (confidence interval or CI, 2.4 to 4.0) , for tramadol it was 3.4 (CI, 2.3 to 6.4), for phenytoin it was 2.1 (CI, 1.5 to 3.6), for carbamazepine it was 3.3 (CI, 2.0 to 9.2), and for GBP it was 3.7 (CI, 2.4 to 8.3). For postherpetic neuralgia, a comparison is available only between tricyclic antidepressants achieving an NNT of 2.5 (CI, 1.7 to 3.3) and GBP 3.2 (CI, 2.4 to 5.0). Those comparisons do not take tolerability or dropout rates from adverse events into consideration (4).

Further to these randomized controlled trials is a large body of literature about GBP use in a variety of other neu-ropathic pain syndromes caused by peripheral nerve trauma or compression, infections, metabolic disturbances, or neurodegeneration. Most of these reports are based on open case series with heterogeneous patient populations.

Trigeminal neuralgia was treated in 13 patients with increasing GBP doses of between 300 and 2,000 mg/day; half of these patients had been unresponsive to previous carbamazepine therapy. In the *de novo* treatment group, GBP was found to be effective in 83% of the patients; 57% in the carbamazepine-refractory group responded (5). Seven patients with multiple sclerosis and chronic, severe , refractory trigeminal neuralgia received GBP doses of between 900 and 2,400 mg/day. Three patients with multiple sclerosis were receiving concomitant baclofen. Six of the seven patients experienced complete pain relief, and no patient discontinued GBP because of adverse events. The onset of the drug's effect occurred after 3 to 4 days, with a maximum effect reached from week 2 onward that was maintained for at least 1 year (6). Neuropathic pain related to acquired immunodeficiency syndrome was treated with GBP in addition to antiretroviral medication, and GBP demonstrated partial efficacy in this condition as well (7).

Neuropathic cancer pain was investigated openly in 22 patients who receiving GBP, 800 to 1,200 mg/day, as an adjunct to stable opioid doses. Assessment of a treatment effect was made 7 to 14 days after stable doses of GBP had been achieved, and the result was a significant reduction of global pain, burning pain, and shooting pain scores. No control group was included in the study design. No new adverse events, aside from mild sedation attributable to GBP, was reported. The authors of this study discussed the option of reducing concomitant opioids, to ease the drug burden of patients with cancer and to improve the overall side effects (8).

A more in-depth evaluation of an effect of GBP on the different components of neuropathic pain was undertaken in 18 patients with postherpetic neuralgia, phantom limb pain, postthoracotomy pain, idiopathic peripheral neuropathy, poststroke central pain, and pain from spinal injury. In this study, GBP doses were titrated up to a maximum of 2,400 mg/day and were maintained for 6 weeks. GBP induced a statistically significant pre–post effect on spontaneous pain, but particularly on paroxysmal pain and evoked pain (brush-induced allodynia, cold-induced allodynia, and hyperalgesia) (9).

SPASTICITY AND PAROXYSMAL SYMPTOMS ASSOCIATED WITH MULTIPLE SCLEROSIS

In 1984, even before the use of GBP was explored in epilepsy, the manufacturer initiated 4-week pilot studies of the drug in spasticity of spinal and supraspinal origin, because GBP was able to relieve muscular rigidity in mice. In those early studies, only individual patients had a moderate benefit, probably because of the low doses (900 mg/day maximum) used at that time. Based on the results, the development program for the use of this drug in spasticity was not continued.

However, a 6-day, placebo-controlled, blinded crossover study using 2,700 mg/day GBP in 21 evaluable patients with multiple sclerosis demonstrated significant beneficial effects in self-rating and observer rating scales. Values on the Kurtzke Expanded Disability Status Scale were not different between active treatment and placebo, a finding that could be attributed to the short-term nature of this trial. Tolerability was not found to be a problem, not even during the rapid forced titration (10).

A longer, but open, study looked at the effects of 600 to 1,200 mg/day GBP given for a follow-up period ≥3 and ≤9 months in 18 evaluable patients with multiple sclerosis who had painful tonic spasms, trigeminal neuralgia, dysesthetic or paresthetic symptoms, and ocular ataxia resistant to previous treatment. Fourteen of the 18 patients experienced complete and sustained recovery within 1 month of the start of treatment, as evaluated by means of a three-point score compared with the baseline value. Mild somnolence occurred in two patients (11). Larger and longer blinded randomized controlled trials with electrophysiologic and functional outcomes would be required to establish definitively GBP's place in disorders associated with spasticity.

RESTLESS LEG SYNDROME

Two open case series investigated the use of GBP in the restless leg syndrome and periodic limb movement disorder of sleep. Three of eight patients receiving a median dose of GBP of 1,163 mg/day for a minimum of 1 week reported ≥75% improvement, compared with pretreatment. Adverse events included dizziness, nausea, and drowsiness, causing two patients to discontinue the trial (12).

Of the initial 71 patients with periodic limb movement disorder of sleep, 48% were rated subjectively improved in terms of sleep depth and continuity, when the GBP dose was titrated ≤1,800 mg/day, with the larger of the divided doses given in the late afternoon. Otherwise rare adverse events, abnormal sensations, and movements are reported in a review of restless leg syndrome and periodic limb movement disorder of sleep (13).

PARKINSON'S DISEASE AND AMYOTROPHIC LATERAL SCLEROSIS

In an acute challenge experiment, 19 patients with Parkinson's disease (Hoehn and Yahr stages 2.5 to 5.0) received six consecutive doses of 400 mg GBP, in addition to dopamin-

ergics, followed by six doses of placebo, or vice versa, in a double-blind, crossover trial. A significant ($p = .0028$) improvement of total score on the Unified Parkinson's Disease Rating Scale was noted in favor of GBP, but not in individual subscales. The most frequent adverse events in patients between 41 and 78 years of age were unsteady gait, dizziness, and sleepiness. The authors of this study discussed the weaknesses of this brief study, such as a potentially unsuitable dose regimen, short exposure, and failure to discriminate among various forms of Parkinsonism. These investigators also stated that other patients who were not in the study did benefit from GBP over several years, whereas others observed a worsening of their disease (14).

In 152 patients with amyotrophic lateral sclerosis who underwent 6 months of treatment with 2,400 mg/day GBP, a nonsignificant trend toward a slower decline in arm strength megascores versus placebo was described, with a median difference of 37% and no effect on vital capacity. The study was initially powered to detect a 50% reduction in arm megascore decline. Compared with placebo, there were significantly more adverse effects, such as light-headedness, drowsiness, and limb swelling, in the GBP-treated group (15).

Later, an open, randomized, natural history–controlled study looked into the effects of GBP, 500 versus 1,000 mg/day, given for 6 to 12 months to a total of 110 patients with definite amyotrophic lateral sclerosis. An additional 121 patients who were receiving other symptomatic treatments were considered the control group. The authors of this study found dose- and treatment duration–dependent effects on average slopes for less decline of muscular limb strength, forced vital capacity, a disease severity score (Norris), and an activities of daily living scale (Functional Rating Scale). Statistical differences are significant when the patients who were treated for longer periods and with higher doses are compared with the natural history control group. No blinding or placebo was involved in this study (16).

HUNTINGTON'S DISEASE AND MISCELLANEOUS MOVEMENT DISORDERS

Four patients with Huntington's disease were reported in an abstract to have received a low dose of GBP, 900 mg/day, for a mean duration of 3 years. Improvement in terms of reduction of choreic movements was measured, as well as severity of Huntington's disease, by the Abnormal Involuntary Movement Scale. In all patients from this open case series, a moderate to good effect on the Abnormal Involuntary Movement Scale without adverse events was noted (17).

Another study treated 12 outpatients with schizoaffective and bipolar disorders and tardive dyskinesia for 1 to 6 years and who had otherwise pharmacoresistant antipsychotic-induced movement disorders; GBP, 600 to 1,200 mg/day, was added to their baseline medication. Ten of 12 patients in this openly treated cohort experienced a clinically relevant benefit after 3 weeks. In additional single patients, a continued effect, particularly on blepharospasm and facial dyskinesias, outlasted the 24-month observation time point, without relevant adverse events, aside from some sedation (18).

A single case report deals with good results of GBP titrated ≤75 mg/kg/day after 6 months in a 13-year-old pediatric patient, presenting with hemichorea and hemiballismus after an embolic stroke. The patient did not complain of dizziness, nausea, or sedation at the time of peak GBP levels (19).

In contrast to the benefits of GBP in a variety of movement disorders, worsening or the new development of abnormal movement patterns when GBP is initiated has been noted and reviewed; all these effects are reversible after dose reduction or withdrawal of GBP. In the case of a 68-year-old patient, the development of paroxysmal dystonic movements in both hands was reported during combined therapy with propranolol and GBP 900 mg/day; the problem resolved immediately after reduction of the propranolol dose to 40 mg/day, a finding suggesting a pharmacodynamic interaction between the two drugs (20).

TREMORS

Besides pain syndromes, GBP is widely used at present in various types of tremors, mainly essential tremor. Eighteen patients with essential tremor completed a placebo-controlled crossover design with 2-week treatment periods of GBP, 1,800 mg/day, added to baseline antitremor medication. Tremor was assessed by examiners who rated tremors in different body parts, using Fahn-Tolosa-Marin Tremor Rating Scales, as well as a global disability rating. Statistical analysis for nonparametric data did not show a difference in any outcome parameters among the baseline, GBP, and placebo values. Two patients from the initial group of 20 randomized dropped out because of adverse events that occurred while they were taking GBP, and seven patients reported fatigue, nausea, or dizziness (21).

In contrast to the previously described add-on therapy, GBP was given as the only antitremor drug to 16 patients with essential tremor in a double-blind, three-way placebo- and propranolol-controlled crossover study (GBP, 1,200 mg/day; propranolol, 120 mg/day). Significant and similar improvements in all outcome measures (Tremor Clinical Rating Scale, self-reported disability scale) were found for both treatment strategies, GBP and propranolol, versus baseline. Accelometric assessments proved not to work methodologically within this trial. The authors of this study concluded that a larger and longer trial would be needed (22).

The call for blinded, well-controlled randomized controlled trials is reiterated in two further articles dealing with the use of GBP in orthostatic tremor in patients who unsuc-

cessfully responded previously to clonazepam. Four, respectively seven, patients were treated with GBP individually at doses between 300 and 2,400 mg/day; immediate effects were mostly investigated, but one patient was observed for ≤22 months. In both open studies, orthostatic tremor was found to be reduced in most patients; the adverse effects were only mild to moderate and were much less severe than these patients had experienced with many other antitremor medications (23,24).

MIGRAINE

Results of studies of patients with migraine are available mainly through abstracts, which do not always describe the study in detail. The largest number of patients with migraine, with or without aura, is reported from a 12-week prophylaxis trial with two imbalanced groups of 99 patients taking between 1,800 and 2,400 mg GBP versus placebo. In a modified intent-to-treat population, the mean baseline migraine headache rate during the last month of treatment compared with baseline values, was 2.9 for the GBP-treated group and 3.4 for the placebo-treated group ($p = .031$). The proportion of patients who had a reduction of migraines of ≥50% was 36% with GBP and 14% with placebo; 16% of the patients taking GBP and 9% taking placebo discontinued the trial because of adverse events. Dizziness (25%), somnolence (24%), and asthenia (22%) were the leading adverse events within the GBP-treated group (25).

In one study, 145 Italian patients with migraine were openly randomized to GBP, either 1,200 or 2,000 mg/day, and were evaluated after weeks 4, 10, and 16. Only 34 of the patients completed the trial, but in the abstract, no reason for the dropout is provided. In both dosage groups, reduction of migraine crisis was the same after weeks 4 and 16 (40% and 65%, respectively) versus baseline. Adverse events included somnolence (26%), asthenia (10%), and dizziness (7%). Rightly, the authors concluded that other studies are necessary (26).

Another cohort of 20 Italian patients with migraine, with or without aura, openly received 600, 900, or 1,200 mg/day GBP for 6 months. A relevant improvement in number of attacks per month, pain intensity, and disability was observed for the 900- and 1,200-mg doses, but not for the 600-mg dose. Tolerability was not a problem (27).

MISCELLANEOUS CONDITIONS

In addition to the previously mentioned categories, case series or anecdotal reports note GBP use in rarer neurologic conditions such as reflex sympathetic dystrophy, central pain, myokymia-cramp syndrome, muscle cramps associated with various diseases, and hemifacial spasms and as adjunctive therapy for idiopathic chronic hiccup. The reported patients usually improved within a dose range of GBP of 1,200 to 2,700 mg/day, in a thrice-daily dose regimen (28).

REFERENCES

1. Backonja M, Beydoun A, Edwards KR, et al. Gabapentin for the symptomatic treatment of painful neuropathy in patients with diabetes mellitus: a randomized controlled trial. *JAMA* 1998; 280:1831–1836.
2. Rowbotham M, Harden N, Stacey B, et al. Gabapentin for the treatment of postherpetic neuralgia: a randomized controlled trial. *JAMA* 1998;280:1837–1842.
3. Morello CM, Leckband SG, Stoner CP, et al. Randomized double-blind study comparing the efficacy of gabapentin with amitriptyline on diabetic peripheral neuropathy pain. *Arch Intern Med* 1999;159:1931–1937.
4. Sindrup SH, Jensen TS. Efficacy of pharmacological treatments of neuropathic pain: an update on effect related to mechanism of drug action. *Pain* 1999;83:389–400.
5. Magnus L. Nonepileptic uses of gabapentin. *Epilepsia* 1999;40 [Suppl 6]:S66–S74.
6. Khan OA. Gabapentin relieves trigeminal neuralgia in multiple sclerosis patients. *Neurology* 1998;51:611–614.
7. Neville MW. Gabapentin in the management of neuropathic pain. *Am J Pain Manage* 2000;10:6–12.
8. Caraceni A, Zecca E, Martini C, et al. Gabapentin as an adjuvant to opioid analgesia for neuropathic cancer pain. *J Pain Symptom Manage* 1999;17:441–445.
9. Attal N, Brasseur L, Parker F, et al. Effects of gabapentin on the different components of peripheral and central neuropathic pain syndromes: a pilot study. *Eur Neurol* 1998;40:191–200.
10. Cutter NC, Scott DD, Johnson JC, et al. Gabapentin effect on spasticity in multiple sclerosis: a placebo-controlled, randomized trial. *Arch Phys Med Rehabil* 2000;81:164–169.
11. Solaro C, Lunardi GL, Capello E, et al. An open-label trial of gabapentin treatment of paroxysmal symptoms in multiple sclerosis patients. *Neurology* 1998;51:609–611.
12. Alder CH. Treatment of restless legs syndrome with gabapentin. *Clin Neuropharmacol* 1997; 20:148–151.
13. Williams DC. Periodic limb movements of sleep and restless legs syndrome. *Va Med Q* 1996;123:260–265.
14. Olson W, et al. Gabapentin for Parkinsonism: a double-blind, placebo-controlled, crossover trial. *Am J Med* 1997;102:60–66.
15. Miller RG, Moore D, Young LA, et al. Placebo-controlled trial of gabapentin in patients with amyotrophic lateral sclerosis. *Neurology* 1996;47:1383–1388.
16. Mazzini L, Mora G, Balzarini C, et al. The natural history and the effects of gabapentin in amyotrophic lateral sclerosis *J Neurol Sci* 1998;160[Suppl 1]:S57–63.
17. Cosentino C, Torres L, Cuba JM. Gabapentin for Huntington's disease. *J Neurol* 1996;243[Suppl 2]:S75–S76.
18. Hardoy MC, Hardoy MJ, Carta MG, et al. Gabapentin as a promising treatment for antipsychotic-induced movement disorders in schizoaffective and bipolar patients. *J Affect Disord* 1999; 54:315–317.
19. Kothare SV, Pollack P, Kulberg AG, et al. Gabapentin treatment in a child with delayed-onset hemichorea/hemiballismus. *Pediatr Neurol* 2000;22:68–71.
20. Palomeras E, Sanz, P, Cano, A, et al. Dystonia in a patient treated with propranolol and gabapentin. *Arch Neurol* 2000;57:570–571.
21. Pahwa R, Lyons K, Hubble JP, et al. Double-blind controlled trial of gabapentin in essential tremor. *Mov Disord* 1998;13:4 65–467.
22. Gironell A, Kulisevsky J, Barbanoj M, et al. A randomized placebo-controlled comparative trial of gabapentin and propranolol in essential tremor. *Arch Neurol* 1999;56:475–580.
23. Onofrj M, Thomas A, Paci C, et al. Gabapentin in orthostatic tremor: results of a double-blind crossover with placebo in four patients. *Neurology* 1998;51:880–882.
24. Evidente VG, Adler CH, Caviness JN, et al. Effective treatment of orthostatic tremor with gabapentin. *Mov Disord* 1998;13:829–831.
25. Mathew NT, Magnus-Miller L, Saper J, et al. Efficacy and safety of gabapentin in migraine prophylaxis. *Cephalgia* 1999;19:380.
26. Jimenez MD, Friera G, Manjon MT. Efficacy and safety of gabapentin in prophylaxis of migraine headache. *Cephalgia* 1999; 19:376.
27. Farinelli M, Betti E, Benedetti O, et al. Gabapentin in drug resistant migraine. *Cephalgia* 1999;19:378.
28. Merren MD. Gabapentin for treatment of pain and tremor:a large case series. *South Med J* 1998;91:739–744.

Antiepileptic Drugs, 5th Edition. Edited by R.H. Levy, R.H. Mattson, B.S. Meldrum, and E. Perucca. Lippincott Williams & Wilkins, Philadelphia © 2002.

GABAPENTIN

CLINICAL EFFICACY AND USE IN PSYCHIATRIC DISORDERS

JOHN H. GREIST

The utility of nonbenzodiazepine anticonvulsants in the treatment of bipolar illness has been shown in controlled studies (1). The notion that anticonvulsants may be useful in psychiatric conditions other than bipolar illness (e.g., anxiety or psychotic disorders) has not enjoyed the same benefit of controlled research. Although claims of anxiolytic effects have been made for phenytoin, carbamazepine, and valproate, little evidence exists to support such use. The improved tolerability of newer anticonvulsant agents has renewed interest in exploring their psychiatric uses.

Gabapentin was introduced in the early 1990s and is of interest for its potential psychotropic effects. Early studies in seizure disorders indicated that gabapentin possessed minimal cognition-impairing effects such as those commonly associated with the older antiepileptic drugs (2–6). Additionally, improvements in mood and well-being among epileptic patients who were taking gabapentin were reported in a retrospective data analysis (7) and were subsequently confirmed in a prospective study (8).

The published open-label reports to date on the utility of gabapentin for the treatment of anxiety and bipolar disorders are noted in Table 32.1. Numerous reports of patient series successfully treated with gabapentin for various psychiatric conditions have been presented at various scientific meetings but are not included here. Despite the multitude of published reports, systematic evaluation of the psychiatric uses of gabapentin has not been carried out, and gabapentin is not approved by any government agency in the United States for such uses.

ANXIETY DISORDERS

Preclinical data gathered early in the development of gabapentin showed anxiolyticlike effects in several animal models (9). Isolated anecdotal reports emerged over the years (10,11) and indicated the successful use of gabapentin to treat anxiety symptoms. Contemporaneously, we conducted two controlled clinical studies to test the hypothesis that gabapentin may be anxiolytic.

The first study (12) compared gabapentin and placebo in outpatients (n = 69) who were diagnosed with social phobia, according to the criteria of the fourth edition of the *Diagnostic and Statistical Manual of Mental Disorders* (DSM-IV), and who were treated for 14 weeks in a randomized, double-blind study design. Gabapentin was administered with doses given in a flexible escalating manner between the range of 900 and 3,600 mg/day. Using the Liebowitz Social Anxiety Scale as the primary measure of efficacy, this study found that patients taking gabapentin showed a significantly greater reduction in Liebowitz Social Anxiety Scale scores than those receiving placebo. The improvement seen with gabapentin was significantly greater than that observed with placebo after 1 week of treatment, and the superiority continued at each subsequent evaluation.

The second study (13) treated outpatients with DSM-IV-diagnosed panic disorder, with or without agoraphobia, in a randomized double-blind study lasting 8 weeks. Gabapentin was given in flexible doses of between 900 and 3,600 mg daily. The primary efficacy measure was the baseline to end point change in the total score of the Panic and Agoraphobia Scale (14), which is a composite measure of five domains of symptomatic and functional impairment in panic disorder. The protocol-specified analysis of efficacy did not show a difference between drug and placebo on the change in Panic and Agoraphobia Scale score. However, the same analysis on a subset of patients with at least a moderate severity of symptoms (as defined by a baseline total Panic and Agoraphobia Scale score of 20 or more) found that the drug-treated group showed a significantly greater improvement than the placebo-treated group.

The results of these studies, along with the experience of clinicians as mentioned in published case reports, provide

John H. Greist, MD: Distinguished Senior Scientist, Madison Institute of Medicine; and Clinical Professor of Psychiatry, University of Wisconsin, Madison, Wisconsin

TABLE 32.1. PUBLISHED REPORTS OF UNCONTROLLED GABAPENTIN USE IN MOOD AND ANXIETY DISORDERS

Authors	Diagnosis	No. Patients	Dose/Regimen	Outcome
Ryback et al., 1997	Bipolar disorder	73	Variable, up to 3,600 mg/day	Good response in 67
Schaffer and Schaffer, 1997	Bipolar disorder	28	33–2,700 mg/day (mean, 539)	Good response in 18
Young et al., 1997	Bipolar depression	15	Flexible dosing	Full or partial response in 8
McElroy et al., 1997	Bipolar disorder (hypomanic, manic, or mixed)	9 consecutive	Adjunctive 300–4,800 mg/day	Moderate or marked improvement in 7 by 1 mo, in 1 by 3 mo; of these eight, six maintained their response at 1–7 mo follow-up
Stanton et al., 1997	Acute mania	1	3,600 mg/day	Marked improvement
Bennett et al., 1997	Bipolar disorder schizoaffective	5	Adjunctive 600–2,400 mg/day	Marked or moderate improvement in 4
Chouinard et al., 1998	Schizophrenia, schizoaffective disorder, bipolar disorder, generalized anxiety disorder	18	Adjunctive 100–4,400 mg/day	Improved sleep and reduced anxiety in all patients
Erfurth et al., 1998	Acute mania	14	1,200–4,800 mg/day alone or in combination	BRMAS 38 to 8 in add-on group (n = 6); 27 to 9 in 4/8 solo group (n = 8)
Soutullo et al., 1998	Acute mania and ADHD	1	1,500 mg/day added on to carbamazepine	Marked response within 1 mo
Ghaemi and Katzow, 1998	Bipolar or unipolar MDD	50	100–5,600 mg/day (mean 1,597 mg/day)	Moderate to marked efficacy in 15 (30%)
Knoll et al., 1998	Bipolar disorder	12	Adjunctive gabapentin, median top dose = 2,400 mg/day	Marked response in 1, moderate response in 7, mild response in 2 and no response in 2
Brown and Hong, 1999	Bipolar disorder with anti-depressant-induced bruxism	1	Adjunctive	Complete resolution of bruxism
Young et al., 1999	Non-rapid-cycling bipolar disorder type I and II	37	Adjunctive, up to 6 mo	Significant reduction in manic and depressive symptoms
Grunze et al., 1999	Bipolar disorder type I	20*	1,200–4,800	BRMAS score declined significantly in patients with moderate mania, but gabapentin was not efficacious in patients with very severe mania
Cabras et al., 1999	Bipolar disorder schizoaffective	25	Adjunctive, flexible dosing (mean dose, 1,440 mg/day)	Positive response in 19 (76%)
Hatzimanolis et al., 1999	Acute mania	2	Adjunctive, flexible dosing	Moderate improvement after 2 wk of treatment
Maurer et al., 1999	MMD with somatoform pain disorder	1	Adjunctive, 1,800 mg/day	Remission of depression and pain
Perugi et al., 1999	Bipolar type I (mixed)	21	300–2,000 mg/day for 8 wk (mean dose, 1,130 mg/day)	Marked improvement in 4, moderate improvement in 6, mild worsening in 1; improvements maintained for 4–12 mo; HAMD decrease significantly
Sokolski et al., 1999	Bipolar disorder (mixed)	10	Adjunctive, flexible dosing	HAMD and BRMAS declined rapidly and significantly over 1 mo; improvement in insomnia
Hardoy et al., 1999	Schizoaffective and bipolar disorder with antipsychotic-induced movement disorder	16	Adjunctive, flexible dosing	14 patients showed improvement of movement disorders
Wang et al., 2000	Bipolar depression	23	Adjunctive, flexible dosing	60% response in mild to moderate depression, little or no response in severe depression
Vieta et al., 2000	Bipolar disorder type I and II	22	Flexible dosing (mean dose, 1,310 mg/day)	Two-point improvement on CGI-BP among 8 of 16 patients who completed 12 wk of treatment; those with anxious or depressive symptoms had the most improvement

ADHD, attention deficit/hyperactivity disorder; MDD, major depressive disorder.

preliminary evidence for the anxiolytic effects of gabapentin. Yet many unanswered questions remain. In addition to confirmation of the controlled trial results, a primary question centers on the dose–response curve in anxiety disorders. The doses used in the controlled trials were adjusted based on response and tolerability in the range of 900 to 3,600 mg daily given in three divided doses. Nearly two-thirds of the patients received doses >3,000 mg daily. Although these doses were well tolerated in both studies, the dose–response curve for anxiolytic effect can be definitively established only by fixed-dose studies. Anecdotal reports from experienced clinicians suggest that much smaller doses, perhaps in the range of 600 to 1,200 mg, may be sufficient to treat anxiety symptoms.

The safety of gabapentin among patients with epilepsy is now well known (15–19), but the safety of the drug in anxious patients is less well described. Both the controlled studies showed a profile of adverse events consistent with that previously reported among epileptic patients. The most frequent adverse events were somnolence and dizziness that dissipated with continued treatment. Fewer data are available on adverse effects associated with cessation of gabapentin treatment. In both controlled anxiety studies, gabapentin was discontinued at the end of the trial by a rapid taper-down over 6 days. No overt withdrawal phenomena were observed, a finding suggesting that, unlike some other anxiolytics, gabapentin may not produce tolerance and withdrawal effects. One case report, however, suggested that rebound anxiety may occur after withdrawal of high-dose gabapentin among patients with obsessive-compulsive disorder (20). Until more data accrue on this issue, following the general clinical principle of withdrawing any antiepileptic agent gradually seems advisable.

MOOD DISORDERS

The data on the use of gabapentin in the treatment of bipolar disorder are more complicated. Several clinical reports first suggested that gabapentin, like other anticonvulsants, may be clinically useful in treating patients with bipolar disorder who are partially responsive to conventional mood stabilizers (21,22). Numerous case series (23–35) were subsequently reported, confirming that therapeutic benefit was associated with the addition of gabapentin to combination drug regimens in patients with bipolar illness who were refractory to other treatments (Table 32.1).

Several of these reports involve patients with acute mania treated with gabapentin alone or in combination with other drugs (36–40). In the treatment of acute mania, the most important contribution comes from an open-label prospective study (36,37) using gabapentin either alone or in combination with other antimanic agents. These two reports involved 20 acutely manic inpatients treated with gabapentin either alone or added to other antimanic drugs.

Clinical symptom severity ratings were collected prospectively using the Bech-Rafaelsen Mania Scale. The authors of this study concluded that patients receiving gabapentin as adjunctive treatment derived greater benefit than those who received it as monotherapy. This finding may suggest that gabapentin treats some component of acute mania (e.g., comorbid anxiety, insomnia) that responds incompletely to traditional antimanic treatments. In this respect, gabapentin may be complementary to, rather than a substitute for, established antimanic agents. This idea is supported by another report of the open-label treatment of 22 patients with type I or II bipolar disorder (41). Of the 16 patients who completed 12 weeks of treatment, eight showed at least a two-point improvement on the Clinical Global Impression (Bipolar). The greatest improvement seemed to occur in patients with anxious and depressive features.

Some data suggest that the best candidates for adjunctive gabapentin treatment may be patients with bipolar depression in the mild to moderate range of severity (35). In this group, the rate of response was noted to be about 60%, whereas patients with more severe symptoms had little or no response.

Two controlled studies of gabapentin in bipolar disorder have been conducted. In a crossover design, Frye et al. (42) tested the utility of high-dose gabapentin (≤4,800 mg/day) among patients with bipolar disorder who were refractory to treatment with conventional mood stabilizer treatment (i.e., lithium, valproate, or carbamazepine). The patients were entered into a crossover study that included three randomized 6-week treatment periods with gabapentin, lamotrigine, or placebo. Only a modest benefit of gabapentin over placebo was demonstrated in the initial parallel-group portion of the study. Overall, the rate of improvement in mood symptoms on gabapentin did not differ from placebo.

Another study (43) involved patients with bipolar disorder (n = 117) treated with lithium, valproate, or the combination of the two and who were still manifesting manic, hypomanic, or mixed manic-depressed symptoms. After a 2-week single-blind placebo stabilization period to adjust the doses of lithium or valproate, patients were randomized to treatment with adjunctive gabapentin (900 to 3,600 mg/day) or placebo for 10 weeks. Their clinical status was rated using the Young Mania Rating Scale, the Hamilton Depression Rating Scale, the Internal States Scale, the NIMH-Life Chart, and the Clinical Global Impression of Change.

The results of this study were surprising in light of the previously published anecdotal reports of the beneficial effects of gabapentin in patients with bipolar disorder. Patients who received adjunctive placebo showed significantly greater reductions in the total Young Mania Rating Scale scores than those receiving adjunctive gabapentin. This difference was not explained by worsening in the gabapentin-treated group but by a larger therapeutic effect in the placebo-treated group. Further data exploration showed that the group randomized to placebo included a large number of patients whose background therapy (mainly lithium) was adjusted during the stabilization period. It is conceivable that this treatment optimization may have produced the greater therapeutic effect seen among patients receiving placebo during the randomized treatment phase. A fuller discussion of the methodologic problems with this study has been published (43).

The discrepancy between anecdotal reports and the controlled studies on the use of gabapentin in bipolar disorder is puzzling. It is possible that the patient population selected for the two controlled studies differed in some fundamental respect from the sort of patients selected by clinicians on a case-by-case basis and included in the published case reports. Alternatively, gabapentin may have a beneficial effect on some component of the bipolar disorder symptom picture (e.g., comorbid anxiety) that is not adequately treated by agents such as lithium and valproate and that was not adequately measured in the controlled studies.

OTHER PSYCHIATRIC CONDITIONS

A few published reports discuss the use of gabapentin for the control of behavioral disorders associated with dementia (44–47). This could be a valuable use for a well-tolerated drug such as gabapentin. Unfortunately, current knowledge on the use of gabapentin in this population lacks support from controlled studies.

Another promising application of gabapentin is enhancing abstinence during treatment of alcohol or cocaine abusers (48). Based on the association between postdetoxification insomnia and the risk of alcoholic relapse, it is proposed that using gabapentin to improve sleep may help to minimize resumption of drinking (49).

CONCLUSION

The data to date suggest that gabapentin is superior to placebo in reducing anxiety symptoms among patients with social phobia and in a subset of patients with panic disorder. The anxiolytic effect of gabapentin was shown in the social phobia study to be apparent as early as the first week of treatment. This speedy effect could be clinically useful, especially among patients requiring more rapid relief than that provided by the antidepressant drugs.

The efficacy of gabapentin in bipolar disorder is unclear. Anecdotal reports involving over 200 patients with bipolar disorder report therapeutic benefit on gabapentin treatment. Yet controlled studies have failed to detect such an effect. Several potential explanations exist for such a discrepancy that can only be resolved through further studies. In summary, gabapentin may be useful in the treatment of

psychiatric symptoms in anxiety and other disorders, but a great deal more controlled research is required before definitive recommendations for such use can be made.

ACKNOWLEDGMENT

Atul C. Pande, MD, graciously reviewed this manuscript, and I appreciate his thoughtful criticisms.

REFERENCES

1. Post RM, Frye MA, Denicoff KD, et al. Beyond lithium in the treatment of bipolar illness. *Neuropsychopharmacology* 1998;19: 206–219.
2. Blum DE. New drugs for persons with epilepsy. *Adv Neurol* 1998;76:57–87.
3. Leach JP, Girvan J, Paul A, et al. Gabapentin and cognition: a double blind, dose ranging, placebo controlled study in refractory epilepsy. *J Neurol Neurosurg Psychiatry* 1997;62:372–376.
4. Martin R, Kuzniecky R, Ho S, et al. Cognitive effects of topiramate, gabapentin, and lamotrigine in healthy young adults. *Neurology* 1999;52:321–327.
5. Meador KJ, Loring DW, Ray PG, et al. Differential cognitive effects of carbamazepine and gabapentin. *Epilepsia* 1999;40:1279–1285.
6. Mortimore C, Trimble M, Emmers E. Effects of gabapentin on cognition and quality of life in patients with epilepsy. *Seizure* 1998;7:359–364.
7. Dimond KR, Pande AC, Lamoreaux L, et al. Effect of gabapentin (Neurontin) [corrected] on mood and well-being in patients with epilepsy [published erratum appears in *Prog Neuropsychopharmacol Biol Psychiatry* 1996;20:1081]. *Prog Neuropsychopharmacol Biol Psychiatry* 1996;20:407–417.
8. Harden CL, Lazar LM, Pick LH, et al. A beneficial effect on mood in partial epilepsy patients treated with gabapentin. *Epilepsia* 1999;40:1129–1134.
9. Singh L, Field MJ, Ferris P, et al. The antiepileptic agent gabapentin (Neurontin) possesses anxiolytic-like and antinociceptive actions that are reversed by D-serine. *Psychopharmacology (Berl)* 1996;127:1–9.
10. Chouinard G, Beauclair L, Belanger MC. Gabapentin: long-term antianxiety and hypnotic effects in psychiatric patients with comorbid anxiety-related disorders [Letter]. *Can J Psychiatry* 1998;43:305.
11. Pollack MH, Matthews J, Scott EL. Gabapentin as a potential treatment for anxiety disorders [Letter]. *Am J Psychiatry* 1998; 155:992–993.
12. Pande AC, Davidson JR, Jefferson JW, et al. Treatment of social phobia with gabapentin: a placebo-controlled study. *J Clin Psychopharmacol* 1999;19:341–348.
13. Pande AC, Pollack MH, Crockatt J, et al. Placebo-controlled study of gabapentin treatment of panic disorder. *J Clin Psychopharmacol* 2000;20:467–471.
14. Bandelow B. Assessing the efficacy of treatments for panic disorder and agoraphobia. II. The Panic and Agoraphobia Scale. *Int Clin Psychopharmacol* 1995;10:73–81.
15. McLean MJ. Gabapentin. *Epilepsia* 1995;36[Suppl 2]:S73–S86.
16. Marson AG, Kadir ZA, Chadwick DW. New antiepileptic drugs: a systematic review of their efficacy and tolerability. *BMJ* 1996; 313:1169–1174.
17. Bourgeois BF. New antiepileptic drugs. *Arch Neurol* 1998; 55:1181–1183.

18. Curry WJ, Kulling DL. Newer antiepileptic drugs: gabapentin, lamotrigine, felbamate, topiramate and fosphenytoin. *Am Fam Physician* 1998;57:513–520.
19. Shorvon S, Stefan H. Overview of the safety of newer antiepileptic drugs. *Epilepsia* 1997;38[Suppl 1]:S45–S51.
20. Cora Locatelli G, Greenberg BD, Martin JD, et al. Rebound psychiatric and physical symptoms after gabapentin discontinuation [Letter]. *J Clin Psychiatry* 1998;59:131.
21. Ryback RS, Brodsky L, Munasifi F. Gabapentin in bipolar disorder [Letter]. *J Neuropsychiatry Clin Neurosci* 1997;9:301.
22. Schaffer CB, Schaffer LC. Gabapentin in the treatment of bipolar disorder [Letter]. *Am J Psychiatry* 1997;154:291–292.
23. Young LT, Robb JC, Patelis Siotis I, et al. Acute treatment of bipolar depression with gabapentin. *Biol Psychiatry* 1997;42:851–853.
24. Young LT, Robb JC, Hasey GM, et al. Gabapentin as an adjunctive treatment in bipolar disorder. *J Affect Disord* 1999;55:73–77.
25. McElroy SL, Soutullo CA, Keck PE Jr, et al. A pilot trial of adjunctive gabapentin in the treatment of bipolar disorder. *Ann Clin Psychiatry* 1997;9:99–103.
26. Bennett J, Goldman WT, Suppes T. Gabapentin for treatment of bipolar and schizoaffective disorders. *J Clin Psychopharmacol* 1997;17:141–142.
27. Ghaemi SN, Katzow JJ, Desai SP, et al. Gabapentin treatment of mood disorders: a preliminary study. *J Clin Psychiatry* 1998;59:426–429.
28. Knoll J, Stegman K, Suppes T. Clinical experience using gabapentin adjunctively in patients with a history of mania or hypomania. *J Affect Disord* 1998;49:229–233.
29. Brown ES, Hong SC. Antidepressant-induced bruxism successfully treated with gabapentin. *J Am Dent Assoc* 1999;130:1467–1469.
30. Cabras PL, Hardoy MJ, Hardoy MC, et al. Clinical experience with gabapentin in patients with bipolar or schizoaffective disorder: results of an open-label study. *J Clin Psychiatry* 1999;60:245–248.
31. Hardoy MC, Hardoy MJ, Carta MG, et al. Gabapentin as a promising treatment for antipsychotic-induced movement disorders in schizoaffective and bipolar patients. *J Affect Disord* 1999;54:315–317.
32. Maurer I, Volz HP, Sauer H. Gabapentin leads to remission of somatoform pain disorder with major depression. *Pharmacopsychiatry* 1999;32:255–257.
33. Perugi G, Toni C, Ruffolo G, et al. Clinical experience using adjunctive gabapentin in treatment-resistant bipolar mixed states. *Pharmacopsychiatry* 1999;32:136–141.
34. Sokolski KN, Green C, Maris DE, et al. Gabapentin as an adjunct to standard mood stabilizers in outpatients with mixed bipolar symptomatology. *Ann Clin Psychiatry* 1999;11:217–222.
35. Wang PW, Winsberg ME, Santosa CM, et al. Open adjunctive gabapentin effective in bipolar depression. *Biol Psychiatry* 2000;47[Suppl]:84S.
36. Erfurth A, Kammerer C, Grunze H, et al. An open label study of gabapentin in the treatment of acute mania. *J Psychiatr Res* 1998;32:261–264.
37. Grunze H, Erfurth A, Amann B, et al. Gabapentin in the treatment of mania. *Fortschr Neurol Psychiatr* 1999;67:256–260.
38. Hatzimanolis J, Lykouras L, Oulis P, et al. Gabapentin as monotherapy in the treatment of acute mania. *Eur Neuropsychopharmacol* 1999;9:257–258.
39. Stanton SP, Keck PE Jr, McElroy SL. Treatment of acute mania with gabapentin [Letter]. *Am J Psychiatry* 1997;154:287.
40. Soutullo CA, Casuto LS, Keck PE Jr. Gabapentin in the treatment of adolescent mania: a case report. *J Child Adolesc Psychopharmacol* 1998;8:81–85.
41. Vieta E, Martinez-Arán A, Nieto E, et al. Adjunctive gabapentin treatment of bipolar disorder. *Eur J Psychiatry* 2000;15:433–437.
42. Frye MA, Ketter TA, Kimbrell TA, et al. A placebo-controlled study of lamotrigine and gabapentin monotherapy in refractory mood disorders. *J Clin Psychopharmacol* 2000;20:607–614.
43. Pande AC, Crockatt JG, Janney CA, et al. Gabapentin in bipolar disorder: a placebo-controlled trial of adjunctive therapy. *Bipolar Disord* 2000;2:249–255.
44. Dallocchio C, Buffa C, Mazzarello P. Combination of donepezil and gabapentin for behavioral disorders in Alzheimer's disease [Letter]. *J Clin Psychiatry* 2000;61:64.
45. Hawkins JW, Tinklenberg JR, Sheikh JI, et al. A retrospective chart review of gabapentin for the treatment of aggressive and agitated behavior in patients with dementias. *Am J Geriatr Psychiatry* 2000;8:221–225.
46. Herrmann N, Lanctot K, Myszak M. Effectiveness of gabapentin for the treatment of behavioral disorders in dementia. *J Clin Psychopharmacol* 2000;20:90–93.
47. Letterman L, Markowitz JS. Gabapentin: a review of published experience in the treatment of bipolar disorder and other psychiatric conditions. *Pharmacotherapy* 1999;19:565–572.
48. Myrick H, Malcolm R, Brady KT. Gabapentin treatment of alcohol withdrawal [Letter]. *Am J Psychiatry* 1998;155:1632.
49. Karam Hage M, Brower KJ. Gabapentin treatment for insomnia associated with alcohol dependence [Letter]. *Am J Psychiatry* 2000;157:151.

GABAPENTIN

ADVERSE EFFECTS

R. EUGENE RAMSAY
FLAVIA M. PRYOR

Gabapentin is a chemical derivative of the inhibitory neurotransmitter γ-aminobutyric acid (GABA). It was originally developed to be a GABA analog that would penetrate the blood–brain barrier.

ANIMAL STUDIES

Preclinical toxicology studies showed gabapentin to be well tolerated in mice and rats in acute doses up to 8,000 mg/kg and with chronic dosing up to 3,000 mg/kg (1). Signs of toxicity (e.g., ataxia and sedation) were noted only at the higher doses. No toxicity was noted in monkeys in doses up to 1,250 mg/kg. Efficacy was evident in rats and mice in doses of 25 to 100 mg/kg. Thus, the studies suggested a very favorable toxicity-to-efficacy ratio.

Pancreatic Tumors

In chronic preclinical studies, a statistically significant increase in the incidence of pancreatic acinar cell tumors was found in male Wistar rats receiving 2,000 mg/kg of gabapentin, but not with lower doses (1,2,3). These tumors were not observed in female rats or mice of either sex. The tumors were low-grade malignancies, did not metastasize, were similar to those seen in concurrent control animals, and did not affect survival (1,2,3). Cellular hyperplasia, carcinoma *in situ*, and locally invasive tumors became evident after the same duration of drug exposure. This is not the pattern of occurrence seen with carcinogenic drugs, where hyperplasia is evident early, followed by carcinoma *in situ*, and then invasive tumors. The rat is not a generally accepted model for human pancreatic cancer and no pancreatic tumors have been reported in patients taking gabapentin (3). The relevance of these tumors to humans is

R. Eugene Ramsay, MD: Professor of Neurology and Psychiatry, Department of Neurology, University of Miami School of Medicine, Miami, Florida

Flavia M. Pryor, RN, BSN: Nurse Researcher, Department of Neurology Service, Miami Veterans Affairs Medical Center, Miami, Florida

questionable given the characteristics of the pancreatic tumors in male rats and the circumstances under which they develop. As a result of the animal studies, clinical trials were halted in the United States in August 1990 while this issue was reviewed further. A National Institutes of Health Advisory Committee reviewed the available information and recommended that the clinical trials be restarted. Trials were restarted in October 1991.

Teratogenesis

Clinical studies of gabapentin in pregnant women have not been conducted. In rats and mice given up to 2,000 mg/kg of gabapentin, delayed skeletal ossification was found; however, fetal weight and subsequent growth and development were unaffected. Doses 25 to 50 times those used in humans resulted in an increased occurrence of hydroureter and hydronephrosis. In these animals, the incidence of major malformations (e.g., clefting and congenital heart, gastrointestinal, or neural tube defects) was the same as in control animals. Maternal toxicity resulted when rabbits were given 1,500 mg/kg. However, no malformations were observed and skeletal ossification was not affected. Gabapentin was not mutagenic *in vitro* in standard assays using bacterial or mammalian cells (1).

CLINICAL ADVERSE EVENTS

Gabapentin's adverse event profile has been compiled from results from clinical trials and long-term follow-up studies (1,3–12). Doses up to 1,800 mg/day were used in the controlled trials and up to 3,600 mg/day in open studies. Since gabapentin has been marketed, doses above 7,000 mg/day have been prescribed. However, the typical upper dosage limit has been 3,600 to 4,800 mg/day. In the controlled clinical trials, gabapentin was used mainly as add-on therapy, and hence a direct causal relationship between the adverse events reported and gabapentin therapy has not

TABLE 33.1. FREQUENCY OF ADVERSE EVENTS BEING REPORTED IN THE CONTROLLED CLINICAL TRIALS WITH THE ADDITION OF EITHER GABAPENTIN OR PLACEBO

	Gabapentin (%)	Placebo (%)
Somnolence	20	9
Dizziness	18	7
Ataxia	13	6
Fatigue	11	5
Tremor	7	3
Diplopia	6	2

been established. The most common adverse events reported were those affecting the central nervous system (CNS) and included somnolence, dizziness, and ataxia (Table 33.1). The median time to onset of the first side effect of any type was 14 days in gabapentin-treated patients and 20 days for those receiving placebo (1,9). In those patients reporting CNS symptoms, the median time of onset was 3 days after initiating gabapentin treatment, compared with a 14-day median onset of CNS symptoms in patients receiving placebo (1,9). Although most patients experienced one or more adverse events, the events were of mild to moderate severity and usually transient, resolving within 2 weeks of onset during continued treatment (1,1,13–15). The median duration of symptoms in the gabapentin treatment group was 14 days, versus 13 days with placebo groups (1). Long-term gabapentin therapy did not result either in an increase in number or in new types of adverse events (1). Although overall, side effects were reported more often in the groups treated with gabapentin, a clear dose–effect relationship was not evident (Figure 33.1). The incidence of somnolence was higher in the placebo than in the 900 mg/day gabapentin group, whereas

the incidence of dizziness was higher in the 900 mg/day than in the 1,200 or 1,800 mg/day gabapentin groups (1,1,9,16). Results from 59 healthy patients older than 65 years of age revealed no evidence for increased frequency of adverse events in this age group compared with younger patients (1).

Few patients withdrew from the controlled clinical trials with gabapentin as a result of side effects (9). Overall, approximately 7% of patients receiving gabapentin withdrew, compared with approximately 3% of those receiving placebo (1,14–16). The most common reason for the gabapentin-treated patients to withdraw was development of CNS symptoms (1,3,5,14,15) (Table 33.2). To evaluate the relative incidence of side effects, Marson et al. (17) collected outcomes on all the placebo-controlled trials involving the new antiepileptic drugs (AEDs). The side effect odds ratios (ratio of outcomes on therapy compared with placebo) ranged across all the drugs from 1.19 to 4.23. Gabapentin's odds ratio of 1.36 was second lowest of all the new AEDs, indicating a low incidence of side effects.

Gabapentin has been compared with carbamazepine (18) and lamotrigine (19) in controlled clinical trials involving patients with newly diagnosed epilepsy. The dropout rate was 0% to 14% for gabapentin (doses of 300, 900, and 1,800 mg/day), compared with 24% for carbamazepine. The dropout rate was similar comparing the outcome of gabapentin and lamotrigine (600 mg/day) (19).

Cognitive effects of AEDs always are of concern. In the controlled clinical trials, anecdotal reports of a feeling of well-being were encountered in patients taking gabapentin. In normal subjects, gabapentin manifests a psychotropic effect compared with placebo (20). This was characterized by improvement in concentration, numerical memory, complex reaction, and reaction time test. A blinded, controlled study was performed in healthy young adults using

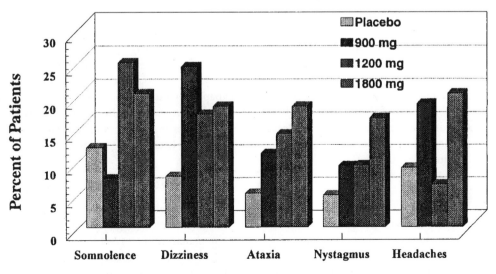

FIGURE 33.1. Incidence of adverse effects with gabapentin.

TABLE 33.2. MOST FREQUENT ADVERSE EVENTS FOR WHICH PATIENTS WITHDREW FROM THE GABAPENTIN CLINICAL TRIALS

	Gabapentin (%)	Placebo (%)
Somnolence	1.12	0.53
Ataxia	1.73	0.35
Dizziness	0.58	0.35
Fatigue	0.58	0
Nausea/vomiting	0.58	0.88
Abnormal thinking	0.34	0.35

topiramate, gabapentin, and lamotrigine (21). Neurocognitive performance was established before and after 2 and 4 weeks of chronic dosing. Gabapentin-treated subjects had no alteration in performance at any testing period. Similar results were reported by Leach et al. (22) comparing 1,200, 1,800, and 2,400 mg/day of gabapentin with placebo added to the existing AED regimen in patients with uncontrolled seizures. Gabapentin has been compared with carbamazepine for their effects on cognitive testing in healthy senior adults (≥65 years of age) (23). Most (15 of 19) of the subjects who dropped out before study's end were taking carbamazepine. A mild effect was evident with both drugs, but performance with gabapentin was better than with carbamazepine in 9 of 11 cognitive measures. A similar comparison was made in healthy young subjects, and the results favored gabapentin over carbamazepine in 22 of the 31 cognitive measures studied (24).

Mood Changes

Gabapentin-induced mood and behavioral changes have been reported in both adults and children (25–29). In children, behavioral changes are characterized by acute onset of aggression, hyperactivity, and impulsive behavior (25–27). All children had chronic epilepsy and static encephalopathy, and many were multiply handicapped. In all cases, these behaviors were reversible either with dose reduction or discontinuation of gabapentin. These side effects, however, are not unique to gabapentin and have been reported with other AEDs, including carbamazepine, valproate, clonazepam, and phenobarbital (30–33). Mood changes characterized by euphoria and behavioral disinhibition have been reported in adults being treated for epilepsy or paresthesias (28,29). In each case, the severity of the mood change has been mild and self-limiting or reversible.

Seizure Exacerbation

Gabapentin has been reported to aggravate seizures in some epileptic patients (34–36). This side effect is not unique to gabapentin. In fact, virtually all AEDs can produce similar effect(s). Specifically, gabapentin may increase typical and atypical absences and worsen or produce myoclonus

(36,37). In reviewing 104 consecutive patients started on gabapentin, 13 cases of myoclonus were found (37). Multifocal myoclonus developed in 10 patients; focal myoclonus contralateral to the epileptic focus developed in 3 of these patients. Exacerbation of preexisting myoclonus was observed in two patients. In all cases, the myoclonus was of mild intensity and did not significantly interfere with daily living. The myoclonus resolved when gabapentin was discontinued. There have been no reports of gabapentin aggravating partial-onset seizures.

Weight Gain

Early clinical trials did not report weight gain associated gabapentin therapy. However, changes in body weight have subsequently been reported with long-term, high-dose gabapentin therapy (38). Of 44 patients [23 men and 21 women; 18 to 54 years of age (mean, 27.2 years)] treated with gabapentin for 12 months, 10 patients gained more than 10% of their baseline weight; 15 patients gained 5% to 10% of baseline; 16 patients had no change; and 3 patients lost 5% to 10% of baseline weight. All patients were receiving at least 1,800 mg/day; 28 of the 44 were receiving dosages 3,000 mg/day. Weight gain also was reported in a retrospective study of 121 epileptic patients (62 men and 59 women; mean age, 36 years) receiving gabapentin for at least 3 months (39). The average gabapentin dose was 2,291 mg/day. Seventy-eight (64%) of patients gained 10 lbs. The greatest weight gain (average, 20.1 lbs.) occurred in those patients discontinuing felbamate (n = 72) compared with those on concomitant valproate (n = 15; average weight gain, 14.7 lbs.). Patients receiving other AEDs (n = 34) gained an average of 7 lbs.

Pedal Edema

In the authors' clinical experience, gabapentin therapy has been associated with pedal edema. This often occurs with relatively low doses (900 to 1,800 mg/day) and improves or resolves with dosage reduction or discontinuing the drug. Pedal edema occurs with approximately the same frequency as with valproate therapy (40,41). Cotherapy with gabapentin and valproate does not seem to increase the frequency with which this side effect is encountered. The mechanism is unclear, and it occurs without evidence for congestive heart failure or low serum protein.

Sexual Dysfunction

Ejaculatory failure and anorgasmia have been reported in patients treated with gabapentin for psychiatric disorders or pain management (42–44). These adverse events are rare and have been reported in men receiving doses as low as 900 mg/day. In each case, symptoms resolved after gabapentin therapy was discontinued. In all cases, the patients were receiving other psychotropic medications. No clear pharmacokinetic or pharmacodynamic drug interaction associated with gabapentin resulting in ejaculatory difficulty has been identified.

SERIOUS ADVERSE EVENTS

Very few potentially serious adverse events requiring discontinuation of gabapentin therapy have been reported in over 2,000 patient exposures in randomized, controlled clinical trials. Those events reported include rash (0.54%), decreased white blood cell counts (WBC; 0.19%), increased blood urea nitrogen (0.09%), decreased platelets (0.09%), and angina or electrocardiographic changes (0.04%) (1). The low incidence of rash compares favorably with an average 5% to 10% incidence of rash requiring discontinuation of therapy with traditional AEDs (45). No patient has experienced a Stevens-Johnson reaction or other severe allergic reaction to gabapentin during clinical trials. Subsequently, only two verified skin reactions from gabapentin have been published (see later).

Systemic Toxicities

Only four patients discontinued therapy owing to low WBC counts, and they were all receiving concurrent AEDs. The overall incidence of WBC <3,000 cells/mm^3 was 8% in patients treated with gabapentin, versus 7% in those patients receiving placebo (1). As might be expected from a drug that does not undergo hepatic metabolism, hepatotoxicity has not been observed (9). No changes in liver function have been observed that required termination of gabapentin therapy (1).

Overdose

Five cases of overdose with gabapentin have occurred. The largest dose was 48.9 g in a 16-year-old, otherwise healthy girl (46). She presented to an emergency department with complaints of dizziness and lethargy. Her highest plasma level was 62 µg/mL, which is approximately three times the level being achieved in clinical use. The patient's symptoms had cleared by 18 hours postingestion. A case of sustained massive overdose also was reported without serious side effects (47). Because of the dose-dependent absorption of gabapentin, overdosing appears unlikely to occur.

Allergic Reactions

Only two verified cases of serious skin reactions from gabapentin have been published (48,49). These patients had significant skin rashes to other AEDs and the reaction to gabapentin was milder than they had previously experienced (48). Considering that over 5 million patients have

been treated with this drug and given the rarity of reported skin reactions, gabapentin appears to have the lowest incidence of allergic reactions of all the AEDs.

OTHER ADVERSE EVENTS

Other case reports of side effects have included choreoathetosis (50,51), dystonia (52), isolated ataxia (53), reversible acute renal allograft dysfunction (54), and worsening of myasthenia gravis (55). A causal relationship with gabapentin therapy is more difficult to determine when there is only a single or very few reported cases of each of these effects.

PHARMACODYNAMIC INTERACTIONS

Few pharmacodynamic interactions have been described with concomitant use of gabapentin. In the authors' clinical experience, visual disturbances consisting oscillopsia and diplopia may be encountered when gabapentin is administered to patients with high plasma levels of carbamazepine. Neurologic examination when the patient is symptomatic reveals the presence of a prominent nystagmus with a downbeat component at the extremes of horizontal gaze and an ataxic gait. This possibly represents a pharmacodynamic interaction between gabapentin and carbamazepine resulting in carbamazepine toxicity. This interaction is similar to that reported with concurrent use of carbamazepine and lamotrigine (56). Morris et al. (57) also noted an increase in fatigue when gabapentin was added to carbamazepine therapy.

TERATOGENESIS

As of March 1997, 38 pregnancies have been verified in women taking gabapentin during their first trimester. All the infants were normal in the eight monotherapy exposures. Pregnancies were electively terminated with no evidence of malformations in the fetuses. Two malformations have been reported—pyloric stenosis and a sixth digit. A third infant was delivered at 26 weeks of gestation and did not survive. Additional clinical experience is needed, but these data suggest a relative lack of teratogenic potential.

SUMMARY

The safety profile of an anticonvulsant is an important consideration. The older AEDs have a significant incidence of side effects that either limit the dosage that can be used or, in some cases, are life threatening. The differences in the usefulness of AEDs often are related to their relative toxicities

(58–60). Gabapentin is very well tolerated, with the CNS symptoms of somnolence, dizziness, and ataxia the most frequently encountered. A very low incidence of potentially serious side effects has been encountered, and no fatalities have been reported that can be attributed to this drug. The adverse effects encountered are dose related and usually transient. The use of a higher dose does produce a somewhat greater incidence of side effects. These usually are transient and tolerated by the patient. The safety and tolerability of gabapentin, along with the absence of pharmacokinetic interactions, are strong advantages in using this drug.

REFERENCES

1. Parke-Davis. Data on file. Morris Plains, New Jersey, 1993.
2. Browne TR, U.S. IaP-DGsg. Long-term efficacy and toxicity of gabapentin. *Neurology* 1993;43:A307(abstr).
3. Browne TR. Efficacy and safety of gabapentin. In: Chadwick DW, ed. *New trends in epilepsy management: the role of gabapentin.* London: Royal Society of Medical Services, 1993: 47–57.
4. Abou-Khalil BW, McLean M, Castro O, et al. Gabapentin in the treatment of refractory partial seizures. *Epilepsia* 1990;31:644 (abstr).
5. Abou-Khalil BW, Shellenberger MK, Anhut H. Two open-label, multicenter studies of the safety and efficacy of gabapentin in patients with refractory epilepsy. *Epilepsia* 1992;33[Suppl 3]: 77–77(abstr).
6. Handforth A, Treiman DM, Norton LC. Effect of gabapentin on complex partial seizure frequency. *Neurology* 1989;39[Suppl 1]: 114(abstr).
7. Leppik IE, Shellenberger K, Anhut H. Two open-label, multicenter studies of the safety and efficacy of gabapentin as add-on therapy in patients with refractory partial seizures. Epilepsia 1992;33[Suppl 3]:117(abstr).
8. Ojemann LM, Wilensky AJ, Temkin NR, et al. Long-term treatment with gabapentin for partial epilepsy. *Epilepsy Res* 1992; 13:159–165.
9. Ramsay RE. Clinical efficacy and safety of gabapentin [Review]. *Neurology* 1994;44:S23–S30; discussion S31–S32.
10. Schear MJ, Wiener JA, Rowan AJ. Long-term efficacy of gabapentin in the treatment of partial seizures. *Epilepsia* 1991;32 [Suppl 3]:6(abstr).
11. Sivenius J, Kalvianen R, Ylinen A, et al. Efficacy of gabapentin in long-term therapy in partial seizures. *Epilepsia* 1990;31:644(abstr).
12. Wiener JA, Schear MJ, Rowan AJ, et al. Safety and effectiveness of gabapentin in the treatment of partial seizures. *Epilepsia* 1990;31:644(abstr).
13. Bruni J, Saunders M, Anhut H, et al. Efficacy and safety of gabapentin: a multicenter, placebo-controlled, double-blind study. *Neurology* 1991;41[Suppl 1]:330–331(abstr).
14. UK Gabapentin Study Group. Gabapentin in partial epilepsy. *Lancet* 1990;335:1114–1117.
15. U.S. Gabapentin Study Group No.5. Gabapentin as add-on therapy in refractory partial epilepsy: a double-blind, placebo-controlled, parallel-group study. *Neurology* 1993;43:2292–2298.
16. Goa KL, Sorkin EM. Gabapentin: a review of its pharmacological properties and clinical potential in epilepsy. *Drugs* 1993; 46:409–427.
17. Marson AG, Kadir ZA, Jutton JL, et al. The new antiepileptic drugs: a systematic review of their efficacy and tolerability. *Epilepsia* 1997;38:859–880(abstr).

18. Murray G, Anhut H, Greiner MJ, et al., and the GBP monotherapy study group 945-77/78. Gabapentin (Neurontin) monotherapy: results of a multicenter study comparing gabapentin and carbamazepine in patients with newly diagnosed partial seizures. *Epilepsia* 1997;38:205(abstr).
19. Brodie MJ, Chadwick DW, Anhut H, et al. Gabapentin versus lamotrigine monotherapy: a double-blind comparison in newly diagnosed epilepsy. *Epilepsia* 2001(abstr).
20. Saletu B, Grunberger J, Linzmayer L. Evaluation of encephalotrophic and psychotrophic properties of gabapentin in man by pharmacy-EEG psychometry. *Int J Clin Pharmacol Ther Toxicol* 1986;24:362–373.
21. Martin R, Kuzniecky R, Ho S, et al. Cognitive effects of topiramate, gabapentin, and lamotrigine in healthy young adults. *Neurology* 1999;52:321–327(abstr).
22. Leach JP, Girvan J, Paul A, et al. Gabapentin and cognition: a double blind, dose ranging, placebo controlled study in refractory epilepsy. *J Neurol Neurosurg Psychiatry* 1997;62:372–376.
23. Martin R, Meador KJ, Turrentine L, et al. Comparative cognitive effects of carbamazepine and gabapentin in healthy senior adults. *Epilepsia* 2001;42:764–771(abstr).
24. Meador KJ, Loring DW, Ray PG, et al. Differential cognitive effects of carbamazepine and gabapentin. *Epilepsia* 1999;40: 1279–1285(abstr).
25. Wolf SM, Shinnar S, Kang H, et al. Gabapentin toxicity in children manifesting as behavioral changes. *Epilepsia* 1995;36: 1203–1205.
26. Tallian K, Nahata M, Lo W, et al. Gabapentin associated with aggressive behavior in pediatric patients with seizures. *Epilepsia* 1996;37:501–502.
27. Lee D, Steingard R, Cesena M, et al. Behavioral side effects of gabapentin in children. *Epilepsia* 1996;37:87–90.
28. Short C, Cooke L. Hypomania induced by gabapentin. *Br J Psychiatry* 1995;166:679–680.
29. Trinka E, Niedermuller U, Thaler C, et al. Gabapentin-induced mood changes with hypomanic features in adults. *Seizure* 2000;9:505–508.
30. Rivinius T. Psychiatric effects of the anticonvulsant regimens. *J Clin Psychopharmacol* 1982;2:165–192.
31. Wolf SM, Forsythe A. Behavior disturbance, phenobarbital and febrile seizures. *Pediatrics* 1978;61:728–731.
32. Committee on Drugs. Behavioral and cognitive side effects of anticonvulsant therapy. *Pediatrics* 1985;76:644–677.
33. Silverstein F, Parrish M, Johnston M. Adverse behavioral reactions in children treated with carbamazepine (Tegretol). *J Pediatr* 1982;101:785–787.
34. Elger CE, Bauer J, Scherrmann J, et al. Aggravation of focal epileptic seizures by antiepileptic drugs. *Epilepsia* 1998;39: S15–S18.
35. Perucca E, Gram LF, Avanzani G, et al. Antiepileptic drugs as a cause of worsening seizures. *Epilepsia* 1998;39:5–17.
36. Genton P. When antiepileptic drugs aggravate epilepsy. *Brain Dev* 2000;22:75–80.
37. Asconape J, Diedrich A, DellaBadia J. Myoclonus associated with the use of gabapentin. *Epilepsia* 2000;41:479–481.
38. DeToledo JC, Toledo C, DeCerce J, et al. Changes in body weight with chronic, high- dose gabapentin therapy. *Ther Drug Monit* 1997;19:394–396.
39. Cahill WT, Mozahem K, Privitera M. Weight changes with the use of gabapentin. *Epilepsia* 1998;39:54–54.
40. Basel-Vanagaite L, Zeharia A, Mimouni M. Edema associated with valproate therapy. *Ann Pharmacother* 1999;33:1370–1371.
41. Ettinger A, Moshe S, Shinnar S. Edema associated with long-term valproate therapy. *Epilepsia* 1990;31:211–213.
42. Labbate LA, Rubey RN. Gabapentin-induced ejaculatory failure and anorgasmia. *Am J Psychiatry* 1999;156:972–972.

43. Clark JD, Elliott J. Gabapentin-induced anorgasmia. *Neurology* 1999;53:2209–2209.

44. Brannon GE, Rolland PD. Anorgasmia in patient with bipolar disorder type I treated with gabapentin. *J Clin Psychopharmacol* 2000;20:379–381.

45. Mattson RH, Cramer JA, Collins JF, et al., DVA Cooperative Study No.264 Group. A comparison of valproate with carbamazepine for the treatment of complex partial seizures and secondarily generalized tonic-clonic seizures in adults. *N Engl J Med* 1992;327:765–771.

46. Fischer JH, Barr AN, Trudeau VL, et al. Lack of serious toxicity following gabapentin overdose. *Neurology* 1994;44:982–983.

47. Verma A, St. Clair EW, Radtke RA. A case of sustained massive gabapentin overdose without serious side effects. *Ther Drug Monit* 1999;21:615–617.

48. DeToledo JC, Minagar A, Lowe M, et al. Skin eruption with gabapentin in a patient with repeated AED-induced Stevens-Johnson's syndrome. *Ther Drug Monit* 1999;21:37–38. 1999.

49. Gonzalez-Sicilia L, Cano A, Serrano M, et al. Stevens-Johnson syndrome associated with gabapentin. *Am J Med* 1998;105:455(abstr).

50. Chudnow RS, Dewey RB, Lawson CR. Choreoathetosis as a side effect of gabapentin therapy in severely neurologically impaired patients. *Arch Neurol* 1997;54:910–912.

51. Buetefisch CM, Gutierrez A, Gutmann L. Choreoathetotic movements: a possible side effect of Neurontin. *Neurology* 1996;46:851–852.

52. Palomeras E, Sanz P, Cano A, et al. Dystonia in a patient treated with propranolol and gabapentin. *Arch Neurol* 2000;57:570–571.

53. Steinhoff BJ, Herrendorf G, Bittermann HJ, et al. Isolated ataxia as an idiosyncratic side-effect under gabapentin. *Seizure* 1997;6:503–504.

54. Gallay BJ, de Mattos AM, Norman DJ. Reversible acute renal allograft dysfunction due to gabapentin. *Transplantation* 2000;70:208–209.

55. Boneva N, Brenner T, Argov Z. Gabapentin may be hazardous in myasthenia gravis. *Muscle Nerve* 2000;38:1204–1208.

56. Besag FM, Berry DJ, Pool F, et al. Carbamazepine toxicity with lamotrigine: pharmacokinetic or pharmacodynamic interaction? *Epilepsia* 1998;39:183–187.

57. Morris GL. Efficacy and tolerability of gabapentin in clinical practice. *Clin Ther* 1995;17:891–900.

58. Homan RW, Miller B, the Veterans Administration Epilepsy Cooperative Study Group. Causes of treatment failure with antiepileptic drugs vary over time. *Neurology* 1987;37:1620–1623.

59. Mattson RH, Cramer JA, Collins JF, et al. Comparison of carbamazepine, phenobarbital, phenytoin, and primidone in partial and secondarily generalized tonic-clonic seizures. *N Engl J Med* 1985;313:145–151.

60. Smith DB, Mattson RH, Cramer JA, et al. Results of a nationwide Veterans Administration Cooperative Study comparing the efficacy and toxicity of carbamazepine, phenobarbital, phenytoin, and primidone. *Epilepsia* 1987;28:S50–S58.

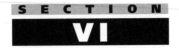

LAMOTRIGINE

LAMOTRIGINE

MECHANISMS OF ACTION

MICHAEL J. LEACH
ANDREW D. RANDALL
ALESSANDRO STEFANI
ATTICUS H. HAINSWORTH

Lamotrigine (LTG, Lamictal: 3,5-diamino-6-[2,3-dichloro-phenyl]-1,2,4-triazine) is emerging as a clinically useful antiepileptic drug in the treatment of refractory partial epilepsy, generalized seizures, typical absence seizures, and Lennox-Gastaut syndrome (5,51). Positive clinical trials with LTG have also been reported for the treatment of mania in bipolar disorder (2,24,35,52), neuropathic pain (20,72), migraine with aura attacks (18), and Huntington's disease (39). Experimental evidence supports the view that the principal mechanism of action of LTG is blockade of both voltage-gated sodium (Na) and calcium (Ca) channels (50,54,68,69,80,83), although other actions have been proposed (17,83).

PRECLINICAL ANTICONVULSANT STUDIES

Many of the clinical utilities for LTG were predicted from animal anticonvulsant studies, with the notable exception of absence seizures. Thus, LTG blocks hindlimb extension after maximal electroshock- and pentylenetetrazole-induced tonic seizures (rodent models of partial and generalized tonic-clonic seizures) (57,80).

Paradigms considered to be predictive for efficacy in absence epilepsy are increased clonus latency in the pentylenetetrazole model (38), the genetic absence epilepsy rat from Strasbourg (GAERS) (73), and genetic mouse variants

Michael J. Leach, PhD: Reader in Pharmacology and Drug Development, Department of Chemical and Life Sciences, University of Greenwich, London, United Kingdom

Andrew D. Randall, MA, PhD: Head of Neurophysiology and Neuropharmacology, Department of Neurology, GlaxoSmithKline Pharmaceuticals, Harlow, Essex, United Kingdom

Alessandro Stefani, MD: Diplomate Neuroscienze, University of Tor Vergata, Rome, Italy

Atticus H. Hainsworth, MA, PhD: Senior Lecturer in Pharmacology, School of Pharmacy, De Montfort University, Leicester, United Kingdom

that have been isolated (6,7). In particular, three voltage-dependent Ca channel subunit mutants—tottering (tg), lethargic (lh), and stargazer (stg)—display cortical spike–wave discharges with characteristics similar to those of human absence epilepsy (6,33). Lh/lh mice appear to have normal presynaptic N and P/Q-type channel densities (63), whereas tg/tg mice, despite lacking P/Q-type channels, have normal synaptic transmission because of a compensatory increase in N-type channel numbers (63) . The action of LTG in tg and stg mice is unreported, but in lh mice, LTG is effective (32). LTG does not increase clonus latency in the pentylenetetrazole model (38), and LTG is ineffective in the GAERS rat, although unlike many other anticonvulsants (e.g., phenytoin, carbamazepine, vigabatrin, gabapentin, tiagabine), LTG does not aggravate the spike–wave discharges in the GAERS model (19). In the lethargic (lh/lh) mouse model, however, LTG (C_{50}, 16 mg/kg) reduced seizure frequency (65% maximal effect), whereas vigabatrin and tiagabine (as in the GAERS model) increased seizure frequency (32).

The rat kindling model is a test for drugs effective against partial epilepsy and secondary generalized seizures. In early studies with cortically kindled rats, LTG reduced both the afterdischarge duration and the number of kindled responses but failed to block the development of kindling (59). LTG also blocked limbic-kindled seizures (60) and secondary generalized but not focal seizures after amygdala kindling (19), although this lack of effect against focal seizures has been attributed to method (19,21). LTG increased the afterdischarge threshold in phenytoin-resistant amygdala-kindled rats (21). This finding is consistent with LTG's clinical efficacy against partial seizures in patients refractory to other drugs (29) and indicates a mechanistic difference between phenytoin and LTG (21).

Despite LTG's broad-spectrum efficacy as an anticonvulsant, ion channel blockers, including LTG, were ineffective against cocaine-induced seizures in mice, in contrast to agents that enhance γ-aminobutyric acid (GABA)–ergic neurotransmission (28). Similarly, LTG did not alter behavioral responses to intranasal cocaine in humans (82).

EFFECT OF LAMOTRIGINE ON RECEPTOR AND BIOCHEMICAL SYSTEMS

LTG does not bind to dopamine (D1, D2), noradrenergic (α1, α2, β), adenosine (A1, A2), muscarinic, or σ sites (42,56). LTG appears to have little direct action on glutamatergic receptors of the α-amino-3-hydroxy-5-methyl-4-isoxazzole propionate and N-methyl-D-aspartate type (Table 34.1) (8,61), a finding suggesting that the anticonvulsant action of LTG is unlikely to involve blockade of ionotropic glutamate receptors (Table 34.1). LTG has also been shown to reduce markers of nitric oxide synthase activity in some preparations (27,49).

Effects on Monoamine Systems

In Balb/c mice, LTG (20 mg/kg) abolished audiogenic seizures and reduced dopamine synthesis, as evidenced by decreased striatal dihydrophenylacetic acid content (>50%) and tyrosine hydroxylase activity (74). By contrast, in C57 BL/6 mice treated with 1-methyl-4-phenyl-1,2,3,6-tetrahydropyridine, in which severe dopamine depletion occurs, LTG (3 mg/kg) coadministered with L-DOPA produced a synergistic improvement in motor behavior (25,67). This potenti-

TABLE 34.1. LAMOTRIGINE ACTIONS IN VITRO

Experimental Paradigm	Lamotrigine Action	Preparation
Neurotransmission		
Veratrine-evoked transmitter efflux	Inhibition, IC_{50} 25 μmol/L for glutamate, 44 μmol/L for GABA	Rat brain slices (42)
	IC_{50} 200 μmol/L	Rat brain synaptosomes (48)
K^+-evoked glutamate efflux	No effect, IC_{50} >300 μmol/L	Rat brain slices (42)
		Synaptosomes (48)
Evoked extracellular field potentials	Inhibited amplitude, IC_{50} 60 μmol/L	Rat cortical slices (10)
Glutamatergic synaptic responses	Inhibited EPSP amplitude, IC_{50} 27 μmol/L, maximal: 60%	Medium spiny neurons, rat striatal slice (8)
	Inhibited EPSP amplitude 50 μmol/L	Rat amygdala neurons (76,77)
	Inhibited frequency of miniature post synaptic currents, IC_{50} <100 μmol/L	Rat cortical neurons, primary culture (46)
	Inhibited frequency of glutamatergic synaptic currents	Rat entorhinal cortical slice (17)
GABAergic synapses	Inhibited frequency, miniature postsynaptic currents, IC_{50} <100 μmol/L	Rat cortical neurons, primary culture (46)
	Increased frequency and amplitude of GABAergic inhibitory currents (50 μmol/L)	Rat entorhinal cortical slice (17)
Paired pulse facilitation (index of presynaptic inhibition)	Enhanced ratio: 1.2, 1.7, 1.5, 1.25 (0, 30, 50, 100 μmol/L)	Glutamatergic EPSPs in rat brain slices (8,76)
Glutamate receptors	No effect on response to 1 mmol/L glutamate (30–100 μmol/L)	Rat striatal medium spiny neurons (8)
	Weak inhibition of AMPA and NMDA responses, IC_{50} >100 μmol/L	Rat cortical wedges (61)
Action potential firing		
Extracellular recording	Inhibited 0 mg induced firing, IC_{50} 140 μmol/L	Rat hippocampal slice (83)
Intracellular recordings	Inhibited evoked spikes, IC_{50} 20 μmol/L	Mouse cultured spinal neurons (11)
	IC_{50} 50 μmol/L maximal: 50% activity dependent (Figure 34.1)	Medium spiny neurons, rat striatal slice (8)
Ion channels		
Sodium currents	IC_{50} 90 μmol/L (V_{hold} –80 mV); activity-dependent inhibition	Mouse neuroblastoma (40)
	IC_{50} 60 μmol/L (V_{hold} –60 mV); ~1 mmol/L (V_{hold} –90 mV); activity-dependent inhibition	Recombinant type IIA Na channels (83,84)
	Residues in helices IIIS6 and IVS6 required for lamotrigine action (Fig. 34.3)	Recombinant Na channel site mutants (85)
Potassium currents	Enhanced? (100 μmol/L)	Pyramidal neurons, rat hippocampal slices (30)
	Weak inhibition (100 μmol/L)	Rat cortical or hippocampal neurons (46,83,84)
	Weak inhibition <10% at 10 μmol/L	Two-pore domain K channels, TREK 1 and TRAAK H (53)
Calcium currents	Spared I- and T-type (100 μmol/L)	GH3 rat pituitary cells (40)
	Inhibited N-; P-type, spared L-type IC_{50} 12 μmol/L (V_{hold} –70 to –40 mV)	Rat cortical pyramidal neurons (69)
	Inhibited amplitude through N-type Ca channel action (50 μmol/L)	Rat amygdala neurons (76)
	Weak inhibition IC_{50} ~1 mmol/L (V_{hold} –90, –60 mV)	Recombinant N-type, α1B (+α2-δ, β1) (83)
	Weak inhibition IC_{50} >300 μmol/L (V_{hold} –90 mV)	Recombinant T-type, α1G, α1I [AHH and ADR, unpublished (see Fig. 34.2)]
	Weak inhibition <10% at 100 μmol/L (V_{hold} –90 mV)	Recombinant R-type human α1E (+β3) (AHH, unpublished)

GABA, γ-aminobutyric acid; NMDA, N-methyl-D-aspartate.

ation of the antiparkinsonian action of L-DOPA is unlikely to occur through LTG action at D1 or D2 receptors (see the preceding discussion on receptor binding data) (42,67).

LTG is a weak inhibitor of 5-hydroxytryptamine (5-HT) uptake into both human platelets and rat brain synaptosomes *in vitro,* and at 20 mg/kg, LTG only partially attenuates the *p*-chloroamphetamine–induced 5-HT syndrome (a measure of 5-HT uptake *in vivo*) in rats (IC$_{50}$ >200 μmol/L) (66) (compare values for ion channel actions in Table 34.1). In children treated with LTG for intractable epilepsy, plasma 5-HT concentrations decreased in seven of 16 children who responded to LTG treatment (36). Urinary 5-HT and 5-hydroxyindoleacetic acid concentrations in these children were unchanged, a finding suggesting that 5-HT catabolism was increased after LTG treatment in some subjects (36). LTG had no effect on 5-HT1A receptor function in humans (64). The foregoing weak and inconsistent effects on 5-HT systems appear unlikely to contribute to the clinical efficacy of LTG in bipolar disorder and mood stabilization (83).

ACTION OF LAMOTRIGINE ON ION CHANNELS

Earlier work demonstrated that LTG inhibits voltage-activated Na channels (11,40,46,56) (Table 34.1). This action is characterized by use dependency (potency of inhibition increasing with action potential firing activity) (Figure 34.1)

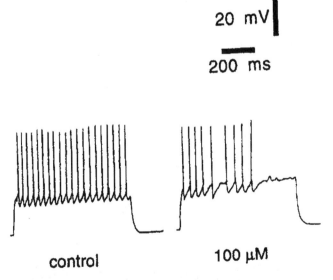

FIGURE 34.1. Activity-dependent inhibition of voltage-activated Na$^+$ channels by lamotrigine (LTG). Na$^+$ channel–dependent action potential firing was induced by injection of a depolarizing current pulse (0.7 nA, 700 milliseconds) in control conditions *(left)* or in the presence of LTG (100 μmol/L) *(right).* Resting potential remained constant at –90 mV. Medium spiny neuron, rat striatal slice (From Calabresi P, Centonze D, Marfia GA, et al. An *in vitro* electrophysiological study on the effects of phenytoin, lamotrigine and gabapentin on striatal neurons. *Br J Pharmacol* 1999;126:689–696, with permission.)

(8,84) and by increased potency at less-negative holding voltages (or resting voltages) (84). We present electrophysiologic information (Table 34.1) that has emerged since the previous review in this series (42).

Calcium Channels

LTG inhibited native high-voltage-activated Ca^{2+} channel populations (69,76), including the ω-conotoxin GVIA-sensitive N-type and ω-agatoxin (100 nmol/L)–sensitive P-type components, but spared the dihydropyridine-sensitive L-type component (69,76). Recombinant α1B subunit-mediated N-type currents, however, were weakly LTG sensitive (Xie and Hagan, *unpublished data,* 1998). Recombinant R-type currents, mediated by α1E subunit-containing channels, were also only weakly inhibited by LTG (A. H. Hainsworth, *unpublished data*) (Table 34.1). Presynaptic Ca channels on nerve terminals that mediate normal synaptic transmission are principally of the P/Q and N types. Inhibition of these channel types by LTG probably accounts for inhibition of neurotransmitter release (41) and inhibition of glutamate-mediated excitatory postsynaptic potentials (8,76,77). This mechanism may also underlie the enhancement produced by LTG (30 to 100 μmol/L) in the paired-pulse facilitation ratio (8,77), a marker for presynaptic inhibition.

Low-voltage-activated currents mediated by recombinant T-type Ca channels of the two isoforms that are highly expressed in brain tissue (α1G, α1I) showed little sensitivity to LTG (Figure 34.2). This finding agrees with earlier work showing that T-type currents in a pituitary cell line were LTG-resistant (40). T-type currents in thalamic neurons have been implicated in the slow-wave discharges characteristic of absence seizures (6,54), partly because of the inhibition of T-type Ca^{2+} currents in thalamic relay neurons by the classic antiabsence drug ethosuximide (14). However, T-type currents in many preparations, including some thalamic neurons, were ethosuximide resistant (14,47,70). Thus, the precise contribution of T-type inhibition to antiabsence therapy appears unclear, but it seems to contribute little to the antiabsence activity of LTG.

Potassium Channels

Negligible inhibition of potassium (K$^+$) currents by LTG is seen in native neuronal populations (46,83). The drug also failed to inhibit recombinant two-pore domain K$^+$ channels of the family thought to underlie background "leak" currents at negative voltages (53).

Sodium Channels

A quantitative study of the holding-voltage dependence and activity dependence of Na channel blockade by LTG

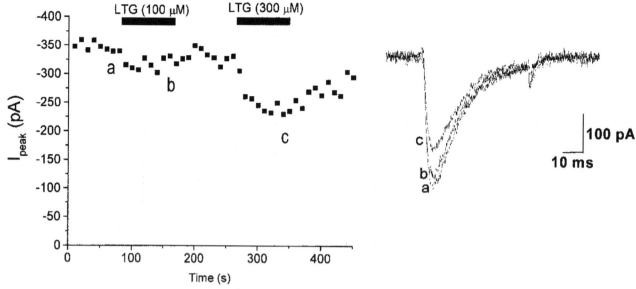

FIGURE 34.2. Weak inhibition of T-type Ca^{2+} channels by lamotrigine (LTG). **A:** Time-course of peak current amplitude in HEK293 cell expressing α1G subunit, exposed to LTG (100, 300 μmol/L, as indicated). **B:** Example current traces at time points marked *a, b,* and *c* in **A.** Holding voltage –90 mV, test pulse –25 mV, 50 milliseconds, applied every 10 seconds. (From A. H. Hainsworth and A. D. Randall, *unpublished data*).

concluded that the drug stabilizes a long-lived inactivated state of the channel, only entered on prolonged depolarization (84). A mutagenesis study has identified residues in the Na channel α1 subunit that are required for inhibition by LTG (85) (Figure 34.3). The S6 helices of the four transmembrane domains in the α1 subunit are thought to line the pore region, at the intracellular end. Point mutation of successive amino acids in the IIIS6 and IVS6 α helices to alanine (a small, neutral amino acid) reveal six residues that significantly influence the potency of LTG blockade. These may form a binding site for LTG within the Na channel pore (85) (Figure 34.3), possibly also including amino acids from the IS6 and IIS6 helices. A combination of Na channel inhibition and N/P/Q-type Ca channel inhibition, all with some degree of voltage dependence and activity dependence, may explain most of the anticonvulsant actions of LTG.

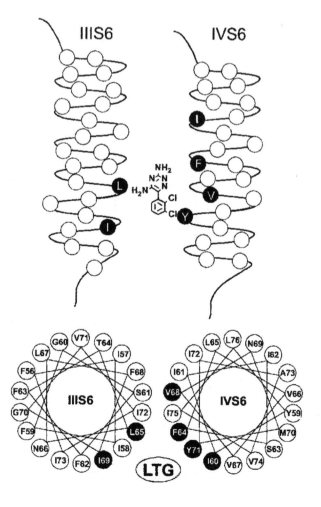

FIGURE 34.3. Regions of the Na^+ channel proposed to form a lamotrigine (LTG) binding site. The pore-forming IIIS6 and IVS6 α helices of type IIA Na^+ channel are shown (from side view and from above); residues affecting LTG sensitivity are *shaded*. (From Yarov-Yarovoy V, Brown J, Sharp E, et al. Molecular determinants of voltage-dependent gating and binding of pore-blocking drugs in transmembrane segment IIIS6 of the Na^+ channel a subunit. *J Biol Chem* 2000, with permission).

OTHER ACTIONS OF LAMOTRIGINE

Neuroprotection

In animal models of cerebral ischemia, LTG and structural analogs (e.g., sipatrigine) are neuroprotective (31,43,55). LTG gives modest neuroprotection at doses usually five- to 10-fold higher than anticonvulsant doses (42,55). LTG (20 mg/kg intravenously) significantly reduced cortical infarct volume after focal ischemia induced by permanent middle cerebral artery occlusion in rats but provided no striatal protection, despite reducing striatal glutamate efflux (42,55). In models of global ischemia, LTG (10 to 50 mg/kg) is neuroprotective in gerbil (41,45,65,81), rat (16), and pig (13). In gerbil, coadminstration with flunarizine, an inhibitor of L- and T-type Ca channel inhibitor, gave a further increase in neuroprotection (45). The drug also ameliorated neuronal damage in 3-nitropropionic acid–intoxicated rats (20 mg/kg) (44) and in a rat *in vitro* model of white matter ischemia (50% reduction in axonopathy at 300 μmol/L) (26). The role of ion channel blockade in neuroprotective processes has been extensively reviewed (9,31,71).

Pain Relief

Neuropathic pain disorders (e.g., postherpetic neuralgia, painful diabetic neuropathy, central poststroke pain syndrome) respond poorly to traditional analgesics, but ion channel-blocking agents have varying degrees of clinical efficacy (1). LTG was effective in treating painful diabetic neuropathy (23), as well as chronic refractory neuropathic pain, particularly in combination with morphine (20), but it had no effect in an acute pain model (37). LTG is analgesic in various rat models of neuropathic pain (4,34,58), and it inhibited mechanical allodynia after nerve injury (10 to 25 mg/kg orally) (4).

Ion channels are strongly implicated in pain relief (12,22,75,78,79), and changes in Na channel expression have been described after peripheral nerve or tissue injury (3,15). The TTX-resistant Na channel PN3/SNS (NaV1.8) found predominantly in small neurons of dorsal root ganglia may play a major role in the sustained repetitive firing of peripheral injured nerves. Antisense knockdown of PN3 mRNA in the dorsal root ganglion prevents hyperalgesia and allodynia after chronic nerve or tissue injury (15,62). Subtype-selective LTG action at peripheral Na channels as a basis for analgesic activity has yet to be reported.

CONCLUSION

LTG is an antiepileptic agent with a broad clinical spectrum of activity, including absence epilepsy and Lennox-Gastaut syndrome. In contrast to other Na channel blockers such as phenytoin, the clinical profile of LTG supports the notion of an additional novel mechanism of action. Data presented in this review now implicate inhibition of Ca conductances (including N and P type) in the anticonvulsant actions of LTG. Although the precise role of high-threshold Ca currents (N type in particular) in relation to epilepsy is not fully understood, we speculate that the antiabsence efficacy of LTG may reflect inhibition of N- and P/Q-type Ca channels in addition to Na channels.

REFERENCES

1. Backonja M-M. Anticonvulsants (antineuropathics) for neuropathic pain syndromes. *Clin J Pain* 2000;16:S67–S72.
2. Berk M. Lamotrigine and the treatment of mania in bipolar disorder. *Eur Neuropsychopharm* 1999;9[Suppl 4]:S119–S123.
3. Bongenhielm U, Nosrat CA, Nosrat I, et al. Expression of sodium channel SNS/PN3 and ankyrin(G) mRNAs in the trigeminal ganglion after inferior alveolar nerve injury in the rat. *Exp Neurol* 2000;164:384–395.
4. Boyce S, Webb J, O'Donnell R, et al. Selective NMDA NR2B antagonists induce antinociception without motordysfunction: correlation with resticted localisation of NR2B subunit in dorsal horn *Neuropharmacology* 1999;38:611–623.
5. Buoni S, Grosse S, Fois A. Lamotrigine in typical absence epilepsy. *Brain Dev* 1999;21:303–306.
6. Burgess DL, Noebels JL. Single gene defects in mice: the role of voltage-dependent calcium channels in absence models. *Epilepsy Res* 1999;36:111–122.
7. Burgess DL, Noebels JL. Calcium channel defects in models of inherited generalised epilepsy. *Epilepsia* 2000;41:1074–1075.
8. Calabresi P, Centonze D, Marfia GA, et al. An in vitro electrophysiological study on the effects of phenytoin, lamotrigine and gabapentin on striatal neurons. *Br J Pharmacol* 1999;126:689–696.
9. Calabresi P, Picconi B, Saulle E, et al. Is pharmacological neuroprotection dependent on reduced glutamate release? *Stroke* 2000; 31:766–773.
10. Calabresi P, Siniscalchi A, Pisani,A, et al. A field potential analysis on the effects of lamotrigine, GP47779 and felbamate in neocortical slices. *Neurology* 1996;47:557–562.
11. Cheung H, Kamp D, Harris E. An in vitro investigation of the action of lamotrigine on neuronal voltage-activated sodium channels. *Epilepsy Res* 1992;13:107–112.
12. Clare JJ, Tate S, Nobbs MS, et al. Voltage gated sodium channels as therapeutic targets, *Drug Discovery Today* 2000;5:506–520.
13. Conroy B, Black D, Lin C, et al. Lamotrigine attenuates cortical glutamate release during global cerebral ischemia in pigs on cardiopulmonary bypass. *Anesthesiology* 1999;90:844–854.
14. Coulter D, Huguenard J, Prince D. Differential effects of petit mal anticonvulsants and convulsants in thalamic neurones: calcium current reduction. *Br J Pharmacol* 1990;100:800–806.
15. Coward K, Plumpton C, Facer P, et al. Immunolocalisation of SNS/PN3 and NaN/SNS2 sodium channels in human pain states. *Pain* 2000;85:41–50.
16. Crumrine R, Bergstrand K, Cooper A, et al. Lamotrigine protects hippocampal CA1 neurons from ischemic damage after cardiac arrest. *Stroke* 1997;28:2230–2237.
17. Cunningham MO, Jones RSG. The anticonvulsant, lamotrigine decreases spontaneous glutamate release but increases spontaneous GABA release in the rat entorhinal cortex. *Neuropharmacology* 2000;39:2139–2146.
18. D'Andrea G,Granella F, Cadaldini M, et al. Effectiveness of lam-

otrigine in the prophylaxis of migraine with aura: an open pilot study. *Cephalalgia* 1999:19:64–66.

19. Dalby NO, Nielsen EB. Comparison of the preclinical anticonvulsant profiles of tiagabine, lamotrigine, gabapentin and vigabatrin. *Epilepsy Res* 1997;28:63–72.

20. Devaulder J, De Laat M. Lamotrigine in the treatment of chronic refractory neuropathic pain. *J Pain Symptom Manage* 2000;19:398–403.

21. Ebert U, Reissmuller E, Loscher W. The new antiepileptic drugs lamotrigine and felbamate are effective in phenytoin-resistant kindled rats. *Neuropharmacology* 2000;39:1893–1903.

22. Eglen RM, Hunter JC, Dray A. Ions in the fire: recent ion-channel research and approaches to pain therapy. *Trends Pharmacol Sci* 1999;20:337–342.

23. Eisenberg E, Alon N, Ishay A, Daoud D, Yarnitsky D. Lamotrigine in the treatment of painful diabetic neuropathy. *Eur J Neurol* 1998;5:167–173.

24. Engle PM, Peck AM. Lamotrigine for the treatment of bipolar disorder. *Ann Pharmacother* 2000;34:258–262.

25. Fredriksson A, Palomo T, Archer T. Effects of co-administartion of anticonvulsant and putative anticonvulsive agents and sub/suprathreshold doses of L-dopa upon motor behaviour of MPTP-treated mice. *J Neural Transm* 1999;106:889–909.

26. Garthwaite G, Brown G, Batchelor A, et al. Mechanisms of ischaemic damage to central white matter axons: a quantitative histological analysis using rat optic nerve. *Neuroscience* 1999;94:1219–1230.

27. Garthwaite G, Goodwin D, Garthwaite J. Nitric oxide stimulates cGMP formation in rat optic nerve axons, providing a specific marker of axon viability. *Eur J Neurosci* 1999;11:4367–4372.

28. Gasior M, Ongard JT, Witkin JM. Preclinical evaluation of newly approved and potential antiepileptic drugs against cocaine-induced seizures. *J Pharmacol Exp Ther* 1999;290:1148–1156.

29. Goa KL, Ross SR, Chrisp P. Lamotrigine: a review of its pharmacological properties and clinical efficacy in epilepsy. *Drugs* 1995;46:152–176.

30. Grunze H, Wegerer JV, Greene R, et al. Modulation of calcium and potassium currents by lamotrigine. *Neuropsychobiology* 1998;38:131–138.

31. Hainsworth AH, Stefani A, Calabresi P, et al. Sipatrigine (BW 619C89) is a neuroprotective agent and a sodium channel and calcium channel inhibitor. *CNS Drug Rev* 2000;6:111–134.

32. Hosford DA, Wang Y. Utility of the lethargic (lh/lh) mouse model of absence seizures in predicting the effects of lamotrigine, vigabatrin, tiagabine,gabapentin, and topiramate against human absence seizures. *Epilepsia* 1997;38:408–414.

33. Hosford DA, Fu-Hsiung L, Wang Y, et al. Studies of the lethargic (*lhlh*) mouse model of absence seizures:regulatory mechanisms and identification of the *lh* gene. In: Delgardo-Escuetta AV, Wilson WA, Olsen RW, et al., eds. Jasper's basic mechanisms of epilepsies, 3rd ed. *Adv Neurol* 1999;79:239–252.

34. Hunter JC, Gogas KR, Hedley LR, et al. The effect of novel antiepileptic drugs in rat experimental models of acute and chronic pain. *Eur J Pharmacol* 1997;324:153–160.

35. Ichim L, Berk M, Brook S. Lamotrigine compared with lithium in mania: a double-blind randomised controlled trial. *Ann Clin Psychiatry* 2000;12:5–10.

36. Jovic NJ, Mirkovic D, Majkic-Singh N, et al. Plasma and urinary serotonin and 5-HIAA in children treated with lamotrigine for intractable epilepsy. *Adv Exp Med Biol* 1999;467:297–302.

37. Klamt JG, Posner J. Effects of lamotrigine on pain-induced chemo-somatosensory evoked potentials. *Anaesthesia* 1999;54:774–777.

38. Koella WP. Animal experimental methods in the study of antiepileptic drugs. In: Frey H-H, Janz D, eds. *Antiepileptic drugs*. Berlin: Springer-Verlag, 1985:283–340.

39. Kremer B, Clark CM, Almqvist EW, et al. Influence of lamotrigine on progression of early Huntington disease: a randomised clinical trial. *Neurology* 1999;53:1000–1011.

40. Lang D, Wang CM, Cooper B. Lamotrigine, phenytoin and carbamazepine interactions on the sodium current in N4TG1 mouse neuroblastoma cells. *J Pharmacol Exp Ther* 1993;266:29–35.

41. Leach M, Baxter M, Critchley M. Neurochemical and behavioural aspects of lamotrigine. *Epilepsia* 1991;32[Suppl 2]:S4–S8.

42. Leach MJ, Lees G, Riddall DR. Lamotrigine: mechanisms of action. In: Levy RH, Mattson RH, Meldrum BS, eds. *Antiepileptic drugs*, 4th ed. New York: Raven Press, 1995:861–869.

43. Leach MJ, Swan JH, Eisenthal D, et al. BW619C89, a glutamate release inhibitor, protects against focal cerebral ischemic damage. *Stroke* 1993;24:1063–1067.

44. Lee W, Shen Y, Chang C. Neuroprotective effect of lamotrigine and MK801 on rat brain lesions induced by 3-nitropropionic acid: evaluation by magnetic resonance imaging and in vivo proton magnetic resonance spectroscopy. *Neuroscience* 2000;95:89–95.

45. Lee Y, Yoon B, Roh J. Neuroprotective effects of lamotrigine enhanced by flunarizine in gerbil global ischemia. *Neurosci Lett* 1999;265:215–217.

46. Lees G, Leach MJ. Studies on the mechanism of action of the novel anticonvulsant lamotrigine (Lamictal) using primary neuroglial cultures from rat cortex. *Brain Res* 1993;612:190–199.

47. Leresche N, Parri H, Erdemli G, et al. On the action of the anti-absence drug ethosuximide in the rat and cat thalamus. *J Neurosci* 1998;18:4842–4853.

48. Lingamaneni R, Hemmings H. Effects of anticonvulsants on veratridine-and KCL-evoked glutamate release from rat cortical synaptosomes. *Neurosci Lett* 1999;276:127–130.

49. Lizasoian I, Knowles R, Moncada S. Inhibition by lamotrigine of the generation of nitric oxide in rat forebrain slices. *J Neurochem* 1995;64:636–642.

50. MacDonald R, Greenfield LJ. Mechanisms of action of new antiepileptic drugs. *Curr Opin Neurol* 1997;10:121–128.

51. Matsuo F. Lamotrigine. *Epilepsia* 1999;40[Suppl 5]:S30–S36.

52. McElroy SL, Keck PE Jr. Pharmacological agents for the treatment of acute bipolar mania. *Biol Psychiatry* 2000;48:539–557.

53. Meadows HJ, Chapman CG, Duckworth DM, et al. The neuroprotective agent sipatrigine (BW619C89) potently inhibits the human tandem pore-domain K+ channels TREK-1 and TRAAK. *Brain Res* 2001.

54. Meldrum BS. Update on the mechanisms of action of antiepileptic drugs. *Epilepsia* 1996;37[Suppl 6]:S4–S11.

55. Meldrum BS, Smith SE, Lekieffre D, et al. Sodium-channel blockade and glutamate release: the mechanism of cerebroprotection by lamotrigine, BW1003C87 and BW619C89. In: Krieglstein J, Oberpichler-Schwenk H, eds. *Pharmacology of cerebral ischaemia*. Stuttgart: WVmbH, 1994:203–209.

56. Meldrum BS, Leach MJ. The mechanisms of action of lamotrigine. *Rev Contemp Pharmacother* 1994;5:107–114.

57. Miller AA, Wheatley P, Sawyer DA, et al. Pharmacological studies on lamotrigine, a novel potential antiepileptic agent drug. I. Anticonvulsant profile in mice and rats. *Epilepsia* 1986;27:483–489.

58. Nakamura-Craig M, Follenfant RL. Analgesic effects of lamotrigine in an experimental model of neuropathic pain. *Br J Pharmacol* 1992;107:337.

59. O'Donnell RA, Miller AA. The effect of lamotrigine upon the development of cortical kindled seizures in the rat. *Neuropharmacology* 1991;30:253–258.

60. Otsuki K, Morimoto K, Sato K, et al. Effects of lamotrigine and conventional antiepileptic drugs on amygdala- and hippocampal-kindled seizures in the rat. *Epilepsy Res* 1998;31:101–112.

61. Phillips I, Martin KF, Thompson KS, et al. Weak blockade of AMPA receptor-mediated depolarisations in the rat cortical wedge by phenytoin but not by lamotrigine or carbamazepine. *Eur J Pharmacol* 1997;337:189–195.

62. Porreca F, Lai J, Bian D, et al. A comparison of the potential role of the tetrodotoxin-insensitive sodium channels, PN3/SNS and NaN/SNS2, in the rat models of chronic pain. *Proc Natl Acad Sci USA* 1999;96:7640–7644.

63. Qian J, Noebels J. Presynaptic Ca^{2+} influx at a mouse central synapse with Ca^{2+} channel subunit mutations. *J Neurosci* 2000; 20:163–170.

64. Shiah IS, Yatham LN, Lam RW, et al. Effects of lamotrigine on the 5-HT1A receptor function in healthy human males. *J Affect Disord* 1998;49:157–162.

65. Shuaib A, Mahmood R, Wishart T, et al. Neuroprotective effects of lamotrigine in global ischemia in gerbils: a histological, *in vivo* microdialysis and behavioral study. *Brain Res* 1995;702: 199–206.

66. Southam E, Kirkby D, Higgins GA, et al. Lamotrigine inhibits monoamine uptake *in vitro* and modulates 5-hydroxytryptamine uptake in rats. *Eur J Pharmacol* 1998;358:19–24.

67. Starr MS, Starr BS, Kaur S. Stimulation of basal and L-DOPA-induced motor activity by glutamate antagonists in animal models of Parkinson's disease. *Neurosci Biobehav Rev* 1997;21:437–446.

68. Stefani A, Spadoni F, Bernardi G. Voltage gated calcium currents: targets for antiepileptic drug therapy? *Epilepsia* 1997;38:959–965.

69. Stefani A, Spadoni F, Siniscalchi A, et al. Lamotrigine inhibits Ca^{2+} currents in cortical neurons: functional implications. *Euro J Pharmacol* 1996;307:113–116.

70. Todorovic S, Lingle C. Pharmacological properties of T-type Ca^{2+} current in adult rat sensory neurons: effects of anticonvulsant and anesthetic agents. *J Neurophysiol* 1998;79:240–252.

71. Urenjak J, Obrenovitch TP. Pharmacological modification of voltage-gated Na^+ channels: a rational and effective strategy against ischemic brain damage. *Pharmacol Rev* 1996;48:21–67.

72. Vadi PP di, Hamann W. The use of lamotrigine in neuropathic pain. *Anaesthesia* 1998;53:808–809.

73. Vergnes M, Marescaux C, Depaulis A. The spontaneous spike and wave discharges in Wistar rats: a model of genetic generalised nonconvulsive epilepsy. In: Avoli M, Gloor P, Kostopoulos G, et al., eds. *Generalised epilepsy: neurobiological approaches.* Boston: Birkhauser, 1990:238–253.

74. Vriend J, Alexiuk NA. Lamotrigine inhibits the in situ activity of tyrosinehydroxylase in striatum of audiogenic seizure-prone and audiogenic seizure-resistant Balb/c mice. *Life Sci* 1997;61: 2467–2474.

75. Wallace MS. Calcium and sodium channel antagonists for the treatment of pain. *Clin J Pain* 2000;16:S80–S85.

76. Wang S-J, Huang C-C, Hsu K-S, et al. Inhibition of N-type calcium currents by lamotrigine in rat amygdala neurones. *Neuroreport* 1996;7:3037–3040.

77. Wang S-J, Huang C-C, Hsu K-S, et al. Presynaptic inhibition of excitatory neurotransmission by lamotrigine in the rat amygdala neurons. *Synapse* 1996;24:248–255.

78. Waxman SG. The molecular pathophysiology of pain: abnormal expression of sodium channel genes and its contributions to hyperexcitability of primary sensory neurons. *Pain* 1999; [Suppl 6]:S133–S140.

79. Waxman SG, Cummins TR, Dib-Hajj S, et al. Sodium channels, excitability of primary sensory neurons, and the molecular basis of pain. *Muscle Nerve* 1999;22:1177–1187.

80. White H. Comparative anticonvulsant and mechanistic profile of the established and newer antiepileptic drugs. *Epilepsia* 1999; 40[Suppl 5]:S2–S10.

81. Wiard R, Dickerson M, Beek O, et al. Neuroprotective properties of the novel antiepileptic lamotrigine in a gerbil model of global cerebral ischemia. *Stroke* 1995;26:466–472.

82. Winther LC, Saleem R, McCance-Katz EF, et al. Effects of lamotrigine on behavioural and cardiovascular responses to cocaine in human subjects. *Am J Drug Alcohol Abuse* 2000;26:47–59.

83. Xie X, Hagan RH. Cellular and molecular actions of lamotrigine:possible mechanisms of efficacy in bipolar disorder. *Neuropsychobiol* 1998;38:119–130.

84. Xie X, Lancaster B, Peakman T, et al. Interaction of the antiepileptic drug lamotrigine with recombinant rat brain type IIA Na^+ channels and with native Na^+ channels in rat hippocampal neurones. *Pflugers Arch* 1995;430:437–446.

85. Yarov-Yarovoy V, Brown J, Sharp E, et al. Molecular determinants of voltage-dependent gating and binding of pore-blocking drugs in transmembrane segment IIIS6 of the Na^+ channel a subunit. *J Biol Chem* 2000.

Antiepileptic Drugs, 5th Edition. Edited by R.H. Levy, R.H. Mattson, B.S. Meldrum, and E. Perucca. Lippincott Williams & Wilkins, Philadelphia © 2002.

LAMOTRIGINE

CHEMISTRY, BIOTRANSFORMATION, AND PHARMACOKINETICS

MAURICE DICKINS
CHAO CHEN

CHEMISTRY

Lamotrigine (3,5-diamino-6-[2,3-dichlorophenyl]-1,2,4-triazine, Lamictal) is synthesized by reacting thionyl chloride with 2,3-dichlorobenzoic acid, yielding an acid chloride derivative, which is converted to the corresponding ketonitrile in the presence of cuprous cyanide. Condensation of the ketonitrile with aminoguanidine under strongly acidic conditions (6 mol/L HNO_3) produced an amidinohydrazone product that readily cyclized in basic conditions to yield lamotrigine (1). Lamotrigine is a weak base with a negative log of dissociation constant (pKa) of 5.5 and a molecular weight of 256.09 (2). In contrast, metabolites of lamotrigine substituted at the N-2 nitrogen such as the N-2 glucuronide are much stronger bases (pKa = 10.6) because of the presence of a quaternary N atom. Lamotrigine is poorly soluble in water (0.17 mg/mL at 25°C) with a log octanol/water partition coefficient (Log P) of 1.19 at pH 7.6. Isethionate and mesylate salts of lamotrigine have been synthesized with greater aqueous solubility.

BIOTRANSFORMATION

Species Differences

The metabolism of lamotrigine occurs predominantly by attack at the N-2 nitrogen atom of the molecule, although there are species differences both in the nature and the extent of metabolism (3). The major human metabolite

seen *in vivo* was the aromatic N-2 glucuronide (4), whereas in the dog, the N-2 methyl derivative was the primary metabolite. In rodents, the N-2 oxide was a significant metabolite, but a substantial proportion of the drug was excreted as the parent molecule. Lamotrigine also undergoes significant metabolism in the guinea pig to the N-2 glucuronide (5); both the rabbit and cynomolgus monkey also produced substantial amounts of the N-2 glucuronide in addition to the aliphatic N-5 glucuronide (6) (Figure 35.1).

In healthy volunteers, the total dose after oral administration of [^{14}C]-labeled lamotrigine over a 1-week period was essentially recovered in the urine, with 71% of the dose as the N-2 glucuronide, 9% as the N-5 glucuronide, 10% as unchanged lamotrigine and 0.1 % as the N-2 methyl metabolite (1). In patients, a similar amount (43% to 87% of the dose) was excreted in the urine, mainly as the N-2 glucuronide (7). The majority (60%) of an intravenous dose of lamotrigine in the guinea pig was recovered in the urine as the N-2 glucuronide metabolite (5). In contrast, 50% of the dose in rats and mice was excreted in the urine as unchanged parent drug, whereas approximately 50% of the dose in the dog was N-2-methyl lamotrigine (1).

Lamotrigine is metabolized in the rat both *in vivo* and in isolated hepatocytes to a glutathione conjugate by epoxidation of the dichlorophenyl ring, although the actual sites of metabolism were not determined (8). *In vivo* metabolites excreted in the bile were the arene oxide intermediate (found as an unstable glutathione conjugate) and the dehydrated glutathione adduct of the parent drug together with the cysteinylglycine and N-acetylcysteine adducts of lamotrigine. Rat hepatocytes produced the glutathione adduct and the N-2 oxide. However, neither rat nor human liver microsomes catalyzed NADPH (reduced form of nicotinamide-adenine dinucleotide phosphate)–dependent irreversible binding to microsomal protein.

Maurice Dickins, PhD: Senior Scientist, Drug Metabolism and Pharmacokinetics, GlaxoSmithKline, Ware, Hertfordshire, United Kingdom

Chao Chen, PhD: Section Head, Pharmacokinetics, Department of Clinical Pharmacology and Experimental Medicine, GlaxoSmithKline, Greenford, Middlesex, United Kingdom

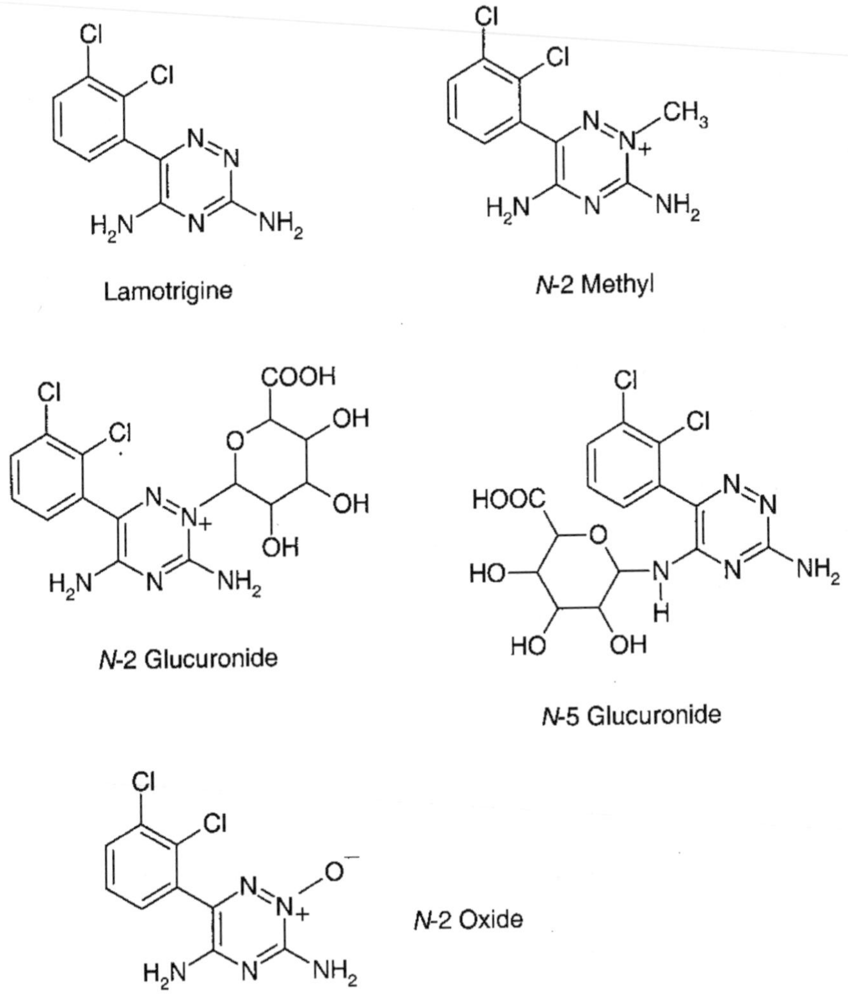

Lamotrigine

N-2 Methyl

N-2 Glucuronide

N-5 Glucuronide

N-2 Oxide

FIGURE 35.1. Structures of lamotrigine and its major metabolites.

Enzymology

N-2 Methyl Metabolite

Metabolism of lamotrigine to the *N*-2 methyl metabolite in the dog was hardly detectable in all other species investigated, including humans. The reaction was catalyzed by a nonspecific methyltransferase found in dog liver (1). Hepatic cytosol preparations from the dog (but not other species) were shown to metabolize lamotrigine to the *N*-2 methyl derivative in the presence of the cofactor *S*-adenosyl methionine. There is a literature precedent for this class of reaction being specific to the dog; the tetrahydroisoquinoline compound SK&F 64139 and related compounds also undergo *N*-methylation in this species (9).

N-2 Glucuronide

Several studies have demonstrated the metabolism of lamotrigine to its *N*-2 glucuronide metabolite using hepatic microsomal preparations. Liver microsomes from rabbits (10), guinea pigs (5), and humans (10,11) all catalyzed the formation of the *N*-2 glucuronide in the presence of the cofactor uridine diphosphate (UDP) glucuronic acid. Isolated hepatocytes from guinea pigs (5) and humans (12) also catalyzed the metabolism of lamotrigine to this metabolite. These findings are in agreement with the known *in vivo* metabolic profile of lamotrigine for these species and suggest that the liver is a major site of metabolism to the *N*-2 glucuronide.

Michaelis constant (K_m) and maximum velocity (V_{max}) values for the formation of lamotrigine *N*-2 glucuronide are similar using both guinea pig and human liver microsomes as the enzyme source: K_m = 2.1 mmol/L (guinea pig) (5) and 2.6 mmol/L (human) (10) ; V_{max} = 252 pmol/min/mg protein (guinea pig) (5) and 650 pmol/min/mg protein (human) (10). More recent data with a greater number of human liver samples (n = 12) produced values of K_m = 5.5±5.2 mmol/L and V_{max} = 960±380 pmol/min/mg protein (11). In this latter study, some liver samples from patients with liver cirrhosis (n = 10) did not show an appreciable change in the kinetics of lamotrigine *N*-2 glucuronidation (K_m = 4.3±2.0 mmol/L; V_{max} = 850±540 pmol/min/mg protein). However, the clearance of lamotrigine *in vivo* was reduced in diseased patients compared with those with normal liver function (see the later discussion of hepatic dysfunction). A reduction in the dose of lamotrigine for patients with liver cirrhosis was advised.

Glucuronidation is a major conjugation reaction that is catalyzed by a number of different isoforms of UDP-glucuronosyltransferase (UGT) (13,14). *N*-glucuronidation is a now a well-established pathway in the human metabolism of drugs with a tertiary amine group (15). Although the substrate specificity of many UGTs is unclear, UGT1A4 has been implicated in the formation of quaternary ammonium–linked glucuronides including lamotrigine (16). A panel of expressed UGT isoforms has been used to investigate the metabolism of 1-phenylimidazole, a model substrate for the quaternary nitrogen–linked glucuronidation reaction (17). Only UGTs 1A3 and 1A4 were capable of catalyzing the formation of 1-phenylimidazole *N*+ glucuronide. However, a significant contribution of UGT1A3 to the overall metabolism of tertiary amines by human liver preparations is unlikely (18), given that the expression of UGT1A3 is very low in human liver (19). Lamotrigine has also been cited as a UGT1A4 substrate in inhibition experiments with the anticonvulsant agent retigabine (20). In this study, retigabine was metabolized to an aliphatic *N*-glucuronide by human liver microsomes and several expressed UGT isoforms including UGT1A1 and 1A4. However, retigabine *N*-glucuronidation by human liver microsomes was inhibited by lamotrigine and not by bilirubin, a substrate for UGT1A1.

The evidence taken together suggests that lamotrigine *N*-2 glucuronidation, the major route of metabolism in humans, is catalyzed by human UGT1A4. This pathway is inhibited by the anticonvulsant drug valproate (21–23), and it is inducible by other anticonvulsants (22,23). Rifampicin has also been shown to increase the clearance of lamotrigine (24). Direct evidence of induction of UGT was shown by measurement of increased production of lamotrigine *N*-2 glucuronide after rifampicin treatment.

HUMAN PHARMACOKINETICS OF LAMOTRIGINE

Absorption

Lamotrigine is available for oral administration as conventional and chewable or dispersible tablets. Although the availability of the formulations and their strengths vary among the regional markets, the conventional tablets exist in 25-, 50-, 100-, 150-, 200-, and 250-mg strengths and the chewable or dispersible tablets exist in 2-, 5-, 25-, and 100-mg strengths. Gelatin oral capsules were used during early clinical testing. Bioequivalency has been demonstrated

among the capsules, the conventional tablets, and the chewable or dispersible tablets. Bioequivalency has also been established when the chewable or dispersible tablets are swallowed whole, chewed, or ingested after dispersion in a small amount of liquid (25). Treatments are considered bioequivalent when the 90% confidence intervals for the geometric least-square mean ratios of the area under the systemic concentration-time profile and of the maximum systemic concentration between the treatments are between 0.8 and 1.25. Because data on individual bioequivalence are currently lacking, patients need close clinical monitoring for toxicity or seizure worsening when they are switched between formulations.

Oral absorption is rapid, with the peak plasma concentration typically appearing between 1 and 3 hours after administration (Table 35.1). The average maximum plasma concentration increased linearly from 0.4 to 3.16 µg/mL after a 30- to 240-mg dose and from 0.58 to 4.63 µg/mL after a 50- to 400-mg dose (26–28). The steady-state maximum plasma concentration also increased dose proportionally from 3.45 to 9.44 µg/mL in healthy subjects receiving once-daily doses of 50 to 150 mg of lamotrigine in addition to concurrent sodium valproate and 0.96 to 3.00 µg/mL in patients receiving twice-daily doses of 50 to 150 mg lamotrigine in addition to concurrent enzyme-inducing anticonvulsants (29,30). Time to the maximum concentration is not altered by concurrent administration of sodium valproate or enzyme-inducing anticonvulsants, and it is dose independent after a single dose in the absence of any other medication or at steady state with these concurrent medications (26,28–30).

Oral absorption is complete. A single 75-mg dose showed an absolute bioavailability of 98±0.05% when the drug was given to eight healthy men and women who also received an equivalent intravenous dose (31). The near-complete oral absorption was supported by an average of 94% urinary recovery of radioactivity from six healthy subjects who ingested 240 mg [^{14}C]-labeled lamotrigine (32). This means that lamotrigine is unlikely to show variable absorption that can sometimes be caused by factors including concurrent medication or meals. Indeed, whereas food consumed at the time of tablet administration slightly delays the occurrence of the peak plasma concentration, it does not alter the peak concentration or the area under the concentration-time curve (27). Therefore, there is no need to control mealtimes when one is taking lamotrigine.

Distribution

After intravenous or oral administration, the plasma concentration of lamotrigine is best characterized by a one-compartment open model with first-order elimination (26,31–34). Weight-normalized volume of distribution after intravenous administration and weight-normalized apparent volume of distribution after oral administration have

TABLE 35.1. MEAN PHARMACOKINETIC PARAMETER VALUES OF LAMOTRIGINE

Subjects	n	Lamotrigine Treatment	T_{max} (hr)	CL/F	V/F (L/kg)	$T_{1/2}$ (hr)	Reference
Healthy subjects	8	75 mg sd i.v.		36.4 (8.3) (mL/min)	1.14 (0.11)	26.7 (6.7)	31
Healthy subjects	8	75 mg sd		38.5 (14) (mL/min)	1.11 (0.13)	26 (8.9)	31
Healthy male subjects	5	30 mg sd	1.9 (1)	31.7 (6.1) (mL/min)	0.87 (0.09)	28.8 (9.6)	26
Healthy male subjects	5	60 mg sd	1.7 (0.6)	29.7 (3.1) (mL/min)	0.88 (0.08)	29.3 (5.4)	26
Healthy male subjects	5	120 mg sd	2.1 (0.9)	30.5 (2.5) (mL/min)	0.9 (0.02)	29.1 (6.0)	26
Healthy male subjects	5	240 mg sd	3.1 (1)	26.6 (3.2) (mL/min)	0.92 (0.1)	35.0 (11.3)	26
Healthy subjects	10	120 mg sd	2.8 (1.3)	41.7 (10.3) (mL/min)	1.2 (0.12)	24.1 (5.7)	26
Healthy subjects	5	60 mg b.i.d. for 10 days		41 (14) (mL/min)	1.12 (0.12)	25.5 (10.2)	26
Healthy male subjects receiving VPA	18	50 mg o.d. for 1 week	1.83 (0.98)	0.17 (0.03) (mL/min/kg)	0.94 (0.10)	74.3 (12.6)	29
Healthy male subjects receiving VPA	18	100 mg o.d. for 1 week	1.96 (1.00)	0.17 (0.04) (mL/min/kg)	0.88 (0.09)	67.6 (14.6)	29
Healthy male subjects receiving VPA	18	150 mg o.d. for 1 week	2.02 (0.96)	0.20 (0.05) (mL/min/kg)	1.03 (0.18)	69.1 (15.8)	29
Healthy male subjects	6	100 mg sd	1.92 (1.02)	0.37 (0.11) (mL/min/kg)	1.12 (0.04)	37.4 (15.7)	21
Healthy male subjects receiving VPA	6	100 mg sd	1.75 (1.13)	0.30 (0.10) (mL/min/kg)	1.15 (0.09)	48.3 (20.8)	21
Patients receiving AEDs including EIs	8	50 mg b.i.d. for 4 days	1.92	1.25 (mL/min/kg)	1.35	13.4	30
Patients receiving AEDs including EIs	8	100 mg b.i.d. for 7 days	1.47	1.23 (mL/min/kg)	1.25	12.3	30
Patients receiving AEDs including EIs	8	150 mg b.i.d. for 13 days	1.75	1.20 (mL/min/kg)	1.47	15.1	30
Patients receiving EIs and VPA	25	Various sd	3.8	0.53 (mL/min/kg)		27	25
Patients receiving AEDs including EIs	9	120 or 240 mg sd				15	34
Patients receiving VPA	4	120 or 240 mg sd				59	34
Patients receiving AEDs including EIs	9	100 mg sd				14.3 (6.9)	33
Patients receiving EIs and VPA	13	100 mg sd				29.6 (10)	33
Healthy male subjects	12	100 mg sd	1.0	23.3 (6.9) (mL/min)		40.9 (11.3)	49
Healthy males receiving bupropion	12	100 mg sd	1.0	23.9 (8.6) (mL/min)		44.6 (13.9)	49
Patients 3–5 yr of age	4	2 mg/kg sd	4.5 (5.1)	0.82 (0.25) (mL/min/kg)	2.08 (0.38)	30.5 (5.6)	50
Patients 6–11 yr of age	8	2 mg/kg sd	3.9 (3.6)	0.55 (0.22) (mL/min/kg)	1.21 (0.25)	33.2 (29.3)	50
Patients 10 mo to 5 yr of age receiving non-EI non-VPA AEDs	7	2 mg/kg sd	5.2	1.2 (mL/min/kg)		19	25
Patients 10 mo to 5 yr of age receiving EIs	10	2 mg/kg sd	3.0	3.6 (mL/min/kg)		7.7	25
Patients 10 mo to 5 yr of age receiving VPA	8	2 mg/kg sd	2.9	0.47 (mL/min/kg)		45	25
Patients 5–11 yr of age receiving EIs	7	2 mg/kg sd	1.6	2.5 (mL/min/kg)		7.0	25
Patients 5–11 yr of age receiving VPA	3	2 mg/kg sd	4.5	0.24 (mL/min/kg)		66	25
Patients 5–11 yr of age receiving EIs and VPA	8	2 mg/kg sd	3.3	0.89 (mL/min/kg)		19	25
Patients with Gilbert's syndrome	7	120 mg sd	3 (1)	30.2 (7.7) (mL/min)		31.2 (7.4)	58
Healthy subjects	9	120 mg sd	3 (1)	44.2 (7.5) (mL/min)		22.8 (4.4)	58
Healthy subjects	11	100 mg sd	2.2 (1.2)	0.50 (0.11) (mL/min/kg)	1.18 (0.20)	28 (4.3)	56
Patients with renal failure	10	100 mg sd	2.1 (1.0)	0.51 (0.30) (mL/min/kg)	1.38 (0.28)	36 (11)	56
Healthy subjects	6	100 mg sd	2.2 (2.9)	38.5 (9.7) (mL/min)	1.2 (0.2)	25.7 (6.4)	57
Patients renally impaired not requiring dialysis	14	100 mg sd	1.8 (1.0)	27.9 (22) (mL/min/kg)	1.3 (0.3)	50.7 (31.3)	57
Patients renally impaired requiring dialysis, off dialysis	6	100 mg sd				59.6 (28.1)	57
Patients renally impaired requiring dialysis, on dialysis	6	100 mg sd				15.5 (12.0)	57

EI, enzyme inducers, which may include carbamazepine, phenytoin, phenobarbital and primidone; VPA, sodium valproate; AED, antiepileptic drugs; sd, single dose; i.v., intravenous; o.d., once daily; b.i.d., twice daily; T_{max}, time of maximum concentration; V/F, apparent volume of distribution; CL/F, oral clearance; $T_{1/2}$, half-life.
Data presented as mean (± standard deviation). Unless otherwise noted, subjects are male or female nonelderly adults receiving no other medication; and lamotrigine is given orally.

been reported to be 1.14 and mostly between 0.9 to 1.5 L/kg, respectively (Table 35.1). Apparent volume of distribution is not altered by concurrent administration of sodium valproate or enzyme-inducing anticonvulsants, and it is dose independent after a single dose in the absence of any other medication or at steady state with these other medications (26,28–30).

Data from *in vitro* experiments show that lamotrigine is approximately 55% protein bound in human plasma at total concentrations from 1 to 10 μg/mL. The low degree of protein binding suggests that protein binding is unlikely to cause interactions between lamotrigine and other drugs. The binding of lamotrigine to plasma proteins does not change in the presence of therapeutic concentrations of phenytoin, phenobarbital, or valproate (25). These *in vitro* results are supported by clinical findings. Plasma protein binding of lamotrigine in patients receiving 150 to 300 mg/day of lamotrigine in the presence of a variety of concurrent medications has been reported to be about 55% (35). Although serum free fraction in a woman maintained on lamotrigine during the 3 months after labor was unchanged (34%), the free fraction in the breast-fed child decreased from 43% at birth to 32% 3 months later (36).

Little information is available on tissue distribution of lamotrigine in humans. In pediatric and young adult patients receiving adjunctive lamotrigine therapy, the cerebrospinal fluid:plasma concentration ratio is 43% (37). Therefore, the cerebrospinal concentration is likely to be similar to plasma-free concentration. The brain tissue and plasma free concentrations found in an epileptic patient undergoing a frontal topectomy at 4 hours after the last lamotrigine dose were 4.2 μg/g and 2.64 μg/mL, respectively, a finding suggesting tissue binding in the brain (38). In a woman undergoing labor, the concentrations in the umbilical cord and plasma were 4.0 and 3.3 μg/mL, respectively (39). The saliva: plasma concentration ratio has been reported to be 0.46 in healthy subjects receiving a single 120- or 240-mg dose or 0.56 in epileptic patients receiving adjunctive therapy at 150 to 300 mg/day (31,35,40). Therefore, the saliva concentration appears to be comparable to the plasma free concentration. Although the strong correlation between saliva and plasma concentrations suggests the potential to use saliva for noninvasive monitoring of the systemic concentrations of lamotrigine, data on the reliability of this approach in clinical practice are currently lacking.

Routes of Elimination

Lamotrigine is metabolized *in vitro* by glucuronic acid conjugation, catalyzed by UGT (10). After oral administration of 240 mg of [^{14}C]lamotrigine (15 μCi) to six healthy subjects, 94% of the radioactivity was recovered in the urine, and 2% was recovered in the feces. The radioactivity in the

urine consisted of unchanged lamotrigine (10%), a 2-*N*-glucuronide (76%), a 5-*N*-glucuronide (10%), a 2-*N*-methyl metabolite (0.14%), and other unidentified minor metabolites (4%) (25).

Lamotrigine is excreted in breast milk. Concentrations of 3.6 to 9.6 μg/mL were found in the milk from a woman maintained on 200 to 300 mg/day treatment during the 3 months after labor. These concentrations were between the total and free serum concentrations measured at the same times. It was estimated that 2 to 5 mg/day was excreted in the milk. The serum concentrations in the breast-fed baby were between 0.75 and 2.79 μg/mL (36). In another case, concentrations of roughly 13 μmol/L were found in the milk of a woman who was receiving 200 mg/day lamotrigine and whose plasma concentrations were 22 μmol/L. The plasma concentration in the breast-fed baby was between 5 and 6 μmol/L (39). Therefore, by breast-feeding, a mother receiving therapeutic doses of lamotrigine can pass a significant amount of the drug to the baby.

Clearance and Half-Life

Healthy Subjects

Clearance after intravenous administration and apparent clearance after oral administration of a single dose have been reported to be 36.4 and typically between 30 and 40 mL/min, respectively (Table 35.1). The plasma half-life usually averages between 24 and 35 hours (Table 35.1). Plasma concentration is dose proportional, and half-life is dose independent after a single dose in the range of 30 to 400 mg (26,28).

There is conflicting information on whether lamotrigine induces its own metabolism. Oral clearance calculated in a single-dose study was almost identical to that obtained at the steady state on day 7 of a multiple-dose study (26). Another study noted a 25% decrease in half-life and a 37% increase in oral clearance on day 14 of 150 mg twice daily compared with values obtained in the same subjects after a single dose (25). Population pharmacokinetic modeling using concentrations collected in monotherapy trials revealed a small (17.3%) but statistically significant increase in oral clearance during long-term administration (41).

Comedicated Epileptic Patients

Valproate decreases oral clearance and increases the half-life of lamotrigine. Weight-normalized oral clearance averaged 0.17 to 0.20 mL/min/kg, and half-life averaged 68 to 74 hours when healthy subjects received steady-state lamotrigine doses of 50, 100, or 150 mg/day in addition to valproate treatment of 500 mg twice daily. Steady-state concentration of lamotrigine was dose proportional (29). In another study, subjects received 100-mg single doses of lamotrigine with or without six doses of 200 mg valproate given at 8-hour intervals. Lower clearance and longer half-life were observed when lamotrigine was administered with valproate. Results from this second study should be treated with caution because valproate concentrations were not at the steady state for the entire duration of the study (21).

Lamotrigine oral clearance is higher and half-life is shorter in patients maintained on anticonvulsants known to induce liver enzymes, including carbamazepine, phenytoin, phenobarbital, and primidone. In patients receiving daily doses of 100 to 300 mg in addition to these enzyme inducers and not valproate, lamotrigine oral clearance averaged 1.20 to 1.25 mL/min/kg, and half-life averaged 12.3 to 15.1 hours. Plasma concentration was again proportional to dose (30). Oral clearance and half-life in patients receiving both enzyme inducers and sodium valproate lie between the corresponding values in the populations receiving enzyme inducers or sodium valproate alone (25,33).

The effects of sodium valproate and enzyme-inducing anticonvulsants on the oral clearance of lamotrigine identified in small studies have been confirmed in population-based pharmacokinetic analysis using plasma concentration data collected in large patient trials (42,43). In addition, methsuximide and oxcarbazepine have also been found to lower lamotrigine blood concentration (44,45).

A few data suggest that topiramate lowers lamotrigine serum concentration (46) and sertraline elevates lamotrigine blood level (47). In healthy male subjects, felbamate, at 1,200 mg twice daily, or bupropion, 150 mg twice daily, did not cause clinically relevant change in the pharmacokinetics of lamotrigine (48,49).

Children

The pharmacokinetics of lamotrigine has been studied in pediatric patients receiving sole and adjunctive therapies. In one study (50), 12 patients aged 3 to 11 years received a 2 mg/kg single dose. Oral clearance and apparent volume of distribution averaged 16.6 mL/min (0.64 mL/min/kg) and 37.7 L (1.5 L/kg), both greater than the corresponding values in adults; and half-life averaged 32 hours, similar to the adult value. Although clearance was greater in the older (≥ 6 years, and heavier) patients (19.0 versus 12.6 mL/min), weight-normalized clearance was lower in the same patients (0.55 versus 0.82 mL/min/kg). This probably reflects the smaller liver size relative to body weight in the older patients. In two other studies, patients aged 10 months to 5 years or 5 to 11 years was each given a 2-mg dose while they received other anticonvulsants (25). Among the younger children, clearance averaged 3.6 or 0.47 mL/min/kg, and half-life averaged 7.7 or 45 hours in those receiving enzyme inducers or those receiving sodium valproate. Among the older children, clearance averaged 2.5 or 0.24 mL/min/kg, and half-life averaged 7.0 or 66 hours in those receiving enzyme inducers or in those receiving sodium valproate. When these results are compared with the values obtained

from children receiving lamotrigine monotherapy (50), it becomes clear that the anticonvulsants carbamazepine, phenytoin, phenobarbital, and primidone, which induce lamotrigine metabolism in adults, and sodium valproate, which inhibits lamotrigine metabolism in adults, have similar effects in children. Further, as in monotherapy (50), weight-normalized clearance is higher in younger children receiving adjunctive lamotrigine therapy.

The effects of the concurrent antiepileptic therapy on lamotrigine oral clearance have been confirmed in population pharmacokinetic analyses including data from seven clinical studies in children >2 years old (51,52). The population analyses have also revealed that weight has more impact on clearance than age. In fact, when clearance is described by a linear model that adequately takes into account the weight effect, clearance is no longer a function of age in the population studied. In other words, children >2 years old with the same weight are expected to have the same clearance even if they are at different ages. Because lamotrigine is predominantly eliminated by glucuronidation, this finding is not inconsistent with the suggestions that the adult level of glucuronidation capacity is achieved by 3 years of age (53,54).

Elderly Patients

A report comparing lamotrigine pharmacokinetics in 12 elderly subjects receiving a 150-mg single dose in one study with that in 12 nonelderly adults receiving the same dose in a different study concluded that apparent clearance was 37% lower and half-life was 6.3 hours longer in the elderly (55). The mean clearance in the elderly (0.39 mL/min/kg) lies within the range of the mean clearance values (0.31 to 0.65 mL/min/kg) obtained from nine studies in nonelderly adults after single doses of 30 to 450 mg (GlaxoSmithKline, *unpublished data*). The similarity in pharmacokinetics between young and elderly subjects was confirmed in a population pharmacokinetic analysis performed on data from 163 subjects receiving lamotrigine monotherapy, among whom 25 were aged 65 to 76 years (41). After a single dose, apparent clearance decreased by 12% from 35 mL/min at the age of 20 years to 31 mL/min at 70 years. The corresponding decrease after 48 weeks of treatment was 10% from 41 to 37 mL/min. Therefore, the pharmacokinetics of lamotrigine in elderly patients does not differ markedly from that in young subjects.

Race

Few data have been reported on the possible difference in lamotrigine clearance among races. Nonlinear mixed-effect pharmacokinetic modeling of the routine blood monitoring data showed that clearance was 28.7% lower in Asians (n = 5) of unspecified geographic origin than in whites (n = 158), and clearance was 25% lower in nonwhites of undocumented ethnic origin (n = 53) than in whites (n = 464). Both findings were statistically significant. Because the clinical trial experience of lamotrigine use was gained primarily from the white population, caution should be exercised when administering the drug to patients of other races.

Gender

Pharmacokinetic differences between the sexes have been investigated by population pharmacokinetic analysis using plasma concentrations obtained in patient trials. Results of nonlinear mixed-effect modeling of pharmacokinetics conclude a lack of statistically significant or clinically relevant difference in clearance, once corrected by weight using proper functions, between men and women receiving lamotrigine monotherapy or adjunctive therapy (41,42). Linear regression showed that lamotrigine concentration was slightly (13.7%) lower in women than in men of equal weight and receiving the same dose (43). Initial assessment in children receiving adjunctive therapy revealed a statistically significant 12% difference in weight-corrected clearance between boys and girls. The difference was not confirmed in a subsequent analysis including more patients (52). Therefore weight-corrected clearance is not markedly different between male and female patients.

Pregnancy

Limited evidence suggests an increase in lamotrigine clearance during pregnancy (39).

Renal Dysfunction

The pharmacokinetics of lamotrigine in subjects with renal function impairment, including those requiring hemodialysis, has been described. In one report, 10 patients with renal failure and 11 normal subjects each took a 200-mg single dose of lamotrigine (56). Although renal clearance of lamotrigine in the patients was much lower than that in the healthy persons, the difference did not cause a clinically relevant difference in total clearance because renal elimination of lamotrigine has only a small contribution to the overall elimination. Clearance of lamotrigine was similar between the two populations, averaging 0.51 mL/min/kg among the patients or 0.51 mL/min/kg among the healthy subjects. Mean half-life was 36 hours among the patients, longer than the 28-hour average among the healthy subjects, a finding reflecting a larger volume of distribution in the patients. In another study, six healthy subjects, 14 patients with moderate to severe renal impairment not requiring hemodialysis, and six patients undergoing hemodialysis each took a 100-mg single dose of lamotrigine (57). Mean clearance of 27.9 mL/min was lower and mean half-life of 50.7 hours was longer in the patients who were not undergoing dialysis compared with the corresponding values of

38.5 mL/min and 25.7 hours in the healthy controls. Mean half-lives in the dialyzed patients were 59.6 hours off dialysis and 15.5 hours during dialysis. Dialysis clearance on two occasions averaged 42.4 and 44.6 mL/min/kg. On average, 17% of the drug was removed by each 4-hour dialysis session. Although hemodialysis may be used as an effective way to reduce the body load of lamotrigine, there does not seem to be a need for a supplement dose immediately after a dialysis session conducted under the conditions used in this study. The daily therapeutic dose for a given patient requiring dialysis depends on the overall clearance, which can be influenced by the dialysis conditions. In light of the findings reported in this study, daily doses required for patients with renal dysfunction may be lower than those for patients with normal renal function.

Hepatic Dysfunction

The pharmacokinetics of lamotrigine after a single 100-mg dose was compared between 24 subjects with liver cirrhosis and 12 healthy subjects. The median oral clearance was 0.31, 0.24, or 0.10 mL/min/kg in patients with grade A, B, or C (Child-Hugh classification) hepatic impairment, respectively, compared with 0.34 mL/min/kg in the healthy controls. Median half-life was 36, 60, and 110 hours in the corresponding patient groups and 32 hours in the controls. It is advised that doses prescribed for patients with liver cirrhosis should be lower than those for patients with normal liver function (25).

Gilbert's Syndrome

Unconjugated hyperbilirubinemia (Gilbert's syndrome) is a disorder of bilirubin metabolism. It is caused by the functional impairment of UGT, which is responsible for the metabolism of bilirubin. Because lamotrigine is eliminated primarily by glucuronidation catalyzed by UGT, the pharmacokinetics of lamotrigine in patients with Gilbert's disease were compared with that in healthy subjects (58). Lamotrigine clearance was 32% lower and half-life was 37% longer in the patients with Gilbert's syndrome than in the healthy controls. The lamotrigine:glucuronide ratio in urine collected during the 168 hours after dose was 0.116 for the healthy subjects and 0.146 for the patients with Gilbert's syndrome, a finding providing mechanistic evidence that lamotrigine glucuronidation is partially impaired in the patients with Gilbert's syndrome. Treating patients with Gilbert's syndrome with lamotrigine should be done carefully.

Relationship between Serum Concentration and Dose

Lamotrigine has linear pharmacokinetics in the dose ranges tested when it is given alone, with enzyme-inducing anticonvulsants, or with sodium valproate (26–30). The maximum concentration, the area under the concentration-time curve, the steady-state average concentration, and the steady-state trough concentration are all proportional to dose. This means that the values of these parameters at any given dose are readily predictable based on the values obtained at any other dose.

Relationship between Serum Concentration and Effect

Lamotrigine was predicted from animal experiments to be clinically effective in the plasma concentration range of 1.5 to 3 μg/mL (40). In this concentration range, lamotrigine has been shown to reduce photosensitivity and interictal spikes in small numbers of patients with epilepsy (34,59). A trend of dose–response correlation observed in one study employing three treatment groups (placebo, 200 to 300 mg/day, and 400 to 500 mg/day) suggested an underlining concentration–response relationship within the dose range included (60). However, the concentration–effect relationship of lamotrigine for seizure control is yet to be established.

Most of the reported efficacy trials required a target maintenance dose or a narrow range of doses, allowed flexibility on the basis of efficacy and tolerance within a dosage window, or adapted a dosing strategy to achieve a trough concentration within the range of 1 to 4 μg/mL. These trial design characteristics are not suitable for identifying any concentration–effect relationship. Attempts, with limited success, were made in many of these trials to identify the correlation between plasma concentration and the measurement of the primary efficacy end point, which is usually seizure frequency, or its change from baseline, during the maintenance phase of the trial.

In a placebo-controlled fixed-dose crossover trial (61), daily doses of lamotrigine were 400 mg for patients receiving enzyme inducers without valproate and 200 mg for patients receiving both. The mean concentration of lamotrigine was 2.2 μg/mL in responders and 2.4 μg/mL in nonresponders. In several reports, lamotrigine dose was determined individually to achieve a peak concentration of 3 μg/mL (33,62) or a trough concentration between 1.5 and 2 μg/mL (63). In all these cases, mean trough concentrations were nearly identical in the responders and the nonresponders. In three studies in which lamotrigine dose adjustment based on clinical effects was allowed, there was a lack of either a correlation between lamotrigine concentration and efficacy (64) or a difference in concentration between responders and nonresponders (65,66). Yet two other reports with dosages targeting concentration ranges of 1 to 3 μg/mL (67) or 1.2 to 2.5 μg/mL (68) showed slightly higher concentrations in the responders and significant correlation between concentration and efficacy. However, these results do not establish any causal relationship, and the narrow concentration range does not allow an adequate definition of the concentration–response relationship. Lamotrigine concentration–effect relationship for seizure control is yet to be established.

One retrospective investigation revealed a large proportion of patients being maintained on lamotrigine concentrations outside the range of 1 to 4 μg/mL and questioned the adequacy of this commonly targeted range (43). Although the exact concentration range, the concentration distribution, and the effectiveness of lamotrigine treatment in these patients were not included in the report, the data indicate potential therapeutic benefits at concentrations outside the range of 1 to 4 μg/mL. In a prospective dose-titration adjunctive therapy study (69), the median trough concentration of lamotrigine at which monthly seizure frequency fell by ≥50% in the responders was 7.9 (2.1 to 15.4) mg/L; and the median trough plasma concentration at which lamotrigine-related side effects appeared was 16 (range, 7.9 to 19.4) mg/L. The therapeutic window was therefore proposed to be 7.9 to 16 mg/L. A retrospective survey has concluded that a proposed therapeutic concentration range of 3 to 14 mg/L is widely accepted and is increasingly applied in clinical practice (70).

REFERENCES

1. Dickins M, Sawyer DA, Morley TJ, et al. Lamotrigine: chemistry and biotransformation. In: Levy RH, Mattson RH, Meldrum BS, eds. *Antiepileptic drugs,* 4th ed. New York: Raven Press, 1995: 871–875.
2. Miller AA, Sawyer DA, Roth B, et al. Lamotrigine. In: Meldrum BS, Porter RJ, eds. *New anticonvulsant drugs.* London: John Libbey, 1986:165–177.
3. Parsons DN, Miles DW. Metabolic studies with BW430C, a novel anticonvulsant. *Epilepsia* 1984;25:656.
4. Sinz MW, Remmel RP. Isolation and characterization of a novel quaternary ammonium-linked glucuronide of lamotrigine. *Drug Metab Dispos* 1991;19:149–153.
5. Remmel RP, Sinz MW. A quaternary ammonium glucuronide is the major metabolite of lamotrigine in guinea pigs: *in vitro* and *in vivo* studies. *Drug Metab Dispos* 1991;19:630–636.
6. Doig MV, Clare RA. Use of thermospray liquid chromatography-mass spectrometry to aid in the identification of urinary metabolites of a novel antiepileptic drug, lamotrigine. *J Chromatogr* 1991;554:181–189.
7. Mikati MA, Schachter SC, Schomer DL, et al. Long term tolerability, pharmacokinetic and preliminary efficacy study of lamotrigine in patients with resistant partial seizures. *Clin Neuropharmacol* 1989;12:312–321.
8. Maggs JL, Naisbitt DJ, Tettey JNA, et al. Metabolism of lamotrigine to a reactive arene oxide intermediate. *Chem Res Toxicol* 2000;13:1075–1081.
9. Fong K-LL, Hwang BY-H. Dog liver *N*-methyltransferase: a drug-metabolizing enzyme. *Biochem Pharmacol* 1983;18: 2781–2786.
10. Magdalou JM, Herber R, Bidault R, et al. *In vitro N*-glucuronidation of a novel antiepileptic drug, lamotrigine, by human liver microsomes. *J Pharmacol Exp Ther* 1992;260: 1166–1173.

11. Furlan V, Demirdjian S, Bourdon O, et al. Glucuronidation of drugs by hepatic microsomes derived from healthy and cirrhotic livers. *J Pharmacol Exp Ther* 1999;289:1169–1175.

12. Odishaw JL, Brouwer KLR, Brouwer KR, et al. A comparison of human liver slices and suspended hepatocytes to examine drug interactions with lamotrigine glucuronidation. *ISSX Proc* 1997; 12:165(abst).

13. Radominska-Pandya A, Czernik PJ, Little JM. Structural and functional studies of UDP-glucuronosyltransferases. *Drug Metab Rev* 1999;31:817–899.

14. Tukey RH, Strassburg CP. Human UDP-glucuronosyltransferases: metabolism, expression and disease. *Annu Rev Pharmacol Toxicol* 2000;40:581–616.

15. Hawes EM. *N*-glucuronidation, a common pathway in human metabolism of drugs with a tertiary amine group. *Drug Metab Dispos* 1998;26:830–837.

16. Green MD, Bishop WP, Tephly TR. Expressed human UGT1.4 protein catalyzes the formation of quaternary ammonium linked glucuronides. *Drug Metab Dispos* 1995;23:299–302.

17. Vashishtha SC, Hawes EM, McKay G, et al. Synthesis and identification of the quaternary ammonium-linked glucuronide of 1-phenylimidazole in human liver microsomes and investigation of the human UDP-glucuronosyltransferases involved. *Drug Metab Dispos* 2000;28:1009–1013.

18. Green MD, Tephly TR. Glucuronidation of amine substrates by purified and expressed UDP-glucuronosyltransferase proteins. *Drug Metab Dispos* 1998;26:860–867.

19. Mojarrabi B, Butler R, Mackenzie PI. cDNA cloning and characterization of the human UDP-glucuronosyltransferase, UGT1A3. *Biochem Biophys Res Commun* 1996;225:785–790.

20. Hiller A, Nguyen N, Strassburg CP, et al. Retigabine *N*-glucuronidation and its potential role in enterohepatic circulation. *Drug Metab Dispos* 1999;27:605–612.

21. Yuen AWC, Land G, Weatherley BC, et al. Sodium valproate acutely inhibits lamotrigine metabolism. *Br J Clin Pharmacol* 1992;33:511–513.

22. Anderson GD. A mechanistic approach to antiepileptic drug interactions. *Ann Pharmacother* 1998;32:554–563

23. Tanaka E. Clinically significant pharmacokinetic drug interactions between antiepileptic drugs. *J Clin Pharm Ther* 1999;24: 87–92.

24. Ebert U, Thong NQ, Oertel R, et al. Effects of rifampicin and cimetidine on pharmacokinetics and pharmacodynamics of lamotrigine in healthy subjects. *Eur J Clin Pharmacol* 2000;56: 299–304.

25. Glaxo Wellcome Inc. Product information of LAMICTAL (lamotrigine) tablets and LAMICTAL (lamotrigine) chewable dispersible tablets. In: *Physicians' desk reference,* 53rd ed. Montvale, NJ: Medical Economics, 1999:A143.

26. Cohen AF, Land GS, Breimer DD, et al. Lamotrigine, a new anticonvulsant: pharmacokinetics in normal humans. *Clin Pharmacol Ther* 1987;42:535–541.

27. Goa KL, Ross SR, Chrisp P. Lamotrigine: a review of its pharmacological properties and clinical efficacy in epilepsy. *Drugs* 1993;46:152–176.

28. Yau MK, Garnett WR, Wargin WA, et al. A single dose, dose proportionality and bioequivalence study of lamotrigine in normal volunteers. *Epilepsia* 1991;32[Suppl 3]:8.

29. Anderson GD, Yau MK, Gidal BE, et al. Bidirectional interaction of valproate and lamotrigine in healthy subjects. *Clin Pharmacol Ther* 1996;60:145—156.

30. Ramsay RE, Pellock JM, Garnett WR, et al. Pharmacokinetics and safety of lamotrigine (Lamictal) in patients with epilepsy. *Epilepsy Res* 1991;10:191–200.

31. Yuen WC, Peck AW. Lamotrigine pharmacokinetics: oral and i.v. infusion in man. *Br J Clin Pharmacol* 1988;26:242P.

32. Yuen AW. Lamotrigine. In: Pisani E, Avanzini G, Richens A, eds. *New epileptic drugs.* Amsterdam: Elsevier Science Publishers, 1991.

33. Jaward S, Yuen WC, Peck AW, et al. Lamotrigine: single-dose pharmacokinetics and initial 1-week experience in refractory epilepsy. *Epilepsy Res* 1987;1:194–201.

34. Binnie CD, van Emde Boas W, Kasteleijn-Nolste-Trenite DGA, et al. Acute effects of lamotrigine (BW430C) in persons with epilepsy. *Epilepsia* 1986;27:248–254.

35. Trnavska Z, Krejcova H, Tkaczykovam Z, et al. Pharmacokinetics of lamotrigine (Lamictal) in plasma and saliva. *Eur J Drug Metab Pharmacokinet* 1991;3:211–215.

36. Rambeck B, Kurlemann G, Stodieck SRG, et al. Concentrations of lamotrigine in a mother on lamotrigine treatment and her newborn child. *Eur J Clin Pharmacol* 1997;51:481–484.

37. Eriksson A, Hoppu K, Nergardh A, et al. Pharmacokinetic interactions between lamotrigine and other antiepileptic drugs in children with intractable epilepsy. *Epilepsia* 1996;37:769–773.

38. Remmel RP, Sinz MW, Graves NW, et al. Lamotrigine and lamotrigine-*N*-glucuronide concentrations in human blood and brain tissue. *Seizure* 1992;1[Suppl A]:P7/34.

39. Tomson T, Ohman I, Vitols S. Lamotrigine in pregancy and lactation: a case report. *Epilepsia* 1997;38:1039–1041.

40. Cohen AF, Ashby L, Crowley D, et al. Lamotrigine (BW430C), a potent anticonvulsant: effects on the central nervous system in comparison with phenytoin and diazepam. *Br J Clin Pharmacol* 1985;20:619–629.

41. Hussein Z, Posner J. Population pharmacokinetics of lamotrigine monotherapy in patients with epilepsy: retrospective analysis of routine monitoring data. *Br J Clin Pharmacol* 1997;43:457–465.

42. Grasela TH, Fiedler-Kelly J, Cox E, et al . Population pharmacokinetics of lamotrigine adjunctive therapy in adults with epilepsy. *J Clin Pharmacol* 1999;39:373–384.

43. May TW, Rambeck B, Jurgens U. Serum concentrations of lamotrigine in epileptic patients: the influence of dose and comedication. *Ther Drug Monit* 1996;18:523–531.

44. May TW, Rambeck B. Influence of oxcarbazepine and methsuximide on lamotrigine concentrations in epileptic patients with or without valproic acid comedication: results of a retrospective study. *Ther Drug Monit* 1999;21:175–181.

45. Besag FMC, Berry DJ, Pool F. Methsuximide lowers LTG blood levels: a pharmacokinetic AED interaction. *Epilepsia* 1998;39 [Suppl 2]:25.

46. Wnuk W, Volanski A, Foletti G. Topiramate decreases lamotrigine concentrations. *Ther Drug Monit* 1999;21:449.

47. Kaufman KR, Gerner R. Lamotrigine toxicity secondary to sertraline. *Seizure* 1998;7:163–165.

48. Colucci R, Glue P, Holt B, et al. Effect of felbamate on the pharmacokinetics of lamotrigine. *J Clin Pharmacol* 1996;36: 634–638.

49. Odishaw J, Chen C. Effects of steady-state bupropion on the pharmacokinetics of lamotrigine in healthy subjects. *Pharmacotherapy* 2000;20:1448–1453.

50. Chen C, Casale EJ, Duncan B, et al. Pharmacokinetics of lamotrigine in children in the absence of other antiepileptic drugs. *Pharmacotherapy* 1999;19:437–441.

51. Chen C, Grasela TH, Phillips L, et al. Population pharmacokinetics of add-on lamotrigine in pediatric patients. *Ann Neurol* 1997;42:508.

52. Chen C. Validation of a population pharmacokinetic model for adjunctive lamotrigine therapy in children. *Br J Clin Pharmacol* 2000;50:135–145.

53. Perucca E. Drug metabolism in pregnancy, infancy and childhood. *Pharmacol Ther* 1987;34:129–143.

54. Besunder JB, Reed MD, Blumer JL. Principles of drug disposition in the neonate: a critical evaluation of the pharmacokinetic-

pharmacodynamic interface. I. *Clin Pharmacokinet* 1988;14: 189–216.

55. Posner J, Holdich T, Crome P. Comparison of lamotrigine pharmacokinetics in young and elderly healthy volunteers. *J Pharm Med* 1991;1:121–128.

56. Wootton R, Soul-Lawton J, Rolan PE, et al. Comparison of the pharmacokinetics of lamotrigine in patients with chronic renal failure and healthy volunteers. *Br J Clin Pharmacol* 1997;43: 23–27.

57. Fillastre JP, Taburet AM, Fialaire A, et al. Pharmacokinetics of lamotrigine in patients with renal impairment: influence of haemodialysis. *Drugs Exptl Clin Res* 1993;19:25–32.

58. Posner J, Cohen AF, Land G, et al. The pharmacokinetics of lamotrigine (BW430C) in healthy subjects with unconjugated hyperbilirubinaemia (Gilbert's syndrome). *Br J Clin Pharmacol* 1989;28:117–120.

59. Jawad S, Oxley J, Yuen WC, et al. The effects of lamotrigine, a novel anticonvulsant, on interictal spikes in patients with epilepsy. *Br J Clin Pharmacol* 1986;22:191–193.

60. Matsuo F, Bergen D, Faught E, et al. Placebo-controlled study of the efficacy and safety of lamotrigine in patients with partial seizures. *Neurology* 1993;43:2284–2291.

61. Smith D, Baker G, Davies G, et al. Outcomes of add-on treatment with lamotrigine in partial seizure. *Epilepsia* 1993;34: 312–322.

62. Binnie CD, Debets RMC, Engelsman M, et al. Double-blind crossover trial of lamotrigine (Lamictal) as add-on therapy in intractable epilepsy. *Epilepsy Res* 1989;4:222–229.

63. Jawad S, Richens A, Goodwin G, et al. Controlled trial of lamotrigine (Lamictal) for refractory partial seizures. *Epilepsia* 1989; 30:356–363.

64. Messenheimer J, Ramsay RE, Willmore LJ, et al. Lamotrigine therapy for partial seizures: a multicenter, placebo-controlled, double-blind, cross-over trial. *Epilepsia* 1994;35:113–121.

65. Bartoni A, Guerrini R, Belmonte A, et al. The influence of dosage, age and comedication on steady-state plasma lamotrigine concentration in epileptic children: a prospective study with preliminary assessment of correlations with clinical response. *Ther Drug Monit* 1997;19:252–260.

66. Kilpatrick ES, Forrest G, Brodie MJ. Concentration-effect and concentration-toxicity relations with lamotrigine: a prospective study. *Epilepsia* 1996;37:534–538.

67. Schapel GJ, Beran RG, Vajda FJE, et al. Double-blind, placebo controlled, crossover study of lamotrigine in treatment resistant partial seizures. *J Neurol Neurosurg Psychiatry* 1993;56:448–453.

68. Loiseau P, Yuen AWC, Duche B, et al. A randomised double-blind placebo-controlled crossover add-on trial of lamotrigine in patients with treatment-resistant partial seizures. *Epilepsy Res* 1990;7:136–145.

69. Schapel GJ, Black AB, Lam EL, et al. Combination vigabatrin and lamotrigine therapy for intractable epilepsy. *Seizure* 1996; 5:51–56.

70. Morris RG, Black AB, Harris AL, et al. Lamotrigine and therapeutic drug monitoring: retrospective survey following the introduction of a routine service. *Br J Clin Pharmacol* 1998;46: 547–551.

LAMOTRIGINE

INTERACTION WITH OTHER DRUGS

WILLIAM R. GARNETT

Drug interactions occur frequently with the first-generation antiepileptic drugs (AEDs), such as phenobarbital, phenytoin, carbamazepine, and valproic acid (2). Therefore, the early development of lamotrigine evaluated the effects of other AEDs on lamotrigine, and these effects were included in the initial study designs. Although it has been demonstrated that other AEDs can increase and decrease the metabolism of lamotrigine, lamotrigine is not metabolized by the cytochrome P450 pathways and is less likely to interfere with the metabolism of other drugs. The low protein binding of lamotrigine also makes it less likely to interact with other drugs. More recently, some pharmacodynamic interactions between lamotrigine and other AEDs that may result in toxicity or synergy have been identified. Therefore, it is important to review the drug interaction profile of lamotrigine.

PHARMACOKINETICS OF LAMOTRIGINE

A review of the clinical pharmacokinetics of lamotrigine is useful in evaluating the potential for and possible mechanisms of the pharmacokinetic drug interactions associated with lamotrigine. Studies in normal volunteers established that lamotrigine reaches a peak concentration (C_{max}) in 1 to 3 hours after an oral dose. An absolute bioavailability of 97.6% was determined by comparing the area under the concentration–time curve (AUC) after intravenous and oral doses. Thus, lamotrigine is rapidly and completely absorbed. Lamotrigine demonstrates linear pharmacokinetics, with AUC and C_{max} increasing proportionally with dose. This indicates that there is no significant autoinduction or saturable metabolism. The half-life of lamotrigine is approximately 22 hours in drug-naive individuals and the clearance is approximately 42 mL/min. Although there is

significant intersubject variability in clearance, there is little intrasubject variability (41). Approximately 70% of a dose of lamotrigine is eliminated by the phase II metabolic pathway (i.e., by glucuronide conjugation) in the liver (21). There is no first-pass metabolism, which means that alterations in liver blood flow do not change metabolism. The metabolism of lamotrigine may be moderately reduced in people with Gilbert's syndrome (21). A population pharmacokinetics study of patients aged 14 to 74 years receiving lamotrigine demonstrated that the apparent oral clearance was not significantly influenced by body weight, age, sex, oral contraceptives, and dose (29). Whereas a mild autoinduction effect (17.3%) and a lower clearance in Asians versus whites (28.7%) have been reported, these effects are not thought to be clinically significant and do not warrant dosage adjustments (29). Renal failure does not alter the pharmacokinetics of lamotrigine (50). Lamotrigine is only approximately 55% bound to plasma proteins, indicating a low potential for displacement with highly (>90 %) protein-bound drugs. The volume of distribution (VD) is approximately 1.1 L/kg (21). The weight-normalized clearance and VD are higher in children. Therefore, children will likely require higher weight-normalized doses at the same dosing frequency to achieve comparable serum concentrations (13) (Table 36.1).

PHARMACOKINETIC EFFECTS OF OTHER DRUGS ON LAMOTRIGINE

Effects of Antiepileptic Drugs on Lamotrigine

Several studies have shown that the clearance of lamotrigine is enhanced by coadministration with AEDs that can induce liver enzymes and reduced by drugs that inhibit liver enzymes (Table 36.2). Armijo et al. used bivariate and multivariate methods to analyze retrospectively the influence of patient age and the use of concomitant AEDs on the lamotrigine concentration-to-dose (C/D) ratio in samples from

William R. Garnett, PharmD: Professor of Pharmacy and Neurology, Deparment of Pharmacy, Virginia Commonwealth University, Medical College of Virginia, Richmond, Virginia

TABLE 36.1. CLINICAL PHARMACOKINETICS OF LAMOTRIGINE

Absorption	C_{max} 1–3 h
Bioavailability	97.6%
Protein binding	55%
Metabolism	Glucuronidation
	No cytochrome P
	No first pass
	More rapid in children
	Mild reduction in Asians
	Mild (17%) autoinduction
$T_{1/2}$	Naive subjects: 22 h
	Enzyme induced: 14 h
	Enzyme inhibited: >60 h

C_{max}, time to maximum plasma concentration; $T_{1/2}$, half-life.

164 patients (3). The lamotrigine C/D ratio increased with age in patients receiving lamotrigine alone, but decreased with age in patients receiving lamotrigine with enzyme inducers. The lamotrigine C/D ratio increased in patients taking valproic acid. The lamotrigine C/D ratio was 10 times lower in patients receiving lamotrigine and inducers than in those receiving lamotrigine and valproic acid.

Bottiger et al. reviewed 149 lamotrigine samples from 104 adult patients to determine the effects of drug interactions on lamotrigine (10). In 20 patients on monotherapy, the C/D ratio was 65 (range, 50 to 84) nmol/L/mg. In 37 patients with concomitant carbamazepine treatment, the C/D ratio was 31 nmol/L/mg, which was less than half that of patients on monotherapy, and in 14 patients on phenytoin, it was even lower (17 nmol/L/mg). In a few patients taking phenobarbital with lamotrigine, the C/D ratio was slightly less than with monotherapy. In the 13 patients taking valproic acid concurrently with lamotrigine, the C/D ratio was significantly increased to 251 nmol/L/mg. In patients taking valproic acid with either carbamazepine or phenytoin and lamotrigine, the C/D ratio was slightly above that of monotherapy for lamotrigine.

Grasela et al. used NONMEN, a population pharmacokinetics computer program, to pool and analyze the plasma concentrations of lamotrigine obtained from the three adult clinical trials conducted in the United States (26). A total of 2,407 lamotrigine plasma concentrations from 527 patients were analyzed to determine the effect of body size, age, sex, race, and use of concomitant AEDs. The population mean apparent oral clearance of lamotrigine in adult patients receiving one concomitant enzyme-inducing AED and not valproic acid was estimated to be 1 mL/min/kg. The clearance of lamotrigine was increased by 13% in patients receiving more than one concomitant enzyme-inducing AED. Lamotrigine did not affect the clearance of other AEDs.

Battino et al. evaluated the effects of age and concomitant treatment on plasma lamotrigine C/D ratios in 482 samples from 106 chronically treated patients with epilepsy (5). A linear C/D relationship was observed in individual patients, but there was no correlation between the administered lamotrigine dose and plasma concentration in the cumulative analysis. Concurrent AED therapy affected the lamotrigine C/D ratio, which was significantly higher in the patients receiving valproic acid and significantly lower in those treated with enzyme-inducing AEDs. The lamotrigine C/D ratios significantly increased with increasing plasma valproic acid concentrations and significantly decreased with increasing phenytoin concentrations. The effect of enzyme-inducing AEDs increased with the number of concomitant drugs.

In a prospective study by Bartoli et al., there was more enzyme induction than inhibition in children 3 to 6 years of age than in older children (4). These investigators evaluated 45 patients 3 to 38 years of age who received lamotrigine as adjunctive therapy for uncontrolled seizures. In the

TABLE 36.2. PHARMACOKINETIC EFFECTS OF OTHER DRUGS ON LAMOTRIGINE

Drug	Effect	Mechanism
AEDs		
Phenytoin	Decrease $t_{1/2}$, increase clearance	Enzyme induction
Carbamazepine	Decrease $t_{1/2}$, increase clearance	Enzyme induction
Phenobarbital	Decrease $t_{1/2}$, increase clearance	Enzyme induction
Methsuximide	Decrease $t_{1/2}$, increase clearance	Enzyme induction
Oxcarbazepine	Decrease $t_{1/2}$, increase clearance	Enzyme induction
Valproic acid	Increase $t_{1/2}$, decrease clearance	Enzyme inhibition
Felbamate	No effect	No effect
Non-AEDs		
Rifampicin	Decrease $t_{1/2}$, increase clearance	Enzyme induction
Acetaminophen	Decrease $t_{1/2}$, increase clearance	Enzyme induction
Sertraline	Decrease $t_{1/2}$, increase clearance	Enzyme induction
Cimetidine	No effect	

AED, antiepileptic drug; $t_{1/2}$, half-life.

patients receiving enzyme-inducing AEDs, the lamotrigine concentrations normalized to a 1 mg/kg daily dosage were lower in children aged 3 to 6 years than in older children, adolescents, and adults. Although valproic acid increased the concentrations of lamotrigine, the age effect was less evident. In any age group, the dose-normalized lamotrigine concentrations were approximately fivefold higher in patients comedicated with valproic acid than in those comedicated with enzyme inducers.

May et al. investigated the influence of carbamazepine, phenytoin, phenobarbital, valproic acid, and combinations of these drugs on the serum concentration of lamotrigine in 588 blood samples taken from 302 patients (35). The lamotrigine serum concentration in relation to lamotrigine dose/body weight [level-to-dose ratio (LDR), in μg/mL/mg/kg] was calculated and compared for different drug combinations. The results showed that comedication had a significant effect on the lamotrigine serum concentrations. The mean LDRs for lamotrigine were 0.32 (lamotrigine + phenytoin), <0.52 (lamotrigine + phenobarbital), ≈0.57 (lamotrigine + carbamazepine), <0.98 (lamotrigine mono), ≈0.99 (lamotrigine + valproic acid + phenytoin), <1.67 (lamotrigine + valproic acid + carbamazepine), ≈1.80 (lamotrigine + valproic acid + phenobarbital), and <3.57 (lamotrigine + valproic acid). The mean lamotrigine concentrations in patients on comedication with valproic acid were approximately two times higher than in patients on lamotrigine monotherapy or on comedication without valproic acid.

Eriksson et al. assessed the interactions of lamotrigine with other AEDs in 31 children (19). The median elimination half-life in patients receiving concomitant valproic acid was 43.3 hours, in patients receiving carbamazepine and/or phenobarbital, it was 14.1 hours, and in patients receiving both valproate and carbamazepine/phenobarbital or other AEDs, it was 28.9 hours.

Valproic acid inhibits the metabolism of lamotrigine. The half-life of a single dose of lamotrigine given to four patients stabilized on valproic acid was 59 ± 26 hours. The half-life of lamotrigine was 69.6 ± 14.8 hours in 18 healthy volunteers who took valproic acid for 70 days and added 50-, 100-, and 150-mg doses of lamotrigine for 7 days in a random fashion (51). In a study of six normal volunteers who received single doses of 100 mg of lamotrigine and six doses of 200 mg of valproic acid every 8 hours beginning 1 hour before the lamotrigine, Yuen et al. reported a 21% decrease in the clearance of lamotrigine, with an increase in the half-life of lamotrigine from 37.4 to 48.3 hours and an increase in the AUC of lamotrigine from 70.9 to 91.8 μg/mL/hr (53). The reduction in elimination occurred within the first hour. C_{max}, t_{max}, and renal elimination were not altered. The proposed mechanism for the interaction was competition between valproic acid and lamotrigine for glucuronidation. The effects detected in this study may not have been maximal because the dose of valproic acid was not at steady state (53). Anderson et al. evaluated the

steady-state pharmacokinetics of lamotrigine and valproic acid with three different doses of lamotrigine in normal volunteers (1). Eighteen normal male volunteers received 500 mg orally of valproic acid twice a day throughout the study. Each subject randomly received 50, 100, and 150 mg of lamotrigine for 1 week each, with a 2-week washout period between lamotrigine treatment periods. Concomitant valproic acid markedly increased the half-life of lamotrigine and decreased lamotrigine clearance without altering the linear pharmacokinetics of lamotrigine (1). In a study using population pharmacokinetics to describe the pharmacokinetics of lamotrigine in developmentally disabled patients, the clearances of lamotrigine as monotherapy, lamotrigine plus inducers, and lamotrigine plus valproic acid were 0.69 ± 0.2, 1.60 ± 0.65, and 0.2 ± 0.05 mL/kg/min, respectively (22). The addition of the valproic acid concentration to the model used to define the clearance of lamotrigine did not significantly improve the estimates of clearance. This suggests that valproic acid inhibition of lamotrigine is maximal within the usually accepted target ranges for valproic acid (22). Kanner and Frey evaluated the clearance of lamotrigine in 28 patients with intractable epilepsy who were treated with a combination of lamotrigine and valproic acid (31). Correlations between lamotrigine clearance and the dose and steady-state concentration of valproic acid demonstrated that the degree of inhibition of lamotrigine clearance is independent of the dose and steady-state concentration of valproic acid (31). Chen also used population pharmacokinetics to establish a basis for dosage recommendations for lamotrigine in children and reported that to achieve the same concentrations, children receiving enzyme-inducing AEDs without valproic acid require higher doses of lamotrigine than those receiving valproic acid (12). Also, heavier children require higher doses (12). May et al. found that valproic acid increases the concentration of lamotrigine by 211% (34). The combination of lamotrigine with enzyme-inducing AEDs and valproic acid reduces some of the effect of valproic acid on the inhibition of lamotrigine metabolism (30). Therefore, if valproic acid is discontinued from the regimen of a patient taking lamotrigine, the concentrations of lamotrigine will decrease, necessitating a dosage increase (Tables 36.3 and 36.4).

Two studies have evaluated the effects of methsuximide on the pharmacokinetics of lamotrigine. Besag et al. evaluated lamotrigine serum levels in 16 patients taking methsuximide before starting or after stopping methsuximide (6). Methsuximide lowered the concentration of lamotrigine in every case, with a mean decrease of 53% (range, 36% to 72%) (6). May et al. retrospectively evaluated 376 blood samples from 222 patients to determine the effects of methsuximide and oxcarbazepine on lamotrigine concentrations (34). Methsuximide was found to have a strong inducing effect on the metabolism of lamotrigine, and decreased the lamotrigine concentration by approximately 70% compared with lamotrigine monotherapy. Methsuximide could

TABLE 36.3. LAMOTRIGINE: ADULT DOSING

	Weeks 1 and 2	Weeks 3 and 4	Usual Maintenance Dosage
With enzyme-inducing AED and no valproic acid	50 mg qd	100 mg bid	300–500 mg/day in two divided doses Escalate dose by 100 mg/day every 1–2 wks
With enzyme-inducing AED and valproic acid	25 mg qod	25 mg qd	100–400 mg/day in one or two divided doses Escalate dose by 25–50 mg/day every 1–2 wk
With valproic acid alone	12.5 mg qod	12.5 mg qd	100–200 mg/day in two divided doses Escalate doses by 12.5–25 mg/day every 2 wk

AED, antiepileptic drug.

attenuate most of the inhibitory effect of valproic acid on the metabolism of lamotrigine. When given with lamotrigine alone, valproic acid increased the lamotrigine concentration by 211%, but the increase was only 8% when methsuximide was given concomitantly with valproic acid and lamotrigine (34).

In addition to finding an effect of methsuximide on the pharmacokinetics of lamotrigine, May et al. found an enzyme-inducing effect of oxcarbazepine, which they estimated to be 29% (34). The enzyme-inducing effect of oxcarbazepine was less than that of carbamazepine, which was 54%. Oxcarbazepine reduced some of the inhibitory effect of valproic acid on the metabolism of lamotrigine. Valproic acid increased the lamotrigine concentration by 211% when given alone, but increased the concentration only by 111% when given with oxcarbazepine (34).

Gidal et al. compared the pharmacokinetics of lamotrigine in six patients concomitantly receiving felbamate with five patients receiving lamotrigine as monotherapy (23). There was no statistically significant difference in either apparent lamotrigine oral clearance (0.026 ± 0.005 L/kg/hr versus 0.0924 ± 0.01 L/kg/hr) or in mean elimination half-life (33.7 ± 7.5 hours versus 40.2 ± 15.05 hours). It was concluded that felbamate did not have a significant effect on lamotrigine pharmacokinetics (23). Glue et al. analyzed the degree of agreement between *in vivo* interaction studies performed in patients with epilepsy and healthy individuals and *in vitro* studies that identified the cytochrome P450 enzymes inhibited by felbamate (25). They found no interactions between felbamate and lamotrigine (25). Colucci et al. administered 1,200 mg of felbamate every 12 hours to normal volunteers who also took 100 mg of lamotrigine every 12 hours for 10 days in a double-blind, randomized, placebo-controlled, two-way crossover study (15). Although there was a 13% increase in C_{max} and a 14% in the AUC of lamotrigine when it was given with felbamate compared with placebo, the 90% confidence intervals of the pharmacokinetic parameters were within the 80% to 125% bioequivalance limits, and it was determined that felbamate had no clinically relevant effects on the pharmacokinetics of lamotrigine (15).

Effects of Nonantiepileptic Drugs on Lamotrigine

Rifampicin is a potent inducer of cytochrome P450 and of the uridine 5'-diphosphate-glucuronyl transferase enzyme systems, and cimetidine is an inhibitor of the cytochrome P450 enzyme system. The effects of these drugs on the pharmacokinetics of lamotrigine were evaluated by Ebert et al. in 10 normal volunteers who received a single 25-mg oral dose of lamotrigine after pretreatment with either 400 mg of cimetidine twice a day, 600 mg of rifampicin once a day, or placebo (17). Rifampicin significantly increased the clearance-over-bioavailability ratio (5.13 ± 1.05 L/hr versus 2.60 ± 0.40 L/hr) and the amount of lamotrigine excreted

TABLE 36.4. LAMOTRIGINE: PEDIATRIC DOSING

	Weeks 1 and 2	Weeks 3 and 4	Usual Maintenance Dosage
With enzyme-inducing AED and no valproic acid	0.6 mg/kg/bid	1.2 mg/kg/bid	5–15 mg/kg/day (maximum 400 mg/day in two divided doses). Escalate dose by 1.2 mg/day every 1–2 weeks. Round down to nearest whole tablet for all doses.
Monotherapy and valproic acid	0.15 mg/kg/bid	0.3 mg/kg/bid	1–5 mg/kg/day (maximum 200 mg/day in one or two divided doses). Escalate dose by 0.3 mg/kg/day every 1–2 weeks. Round down to nearest whole tablet for all doses.
With valproic acid	0.2 mg/kg/day	0.5 mg/kg/day	1–5 mg/kg/day

AED, antiepileptic drug.

as glucuronide (12.12 ± 0.94 mg versus 8.90 ± 0.77 mg) compared with placebo, whereas both the half-life (14.1 ± 1.7 hours versus 23.8 ± 2.1 hours) and the AUC (396.24 ± 60.18 μg/mL/min versus 703.99 ± 82.31 μg/mL/min) were significantly decreased compared with placebo. Cimetidine did not alter the pharmacokinetics of lamotrigine. The authors concluded that rifampicin induced the enzymes responsible for the glucuronidation of lamotrigine, but that cimetidine had negligible effects (17).

Because both lamotrigine and acetaminophen are metabolized by hepatic glucuronidation, the potential for an interaction exists. A study was done in eight normal volunteers who took a single 300-mg dose of lamotrigine before and after taking acetaminophen 900 mg three times a day for 11 days. There was a 15% increase in the clearance of lamotrigine, a 15% decrease in the half-life, and a 20% decrease in the AUC after acetaminophen treatment (16). This suggests that acetaminophen may stimulate the metabolism of lamotrigine. However, the differences are small and within the intersubject differences.

Kaufman and Gerner reported two patients who had sertraline added to their lamotrigine regimen (32). In the first case, a 25-mg dose of sertraline that did not produce detectable blood levels of sertraline or its metabolite resulted in a doubling of the concentration of lamotrigine, with symptoms of side effects. In the second case, a 25-mg reduction in the dose of sertraline resulted in a 50% reduction in the concentration of lamotrigine despite a 33% increase in the lamotrigine dosage. The authors hypothesize that sertraline inhibits the glucuronidation of lamotrigine (32).

PHARMACOKINETIC EFFECTS OF LAMOTRIGINE ON OTHER DRUGS

Effect of Lamotrigine on Other Antiepileptic Drugs

The potential for lamotrigine to induce mixed-function oxygenase enzymes was evaluated in normal volunteers (39). In a randomized, double-blind, parallel-group study, nine normal volunteers received 100 mg of lamotrigine twice a day for 14 days and nine subjects received placebo. The clearance of antipyrine, the 48-hour urinary excretion of 6-β-hydroxycortisol, and the plasma γ-glutamyl transferase concentrations were assessed before treatment, within 24 hours of the last dose, and 14 days later. There were no significant changes in the clearance of antipyrine or 6-β-hydroxycortisol, and no significant changes in the plasma γ-glutamyl transferase concentrations. The authors concluded that it is unlikely that lamotrigine induces mixed-function oxygenase enzymes to an extent that would result in drug interactions (39). Lamotrigine is only approximately 56% protein bound, and it is unlikely to alter the binding of other highly protein-bound drugs (e.g., phenytoin, valproic acid) or to be affected by them. This was confirmed in an *in vitro* study using equilibrium dialysis (36). The binding of lamotrigine was constant over the concentration of 1 to 3 μg/mL and was unaffected by concentrations of phenytoin, phenobarbital, or valproic that were in the target range (36).

Data collected during the clinical trials of lamotrigine showed no changes in the concentrations of carbamazepine, phenytoin, valproic acid, primidone, phenobarbital, or clobazam (Table 36.5). In the NONMEN analysis of the 2,407 samples from the 527 patients in the three adult trials of lamotrigine in the United States, it was documented that lamotrigine had no effect on the plasma levels of phenytoin or carbamazepine (26). In the previously mentioned study by Eriksson et al. (19), there were no clinically important changes in the plasma levels of carbamazepine, valproic acid, ethosuximide, or phenobarbital after the addition of lamotrigine. There was a reduction in the plasma concentration of clonazepam when lamotrigine was added (19).

There have been anecdotal reports of an increase in the concentration of carbamazepine or carbamazepine-10,11-epoxide in patients receiving lamotrigine. Warner et al. reported that the concentration of carbamazepine increased from 28 ± 6 μmol/L before lamotrigine therapy to 32 ± 10 μmol/L after lamotrigine (48). The carbamazepine epoxide concentrations also increased from 5.6 ± 2.5 μmol/L to 7.9 ± 3.5 μmol/L. However, there was a wide range of epoxide

TABLE 36.5. PLASMA ANTIEPILEPTIC DRUG CONCENTRATIONS POOLED ACROSS FOUR STUDIES

	No. of Patients	Mean During PLO (μg/mL)	Mean During LTG (μg/mL)	Mean Difference	95% Interval Estimate of Difference
Carbamazepine	62	6.9	7.0	−0.1	−0.5, 0.3
Phenytoin	33	12.9	12.0	0.9	−0.6, 2.5
Sodium valproate	22	63.7	64.1	−0.4	−5.9, 4.4
Primidone	13	6.8	6.4	0.4	−0.2, 1.2
Phenobarbital	11	18.4	16.7	1.7	−0.7, 3.5
Phenobarbital (derived from primidone metabolism)	11	18.3	17.7	0.5	−0.9, 1.8
Clobazam	9	55.6	55.8	−0.2	−19.4, 19.1

PLO, placebo; LTG, lamotrigine.

concentrations (48). Graves et al. reported three case histories in which there was an increase in the epoxide metabolite without a change in the parent carbamazepine concentration (27). Potter and Donnelly reported that phenytoin and lamotrigine caused a relative increase in the carbamazepine-10,11-epoxide concentration and a significant decrease in the ratio of carbamazepine to the epoxide (from 5 to 3) (40). If valproic acid also was present, the concentration of parent and metabolite increased significantly, causing potential toxicity (40). However, more controlled trials have failed to demonstrate an effect of lamotrigine or its metabolite (44). In one study, 11 patients taking carbamazepine took lamotrigine or placebo in a controlled crossover study. The carbamazepine concentrations were 8.3 µg/mL during the lamotrigine period and 8.7 µg/mL during the placebo period. The carbamazepine epoxide concentrations were 2.0 µg/mL during the lamotrigine period and 2.1 µg/mL during the placebo period. None of the differences was statistically significant (45). In another placebo-controlled study, Stolarek et al. evaluated the plasma concentrations of carbamazepine and epoxide in 22 patients during the placebo period and during the period when lamotrigine was added to the patients' regimen (47). They found no significant changes in the concentrations of either carbamazepine or its metabolite (47). More recently, Besag et al. evaluated the concentrations of carbamazepine and its active epoxide metabolite in 47 patients with escalating doses of lamotrigine. There was no significant change in the serum concentrations of either the parent drug or its metabolite (8). Eriksson and Boreus also failed to find a change in the concentration of carbamazepine or carbamazepine-10,11-epoxide (18). They studied 11 children and 3 adolescents who had been treated for more than 1 year with carbamazepine when lamotrigine was titrated as concomitant therapy. Lamotrigine had no effect on mean carbamazepine concentrations, but lamotrigine decreased the carbamazepine-10,11-epoxide concentrations slightly (6.4 ± 2.6 µmol/L to 4.9 ± 2.4 µmol/L) (18). Pisani et al. compared the pharmacokinetics of a single dose of carbamazepine-10,11-epoxide in 10 patients on chronic monotherapy with lamotrigine and in 10 normal volunteers (38). The pharmacokinetic parameters of the epoxide in the patients were similar to those in the normal volunteers, indicating that lamotrigine had no effect on the disposition of carbamazepine-10,11-epoxide (38). Gidal et al. evaluated the apparent oral clearance of carbamazepine and the steady-state ratio of carbamazepine epoxide to carbamazepine in nine patients with epilepsy before and after the initiation of adjunctive treatment with lamotrigine (24). The apparent oral clearance of carbamazepine did not change after the initiation of lamotrigine (5.58 ± 1.60 L/hr versus 5.81 ± 1.74 L/hr), and the ratio of carbamazepine epoxide to carbamazepine did not change (0.241 ± 0.082 versus 0.232 ± 0.082) (24). Thus, there is no clear evidence that lamotrigine affects the concentrations of carba-

mazepine or its metabolite. The data from controlled trials support the notion that there is no significant pharmacokinetic interaction between lamotrigine and carbamazepine.

The study by Anderson et al. was a bidirectional study of the interaction between valproic acid and lamotrigine (1). In addition to finding that valproic acid significantly increased the half-life and decreased the clearance of lamotrigine, it also was reported that lamotrigine caused a 25% decrease in the steady-state valproic acid plasma concentration. The oral clearance of valproic acid was increased from 7.2 ± 1.1 mL/hr/kg before lamotrigine treatment to 9.0 ± 2.0 mL/hr/kg on day 28 of lamotrigine therapy. There was no change in the formation of the metabolite of valproic acid believed to be hepatotoxic (1).

Effect of Lamotrigine on Nonantiepileptic Drugs

Because enzyme-inducing AEDs can cause oral contraceptive failure, an interaction between lamotrigine and oral contraceptives was evaluated in 12 healthy women taking an oral contraceptive containing ethinyl estradiol and levonorgestrel. The subjects took lamotrigine 150 mg/day for 14 days. There were no significant changes in the mean plasma concentrations of ethinyl estradiol or levonorgestrel or in the urinary excretion of 6-β-hydroxycortisol (28). Thus, there is no interaction between lamotrigine and oral contraceptives.

Chen et al. studied 20 normal volunteers who took 2 g of lithium gluconate anhydrous every 12 hours for 5 days and in the morning of the sixth day with or without 100 mg of lamotrigine. Lamotrigine did not cause any significant changes in the pharmacokinetics of lithium as determined by noncompartmental methods (14).

PHARMACODYNAMIC INTERACTIONS WITH LAMOTRIGINE

Toxic

Warner et al. (48) and Graves et al. (27) published anecdotal case reports of patients who experienced carbamazepine side effects when lamotrigine was added, which they attributed to an increase in the carbamazepine or epoxide concentration. However, although there is an increase in central nervous system (CNS) side effects when lamotrigine is added to the regimen of a patient taking carbamazepine, there is a lack of controlled data to support a pharmacokinetic interaction between lamotrigine and carbamazepine. It has been postulated that the increase in CNS side effects is related to an interaction at the receptor site (i.e., a pharmacodynamic drug interaction) (Table 36.6) (49). Besag et al. evaluated the effect of escalating doses of lamotrigine in 47 patients taking carbamazepine (8). Although they did not find a change in the concentration of carbamazepine or

TABLE 36.6. PHARMACODYNAMIC DRUG INTERACTIONS WITH LAMOTRIGINE

Combination	Effect	Management
Increased toxicity		
Carbamazepine plus lamotrigine	Increased central nervous system side effects	Decrease dose of carbamazepine
Valproic acid plus lamotrigine	Increased skin rash	Slow dosage titration of lamotrigine
Synergy		
Valproic acid plus lamotrigine	Increased seizure control	Titrate dose to patient response

its epoxide, they did find that nine patients demonstrated clinical signs of CNS toxicity (e.g., diplopia and dizziness). The concentrations of lamotrigine were below those normally associated with CNS side effects. In seven of the nine patients experiencing toxicity, the carbamazepine concentration was >8 mg/L on the initiation of lamotrigine. The authors concluded that CNS toxicity is likely if the carbamazepine concentration is >8 mg/L when lamotrigine is added, and that the mechanism is a result of a pharmacodynamic interaction at the receptor site. They advised clinicians to be prepared to decrease, but not stop, the dose of carbamazepine when lamotrigine is added (8). Eriksson and Boreus evaluated 11 children taking carbamazepine who received lamotrigine as add on therapy (18). Two of these children developed diplopia, two experienced agitation, and one experienced an increase in seizures. None of these children had an increase in carbamazepine or carbamazepine epoxide concentrations. The authors also concluded that the increase in side effects seen with the addition of lamotrigine to the regimen of patients taking carbamazepine is the result of a pharmacodynamic effect (18). Therefore, clinicians should monitor patients on carbamazepine carefully when lamotrigine is added, and be prepared to decrease the dose.

The most serious adverse reaction associated with lamotrigine is skin rash (33) (Table 36.6). This rash typically is maculopapular and appears in the first 4 weeks of therapy. However, it may progress to Stevens-Johnson syndrome (SJS) (43) or to toxic epidermal necrolysis (TEN) (9), which has been associated with death (46). Using a case-controlled methodology, Rzany et al. determined that 73 of 352 (21%) patients with SJS/TEN were taking an AED, whereas only 28 of 1,579 (2%) of the control group reported taking an AED (43). For individual AEDs, the univariate relative risk of SJS/TEN for 8 weeks or less of use was 57 for phenobarbital, 91 for phenytoin, 120 for carbamazepine, 25 for lamotrigine, and 24 for valproic acid (43). The incidence of rash is higher in patients who initiate lamotrigine therapy at a high dose, have a rapid dose escalation, and are taking valproic acid. Conversely, the rate of skin rash is lower in patients taking enzyme-inducing agents (52). Presumably, valproic acid increases the incidence of skin rash because it significantly increases the half-life and decreases the clearance of lamotrigine (2). The combination of lamotrigine and valproic acid also may be associated with an increase in

tremor (42). The association of lamotrigine-induced skin rash with the use of valproic acid is not a *sine qua non* for not using the drugs in combination. In fact, there are data indicating that the two drugs are synergistic when used together (11). However, the initial dose of lamotrigine should be low and the rate of titration should be slow in a patient taking valproic acid (7) (Tables 36.3 and 36.4).

Synergistic

Numerous trials document that when lamotrigine is added to other AEDs there is a reduction in seizure frequency, and lamotrigine appears to be a broad-spectrum AED (33). However, there appears to be a synergistic response to the combination of lamotrigine and valproic acid. Ferrie and Panayiotopoulos reported the case of a 13-year-old patient with refractory myoclonic epilepsy who achieved seizure control only when lamotrigine was combined with valproic acid. They attributed this to a specific pharmacodynamic interaction (20). Brodie and Yuen published the results of a large, multicenter European trial of lamotrigine in 347 patients who had not achieved complete seizure control on valproic acid, carbamazepine, phenytoin, or phenobarbital as monotherapy (11). The response rate was better in patients with idiopathic tonic-clonic seizures (61%) than in patients with partial seizures (43%). The addition of lamotrigine to patients taking valproic acid resulted in a significantly better response (64%) than when added to carbamazepine (41%) or phenytoin (38%). A slow rate of dosage titration was associated with lower incidences of skin rash and patient withdrawal. The increased response for the combination of lamotrigine and valproic acid was better for both tonic-clonic and partial seizures. They stated that their data supported a therapeutic synergy between lamotrigine and valproic acid (11). Pisani et al. assessed the comparative therapeutic value of valproic acid, lamotrigine, and the combination of the two in 20 patients with complex partial seizures resistant to other AEDs (37). Patients were started on valproic acid and then given lamotrigine and then the combination for 3 months. The patients progressed to the next treatment only if they failed to respond to the previous treatment. There was a >50% reduction in seizure frequency in 3 of 20 patients given valproic acid and in 4 of 17 patients given lamotrigine. In the other 13 patients who were given the combination of lamotrigine and valproic acid, 4 became seizure free and 4 had a 62% to 78% reduction in seizure frequency. In the patients responding to the combination, the doses and peak serum concentration of lamotrigine and valproic acid were lower than those during separate administration of either drug. These data also support a synergistic effect between lamotrigine and valproic acid (37) (Table 36.6).

SUMMARY

Lamotrigine is not highly protein bound and is predominantly metabolized by glucuronidation pathways in the liver. Although lamotrigine has a mild stimulating effect on glucuronosyl transferase enzymes, it has no effect of cytochrome P450 isoenzymes. Therefore, the pharmacokinetics of lamotrigine support a reduced potential for drug interactions (2). Enzyme-inducing drugs (e.g., carbamazepine and phenytoin) increase the clearance and decrease the half-life of lamotrigine, whereas valproic acid significantly decreases the clearance and increases the half-life of lamotrigine. If phenytoin, carbamazepine, or valproic acid is given in combination with lamotrigine and then discontinued, the concentration of lamotrigine will increase when the inducers are removed and decrease when the inhibitor is removed. The addition of lamotrigine to patients taking valproic acid should begin with a very low dose, and the dose should be titrated very gradually. If valproic acid is discontinued in a patient taking lamotrigine, the concentration of lamotrigine will decrease and an increase in dose may be necessary. Clinicians should be prepared to reduce, but not stop, the dose of carbamazepine when lamotrigine is added to a patient's regimen because of a pharmacodynamic effect. A synergistic effect may exist with the combined use of lamotrigine and valproic acid. The drug interactions of lamotrigine can be anticipated and patients can be dosed and monitored carefully to maximize the use of lamotrigine. It is wise to monitor carefully any patient who is taking any other medication at the time lamotrigine is added, as well as patients who are taking lamotrigine in whom other drugs are added or discontinued.

REFERENCES

1. Anderson GD, Yau MK, Gidal BE, et al. Bidirectional interaction of valproate and lamotrigine in healthy subjects. *Clin Pharmacol Ther* 1996;60:145–156.
2. Anderson GD. A mechanistic approach to antiepileptic drug interactions. *Ann Pharmacother* 1998;32:554–563.
3. Armijo JA, Bravo J, Cuadrado A, et al. Lamotrigine serum concentration-to-dose ratio: influence of age and concomitant antiepileptic drugs and dosage implications. *Ther Drug Monit* 1999;21:183–190.
4. Bartoli A, Guerrini R, Belmonte A, et al. The influence of dosage, age, and comedication on steady state plasma lamotrigine concentrations in epileptic children: a prospective study with preliminary assessment of correlations with clinical response. *Ther Drug Monit* 1997;19:252–260.
5. Battino D. Lamotrigine plasma concentrations in children and adults: influence of age and associated therapy. *Ther Drug Monit* 1997;19:620–627.
6. Besag FM, Berry DJ, Pool R. Methsuximide lowers lamotrigine blood levels: a pharmacokinetic antiepileptic drug interaction. *Epilepsia* 2000;41:624–627.
7. Besag FM. Lamotrigine in the treatment of epilepsy in people with intellectual disability. *J Intellect Disabil Res* 1998;42[Suppl 1]:50–56.
8. Besag FM, Berry DJ, Pool F, et al. Carbamazepine toxicity with lamotrigine: pharmacokinetic or pharmacodynamic interaction? *Epilepsia* 1998;39:183–187.
9. Bhushan M, Brooke R, Hewitt-Symonds M, et al. Prolonged toxic epidermal necrolysis due to lamotrigine. *Clin Exp Dermatol* 2000;25:349–351.
10. Bottiger Y, Svensson JO, Stahle L. Lamotrigine drug interactions in a TDM material. *Ther Drug Monit* 1999;21:171–174.
11. Brodie MJ, Yuen AW. Lamotrigine substitution study: evidence for synergism with sodium valproate? 105 Study Group. *Epilepsy Res* 1997;26:423–432.
12. Chen C. Validation of a population pharmacokinetic model for adjunctive lamotrigine therapy in children. *Br J Clin Pharmacol* 2000;50:135–145.
13. Chen C, Casale EJ, Duncan B, et al. Pharmacokinetics of lamotrigine in children in the absence of other antiepileptic drugs. *Pharmacotherapy* 1999;19:437–441.
14. Chen C, Veronese L, Yin Y. The effects of lamotrigine on the pharmacokinetics of lithium. *Br J Clin Pharmacol* 2000;50:193–195.
15. Colucci R, Glue P, Holt B, et al. Effect of felbamate on the pharmacokinetics of lamotrigine. *J Clin Pharmacol* 1996;36:634–638.
16. Depot M, Powell JR, Messenheimer JA Jr, et al. Kinetic effects of multiple oral doses of acetaminophen on a single oral dose of lamotrigine. *Clin Pharmacol Ther* 1990;48:346–355.
17. Ebert U, Thong NQ, Oertel R, et al. Effects of rifampicin and cimetidine on pharmacokinetics and pharmacodynamics of lamotrigine in healthy subjects. *Eur J Clin Pharmacol* 2000;56:299–304.
18. Eriksson AS, Boreus LO. No increase in carbamazepine-10,11-epoxide during addition of lamotrigine treatment in children. *Ther Drug Monit* 1997;19:499–501.
19. Eriksson AS, Hoppu K, Nergardh A, et al. Pharmacokinetic interactions between lamotrigine and other antiepileptic drugs in children with intractable epilepsy. *Epilepsia* 1996;37:769–773.
20. Ferrie CD, Panayiotopoulos CP. Therapeutic interaction of lamotrigine and sodium valproate in intractable myoclonic epilepsy. *Seizure* 1994;157–159.
21. Garnett WR. Lamotrigine: pharmacokinetics. *J Child Neurol* 1997;12[Suppl 1]:S10–S15.
22. Gidal BE, Anderson GD, Rutecki PR, et al. Lack of valproate concentration on lamotrigine pharmacokinetics in developmentally disabled patients with epilepsy. *Epilepsy Res* 2000;42:23–31.
23. Gidal BE, Kanner A, Maly M, et al. Lamotrigine pharmacokinetics in patients receiving felbamate. *Epilepsy Res* 1997;27:1–5.
24. Gidal BE, Rutecki P, Shaw R, et al. Effect of lamotrigine on carbamazepine epoxide/carbamazepine serum concentration ratios in adult patients with epilepsy. *Epilepsy Res* 1997;28:207–211.
25. Glue P, Banfield CR, Perhack JL, et al. Pharmacokinetic interactions with felbamate: in vitro-in vivo correlation. *Clin Pharmacokinet* 1997;33:214–224.
26. Grasela TH, Fiedler-Kelly J, Cox E, et al. Population pharmacokinetics of lamotrigine adjunctive therapy in adults with epilepsy. *J Clin Pharmacol* 1999;39:373–384.
27. Graves NM, Ritter FJ, Wagner ML, et al. Effect of lamotrigine

on carbamazepine epoxide concentrations. *Epilepsia* 1991;32 [Suppl 3]:13.

28. Holdich T, Whiteman P, Orme M, et al. Effect of lamotrigine on the pharmacology of the combined oral contraceptive pill. *Epilepsia* 1991;32[Suppl 1]:96.

29. Hussein Z, Posner J. Population pharmacokinetics of lamotrigine monotherapy in patients with epilepsy: retrospective analysis of routine monitoring data. *Br J Clin Pharmacol* 1997;43: 457–465.

30. Jawad S, Richens A, Goodwin G, et al. Controlled trial of lamotrigine (Lamictal) for refractory partial seizures. *Epilepsia* 1989; 30:356–363.

31. Kanner AM, Frey M. Adding valproate to lamotrigine: a study of their pharmacokinetic interaction. *Neurology* 2000:55:588–591.

32. Kaufman KR, Gerner R. Lamotrigine toxicity secondary to sertraline. *Seizure* 1998;7:163–165.

33. Matsuo F. Lamotrigine. *Epilepsia* 1999;40[Suppl 5]:S30–S36.

34. May TW, Rambeck B, Jurgens U. Influence of oxcarbazepine and methsuximide on lamotrigine concentrations in epileptic patients with and without valproic acid comedication: results of a retrospective study. *Ther Drug Monit* 1999;21:175–181.

35. May TW, Rambeck B, Jurgens U. Serum concentrations of lamotrigine in epileptic patients: the influence of dose and comedication. *Ther Drug Monit* 1996;18:523–531.

36. Miller AA, Sawyer DA, Roth B, et al. Lamotrigine. In: Meldrum BS, Porter RJ, eds. *New anticonvulsant drugs*. London: John Libbey, 1986.

37. Pisani F, Oteri G, Russo MF, et al. The efficacy of valproate-lamotrigine comedication in refractory complex partial seizures: evidence for a pharmacodynamic interaction. *Epilepsia* 1999;40: 1141–1146.

38. Pisani F, Xiao B, Fazio A, et al. Single dose pharmacokinetics of carbamazepine-10,11-epoxide in patients with lamotrigine monotherapy. *Epilepsy Res* 1994;19:245–248.

39. Posner J, Webster H, Yuen AWC. Investigation of the ability of lamotrigine, a novel antiepileptic drug, to induce mixed function oxygenase enzymes. *Br J Clin Pharmacol* 1991;32:658P.

40. Potter JM, Donnelly A. Carbamazepine-10,11-epoxide in therapeutic drug monitoring. *Ther Drug Monit* 1998;20: 652–657.

41. Ramsey RE, Pellock JM, Garnett WR, et al. Pharmacokinetics and safety of lamotrigine (Lamictal) in patients with epilepsy. *Epilepsy Res* 1991;10:191–200.

42. Reutens DC, Duncan JS, Patsalos PN. Disabling tremor after lamotrigine with sodium valproate. *Lancet* 342:185–186.

43. Rzany B, Correia O, Kelly JP, et al. Risk of Stevens-Johnson syndrome and toxic epidermal necrolysis during first weeks of antiepileptic therapy: a case-controlled study: Study Group of the International Case Control Study on Severe Cutaneous Adverse Reactions. *Lancet* 53:2190–2194.

44. Schapel GJ, Dollman W, Beran RG, et al. No effect of lamotrigine on carbamazepine and carbamazepine epoxide concentration. *Epilepsia* 1991;32[Suppl 1]:58.

45. Schapel GJ, Beran RG, Vajda FJE, et al. Double blind, placebo controlled, crossover study of lamotrigine in treatment resistant partial seizures. *J Neurol Neurosurg Psychiatry* 1992;56:448–453.

46. Sterker M, Berrouschot J, Schneider D. Fatal course of toxic epidermal necrolysis under treatment with lamotrigine. *Int J Clin Pharmacol* 1995;33:595–597.

47. Stolarek I, Blacklaw J, Thompson GG, et al. Vigabatrin and lamotrigine: synergism in refractory epilepsy? *Epilepsia* 1993;34 [Suppl 2]:108–109.

48. Warner T, Patsalos PN, Prevett M, et al. Lamotrigine-induced carbamazepine toxicity: an interaction with carbamazepine-10,11-epoxide. *Epilepsy Res* 1992;11:147–150.

49. Wolf P. Lamotrigine: preliminary clinical observations on pharmacokinetics and interactions with traditional antiepileptic drugs. *J Epilepsy* 1992;5:73–79.

50. Wooton R, Soul-Lawton J, Rolan PE, et al. Comparison of the pharmacokinetics of lamotrigine in patients with chronic renal failure and healthy volunteers. *Br J Clin Pharmacol* 1997;43:23–27.

51. Yau MK, Wargin WA, Wolf KB, et al. Effect of valproate on the pharmacokinetics of lamotrigine at steady state. *Epilepsia* 1992; 33[Suppl 3]:82.

52. Yuen AWC. Safety issues. In: Richens A, ed. *Clinical update on lamotrigine: a novel antiepileptic agent*. Tunbridge Wells, UK: Wells Medical, 1992:69–75.

53. Yuen AW, Land G, Weatherley BC, et al. Sodium valproate acutely inhibits lamotrigine metabolism. *Br J Clin Pharmacol* 1992;33:511–513.

Antiepileptic Drugs, 5ᵗʰ Edition. Edited by R.H. Levy, R.H. Mattson, B.S. Meldrum, and E. Perucca. Lippincott Williams & Wilkins, Philadelphia © 2002.

LAMOTRIGINE

CLINICAL EFFICACY AND USE IN EPILEPSY

LINDA J. STEPHEN
MARTIN J. BRODIE

In the 1960s, some antiepileptic drugs were observed to give rise to abnormalities in folate metabolism, and later folate itself was shown to be proconvulsant in rodents. Around that time, Reynolds and colleagues proposed that antifolate drugs would have anticonvulsant properties (1). Lamotrigine, a phenyltriazine compound among a group having antifolate properties, was born out of this suggestion. Lamotrigine is now licensed worldwide for use as monotherapy in adults and as add-on treatment in adults and children for partial and generalized tonic-clonic seizures and for seizures associated with Lennox-Gastaut syndrome.

CLINICAL EFFICACY

Evidence from Randomized, Controlled Clinical Trials

Partial-Onset Seizures

Eleven placebo-controlled, double-blind, crossover, and parallel-group trials (Table 37.1) involving 1,052 patients have confirmed the efficacy of lamotrigine for partial seizures with or without secondary generalization (2–12).

In the preliminary report by Binnie and colleagues (2), 10 patients with treatment-resistant partial seizures were recruited and all completed the study. There was a significant decrease in seizure counts with lamotrigine compared with placebo. Six noted a decrease in seizure frequency of at least 50% on lamotrigine, with one patient remaining seizure free throughout the 7-day treatment period.

Linda J. Stephen, MBChB, MRCGP: Honorary Clinical Teacher, Department of Medicine and Therapeutics, University of Glasgow; and Deputy Director, Epilepsy Unit, Western Infirmary, Glasgow, Scotland, United Kingdom

Martin J. Brodie, MD: Professor of Medicine and Clinical Pharmacology, University Department of Medicine and Therapeutics, Glasgow, Scotland, United Kingdom

Jawad and colleagues (3) maintained trough levels of lamotrigine between 1.5 and 2 mg/L. They found a significant reduction in seizure days and number of seizures among their 21 patients over 12 weeks of therapy. Two-thirds of patients had their total seizure count more than halved. Seventy-five percent of patients with partial seizures responded to lamotrigine, compared with 44% with secondary generalization.

In Binnie and colleagues' later study (4), 30 patients were given lamotrigine as add-on therapy. In seven patients, the lamotrigine dosage was reduced, mostly because of headache and dizziness. Twelve patients had their total seizure count reduced by more than 25% with lamotrigine, compared with only four taking placebo. Twenty of the 22 patients with partial seizures noted an improvement in seizure numbers. This exceeded 50% in just two.

The results from Sander and colleagues' study (5) were the least conclusive. Eighteen of 21 patients completed the trial. There was an overall reduction in seizure numbers, which was greater for secondary generalized events in the later stages of the lamotrigine treatment period. Partial seizures appeared unaffected. Tolerability was not a problem, with similar numbers of adverse events reported on lamotrigine and placebo. Modest efficacy, however, was most likely due to a combination of low-dose lamotrigine and severity of the epilepsy.

Loiseau and coworkers (6) found that over an 8-week period, 15 of 23 patients reported a reduction in total seizures while taking lamotrigine compared with placebo. Fourteen had the frequency of their partial seizures reduced, eight by more than 50%.

Over a 6-month treatment period, Matsuo and colleagues (7) studied 216 patients. Equal numbers were randomized to 300 or 500 mg/day of lamotrigine or placebo. Efficacy was greatest in the 500-mg arm, with a reduction in median seizure frequency of 36%. Patients taking placebo had a reduction of 8%, and those on 300 mg, 20%. One-third of patients taking 500 mg/day experienced a

TABLE 37.1. PLACEBO-CONTROLLED EFFICACY TRIALS WITH ADJUNCTIVE LAMOTRIGINE

Reference	Patients Recruited	Patients Completed	Duration of Treatment (wk)	Dose range (mg/day)	Decrease in Total Seizure Frequency (%)	Patients with >50% Decrease in Total Seizures	Patients with >50% Decrease in Generalized Seizures	Patients with >50% Decrease in Other Seizure Types
Binnie et al., 1987	10[a]	10	1	100–300	NA	60	5/5 (100%)	5/8 (62.5%)[c]
Jawad et al., 1989	24[a]	21	12	75–400	59 (median)	66	7/15 (47%)	12/17 (71%)[c]
Binnie et al., 1989	34[a]	30	12	50–150 (VPA) 50–400 (non-VPA)	17 (median)	7	2/19 (9%)	2/20 (10%)[c]
Sander et al., 1990	21[a]	18	12	100–300	18 (mean)	11	NA	NA
Loiseau et al., 1990	25[a]	23	8	75–300	23 (median)	30	NA	8/23 (35%)[c]
Matsuo et al., 1993	216[b]	191	24	300 500	20 (median) 36 (median)	20 34	NA NA	NA NA
Schapel et al., 1993	41[a]	41	12	150 (VPA) 300 (non-VPA)	24 (median)	22	9/32 (28%)	8/41 (20%)[c]
Smith et al., 1993	81[a]	62	18	100–400	30 (mean)	18	10/36 (28%)	12/62 (19%)[c]
Messenheimer et al., 1994	98[a]	88	14	100–400	25 (median)	20	NA	NA
Schachter et al., 1995	446[b]	374	24	100–500	NA	NA	NA	NA
Boas et al., 1996	56[a]	38	12	75–400	30 (mean)	24	12/19 (63%)	10/46 (22%)[c]
Beran et al., 1998	26[a]	22	8	75 (VPA) 150 (non-VPA)	NA	NA	7/14 (50%)	5/15 (33%)[d]

NA, data not available; VPA, valproic acid.
[a]Crossover trials.
[b]Parallel groups.
[c]Partial seizures.
[d]Absence seizures.

≥50% reduction in seizure number, and one-fourth of these patients had a similar reduction in seizure days. Frequency of partial seizures was significantly reduced compared with baseline in patients taking 500 mg lamotrigine. Thirteen patients on active treatment were withdrawn as a result of adverse events, most of whom were in the 500-mg arm.

Schapel and colleagues (8) undertook 12 weeks of treatment with lamotrigine and matched placebo in 41 patients, all of whom completed the study. Those on enzyme-inducing antiepileptic drugs were titrated to 300 mg lamotrigine daily; those on sodium valproate and an enzyme inducer received 150 mg/day. Twenty-six patients reported a decrease in total seizure numbers, by more than half in nine (22%). Overall, 20% and 47% of patients with partial and secondary generalized seizures had these reduced by more than 50% with lamotrigine, compared with 16% on placebo. Although the decrease in secondary generalized seizures did not reach statistical significance, it became more marked when patients with less than four seizures a month were excluded.

Smith and coworkers (9) reported 18-week lamotrigine and placebo treatment periods. Of 81 patients recruited, 62 completed the trial. Lamotrigine dosages were relatively high compared with other crossover studies—200 mg/day for patients on non–enzyme-inducing drugs and 400 mg/day for those taking enzyme-inducing antiepileptic drugs. Eleven patients withdrew because of adverse events, mostly headache, diplopia, and dizziness. Eighteen of the completing patients had a modest response, reporting a reduction in total seizures of 25% to 49% compared with placebo. A further 11 were regarded as responders (reduction >50%). On analysis by seizure type, 12 of 62 patients experienced a significant reduction in partial seizures, with 10 of 36 demonstrating a similar response for secondary generalized seizure frequency. Seizure severity was ameliorated by lamotrigine. For the first time, quality-of-life factors were monitored in an antiepileptic drug study. Although most of the tests revealed no difference between lamotrigine and placebo, there were significant improvements in mastery (perceived internal control) and happiness scores. Forty-two of the completing patients chose to remain on lamotrigine, some despite little change in seizure pattern.

Messenheimer and colleagues (10) undertook a study comparing 14 weeks of lamotrigine treatment with placebo. A total of 98 patients, 75% of whom were taking carbamazepine, entered the trial. Lamotrigine dosage was titrated to a maximum of 400 mg/day. Efficacy data were evaluated in 88 patients, 44% of whom had a >25% decrease and 20% of whom had a ≥50% decrease in seizure frequency on lamotrigine compared with placebo. The number of seizure days was reduced by 18% during the active treatment period.

Schachter and colleagues (11) conducted the largest American parallel group study in 446 patients, 112 of whom received placebo. The remaining 334 took up to 500 mg/day of lamotrigine for 6 months. Efficacy data were scanty, although investigators rated 65% of patients who received lamotrigine "improved" compared with 35% of those on placebo. The withdrawal rate was 8% for both groups because of side effects.

Boas and colleagues (12) assessed the antiepileptic effect of lamotrigine in 56 patients over a 12-week period. Those not receiving sodium valproate were titrated to 400 mg lamotrigine daily and those taking valproate to 200 mg/day. Thirty-eight patients completed the study. Significant reductions in mean seizure count (30.3%) and in mean seizure days (27.5%) occurred with lamotrigine. Two patients withdrew from the active treatment arm because of lack of efficacy, and six because of adverse effects.

Generalized Seizures

Beran and colleagues (13) performed the first double-blind, placebo-controlled, crossover study of adjunctive lamotrigine in 26 patients with generalized epilepsies (Table 37.1). Twenty-one had idiopathic generalized epilepsy, two had symptomatic epilepsy, and three patients were unclassifiable. Twenty-two patients were included in the efficacy analysis, with tonic-clonic and absence seizure rates being at least halved in 50% and 30%, respectively, compared with placebo. Two patients had myoclonic seizures, one of whom became worse and the other experiencing no change.

Monotherapy Studies

Four randomized, comparative trials have supported the efficacy of lamotrigine as monotherapy for partial-onset and generalized tonic-clonic seizures in adults (14–16) and in elderly patients (17) with newly diagnosed epilepsy (Table 37.2).

Brodie and colleagues (14) randomized 260 patients with partial-onset or primary generalized tonic-clonic seizures to receive lamotrigine or carbamazepine during 48 weeks of treatment in a double-blind study. Baseline seizure counts were similar for both treatment arms. No significant difference was noted for seizure freedom at 6 weeks or in time to first seizure, but patients taking lamotrigine were significantly more likely to remain on antiepileptic medication than their carbamazepine-treated counterparts. More patients on carbamazepine withdrew because of rash (13% carbamazepine; 9% lamotrigine) and other side effects. Somnolence was significantly more common in carbamazepine-treated patients.

Ruenanen and coworkers (15) studied the efficacy of lamotrigine and carbamazepine in a randomized open-label trial. In equal numbers, 343 patients were randomized to receive lamotrigine 100 mg/day, lamotrigine 200 mg/day, or carbamazepine 600 mg/day. After 30 weeks of treatment, data from the 223 completers were analyzed. A higher pro-

TABLE 37.2. RANDOMIZED COMPARATIVE MONOTHERAPY TRIALS OF LAMOTRIGINE IN PATIENTS WITH NEWLY DIAGNOSED PARTIAL-ONSET AND GENERALIZED TONIC-CLONIC SEIZURES

Reference	Comparative Antiepileptic Drug	Dose Range (mg/day)	Patients Recruited	Patients Completed	Duration of Treatment (wk)	Seizure Freedom Comparison at 6 Wk	Time to First Seizure	Time to Withdrawal
Brodie et al., 1995	CBZ	LTG 100–300 CBZ 300–1400	260[a] 131 LTG 129 CBZ	151 85 (65%) LTG 66 (51%) CBZ	48	No significant difference	No significant difference	Significantly longer for LTG patients
Reunanen et al., 1996	CBZ	LTG 100 LTG 200 CBZ 600	343[b] 115 LTG 100 mg 111 LTG 200 mg 117 CBZ	223 71 (61.7%) LTG 100 mg 76 (68.5%) LTG 200 mg 76 (64.7%) CBZ	30	No significant difference	No significant difference	No significant difference
Steiner et al., 1999	PHT	LTG NA-400 PHT NA-600	181[a] 86 LTG 95 PHT	174 81 (94%) LTG 93 (98%) PHT	48	No significant difference	Cumulative trend favored LTG	PHT favored during titration period
Brodie et al., 1999	CBZ[c]	LTG 75–300 CBZ 200–800	150[a] 102 LTG 48 CBZ	92 72 (71%) LTG 20 (42%) CBZ	24	No significant difference	NA	Significantly longer for LTG patients (p < .001)

CBZ, carbamazepine; LTG, lamotrigine; NA, data not available; PHT, phenytoin.
[a]Double-blind trial.
[b]Open-label trial.
[c]Elderly patients.

portion of patients taking 200 mg/day of lamotrigine (60.4%) remained seizure free for the last 24 weeks compared with those taking 100 mg/day (51.3%) and carbamazepine (54.7%). There were no differences among the three study arms in the number of patients seizure free at 6 weeks, in time to first seizure, or in time to treatment withdrawal.

Steiner and coworkers (16) compared lamotrigine and phenytoin monotherapy in 181 patients. The efficacy analysis included 81 patients taking lamotrigine and 93 on phenytoin. There was no significant difference during the last 24 and 40 weeks of treatment in the percentage of patients remaining on treatment and seizure free, the numbers of seizures, and the changes in seizure frequency from baseline. Time to first seizure analysis favored lamotrigine for all seizure types considered together. Time to study discontinuation showed a trend favoring phenytoin during the titration period, but not subsequently. A total of 31 patients were discontinued because of adverse events, 13 (15%) with lamotrigine and 18 (19%) with phenytoin.

To compare efficacy of lamotrigine and carbamazepine in elderly patients, Brodie and associates (17) randomized 150 patients aged 65 years and older to receive lamotrigine or carbamazepine in a 2:1 ratio. The study was completed by 71% of lamotrigine-treated patients and 42% of those taking carbamazepine. There was no statistical difference in seizure freedom rates at 6 weeks, but analysis excluded the 58% of patients on carbamazepine who withdrew prematurely. A higher percentage of patients on lamotrigine remained seizure free for the last 4 months because of the greater dropout rate in the carbamazepine arm (lamotrigine 39%, carbamazepine 21%). Of those discontinuing, 42% on carbamazepine and 18% taking lamotrigine did so because of adverse events. Significantly fewer patients on lamotrigine (3%) withdrew because of rash compared with those taking carbamazepine (19%). Significantly more patients taking carbamazepine reported somnolence.

A double-blind, double-dummy, active-control study was undertaken by Gilliam and colleagues (18) to evaluate the efficacy and safety of lamotrigine as monotherapy. In equal numbers, 156 patients taking carbamazepine or phenytoin were randomly assigned to receive adjunctive lamotrigine or sodium valproate during 20 weeks' treatment. Lamotrigine was titrated to 500 mg/day or the maximally tolerated dosage over 3 weeks. Sodium valproate was titrated over 8 days to 1,000 mg/day or the maximally tolerated dosage. Initial antiepileptic medications were then withdrawn. Significantly more patients taking lamotrigine (56%) completed the study compared with those on valproate (20%). The time to escape was statistically longer in lamotrigine-treated patients. The lamotrigine daily dosage of 500 mg was achieved in 95% of patients treated for at least 5 weeks.

To compare adjunctive treatment and withdrawal to monotherapy with lamotrigine or carbamazepine, Fakhoury

and associates (19) randomized 143 patients with uncontrolled epilepsy to receive the drugs in a 2:1 ratio as add on therapy. Each drug was added over 12 weeks, after which existing therapy was withdrawn. Patients taking monotherapy remained on lamotrigine for longer, with more becoming seizure free or having a reduction in seizure frequency. Fewer lamotrigine-treated patients withdrew because of drug-related adverse events.

Gazda and colleagues (20) compared adjunctive treatment and monotherapy with lamotrigine and sodium valproate in 154 patients with uncontrolled epilepsy. Patients were randomized in a 2:1 ratio to receive lamotrigine or valproate. The drugs were added to current therapy for 12 weeks, after which existing treatment was withdrawn and patients entered an 8-week monotherapy phase. After conversion to monotherapy, seizure freedom and reduction rates were greater for lamotrigine than for valproate. More patients on lamotrigine were successfully withdrawn to monotherapy.

Martinez and coworkers (21) compared lamotrigine with conventional antiepileptic monotherapies in 115 patients who had failed on carbamazepine, phenytoin, or sodium valproate. Fifty-seven patients were randomized to be converted from their original antiepileptic drugs to lamotrigine and 58 were randomized to receive carbamazepine, phenytoin, or sodium valproate, according to the physician's choice. More patients on lamotrigine (65%) completed the study than those taking conventional antiepileptic drugs (57%), with the former having improvements in seizure frequency, seizure intensity, intellectual functioning, adverse events, overall status, and global self-assessment. The extent of reduction in seizure frequency was comparable in both groups.

Children: Partial-Onset Seizures

Two placebo-controlled studies of lamotrigine in children with partial-onset seizures have been conducted (22,23).

Schlumberger and colleagues (22) evaluated the efficacy of adjunctive lamotrigine in 120 children, 63% of whom had learning disabilities, over 3 months to 3 years. Sixty patients participated in a single-blind study, receiving placebo for 1 month before switching to lamotrigine in a dose-ranging phase. Patients were started on 0.5, 1, or 2 mg/kg/day according to whether they were taking enzyme-inhibiting, balanced, or enzyme-inducing comedication, respectively. The dosage was doubled during the second month, tripled during the third, and increased thereafter if required. Of the other 60 children in whom efficacy was evaluated, 23 participated in a pharmacokinetic study and 37 received lamotrigine on a compassionate basis with dosing schedules based on results from the single-blind study. No difference was seen between baseline and placebo in the single-blind study. Fourteen patients, 13 with generalized epilepsy, became seizure free for more than 6 months. Treatment could be reduced to monotherapy in 12 patients, 11 of whom had generalized epilepsy. Ten remained seizure free. The best results were obtained for the nine patients with absence epilepsy, of whom three became seizure free, four had a >50% improvement, and none worsened. Of the 10 patients with the Lennox Gastaut syndrome, 3 became seizure free, 3 had a >50% improvement, and none worsened.

Duchowny and colleagues (23) examined the efficacy and safety of adjunctive lamotrigine in 201 children and adolescents with partial-onset seizures during a placebo-controlled, parallel-group trial. After a 6-week titration period, patients received an unchanged dosage of lamotrigine or placebo for 12 weeks. A total of 167 patients completed the study, 84 on lamotrigine and 83 on placebo. Patients taking lamotrigine had a significant reduction in partial and secondary generalized seizure numbers from baseline (44%) compared with those on placebo (13%). Significantly more patients with partial and secondary generalized seizures taking lamotrigine had at least a 50% reduction in seizure frequency and seizure-free days compared with placebo. Adverse events were no different from those reported in adults.

Children: Generalized Seizures

Eriksson and coworkers (24) undertook a randomized, double-blind, crossover study of adjunctive lamotrigine in 30 children and adolescents with refractory generalized epilepsy. Twenty had the Lennox-Gastaut syndrome. After an 8-week baseline phase, lamotrigine was added to current antiepileptic drugs during a 2- to 12-month open-label phase. At the end of this time, children who had a ≥50% reduction in seizure frequency, seizure severity or both, or definite improvements in behavior, motor skills, or both were classified as responders. These children entered two 12-week double-blind phases during which their previous dosage of lamotrigine or placebo was administered in random order. The open phase was completed by 27 patients, all of whom had a significantly lower monthly seizure rate compared with baseline. Atypical absences and myoclonic events were excluded from analysis because of difficulty in counting them. Lamotrigine was found to be significantly more effective than placebo. A total of 17 children were classified as responders, with 7 having a ≥50% reduction in seizure frequency and 2 having a ≥75% reduction. Fifteen children completed the double-blind phase, showing a ≥50% reduction in seizure frequency on lamotrigine. One child became seizure-free and one had a ≥75% reduction in seizures. Seven of the 20 patients with the Lennox-Gastaut syndrome had a >50% reduction in seizure frequency, with 2 becoming seizure free and 3 having a >75% decrease in seizures. Eight (47%) of the 17 children with tonic-clonic seizures, 6 (55%) of 11 with atonic seizures, and 13 (62%) of 21 with tonic seizures had a >50% reduction in seizure frequency.

Children: Monotherapy Studies

To evaluate whether lamotrigine monotherapy was efficacious and safe for children with typical absence epilepsy, Frank and colleagues (25) undertook a study in 45 newly diagnosed children using an enrichment design. Patients received escalating doses of open-label medication for ≥5 weeks, with the 29 who became seizure free subsequently being randomized in a double-blind phase to receive lamotrigine or placebo for ≥10 weeks. This phase was completed by 28 patients, 14 each taking lamotrigine and placebo. During the double-blind phase, significantly more patients on lamotrigine (64%) became seizure free compared with those taking placebo (21%). Overall, 30 (71%) of the 42 patients who completed the dose escalation phase became seizure free at a median lamotrigine dosage of 5 mg/kg/day (range, 2 to 15 mg/kg/day). Twenty-two patients who continued to seize on 7 mg/kg/day had their dosage increased to a maximal dosage of 15 mg/kg/day and, of these, 18 (82%) became seizure free.

Lennox-Gastaut Syndrome

Motte and colleagues (26) undertook a double-blind study of adjunctive lamotrigine in 169 children and adults with the Lennox-Gastaut syndrome. During a 4-week baseline period, all patients received placebo together with their standard antiepileptic drug regimens. In total, 169 eligible patients entered a 16-week treatment period, receiving either active drug or placebo. The study was completed by 148 patients. The median reduction in seizure count from baseline for those taking lamotrigine (34%) was significantly greater than for those taking placebo (9%). Statistically more lamotrigine-treated patients had a reduction of at least 50% in the frequency of all types of major seizures, drop attacks, and tonic-clonic seizures. No significant difference was found for atypical absences. Three patients taking lamotrigine withdrew because of adverse events, one because of worsening seizures and two, who also were taking sodium valproate, because of rash.

Patients with Learning Disabilities

An interim analysis from Veendrick-Meekes and colleagues (27) reports on their placebo-controlled trial of adjunctive lamotrigine in 48 adults with learning disabilities. Seizure counts more than halved in 30 (37%) of the patients on lamotrigine compared with 18 (22%) of those taking placebo. Seizure freedom occurred in 11% of lamotrigine patients, but in none on placebo. Investigator global evaluation showed that 52% of patients on lamotrigine improved, 41% had no change, and 7% deteriorated, compared with those on placebo, of whom 6% improved, 88% had no change, and 6% deteriorated. Using the Hague Seizure Severity Scale, carers reported a significant decrease in seizure severity in lamotrigine-treated patients compared with those taking placebo.

Evidence from Other Studies

Partial-Onset and Generalized Seizures

A number of open-label studies with lamotrigine in patients with a variety of seizure types have played a valuable role in exploring dose requirements and identifying common side effects.

Jawad and coworkers (28) gave 23 patients adjunctive lamotrigine for 7 days. Of the 20 who completed the study, 18 took 2 other drugs, the remainder receiving 3. Eight patients (40%) had a reduction in seizure frequency exceeding 50%, whereas a similar number noted a less striking improvement.

Sander and colleagues' open-label study (29) also supported efficacy for adjunctive lamotrigine. A total of 104 patients completed 12 months of treatment with lamotrigine, with 25% experiencing a reduction in seizure count by more than half. The dropout rate was 15%. Six to 8 years later, these patients were followed up (30). It was reported that 21% had a >50% reduction in seizure frequency, with only one being seizure free.

Timmings and Richens (31) reviewed records from 82 patients started on lamotrigine. The drug was withdrawn in 22 because of lack of efficacy or adverse events. Of the remaining patients, 19 had primary generalized epilepsy, 29 had partial-onset seizures, and 12 had mixed or unclassifiable seizure types. Seizure frequency more than halved in 79% of patients with primary generalized epilepsy and in 48% of those with partial-onset seizures. Six patients became seizure free. Concomitant antiepileptic drugs could be successfully withdrawn in 33%.

Stewart and associates (32) reported results in 72 patients with refractory epilepsy, 63 with partial-onset, 4 with primary generalized, and 5 with unclassifiable seizures. The addition of lamotrigine resulted in 30% of those with partial-onset seizures having a ≥50% improvement in seizure control, with one patient becoming seizure free. Two patients with primary generalized seizures had their seizures abolished and two had a >75% improvement in control.

Cocito and colleagues (33) gave add-on lamotrigine to 13 patients with refractory partial-onset seizures and to 3 with uncontrolled primary generalized epilepsy. Ten patients completed 1 year of treatment, with six having their seizure frequency more than halved compared with baseline.

Schapel and Chadwick (34) undertook a retrospective analysis comparing the efficacy and tolerability of adjunctive lamotrigine and vigabatrin in 333 patients with refractory epilepsy. One hundred sixteen patients were exposed to lamotrigine only, 108 to vigabatrin only, and 109 to both drugs, together or in combination. Lamotrigine was con-

tinued in preference to vigabatrin by 36 patients, and vigabatrin was continued in preference to lamotrigine by 17 patients. Both drugs were continued in combination by 31 patients. After 40 months, the probability of patients remaining on lamotrigine was 57%, and on vigabatrin, 43%. With lamotrigine, 10% of patients became seizure free, and 45% had a 50% improvement in seizure frequency.

Buchanan (35) followed up 200 patients of all ages with different seizure types who had taken lamotrigine for at least 6 months. Introduction of the drug resulted in seizure freedom for 70 (35%) patients, with 54% of those with primary generalized and 26% of those with partial-onset seizures becoming seizure free. Of the 67 patients with cerebral palsy or brain injury, 67% were reported to have a marked improvement in alertness, cognition, and quality of life. Eleven (73%) patients with juvenile myoclonic epilepsy were seizure free, although 13 patients switched to lamotrigine because of side effects rather than poor control. Of patients with absences or tonic-clonic seizures, 18 (69%) became fully controlled. One (14%) patient with tonic seizures and three (21%) with the Lennox-Gastaut syndrome became seizure free.

Kilpatrick and colleagues (36) undertook a prospective study of adjunctive lamotrigine in 27 patients with newly diagnosed and 42 patients with refractory epilepsy. Overall, 26 patients had idiopathic generalized and 43 had partial-onset seizures. The drug was started in a dosage of 25 or 50 mg/day with an increase in 50-mg monthly increments until seizure freedom or unacceptable side effects occurred. The study was completed by 50 patients, 32 of whom became seizure free on a median lamotrigine dose of 200 mg (range, 50 to 850 mg). No useful concentration–toxicity effect relationship was demonstrated.

Gericke and coworkers (37) examined the efficacy of lamotrigine as add-on therapy or monotherapy in 46 patients with idiopathic generalized epilepsy. Lamotrigine was started because of poor seizure control, and concomitant antiepileptic drugs were withdrawn if patients subsequently developed side effects. After 5 months' follow-up, 32 (70%) patients became seizure free—9 of 12 (75%) with childhood absence epilepsy, 10 of 12 (83%) with juvenile absence epilepsy, 7 (50%) with juvenile myoclonic epilepsy, 3 (60%) as with generalized tonic-clonic seizures on awakening, and 3 (100%) with photosensitive epilepsy. An improvement of >50% was seen in one-fourth. Patients who were not controlled had either absences with a mild atonic component, absences with eyelid myoclonia, a long-standing history of epilepsy, or poor compliance. In seven patients with juvenile myoclonic epilepsy, tonic-clonic and absence seizures were abolished, but myoclonic seizures persisted. Eleven of the 16 patients on lamotrigine monotherapy became seizure free, 3 with childhood absence epilepsy, 4 with juvenile absence epilepsy, 2 with juvenile myoclonic epilepsy, and 2 with pure photosensitive epilepsy.

Collins and coworkers (38) conducted a retrospective review of 61 patients with uncontrolled partial-onset seizures, comparing add-on treatment with lamotrigine in 37, gabapentin in 36, topiramate in 28, and vigabatrin in 26. The median time to 50% dropout was >43 months for lamotrigine, compared with 13, 28, and 26 months for gabapentin, topiramate, and vigabatrin, respectively. Sixty percent of patients taking lamotrigine, 19% of those on gabapentin, 50% of those on topiramate, and 27% of those on vigabatrin continued on treatment.

Faught (39) reported that four adult patients with startle-induced seizures who had been resistant to almost every other antiepileptic drug improved with lamotrigine.

Status Epilepticus

A report of its intravenous use in status epilepticus suggests that lamotrigine also possesses acute anticonvulsant properties (40). This also may be the case in children. Besag (41) studied the use of lamotrigine in 12 children with intermittent nonconvulsive status epilepticus using an automatic spike-and-wave recording system. Half the patients had a significant reduction in seizure frequency over a 48-week period. A decrease in episode frequency of 80% or more was reported. Increased well-being was postulated to be due to a reduction in subclinical seizures.

Children: Partial-Onset Seizures

A number of open-label trials of lamotrigine in children have been performed. Several studies have included children with different seizure types and those with and without learning disabilities.

Battino and coworkers (42) administered adjunctive lamotrigine over a 12-month period to 14 children with refractory epilepsy, half of whom had structural brain lesions. Of the seven patients who completed the study, two became seizure free, four had their seizure frequency more than halved, and one had no change.

Uvebrant and Bauzienè (43) treated 50 children and adolescents with adjunctive lamotrigine. Several had multiple seizure types, with 40 (36%) having partial-onset seizures and 71 (64%) having generalized epilepsy. Eight children had infantile spasms, eight had the Lennox-Gastaut syndrome, four had myoclonic astatic epilepsy, three had electrical status epilepticus during slow sleep (ESES), two had gelastic epilepsy with hypothalamic hamartoma, and two had absence seizures. Children were followed up for 4 to 35 months (mean 14 months), after which 30 continued on lamotrigine. Five (11%) of these became seizure free and 16 (36%) had more than a 30% improvement in their seizure frequency. The situation did not improve in 24 (53%). Myoclonic, tonic, and tonic-clonic seizures were the most resistant. Seizure frequency in 60% of the children with the Lennox-Gastaut syndrome improved by more than

half. One of the two children with gelastic epilepsy improved, as did one with myoclonic astatic epilepsy. None of those with ESES improved. Fifty-three percent of parents reported an improvement in the mental state of their child.

Besag and coworkers (44) analyzed pooled data from five open add-on studies of adjunctive lamotrigine in 285 children with refractory epilepsy. Most had two or more seizure types. Assessments were made at the end of four 12-week treatment periods. Seizure frequency was reduced by 50% or more in one-third of patients. Lamotrigine was effective in partial, generalized tonic-clonic, myoclonic, and atonic seizures, but was particularly so for typical and atypical absences.

After this study, Besag and colleagues (45) evaluated the safety, tolerability, and efficacy of lamotrigine at 2 or 3 years in 155 children and adolescents with epilepsy who had already completed a 12-month add-on trial. Patients entered the study on their optimal dose of lamotrigine from the previous trial. Twenty-two were on monotherapy. Change in seizure control was evaluated using a numerical scale of 1 (marked deterioration) to 7 (marked improvement). The study was completed by 109 patients. The overall percentage with improved or unchanged seizure control was maintained throughout the trial, ranging from 73% to 80% and 11% to 16%, respectively. Thirteen of the 22 patients on monotherapy remained on lamotrigine.

Herranz and coworkers (46) reported on efficacy and tolerability of adjunctive lamotrigine over a period of 144 weeks in 13 children with refractory epilepsy. Seven patients continued on lamotrigine, two becoming seizure free and four having a >50% reduction in seizure frequency.

Buoni and colleagues (47) studied the response to lamotrigine in 63 children with drug-resistant epilepsies over 1 to 3 years. Sixteen (25%) patients, six with typical absence seizures, four with myoclonic astatic seizures, three with the Lennox-Gastaut syndrome, and three with complex partial seizures, became seizure free. A significant long-standing response to lamotrigine treatment occurred in six (10%) children. Eleven (17.4%) patients showed an initial unsustained improvement. No response occurred in 30 (47.6%) patients.

Three studies compared outcomes in children taking adjunctive lamotrigine and vigabatrin (48–50).

Schapel and colleagues (48) surveyed 109 children with poorly controlled epilepsy treated with add-on lamotrigine or vigabatrin. Localization-related epilepsy was present in 65%, with the remainder having generalized seizures. There were 79 patient exposed to lamotrigine and 86 with vigabatrin. Forty-two patients received lamotrigine, 52 received vigabatrin, and 20 were treated with both drugs simultaneously. Fifteen patients were treated with both drugs serially, 12 continuing on lamotrigine and 3 continuing on vigabatrin. It was estimated from a Kaplan-Meier curve that 71% and 62% of patients would be expected to take lamotrigine or vigabatrin, respectively, after 40 months. Seizure control had improved by 50% or more in 65% of patients on lamotrigine and in 58% of patients on vigabatrin. Lamotrigine was more successful than vigabatrin for generalized seizures, with the converse found for partial seizures. The drugs appeared equally effective for the Lennox-Gastaut syndrome, but more patients with myoclonic astatic epilepsy improved with lamotrigine. All five patients with epilepsy with myoclonic absences responded to lamotrigine.

Bélanger and colleagues (49) reviewed medical records from 105 children with a variety of seizure types and syndromes who had been prescribed lamotrigine, vigabatrin, or both for at least 1 year. Fifty-eight patients had generalized epilepsy, including 23 with infantile spasms. Forty-seven patients had localization-related epilepsy. Of these, 42 had lamotrigine added to their antiepileptic drug regimen, whereas 83 received vigabatrin. Eight patients received both drugs. The authors concluded that lamotrigine was more effective for generalized epilepsies and vigabatrin was significantly more effective in partial epilepsies. Lamotrigine was statistically more efficacious in children whose electroencephalograms (EEGs) showed a primary generalized pattern compared with those with multifocal spikes or secondarily generalized activity.

Dimova and Korinthenberg (50) undertook a retrospective comparison of the efficacy and side effects of add-on lamotrigine and vigabatrin in 134 children with refractory partial-onset and primary generalized seizures. Lamotrigine was given to 57 patients. A >50% reduction in seizure frequency was observed in 33% on lamotrigine and 41% on vigabatrin for patients with partial-onset seizures, and in 34% of patients on lamotrigine and 33% of patients on vigabatrin for those with generalized seizures.

Children: Generalized Seizures

Buchanan (51) examined the use of lamotrigine in 12 girls with juvenile myoclonic epilepsy who either had side effects with or did not wish to take sodium valproate. Four were seizure free at the start of the study. Attempts to withdraw sodium valproate were made in the seven patients taking this drug. Five patients became completely controlled on lamotrigine monotherapy. Five patients remained on a combination of valproate and lamotrigine. Reduction in valproate led to breakthrough of myoclonic jerks in three.

Farrell and colleagues (52) evaluated the efficacy and adverse effects of adjunctive lamotrigine in 56 children with uncontrolled generalized epilepsies, 46 of whom had learning disabilities and 36 of whom had two or more seizure types. Patients were reviewed at three monthly intervals for 25 weeks. Six (11%) patients became seizure free and 24 (43%) had a >50% reduction in seizure frequency. Three of the 15 children with the Lennox-Gastaut syndrome became seizure free and 8 had a >50% improvement in their seizure frequency.

Buoni and colleagues (53) studied the effects of lamotrigine in 15 children with absence epilepsy. Five already were taking sodium valproate, three were taking sodium valproate and ethosuximide, and seven had untreated seizures. Patients were followed up from 1.8 to 4.3 years. Absence seizures became controlled in all patients started on lamotrigine monotherapy, although rash led to treatment withdrawal in one. Seizure control in the others was significantly more likely with lamotrigine and sodium valproate duotherapy, compared with lamotrigine monotherapy. Normalization of the surface EEG with lamotrigine occurred in 13 patients.

Infantile Seizures

Lamotrigine has demonstrated efficacy for seizures in infants.

Veggiotti and colleagues (54) studied 30 infants with refractory infantile spasms who had lamotrigine added to their antiepileptic drug regimen. After 3 months' treatment, spasms had ceased in 5 (16.6%) patients also taking sodium valproate, improved in 4 (13.3%), worsened in 2 (6.6%) and remained unchanged in 19 (63.5%). Asymmetric spasms were significantly associated with a favorable outcome.

Barr and coworkers (55) reported that a newborn infant with seizures of unknown etiology refractory to conventional antiepileptic drugs had a rapid and sustained cessation with lamotrigine 4.4 mg/kg/day. The drug was well tolerated and allowed discontinuation of phenobarbital and phenytoin, leaving the neonate on lamotrigine and vigabatrin.

Patients with Learning Disabilities

Timmings and Richens (56) reported on 11 patients with the Lennox-Gastaut syndrome who had been treated with adjunctive lamotrigine for 3 months. Ten (91%) patients had a ≥50% improvement in seizure frequency, with one becoming seizure free. The drug was well tolerated, allowing withdrawal of other antiepileptic drugs in six patients.

Buchanan (57) studied the outcomes of 6 months of add-on lamotrigine in 34 children and adults with brain injury. Overall, 35.3% of patients became seizure free and 76.6% had a >50% reduction in seizure frequency.

Donaldson and associates (58) conducted a retrospective review of adjunctive lamotrigine in 16 adults and children with the Lennox-Gastaut syndrome over 18 months. Efficacy data were derived from 15 patients, 53% of whom experienced a >50% reduction in total seizure frequency, with 20% having a >90% reduction. At the end of the study, 53% of parents reported that their child's quality of life was much or very much improved, 33% reported minimal improvement or no change, and 13% said that quality of life had worsened since lamotrigine had been initiated. Myoclonic seizures were the least responsive.

Bhaumik and coworkers (59) undertook a retrospective analysis of outcomes for adults with learning disabilities treated with lamotrigine, vigabatrin, and gabapentin. Twenty-five treatment episodes were identified for lamotrigine, with 10 patients on monotherapy. Nine (36%) patients experienced a >50% reduction in seizure frequency.

Huber and colleagues (60) studied the effect of add-on lamotrigine in 125 patients with refractory seizures and multiple additional handicaps during a mean treatment period of 21.9 months. Lamotrigine was continued by 71.4% of patients, one-third of whom had a ≥50% reduction in their seizure frequency. Responder rates were 35.6% for patients with focal epilepsies, 26.7% for patients with generalized epilepsies, and 22.4% for patients with both. Patients taking concomitant valproate (51.5%) were significantly more likely to respond than those not taking the drug (20.7%).

Coppola and Pascotto (61) studied the outcome of 7 months of adjunctive lamotrigine in 37 children and adolescents with refractory epilepsy and mental delay. Thirteen (35.1%) patients showed a >50% decrease in seizure frequency. Of the eight (21.6%) patients who became seizure free, four had typical absences, two atypical absences, and two atonic seizures. The authors commented that lamotrigine seemed to be more efficacious in patients with a shorter duration and later onset of epilepsy.

Gidal and associates (62) retrospectively analyzed the efficacy of adjunctive lamotrigine in 44 institutionalized, developmentally disabled patients with epilepsy. Twenty-four patients had generalized seizures, 15 had partial seizures, and 5 were classified as having mixed seizure disorders. A significant reduction in total and generalized seizures occurred. A decrease in seizures of >75% was seen in 14 (32%) patients.

Lamotrigine has been reported to be efficacious in Rett's syndrome (63,64). Uldall and colleagues (63) gave the drug to four girls with the syndrome who all improved with a >50% reduction in seizures. Stenbom and associates (64) also found that four girls with Rett's syndrome had improved behavior, mood, and alertness on lamotrigine.

MODE OF USE

Indications

Lamotrigine is available as adjunctive treatment for partial seizures, primary and secondary generalized seizures, and seizures associated with the Lennox-Gastaut syndrome for adults and children 2 years of age and older. The drug also is licensed as monotherapy for these indications in adults.

Dosing Recommendations

Starting Dose and Titration Rate

Recommended dosing schedules for lamotrigine are outlined in Table 37.3. Long-term studies have revealed no evidence of tolerance (65). The low starting dose and slow titration rate for adjunctive therapy depend on existing treatment, the aim of which is to reduce the likelihood of rash (66). Tablets containing 25, 50, 100, and 200 mg lamotrigine are available. Dispersible chewable tablets containing 5, 25, and 100 mg provide an alternative preparation for children and for patients who have difficulty swallowing. These also can be dispersed in water. Lamotrigine usually is prescribed twice daily, but a single daily dose can be used in patients taking the drug with sodium valproate or as monotherapy.

Initial Target and Optimal Range of Maintenance Dosages

Seizures are controlled in most patients receiving monotherapy at dosages of 100 to 300 mg/day, although some need higher amounts. Higher dosages of 400 to 800 mg/day may be required in refractory epilepsy when lamotrigine is used with an enzyme-inducing antiepileptic drug. Substantially lower dosages of 50 to 200 mg/day are advised when lamotrigine is combined with sodium valproate. Withdrawal of enzyme-inducing antiepileptic drugs causes a rise in circulating concentrations of lamotrigine, whereas discontinuing sodium valproate produces a fall.

TABLE 37.3. LAMOTRIGINE DOSAGE SCHEDULES

Antiepileptic Drug Group	Weeks 1–2	Weeks 3–4	Increase Per 1–2 Weeks	Maintenance
Adult on monotherapy	25 mg/day	50 mg/day	50–100 mg/day	100–200 mg/day[a]
Adult on enzyme-inducer(s)	50 mg/day	100 mg/day	100 mg/day	300–500 mg/day[a]
Adult on valproate	12.5 mg/day	25 mg/day	25–50 mg/day	100–200 mg/day[a]
Child on enzyme inducer(s)	0.6 mg/kg/day	1.2 mg/kg/day	1.2 mg/kg/day	5–15 mg/kg/day[a]
Child on valproate	0.15 mg/kg/day	0.3 mg/kg/day	0.3 mg/kg/day	1–5 mg/kg/day[a]

[a]Higher doses can be tried if seizures persist and the patient is tolerating the drug without complaint.

CURRENT ROLE IN EPILEPSY MANAGEMENT

Lamotrigine has a broad range of efficacy against partial-onset and primary generalized seizures and seizures associated with the Lennox-Gastaut syndrome. The drug is widely prescribed as monotherapy and add-on treatment for these indications in adults and as adjunctive therapy in children. Its efficacy for tonic-clonic and typical absence seizures is better documented than for juvenile myoclonic epilepsy and other myoclonic syndromes. Because lamotrigine does not influence the metabolism of lipid-soluble drugs such as warfarin and the combined oral contraceptive pill, its use with other agents generally is straightforward. It usually is well tolerated and has a wide therapeutic ratio.

Lamotrigine's ability to suppress interictal spiking may be a factor in improving well-being (41). A double-blind comparison with carbamazepine in newly diagnosed epilepsy supported better health-related quality-of-life scores with lamotrigine (67). Other workers have shown better mood and quality of life in patients receiving lamotrigine than sodium valproate as monotherapy (68,69). In another study, randomly switching poorly controlled patients from carbamazepine, phenytoin, or valproate to one of these drugs or lamotrigine resulted in lamotrigine-treated patients having better cognitive functioning, energy, and other life-style factors (70). Improved behavior also has been observed when the drug was used in patients with learning disabilities (71).

The combination of lamotrigine and sodium valproate appears particularly efficacious for partial or tonic-clonic seizures (72,73). This effect also has been noted in patients with generalized absence or myoclonic seizures (74–76). The use of lamotrigine with topiramate or vigabatrin also has been reported to enhance its effectiveness (77–79).

No significant relationship has been found between lamotrigine plasma levels and its pharmacologic effect (36,80). A tentative concentration range of 2 to 4 mg/L was originally suggested (80,81). A wider range of 3 to 14 mg/L has been mooted more recently (82). Some patients, however, can tolerate lamotrigine concentrations of up to 18 mg/L, whereas side effects develop in others at levels of approximately 1 mg/L (36). Routine monitoring of lamotrigine concentrations therefore is not recommended. Exceptions may be during pregnancy and when switching patients to lamotrigine from carbamazepine, phenytoin, or sodium valproate (83).

USE IN SPECIAL POPULATIONS

The Elderly

Lamotrigine is effective and well tolerated in elderly patients (17). Because it does not induce hepatic enzymes, it can be used safely with drugs metabolized by monooxygenase and conjugation enzyme systems. Lamotrigine clearance is unaffected by renal impairment (84). Because peak concentrations can be elevated, older patients may respond to lower doses (85). As monotherapy, lamotrigine can be started at 25 mg/day for 2 weeks, increasing to 25 mg twice daily for 2 weeks, and 50 mg twice daily thereafter (17). If add-on treatment is required, combining lamotrigine with low-dose sodium valproate can be particularly effective (86).

Women

Lamotrigine is a good initial choice for young women with epilepsy because it has a wide spectrum of activity, is well tolerated, and does not interact with the combined oral contraceptive pill (87). Although not recommended for use in pregnancy, lamotrigine has not produced malformations in animal models sensitive to the teratogenic effects of sodium valproate and carbamazepine (88). Encouraging interim results from an 8-year study have shown the rate of birth defects in 79 live births from women exposed to lamotrigine monotherapy in the first trimester to be 3.8% (89). This is consistent with the frequency of major malformations expected in the general population (2.2%) and in women with epilepsy (6% to 9%).

Because the clearance of lamotrigine is increased in pregnancy, women should be monitored carefully during this time in case dose adjustment is required (90,91). Plasma concentrations tend to normalize after delivery (90,92). Because lamotrigine has antifolate properties, all women planning a pregnancy should be prescribed folic acid 5 mg/day until at least 12 weeks' gestation (88).

Children

Children tolerate lamotrigine well, although the incidence of rash is higher than in adults (66,93). For this reason, the drug should be introduced at low dosage and titrated slowly, especially if combined with sodium valproate (Table 37.3). Lamotrigine is not licensed as monotherapy in this age group, but good tolerability and efficacy against a range of generalized seizures make it a useful adjunct in a wide range of childhood epilepsies, including seizures associated with the Lennox-Gastaut and other syndromes. The drug also may be effective for infantile seizures, particularly when combined with sodium valproate.

Patients with Learning Disabilities

Because of its wide spectrum of activity and potential to improve mental state, lamotrigine can be useful for patients with learning disabilities (94). In addition, the drug has proved effective in some patients with Rett's syndrome. A low, slow titration schedule is recommended. Combining the drug with sodium valproate or topiramate can be efficacious in controlling refractory seizures (86,95).

PRECAUTIONS

Lamotrigine usually is well tolerated, with rash being the most serious side effect. Most rashes are mild, but some patients have experienced severe, life-threatening skin eruptions with systemic toxicity. There is good evidence to suggest that a low starting dose with a slow titration schedule (Table 37.3) helps to minimize risk, especially in patients taking sodium valproate. If rash does occur, the drug should be withdrawn immediately and the patient monitored closely. Reintroduction at very low dosage may be possible at a later date, but this requires close supervision and should not be undertaken if the initial reaction was severe (96).

Some patients taking carbamazepine experience headache, dizziness, ataxia, and diplopia when lamotrigine is introduced. This is thought to be the result of a pharmacodynamic interaction between the two drugs (72,77,97). Symptoms usually resolve with a reduction in the carbamazepine dose.

Like other antiepileptic drugs, lamotrigine appears to exacerbate seizures in a small number of patients (98). In particular, there is evidence to suggest that the drug may aggravate severe myoclonic epilepsy (99–102). A paradoxical reaction also was noted in a child with benign childhood epilepsy with centrotemporal spikes who became worse on lamotrigine (103). If exacerbation of seizures does occur, lamotrigine should be rapidly withdrawn.

CONTRAINDICATIONS

Because lamotrigine is metabolized in the liver, it is sensible to avoid its use in patients with end-stage hepatic impairment. Children with severe myoclonic epilepsy should not receive the drug.

CONCLUSION

Lamotrigine is a broad-spectrum antiepileptic drug that has been in widespread clinical use since the early 1900s. It has efficacy for most seizure types in adults and children, although it may worsen severe myoclonic epilepsy. The drug is useful in patients with coexistent learning disabilities. Its good tolerability makes it suitable as an alternative to traditional antiepileptic drugs as a first-line agent for adolescents and adults with newly diagnosed epilepsy. In polytherapy regimens, the drug is particularly effective when combined with sodium valproate. Outcomes from pregnant women taking lamotrigine hold out the possibility that it will prove to be nonteratogenic. Monotherapy trials in children and quality-of-life studies are underway, with encouraging preliminary results.

REFERENCES

1. Reynolds EH, Milner G, Matthews DM, et al. Anticonvulsant therapy, megaloblastic haemopoiesis and folic acid metabolism. *QJM* 1966;35:521–537.
2. Binnie CD, Beintema DJ, Debets RMC, et al. Seven day administration of lamotrigine in epilepsy: placebo-controlled add-on trial. *Epilepsy Res* 1987;1:202–208.
3. Jawad S, Richens A, Goodwin G, et al. Controlled trial of lamotrigine (Lamictal) for refractory partial seizures. *Epilepsia* 1989;30:356–363.
4. Binnie CD, Debets RMC, Engelsman M, et al. Double-blind crossover trial of lamotrigine (Lamictal) as add-on therapy in intractable epilepsy. *Epilepsy Res* 1989;4:222–229.
5. Sander JWAS, Patsalos PN, Oxley JR, et al. A randomised double-blind placebo-controlled add-on trial of lamotrigine in patients with severe epilepsy. *Epilepsy Res* 1990;6:221–226.
6. Loiseau P, Yuen AWC, Duché B, et al. A randomised double-blind placebo-controlled, crossover, add-on trial of lamotrigine in patients with treatment-resistant partial seizures. *Epilepsy Res* 1990;7:136–145.
7. Matsuo F, Bergen D, Faught E, et al. Placebo-controlled study of the efficacy and safety of lamotrigine in patients with partial seizures. *Neurology* 1993;43:2284–2291.
8. Schapel GJ, Beran RG, Vajda FJE, et al. Double-blind, placebo-controlled, crossover study of lamotrigine in treatment resistant partial seizures. *J Neurol Neurosurg Psychiatry* 1993;56: 448–453.
9. Smith D, Baker G, Davies G, et al. Outcomes of add-on treatment with lamotrigine in partial epilepsy. *Epilepsia* 1993;34: 312–322.
10. Messenheimer J, Ramsay RE, Willmore LJ, et al. Lamotrigine therapy for partial seizures: a multicentre, placebo-controlled, double-blind, cross-over trial. *Epilepsia* 1994;35:113–121.
11. Schachter SC, Leppik IE, Matsuo F, et al. Lamotrigine: a six-month, placebo-controlled, safety and tolerance study. *J Epilepsy* 1995;8:201–209.
12. Boas J, Dam M, Friis ML et al. Controlled trial of lamotrigine (Lamictal®) for treatment-resistant partial seizures. *Acta Neurol Scand* 1996;94:247–252.
13. Beran RG, Berkovic SF, Dunagan FM, et al. Double-blind, placebo-controlled, crossover study of lamotrigine in treatment-resistant generalised epilepsy. *Epilepsia* 1998;39:1329–1333.
14. Brodie MJ, Richens A, Yuen AWC, et al. Double-blind comparison of lamotrigine and carbamazepine in newly diagnosed epilepsy. *Lancet* 1995;345:476–479.
15. Ruenanen M, Dam M, Yuen AWC. A randomised open multi-centre comparative trial of lamotrigine and carbamazepine as monotherapy in patients with newly diagnosed or recurrent epilepsy. *Epilepsy Res* 1996;23:149–155.
16. Steiner TJ, Dellaportas CI, Findley LJ, et al. Lamotrigine monotherapy in newly diagnosed untreated epilepsy: a double-blind comparison with phenytoin. *Epilepsia* 1999;40:601–607.
17. Brodie MJ, Overstall PW, Giorgi L et al. Multicentre, double-blind, randomised comparison between lamotrigine and carbamazepine in elderly patients with newly diagnosed epilepsy. *Epilepsy Res* 1999;37:81–87.
18. Gilliam F, Vazquez B, Sackellares JC, et al. An active-control trial of lamotrigine monotherapy for partial seizures. *Neurology* 1998;51:1018–1025.
19. Fakhoury T, Gazda S, Nanry KP, et al. Comparison of monotherapy with lamotrigine versus carbamazepine in patients with uncontrolled epilepsy with a broad range of seizure types. *Epilepsia* 2000;41[Suppl 7]:107(abstr).

20. Gazda S, Fakhoury T, Nanry KP, et al. Comparison of monotherapy with lamotrigine in patients with uncontrolled epilepsy with a broad spectrum of seizure types. *Epilepsia* 2000; 41[Suppl 7]:107(abstr).

21. Martinez W, Kaminow L, Nanry KP, et al. Evaluation of lamotrigine versus carbamazepine, phenytoin or divalproex sodium as monotherapy for epilepsy patients who failed or could not tolerate previous antiepileptic drug therapy. *Epilepsia* 2000;41 [Suppl 7]:100(abstr).

22. Schlumberger E, Chavez F, Palacios L, et al. Lamotrigine in treatment of 120 children with epilepsy. *Epilepsia* 1994;35: 359–367.

23. Duchowny M, Pellock JM, Graf WD, et al. A placebo-controlled trial of lamotrigine add-on therapy for partial seizures in children. *Neurology* 1999;53:1724–1731.

24. Eriksson AS, Nergårdh A, Hoppu K. The efficacy of lamotrigine in children and adolescents with refractory generalised epilepsy: a randomised, double-blind, cross-over study. *Epilepsia* 1998;39:495–501.

25. Frank LM, Enlow T, Holmes GL, et al. Lamictal (lamotrigine) monotherapy for typical absence seizures in children. *Epilepsia* 1999;40:973–979.

26. Motte J, Trevathan E, Arvidsson JVF, et al. Lamotrigine for generalised seizures associated with the Lennox-Gastaut syndrome. *N Engl J Med* 1997;337:1807–1812.

27. Veendrick-Meekes MJBM, Beun AM, Carpay JA, et al. Use of lamotrigine as adjunctive therapy in patients with mental retardation and epilepsy: an interim analysis of a double-blind study with evaluation of behavioural effects. *Epilepsia* 2000;41 [Suppl]:97(abstr).

28. Jawad S, Yuen AWC, Peck AW, et al. Lamotrigine: single dose pharmacokinetics and initial 1 week experience in refractory epilepsy. *Epilepsy Res* 1986;1:194–201.

29. Sander JWAS, Trevisol-Bittencourt PC, Hart YM, et al. The efficacy and long-term tolerability of lamotrigine in the treatment of severe epilepsy. *Epilepsy Res* 1990;7:226–229.

30. Walker MC, Li LM, Sander JWAS. Long term use of lamotrigine and vigabatrin in severe refractory epilepsy: audit of outcome. *BMJ* 1996;313:1184–1185.

31. Timmings PL, Richens A. Lamotrigine in primary generalised epilepsy. *Lancet* 1992;339:1300–1301.

32. Stewart J, Hughes E, Reynolds EH. Lamotrigine for generalised epilepsies. *Lancet* 1992;340:1223.

33. Cocito L, Maffini M, Loeb C. Long-term observations on the clinical use of lamotrigine as add-on drug in patients with epilepsy. *Epilepsy Res* 1994;19:123–127.

34. Schapel G, Chadwick D. A survey comparing lamotrigine and vigabatrin in everyday clinical practice. *Seizure* 1996;5: 267–270.

35. Buchanan N. Lamotrigine: clinical experience in 200 patients with epilepsy with follow-up to four years. *Seizure* 1996;5: 209–214.

36. Kilpatrick ES, Forrest G, Brodie M. Concentration-effect and concentration-toxicity relations with lamotrigine: a prospective study. *Epilepsia* 1996;37:534–538.

37. Gericke CA, Picard F, de Saint-Martin A, et al. Efficacy of lamotrigine in idiopathic epilepsy syndromes. *Epileptic Dis* 1999;1: 159–165.

38. Collins TL, Petroff OAC, Mattson RH. A comparison of four new antiepileptic medications. *Seizure* 2000;9:291–293.

39. Faught E. Lamotrigine for startle-induced seizures. *Seizure* 1999;8:361–363.

40. Pisani F, Gallitto G, Di Perri R. Could lamotrigine be useful in status epilepticus? A case report. *J Neurol Neurosurg Psychiatry* 1991;54:845–846.

41. Besag FMC. Lamotrigine in the management of subtle seizures. *Rev Contemp Pharmacother* 1994;5:123–131.

42. Battino D, Buti D, Croci D, et al. Lamotrigine in resistant childhood epilepsy. *Neuropediatrics* 1993;24:332–336.

43. Uvebrant P, Bauzienè R. Intractable epilepsy in children: the efficacy of lamotrigine treatment, including non-seizure-related benefits. *Neuropediatrics* 1994;25:284–289.

44. Besag FMC, Wallace SJ, Dulac O, et al. Lamotrigine for the treatment of epilepsy in childhood. *J Pediatr* 1995;127: 991–997.

45. Besag FMC, Dulac O, Alving J, et al. Long-term safety and efficacy of lamotrigine (Lamictal®) in paediatric patients with epilepsy. *Seizure* 1997;6:51–56.

46. Herranz JL, Arteaga R, Armijo JA. Three-year efficacy and tolerability of add-on lamotrigine in treatment-resistant epileptic children. *Clin Drug Invest* 1996;11:214–223.

47. Buoni S, Grosso S, Fois A. Lamotrigine treatment in childhood drug resistant epilepsy. *J Child Neurol* 1998;13:163–167.

48. Schapel GJ, Wallace SJ, Gordon GS. A survey of lamotrigine and vigabatrin in children with severe epilepsy. *Seizure* 1997; 6:479–483.

49. Bélanger S, Coulombe G, Carmant L. Role of vigabatrin and lamotrigine in treatment of childhood epileptic syndromes. *Epilepsia* 1998;39:878–883.

50. Dimova PS, Korinthenberg R. Efficacy of lamotrigine and vigabatrin in drug-resistant epilepsies of childhood. *Pediatr Neurol* 1999;21:802–807.

51. Buchanan N. The use of lamotrigine in juvenile myoclonic epilepsy. *Seizure* 1996;5:149–151.

52. Farrell K, Connolly MB, Munn R, et al. Prospective, open-label, add-on study of lamotrigine in 56 children with intractable generalised epilepsy. *Pediatr Neurol* 1997;16:201–205.

53. Buoni S, Grosso S, Fois A. Lamotrigine in typical absence epilepsy. *Brain Dev* 1999;21:303–306.

54. Veggiotti P, Cieuta C, Rey E, et al. Lamotrigine in infantile spasms. *Lancet* 1994;244:1375–1376.

55. Barr PA, Buettiker VE, Antony JH. Efficacy of lamotrigine in refractory neonatal seizures. *Pediatr Neurol* 1999;20:161–163.

56. Timmings PL, Richens A. Lamotrigine as an add-on drug in the management of Lennox-Gastaut syndrome. *Eur Neurol* 1992; 32:305–307.

57. Buchanan N. The efficacy of lamotrigine on seizure control in 34 children, adolescents and young adults with intellectual and physical disability. *Seizure* 1995;4:233–236.

58. Donaldson JA, Glauser TA, Olberding LS. Lamotrigine adjunctive therapy in childhood epileptic encephalopathy (the Lennox Gastaut syndrome). *Epilepsia* 1997;38:68–73.

59. Bhaumik S, Branford C, Duggirala C, et al. A naturalistic study of the use of vigabatrin, lamotrigine and gabapentin in adults with learning disabilities. *Seizure* 1997;6:127–133.

60. Huber B, May T, Seidel M. Lamotrigine in multihandicapped therapy-resistant epileptic patients. *Clin Drug Invest* 1998; 16:263–277.

61. Coppola G, Pascotto A. Lamotrigine as add-on drug in children and adolescents with refractory epilepsy and mental delay: an open trial. *Brain Dev* 1997;19:398–402.

62. Gidal BE, Walker JK, Lott RS, et al. Efficacy of lamotrigine in institutionalised developmentally disabled patients with epilepsy: a retrospective evaluation. *Seizure* 2000;9:131–136.

63. Uldall P, Hansen FJ, Tonnby B. Lamotrigine in Rett syndrome. *Neuropediatrics* 1993;24:339–340.

64. Stenbom Y, Tonnby B, Hagberg B. Lamotrigine in Rett syndrome: treatment experience from a pilot study. *Eur Child Adolesc Psychiatry* 1998;7:49–52.

65. Mullens EK. Clinical experience with lamotrigine monotherapy

in adults with newly diagnosed epilepsy. *Clin Drug Invest* 1998; 16:125–133.

66. Guberman AH, Besag FMC, Brodie MJ, et al. Lamotrigine-associated rash: risk/benefit considerations in adults and children. *Epilepsia* 1999;40:985–991.

67. Gillham R, Kane K, Bryant-Comstock L, et al. A double-blind comparison of lamotrigine and carbamazepine in newly diagnosed epilepsy with health-related quality of life as an outcome measure. *Seizure* 2000;9:375–379

68. Edwards K, Kalogjera-Sackellares D, Sackellares C, et al. Lamotrigine monotherapy improves mood in epilepsy: a randomised double-blind comparison with valproate. *Epilepsia* 2000;41[Suppl 7]:104(abstr).

69. Kalogjera-Sackellares D, Sackellares JC, Kwong WJ, et al. Quality of life improvements with lamotrigine monotherapy: a randomised double-blind comparison with valproate. *Epilepsia* 2000;41[Suppl 7]:116(abstr).

70. Nanry K, Li H, Martinez W, et al. Epilepsy patients switched from older antiepileptic drugs to lamotrigine monotherapy show improvement in quality of life. *Epilepsia* 2000;41[Suppl 7]:176(abstr).

71. McKee J, Sunder T, Vuong A, et al. Lamotrigine adjunctive therapy improves behaviour in persons with refractory epilepsy and mental retardation. *Epilepsia* 2000;41[Suppl 7]:91(abstr).

72. Brodie MJ, Yuen AWC, the 105 Study Group. Lamotrigine substitution study: evidence for synergism with sodium valproate? *Epilepsy Res* 1997;26:423–432.

73. Pisani F, Oteri G, Russo MF, et al. The efficacy of valproate-lamotrigine comedication in refractory complex partial seizures: evidence for a pharmacodynamic interaction. *Epilepsia* 1999; 40:1141–1146.

74. Panayiotopoulos CP, Ferrie CD, Knott C, et al. Interaction of lamotrigine with sodium valproate. *Lancet* 1993;341:445.

75. Ferrie CD, Panayiotopoulos CP. Therapeutic interaction of lamotrigine and sodium valproate in intractable myoclonic epilepsy. *Seizure* 1994;3:157–159.

76. Ferrie CD, Robinson RO, Knott C, et al. Lamotrigine as an add-on drug in typical absence seizures. *Acta Neurol Scand* 1995;91:200–202.

77. Stolarek I, Blacklaw J, Forrest G, et al. Vigabatrin and lamotrigine in refractory epilepsy. *J Neurol Neurosurg Psychiatry* 1994; 57:921–924.

78. Stephen LJ, Sills GJ, Brodie MJ. Lamotrigine and topiramate may be a useful combination. *Lancet* 1998;351:58–59.

79. Deckers CLP, Czuczwar SJ, Hekster YA, et al. Selection of antiepileptic drug polytherapy based on mechanisms of action: the evidence reviewed. *Epilepsia* 2000;41:1364–1374.

80. Bartoli A, Guerrini R, Belmonte A, et al. The influence of dosage, age and co-medication on steady-state plasma lamotrigine concentrations in epileptic children: a prospective study with preliminary assessment of correlations with clinical response. *Ther Drug Monit* 1997;19:252–260.

81. Rambeck B, Wolf P. Lamotrigine clinical pharmacokinetics. *Clin Pharmacokinet* 1993;25:433–443.

82. Morris RG, Black RB, Harris AL, et al. Lamotrigine and therapeutic drug monitoring: retrospective survey following the introduction of a new service. *Br J Clin Pharmacol* 1998;45:547–551.

83. Tomson T, Johannessen SI. Therapeutic monitoring of new antiepileptic drugs. *Eur J Clin Pharmacol* 2000;55:697–705.

84. Wootton R, Soul-Lawton J, Rolan PE, et al. Comparison of the pharmacokinetics of lamotrigine in patients with chronic renal failure and healthy volunteers. *Br J Clin Pharmacol* 1997;43: 23–28.

85. Posner J, Holdich T, Crome P. Comparison of lamotrigine pharmacokinetics in young and elderly healthy volunteers. *J Pharm Med* 1991;1:121–128.

86. Stephen LJ, Brodie MJ. Epilepsy in elderly people. *Lancet* 2000;355:1441–1446.

87. Brodie MJ, French JA. Management of epilepsy in adolescents and adults. *Lancet* 2000;356:323–329.

88. Crawford P, Appleton R, Betts T, et al. Best practice guidelines for the management of women with epilepsy. *Seizure* 1999; 8:201–217.

89. Tennis P, Eldridge RR. Eight-year interim results of the lamotrigine pregnancy registry. Lamotrigine clinical research update [Glaxo-Wellcome]. Annual meeting of the American Epilepsy Society, Los Angeles, 2000.

90. Tomson T, Öhman I, Vitols S. Lamotrigine in pregnancy and lactation: a case report. *Epilepsia* 1997;38:1039–1041.

91. Sathanandar ST, Blesi K, Tran T, et al. Lamotrigine clearance increases markedly during pregnancy. *Epilepsia* 2000;41[Suppl 7]:246(abstr).

92. Öhman I, Vitols S, Tomson T. Lamotrigine in pregnancy: pharmacokinetics during delivery, in the neonate, and during lactation. *Epilepsia* 2000;41:709–713.

93. Faught E, Morris G, Jacobson M, et al. Adding lamotrigine to valproate: incidence of rash and other adverse effects. *Epilepsia* 1999;40:1135–1140.

94. Hannah JA, Brodie MJ. Treatment of seizures in patients with learning disabilities. *Pharmacol Ther* 1998;78:1–8.

95. Hannah JA, Brodie MJ. Epilepsy and learning disabilities: a challenge for the next millennium? *Seizure* 1998;7:3–13.

96. Besag FMC. Approaches to reducing the incidence of lamotrigine-induced rash. *CNS Drugs* 2000;13:21–33.

97. Besag FMC, Berry DJ, Pool F, et al. Carbamazepine toxicity with lamotrigine: pharmacokinetic or pharmacodynamic interaction? *Epilepsia* 1998;39:183–187.

98. Perucca E, Gram L, Avanzini G, et al. Antiepileptic drugs as a cause of worsening seizures. *Epilepsia* 1998;39:5–17.

99. Wallace SJ. Myoclonus and epilepsy in childhood: a review of treatment with valproate, ethosuximide, lamotrigine and zonisamide. *Epilepsy Res* 1998;29:147–154.

100. Guerrini R, Dravet C, Genton P, et al. Lamotrigine and seizure aggravation in severe myoclonic epilepsy. *Epilepsia* 1998;39: 508–512.

101. Guerrini R, Belmonte A, Parmeggiani L, et al. Myoclonic status epilepticus following high-dosage lamotrigine therapy. *Brain Dev* 1999;21:420–424.

102. Jansky J, Rásonyi G, Halász P, et al. Disabling erratic myoclonus during lamotrigine therapy with high serum levels: report of 2 cases. *Clin Neuropharmacol* 2000;23:86–89.

103. Catania S, Cross H, de Sousa C, et al. Paradoxic reaction to lamotrigine in a child with benign focal epilepsy of childhood with centrotemporal spikes. *Epilepsia* 1999;40:1657–1660.

Antiepileptic Drugs, 5th Edition. Edited by R.H. Levy, R.H. Mattson, B.S. Meldrum, and E. Perucca. Lippincott Williams & Wilkins, Philadelphia © 2002.

LAMOTRIGINE

EFFICACY AND USE IN PSYCHIATRIC DISORDERS

MELVIN D. SHELTON
JOSEPH R. CALABRESE

During clinical trials in the development of lamotrigine as an antiepileptic drug, it was observed that patients demonstrated improvements in mood and sense of well-being. There are theoretical reasons to suppose that lamotrigine might possess mood-stabilizing properties; mood swings may be associated with the kindling process, as are seizures. Bipolar disorders are defined as cyclic affective patterns comprising different combinations of mania, hypomania, depression, mixed states (coincident mania and depression), and rapid cycling (four or more cycles per year). These different mood states are not equally amenable to treatment; bipolar depression and rapid-cycling bipolar disorder are particularly treatment refractory. The first prospective, randomized, placebo-controlled study of lamotrigine monotherapy in bipolar-I depressed patients has shown that patients receiving 200 mg and 50 mg daily showed significant improvement compared with placebo on several measures of depression. In the first double-blind maintenance study of lamotrigine and the first controlled study of any medication in a cohort of patients with rapid-cycling bipolar disorder, results indicated lamotrigine was a useful treatment for those patients with bipolar II disorder. Lamotrigine has not been shown to have clear efficacy in the treatment of mania or unipolar depression. A series of controlled studies investigating the use of lamotrigine in bipolar disorder is ongoing.

There are theoretical reasons to postulate that antiepileptic drugs (AEDs) might be effective in the treatment of mood disorders. Post and colleagues have suggested that mood instability leading to bipolar affective disorder (BAD) may be causally related, as are seizures, to progressive neural kindling (1). The *Diagnostic and Statistical Manual for Mental Disorders*, 4th edition, Text Revision (DSM-IV-TR) (2) describes bipolar disorder as a recurrent condition with a lifetime prevalence of approximately 0.4% to 1.6% in community samples. Patients with the disorder experience marked mood fluctuations, which have been described as type I (BP-I, showing depressions, possibly euthymias and manias), type II (BP-II, with depressions, possibly euthymias, and hypomanias, but not manias), and mixed states (simultaneously meeting criteria for both depression and mania). In men, the first episode is likely to be manic, and the proportion of manias to depressions is 1:1 or higher. In women, the index episode is likely to be depressive, and depressive episodes predominate during the course of the disorder (2). The sex ratio in patients with BP-I is equal; female patients with BP-II are more common (3). Any of these three variants may show a rapid cycling course (RC), defined as four or more mood states (i.e., at least two full bipolar cycles) per year (2). Patients with RC, comprising 13% to 20% of patients with bipolar disorder (4), are more likely to be female (5). There is evidence of ultrarapid cycling, with cycle periods as short as several days, and ultradian cycling, with periods of less than 24 hours (6). RC patients were initially identified by Dunner and Fieve as having poor prognoses, and poor responses to treatment with lithium (7), the earliest pharmacologic gold standard for treatment of bipolar disorder. It appears that only approximately 50% of patients with bipolar spectrum disorder, 30% to 40% of patients with mixed-state disorder, and 20% to 30% of patients with RC bipolar disorder respond to lithium treatment. Lithium as a first-line mood stabilizer has been joined by carbamazepine and divalproex. Like lithium, they appear to be less effective in the depressed phase of the illness, particularly in patients with RC bipolar disorder (8). Antidepressant medications are useful, but run the risk of inducing hypomania, mania, or increased cycle frequency (9). Because there are no published reports of any single mood stabilizer equally effica-

Melvin D. Shelton, MD, PhD: Clinical Trials Section, Mood Disorders Program; and Assistant Professor of Psychiatry, Case Western Reserve University School of Medicine, University Hospitals of Cleveland, Cleveland, Ohio

Joseph R. Calabrese, MD: Professor of Psychiatry, Department of Psychiatry, Case Western Reserve University School of Medicine; and Director, Mood Disorders Program, Department of Psychiatry, University Hospitals of Cleveland, Cleveland, Ohio

cious in all phases of bipolar illness, polypharmacotherapy has been increasingly used (10,11). Clearly, there is a need for such a mood stabilizer.

LAMOTRIGINE AS A MOOD STABILIZER

Initial findings (12) of the efficacy of lamotrigine in the treatment of intractable seizures gave anecdotal evidence of mood improvement in treated patients. These findings were extended (13) in a study of 81 lamotrigine-treated patients with mixed epilepsy. The primary efficacy variable was seizure frequency; a secondary measure was quality of life. Although the quality-of-life examination was methodologically limited, there was evidence that patients thought of themselves as both happier and more in control of their situation, and that they experienced improvements in self-esteem. These reports led to closer scrutiny of the drug's effects in patients with mood disorders, especially bipolar affective disorder (13–18).

There have been approximately 16 open studies of lamotrigine's efficacy as a mood stabilizer. The largest of these (18) was published in 1999. A 48-week prospective, open-label trial was conducted using lamotrigine as monotherapy (n = 15) or as an adjuvant (n = 60) in patients with BP-I and BP-II. Depressed patients exhibited a 42% improvement in scores on the Hamilton Depression Rating Scale (HAMD); patients with mania, hypomania, or mixed states showed a 74% improvement in scores on the Mania Rating Scale from the Schedule for Affective Disorders, Change Version (MRS). Eighty percent of nondepressed patients showed a marked response to treatment; only 60% of depressed patients showed similar improvement.

CONTROLLED STUDIES

The first randomized, placebo-controlled, parallel-group trial evaluating the efficacy of lamotrigine monotherapy in the treatment of bipolar disorder has been completed (19). One hundred ninety-five adult outpatients diagnosed with BP-I depression and moderately to severely depressed at study entry were randomized to either 50 mg (LTG50, 63 patients) or 200 mg (LTG200, 66 patients) daily of lamotrigine, or to placebo (66 patients) at 15 U.S. centers and 6 centers in Australia, the United Kingdom, and France. Treatment groups were stratified to detect any lithium effect on subsequent lamotrigine treatment. Lamotrigine dosing was titrated according to the protocol depicted in Figure 38.1. The test instruments were the HAMD, MRS, Clinical Global Impression—Severity (CGI-S), and the Montgomery-Asberg Rating Scale for Depression (MADRS).

Lamotrigine was significantly more effective than placebo on most outcome measures. Patients on LTG200 showed significant improvement by all measures except for

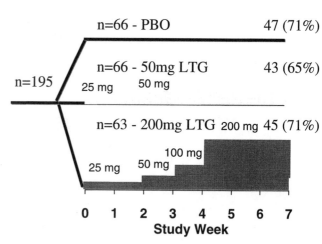

FIGURE 38.1. Lamotrigine at 50 and 200 mg/day versus placebo. (From Calabrese J, Bowden C, Sachs G, et al. A double-blind, placebo-controlled study of lamotrigine monotherapy in outpatients with bipolar I depression. *J Clin Psychiatry* 2000;20:607–614, with permission.)

the 31-item HAMD [observed and last observation carried forward (LOCF) analysis] and the LOCF analysis of the 17-item HAMD. Over 50% of the LTG200 patients met response criteria for the HAMD-17, Clinical Global Impression—Intensity (CGI-I), and MADRS. On the latter two instruments, the degree of improvement was nearly twice that shown by patients in the placebo arm, and the difference reached statistical significance ($p < .05$). Patients in the LTG50 group showed less robust improvement than the LTG200 group (Figure 38.2). By design, both groups received the same lamotrigine doses for the first 3 weeks of treatment; the pooled patients on lamotrigine showed significant improvement over placebo by the end of week 3.

Two frequent impediments to successful treatment of patients with mood stabilizers are (a) idiopathic switches to mania, hypomania, or mixed states; and (b) poor medica-

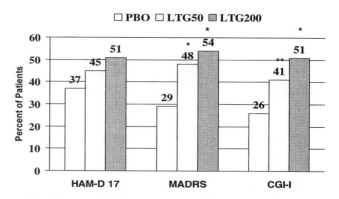

FIGURE 38.2. Percentage of patients on placebo, lamotrigine 50 mg/day (LTG50), and lamotrigine 200 mg/day (LTG200) meeting end point response criterion (see text). (From Calabrese J, Bowden C, Sachs G, et al. A double-blind, placebo-controlled study of lamotrigine monotherapy in outpatients with bipolar I depression. *J Clin Psychiatry* 2000;20:607–614, with permission.)

tion compliance secondary to intolerable side effects. In this study, approximately 5% of patients cycled into a manic, hypomanic, or mixed state. In contrast, switch rates as high as 25% for monoamine oxidase inhibitors and 21% for tricyclic antidepressants have been reported. (17). In each group, over 91% of patients were over 70% medication compliant. There also was no intergroup difference in the number of study withdrawals due to adverse effects.

LAMOTRIGINE IN RAPID CYCLING BIPOLAR DISORDER

As noted previously, the RC variant of bipolar disorder was initially identified as a characteristic of patients resistant to lithium treatment (7), so the development of a more effective mood stabilizer for use in this population is desirable. The first controlled, prospective study of adult RC patients has been published; it also is the first double-blind maintenance study of lamotrigine (20). Three hundred twenty-four patients entered treatment at 24 U.S. (n = 292) and three Canadian (n = 32) sites. The initial phase of the study was an open-label stabilization phase; the second phase was double-blind, placebo-controlled, and randomized (Figure 38.3). After screening, patients entered a 6-week titration to a target dosage of 100 to 300 mg daily. Flexible dosing was permitted to allow for differences in tolerability. During the first 4 weeks of treatment, patients were permitted addi-

tional psychotropic medications for acute episodes; over 4 to 8 weeks, all other psychotropics were tapered. To meet randomization criteria, subjects scored 14 or less on the HAMD, 12 or less on the MRS, and remained compliant on lamotrigine 100 mg/day, all over a 2-week period.

Patients successfully negotiating the taper of psychotropics while retaining affective stability were offered advancement to the 26-week randomized phase, in which they underwent discontinuation of open-label lamotrigine and double-blind 1:1 randomization to lamotrigine or placebo treatment. In contrast to the monotherapy study, this study was open to patients with either BP-I or BP-II, and groups were appropriately stratified. As in the preliminary phase, lamotrigine dosing was flexible, and ranged from 100 to 500 mg/day. Use of up to 2 mg/day of lorazepam was permitted for agitation, hostility, and insomnia. The primary outcome variable was time to pharmacologic intervention to prevent a mood episode. A secondary outcome variable was survival time in study, that is, time to premature discontinuation for any reason. Secondary test instruments were the HAMD, MRS, CGI-S, and Global Assessment Scale.

The lamotrigine and placebo groups did not differ significantly in time to intervention; however, mean survival times were 18 weeks for lamotrigine and 12 weeks for placebo. The mean group survival times were 14 weeks for lamotrigine and 8 weeks for placebo; the difference was significant ($p < .05$). Figure 38.4 summarizes the differences in

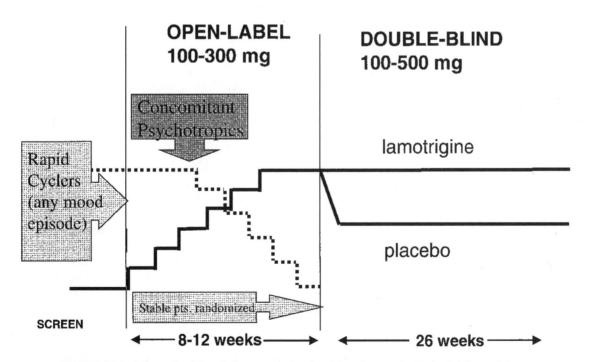

FIGURE 38.3. Schema for lamotrigine versus placebo comparison study. (From Calabrese J, Suppes T, Bowden C, et al. A double-blind, placebo-controlled prophylaxis study of lamotrigine in rapid-cycling bipolar disorder. *J Clin Psychiatry* 2000;61:841–850, with permission.)

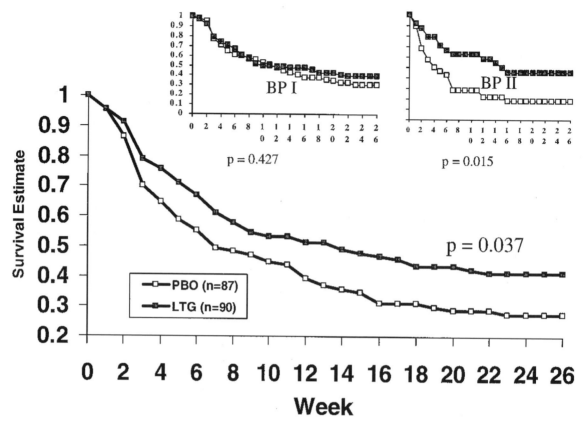

FIGURE 38.4. Kaplan-Meier curves for survival time in study for bipolar disorder type I (BP-I), bipolar disorder type II (BP-II), and BP-I = BP-II groups. (From Calabrese J, Suppes T, Bowden C, et al. A double-blind, placebo-controlled prophylaxis study of lamotrigine in rapid-cycling bipolar disorder. *J Clin Psychiatry* 2000;61:841–850, with permission.)

response between patients with BP-I and BP-II disorder. There was no significant difference in lamotrigine versus placebo group survival times for patients with BP-I. For patients with BP-II, there was a trend toward significance in the time to intervention analysis, and a significant difference ($p < .015$) in the median survival in study times (lamotrigine 17 weeks, placebo 7 weeks).

Figure 38.4 summarizes findings from the 6-month stability data. The percentage of patients with BP-I stable for 6 months was not significantly different between lamotrigine and placebo groups (39% and 31%, respectively), but was significantly different (46% and 18%, respectively; $p < .04$) for patients with BP-II. Median survival time in study for patients with BP-I was not significantly different for those in lamotrigine and placebo groups; the mean for patients with BP-II was 17 weeks for lamotrigine and 7 weeks for placebo. However, these differing survival times may have been due to intergroup differences in placebo response rates. Thirty-seven of 60 patients stable for 6 months without relapse were in the lamotrigine group; this constituted 41% of the lamotrigine group. Twenty-three of 60 stable patients were in the placebo

group; this was 26% of the placebo sample. The difference was significant ($p < .03$).

This study design had limitations in addition to the elevated BP-I placebo response rate. Because of the lack of previous lamotrigine monotherapy data in this population, the primary outcome measure study was discovered retrospectively to have been underpowered to detect the observed differences, although secondary measures were not. The abrupt discontinuation of lamotrigine at randomization may have produced artifactual affective changes, and the immediate intervention to prevent relapse prevented measurement of actual time to full relapse.

Comparisons between lamotrigine's efficacy in unipolar and in bipolar depression are of interest. There is one case report (21) of efficacious lamotrigine monotherapy in unipolar depression, and a report of two patients receiving effective lamotrigine adjuvant therapy (22). During development (Glaxo-Smith Kline, Research Triangle Park, North Carolina, data on file), evidence supported antidepressant activity in unipolar disorder. However, this conclusion was weakened by differences in the LOCF and observed analyses, and by a high placebo response rate. In a randomized, double-blind, crossover trial, Frye and colleagues (23) studied lamotrigine and gabapentin monotherapy of patients with BP-I (n = 13), BP-II (n = 15), RC (n = 21), and unipolar depression (n = 10). Forty-five percent of lamotrigine-treated patients were assessed as improved or very much improved on the CGI. Response for patients with unipolar disorder (29%) was less than that for patients with bipolar disorder. In this study, more patients with BP-I (73%) improved than those with BP-II (47%). This result must be interpreted carefully, however, because the measure of improvement was of overall clinical impression of illness rather than a straightforward measurement of depression. Lamotrigine also has been evaluated in the acute management of mania (18). In a placebo-controlled designs using lamotrigine treatment as monotherapy and as add-on therapy, minimal efficacy was observed; lamotrigine was well tolerated in this study and did not worsen the symptoms of mania.

Additional evidence supporting the premise that lamotrigine might be expected to be more effective in patients with BP-II than in those with BP-I has been offered in several studies. The most recent examination of the question is the multisite study referred to previously (21): 57% of subjects were depressed at study entry, compared with 21% manic/hypomanic, 18% euthymic, and 5% mixed. Also in that study, a high percentage of both the lamotrigine and control groups (37% and 45%, respectively) reached study end point because of depression. Because depression appears to be a hallmark of BP-II disorder, it is reasonable to postulate that patients with BP-II disorder may respond to lamotrigine treatment. The issue of whether lamotrigine is more efficacious in BP-I or BP-II disorder awaits results of further controlled studies. However, the cumulative results of the studies done so far provide evidence that lamotrigine is effective in the acute management of the depressed phase of BP-I depression, and effective in the long-term stabilization of mood in patients with RC bipolar disorder.

REFERENCES

1. Post R, Weiss S, Pert A. Differential effects of carbamazepine and lithium on sensitization and kindling. *Prog Neuropsychopharmacol Biol Psychiatry* 1984;8:425–434.
2. American Psychiatric Association. *Diagnostic and statistical manual of mental disorders*, 4th ed, text revision. Washington, DC: American Psychiatric Association, 2000.
3. Goodwin F, Jamison K. *Manic-depressive illness*. New York: Oxford University Press, 1990.
4. Bauer M, Calabrese J, Dunner D, et al. Multisite data reanalysis of the validity of rapid cycling as a course modifier for bipolar disorder in DSM-IV. *Am J Psychiatry* 1994;151:506–515.
5. Coryell W, Endicott J, Keller M. Rapidly cycling affective disorder: demographics, diagnosis, family history, and course. *Arch Gen Psychiatry* 1992;49:126–131.
6. Kramlinger K, Post R. Ultra-rapid and ultradian cycling in bipolar affective illness. *Br J Psychiatry* 1996;168:214–323.
7. Dunner D, Fieve R. Clinical factors in lithium prophylaxis failure. *Arch Gen Psychiatry* 1974;30:229–233.
8. Calabrese J, Bowden C, Woyshville M. Lithium and anticonvulsants in bipolar disorder. In: Bloom F, Kupfer D, eds. *Psychopharmacology: the fourth generation of progress*. CD-ROM Version 3, http://www.acnp.org/citations/GN401000106, 2000.
9. Post R, Denicoff K, Leverich G, et al. Drug-induced switching in bipolar disorder: epidemiology and therapeutic implications. *CNS Drugs* 1997;8:352–365.
10. Frye M, Ketter K, Leverich G, et al. The increasing use of polypharmacotherapy for refractory mood disorders: 22 years of study. *J Clin Psychiatry* 2000;61:9–15.
11. Shelton M, Calabrese J. Current concepts in rapid cycling bipolar disorder. *Curr Psychiatry Rep* 2000;2:310–315.
12. Jawad S, Richens A, Goodwin G, et al. Controlled trial of lamotrigine (Lamictal) for refractory partial seizures. *Epilepsia* 1989; 30:656–653.
13. Smith D, Chadwick D, Baker G, et al. Seizure severity and the quality of life. *Epilepsia* 1993;34[Suppl 5]:S31–S35.
14. Calabrese J, Fatemi S, Woyshville M. Antidepressant effects of lamotrigine in rapid cycling bipolar disorder. *Am J Psychiatry* 1996;153:1236.
15. Fogelson D, Sternback H. Lamotrigine treatment of refractory bipolar disorder. *J Clin Psychiatry* 1997;58:271–273.
16. Kusumakar V, Yatham L. An open study of lamotrigine in refractory bipolar depression. *Psychiatry Res* 1997;72:145–148.
17. Sporn J, Sachs G. The anticonvulsant lamotrigine in treatment-resistant manic-depressive illness. *J Clin Psychopharmacol* 1997; 17:185–189.
18. Calabrese, J, Bowden C, McElroy S, et al. Spectrum of activity of lamotrigine in treatment refractory bipolar disorder. *Am J Psychiatry* 1999;156:1019–1023.
19. Calabrese, J, Bowden C, Sachs G, et al. A double-blind placebo-controlled study of lamotrigine monotherapy in outpatients with bipolar I depression. *J Clin Psychiatry* 1999;60:2:79–88.
20. Calabrese J, Suppes T, Bowden C, et al. A double-blind, placebo-controlled, prophylaxis study of lamotrigine in rapid cycling bipolar disorder. *J Clin Psychiatry* 2000;61:841–850.
21. Rapport D, Calabrese J, Clegg K, et al. Lamotrigine in unipolar major depression. *Prim Psychiatry* 1999;6(4):41–42.
22. Maltese, T. Adjunctive lamotrigine treatment for major depression. *Am J Psychiatry* 1999;156:1833.
23. Frye M, Ketter T, Kimbrell, et al. A placebo-controlled evaluation of lamotrigine and gabapentin monotherapy in refractory mood disorders. *J Clin Psychopharmacol* 2000;20:607–614.

LAMOTRIGINE

ADVERSE EFFECTS

FRANCESCO PISANI
ALAN RICHENS

Lamotrigine was introduced to its first market in the Republic of Ireland in 1991 and, at the time of writing, 10 years of postmarketing experience has been gained. It is estimated that at May 1, 2000, approximately 11,000 adults and 2,000 children (<12 years of age) in clinical trials and more than 1,000,000 patients worldwide have received lamotrigine, with >583,000 patient-years of experience accumulated (1). Lamotrigine was developed as a member of a series of phenyltriazine compounds with dihydrofolate reductase–inhibiting activity, although in the case of lamotrigine, the latter property is weak and does not appear to create adverse effects in humans. Toxicity studies in rodents, marmosets, and cynomolgus monkeys have shown that the dose of lamotrigine required to produce an anticonvulsant effect is well below that needed to cause toxic effects, such as decreased locomotor activity, ataxia, and reflex impairment (2). Carcinogenicity, reproductive toxicity, and mutagenicity tests have demonstrated no toxic effects.

In general, lamotrigine is well tolerated and the general safety assessment measures usually evaluated in most clinical trials, including the routine measurement of vital signs, clinical chemistry, and hematologic parameters, as well as urinalysis and electrocardiography, were not modified by the use of lamotrigine. Unlike other conventional antiepileptic drugs, such as phenytoin and carbamazepine, long-term use of lamotrigine does not seem to affect peripheral nerve function (3).

MOST COMMONLY OBSERVED ADVERSE EFFECTS

During the phase I clinical development of lamotrigine, a battery of psychomotor, autonomic, sensory, and subjective

---

Francesco Pisani, MD: Associate Professor of Neurology, Department of Neurosciences, Psychiatric and Anaesthesiological Sciences, University of Messina, Messina, Italy

Alan Richens, MD, PhD: Emeritus Professor of Pharmacology and Therapeutics, Department of Pharmacology and Therapeutics, University of Wales College of Medicine, Cardiff, United Kingdom

tests was used in healthy volunteers, with an emphasis on saccadic eye movements, to compare the central nervous system (CNS) effects of lamotrigine with some established drugs, namely, phenytoin and diazepam (4), and carbamazepine (5). Phenytoin and diazepam were found to impair smooth-pursuit eye movements, reduce peak saccade velocity (diazepam only), impair adaptive tracking, and cause drowsiness, but lamotrigine had none of these effects. Carbamazepine impaired smooth pursuit, reduced peak saccade velocity, impaired adaptive tracking, and increased body sway in single doses of 400 and 600 mg, whereas lamotrigine again had none of these effects in doses of 150 and 300 mg. It was predicted from these studies that lamotrigine would be well tolerated in patients at the doses used. These doses subsequently were shown to suppress interictal spikes (6) and photosensitivity (7), and therefore the findings in volunteers were thought to be relevant to subsequent clinical trials.

Central Nervous System Side Effects

Dose Dependency, Incidence, and Prevalence

The first definitive efficacy trials of lamotrigine in patients were conducted in four centers and included a total of 92 patients (8–11). The trials were of a crossover design, and either lamotrigine or placebo was added to existing therapy in a randomized order for 8 to 12 weeks in patients with refractory epilepsy. The dose of lamotrigine ranged from 50 to 400 mg/day and was adjusted according to the background therapy to allow for the inducing effect of some of the conventional antiepileptic drugs and the inhibitory effect of valproate on the metabolism of lamotrigine (Chapter 37). The most commonly recorded adverse events are given in Table 39.1. Although they were seen more frequently when patients were on lamotrigine rather than placebo, in no case was the difference statistically significant (12). However, with ataxia, the confidence intervals (CIs) intercepted zero, indicating a difference of borderline significance.

A similar spectrum of adverse reactions was seen in an Australian double-blind, crossover study in which doses of

TABLE 39.1. INCIDENCE OF ADVERSE EVENTS IN PATIENTS TREATED WITH LAMOTRIGINE OR PLACEBO, AND THE 95% CONFIDENCE INTERVAL OF THE DIFFERENCE BETWEEN THE INCIDENCE RATES, BASED ON A METAANALYSIS OF FOUR DOUBLE-BLIND, PLACEBO-CONTROLLED, CROSSOVER, ADD-ON STUDIES INVOLVING A TOTAL OF 92 PATIENTS

Adverse Experience	Incidence (%)		
	Lamotrigine	Placebo	95% Confidence Interval for Difference
Asthenia	17	13	−12; 4
Diplopia	15	12	−13; 6
Headache	13	7	−14; 1
Somnolence	13	12	−9; 7
Ataxia	12	4	−15; 0
Dizziness	9	8	−9; 7
Nausea	4	3	−7; 5
Nervousness	4	2	−7; 3

Modified from Betts T, Goodwin O, Withers RM, et al. Human safety of lamotrigine. *Epilepsy Res* 1991;32[Suppl 2]:S17–S21, with permission.

up to 300 mg of lamotrigine daily or placebo were added to the background therapy in 41 patients with partial seizures (13). Dizziness was significantly more common with lamotrigine treatment (11%) than with placebo (0%). A further double-blind, crossover, add-on study (14) in 81 patients showed a significantly higher incidence of ataxia, diplopia, nausea and vomiting, blurred vision, and insomnia with lamotrigine in doses of up to 400 mg/day.

Experience in the United States is similar to that in Europe. In a large multicenter study, lamotrigine or placebo was added to the existing therapy in outpatients with partial epilepsy (15). Patients were randomized in a 3-to-1 ratio to receive lamotrigine in doses of up to 500 mg/day or placebo, respectively. Patients receiving valproate were excluded. Follow-up lasted for 24 weeks. The adverse event profiles in 334 patients treated with lamotrigine and 112 treated with placebo are given in Table 39.2. The high incidence of adverse events on adding placebo should be noted, highlighting the need for a placebo control in assessing the adverse reaction profile of a new antiepileptic drug. Headache, for example, occurred in just over one-third of lamotrigine-treated patients, but the incidence with placebo was virtually identical. Significant differences were seen, however, for dizziness, diplopia, ataxia, blurred vision, and somnolence. There was evidence in this trial that the incidence of some CNS adverse effects was dose related.

Systematic reviews (16–18), including subsequent studies and a larger number of patients, have confirmed the foregoing CNS toxicity profile of lamotrigine and have indicated that the most frequently occurring side effects (i.e. >5% of patients) during lamotrigine therapy at doses of up to 500 mg/day are dizziness, diplopia, ataxia, blurred vision, headache, and nausea or vomiting. It is not known whether the latter two effects are due to a central or peripheral action of the drug.

The CNS adverse effects with lamotrigine often are mild, do not require drug withdrawal, and lessen over time. Con-

sequently, the proportion of patients in whom withdrawal of lamotrigine is necessary for a particular event is much smaller than the overall incidence of the event (Table 39.3). In the analysis of Betts (19), less than 1% of patients had to discontinue lamotrigine for any one CNS adverse event, and in the U.S. trial (15), the proportion of patients withdrawn from the study because of adverse events was identical in both the lamotrigine- and the placebo-treated groups (i.e., 8%). In a recent meta-analysis (16), the overall odds ratio (ratio of incidence with the drug to incidence with placebo) for discon-

TABLE 39.2. ADVERSE EVENTS OCCURRING IN U.S. PLACEBO-CONTROLLED EVALUATION OF THE SAFETY OF LAMOTRIGINE (EVENTS REPORTED IN 10% OR MORE PATIENTS)

Adverse Events	Number (%) of Patients	
	Lamotrigine (n = 334)	Placebo (n = 112)
Dizziness	168 (50)[a]	20 (18)
Headache	125 (37)	40 (36)
Diplopia	109 (33)[a]	12 (11)
Ataxia	80 (24)[a]	5 (5)
Blurred vision	77 (23)[a]	10 (9)
Nausea	73 (22)	17 (15)
Rhinitis	58 (17)	21 (19)
Somnolence	46 (14)[a]	8 (7)
Pharyngitis	42 (13)	13 (12)
Coordination abnormality	39 (12)	7 (6)
Flu syndrome	38 (11)	10 (9)
Cough	35 (10)	9 (8)
Rash	34 (10)	6 (5)
Dyspepsia	32 (10)	6 (5)
Vomiting	32 (10)	10 (9)

[a]Statistically significantly greater than with placebo.
Modified from Schachter SC, Leppik IE, Matsuo F, et al. A multicentre, placebo-controlled evaluation of the safety of lamotrigine (Lamictal) as add-on therapy in outpatients with partial seizures. *Epilepsy Res* 1992;33[Suppl 3]:1–19, with permission.

TABLE 39.3. ADVERSE EVENTS LEADING TO WITHDRAWAL OF LAMOTRIGINE IN 1,920 PATIENTS INCLUDED IN OPEN-LABEL AND DOUBLE-BLIND STUDIES.

Adverse Event	Number (%) of Patients
Rash	54 (2.8)
Headache	15 (0.8)
Ataxia	12 (0.6)
Diplopia	11 (0.6)
Nausea	11 (0.6)
Blurred vision	10 (0.5)
Dizziness	9 (0.5)
Asthenia	9 (0.5)
Vomiting	9 (0.5)
Somnolence	6 (0.3)
Insomnia	6 (0.3)
Depression	5 (0.3)
Psychosis	4 (0.2)
Increased seizures	4 (0.2)
Total number of patients withdrawn	150 (7.8)

Modified from Betts T. Safety of lamotrigine. In: Richens A, ed. *Clinical update on lamotrigine: a novel antiepileptic agent.* Tunbridge Wells, UK: Wells Medical 1992:61–68, with permission.

tinuation for any reason was 1.19 (95% CI, 0.79 to 1.79). This value, slightly above unity, indicates that the difference between lamotrigine and placebo is very small. Lower values, as reported in open observational studies, probably are due to the fact that in these studies the dose of lamotrigine could be modified and rapidly adjusted to the clinical situation without any adherence to the specific rigid protocols that are typical of controlled studies.

Few published data are available regarding the correlation between lamotrigine dose or plasma concentration and CNS adverse effects. Based on current knowledge, this correlation seems to be poor for most of the aforementioned effects (13,20,21).

Experience with lamotrigine monotherapy is increasing since a number of monotherapy comparative studies have been completed (22–25). Fifteen countries have approved lamotrigine in monotherapy in adults and six in childhood (i.e., <12 years of age). In two double-blinded, randomized, placebo-controlled, parallel-group studies, lamotrigine was better tolerated than carbamazepine (22) or phenytoin (25). In fact, the withdrawal rate due to adverse events (including rash) was 14% to 15% with 100 to 400 mg/day lamotrigine (plasma concentrations within the target range of 2 to 4 mg/L), this value being lower than that of carbamazepine (27%, daily dose 300 to 1,400 mg , median plasma concentration 8.3 mg/L, target range 4 to 10 mg/L) and phenytoin (19%, modal and maximal daily doses 300 and 600 mg, mean plasma level 13.4 mg/L, target range 10 to 20 mg/L).

Time Dependency

Usually, add-on therapy with lamotrigine is well tolerated. In most clinical trials, as great as 30% to 40% of treatment-emergent adverse events, typically the most frequent on CNS, was judged by the investigators to be reasonably attributable to lamotrigine (17). These effects develop during the first 4 to 6 weeks of treatment and tend to lessen or resolve over time or after dosage adjustment.

Risk Factors

It is general experience that some CNS side effects occur more frequently when lamotrigine is added to carbamazepine (dizziness and diplopia) (15,26,27) or to valproate (hand tremor) (28,29). Adding a new drug to existing therapy can cause adverse reactions by pharmacokinetic or pharmacodynamic interaction with the baseline drugs. Lamotrigine causes little in the way of pharmacokinetic interactions with other drugs, although enzyme inducers and valproate influence its own metabolism (Chapter 37). Available data suggest that lamotrigine does not cause substantial changes in plasma levels of carbamazepine and its active metabolite, carbamazepine 10,11-epoxide, and therefore the dizziness and diplopia associated with a combination of the two drugs is thought to be a pharmacodynamic phenomenon. Hand tremor occurring when lamotrigine and valproate are taken in combination has been observed to be unrelated to plasma drug concentrations (29), and also may be the result of a pharmacodynamic interaction.

Use in Children

Messenheimer and colleagues (30) analyzed the safety data of lamotrigine in 1,096 children who took part in controlled clinical trials. CNS adverse effects were quantitatively and qualitatively similar to those described for adults. Similar results were obtained in a large, placebo-controlled, add-on study in the United States (31). Childhood, therefore, does not seem to be a particular risk factor for lamotrigine-induced CNS adverse effects.

Use in Elderly

Lamotrigine is largely metabolized in the liver to a glucuronide conjugate. This pathway has a large capacity and therefore is little affected by the processes involved in aging. The plasma elimination half-life was found to be no different in a group of elderly subjects compared with young adults (32). On the other hand, changes that occur in the brain as a result of aging may make the elderly more susceptible to the adverse effects of antiepileptic drugs. In a multicenter, double-blind, monotherapy study comparing 75 to 500 mg/day lamotrigine versus 200 to 2,000 mg/day carbamazepine treatment in newly diagnosed patients, the rate of dropout due to adverse events was twofold higher for carbamazepine—42%, versus 18% for lamotrigine (33). This was in part the consequence of lower rash and somnolence rates with lamotrigine (rash: lamotrigine 3%, carbamazepine 19%, 95% CI 7% to 25%; somnolence: lamotrigine 12%, carbamazepine 29%, 95% CI 4% to 30%).

Advice Concerning Precautions and Management

As stated previously, most of the CNS adverse effects of lamotrigine lessen or resolve over time and therefore do not require any particular treatment. Adherence to the recommended starting doses and to the indicated dose escalation (Table 39.4), especially in patients receiving carbamazepine or valproate (see previous discussion), is a good precaution to avoid increases both in the incidence and in the intensity of these side effects.

Lamotrigine may have beneficial side effects on CNS function. A number of investigators have observed that a small proportion of patients, particularly those with a learning disability, seem much brighter and more responsive when taking lamotrigine. Smith et al. (14) included a health-related quality-of-life measure in their placebo-controlled, crossover study in 81 patients with partial epilepsy. Although only 11 patients experienced at least a 50% reduction in seizure frequency, no fewer than 41 elected to continue with lamotrigine at the end of the trial, indicating that factors other than seizure control influenced their decision. A significant improvement was seen in the subscales for happiness and mastery, suggesting that effects on mood and attitude might be an additional benefit with lamotrigine. Overall, lamotrigine has proven to exhibit a favorable profile on health-related quality-control measures (14,34).

Rash

The most common hypersensitivity reaction to lamotrigine is a simple morbilliform skin rash, typically maculopapular, most frequently with no evidence of systemic involvement. Other reported rash types include angioedema, erythema, petechiae, purpura, pustular and vesicular rashes, and urticaria. Rash also is the most frequent side effect leading to lamotrigine discontinuation and, although rarely serious, it represents an annoying adverse effect of lamotrigine. Rash is not a new concern of antiepileptic therapy because some of the most commonly used conventional antiepileptic drugs, like carbamazepine and phenytoin, exhibit this adverse effect. In recent reviews (17,35), in fact, the inci-

dence of rash in monotherapy showed similar values for lamotrigine (~14%, discontinuation rate ~6%), carbamazepine (~15%, discontinuation rate ~9%), and phenytoin (~12%, discontinuation rate ~5%).

Dose Dependency, Incidence, and Prevalence

The incidence of skin rashes has been evaluated in different systematic reviews of double-blind, placebo-controlled trials (17,18,35,36). The proportion of adult patients experiencing skin rash after addition of placebo in most of the studies analyzed was approximately one-half of that associated with addition of lamotrigine, and ultimately the real incidence of lamotrigine rashes, as indicated by the difference between the drug and placebo, was ~5% (18,36). Table 39.5 shows the results obtained by one of the earlier reviews (36) in which the proportion of patients withdrawn from a trial because of the occurrence of a skin rash was 1.7%. There was, however, a wide range of variation, up to >20-fold, because they are greatly influenced by a number of factors. Overall, it is possible that up to ~3% of patients were withdrawn when data from open-label and controlled trials were combined (19) (Table 39.3). Among those factors influencing the incidence of rash, it has become clear with further experience that the size of the initial dose of lamotrigine and the rate of escalation in dose are two of the most important.

Yuen (36) found a rash rate of 2.1% in patients whose plasma lamotrigine concentration was greater than 1.4 mg/L when measured 2 weeks after initiation of therapy, whereas the rate was only 0.6% when plasma concentrations were below this level. Data from monotherapy studies (17) showed that the withdrawal rates due to rash progressively increased in line with the lamotrigine dose in the first week of treatment, from ~2% at 25 mg/day up to ~40% at 200 mg/day. Similarly, discontinuation rates due to rash ranged from ~2% at a mean daily lamotrigine dose of <100 mg achieved during the first 5 weeks of treatment up to ~13% at a mean dose of ~400 mg/day. This relationship is not unique with antiepileptic drugs, because both phenytoin and carbamazepine are more likely to cause rashes when the starting dose is high (37).

TABLE 39.4. STARTING AND MAINTENANCE DOSE OF LAMOTRIGINE IN ADULTS AND CHILDREN

Concomitant Therapy	Weeks 1–2	Weeks 3–4	Maintenance Dose
Adults and children >12 yr			
Valproic acid	25 mg on alternate days	25 mg	100–200 mg
Nil	25 mg	50 mg	100–200 mg
Inducing antiepileptic drugs	50 mg	100 mg	200–400 mg
Children 2–12 yr			
Valproic acid	0.2 mg/kg	0.5 mg/kg	1–5 mg/kg
Nil	0.5 mg/kg	1 mg/kg	2–8 mg/kg
Inducing antiepileptic drugs	2.0 mg/kg	5 mg/kg	5–15 mg/kg

TABLE 39.5. INCIDENCE OF SKIN RASH IN DOUBLE-BLIND-PLACEBO-CONTROLLED STUDIES.

	Lamotrigine	Placebo	Difference
Number of patients	890	559	—
Incidence of rash (%)	10.5	5.2	5.3
Withdrawn due to rash (%)	1.9	0.2	1.7

Modified from Yuen AWC. Safety issues. In: Richens A, ed. *Clinical update on lamotrigine: a novel antiepileptic agent.* Tunbridge Wells, UK: Wells Medical 1992:69–75, with permission.

Time Dependency

Skin rash with lamotrigine typically occurs within the first 4 to 8 weeks of treatment, occasionally up to 12 weeks, and only rarely after that. Usually, in the absence of systemic involvement, it resolves on discontinuing the drug without any further therapeutic intervention. The fact that it is an immediate immune-mediated hypersensitivity reaction was demonstrated by substantial increases in the percentage of activated T-helper and activated T-suppressor lymphocytes, a slight increase in the percentage of B lymphocytes, and a greater increase in the serum concentration of immunoglobulin E (IgE) in two children immediately after the first manifestation of a rash (38). In one of these children, reevaluation of immunity 20 days after the rash appeared and lamotrigine had been discontinued showed normal proportions of lymphocytes with a parallel decrease in the serum IgE concentration. In another case, a severe hypersensitivity reaction to lamotrigine developed in a man on combination lamotrigine and valproate therapy; skin tests were found to be negative, whereas lymphocyte stimulation tests *in vitro* were positive on two occasions with lamotrigine (39). Obviously, one of the goals of future immunologic studies is identification of susceptible patients.

Risk Factors

Several risk factors for the development of skin rash with lamotrigine have been identified, including high starting dose and rapid dose escalation (see previous discussion), the presence of valproate in the baseline therapy, pediatric age range, and, possibly, a previous history of allergic reactions. Most rashes recorded in clinical trials with lamotrigine were mild and judged to be nonserious by the investigators, although distinguishing the degree of severity of a given eruption and establishing causality with confidence may not be easy in clinical practice (40).

The incidence of skin rash when lamotrigine was added on to the therapy of patients receiving valproate alone was seen to be in the order of ~13% to 20%; up to ~5% to 14% of patients discontinued the drug, and ~1% to 4 % were hospitalized (17). The lowest incidence usually was associated with the lowest lamotrigine dose. It is unclear whether the occurrence of skin rash in patients comedicated with lamotrigine and valproate is mediated through inhibition of lamotrigine metabolism by valproate (Chapter 37) or through other pathogenetic mechanisms. However, in a recent, large postmarketing survey (41), skin rash occurred in ~14% of patients, with approximately one-half requiring drug discontinuation, but no difference was detected attributable to the presence or absence of valproate in the baseline therapy and, according to the authors, this might have been a consequence of very low initial doses of lamotrigine. Severe rash requiring hospitalization has been reported to occur in <1% of patients in the absence of valproate, and in 1% to 4% when lamotrigine is associated to this drug (17,35). By contrast, when lamotrigine was added on to enzyme-inducing drugs, the incidence of rash was lower than when the drug was used in monotherapy, as was the number of patients who discontinued lamotrigine because of skin rash (17). This protective effect is explained by induction of lamotrigine metabolism, resulting in lower plasma levels of the drug.

Pediatric trials with lamotrigine usually have shown greater incidence of skin rash compared with adult trials, ~12% to 13% with a discontinuation rate of ~5% (17,35,42). Similarly, the proportion of children requiring hospitalization was threefold higher than in adults (0.9% versus 0.3%) (17,35). Two recent trials, however, a randomized, placebo-controlled study (31) and a retrospective investigation (43), have reported a lower incidence (~2%) of rash leading to lamotrigine discontinuation, and this is similar to the incidence observed in adult populations (17,35,36).

Advice Concerning Precautions and Management

If a rash occurs after starting lamotrigine, the drug should be immediately withdrawn because there is evidence that progression to a more serious rash may occur if therapy is continued (35). When a more severe rash occurs and it is accompanied by other manifestations of hypersensitivity, namely, lymphadenopathy, general malaise, fever, and eosinophilia, the need for admission to hospital with prospective administration of intravenous fluids and steroid therapy should be considered. Clearly, because the initial dose and the dose titration play a crucial role in triggering skin rash, it is good practice to prescribe a low starting dose. After 2 weeks, the dose can be doubled; after a further 2 weeks, it can be titrated to an effective maintenance dose. Details of the manufacturer's recommendations for adults and children, in the presence or absence of valproate, are given in Table 39.4. Patients who experienced a previous rash may be considered for rechallenge with lamotrigine if the therapeutic response to the drug was satisfactory (44).

LESS COMMON, BUT CLINICALLY RELEVANT ADVERSE EFFECTS

Less common effects reported with lamotrigine include diarrhea, dyspepsia, rhinitis, tremor, depression, psychosis, increased seizures, and, especially in children, infection, fever, pharyngitis, abdominal pain, influenza-like symptoms, bronchitis, and cough (17,18,30,36). Usually, the incidence of these effects is <10%, the intensity is mild, and discontinuation of lamotrigine is needed in <1% of the patients. For most of these effects, the causative relation to the drug treatment is not clearly proven and, in any case, they resolve over time or with dosage adjustment. In only a minority of patients is it necessary to discontinue the drug. Insomnia, for example, has been reported to occur in 7 of 109 patients exposed to lamotrigine, to be a dose-dependent effect, and to require drug discontinuation in 5 patients (45).

A paradoxical increase in seizures, an effect that almost always needs drug discontinuation, has been reported to occur in 1.5% of patients in lamotrigine add-on studies and in 2.2% in monotherapy studies (17). The incidence has been seen to be much higher (i.e., up to 30% to 40%) in children with severe myoclonic epilepsy (46). Drug-induced exacerbation of seizures is not a new problem with antiepileptic drug therapy. Carbamazepine, phenytoin, some benzodiazepines, and, among the more recent drugs, vigabatrin and gabapentin have been reported to precipitate seizures (47). Analysis of literature reports showed that the phenomenon is mediated by at least two distinct mechanisms: (a) a nonspecific drug intoxication, possibly consequent to an excessive dose or to complex drug combinations; and (b) a specific primary action of the drug in certain types of seizures or particular syndromes (47).

A mild hand tremor occurs in a minority of patients on lamotrigine therapy, and is more common when lamotrigine is combined with sodium valproate (28,29).

Isolated cases of encephalopathy (48), tic disorder (49), pseudolymphoma (50), hepatic involvement (51,52) or adverse hematologic effects such as leukopenia (53), anemia (54), or agranulocytosis (55) have been described in the literature. All the patients involved recovered completely after discontinuation of lamotrigine.

POTENTIALLY LIFE-THREATENING ADVERSE EFFECTS

When systemic manifestations of hypersensitivity, such as general malaise, fever, and eosinophilia, occur and are associated with a rapidly developing, blistering rash and involvement of mucous membranes or even signs of involvement of internal organs, urgent admission to hospital is essential. Two potentially life-threatening disorders

have been reported in a small number of patients started on lamotrigine, the Stevens-Johnson syndrome (SJS) and Lyell's syndrome, or toxic epidermal necrolysis (TEN). These are known to be a rare complication of other antiepileptic drug therapy, including phenytoin, carbamazepine, and valproate (56) and, in some cases, they represent the cutaneous manifestation of a condition that has been labeled the *antiepileptic drug hypersensitivity syndrome*. This syndrome is characterized by the hallmark features of fever, internal organ involvement with lymphadenopathy, and cutaneous reactions.

With lamotrigine, severe rashes, including SJS and TEN, have been reported in approximately 1 in 1,000 to 10,000 adult patients after short-term (within 4 to 8 weeks) exposure to lamotrigine (35,57–59). These values are lower that those with carbamazepine, phenytoin, and phenobarbital, and are similar to those found with valproate (59). Analysis of the literature data suggests that the risk factors for these rare and life-threatening adverse effects are the same as those influencing skin rash (see page 412, Risk Factors).

During the phase III trials program, three patients were reported to have died of disseminated intravascular coagulation and multiorgan failure, but an evaluation of case records of these patients suggested that their condition was the result of seizures rather than treatment with lamotrigine (60). Multiorgan failure is a recognized complication of status epilepticus, and lamotrigine was shown not to affect the coagulation pathways in humans or in a rat model (36). Although a few further cases suggesting induction by lamotrigine have been reported (61–63), the existence of a true causative relationship with lamotrigine therapy still requires further careful investigation.

A case of a child who died of fulminant hepatic failure associated with pulmonary embolism has been described (64).

In early trials, there was concern about the occurrence of sudden, unexpected death among patients receiving lamotrigine. Further analysis has shown, however, that the incidence of this event is within the expected range for the population at risk (65).

MANIFESTATIONS AND MANAGEMENT OF OVERDOSE

Lamotrigine overdose has been described infrequently. In one report (66), a patient inadvertently received four daily doses of lamotrigine, 2,700 mg each, after which he presented with periorbital edema and discrete and confluent blanching red macules and papules involving the face, trunk, and extremities. Laboratory tests revealed leukocytosis, hepatitis, and acute renal failure. All these clinical signs and laboratory abnormalities disappeared after discontinuation of lamotrigine. The same resolution, without any complication, was observed in a case of self-poisoning with lamotrigine (67). A case of lamotrigine overdose also has been described in childhood (68). After ingesting sixteen 50-mg tablets of lamotrigine, a 2-year-old boy had generalized tonic-clonic seizures, tremor of limbs, ataxia, muscle weakness, and hypertonia without any abnormality of vital signs, electroencephalogram, and laboratory tests. Treatment included midazolam and gastric lavage followed by activated charcoal and fluid loads. Symptoms resolved within 24 hours without any other complication. The patient's lamotrigine plasma concentration was 3.8 mg/L.

PREGNANCY

Clinical experience in pregnancy is limited at the time of writing. An analysis in March 2000 of 335 pregnancies during which lamotrigine was being administered (98 as monotherapy) is shown in Table 39.6 (data on file from Glaxo-Wellcome). One hundred sixty-two pregnancies went to term with births without any malformation (76 mothers on monotherapy). Most of the other pregnancies (39, of which 14 were on monotherapy) were terminated by elective abortion.

Of the three malformed neonates from mothers exposed to lamotrigine alone, one presented with an esophageal malformation corrected by surgical intervention, another one with cleft palate, and the third with talipes equinovarus. Malformations occurring in neonates from mothers treated with lamotrigine associated with other conventional antiepileptic drugs have included facial dysmorphisms, cardiac malformations, malformations of the neural tube, extra digits, and others.

Based on these limited data, there is little to suggest that lamotrigine has a major teratogenic effect, but much greater experience, running to several hundred pregnancies, will be necessary before its safety can be assured. In view of the known teratogenic effects of established antiepileptic drugs,

there is no good reason for avoiding lamotrigine during pregnancy.

CONCLUSION

In conclusion, 10 years of marketing experience with lamotrigine indicates that the most common adverse effects of lamotrigine are on the CNS , appearing soon after lamotrigine treatment is started, and rarely requiring lamotrigine discontinuation. Skin rashes occur in approximately 5% of patients treated with the drug, but their incidence can be minimized by starting with a low dose and escalating it slowly. The rashes usually are mild, although rarely they can be serious and life threatening. Although there is no evidence of a major teratogenic effect, the safety of lamotrigine in pregnancy cannot be fully assessed by the experience to date.

REFERENCES

1. Glaxo-Wellcome. *Lamictal Advisory Board briefing document.* Glaxo-Wellcome, May 1, 2000.
2. Miller AA, Wheatley PL, Sawyer DA, et al. Pharmacological studies on lamotrigine, a novel potential antiepileptic drug: I. anticonvulsant profile in mice and rats. *Epilepsy Res* 1986; 27:483–489.
3. Pisani F, Nicolosi C, Macaione V, et al. Long-term lamotrigine therapy does not affect peripheral nerve function. *Epilepsia* 1999; 40:252–253.
4. Cohen AF, Ashby L. Crowley D, et al. Lamotrigine, a potential anticonvulsant: effects on the CNS in comparison with phenytoin and diazepam. *Br J Clin Pharmacol* 1985;20:619–629.
5. Hamilton MI, Cohen AF, Yuen AWC, et al. Carbamazepine and lamotrigine in healthy volunteers: relevance to early tolerance and clinical trial dosage. *Epilepsy Res* 1993;34:166–173.
6. Jawad S, Oxley J, Yuen WC, et al. The effect of lamotrigine, a novel anticonvulsant, on interictal spikes in patients with epilepsy. *Br J Clin Pharmacol* 1986;22:191–193.
7. Binnie CD, Von Emde Boas W, Kasteleijn-Nolst Trenite DGA, et al. Acute effects of lamotrigine (BW43OC) in persons with epilepsy. *Epilepsia* 1986;27:248–254.
8. Binnie C, Debets R, Engelman M, et al. Double-blind, crossover trial of lamotrigine (Lamictal) as add-on therapy in intractable epilepsy. *Epilepsy Res* 1989;4:222–229.
9. Jawad S, Richens A, Yuen AWC. Controlled trial of lamotrigine for refractory partial epilepsy. *Epilepsia* 1989;30:356–363.
10. Loiseau P, Yuen W, Duche B, et al. A randomized double-blind, placebo-controlled, cross-over, add-on trial of lamotrigine in patients with treatment-resistant partial seizures. *Epilepsy Res* 1990;7:136–145.
11. Sander J, Patsalos P, Oxley J, et al. A randomized, double-blind, placebo-controlled, add-on trial of lamotrigine in patients with severe epilepsy. *Epilepsy Res* 1990;6:221–-226.
12. Betts T, Goodwin O, Withers RM, et al. Human safety of lamotrigine. *Epilepsy Res* 1991;32[Suppl 2]:S17–S21.
13. Schapel GJ, Beran RG, Vajda FJE, et al. Double-blind placebo controlled crossover study on lamotrigine in treatment resistant partial seizures. *J Neurol Neurosurg Psychiatry* 1993;56;448–453.
14. Smith D, Baker G, Davies G, et al. Outcomes of add-on treat-

TABLE 39.6. PREGNANCIES OCCURRING IN PATIENTS RECEIVING LAMOTRIGINE

	Lamotrigine Only	Lamotrigine and Antiepileptic Drugs
Births		
Normal	76	186
Abnormal	3	14
Abortion		
Spontaneous	4	9
Elective[a]	14	25
Abnormal	0	2
Fetal death[b]	1	1
Total	98	237

[a]For causes different from ascertainment of fetal malformations.
[b]Without demonstrated fetal malformations.
From Glaxo-Wellcome database, March 31, 2000, with permission.

ment with lamotrigine in partial epilepsy. *Epilepsia* 1993:34: 312–322.

15. Schachter SC, Leppik IE, Matsuo F, et al. A multicentre, placebo-controlled evaluation of the safety of lamotrigine (Lamictal) as add-on therapy in outpatients with partial seizures. *Epilepsy Res* 1992;33[Suppl 3]:1–19.

16. Marson AG, Kadir ZA, Chadwick DW. New antiepileptic drugs: a systematic review of their efficacy and tolerability. *BMJ* 1996; 313:1169–1174.

17. Messenheimer J, Mullens EL, Giorgi L, et al. Safety review of adult clinical trial experience with lamotrigine. *Drug Saf* 1998; 18:281–296.

18. Cramer J, Fisher R, Ben-Menachem E, et al. New antiepileptic drugs: comparison of key clinical trials. *Epilepsia* 1999;40: 590–600.

19. Betts T. Safety of lamotrigine. In: Richens A, ed. *Clinical update on lamotrigine: a novel antiepileptic agent.* Tunbridge Wells, UK: Wells Medical, 1992:61– 68.

20. Kilpatrick ES, Forrest G, Brodie MJ. Concentration-effect and concentration-toxicity relations with lamotrigine: a prospective study. *Epilepsia* 1996;37:534–538.

21. Morris RG, Black AB, Harris AL, et al. Lamotrigine and therapeutic drug monitoring: retrospective survey following the introduction of a routine service. *Br J Clin Pharmacol* 1998;46: 547–551.

22. Brodie MJ, Richens A, Yuen AW. Double-blind comparison of lamotrigine and carbamazepine and lamotrigine in newly diagnosed epilepsy: UK Lamotrigine/Carbamazepine Monotherapy Trial Group. *Lancet* 1995;345:476–479.

23. Reunanen M, Dam M, Yuen AW. A randomised open multicentre comparative trial of lamotrigine and carbamazepine as monotherapy in patients with newly diagnosed or recurrent epilepsy. *Epilepsy Res* 1996;23:149–155.

24. Gilliam F, Wazquez B, Sackellares JC, et al. An active-control trial of lamotrigine monotherapy for partial seizures. *Neurology* 1998;51:1018–1025.

25. Steiner TJ, Dellaportas CI, Findley LJ, et al. Lamotrigine monotherapy in newly diagnosed untreated epilepsy: a double-blind comparison with phenytoin. *Epilepsia* 1999;40:601–607.

26. Matsuo F, Bergen D, Faught E, et al. Placebo-controlled study of the efficacy and safety of lamotrigine in patients with partial seizures. *Neurology* 1993;43:2284–2291.

27. Messenheimer J, Ramsay RE, Willmore U, et al. Lamotrigine therapy for partial seizures: a multicenter, placebo-controlled, double-blind, cross-over trial. *Epilepsia* 1994;35:113–121.

28. Reutens DC, Duncan JS, Patsalos PN. Disabling tremor after lamotrigine with sodium valproate. *Lancet* 1993;542:185–186.

29. Pisani F, Oteri G, Russo MF, et al. The efficacy of valproate-lamotrigine comedication in refractory complex partial seizures: evidence for a pharmacodynamic interaction. *Epilepsia* 1999;40:1141–1146.

30. Messenheimer A, Giorgi L, Risner ME. The tolerability of lamotrigine in children. *Drug Saf* 2000;22:303–312.

31. Duchowny M, Pellock JM, Graf WD, et al. A placebo-controlled trial of lamotrigine add-on therapy for partial seizures in children: Lamictal Pediatric Partial Seizure Study Group. *Neurology* 1999;53:1724–1731.

32. Posner J, Holdich T, Crome P. Comparison of lamotrigine pharmacokinetics in young and elderly healthy volunteers. *J Pharm Med* 1991:1:121–128.

33. Brodie MJ, Overstall PW, Giorgi L, et al. Multicentre, double-blind, randomised comparison between lamotrigine and carbamazepine in elderly patients with newly diagnosed epilepsy. *Epilepsy Res* 1999;37:81–87.

34. Gillham R, et al. A double blind comparison of lamotrigine and carbamazepine in newly diagnosed epilepsy with health related quality of life as an outcome measure. *Seizure* 2000;9:375–379.

35. Guberman AH, Besag FM, Brodie, et al. Lamotrigine-associated rash: risk/benefit considerations in adults and children. *Epilepsia* 1999;40:985–991.

36. Yuen AWC. Safety issues. In: Richens A, ed. *Clinical update on lamotrigine: a novel antiepileptic agent.* Tunbridge Wells, UK: Wells Medical, 1992:69–75.

37. Chadwick D, Shaw M, Foy P, et al. Serum anticonvulsant concentrations ad the risk of drug induced skin eruptions. *J Neurol Neurosurg Psychiatry* 1984;47:642–644.

38. Iannetti P, Raucci U, Zuccaro P, et al. Lamotrigine hypersensitivity in childhood epilepsy. *Epilepsia* 1998;39:502–507

39. Schaub N, Bircher AJ. Severe hypersensitivity syndrome to lamotrigine confirmed by lymphocyte stimulation in vitro. *Allergy* 2000;55:191–193.

40. Roujeau JC, Stern RS. Severe adverse cutaneous reactions to drugs. *N Engl J Med* 1994;331:1272–1285.

41. Faught E, Morris G, Jacobson M, et al. Adding lamotrigine to valproate: incidence of rash and other adverse effects. Postmarketing Antiepileptic Drug Survey (PADS) Group. *Epilepsia* 1999; 49:1135–1140.

42. Dooley J, Camfield P, Gordon K, et al. Lamotrigine-induced rash in children. *Neurology* 1996;46:240–242.

43. Barron TF, Hunt SL, Hoban TF, et al. Lamotrigine monotherapy in children. *Pediatr Neurol* 2000;23:160–163.

44. Tavernor SJ, Wong IC, Newton R, et al. Rechallenge with lamotrigine after initial rash. *Seizure* 1995;4:67–71.

45. Sadler M. Lamotrigine associated with insomnia. *Epilepsia* 1999;40:322–325.

46. Guerrini R, Dravet E, Genton P, et al. Lamotrigine and seizure aggravation in severe myoclonic epilepsy. *Epilepsia* 1998;39: 508–512.

47. Perucca E, Gram L, Avanzini G, et al. Antiepileptic drugs as a cause of worsening seizures. *Epilepsia* 1998;39:5–17.

48. Hennessy MJ, Wiles CM. Lamotrigine encephalopathy. *Lancet* 1996;347:974–975.

49. Sotero de Menezes MA, Rho JM, Murphy P, et al. Lamotrigine-induced tic disorder: report of five pediatric cases. *Epilepsia* 2000;41:862–867.

50. Pathak P, McLachian RS. Drug-induced pseudolymphoma secondary to lamotrigine. *Neurology* 1998;50:1509–1510.

51. Arnon R, De Vivo D, Defelice AR, et al. Acute hepatic failure in a child treated with lamotrigine. *Pediatr Neurol* 1998;18: 251–251.

52. Fayad M, Choueiri R, Mikati M. Potential hepatotoxicity of lamotrigine. *Pediatr Neurol* 2000;22:49–52.

53. Nicholson RJ, Kelly KP, Grant IS. Leucopenia associated with lamotrigine. *BMJ* 1995;310:504.

54. Esfahani FE, Dasheiff RM. Anemia associated with lamotrigine. *Neurology* 1997;49:306–307.

55. De Camargo OA, Bode H. Agranulocytosis associated with lamotrigine. *BMJ* 1999;318:1179.

56. Tennis P, Stern RS. Risk of cutaneous disorders after initiation of use of phenytoin, carbamazepine, or sodium valproate: a record linkage study. *Neurology* 1997;49:542–546.

57. Richens A. Safety of lamotrigine. *Epilepsia* 1994;35:S37–S40.

58. Schlienger RG, Shapiro LE, Shear NH. Lamotrigine-induced severe cutaneous adverse reactions. *Epilepsia* 1998;39[Suppl 7]: 22–26.

59. Rzany B, Correia O, Kelly JP, et al. Risk of Stevens-Johnson syndrome and toxic epidermal necrolysis during first weeks of antiepileptic therapy: a case-control study: Study Group of the International Case Control Study on Severe Cutaneous Adverse Reactions. *Lancet* 1999;353:2190–2194.

60. Yuen AWC, Bihari DJ. Multiorgan failure with disseminated intravascular coagulation in severe convulsive seizures. *Lancet* 1992;340:618.

61. Schaub JE, Williamson PJ, Barnes EW, et al. Multisystem adverse reaction to lamotrigine. *Lancet* 1994;344:281.

62. Chattergoon DS, McGuigan MA, Koren G, et al. Multiorgan dysfunction and disseminated intravascular coagulation in children receiving lamotrigine and valproic acid. *Neurology* 1997;49: 1442–1444.

63. Wadelius M, Karlsson T, Wadelius E, et al. Lamotrigine and toxic epidermal necrolysis. *Lancet* 1996;348:1392.

64. Makin AJ, Fitt S, Williams R, et al. Fulminant hepatic failure induced by lamotrigine. *BMJ* 1995;311:292.

65. Leestma JE, Annegers JF, Brodie MJ, et al. Incidence of sudden unexplained death in the Lamictal (lamotrigine) clinical development program. *Epilepsia* 1994;35:12.

66. Mylonakis E, Vittorio CC, Hollik DA, et al. Lamotrigine overdose presenting as anticonvulsant hypersensitivity syndrome. *Ann Pharmacother* 1999;33:557–559.

67. Buckley NA, Whyte IM, Dawson AH. Self-poisoning with lamotrigine. *Lancet* 1993; 342:1552–1553.

68. Briassoulis G, Kalabalikis P, Tamiolaki M, et al. Lamotrigine childhood overdose. *Pediatr Neurol* 1998;19:239–242.

Antiepileptic Drugs, 5th Edition. Edited by R.H. Levy, R.H. Mattson, B.S. Meldrum, and E. Perucca. Lippincott Williams & Wilkins, Philadelphia © 2002.

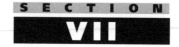

LEVETIRACETAM

LEVETIRACETAM

MECHANISMS OF ACTION

DORU GEORG MARGINEANU
HENRIK KLITGAARD

Levetiracetam [LEV; ucb L059; (S)-α-ethyl-2-oxo-pyrrolidine acetamide; Figure 40.1] is the (S)-enantiomer of the ethyl analog of piracetam (Figure 40.1), synthesized during a follow-up chemical program aimed at identifying a second-generation nootropic drug. Consequently, the initial pharmacologic studies with LEV explored its ability to facilitate cholinergic neurotransmission (1). However, *in vivo* results demonstrated an unexpected potent ability of LEV to suppress seizures in the audiogenic-susceptible mouse (2), unlike piracetam, which was only weakly active. Further testing in the same model has shown that LEV remains active after injection directly into the brain, whereas both its (R)-enantiomer (ucb L060; Figure 40.1) and the main metabolite of LEV (ucb L057; Figure 40.1) lack activity in this model (2,3), suggesting that the observed seizure suppression relates to a specific central action of the parent compound.

Adjunctive therapy with LEV (Keppra, UCB S.A., Braine-l'Allend, Belgium) was recently proven effective and very well tolerated in controlling refractory partial seizures in adults (4). This resulted in a marketing authorization from the U.S. Food and Drug Administration in December 1999 and from the European Medicines Evaluation Agency (EMEA) in September 2000. However, the current understanding of the antiepileptic mechanisms of LEV is at an early stage because it is a molecule unrelated to established antiepileptic drugs (AEDs).

The prevailing consensus that cell biology provides the ultimate conceptual frame for understanding the physiopathology of disease has stimulated the search at the cellular level for the abnormalities that underlie seizures (5). This obviously is legitimate, but complicated by the fact that epilepsy is a brain pathologic condition of large neuronal populations. The main cellular mechanisms that are thought to account for the antiseizure activities of the established AEDs refer to either (a) facilitation of inhibitory γ-aminobutyric acid (GABA)-ergic neurotransmission; (b) inhibition of excitatory glutamate receptors; or (c) block of voltage-gated Na^+ or Ca^{2+} channels. This chapter reviews the effects of LEV on these and other mechanisms presumed to be of antiepileptic relevance.

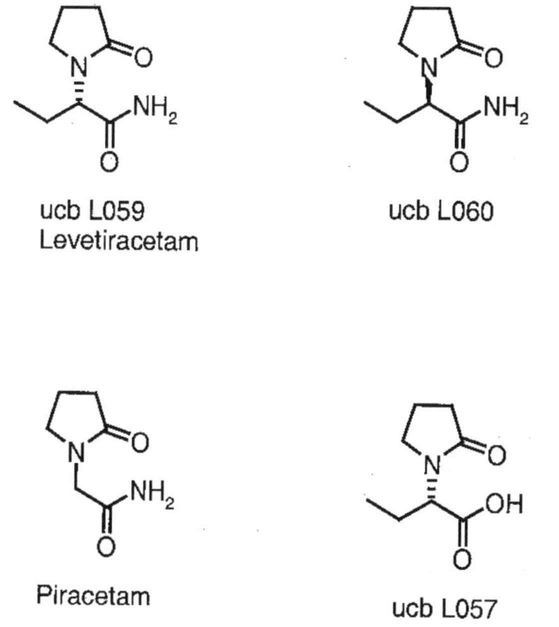

FIGURE 40.1. Chemical structures of levetiracetam and of its (R)-enantiomer, ucb L060, along with the pyrrolidine compound, piracetam, and the main metabolite of levetiracetam, ucb L057.

Doru Georg Margineanu, PhD: Senior Scientist, Preclinical CNS Research, UCB S.A. Pharma Sector, Braine-l'Alleud, Belgium

Henrik Klitgaard, PhD: Director, Preclinical CNS Research, UCB S.A. Pharma Sector, Braine-l'Alleud, Belgium

EFFECTS IN ANIMAL MODELS OF SEIZURES AND EPILEPSY

LEV differs from other known AEDs by a lack of anticonvulsant activity in the two classic screening tests for AEDs in mice and rats, the maximal electroshock seizure (MES) and pentylenetetrazol (PTZ) models (3,6). Testing in other seizure paradigms in rodents has confirmed a weak anticonvulsant activity in threshold tests involving acute electrical or chemical stimulation (6), and only modest protection was observed against acute seizures induced by submaximal doses of chemoconvulsants (2). This is in contrast to the potent seizure suppression observed in animal models of chronic epilepsy, involving genetic and kindled animals with spontaneous, recurrent seizures or with seizures showing a phenomenology similar to human epileptic seizures.

A striking example is the potent seizure protection afforded by LEV in corneal electroshock– and PTZ-kindled mice and the absence of anticonvulsant activity against MES and PTZ seizures in normal mice (Table 40.1). This observation is supported further by results with fully amygdala-kindled rats (6), phenytoin-resistant amygdala-kindled rats (7), and hippocampal-kindled rats (8), confirming that LEV provides dose-dependent protection against several seizure parameters in kindled animals, including motor seizure severity and the duration of motor seizures and afterdischarges. Likewise, results with LEV in genetic animal models of epilepsy also revealed a suppression of several seizure parameters, including protection against postural stimulation–induced seizures in epilepsy-like mice (9), seizures induced by acoustic stimulation in mice (2) and rats (10), and spontaneous spike-and-wave discharges (SWDs) in the Genetic Absence Epilepsy Rat from Strasbourg (GAERS) model (10).

The behavioral alterations induced by LEV do not differ between normal and kindled animals, showing only mild sedative and ataxic properties, and no psychotomimetic effects (2,3,6). Likewise, LEV is devoid of negative impact on cognitive performance in normal and kindled rats (11). Sedation and muscle relaxation occur only at doses above 1,000 mg/kg, showing that LEV has a low adverse effect potential in rodents. Combined with its potent seizure protection, this results in an unusually high safety margin for LEV in animal models mimicking both partial and generalized epilepsy (Figure 40.2).

Among the major AEDs in clinical use, only valproate and phenobarbital appear to suppress kindling acquisition, but do so only at doses associated with adverse effects (12). LEV has been reported to inhibit the development of PTZ kindling in mice (2) and amygdala kindling in rats (13) at doses devoid of adverse effects. Afterdischarges recorded from amygdala in animals previously treated with LEV remained significantly shorter compared with vehicle controls in the latter study, despite cessation of LEV treatment and continued amygdala stimulations. This observation led to several experimental approaches that currently are assessing the antiepileptogenic potential of LEV.

Taken together, these findings suggest that LEV is devoid of anticonvulsant activity in traditional seizure screening models, but reveals a potent broad-spectrum activity with a wide safety margin in animal models of chronic epilepsy reflecting both partial and generalized epilepsy. This preferential action in animal models of chronic epilepsy markedly distinguishes LEV from classical AEDs (Table 40.1).

TABLE 40.1. EFFECTS OF LEVETIRACETAM VERSUS CLASSIC ANTIEPILEPTIC DRUGS ON SUPRAMAXIMAL ELECTROSHOCK, MAXIMAL SUBCUTANEOUS PENTYLENETETRAZOL, CORNEAL ELECTROSHOCK-KINDLED AND PENTYLENETETRAZOL-KINDLED SEIZURES IN MICE[a]

Antiepileptic Drug	ED$_{50}$ (mgkg i.p.)			
	MES	s.c. PTZ	Electroshock Kindling	PTZ Kindling
Levetiracetam	>540	>540	7 (2–10)	36 (15–96)
Valproate	188 (154–216)	106 (64–170)	66 (52–83)	147 (116–189)
Phenobarbital	12 (9–16)	11 (7–18)	12 (8–17)	5 (3–7)
Clonazepam	>3	0.02 (0.01–0.04)	0.03 (0.02–0.05)	0.03 (0.02–0.04)
Ethosuximide	>452	126 (78–196)	>254	117 (99–161)
Carbamazepine	6 (5–9)	>42	6 (4–10)	17 (8–28)
Phenytoin	6 (4–10)	>45[b]	6 (1–16)	38 (22–171)

i.p., intraperitoneally; MES, supramaximal electroshock; s.c. PTZ, subcutaneous pentylenetetrazol.
[a]Values given are ED$_{50}$values, i.e. the doses protecting 50% of the animals, with associated 95% confidence intervals. All compounds were administered at their optimal pretreatment times.
Protection against clonic convulsions occurred in a significant ($p < .05$) proportion of the animals.
From Klitgaard H, Matagne A, Gobert J, et al. Evidence for a unique profile of levetiracetam in rodent models of seizures and epilepsy. *Eur J Pharmacol* 1998;353:191–206, with permission from Elsevier Science.

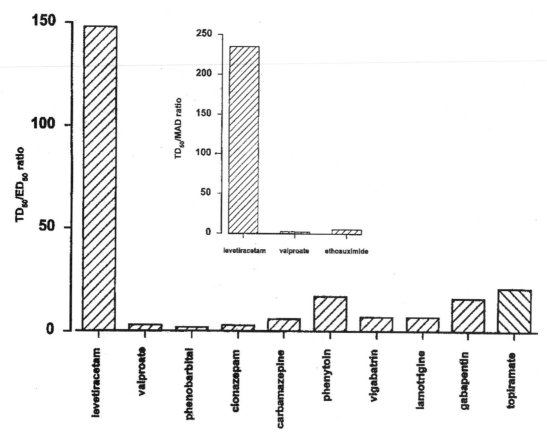

FIGURE 40.2. Safety margins of levetiracetam versus other antiepileptic drugs in corneally kindled mice (main graph) and versus valproate and ethosuximide in Genetic Absence Epilepsy Rat from Strasbourg (GAERS) animals (*inset*). The safety margins are expressed as the ratios of the median toxic dose (TD_{50}) value for Rotorod impairment and either the protective median effective dose (ED_{50}) value against motor seizures, in corneally kindled mice, or the minimum active dose (MAD) reducing significantly the duration of spontaneous spike-and-wave discharges in GAERS rats. For topiramate, the protective ED_{50} value in the maximal electroshock seizure test and the TD_{50} value for Rotorod impairment in normal mice were used owing to the lack of effect of this drug against corneally kindled seizures. (From Klitgaard H, Matagne A, Gobert J, et al. Evidence for a unique profile of levetiracetam in rodent models of seizures and epilepsy. *Eur J Pharmacol* 1998;353:191–206, with permission from Elsevier Science.)

EFFECTS ON NORMAL AND EPILEPTIFORM ELECTROPHYSIOLOGIC RESPONSES

Electrophysiologic recordings, performed both *in vivo* and *in vitro*, consistently showed an absence of any intrinsic effect of LEV on normal neural responses and neuronal characteristics. An early report of the anticonvulsant profile of LEV in rodents (2) indicated that LEV did not change the baseline electroencephalogram (EEG), unlike clonazepam, which increased the proportion of lower-frequency background activity (in rats injected with PTZ to induce SWDs; see later). Similarly, in the GAERS model of absence seizures, LEV left the baseline EEG trace normal, whereas it markedly suppressed the SWDs (see later) (10). Finally, in urethane-anesthetized rats, LEV did not modify

the field potentials recorded in hippocampal CA3 area, in response to commissural stimulation (14).

In agreement with these *in vivo* observations, it also was reported that LEV, perfused for 20 minutes at a concentration of 10 μmol/L, did not alter basic cell characteristics or normal synaptic transmission in pyramidal neurons in the CA3 area of rat hippocampal slices (15), whereas it suppressed epileptiform activity (see later). That study lists no effects of LEV on membrane potential, input resistance, amplitude, duration at half-amplitude and area of the action potential evoked by stimulation of commissural afferents, amplitudes of fast and slow after-hyperpolarizations, amplitudes of excitatory (EPSP) and fast inhibitory (IPSP) postsynaptic potentials evoked by subthreshold stimulation, area of EPSP and amplitudes of fast and slow

IPSPs evoked by suprathreshold stimulation, and amplitudes of baclofen-induced hyperpolarization and (1S,3R)-ACPD- and *N*-methyl-D-aspartate (NMDA)–induced depolarizations [Table 1 in Birnstiel et al., (15)].

The absence of effect of LEV on normal electrophysiologic responses is in contrast to its clear-cut effects on epileptiform electrophysiologic responses, both *in vitro* and *in vivo*. A perfusion of LEV at 10 μmol/L for 20 minutes markedly inhibited the development of epileptiform bursting induced by the GABA$_A$ receptor antagonist bicuculline methiodide (BMI) in CA3 pyramidal neurons from rat hippocampal slices (15). LEV (3 to 100 μmol/L) added to the perfusion medium 30 minutes after BMI caused a concentration-dependent decrease in the area of the bursts, without altering the after-hyperpolarization that follows the bursts. LEV (10 μmol/L) significantly reduced the frequency of the spontaneous bursting induced by application of NMDA, 10 or 15 μmol/L, in CA3 pyramidal neurons from rat hippocampal slices *in vitro*, although no consistent effect was observed on the size of the bursts (15). In another study, LEV (200 and 400 μmol/L) significantly reduced the length of the seizure-like population bursts recorded extracellularly in the CA1 area of rat hippocampal slices that were bathed in a medium with bicuculline and increased potassium (16). These *in vitro* effects of LEV against epileptiform discharges induced by BMI (or bicuculline) agree with the action of the drug when administered systemically (3.2 to 32 μmol/kg intravenously) to inhibit the epileptiform effect of BMI (applied locally, through the recording microelectrode) on the field potentials recorded in the hippocampal CA3 area of anesthetized rats (17).

We have shown that LEV (32 and 100 μmol/L) consistently diminished the epileptiform field potentials recorded in the CA3 area of rat hippocampal slices that were bathed in an epileptogenic medium containing increased (7.5 mmol/L) potassium and lowered (0.5 mmol/L) calcium (18). LEV, along with the classic AEDs valproate, clonazepam, and carbamazepine, reduced the number of repetitive population spikes evoked by single stimuli when the slices were in the epileptogenic medium, whereas it differed from these reference AEDs in its specific ability to reduce population spike amplitude (i.e., to antagonize neuronal hypersynchronization). In agreement with this, an electrographic study in rats has shown that LEV [17 mg/kg intraperitoneally (i.p.)] also differed from reference AEDs in not interfering with the onset of spike-and-burst discharges in the hippocampus induced by systemic administration of pilocarpine. Instead, LEV selectively inhibited the synchronization necessary for their propagation to the cortex. Likewise, LEV (170 mg/kg i.p.) had no impact on the appearance of kainic acid–induced spike-and-burst discharges in the hippocampus, but it retarded their generalization to the cortex (19).

In vivo demonstration of LEV's effect on epileptiform EEG activity was observed in several rat models of epilepsy. LEV (17 mg/kg i.p.) reduced the cumulative duration of SWDs induced in rats by a subconvulsant dose of PTZ (2). In GAERS rats, LEV markedly reduced the cumulative duration of spontaneous SWDs to between 15% and 30% of the predrug level, with a dose as low as 5.4 mg/kg i.p. and no further incremental effect at higher doses (10). As mentioned previously, a prominent effect of LEV against electrographic epileptiform discharges *in vivo* is to reduce the duration of the afterdischarges recorded in amygdala-kindled rats, observed with both acute (13 to 108 mg/kg i.p.) (6) and chronic (13 to 54 mg/kg/day i.p.) (13) administration of the drug.

Table 40.2 summarizes the main currently reported effects of LEV on epileptiform discharges, both *in vivo* and

TABLE 40.2. EFFECTS OF LEVETIRACETAM ON EPILEPTIFORM ELECTROPHYSIOLOGIC EVENTS, RECORDED IN RAT EPILEPSY MODELS, REPORTED TO DATE IN FULL-LENGTH ARTICLES

Animal Model	Electrophysiologic Recording	Reported Action of Levetiracetam	References
In vivo			
Freely moving rats	Electroencephalogram	Inhibition of pentylenetetrazol-induced spike-and-wave discharges	2
		Inhibition of spontaneous spike-and-wave discharges in GAERS rats	10
		Reduction of afterdischarge duration in amygdala-kindled rats	6, 13
Anesthetized rats	Evoked field potentials	Inhibition of bicuculline-induced increases in amplitude of hippocampal population spikes	14, 17
In vitro			
Rat hippocampal slices	Evoked field potentials	Reduction of the amplitudes and the number of repetitive population spikes induced by a "high K$^+$–low Ca^{2+}" perfusion fluid	18
	Action potentials (intracellular recordings) in pyramidal neurons	Inhibition of bicuculline-induced bursts of action potentials and of the frequency of bursting induced by *N*-methyl-D-aspartate	15

GAERS, genetic absence epilepsy rat from Strasbourg.

in vitro. Several of these effects were not dose or concentration dependent, suggesting that the antiepileptic action of the drug may involve multiple mechanisms.

BRAIN-SPECIFIC BINDING OF [³H]LEVETIRACETAM

A specific [³H]LEV binding site (LBS), which is saturable, reversible, and stereoselective, has been reported to exist in rat brain membranes (20–22). LBS appears to be located in brain structures, with high densities in the cortex, hippocampus, and cerebellum, whereas it was not detected in a range of peripheral tissues (Figure 40.3). [³H]LEV was reported to label a single class of binding sites in hippocampal membranes, with modest affinity (K_d = 780 ± 115 nmol/L) and high binding capacity (B_{max} = 9.1 ± 1.2 pmol/mg protein) (22). The rank order of affinity for LBS of the (*S*)-stereoisomer homologs of LEV appeared well correlated with their anticonvulsant activity against the expression of tonic convulsions in the audiogenic mouse test (Figure 40.3, inset). This correlation suggests a possible functional role for LBS in the antiepileptic mechanisms of LEV.

LEV, up to 10 µmol/L, did not displace known radioligands from a large variety of binding sites presumed to be related to altered neural excitability (22). Thus, no affinity was observed for opiate, adenosine, adrenergic, cholinergic, dopaminergic, serotonergic, histaminergic, glutamatergic, $GABA_B$, and $GABA_A$/benzodiazepine receptors. Monoamine reuptake sites, peptide-specific receptors, second messenger systems such as adenylate cyclase and protein kinase C, and different ion channel proteins likewise were unaffected. Neither phenytoin, carbamazepine, sodium valproate, phenobarbital, nor the benzodiazepines, diazepam and clonazepam, displayed any relevant affinity for the LBS. However, the anticonvulsants ethosuximide and pentobarbital, and the GABA-related convulsants, PTZ and bemegride, were effective at concentrations comparable with active drug concentrations *in vivo* (22). Sacaan and Lloyd (21) reported that the T-type calcium channel antagonist amiloride inhibited the binding of [³H]LEV, and the anticonvulsants trimethadione and dimethadione displaced the binding of [³H]LEV with inhibitory concentration 50% (IC_{50}) values close to their anticonvulsant plasma levels. However, the affinity of dimethadione for LBS was shown by Noyer et al. (22) to correspond to a pK_i ≤2.0, suggesting a very low affinity for the LBS.

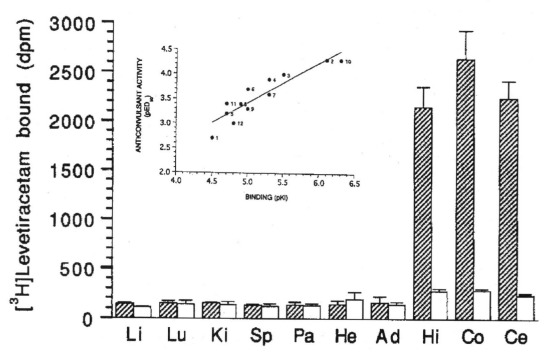

FIGURE 40.3. Binding of [³H]levetiracetam in rat brain (Hi, hippocampus; Co, cortex; Ce, cerebellum) and peripheral tissues (Li, liver; Lu, lung; Ki, kidney; Sp, spleen; Pa, pancreas; He, heart; Ad, adrenals). The *hatched columns* indicate the total binding and the *open columns* indicate the nonspecific binding. The *inset* shows the correlation of the anticonvulsant activity of (*S*)-homologs of levetiracetam in the audiogenic mouse with their affinity at the [³H]levetiracetam binding site. Points 1 and 2 on the plot represent piracetam and levetiracetam, respectively. [From Noyer M, Gillard M, Matagne A, et al. The novel antiepileptic drug levetiracetam (ucb L059) appears to act via a specific binding site in CNS membranes. *Eur J Pharmacol* 1995;286:137–146, with permission from Elsevier Science.]

In summary, stereoselective, reversible, low-affinity, high-capacity binding of LEV was identified in rat brain membranes, on a specific site not present in peripheral tissues and distinct from binding sites known to alter neuronal excitability. Intense investigations are in progress at UCB Pharma to isolate this binding site and help to further the understanding of its possible role in the antiepileptic mechanism of LEV.

EFFECTS ON NEUROTRANSMITTER SYSTEMS

Ionotropic Inhibitory Receptors

Systemic administration of LEV at doses known to suppress seizures in the rat (1.7 to 170 mg/kg i.p.) was reported to induce alterations in GABA metabolism and turnover in several brain regions (23). LEV, 170 mg/kg i.p., increased the activity of the GABA-degrading enzyme GABA aminotransferase (GABA-T) in 7 of 12 brain regions studied, but the effect was short-lived (~15 minutes) and it was observed only at this relatively high dose. In the striatum, the significant increase in GABA-T activity, observed 15 minutes after LEV 170 mg/kg i.p., was associated with a decrease in activity of the GABA-synthesizing enzyme glutamic acid decarboxylase (GAD), leading to a significant reduction in regional GABA turnover. This was followed, however, by a pronounced increase in striatal GABA turnover, and the activities of both GABA-T and GAD were nearly normalized 60 minutes after LEV, in all brain regions. The reduction of GABAergic activity in the striatum has been reported to be anticonvulsant (24) because a disinhibited striatal output enhances inhibition in the substantia nigra pars reticulata, which receives a strong GABAergic input from the striatum and is known to control seizure propagation (25). Indeed, Löscher et al. (23) recorded decreased spontaneous firing of nondopaminergic, presumably GABAergic neurons in the substantia nigra pars reticulata after LEV 170 mg/kg i.p. administration. However, because LEV induced both increases and decreases in GABA-T and GAD activities and did not alter either GABA-T or GAD activities *in vitro*, Löscher et al. (23) inferred that the enzyme alterations they found were not direct effects of LEV, but possibly indirect consequences of postsynaptic changes. Moreover, the fact that GABA turnover was normalized 60 minutes after LEV casts serious doubts on the anticonvulsant relevance of the regional alterations in GABA turnover for the antiepileptic action of LEV, because the time of the peak effect of LEV was previously reported from the same laboratory to be 60 minutes in both mice and rats (6). Furthermore, neurochemical studies in mouse brains (26) indicated that LEV (up to 300 mg/kg i.p.; single/multiple doses) had no effect on the concentrations of GABA, glutamate, and glutamine, and on the activities of GAD and GABA-T. Also, the same group reported that a 1-hour exposure to LEV had no effect on GABA transport and metabolism in rat astrocyte culture (27). Accordingly, these authors concluded that it is

unlikely that the action of LEV would be mediated through the GABAergic system (26,27).

LEV produced only minor and contrasting effects on GABA-induced currents recorded by whole-cell patch-clamp methods in cultured rat cerebellar granule and hippocampal neurons (28). They consisted of a small reduction in the peak amplitude and a prolongation of the decay phase. However, these effects were significant only at LEV concentrations beyond 100 μmol/L. Interestingly, LEV potently suppressed (median effective dose = 1 – 10 μmol/L) the inhibitory effects of several negative allosteric modulators (Zn^{2+}, β-carbolines, chlordiazepam) on GABA-gated currents in cultured rat hippocampal and cerebellar granule neurons and glycine-gated currents in spinal cord neurons (28). These results are remarkable in view of the hypothesis that suggests that the hyperexcitability characteristics of the epileptic hippocampus may be associated with circuit and cellular alterations in dentate granule cells (DGCs). These involve changes both in the subunit expression pattern of GABA$_A$ receptors, rendering them more sensitive to inhibition by Zn^{2+}, and in sprouting of Zn^{2+}-containing DGC axons (mossy fibers) back onto the inner molecular layer of the dentate gyrus (29). This creates an environment in which excessive Zn^{2+} is released during repetitive activation of DGCs and is purported to result in a pathologic lowering of inhibition as well as an enhanced seizure propensity in the epileptic hippocampus.

Ionotropic Excitatory Receptors

Single and repeated systemic administrations of LEV (1 to 300 mg/kg i.p.) were reported to have no effect on glutamine synthetase, a key enzyme in the regulation of glutamate neurotransmission, in mouse brain (30).

LEV at high concentrations (IC$_{50}$ = 268 μmol/L) inhibited the α-amino-3-hydroxy-5-methylisoxazole-4-propionic acid (AMPA)–gated current in cultured rat hippocampal neurons, although it was without effect on the currents gated by either NMDA or kainate. The inhibition by LEV of α-amino-3-hydroxy-5-methylisoxazole-4-propionic acid–gated currents, however, seems to lack antiseizure relevance in view of the relatively high concentration at which it was observed and because LEV is ineffective in suppressing the clonic convulsions induced *in vivo* by AMPA, kainic acid, or NMDA (31).

Dopaminergic System

A neurochemical study in the rat (32) has reported that systemic pretreatment with LEV (17 mg/kg i.p.) prevented an increase in the extracellular levels of dopamine and its metabolites (dihydroxyphenylacetic acid and homovanillic acid) induced by a subconvulsant dose of bicuculline (3 mg/kg i.p.). This appears to be an indirect effect of the ability of LEV to inhibit the epileptiform modifications induced by bicuculline described previously because the same study showed only a minimal effect of LEV against haloperidol-induced enhancement of the release of dopamine and its metabolites.

EFFECTS ON NEURONAL VOLTAGE-GATED IONIC CURRENTS

Na$^+$ Current

LEV (up to 1 mmol/L) did not inhibit or modify the biophysical properties (steady-state activation and inactivation, time to peak, fast kinetics of inactivation, and recovery from steady-state inactivation) of the tetrodotoxin (TTX)-sensitive, inward, voltage-dependent Na$^+$ current, recorded in the whole-cell configuration of the patch-clamp technique, in cultured rat cortical neurons (33).

Ca^{2+} Currents

LEV (32 and 100 μmol/L) did not inhibit or modify the biophysical properties of the low-voltage–activated (T-type) Ca^{2+} current, recorded in the whole-cell configuration of the patch-clamp technique, in pyramidal neurons from the CA1 area of rat hippocampal slices (34). On the other hand, LEV (32 μmol/L) depressed high-voltage–activated Ca^{2+} currents in visually identified pyramidal neurons from

rat hippocampal slices (35) (with inhibition becoming significant after a 30-minute perfusion of the drug). The type of LEV-sensitive Ca^{2+} channel and the antiepileptic relevance remain to be established.

K$^+$ Currents

One study (36) reports that LEV produced a significant inhibition (≈30%) of the delayed rectifier potassium current (I_K) in isolated hippocampal neurons from both rat (IC$_{50}$ 5 μmol/L) and guinea pig (IC$_{50}$ 45 μmol/L). The blocking of I_K by LEV appeared irreversible and voltage independent. Furthermore, the same study reports a broadening of the secondary action potentials produced by long-step depolarizations, entailing a decrease (≈20%) in the area of the depolarization-induced action potentials. This suggests that a moderate block of the I_K currents may reduce the generation of repetitive action potentials and thereby contribute to the antiepileptic mechanism(s) of LEV.

MECHANISMS OF LEVETIRACETAM: CURRENT PERSPECTIVE

The cellular-level effects of LEV on neurons, reported or hypothesized to date, are summarized in Table 40.3. It

TABLE 40.3. EFFECTS OF LEVETIRACETAM ON NEUROTRANSMITTER RECEPTORS AND NEURONAL ION CHANNELS

Target	Action of Levetiracetam	Reference	Comments
GABA-associated			
GABA metabolism or turnover	Local alterations in rat brain	23	Only at high doses; short lasting; disparate between areas
	No effect in mouse brain	26	
	No effect *in vitro*	23, 27	
GABA-gated current	Prolongation of the decay	28	Significant only at ≥100 μmol/L
	No consistent effect on the amplitude	28	
GABA- and glycine-gated currents	Suppression of inhibition by negative modulators (e.g., Zn^{2+}, β-carbolines)	28	EC$_{50}$ = 1–10 μmol/L
Glutamate-associated			
Glutamate metabolism	No effect in mouse brain	26, 30	
AMPA-gated current	Inhibition	31	IC$_{50}$ = 268 μmol/L, no effect *in vivo*
N-methyl-D-aspartate–gated current	No effect	31	
Kainate-gated current	No effect	31	
Voltage-gated ion channels			
Na$^+$ current	No effect	33	
Low-voltage-gated Ca^{2+} current	No effect	34	In hippocampal neurons
High-voltage-gated Ca^{2+} currents	Inhibition	35	In hippocampal neurons
K$^+$ currents	Inhibition of the delayed rectifier (I_K) current	36	Maximal effect(≈30%) at 30 μmol/L, IC$_{50}$ 5–45 μmol/L, entailing a broadening of secondary action potentials
Ca^{2+} -dependent mechanisms, Potentially involving intraneuronal effects	Hypothesized to account for a non-GABA$_A$–related antibiculline effect of levetiracetam	17, 37, 38	No direct proof (only indirect indications) to date

AMPA, α-amino-3-hydroxy-5-methylisoxazole-4-propionic acid; EC$_{50}$, median effective concentration; GABA, γ-aminobutyric acid, I$_k$; IC$_{50}$, inhibitory concentration of 50.

appears that two conclusions can be substantiated: (a) no existing data favor ascribing to LEV any conventional modulation of the three main mechanisms currently accepted for the established AEDs (GABAergic facilitation or inhibition of either Na^+ currents or low-voltage–activated Ca^{2+} currents), implying that the antiepileptic mechanism(s) of LEV must be novel; and (b) the actions of LEV on neurons, established to date, appear multiple, mild, and of a modulatory type, rather than expressing a straightforward dose-dependent inhibition/activation of one single cellular effect.

LEV appears able to control pathologic neuronal hyperexcitability through a modulatory inhibition of neuronal high-voltage Ca^{2+} currents, a prolongation of the hyperpolarizing GABA-gated currents, and an inhibition of the AMPA-gated current. However, although the inhibition of Ca^{2+} currents was observed at a clinically relevant concentration, the other two effects of LEV appeared only at relatively high concentrations *in vitro*. Two other cellular effects of LEV, namely, the suppression of the inhibition by Zn^{2+} and other negative allosteric modulators of both GABA- and glycine-gated currents, and the broadening/delaying of secondary action potentials on inhibition of the I_K current, seem of particular potential interest for the basic understanding of epileptic pathophysiology.

The "sprouted mossy fiber/Zn^{2+}–sensitive $GABA_A$ receptor" hypothesis, recently proposed [for reviews, see Coulter (29,39)], postulates that epileptogenesis may involve sprouting of Zn^{2+}-containing mossy fiber terminals, which innervate DGCs containing $GABA_A$ receptors with an altered subunit composition, rendering them more sensitive to inhibition by Zn^{2+}. When repetitive stimulation results in enhanced release of Zn^{2+}, this in turn may diffuse to and block these "epileptic" $GABA_A$ receptors on DGCs. This would induce a vicious cycle of disinhibition that may result in aberrant activity, triggering epileptiform discharges in the epileptic hippocampus. LEV may reverse this process by its ability to suppress the inhibitory effects of Zn^{2+} and other negative allosteric modulators on both GABA- and glycine-gated currents (28). These attributes of LEV may represent a novel mechanism that could contribute substantially to its antiseizure action as well as to its potential antiepileptogenic properties, such as those observed in the kindling model (13).

The unexpected possibility of obtaining an antiepileptic effect that involves a reduction of repetitive neuronal firing upon delaying membrane repolarization through the inhibition of a potassium current (36) seems likely to attract the further attention of epileptologists. If confirmed, this would represent a completely novel antiepileptic mechanism.

At this stage, it is not possible to formulate a unified mechanism of action for LEV, especially because the molecular nature of its brain-specific binding site remains to be characterized, and further cellular effects of LEV are likely to be identified. Thus, the robust anti-BMI effect of LEV

on hippocampal neurons, which appeared not be associated with the $GABA_A$ receptor (17), is mimicked by thapsigargin (38), a blocker of Ca^{2+}-adenosine triphosphatase in the endoplasmic reticulum. This suggested that putative Ca^{2+}-dependent actions of LEV to downregulate neuronal excitability might involve not only the membrane channels, but intraneuronal effects. This possibility needs further exploration. Likewise, it remains to be investigated whether (and, if so, which) nonsynaptic desynchronizing effects might be involved in the distinct ability of LEV to antagonize neuronal hypersynchronization (18). Finally, the near-absence of an effect of LEV on normal neural responses, together with its antiepileptic efficacy, seem to legitimize the hope that forthcoming progress in understanding the mechanisms of this drug also might shed some light on the pathologic states it treats.

REFERENCES

1. Wülfert E, Hanin I, Verloes R. Facilitation of calcium-dependent cholinergic function by ucb L059, a new "second generation" nootropic agent. *Psychopharmacol Bull* 1989;25:498–502.
2. Gower A, Noyer M, Verloes R, et al. ucb L059, a novel anti-convulsant drug: pharmacological profile in animals. *Eur J Pharmacol* 1992;222:193–203.
3. Klitgaard H, Matagne A, Gobert J, et al. Evidence for a unique profile of levetiracetam in rodent models of seizures and epilepsy. *Eur J Pharmacol* 1998;353:191–206.
4. Cereghino JJ, Biton V, Abou-Khalil B, et al. Levetiracetam for partial seizures: results of a double- blind, randomized clinical trial. *Neurology* 2000;55:236–242.
5. McNamara JO. Cellular and molecular basis of epilepsy. *J Neurosci* 1994;14:3413–3425.
6. Löscher W, Hönack D. Profile of ucb L059, a novel anticonvulsant drug, in models of partial and generalized epilepsy in mice and rats. *Eur J Pharmacol* 1993;232:147–158.
7. Löscher W, Reissmüller E, Ebert U. Anticonvulsant efficacy of gabapentin and levetiracetam in phenytoin-resistant kindled rats.*Epilepsy Res* 2000;40:63–77.
8. Matagne A, Klitgaard H. Levetiracetam protects against seizures in fully hippocampal-kindled rats. *Epilepsia* 1999;40[Suppl 7]:137.
9. De Deyn PP, Kabuto H, D'Hooge R, et al. Protective effect of ucb L059 against postural stimulation-induced seizures in EL mice. *Neurosciences* 1992;18[Suppl 2]:187–192.
10. Gower A, Hirsch E, Boehrer A., et al. Effects of levetiracetam, a novel antiepileptic drug, on convulsant activity in two genetic rat models of epilepsy. *Epilepsy Res* 1995;22:207–213.
11. Lamberty Y, Margineanu DG, Klitgaard H. Absence of negative impact of levetiracetam on cognitive function and memory in normal and amygdala-kindled rats. *Epilepsy Behav* 2000;1: 333–342.
12. Silver JM, Shin C, McNamara JO. Antiepileptogenic effects of conventional anticonvulsants in the kindling model of epilepsy. *Ann Neurol* 1991;29:356–363.
13. Löscher W, Hönack D, Rundfeldt C. Antiepileptogenic effects of the novel anticonvulsant levetiracetam (ucb L059) in the kindling model of temporal lobe epilepsy. *J Pharmacol Exp Ther* 1998;284:474–479.
14. Margineanu DG, Wülfert E. ucb L059, a novel anticonvulsant, reduces bicuculline-induced hyperexcitability in rat hippocampal CA3 in vivo. *Eur J Pharmacol* 1995;286:321–325.

15. Birnstiel S, Wülfert E, Beck SG. Levetiracetam (ucb L059) affects in vitro models of epilepsy in CA3 pyramidal neurons without altering normal synaptic transmission. *Naunyn Schmiedebergs Arch Pharmacol* 1997;356:611–618.
16. Doheny HC, Whittington MA, Jefferys JGR, et al. Levetiracetam inhibits bicuculline/potassium induced seizure like events in vitro. *Eur J Neurosci* 1998;[Suppl 10]:39.
17. Margineanu DG, Wülfert E. Inhibition by levetiracetam of a non-GABA$_A$ receptor-associated epileptiform effect of bicuculline in rat hippocampus. *Br J Pharmacol* 1997;122:1146–1150.
18. Margineanu DG, Klitgaard H. Inhibition of neuronal hyper-synchrony *in vitro* differentiates levetiracetam from classical antiepileptic drugs. *Pharmacol Res* 2000;42:281–285.
19. Klitgaard H. Levetiracetam counteracts propagation of epileptiform activity induced by systemic administration of pilocarpine and kainic acid to rats *in vivo*. *Epilepsia* 1999;40[Suppl 7]:138.
20. Gillard M, Noyer M, Henichart J-P, et al. The novel antiepileptic drug levetiracetam (ucb L059) appears to act via a specific binding site in CNS membranes. *Br J Pharmacol* 1994;112[Suppl]:615P.
21. Sacaan AI, Lloyd GK. The binding of the anticonvulsant levetiracetam to rat brain membranes distinguishes a novel site relevant to antiepileptic drug activity. *Neuropsychopharmacology* 1994;10[Suppl, Pt 2]:133S.
22. Noyer M, Gillard M, Matagne A, et al. The novel antiepileptic drug levetiracetam (ucb L059) appears to act via a specific binding site in CNS membranes. *Eur J Pharmacol* 1995;286:137–146.
23. Löscher W, Hönack D, Bloms-Funke P. The novel antiepileptic drug levetiracetam (ucb L059) induces alterations in GABA metabolism and turnover in discrete areas of rat brain and reduces neuronal activity in substantia nigra pars reticulata. *Brain Res* 1996;735:208–216.
24. Turski L, Cavalheiro EA, Calderazzo-Filho LS, et al. The basal ganglia, the deep piriform cortex, and seizure spread: bicuculline is anticonvulsant in the rat striatum. *Proc Natl Acad Sci U S A* 1989;86:1694–1697.
25. Gale K. Progression and generalization of seizure discharge: anatomical and neurochemical substrates. *Epilepsia* 1988;29[Suppl 2]:S15–S34.
26. Sills GJ, Leach JP, Frazer CM, et al. Neurochemical studies with the novel anticonvulsant levetiracetam in mouse brain. *Eur J Pharmacol* 1997;325:35–40.
27. Frazer CM, Sills GJ, Butler E, et al. Levetiracetam fails to influence GABA transport and metabolism in rat astrocyte culture. *Epilepsia* 1997;38[Suppl 3]:177.
28. Rigo JM, Nguyen L, Rocher V, et al. Levetiracetam: novel modulation of ionotropic inhibitory receptors. *Epilepsia* 2000;41[suppl]:35.
29. Coulter DA. Chronic epileptogenic cellular alterations in the limbic system after status epilepticus. *Epilepsia* 1999;40[Suppl 1]:S23–S33.
30. Frazer CM, Sills GJ, Forrest G, et al. Effects of anti-epileptic drugs on glutamine synthetase activity in mouse brain. *Br J Pharmacol* 1999;126:1634–1638.
31. Hans G, Rigo JM, Crommen J, et al. Levetiracetam: no relevant effect on ionotropic excitatory glutamate receptors. *Epilepsia* 2000;41[Suppl]:37.
32. Zhang X, Wülfert E, Hanin I. Effects of ucb L059, a potential anticonvulsant agent, on release of dopamine and its metabolite from cerebral ventricular perfusate induced by bicuculline and haloperidol in rats. *Pharmacologist* 1993;35(3):187.
33. Zona C, Marchetti C, Margineanu DG. The novel antiepileptic drug candidate levetiracetam does not modify the biophysical properties of the Na$^+$ channel in rat cortical neurons in culture. *Soc Neurosci Abstr* 1999;25:1868.
34. Niespodziany I, Klitgaard H, Margineanu DG. Levetiracetam had no effect on low-voltage-activated Ca^{2+} current in rat CA1 hippocampal neurons. *Neurology* 2000;54[Suppl 3]:A307–A308.
35. Niespodziany I, Klitgaard H, Margineanu DG. Levetiracetam: modulation of high-voltage-activated Ca^{2+}current in CA1 pyramidal neurons of rat hippocampal slices. *Epilepsia* 2000;31[Suppl]:347.
36. Madeja M, Margineanu DG, Klitgaard H. Effect of levetiracetam on voltage-gated potassium channels: a novel antiepileptic mechanism of action? *Epilepsia* 2001;42[Suppl 2]:19.
37. Margineanu DG, Wülfert E. ucb L059, a novel anticonvulsant, reduces bicuculline-induced neuronal hyperexcitability, possibly through Ca-dependent mechanisms. *Pharmacol Res* 1995;31S:347.
38. Wülfert E, Margineanu DG. Thapsigargin inhibits bicuculline-induced epileptiform excitability in rat hippocampal slices. *Neurosci Lett* 1998;243:141–143.
39. Coulter DA. Mossy fiber zinc and temporal lobe epilepsy: pathological association with altered "epileptic" gamma-aminobutyric acid A receptors in dentate granule cells. *Epilepsia* 2000;41[Suppl 6]:S96–S99.

Antiepileptic Drugs, 5th Edition. Edited by R.H. Levy, R.H. Mattson, B.S. Meldrum, and E. Perucca. Lippincott Williams & Wilkins, Philadelphia © 2002.

LEVETIRACETAM

CHEMISTRY, BIOTRANSFORMATION, PHARMACOKINETICS, AND DRUG INTERACTIONS

PHILIP N. PATSALOS

Levetiracetam is derived from a series of nootropic drugs and is the (S)-enantiomer of the ethyl analog of piracetam. It is structurally unrelated to other antiepileptic drugs and has unique preclinical and clinical profiles. Because levetiracetam is ineffective in the classic screening models for acute seizures, its antiepileptic efficacy was nearly overlooked. Its potent anticonvulsant effects against a variety of seizure types in animal models of chronic epilepsy combined with its significant clinical efficacy and highly favorable therapeutic index, suggest that levetiracetam will be a useful antiepileptic drug (1,2).

CHEMISTRY AND METABOLIC SCHEME

Levetiracetam, (S)-α-ethyl-2-oxo-1-pyrrolidine acetamide (Figure 41.1), has a molecular weight of 170.21 and an empirical formula of $C_8H_{14}N_2O_2$. It is a white to off-white powder with a bitter taste and faint odor. Levetiracetam is highly soluble in water (104.0 g/100 mL), freely soluble in chloroform (65.3 g/100 mL) and methanol (53.6 g/100 mL), soluble in ethanol (16.5 g/100 mL), sparingly soluble in acetonitrile (5.7 g/100 mL), and practically insoluble in n-hexane. It is formulated for clinical use as 250-, 500-, and 1,000-mg film-coated tablets. Blood concentrations of levetiracetam can be measured either by using gas chromatography with nitrogen-phosphorus detection after solid-phase extraction or by isocratic high-performance liquid chromatography with ultraviolet detection after extraction with dichloromethane (3,4).

Philip N. Patsalos, FRCPath, PhD: Senior Lecturer in Clinical Pharmacology, Department of Clinical and Experimental Epilepsy, Institute of Neurology; and Director, Department of Pharmacology and Therapeutics Unit, National Hospital of Neurology and Neurosurgery, London, United Kingdom

ABSORPTION

Absorption of levetiracetam after oral ingestion of doses ranging from 250-mg to 5,000-mg is rapid, linear, and almost complete (>95%), with peak plasma concentrations (C_{max}) occurring approximately 1 hour later (T_{max}). Although an intravenous formulation of levetiracetam is not available, absolute oral bioavailability is considered to be essentially 100%, and the extent of absorption is independent of dose. A study comparing 500-mg tablets and two 250-mg capsules of levetiracetam in healthy volunteers after single and multiple doses has shown that the two formulations are bioequivalent. Levetiracetam can be ingested without regard to meal times because although food coingestion slows the rate of levetiracetam absorption, the extent is unaffected (5).

DISTRIBUTION

In humans and in the rat, levetiracetam is not bound to plasma proteins. The volume of distribution of levetiracetam is approximately 0.5 to 0.7 L/kg. Steady-state plasma concentrations are reached within 48 hours. Human tissue distribution data are not available. In the rat, mouse, rabbit, and dog, levetiracetam rapidly distributes into tissues with concentrations approximating those in blood, with the exception of lower concentrations in the lens and adipose tissue and higher levels in the kidneys. In rats, levetiracetam rapidly and readily crosses the blood–brain barrier to enter both brain extracellular and cerebrospinal fluid compartments (6,7). Levetiracetam brain concentration increases linearly and dose-dependently and does not display brain region specificity, as indicated by its comparable distribution in the extracellular fluid of the hippocampus and frontal cortex (7).

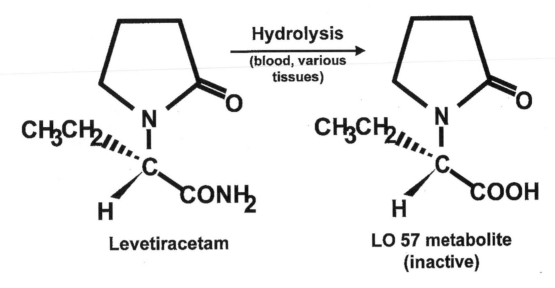

FIGURE 41.1. The chemical structure of levetiracetam [(S)-α-ethyl-2-oxo-1-pyrrolidine acetamide] and its primary pharmacologically inactive metabolite, L057.

ROUTES OF ELIMINATION

The major route of elimination of levetiracetam is renal (Table 41.1). Clearance is rapid, so that within 48 hours approximately 93% of an oral dose is eliminated. It undergoes minimal metabolism (hydrolysis of the acetamide group) to three inactive metabolites: one major carboxylic acid metabolite (L057; 24% of dose; Figure 41.1) and two minor metabolites (~3% of dose). Other unknown components account for 0.6% of the dose. Thus, approximately 66% of an administered dose is recovered as unchanged levetiracetam in urine, whereas the inactive metabolites account

for 27%. The metabolic pathway of the two minor inactive metabolites has not yet been determined. Hepatic autoinduction is not a feature of levetiracetam metabolism (8). Enantiomeric interconversion has not been observed for levetiracetam or its primary metabolite in the dog (9). Whether enantiomer interconversion occurs in humans is unknown.

ROUTES OF EXCRETION

As mentioned previously, the major route of elimination for levetiracetam is through urine (66% of administered dose is eliminated unchanged and 27% is excreted in urine as inactive metabolites) (10). Excretion by the fecal route accounts for only 0.3% of administered dose. Renal clearance of levetiracetam occurs at a rate of 40 mL/min/1.73 m² (0.6 mL/min/kg), indicating excretion by glomerular filtration and partial subsequent tubular reabsorption. Renal clearance of the primary metabolite L057 is approximately 4.2 mL/min/kg, indicating active tubular secretion in addition to glomerular filtration.

CLEARANCE AND HALF-LIFE

Healthy Subjects

The elimination half-life of levetiracetam in healthy, young volunteers ranges from 6 to 8 hours, and is independent of dose or frequency of administration (5).

Comedicated Epileptic Patients

In patients taking enzyme-inducing antiepileptic drugs (phenytoin, phenobarbitone, primidone, or carbamaze-

TABLE 41.1. PHARMACOKINETIC CHARACTERISTICS OF LEVETIRACETAM

Parameter	Value
Time to maximum plasma concentration	1.3 h
Bioavailability	>95%
Volume of distribution	0.5–0.7 L/kg
Plasma protein binding	0%
Half-life	
Healthy adult subjects[a]	6–8 h
Elderly subjects	10–11 h
Patients with epilepsy[a]:	
Adults	6–8 h
Children	5–7 h
Clearance (adults)	40 mL/min/1.73 m²(0.6 mL/min/kg)
Metabolism	Minimal: in blood to the inactive deaminated metabolite L057
Route of elimination	Renal

[a]Patients taking various hepatic enzyme inducing antiepileptic drugs and including valproic acid, which is a known hepatic enzyme inhibitor.

pine) or valproic acid, the elimination half-life of levetiracetam is comparable with that of subjects receiving levetiracetam alone. During the clinical evaluation of levetiracetam, patients comedicated with tiagabine, topiramate, oxcarbazepine, or zonisamide were excluded, and thus the effects of these antiepileptic drugs on the elimination half-life of levetiracetam are unknown.

Children

In a series of 24 children (aged 6 to 12 years) with partial-onset seizures, the elimination half-life of levetiracetam (after a single oral dose of 20 mg/kg) was 5–7 hours and was independent of sex (11). The half-life of the L057 metabolite was approximately 8 hours. C_{max} and area under the curve (AUC) values (adjusted to a dose of 1 mg/kg) were approximately 30% to 40% lower than that in adults, although the renal clearance was similar. The apparent total body clearance was approximately 30% to 40% higher than that in adults. Over a 24-hour interval, 52% of the administered dose was excreted in urine as levetiracetam and 9% as L057. Based on these data, a maximum maintenance dosage equivalent to 130% to 140% of the usual adult dose is recommended.

Elderly Subjects

The elimination half-life of levetiracetam in the elderly increases to between 10 and 11 hours (12,13). A study of 16 elderly subjects (mean age, 77 years; range, 61 to 88 years) receiving 1,000 mg/day for 10 consecutive days suggests that the longer half-life of levetiracetam is in fact the consequence of a reduction in creatinine clearance consequent to an age-related decline in renal function (5). Thus, it is appropriate for levetiracetam dose to be adjusted in elderly patients according to their creatinine clearance.

Patients with Renal Impairment

Because the renal clearance of levetiracetam and its metabolite L057 correlate directly with creatinine clearance, the elimination half-life of levetiracetam is increased in patients with renal impairment and in patients with severe hepatic impairment and concurrent renal impairment (hepatorenal syndrome) (12,13). At steady-state, the C_{max} of levetiracetam is higher than that of healthy subjects. AUC values increase with decreasing renal function, so that in patients with mildly to moderately impaired renal function, values can be nearly twice those with normal renal function. Also, the elimination half-life of levetiracetam is prolonged. In patients with very mild to moderately severe renal impairment (creatinine clearance = 20 to 89 mL/min/1.73 m^2), total clearance has been observed to decrease by 35% to

60%. Thus, dosage should be reduced in patients with impaired renal function.

In a series of five patients with anuric end-stage renal disease undergoing hemodialysis, the pharmacokinetic profiles of levetiracetam and L057 over 104 hours after a single 500-mg dose were determined (14). Levetiracetam was rapidly and completely absorbed after a single 500-mg dose. However, clearance was only 30% of that in healthy subjects, and during dialysis its elimination half-life was approximately 3 hours, whereas in the periods between dialysis its half-life was 25 hours. Dialyzer extraction efficiency was high, leading to the removal of 50% of levetiracetam during a 4-hour session. L057 also was rapidly removed from plasma. Therefore, for patients with end-stage renal disease maintained on hemodialysis, levetiracetam should be supplemented by 30% to 50% of the usual daily dose on dialysis days.

Patients with Hepatic Impairment

The pharmacokinetics of levetiracetam and L057 are unaffected by mild to moderate hepatic impairment (15). This is consistent with the fact that the liver contributes little to the metabolism of levetiracetam. In patients with severe hepatic impairment, levetiracetam and L057 elimination half-life and AUC values were observed to be increased twofold to threefold, and the total-body clearance of levetiracetam was reduced by >50%. However, these changes are most likely the consequence of concurrent mild to moderate renal impairment (hepatorenal syndrome) rather than liver impairment *per se*. Thus, dosage adjustments may not be necessary in patients with hepatic impairment.

RELATIONSHIP BETWEEN SERUM CONCENTRATION AND DOSE

In healthy volunteers, levetiracetam C_{max} and AUC values increase dose-dependently and linearly in the range of 500 to 5,000-mg (5). In multiple dose-ranging studies, levetiracetam has exhibited predictable, linear, and dose-proportional steady-state pharmacokinetics, with steady-state concentrations occurring within 2 days of initiation of dosing. After a single 1,000-mg and repeated 1,000-mg twice-daily doses, levetiracetam plasma C_{max} values typically are 23 and 43 µg/mL, respectively.

RELATIONSHIP BETWEEN PLASMA CONCENTRATION AND EFFECT

The relationship between levetiracetam plasma concentration and its antiepileptic activity or its adverse effects profile has not been formally investigated.

INTERACTION PROFILE

The interaction potential of levetiracetam has been extensively investigated in studies conducted *in vitro*, in healthy volunteers, and in patients with epilepsy. Because levetiracetam is not metabolized in the liver or bound to plasma proteins, it has a very low potential for drug interactions (16). However, drugs excreted by tubular secretion potentially may interact with both levetiracetam and L057 because both undergo tubular secretion.

Because by far the most clinically significant pharmacokinetic drug–drug interactions involve the induction or inhibition of cytochrome P450 (CYP) enzymes (17,18), the effect of levetiracetam on the activity of hepatic CYP enzymes was investigated using *in vitro* human liver microsomal markers (19). Levetiracetam and its primary metabolite, L057, at concentrations exceeding five times the plasma therapeutic concentration, were evaluated for their potential inhibitory effect on 11 different drug-metabolizing enzymes [CYP3A4, CYP1A2, CYP2C19, CYP2E1, CYP2C9, CYP2D6, epoxide hydrolase, uridine 5′-diphospho-glucuronyltransferase*1 (UGT1*6), UGT1*1, and UGT(pl 6.2)]. Enzyme activities were unaffected. Furthermore, using primary cultures of rat hepatocytes, levetiracetam did not induce CYP activity (19). These results suggest that levetiracetam is unlikely to produce clinically relevant interactions through the induction or inhibition of CYP- or UGT-mediated reactions.

Antiepileptic Drugs

Levetiracetam does not appear to interact with other antiepileptic drugs, and overall the pharmacokinetic parameters of levetiracetam during polytherapy with antiepileptic drugs are comparable to those of subjects receiving levetiracetam alone (20). In various add-on clinical studies of levetiracetam, plasma concentrations of antiepileptic drugs were compared before and during administration of levetiracetam (13,21–25). Meta-analysis has revealed that levetiracetam does not affect the concentrations of carbamazepine, clobazam, clonazepam, diazepam, gabapentin, lamotrigine, phenobarbital, phenytoin, primidone, valproic acid, and vigabatrin. However, in one study, the addition of levetiracetam to the polytherapy regimens of patients with epilepsy resulted in a 27% to 52% increase in phenytoin concentrations, with one patient requiring a reduction in the dosage of phenytoin because of neurotoxicity (13). Because phenytoin is a commonly prescribed antiepileptic drug, its interaction potential with levetiracetam has been investigated further using a sensitive technique that employs deuterium-labeled phenytoin (26). Six male patients taking phenytoin as monotherapy for the treatment of their epilepsy were investigated; however, no interactions between levetiracetam and phenytoin were observed.

In a formal study of 16 healthy volunteers designed to investigate the effect of valproic acid (a potent inhibitor of hepatic metabolism) on the pharmacokinetics of levetiracetam, it was observed that valproic acid did not affect the extent of oral absorption or the metabolism and urinary excretion of levetiracetam (27).

The interaction potential between levetiracetam and felbamate, tiagabine, topiramate, and zonisamide has not been investigated.

Other Drugs

Numerous studies have been undertaken to determine possible interactions between levetiracetam and various commonly used drugs, including warfarin, digoxin, the oral contraceptives ethinylestradiol and levonorgestrel, and probenecid (5). Coadministration of levetiracetam (2,000 mg/day) with warfarin did not affect the pharmacokinetics or pharmacodynamics of warfarin, as determined by measuring prothrombin time. Conversely, the pharmacokinetics of levetiracetam were unaffected by warfarin.

The pharmacokinetics of digoxin and levetiracetam were assessed using a double-blind, placebo-controlled, two-way crossover design in 11 healthy adults (7 male) (28). Electrocardiograms also were recorded. At the doses investigated, no relevant pharmacokinetic or pharmacodynamic interactions were observed between levetiracetam (2,000 mg/day) and digoxin (0.25 mg/day).

Contraceptive efficacy appears not to be affected by levetiracetam (29). Coadministration of levetiracetam (500 mg twice daily) and a low-dose monophasic oral contraceptive (0.3 mg ethinylestradiol, 0.15 mg levonorgestrel) in 18 women over 21 days did not alter plasma estrogen or progesterone values or bleeding patterns compared with placebo.

Concomitant administration of levetiracetam (2,000 mg/day) both as single doses and multiple doses with probenecid (500 mg four times daily) did not affect the pharmacokinetic parameters of levetiracetam (5). However, the plasma concentration of its primary metabolite, L057, increased 2.5-fold consequent to a 61% decrease in tubular secretion. Although the clinical relevance of elevated concentrations of L057 is not known, caution is warranted with concurrent use of levetiracetam and probenecid. The effect of levetiracetam on probenecid has not been studied. Furthermore, the interaction potential between levetiracetam and other drugs undergoing tubular secretion has not been investigated.

SUMMARY

Pharmacokinetic studies of levetiracetam have been conducted in healthy volunteers, in patients of all ages with epilepsy, and in certain special populations. Results of these studies indicate that levetiracetam has a favorable pharmacokinetic profile characterized by excellent oral absorption and bioavailability and a mean elimination half-life of 7 hours. Levetiracetam is not bound to plasma proteins and is not metabolized in the liver, so it is not expected to be associated with significant pharmacokinetic interactions. Indeed, to date, no clinically relevant interactions with levetiracetam have been identified. Because levetiracetam is primarily excreted unchanged in urine, dosage adjustments are necessary for patients with moderate to severe renal impairment.

REFERENCES

1. Klitgaard H, Matagne A, Gobert J, et al. Evidence for a unique profile of levetiracetam in rodent models of seizures and epilepsy. *Eur J Pharmacol* 1988;353:191–206.
2. Löscher W, Hönack D, Rundfeldt C. Antiepileptogenic effects of the novel anticonvulsant levetiracetam (ucb L059) in the kindling model of temporal lobe epilepsy. *J Pharmacol Exp Ther* 1998;284:474–479.
3. Vermeij TAC, Edelbroek PM. High-performance liquid chromatographic and megabore gas-liquid chromatographic determination of levetiracetam (ucb L059) in human serum after solid-phase extraction. *J Chromatogr Biomed Appl* 1994;662:134–139.
4. Ratnaraj N, Doheny HC, Patsalos PN. A micromethod for the determination of the new antiepileptic drug levetiracetam (UCB L059) in serum or plasma by high performance liquid chromatography. *Ther Drug Monit* 1996;18:154–157.
5. Patsalos PN. Pharmacokinetic profile of levetiracetam: toward ideal characteristics *Pharmacol Ther* 2000;85:77–85.
6. Doheny HC, Ratnaraj N, Whittington MA, et al. Blood and cerebrospinal fluid pharmacokinetics of the novel anticonvulsant levetiracetam (ucb L059) in the rat. *Epilepsy Res* 1999;34:161–168.
7. Tong X, Patsalos PN. A microdialysis study of the novel antiepileptic drug levetiracetam: extracellular pharmacokinetics and effect on taurine in rat brain. *Br J Pharmacol* 2001;133:867–74.
8. Doheny HC, Whittington MA, Jeffrey JGR, et al. A comparison of the efficacy of carbamazepine and the novel antiepileptic drug levetiracetam in the tetonus toxin model of focal complex partial epilepsy. *Br J Pharmacol* 20002 (*in press*).
9. Isoherranen N, Yagen B, Roder M, et al. Pharmacokinetics of levetiracetam and its enantiometer (R) α-ethyl-2-oxo-pyrrolidine acedtamide in dogs. *Epilepsia* 2000;42(7);825–30.
10. Walker MC, Patsalos PN. Clinical pharmacokinetics of new antiepileptic drugs. *Pharmacol Ther* 1995;67:351–384.
11. Pellock J, Glauser T, Bebin M. et al. Single dose pharmacokinetics of levetiracetam in pediatric patients with partial epilepsy. *Epilepsia* 1999;40[Suppl 2]:238–239(abstr).
12. Edelbroek PM, de Wilde-Ockeloen JM, Kasteleijn-Nolst Trenité DGA, et al. Evaluation of the pharmacokinetic and neuropsychometric parameters in chronic comedicated epileptic patients

13. of three increasing dosages of a novel antiepileptic drug, UCB L059 250-mg capsules per os each dose for one week followed by two-weeks of placebo. *Epilepsia* 1993;34[Suppl 2]:7(abstr).
13. Sharief MK, Singh P, Sander JWAS, et al. Efficacy and tolerability study of ucb L059 in patients with refractory epilepsy. *J Epilepsy* 1996;9:106–112.
14. Baltes E, Coupez R. Levetiracetam dose adjustment for patients on hemodialysis. *Epilepsia* 2000;41[Suppl 7]:254(abstr).
15. Brockmoller J, Thomsen T, Eckl K, et al. Levetiracetam: Liver impairment does not influence its pharmacokinetic profile. *Epilepsia* 2000;41[Suppl 6]:150(abstr).
16. Patsalos PN. Phenobarbitone to gabapentin: a guide to 82 years of anti-epileptic drug pharmacokinetic interactions. *Seizure* 1994;3:163–170.
17. Patsalos PN. The new generation of anti-epileptic drugs. In: Bowman WC, Fitzgerald JD, Taylor JB, eds. *Emerging drugs: the prospect for improved medicines*, vol 4. London: Ashley Publications, 1999:87–106.
18. Browne TR. Pharmacokinetics of antiepileptic drugs. *Neurology* 1998;51[Suppl 4]:S2–S7.
19. Nicolas JM, Collart P, Gerin B, et al. In vitro evaluation of potential drug interactions with levetiracetam, a new antiepileptic agent. *Drug Metab Dispos* 1999;27:250–254.
20. Perucca E, Baltes E, Ledent E. Levetiracetam: absence of pharmacokinetic interactions with other antiepileptic drugs (AEDs). *Epilepsia* 2000;41[Suppl 6]:150(abstr).
21. Ben-Menachem E, Falteru U. Efficacy and tolerability of levetiracetam 3000 mg/day in patients with refractory partial seizures: a multicentre, double-blind, responder-selected study evaluating monotherapy. *Epilepsia* 2000;41:1276–1283.
22. Betts T, Waegemans T, Crawford P. A multicentre, double-blind, randomized, parallel group study to evaluate the tolerability and efficacy of two oral doses of levetiracetam, 2000 mg daily and 4000 mg daily, without titration in patients with refractory epilepsy. *Seizure* 2000;9:80–87.
23. Cereghino J, Biton V, Abou-Khalil B, et al. Levetiracetam for partial seizures: results of a double-blind, randomized clinical trial. *Neurology* 2000;55:236–242.
24. Grant R, Shorvon SD. Efficacy and tolerability of 1000–4000 mg per day of levetiracetam as add-on therapy in patients with refractory epilepsy. *Epilepsy Res* 2000;42:89–95.
25. Shorvon SD, Lowenthal A, Janz D, et al. Multicentre double-blind, randomized, placebo-controlled trial of levetiracetam as add-on therapy in patients with refractory partial seizures. *Epilepsia* 2000;41:1179–1186.
26. Browne TR, Szabo GK, Leppik IE, et al. Absence of pharmacokinetic drug interaction of levetiracetam with phenytoin in patients with epilepsy determined by new technique. *J Clin Pharmacol* 2000;40:590–595.
27. Browne TR, Baltes E. Valproate does not alter levetiracetam pharmacokinetics. *Epilepsia* 2000;41[Suppl 7]:99(abstr).
28. Levy RH, Ragueneau-Majlessi I, Baltes E. Repeated administration of the novel antiepileptic agent levetiracetam does not alter digoxin pharmacokinetics and pharmacodynamics in healthy volunteers. *Epilepsia* 2000;46:93–99.
29. Giuliano RA, Hiersemenzel R, Baltes E, et al. Influence of a new antiepileptic drug (levetiracetam, ucb L059) on the pharmacokinetics and pharmacodynamics of oral contraceptives. *Epilepsia* 1996;37[Suppl 4]:90(abstr).

LEVETIRACETAM

CLINICAL USE

ILO E. LEPPIK

Levetiracetam (LEV) is a new antiepileptic drug (AED) approved in Switzerland in late 1999 and in the United States in November 1999. Approvals in other countries have followed, and LEV is becoming more widely available. Most of the available literature on LEV is based on three studies performed for registration. Its efficacy has been tested mostly in localization-related epilepsies. However, it may have a broader applicability.

EFFICACY

Early evidence of the clinical efficacy of LEV was obtained from several phase I and phase II studies (1–6). These studies explored doses of 1,000 to 4,000 mg/day in various titration schedules. One study was an open dose-escalation model in 29 patients who received placebo for 4 weeks (baseline) followed by LEV 1,000 mg/day for 2 weeks, 2,000 mg/day for 2 weeks, 3,000 mg/day for 4 weeks, and, finally, 4,000 mg/day for 4 weeks. Twenty-seven of the 29 patients completed the study, and a substantially lower median seizure frequency was observed at all dosing periods. Placebo seizure frequency was 2.06 seizures per week, compared with 1, 1.5, 1, and 0.75 for the respective LEV doses. Somnolence and asthenia were most frequent with the 4,000-mg/day dose, suggesting that this may represent the upper limit in some patients (4). These early studies were influential in leading to the use of doses of 1,000 to 3,000 mg/day in the pivotal studies (7).

The efficacy of LEV as adjunctive therapy for localization-related epilepsy has been established by three pivotal, multicenter studies in the United States and Europe (8–10). These double-blind, placebo-controlled studies involved a total of 904 adult patients and constitute the core data for the approvals granted by various regulatory agencies. These studies also provided information regarding effectiveness for specific seizures types and quality-of-life issues. These

three studies used similar patient populations and protocols, but differed in some details. Other studies on the effects of LEV are becoming available.

Pivotal Adjunctive Therapy Studies

One pivotal study (study 1) was performed in the United States (9) and two in Europe (8,10) (Table 42.1). The major differences between these involved dose regimens. In the U.S. study, final doses of LEV of 1,000 or 3,000 mg/day were compared with placebo. In the first European study (study 2), doses of 1,000 or 2,000 mg/day were compared with placebo (10). In the second European study (study 3), doses of 3,000 mg/day were compared with placebo, and titration to monotherapy was evaluated (8).

Study 1

The U.S. study was a multicenter, randomized, add-on, double-blind, placebo-controlled, parallel-group trial that compared placebo, LEV 1,000 mg/day, and LEV 3,000 mg/day in patients with refractory partial epilepsy (9). Patients were enrolled from September 1994 to March 1996. The study consisted of a selection visit; a 12-week, single-blind, placebo baseline period; a 4-week double-blind drug titration period; a 14-week double-blind treatment period; and an 8-week double-blind study medication withdrawal period, or the possibility of entering an open follow-up study. During the 12-week placebo baseline period, eligible patients stabilized on one or two appropriate AEDs at usual plasma concentrations were evaluated to determine whether they met all randomization criteria. Overall, 32% of patients were receiving one AED, 62% two AEDs, and 6% three or more AEDs. Patients had been stabilized on carbamazepine (57%), phenytoin (44%), gabapentin (28%), valproate (26%), phenobarbital (9%), primidone (6%), lamotrigine (5%), and "other" (7%) as one of their AEDs.

Randomization was in blocks by study site. Each patient was assigned a unique treatment number, which corre-

Ilo E. Leppik, MD: Director of Research, MINCEP Epilepsy Care, Minneapolis, Minnesota

TABLE 42.1. OVERVIEW OF THE THREE PIVOTAL STUDIES[a]

	Study 1 (9)	Study 2 (10)	Study 3 (8)
Minimum duration of intractable epilepsy before entry	2	2	1
Number of concomitant antiepileptic drugs	1–2	1–2	1
Minimum seizure frequency	12/12 wk	4/4 wk	2/4 wk
Levetiracetam dosage (maintenance, mg/d)	1,000; 3,000	1,000; 2,000	3,000
Conversion to monotherapy	No	No	Yes
Length of evaluation after titration	14 wk	12 wk	14 wk[b]

[a]All studies included patients from 16 to 65 or 70 years of age, required a stable regimen of the other antiepileptic drugs for at least 1 month, and excluded progressive neurological disorders and recent participation in other studies of antiepileptic drugs in the last 4 weeks.
[b]Followed by 12 weeks of conversion to monotherapy and 12 weeks of evaluation on monotherapy.

sponded to the blinded, randomized treatment, and each investigator was allocated treatment numbers in chronologic study entry order. Study medication was provided as identical white, film-coated, scored tablets containing either 166.5 mg LEV, 500 mg LEV, or placebo. LEV dosage was escalated at 2-week intervals during the 4-week, double-blind, dose titration period to the dose assigned at randomization. For the 1,000-mg/day group, dosages of LEV were 333 mg/day for 2 weeks, then 666 mg/day for 2 weeks and 1,000 mg/day started on the first visit of the evaluation period. The 3,000-mg/day group received 1,000 mg/day for two weeks, 2,000 mg/day for the next 2 weeks, then 3,000 mg/day. At the end of the 14-week treatment period, patients and investigators were given the option of entering a 1-year, open-label LEV continuation study. For patients choosing not to enter the follow-up study, LEV was withdrawn at a maximum of 500 mg/week during an 8-week study withdrawal period.

The primary efficacy variable was the mean number of partial seizures per week computed over the entire 14-week evaluation period. Secondary efficacy variables were median percentage reduction compared with baseline, responder rate (number of patients with a minimum of 50% reduction from baseline in partial seizure frequency), and number of seizure-free patients.

Of 385 enrolled patients, 91 were determined to be ineligible and were never randomized. The most common reasons for not randomizing patients were failure to fulfill selection criteria (33 patients), consent withdrawn (19 patients), adverse events not related to study (14 patients), and protocol violation (12 patients). Of the 294 intent-to-treat (ITT; randomized) patients, 95 were in the placebo group, 98 in the LEV 1,000-mg/day group, and 101 in the LEV 3,000-mg/day group.

Of the 294 ITT patients, 285 completed the titration period, 268 (91.2%) completed the 14-week observation period, and 266 chose to enter the open-label, follow-up study. Premature study discontinuations during the dose titration and observation periods included 12 of 98 patients (12.2%) in the LEV 1,000-mg/day group, 8 of 101 patients

(7.9%) in the LEV 3,000-mg/day group, and 6 of 95 patients (6.3%) in the placebo group.

The primary efficacy analysis of partial seizure frequency during the evaluation period was based on the 285 patients who completed the titration period. The percentage reduction in partial seizure frequency over placebo was 20.9% in the LEV 1,000-mg/day group and 27.7% in the LEV 3,000-mg/day group ($p < .001$ for both LEV groups).

Notably, reductions in partial seizure frequency over placebo were higher for both LEV groups at each evaluation visit ($p \leq .016$). The median percentage reduction (and median absolute reduction) from baseline in partial seizure frequency also was greater in patients receiving LEV than placebo: 32.5% (0.81 seizures/week) with LEV 1,000 mg/day and 37.1% (0.98 seizures/week) with LEV 3,000 mg/day, versus 6.8% (0.13 seizures/week) with placebo ($p < .001$).

The 50% responder rate using the ITT population (294) was 37.1% ($p < .001$) for the LEV 1,000-mg/day group, 39.8% ($p < .001$) for the LEV 3,000-mg/day group, and 7.4% for the placebo group. The 75% and 90% responder rates calculated for the 285 patients who had completed titration are presented in Table 42.2.

Three patients receiving LEV 1,000 mg/day (not significant) and eight receiving 3,000 mg/day ($p = .01$) compared with none receiving placebo were seizure free during the entire 14-week evaluation period. The percentage of placebo-treated patients experiencing a >25% increase in partial seizure frequency was approximately twice that of LEV-treated patients: 13.8% (13 of 94 patients) for LEV 1,000 mg/day and 12.2% (12 of 98 patients) for LEV 3,000 mg/day, versus 25.8% (24 of 93 patients) for placebo (9).

Seizure reduction was notable for all seizure subtypes, with significant reduction in complex partial (type IB) seizures and secondarily generalized (type IC) seizures for the LEV 1,000- and 3,000-mg/day groups.

Of the 268 patients completing the study, 266 chose to continue in a long-term follow-up study. Of these, 148 were still on LEV 2 years later, and their median percentage

TABLE 42.2. RESPONDER RATES FOR THE THREE PIVOTAL STUDIES

	Study 1 (9)			Study 2 (10)			Study 3 (8)	
	Placebo (n = 95)	LEV 1,000 (mg/day) (n = 98)	LEV 3,000 mg/day (n = 101)	Placebo (n = 111)	LEV 1,000 (mg/day) (n = 106)	LEV 2,000 mg/day (n = 105)	Placebo (n = 104)	LEV 3,000 mg/day (n = 180)
Percentage reduction in seizure frequency over placebo	—	26.1%[a,b]	30.1%[a,b]—	16.4[c]	17.7[c]	—	23.0%[a]	
Responder rate (% reduction from baseline)								
≥50%	7.4[b]	37.1%[a,b]	39.8%[a,b]	10.4%	22.8%	31.6%	16.7%	42.1%
≥75%	1.1%[d]	13.4%[a,d]	19.8%[d]	1.8%	8.5%	16.2%	4.8%	23.9%
≥90%	0[d]	8.3%[d]	10.9%[d]	0.9%	4.7%	6.7%	0	12.2%
100%	0[d]	4.1%[d]	5.9%[d]	0.9%	5%	2%	0	8.2%

[a]$p < .001$ vs. placebo.
[b]Based on 294 intent-to-treat subjects (18-wk titration and evaluation period).
[c]$p < .01$.
[d]Based on the 285 subjects who completed titration.

reduction in seizure frequency compared with their baseline was 73% at 2 years (9).

Study 2

This study was a randomized, double-blind, placebo-controlled, parallel-group study at 61 sites in Belgium, France, Germany, Luxembourg, Switzerland, and the United Kingdom (11). LEV was evaluated against placebo at doses of 1,000 mg/day (500 mg twice daily) and 2,000 mg/day (1,000 mg twice daily) as add-on therapy. LEV was started at 500 mg twice daily in both groups, and increased to 1,000 mg twice daily after 2 weeks in the 2,000-mg/day group.

The primary efficacy variable was the mean number of partial seizures per week computed during the evaluation period (i.e., seizure frequency). Secondary efficacy variables included the seizure frequency by seizure type and subtype, the responder rate, and the incidence of seizure-free patients.

Three hundred ninety-two patients were screened and 324 patients were randomized. All randomized patients became part of the ITT population: 112 in the placebo group, 106 in the group receiving LEV 1,000 mg/day, and 106 in the group receiving LEV 2,000 mg/day. Two hundred seventy-eight patients completed the study period. Dropout rates were 13% in the placebo group, 11% in the 1,000-mg/day group, and 18% in the 2,000-mg/day group. Across all treatment groups, the mean duration of epilepsy was 24 years and the mean age of epilepsy onset was 14 years. For more than half of the patients (57%), the cause of epilepsy was cryptogenic. At baseline, 31% of patients had simple partial seizures, 83% had complex partial seizures, and 26% had partial seizures with secondary generalization; 7% had generalized seizures or unclassified epileptic seizures. Baseline seizure frequency was compara-

ble between groups. The number of AEDs taken by patients at baseline and throughout the study was similar among treatment groups. Most patients' conditions had been stabilized on carbamazepine (72%), phenytoin (22%), or valproate (21%). Among newer agents, the most frequently prescribed were vigabatrin (18%), lamotrigine (12%), and gabapentin (2%).

LEV significantly decreased the seizure frequency compared with placebo, with reductions over placebo of 16.4% for the 1,000-mg/day group [98% confidence interval (CI), 2.7% to 28.1%; $p = .006$] and 17.7% (98% CI, 4.1% to 29.4%; $p = .003$) for the 2,000-mg/day group. The median percentage reductions in seizure frequency from baseline were 6.1% for placebo, 17.7% for LEV 1,000 mg/day, and 26.5% for LEV 2,000 mg/day; no significant difference was identified between the two doses of LEV.

The median reductions in simple partial seizure frequency from baseline were 9.1%, 38.1%, and 46.3%, respectively, for the placebo group, the 1,000-mg group, and the 2,000-mg group. For patients with complex partial seizures, the median reductions from baseline in frequency of complex partial seizures were 9.1%, 12.4%, and 24.4%, respectively. Median secondarily generalized seizure frequency increased by 16.8% in the placebo group but decreased by 37.4% in the 1,000-mg group and 28.2% in the 2,000-mg group.

A significant difference in the responder rate was found between the placebo and treatment groups ($p = .004$). More patients treated with LEV 1,000 mg/day (22.8%, $p = .019$ versus placebo) or 2,000 mg/day (31.6%, $p < .001$ versus placebo) could be categorized as treatment responders than in the placebo group (10.4%). The number of patients needed to treat to get a responder with a ≥50% reduction in seizure frequency during treatment with LEV was 6.9 (95% CI, 4.3 to 17.9) for the 1,000-mg group and 3.5 (95% CI, 2.6 to 5.4) for the 2,000-mg group. In addition,

3.7% of patients in the placebo group experienced a ≥75% reduction in seizure frequency, compared with 10.9% ($p = .03$) for the 1,000-mg group and 16.8% ($p = .001$ for the 2,000-mg group. Five patients (5.0%) in the 1,000-mg group and two patients (2.0%) in the 2,000-mg group were seizure free during the evaluation period, compared with one patient (0.9%) in the placebo group who reported no seizures until study withdrawal at day 29.

Study 3

This European, multicenter (47 institutions), randomized, double-blind, parallel-group, responder-selected study evaluated LEV 3,000 mg/day against placebo (8). Patients were recruited between June 1995 and May 1998, and a total of 343 were enrolled. This was a two-phase study, with evaluation of the target dose followed by withdrawal to monotherapy. Patients were evaluated on the target dose for 12 weeks (add-on evaluation period) after a 4-week titration period. During the following 2 weeks of the add-on evaluation period, investigators prepared a seizure profile of each patient using information obtained in the baseline and add-on phase and forwarded the profile to a central evaluator who determined which patients met the entry criteria for the monotherapy phase of the study.

The most frequently prescribed AEDs were carbamazepine (74%), lamotrigine (9%), valproate (8%), and phenytoin (6%). The main efficacy variable for the add-on phase of the study was seizure frequency, reported as the median number of partial seizures per week, and the responder rate (i.e., the proportion of patients with a reduction in partial seizure frequency of ≥50% compared with baseline).

Efficacy and safety analyses were conducted on the ITT population, which included all patients who were randomized and took at least one dose of study medication. For the monotherapy portion of the study, the primary efficacy assessment (i.e., the percentage of patients who completed the monotherapy phase relative to the number of patients randomized to study medication) was analyzed using Fisher's exact test.

Of the 343 enrolled, 286 patients were eligible for randomization to LEV or placebo (181 to LEV, 105 to placebo) and comprised the ITT study population. The percentage of patients completing the add-on phase was similar in both treatment groups (placebo, n = 90, 85%; LEV, n = 149, 82%). The median partial seizure frequency was significantly lower in patients treated with LEV (1.06 seizures/week) compared with placebo (1.75 seizures/week) during the add-on phase. Likewise, the median percentage reduction in partial seizure frequency from baseline to the add-on phase was 39.9% with LEV compared with 7.2% with placebo ($p < .001$). the responder rate was significantly higher with LEV than placebo (42.1% versus 16.7%, $p < .001$), with the odds of achieving a ≥50% reduction in

seizure frequency 3.6 times greater. In addition, 8.2% (14/171) of LEV-treated patients remained seizure free during the add-on evaluation period, compared with only 1 patient in the placebo group ($p = .012$). The number of patients needed to treat to obtain one responder due to LEV effect was 3.9 (95% CI, 2.8 to 6.6) (12). The number of patients needed to treat to obtain one seizure-free patient due to LEV effect was 13.9 (95% CI, 8.5 to 37.4). Monotherapy results are discussed later in this chapter.

Pooled Analyses

After the three pivotal studies were completed, a pooled efficacy analysis of the 589 LEV-treated patients (all doses and seizure types) and 310 placebo-treated patients who had baseline and add-on treatment data was done (13). Overall, there was a 31.3% median decrease in the number of seizures per week in all LEV-treated patients compared with a 5.4% decrease in the placebo group ($p < .001$). The overall ≥50% responder rate was 35.0% (206 of 589) for LEV-treated patients compared with 9.4% for placebo ($p < .001$). This responder rate was dose dependent, with the responder rate being 28.6% for the 1,000-mg/day dose, 35.2% for 2,000 mg/day, and 39.5% for 3,000 mg/day (13).

Additional evaluation was performed by seizure type: IA (simple partial), IB (complex partial), and IC (secondarily generalized), using the International League Against Epilepsy classification system (14). The efficacy of LEV on IC seizures over and above the ability to reduce all partial seizures was analyzed in all patients with IC seizures during baseline or the evaluation period (15). The ratio of secondarily generalized seizure frequency per week over partial seizure frequency per week was calculated for each patient both for the baseline and evaluation periods. Treatment was considered to have a greater ability to reduce IC seizures over and above all partial seizures if (Equation 1):

$$\frac{IC\ baseline}{(IA + IB + IC)\ baseline} > \frac{IC\ evaluation}{(IA + IB + IC)\ evaluation}$$

A logistic regression model taking into account treatment and study was used to compare treatment groups with respect to secondarily generalized seizure success rate. The median percentage seizure reduction from baseline was 42.7% for simple partial seizures, 36.1% for complex partial seizures, and 68.5% for secondarily generalized seizures ($p < .05$ for all seizure types versus placebo).

The percentage of patients successfully treated for secondarily generalized seizures (ratio less during evaluation versus baseline) was significantly greater in the LEV group (59%) than in the placebo group (44.9%). The odds of successful treatment of secondarily generalized seizures with LEV therapy were 1.83 (95% CI, 1.10 to 3.05) times higher than the odds of successful treatment with placebo (15).

Monotherapy

The major study of monotherapy completed to date was the second phase of the second European study (study 3 in this chapter) (8). Only patients who responded to LEV or placebo during the add-on phase were eligible for entry into the monotherapy phase. The following criteria (relative to baseline) must have been met: (a) ≥50% reduction in partial seizures or ≥35% reduction in simple partial seizures (type IA) provided that complex partial seizures (type IB) were reduced by ≥50% and secondary generalized seizures (type IC) were not higher than baseline; (b) no doubling of IB or IC seizure frequency; and (c) no type IC seizures during add-on phase if not present during baseline.

In the first half of the monotherapy phase, the dose of the standard AED was withdrawn gradually over a period of up to 12 weeks (downtitration period), while the dose of the study medication remained constant. The latter half was the monotherapy evaluation phase, in which patients received only study medication for up to 12 weeks. Patients were withdrawn from the monotherapy phase if they met one of the following escape criteria relative to baseline: (a) doubling of monthly type IB or IC seizure frequency, (b) occurrence of status epilepticus, or (c) emergence of type IC seizures if none occurred during baseline.

For ethical reasons, the study was designed under the assumption that no more than 10% of patients taking placebo would fulfill the responder selection criteria. When a total of nine placebo responders was reached, for ethical reasons, each subsequent placebo responder was switched to LEV for the monotherapy phase without breaking the blind. These patients were analyzed as if they were still taking placebo.

The primary efficacy variable of the study was the percentage of patients who completed the monotherapy phase relative to the number of patients randomized to receive study medication. Except for the primary efficacy assessment, no statistical comparison between treatment groups was performed in the monotherapy phase because the placebo group was established solely to maintain the double-blind status of the study and not to be used as a comparative group.

Of the 239 patients who completed the add-on phase, 86 patients were eligible to enter the monotherapy phase of the study (placebo, n = 17, 16.2%; LEV, n = 69, 38.1%). For ethical purposes, 8 of the 17 patients taking placebo were switched to treatment with LEV, but for analysis, they remained in the placebo group. Twenty-five patients (placebo, n = 5; LEV, n = 20) were withdrawn during the downtitration period mostly because they met escape criteria (placebo, n = 2; LEV, n = 11). Forty-nine of the 69 (70%) patients receiving LEV were successfully downtitrated to LEV monotherapy. In these patients, the median absolute reduction in partial seizure frequency from baseline to the monotherapy evaluation period was 0.61 (*p* = .012), with a 73.8% median percentage reduction in partial seizure frequency (*p* = .037).

Of the ITT population, 19.9% (36/181) of patients randomized to LEV treatment completed the study, compared with only 9.5% (10/105) in the placebo group (*p* = .029). The odds of completing the study were 2.36 times higher for LEV than placebo. Of note, 4 of the 10 patients in the placebo group who completed the study had been switched to treatment with LEV at the start of the monotherapy phase for ethical reasons.

Compared with the add-on phase, a slightly higher frequency of seizures was reported during the monotherapy evaluation period (median increase = 0.04). In addition, the 50% responder rate during this treatment period was 59.2%. Nine of 49 patients (18.4%) taking LEV were completely seizure free throughout the 12-week monotherapy evaluation period. Of these nine patients, six had been seizure free since the uptitration period, a total interval of 31 to 39 weeks. In the placebo group, three patients were seizure free throughout the 12-week monotherapy evaluation period. One of these patients had received placebo during the add-on phase and became seizure free during the 12-week monotherapy evaluation period subsequent to his switch to LEV in the monotherapy phase.

Other Seizure Types

Animal studies suggest that LEV should have a broad spectrum of action in human epilepsy (16). However, few clinical reports are available yet. One review of participants of various open-label studies of LEV found 13 who had juvenile myoclonic epilepsy and had not responded to valproate and lamotrigine. Twelve had suppression of seizures by 50% or more, and 6 of 13 became seizure free for the duration of the various studies, with a mean of 36 months (17). In one study of photosensitive epilepsy, LEV was found to be effective in blocking the induced epileptiform response (5). Because LEV is structurally related to piracetam, it has been suggested that it may be effective in myoclonic syndromes (18). To date, six patients with myoclonus treated with LEV have been reported. In one report, three patients with debilitating myoclonus (one with postanoxic myoclonus, two with Unverricht-Lundborg disease) were treated with LEV 4,000 mg/day as the initial dose with no titration. All three patients had a dramatic reduction of myoclonus. However, because LEV was an investigational drug, it was replaced by piracetam (19). Three additional patients with posthypoxic or postencephalitic myoclonus successfully treated with LEV have been reported (20).

CLINICAL USE ISSUES

Initiation of Treatment

In most studies, LEV had been titrated to higher dosages. In the U.S. phase III studies, the treatment groups were divided into low-dose titration (333 mg/day, 666 mg/day, and 3,000 mg/day) or high-dose titration (1,000 mg/day, 2,000 mg/day, and 3,000 mg/day). There appears to be no differences in dropout rate or adverse event reports between these groups. One study was specifically designed to address this issue and involved 119 subjects who received 1,000 mg twice daily (2,000 mg/day) or 2,000 mg twice daily (4,000 mg/day) immediately. The overall responder rate (≥50% reduction in seizures compared with baseline) was 43.0% (21). Both 2,000-mg and 4,000-mg doses were well tolerated, with similar side effect profiles and discontinuation rates. Labeling in the United States recommends initiation with 500 mg twice daily with dosage increases based on clinical response (22). However, in clinical practice involving less refractory patients, some individuals do not tolerate these initial dosages and slower titration may be needed (Leppik, personal observation).

Onset of antiseizure activity is rapid after the initiation of LEV. Data from the three phase III trials were evaluated to determine the proportion of seizure-free days after initiation of treatment. The percentage of patients having a seizure-free day was increased by 11% to 20% compared with placebo ($p < .001$) 1 day after initiation, and similar increases were seen if a 3- or 7-day period was used (23). A similar rapid onset was observed for the patients with myoclonus (19).

Special Populations

Studies performed for the purpose of registration have narrow entry criteria that often exclude or limit children, women of childbearing potential, and persons with medical illnesses. Some information regarding these populations has been obtained from various smaller open-label studies (24).

Pediatric Population

A safety, tolerability, and pharmacokinetic study of LEV in pediatric patients with epilepsy was conducted at six sites in the United States (25,26). Twenty-four patients were enrolled (15 boys, 9 girls) with a mean age of 9.4 years (range, 5.6 to 12.6 years), and all had partial seizures with or without secondary generalized seizures. In this add-on study, all patients were taking a steady regimen of one other AED. LEV was administered as a single dose of approximately 20 mg/kg on day 1 of active treatment and then, starting on day 2, LEV was given every 12 hours beginning at approximately 10 mg/kg/day. Dosages were escalated to ~40 mg/kg/day (in equal doses twice daily), in 2-week increments, with a safety evaluation before each dosage escalation (25). The 40-mg/kg/day dosage would equal 3,000 mg/day LEV in an adult patient weighing approximately 75 kg.

Pharmacokinetic data were obtained after the initial administration of 20 mg/kg (26). Titration was followed by an 8-week evaluation period. The clearance of LEV was

30% to 40% higher in these children than in adults, and the half-life was correspondingly shorter (~6 hours). The preliminary recommendation from this study is that the maintenance dose of LEV in children should be 30% to 40% higher on a weight basis than the recommended maintenance dose in adults. Although efficacy was observed, results from ongoing studies involving larger numbers of subjects of the efficacy of LEV in children are needed.

Elderly

One study was conducted in 16 hospitalized elderly volunteers (5 men and 11 women) (11). Plasma concentration and urinary excretion of LEV were studied after a single 500-mg dose and also after 500 mg twice daily for 10 days. Creatinine clearance (ClCr) was diminished but higher than 30 mL/min/1.73 m^2 in all subjects (range = 30.1 to 73.9 mL/min/1.73 m^2). After a single 500-mg oral dose of LEV, plasma half-life was longer (10.3 ± 1.7 hours) compared with that seen in young adult volunteers (7.7 hours). After multiple dosing, plasma half-life was 10.4 ± 1.8 hours.

Results indicated that although clearance was reduced and half-life prolonged in these elderly subjects, these effects were entirely attributable to reduced renal function.

Renal Impairment

Three studies have been done to assess LEV in patients with impaired renal function: a single-dose study, a multiple-dose study, and a study in patients with end-stage renal disease. A single-dose study of LEV was conducted in 11 subjects (6 men and 5 women) with varying degrees of renal function (11). Two of the subjects had normal renal function (ClCr ≥ 90 mL/min/1.73 m^2). The other nine subjects had mild, moderate, or severe impairment (ClCr range = 5.6 to 84 mL/min/1.73 m^2). The dose of LEV was 500 mg. The renal clearance of LEV was directly proportional to the ClCr. The half-life of the drug ranged from 10.4 hours in those with mild impairment to 24.1 hours in those with severe impairment.

In a follow-up to the single-dose study, patients with renal insufficiency were administered multiple doses of LEV (11). Twenty-one patients were enrolled (14 men and 7 women), 5 of whom had normal renal function (ClCr ≥ 90 mL/min/1.73 m^2). The remaining patients had varying degrees of renal impairment (ClCr = 13 to 80 mL/min/1.73 m^2). The mean age was 57.9 years (range, 21 to 77 years). A single dose of LEV was administered on the first day of the study. Patients with ClCr ≥ 40 mL/min/1.73 m^2 received a single 1,000-mg dose of LEV; subjects with poorer renal function received a single dose of 500 mg. On days 2 to 9, patients with ClCr ≥ 40 mL/min/1.73 m^2 received a 2,000-mg dose of LEV (1,000 mg twice daily), whereas subjects with poorer renal function received 1,000 mg (500 mg twice daily). Total-body clearance was reduced in patients with renal impairment and was proportional to ClCr. Multiple dosing did not affect the pharmacokinetic parameters.

A study of five patients with end-stage renal disease undergoing dialysis (two male and three female; mean age = 58.4 years, range = 36 to 72 years) also was conducted (11). A single dose of 500 mg of LEV was administered to each subject immediately after a 4-hour dialysis. As expected, the half-life of the drug was prolonged, to an average of 24.6 hours, and the principal inactive metabolite of LEV, UCB L057, accumulated during the interdialysis period. After dialysis, the plasma LEV and metabolite concentration was reduced by approximately 50%.

These three studies in patients with impaired renal function indicate that LEV dosing must be individualized according to the patient's renal function status.

LONG-TERM EFFICACY

Follow-up evaluations of persons participating in various LEV studies have provided information regarding long-term efficacy. A total of 1,442 patients with refractory epilepsy (median age 36.0 years, range 7 to 78 years) were exposed to LEV. The mean duration of treatment was 537 (standard deviation, 492) days, and the median LEV dosage was 3,000 mg/day. The LEV retention rate was estimated to be 58% after 1 year, 43% after 2 years, and 36% after 3 years. In the 970 patients with a baseline evaluation, the median seizure reduction under LEV treatment was 37.8% (evaluation period, 1 week to 5 years). At least a 50% seizure reduction was seen in 38.5% of patients, and 19.2% had at least a 75% seizure reduction. From the 599 patients with an exposure to treatment exceeding 1 year, 67 (11.2%) because seizure free for at least 1 year. No tolerance to the effects of LEV has been noted (23).

Data of all patients with epilepsy exposed to LEV during the developmental program of the drug were analyzed. The retention rate was analyzed using the Kaplan-Meier method. A Cox regression model was used to identify predictors of a higher retention. Data collected through a cut-off date of June 30, 1999 have been presented (27). A total of 1,422 patients with refractory epilepsy were exposed to LEV (median age, 36 years, range 5 to 78 years); the median dose was 3,000 mg/day. The mean duration of exposure was 622 days (range, 1 to 2,984 days). Forty percent of patients were still being treated at the end of the observation period. In 16% of patients, the treatment was terminated because of adverse events, in 18% because of lack or loss of efficacy. The LEV retention rate was estimated to be 60% after the first year, 37% after 3 years, and 32% after 5 years. The median seizure reduction from baseline was 40%. Thirty-nine percent of patients had a seizure reduction of 50% or more, 20% of patients of 75% or more. Thirteen percent of patients were seizure free for at

least 6 months and 8% for at least 1 year in ITT analysis. If the analysis was restricted to patients who effectively were exposed to LEV treatment exceeding 6 months, seizure freedom for at least 6 months was observed in 17% of patients. The drug was usually well tolerated, and adverse events were mainly central nervous system related and mild, including somnolence and dizziness. There was no evidence for idiosyncratic side effects. No tolerance to the effects of LEV has been noted. The Cox regression model identified four factors that were correlated with higher retention rates: (a) higher maintenance doses of LEV, (b) lower starting doses of LEV, (c) presence of convulsive seizures, and (d) lower number of concomitant AEDs. Factors that did not significantly influence retention on LEV were age at onset of epilepsy, duration of epilepsy, history of status epilepticus, and history of withdrawal seizures. These data indicate that LEV is an effective and well tolerated new AED. The long-term retention rate and percentage of seizure freedom in patients with refractory epilepsy seem to be higher than those of other new AEDs.

SURROGATE MEASURES OF EFFICACY
Quality of Life

Although efficacy as measured by seizure frequency is the principal outcome evaluated in studies, of great importance to the patient is the change in quality of life made possible by a new treatment. The ultimate effectiveness of a drug when used in typical clinical situations encompasses the patient's perception of its modulation of the overall health status. The U.S. phase III study incorporated the QOLIE-31 battery (31-item Quality of Life in Epilepsy) and was completed by 246 of the 294 patients enrolled (28). Overall, "seizure-worry" cognitive functioning, and overall QOL scores improved compared with placebo ($p < .0003$; $p < 0.04$; and $p < 0.01$, respectively). The improvements were most marked for persons who were responders (28). A shorter form, QOLIE-10, compares well with the longer version and may be more useful in clinical settings (12).

Seizure-Free Days

Another measure of improvement is the evaluation of seizure-free days. Of 904 patients, 846 with evaluable data were considered in the analysis of seizure-free days: 189 at 1,000 mg/day, 90 at 2,000 mg/day; 269 at 3,000 mg/day, and 298 on placebo. A seizure-free day was defined as a reported day without seizures. The mean proportion of seizure-free days per year was defined as the proportion of days without seizure computed over a period of time and extrapolated to a per year value. The increase in days without seizure was examined during the evaluation period and compared with baseline. Patient diaries were used as data sources for seizure dates and characteristics. Treatment effect was tested in each individual study and in a pooled analysis, using an analysis of variance with baseline as covariate. Results were confirmed by a nonparametric Wilcoxon test. In the three individual studies and in the pooled analysis, the increase in seizure-free days was statistically significant at all LEV doses over placebo. Considering the impact on days with seizure, the pooled analysis reveals that from an adjusted baseline of 105.8 seizure days per year, patients experienced a 14.7-days/year (13.9%) decrease for LEV 1,000 mg/day, a 19-days/year (17.9%) decrease for LEV 2,000 mg/day, and a 20.2-days/year (19.1%) decrease for LEV 3,000 mg/day in the number of days with seizures ($p < .0001$ for analysis of covariance). The treatment effect was confirmed by the results of the Wilcoxon test ($p < .0001$) (29).

CONCLUSION

Levetiracetam has proven efficacy in the treatment of localization-related epilepsies. Dosages of 1,000 to 3,000 mg/day have been thoroughly evaluated in placebo-controlled trials. In clinical use, higher dosages may be found to be useful. At present, LEV does not have a monotherapy indication in the United States, but in some persons, withdrawal to monotherapy may be a useful approach. It appears to maintain antiseizure activity for extended periods. Further studies in absence and myoclonic disorders are needed, but preliminary observations are favorable for broader use (30).

ACKNOWLEDGMENTS

Supported in part by NIH grant P50 NS16308. The author thanks Liliane Dargis for word processing.

REFERENCES

1. Chevalier Y, Grant R, Sander JWAS, et al. Twelve week add-on, increasing dose (1,000–4,000 mg/day) multicenter pilot study of ucb L059 in epileptic patients. *Epilepsia* 1995;36[Suppl 3]:S153.
2. Creech J, Abou-Khalil BW, Fakhoury T, et al. Levetiracetam in intractable partial epilepsy: efficacy of add-on therapy and patient retention. *Epilepsia* 1999;40[Suppl 7]:148.
3. Dreifuss F, Cereghino J, Debrabandere L, et al. Multicenter, double-blind, placebo-controlled trial of ucbL059 (500 mg b.i.d. and 1500 mg b.i.d.) as add-on therapy in patients with refractory partial epilepsy. *Epilepsia* 1996;37[Suppl 5]:204.
4. Grant R, Shorvon SD. Efficacy and tolerability of 1000–4000 mg per day of levetiracetam as add-on therapy in patients with refractory epilepsy. *Epilepsy Res* 2000;42:89–95.
5. Kastelijn-Nolst Trenite DGA, Marescaux C, Stodieck S, et al. Photosensitive epilepsy: a model to study the effects of antiepileptic drugs. Evaluation of the piracetam analogue, levetiracetam. *Epilepsy Res* 1996;25:225–230.
6. Van Rijckevorselk K, Debrabandere L, Deberdt W. Evaluation of the efficacy and tolerability of UCB L059 in refractory epileptic patients with complex partial seizures: a 12 week, single blind, add-on, rising dose study. *Epilepsia* 1996;37[Suppl 5]:169.
7. Dooley M, Plosker GL. Levetiracetam: a review of its adjunctive use in the management of partial onset seizures. *Drugs* 2000; 60:871–893.
8. Ben-Menachem E, Falter U, for the European Levetiracetam Study Group. Efficacy and tolerability of levetiracetam 3000 mg in patients with refractory partial seizures: a multicenter, double-blind, responder-selected study evaluating monotherapy. *Epilepsia* 2000;41:1276–1283.
9. Cereghino JJ, Biton V, Abou-Khalil B, et al., and the United States Levetiracetam Study Group. Levetiracetam for partial seizures: results of a double-blind, randomized clinical trial. *Neurology* 2000;55:236–242.
10. Shorvon SD, Lowenthal A, Janz D, et al., for the European Levetiracetam Study Group. Multicenter double-blind, randomized, placebo-controlled trial of levetiracetam as add-on therapy in patients with refractory partial seizures. *Epilepsia* 2000;41: 1179–1186.
11. UCB Pharma. Data on file.
12. Cramer JA, Arrigo C, Van Hammee G, et al. Comparison between the QOLIE-31 and derived QOLIE-10 in a clinical trial of levetiracetam. *Epilepsy Res* 2000;41:29–38.
13. Privitera M. Efficacy of levetiracetam: a review of three pivotal clinical trials. *Epilepsia* 2001 (*in press*).
14. Commission on Classification and Terminology of the International League Against Epilepsy. Proposal for the classification of epilepsy and epileptic syndromes. *Epilepsia* 1989;30:389–399.
15. Nohria V, Leppik IE, Verdru P, et al. Levetiracetam: evaluation of success rate in secondarily generalized seizures (type IC) in addition to activity in partial seizures (type I). *Neurology* 1999;52 [Suppl 2]:A247.
16. Jain KK. An assessment of levetiracetam as an anti-epileptic drug. *Expert Opin Invest Drugs* 2000;9:1611–1624.
17. Smith K, Betts T, Pritchett L. Levetiracetam, a promising option for the treatment of juvenile myoclonic epilepsy. Presented at the 4th European Congress on Epileptology, Firenze, Italy, October 7, 2000.
18. Genton P, Van Vleymen B. Piracetam and levetiracetam: close structural similarities but different pharmacological and clinical profiles. *Epileptic Dis* 2000;2:99–105.
19. Genton P, Gelisse P. Antimyoclonic effect of levetiracetam. *Epileptic Dis* 2000;2:209–212.
20. Krauss GL, Bergin A, Kramer RE, et al. Suppression of posthypoxic and post-encephalitic myoclonus with levetiracetam. *Neurology* 2001;56:411–412.
21. Betts T, Waegemans T, Crawford P. A multicentre, double-blind, randomized, parallel group study to evaluate the tolerability and efficacy of two oral doses of levetiracetam, 2000 mg daily and 4000 mg daily, without titration in patients with refractory epilepsy. *Seizure* 2000;9:80–87.
22. *Physicians' Desk Reference*, 55th ed. Montvale, NJ: Medical Economics Company, 2001.
23. French J, Privitera M, Arrigo C, et al. Rapid onset of action of levetiracetam in refractory epileptic patients. *Neurology* 2000;54 [Suppl 3]:A83.
24. French J. Use of levetiracetam in special populations. *Epilepsia* 2001 (*in press*).
25. Glauser T. Open-label efficacy and safety of levetiracetam in pediatric patients with partial-onset seizures. Presented at the Annual Meeting of the American Epilepsy Society, Orlando, FL, December 7, 1999.
26. Pellock J, Glauser T, Bebin M, et al. Single-dose pharmacokinet-

ics of levetiracetam in pediatric patients with partial epilepsy. Presented at the Annual Meeting of the American Epilepsy Society, Orlando, FL, December 7, 1999.

27. Krakow K, Otoul C, l'Alleud B, et al. Long-term efficacy and tolerability of levetiracetam (LEV) in refractory epilepsy. *Neurology* 2000;54[Suppl 3]:A83.

28. Cramer JA, Arrigo C, Van Hammee G, et al., for the N132 Study Group. Effect of levetiracetam on epilepsy-related quality of life. *Epilepsia* 2000;41:868–874.

29. Leppik I, Morrell M, Bigdeli M, et al. Seizure-free days gained with levetiracetam in refractory epileptic patients. *Neurology* 2000;54[Suppl 3]:A307.

30. Leppik I. The place of levetiracetam in the treatment of epilepsy. *Epilepsia* 2001 (*in press*).

Antiepileptic Drugs, 5th Edition. Edited by R.H. Levy, R.H. Mattson, B.S. Meldrum, and E. Perucca. Lippincott Williams & Wilkins, Philadelphia © 2002.

LEVETIRACETAM

ADVERSE EXPERIENCES

VICTOR BITON

Levetiracetam, or ucb L059, was approved by the U.S. Food and Drug Administration in November 1999 as add-on therapy for the treatment of partial seizures in adults, and is marketed under the trade name Keppra (UCB Pharmaceuticals, Hampton, VA). Recommended dosages are 1,000 to 3,000 mg/day, given twice daily. Levetiracetam is the (S)-enantiomer of α-ethyl-2-oxo-1-pyrrolidine acetamide, structurally and pharmacologically a novel compound with respect to other antiepileptic drugs. It is chemically related to piracetam, a drug marketed in Europe for many years.

The toxicity profile of levetiracetam has been characterized after single and repeat intravenous (i.v.) and oral administration in mice, rats, and dogs. Repeat oral administration of levetiracetam in dosages of up to 1,800 mg/kg/day in rats and 1,200 mg/kg/day in dogs is well tolerated. Clinical signs are minimal across studies and species, with the most consistent observations being neuromuscular effects, salivation, and, in dogs, emesis. Only in the rodent were treatment-related changes in the liver and kidney reported; these are species specific and are not of toxicologic concern to humans. Studies in neonatal or juvenile animals do not indicate any greater potential for toxicity compared with adult animals. Investigations involving administration of ucb L057, the major human metabolite, and ucb L060 [the (R)-enantiomer] indicate a low potential for toxicity in animals. Levetiracetam is neither carcinogenic nor mutagenic; although no evidence for carcinogenicity was seen, the potential for a carcinogenic response has not been fully evaluated in mice. As discussed elsewhere in this chapter, the drug is not teratogenic.

The clinical development of levetiracetam began in the early 1980s. Before its approval, comprehensive safety data were obtained in 3,347 subjects exposed to levetiracetam. The primary focus of this review of the safety of levetiracetam is its use in the 1,422 (primarily adult) patients with epilepsy who participated in clinical trials. Overall, the median levetiracetam dosage was 3,000 mg/day, with treatment continuing on average for approximately 1 year, and for up to 8 years. A total of 769 of these patients received levetiracetam 1,000 to 4,000 mg/day in one of four placebo-controlled studies of approximately 6 months' duration (1–4). The dosage and duration of exposure in placebo-controlled trials are illustrated in Figure 43.1.

Given levetiracetam's structural relationship to piracetam, early development efforts were in diverse indications relating to cognition, anxiety, and prevention of deep vein thrombosis. The dosages used in the 1,559 patients who participated in these studies in general were lower than those in patients with epilepsy, and the durations of treatment were shorter. Three hundred sixty-seven volunteers have participated in clinical pharmacology studies, including geriatric patients and subjects with hepatic or renal impairment. The safety profile in these studies is consistent with that observed in the epilepsy trials.

Levetiracetam has been available for use in the United States since April 2000. It was launched internationally in September 2000. It is estimated that approximately 38,000 patients have used this medication during the first 6 months of commercial use, a 25-fold increase in exposure relative to the investigational stage. To date, no new treatment-related adverse events have been identified during this broader use.

MOST COMMONLY OBSERVED ADVERSE EFFECTS

Adverse Events

Adverse events associated with levetiracetam pertain primarily to the central nervous system. In placebo-controlled studies, the most common such events were somnolence, asthenia, and dizziness. Vertigo, although infrequent, occurred in significantly more levetiracetam-treated patients. Headache and accidental injury also were common adverse effects, but occurred with a comparable or

Victor Biton, MD: Director, Arkansas Epilepsy Program, Little Rock, Arkansas

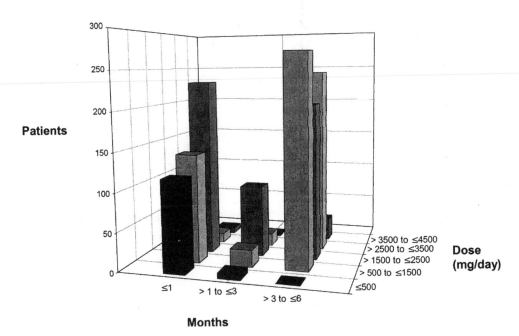

FIGURE 43.1. Dose and duration of exposure to levetiracetam in placebo-controlled studies in patients with epilepsy.

higher frequency before treatment and in placebo-treated patients. The incidence of treatment-emergent adverse events that occurred in at least 3% of the levetiracetam-treated patients is summarized in Table 43.1.

Psychiatric events commonly are reported in patients with epilepsy, often related to the disease itself or the effects of antiepileptic medication. The overall incidence of psychiatric adverse experiences in placebo-controlled studies of

TABLE 43.1. MOST COMMON ADVERSE EXPERIENCES IN PLACEBO-CONTROLLED EPILEPSY TRIALS: LIMITED TO THOSE REPORTED BY ≥3.0% LEVETIRACETAM-TREATED ADULT PATIENTS AND OCCURRING MORE OFTEN THAN WITH PLACEBO

	Levetiracetam (n = 769)	Placebo (n = 439)
Body as a whole		
Asthenia	113 (14.7%)	40 (9.1%)
Headache	105 (13.7%)	59 (13.4%)
Infection	103 (13.4%)	33 (7.5%)
Pain	52 (6.8%)	26 (5.9%)
Digestive system		
Nausea	34 (4.4%)	19 (4.3%)
Nervous system		
Depression	31 (4.0%)	10 (2.3%)
Dizziness	68 (8.8%)	18 (4.1%)
Insomnia	24 (3.1%)	11 (2.5%)
Nervousness	30 (3.9%)	8 (1.8%)
Somnolence	114 (14.8%)	37 (8.4%)
Respiratory system		
Pharyngitis	47 (6.1%)	17 (3.9%)
Rhinitis	34 (4.4%)	11 (2.5%)

levetiracetam in adult patients with epilepsy is within the expected range for patients with epilepsy. Nonpsychotic behavioral symptoms were the most common, occurring in approximately 13% of the patients (compared with 6% in the placebo-treated group). Individual events that were significantly more common with levetiracetam treatment were nervousness, emotional lability, and hostility. Sleep disorders, including abnormal dreams and insomnia, occurred less frequently (4% levetiracetam-treated patients, compared with 3% of placebo-treated patients).

Adverse events reflective of cognition (such as amnesia, confusion, and thinking abnormal) occurred in 3% to 4% of patients, regardless of treatment group. Although an infrequent event, significantly more levetiracetam-treated patients reported amnesia (2%, compared with <1% in placebo-treated patients).

A significantly higher incidence of infections was observed in the levetiracetam-treated patients (approximately 13%, compared with 7% of patients in the placebo group). These were primarily mild infections, such as common colds and upper respiratory infections, and did not interrupt treatment. There was not an increase in the incidence of other infections. The underlying cause is unclear and the symptoms were not related to changes in white blood cell or neutrophil counts.

Few patients discontinued double-blind treatment as a result of an adverse event (11% of levetiracetam-treated patients and 8% of placebo-treated patients). For the levetiracetam-treated group, the most frequent reasons for dose reduction or discontinuation were somnolence, dizziness, asthenia, and headaches. Convulsions also were a frequent cause, 3% in both treatment groups. Table 43.2 describes

TABLE 43.2. ADVERSE EXPERIENCES THAT RESULTED IN ≥0.5% LEVETIRACETAM-TREATED PATIENTS DISCONTINUING OR HAVING A DOSE REDUCTION

	Levetiracetam (n = 769)	Placebo (n = 439)
Body as a whole		
Accidental injury	6 (0.8%)	3 (0.7%)
Asthenia	10 (1.3%)	3 (0.7%)
Headache	8 (1.2%)	2 (0.5%)
Digestive system		
Nausea	7 (0.9%)	2 (0.5%)
Nervous system		
Ataxia	7 (0.9%)	1 (0.2%)
Dizziness	11 (1.4%)	0
Emotional lability	4 (0.5%)	1 (0.2%)
Hostility	4 (0.6%)	1 (0.3%)
Nervousness	5 (0.7%)	0
Personality disorder	4 (0.5%)	0
Somnolence	34 (4.4%)	7 (1.6%)
Mental slowing	5 (0.7%)	1 (0.2%)
Special senses		
Diplopia	4 (0.5%)	0

the incidence of adverse experiences resulting in 0.5% or more patients in the levetiracetam treatment group discontinuing or having a dose reduction.

Clinical Laboratory and Other Objective Studies

In the double-blind, placebo-controlled studies, levetiracetam treatment did not affect any of the five parameters of liver functions that were measured. These included aspartate aminotransferase, alanine aminotransferase, γ-glutamyl transferase, total bilirubin, and alkaline phosphatase. No effects were found on any other serum biochemistry parameter. There were no treatment-related effects on hematology parameters. Although there were statistically significant differences noted between the levetiracetam and placebo treatment groups, with lower hemoglobin, hematocrit, and neutrophil count in patients receiving levetiracetam, the magnitudes of change were not clinically meaningful. Furthermore, abnormalities were not associated with clinical consequences.

There were no treatment-related effects noted on physical or neurologic examination. Similarly, vital sign measurements did not reveal any treatment-related effects. Specifically with respect to body weight, there was no statistically significant change from baseline in the levetiracetam treatment group.

Electrocardiograms were obtained on 567 patients who received levetiracetam and 298 patients who received placebo in the double-blind, placebo-controlled epilepsy studies. There was no apparent effect of levetiracetam on the PR, QRS, or QTC intervals.

Dose Dependency

In the recommended adult dosage range, 1,000 to 3,000 mg/day, there is no clear dose–response relationship for adverse events. Adverse events occurring in 3% or more of patients in placebo-controlled studies are summarized by dosage in Table 43.3; only those events occurring more often among levetiracetam-treated patients are included. In

TABLE 43.3. ADVERSE EXPERIENCES BY RANDOMIZED DOSE IN PLACEBO-CONTROLLED EPILEPSY TRIALS: LIMITED TO THOSE OCCURRING IN ≥3.0% OF LEVETIRACETAM PATIENTS OVERALL, AND OCCURRING MORE OFTEN THAN WITH PLACEBO

	By Dose (mg/d)			
	1,000 (n = 298)	2,000 (n = 244)	3,000 (n = 282)	4,000 (n = 38)
Body as a whole				
Asthenia	32 (10.7%)	41 (16.8%)	38 (13.5%)	5 (13.2%)
Headache	48 (16.1%)	30 (12.3%)	29 (10.3%)	3 (7.9%)
Infection	42 (14.1%)	17 (7.0%)	39 (13.8%)	6 (15.8%)
Pain	26 (8.7%)	5 (2.0%)	20 (7.1%)	1 (2.6%)
Digestive system				
Nausea	15 (5.0%)	6 (2.5%)	8 (2.8%)	5 (13.2%)
Nervous system				
Depression	10 (3.4%)	11 (4.5%)	8 (2.8%)	3 (7.9%)
Dizziness	25 (8.4%)	12 (4.9%)	27 (9.6%)	4 (10.5%)
Insomnia	7 (2.3%)	4 (1.6%)	11 (3.9%)	2 (5.3%)
Nervousness	8 (2.7%)	10 (4.1%)	11 (3.9%)	2 (5.3%)
Somnolence	37 (12.4%)	31 (12.7%)	30 (10.6%)	17 (44.7%)
Respiratory system				
Pharyngitis	22 (7.4%)	15 (6.1%)	10 (3.5%)	2 (5.3%)
Rhinitis	22 (7.4%)	3 (1.2%)	9 (3.2%)	1 (2.6%)

TABLE 43.4. INCIDENCE OF ADVERSE EXPERIENCES BY ONSET: LIMITED TO EVENTS REPORTED IN ≥5.0% OF LEVETIRACETAM-TREATED PATIENTS OVERALL AND OCCURRING MORE OFTEN THAN WITH PLACEBO

	By Categorization of Onset			
	1 Day–≤4 Wk (n = 769)	>4 Wk–≤3 Mo (n = 732)	>3 Mo–≤6 Mo (n = 679)	6 Mo–≤1 Yr (n = 90)
Body as a whole				
Asthenia	69 (9.0%)	28 (3.8%)	21 (3.1%)	2 (2.2%)
Headache	58 (7.5%)	38 (5.2%)	29 (4.3%)	5 (5.6%)
Infection	26 (3.4%)	46 (6.3%)	37 (5.4%)	4 (4.4%)
Pain	14 (1.8%)	23 (3.1%)	17 (2.5%)	2 (2.2%)
Nervous system				
Dizziness	37 (4.8%)	32 (4.4%)	8 (1.2%)	1 (1.1%)
Somnolence	90 (11.7%)	19 (2.6%)	9 (1.3%)	4 (4.4%)
Respiratory system				
Pharyngitis	12 (1.6%)	21 (2.9%)	14 (2.1%)	2 (2.2%)

the clinical pharmacology studies in healthy volunteers encompassing dosages up to 5,000 mg, somnolence and asthenia were dose related. In the placebo-controlled clinical trials in patients with epilepsy, the incidences of somnolence and nausea were higher at the highest dosage studied, 4,000 mg/day. However, these patients were randomized directly to this dosage without uptitration as is recommended.

Convulsions were more common at the lowest dosages (7% at dosages of 1,000 and 2,000 mg/day, 5% at a dosage of 3,000 mg/day, and 3% at a dosage of 4,000 mg/day). This event does not appear on Table 43.3 because it was more common in placebo-treated patients overall (7%).

Time Dependency

Somnolence, asthenia, and dizziness tended to occur early in treatment. Less frequent events that also may occur more often early in the treatment are anorexia, dry mouth, nausea, ataxia, nervousness, abnormal thinking, vertigo, amblyopia, and diplopia. The time course of onset of the side effects that

TABLE 43.5. MOST COMMON ADVERSE EXPERIENCES (≥5.0%) WITH ONSET BETWEEN 1 AND 2 YEARS

	Exposed ≥1 Year (n = 674)
Body as a whole	
Accidental injury	109 (16.2%)
Asthenia	35 (5.2%)
Back pain	38 (5.6%)
Flu syndrome	35 (5.2%)
Headache	80 (11.9%)
Infection	87 (12.9%)
Pain	42 (6.2%)
Nervous system	
Convulsiond	79 (11.7%)
Dizziness	31 (4.6%)
Respiratory system	
Pharyngitis	38 (5.6%)

were reported in more than 5% of the patients in the levetiracetam treatment group is described in Table 43.4.

There are no adverse events that are uniquely associated with long-term treatment. Adverse events with an onset after at least 1 year of treatment are presented in Table 43.5; the table is limited to those events with an incidence of 5% or greater. Clinical laboratory results also were reviewed for evidence of abnormalities associated with long-term treatment. None was identified. There were no apparent long-term effects on body weight.

Risk Factors

No demographic or concomitant disease factors have been identified that pose an added risk to the use of levetiracetam. The safety profiles by sex and ethnicity have been compared and no differences have been found. Patients also have been categorized on the basis of other medical diagnoses, including psychiatric diagnoses, and no risk factors have been identified. Clinical pharmacology studies have been conducted in patients with hepatic or renal impairment. The safety profile in these patients is similar to that seen in other patient populations.

Levetiracetam is tolerated well in pediatric patients, but less so than in adult patients. A total of 29 pediatric epilepsy patients between the ages of 5 and 12 years of age have been treated with levetiracetam in open-label studies. The mean dosage was 1,271 mg/day (median of 1,000 mg/day); when body weight is taken into consideration, doses are similar to those used by adults. The types of adverse events reported in children are similar to those reported by adults, but occur with an apparently higher incidence in children.

No clinically meaningful drug interactions have been identified, either on the basis of formal pharmacokinetic interaction studies or on review of the safety profile in the placebo-controlled clinical trials in patients with epilepsy. Pharmacokinetic studies have evaluated interactions between levetiracetam and phenytoin, digoxin, oral contraceptives, warfarin, and probenecid. A population pharmacokinetics approach also has been used to identify pharmacokinetic interactions with other antiepileptic drugs. Adverse event profiles were reviewed by categorizing patients by concomitant antiepileptic drug and also by the more commonly used concomitant medications.

PRECAUTIONS

Levetiracetam is primarily excreted renally by glomerular filtration and active secretion, and hence pharmacokinetic half-life is prolonged in patients with renal impairment. Although no undue adverse events have been observed in the small number of patients with renal impairment studied, dose adjustments are recommended as a precautionary measure for patients with creatinine clearance of less than 60 mL/min.

In animal studies, levetiracetam has been shown to cross the placenta and is present in excreted milk. There is limited experience with the use of levetiracetam in pregnant women, and such use should be considered only in those cases where the benefit clearly outweighs the risk. There were 16 documented pregnancies in women who received levetiracetam during the course of clinical development, 6 of which resulted in live births. All deliveries and infants were characterized as normal; to date, the oldest children (twins) are approximately 7 years of age (delivered in December of 1994). Of the seven abortions (spontaneous, elective, or due to an ectopic pregnancy), one of the fetuses had possible trisomy. Studies in rats at dosages up to 1,800 mg/kg/day have not identified any effects of levetiracetam representing a risk to human fertility. Similarly, maternal treatment during gestation and lactation did not affect survival, growth, and development of the offspring. No fetal abnormalities were noted in the rat teratology studies at dosages up to 3,600 mg/kg/day, although fetal growth was slightly retarded and rib numbers were slightly altered at the highest dose. At this high dose, mild maternal toxicity was noted, as demonstrated by a slightly lower body weight gain at the end of pregnancy. In one of three rabbit teratology studies, there was a twofold increase in incidence of spontaneously occurring abnormalities at 1,800 mg/kg/day, a markedly maternally toxic dose; this was not seen in the other two studies.

LESS COMMON, BUT CLINICALLY RELEVANT ADVERSE EVENTS

Less common, but clinically significant adverse events observed during treatment with levetiracetam include psychotic events and allergic reactions.

Twenty-three patients (0.7%) receiving levetiracetam in all studies reported delusions, hallucinations, manic reactions, paranoid reaction, or psychotic depression. Nineteen of those 23 patients participated in the epilepsy studies. In approximately one-half of the patients, these events required dose reduction or discontinuation from therapy. During the initial postmarketing use, the types of psychiatric events spontaneously reported were abnormal behavior, aggression, anger, autoaggression, anxiety, confusion, depressed mood, depression, hallucinations, hostility, irritability, mood alteration, nervousness, and restlessness.

Allergic reactions are not commonly associated with this treatment. In placebo-controlled trials, there was no difference between levetiracetam and placebo in the incidence of rashes, urticaria, and other dermatologic manifestations of allergy (6% of patients in each treatment group). In all 3,347 patients exposed to levetiracetam during the development program, only 7 cases of severe allergic events occurred. Eleven patients discontinued levetiracetam therapy owing to an allergic event, and in most cases the event resolved on discontinuation. No allergic reactions have been spontaneously reported during the initial period of commercialization.

To date, taking into consideration the initial 6 months of commercial use, no other rare but serious events have been identified.

POTENTIALLY LIFE-THREATENING ADVERSE EVENTS

The overall mortality rate associated with epilepsy is two to three times that of the general population. No adverse events associated with levetiracetam use have been identified, either during the course of clinical development or subsequent to marketing, that represent an added life-threatening risk.

Nine levetiracetam-treated patients with epilepsy died who had otherwise been in good health. The deaths were not attributed to seizures or to any other medical cause and therefore are consistent with a syndrome known as *sudden and unexplained death in epilepsy patients* (SUDEP). The overall SUDEP rate, 3.7, is lower than that for placebo-treated patients (6.8), and is similar to that seen in similar drug development programs such as lamotrigine, gabapentin, and tiagabine.

Eleven suicide attempts and one successful suicide were reported during clinical trials with patients with epilepsy receiving levetiracetam. Approximately one-half of these patients reported a previous history of psychiatric problems. This incidence is similar to that seen with other newer antiepileptic drugs.

MANIFESTATIONS AND MANAGEMENT OF OVERDOSE

Oral dosages of levetiracetam up to 5,000 mg/kg/day in the mouse and rat were not lethal and were associated with only transient clinical signs. In dogs, emesis is a dose-limiting effect. Single-dose escalation to 2,000 mg/kg orally in monkeys resulted in transient behavioral observations indicative of central nervous system depression, nausea, and emesis; all signs disappeared within 24 hours.

There have been no true toxic overdoses with levetiracetam. The highest known dosage of levetiracetam received in the clinical development program was 6,000 mg/day. Other than drowsiness, no adverse sequelae were reported. Consistent with its primarily renal excretion, levetiracetam has been shown to be efficiently removed by hemodialysis. Although there is no clinical experience in overdose, this may be a useful option in the management of such cases should clinical symptoms warrant.

CONCLUSION

Levetiracetam is well tolerated and without significant risks when used as add-on treatment in patients with partial seizures. There are no significant side effects when treatment is initiated at clinically efficacious doses. The overall incidence of adverse events is low, with the most commonly reported events being transient somnolence, asthenia, and dizziness. Nonpsychotic psychiatric events such as nervousness, emotional lability, and hostility also are associated with levetiracetam treatment. These events occur infre-

quently; however, approximately one-half of the patients experiencing these events required a dose reduction or discontinuation of levetiracetam. More rarely, psychotic events may occur. Allergic reactions are uncommon. Levetiracetam is notable for its lack of effect on clinical laboratory parameters and its lack of drug interactions. No adverse events have been identified that are specific to long-term use. Levetiracetam is not teratogenic, and based on limited clinical experience, no birth defects have been reported.

REFERENCES

1. Cereghino JJ, Biton V, Abou-Khalil MD, et al. Levetiracetam for partial seizures: results of a double-blind, randomized clinical trial. *Neurology* 2000;55:236–242.
2. Shorvon SD, Lowenthal A, Janz D, et al. Multicenter double blind, randomized, placebo-controlled trial of levetiracetam as add-on therapy in patients with refractory partial seizures. *Epilepsia* 2000;41:1179–1186.
3. Betts T, Waegemans T, Crawford P. A multicentre, double-blind, randomized, parallel group study to evaluate the tolerability and efficacy of two oral doses of levetiracetam, 2000 mg/day and 4000 mg/daily, without titration in patients with refractory epilepsy. *Seizure* 2000;9:80–87.
4. Ben-Menachem E, Falter U. Efficacy and tolerability of levetiracetam 3000 mg daily in patients with refractory partial seizures: a multicenter, double-blind, responder-selected study evaluating monotherapy. *Epilepsia* 2000;41:1276–1283.

Antiepileptic Drugs, 5ᵗʰ Edition. Edited by R.H. Levy, R.H. Mattson, B.S. Meldrum, and E. Perucca. Lippincott Williams & Wilkins, Philadelphia © 2002.

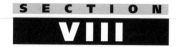

SECTION

VIII

OXCARBAZEPINE

OXCARBAZEPINE

MECHANISMS OF ACTION

MICHAEL J. MCLEAN

Detailed mechanistic information could help to resolve two issues that affect the use of oxcarbazepine (10,11-dihydro-10-oxo-carbamazepine; Trileptal, Novartis, East Hanover, NJ). First, oxcarbazepine is indicated as first-line therapy for the treatment of partial and secondarily generalized tonic-clonic seizures [see full prescribing information (3,17,60,61)]. The percentage of patients achieving complete seizure control on oxcarbazepine was comparable with that of patients taking carbamazepine (60). At the 10 position of the central 7-membered ring, oxcarbazepine has a keto group that is rapidly converted to an active monohydroxy derivative in humans (63). Carbamazepine differs structurally in having a 10,11 double bond that is converted to an active epoxide (15). Thus, oxcarbazepine achieves significant efficacy with one active compound, whereas the efficacy of carbamazepine results from two active compounds. Pharmacokinetic considerations aside, it would be useful to know whether different profiles of cellular actions account for the comparable efficacy of these two compounds. Pharmacologic differentiation would provide a rational basis for considering oxcarbazepine and carbamazepine to be distinct therapeutic agents.

Second, there is a trend toward treating disorders other than epilepsy with antiepileptic drugs. In this regard, three tricyclic compounds are notable. Amitriptyline, a tertiary amine antidepressant, is effective in migraine prophylaxis (19). It also has been shown to relieve the pain of postherpetic neuralgia (35,77) and painful diabetic neuropathy independent of effects on mood (33,34). In addition to antiepileptic effects, carbamazepine is effective in the treatment of trigeminal neuralgia (8,27), painful diabetic neuropathy (20,56), and bipolar disorder (12,37). Oxcarbazepine and its monohydroxy derivative have both been shown to be effective in the treatment of trigeminal neuralgia (16,81) and of affective and schizoaffective symptoms of patients with mood disorders (14,26,42,71). A distinctive

mechanistic profile could help to choose among therapeutic agents for selected patients.

Known cellular actions of oxcarbazepine and its monohydroxy derivative are examined here in an effort to focus on these two questions.

BLOCKADE OF SODIUM-DEPENDENT ACTION POTENTIAL FIRING

Oxcarbazepine and its monohydroxy derivative limited sustained, high-frequency repetitive firing (SRF) of sodium-dependent action potentials of cultured mouse spinal cord neurons equipotently at concentrations between 10^{-8} and 10^{-6} mol/L (75). This is lower than maximum plasma (up to 60 µmol/L) and tissue concentrations achieved after chronic use (presumably as high as 60 µmol/g) (22), suggesting that this is a therapeutically relevant mechanism of action. The experimental paradigm for showing this effect on a single neuron is shown at the top of Figure 44.1. In the control state, SRF is elicited by depolarizing current pulses applied intracellularly (PRE in Figure 44.1). Then, in the presence of the drug, depolarizing steps were applied to examine firing (DRUG in Figure 44.1). In the example shown, action potential amplitude diminishes in parallel with declining maximal rate of rise (top trace), an indirect reflection of inward sodium current generating the upstroke of the action potential, until firing ceases for the remainder of the depolarizing step. Passage of hyperpolarizing current into the neuron led to restoration of SRF in the continuing presence of the drug, indicative of the voltage dependence of the block. After washout of the drug (POST in Figure 44.1), SRF was restored at transmembrane potentials near to or less negative than the resting potential, demonstrating reversibility of the voltage-sensitive block. In population studies, oxcarbazepine, the monohydroxy derivative, and carbamazepine reduced the percentage of neurons with SRF in a concentration-dependent manner (Figure 44.1, bottom) (38,75). The concentration dependence of this effect for car-

Michael J. McLean, MD, PhD: Department of Neurology, Vanderbilt University Medical Center, Nashville, Tennessee

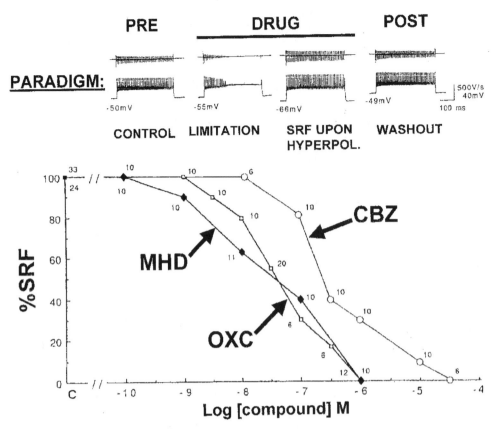

FIGURE 44.1. Top: An experimental paradigm for showing effects of oxcarbazepine (OXC), its monohydroxy derivative (MHD), and carbamazepine (CBZ) on sodium-dependent action potential firing. PRE: Control trace showing sustained repetitive firing (SRF) elicited by an intracellularly applied depolarizing current pulse. DRUG: During superfusion with an effective concentration of a drug, firing was limited at less negative resting potentials (–55 mV) but was restored by hyperpolarization (–66 mV), indicating voltage dependence of the block. POST: After washout, repetitive firing was sustained throughout depolarizing pulses at the original resting potential. Calibrations at right apply to all traces. **Bottom:** Concentration dependence of limitation of SRF. Percentage of neurons with SRF (ordinate) versus drug concentration is shown.

bamazepine was shifted to the right compared with the other two drugs (Figure 44.1, bottom) (39,75). Carbamazepine has been shown to block sodium current directly in a number of preparations (51,52,64,73), including the slow sodium currents of pain-processing neurons (57,67). Oxcarbazepine and its monohydroxy derivative have not been shown to block sodium current directly, but are assumed to do so based on voltage- and use-dependent limitation of action potential firing, and by analogy with carbamazepine (75). Amitriptyline also has been reported to block sodium current by affecting both activation and inactivation kinetics in bovine chromaffin cells (2,47,48), in human embryonic kidney cells expressing human cardiac sodium channels (43), and in dorsal root ganglion cells (47,67).

CALCIUM CHANNEL BLOCKADE

The monohydroxy derivative of oxcarbazepine reduced glutamatergic synaptic transmission and high-voltage–acti-

vated, N-type calcium currents in cortical and striatal neurons (6,69). Carbamazepine had only minor effects on high-voltage–activated calcium currents in neurons isolated from human hippocampus (62) and neocortex (59) obtained at epilepsy surgery. Amitriptyline relaxed smooth muscle cells isolated from human mesenteric arteries at supratherapeutic concentrations (72) and decreased motility of human vas deferens smooth muscle cells at concentrations slightly higher than the therapeutic range (40). These findings suggest an L-type blocking action of amitriptyline, but effects on neuronal L-calcium channels have not been clearly demonstrated at therapeutically relevant concentrations.

POTASSIUM CURRENTS

Enhancement of hyperpolarizing potassium currents could contribute to anticonvulsant, pain-relieving, and mood-stabilizing effects of antiepileptic drugs. Both enantiomers of the monohydroxy derivative blocked penicillin-induced bursting in hippocampal slices. This effect was prevented by the potassium channel blocker, 4-aminopyridine. These findings suggested that the monohydroxy derivative blocked bursting by increasing a hyperpolarizing potassium current (Olpe et al., unpublished results). Carbamazepine had similar effects on penicillin-induced bursting (45) and enhanced a voltage-sensitive potassium current in rat cortical neurons in cell culture (82). Amitriptyline opened several types of potassium channels (voltage-gated, adenosine triphosphate–activated, and Ca^{2+}-activated) that could contribute to analgesic efficacy (18). However, blockade of certain cardiac potassium channels may contribute to the arrhythmogenic potential of amitriptyline (11,25). Potassium channel blockade by amitriptyline in the central nervous system also could be proconvulsant in some instances. Interestingly, amitriptyline has anticonvulsant effects in some experimental models (10,30,79), but is associated with seizures in some patients, especially at high concentrations (50).

NMDA RECEPTORS

The importance of glutamatergic hyperexcitability, particularly that mediated by the *N*-methyl-D-aspartate (NMDA) type of receptors, to human (65,66) and animal (41) epileptogenesis is well documented. The monohydroxy derivative of oxcarbazepine, the principal active anticonvulsant metabolite of oxcarbazepine, decreased stimulation-evoked field potentials elicited from hippocampal slices in buffers containing low magnesium concentration to enhance the NMDA component of this potential (6,7). This occurred at concentrations of 10 to 100 μmol/L monohydroxy derivative. Assuming that total-brain concentrations of the monohydroxy derivative could reach 60 μmol/L, the peak plasma concentration obtained in epileptic patients receiving repeated doses (22), up to 30% of the NMDA-mediated field potential could be blocked.

Therapeutically relevant concentrations of carbamazepine (including concentrations in brain with chronic administration) blocked NMDA-activated current in cultured spinal cord neurons (28), inhibited NMDA-elicited calcium influx into rat cerebellar granule cells (9,24,53), inhibited NMDA-induced depolarizations in cortical wedges from epileptic mice (29) and blocked glutamato release (44).

Amitriptyline blocked NMDA-induced toxicity but not NMDA-induced elevation of extracellular glutamate in cerebellar granule cells at supratherapeutic concentrations (36). NMDA-induced currents in *Xenopus* oocytes injected with rat brain RNA were only slightly blocked by high concentrations of amitriptyline (70,76). At concentrations near the top of the therapeutically useful range, amitriptyline reduced NMDA-induced intracellular calcium elevations (5). Pretreatment with amitriptyline intrathecally prevented

hyperalgesia produced by NMDA in rats (13). These findings suggest that some benefit of amitriptyline, particularly for the treatment of pain, may result from NMDA antagonism. However, oxcarbazepine, its monohydroxy derivative, and carbamazepine seem to have greater NMDA-blocking capabilities.

Figure 44.2 shows the results of pressure application of 10^{-5} mol/L glutamate in magnesium-free buffer to cultured spinal cord neurons, to enhance the NMDA component of the response. The neurons depolarized and fired continuously throughout the application (Control, top row). The monohydroxy derivative and carbamazepine blocked the depolarization and firing at concentrations that might be reached in brain with chronic administration. A relatively high concentration of amitriptyline (near top of the antidepressant range) limited action potential firing, but did not diminish the depolarization significantly. This suggests that there may be differences in concentration dependence of blockade of the NMDA component by these three tricyclic drugs that determine the extent to which NMDA blockade contributes to their therapeutic clinical utility.

SEROTONIN

Blockade of the serotonin (5-HT) transporter with a resultant increase in interstitial serotonin concentrations is thought to contribute to the antidepressant effect of amitriptyline (58). Carbamazepine at therapeutically relevant concentrations also may increase interstitial serotonin by enhancing release and by modestly blocking the transporter at higher concentrations (80). The increase in interstitial serotonin concentrations may contribute to antiepileptic efficacy of carbamazepine by stimulating γ-aminobutyric acid (GABA)-ergic interneurons bearing 5-HT3–type receptors (55) or by activation of inhibitory serotonin receptors. Oxcarbazepine has not been reported to alter extracellular serotonin concentrations or serotonin receptor profiles.

GABA RECEPTORS

The importance of GABA-mediated inhibition in controlling seizures has been well documented (46), and $GABA_A$ receptors are the target of several antiepileptic drugs (31). Carbamazepine did not alter $GABA_A$- or $GABA_B$-mediated responses of hippocampal CA3 neurons at concentrations up to 500 μmol/L (supratherapeutic) (4). Also, carbamazepine did not change the amplitude of responses to GABA applied by electrophoresis to cultured spinal cord neurons (38). Blockade of peripheral benzodiazepine receptors by Ro 5-4864, but not blockade of central benzodiazepine receptors by Roche compound (Ro) 15-1788, prevented the anticonvulsant effect of carbamazepine in amygdala-kindled rats (78). Carbamazepine and phenytoin potenti-

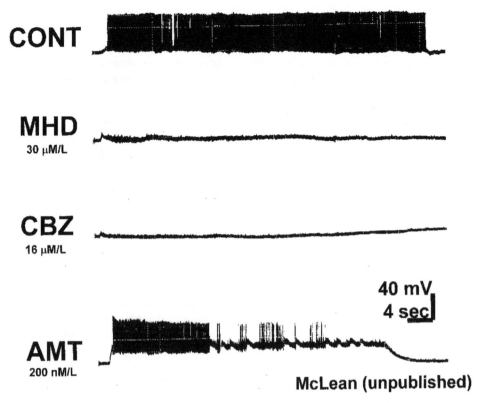

FIGURE 44.2. Effects of tricyclic compounds on glutamate-induced depolarization and action potential firing in cultured spinal cord neurons. Glutamate (10^{-5} mol/L) was applied in magnesium-free buffer to emphasize the NMDA component of the response. **Top row:** Control (CONT) response to a 50-second application of glutamate by pressure ejection from a micropipette positioned near the neuron under study. **Middle rows:** The monohydroxy derivative of oxcarbazepine (MHD) and carbamazepine (CBZ) blocked depolarization and action potential firing at concentrations that might be reached in the brain during chronic administration. **Bottom row:** Amitriptyline (AMT) limited firing but did not reduce glutamate-induced depolarization substantially at a high therapeutically relevant concentration encountered in treatment of depression. Concentrations are shown below drugs. Calibrations at lower right apply throughout. (*Unpublished data.*)

ated the response of GABA$_A$ receptors expressed in human embryonic kidney cells and in cultured rat cortical neurons as long as the recombinant receptors included α1, α3, or α5 subunit isoforms (23). Thus, there is mixed evidence for effects of carbamazepine in different systems. It is possible that concentration dependence of effects determines the contribution of GABA$_A$ receptor–mediated effects to the anticonvulsant efficacy of carbamazepine.

There is little information about the effects of amitriptyline on GABA receptors. Blockade of GABA$_A$ receptors could contribute to proconvulsant effects of amitriptyline under some conditions (32).

There are no reports of oxcarbazepine effects on GABA receptors or GABA concentrations in brain.

ACETYLCHOLINE RECEPTORS

Anticholinergic side effects of amitriptyline can limit therapeutic utility (21). These include reduced activity of blad-

der and gut smooth muscle leading to urinary retention and constipation, pseudodementia, and cardiac arrhythmias. Amitriptyline blocked cloned muscarinic receptors (68) and reduced acetylcholine binding to muscarinic receptors (54).

Carbamazepine-induced urinary retention also is likely to result from muscarinic cholinergic blockade. Its interaction with cholinoreceptors may be indirect. Carbamazepine uncouples muscarinic receptors and β-adrenergic receptors from G proteins (1). Mutant nicotinic cholinergic receptors that are associated with autosomal dominant nocturnal frontal lobe epilepsy are more sensitive to carbamazepine than are human native nicotinic receptors (49).

There are no reports of effects of oxcarbazepine or its monohydroxy derivative on cholinergic neurotransmission.

DISCUSSION

Based on a series of indirect assays, the mechanistic profile of oxcarbazepine and its monohydroxy derivative at therapeutically relevant concentrations is likely to include a variety of actions. Sodium channel blockade could interrupt high-frequency repetitive firing of neurons; N-calcium channel blockade is expected to damp synaptic activity diffusely; opening of potassium channels should reduce burst activity; and blockade of NMDA receptor–mediated activity could limit hyperexcitability. All of these actions could contribute to the broad clinical utility of oxcarbazepine outlined in the introductory paragraphs of this chapter.

At face value, the mechanistic profiles of action of carbamazepine and amitriptyline appear to overlap that of oxcarbazepine substantially (Figure 44.3), but differences appear on closer inspection. Limitation of firing of sodium-dependent action potentials by oxcarbazepine and the monohydroxy derivative occurred at lower concentrations than with carbamazepine. However, the N-calcium effect of the monohydroxy derivative differentiates it further from carbamazepine. Potassium channel and NMDA receptor effects seem comparable with those of carbamazepine. In the absence of comparative data, no difference in effects on GABA and cholinergic receptors or on serotonin levels can be assumed. The sodium channel blocking action of amitriptyline rivals that of oxcarbazepine and carbamazepine in terms of occurrence at concentrations in the therapeutic range. A combination of antimuscarinic cholinergic activity, blockade of certain potassium conductances, and possibly GABA$_A$ receptor antagonism confers cardiac arrhythmogenic and proconvulsant effects in some cases. In the balance, this profile disqualifies amitriptyline as an anticonvulsant. Serotonergic actions of amitriptyline and carbamazepine may be important for pain control, and the serotonin-releasing effect of carbamazepine is essential for anticonvulsant effects in the genetically epilepsy-prone rat (80). It would be of considerable interest to know if oxcarbazepine and the monohydroxy derivative affect interstitial serotonin levels in the nervous system. This action, N-calcium channel blockade, and some pharmacokinetic properties (e.g., less induction of hepatic enzymes and fewer drug–drug interactions) could make oxcarbazepine preferable to carbamazepine in some instances.

The ability of the monohydroxy derivative and carbamazepine to block glutamate responses (Figure 44.2) begs for further mechanistic resolution to differentiate the two drugs. The potency of oxcarbazepine and carbamazepine in

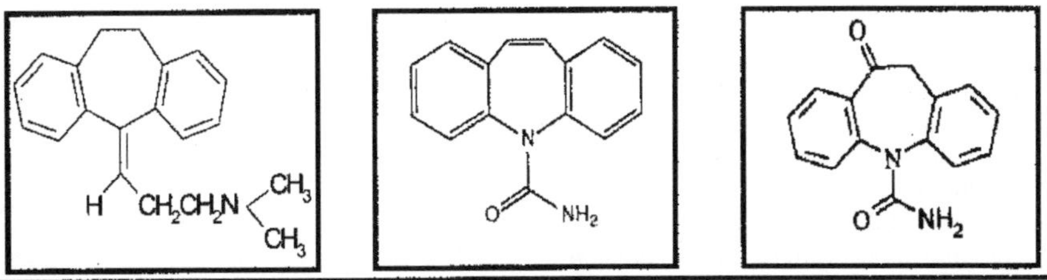

	AMITRIPTYLINE	**CARBAMAZEPINE**	**OXCARBAZEPINE**
Na⁺ channel block	✓	✓	✓
K⁺ channel effect	BLOCK	Incr.?	Incr.?
Ca⁺⁺ channel block	✓, L-type	✓, L-type	✓, MHD blocks N-type
NMDAr block	✓	✓	✓
Incr. extracellular 5-HT	✓ 5-HT and NE reuptake inhib.	✓ Incr. 5-HT release	???
AChR block	✓, major	✓, minor	???

FIGURE 44.3. Tricyclic compounds.

inhibiting glutamate release was comparable with that of lamotrigine (74). Clarification of monohydroxy derivative effects on glutamate receptor–mediated activities also could clarify situations in which oxcarbazepine might be selected over lamotrigine for a variety of conditions.

In conclusion, current knowledge of the mechanistic profile of oxcarbazepine does not provide a simple formula for selection over other antiepileptic drugs. There are some subtle differences from carbamazepine. Multiple known actions of oxcarbazepine and its monohydroxy derivative provide a rationale for utility in the treatment of a broad range of clinical disorders, including epilepsy, neuropathic pain, and mood disorders. However, there still is much to learn about these compounds mechanistically.

REFERENCES

1. Avissar S, Schreiber G, Aulakh CS, et al. Carbamazepine and electroconvulsive shock attenuate beta-adrenergic and muscarinic cholinoceptor coupling to G proteins in rat cortex. *Eur J Pharmacol* 1990;189:99–103.

2. Barber MJ, Starmer CF, Grant AO. Blockade of cardiac sodium channels by amitriptyline and diphenylhydantoin: evidence for two use-dependent binding sites. *Circ Res* 1991;69:677–696.

3. Barcs G, Walker EB, Elger CE, et al. Oxcarbazepine placebo-controlled, dose-ranging trial in refractory partial epilepsy. *Epilepsia* 2000;41:1597–1607.

4. Bonnet U, Bingmann D. Missing action of carbamazepine on postsynaptic GABA-responses of hippocampal CA3-neurons (slice, guinea pig). *Eur Neuropsychopharmacol* 1998;8:353–356.

5. Cai Z, McCaslin PP. Amitriptyline, desipramine, cyproheptadine and carbamazepine, in concentrations used therapeutically, reduce kainate- and N-methyl-D-aspartate-induced intracellular Ca²⁺ levels in neuronal culture. *Eur J Pharmacol* 1992;219:53–57.

6. Calabresi P, DeMurtas M, Stefani A, et al. Action of GP 47779, the active metabolite of oxcarbazepine, on the corticostriatal system: I. modulation of corticostriatal synaptic transmission. *Epilepsia* 1995;36:990–996.

7. Calabresi P, Siniscalchi A, Pisani A, et al. A field potential analysis on the effects of lamotrigine, GP 47779, and felbamate in neocortical slices. *Neurology* 1996;47:557–562.

8. Campbell FG, Graham JG, Zilkha KJ. Clinical trial of carbamazepine (Tegretol) in trigeminal neuralgia. *J Neurol Neurosurg Psychiatry* 1966;29:265–267.

9. Crowder JM, Bradford HF. Common anticonvulsants inhibit Ca²⁺ uptake and amino acid neurotransmitter release in vitro. *Epilepsia* 1987;28:378–382.

10. Dailey JW, Reith MEA, Steidley KR, et al. Carbamazepine-induced release of serotonin from rat hippocampus in vitro. *Epilepsia* 1998;39:1054–1063.

11. Dreixler JC, Jenkins A, Cao YJ, et al. Patch-clamp analysis of anesthetic interactions with recombinant SK2 subtype neuronal calcium-activated potassium channels. *Anesthesia and Analgesia* 2000; 90(3):727-732.

12. Dunn RT, Frye MS, Kimbrell TA, et al. The efficacy and use of anticonvulsants in mood disorders. *Clin Neuropharmacol* 1998;21:215–235.

13. Eisenach JC, Gebhart GF. Intrathecal amitriptyline acts as an N-methyl-D-aspartate receptor antagonist in the presence of inflammatory hyperalgesia in rats. *Anesthesiology* 1995;83:1046–1054.

14. Emrich HM. Studies with oxcarbazepine (Trileptal®) in acute mania. *Int J Clin Psychopharmacol* 1990;5[Suppl 1]:83–88.

15. Faigle JW, Menge GP. Pharmacokinetic and metabolic features of oxcarbazepine and their clinical significance: comparison with carbamazepine. *Int J Clin Psychopharmacol* 1990;5[Suppl 1]:73.

16. Farago F. Trigeminal neuralgia: its treatment with two new carbamazepine analogues. *Eur Neurol* 1987;26:73–83.

17. Friis ML, Kristensen O, Boas J, et al. Therapeutic experiences with 947 epileptic outpatients in oxcarbazepine treatment. *Acta Neurol Scand* 1993;87:224.

18. Galeotti N, Ghelardini C, Capaccioli S, et al. Blockade of clomipramine and amitriptyline analgesia by an antisense oligonucleotide to mKv1.1, a mouse Shaker-like K+ channel. *Eur J Pharmacol* 1997; 330(1):15-25.

19. Gomersall JD, Stuart A. Amitriptyline in migraine prophylaxis: changes in pattern of attacks during a controlled trial. *J Neurol Neurosurg Psychiatry* 1973;36:684.

20. Gomez-Perez FJ, Choza R, Rios JM, et al. Nortriptyline-fluphenazine vs. carbamazepine in the symptomatic treatment of diabetic neuropathy. *Arch Med Res* 1996;27:525–529.

21. Goodman Baldessarini R. Drugs and the Treatment of Psyciatric Disorders. In: *Goodman and Gilman's the Pharmacological Basis of Therapeutics*, 10th edition. Edited by JG Hardman and LE Limbird, consulting editor, AG Gilman. McGraw-Hill; New York, 2001, 466.

22. Gram L, Philbert A. Oxcarbazepine. In: Meldrum BS, Porter RJ, eds. *New anticonvulsant drugs*. London: John Libbey, 1986: 229–235.

23. Granger P, Biton B, Faure C, et al. Modulation of the gamma-aminobutyric acid type A receptor by the antiepileptic drugs carbamazepine and phenytoin. *Mol Pharmacol* 1995;47:1189–1196.

24. Hough CJ, Irwin RP, Gao XM, et al. Carbamazepine inhibition of N-methyl-D-aspartate-evoked calcium influx in rat cerebellar granule cells. *J Pharmacol Exp Ther* 1996;276:143–149.

25. Jo SH, Youm JB, Lee CO, et al. Blockade of the HERG human cardiac K(+) channel by the antidepressant drug amitriptyline. *Br J Pharmacol* 2000;129:1471–1480.

26. Kiguchi S, Ichikawa K, Kojima M. Suppressive effects of oxcarbazepine on tooth pulp-evoked potentials recorded at the trigeminal spinal tract nucleus in cats. *Clin Exp Pharmacol Physiol* 2001; 28:169–175.

27. Killian JM, Fromm GH. Carbamazepine in the treatment of neuralgia: use and side effects. *Arch Neurol* 1968;19:129–136.

28. Lampe H, Bigalke H. Carbamazepine blocks NMDA-activated currents in cultured spinal cord neurons. *Neuroreport* 1990;1: 26–28.

29. Lancaster JM, Davies JA. Carbamazepine inhibits NMDA-induced depolarizations in cortical wedges prepared from DBA/2 mice. *Experientia* 1992;48:751–753.

30. Luchins DJ, Oliver AP, and Wyatt RJ. Seizures with antidepressants: an in vitro technique to assess relative risk. *Epilepsia* 1984; 25(1): 25-32.

31. Macdonald R. L. Is there a mechanistic basis for rational polypharmacy? *Epilepsy Res* 1996, Suppl. 11:79-93.

32. Malatynska E, Knapp RJ, Ikeda M, et al. Antidepressants and seizure-interactions at the GABA-receptor chloride-ionophore complex. *Life Sci* 1988;43:303–307.

33. Max M.B, Culnane M, Schafer SC, et al. Amitriptyline relieves diabetic neuropathy pain in patients with normal or depressed mood. *Neurology* 1987;37:589–594.

34. Max MB, Lynch SA, Muir J, et al. Effects of desipramine, amitriptyline and fluoxetine on pain in diabetic neuropathy. *N Engl J Med* 1992;326:1250–1256.

35. Max MB, Schafer SC, Culnane M. Amitriptyline but not lorazepam, relieves postherpetic neuralgia. *Neurology* 1988;38: 1427–1452.

36. McCaslin PP, Yu XZ, Ho IK, et al. Amitriptyline prevents N-methyl-D-aspartate (NMDA)-induced toxicity, does not prevent

NMDA-induced elevations of extracellular glutamate, but augments kainate-induced elevations of glutamate. *J Neurochem* 1992;59:401–405.

37. McElroy SL, Keck PE. Pharmacologic agents for the treatment of acute bipolar mania. *Biol Psychiatry* 2000;48:539–555.

38. McLean MJ, Macdonald RL. Carbamazepine and 10,11-epoxy-carbamazepine produce use- and voltage-dependent limitation of rapidly firing action potentials of mouse central neurons in cell culture. *J Pharmacol Exp Ther* 1986;238:727–739.

39. McLean MJ, Schmutz M, Wamil AW, et al. Oxcarbazepine: mechanisms of action. *Epilepsia* 1994;35[Suppl 3]:S5–S9.

40. Medina P, Segarra G, Ballester R, et al. Effects of antidepressants in adrenergic neurotransmission of human vas deferens. *Urology* 2000;55:592–597.

41. Mody I, Heinemann U. NMDA receptors of dentate gyrus granule cells participate in synaptic transmission following kindling. *Nature* 1987;326:701–709.

42. Müller AA, Stoll K-D. Carbamazepine and oxcarbazepine in the treatment of manic syndromes: studies in Germany. In: Emrich HM, Okuma T, Müller AA, eds. *Anticonvulsants in affective disorders.* Elsevier Science Publishers BV, 1984.

43. Nau C, Seaver M, Wang S-Y, et al. Block of human heart hH1 sodium channels by amitriptyline. *J Pharmacol Exp Ther* 2000;292:1015–1023.

44. Okada M, Kawata Y, Mizuno K, et al. Interaction between Ca^{2+}, K^+, carbamazepine and zonisamide on hippocampal extracellular glutamate monitored with a microdialysis electrode. *Br J Pharmacol* 1998;124:1277–1285.

45. Olpe H, Kolb CN, Hausdorf A, et al. 4-Aminopyridine and barium chloride attenuate the antiepileptic effect of carbamazepine in hippocampal slices. *Experientia* 1991;47:254–257.

46. Olsen RW, DeLorey TM. GABA and glycine. In: Siegel GJ, Agranoff BW, Albers RW, et al., eds. *Basic neurochemistry: molecular, cellular and medical aspects,* 6th ed. Philadelphia: Lippincott Williams & Wilkins, 1999:335–346.

47. Pancrazio J, Kamatchi GL, Roscoe AK, et al. Inhibition of neuronal Na^+ channels by antidepressant drugs. *J Pharmacol Exp Ther* 1998;284:208–214.

48. Park T-J, Shin S-Y, Suh B-C, et al. Differential inhibition of catecholamine secretion by amitriptyline through blockage of nicotinic receptors, sodium channels, and calcium channels in bovine adrenal chromaffin cells. *Synapse* 1998;29:248–256.

49. Picard F, Bertrand S, Steinlein OK, et al. Mutated nicotinic receptors responsible for autosomal dominant nocturnal frontal lobe epilepsy are more sensitive to carbamazepine. *Epilepsia* 1999;40:1198–209.

50. Preskorn SH and Fast GA. Tricyclic antidepressant-induced seizures and plasma drug concentration. *J Clin Psychiatry*, 1992;53(5):160-162.

51. Ragsdale DS, Scheuer T, Catteral WA. Frequency and voltage-dependent inhibition of type IIA Na+ channels, expressed in a mammalian cell line, by local anesthetic, antiarrhythmic, and anticonvulsant drugs. *Mol Pharmacol* 1991;40:756.

52. Reckziegel G, Beck H, Schramm J, et al. Carbamazepine effects on Na^+ currents in human dentate granule cells from epileptogenic tissue. *Epilepsia* 1999;40:401–407.

53. Reichlin S, Mothon S. Carbamazepine and phenytoin inhibit somatostatin release from dispersed cerebral cells in culture. *Ann Neurol* 1991;29:413–417.

54. Richelson E, Nelson A. Antagonism by antidepressants of neurotransmitter receptors of normal human brain in vitro. *J Pharmacol Exp Ther* 1984;230:94–102.

55. Ropert N, Guy N. Serotonin facilitates GABAergic transmission in the CA1 region of rat hippocampus in vitro. *J Physiol (Lond)* 1991;441:121–136.

56. Rull J, Quibrera R, Gonzalez-Millan H, et al. Symptomatic treatment of peripheral diabetic neuropathy with carbamazepine: double blind crossover trial. *Diabetologia* 1969;5:215–218.

57. Rush AM, Elliott JR. Phenytoin and carbamazepine: differential inhibition of sodium currents in small cells from adult rat dorsal root ganglia. *Neurosci Lett* 1997;226:95–98.

58. Sanchez C, Hyttel J. Comparison of the effects of antidepressants and their metabolites on reuptake of biogenic amines and on receptor binding. *Cell Mol Neurobiol* 1999;19:467–489.

59. Sayer RJ, Brown AM, Schwindt PC, et al. Calcium currents in acutely isolated human neocortical neurons. *J Neurophysiol* 1993;69:1596–1606.

60. Scandinavian Oxcarbazepine Study Group. A double-blind study comparing oxcarbazepine and carbamazepine in patients with newly diagnosed, previously untreated epilepsy. *Epilepsy Res* 1989;3:70.

61. Schachter SC, Vazques B, Fisher RS, et al. Oxcarbazepine: double-blind, randomized, placebo-controlled, monotherapy trial for partial seizures. *Neurology* 1999;52:732–737.

62. Schumacher TB, Beck H, Steinhauser C, et al. Effects of phenytoin, carbamazepine, and gabapentin on calcium channels in hippocampal granule cells from patients with temporal lobe epilepsy. *Epilepsia* 1998;39:355–363.

63. Schutz M, Brugger F, Gentsch C, et al. Oxcarbazepine: preclinical profile and putative mechanism of action. *Epilepsia* 1994;35[Suppl 5]:S5–S9.

64. Schwarz JR, Grigat G. Phenytoin and carbamazepine: potential- and frequency-dependent block of Na currents in mammalian myelinated nerve fibers. *Epilepsia* 1989;30:286.

65. Schwartzkroin PA. Cellular electrophysiology of human epilepsy. *Epilepsy Res* 1994;17:185–192.

66. Schwartzkroin PA. Origins of the epileptic state. *Epilepsia* 1997;38:853–858.

67. Song J-H, Ham S-S, Shin Y-K, et al. Amitriptyline modulation of Na^+ channels in rat dorsal root ganglion neurons. *Eur J Pharmacol* 2000;401:297–305.

68. Stanton T, Bolden-Watson C, Cusack B, et al. Antagonism of the five cloned human muscarinic cholinergic receptors expressed in CHO-K1 cells by antidepressants and antihistamines. *Biochem Pharmacol* 1993;45:2352–2354.

69. Stefani A, Pisani A, DeMurtas M. Action of GP 47779, the active metabolite of oxcarbazepine, on the corticostriatal system: II. modulation of high-voltage-activated calcium currents. *Epilepsia* 36:997–1002.

70. Tohda M, Urushihara H, Nomura Y. Inhibitory effects of antidepressants on NMDA-induced currents in *Xenopus* oocytes injected with rat brain RNA. *Neurochem Int* 1995;26:53–58.

71. Velikonja M, Heinrich K. Effect of oxcarbazepine (CG 47.680) on affective and schizoaffective symptoms: a preliminary report. In: Emrich HM, Okuma T, Muller AA, eds. *Anticonvulsants in affective disorders.* Elsevier Science Publishers BV, Amsterdam, 1984, pp. 209–210.

72. Vila JM, Medina P, Segarra G, et al. Relaxant effects of antidepressants on human isolated mesenteric arteries. *Br J Clin Pharmacol* 1999;48:223–229.

73. Vreugdenhil M, Wadman WJ. Modulation of sodium currents in rat CA1 neurons by carbamazepine and valproate after kindling epileptogenesis. *Epilepsia* 1999;40:1512–1522.

74. Waldmeier PC, Baumann PA, Wicki P, et al. Similar potency of carbamazepine, oxcarbazepine, and lamotrigine in inhibiting the release of glutamate and other neurotransmitters. *Neurology* 1995;45:1907–1913.

75. Wamil A, Schmutz M, Portet C, et al. Effects of oxcarbazepine and 10-hydroxycarbazepine on action potential firing and generalized seizures. *Eur J Pharmacol* 1994;271:301–308.

76. Watanabe Y, Saito H, Abe K. Tricyclic antidepressants block NMDA receptor-mediated synaptic responses and induction of

long-term potentiation in rat hippocampal slices. *Neuropharmacology* 1993;32:479–486.

77. Watson CP, Evans RJ, Reed K, et al. Amitriptyline versus placebo in postherpetic neuralgia. *Neurology* 1982;32:671–673.

78. Weiss SR, Post RM, Patel J, et al. Differential mediation of the anticonvulsant effects of carbamazepine and diazepam. *Life Sci* 1985;36:2413–2419.

79. Yacobi R and Burnham WM. The effect of tricyclic antidepressant of cortex- and amygdala-kindled seizures in the rat. *Can J Neurol Sci* 1991; 18(2):132-136.

80. Yan Q-S, Mishra PK, Burger RL, et al. Evidence that carbamazepine and antiepilepsirine may produce a component of their anticonvulsant effects by activating serotonergic neurons in genetically epilepsy-prone rats. *J Pharmacol Exp Ther* 1992;261:652–659.

81. Zakrzewska JM, Patsalos PN. Oxcarbazepine: a new drug in the management of intractable trigeminal neuralgia. *J Neurol Neurosurg Psychiatry* 1989;52:472–476.

82. Zona C, Tancredi V, Palma E, et al. Potassium currents in rat cortical neurons in culture are enhanced by the antiepileptic drug carbamazepine. *Can J Physiol Pharmacol* 1990;68:545–547.

OXCARBAZEPINE

CHEMISTRY, BIOTRANSFORMATION, AND PHARMACOKINETICS

MEIR BIALER

Oxcarbazepine (OXC), 10,11-dihydro-10-oxo-carbamazepine or 10-oxo-carbazepine (Figure 45.1) is a 10-keto analog of carbamazepine (CBZ). OXC is a new antiepileptic drug (AED) that has been approved worldwide for the treatment of different kinds of partial-onset seizures and generalized tonic-clonic seizures (1–5). OXC was developed as a "second-generation" and follow-up compound to CBZ (1,2). The main advantage of OXC is its nonoxidative metabolic pathway, which implies lower induction potential and fewer drug interactions (3–5). Whereas CBZ undergoes oxidative metabolism to carbamazepine-10,11-epoxide (CBZ-E), OXC is rapidly and extensively reduced by cytosolic enzymes in the liver to its monohydroxylated derivative (MHD) (2) (Figure 45.1). Whereas CBZ metabolism to CBZ-E is mediated by cytochrome P450 (CYP) isoforms CYP3A4 and CYP2C8 (6) and is highly susceptible to induction and drug interactions, the biotransformation of OXC to MHD is catalyzed by reductases that are much less subject to enzyme induction (7–9). Thus, OXC can be regarded a soft drug analog of CBZ owing to its lack of oxidative metabolism (10). However, OXC is not only a soft drug analog of CBZ but a prodrug of MHD because in humans it undergoes an extensive presystemic first-pass conversion to MHD. Therefore, in humans MHD is in essence the active entity of OXC. In a study conducted in rats, no marked difference in anticonvulsant activity was found between CBZ, OXC, and racemic MHD (11,12).

CHEMISTRY AND METABOLIC SCHEME

Synthetic and Analytical Chemistry

OXC is a neutral lipophilic compound (molecular weight 252.3) with a melting point of 215°C to 216°C and low water solubility. The compound is prepared by hydrolysis of 10-methoxycarbazepine in dilute hydrochloric or sulfuric acid (13). The starting material, 10-methoxycarbazepine, is produced by reacting 10-methoxy-5H-dibenz[b,f]azepine with phosgene in toluene to give the 10-methoxy-5H-dibenzo[b,f]azepine-5-carbonyl chloride, which is then converted in ethanol with ammonia to the amide (13).

Methods of Determination

OXC is a prodrug of MHD, which is the principal active entity of OXC. Consequently, the published methods of determination for OXC actually measure plasma levels of MHD and in some cases OXC as well. The first methods were nonstereoselective high-performance liquid chromatography (HPLC) methods with a limit of quantification (LOQ) of 2 µmol/L or 0.5 mg/L (14,15). von Unruh et al. described a nonstereoselective gas chromatographic assay for OXC and its metabolites (16). Flesch et al. were the first to describe a stereoselective (enantioselective) method for the simultaneous determination of the two enantiomers, (S)-MHD and (R)-MHD, with an LOQ of 0.1 mg/L (17). Volosov et al. published an enantioselective HPLC method for monitoring the enantiomers of MHD and its metabolite carbamazepine-10,11-trans-dihydrodiol (DHD; Figure 45.1) (18). This method had a precision better than 15% for all analytes and a LOQ of 0.1 mg/L (serum) and 0.2 mg/L (urine) for each MHD enantiomer, and 0.4 mg/L (urine) for each of the DHD enantiomers. No enantiomeric interconversion occurred during the procedure of this assay. This method allows reliable determination of the MHD and DHD enantiomers in human urine

Meir Bialer, PhD, MBA: David H. Eisenberg Professor of Pharmacy, Department of Pharmaceutics, School of Pharmacy, Faculty of Medicine, The Hebrew University of Jerusalem, Jerusalem, Israel

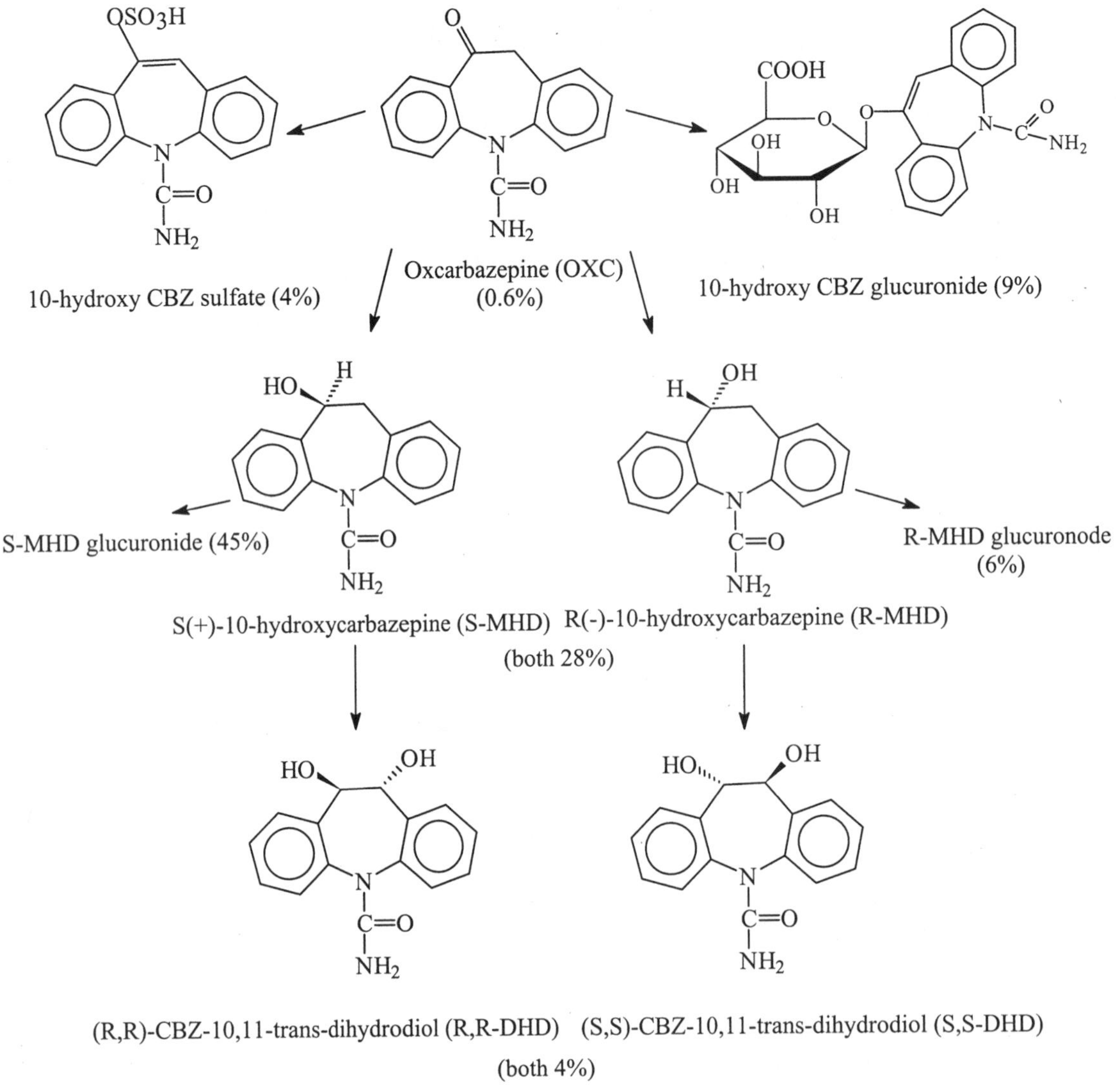

FIGURE 45.1. Metabolic scheme of oxcarbazepine (OXC). %, percentage of dose excreted in the urine. (From Schutz H, Feldmann KF, Faigle JW, et al. The metabolism of 14C-oxcarbazepine in man. *Xenobiotica* 1986;8:769–778, with permission.)

and was used recently in enantioselective pharmacokinetic studies of MHD in humans and dogs (19–21).

Metabolic Scheme

OXC undergoes rapid presystemic metabolic 10-keto reduction, mediated by cytosol arylketone reductase, to MHD (Figure 45.1), which is then partly conjugated with glucuronic acid and partly biotransformed to DHD before excretion in the urine (22–26). The first-pass reduction of OXC to MHD in humans is stereoselective, resulting in approximately a 1:4 area under the concentration–time curve (AUC) ratio between (*R*)-MHD and (*S*)-MHD (17,19,24,27). Because the phase II metabolite DHD has two chiral centers at positions 10 and 11, its *trans*-configu-

ration exists in two enantiomeric forms, (*R*)-DHD and (*S*)-DHD (Figure 45.1) (19).

ABSORPTION

Bioavailability

OXC given orally as a tablet is almost completely absorbed in humans, and peak plasma concentrations of OXC and MHD occur 1 to 3 hours and 4 to 6 hours after dosing, respectively (3,7). The peak plasma concentration of (racemic) MHD was approximately five times higher than that of OXC, and the AUC of OXC was less than 4% of that of MHD (7,25,26,28,29). Oral doses of racemic MHD produced the same plasma profile as OXC (3).

TABLE 45.1. MEAN (± SD) PHARMACOKINETIC PARAMETERS OF OXCARBAZEPINE (OXC) AND THE TWO ENANTIOMERS OF 10-HYDROXYCARBAZEPINE (MHD) IN HUMANS

	OXC	Reference	R-MHD	S-MHD	Reference
CL (L/h)			42 ± 0.9	3.0 ± 0.7	27
CL/F (L/h)	162 ± 76 (single dose)	26[a]			
	109 ± 32 (multiple dose)				
Vβ (L)			11.7	13.8	27[b]
Vβ/F (L)	525 ± 599	26[a]			
t ½ (h)	3.7 ± 4.0 (single dose)	26[a]	9.0 ± 1.5 (i.v.)	10.6 ± 2.6 (i.v.)	27
	3.1 ± 1.5 (multiple dose)		16 ± 28 (OXC, p.o.)	11 ± 1.5 (OXC, p.o.)	
CL_r (L/h)			0.9 ± 0.2 (i.v.)	0.9 ± 0.2 (i.v.)	27
			1 ± 0.3 (OXC, p.o.)	1.1 ± 0.3 (OXC, p.o.)	27
			0.7 ± 0.5	1.2 0.8 ± 0.4	19
f_e (%)	0.6	24	12 ± 1.9 (i.v.)	16 ± 3.1 (i.v.)	27
			4.5 ± 1.3 (OXC, p.o.)	22 ± 4.3 (OXC, p.o.)	27
			2.7 ± 1.7 (OXC, p.o.)	14 ± 6.8 (OXC, p.o.)	19
F (%)				89 (OXC, p.o.)	27[b]
MRT (h)			21 ± 3.9 (OXC, p.o.)	23 ± 5.7 (OXC, p.o.)	19
C_{max} (mg/L)	1.1 ± 0.2	25	1 ± 0.26 (OXC, p.o.)	4.5 ± 0.9 (OXC, p.o.)	19
(OXC dose, 600 mg)	1.7 ± 0.5	28			
	1.7 ± 0.7	29			
t_{max} (h)	1.3 ± 0.2	25	5.5 ± 2.3 (OXC, p.o.)	6.0 ± 21 (OXC, p.o.)	19
CL_f (L/h)			0.35 ± 0.2 (OXC, p.o.)	0.48 ± 0.2 (OXC, p.o.)	19

CL, total body clearance; CL/F, oral clearance; Vβ, volume of distribution, Vβ/F, oral volume of distribution; CL_r, renal clearance; f_e, fraction excreted unchanged in the urine; F, oral availability or absolute bioavailability of racemic MHD after oral administration of OXC; MRT, mean residence time of MHD after oral administration of OXC; C_{max}, peak serum or plasma concentration; t_{max}, time to reach C_{max}; CL_f, formation clearance of MHD-glucuronide; MHD, 10-hydroxycarbazepine; OXY, oxcarbazepine; i.v., intravenously; p.o., orally.
[a]The data from reference 26 are in patients with epilepsy who are receiving polytherapy, whereas the data in reference 19, 23, 24, and 27–29 are in healthy subjects.
[b]These parameters were calculated from reference 27.

When OXC was taken with a fat- and protein-rich breakfast, the AUC of MHD increased by 16% and the peak plasma concentration by 23% (30). In one study, 12 healthy (6 male and 6 female) adult volunteers received OXC orally (300-mg tablet) and racemic MHD intravenously (i.v.; 250 mg infused over 30 minutes) (27). After i.v. administration of racemic MHD, the mean [± standard deviation (SD)] AUC values of (*R*)-MHD and (*S*)-MHD were 120 ± 26 μmol/L/hr and 167 ± 37 μmol/L/hr., respectively (27). After oral administration of OXC to the same healthy subjects, the enantiomeric ratio of the mean AUC values of (*S*)-MHD (241 ± 55 μmol/L/hr) over (*R*)-MHD (64 ± 20 μmol/L/hr) equaled 3.8 (27). An enantiomeric AUC ratio of 4.9 was obtained after oral administration of OXC (600 mg) to 12 healthy Chinese subjects (19). These two studies demonstrate an enantiospecific metabolic reduction of the prochiral carbonyl group of OXC in its biotransformation to MHD (19,27). The ratio (normalized to the dose) of the total AUC values for both MHD enantiomers obtained after oral (OXC) and i.v. (racemic MHD) administration (27) to the same subjects gives a mean absolute bioavailability (oral availability) value of 89% (Table 45.1). The oral availability of MHD after oral and i.v. administration (400 mg) of racemic MHD to six dogs

was 78% ± 21% and 79% ± 27% for (*R*)-MHD and (*S*)-MHD, respectively (20).

Formulations and Routes of Administration

OXC is commercially available (Trileptal; Novartis, Summit, NJ) as a regular film-coated, divisible tablet at dosage strengths of 150, 300, and 600 mg and as an oral suspension at a concentration of 60 mg/mL. Because of its water insolubility, there are no parenteral preparations of OXC. However, MHD is being developed in its racemic form as a new AED for parenteral administration to supplement OXC oral therapy because of its better water solubility compared with OXC and CBZ.

DISTRIBUTION

Calculations of MHD volume of distribution (Vβ) based on the only published study where racemic MHD was administered intravenously (250 mg) to six healthy subjects yielded mean values of 11.7 L and 13.8 L for (*R*)-MHD and (*S*)-MHD, respectively (27) (Table 45.1). Higher Vβ values were obtained after i.v. administration (400 mg) of racemic MHD to six dogs: 25 ± 6 L for (*R*)-MHD and 47 ± 14 L for (*S*)-MHD (20). The apparent volume of distribution (Vβ/F) of OXC obtained after its oral administration (600 mg) to eight healthy subjects was very high and variable, 12.5 ± 12.9 L/kg (26) (Table 45.1).

The plasma protein binding of MHD is approximately 40% and is constant at clinically relevant concentration ranges of 20 to 150 μmol/L (31). OXC is approximately 60% bound at a plasma concentration range of 0.2 to 11.4 μmol/L. OXC and MHD are excreted in breast milk, with a milk–plasma concentration ratio of 0.5 (32,33). OXC and MHD cross the placenta. The transfer of OXC through the perfused placenta was quicker than the transfer of antipyrine, whereas the transfer of MHD was slower (34). OXC is biotransformed to some extent in human placenta *in vitro*, suggesting that the placenta also might be a metabolic site for OXC *in vivo* (34). As neutral lipophilic compounds, OXC and MHD pass rapidly through biologic membranes, including the blood–brain barrier (1).

ROUTES OF ELIMINATION

OXC undergoes rapid and extensive metabolism to MHD by a stereoselective biotransformation mediated by a cytosolic, nonmicrosomal, and noninducible arylketone reductase. MHD is eliminated from the body by metabolism, and the metabolic scheme of OXC and MHD is depicted in Figure 45.1 (24). Each of the formed MHD enantiomers is excreted in the urine or undergoes glucuronide conjugation or subsequent oxidation to the respective DHD enantiomers (19,24) (Figure 45.1). After oral administration (600 mg) of OXC to 12 healthy subjects, approximately 27% of the molar dose of OXC was recovered (free and conjugated) in the urine (within 48 hours after dosing) as the enantiomers of MHD: (*R*)-MHD 4.0% ± 2.1% and (*S*)-MHD 22.6% ± 8.2% (19). The urinary recovery of the DHD enantiomers accounts for less than 1%, mostly in unconjugated form.

After oral administration (400 mg) of ^{14}C-labeled MHD to two healthy subjects, most of the dose (94.6% and 97.1%) was excreted in the urine within 6 days after dosing. Fecal excretion in the two studied subjects accounted for 4.3% and 1.9%, respectively (24). In this study, 28% and 71% of the dose was excreted in the urine as free and conjugated MHD enantiomers, respectively (24). Analysis of the diastereoisomeric MHD glucuronide shows that approximately 6% is accounted for by (*R*)-MHD glucuronide and approximately 45% by (*S*)-MHD glucuronide (Figure 45.1). Approximately 4% and 9% of the dose appeared in the urine as sulfate and glucuronide conjugates, respectively, of 10-hydroxy carbamazepine (24). Thus, the involvement of the CYP isozyme family in the metabolism of OXC is quite minimal and is limited to the

formation of DHD. Consequently, to date there have been no reports of genetic polymorphism in OXC metabolism.

CLEARANCE AND HALF-LIFE

The half-life of OXC is 1 to 3.7 hours, and its AUC after oral administration to healthy subjects amounted to 2% to 4% of the AUC for MHD, indicating that OXC has a high oral clearance value of 2.4 ± 1.1 L/hr/kg (25,26,28,29). After multiple dosing to six epileptic patients (daily dose, 1.5 to 2.4 g), the oral clearance (mean ± SD) of OXC was 1.6 ± 0.5 L/hr/kg and its half life was 3.1 ± 1.5 hours (26). After i.v. administration (250 mg infused over 30 minutes) of racemic MHD to 12 healthy subjects, the clearance (calculated from the AUC data) and half-life of (*R*)-MHD and (*S*)-MHD were 4.2 ± 0.9 L/hr and 9.0 ± 1.5 hours, and 3.0 ± 0.7 L/hr and 10.6 ± 2.6 hours, respectively (27) (Table 45.1). After oral administration of OXC (300 mg) to the same 12 healthy subjects, the half-life values for (*R*)-MHD and (*S*)-MHD were 15.8 ± 2.8 hours and 11.2 ± 1.5 hours, respectively (27).

In another study, the half-life of MHD enantiomers obtained after oral administration of OXC (600 mg) to 12 Chinese healthy subjects was 11.9 ± 3.3 hours and 13.0 ± 4.1 hours for (*R*)-MHD and (*S*)-MHD, respectively (19). The renal clearance of the two MHD enantiomers ranged between 0.7 to 1.1 L/hr, with no enantioselectivity (19,27). After i.v. administration of racemic MHD to healthy subjects, 12% and 16% of the dose was excreted in the urine as (*R*)-MHD and (*S*)-MHD, respectively (27). After oral administration of OXC to healthy subjects, 4% and 23% of the dose was excreted in the urine as (*R*)-MHD and (*S*)-MHD, respectively (19,27).

When MHD is given i.v., the AUC of (*S*)-MHD is 40% higher than that of (*R*)-MHD because its clearance is significantly smaller than that of its enantiomer. After oral administration of OXC, the enantioselective pharmacokinetics of MHD are much more profound because of enantioselective presystemic metabolic ketoreduction of the prochiral carbonyl group of the OXC molecule (Figure 45.2). The enantiomeric serum concentrations ratio of (*S*)-MHD over (*R*)-MHD increases from a value of 3 at 1 hour after dosing to 5.8 at 48 hours after dosing (19) (Figure 45.2). The observation that the ratio between the (*S*)- and (*R*)-enantiomers in serum increased over time shows that differences in elimination (clearance) of the enantiomers contribute to the higher serum levels of (*S*)-MHD. However, differences in clearance are too small (40%) to explain the striking difference (400%) in the AUC values of MHD enantiomers after oral administration of OXC. Indeed, the observation that at the first sampling time (1 hour after dosing) the concentration of (*S*)-MHD was three times greater than that of (*R*)-MHD (Figure 45.2) strongly suggests that the differences in their kinetic profiles are related mainly to

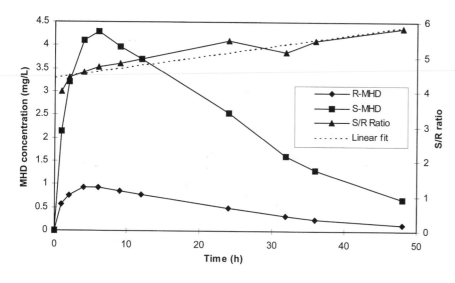

FIGURE 45.2. Mean serum concentrations of (*S*)- and (*R*)-10-hydroxycarbazepine (MHD) and (*S*)/(*R*) ratios in serum after a single oral dose of 600 mg oxcarbazepine (OXC) to 12 healthy Chinese subjects. (From Volosov A, Xiaodong S, Perucca E, et al. Enantioselective pharmacokinetics of 10-hydroxycarbazepine after oral administration of oxcarbazepine to Chinese subjects. *Clin Pharmacol Ther* 1999;66:547–553, with permission.)

stereoselectivity in the formation clearance of MHD after oral administration of OXC.

There are no reports on MHD clearance in comedicated epileptic patients, children, or the elderly. The half-life of MHD was similar in patients and healthy subjects (7). In healthy subjects aged 60 to 82 years, the AUC and peak plasma concentration values of MHD were significantly higher than in younger adults, probably because of the diminished creatinine clearance in older persons (35). MHD concentrations in children 6 to 18 years of age are similar to those observed in adults, but those reported in children 2 to 5 years of age have been lower (36,37).

Hepatic impairment has no effect on the pharmacokinetics of OXC and MHD. However, MHD plasma levels increased significantly in patients with creatinine clearance of 30 mL/min. In this group of patients, the dosage of OXC should be reduced by 50% and the dosage titration should be prolonged (38).

RELATIONSHIP BETWEEN SERUM CONCENTRATION AND DOSE

Studies in healthy subjects and epileptic patients showed a linear, proportional relationship between daily doses of OXC and serum concentrations of MHD (3,39). After oral administration of MHD (600 mg) to healthy subjects, serum levels of (*S*)-MHD and (*R*)-MHD ranged from 1 to 4.5 mg/L and 0.2 to 1 mg/L, respectively (19). In other (nonstereospecific) studies, the peak plasma concentration of MHD and OXC obtained after oral administration of a single 600-mg dose of OXC to healthy subjects ranged from 5.4 to 8.9 mg/L (MHD) and 1.1 to 1.7 mg/L (OXC) (26,28,29,37,40) (Table 45.1). After multiple dosing OXC (300 mg twice daily) to 24 young (18 to 32 years of age) and old (60 to 81 years of age) healthy subjects, the accumulation of MHD was found to be more than expected

based on linear pharmacokinetics (35). No significant difference was observed between male and female volunteers. The following MHD plasma levels (mean ± SD) were obtained in this study: young men, 8.5 ± 2 mg/L; elderly men, 12 ± 1.2 mg/L; young women, 9.3 ± 1.1 mg/L; and elderly women, 11.7 ± 2.0 mg/L. The peak-to-trough fluctuation of (racemic) MHD ranged from 22% to 43% (35).

According to the manufacturer's prescribing information, treatment with OXC was well tolerated in epileptic patients receiving dosages of 1,200 mg/day. At dosages of 2,400 mg/day, more than 65% of the patients discontinued treatment mainly because of central nervous system–related side effects. Consequently, assuming linear kinetics, it is expected that OXC daily doses of 1,200 mg will yield MHD steady-state plasma levels in a range of 12 to 25 mg/L.

RELATIONSHIP BETWEEN SERUM CONCENTRATION AND EFFECT

In a review article on therapeutic drug monitoring of major AEDs, the target range of MHD plasma concentrations associated with antiepileptic effect was reported to be 5 to 50 mg/L or 20 to 200 µmol/L (41).

CONCLUSION

OXC is a soft drug analog of CBZ and a prodrug to MHD. Thus, MHD is the active entity in OXC therapy. Because of species differences in the pharmacokinetics of OXC, this finding was discovered in the late stages of OXC development. Otherwise, it might be worthwhile from a pharmacokinetic and biopharmaceutic standpoint to develop MHD (in its racemic or stereospecific form) rather than OXC. The two enantiomers of MHD showed similar median effective dose (ED$_{50}$) values in animal models for anticonvulsant activity (11,12). The stereoselective pharmacokinetics of MHD in dogs (20,21) and humans (19,27) and the different pharmacokinetic profile and exposure between animals and humans suggest that the *in vivo* anticonvulsant activity of MHD be assessed in terms of median effective concentration (EC_{50}) rather than ED_{50}. Only after a comparative analysis of the EC_{50}s and the toxicologic profile of the two MHD enantiomers, as well as a thorough stereospecific pharmacokinetic–pharmacodynamic evaluation, can a decision be made regarding the possible development of an individual MHD enantiomer as a new drug candidate.

REFERENCES

1. Dam M, Ostergaard LH. Oxcarbazepine. In: Levy RH, Mattson RH, Meldrum BS, eds. *Antiepileptic drugs*, 4th ed. New York: Raven Press, 1995:987–995.
2. Grant SM, Faulds D. Oxcarbazepine: a review of its pharmacology and therapeutic potential in epilepsy, trigeminal neuralgia and affective disorders. *Drugs* 1992;43:873–888.
3. Lloyd P, Flesch G, Dieterle W. Clinical pharmacology and pharmacokinetics of oxcarbazepine. *Epilepsia* 1994;35[Suppl 3]: S10–S13.
4. Perucca E. The new generation of antiepileptic drugs: advantages and disadvantages. *Br J Clin Pharmacol* 1996;42:531–543.
5. Baruzzi A, Albani F, Riva R. Oxcarbazepine: pharmacokinetic interactions and their clinical relevance. *Epilepsia* 1994;35[Suppl 3]:S14–S19.
6. Kerr BM, Thummel KE, Wurden CJ, et al. Human liver carbamazepine metabolism: role of CYP3A4 and CYP2C8 in 10,11-epoxide formation. *Biochem Pharmacol* 1994;47:1969–1979.
7. Schachter SC. Oxcarbazepine. In: Eadie MJ, Vajda FJE, eds. *Antiepiletic drugs: pharmacology and therapeutics. Handbook of experimental pharmacology.* Berlin: Springer-Verlag, 1999: 319–330.
8. Spina E, Pisani F, Perucca E. Clinically significant pharmacokinetic drug interactions with carbamazepine. *Clin Pharmacokinet* 1996;31:198–214.
9. Leach JP, Blacklaw J, Jamieson V, et al. Mutual interaction between remacemide hydrochloride and carbamazepine: two drugs with active metabolites. *Epilepsia* 1996;37:1100–1106.
10. Bodor N. Soft drugs. In: *Encyclopedia of human biology.* San Diego: Harcourt Brace Jovanovich, 1991;7:101–107.
11. Kubova H, Mares P. Anticonvulsant action of oxcarbazepine, hydroxycarbamazepine, and carbamazepine against metrazol-induced motor seizures in developing rats. *Epilepsia* 1993;34: 188–192.
12. Schmutz M, Ferrat T, Heckendorn R, et al. GP47779, the main human metabolite of oxcarbazepine (Trileptal), and both enantiomers have equal anticonvulsant activity. *Epilepsia* 1993;34 [Suppl 2]:122.
13. U.S. Patent 3,642,775, W. Schindler assigned to Ciba Geigy, 1972.
14. Elyas AA, Goldberg VD, Patsalos PN. Simple and rapid micro-analytical high-performance liquid chromatographic technique for the assay of oxcarbazepine and its primary active metabolite 10-hydroxycarbazepine. *J Chromatogr Biomed Appl* 1990;528:473–479.
15. Hartley R, Green M, Lucock MD, et al. Solid phase extraction of oxcarbazepine and its metabolites from plasma for analysis by

16. high performance liquid chromatography. *Biomed Chromatogr* 1991;5:212–215.
16. von Unruh GE, Paar WD. Gas chromatographic assay for oxcarbazepine and its main metabolites in plasma. *J Chromatogr Biomed Appl* 1985;345:67–76.
17. Flesch G, Francotte E, Hell F, et al. Determination of the R-(−) and S-(+) enantiomers of the monohydroxylated metabolite of oxcarbazepine in human plasma by enantioselective high-performance liquid chromatography. *J Chromatogr* 1992;581:147–151.
18. Volosov A, Bialer M, Xiaodong, et al. Simultaneous stereoselective high-performance liquid chromatographic determination of 10-hydroxycarbazepine and its metabolite carbamazepine-10,11-trans-dihydrodiol in human urine. *J Chromatogr B Biomed Sci Appl* 2000;738:419–425.
19. Volosov A, Xiaodong S, Perucca E, et al. Enantioselective pharmacokinetics of 10-hydroxycarbazepine after oral administration of oxcarbazepine to Chinese subjects. *Clin Pharmacol Ther* 1999;66:547–553.
20. Volosov A, Sintov A, Bialer M. Stereoselective pharmacokinetic analysis of the antiepileptic 10-hydroxycarbazepine in dogs. *Ther Drug Monit* 1999;21:219–223.
21. Volosov A, Yagen B, Bialer M. Comparative stereoselective pharmacokinetic analysis of 10-hydroxycarbazepine after oral administration of its individual enantiomers and racemic mixture to dogs. *Epilepsia* 2000;41:1107–1110.
22. Feldmann KF, Dorhofer G, Faigle JW, et al. Pharmacokinetics and metabolism of GP 47779, the main human metabolite of oxcarbazepine (GP 47680) in animals and human volunteers. *Adv Epileptol* 1981:89–96.
23. Feldmann KF, Brechbuhler S, Faigle JW, et al. Pharmacokinetics and metabolism of GP 47680, a compound related to carbamazepine, in animals and man. *Adv Epileptol* 1978:290–294.
24. Schutz H, Feldmann KF, Faigle JW, et al. The metabolism of 14C-oxcarbazepine in man. *Xenobiotica* 1986;8:769–778.
25. Tarata A, Galimberti CA, Mani R, et al. The pharmacokinetics of oxcarbazepine and its active metabolite 10-hydroxy-carbazepine in healthy subjects and epileptic patients treated with phenobarbital and valproic acid. *Br J Clin Pharmacol* 1993;36:366–368.
26. Dickinson RG, Hooper WD, Dunstan PR, et al. First dose and stead-state pharmacokinetics of oxcarbazepine and its 10-hydroxy metabolite. *Eur J Clin Pharmacol* 1989;37:69–74.
27. Flesch G, Czendlik C, Ehrhart F, et al. Pharmacokinetics of two enantiomers of the monohydroxy derivative of oxcarbazepine in man. *Eur J Pharm Sci* 1999;8:xxii(abstr).
28. Keranen T, Jolkkonen J, Jensen PK, et al. Absence of interaction between oxcarbazepine and erythromycin. *Acta Neurol Scand* 1992;86:120–123.
29. Keranen T, Jolkkonen J, Klosterskov-Jensen P, et al. Oxcarbazepine does not interact with cimetidine in healthy volunteers. *Acta Neurol Scand* 1992;85:239–242.
30. Degen PH, Flesch G, Cardot JM, et al. The influence of food on the disposition of the antiepileptic oxcarbazepine and its major metabolites in healthy volunteers. *Biopharm Drug Dispos* 1994; 15:519–526.
31. Patsalos PN, Elyas AA, Zakrewska JM. Protein binding of oxcarbazepine and its primary active metabolite, 10-hydroxy carbazepine, in patients with trigeminal neuralgia. *Eur J Clin Pharmacol* 1990;39:413–415.
32. Bulau P, Paar WD, von Unruh GE. Pharmacokinetics of oxcarbazepine and 10-hydroxycarabazepine in the newborn child of an oxcarbazepine-treated mother. *Eur J Clin Pharmacol* 1988;34: 311–313.
33. Bar-Oz B, Nulman I, Koren G, et al. Anticonvulsant and breast feeding: a critical review. *Pediatr Drugs* 2000;2:113–126.

34. Pienmimaki P, Lampeal E, Hakkola J, et al. Pharmacokinetics of oxcarbazepine and carbamazepine in human placenta. *Epilepsia* 1997;38:309–316.

35. van Heiningen PNM, Eve MD, Oosterhuis B, et al. The influence of age on the pharmacokinetics of the antiepileptic agent oxcarbazepine. *Clin Pharmacol Ther* 1991;50:410–419.

36. Sallas W, Hossain M, D'Souza J. Population pharmacokinetic analysis of oxcarbazepine (Trileptal) in children with epilepsy. *Epilepsia* 1999;40[Suppl 7]:102(abstr).

37. Schachter SC. The next wave of anticonvulsants: focus on levetiracetam, oxcarbazepine and zonisamide. *CNS Drugs* 2000;14:229–249.

38. Rouan MC, Lecaillon JB, Godbillon J, et al. The effect of renal impairment on the pharmacokinetics of oxcarbazepine and its metabolites. *Eur J Clin Pharmacol* 1994;47:161–167.

39. Augusteijn R, van Parys JAP. Oxcarbazepine (Trileptal, OXC): dose concentration relationship in patients with epilepsy. *Acta Neurol Scand Suppl* 1990;133:37.

40. Jung H, Noguez A, Mayet L, et al. The distribution of 10-hydroxy carbazepine in blood compartments. *Biopharm Drug Dispos* 1997;18:17–23.

41. Glauser TA, Pippenger CE. Controversies in blood-level monitoring: reexamining its role in the treatment of epilepsy. *Epilepsia* 2000;41[Suppl 8]:S6–S15.

Antiepileptic Drugs, 5th Edition. Edited by R.H. Levy, R.H. Mattson, B.S. Meldrum, and E. Perucca. Lippincott Williams & Wilkins, Philadelphia © 2002.

OXCARBAZEPINE

INTERACTIONS WITH OTHER DRUGS

FIORENZO ALBANI
ROBERTO RIVA
AGOSTINO BARUZZI

GENERAL CONSIDERATIONS

Antiepileptic drug (AED) interactions are relatively common and represent a frequent clinical problem during epilepsy treatment (1,2). Oxcarbazepine (OXC) is an AED chemically related to carbamazepine (CBZ), but shows a completely different metabolic profile. After oral administration in humans, OXC undergoes rapid and almost quantitative enzymatic reduction to form its active metabolite, 10,11-dihydro-10-hydroxycarbazepine (monohydroxy derivative, MHD). Only minimal amounts of the parent drug are found in peripheral blood (3). Elimination of MHD occurs through direct renal excretion, glucuronidation, and, marginally, hydroxylation to a dihydroxy derivative (DHD) (3). Only the latter reaction depends on microsomal cytochrome P450 (CYP450) enzymes, suggesting that interference with oxidative metabolism, usually the most common source of pharmacokinetic interactions, should be of minor relevance. Studies on the enzyme-inducing properties of OXC treatment, tested in most cases using antipyrine as a probe, have been reviewed previously (4). In brief, OXC seems to have only a modest inducing action, possibly more evident at high doses or related to induction of specific isoforms of CYP450 enzymes (2–4). Another common source of pharmacokinetic interactions for AEDs is at the level of competitive plasma protein binding (1,2). These interactions, however, seldom are clinically relevant, and in the case of OXC are unlikely to occur to any significant extent because the main active substance (MHD) is only approximately 40% plasma protein bound (3).

Fiorenzo Albani, PharmD: Research Assistant, Department of Neurological Sciences, University of Bologna, Bologna, Italy
Roberto Riva, MD: Senior Researcher, Department of Neurological Sciences, University of Bologna, Bologna, Italy
Agostino Baruzzi, MD: Professor of Neurology, Department of Neurological Sciences, University of Bologna, Bologna, Italy

To define better the clinical relevance of OXC drug interactions, some reference to other AEDs is made thoroughly this review.

EFFECTS OF OXCARBAZEPINE ON ANTIEPILEPTIC DRUGS

Information about OXC effects on the kinetics of other AEDs derives from a few specific studies and from AED plasma concentration data collected during polytherapy clinical studies. Houtkooper et al. (5) reported that the substitution of OXC for CBZ given in association with valproic acid (VPA) or phenytoin (PHT), at constant dosages, increased VPA and PHT plasma concentrations by 20% to 30%. Battino et al. (6) reported similar data on total and free VPA concentrations in young epileptic patients. Total or partial deinduction is the probable cause of these effects. Therefore, when OXC is substituted for an inducing drug in polytherapy, the clinical status of the patient and the plasma concentrations of other AEDs should be closely monitored.

McKee et al. (7) studied the effect of OXC on the steady-state concentrations of CBZ, VPA, and PHT in 3 groups of 12 chronically treated patients, both after single-dose administration (OXC 600 mg) and after 1-week treatment (OXC 300 mg three times daily), compared with placebo. Median areas under the conentration curve (AUCs) for CBZ, VPA, and PHT during a dosage interval (12 hours) did not differ significantly after treatment with OXC and placebo, although a trend for reduced CBZ AUC and increased PHT AUC was observed.

Analyzing data collected in two large, controlled clinical trials, Hossain et al. (8) reported that plasma concentrations of phenobarbital (PB) increased (+14%) and those of CBZ were reduced (−15%) during OXC coadministration. More clinically relevant is the observation of a mean 40% increase in PHT concentrations for MHD plasma levels above 43 µg/mL (8).

In a series of 14 patients treated with OXC and lamotrigine (LTG), the LTG level-to-dose ratio (LDR) was 33% less with respect to LTG monotherapy (9). Given LTG's pharmacokinetic characteristics (2), an involvement of enzymes responsible for LTG glucuroconjugation may be suspected. For comparison, the LTG LDR in patients cotreated with CBZ was approximately 50% less.

EFFECTS OF OXCARBAZEPINE ON OTHER DRUGS

The interaction of AEDs with oral anticoagulants often is of clinical importance (1). The influence of OXC on the anticoagulant effect of warfarin was investigated in 10 healthy volunteers (10). A dose of 900 mg administered daily for a week, after a warfarin titrating period of 3 weeks, did not significantly modify warfarin action as measured by prothrombin time (mean Quick values 36.6% at baseline, 38.1% after OXC). The authors concluded that when coadministration of warfarin is required, OXC offers a clinical advantage over other AEDs, such as PB, PHT, and CBZ. However, no data in patients are available.

The clinical significance of AED interaction with oral contraceptives also is well known (1,11), and the potential effects of OXC have been investigated. In a preliminary study (12), OXC 900 mg/day added for a month to a stable oral contraceptive regimen (low-dose, triphasic) reduced the bioavailability of ethinylestradiol (EE) and levonorgestrel (LN) by 48% and 32%, respectively, in the 10 healthy women who completed the protocol. These data were confirmed in a crossover, placebo-controlled study in 22 healthy women receiving a high-dose, fixed-ratio combination of EE (50 μg) and LN (250 μg) (13), where $AUCs_{0-24}$ of EE and LN were decreased by 47% during OXC treatment at 1,200 mg/day. It has been suggested that OXC selectively induces the CYP3A-mediated metabolism responsible for the major EE and LN metabolic pathways (10–12). In the study by Klosterskov Jensen et al. (12), breakthrough bleeding, a clinical consequence of reduced hormone bioavailability and an indication of diminished contraceptive efficacy, showed an incidence of 15%, which was considerably higher than that observed when the same oral contraceptives were used without associated drugs. Similarly, of six women receiving OXC in combination with an oral low-dose contraceptive containing 30 μg of EE, four had breakthrough bleeding with OXC (14). In 59 patients treated with CBZ, 37 (63%) had the same adverse effect (14). Therefore, the same cautions exercised with enzyme-inducing AEDs possibly apply to OXC as well.

Felodipine, a calcium antagonist, undergoes extensive first-pass oxidative hepatic metabolism and normally has an oral absolute bioavailability of 15%. Drug-inducing AEDs reduce this bioavailability to less than 1% (15). A study performed in eight volunteers, however, reported a 28% relative reduction in felodipine bioavailability (absolute value ~10%), when OXC (900 mg/day) was coadministered for 1 week (16). The clinical relevance of this interaction in patients is not defined.

EFFECTS OF ANTIEPILEPTIC DRUGS ON OXCARBAZEPINE

An early retrospective study showed that enzyme-inducing drugs such as PB and PHT do not induce MHD formation but can increase its oxidative conversion to DHD. This has been considered to be clinically insignificant and to represent a minor pathway in OXC metabolism (17). The ratio between MHD concentrations (milligrams per liter) and the OXC oral doses (milligrams per kilogram), however, was lower in a group of adult patients receiving comedication with enzyme-inducing drugs (mean value, 0.74) compared with patients receiving OXC alone (mean value, 0.94), indicating that some interaction with enzyme-inducing comedication may occur (18). When OXC was combined with VPA, the ratio was 0.93, similar to that found in monotherapy (18).

These preliminary data have been substantially confirmed by specific studies. Tartara et al. (19) reported a comparison of OXC and MHD kinetics after acute administration in normal subjects and in patients treated with other AEDs. Three groups of eight subjects (drug-free healthy control subjects or epileptic patients on chronic treatment with either PB or VPA alone) each received a single oral dose of OXC 600 mg. Plasma concentrations of OXC and MHD were followed for up to 48 hours. The AUCs of OXC and MHD were significantly lower in patients receiving PB than in control subjects, whereas no differences were found between patients receiving VPA and control subjects.

In the study already mentioned, McKee et al. (7) reported the effect of CBZ, VPA, and PHT on OXC pharmacokinetics in 3 groups of 12 patients each, both after single-dose administration (OXC 600 mg) and after 1-week treatment (OXC 300 mg three times daily), compared with placebo. A group of seven otherwise untreated patients served as control, receiving active treatment (OXC) only. MHD AUCs at steady state were lower in PHT- and CBZ-treated patients with respect to control subjects (approximately one-third less). In CBZ-treated patients the difference reached statistical significance ($p < .05$). Possible explanations were a small induction effect on MHD metabolism or the induction of an alternative pathway of OXC biodegradation. Values for patients on VPA cotherapy were similar to those for control subjects.

In a small series of patients, May et al. (20) reported comparable mean values for MHD LDR after treatment with OXC in monotherapy or with VPA cotreatment. The MHD free fraction during VPA cotherapy was slightly but significantly higher (64% versus 56.7% in monotherapy). Interestingly, two patients receiving methsuximide had the lowest MHD LDR: <50% with respect to monotherapy.

Overall, these data suggest that enzyme-inducing AEDs such as PB, PHT, and CBZ cause only modest modifications of OXC pharmacokinetics in most cases; the interaction, however, may be clinically relevant in some patients. The association with VPA should not require any adjustment of OXC dosages.

The effect of felbamate (FBM) on OXC kinetics was assessed in 18 healthy volunteers (21). Subjects received OXC, 1,200 mg/day, on an open basis in combination with placebo or FBM, 2,400 mg/day, for two 10-day treatments periods. FBM had no significant effects on MHD plasma or urine pharmacokinetics compared with placebo. However, DHD maximum plasma concentration and AUC_{0-12} values as well as DHD urinary excretion (free and total) were significantly increased, probably as a consequence of the induction of oxidative metabolism of MHD. The authors considered the effects of FBM on OXC pharmacokinetics not clinically relevant.

EFFECTS OF OTHER DRUGS ON OXCARBAZEPINE

Most data on the effects of other, non-AED drugs on OXC derive from preclinical studies in healthy volunteers. Verapamil inhibits the metabolism of CBZ to an extent that can produce clinical manifestations of CBZ neurotoxicity (1). The potential interaction of verapamil and OXC was studied in 10 healthy volunteers (22). After titration of OXC to 900 mg/day, verapamil (240 mg/day) was administered for 1 week. The main result was a 20% decrease of the MHD AUC compared with baseline, an effect that remains to be explained. This interaction, however, is likely to be clinically negligible in most cases. Cimetidine interacts with many drugs (23), inhibiting their metabolism and causing clinical

toxicity in some cases. The cimetidine–OXC interaction was studied in eight healthy volunteers: cimetidine treatment 800 mg/day for 1 week did not significantly modify the pharmacokinetics of OXC or MHD (24). Erythromycin is a macrolide antibiotic frequently implicated in clinically relevant pharmacokinetic drug interactions (25). Results of an eight-volunteer study indicated that a week of erythromycin therapy (1,000 mg/day) had no major influence on the pharmacokinetic parameters of OXC and MHD (26).

Dextropropoxyphene can interfere with AEDs (1), but the clinical significance of individual interactions varies. The effects of dextropropoxyphene on the kinetics of OXC and its metabolites were reported in a study in eight patients receiving chronic OXC treatment (27). Plasma concentrations of MHD were not significantly affected by dextropropoxyphene (195 mg/day for 1 week), even if the DHD concentrations were reduced as a possible consequence of inhibited MHD oxidation.

Clinically significant interactions have been described between viloxazine and AEDs (1). In a study in six epileptic patients receiving chronic OXC monotherapy (1,500 ± 465 mg/day), a 10-day add-on treatment with viloxazine did not modify OXC plasma concentrations, whereas MHD concentrations were increased by 11% and DHD concentrations decreased by an average of 31% (28). No adverse effects were reported in any patients. These results suggest that viloxazine coadministration causes a very modest inhibition of MHD oxidation and that viloxazine can be used safely in depressed epileptic patients receiving OXC treatment.

CONCLUSION

Table 46.1 summarizes the published data on OXC interactions. In general, OXC shows a favorable profile, with a

TABLE 46.1. PHARMACOKINETIC INTERACTIONS OF OXCARBAZEPINE

Interaction	Effect	Subjects	Reference
Effect of oxcarbazepine on:			
Phenytoin	Increased concentrations	Patients	7, 8
Phenobarbital	Increased concentrations	Patients	8
Valproate	No relevant effect	Patients	7
Carbamazepine	Reduced concentrations	Patients	7, 8
Lamotrigine	Reduced concentrations	Patients	9
Warfarin	No effect	Healthy volunteers	10
Oral contraceptives	Significant metabolic induction	Healthy volunteers	12–14
Felodipine	Bioavailability reduction	Healthy volunteers	16
Effect on oxcarbazepine by:			
Phenobarbital; phenytoin and carbamazepine	MHD AUC reduction of 25%	Patients	7, 18, 19
Valproate	No relevant effect	Patients	7, 19, 20
Felbamate	No relevant effect	Patients	21
Verapamil	MHD AUC reduction of 20%	Healthy volunteers	22
Cimetidine	No relevant effect	Healthy volunteers	24
Erythromycin	No relevant effect	Healthy volunteers	26
Dextropropoxyphene	No relevant effect	Patients	27
Viloxazine	No relevant effect	Patients	28

AUC, area under plasma concentration curve; MHD, monohydroxy derivative; 10,11-dihydro-10-hydroxycarbazepine.

limited capacity to affect disposition of other AEDs in a clinically relevant fashion. Only the observed reduction of LTG concentrations and, possibly, the increase in PHT concentrations may require a dose adjustment. The effects of OXC on the clinical efficacy of other drugs should be a minor problem except for the possibly reduced efficacy of oral contraceptives.

On the other hand, the substitution of an inducing agent with OXC should be carefully monitored because of potentially significant deinduction, and the oral doses of associated drugs may need to be adjusted.

Plasma concentrations of OXC are moderately affected by enzyme-inducing AEDS like PB, PHT, and CBZ, and no relevant interactions were observed with VPA and FBM. The modifications of OXC kinetics caused by other drugs seem of little, if any, clinical significance.

REFERENCES

1. Patsalos PN, Duncan JS. Antiepileptic drugs: a review of clinically significant drug interactions. *Drug Saf* 1993;9:156–184.
2. Riva R, Albani F, Contin M, et al. Pharmacokinetic interaction between antiepileptic drugs. *Clin Pharmacokinet* 1996;31: 470–493.
3. Tecoma ES. Oxcarbazepine. *Epilepsia* 1999;40[Suppl 5]: S37–S46.
4. Baruzzi A, Albani F, Riva R. Oxcarbazepine: pharmacokinetic interactions and their clinical relevance. *Epilepsia* 1994;35[Suppl 3]:14–19.
5. Houtkooper MA, Lammertsma A, Meyer JWA, et al. Oxcarbazepine (GP 47680): a possible alternative to carbamazepine? *Epilepsia* 1987;28:693–698.
6. Battino D, Croci D, Granata T, et al. Changes in unbound and total valproic acid concentrations after replacement of carbamazepine with oxcarbazepine. *Ther Drug Monit* 1992;14: 376–379.
7. McKee PJ, Blacklaw J, Forrest G, et al. A double-blind, placebo-controlled interaction study between oxcarbazepine and carbamazepine, sodium valproate and phenytoin in epileptic patients. *Br J Clin Pharmacol* 1994;37:27–32.
8. Hossain M, Sallas W, Gasparini M, et al. Drug-drug interaction profile of oxcarbazepine in children and adults. *Neurology* 1999;52[Suppl 2]:A525(abstr).
9. May TW, Rambeck B, Jurgens U. Influence of oxcarbazepine and methsuximide on lamotrigine concentrations in epileptic patients with and without valproic acid comedication: results of a retrospective study. *Ther Drug Monit* 1999;21:175–181.
10. Kramer G, Tettenborn B, Klosterskov Jensen P, et al. Oxcarbazepine does not affect the anticoagulant activity of warfarin. *Epilepsia* 1992;33:1145–1148.
11. Wilbur K, Ensom MHH. Pharmacokinetic drug interactions between oral contraceptives and second-generation anticonvulsants. *Clin Pharmacokinet* 2000;38:355–365.
12. Klosterskov Jensen P, Saano V, Haring P, et al. Possible interaction between oxcarbazepine and an oral contraceptive. *Epilepsia* 1992;33:1149–1152.
13. Fattore C, Cipolla G, Gatti G, et al. Induction of ethinylestradiol and levonorgestrel metabolism by oxcarbazepine in healthy women. *Epilepsia* 1999;40:783–787.
14. Sonnen AEH. Oxcarbazepine and oral contraceptives. *Acta Neurol Scand Suppl* 1990;133:37(abstr).
15. Capewell S, Freestone S, Critchley JAJH, et al. Reduced felodipine bioavailability in patients taking anticonvulsants. *Lancet* 1988;2:480–482.
16. Zaccara G, Gangemi PF, Bendoni L, et al. Influence of single and repeated doses of oxcarbazepine on the pharmacokinetic profile of felodipine. *Ther Drug Monit* 1993;15:39–42.
17. Kumps A, Wurth C. Oxcarbazepine disposition: preliminary observations in patients. *Biopharmacol Drug Dispos* 1990;11: 365–370.
18. van Parys JAP, Meijer JWA, Segers JP. Dose-concentration proportionality in epileptic patients stabilized on oxcarbazepine: effects of co-medication. *Epilepsia* 1991;32[Suppl 1]:70(abstr).
19. Tartara A, Galimberti CA, Manni R, et al. The pharmacokinetic profile of oxcarbazepine and its active metabolite 10-hydroxycarbazepine in normal subjects and in epileptic patients treated with phenobarbitone or valproic acid. *Br J Clin Pharmacol* 1993;36: 366–368.
20. May TW, Rambeck B, Salke-Kellermann A. Fluctuations of 10-hydroxy-carbazepine during the day in epileptic patients. *Acta Neurol Scand* 1996;93:393–397.
21. Hulsman JA, Rentmeester TW, Banfield CR, et al. Effects of felbamate on the pharmacokinetics of the monohydroxy and dihydroxy metabolites of oxcarbazepine. *Clin Pharmacol Ther* 1995; 58:383–389.
22. Kramer G, Tettenborn B, Flesch G. Oxcarbazepine-verapamil drug interaction in healthy volunteers. *Epilepsia* 1991;32[Suppl 1]:70–71.
23. Somogyi A, Muirhead M. Pharmacokinetic interactions of cimetidine. *Clin Pharmacokinet* 1987;12:321–366.
24. Keranen T, Jolkkonen J, Klosterskov Jensen P, et al. Oxcarbazepine does not interact with cimetidine in healthy volunteers. *Acta Neurol Scand* 1992;85:239–242.
25. Periti P, Mazzei T, Mini E, Novelli A. Pharmacokinetic drug interactions of macrolides. *Clin Pharmacokinet* 1992;23: 106–131.
26. Keranen T, Jolkkonen J, Jensen PK, et al. Absence of interaction between oxcarbazepine and erythromycin. *Acta Neurol Scand* 1992;86:20–23.
27. Mogensen PH, Jorgensen L, Boas J, et al. Effects of dextropropoxyphene on the steady-state kinetics of oxcarbazepine and its metabolites. *Acta Neurol Scand* 1992;85:14–17.
28. Pisani F, Fazio A, Oteri G, et al. Effects of the antidepressant drug viloxazine on oxcarbazepine and its hydroxylated metabolites in patients with epilepsy. *Acta Neurol Scand* 1994;90: 130–132.

OXCARBAZEPINE

CLINICAL EFFICACY AND USE IN EPILEPSY

STEVEN C. SCHACHTER

The available treatments for seizures dramatically increased during the 1990s—the decade of the brain. Although the chemical structures of most new antiepileptic drugs (AEDs) are distinctly different from available therapies, others share structural similarities. Two drugs that are similar in structure may have identical actions, such as fosphenytoin and phenytoin (PHT). Alternatively, two structurally similar drugs may have different metabolic pathways, and therefore potentially different clinical profiles.

Carbamazepine (CBZ) is a first-line drug for partial seizures (1); however, its use is limited in some patients by toxicity or ineffectiveness. Oxcarbazepine (OXC), a 10-keto analog of CBZ, is primarily metabolized by reduction, whereas CBZ undergoes oxidation to the 10,11-CBZ epoxide, as discussed in Chapter 45. The epoxide probably accounts for some of the toxicity associated with CBZ (2).

This chapter reviews the efficacy and clinical status of OXC for the treatment of seizures.

EFFICACY

Monotherapy Studies

Five studies compared the efficacy of OXC as monotherapy with that of other first-line AEDs (Table 47.1). The first controlled comparative trial of OXC monotherapy enrolled 40 patients with a variety of epilepsy syndromes who had refractory seizures or unwanted side effects on PHT monotherapy (3). Patients were converted from PHT monotherapy to either OXC or CBZ and dosed to clinical effect for 48 to 50 weeks. This double-blind, parallel-group study showed equivalent efficacy for OXC (600 to 900 mg/day) and CBZ (400 to 800 mg/day). Similarly, Dam et al. dosed OXC and CBZ to clinical effect in a parallel-

Steven C. Schachter, MD: Associate Professor, Department of Neurology, Harvard Medical School; and Director of Clinical Trials, Beth Israel Deaconess Medical Center, Boston, Massachusetts

group, double-blind study of 235 patients with newly diagnosed partial-onset or primary generalized seizures and found equivalent efficacy over 48 weeks of treatment (4).

Three other multicenter, randomized, double-blind, parallel-group, monotherapy trials of OXC in patients with newly diagnosed or previously untreated partial-onset or primary generalized seizures have been performed (Table 47.2). One study compared OXC with valproate (VPA) (5) and the other two compared OXC with PHT—one in adults (6) and one in children and adolescents (7). Each of these studies had a retrospective baseline period; patients had to have at least two seizures separated by more than 48 hours in the preceding 6 months to qualify. Randomization was 1:1. Blinded treatment was administered three times daily and titrated over 8 weeks based on clinical response.

In the OXC versus VPA study, randomized patients were titrated to between 900 and 2,400 mg daily for both AEDs. In the other two studies, OXC and PHT dosages were 450 to 2,400 mg daily and 150 to 800 mg daily, respectively.

In the OXC versus VPA study, 249 patients aged 15 to 65 years were randomized. The groups were well matched with respect to age, sex, seizure type, and duration of epilepsy. Nearly 62% of the patients had partial seizures as their predominant seizure type; the others had generalized seizures without focal onset. Although this was a study of newly diagnosed patients, the mean duration of epilepsy was approximately 180 weeks.

In the adult OXC versus PHT study, 287 patients aged 15 to 91 years were randomized. The treatment groups were well matched. Most patients (63%) had partial seizures as their main seizure type (59% of OXC- and 68% of PHT-treated patients); the rest had generalized seizures without partial onset. The mean duration of epilepsy was 95 and 89 weeks for the OXC- and PHT-treated patients, respectively. Patients were previously untreated for their seizures.

In the pediatric OXC versus PHT study, 193 patients aged 5 to 17 years were randomized. The treatment groups were well matched. Most patients (78%) had partial seizures as their main seizure type; the rest had generalized seizures with-

TABLE 47.1. LARGE CONTROLLED CLINICAL TRIALS OF OXCARBAZEPINE

Study Design	Number of Trials (Reference)
Monotherapy: comparative in newly treated patients	4 (4–7)
Monotherapy: comparative in chronically treated patients	1 (3)
Monotherapy: low-dose vs. high-dose	2 (11, 12)
Monotherapy: placebo controlled	1 (23)
Add-on: adult	1 (16)
Add-on: pediatric	1 (17)
Total	10

out partial onset. The mean duration of epilepsy was 30 and 38 weeks for the OXC- and PHT-treated patients, respectively. Patients were previously untreated for their seizures.

In each of these studies, the primary efficacy variable was the proportion of seizure-free patients who had at least one seizure assessment during the maintenance period (Table 47.3). Efficacy was evaluated during a 48-week maintenance period.

In the OXC versus VPA study, 212 patients (85% of those randomized) were included in the efficacy analysis. Slightly more than half of the patients in each treatment group remained seizure free during the maintenance period; there was no statistically significant treatment difference. Similarly, there was no treatment difference in the percentage of patients with partial-onset seizures who were seizure free (46% and 48% for OXC and VPA, respectively) or the proportion of patients with primary generalized seizures who were seizure free (72% and 62%, respectively). A greater proportion of VPA-treated patients with secondarily generalized seizures as their main seizure type were seizure free compared with OXC-treated patients, although the number of patients in each treatment arm was low. Six patients in each treatment group discontinued treatment prematurely because of lack of efficacy.

TABLE 47.2. MONOTHERAPY DOUBLE-BLIND COMPARATIVE TRIALS IN NEWLY TREATED PATIENTS.

Comparator	n[a]	Age (Yr)	Seizure Types	Duration (Wk)
Phenytoin[b]	193	5–18	Partial/GTC	56
Phenytoin[c]	287	16–65	Partial/GTC	56
Valproate[d]	249	15–65	Partial/GTC	56
Carbamazepine[e]	235	14–63	Partial/GTC	56

GTC, generalized tonic-clonic seizures; partial, partial-onset seizures.
[a]Total number in both treatment groups.
[b]Guerreiro et al. (7).
[c]Bill et al. (6).
[d]Christie et al. (5).
[e]Dam et al. (4).

TABLE 47.3. MONOTHERAPY DOUBLE-BLIND COMPARATIVE TRIALS IN NEWLY TREATED PATIENTS: SEIZURE-FREE RATES FOR THE 48-WEEK TREATMENT PERIOD

Reference	Proportion Seizure Free (%)
Phenytoin[a]	60
Oxcarbazepine	61
Phenytoin[b]	58
Oxcarbazepine	59
Valproate[c]	54
Oxcarbazepine	57
Carbamazepine[d]	60
Oxcarbazepine	52

[a]Guerreiro, et al. (7).
[b]Bill, et al. (6).
[c]Christie, et al. (5).
[d]Dam, et al. (4).

In the adult OXC versus PHT study, 237 patients (83% of those randomized) were included in the efficacy analysis. Overall, nearly 60% of patients in each treatment group were seizure free during the maintenance period; there was no statistically significant treatment difference. Similarly, there was no treatment difference in the percentage of patients with partial-onset seizures who were seizure free (56% and 53% for OXC and PHT, respectively) or the proportion of patients with primary generalized seizures who were seizure free (64% and 68%, respectively). One patient in each treatment group discontinued treatment prematurely because of lack of efficacy.

In the pediatric OXC versus PHT study, 158 patients (82% of those randomized) were included in the efficacy analysis. Nearly 60% of patients in each treatment group were seizure free during the maintenance period; there was no statistically significant treatment difference. Similarly, there was no treatment difference in the percentage of patients with partial-onset seizures who were seizure free (60% and 62% for OXC and PHT, respectively) or the proportion of patients with primary generalized seizures who were seizure free (59% and 54%, respectively). Four OXC- and three PHT-treated patients discontinued treatment prematurely because of lack of efficacy.

Although informative clinically, these comparative monotherapy studies lacked true control groups. This problem was addressed by another monotherapy trial design, the inpatient presurgical design (8). An impressive degree of seizure reduction was seen in an open-label pilot trial of OXC monotherapy in presurgical patients (9); therefore, a placebo-controlled trial of OXC monotherapy was performed (10), the first placebo-controlled trial of OXC (Figure 47.1). This multicenter, double-blind, randomized, two-arm, parallel monotherapy trial compared OXC 1,200 mg twice daily with placebo in inpatients with refractory partial seizures who had undergone complete taper-off of

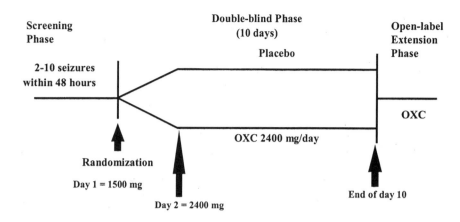

FIGURE 47.1. Oxcarbazepine (OXC) monotherapy inpatient presurgical study design. (From Schachter SC, Vazquez B, Fisher RS, et al. Oxcarbazepine: double-blind, randomized, placebo-control, monotherapy trial for partial seizures. *Neurology* 1999;52: 732–737, with permission.)

AEDs and completed a presurgical evaluation. Patients exited the trial after completing the 10-day treatment period or after experiencing four partial seizures, two new-onset secondarily generalized seizures, serial seizures, or status epilepticus, whichever came first.

One hundred two patients were randomized at 10 sites. The 56 men and 46 women were from 11 to 62 years of age and had an average of 4.6 partial seizures during a 48-hour period before randomization. Therapeutic dosages of OXC were reached with a 24-hour titration scheme. The primary efficacy variable, time to meeting one of the exit criteria, was statistically significant in favor of OXC ($p = .0001$; Figure 47.2). The secondary efficacy variables, percentage of patients who met one of the exit criteria and total partial seizure frequency from the 2nd through 10th day of double-blind treatment, also were statistically significant in favor of OXC. Thirteen of the 51 OXC-treated patients (25%) remained seizure free throughout the entire 10-day treatment period, compared with only 1 placebo-treated patient (2%).

Two outpatient, double-blind OXC monotherapy studies compared seizure frequencies in patients with medically refractory partial epilepsy (11,12). In both studies, one group of patients was randomized to OXC 2,400 mg/day and the other group was randomized to tapering dosages of OXC down to 300 mg/day. The primary efficacy outcome in both studies was time to meeting one of four exit criteria: twofold increase in partial seizure frequency in any 28-day treatment period relative to baseline; a twofold increase in the highest consecutive 2-day partial seizure frequency relative to baseline; occurrence of a single generalized seizure if none occurred in the previous 6 months; or prolongation or worsening of seizures requiring intervention. In each study, there was a significant difference in time to exit in favor of the high-dose OXC group.

Add-on Trials; Open-Label, Long-Term Trials; and Retrospective Studies

A double-blind, randomized, crossover study compared OXC with CBZ as add-on therapy in 48 institutionalized patients with refractory epilepsy (13). The mean daily doses of OXC and CBZ were 2,628 mg and 1,302 mg, respectively. Patients with tonic-clonic or clonic seizures had significantly fewer seizures when treated with OXC compared with CBZ, although no significant treatment differences were seen in frequencies of partial or myoclonic seizures. Serum concentrations of concomitant AEDs were not controlled; PHT and VPA concentrations were higher during OXC treatment compared with CBZ and could have contributed to the treatment effect. Another crossover study

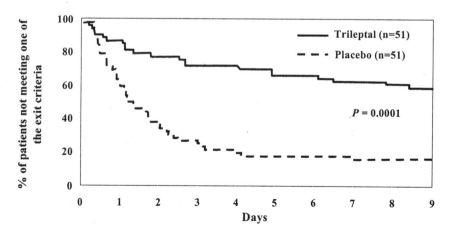

FIGURE 47.2. Oxcarbazepine (OXC) monotherapy inpatient presurgical study. Time to exit: OXC vs. placebo. Day 0 = first day of full-dose (1,200 mg/day) treatment. Schachter SC, Vazquez B, Fisher RS, et al. Oxcarbazepine: double-blind, randomized, placebo-control, monotherapy trial for partial seizures. *Neurology* 1999;52:732–737, with permission.

TABLE 47.4. ADULT ADD-ON OXCARBAZEPINE STUDY: INTENT-TO-TREAT RESPONSE

Treatment	Median Reduction in Seizure Frequency (%)	≥50% Seizure Reduction (%)	Seizure Free (%)
Placebo	8	13	0.6
Oxcarbazepine 300 mg b.i.d.	26[a]	27[b]	3
Oxcarbazepine 600 mg b.i.d.	40[a]	42[b]	10
Oxcarbazepine 1,200 mg b.i.d.	50[a]	50[b]	22

[a]$p \leq .0001$.
[b]$p < .001$.
From Barcs G, Walker EB, Elger CE, et al. Oxcarbazepine placebo-controlled, dose-ranging trial in refractory partial epilepsy. *Epilepsia* 2000;41:1597–1607, with permission.

compared OXC with CBZ as add-on therapy in 16 patients with at least one seizure per month and found 90% reduction in seizure frequency for both treatment groups (14).

Van Parys and Meinardi treated 260 patients with open-label OXC for a total of 935 patient-years of exposure (15). Among 89 patients whose treatment was changed to OXC because CBZ treatment had been ineffective, 8 (9%) became seizure free and 36 others (40%) showed substantial improvement in seizure frequency.

A double-blind, multicenter, randomized, placebo-controlled trial assessed the efficacy and safety of three different doses of adjunctive OXC (600, 1,200, and 2,400 mg/day) compared with placebo in adults with medically refractory partial seizures (16) (Table 47.4). Nearly three-fourths of the enrolled patients were taking CBZ as a concomitant AED. The primary efficacy variable was percentage change in seizure frequency per 28 days relative to baseline. The median reduction in seizure frequency was 26%, 40%, 50%, and 8% for patients receiving 600, 1,200, or 2,400 mg/day OXC or placebo, respectively (all OXC groups $p < .0001$). Further, among patients in the 600-, 1,200-, or 2,400-mg/day OXC groups, 27%, 42%, and 50%, respectively, had >50% reduction in seizure frequency compared with 13% for placebo (all $p < .001$). A separate analysis of patients who took concomitant CBZ showed percentage reductions in seizure frequency of 22%, 40%, and 50% for 600, 1,200, and 2,400 mg/day OXC, respectively. These findings suggest that the addition of OXC to maximally tolerated dosages of CBZ is as likely to result in seizure improvement as the addition of OXC to regimens not containing CBZ.

A double-blind, multicenter, randomized, placebo-controlled trial assessed the efficacy and safety of adjunctive OXC (6 to 50 mg/kg/day) versus placebo in children aged 3 to 17 years with partial seizures refractory to other AEDs (17). In approximately half the enrolled patients, CBZ was a concomitant AED. OXC-treated patients (n = 138) experienced a 35% median reduction from baseline in partial seizure frequency, compared with 9% for placebo-treated patients (n = 129; $p = .0001$). Further, 41% of patients treated with OXC had at least a 50% reduction in partial seizure frequency compared with baseline versus 22% of placebo-treated patient ($p = .0005$). Five OXC-treated patients and one patient on placebo were seizure free dur-

ing the 98-day double-blind treatment period. The efficacy of the combination of CBZ and OXC was not reported or compared with combinations of OXC with other AEDs

Two retrospective open studies evaluated the effectiveness of OXC in children (18,19). Borusiak et al. assessed the efficacy of OXC as monotherapy or add-on therapy in 46 children (mean age, 10.3 years; mean duration of epilepsy, 7.2 years) (18). The mean dose of OXC during chronic treatment was 56.7 mg/kg/day. Twelve children discontinued OXC because of insufficient seizure control. Among those children remaining on treatment for 1 year, 19 had at least 50% reduction in seizure frequency and 4 were seizure free.

In the other study, chart analysis of 53 children younger than 7 years of age with seizures refractory to one or more AEDs showed that young children needed a higher dose per body weight of OXC than adults: the mean maximum OXC dose was 50 mg/kg/day (range, 21 to 86 mg/kg/day) (19). Twelve of 44 (27%) children with localization-related epilepsy became seizure free and an additional 16 (36%) had at least 50% seizure reduction. None of the children with generalized epilepsy became seizure free.

DOSAGE AND ADMINISTRATION

OXC is available as 300- and 600-mg scored tablets and can be taken with or without food. The recommended dosage as monotherapy in adults is 600 to 1,200 mg/day in two divided doses; higher dosages may be necessary when used as polytherapy in patients with refractory seizures. Adult patients with new-onset seizures can be initiated at 150 mg/day; the dosage can be increased by 150 mg every 2 to 4 days until the target dose is reached. Higher starting doses and faster titration rates are feasible in selected patients, although dose-related neurotoxicity may limit the titration rates in some patients. Children should be initiated at 8 to 10 mg/kg/day; dosages can be increased weekly by 8 to 10 mg/kg/day to clinical effect.

In clinical practice, OXC often is substituted for CBZ. Dam suggests that the full maintenance dose of OXC (at 1.5 times the CBZ dose, somewhat less in the elderly) be started as CBZ is abruptly discontinued (20). Others have advocated a slower transition strategy by starting OXC at low dose, with graduated increments as tolerated while CBZ is slowly tapered (21). OXC dosage reductions may be necessary once enzyme-inducing AEDs are fully discontinued if signs or symptoms of neurotoxicity develop.

There is a linear relationship between daily OXC dose and serum concentrations of the active metabolite (MHD) (22). However, the correlation between MHD concentrations and likelihood of efficacy varies widely among patients; therefore, the principal uses for MHD assays are to verify compliance and establish the therapeutic MHD concentration for individual patients.

REGULATORY STATUS AND INDICATIONS

OXC was synthesized in 1963 and first marketed in Denmark, Argentina, and Mexico in 1990. OXC now is registered in over 60 countries worldwide under the brand name Trileptal (Novartis, Summit, NJ) as monotherapy and add-on treatment for partial seizures with or without secondary generalized seizures and primary generalized tonic-clonic seizures. The U.S. Food and Drug Administration cleared OXC for marketing in the United States in February 2000 for use as monotherapy or adjunctive therapy in the treatment of partial seizures (simple partial, complex partial, secondarily generalized) in adults with epilepsy and as adjunctive therapy in the treatment of partial seizures in children 4 to 16 years of age with epilepsy.

The patient exposure currently is estimated to exceed 250,000 patients and 200,000 patient-years based on drug sales and an assumed average daily dose of 1,200 mg.

CONCLUSION

Despite their structural similarities, OXC and CBZ exhibit many differences and should be considered as distinct drugs. The chemical structures, pharmacokinetics, and metabolic pathways of their active metabolites are different; and their drug–drug interactions, side effect profiles, effects on laboratory values, and titration and dosing are distinctly different. Although their overall efficacy profiles are similar, seizures in some patients respond to one drug and not the other in controlled trials and open clinical experience. Hence, patients with partial-onset seizures that are refractory to CBZ may benefit from a trial of OXC, and vice-versa.

OXC shows comparable efficacy to PHT and VPA in addition to CBZ as monotherapy for partial-onset seizures. Adjunctive OXC affords incremental seizure control that is dose dependent, even for patients whose other AEDs include CBZ or whose seizures failed to respond to CBZ in the past.

Physicians will be reassured by the extensive previous clinical experience with this compound and unusually broad portfolio of clinical studies. OXC is an important treatment option for patients with epilepsy that should be considered first-line therapy for partial-onset seizures. Because only a limited number of intravenous AEDs are available, studies of the feasibility and efficacy of an intravenous formulation of MHD are warranted.

REFERENCES

1. Mattson RH, Cramer JA, Collins JF, et al. Comparison of carbamazepine, phenobarbital, phenytoin, and primidone in partial and secondarily generalized tonic-clonic seizures. *N Engl J Med* 1985;313:145–151.
2. Theodore WH, Narang PK, Holmes MD, et al. Carbamazepine and its epoxide: relation of plasma levels to toxicity and seizure control. *Ann Neurol* 1989;15:194–196.
3. Reinikainen KJ, Keranen T, Halonen T, et al. Comparison of oxcarbazepine and carbamazepine: a double-blind study. *Epilepsy Res* 1987;1:284–289.
4. Dam M, Ekberg R, Løying Y, et al. A double-blind study comparing oxcarbazepine and carbamazepine in patients with newly diagnosed, previously untreated epilepsy. *Epilepsy Res* 1989; 3:70–76.
5. Christe W, Kramer G, Vigonius U, et al. A double-blind controlled clinical trial: oxcarbazepine versus sodium valproate in adults with newly diagnosed epilepsy. *Epilepsy Res* 1997;26:451–460.
6. Bill PA, Vigonius U, Pohlmann H, et al. A double-blind controlled clinical trial of oxcarbazepine versus phenytoin in adults with previously untreated epilepsy. *Epilepsy Res* 1997;27:195–204.
7. Guerreiro MM, Vigonius U, Pohlmann H, et al. A double-blind controlled clinical trial of oxcarbazepine versus phenytoin in children and adolescents with epilepsy. *Epilepsy Res* 1997;27:205–213.
8. Pledger GW, Krämer LD. Clinical trials of investigational antiepileptic drugs: monotherapy designs. *Epilepsia* 1991;32: 716–721.
9. Fisher RS, Eskola J, Blum D, et al. Open-label, pilot study of oxcarbazepine for inpatients under evaluation for epilepsy surgery. *Drug Dev Res* 1996;38:43–49.
10. Schachter SC, Vazquez B, Fisher RS, et al. Oxcarbazepine: double-blind, randomized, placebo-control, monotherapy trial for partial seizures. *Neurology* 1999;52:732–737.
11. Sachdeo R, Beydoun A, Schachter S, et al. Safety and efficacy of oxcarbazepine monotherapy. *Neurology* 1998;50:A200.
12. Beydoun A, Sachdeo RC, Rosenfeld WE, et al. Oxcarbazepine monotherapy for partial-onset seizures: a multicenter, double-blind, clinical trial. *Neurology* 2000;54:2245–2251.
13. Houtkooper MA, Lammertsma A, Meyer JWA, et al. Oxcarbazepine (GP 47680): a possible alternative to carbamazepine? *Epilepsia* 1987;28:693–698.
14. Bulau P, Stoll KD, Froscher W. Oxcarbazepine versus carbamazepine. *Adv Epileptol* 1987:531–536. In: Wolf P, Dam M, Jang D, eds. *Advances in Epileptology. XVth epilepsy international symposium.* New York, Raven Press, 531–536.
15. Van Parys JAP, Meinardi H. Survey of 260 epileptic patients treated with oxcarbazepine (Trileptal) on a named-patient basis. *Epilepsy Res* 1994;19:79–85.
16. Barcs G, Walker EB, Elger CE, et al. Oxcarbazepine placebo-controlled, dose-ranging trial in refractory partial epilepsy. *Epilepsia* 2000;41:1597–1607.
17. Glauser TA, Nigro M, Sachdeo R, et al. Adjunctive therapy with oxcarbazepine in children with partial seizures. *Neurology* 2000; 54:2237–2244.
18. Borusiak P, Korn-Merker E, Holert N, et al. Oxcarbazepine treat-

ment of childhood epilepsy: a survey of 46 children and adolescents. *JEpilepsy* 1998;11:355–360.

19. Gaily E, Granstrom M-L, Liukkonen E. Oxcarbazepine in the treatment of early childhood epilepsy. *J Child Neurol* 1997; 12:496–498.

20. Dam M. Practical aspects of oxcarbazepine treatment. *Epilepsia* 1994;35[Suppl 3]:523–525.

21. Schmidt D, Sachdeo R. Oxcarbazepine for treatment of partial epilepsy: a review and recommendations for clinical use. *Epilepsy Behav* 2000;1:396–405.

22. Augusteijn R, van Parys JAP. Oxcarbazepine (Trileptal, OXC): dose–concentration relationship in patients with epilepsy. *Acta Neurol Scand Suppl* 1990;133:37.

23. Schachter SC, Vazquez B, Fisher RS, et al. Oxcarbazepine: double-blind, randomized, placebo-control, monotherapy trial for partial seizures. *Neurology* 1999;52:732–737.

Antiepileptic Drugs, 5th Edition. Edited by R.H. Levy, R.H. Mattson, B.S. Meldrum, and E. Perucca. Lippincott Williams & Wilkins, Philadelphia © 2002.

OXCARBAZEPINE

CLINICAL EFFICACY AND USE IN PSYCHIATRIC DISORDERS

MICHAEL R. TRIMBLE

There is a considerable literature on the use of antiepileptic drugs for the management of psychiatric disorders; an introduction to this subject is given in Chapter 25. It was therefore to be expected with the introduction of oxcarbazepine, which has a clinical profile similar to that of carbamazepine, that it, too, would be tried in the management of disorders other than epilepsy, particularly for psychiatric syndromes.

The investigations with oxcarbazepine were carried out mainly over a decade ago, and there are few trials from which to draw any conclusions. However, this is a review of the published data, and most of the research has been conducted in patients with affective disorders.

CLINICAL TRIALS OF OXCARBAZEPINE IN AFFECTIVE DISORDERS

The studies reviewed here are all summarized in Table 48.1.

Acute Mania

The first study was that of Emrich et al. (1). The effects of sodium valproate were compared with the effects of oxcarbazepine, and all patients were said to have a maniform psychosis. The design was double-blind, placebo-controlled trial with an A-B-A design. The evaluations were carried out using the In-patient Multi-dimensional Psychiatric Scale (IMPS), and all patients had clinical evaluations. The doses of oxcarbazepine were 1,800 to 2,100 mg/day, and at the end of an unspecified treatment period, a 49.9% improvement in the IMPS score was recorded.

Based on the relative success of this pilot investigation, Emrich presented data on a more extended multicenter trial of 42 patients with acute mania, oxcarbazepine (n = 19)

Michael R. Trimble, MD: Professor of Behavioral Neurology, Department of Neurology, Institute of Neurology, London, United Kingdom

being compared with haloperidol (2). The data from this study are shown in Figure 48.1. Although initially the improvements seemed to be more rapid with haloperidol, after 2 weeks the results with both drugs were comparable. The dose of oxcarbazepine was increased during the course of the study, the mean dose being 2.4 g/day. The equivalent dose of haloperidol was 15 mg. Ten percent of patients taking oxcarbazepine experienced unwanted effects, in comparison with 35% of those taking haloperidol. The Physicians' Global Rating Scale over the treatment course was good to excellent for carbamazepine in 94% of those studied in comparison with 83% taking haloperidol. It was moderate to poor in five patients receiving haloperidol and only one patient taking oxcarbazepine.

In a further study, 28 patients receiving oxcarbazepine were compared with 24 receiving lithium over a similar time course. After 2 weeks, there was no difference in the response rate. In this study, a lower dose of oxcarbazepine was reached (1.4 g/day), the mean dose of lithium being 1.1 g. When comparing adverse effects, 28% of patients receiving oxcarbazepine and 18.5% of patients taking lithium reported such effects; however, the tolerability according to the Physician's Global Evaluation was the same for both drugs. An excellent or good response to oxcarbazepine was reported in 93% of cases, compared with 92% in patients taking lithium. There were 3.4% poor responders with oxcarbazepine and 8.3% with lithium. From these data, the authors concluded that oxcarbazepine was as effective as lithium in the management of acute mania and had some advantage with regard to tolerability.

Mueller et al. (3) pointed out that the tolerability of oxcarbazepine was good, and it was better in comparison with carbamazepine in patients with epilepsy or trigeminal neuralgia. These investigators performed a trial in patients with acute mania. This was an open study of 48 patients treated for 10 to 86 days. The doses varied between 600 and 1,800 mg/day, and 83% of patients were said to have had a very good response.

TABLE 48.1. STUDIES OF OXCARBAZEPINE IN AFFECTIVE DISORDERS

	Number of Patients	Diagnosis	Design	Dose	Duration	Results
Emrich, 1984	7 Oxc 5 placebo	Mania	A-B-A	1,800–2,100	Variable	80% Oxc improved
Mueller and Stoll, 1984	10	Mania	vs. haloperidol	900–1,200	2 wk	Oxc = haloperidol
Emrich, 1990	19	Mania	vs. haloperidol	600–2,400	2 wk	Oxc = haloperidol Oxc < side effects
Emrich, 1990	28	Mania	vs. lithium	1,400	2 wk	Oxc = lithium Oxc < side effects
Mueller et al., 1985	48	Mania	Open	600–800	10–86 d	83% good response
Greil et al., 1985	9	Prophylaxis	Open	600–1,200	2–11 mo	Oxc well tolerated
Cabrera et al., 1986	8	Prophylaxis	vs. lithium	≤1,350	22 wk	Oxc = lithium
Wildegrube et al., 1990	8	Prophylaxis	vs. lithium	2,400	33 wk	Lithium < Oxc

Oxc, oxcarbazepine.

These investigators then carried out a double-blind study of oxcarbazepine (900 to 1,200 mg/day), comparing it with haloperidol (15 to 20 mg/day), with 10 patients in each group. The change in mood was rated using the Bech-Rafaelson Mania Scale. The results were equivalent, with a slightly faster onset of action in the oxcarbazepine-treated group. The authors considered carbamazepine and oxcarbazepine to be effective for the treatment of acute mania, but they considered that oxcarbazepine would be better tolerated. They specified the antimanic action of oxcarbazepine as not one of sedation, but rather suggested a more direct action on psychopathologic symptoms.

Prophylaxis of Bipolar Disorders

There are even fewer studies of oxcarbazepine in the longer-term management of bipolar disorders than the acute studies or the data on carbamazepine. An early study was carried out by Greil et al. (4). These investigators conducted an open pilot study on nine patients and commented on the good tolerability of oxcarbazepine in doses up to 1,200 mg/day, but they were unable to say anything about the clinical effectiveness of the drug.

Wildgrube (5) incorporated 18 patients with a diagnosis of bipolar affective disorders, unipolar mania, or schizoaffective psychoses into a study randomly allocating them to lithium or oxcarbazepine; another five patients were treated with oxcarbazepine after unsatisfactory treatment with lithium. During the course of the trial, the dose of oxcarbazepine was increased to a maximum of 2,400 mg/day. The patients were rated using the Bech-Rafaelson Rating Scale, and the maximum period of observation in this study was 2 years and 9 months.

From the initial group, the results of eight patients taking oxcarbazepine and of seven taking lithium were compared. The lithium-treated patients were younger (mean age, 31 years) than the oxcarbazepine-treated patients (mean age, 44 years). Further, the oxcarbazepine-treated patients had a longer history of bipolar disorder than did the patients who were taking lithium. As noted, some of the oxcarbazepine-treated patients were lithium nonresponders.

The study proved disappointing, in that six of nine oxcarbazepine-treated patients and three of nine lithium-treated patients dropped out of the study. The conclusion, noting the number of manic and depressive relapses in patients, was that oxcarbazepine was less effective than

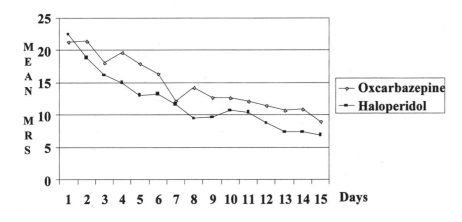

FIGURE 48.1. Oxcarbazepine in acute mania. Mean mania rating scale values during 15 days of therapy using oxcarbazepine or haloperidol in 19 manic patients in each group. (Rating according to Bech P, Bolung TG, Kramp P, et al. The Bech-Rafaelson mania scale and the Hamilton depression scale. *Acta Psychiatric Scandanavica* 1979;59: 420–430.) [From Emrich HM. Studies with oxcarbazepine in acute mania. *Int Clin Psychopharmacol* 1990;5(Suppl 1):83–88, with permission.]

lithium, although the problem with patient recruitment and dropout was obvious, and few reliable conclusions could be drawn.

Cabrera et al. (6) compared the prophylactic effects of oxcarbazepine and lithium; two small groups were tested. One was randomized, and the other was nonrandomized. Essentially fewer episodes of affective disorder were seen after the initiation of oxcarbazepine, when compared with before. In comparison with lithium, fewer adverse reactions occurred.

OXCARBAZEPINE IN OTHER PSYCHIATRIC DISORDERS

The only other population examined with oxcarbazepine comprised patients with aggressive disorders, but the results of these trials have not been published in full. Vartiainen et al. (7) studied 16 chronically psychotic patients who had been receiving carbamazepine for aggressive behavior. This was a 16-week open study, and the patients were given carbamazepine for 8 weeks, followed by the oxcarbazepine substitution. The clinical state was measured using the Global Aggression Scale. These investigators reported that the antiaggressive effects of the oxcarbazepine and carbamazepine were equivalent, but they noted that oxcarbazepine had fewer side effects. Concomitant haloperidol, which was also being prescribed, led to an increase in serum levels of oxcarbazepine in two patients.

CONCLUSION

The data on the effects of oxcarbazepine on psychopathology are limited. There are no studies in patients with epilepsy in which mood has been monitored, and the few studies in psychiatric patients are mostly in acute mania. However, it is known form the studies on epilepsy (Chapter 47), that oxcarbazepine is well tolerated, better so than carbamazepine, and it seems likely that this favorable profile would have benefit for patients with psychopathology, irrespective of whether they have epilepsy.

In the studies reviewed here, >80% of the patients given oxcarbazepine for affective disorders were reported to have a favorable response, and this finding compares well with lithium comparisons (~55% to 80%). Further studies are needed to clarify the role of oxcarbazepine for prophylaxis of bipolar disorder and to establish its utility for some other conditions in which carbamazepine has been shown to be of value, such as schizoaffective disorder and a variety of aggressive syndromes.

REFERENCES

1. Emrich HM, Dose M, Von Zerssen D. Action of sodium valproate and oxcarbazepine in patients with affective disorders. In: Emrich HM, Okuma T, Muller A, eds. *Anticonvulsants in affective disorders.* Amsterdam: Elsevier, 1984:45–55.
2. Emrich HM. Studies with oxcarbazepine in acute mania. *Int Clin Psychopharmacol* 1990;5[Suppl 1]:83–88.
3. Mueller AA, Klaus D, Wendt S. Oxcarbazepine in acute mania. In: Pichot P, ed. *The state of the art,* vol 3: *Pharmacopsychiatry.* London: Plenum Press, 1985:495–500.
4. Greil W, Krueger R, Rossnagl G, et al. Prophylactic treatment of affective disorders with carbamazepine and oxcarbamazepine: an open clinical trial. In: Pichot P, Berner P, Wolf R, et al., eds. *Psychiatry: the state of the art.* New York: Plenum Press, 1985:491–494.
5. Wildgrube C. Case studies on prophylactic long-term effects of oxcarbazepine in recurrent affective disorders. *Int Clin Psychopharmacol* 1990;5[Suppl 1]:89–94.
6. Cabrera JF, Muehlbauer HD, Schley J, et al. Long term randomised clinical trial of oxcarbazepine versus lithium in bipolar disorder and schizoaffective disorders: preliminary results. *Pharmacopsychiatry* 1986;19:282–283.
7. Vartiainen, H, Tiihoneen J, Hakola P. Carbamazepine and oxcarbazepine in the treatment of aggressive behaviour. *Psychopharmacology (Berl)* 1994;114:13(abst).
8. Bech P, Bolung TG, Kramp P, et al. the Bech-Rafaelson mania scale and the Hamilton depression scale. *Acta Psychiatric Scandanavica* 1979;59:420–430.

OXCARBAZEPINE

ADVERSE EFFECTS

GÜNTER KRÄMER

Whereas up to now all new antiepileptic drugs have failed to demonstrate superior efficacy in comparison with the established drugs, the risk:benefit ratio of at least some compounds has advantages. For oxcarbazepine (OXC), a ketoderivative of carbamazepine (CBZ), it is of special clinical interest that there is no major hepatic enzyme induction and no active epoxide metabolite, to which at least some of the adverse effects of CBZ have been attributed (1). Although OXC has a tolerability profile similar to that of CBZ, it is associated with a lower incidence of serious adverse effects such as severe allergic reactions (2,3). After >450,000 patient-years up to 2001 (4) and >20 years of experience with OXC (5,6), the spectrum of adverse effects is well known, and the risk of emerging new severe or potentially life-threatening adverse effects is likely to be low (7,8).

MOST COMMONLY OBSERVED ADVERSE EFFECTS

The data are presented for adults and children and for monotherapy or add-on-therapy. Hyponatremia is discussed separately.

Adults with Monotherapy

The most commonly observed adverse effects (>10% of patients) associated with OXC monotherapy in adults are somnolence or sedation, headache, dizziness, nausea, vomiting, fatigue, abnormal vision, and diplopia. In general, OXC was well tolerated in five clinical monotherapy trials in comparison with phenytoin (PHT), valproate (VPA), or placebo (9–13) (Table 49.1). Although ≤90% of the patients who received at least one dose of OXC reported adverse experiences, <10% withdrew from treatment because of these effects. Reasons for premature discontinuation included rash (9–13), postictal psychosis (9,13),

ataxia (9), suicide attempt with OXC (10), or headache and dizziness (11,12). However, in one trial, all dropouts occurred during the tapering phase in which concomitant antiepileptic drugs were discontinued and before OXC monotherapy was reached (9).

The time to premature discontinuation of treatment because of adverse experiences was significantly in favor of OXC compared with PHT (p = .02) in one study (10), but there was no significant difference compared with VPA (11). Overall, OXC was better tolerated than PHT (particularly with respect to gum hyperplasia, tremor, diplopia, and nystagmus), and VPA (particularly with respect to tremor, weight gain, alopecia, and headache).

In a retrospective analysis of 947 outpatients with epilepsy, as few as 33% of OXC treated patients reported adverse effects, with 18% discontinuing treatment prematurely (14). Most patients (93%) were aged ≥15 years and received OXC at an average dosage of 18 mg/kg/day as monotherapy (n = 597) for a mean duration of 23 months. Among the patients who received OXC as monotherapy, rash (7%), fatigue (5%), dizziness (4%), and sedation (4%) were the most common side effects. Half of the patients who experienced rash had previously had allergic reactions to CBZ (see the later discussion of skin rashes in this chapter). Central nervous system–related adverse effects associated with OXC monotherapy were usually moderate and less frequent than those in patients receiving adjunctive therapy, yet they were more often rated as severe (in 26% versus 15% of patients). The rate of discontinuation of treatment because of adverse effects was similar in both groups (14).

Two controlled double-blind comparisons of OXC with CBZ with equipotent dosages (OXC:CBZ = 1.5:1) in patients with epilepsy indicated a similar incidence of adverse reactions for both drugs (15,16). However, in the largest randomized comparison to date, OXC was associated with significantly fewer severe adverse effects, defined as events requiring drug withdrawal (14% for OXC versus 26% for CBZ). Rash was the most severe adverse effect in 16 of 25 patients withdrawn from CBZ and in nine of 13 patients withdrawn from OXC (17).

Günter Krämer, MD: Medical Director, Swiss Epilepsy Center, Zurich, Switzerland

TABLE 49.1. PERCENTAGES OF PATIENTS WHO EXPERIENCED ADVERSE EVENTS IN RANDOMIZED MONOTHERAPY PARALLEL-GROUP TRIALS COMPARING OXCARBAZEPINE WITH PHENYTOIN, VALPROATE, AND PLACEBO

	Reference									
	Beydoun et al. (9)		Bill et al. (10)		Christe et al. (11)		Sachdeo et al. (12)		Schachter et al. (13)	
Adverse Events	OXC (2,400 mg/d[a], n = 41)	OXC (300 mg/day[a], n = 46)	OXC[b] (n = 136)	PHT[b] (n = 142)	OXC[c] (n = 128)	VPA[c] (n = 121)	OXC[d] (n = 32)	PL (n = 35)	OXC[e] (n = 51)	PL[e] (n = 51)
Somnolence	29.3	4.3	30.1	28.9	14.8	19.8	6.3	11.4	16	0
Headache	22.0	8.7	14.7	19.0	10.2	17.4	15.6	11.4	20	20
Dizziness	46.3	8.7	13.2	15.5	10.2	11.6	25.0	2.9	18	12
Nausea	29.3	8.7	9.6	11.3	8.6	11.6	12.5	17.1	20	6
Vomiting	22.0	4.3							10	4
Fatigue	39.0	8.7			12.5	15.7	21.9	14.3	10	2
Rash	12.2	4.3	8.8	11.3					18[f]	8[f]
Gum hyperplasia			1.5	12.7						
Tremor			2.9	7.0	3.9	15.7				
Diplopia	19.5	0	0.7	7.7					12	0
Apathy					11.5	10.6				
Weight gain					12.5	21.5				
Alopecia					8.6	17.4				
Abnormal vision	17.1	2.2								

OXC, oxcarbazepine; PHT, phenytoin; PL, placebo; VPA, valproate.
Only events occurring in at least 10% of patients in at least one arm of the trial are reported.
[a]OXC 2,400 or 300 mg/day in adults with refractory partial or generalized seizures (short-term trial).
[b]OXC 600 to 2,100 mg/day or PHT 100 to 650 mg/day in previously untreated adults with partial seizures.
[c]OXC 450 to 2,400 mg/day or PHT 150 to 800 mg/day in previously untreated adults with partial seizures.
[d]OXC 1,200 mg/day or PL in untreated patients with recent onset epilepsy (short-term trial).
[e]OXC 2,400 mg/day or PL in patients with refractory partial and/or generalized seizures (short-term trial).
[f]These patients experienced pruritus.

Adults with Add-on Therapy

The most commonly reported adverse effects in adults with OXC add-on therapy are dizziness, somnolence, sedation, headache, fatigue, nausea, vomiting, ataxia, nystagmus, and abnormal gait.

OXC was well tolerated in two retrospective studies involving the long-term use of OXC adjunctive therapy (14,18). In 757 predominantly adult patients (age range, 7 to 91 years) with severe focal (66%) and/or generalized seizures, as few as 100 adverse effects were reported, which were severe in 0.9% of patients, and only 10 patients (1.3%) discontinued treatment because of them. Most patients were treated for 2 to 6 years, with dosages between 150 and 3,600 mg/day (18). Along with dizziness, headache, nausea, and vomiting, hyponatremia was also a common adverse effect (see later).

In a long-term monitoring study, 164 patients who had previously been treated with CBZ were switched to OXC therapy (monotherapy and adjunctive therapy were not differentiated) because of adverse effects and/or intolerability during CBZ therapy (19). Eighteen percent became free of adverse effects, and in 60% of the patients, symptoms became tolerable. The adverse effects most likely to resolve on switching to OXC were undetermined skin reactions (rashes, pruritus, eczema), allergic reactions, and a combination of malaise, dizziness, and headache.

In a large randomized, four-arm, double-blind, placebo-controlled parallel trial with three different OXC doses in 694 patients (15 to 65 years of age) with at least four seizures per month (20), the most common adverse effects were related to the central nervous system (dizziness, headache, somnolence, ataxia, nystagmus, abnormal gait) and the digestive system (nausea, vomiting, abdominal pain). The highest adjunctive dosage of OXC (2,400 mg/day) was associated with a very high proportion of patients (>65%) discontinuing treatment, mainly because of central nervous system–related adverse events. However, treatment was well tolerated in patients receiving OXC 1,200 mg/day (20).

A Cochrane review calculated the overall odds ratio and corresponding confidence interval (CI) for treatment withdrawal in the two largest add-on trials representing 961 randomized patients—694 adults (20) as well as 267 children (21); see later for details—as 2.17 (95% CI, 1.59, 2.97). The significantly associated figures for individual adverse effects were 4.32 for diplopia (99% CI, 2.65, 7.04), 3.05 for dizziness (99% CI, 1.99, 4.67), 2.93 for ataxia (99% CI, 1.72, 4.99), 2.88 for nausea (99% CI 1.77, 4.69), 2.55 for somnolence (99% CI, 1.84, 3.55), and 1.80 for fatigue (99% CI, 1.02, 3.19) (22).

In the context of polytherapy, OXC has a lower enzyme-inducing activity compared with CBZ, PHT, or barbiturates. When one of the latter drugs is substituted with OXC, cessation of enzyme induction may lead to increased serum levels of certain comedications, with possible signs of intoxication. For example, in a study in patients receiving haloperidol, chlorpromazine, or clozapine, replacement of

CBZ with OXC resulted within 2 to 4 weeks in a 28% to 200% increase in the plasma concentrations of these antipsychotic agents (all of which are known to be lowered by CBZ) and in the appearance of extrapyramidal symptoms (23).

Children with Monotherapy

In three of the five randomized, controlled trials that have studied effectiveness and tolerability in pediatric patients, OXC was initiated as monotherapy (12,13,24), the patients of another trial were converted to monotherapy with OXC (9), and the remaining trial was an add-on study in refractory patients (21). However, only two studies were restricted to pediatric patients (21,24), whereas the others involved adult patients as well. Common adverse effects in previously untreated children receiving OXC monotherapy are similar to those in adults: somnolence, headache, dizziness, nausea, apathy, and rash.

In a multicenter, randomized, double-blind, parallel-group trial comparing OXC with PHT in 193 children and adolescents with newly diagnosed epilepsy with at least two seizures in the last 6 months, the primary tolerability variable was a comparison of the time to premature discontinuation because of adverse effects (24). This was significantly longer for OXC (p = .002). OXC was better tolerated than PHT, particularly with respect to nervousness, dizziness, gum hyperplasia, hypertrichosis, and ataxia. In total, 82.3% of patients reported adverse experiences while receiving OXC compared with 89.4% of the PHT-treated group. Of these patients, two receiving OXC discontinued treatment because of rash, and 14 PHT recipients were withdrawn from treatment because of hypertrichosis, gingival hypertrophy, or rash. The physician's and patient's overall assessments of tolerability were significantly better in the OXC-treated group (p = .001 for physicians and p = .038 for patients).

Children with Add-on Therapy

The most common adverse events experienced by children (aged 1.2 to 17.9 years) undergoing add-on therapy with OXC were somnolence, headache, dizziness, vomiting, nausea, diplopia, fever, and ataxia (21,25). In a multinational, multicenter, placebo-controlled, double-blind, parallel-group trial evaluation of the efficacy and tolerability of OXC as adjunctive therapy (30 to 46 mg/kg/day) to stable doses of up to two standard antiepileptic drugs, 267 children and adolescents (between 3 and 17 years of age) with inadequately controlled partial seizures were randomized (21). Ninety-one percent of patients receiving OXC and 82% of those receiving placebo reported adverse events. Fourteen patients (10%) receiving OXC discontinued treatment prematurely (mainly because of nausea, vomiting, and rash) compared with 3% of the patients receiving placebo. Rash occurred in 4% of the OXC group and in 5% of the

placebo group, and two of the four patients who discontinued OXC treatment because of maculopapular and erythematous rash received CBZ as concomitant medication (21).

Hyponatremia

Hyponatremia is usually defined as a serum sodium level <135 mmol/L and is a well-known adverse effect of CBZ and OXC (16). In clinical studies, the incidence of this effect varies between 5% and 40% for CBZ (26) and between 23% (14) and 73.3% (27) for OXC. In most patients, hyponatremia is asymptomatic, and discontinuation of OXC is only rarely necessary. Clinical symptoms of acute hyponatremia usually occur with sodium levels <125 mmol/L and may include headache, nausea, vomiting, tremor, delirium, increased seizure frequency, and coma (28). The symptoms of chronic hyponatremia are more subtle and include anorexia, cramps, personality changes, gait disturbance, stupor, nausea, and vomiting, but the condition may be accompanied by increased seizures and psychosis as well (29).

In a large retrospective series of OXC therapy (14), a shift to abnormal (not further defined) serum sodium levels was observed in 23% of the 350 patients (from a total population of 947) with available laboratory test data. However, only four patients (0.4% of the total population) discontinued treatment because of hyponatremia.

The manufacturer's prescribing information states that hyponatremia with a serum sodium <125 mmol/L developed in 2.5% of OXC-treated patients in the 14 controlled monotherapy and adjunctive therapy studies conducted to date, compared with no patients who received placebo or active controls (CBZ, phenobarbital, PHT, or VPA). Most hyponatremic patients were asymptomatic, but patients in clinical trials were frequently monitored, and some had their OXC dosage reduced or discontinued. The manufacturer's database included records of 1,966 patients with epilepsy aged between 2 and 88 years who had been treated for 20 months with OXC 600 to 1,800 mg/day (4). Serum sodium levels were <135 mmol/L in 423 patients (21.5%) and <125 mmol/L in 54 patients (2.7%). Generally, patients with hyponatremia recovered once OXC therapy was stopped. The incidence of symptoms suggestive of hyponatremia was similar among all patients, irrespective of sodium levels (4).

In a study of 15 patients with epilepsy refractory to multidrug therapy in which OXC was substituted for CBZ, mean plasma sodium levels decreased from 137.5 to 128.5 mmol/L. Imposed restriction of fluid intake may have minimized the degree of hyponatremia in these patients (27). In another study, serum sodium levels decreased significantly in six of 10 male patients changed from CBZ to OXC (30). Although it had been proposed that both drugs cause an increase in plasma arginine vasopressin secretion or have a direct tubular effect in the kidney, this study suggested that

OXC-induced hyponatremia is not caused by changes in serum aldosterone or atrial natriuretic peptide.

The degree of hyponatremia seems to be related to the dose and to the serum concentration of the active monohydroxy derivative (MHD) of OXC, with an increased incidence at OXC doses >25 to 30 mg/kg per day (27,31,32). Increasing age has also been identified as a risk factor for OXC-induced hyponatremia. In an analysis of the manufacturer's database (33), marked hyponatremia (sodium levels <125 mmol/L) increased with age from 0% at <6 years and 0.5% between 6 and 17 years to 3.4% between 18 and 64 years and 7.3% at >65 years. In a study of 144 randomly selected patients with epilepsy (3), female patients were found to have lower serum sodium levels than male patients (monotherapy: 134 versus 137.6 mmol/L, $p < .05$; adjunctive therapy 131.3 versus 137.9 mmol/L, $p < .001$). Other authors described an increased incidence of hyponatremia in patients receiving polytherapy (34) or in patients taking sodium-lowering drugs such as diuretics (35). Because in monotherapy trials the incidence of hyponatremia was highest in a 10-day study with a 2-day titration period (13), fast titration may be another risk factor (3).

Appropriate management of symptomatic OXC-induced hyponatremia includes restriction of fluids and dose reduction or discontinuation. In case of discontinuation, switch to CBZ or PHT is preferable. Rapid correction of hyponatremia with hypertonic saline is rarely if ever required and is associated with risks greater than those of hyponatremia itself (7). There is no evidence of the effectiveness of additional intake of sodium chloride in the prevention or amelioration of hyponatremia. Some clinicians routinely monitor serum sodium in patients on OXC and regard values of <130 mmol/L as unacceptable (36).

Skin Rashes

The incidence of allergic rashes for OXC is lower than for CBZ (15,37). In the prospective Scandinavian multicenter study, rashes led to early discontinuation in 10% of patients given OXC and in 16% of those given CBZ, despite low starting doses of both drugs (OXC, 300 mg; CBZ, 200 mg) and a slow titration rate (17). Cross-allergies in patients with known rashes from CBZ are in the range of 25% to 31% (19,38,39), and this does not exclude the possibility of three consecutive patients' experiencing a cross-reaction (12). Most rashes occurs in the first month of treatment. Some authors have recommended patch tests or lymphocyte proliferation assays before starting OXC in patients with known CBZ-induced skin problems (19,32). Finally, successful desensitization has been described in a patient with a rash caused by OXC (41).

Effects on Cognition

The cognitive side effects of OXC have been little investigated up to now. In a study in patients undergoing initiation of antiepileptic drug treatment, no cognitive function changes were detected 4 months after starting OXC monotherapy compared with baseline (12). In another study in patients receiving long-term OXC monotherapy, cognitive side effects were similar to those seen in patients taking PHT (43).

In a double-blind, three-phase, crossover study, 12 healthy volunteers received OXC 150 mg twice daily, OXC

TABLE 49.2. PERCENTAGES OF PATIENTS WHO EXPERIENCED ADVERSE EVENTS IN A RANDOMIZED, PLACEBO-CONTROLLED, PARALLEL-GROUP TRIAL COMPARING DIFFERENT DOSAGES OF OXCARBAZEPINE GIVEN AS ADJUNCTIVE THERAPY IN ADULTS WITH REFRACTORY PARTIAL EPILEPSY

Adverse Event	OXC (600 mg/day, n = 168)	OXC (1,200 mg/day, n = 177)	OXC (2,400 mg/day, n = 174)	PL (n = 173)
Reporting an adverse event	83.9	90.4	97.7	76.3
Dizziness	25.0	31.6	42.5	12.7
Headache	32.1	27.1	23.0	23.7
Somnolence	19.6	27.1	32.2	11.6
Ataxia	9.5	17.5	32.2	5.2
Nystagmus	6.5	20.3	23.6	4.0
Abnormal gait	5.4	9.6	14.9	1.2
Tremor	3.6	7.9	14.4	4.0
Vomiting	13.1	24.9	33.3	4.6
Nausea	14.9	24.3	28.2	8.1
Abdominal pain	9.5	12.4	8.0	4.6
Diplopia	13.7	30.5	39.1	4.6
Abnormal vision	6.5	13.6	17.2	4.0
Vertigo	6.5	11.3	13.8	2.3
Fatigue	14.9	11.9	14.9	6.9
Viral infection	11.9	9.6	5.7	13.9

OXC, oxcarbazepine; PL, placebo.
Only events occurring in at least 10% of patients in at least one arm of the trial are reported (20).

300 mg twice daily, or placebo for 1 week each. In this study, OXC was associated with a slight stimulant effect, documented by improved performance on a focused attention task, increased manual writing, and enhanced alertness and clearheadedness (44). By contrast, in patients with epilepsy, increased sedation and decreasing test results were observed 2 to 6 hours after intake of OXC (45). However, as already stated, other studies did not find significant changes after 4 months of OXC monotherapy (42) or after 6 to 12 months monotherapy in comparison with PHT (43).

Dose Dependency

For some adverse effects of OXC, a dose dependency has been described. In the large add-on trial in adults comparing 600 mg, 1,200 mg, and 2,400 mg/day OXC (20), most of the adverse effects were dose related; these included dizziness, diplopia, somnolence, vomiting, nausea, ataxia, nystagmus, abnormal vision, vertigo, and abnormal gait (Table 49.2). In a survey of children and adolescents treated with OXC, it was stated that adverse effects appeared in most patients at blood levels of MHD ~35 to 40 mg/L (25). As discussed earlier, the incidence of hyponatremia is also related to OXC dose and serum drug levels (27,31,32).

Time Dependency

With the exception of the well-known prevalence of allergic rashes during the initiation of treatment, there are no other data on a time dependency of adverse effects of OXC.

LESS COMMON BUT CLINICALLY RELEVANT ADVERSE EFFECTS

Less common adverse effects of OXC include, in alphabetic order, abdominal pain, acne, agitation, alopecia, apathy, diarrhea, gum hyperplasia, laboratory abnormalities, nervousness, oculogyric crises, respiratory distress, tremor, and weight gain.

With the exception of hyponatremia, OXC-induced laboratory abnormalities are rare and are less common in comparison to CBZ (4,46). Single cases of pancytopenia and thrombopenia have been observed (47). As far as liver function tests are concerned, a trend toward slightly elevated values has been described by some investigators (14,16,48). In an open long-term study comparing OXC with CBZ and VPA in young girls with epilepsy, OXC as well as the other drugs did not affect linear growth or pubertal development, and OXC was not associated with weight gain. However, although fasting serum insulin and insulinlike growth factor binding protein 1 or 3 were not influenced by OXC (14.2 to 33.2 mg/kg/day), the levels of plasma insulinlike growth factor I (IGF-I) were increased, and this was attributed to increased hepatic synthesis of IGF-I. The

clinical significance of this observation remains to be established (49). OXC induces the metabolism of steroid hormones such as ethinylestradiol and levonorgestrel (50).

After a switch from CBZ to OXC, a normalization of several laboratory values can be observed. This can be the case for some sex hormones such as dehydroepiandrosterone sulfate and sex hormone-binding globulin (SHBG) (51), serum thyroxine, free thyroxine and thyrotropin (52,53), total cholesterol (54), serum γ-glutamyltransferase activity, erythrocyte folate, serum vitamin B_{12} levels, white blood cell count, and mean corpuscular volume of erythrocytes (55). OXC has been reported to increase the serum concentrations of testosterone, gonadotropins, and SHBG in men with epilepsy (56).

Oculogyric crises can be a particularly unusual side effect of both CBZ and OXC. A 31-year-old man developed oculogyric crises after starting treatment with OXC, and the frequency of these episodes correlated with the dosage of the drug (57). Similar episodes had occurred in the past after exposure to CBZ. The patient was implanted a vagus nerve stimulator, whose use led to disappearance of the oculogyric crises.

A computerized analysis of saccadic and smooth-pursuit eye movements in a double-blind crossover study after single doses of 600 mg OXC or 400 mg CBZ in six healthy male volunteers demonstrated that OXC had weaker effects on the maximum saccade peak velocity and the typical target velocity (58).

POTENTIALLY LIFE-THREATENING ADVERSE EFFECTS

According to the manufacturer's database, serious adverse effects were observed in 326 of 2,486 (13.1%) OXC-treated patients with epilepsy, resulting in a total of 411 events. Disorders of gait, balance and coordination, hyponatremia, seizures, and rash were the adverse events most frequently considered to be related to OXC (4).

MANIFESTATIONS AND MANAGEMENT OF OVERDOSE

A total of six patients (all suicide attempts) took overdoses of OXC during the clinical trials, the maximum estimated dose taken being 24 g (4). Symptoms of overdose include somnolence, dizziness, nausea, vomiting, hyperkinesia, hyponatremia, ataxia, and nystagmus. All patients recovered with symptomatic and supportive treatment. There is no specific antidote. Removal of the drug by gastric lavage and/or inactivation by administering activated charcoal should be considered.

Because of only minor removal of the major OXC metabolite MHD during a series of six plasmaphereses in a

13-year-old boy taking 2,550 mg OXC/day (mean amount of MHD removed per plasmapheresis of less than 80 mg, or 3% to 4% of the daily dose), plasmapheresis was considered to be unlikely to be of therapeutic benefit in the treatment of OXC overdose (59).

PREGNANCY

The clinical experience with OXC in pregnant women is minimal up to now, and therefore the teratogenic potential of this drug in humans is virtually unknown. Up to 2001, 47 pregnancies have been documented in the manufacturer's database. There were 25 pregnancies reported in the primary database, two in named patient programs and 20 in postmarketing experience after exposure to OXC *in utero*. Of these 47 pregnancies, delivery of 20 healthy babies was documented. There were 13 abortions, five infants with malformations (three lip-facial-palatal clefts, a facial dysmorphia, and a case with unspecific cardiac abnormalities), and the outcome *was* unknown for the remaining seven (4).

USE IN SPECIAL POPULATIONS

Limited experience with OXC in treatment of early childhood epilepsy did not result in any special adverse effects. Hyponatremia (<132 mmol/L) was observed in 15% in a series of 53 children <7 years old; all but two patients were asymptomatic and needed no dose adjustments. Based on their observations, the authors of this study suggested that the risk of symptomatic hyponatremia may increase when children contract an infection or have prolonged seizures (60).

In a retrospective analysis of 40 children and adolescents with intellectual disability, most of whom were receiving polytherapy, OXC was associated with adverse effects in 16 (40%) patients, which led to dose reduction or discontinuation in eight (20%). Hyponatremia (defined as at least one level <132 mmol/L) was observed in 24% (61).

A 28-year-old patient with porphyria cutanea tarda who could not tolerate CBZ (resulting in elevation of transaminases as well as pruritus and erythema) was successfully treated with OXC (62). Because OXC retains some enzyme inducing activity, however, great caution should be used in prescribing this drug in patients with porphyrias.

Because the incidence of symptomatic OXC-induced hyponatremia is increased in elderly patients (especially women), in patients comedicated with diuretics, desmopressin, or nonsteroidal antiinflammatory agents, and in patients with renal disease, OXC is not a drug of first choice for these populations. If it is used, serum sodium concentrations should be monitored, at least in those patients at special risk or with symptoms likely related to hyponatremia (e.g., somnolence, nausea, vomiting, headache, confusion) (63).

CONCLUSION

Mainly because of its improved tolerability OXC, is a good candidate to replace CBZ as a drug of first choice in the treatment of focal seizures with or without secondary generalization. Direct comparisons of OXC and CBZ in patients with newly diagnosed epilepsy indicate that the two compounds are equally effective, but OXC may be associated with fewer adverse effects. Allergic skin reactions are less common with OXC, and the reduced propensity of OXC to induce oxidative metabolism may facilitate the attainment of therapeutic serum concentrations of comedications vulnerable to enzyme induction such as VPA. A systematic review and meta-analysis comparing the results of add-on trials of OXC and the other new antiepileptic drugs levetiracetam, remacemide, and zonisamide in drug-resistant localization-related epilepsy in children and adults ranked OXC as second after levetiracetam in terms of favorable responder and withdrawal rates (64). The only disadvantage of OXC in comparison with CBZ regarding adverse effects is the more pronounced hyponatremia. In addition, physicians in those European and other countries where a new formulation has recently been introduced have to be aware of the risk of increased adverse effects resulting from faster absorption and higher serum drug concentrations (65).

REFERENCES

1. Patsalos PN, Sander JWAS. Newer antiepileptic drugs: towards an improved risk-benefit ratio. *Drug Saf* 1994;11:37–67.
2. Grant SM, Faulds D. Oxcarbazepine: a review of its pharmacology and therapeutic potential in epilepsy, trigeminal neuralgia and affective disorders. *Drugs* 1992;43:873–888.
3. Wellington K, Goa KL. Oxcarbazepine: an update of its efficacy in the management of epilepsy. *CNS Drugs* 2001;15:137–163.
4. Novartis Pharmaceuticals. Data on file. Basel, 2001.
5. Rai PV. Clinical trial for the estimation of anticonvulsive properties and side reactions of a new drug: ketocarbamazepine. In: Wada JA, Penry JK, eds. *Advances in epileptology: the Xth Epilepsy International Symposium*. New York: Raven Press, 1980:357 (abst).
6. Krämer G. Oxcarbazepin: ein neues Antiepileptikum zur Mono- und Kombinationstherapie. *Aktuelle Neurol* 2000;27.
7. Schmidt D, Sachdeo R. Oxcarbazepine for treatment of partial epilepsy: a review and recommendations for clinical use. *Epilepsy Behav* 2000;1:306–405.
8. Schmidt D, Arroyo S, Baulac M, et al. Recommendations on the clinical use of oxcarbazepine in the treatment of epilepsy: a consensus view. *Acta Neurol Scand* 2001;104:167–170.
9. Beydoun A, Sachdeo RC, Rosenfeld WE, et al. Oxcarbazepine monotherapy for partial-onset seizures: a multicenter, double-blind, clinical trial. *Neurology* 2000;54:2245–2251.
10. Bill PA, Vigonius U, Pohlmann H, et al. A double-blind controlled clinical trial of oxcarbazepine versus phenytoin in adults with previously untreated epilepsy. *Epilepsy Res* 1997;27: 195–204.
11. Christe W, Krämer G, Vigonius U, et al. A double-blind controlled clinical trial: oxcarbazepine versus sodium valproate in

adults with newly diagnosed epilepsy. *Epilepsy Res* 1997;26:451–460.

12. Sachdeo RC, Edwards K, Hasegawa H, et al. Safety and efficacy of oxcarbazepine 1200 mg/day in patients with recent onset partial epilepsy. *Neurology* 1999;52[Suppl 2]:A391(abst).

13. Schachter SC, Vazquez B, Fisher RS, et al. Oxcarbazepine: a double blind, randomized, placebo-control, monotherapy trial in patients with epilepsy after presurgical evaluation of refractory partial seizures. *Neurology* 1999;52:732–737.

14. Friis, ML, Kristensen O, Boas J, et al. Therapeutic experiences with 947 epileptic out-patients in oxcarbazepine treatment. *Acta Neurol Scand* 1993;87:224–227.

15. Houtkooper MA, Lammertsma, A, Meyer JWA, et al. Oxcarbazepine (GP 47.680): a possible alternative to carbamazepine? *Epilepsia*1987;25:693–698.

16. Reinikainen KJ, Keränen T, Halonen T, et al.. Comparison of oxcarbazepine and carbamazepine: a double blind study. *Epilepsy Res* 1987;1:284–289.

17. Dam M, Ekberg R, Løyning Y, et al. A double-blind study comparing oxcarbazepine and carbamazepine in patients with newly diagnosed, previously untreated epilepsy. *Epilepsy Res* 1989;3:70–76.

18. Suter P, Nungässer A. Long-term data of patients treated with oxcarbazepine in Switzerland on a named-patient basis. *Epilepsia* 1996;37[Suppl 4]:88–89(abst).

19. van Parys JAP, Meinardi H. Survey of 260 patients treated with oxcarbazepine (Trileptal) on a named-patient basis. *Epilepsy Res* 1994;19:79–85.

20. Barcs G, Walker EB, Elger CE, et al. Oxcarbazepine placebo-controlled dose-ranging trial in refractory partial epilepsy. *Epilepsia* 2000;41:1597–1607.

21. Glauser TA, Nigro M, Sachdeo R, et al. Adjunctive therapy with oxcarbazepine in children with partial seizures. *Neurology* 2000;54:2237–2244.

22. Castillo S, Schmidt DB, White S. Oxcarbazepine add-on for drug resistant partial epilepsy (Cochrane Review). In: *Cochrane Library* 1:2001. Oxford, updated software. Abstract available from the internet: *www.update-software.com/abstracts/ab002028.htm*

23. Raitasuo V, Lehtovaara R, Huttunen MO. Effect of switching from carbamazepine to oxcarbazepine on the plasma levels of neuroleptics. *Psychopharmacology* 1994;116:115–116..

24. Guerreiro MM, Vigonius U, Pohlmann H, et al. A double-blind controlled clinical trial of oxcarbazepine versus phenytoin in children and adolescents with epilepsy. *Epilepsy Res* 1997;27:205–213.

25. Borusiak P, Korn-Merker E, Holert N, et al. Oxcarbazepine in treatment of childhood epilepsy: a survey of 46 children and adolescents. *J Epilepsy* 1998;11:355–360.

26. van Amelsvoort T, Bakshi R, Devaux CB, et al. Hyponatremia associated with carbamazepine and oxcarbazepine therapy: a review. *Epilepsia* 1994;35:181–188.

27. Pendlebury SC, Moses DK, Eadie MJ. Hyponatraemia during oxcarbazepine therapy. *Hum Toxicol* 1998;8:337–344.

28. Steinhoff BJ, Stoll K-D, Stodieck SRG, et al. Hyponatremic coma under oxcarbazepine therapy. *Epilepsy Res* 1992;11:67–70.

29. Johannessen AC, Nielsen OA. Hyponatremia induced by oxcarbazepine. *Epilepsy Res* 1987;1:155–156.

30. Isojärvi JIT, Huuskonen UEJ, Pakarinen AJ, et al. The regulation of serum sodium after replacing carbamazepine by oxcarbazepine. *Epilepsia* 2001;42:741–745.

31. Nielsen OA, Johannessen AC, Bardrum B. Oxcarbazepine-induced hyponatremia, a cross-sectional study. *Epilepsy Res* 1988;2:269–271.

32. Zakrzewska JM, Ivanyi L. *In vitro* lymphocytic proliferation by carbamazepine, carbamazepine-10,11-epoxide, and oxcarbaze-

pine in the diagnosis of drug-induced hypersensitivity. *J Allergy Clin Immunol* 1988;82:110–115.

33. Sachdeo RC, Wassertein AD, D'Souza J. Oxcarbazepine (Trileptal) effect on serum sodium. *Epilepsia* 1999;40[Suppl 7]:103.

34. Huuskonen UEJ, Pakarinen AJ, Moilanen E, et al. The role of gender and drug metabolites in carbamazepine- or oxcarbazepine-related hyponatremia. *Epilepsia* 1998;39[Suppl 6]:126 (abst).

35. Huuskonen UEJ, Isojärvi JIT. Antiepileptic drugs and serum sodium. *Epilepsia* 1997;38[Suppl 8]:89–90(abst).

36. Dasheiff R. Letter to the editor. *Seizure* 2000;9:372.

37. Dam M, Østergaard LH. Oxcarbazepine (other antiepileptic drugs). In: Levy RH, Matson RH, Meldrum BS, eds. *Antiepileptic drugs,* 4th ed. New York: Raven Press, 1995:987–995.

38. Dam M, Jakobsen K (Danish Oxcarbazepine Study Group). Oxcarbazepine in patients hypersensitive to carbamazepine. *Acta Neurol Scand* 1984;70:223(abst).

39. Jensen NO, Danish Oxcarbazepine Study Group: Oxcarbazepine in patients hypersensitive to carbamazepine. In: *Book of abstracts: 16th Epilepsy International Congress.* Hamburg, 1985(abst).

40. Beran RG. Cross-reactive skin eruption with both carbamazepine and oxcarbazepine. *Epilepsia* 1993;34:163–165.

41. Watts D, Bird J. Oxcarbazepine sensitivity treated by desensitivation [Letter]. *J Neurol Neurosurg Psychiatry* 1991;54:376.

42. Sabers A, Møller A, Dam M, et al. Cognitive function and anticonvulsant therapy: effect of monotherapy in epilepsy. *Acta Neurol Scand* 1995;92:19–27.

43. Aikia M, Kälviäinen R, Sivenius J, et al. Cognitive effects of oxcarbazepine and phenytoin monotherapy in newly diagnosed epilepsy: one year follow-up. *Epilepsy Res* 1992;11:199–203.

44. Curran HV, Java R. Memory and psychomotor effects of oxcarbazepine in healthy human volunteers. *Eur J Clin Pharmacol* 1993;44:529–533.

45. Gillham RA, McKee PJW, Brodie MJ. Oxcarbazepine and cognitive function after a single dose and during a double-blind placebo-controlled cross-over study. *Epilepsia* 1993;34[Suppl 2]:122(abst).

46. Klosterskov Jensen P. Oxcarbazepine (Trileptal) in anti-epileptic polytherapy. *Behav Neurol* 1990;3[Suppl 1]:35–39.

47. Ciba Geigy. *Trileptal. Oxcarbazepine: a first line antiepileptic (product information).* Basel: Ciba–Geigy, 1994.

48. Bülau P, Stoll KD, Fröscher W. Oxcarbazepine versus carbamazepine. In: Wolf P, Dam M, Janz D, et al., eds. *Advances in epileptology. XVIth Epilepsy International Symposium.* New York: Raven Press, 1987:531–536.

49. Rättyä J, Vainionpää L, Knip M, et al. The effects of valproate, carbamazepine, and oxcarbazepine on growth and sexual maturation in girls with epilepsy. *Pediatrics* 1999;103:588–593.

50. Fattore C, Cipolla G, Gatti G, et al. Induction of ethinylestradiol and levonorgestrel metabolism by oxcarabazepine in healthy women. *Epilepsia* 1999;40:783–787.

51. Isojärvi JIT, Pakarinen AJ, Rautio A, et al. Serum sex hormone levels after replacing carbamazepine with oxcarbazepine. *Eur J Clin Pharmacol* 1995;47:461–464.

52. Isojärvi JIT, Airaksinen KEH, Mustonen JN, et al. Thyroid and myocardial function after replacement of carbamazepine by oxcarbazepine. *Epilepsia* 1995;36:810–816.

53. Payne TA, Kothary S, Varma NK, et al. Serum sodium and thyroid function after replacement of carbamazepine with oxcarbazepine. *Epilepsia* 1997;38[Suppl 8]:94(abst).

54. Isojärvi JIT, Pakarinen AJ, Rautio A, et al. Liver enzyme induction and serum lipid levels after replacement of carbamazepine with oxcarbazepine. *Epilepsia* 1994;35:1217–1220.

55. Isojärvi JIT, Pakarinen AJ, Myllylä VV. Basic haematological parameters, serum gamma-glutamyl-transferase activity, and erythrocyte folate and serum vitamin B$_{12}$ levels during carbamazepine and oxcarbazepine therapy. *Seizure* 1997;6:207–211.

56. Rättyä J, Turkka J, Pakarinen AJ, et al. Reproductive effects of valproate, carbamazepine, and oxcarbazepine in men with epilepsy. *Neurology* 2001;56:31–36.

57. Gatzonis SD, Georgaculias N, Singounas E, et al. Elimination of oxcarbazepine-induced oculogyric crisis following vagus nerve stimulation. *Neurology* 1999;52:1918–1919.

58. Zaccara G, Gangemi PF, Messori A, et al. Effects of oxcarbazepine and carbamazepine on the central nervous system: computerised analysis of saccadic and smooth-pursuit eye movements. *Acta Neurol Scand* 1992;85:425–429.

59. Christensen J, Balslev T, Villadsen J, et al. Removal of 10-hydroxycarbazepine by plasmapheresis. *Ther Drug Monit* 2001;23:374–379.

60. Gaily E, Granström M-L, Liukkonen E. Oxcarbazepine in the treatment of early childhood epilepsy. *J Child Neurol* 1997;12:496–498.

61. Gaily E, Granström M-L, Liukkonen E. Oxcarbazepine in the treatment of epilepsy in children and adolescents with intellectual disability. *J Intellect Disabil Res* 1998;42[Suppl 1]:41–45.

62. Gaida-Hommernick B, Rieck K, Runge U. Oxcarabzepine in focal epilepsy and hepatic porphyria: a case report. *Epilepsia* 2001;42:793–795.

63. Arroyo S, Krämer G. Treating epilepsy in the elderly: safety considerations. *Drug Saf* 2001;18.

64. Marson AG, Hutton JL, Leach JP, et al. Levetiracetam, oxcarbazepine, remacemide and zonisamide for drug resistant localization-related epilepsy: a systematic review. *Epilepsy Res* 2001;46:259–270.

65. Edelbroek PM, Augustijn PB, de Haan GJ, et al. Change in oxcarbazepine (Trileptal) formulation is associated with more side effects and higher blood concentrations. *J Neurol Neurosurg Psychiatry* 2001;71:708–709.

Antiepileptic Drugs, 5th Edition. Edited by R.H. Levy, R.H. Mattson, B.S. Meldrum, and E. Perucca. Lippincott Williams & Wilkins, Philadelphia © 2002.

PHENOBARBITAL AND OTHER BARBITURATES

PHENOBARBITAL AND OTHER BARBITURATES

MECHANISMS OF ACTION

RICHARD W. OLSEN

The mechanism of action of phenobarbital has proved difficult to pinpoint. This is primarily because of the low potency of the drug and its myriad effects at concentrations and doses not much higher than those needed for the desired action, in this case, antiepileptic efficacy. Like many other central nervous system (CNS) depressants, phenobarbital has anxiolytic, anticonvulsant, sedative-hypnotic, and anesthetic effects, depending on dose. A continuum of depression is produced, with coma at the high end of the concentration–effect curve. Fatal overdose results from respiratory depression (1–3). Many of these CNS depressants, including barbiturates, are able to enhance γ-aminobutyric acid (GABA)–mediated inhibitory synaptic transmission at relevant doses (1,4,5). Some categories of CNS depressants have reasonably potent effects on a variety of excitable tissues, and barbiturates, in particular, have many effects at concentrations near or at those relevant for seizure suppression. The barbiturates have been reported to inhibit action potentials, neurotransmitter release, voltage-regulated calcium channels, and glutamate-mediated excitatory synaptic transmission and to enhance GABA-mediated inhibitory synaptic transmission (3). At high concentrations, barbiturates inhibit many sorts of membrane ion channels and transporter functions and reduce cellular metabolism at the level of mitochondria or membrane ion gradients (6).

A unifying mechanism of action must be consistent with the anatomic and physiologic effects of the drug at the clinically relevant concentration, and it must be quantitatively consistent with the action of the drug and structural analogs at every cellular and molecular assay possible to test (7). A unifying mechanism must also explain phenobarbital's selective utility in long-term epilepsy therapy over that of drugs with a similar pharmacologic profile, including other barbiturates. The GABA$_A$ receptor (GABAR) theory for the

CNS depressant actions of phenobarbital and related compounds' anticonvulsant action was one possibility considered in earlier reviews (8–10). The GABAR target for barbiturate action, including anticonvulsant effects, has been the dominant theory since about that time (4,11), and it has been accepted by several textbook authorities (2,12). Figure 50.1 describes a schematic GABAR target for phenobarbital (5). Although the author of a chapter on this topic in the first edition of *Psychopharmacology: A Generation of Progress,* supported the selective action of barbiturates on synaptic transmission, especially inhibitory (13), the authors of this topic in the previous edition of this book (3), although favoring the GABAR theory, were not thoroughly convinced. They did conclude that "many of the actions already mentioned might suppress seizures if exerted selectively in a part of the nervous system especially important for seizure elaboration." In a review on the mechanism of action of anticonvulsants, the GABAR enhancement hypothesis for phenobarbital action was given only equal consideration with blockade of voltage-regulated sodium channels and blockade of glutamate-mediated excitatory synapses (14). Although there is actually a paucity of new data on the topic, the existing data have solidified on this point, and the GABAR theory is even more generally accepted. However, the discovery of a family of genes for virtually every protein in the body including ion channels has left open the possibility that some subtype of ion channel may fit the phenobarbital action site, whereas its general category of channel previously had been discarded on the evidence.

The mechanism of action of a drug is generally determined by comparing a series of compounds of related structure for relative potency *in vivo* for the desired effect versus relative potency *in vitro* for a candidate mechanism. This is called *structure-activity relationships.* All compounds must correlate in activity unless there is some explanation for exceptions. Usually, stereoisomers and closely related chemical structures with differing pharmacologic effects are use-

Richard W. Olsen, PhD: Professor, Department of Molecular and Medical Pharmacology, University of California, Los Angeles School of Medicine, Los Angeles, California

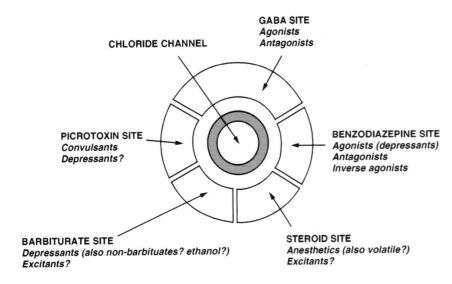

FIGURE 50.1. Schematic donut model of GABAR protein, indicating multiple functional domains including barbiturate binding site, GABA binding site, chloride channel, and sites for other modulatory drugs. No subunit structure (composition, stoichiometry, or wheel arrangement) for the protein is implied. (From Macdonald RL, Olsen RW. GABA$_A$ receptor channels. *Annu Rev Neurosci* 1994;17:569–602, with permission.)

ful in distinguishing mechanisms. In addition to the barbiturates, CNS depressants with a similar pharmacologic action include the neuroactive steroids (alphaxalone, an anesthetic), pyrazolopyridines (etazolate, an anxiolytic), chlormethiazole (an anticonvulsant), etomidate (anesthetic), loreclezole (anxiolytic), and the pyrazinones (15–20). A problem with this approach is the lack of exact correlation between efficacy of these drugs as hypnotics (for which there is much literature) and as anticonvulsants (much less literature), and for long-term therapy in clinical epilepsy (very little literature).

PHENOBARBITAL AND SEIZURES

Phenobarbital (Figure 50.2) is an effective anticonvulsant against many kinds of seizure and certain clinical epilepsy subsyndromes (Chapters 53 and 54). Phenobarbital shows anticonvulsant activity against tonic-clonic and focal seizures (2,3,21–24). Phenobarbital is ineffective against absence or atonic seizures or infantile spasms, or it may even worsen them. Primidone (Figure 50.2) is approved for treatment of grand mal and focal epilepsy. Its action is identical to that of phenobarbital, and its principal metabolite is phenobarbital. The action of the parent compound primi-

done is questionable (25). Other barbiturates approved for use in epilepsy in the United States are mephobarbital and metharbital, considered to be essentially equivalent to phenobarbital. Earlier comparisons of the chemical structure of barbiturates and other antiepileptic medications such as phenytoin and ethosuximide suggested that the common heterocyclic ring structure (2) would be consistent with a unified mechanism of action. This concept has been abandoned with the realization that the three sorts of compounds—barbiturates, hydantoins, and ethosuximide—affect different sorts of seizures with different mechanisms of action. A discussion of barbiturate use in neurology should also note the *Wada test,* in which intracarotid injection of amobarbital is used to determine the lateralization of cerebral speech dominance, especially in patients with focal epilepsy who are under consideration for temporal lobectomy (26).

NEUROPROTECTION, STATUS EPILEPTICUS, AND PROTECTIVE COMA

CNS depressants are able to reduce excitotoxic cell damage associated with ischemic events including stroke, heart attack, and status epilepticus. These include the GABA-

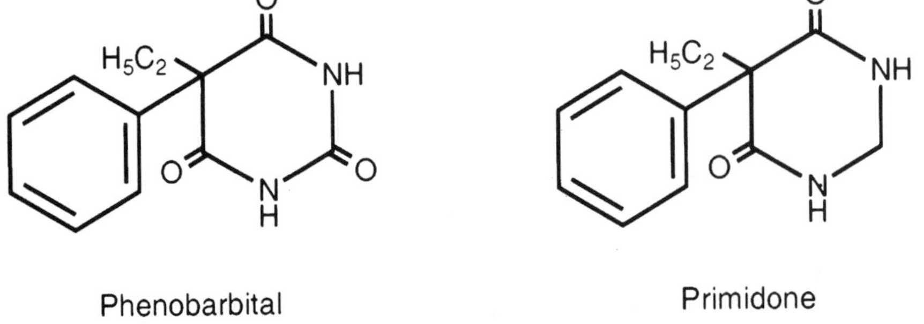

Phenobarbital

Primidone

FIGURE 50.2. Chemical structures of phenobarbital and primidone.

enhancing types of drugs. Barbiturates are therefore prototypic neuroprotective agents (2). Generalized convulsive status epilepticus is treated as an emergency with intravenous benzodiazepine, or phenytoin, or phenobarbital. If these fail, general anesthesia with pentobarbital, with intubation and ventilatory support, may be used (27). The success of barbiturate coma for treatment of status epilepticus typifies the utility of these agents in dangerous clinical situations (28).

PHYSIOLOGIC EFFECTS OF PHENOBARBITAL

Phenobarbital and related compounds have effects on excitable membranes of neurons and muscle, on ion channels, on neurotransmitter release, and on postsynaptic potentials (29). Blockade of neuronal firing, especially repetitive firing, is produced by high doses of barbiturates (30–32); most sodium and potassium channels are weakly inhibited, although the TASK-1 channel is sensitive to anesthetics (33). In general, synaptic transmission is more sensitive than action potential inhibition (34). Inhibition of neurotransmitter release (35,36) is probably the result of

blockade of several types of voltage-gated calcium channels (37–40). Some of these calcium channels remain candidates for the mechanism of action of phenobarbital. At the postsynaptic level, barbiturates have been observed to inhibit excitatory glutamate receptor channels (41,42). The best correlation for barbiturate action has been found for enhancement of GABA-mediated inhibitory synaptic transmission, in particular at the level of the GABAR (4,13,43–48). Figure 50.3 shows an example (49) of enhancement of GABAR single channel currents by diazepam and phenobarbital.

BIOCHEMICAL INTERACTIONS OF BARBITURATES WITH GABAR AND COMPARISON WITH PHYSIOLOGY

The same CNS depressant barbiturates and nonbarbiturates with similar pharmacology, such as pyrazolopyridines, etomidate, chlomethoxide, and neuroactive steroids, that enhanced GABAR at the cellular level were able to enhance GABAR function using the neurochemical assay of GABA-activated ^{36}chloride flux in brain slices, cultured neurons, or brain

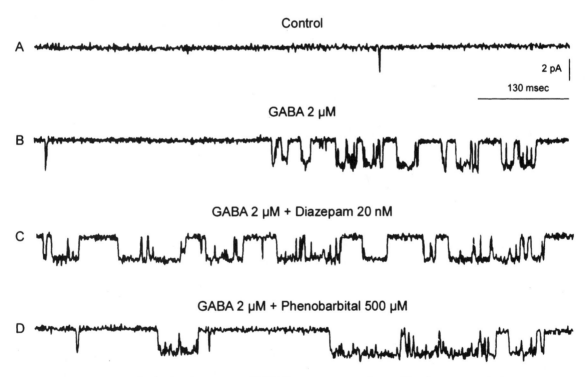

FIGURE 50.3. Single GABA$_A$ receptor (GABAR) currents are enhanced by diazepam and phenobarbital. "Outside-out" patch clamp recordings from mouse spinal cord primary cultured neurons. Membranes were voltage clamped at –75 mV, and the chloride equilibrium potential was 0 mV. **A:** Spontaneous currents in the absence of GABA. **B:** GABA-evoked bursts of firing. **C:** GABA-evoked opening and burst frequencies are increased by diazepam. **D:** Phenobarbital also increases GABAR currents by increasing the average open and burst duration but not the frequency of opening. (From Macdonald RL, Twyman RE. Biophysical properties and regulation of GABA$_A$ receptor channels. *Semin Neurosci* 1991;3:219–235, with permission.)

homogenates (membrane-bound vesicles called synaptoneurosomes or microsacs) (50–52). The correlation of enhancement of GABAR function in flux assays, electrophysiology experiments, and action *in vivo* as sedatives and anesthetics was very high (1,11,15,16,48,53), for a series of barbiturates and nonbarbiturates, including stereoisomers in both categories, such as etomidate isomers, and (+) and (−) pentobarbital, as well as the *N*-methylbarbiturates series (47,54).

These *in vitro* functional studies actually followed, in time, cell-free homogenate radioligand binding assays demonstrating that the active barbiturates allosterically modulated three different sites on the GABAR receptor–chloride ionophore complex. We first observed barbiturates to inhibit binding of the chloride channel blocker picrotoxinin (55), followed by discovery of enhancement of benzodiazepine binding (56,57), enhancement of GABA enhancement of benzodiazepine binding (58), and enhancement of GABA binding (59–61). Further, the barbituratelike pyrazolopyridines show a similar modulation of these binding sites (62,63), as do etomidate and some related nonbarbiturates (47,64,65). Finally, the allosteric effect of barbiturates is sensitive to efficacy: compounds that are positive modulators of GABAR function and agonist binding are also negative modulators of antagonists and inverse agonists at the GABA and benzodiazepine sites (66). These studies establish a clear mechanism of action of barbiturates as CNS depressants by virtue of enhancing GABAR-mediated inhibitory synaptic transmission (16,48). In addition, the purification of the GABAR protein reveals that the GABA, benzodiazepine, barbiturate, and other anesthetic binding sites are all on the same protein (67). Molecular cloning of GABAR proteins confirms that the allosteric binding sites are indeed carried by the GABA-binding protein–chloride ion channel complex (68).

Some barbiturates, such as cyclohexylidene ethylbarbiturate and dimethyldibutylbarbiturate (DMBB), are relatively potent convulsants. The (+) isomer of DMBB and the (+) isomer of pentobarbital are more potent as convulsants than the (−) isomers. However, this excitatory activity is not the result of inhibition of GABAR but rather of action at another, still unknown, target. Thus, both isomers of both DMBB and pentobarbital are enhancers of GABAR function and modulate binding accordingly, with the (−) isomers more potent. If one uses the racemic mixture, in the case of pentobarbital, the (−) isomer depressant effect, through GABAR enhancement, predominates over the (+) isomer convulsant activity at a non-GABAR site. For DMBB, however, the (+) isomer excitatory activity (non-GABAR) predominates over its (−) isomer GABAR enhancement. Conversely, some isomeric barbiturates, such as (+)*N*-methylphenylpropyl barbiturate (MPPB) (54), may be antagonists of those barbiturates including (−) MPPB that enhance GABA. Thus, variable efficacy at this site may be possible (18).

The actual functional domains within the GABAR protein for action of various ligands can be determined by comparing the sequence of receptor subunits differing in sensitivity to the drugs, such as barbiturates. Thus, the retinal subunit ρ is insensitive to barbiturate enhancement, whereas the usual GABAR subunits α, β, and γ are all sensitive. The use of chimeras and site-directed mutagenesis allowed identification of a single residue at the extracellular end of membrane-spanning region 3 (TM3) that is necessary for barbiturate enhancement of GABAR function: replacement of the ρ residue (W328) with that from β1 (M) endues the ρ receptor with barbiturate sensitivity (69). Similarly, replacement of the single residue G219 at the extracellular end of the membrane-spanning region 1 (TM1) with the ρ residue F leads to the loss of barbiturate sensitivity (70). A residue at the extracellular end of TM2 (β1S265) has also been shown to be essential for the action of volatile anesthetics and alcohols (71). It is not yet known whether these amino acids form actual binding pockets for the modulatory drugs or whether these residues are needed for allosteric coupling; these studies are consistent with the notion that barbiturates act directly on the GABAR protein.

PHENOBARBITAL VERSUS PENTOBARBITAL

Although the evidence of a GABAR mechanism for the sedative actions of barbiturates is substantial, it may not be so clear for the anticonvulsant actions. This is highlighted by the difference between phenobarbital and pentobarbital. Pentobarbital is about 10 times more potent than phenobarbital in enhancing GABAR and as a sedative-hypnotic agent. Pentobarbital is also a more potent anticonvulsant than phenobarbital, but not as different, relatively speaking, as the difference in sedation potency. Thus, a much more sedative dose of pentobarbital is needed for the same degree of seizure protection as afforded by a relatively unsedative dose of phenobarbital. This leads to phenobarbital's and not pentobarbital's clinical effectiveness in treatment of certain clinical seizures. This cannot be explained by differences in pharmacokinetics. Could this be explained by GABAR heterogeneity, possibly involving differential brain regional circuitry? For example, pentobarbital enhances GABAR binding in total brain homogenates as well as all brain regions in tissue section autoradiography assays, although the extent of the effect varies, because of subunit composition (72). Phenobarbital modulates binding kinetics (73) in total brain homogenates without enhancing the equilibrium affinity (74), but brain regional studies show that phenobarbital does enhance GABAR binding affinity in some regions (72). It seems feasible that these differences in the interaction of the two barbiturates with GABAR binding reflect slightly different molecular mechanisms of modulation of GABAR function (Figure 50.4). Thus, some evidence supports the receptor subtype explanation, but it is not clear whether this explanation is sufficient *in vivo*. If not, is it necessary to postulate different targets for the anticonvulsant actions of barbiturates?

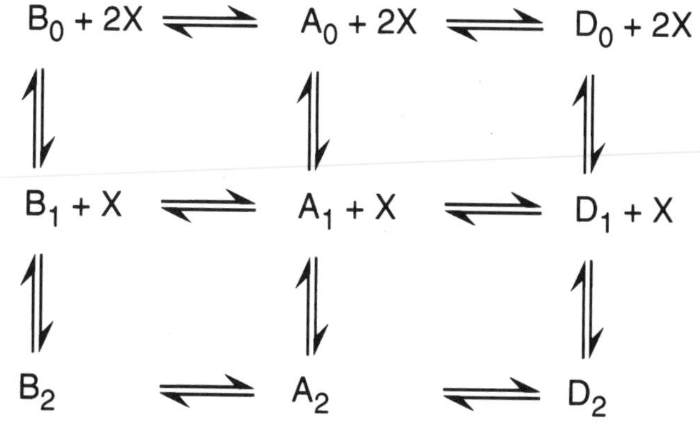

$$B_0 + 2X \rightleftharpoons A_0 + 2X \rightleftharpoons D_0 + 2X$$

$$\updownarrow \qquad\qquad \updownarrow \qquad\qquad \updownarrow$$

$$B_1 + X \rightleftharpoons A_1 + X \rightleftharpoons D_1 + X$$

$$\updownarrow \qquad\qquad \updownarrow \qquad\qquad \updownarrow$$

$$B_2 \rightleftharpoons A_2 \rightleftharpoons D_2$$

FIGURE 50.4. Allosteric three-state model of GABAR. The receptor-channel protein exists in three conformations: *B* for basal, a closed channel state highly favored in absence of agonist GABA or modulator (e.g., phenobarbital); *A* for active, the open state of the channel, highly favored by binding of X (agonist or modulatory drug such as phenobarbital); and *D*, the desensitized state, closed even when bound by X. Either an agonist such as GABA or a modulator such as phenobarbital can directly promote channel opening in the absence of the other, or the two can work cooperatively to promote channel open state. Conversely, modulators such as the benzodiazepines can only modify the kinetics of the steps (including X) but cannot by themselves promote open channel state. Additional conformational states and kinetics constants present in many models are omitted here to emphasize the major states. (From references 5, 49, 73, and 75, with permission.)

This uncertainty motivates analysts to question the GABAR hypothesis for the *anticonvulsant* action of *phenobarbital*, despite convincing evidence for the GABAR mechanism in the sedative action of barbiturates in general. I believe, however, that the GABAR mechanism is still the most likely for the anticonvulsant action of phenobarbital.

BARBITURATES VERSUS BENZODIAZEPINES

If the pharmacologic actions of barbiturates are the result of enhancement of GABAR, one may ask why their effects differ from those of the benzodiazepines, accepted GABAR-enhancing agents. The benzodiazepines do not produce general anesthesia as barbiturates do. The sedative-hypnotic efficacy of barbiturates, which among their many actions is probably the one most clearly related to GABAR, is greater than that of the benzodiazepines. Thus, the benzodiazepines are less able to induce coma and fatal overdose. Further, the anticonvulsant efficacies of the benzodiazepines and the barbiturates differ for several classes of seizures. These differences may result, at least partially, from other, non-GABAR mechanisms of action for high doses of barbiturates, such as the inhibition of mitochondrial function (6). However, feasible explanations at the GABAR level also have been proposed. Because benzodiazepines do not act on all GABAR subtypes, the more "nonspecific" actions of barbiturates to enhance all GABAR could explain their differences. Further, the molecular details of the modula-

tion of GABAR channel function by the two classes of drugs has been shown to differ: benzodiazepines apparently enhance the affinity of GABA for the receptor and thus increase the frequency of channel opening triggered by the neurotransmitter (Figures 50.3 and 50.4). Barbiturates increase the open time of the channel activated by GABA, thus affecting the kinetics of the channel opening and closing to a greater degree than the apparent GABA affinity obtained from the dose–response curve for channel opening (Figures 50.3 and 50.4) (44,49). Further, the benzodiazepines do not directly open the GABAR channels, but only enhance those activated by GABA, whereas barbiturates at high doses directly activate the channels (19). Although direct channel activation probably is not the mechanism of the anticonvulsant action, it could explain the differences between the two classes of drugs.

In Figure 50.4, the GABAR channel is described by a multiple conformational state allosteric protein model, originally developed for the related nicotinic acetylcholine receptor at the neuromuscular junction (5,49,73,75,76). This includes the following: the *Basal* state "B," unoccupied by GABA or modulatory drug; the *Active* state "A," with channel open; and the *Desensitized* state "D," with channel closed despite ligand occupancy. Each conformational state can have zero, one, or two molecules of X bound. Ligand X can be GABA or a modulator such as phenobarbital or a neurosteroid, but not a benzodiazepine. Barbiturates and benzodiazepines affect the transitions between these states at different points in the scheme. Benzodiazepines come in earlier and do not themselves directly activate channels, but they increase frequency of channel opening with apparent increase in GABA binding affinity. Barbiturates can increase open time by favoring later states of "A." They can promote channel opening with or without GABA present. Although they increase GABA binding affinity at equilibrium (59,75), this may favor a nonconducting desensitized state "D." These small differences in mode of action could result in different physiologic effects; for example, the benzodiazepines may act selectively on those GABAR synapses with heavy activity, as in a seizure, while having little effect on more GABAR with more normal slow firing activity. Barbiturates, in this theory, would indiscriminately enhance all GABARs (77). This difference could explain differences in efficacy versus different seizure subtypes for the two classes of drugs. Most evidence, then, would allow both types of drug to produce their anticonvulsant actions through GABAR mechanisms. It remains possible that some of the antiepileptic effects of phenobarbital may involve additional mechanisms, as mentioned earlier.

ACKNOWLEDGMENTS

This work is supported by National Institutes of Health grants NS28772 and NS35985. I thank Drs. M.K. Ticku and R.L. Macdonald for their helpful discussions.

REFERENCES

1. Olsen RW. Barbiturates. In: Firestone L, ed. Molecular basis of drug action in anesthesia. *Int Anesthesiol Clin* 1988;26:254–261.
2. Porter RJ, Meldrum BS. Antiepileptic drugs. In: Katzung BG, ed. *Basic and clinical pharmacology*, 5th ed. Norwalk, CT: Appleton & Lange, 1992:331–349.
3. Prichard JW, Ransom BR. Phenobarbital: mechanisms of action. In: Levy RH, Mattson RH, Meldrum BS, eds. *Antiepileptic drugs*, 4th ed. New York: Raven Press, 1995:359–369.
4. Macdonald RL, Barker JL. Different actions of anticonvulsant and anesthetic barbiturates resolved by use of cultured mammalian neurons. *Science* 1978;200:775–777.
5. Macdonald RL, Olsen RW. GABA$_A$ receptor channels. *Annu Rev Neurosci* 1994;17:569–602.
6. Seeman P. Membrane actions of anesthetics and tranquilizers. *Pharmacol Rev* 1972;24:583–656.
7. Bikker JA, Kubanek J, Weaver DF. Quantum pharmacologic studies applicable to the design of anticonvulsants: theoretical conformational analysis and structure-activity analysis of barbiturates. *Epilepsia* 1994;35:411–425.
8. Prichard JW. Barbiturates: physiological effects. I. *Adv Neurol* 1980;27:505–522.
9. Ho IK, Harris RA. Mechanism of action of barbiturates. *Annu Rev Pharmacol Toxicol* 1981;21:83–111.
10. Richter JA, Holtman JR Jr. Barbiturates: their *in vivo* effects and potential biochemical mechanisms. *Prog Neurobiol* 1982;18:275–319.
11. Olsen RW. GABA-benzodiazepine-barbiturate receptor interactions. *J Neurochem* 1981;37:1–13.
12. Goth A. *Medical pharmacology*, 11th ed. Toronto: CV Mosby, 1984:281–318.
13. Nicoll RA. Selective actions of barbiturates on synaptic transmission. In: Killam KF, ed. *Psychopharmacology: a generation of progress*. New York: Raven Press, 1978:1337–1348.
14. Deckers CLP, Czuczwar SJ, Hekster YA, et al. Selection of antiepileptic drug polytherapy based on mechanisms of action: the evidence reviewed. *Epilepsia* 2000;41:1364–1374.
15. Huidobro-Toro JP, Bleck V, Allan AM, et al. Neurochemical actions of anesthetic drugs on the γ-aminobutyric acid receptor-chloride channel complex. *J Pharmacol Exp Ther* 1987;242:963–969.
16. Olsen RW, Sapp DW, Bureau MH, et al. Allosteric actions of CNS depressants including anesthetics on subtypes of the inhibitory GABA$_A$ receptor-chloride channel complex. *Ann NY Acad Sci* 1991;625:145–154.
17. Im HK, Im WB, Judge TM, et al. Substituted pyrazinones, a new class of allosteric modulators for GABA$_A$ receptors. *Mol Pharmacol* 1993;44:468–472.
18. Maksay G, Ticku MK. Dissociation of [^{35}S]TBPS binding differentiates convulsant and depressant drugs that modulate GABAergic transmission. *J Neurochem* 1985;44:480–486.
19. Hales TG, Olsen RW. Basic pharmacology of intravenous induction agents. In: Bowdle TA, Horita A, Kharasch ED, eds. *The pharmacological basis of anesthesiology: basic science and practical applications*. New York: Churchill Livingstone, 1994:295–306.
20. Olsen RW, Gordey M. GABA$_A$ receptor chloride ion channels. In: Endo M, Kurachi Y, Mishina M, eds. *Handbook of experimental pharmacology*, vol 147: *Pharmacology of ionic channel function: activators and inhibitors*. Heidelberg: Springer-Verlag, 2000:499–517.
21. Straw RN, Mitchell CL. Effect of phenobarbital on cortical afterdischarge and overt seizure patterns in the rat. *Neuropharmacology* 1966;5:323–330.
22. Killam EK. Measurement of anticonvulsant activity in the *Papio papio* model of epilepsy. *Fed Proc* 1976;35:2265–2269.
23. Mares P, Kolinova M, Fischer J. The influence of pentobarbital upon cortical epileptogenic focus in rats. *Arch Int Pharmacodyn Ther* 1977;226:313–323.
24. Rastogi SK, Ticku MK. Involvement of GABAergic mechanism in the anticonvulsant effect of pentobarbital against maximal electroshock-induced seizures in rats. *Pharmacol Biochem Behav* 1985;22:141–146.
25. Gallagher BB, Smith DB, Mattson RH. The relationship of the anticonvulsant properties of primidone to phenobarbital. *Epilepsia* 1970;11:293–301.
26. Wada J, Rasmussen TB. Intracarotid injection of sodium amytal for the localization of cerebral speech dominance: experimental and clinical observations. *J Neurosurg* 1960;17:226–282.
27. Engel J. *Seizures and epilepsy*. Philadelphia: FA Davis, 1989.
28. Theodore WH. Barbiturates reduce human cerebral glucose metabolism. *Neurology* 1986;36:60–67.
29. Richards CD. On the mechanisms of barbiturate anaesthesia. *J Physiol (Lond)* 1972;227:749–768.
30. Blaustein MP. Barbiturates block sodium and potassium conductance increases in voltage-clamped lobster axons. *J Gen Physiol* 1968;51:293–307.
31. Carlen PL, Gurevich N, O'Beirne M. Electrophysiological evidence for increased calcium-mediated potassium conductance by low-dose sedative hypnotic drugs. In: Rubin EP, Weiss D, Putney VW, eds. *Calcium in biological systems*. New York: Plenum Press, 1985:193–200.
32. Roth SH, Tan K, MacIver B. Selective and differential effects of barbiturates on neuronal activity. In: Roth SH, Miller KW, eds. *Molecular and cellular mechanisms of anaesthetics*. New York: Plenum Press, 1986:43–56.
33. Sirois JE, Lei Q, Talley EM, et al. The TASK-1 two-pore domain K$^+$ channel is a molecular substrate for neuronal effects of inhalation anesthetics. *J Neurosci* 2000;20:6347–6354.
34. Nicoll RA, Eccles JC, Oshima T, et al. Prolongation of hippocampal inhibitory postsynaptic potentials by barbiturates. *Nature* 1975;258:625–627.
35. Killam EK. Drug action on the brain-stem reticular formation. *Pharmacol Rev* 1962;14:175–224.
36. Haycock JW, Levy WB, Cotman CW. Pentobarbital depression of stimulus-secretion coupling in brain-selective inhibition of depolarization-induced calcium-dependent release *Biochem Pharmacol* 1977;26:159–161.
37. Elrod SV, Leslie SW. Acute and chronic effects of barbiturates on depolarization-induced calcium influx into synaptosomes from rat brain regions. *J Pharmacol Exp Ther* 1979;212:131–136.
38. Blaustein MP, Ector AC. Barbiturate inhibition of calcium uptake by depolarized nerve terminals *in vitro*. *Mol Pharmacol* 1975;11:369–378.
39. Heyer EJ, Macdonald RL. Barbiturate reduction of calcium-dependent action potentials: correlation with anesthetic action. *Brain Res* 1982;236:157–171.
40. ffrench-Mullen JMH, Barker JL, Rogawski MA. Calcium current block by (−)-pentobarbital, phenobarbital, and CHEB but not (+)-pentobarbital in acutely isolated hippocampal CA1 neurons: comparison with effects on GABA-activated Cl$^-$ current. *J Neurosci* 1993;13:3211–3221.
41. Teichberg VI, Tal N, Goldberg O, et al. Barbiturates, alcohols and the CNS excitatory neurotransmission: specific effects on the kainate and quisqualate receptors. *Brain Res* 1984;291:285–292.
42. Sawada S, Yamamoto C. Blocking action of pentobarbital on receptors for excitatory amino acids in the guinea pig hippocampus. *Exp Brain Res* 1985;59:226–231.
43. Bowery NG, Dray A. Reversal of the action of amino acid antag-

onists by barbiturates and other hypnotic drugs. *Br J Pharmacol* 1978;63:197–215.

44. Macdonald RL, Barker JL. Anticonvulsant and anesthetic barbiturates: different postsynaptic actions on cultured mammalian neurons. *Neurology* 1979;29:432–447.

45. Scholfield CN. A barbiturate-induced intensification of the inhibitory potential in slices of guinea pig olfactory cortex. *J Physiol (Lond)* 1978;275:559–566.

46. Schulz DW, Macdonald RL. Barbiturate enhancement of GABA-mediated inhibition and activation of chloride ion conductance. *Brain Res* 1981;209:177–188.

47. Dunwiddie TV, Worth TS, Olsen RW. Facilitation of recurrent inhibition in rat hippocampus by barbiturate and related non-barbiturate depressant drugs. *J Pharmacol Exp Ther* 1986;238:564–575.

48. Olsen RW, Fischer JB, Dunwiddie TV. Barbiturate enhancement of GABA receptor binding and function as a mechanism of anesthesia. In: Roth S, Miller K, eds. *Molecular and cellular mechanisms of anaesthetics.* New York: Plenum Press, 1986:165–177.

49. Macdonald RL, Twyman RE. Biophysical properties and regulation of GABA$_A$ receptor channels. *Semin Neurosci* 1991;3:219–235.

50. Wong, EHF, Leeb-Lundberg LMF, Teichberg VI, et al. γ-Aminobutyric acid activation of ^{36}Cl$^-$ flux in hippocampal slices and its potentiation by barbiturates. *Brain Res* 1984;303:267–275.

51. Schwartz RD, Jackson JA, Weigert D, et al. Characterization of barbiturate-stimulated chloride efflux from rat brain synaptoneurosomes. *J Neurosci* 1985;5:2963–2970.

52. Allan AM, Harris RA. Anesthetic and convulsant barbiturates alter γ-aminobutyric acid stimulated chloride flux across brain membranes. *J Pharmacol Exp Ther* 1986;238:763–768.

53. Olsen RW. Drug interactions at the GABA receptor-ionophore complex. *Annu Rev Pharmacol Toxicol* 1982;22:245–277.

54. Knabe J, Rummel W, Buch HP, et al. Optisch aktive Barbiturate: Synthese, Konfiguration und pharmacologische Wirkung. *Arzneimittelforschung* 1978;28:1048–1056.

55. Ticku MK, Olsen RW. Interaction of barbiturates with dihydropicrotoxinin binding sites in mammalian brain. *Life Sci* 1978;22:1643–1652.

56. Leeb-Lundberg F, Snowman A, Olsen RW. Barbiturate receptors are coupled to benzodiazepine receptors. *Proc Natl Acad Sci USA* 1980;77:7468–7472.

57. Ticku MK. Interaction of depressant, convulsant, and anticonvulsant barbiturates with the [^{3}H]diazepam binding site of the benzodiazepine-GABA-receptor-ionophore complex. *Biochem Pharmacol* 1981;30:1573–1579.

58. Skolnick P, Paul SM, Barker JL. Pentobarbital potentiates GABA-enhanced [^{3}H]-diazepam binding to benzodiazepine receptors. *Eur J Pharmacol* 1980;65:125–l27.

59. Olsen RW, Snowman AM. Chloride-dependent barbiturate enhancement of GABA receptor binding. *J Neurosci* 1982;2:1812–1823.

60. Whittle SR, Turner AJ. Differential effects of sedative and anticonvulsant barbiturates on specific [^{3}H]GABA binding from rat brain cortex. *Biochem Pharmacol* 1982;31:2891–2895.

61. Willow M, Johnston GAR. Pharmacology of barbiturates: electrophysiological and neurochemical studies. *Int Rev Neurobiol* 1983;24:15–49.

62. Leeb-Lundberg F, Snowman A, Olsen RW. Perturbation of benzodiazepine receptor binding by pyrazolopyridines involves picrotoxinin-barbiturate receptor sites. *J Neurosci* 1981;1:471–477.

63. Supavilai P, Karobath M. Action of pyrazolopyridines as modulators of [^{3}H]flunitrazepam binding to the benzodiazepine receptor complex of the cerebellum. *Eur J Pharmacol* 1981;70:183–193.

64. Ashton D, Geerts R, Waterkeyn C, et al. Etomidate stereospecifically stimulates forebrain, but not cerebellar [^{3}H]diazepam binding. *Life Sci* 1981;29:2631–2636.

65. Wong DT, Rathbun RC, Bymaster FP, et al. Enhanced binding of radioligands to receptors of γ-aminobutyric acid and benzodiazepine by a new anticonvulsive agent, LY81067. *Life Sci* 1983;33:917–923.

66. Wong EHF, Snowman AM, Leeb-Lundberg LMF, et al. Barbiturates inhibit GABA antagonist and benzodiazepine inverse agonist binding. *Eur J Pharmacol* 1984;102:205–212.

67. King RG, Nielsen M, Stauber GB, et al. Convulsant/barbiturate activities on the soluble GABA/benzodiazepine receptor complex. *Eur J Biochem* 1987;169:555–562.

68. Schofield PR, Darlison MC, Fujita N, et al. Sequence and functional expression of the GABA$_A$ receptor shows a ligand-gated receptor super-family. *Nature* 1987;328:221–227.

69. Amin J. A single hydrophobic residue confers barbiturate sensitivity to γ-aminobutyric acid type C receptor. *Mol Pharmacol* 1999;55:411–423.

70. Carlson BX, Engblom AC, Kristiansen U, et al. A single glycine residue at the entrance to the first membrane-spanning domain of the γ-aminobutyric acid type A receptor β2 subunit affects allosteric sensitivity to GABA and anesthetics. *Mol Pharmacol* 2000;57:474–484.

71. Mihic SJ, Ye Q, Wick MJ, et al. Sites of alcohol and volatile anesthetic action on GABA$_A$ and glycine receptors. *Nature* 1997;389:385–389.

72. Bureau MH, Olsen RW. GABA$_A$ receptor subtypes: ligand binding heterogeneity demonstrated by photoaffinity labeling and autoradiography. *J Neurochem* 1993;61:1479–1491.

73. Edelstein SJ, Changeux JP. Allosteric transitions of the acetylcholine receptor. *Adv Protein Chem* 1998;51:121–184.

74. Leeb-Lundberg F, Olsen RW. Interaction of barbiturates of various pharmacological categories with benzodiazepine receptors. *Mol Pharmacol* 1982;21:320–328.

75. Srinivasan S, Sapp DW, Tobin AJ, et al. Biphasic modulation of GABA$_A$ receptor binding by steroids suggests functional correlates. *Neurochem Res* 1999;24:1363–1372.

76. Yang JS, Olsen RW. γ-Aminobutyric acid receptor binding in fresh mouse brain membranes at 22°C: ligand-induced changes in affinity. *Mol Pharmacol* 1987;32:266–277.

77. Haefely W, Polc P, Schaffner R, et al. Facilitation of GABAergic transmission by drugs. In: Krogsgaard-Larsen P, Scheel-Kruger J, Kofod G, eds. *GABA neurotransmitters.* Copenhagen: Munksgaard, 1979:357–375.

PHENOBARBITAL AND OTHER BARBITURATES

CHEMISTRY, BIOTRANSFORMATION, AND PHARMACOKINETICS

GAIL D. ANDERSON

CHEMISTRY AND METABOLIC SCHEME

Phenobarbital is 5-ethyl-5-phenylbarbituric acid, a substituted barbituric acid with a molecular weight of 232.23 (Figure 51.1). The free acid of phenobarbital is a white crystalline material with a melting point of 176°C. Phenobarbital is only sparingly soluble in water (1 g in 1000 mL). In addition to the low aqueous solubility, phenobarbital also has a relatively low lipid solubility. It is soluble in organic solvents such as chloroform (1 g in 40 mL), diethylether (1 g in 15 mL), and ethanol (1 g in 10 mL). The sodium salt is freely soluble in water and is used in the formulations for intravenous or intramuscular administration (1).

Phenobarbital is a weak acid with a negative log of dissociation constant (pKa) of 7.3, approximately the same as physiologic pH. Therefore, changes in the ratio of ionized to nonionized phenobarbital that occur within the normal range of physiologic pH (7.35 to 7.45) can alter both the distribution and the excretion of the drug (Table 51.1).

ABSORPTION

Bioavailability. After oral and intramuscular administration, the absorption of phenobarbital is essentially complete, with greater than 95% bioavailability (1–3). The time to peak plasma concentrations after oral administration ranges from 0.5 to 4 hours (1–5). Peak concentrations appear 2 to 8 hours after an intramuscular injection (1,3). Rectal administration of phenobarbital sodium parenteral solution resulted in a mean bioavailability of 90% and a time to peak concentration of 4.4 hours (6).

In a group of newborn infants given a single dose of phenobarbital, the time to peak concentrations ranged from 1.5 to 6 hours (7). Absorption of phenobarbital was delayed

Gail D. Anderson, PhD: Professor, Department of Pharmacy, University of Washington, Seattle, Washington

in a group of malnourished children compared with healthy children (5.6 hours versus 1.0 hour); however, the maximum concentration obtained was not different, a finding suggesting no differences in bioavailability (8).

Administration of activated charcoal can be used to decrease the equilibrium of phenobarbital across the gastrointestinal tract in cases of overdose. Several studies have demonstrated an increase in total body clearance and reduction of the elimination half-life (t½) of phenobarbital by a factor of two- to 10-fold with the administration of charcoal (9–13).

Formulations and Routes of Administration. Phenobarbital is available in tablets, capsules, extentabs, elixir, and a parenteral formulation for oral, rectal, intramuscular, and intravenous routes of administration.

DISTRIBUTION

After intravenous administration, phenobarbital distributes into the body in two phases, which can be characterized by a two-compartmental mathematical model (1,2,14). Studies in animals have demonstrated that the early distribution includes liver, kidney, and heart. During the late phase, phenobarbital distributes to brain, muscle, and intestine. The average volume of distribution of phenobarbital ranges from 0.54 to 0.73 L/kg in adults (1,15,16). Newborns and young infants have a larger average volume of distribution, ranging from 0.8 to 1 L/kg (17–23). This corresponds to a relatively larger extracellular fluid volume in neonates (24). In older infants and children, the average volume of distribution is similar to that in adults, ranging from 0.57 to 0.70 L/kg (7,25,26). Because of the low lipid solubility, phenobarbital does not distribute into fat, and loading doses of phenobarbital are usually calculated using ideal body weight or lean body mass (27). However, a case report suggested that using ideal body weight to calculate the load-

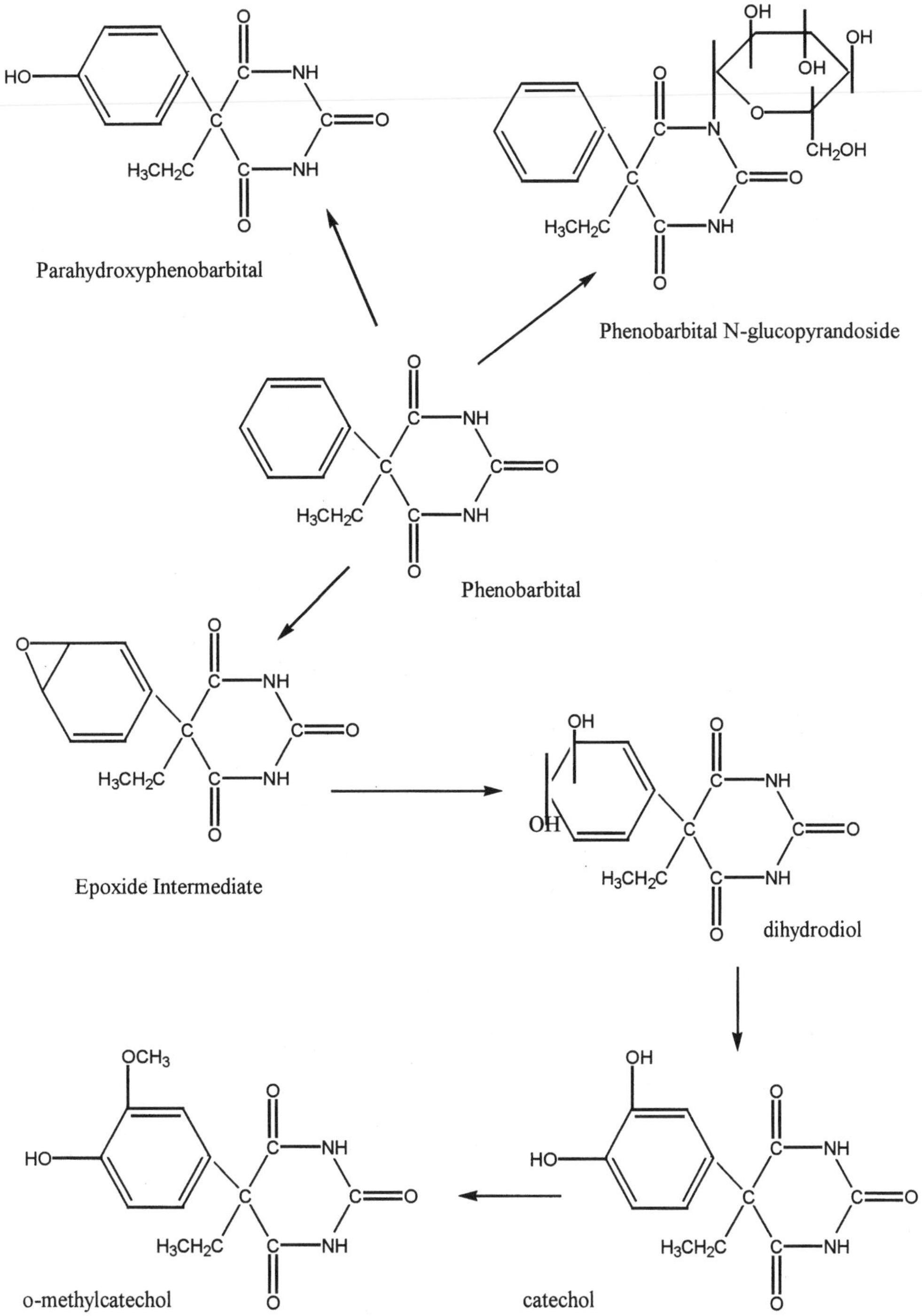

FIGURE 51.1. The main biotransformation pathways of phenobarbital.

ing dose in a patient whose total body weight was greater than 300% ideal body weight significantly underestimated the loading dose needed to provide therapeutic plasma concentrations of phenobarbital (28).

Plasma Protein Binding. Phenobarbital is approximately 55% bound to albumin in adults (4,29–31) and children (30,32). In neonates, phenobarbital binding is reduced, presumably because of relatively low albumin concentrations at birth; binding is 57% to 64% in neonates without hyperbilirubinemia and 70% to 72% in neonates with hyperbilirubinemia (30,33). No data are available regarding protein binding in the elderly patient population, in whom an age-related decline in albumin often occurs (34).

TABLE 51.1. PHENOBARBITAL PHARMACOKINETICS[a]

Population	T$_{max}$ (hr)	F	V (L/kg)	Fraction Bound (%)	Half-life (hr)	Clearance (mL/hr/kg)	Reference
Neonates	p.o.: 1.5–6	1.0	0.8–1.0	36–43	43–217	2.7–10.7	7, 21, 23–25, 75, 94–96
Infants (1–12 mo)	—	—	0.6 ± 0.07	—	63.2 ± 4.2	—	25
Children	1.5–6	1.0	0.57–0.70	55 (46–63)	37–198	5.3–11.3	7, 25, 32, 97, 108
Adults: monotherapy	p.o. 0.5–4	1.0	0.55–0.73	47 (41–56)	75–126	2.1–4.9	1–6, 14, 29, 71, 88, 91
	i.m. 2	1.0					
	Rectal: 4.4	0.9					
Adults: polytherapy with inducers	—	—	—	48 ± 0.5	77–128	3.1–5.3	1, 4
Children: polytherapy with inducers	—	—	—	—	—	6.8 (5.6–8.0)	93, 97
Adults: polytherapy with valproate	—	—	0.55–0.69	44	94–184	2.6–4.8	71, 88
Children: polytherapy with valproate	—	—	—	—	—	5.0 (4.0–6.0)	93
Elderly	—	—	—	—	—	2.5	98
Liver disease							
Cirrhosis	—	—	—	—	130 ± 15		99
Acute hepatitis				104 (60–127)			

F, bioavailability; T$_{max}$, time to maximum plasma concentration; V, volume.
[a]Values reported as mean ± standard deviation and/or range in different populations.

Cerebrospinal Fluid, Brain, and Other Tissues. Cerebrospinal fluid (CSF) concentrations of phenobarbital are similar in infants and adults. In infants, CSF levels are 44% to 57% (7), and in adults, they are 43% to 60% (29,35) of plasma concentrations. Thus, CSF concentrations correlate with unbound phenobarbital serum levels (29). Brain penetration of phenobarbital is relatively slow. Animal studies have demonstrated that maximal entry takes 12 to 60 minutes (36–38). During prolonged status epilepticus, brain uptake is increased, presumably by disruption of the blood–brain barrier (39). The reported concentrations of phenobarbital in surgically removed human epileptic brain tissues relative to plasma concentrations vary from 0.35 to 1.13 (40–43). The brain:plasma phenobarbital concentration ratio in a group of newborns who died while receiving phenobarbital was 0.71±0.21 (19). The ratio of phenobarbital in gray to white matter ranged from 0.86 to 1.11 in this group of newborns, similar to values found in adults (40,42,43). In another group of 11 premature and full-term babies, infants, and children (44), the brain:serum phenobarbital concentration ratio was 0.82±0.22. Phenobarbital concentrations in brain were significantly less than other organs including liver, kidney, spleen, pancreas, and lung (44). A study that evaluated postmortem concentrations of phenobarbital in different regions of the brains from 39 patients with epilepsy determined that the concentrations of phenobarbital in all regions of the cortex and cerebellum were largely comparable (45). Phenobarbital concentrations in the frontal cortex were 1.4 times higher and 2.1 times higher than the total and unbound phenobarbital concentrations in serum, respectively.

Unbound phenobarbital distributes into saliva, with saliva:total phenobarbital serum concentration ratios ranging from 0.21 to 0.52 (32,35,46–50). Two studies have demonstrated that the distribution of phenobarbital into saliva depends on salivary pH (4,51); however, other studies have not found an effect of pH (32,50). In spite of the contradictory results, when equations incorporate the relative ratio of phenobarbital pKa to the salivary pH, there is an excellent correlation between salivary and unbound serum concentrations (4,51).

Transplacental Passage. Phenobarbital distributes across the placenta and accumulates in fetal liver and brain (52–54). At the time of delivery, infants of mothers who have received phenobarbital have equivalent serum concentrations (55–63). In one of the studies, the placental passage of phenobarbital was evaluated in three groups of mothers and infants based on duration of phenobarbital treatment (63). Infants of mothers with epilepsy treated for 229±57 days, mothers treated for gestational hypertension and preeclampsia for 10±16 days, and mothers given prophylaxis of intraventricular hemorrhage in premature birth treated for 3.3±21 days were compared. Phenobarbital arterial cord concentrations were 100±2.8%, 89±21%, and 77±16% compared with the maternal concentrations for the three groups, respectively. In addition, a lower percentage of phenobarbital was found in infants with lower cord arterial pH values at birth.

Breast Milk. Phenobarbital is secreted into breast milk, with concentrations in breast milk 30% to 40% of maternal serum concentrations (58,64). Phenobarbital is slowly eliminated by the infants, with resulting infant serum concentrations that may reach or exceed maternal concentrations (58,60,65). Excess sedation, poor suckling and body-weight gain, and a high incidence of vomiting have resulted in a recommendation by the American Academy of Pediatrics that phenobarbital be used with caution during lactation (66).

ROUTES OF ELIMINATION

Phenobarbital is eliminated from the body by hepatic metabolism and renal excretion of unchanged drug.

Biotransformation. In the liver, phenobarbital is metabolized to two major metabolites, *p*-hydroxyphenobarbital (PBOH), which partially undergoes sequential metabolism to a glucuronic acid conjugate, and 9-D-glucopyranosylphenobarbital, an *N*-glucoside conjugate (PNG). Minor metabolism includes a dihydrodiol, catechol, and *p*-methylcatechol (Figure 51.l).

p*Hydroxyphenobarbital.* Butler (67) first reported the formation of PBOH from phenobarbital in the dog, and it was later confirmed in humans (11,19,68,69) that PBOH was a major metabolite. A substantial fraction of the PBOH is then conjugated with glucuronic acid to form PBOH glucuronide. In studies in patients treated with phenobarbital, an average of 55% (range, 30% to 87%) of the PBOH found was excreted as the *O*-glucuronide (29,70,71).

There is a large intersubject variability in the fraction of the phenobarbital dose that is metabolized by aromatic hydroxylation to PBOH. Several single-dose studies have reported a range of 8% to 34% of the dose recovered in urine as total PBOH (70,72–74). Steady-state experiments found that 6% to 40% of the phenobarbital daily dose was total PBOH (70,71,75,76).

Kadar et al. (69) found a wide range of total PBOH excreted in four children (aged 4 to 15 years). Total PBOH accounted for a range of 4.4% to 32.1%, with 38% to 61% conjugated with glucuronic acid. There was no apparent correlation between the age of the child and the percentage of either total or conjugated PBOH. Boreus (75) found that in four neonates, 15% of the phenobarbital dose was total PBOH, with 33% conjugated with glucuronic acid. These authors concluded that the neonates had a decreased ability to conjugate PBOH. However, because of the lack of pharmacologic activity of PBOH, (67,77) this difference would not be clinically significant.

N-Glucosidation. Glucosidation is an uncommon detoxication pathway in mammals; however, 9-D-glucopyranosylphenobarbital is a quantitatively significant metabolite of phenobarbital (PNG). Tang et al. (73) administered a mixture of ^{14}C-labeled and ^{15}N-labeled phenobarbital to two normal volunteers. Thin-layer chromatography of 16-day urine identified the *N*-glucoside conjugate of phenobarbital after comparison with a synthetic standard. In five volunteers, phenobarbital *N*-glucoside accounted for 26% (range, 24% to 30%) of the phenobarbital dose (39,40,73,74). Bhargava et al. (78) examined randomly collected urine samples from eight patients treated with phenobarbital monotherapy. PNG was detected in all but one patient. Bernus et al. (76) found 14% (range, 0% to 34%) excreted as PNG in 14 patients treated with phenobarbital.

In one study in four children, PNG accounted for 6% to 22.4% of the dose (69). Bhargava and Garrettson (79) also studied the development of phenobarbital metabolism in four neonates by analyzing serial single daily voided urines. The *N*-glucosidation pathway was not active at birth, and onset had not occurred until after 2 weeks of age. In one infant, by day 20, PNG accounted for 50% of the drug and metabolites in the urine sample. In the other infants, PNG was still not apparent when urine collections ended at days 14 and 16. Subsequent studies have demonstrated that PNG is subject to decomposition under physiologic conditions of temperature and pH. Unless the urine collected for analysis is acidified immediately before storage, decomposition may occur, and the percentage of PNG will be underestimated (80).

Minor Metabolites. The phenobarbital epoxide could also spontaneously or enzymatically yield the corresponding dihydrodiol (Figure 51.1). Harvey et al.(81) were able to obtain gas chromatography–mass spectrometry evidence that the dihydrodiol was present in rat, guinea pig, and human urine in small amounts. Theoretically, oxidation of the dihydrodiol could yield the corresponding catechol. This substance has been tentatively identified in rat and human urine by gas chromatography–mass spectrometry analysis (82). The 4-hydroxy 3-methoxy derivative of phenobarbital (*O*-methylcatechol) has been isolated from human urine, and its structure was confirmed by comparison with a synthetic standard. In six normal volunteers who received a single dose of phenobarbital, approximately 1% of the dose was recovered as this metabolite (83).

Isozymes. Cytochrome P450 2C9 (CYP2C9) plays a major role in the metabolism of phenobarbital to PBOH with minor metabolism by CYP2C19 and CYP2E1 (84). There are no data on the identity of the uridine diphosphate glucuronosyltransferase enzyme that is responsible for the formation of PNG.

Genetics. The effect of CYP2C19 polymorphism on the plasma clearance of phenobarbital was studied in a group of Japanese patients receiving phenobarbital treatment (85). Patients who were homozygous for the CYP2C19*3 or CYP2C19*2 genotype (the CYP2C19 poor metabolizers), had a 19% decreased clearance compared with the wild-type homozygous CYP2C19*1. There was also a trend of decreased plasma clearance in heterozygous extensive metabolizers compared with homozygous extensive metabolizers.

A set of twins exhibiting a genetic deficiency in the formation of the metabolite now known as amobarbital *N*-D-glucopyranoside has been reported (86), a finding suggesting that a deficiency in the enzymes responsible for the formation of PNG may also occur. There is also limited evidence that some patients do not form PNG. Of the three series of patients evaluated for urinary excretion of PNG, two identified patients without PNG. Bhargava et al. (78) identified one of seven patients and Bernus et al. (76) found two of 14 without detectable urinary excretion of PNG.

Biliary and Renal Excretion. There is considerable intersubject and intrasubject variability in the amount of phenobarbital excreted unchanged in the urine. Single-dose studies (30,31,72–74,87) in which urine was collected for a minimum of 15 days reported a range of 9% to 33% (average, 23%) of the phenobarbital dose excreted as unchanged drug. Steady-state studies found that the fraction of the dose excreted unchanged in urine averaged 22% (range, 7% to 55%) in four different studies (70,71,76,88).

Boreus et al. (75) showed that the 8-day urinary excretion of unchanged phenobarbital after a single dose in four newborn infants (17%) was similar to that in two adult volunteers (16%). Similarly, in four critically injured children (ages 5, 7, 10, and 15 years), Kadar et al. (69) found a range of 17.8% to 23.1% excreted as unchanged drug.

The renal clearance of phenobarbital depends on both urine flow (29,70,71,89) and urine pH (89), resulting from the lipophilicity and pKa (7.3) of this drug. This phenomenon may explain some of the intersubject variability found in the fraction of dose excreted unchanged in urine. After a drug is filtered by the glomerulus and possibly is actively secreted into the tubule, it may be subject to passive reabsorption. Drug reabsorption takes place primarily in the distal tubule, where the tubule membranes favor the movement of lipid-soluble and un-ionized compounds. The efficient reabsorption of water from the proximal tubule and loop of Henle results in a large concentration gradient between drug in the distal tubule and drug in the plasma. Increasing urine flow decreases this concentration gradient, resulting in a decrease in passive reabsorption. Small changes in urine pH can cause large increases or decreases in the percentage of an un-ionized weak acid (pK$_1$ 3.0 to 7.5) such as phenobarbital subject to passive reabsorption.

Waddell and Butler (89) first demonstrated the effect of urine flow and urine pH on phenobarbital renal clearance in an anesthetized dog model in which diuresis was induced. Kapetanovic et al. (71) studied three epileptic patients receiving prolonged phenobarbital therapy. Twenty-four-hour serial urine samples were collected (n = 26). These investigators found a direct linear correlation between urine flow and urinary excretion of unchanged phenobarbital (*r* = .913) over a fourfold range of urine flow. In a group of 20 epileptic patients, Lous (29) demonstrated the same linear correlation between urine flow and phenobarbital renal clearance but

also observed that the phenobarbital renal clearance was independent of phenobarbital concentration in the therapeutic range. The dependence of phenobarbital renal clearance on urine flow and urine pH has provided the basis for the use of urine alkalization and diuresis in patients who have had a phenobarbital overdose (89,90).

CLEARANCE AND HALF-LIFE

Healthy Subjects. The elimination t½ of phenobarbital has been determined in numerous studies and ranges from 75 to 126 hours in healthy subjects and in patients receiving monotherapy (1–5,14,29,91). Total plasma clearance ranges from 2.1 to 4.9 mL/hr/kg (1,2,14,91).

Comedicated Epileptic Patients. Because phenobarbital is eliminated by multiple pathways (CYP450, *N*-glucosidation, and renal elimination of unchanged drug), the effect of enzyme inducers should be minimal. In a study of three patients receiving concurrent carbamazepine, the t½ of phenobarbital was 110, 122, and 128 hours, compared with 77, 83, and 98 hours in another three patients receiving concurrent phenytoin. However, neither was significantly different from the t½ in six normal subjects (75 to 126 hours) (1). Valproate significantly decreases the plasma clearance of phenobarbital by inhibiting the formation of both PNG and PBOH (71,88,92). A population study in South African children reported mean phenobarbital clearances of 7.6, 5.0, and 6.8 mL/hr/kg in children receiving phenobarbital monotherapy, polytherapy with valproate, or polytherapy with carbamazepine or phenytoin, respectively (93).

Children. Newborns receiving phenobarbital for the treatment of neonatal seizures have a t½ ranging from 43 to 217 hours (7,21,24,25,94–96) and a total clearance of 2.7 to 10.7 mL/hr/kg (21,94). Phenobarbital clearance in asphyxia in neonates (22) was significantly lower (4.1 mL/hr/kg) compared with nonasphyxiated neonates (8.7 mL/h/kg). In children receiving phenobarbital, the t½ ranged from 37 to 198 hours (7,25). In a study of nine pediatric patients, the clearance in the children, ages 8 months to 4 years, was significantly greater than that reported in adults and ranged from 5.3 to 14.1 mL/hr/kg (97).

Elderly Patients. There is no information of the absorption, volume of distribution, or t½ of phenobarbital in elderly patients. Total clearance of phenobarbital was significantly reduced in a group of patients >40 years old (2.5 ml/hr/kg) compared with patients 15 to 40 years old (4.9 mL/hr/kg) (98).

Comorbid Conditions. The t½ of phenobarbital was prolonged in a group of patients with liver cirrhosis (130±15 hours) compared with a group of healthy subjects (86±3 hours). In patients with acute hepatitis, the t½ tended to be longer (60 to 127 hours) but was not significantly different from that of controls (99).

RELATIONSHIP BETWEEN SERUM CONCENTRATION AND DOSE

Large population studies have identified age and cotherapy as the primary determinants of the serum concentration:dose ratio. In an evaluation of data obtained from 536 patients receiving phenobarbital monotherapy, Duran et al. (100) found a decrease of the concentration:dose ratio with increasing age from <3 years, 3 to 6 years, 7 to 9 years, 10 to 14 years, and 15 to 18 years, with corresponding increasing concentration to dose ratios of 3.87±0.15, 4.65±0.16, 6.13±0.29, 7.54±0.73, and 10±1.1, respectively. A similar relationship with age was found in studies by Eadie et al. (98) in a group of 121 patients and by Suzuki et al. in a group of 438 patients (101).

Suzuki et al. (101) found that the concentration:dose ratio was higher in patients receiving phenobarbital in combination with other drugs mainly including phenytoin, valproate, and carbamazepine. Similar results were noted by Yukawa et al. (102) in a population study of 349 pediatric and adult patients with epilepsy in whom polytherapy with valproate or carbamazepine increased the concentration:dose ratio. Botha et al. reported that polytherapy with valproate, phenytoin, or carbamazepine resulted in an increase in the concentration:dose ratio (93).

Eadie et al. (98) demonstrated that sex was a determinant of the concentration:dose ratio only for children <5 years of age; boys required a higher dose (mg/kg) than girls. Sex was not found to be a factor in the other studies (100,101).

RELATIONSHIP BETWEEN SERUM CONCENTRATION AND EFFECT

The recommended therapeutic range for phenobarbital is 10 to 40 μg/mL; however, neither the concentration effect nor the concentration–toxicity relationship is well defined (103). The range is based on studies largely in adults (104–106). Schmidt et al. (106) showed that the therapeutic range varied according to seizure type. Significantly higher phenobarbital plasma concentrations were necessary to control simple or partial complex seizures with or without secondarily generalized seizures (38±6 μg/mL.) than generalized tonic-clonic seizures only (18±10 μg/mL.). Tolerability to the sedative adverse effects of phenobarbital alters the relationship of concentration with toxicity. Initial doses at very low phenobarbital concentration can cause excessive sedation and ataxia; however, over several weeks, tolerability to much higher phenobarbital concentrations can occur (107).

REFERENCES

1. Wilensky AJ, Friel PN, Levy RH, et al. Kinetics of phenobarbital in normal subjects and epileptic patients. *Eur J Clin Pharmacol* 1982;23:87–92.
2. Nelson E, Powell JR, Conrad K, et al. Phenobarbital pharmacokinetics and bioavailability in adults. *J Clin Pharmacol* 1982; 22:141–148.
3. Viswanathan CT, Booker HE, Welling PG. Bioavailability of oral and intramuscular phenobarbital. *J Clin Pharmacol* 1978; 18:100–105.
4. Nishihara K, Katsuyoski U, Saitoh Y, et al. Estimation of plasma unbound phenobarbital concentration by using mixed saliva. *Epilepsia* 1979;20:37–45.
5. Barzaghi N, Gatti G, Manni R, et al. Comparative pharmacokinetics and pharmacodynamics of eterobarbital and phenobarbital in normal volunteers. *Eur J Drug Metabol Pharmacokinet* 1991;16:81–87.
6. Graves NM, Homes GB, Kriel RL, et al. Relative bioavailability of rectally administered phenobarbital sodium parenteral solution. *DICP* 1989;23:565–568.
7. Jalling B. Plasma and cerebrospinal fluid concentrations of phenobarbital in infants given single doses. *Dev Med Child Neurol* 1974;11:781–793.
8. Syed GB, Sharma DB, Raina RK. Pharmacokinetics of phenobarbitone in protein energy malnutrition. *Dev Pharmacol Ther* 1986;9:317–322.
9. Berg JM, Berlinger WG, Goldberg MJ, et al. Acceleration of the body clearance of phenobarbital by oral activated charcoal. *N Engl J Med* 1982;307:642–644.
10. Goldberg MJ, Berlinger WG. Treatment of phenobarbital overdose with activated charcoal. *JAMA* 1982;247:2400–2401.
11. Neuvonen PJ, Elonen E. Effect of activated charcoal on absorption and elimination of phenobarbitone, carbamazepine and phenylbutazone in man. *Eur J Clin Pharmacol* 1980;17:51–57.
12. Veerman M, Espejo MG, Christopher MA, et al. Use of activated charcoal to reduce elevated serum phenobarbital concentration in a neonate. *Clin Toxicol* 1991;29:53–58.
13. Berg MJ, Rose JQ, Wurster DE, et al. Effect of charcoal and sorbitol-charcoal suspension on the elimination of intravenous phenobarbital. *Ther Drug Monit* 1987;9:41–47.
14. Browne TR, Evans JE, Szabo GK, et al. Studies with stable isotopes. II. Phenobarbital pharmacokinetics during monotherapy. *J Clin Pharmacol* 1985;25:51–58.
15. Berg JM, Rose JQ, Wurster DE, et al. Effect of charcoal and sorbitol-charcoal suspension on the elimination of intravenous phenobarbital. *Ther Drug Monit* 1987;9:41–47.
16. Svensmark O, Buchthal F. Accumulation of phenobarbital in man. *Epilepsia* 1963;4:199–206.
17. Painter MJ, Pippenger C, et al. Phenobarbital and diphenylhydantoin levels in neonates with seizures. *Pediatrics* 1978;92: 315–319.
18. Painter MJ, Pippenger C, et al. Phenobarbital and phenytoin blood levels in neonates. *Pediatrics* 1977;92:315–319.
19. Painter MJ, Pippenger C. Phenobarbital and phenytoin in neonatal seizures: metabolism and tissue distribution. *Neurology* 1981;31:1107–1112.
20. Jalling B. Plasma concentrations of phenobarbital in the treatment of seizures in the newborn. *Acta Paediatr Scand* 1975;64: 514–524.
21. Fischer JH, Lockman LA, Zaske D, et al. Phenobarbital maintenance doses requirements in treating neonatal seizures. *Neurology* 1981;31:1042–1044.
22. Gal P, Erkan NV, et al. The influence of asphyxia on phenobarbital dosing requirements in neonates. *Dev Pharmacol Ther* 1984;7:145–152.

23. Lockman LA, Kriel RL, Zaske D, et al. Phenobarbital dosage for control of neonatal seizures. *Neurology* 1979;29:1445–1449.

24. Grasela THJ, Donn SM. Neonatal population pharmacokinetics of phenobarbital derived from routine clinical data. *Dev Pharmacol Ther* 1985;8:374–383.

25. Heimann G, Gladtke E. Pharmacokinetics of phenobarbital in childhood. *Eur J Clin Pharmacol* 1977;12:305–310.

26. Brachet-Liermain A, Gouteres F, Aicardia J. Absorption of phenobarbital after the intramuscular administration of single doses in infants. *J Pediatr* 1975;87:624–626.

27. Dodson WE, Rust RS. Phenobarbital: absorption, distribution and excretion. In: Levy RH, Mattson RH, Meldrum BS, eds. *Antiepileptic drugs,* 4th ed. New York: Raven Press, 1994.

28. Wilkes L, Danziger LH, Rodvold KA. Phenobarbital pharmacokinetics in obesity: a case report. *Clin Pharmacokinet* 1992; 22:481–484.

29. Lous P. Blood serum and cerebrospinal fluid levels and renal clearances of phenemal in treated epileptics. *Acta Pharmacol Toxicol* 1954;10:166–177.

30. Ehrnebo M, Agurell S, Jalling B, et al. Age differences in drug binding by plasma proteins: studies on human foetuses, neonates and adults. *Eur J Clin Pharmacol* 1971;3:189–193.

31. Goldbaum LR, Smith PK. The interaction of barbituates with serum albumin and its possible relation to their disposition and pharmacological actions. *J Pharmacol Exp Ther* 1954;111: 197–209.

32. Tokugawa K, Ueda K, Fujito H, et al. Correlation between the saliva and free serum concentration of phenobarbital in epileptic children. *Eur J Pediatr* 1986;145:401–402.

33. Morselli PL, Franco-Morselli R, Bossi L. Clinical pharmacokinetics in newborns and infants: age-related differences and therapeutic implications. *Clin Pharmacokinet* 1980;5:485–527.

34. Veering BT, Burm AG, Souveijn JH, et al. The effect of age on serum concentrations of albumin and alpha 1-acid glycoprotein. *Br J Clin Pharmacol* 1990;29:201–206.

35. Schmidt D, Kupferberg H. Diphenylhydantoin, phenobarbital, and primidone in saliva, plasma, and cerebrospinal fluid. *Epilepsia* 1975;16:735–741.

36. Engasser JM, Sarahan F, Falcoz C, et al. Distribution, metabolism, and elimination of phenobarbital in rats: physiologically based pharmacokinetic model. *J Pharm Sci* 1981;70: 1233–1238.

37. Mayer S, Maickel RP, Brodie BB. Kinetics of penetration of drugs and other foreign compounds in cerebrospinal fluid and brain. *J Pharmacol Exp Ther* 1959;127:205.

38. Ramsay RE, Hammond EJ, Perchalski RJ, et al. Brain uptake of phenytoin, phenobarbital and diazepam. *Arch Neurol* 1979;36: 535–539.

39. Simon RP, Copeland JR, Benowitz NL, et al. Brain phenobarbital uptake during prolonged status epilepticus. *J Cereb Blood Flow Metab* 1987;7:783–788.

40. Harvey CD, Sherwin AL, Van Der Kleijn E. Distribution of anticonvulsant drugs in gray and white matter of human brain. *Can J Neurol Sci* 1977;4:89–92.

41. Houghton GW, Richens A, Toseland PA, et al. Brain concentrations of phenytoin, phenobarbital and primidone in epileptic patients. *Eur J Clin Pharmacol* 1975;9:73–78.

42. Sherwin AL, Eisen AA, Sagolowski CD. Anticonvulsant drugs in human epileptogenic brain. *Arch Neurol* 1973;29:73.

43. Vajda F, Williams FM, Davidson S, et al. Human brain, cerebrospinal fluid, and plasma concentrations of diphenylhydantoin and phenobarbital. *Clin Pharmacol Ther* 1974;15: 597–603.

44. Onishi S, Ohki Y, Nishimura Y, et al. Distribution of phenobarbital in serum, brain and other organs from pediatric patients. *Dev Pharmacol Ther* 1984;7:153–159.

45. Rambeck B, Schnabel R, May T, et al. Postmortem concentra-

46. Cook C, Amerson E, Poole W, et al. Phenytoin and phenobarbital concentrations in saliva and plasma measured by radioimmunoassay. *Clin Pharmacol Ther* 1975;18:742–747.

47. Horning MG, Brown L, Nowlin J, et al. Use of saliva for therapeutic drug monitoring. *Clin Chem* 1977;23:157–164.

48. Troupin AS, Friel PN. Anticonvulsant level in saliva, serum and cerebrospinal fluid. *Epilepsia* 1975;16:223–227.

49. Goldsmith RF, Ouvrier RA. Salivary anticonvulsant levels in children: a comparison of methods. *Ther Drug Monit* 1981;3: 151–157.

50. Friedman IM, Litt IF, et al. Saliva phenobarbital and phenytoin concentrations in epileptic adolescents. *J Pediatr* 1981;98: 645–647.

51. McAuliffe JJ, Sherwin AL, Leppik IE, et al. Salivary levels of anticonvulsants: a practical approach to drug monitoring. *Neurology* 1977;27:409–413.

52. Plomann L, Persson BH. On the transfer of barbituates to the human fetus and their accumulation in some of its vital organs. *J Obstet Gynecol* 1957;64:706–711.

53. Persson BH. Studies on the accumulation of certain barbituates in the brain of the human fetus. *Acta Obstet Gynecol* 1960;39: 88–99.

54. Nau H, Kuhnz W, Egger HJ, et al. Anticonvulsants during pregnancy and lactation: transplacental, maternal and neonatal pharmacokinetics. *Clin Pharmacokinet* 1982;7:508–543.

55. Boreus LO, Jalling B, Wallin A. Plasma concentrations of phenobarbital in mother and child after combined prenatal and postnatal administration for prophylaxis of hyperbilirubinemia. *J Pediatr* 1978;93:695–698.

56. Bossi L, Battino D, Caccamo ML, et al. Pharmacokinetics and clinical effects of antiepileptic drugs in newborns of chronically treated epileptic mothers. In: Janz D, Dam M, Richens A, et al., eds. *Epilepsy, pregnancy, and the child.* New York: Raven Press; 1982:373–381.

57. Jalling B, Boreus LO, Kallberg N, et al. Disappearance from the newborn of circulating prenatally administered phenobarbital. *Eur J Clin Pharmacol* 1973;6:234–238.

58. Kuhnz W, Koch S, Helge H, et al. Primidone and phenobarbital during lactation period in epileptic women: total and free drug serum levels in the nursed infants and their effect on neonatal behavior. *Dev Pharmacol Ther* 1988;11:147–154.

59. Melchior JC, Svensmark O, Trolle D. Placental transfer of phenobarbitone in epileptic women, and elimination in newborns. *Lancet* 1967;11:860–861.

60. Nau H, Rating D, Hauser I, et al. Placental transfer and pharmacokinetics of primidone and its metabolites, phenobarbital, PEMA and hydroxyphenobarbital in neonates and infants of epileptic mothers. *Eur J Clin Pharmacol* 1980;18:18–42.

61. Rating D, Nau H, Kuhnz W, et al. Antiepileptika in der neugeborenenperiode. *Monatsschr Kinderheilkd* 1983;131:6–12.

62. Shankaran S, Cepeda E, Ilagan N, et al. Pharmacokinetic basis for antenatal dosing of phenobarbital for the prevention of neonatal intracerebral hemorrhage. *Dev Pharmacol Ther* 1986; 9:171–177.

63. De Carolis MP, Romagnoli C, Frezza S, et al. Placental transfer of phenobarbital: What is New? *Dev Pharmacol Ther* 1992;19: 19–26.

64. Kaneko S, Suzuki K, Sato T, et al. The problems of antiepileptic medication in the neonatal periods: is breastfeeding advisable? In: Janz D, Dam M, Richens A, et al., eds. *Epilepsy, pregnancy, and the child.* New York: Raven Press, 1982:343–348.

65. Hagg S, Spigset O. Anticonvulsant use during lactation. *Drug Saf* 2000;22:425–440.

66. American Academy of Pediatrics Committee on Drugs. The transfer of drugs and other chemicals into human milk. *Pediatrics* 1994;93:137–150.
67. Butler TC. The metabolic hydroxylation of phenobarbital. *J Pharmacol Exp Ther* 1956;116:326–336.
68. Curry AS. Curry AS. A note on a urinary metabolite of phenobarbitone. *J Pharm Pharmacol* 1955;7:1072–1073.
69. Kadar D, Tang BK, Conn AW. The fate of phenobarbitone in children in hypothermia and at normal body temperature. *Can Anaesth Soc J* 1982;29:16–23.
70. Whyte MP, Dekaban AS. Metabolic fate of phenobarbital: a quantitative study of p-hydroxyphenobarbital elimination in man. *Drug Metab Dispos* 1977;5:63–70.
71. Kapetanovic IM, Kupferberg HJ, Porter RJ, et al. Mechanism of valproate/phenobarbital interaction in epileptic patients. *Clin Pharmacol Ther* 1981;29:480–486.
72. Raven-Jonsen A, Lundin M, Secher O. Excretion of phenobarbitone in urine after intake of large doses. *Acta Pharmacol Toxicol (Kbh)* 1968;27:193–201.
73. Tang BK, Kalow W, Grey AA. Metabolic fate of phenobarbital in man: N-glucoside formation. *Drug Metab Dispos* 1979;7:315–318.
74. Tang BK, Yilmaz B, Kalow W. Determination of phenobarbital, p-hydroxyphenobarbital and phenobarbital-N-glucoside in urine by gas chromatography chemical ionization mass spectrometry. *Biomed Mass Spectrom* 1983;11:462–465.
75. Boreus LO, Jalling B, Kallberg N. Phenobarbital metabolism in adults and in newborn infants. *Acta Paediatr Scand* 1978;67:193–200.
76. Bernus I, Dickinson RG, Hooper WD, et al. Urinary excretion of phenobarbitone and its metabolites in chronically treated patients. *Eur J Clin Pharmacol* 1994;46:473–475.
77. Danhof M, Levy G. Kinetics of drug action in disease states. I. Effect of infusion rate on phenobarbital concentrations in serum, brain and cerebrospinal fluid of normal rats at onset of loss of righting reflex. *J Pharmacol Exp Ther* 1984;229:44–50.
78. Bhargava VO, Soine WH, Garrettson LK. High performance liquid chromatographic analysis of 1-(D-glucopyranosyl)-phenobarbital in urine. *J Chromatogr* 1985;343:219–223.
79. Bhargava VO, Garrettson LK. Development of phenobarbital glucosidation in the human neonate. *Dev Pharmacol Ther* 1988;11:8–13.
80. Vest FB, Soine WH, Westkaemper RB, et al. Stability of phenobarbital N-glucoside: identification of hydrolysis products and kinetics of decomposition. *Pharm Res* 1989;6:458–465.
81. Harvey DU, Glazner L, Stratton G, et al. Detection of a 5-(3,4-dihydroxy-1,5-cyclohexadien-1-yl)-metabolite of phenobarbital and mephobarbital in rat, guinea pig, and human. *Res Commun Chem Pathol Pharmacol* 1972;3:557–565.
82. Horning EC, Horning MG. Metabolic profiles: gas phase methods for analysis of metabolites. *Clin Chem* 1971;17:802–809.
83. Treston AM, Philippides A, Jacobsen NW, et al. Identification and synthesis of O-methylcatechol metabolites of phenobarbital and some n-alkyl derivatives. *J Pharm Sci* 1987;76:496–501.
84. Hargraves JA, Howald WN, Racha JK, et al. Identification of enzymes responsible for the metabolism of phenobarbital. *Int Soc Stud Xenobiot Proc* 1996;10:259(abst).
85. Mamiya K, Hadama A, Yukawa E, et al. CYP2C19 polymorphism effect on phenobarbitone. Pharmacokinetics in Japanese patients with epilepsy: analysis by population pharmacokinetics. *Eur J Clin Pharmacol* 2000;55:821–825.
86. Tang BK, Kalow W, Grey AA. Amobarbital metabolism in man: N-glucoside formation. *Res Commun Chem Pathol Pharmacol* 1978;21:45–53.
87. Remmer H, Siegert M. Kumulation and elimination von phenobarbital. *Naunyn Schmiedebergs Arch Exp Pathol Pharmakol* 1962;243:479–494.
88. Patel IH, Levy RH, Cutler RE. Phenobarbital-valproic acid interaction. *Clin Pharmacol Ther* 1980;27:515–521.
89. Waddell WJ, Butler TC. Distribution and excretion of phenobarbital. *J Clin Invest* 1957;36:1217–1226.
90. Gary NE, Tresznewsky O. Barbiturates and a potpourri of other sedatives, hypnotics and tranquilizers. *Heart Lung* 1983;12:122–127.
91. Pullar T, Kumar S, Chrystyn H, et al. The prediction of steady-state phenobarbitone concentrations (following low-dose phenobarbitone) to refine its use as an indicator of compliance. *Br J Clin Pharmacol* 1991;32:329–333.
92. Bernus I, Dickinson G, Hooper WD, et al. Inhibition of phenobarbitone N-glucosidation by valproate. *Br J Clin Pharmacol* 1994;38:411–416.
93. Botha JH, Gray AL, Miller R. Determination of phenobarbitone population clearance values for South African children. *Eur J Clin Pharmacol* 1995;48:381–383.
94. Donn SM, Grasela THJ, Goldstein GW. Safety of a higher loading dose of phenobarbital in the term newborn. *Pediatrics* 1985;75:1061–1064.
95. Pitlick W, Painter M, Pippenger C. Phenobarbital pharmacokinetics in neonates. *Clin Pharmacol Ther* 1978;23:346–350.
96. Taburet AM, Chamouard C, Aymard P, et al. Phenobarbital protein binding in neonates. *Dev Pharmacol Ther* 1982;4[Suppl 1]:129–134.
97. Davis AG, Mutchie KD, Thompson JA, et al. Once-daily dosing with phenobarbital in children with seizure disorders. *Pediatrics* 1981;68:824–827.
98. Eadie MJ, Lander CM, Hooper W, et al. Factors influencing plasma phenobarbitone levels in epileptic patients. *Br J Clin Pharmacol* 1977;4:541–547.
99. Alvin J, McHorse T, Hoyumpa A, et al. The effect of liver disease in man on the disposition of phenobarbital. *J Pharmacol Exp Ther* 1975;192:224–235.
100. Duran JA, Sanchez A, Serrano MI, et al. Phenobarbital plasma/level dose ratio in monotherapy: influence of age, sex and dose. *Methods Find Exp Clin Pharmacol* 1988;10:337–340.
101. Suzuki K, Cox S, Hayes J, et al. Phenobarbital doses necessary to achieve "therapeutic" concentrations in children. *Dev Pharmacol Ther* 1991;17:79–87.
102. Yukawa E, To H, Ohdo S, et al. Detection of drug-drug interaction on population-based phenobarbitone clearance using nonlinear mixed-effects modeling. *Eur J Clin Pharmacol* 1998;54:69–74.
103. Theodore W. Rational use of antiepileptic drug levels. *Pharmacol Ther* 1992;54:297–305.
104. Buchthal F, Svensmark O, Simonsen H. Relation of EEG and seizures to phenobarbital in serum. *Arch Neurol* 1968;19:567–672.
105. Feely M, O'Callagan M, Duggan B, et al. Phenobarbitone in previously untreated epilepsy. *J Neurol Neurosurg Psychiatry* 1980;43:365–368.
106. Schmidt D, Einicke I, Haenel F. The influence of seizure type on the efficacy of plasma concentrations of phenytoin, phenobarbital and carbamazepine. *Arch Neurol* 1986;43:263–265.
107. Cramer JA, Mattson RH. Phenobarbital: Toxicity. In: Levy RH, Mattson RH, Meldrum BS, ed. *Antiepileptic drugs,* 4th ed. New York: Raven Press, 1994:409–420.
108. Garrettson LK, Dayton PG. Disappearance of phenobarbital and diphenylhydantoin from serum of children. *Clin Pharmacol Ther* 1970;11:674–679.

PHENOBARBITAL AND OTHER BARBITURATES

INTERACTIONS WITH OTHER DRUGS

J. STEVEN LEEDER

The potential for drug–drug interactions continues to be an important consideration when phenobarbital is included in a given patient's pharmacotherapeutic regimen. Although alterations in drug pharmacokinetics and pharmacodynamics are theoretically possible, almost all documented, clinically relevant drug–drug interactions involving phenobarbital result in pharmacokinetic changes in the concomitantly administered medication. The nature and extent of the pharmacokinetic interactions are best documented through evaluation of parameters such as total body clearance, area under the blood, plasma, or serum concentration–time curves (AUC), distribution volume, elimination half-life, and peak or steady-state plasma concentrations.

Because most drug interactions involving phenobarbital occur at the level of drug biotransformation, the potential for a clinically significant interaction increases if drug elimination is highly dependent on a single metabolic pathway that is subject to modulation by phenobarbital. Furthermore, each individual patient has his or her own unique complement of individual cytochrome P450 (CYP) or glucuronosyl transferase isoforms, and as a consequence, the combination of phenobarbital and drug X may result in lower concentrations of drug X in some patients but may not be associated with any discernible effect in others. Likewise, additional factors such as drug dosages, diet, smoking or alcohol intake, and disease conditions all contribute to the variability in clinical manifestations of a particular drug interaction with phenobarbital.

Considerable progress has been made in evaluating potential drug–drug interactions in humans both *in vitro* and *in vivo*. This chapter is largely restricted to information that has been generated by clinical studies conducted in human subjects or through the use of human-derived experimental systems.

J. Steven Leeder, PharmD, PhD: Associate Professor, Department of Pediatrics and Pharmacology, University of Missouri, Kansas City; and Chief, Section of Developmental Pharmacology and Experimental Therapeutics, Children's Mercy Hospital and Clinics, Kansas City, Missouri

PHARMACOKINETIC DRUG INTERACTIONS

Effects of Other Drugs on Phenobarbital Kinetics

Absorption. Phenobarbital is essentially completely absorbed after oral administration (1), and few, if any, interactions leading to impaired absorption have been reported. Conversely, several studies have documented the utility of activated charcoal in limiting systemic exposure after a phenobarbital overdose. Although absorption of orally administered phenobarbital is reduced by activated charcoal administered in close temporal proximity to the phenobarbital dose (2), several studies also report that the clearance of intravenous phenobarbital is enhanced 60% to 270% by charcoal administered in repeated doses over 36 to 96 hours while half-lives are decreased 2.5- to eightfold (3–5). Studies in rabbits attribute this effect to the ability of the activated charcoal to disrupt phenobarbital enterohepatic recirculation (6).

Distribution. Binding of phenobarbital to plasma proteins is approximately 50% (7), and so clinically significant interactions resulting from displacement from protein binding sites are not anticipated.

Biotransformation. Preliminary data attribute the *p*-hydroxylation of phenobarbital primarily to the CYPs CYP2C9 and CYP2C19 (8). As a result, coadministration of drugs that either induce or inhibit these CYP isoforms has the potential to modulate phenobarbital pharmacokinetics to a clinically significant extent. For example, addition of chloramphenicol to phenobarbital therapy has been reported to reduce phenobarbital clearance by 40% (9). Because polypharmacy is a common feature of antiepileptic drug therapy, there is an increased potential for drug–drug interactions. Some of the more clinically important interactions are discussed in the following paragraph and are summarized in Table 52.1.

TABLE 52.1. EFFECT OF CONCURRENTLY ADMINISTERED DRUGS OR TREATMENTS ON THE CLEARANCE OF PHENOBARBITAL

Causative Agent	Change in Clearance	References
Activated charcoal	↑ 60–270%	3–5
Carbamazepine	No change	11
Felbamate	↓ 24%	12
Phenytoin	No change	10, 11
Valproic acid	↓ 25%	14–17

Carbamazepine. The addition of carbamazepine to patients treated with primidone is reported to result in increased concentrations of the active metabolite, phenobarbital (10). Because concurrent carbamazepine therapy apparently does not affect phenobarbital clearance *per se* (11), the increased phenobarbital concentrations can be attributed to formation from primidone rather than to reduced phenobarbital clearance. The enzymes responsible for primidone biotransformation to phenobarbital have not been identified.

Felbamate. Felbamate, an inhibitor of CYP2C19 but not of CYP2C9 *in vitro* (12), also has been reported to decrease phenobarbital clearance *in vivo*. The addition of a 9-day course of felbamate (2,400 mg/day) to healthy volunteers receiving phenobarbital, 100 mg daily for 28 days, reduced phenobarbital clearance by 24% from baseline values; no such effect was observed in a parallel group receiving placebo instead of felbamate. The change in phenobarbital clearance was largely (~55%) attributed to a reduction in the formation of *p*-hydroxyphenobarbital, a finding consistent with a role for CYP2C19 in mediating this pathway of phenobarbital elimination (13).

Valproic Acid. Valproic acid is associated with a relatively predictable decrease in phenobarbital clearance that manifests initially as drowsiness and increasing somnolence and other signs of concentration-dependent toxicity. Based on single-dose pharmacokinetic studies and studies conducted at steady-state phenobarbital concentrations, valproic acid treatment is associated with an approximately 25% reduction in phenobarbital clearance and a 50% longer half-life (14–17), attributed to decreased biotransformation to *p*-hydroxyphenobarbital (15,18). Increases in phenobarbital serum concentrations appear to be greater in pediatric patients (112.5%) compared with adults (50.9%) (19), and the extent of the interaction is characterized by considerable interindividual variability; reports indicate that between 50% and 80% of patients may require a reduction in phenobarbital dose (14,19). Concurrent administration of valproic acid and primidone is associated with an increase in the phenobarbital:primidone ratio consistent with an inhibitory effect on further biotransformation of phenobarbital (20).

Phenytoin. Phenytoin has been observed to have no effect or to significantly increase plasma phenobarbital concentrations (10,11, 21). When plasma phenobarbital concentrations are derived from primidone, it appears that coadministration of phenytoin and carbamazepine can be expected ultimately to increase phenobarbital levels (10,22). In one study, derived phenobarbital concentrations were 30.6±2.9 mg/L in the presence of phenytoin versus 14.4±3.3 mg/L in its absence, but whether this finding represents increased conversion of primidone to phenobarbital or inhibition of phenobarbital biotransformation has not been unequivocally resolved (22). Overall, the data suggest that phenytoin is less likely to increase phenobarbital concentrations than either valproic acid or felbamate.

Effects of Phenobarbital on the Kinetics of Other Drugs

Almost all clinically significant drug–drug interactions involving phenobarbital are the result of induction, and most involve the CYPs. The effects of phenobarbital on the pharmacokinetics of concomitantly administered medications are summarized in Table 52.2.

Phenobarbital Induction of Drug-Metabolizing Enzymes in Humans

Phenobarbital, a pleiotropic agent that, among other effects, causes proliferation of hepatic smooth endoplasmic reticulum, has been recognized as a prototypical inducer for a group of structurally diverse compounds since the 1960s (23). Extensively studied in rodents and rodent-based sys-

TABLE 52.2. EFFECT OF PHENOBARBITAL ON THE APPARENT ORAL CLEARANCE OF CONCURRENTLY ADMINISTERED DRUGS

Affected Drug	Change in Clearance	References
Carbamazepine	↑ 15–50%	47–49
Cimetidine	↑ 15%	73
Cyclosporine	↑ 70%	83
Dexamethasone	↑ 87%	79
Felodipine	↑ 8–9-fold	71
Lamotrigine	↑ ~50%	53–56
Losartan	No change	105
Metronidazole	↑ ~30%	86
Nifedipine	↑ 270%	72
Nimodipine	↑ 9-fold	70
Phenytoin	No change	50, 51
Prednisolone	↑ 44%	77
Teniposide	↑ 200–300%	89
Theophylline	↑ 35–40%	94, 95
Valproic acid	↑ 10–25%	57–59
Verapamil	↑ 200–500%	69
S-Warfarin	↑ 50%	97
R-Warfarin	↑ 65%	97

tems, induction of members of the CYP2A, CYP2B, CYP2C, and CYP3A subfamilies by phenobarbital is now well characterized (24).

Studies in human-based experimental systems are consistent with induction of CYP2B6, CYP2C8, CYP2C9, and CYP3A4. For example, 48-hour exposure of cultured human hepatocytes to 3.2 mmol/L phenobarbital produced a modest (1.4- to 1.8-fold) increase in CYP2C8/9 immunoreactive protein and no change in CYP3A4 protein (25,26), whereas 2.0- to 2.5-fold increases in testosterone hydroxylation in the 16α- and 16β-positions with smaller increases in 2β- and 6β-hydroxylated metabolites suggest moderate induction of the human CYP3A and CYP2C subfamilies (27). Chang et al. (27a) observed increases in immunoreactive CYP2B6, CYP2C8, CYP2C9, and CYP3A4 proteins after phenobarbital treatment (2 mmol/L, 96 hours), whereas CYP1A1 and CYP1A2 expression was not affected. Studies with replicating human hepatoma cell lines indicate that phenobarbital also induces CYP3A7, but not CYP3A5, messenger RNA, and immunoreactive protein (28). Nevertheless, phenobarbital is less potent as an inducer of CYP activity than dexamethasone or rifampin. Induction of glucuronosyl transferase (29,30), glutathione *S*-transferase α (31), and epoxide hydrolase (32) activities by phenobarbital *in vitro* has also been reported.

The degree of CYP induction observed in primary cultures of human hepatocytes is highly variable. Although some variability is a consequence of the range of culture conditions employed in different laboratories, the use of standardized conditions reveals that induction of CYP activities by phenobarbital and other inducers is highly reproducible in multiple laboratories (33). A more important issue is considerable intersubject variability in the extent of induction observed *in vitro,* consistent with the variability observed *in vivo.*

In vivo, phenobarbital and phenytoin treatment of epileptic children resulted in four- to sevenfold greater 6β-hydroxycortisol:cortisol ratios in urine, a marker of CYP3A activity (34), relative to age-matched controls (35,36). These and other studies (37–39) are consistent with induction of CYP3A activity by phenobarbital in humans, and most drug interactions in which it is involved can be attributed to this factor. Because of the long half-life of the drug, however, maximum effect may not be observed until after 10 to 14 days of therapy.

Mechanism of Induction

Phenobarbital has moderate activity as an activator of the pregnane X receptor (PXR), the orphan nuclear receptor that plays an important role in the transcriptional regulation of the *CYP3A4* gene by prototypical inducers such as dexamethasone, rifampin, and clotrimazole (40). The heterodimer formed between PXR and the 9-*cis* retinoic acid receptor (RXR) binds to specific nucleotide sequences that are organized as an everted repeat separated by six nucleotides (ER-6; TGAACT-N$_6$-AGGTCA). These binding sites are located ≤8,000 base pairs upstream of the *CYP3A4* gene transcription start site (41).

Induction of the *CYP2B6* gene by phenobarbital appears to be mediated by an additional orphan nuclear receptor, the constitutive androstane receptor (CAR), which also heterodimerizes with RXR. CAR-mediated transcriptional activity is stereospecifically inhibited by 5α-reduced steroids with a 3α-hydroxyl group, specifically androstanol and androstenol, by promoting the release of coactivators (e.g., steroid receptor coactivator-1; SRC-1) from the ligand-binding domain of the receptor (42). Induction by phenobarbital is thought to represent release (or derepression) of CAR from the usual state of inhibition by endogenous steroids (Figure 52.1) (43). Although helpful, this model likely is an oversimplification because supraphysiologic concentrations of androstanol are required for inhibition of CAR, and more recent data implicate either a phenobarbital metabolite that can bind directly to CAR or an indirect mechanism involving phosphorylation to account for the induction process (44).

Interactions with Other Antiepileptic Drugs

Carbamazepine. In general, phenobarbital increases carbamazepine clearance, and higher doses are required to maintain carbamazepine concentrations at prephenobarbital levels (45). Epileptic patients receiving both agents display lower steady-state carbamazepine concentrations and higher carbamazepine-epoxide concentrations relative to patients receiving carbamazepine monotherapy (46), although the differences (10% to 15% changes) are generally modest (47). Pediatric patients concurrently treated with phenobarbital had 15% lower carbamazepine concentrations (25.2±5.9 µmol/L versus 29.8±8.8 µmol/L) despite receiving higher total carbamazepine doses (21.1±8.1 versus 18.4±7.2 mg/kg/day) than children treated with carbamazepine alone (48). More extensive reviews of the phenobarbital–carbamazepine interaction indicate that steady-state carbamazepine concentrations may decrease as much as 50%, whereas carbamazepine–epoxide concentrations remain unchanged during combination therapy with phenobarbital (49).

Phenytoin. Because phenobarbital and phenytoin have similar induction profiles and are subject to biotransformation by the same enzymes (CYP2C9 and glucuronosyl transferases), the possibility of induction and competitive inhibition exists. The net outcome of an interaction between the two drugs in a given individual will therefore reflect which, if either, mechanism predominates. For example, phenytoin clearance, half-life, or volume of distribution was not significantly altered at 4 and 12 weeks after the initiation of phenobarbital in one study (50). Further-

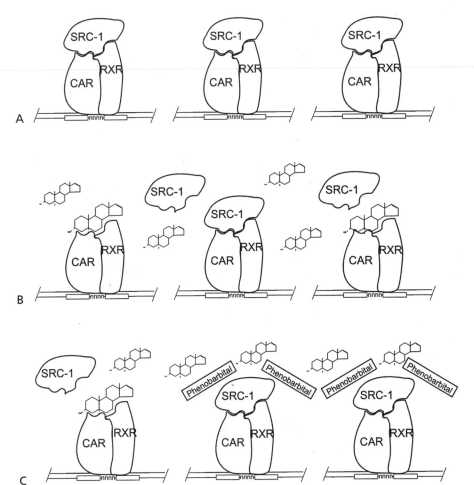

FIGURE 52.1. Proposed mechanism for phenobarbital induction. **A:** The constitutive androstane receptor (CAR) forms a heterodimer with the retinoic acid X receptor (RXR) and bids to a direct repeat separated by four nucleotides (DR-4 motif). Addition of a coactivator (SRC-1) completes the functional transcription unit. **B:** Endogenous 5α-androstanes (androstenol) inhibit CAR transcriptional activity by dissociation of the CAR-RXR-DNA complex from the nuclear receptor activator SRC-1. The degree to which this situation exists determines "normal" constitutive activity. **C:** In the presence of phenobarbital-type inducers, the binding of inhibitory androstanes to CAR-RXR is abolished. The CAR-RXR-DNA complex is then able to interact with the coactivator SRC-1 and reconstitute the functional transcription unit. Thus, phenobarbital induction represents "de-repression" or a reversal of androstane repression. (Adapted from Forman BM, Tzameli I, Choi H-S, et al. Androstane metabolites bind to and deactivate the nuclear receptor CAR-b. *Nature* 1998;395:612–615; and Sueyoshi T, Kawamoto T, Zelko I, et al. The repressed nuclear receptor CAR responds to phenobarbital in activating the human *CYP2B6* gene. *J Biol Chem* 1999;274:6043–6046.)

more, there were no significant differences in the urinary recovery of unchanged phenytoin, its major *p*-hydroxylated metabolite, or the dihydrodiol metabolite in the presence and absence of phenobarbital. Diamond and Buchanan (51) used single point determinations of phenytoin concentration to determine that the addition of phenobarbital to, or the removal of phenobarbital from, a stable regimen of phenytoin produced no change in phenytoin concentrations. However, because phenytoin is subject to saturable metabolism, inhibition by phenobarbital may be more likely to occur under conditions in which maximum induction has been achieved and phenytoin concentrations are in the high therapeutic range (49).

Lamotrigine. *N*-glucuronidation accounts for most (~80%) lamotrigine clearance in humans (52). Several pharmacokinetic studies (53–55) indicate that the lamotrigine half-life is shorter (~14 hours) in the presence of a CYP-inducing anticonvulsant such as phenobarbital, phenytoin, or carbamazepine compared with the combination of lamotrigine and valproic acid (40 to 45 hours) or triple therapy of lamotrigine plus an inducing anticonvulsant and valproic acid (~30 hours). Data from a therapeutic

drug monitoring service (56) provide further indirect evidence of induction of lamotrigine clearance. In this study, the lamotrigine serum concentration:dose ratio reportedly was lower in patients receiving the drug in combination with phenobarbital (ratio = 0.52), phenytoin (0.32), or carbamazepine (0.57), compared with monotherapy (0.98, *p* < .05). In the absence of metabolite data, however, alternative mechanisms for lower lamotrigine concentrations may also be operative.

Valproic Acid. In addition to the inhibitory effects of valproic acid on phenobarbital clearance, phenobarbital increases valproic acid clearance approximately 10% (57). Population-based kinetic studies also indicate that, compared with valproic acid monotherapy, serum concentrations of valproic acid are 25% lower when the drug is given with phenobarbital (58). Studies in children reveal similar results, although the effect of phenobarbital and other CYP inducers on valproic acid clearance is reported to be more pronounced and variable relative to that observed in adults (59).

An additional consideration with respect to phenobarbital interactions with valproic acid therapy is the role of induction by phenobarbital and other CYP-inducing antiepileptic drugs (carbamazepine and phenytoin) as risk factors for valproic acid–associated hepatotoxicity, primarily in young children. Retrospective studies of valproic acid–associated hepatotoxicity in the United States identified polytherapy with enzyme inducing antiepileptic medications as well as patient age <2 years, developmental delay, and coincident metabolic disorders as important risk factors for developing this adverse event (60–62). Although valproic acid–associated hepatotoxicity may occur at any age, data collected between 1978 and 1986 indicate that the risk of fatal hepatotoxicity is highest in children <2 years of age receiving concurrent anticonvulsant therapy; in these children, the incidence of this complication was estimated to be approximately 1:500 (60,61). This represents a 16-fold increase in risk relative to children of the same age receiving valproic acid monotherapy (1:8,000). Comparative estimates of risk for older children aged 3 to 10 years were 1:11,000 during monotherapy and 1:6,000 during polytherapy. Other studies confirmed polytherapy as a risk factor but found little difference in risk between younger (<3 years of age) and older children (3 to 6 years of age) (63,64).

CYP isoforms are responsible for the formation of the potentially reactive metabolite, 4-ene-valproic acid, and this activity is inducible by phenobarbital (65). Further work has specifically implicated CYP2C9 and, to a lesser extent, CYP2A6 in the formation of 4-ene-valproic acid in humans (66). Induction of CYP2A6 and CYP2C9 activities by phenobarbital has not been as rigorously evaluated as has CYP3A4 activity, although modest increases in CYP2C immunoreactive proteins have been observed after phenobarbital treatment of cultured primary human hepatocytes (27,67). Given the comparative variabilities of CYP2A6 activity (30-fold) and CYP2C9 activity (less than fivefold) in human liver microsomes (68), it has been proposed that CYP2C9 may be responsible for most constitutive VPA 4-ene-desaturation, whereas CYP2A6 plays a greater role during polytherapy with anticonvulsants (66). Nevertheless, phenobarbital treatment represents a significant risk factor for the development of valproic acid–associated hepatotoxicity, particularly in children <2 years of age.

Other Antiepileptic Agents. Approximately 50% to 100% increases in dose are recommended for ethosuximide, felbamate, topiramate, zonisamide, and tiagabine when phenobarbital is added to the treatment regimen (49).

Interactions with Other Medications

Calcium Channel Blockers. The apparent clearance of a single oral dose of verapamil was reported to be increased fivefold after a 21-day course of phenobarbital. When verapamil was administered intravenously, total drug clearance was increased 200%, whereas free drug clearance was unchanged (69). In a study that considered the effect of the CYP-inducing antiepileptic drugs carbamazepine, pheny-

toin, and phenobarbital collectively on the disposition of nimodipine, significantly (90%) lower peak concentration and AUC values and a 57% shorter half-life were observed in the anticonvulsant-treated group (70). A similar evaluation of felodipine suggested a reduction in peak concentration and AUC by 82% and 94%, respectively (71). In a study in which a single dose of nifedipine was used as a phenotyping probe for CYP3A4 activity, its clearance was increased by 270% (72). Collectively, the data indicate that bioavailability of calcium channel antagonists is considerably compromised by concurrent administration of phenobarbital, possibly because of induction of intestinal CYP3A isoforms.

Cimetidine. Long-term phenobarbital administration (100 mg/day for 21 days) increased total body clearance of intravenous cimetidine by an average of 18%, an effect that was largely the result of a 37% increase in nonrenal clearance that was accompanied by increased renal excretion of the sulfoxide metabolite of cimetidine. In the same study, the AUC of orally administered cimetidine was reduced by 15% by the same phenobarbital treatment regimen. The amount of cimetidine and its sulfoxide metabolite excreted in urine were reduced by ~30%, a finding consistent either with impaired absorption or, more likely, with induction of intestinal drug biotransformation (73).

Clozapine. Phenobarbital treatment was associated with 33% lower plasma clozapine concentrations in a group of patients with schizophrenia compared with a control group matched for sex, age, and body weight who were treated with clozapine alone. Concentrations of clozapine *N*-oxide were increased more than twofold in the phenobarbital-treated group compared with the control group, whereas norclozapine concentrations did not differ between the two groups (74). These results are consistent with induction of CYP3A4, the CYP isoform primarily responsible for *N*-oxidation of clozapine (75,76).

Corticosteroids. In a study comparing the pharmacokinetics of prednisolone in subjects receiving phenobarbital and phenytoin, alone or in combination, versus controls receiving no concurrent medications, prednisolone half-life was significantly shorter (32%) and total body clearance was significantly greater (44%) in the anticonvulsant-treated group, whereas volume of distribution and protein binding were unchanged. Additionally, patients receiving anticonvulsants had more than a twofold mean elevation in their early morning hydrocortisone peak concentrations, a finding suggesting that the concurrent administration of anticonvulsant enzyme inducer with an exogenously administered corticosteroid resulted in less suppression of the hypothalamic-pituitary-axis and a more normal circadian rhythm of endogenous steroid production (77). Similarly, prednisolone half-life was 25% shorter in patients with rheumatoid arthritis and was accompanied by symptoms of disease exacerbation (e.g., articular index worsened by 31%, pain score doubled, duration of morning stiffness increased 117%) with the addition of phenobarbital (78).

In 16 asthmatic patients before and 3 weeks after the initiation of phenobarbital, the half-life of intravenously administered dexamethasone decreased significantly (45%) and clearance increased significantly (87%) over prephenobarbital values (79). The authors also described three subjects in whom pulmonary function, eosinophilia, and clinical degree of bronchospasm deteriorated while they received phenobarbital, with subsequent improvement in these measurements on discontinuation of the drug. Similar changes in pharmacokinetic parameters have been reported for intravenously administered methylprednisolone, although changes in the pharmacokinetics of the more water-soluble methylprednisolone sodium hemisuccinate were less dramatic (80). The clinical significance of enzyme induction is most evident in transplant recipients in whom evidence of decreased graft survival and increased risk of graft failure have been demonstrated in patients receiving anticonvulsant enzyme inducers compared with control transplant recipients receiving no such agents (81).

Cyclosporine. Phenobarbital therapy has the potential to produce clinically significant changes in cyclosporine pharmacokinetics. Subtherapeutic cyclosporine concentrations were observed in a pediatric transplant recipient who was receiving concurrent phenobarbital treatment, but these concentrations increased as the dose of phenobarbital was reduced (82). Similarly, a 70% reduction in the clearance of cyclosporine (from 12.6 to 3.8 mL/min/kg) was observed when phenobarbital was discontinued from the regimen of a pediatric renal transplant recipient (83).

Metronidazole. Several authors report failure of metronidazole treatment in cases of vaginal trichomoniasis and giardiasis when phenobarbital is prescribed concurrently. Consequently, an increase in dose is necessary to effect a microbiologic cure (84,85). In a crossover study of six patients with chronic disease, metronidazole AUC and half-life were significantly decreased by 30% and 23%, respectively. No significant difference in apparent volume of distribution was observed, although the AUC of the hydroxy metabolite was increased by 29% (86).

Oral Contraceptives. The potential for decreased efficacy of oral contraceptive therapy secondary to the use of enzyme-inducing anticonvulsants has been recognized since 1980 (87,88). This interaction has frequently been attributed to enhanced metabolism of both estrogenic and progestin components, but alterations in protein binding, specifically serum hormone binding globulin, also appear to be involved. In a prospective evaluation of plasma ethynyl estradiol concentrations in the presence and absence of phe-

nobarbital, two of four subjects demonstrated 64% and 72% reductions from baseline values. However, the overall change for all subjects was not statistically significant, given only a moderate decrease in the third subject and an increase in ethynyl estradiol concentrations in the fourth. In contrast, serum hormone binding globulin capacity increased 15% to 49% in all subjects after the administration of phenobarbital. Of clinical interest, breakthrough bleeding developed in the women who demonstrated reductions in plasma ethynyl estradiol concentrations (87). Thus, a pharmacodynamic interaction can be expected with the concurrent administration of oral contraceptives and phenobarbital; however, whether this is a result of alterations in metabolism or a consequence of altered protein binding remains to be elucidated.

Teniposide. Long-term treatment with CYP-inducing antiepileptic agents, including phenobarbital, increases the systemic clearance of the epipodophyllotoxin chemotherapeutic agent teniposide in pediatric patients with leukemia. Compared with control patients matched for age at diagnosis, sex, and race but not receiving antiepileptic drug therapy, teniposide clearance was two- to threefold higher in the treated patients (89). The dramatic reduction in systemic teniposide exposure has been associated with reduced efficacy as measured by significantly worse event-free survival, hematologic relapse, and CNS relapse with hazard ratios ranging from 2.67 to 3.4 (90). The mechanism of this interaction likely involves induction of CYP3A4 (possibly CYP3A5 as well), the CYP primarily responsible for *O*-demethylation of teniposide and etoposide to form their respective catechol metabolites (91). Thus, a similar interaction between phenobarbital, phenytoin, or carbamazepine and etoposide may also be anticipated.

Theophylline. Although theophylline disposition is generally considered to be the result of CYP1A2-mediated biotransformation (92,93), evidence suggests that phenobarbital increases its clearance in older children and adults. In one crossover study with six subjects, theophylline clearance increased 34% after phenobarbital coadministration (94). In seven pediatric patients with asthma, theophylline clearance increased by 42%, and average steady-state concentrations decreased by 30% (95). In contrast, no change in the clearance and dose requirements of aminophylline were observed in premature neonates receiving the agent alone or in combination with phenobarbital (96).

Warfarin. In three subjects administered *R*-warfarin or *S*-warfarin on separate occasions before and concurrently with phenobarbital, the clearance of each enantiomer increased by 65% and 50%, respectively, and was accompanied by approximately 40% decreases in half-lives (97). The increased warfarin clearance has also been observed to result in an approximately 25% decrease in prothrombin time over a 3-week period (98). CYP2C9 appears to be the principal form of human hepatic CYP modulating levels of the pharmacologically more active *S*-enantiomer with a minor contribution from CYP3A4, whereas CYP3A4 and CYP1A2 are primary determinants of *R*-warfarin biotransformation (99). The lack of stereospecificity suggests that multiple CYP pathways are induced, whereas the decreased pharmacologic effects are consistent with CYP2C9 induction. Regardless of CYP isoforms induced, studies with phenobarbital and other barbiturates indicate that induction may persist for 3 or 4 weeks after drug discontinuation (100).

Interactions between Phenobarbital and Nutrients

Folic Acid. The role of reduced folic acid levels and adverse fetal outcomes, such as neural tube defects, is well documented (101,102). Mean serum folate concentrations were found to be significantly lower in patients treated with phenobarbital (3.91±1.73 ng/mL, $p < .01$) and carbamazepine (3.85±1.02 ng/mL, $p < .01$) compared with age-matched controls not treated with antiepileptic agents (5.14±1.88 ng/mL). Neither valproic acid nor zonisamide was associated with folate depletion (103). In addition to maintaining pregnant patients seizure free with the lowest possible dose of antiepileptic agents, folic acid supplementation (5 mg/day) should be implemented 3 months before conception (101,102).

SUMMARY

As a general rule, phenobarbital has the potential to increase the clearance of any drug that is primarily dependent on CYP3A4 activity (and possibly CYP2C9 activity) for most of its elimination from the body. However, there are also cases in which these anticonvulsants have been reported to induce the metabolism of drugs primarily metabolized by CYP isoforms other than CYP3A4. For example, phenobarbital has been reported to increase desipramine clearance by 30% and to produce a comparable increase in 2-hydroxydesipramine formation, a CYP2D6-dependent metabolite (104). However, no convincing evidence of CYP2D6 induction by "enzyme-inducing" anticonvulsants is available that would allow the "induction" to be attributed to CYP2D6. Therefore, one must recognize that each individual patient has his or her own unique complement of CYP isoforms expressed in their liver and other tissues, and the potential consequences of induction in that patient will depend on the CYP isoforms that are quantitatively most important for the disposition of the drug in question. Recognition that additional factors such as the therapeutic index of the drug in question, the presence and contribution of numerous competing drug biotransformation pathways, and the pharmacologic or toxicologic potential of the metabolites produced also contribute to the overall clinical significance of a drug–drug interaction will help to minimize unexpected adverse responses in patients when enzyme-inducing anticonvulsants such as phenobarbital are added to existing treatment regimens.

REFERENCES

1. Nelson E, Powell JR, Conrad K, et al. Phenobarbital pharmacokinetics and bioavailability in adults. *J Clin Pharmacol* 1982;22:141–148.
2. Neuvonen PJ, Elonen E. Effect of activated charcoal on absorption and elimination of phenobarbitone, carbamazepine and phenylbutazone in man. *Eur J Clin Pharmacol* 1980;17:51–57.
3. Berg MJ, Berlinder WG, Goldberg MJ, et al. Acceleration of the body clearance of phenobarbital by oral activated charcoal. *NEngl J Med* 1982;307:642–644.
4. Berg MJ, Rose JQ, Wurster DE, et al. Effect of charcoal and corbitol-charcoal suspension on the elimination of intravenous phenobarbital. *Ther Drug Monit* 1987;9:41–47.
5. Frenia ML, Schauben JL, Wears RL, et al. Multiple-dose activated charcoal compared to urinary alkalinization for the enhancement of phenobarbital elimination. *J Toxicol Clin Toxicol* 1996;34:169–175.
6. Wakabayashi Y, Maruyama S, Hachimura K, et al. Activated charcoal interrupts enterohepatic circulation of phenobarbital. *J Toxicol Clin Toxicol* 1994;32:419–424.
7. Nishihara K, Kaysuyoski U, Saitoh Y, et al. Estimation of plasma unbound phenobarbital concentration by using mixed saliva. *Epilepsia* 1979;20:37–45.
8. Hargreaves JA, Howald WN, Racha JK, et al. Identification of enzymes responsible for the metabolism of phenobarbital. *ISSX Proc* 1996;10:259.
9. Koup JR, Gibaldi M, McNamara P, et al. Interaction of chloramphenicol with phenytoin and phenobarbital. *Clin Pharmacol Ther* 1978;24:571–575.
10. Callaghan N, Feely M, Duggan F, et al. The effect of anticonvulsant drugs which induce liver microsomal enzymes on derived and ingested phenobarbitone levels. *Acta Neurol Scand* 1977;56:1–6.
11. Eadie MJ, Lander CM, Hooper WD, et al. Factors influencing plasma phenobarbitone levels in epileptic patients. *Br J Clin Pharmacol* 1977;4:541–547.
12. Glue P, Banfield CR, Perhach JL, et al. Pharmacokinetic interactions with felbamate: *in vitro–in vivo* correlation. *Clin Pharmacokinet* 1997;33:214–224.
13. Reidenberg P, Glue P, Banfield C. Effects of felbamate on the pharmacokinetics of phenobarbital. *Clin Pharmacol Ther* 1995;58:279–287.
14. Wilder BJ, Willmore LJ, Bruni J, et al. Valproic acid: interaction with other anticonvulsant drugs. *Neurology* 1978;28:892–896.
15. Patel IH, Levy RH, Cutler RE. Phenobarbital-valproic acid interaction. *Clin Pharmacol Ther* 1980;27:515–521.
16. Kapetanovic IM, Kupferberg HJ, Porter RJ, et al. Mechanisms of valproate-phenobarbital interaction in epileptic patients. *Clin Pharmacol Ther* 1981;29:480–486.
17. Yukawa E, To H, Ohdo S, et al. Detection of a drug–drug interaction on population-based phenobarbitaone clearance using nonlinear mixed-effects modeling. *Eur J Clin Pharmacol* 1998;54:69–74.
18. Bruni J, Wilder BJ, Perchalski RJ, et al. Valproic acid and plasma levels of phenobarbital. *Neurology* 1980;30:94–97.

19. Fernandez de Gatta MR, Alonso Gonzalez AC, Garcia Sanchez MJ, et al. Effect of sodium valproate on phenobarbital serum levels in children and adults. *Ther Drug Monit* 1986;8:416–420.

20. Yukawa E, Higuchi S, Aoyama T. The effect of concurrent administration of sodium valproate on serum levels of primidone and its metabolite phenobarbital. *J Clin Pharmacol Ther* 1989;14:387–392.

21. Gambie D, Johnson R. The effects of phenytoin on phenobarbitone and primidone metabolism. *J Neurol Neurosurg Psychiatr* 1981;44:148–151.

22. Fincham R, Schottelius D, Sahs A. The influence of diphenylhydantoin on primidone metabolism. *Arch Neurol* 1974;30:259–262.

23. Conney AH. Pharmacological implications of microsomalenzyme induction. *Pharmacol Rev* 1967;19:317–366.

24. Waxman DJ, Azaroff L. Phenobarbital induction of cytochrome P-450 gene expression. *Biochem J* 1992;281:577–592.

25. Morel F, Beaune P, Ratanasavanh D, et al. Effects of various inducers on the expression of cytochromes *P-450* IIC8, 9, 10 and IIIA in cultured adult human hepatocytes. *Toxicol In Vitro* 1990;4:458–460.

26. Morel F, Beaune PH, Ratanasavanh D, et al. Expression of cytochrome P-450 enzymes in cultured human hepatocytes. *Eur J Biochem* 1990;191:437–444.

27. Donato MT, Gómez-Lechón MJ, Castell JV. Effect of model inducers on cytochrome P450 activities of human hepatocytes in primary culture. *Drug Metab Dispos* 1995;23:553–558.

27a. Chang TKH, Yu L, Maurel O, Waxman DJ. Enhanced cyclophosphamide and ifosfamide activation in primary human hepatocyte cultures: response to cytochrome P-450 inducers and autoinduction by oxazaphosphorines. *Cancer Res* 1997;57:1946–1954.

28. Schuetz EG, Schuetz JD, Strom SC, et al. Regulation of human liver cytochromes P-450 in family 3A in primary and continuous culture of human hepatocytes. *Hepatology* 1993;18:1254–1262.

29. Bock KW, Bock-Hennig BS. Differential induction of human liver UDP-glucuronosyltransferase activities by phenobarbital-type inducers. *Biochem Pharmacol* 1987;36:4137–4143.

30. Doostdar H, Grant MH, Melvin WT, et al. The effects of inducing agents on cytochrome P450 and UDP-glucuronsyltransferase activities in human HepG2 hepatoma cells. *Biochem Pharmacol* 1993;46:629–635.

31. Morel F, Fardel O, Meyer DJ, et al. Preferential increase of glutathione *S*-transferase class a transcripts in cultured human hepatocytes by phenobarbital, 3-methylcholanthrene, and dithiolethiones. *Cancer Res* 1993;53:231–234.

32. Hassett C, Laurenzana EM, Sidhu JS, et al. Effects of chemical inducers on human microsomal epoxide hydrolase in primary hepatocyte cultures. *Biochem Pharmacol* 1998;55:1059–1069.

33. Li AP, Maurel P, Gomez-Lechon MJ, et al. Preclinical evaluation of drug–drug interaction potential: present status of the application of primary human hepatocytes in the evaluation of cytochrome P450 induction. *Chem Biol Interact* 1997;107:5–16.

34. Ged C, Rouillon JM, Pichard L, et al. The increase in urinary excretion of 6 beta-hydroxycortisol as a marker of human hepatic cytochrome P450IIA induction. *Br J Clin Pharmacol* 1989;28:373–387.

35. Saenger P, Forster E, Kream J. 6β-Hydroxycortisol: a noninvasive indicator of enzyme induction. *J Clin Endocrinol Metab* 1981;52:381–384.

36. Saenger P. 6β-Hydroxycortisol in random urine samples as an indicator of enzyme induction. *Clin Pharmacol Ther* 1983;34:818–821.

37. Ohnhaus EE, Breckenridge AM, Park BK. Urinary excretion of 6β-hydroxycortisol and the time course measurement of induction of man. *Eur J Clin Pharmacol* 1989;36:39–46.

38. Eichelbaum M, Mineshita S, Ohnhaus EE, et al. The influence of enzyme induction of polymorphic sparteine oxidation. *Br J Clin Pharmacol* 1986;22:49–53.

39. Leclercq V, Desager JP, Horsmans Y, et al. Influence of rifampicin, phenobarbital and cimetidine on mixed function monooxygenase in extensive and poor metabolizers of debrisoquine. *Int J Clin Pharmacol Ther Toxicol* 1989;27:593–598.

40. Lehmann JM, McKee DD, Watson MA, et al. The human orphan nuclear receptor PXR is activated by compounds that regulate *CYP3A4* gene expression and cause drug interactions. *J Clin Invest* 1998;1998:1016–1023.

41. Goodwin B, Hodgson E, Liddle C. The orphan human pregnane X receptor mediates the transcriptionalactivation of *CYP3A4* by rifampicin through a distal enhancer module. *Mol Pharmacol* 1999;56:1329–1339.

42. Forman BM, Tzameli I, Choi H-S, et al. Androstane metabolites bind to and deactivate the nuclear receptor CAR-β. *Nature* 1998;395:612–615.

43. Sueyoshi T, Kawamoto T, Zelko I, et al. The repressed nuclear receptor CAR responds to phenobarbital in activating the human *CYP2B6* gene. *J Biol Chem* 1999;274:6043–6046.

44. Moore LB, Parks DJ, Jones SA, et al. Orphan nuclear receptors constitutive androstane receptor and pregnane X receptor share xenobiotic and steroid ligands. *J Biol Chem* 2000;275:15122–15127.

45. Christiansen J, Dam M. Influence of phenobarbital and diphenylhydantoin on plasma carbamazepine levels in patients with epilepsy. *Acta Neurol Scand* 1973;49:543–546.

46. Ramsay R, McManus D, Guterman A, et al. Carbamazepine metabolism in humans: effect of concurrent anticonvulsant therapy. *Ther Drug Monit* 1990;12:235–241.

47. Liu H, Delgado MR. Interactions of phenobarbital and phenytoin with carbamazepine and its metabolites' concentrations, concentration ratios, and level/dose ratios in epileptic children. *Epilepsia* 1995;36:249–254.

48. Riva R, Contin M, Albani F, et al. Free concentration of carbamazepine and carbamazepine-10,11-epoxide in children and adults: influence of age and phenobarbitone co-medication. *Clin Pharmacokinet* 1985;10:524–531.

49. Riva R, Albani F, Contin M, et al. Pharmacokinetic interactions between antiepileptic drugs: clinical considerations. *Clin Pharmacokinet* 1996;31:470–493.

50. Browne T, Szabo G, Evans J, et al. Phenobarbital does not alter phenytoin steady-state serum concentration or pharmacokinetics. *Neurology* 1988;38:639–642.

51. Diamond W, Buchanan R. A clinical study of the effect of phenobarbital on diphenylhydantoin plasma levels. *J Clin Pharmacol* 1970;10:306–311.

52. Rambeck B, Wolf P. Lamotrigine clinical pharmacokinetics. *Clin Pharmacokinet* 1993;25:433–443.

53. Binnie CD, van Emde Boas W, Kasteleijn-Nolste-Trenite DG, et al. Acute effects of lamotrigine (BW430C) in persons with epilepsy. *Epilepsia* 1986;27:248–254.

54. Jawad S, Yuen WC, Peck AW, et al. Lamotrigine: single-dose pharmacokinetics and initial 1 week experience in refractory epilepsy. *Epilepsy Res* 1987;1:194–201.

55. Eriksson AS, Hoppu K, Nergårdh A, et al. Pharmacokinetic interactions between lamotrigine and other antiepileptic drugs in children with intractable epilepsy. *Epilepsia* 1996;37:769–773.

56. May TW, Rambeck B, Jurgens U. Serum concentrations of lam-

otrigine in epileptic patients: the influence of dose and comedication. *Ther Drug Monitor* 1996;18:523–531.

57. Yukawa E, To H, Ohdo S, et al. Population-based investigation of valproic acid relative clearance using nonlinear mixed effects modeling: influence of drug–drug interaction and patient characteristics. *J Clin Pharmacol* 1997;37:1160–1167.

58. May T, Rambeck B. Serum concentration of valproic acid: influence of dose and comedication. *Ther Drug Monit* 1985;7:387–390.

59. Cloyd JC, Fischer JH, Kriel RL, et al. Valproic acid pharmacokinetics in children. IV. Effects of age and antiepileptic drugs on protein binding and intrinsic clearance. *Clin Pharmacol Ther* 1993;53:22–29.

60. Dreifuss FE, Santilli N, Langer DH, et al. Valproic acid hepatic fatalities: a retrospective review. *Neurology* 1987;37:379–385.

61. Dreifuss FE, Langer DH, Moline KA, et al. Valproic acid hepatic fatalities. II. US experience since 1984. *Neurology* 1989;39:201–207.

62. Bryant AE, Dreifuss FE. Valproic acid hepatic fatalities. III. U.S. experience since 1986. *Neurology* 1996;46:465–469.

63. Scheffner D, König S, Rauterberg-Ruland I, et al. Fatal liver failure in 16 children with valproate therapy. *Epilepsia* 1988;29:530–542.

64. König SA, Siemes H, Bläker F, et al. Severe hepatotoxicity during valproate therapy: an update and report of eight new fatalities. *Epilepsia* 1994;35:1005–1015.

65. Rettie AE, Rettenmeier AW, Howald WN, et al. Cytochrome P-450-catalyzed formation of D^4-VPA, a toxic metabolite of valproic acid. *Science* 1987;235:890–893.

66. Sadeque AJM, Fisher MB, Korzekwa KR, et al. Human CYP2C9 and CYP2A6 mediate formation of the hepatotoxin 4-ene-valproic acid. *J Pharmacol Exp Ther* 1997;283:698–703.

67. Chang TKH, Maurel P, et al. Enhanced cyclophosphamide and ifosfamide activation in primary human hepatocyte cultures: response to cytochrome P-450 inducers and autoinduction by oxazaphosphorines. *Cancer Res* 1997;57:1946–1954.

68. Wrighton SA, Brian WR, Sari M-A, et al. Studies on the expression and metabolic capabilities of human liver cytochrome P450IIIA5 (HLp3). *Mol Pharmacol* 1990;38:207–213.

69. Rutledge DR, Pieper JA and Mirvis DM. Effects of chronic phenobarbital on verapamil disposition in humans. *J Pharmacol Exp Ther* 1988;246:7–13.

70. Tartara A, Galimberti C, Manni R, et al. Differential effects of valproic acid and enzyme-inducing anticonvulsants on nimodipine pharmacokinetics in epileptic patients. *Br J Clin Pharmacol* 1991;32:335–340.

71. Capewell S, Freestone S, Critchley J, et al. Reduced felodipine bioavailability in patients taking anticonvulsants. *Lancet* 1988, 480–482.

72. Schellens JH, van der Wart JH, Brugman M, et al. Influence of enzyme induction and inhibition on the oxidation of nifedipine, sparteine, mephenytoin and antipyrine in humans as assessed by a "cocktail" study design. *J Pharmacol Exp Ther* 1989;249:638–645.

73. Somogyi A, Thielscher S, Gugler R. Influence of phenobarbital on cimetidine kinetics. *Eur J Clin Pharmacol* 1981;19:343–347.

74. Facciolà G, Avenoso A, Spina E, et al. Inducing effect of phenobarbital on clozapine metabolism in patients with chronic schizophrenia. *Ther Drug Monit* 1998;20:628–630.

75. Eiermann B, Engel G, Johansson I, et al. The involvement of CYP1A2 and CYP3A4 in the metabolism of clozapine. *Br J Clin Pharmacol* 1997;44:439–446.

76. Tugnait M, Hawes EM, McKay G, et al. Characterization of the human hepatic cytochromes P450 involved in the *in vitro* oxidation of clozapine. *Chem Biol Interact* 1999;118:171–189.

77. Gambertoglio J, Holford N, Kapusnik J, et al. Disposition of total and unbound prednisolone in renal transplant patients receiving anticonvulsants. *Kidney Int* 1984;25:119–123.

78. Brooks P, Buchanan W, Grove M, et al. Effects of enzyme induction on metabolism of prednisolone: clinical and laboratory study. *Ann Rheum Dis* 1976;35:339–343.

79. Brooks S, Werk E, Ackerman S, et al. Adverse effects of phenobarbital on corticosteroid metabolism in patients with bronchial asthma. *N Engl J Med* 1972;286:1125–1128.

80. Stjernholm M, Katz F. Effects of diphenylhydantoin, phenobarbital, and diazepam on the metabolism of methylprednisolone and its sodium succinate. *J Clin Endocrinol Metab* 1975;41:887–893.

81. Wassner S, Pennisi A, Malekzadeh M, et al. The adverse effect of anticonvulsant therapy on renal allograft survival: a preliminary report. *J Pediatr* 1976;88:134–137.

82. Carstensen H, Jacobsen N, Dieperink H. Interaction between cyclosporin A and phenobarbitone. *Br J Clin Pharmacol* 1986;21:550–551.

83. Burckart G, Venkataramanan R, Starzl T, et al. Cyclosporin clearance in children following organ transplantation. *J Clin Pharmacol* 1984;24:412(abst).

84. Mead P, Gibson M, Schentag J, et al. Possible alteration of metronidazole metabolism by phenobarbital. *N Engl J Med* 1982;306.

85. Gupte S. Phenobarbital and metabolism of metronidazole. *N Engl J Med* 1983;308:529.

86. Eradiri O, Jamali F, Thomson A. Interaction of metronidazole with phenobarbital, cimetidine, prednisone, and sulfasalazine in Crohn's disease. *Biopharm Drug Dispos* 1988;9:219–227.

87. Back D, Bates M, Bowden A, et al. The interaction of phenobarbital and other anticonvulsants with oral contraceptives. *Contraception* 1980;22:495–503.

88. Shane-McWorter L, Cerveny JD, MacFarlane LL, et al. Enhanced metabolism of levonorgestrel during phenobarbital treatment and resultant pregnancy. *Pharmacotherapy* 1998;18:1360–1364.

89. Baker DK, Relling MV, Pui C-H, et al. Increased teniposide clearance with concomitant anticonvulsant therapy. *J Clin Oncol* 1992;10:311–315.

90. Relling MV, Nemec J, Schuetz EG, et al. O-Demethylation of epipodophyllotoxins is catalyzed by human cytochrome P450 3A4. *Mol Pharmacol* 1994;45:352–358.

91. Relling MV, Pui CH, Sandlund JT, et al. Adverse effect of anticonvulsants on efficacy of chemotherapy for acute lymphoblastic leukaemia. *Lancet* 2000;356:285–290.

92. Sarkar MA, Hunt C, Guzelian PS, et al. Characterization of human liver cytochromes P-450 involved in theophylline metabolism. *Drug Metab Dispos* 1992;20:31–37.

93. Zhang Z-Y, Kaminsky LS. Characterization of human cytochromes P450 involved in theophylline 8-hydroxylation. *Biochem Pharmacol* 1995;50:205–211.

94. Landay R, Gonzalez M, Taylor J. Effect of phenobarbital on theophylline disposition. *J Allergy Clin Immunol* 1978;62:27–29.

95. Saccar C, Danish M, Ragni M, et al. The effect of phenobarbital on theophylline disposition in children with asthma. *J Allergy Clin Immunol* 1985;75:716–719.

96. Kandrotas R, Cranfield T, Gal P, et al. Effect of phenobarbital administration on theophylline clearance in premature neonates. *Ther Drug Monit* 1990;12:139–143.

97. Orme M, Breckenridge A. Enantiomers of warfarin and phenobarbital. *New Engl J Med* 1976;295:1482.

98. Udall J. Clinical implications of warfarin interactions with five sedatives. *Am J Cardiol* 1975;35:67–71.

99. Rettie AE, Korzekwa KR, Kunze KL, et al. Hydroxylation of

warfarin by human cDNA-expressed ctochrome P-450: A role for P-4502C9 in the etiology of (*S*)-warfarin-drug interactions. *Chem Res Toxicol* 1992;5:54–59.

100. Cropp JS, Bussey HI. A review of enzyme induction of warfarin metabolism with recommendations for patient management. *Pharmacotherapy* 1997;17:917–928.

101. Lewis DP, Van Dyke DC, Stumbo PJ, et al. Drug and environment factors associated with adverse pregnancy outcomes. I. Antiepileptic drugs, contraceptives, smoking and folate. *Ann Pharmacother* 1998;32:802–817.

102. Nulman I, Laslo D, Koren G. Treatment of epilepsy in pregnancy. *Drugs* 1999;57:535–544.

103. Kishi T, Fujita N, Eguchi T, et al. Mechanism for reduction of serum folate by antiepileptic drugs during prolonged therapy. *J Neurol Sci* 1997;145:109–112.

104. Spina E, Avenoso A, Campo G, et al. Phenobarbital induces the 2-hydroxylation of desipramine. *Ther Drug Monit* 1996;18:60–64.

105. Goldberg MR, Lo MW, Deutsch PJ, et al. Phenobarbital minimally alters plasm concentrations of losartan and its active metabolite E-3174. *Clin Pharmacol Ther* 1996;59:268–274.

PHENOBARBITAL AND OTHER BARBITURATES

CLINICAL EFFICACY AND USE IN EPILEPSY

MICHEL BAULAC

The longevity of phenobarbital is extraordinary, in the way in which it continues to coexist with successive generations of antiepileptic drugs introduced to the market throughout the twentieth century. Although phenobarbital was previously used as a hypnotic and a tranquilizer, its antiepileptic properties were discovered in 1912, and it became a major first-line drug in the years between World War I and World War II. Then it lost ground progressively as newer drugs took its place, but it nevertheless remained among the most frequently used antiepileptic drugs in Europe. Phenobarbital is still a first-choice drug in developing countries for evident reasons of availability and cost. Even though this drug has been used as an antiepileptic agent for 90 years, evaluating its benefit:risk ratio remains relatively difficult, particularly because very few studies comply with the current standards, and comparisons with other antiepileptic drugs are not available in all clinical situations. Reports are sometimes conflicting, and most of the current knowledge relies on clinical experience. Phenobarbital presents broad-spectrum antiepileptic activity against all seizure types, except absences. Its efficacy appears, in the few comparative studies, either equivalent to or only slightly inferior to that of the other major established agents. However, its potential for inducing sedation and cognitive and behavioral changes limits its clinical use, particularly in children and in countries where many other therapeutic options are available. However, the advantages of phenobarbital remain: single daily dose, predictable pharmacokinetics, low systemic toxicity, and low cost. Furthermore, with its parenteral formulations, phenobarbital continues to occupy an important place in the treatment of status epilepticus. It can be anticipated, however, that the latest generation of antiepileptic drugs, introduced in the 1990s, will further reduce interest in phenobarbital, especially at a time when the emphasis is on improved safety and tolerability.

SPECTRUM OF EFFICACY

Phenobarbital is widely used in the treatment of localization-related epilepsies; it is effective against simple partial, complex partial, and secondarily generalized seizures (1–3). It is also efficacious against some seizure types of the generalized epilepsies, particularly generalized tonic-clonic, tonic, and clonic seizures. It is ineffective against, and may even aggravate, absence seizures, although it phenobarbital sometimes coprescribed with ethosuximide in patients with absence epilepsy to control concomitantly occurring generalized tonic-clonic seizures. Phenobarbital is also widely used in special situations such as neonatal seizures and generalized tonic-clonic status epilepticus.

CONTROLLED TRIALS IN ADULTS

The assessment of phenobarbital's efficacy is largely based on clinical practice, and relatively little information can be obtained from controlled trials. Among the rare publications, one of the most significant is by Mattson et al. (1). In a multicenter, double-blind trial, the efficacy and tolerability of carbamazepine, phenytoin, phenobarbital, and primidone were compared in 622 adults. These patients were randomly assigned to one of these drugs and were followed-up for 2 years or until the drug failed to control seizures or caused unacceptable adverse effects. Patients had been previously untreated (58%) or undertreated, and they had simple or complex partial seizures (265 patients) or secondarily generalized tonic-clonic seizures (357 patients) as their predominant seizure type. The overall treatment success rate, expressed in terms of retention on the allocated treatment, was highest with carbamazepine or phenytoin, it was intermediate with phenobarbital, and it was lowest with primidone. Differences in failure rates were mostly explained by the poorer tolerability of primidone and phenobarbital. Phenobarbital was as effective as the three other drugs in patients with tonic-clonic seizures, but carbamazepine was significantly more effective in the treatment of partial

Michel Baulac, MD: Hôpital de la Salpetriere, Bat. P. Castaigne, Paris, France

seizures. There was no statistical difference between phenobarbital and the other drugs with regard to the number of seizures in all patients at 12, 24, and 36 months, and there was also no difference between the time that therapeutic levels were achieved and the first recurrence of seizures. Total seizure control was obtained only in 30% of the patients during the first 12 months, a finding that underlines that the population enrolled in this study was different from the usual populations of patients with newly diagnosed epilepsy in whom the expectancy for seizure control is higher, 47% with a first drug (4). Complete control of tonic-clonic seizures was similar (carbamazepine, 48%; phenytoin, 43%; phenobarbital, 43%; and primidone, 45%). The complete control of partial seizures, however, was significantly better with carbamazepine than with phenobarbital (33%) or primidone (26%) at 18 months.

Another prospective randomized pragmatic trial assessed the comparative efficacy and toxicity of four major antiepileptic drugs, used as monotherapy in patients with newly diagnosed epilepsy (5). Between 1981 and 1987, 243 patients aged ≥16 years, with a minimum of two previously untreated tonic-clonic seizures or partial seizures with or without secondary generalization, were randomly allocated to treatment with phenobarbital, phenytoin, carbamazepine, or sodium valproate. The protocol was designed to conform with standard clinical practice. Efficacy was assessed by time to first seizure after the start of treatment and time to enter 1-year remission. The overall outcome with all of the four drugs was good, with 27% remaining seizure free and 76% entering 1-year remission by 3 years of follow-up. No significant differences among the four drugs were found for either measure of efficacy at 1, 2, or 3 years of follow-up, but this observation should be interpreted cautiously in view of the small sample size in each group. The overall incidence of unacceptable side effects, necessitating withdrawal of the randomized drug, was 10%. However, for the individual drugs, phenobarbital (22%) was more likely to be withdrawn than phenytoin (3%), carbamazepine (11%), and sodium valproate (5%). Some other studies have compared phenobarbital with carbamazepine, phenytoin, or primidone. Marjerrison et al. (6) compared phenobarbital and carbamazepine in 21 adult patients hospitalized on a long-term basis. One-half of the previous anticonvulsant and antipsychotic medication dose was replaced by a proportionate dose of double-blind capsule of either phenobarbital or carbamazepine. After 2 months, a crossover to the compound was effected and was maintained for 4 more months. No significant difference in the number of seizures per patient during the final months of each drug treatment phase was noted. White et al. (7), in a short double-blind study, found similar efficacy of phenobarbital, phenytoin, and primidone in 20 adult inpatients with partial seizures. All three drugs were more effective than placebo. Cereghino et al. (8) compared these three drugs in a prospective crossover double-blind study performed in 45 institutionalized drug-resistant adult patients with mainly focal and secondarily generalized tonic-clonic seizures. During each of the three 21-day treatment periods, one-third of the patients were assigned to receive phenobarbital (300 mg/day), one-third phenytoin (300 mg/day), and the other one-third carbamazepine (1,200 mg/day), as replacement for previous medication. In these patients, phenobarbital was equal in efficacy to carbamazepine or phenytoin. Benassi et al. (9) compared phenobarbital, phenytoin, and carbamazepine in a prospective double-blind crossover design in 18 patients with complex partial seizures and previous multiple-drug treatment. Phenobarbital and carbamazepine were more active than phenytoin and were associated with an improvement in 61%, 67%, and 32% of the cases, respectively.

CONTROLLED TRIALS IN CHILDREN

Mitchell and Chavez (2) administered phenobarbital or carbamazepine to 39 children with newly diagnosed partial seizures on a single-blind basis for 12 months. Dosage was adjusted to produce serum levels ranging from 15 to 24 μg/mL for phenobarbital and from 4 to 7 μg/mL for carbamazepine. Cognitive function and behavior were evaluated at the onset of the study and at 6- and 12-month follow-ups. There were no significant differences in outcome between the two groups; although carbamazepine caused more systemic problems (two rashes, one case of granulocytopenia), there was a nonstatistically significant trend toward better seizure control with carbamazepine. A long-term, randomized, open-label trial compared the efficacy and toxicity of four standard antiepileptic drugs used as monotherapy in children with newly diagnosed epilepsy (10a). Between 1981 and 1987, 167 children aged 3 to 16 years, who had had at least two previously untreated tonic-clonic or partial seizures, with or without secondary generalization, were randomly allocated to treatment with phenobarbital, phenytoin, carbamazepine, or sodium valproate. Six of the first 10 children randomized to phenobarbital had to be withdrawn from the study because of unacceptable, mostly behavioral, side effects, and it was considered unethical to assign further patients to phenobarbital treatment. More recently, phenobarbital was compared with phenytoin and with sodium valproate in a 2-year double-blind trial in 151 children (aged 4 to 12 years) with newly diagnosed epilepsy in India (10b). All children had generalized tonic-clonic seizures. The three drugs were equally effective in controlling seizures, but phenobarbital caused hyperactivity problems more frequently and was considered as a possible first-choice treatment only in preschool children.

MODE OF USE

Indications

Although in the past phenobarbital was widely employed as a sedative and tranquilizer, in many countries it is now used almost exclusively for the treatment of epilepsy. The drug is employed in the following indications:

1. Generalized epilepsies, but within this category mainly for tonic, clonic, and tonic-clonic seizures. Phenobarbital is ineffective against absence seizures and may even aggravate them (10c). Valproate and lamotrigine are usually considered to be the preferred agents for generalized epilepsies; phenobarbital and its derivatives are considered as second-line agents with reasonable efficacy, but, for most patients, less desirable toxicity profiles, particularly with regard to the effect of sedation and, in children, behavioral disturbances.

2. Partial or localization-related epilepsies, whether or not the seizures become secondarily generalized. In this situation, phenobarbital has reasonable efficacy, but some trials suggest that it may be slightly less effective than carbamazepine, phenytoin, or valproate, and with a rather less acceptable toxicity profile.

3. Convulsive status epilepticus. In these patients, intravenous benzodiazepines (e.g., diazepam, lorazepam, clonazepam) and phenytoin (or fosphenytoin) are usually the preferred agents. Phenobarbital, however, is a possible first-line alternative, and it can be effective when other therapies fail (11). It produces temporary sedation, but this is an acceptable price to pay for control of a life-threatening situation such as status epilepticus.

4. Neonatal seizures, for which phenobarbital and phenytoin are the agents usually recommended. This is partly because both are marketed in preparations suitable for parenteral use, and in neonates it is often necessary to administer antiepileptic therapy by injection.

In terms of age range, phenobarbital may be used in all categories of patients. Besides the specific situations of neonatal seizures and status epilepticus, adults should remain the main target group for the long-term management of epilepsy with phenobarbital. The potential of phenobarbital for cognitive or behavioral adverse effects in children is of particular concern, because it may compromise learning capabilities, and therefore the use of this drug should be restricted whenever possible. Elderly patients also have substantial risks of insidious cognitive impairment or rheumatologic complications. Moreover, the potential for interactions with other treatments frequently prescribed in this age range, with a high rate of multiple disorders, often makes the use of phenobarbital suboptimal.

In terms of regulatory approval, the indications for phenobarbital rely on the proof of time and clinical experience. The drug may be used as monotherapy or polytherapy.

Dosing Recommendations

Starting Dosage and Titration

Except in urgent or relatively urgent situations in which temporary sedation may be acceptable for achieving seizure control, phenobarbital and other barbiturates are best introduced into therapy gradually. There are no specifically recommended procedures for this titration. It largely depends on the urgency of the need to control seizures, expectations about tolerability, and the size of the target dose for an individual patient. Patients should be made aware of potential early sedative effects and should be informed that these effects can be minimized with gradual titration of the drug.

In general, titration may be completed in 6 to 12 weeks. One-third of the expected maintenance daily dose may be prescribed for the first 2 or 3 weeks, after which the dose may be doubled if tolerability is acceptable. A further increment in dose is made 2 or 3 weeks after that, with perhaps a final increment another 2 or 3 weeks later. If this policy is followed, drug doses will be increased only when there has been time for steady-state conditions to apply at the previous dose. In patients whose seizures are frequent during the titration phase, no further dose increment will be necessary if seizures become fully controlled. Nor are doses increased if mild but tolerable adverse effects are present and too little time has passed since the last dose increment for the drug's effectiveness to be known. Some of the side effects, particularly sedation, may disappear when treatment is continued, owing to pharmacodynamic tolerance. The plasma concentrations of the drug may be measured after steady state has been achieved at the final target dose, so long as no adverse effects suggest that the dose needs to be reduced irrespective of the plasma concentration. The plasma phenobarbital concentration may serve as a provisional therapeutic concentration for the particular patient if the seizures appear fully controlled at that time or as a guide to the magnitude of further increases in dose likely to be tolerated if the seizures are not yet controlled. When rapid efficacy is needed, a loading dose of twice the usual daily maintenance dose, given for 4 days, brings the serum concentration to the steady-state value within 3 days.

Maintenance Dosage

The maintenance doses of phenobarbital that should be targeted initially range from 1 to 2.5 mg/kg/day in adults. Young adults 16 to 40 years old are generally treated with higher daily doses, 1.75 mg/kg on average, than adults >40 years old, in whom average daily doses of 1 mg/kg, or sometime less, may be sufficient. The drug may be given conveniently once daily at bedtime. At an early stage of therapy, if a standard dose as a function of age and body weight has been reached and is tolerated comfortably, or if plasma phenobarbital levels of ~15 μg/mL have been achieved, it is reasonable to make no further change in dose until the patient's clinical response becomes clear in time. In cases of seizure recurrence, delayed-onset adverse reactions, or modification of a concomitant medication susceptible of interactions, the phenobarbital dosage may need to be adjusted.

In children, because of changing pharmacokinetics, mainly shorter half-life values than in adults, maintenance dosages per body weight are generally higher. Specific indications for use of phenobarbital for the different seizure types in children are similar to those for adults, with a few exceptions. Rossi (16) studied the dosage of phenobarbital relative to age in children to achieve steady-state concentrations of 10 to 25 µg/mL. Infants from 2 months to 1 year of age require 2.31±0.74 mg/kg, children aged 1 to 3 years require 3.5±0.99 mg/kg, and children from 3 to 6.5 years of age require 4.79±1.31 mg/kg to achieve these plasma concentrations.

Optimal Range of Plasma Phenobarbital Concentrations

It is well known that the statistical concept of therapeutic drug concentrations has serious limitations and must be used cautiously. In the case of phenobarbital, the range of therapeutic concentrations is relatively broad. From a large sample of patients, Booker (12) concluded that the patients who respond to treatment with phenobarbital will do so with plasma levels between 10 and 40 µg/mL. In a study in untreated patients, Buchtal et al. (13) administered phenobarbital in small doses that were gradually increased and showed that the clinical response occurred at an average level of 10 µg/mL. Because of the long half-life of phenobarbital, its plasma concentrations show very little fluctuation during interdose intervals. Hence, predose measurement of the drug's plasma concentration rarely offers advantages over measurements carried out at any stage of the dosage interval, so long as steady-state conditions apply.

Many epileptic patients are completely seizure free with astonishingly low phenobarbital plasma levels. Prescribing higher doses in such patients is unnecessary. Conversely, a few patients may benefit from doses producing very high levels without significant toxicity. Like other drugs, phenobarbital must sometimes be increased to the maximum tolerated dose before being considered ineffective. In fact, in patients with uncontrolled epilepsy, higher plasma levels are found than in patients with controlled epilepsy (13–15). With staged progressive increments of phenobarbital doses, patients may remain free of adverse effects at plasma phenobarbital concentrations of ≥40 µg/mL, although by levels of 50 µg/mL, most patients experience some degree of mental dullness. The phenobarbital dose corresponding to these plasma drug concentrations may be 250 to 300 mg/day. However, one must be very attentive in the long term because adverse effects at these dose ranges, if not apparent at the beginning, may develop very insidiously later. The optimal phenobarbital dose and plasma concentration may vary with the type of syndrome or seizure. Schmidt et al. (3) found that higher concentrations were necessary for controlling partial seizures (37 µg/mL) than for controlling generalized tonic-clonic seizures alone (18 µg/mL).

Current Role in Epilepsy Management

In wealthy countries, a paradox exists in that phenobarbital is still widely used despite acknowledgment that it has no superiority in efficacy as compared with other antiepileptic drugs. Its broad spectrum of efficacy and indications make phenobarbital an easy product to prescribe, especially by nonexperts. Moreover, life-threatening adverse effects and blood or liver toxicity are very rare. All this ensures steady confidence with this compound in a disease context, epilepsy, in which many practitioners do not feel always very comfortable.

Even in specialists' practice, phenobarbital has a place among therapeutic options (17). It may be chosen as add-on drug when several attempts at polytherapy have failed, particularly in patients with refractory primarily or secondarily generalized tonic-clonic seizures. Phenobarbital may be used in combination with any of the marketed antiepileptic drugs, whether old or new. However, dose adjustments of concomitant antiepileptic drugs are often required.

The patient's choice also is important. Many patients initially treated with phenobarbital as monotherapy prefer continuing with it even when it is proposed that they switch to a more recent drug, with a better benefit:risk ratio, that is theoretically more appropriate to their epileptic syndrome. Reasons for the preference are multiple, including fear of change, which is not specific to phenobarbital, as well as the advantage of a single daily dose and the strong, yet erroneous, belief that taking the drug at night will not interfere with their daily activities.

Besides some specific situations such as neonatal seizures or status epilepticus, practitioners may choose phenobarbital for the long-term management of specific categories of patients. For example, because of its relatively long half-life, phenobarbital may offer better protection against seizures in patients who are prone to short periods of noncompliance with therapy, for example, patients with alcoholism. In patients temporarily unable to take oral treatment, phenobarbital can be given by daily intramuscular injection or intravenous infusion in the same dose as the clinically therapeutic oral dose until oral therapy can be resumed (18,19).

The foremost reasons for the important place still occupied by phenobarbital treatment are its low cost and its worldwide availability. Phenobarbital is recommended by the World Health Organization as the first-line drug for the treatment of epilepsies in developing countries (20). Its broad spectrum is well suited to treating patients in places with no neurologists or electroencephalographic facilities. However, concerns exist about the suitability of phenobarbital as an antiepileptic drug for children, owing to its adverse effects on cognition and behavior. A randomized comparison of phenobarbital and phenytoin, aiming at the detection of behavioral side effects, showed similar acceptability of the two drugs as monotherapy for childhood epilepsy in rural India (21), even though it has been argued that phenytoin is also a nonideal choice for pediatric epilepsies (22). Another study in India concluded that phenobarbital is not the ideal treatment for school-age children (10b), but cost and drug availability considerations may not allow alternative choices for many patients who live in the developing world.

Use in Special Populations

Neonatal Seizures

Seizures occur in 1% to 2% of neonates admitted to intensive care units. Treatment is usually with either phenobarbital or phenytoin, but phenobarbital is most frequently chosen (23–27). This choice is not based on its proven superiority but is founded on many years of familiarity with this drug among pediatricians. Analysis of the literature is difficult because many neonatal motor events, clinically classified as seizures, are unaccompanied by electrical seizure activity and are the result of non–seizure-related abnormal neonatal movements (28,29). Conversely, not all true neonatal seizures are recorded with surface scalp electroencephalograms (24). Most studies describing the efficacy of phenobarbital in the treatment of neonatal seizures used purely clinical criteria for diagnosis and assessment of outcome, whereas it is clear that use of videoelectroencephalographic monitoring for proper diagnosis and assessment will certainly improve our current knowledge. Three series show very close agreement regarding the efficacy of phenobarbital as the initial agent in the treatment of neonatal seizures. Lockman et al. (24), in a study of 39 neonates with loading doses of approximately 20 mg/kg, noted seizure control in 32% of the infants. Van Orman and Darrvish (27), in a study of 81 neonates who had received loading doses of phenobarbital at 15 to 20 mg/kg, in combination with phenytoin, noted seizure control in 33% of this population. Painter et al. (26), in a study of 77 neonates, noted that 36% of the study population had their seizures controlled after loading doses of 15 to 20 mg/kg of phenobarbital. Gal et al. (23), however, reported efficacy of 85% in 71 neonates in whom phenobarbital was used as monotherapy, and doses ≤40 mg/kg were given to achieve or surpass plasma concentrations of 40 mg/mL. The lack of specific seizure definition, electrically or clinically, in all these series makes the interpretations of the differences difficult.

One publication reported a series of 59 neonates with seizures that were confirmed by electroencephalography (30). The neonates were randomly assigned to receive either phenobarbital or phenytoin intravenously, at doses sufficient to achieve a free plasma concentration of 25 µg/mL for phenobarbital and 3 µg/mL for phenytoin. Neonates whose seizures were not controlled by the assigned drug were then treated with both drugs. Seizure control was assessed by electroencephalographic criteria. Seizures were controlled in 13 of the 30 neonates assigned to receive phenobarbital (43%) and in 13 of the 29 neonates assigned to receive phenytoin (45%). When combined treatment was considered, seizure control was achieved in 17 (57%) of the

neonates assigned to received phenobarbital first and 18 (62%) of those assigned to receive phenytoin first. The severity of the seizures was a stronger predictor of the success of treatment than was the assigned agent. Neonates with mild seizures or with seizures that were decreasing in severity before treatment were more likely to have their seizures end, regardless of the treatment assignment. The conclusion is that phenobarbital and phenytoin are equally but incompletely effective as anticonvulsants in neonates. With either drug given along, the seizures were controlled in fewer than half of the neonates.

Although all the potential toxicities of phenobarbital are important, its cardiovascular effects and effects on brain growth are of greater immediate concern in neonates (31). However, investigators have reported that high-dose phenobarbital therapy in term newborn infants with severe perinatal asphyxia may improve neurologic outcome (32). In a randomized, prospective study with a 3-year follow-up, phenobarbital, when administered in a dose of 40 mg/kg intravenously, appeared to be safe and was associated with a 27% reduction in the incidence of seizures and a significant improvement in neurologic outcomes at 3 years of age.

Febrile Seizures

Febrile seizures are the most common seizure disorder in childhood, occurring in 2% to 5% of children. Investigators agree (33,34) that although evidence indicates that continuous antiepileptic therapy with phenobarbital or valproic acid is effective in reducing the risk of seizure recurrence, the potential side effects associated with continuous antiepileptic therapy outweigh the relatively minor risks associated with simple febrile seizures. As such, long-term treatment is not recommended, although intermittent prophylactic use of rectal diazepam may be considered on a case-by-case basis.

Anticonvulsant prophylaxis, however, could be considered in patients with neurologic abnormalities, prolonged (>15 minutes) or focal seizures, high rate of recurrences, febrile seizures associated with transient or permanent neurologic deficits, or a family history of nonfebrile seizures. Even when two of these risk factors are present, only 13% of children develop epilepsy, and 87% of this high-risk group do not. If phenobarbital is chosen for prophylaxis in the treatment of seizures, it should not be used intermittently; it must be administered daily. Faero et al. (35) compared 59 patients <3 years old with 172 untreated children of the same age. Of 27 children who maintained plasma levels of 16 to 30 µg/mL, only one (4%) developed a new febrile seizure compared with seven (22%) of 33 children who maintained plasma levels between 8 and 15 µg/mL. The rate of febrile seizure development in the untreated population was 20%.

A retrospective meta-analytic review was conducted to assess the efficacy of various medications in the prevention of recurrent febrile seizures (36). Forty-five articles were taken into account, but only nine trials were randomized and were placebo controlled, four using phenobarbital, three using diazepam, one using pyridoxine, and one using phenytoin. In one of the phenobarbital trails, sodium valproate was also compared with placebo. The risk of recurrence was significantly lower in children receiving continuous phenobarbital therapy than in those receiving placebo (odds ratio, 0.54; 95% confidence interval [CI], 0.33 to 0.90). The odds ratio for recurrences in the sodium valproate group was 0.09 (95% CI, 0.01 to 0.78). No difference in the risk for recurrences was found between children receiving intermittent diazepam and those receiving placebo (odds ratio, 0.81; 95% CI, 0.54 to 1.22). The risk of recurrences in children receiving pyridoxine or phenytoin did not differ from the risk among children receiving placebo. In a number-needed-to-treat analysis, four children would have to be treated with sodium valproate (95% CI, 2 to 11) or eight children would have to be treated with phenobarbital (95% CI, 5 to 27), continuously, to prevent one febrile seizure. As discussed earlier, however, neither phenobarbital nor valproate is recommended because the risk of adverse effects outweighs the benefits in an unselected population of children with febrile seizures. Although a prospective population-based case-control study found that neither febrile seizures nor phenobarbital affected behavior, school performance, and neurocognitive attention outcomes adversely (37), another report suggested that early phenobarbital treatment for simple febrile seizures may lead to late cognitive effects (38). Possibly, long-term impairment of developmental skills (language, verbal) was triggered during the period of treatment.

Status Epilepticus

Although generalized convulsive status epilepticus is a life-threatening emergency, the best initial drug treatment is uncertain. Phenobarbital is known to have advantages and disadvantages in the treatment of status epilepticus. Its anticonvulsant action is long, thus allowing use in subsequent long-term therapy, but adverse effects are considerable and include respiratory depression, excessive sedation, and hypotension. Theoretically, phenobarbital achieves a maximum brain:plasma ratio much more slowly than does diazepam, and the response time in the treatment of status epilepticus therefore may be considerably slower. Although current trends favor the combination of diazepam or lorazepam with phenytoin (39), several studies have shown that the effectiveness of phenobarbital may be as good as, if not better than, the other options. In a randomized, nonblinded clinical trial evaluating 36 consecutive patients with generalized convulsive status epilepticus, Shaner et al. (40) compared phenobarbital with a combination of diazepam and phenytoin. There were 18 episodes of status epilepticus in each treatment group. Phenobarbital was initially admin-

istered intravenously at a rate of 100 mg/min until a dose of 10 mg/kg was achieved. If the patient continued to convulse 10 minutes after treatment was initiated, phenytoin was administered intravenously, and additional phenobarbital was delivered. In the other treatment group, diazepam was infused at 2 mg/min intravenously, and phenytoin was administered simultaneously at a rate of 40 mg/min until a loading dose of 18 mg/kg was achieved. If the patient continued to convulse after delivery of an initial 20-mg dose of diazepam, a continuous diazepam infusion was administered. Convulsions were controlled in all 36 patients within 7 hours. The median cumulative convulsion time, however, was shorter for those patients receiving phenobarbital (5 minutes) than for those receiving the combination of diazepam and phenytoin (9 minutes). Sixteen of the 18 patients (89%) treated with phenobarbital exhibited clinical convulsive activity for <10 minutes, and no patient demonstrated activity for >25 minutes. Ten of 18 patients (56%) in the diazepam–phenytoin group convulsed for <10 minutes, and five experienced a cumulative convulsion time of >25 minutes. The frequency of complications (i.e., arrhythmias, hypotension, and need for intubation) was similar among the two regimens. Sixteen of 18 patients required phenobarbital doses <12 mg/kg. Eleven of 18 cases were controlled with phenobarbital alone at a mean serum concentration of 18.3 μg/mL. Statistical evaluation did not demonstrate a dramatic difference between the phenobarbital and diazepam–phenytoin groups, but 95% CIs demonstrated that the mean cumulative convulsion time for the phenobarbital regimen was between 0 and 14 minutes less than that of the diazepam–phenytoin regimen.

Orr et al. (41) also noted a higher incidence of intubation with attendant complications in children receiving diazepam compared with those receiving phenobarbital for acute seizures. The response time of seizure control was no different between phenobarbital and diazepam. Rather than the postulated 20-minute response latency noted by some investigators, Shaner et al. (40) noted a median response time to phenobarbital of 5.5 minutes. The finding is in keeping with experimental data demonstrating that although maximum brain:plasma ratios of phenobarbital may be achieved only after 60 minutes after administration, effective brain concentration of phenobarbital are achieved within 3 minutes (42,43). A comparison of four treatments for generalized convulsive status epilepticus was conducted by the Veterans Affairs Status Epilepticus Cooperative Study Group (44), in a 5-year randomized, double-blind, multicenter trial of four intravenous regimens: diazepam (0.15 mg/kg body weight) followed by phenytoin (18 mg/kg body weight), lorazepam (0.1 mg/kg), phenobarbital (15 mg/kg), and phenytoin (18 mg/kg). Five hundred eighteen patients were classified as having either overt generalized status epilepticus (defined as easily visible generalized convulsions) or subtle status epilepticus (indicating by coma and ictal discharges on the electroencephalogram, with or without subtle convulsive movements such as rhythmic muscle twitches or tonic eye deviation). Treatment was considered successful when all motor and electroencephalographic seizure activity ceased within 20 minutes after beginning the drug infusion and there was no return of seizure activity during the next 40 minutes. In the group of overt generalized convulsive status epilepticus, lorazepam was successful in 64.9% of those assigned to receive it, phenobarbital in 58.2%, diazepam plus phenytoin in 55.8%, and phenytoin in 43.6% (p = .02 for the overall comparison among the four groups). Lorazepam was significantly superior to phenytoin in a pairwise comparison (p = .002). Among the 134 patients with a verified diagnosis of subtle generalized convulsive status epilepticus, no significant differences among the treatments were detected (range of success rates, 7.7% to 24.2%). In an intention-to-treat analysis, the differences among treatment groups were not significant, either among the patients with overt status epilepticus (p = .12) or among those with subtle status epilepticus (p = .91). There were no differences among the treatments with respect to recurrence during the 12-hour study period, the incidence of adverse reactions, or the outcome at 30 days. Thus, phenobarbital is not less efficacious than lorazepam or diazepam plus phenytoin as initial intravenous treatment for overt generalized convulsive status epilepticus. Although benzodiazepines may be easier to use, and in spite of some theoretic limitations, phenobarbital may be as effective as any other treatment regimen in the therapy of status epilepticus.

Discontinuation of Therapy

Because phenobarbital has a relatively long half-life, even if intake of the drug is ceased abruptly, the antiepileptic effect should decline progressively during 1 or 2 weeks, and this should alleviate the risk of withdrawal seizures. Nevertheless, most clinicians prefer to withdraw barbiturates gradually during a period of some weeks or months, unless there is a good medical reason for ridding the body of the drug as quickly as possible, for example, because of a serious idiosyncratic adverse effect. Thus, the dose may be reduced by 25% of its initial value each month for 4 months or by 33% each month for 3 months. The effects on seizure recurrence of slow phenobarbital withdrawal have been assessed, in comparison with other antiepileptic drugs (45). Patients were randomized to either continued treatment or slow drug withdrawal. This study did not support the contention that barbiturates are more likely to be associated with withdrawal seizures, as compared with carbamazepine or phenytoin.

Contraindications and Precautions

Phenobarbital is contraindicated in persons with histories of previous hypersensitivity reactions to the agent and in patients with porphyria. Barbiturates should be used with

cautions in persons with medically important disorders treated with therapeutic agents whose clearances are likely to be altered by the administration of an inducing agent such as phenobarbital. An example would be persons receiving oral anticoagulant therapy. Some of the alternative antiepileptic drugs (phenytoin, carbamazepine) possess similar disadvantages. Phenobarbital should also be used cautiously in persons with hepatic insufficiency and in elderly patients. In both these populations, lower-than-usual doses may be indicated (18).

REFERENCES

1. Mattson R, Cramer J, Collins J, et al. Comparison of carbamazepine, phenobarbital, phenytoin and primidone in partial and secondarily generalized tonic-clonic seizures. *N Engl J Med* 1985;313:145–151.
2. Mitchell W, Chavez J. Carbamazepine versus phenobarbital for partial onset seizures in children. *Epilepsia* 1987;28:56–60.
3. Schmidt D, Einicke I, Haenel F. The influence of seizure type on the efficacy of plasma concentration of phenytoin, phenobarbital and carbamazepine. *Arch Neurol* 1986;43:263–265.
4. Kwan P, Brodie MJ. Early identification of refractory epilepsy. *N Engl J Med* 2000;342:314–319.
5. Heller AJ, Chesterman P, Elwes RD, et al. Phenobarbital, phenytoin, carbamazepine, or sodium valproate for newly diagnosed adult epilepsy: a randomized comparative monotherapy trail. *J Neurol Neurosurg Psychiatry* 1995;58:44–50.
6. Marjerrison G, Jedlicki SM, Kedgh RP, et al. Carbamazepine: behavioural anticonvulsant and EEG effects in chronically hospitalized epileptics. *Dis Nerv Syst* 1968;29:133–136.
7. White PT, Plott D, Norton J. Relative anticonvulsant potency of primidone. *Arch Neurol* 1966;14:31–35.
8. Cereghino JJ, Brock JT, Van Meter JC, et al. The efficacy of carbamazepine combinations in epilepsy. *Clin Pharmacol Ther* 1975;18:733–741.
9. Benassi E, Loeb C, Desio G, et al. Carbamazepine, diphenylhydantoin, phenobarbital: a prospective trial in 18 temporal lobe epileptics. In: Johannessen SI, Morselli PL, Pippenger CE, et al., eds. *Antiepileptic therapy: advances in drug monitoring.* New York: Raven Press, 1980:195–202.
10a. de Silva M, MacArdle B, McGowan M, et al. Randomised comparative monotherapy trial of phenobarbitone, phenytoin, carbamazepine, or sodium valproate for newly diagnosed childhood epilepsy. *Lancet* 1996;347:709–713.
10b. Thilothammel N, Banu K, Ratnam RS. Comparison of phenobarbitone, phenytoin with sodium valproate: randomized, double-blind study. *Ind Pediatr* 1996;33:549–555.
10c. Perucca E, Gram L, Avanzini G, et al. Antiepileptic drugs as a cause of worsening of seizures. *Epilepsia* 1998;39:5–17.
11. Crawford TO, Mitchell WG, Fishman LS, et al. Very-high-dose phenobarbital for refractory status epilepticus in children. *Neurology* 1988;39:1035–1040.
12. Booker HE. Phenobarbital: relation of plasma concentration to seizure control. In: Woodbury DM, Penry JK, Pippenger DE, eds. *Antiepileptic drugs.* New York: Raven Press, 1982:241–350.
13. Buchthal F, Lennox-Buchtal MA. Relation of serum concentration to control of seizures. In: Woodbury DM, Penry JK, Pippenger DE, eds. *Antiepileptic drugs.* New York: Raven Press, 1982:335–343.
14. Loiseau P, Brachet A, Henry P. Dosage du phenobarbital sanguine chez 250 épileptiques. *Bordeaux Med* 1975;1:27–38.

15. Travers RD, Reynolds EH, Gallagher BB. Variation in response to anticonvulsants in a group of epileptic patients. *Arch Neurol* 1972;27:29–33.

16. Rossi LN, Nino LM, Principi N. Correlation between age and plasma level/dosage ratio for phenobarbital in infants and children. *Acta Pediatr Scand* 1979;68:431–434.

17. Lernam-Sagie T, Lerman P. Phenobarbital still has a role in epilepsy treatment. *J Child Neurol* 1999;14:820–821.

18. Eadie MJ. Phenobarbital and other barbiturates. In: Engel J, Pedley T, eds. *Epilepsy: a comprehensive textbook.* Philadelphia: Lippincott–Raven, 1997:1547–1555.

19. Mattson RH. Parenteral antiepileptic/anticonvulsant drugs. *Neurology* 1996;46[Suppl 1]:S8–S13.

20. World Health Organization. *Initiate of support to people with epilepsy.* Geneva: World Health Organization, 1990.

21. Pal DK, Das T, Chaudhury G, et al. Randomised controlled trial to assess acceptability of phenobarbital for childhood epilepsy in rural India. *Lancet* 1998;351:19–23.

22. Trevathan E, Medina MT, Madrid A. Antiepileptic drugs in developing countries. *Lancet* 1998;351:1201–1211.

23. Gal P, Tobock J, Boer H, et al. Efficacy of phenobarbital monotherapy in treatment of neonatal seizures: relationship to blood levels. *Neurology* 1982;32:1401–1404.

24. Lockman LA, Kriel R, Zaske D. Phenobarbital dosage for control of neonatal seizures. *Neurology* 1979;29:1445–1449.

25. Painter MJ, Minnigh B, Gaus L, et al. Neonatal phenobarbital and phenytoin binding profiles. *J Clin Pharmacol* 1994;34:312–317.

26. Painter MJ, Pippenger CE, Wasterlain C, et al. Phenobarbital and phenytoin in neonatal seizures: metabolism and tissue distribution. *Neurology* 1981;31:1107–1112.

27. Van Orman CB, Darrvish HZ. Efficacy of phenobarbital in neonatal seizures. *Can J Neurol Sci* 1985;12:95–99.

28. Mizrahi E, Kelloway P. Characterization and classification of neonatal seizures. *Neurology* 1987;37:1837–1844.

29. Weiner S, Painter MJ, Geva D, et al. Neonatal seizures: electroclinical dissociation. *Pediatr Neurol* 1991;7:363–368.

30. Painter MJ, Scher MS, Stein AD, et al. Phenobarbital compared with phenytoin for the treatment of neonatal seizures. *N Engl J Med* 1999;341:485–489.

31. Dessens AB, Cohen-Kettenis PT, Mellenbergh GJ, et al. Associate of prenatal phenobarbital and phenytoin exposure with small head size at birth and with learning problems. *Acta Paediatr* 2000;89:533–541.

32. Hall RT, Hall FK, Daily DK. High-dose phenobarbital therapy in term newborn infants with severe perinatal asphyxia: a randomized, prospective study with three-year follow-up. *J Pediatr* 1998;132:345–348.

33. Freeman J. Febrile seizures: a consensus of their significance, evaluation and treatment. *Pediatrics* 1980;66:1009.

34. Baumann RJ, Duffner PK. Treatment of children with simple febrile seizures: the AAP practice parameter. *Pediatr Neurol* 2000;23:11–17.

35. Faero O, Kastrup KW, Nielsen E, et al. Successful prophylaxis of febrile convulsions with phenobarbital. *Epilepsia* 1972;13:279–285.

36. Rantala H, Tarkka R, Uhari M. A meta-analytic review of the preventive treatment of recurrences of febrile seizures. *J Pediatr* 1997;131:922–925.

37. Chang YC, Guo NW, Huang CC, et al. Neurocognitive attention and behavior outcome of school-age children with a history of febrile convulsions: a population study. *Epilepsia* 2000;41:412–420.

38. Sulzbacher S, Farwell JR, Tmekin N, et al. Late cognitive effects of early treatment with phenobarbital. *Clin Pediatr* 1999;38:387–394.

39. Ramsey RE. Treatment of status epilepticus. *Epilepsia* 1993;34[Suppl 1]:571–581.

40. Shaner MD, McCurdy S, Herring M, et al. Treatment of status epilepticus: a prospective comparison of diazepam and phenytoin versus phenobarbital and optional phenytoin. *Neurology* 1988;38:202–207.

41. Orr R, Dimand R, Venkataraman S, et al. Diazepam and intubation in emergency treatment of seizures in children. *Ann Emerg Med* 1991;20:1009–1013.

42. Leppik IE, Sherwin AL. Intravenous phenytoin and phenobarbital: anticonvulsant action, brain content, and plasma binding in the rat. *Epilepsia* 1979;20:201–207.

43. Ramsey RE, Hammond EJ, Perchalski RJ, et al. Brain uptake of phenytoin, phenobarbital and diazepam. *Arch Neurol* 1979;36:535–539.

44. Treiman DM, Meyers PD, Walton NY, et al. A comparison of four treatments for generalized convulsive status epilepticus: Veterans Affairs Status Epilepticus Cooperative Study Group. *N Engl J Med* 1998;339:792–798.

45. Chadwick D. Does withdrawal of different antiepileptic drugs have different effects on seizure recurrence? Further results from the MRC Antiepileptic Drug Withdrawal Study. *Brain* 1999;122;441–448.

PHENOBARBITAL AND OTHER BARBITURATES

CLINICAL EFFICACY AND USE IN NONEPILEPTIC DISORDERS

ETTORE BEGHI

The mechanisms of action of barbiturates include enhancement of γ-aminobutyric acid (GABA)–ergic inhibition and, at high concentrations, limitation of high-frequency repetitive firing of action potentials. These drugs enhance ionic currents by interactions with $GABA_A$ receptor. Phenobarbital (PB) and primidone (PRM) may act synergistically in reducing sustained, high-frequency, repetitive firing. Barbiturates are also known to decrease excitatory amino acid release and postsynaptic response by blocking the excitatory glutamate response (1). Some of these actions may contribute to potential therapeutic activity in certain neurologic disorders other than epilepsy, even though the precise mechanisms by which barbiturates act in various conditions remain poorly understood.

ESSENTIAL TREMOR

Essential tremor is a common condition characterized by oscillating movements caused by alternative contraction of agonist and antagonist muscles. All somatic muscles may be affected, and tremor is typically of the postural type. Propranolol and other β-receptor blocking agents have clear efficacy in the treatment of essential tremor, mostly hand tremor (2). However, the use of β-adrenergic blockers may be followed by bradycardia, hypotension, fatigue, nausea, diarrhea, impotence, and depression, which occasionally require drug withdrawal. β-Adrenergic blockers are also contraindicated in several conditions such as obstructive lung disease, heart block, and peripheral vascular disease, all of which are relatively

Ettore Beghi, MD: Chief, Neurophysiology Unit, "San Gerardo" Hospital, Monza, Italy; and Head, Neurological Disorders Laboratory, Institute for Pharmacological Research "Mario Negri," Milano, Italy

common in elderly patients, in whom essential tremor is more prevalent.

PRM has been extensively investigated in essential tremor in randomized clinical trials (3–10) and in open studies. The drug was used in daily doses ranging from 50 to 1,000 mg. The efficacy of treatment was tested clinically, and tremor reduction was also assessed with an accelerometer. Different daily doses of PRM (250, 750, and 1,000 mg) were similarly effective. In the only study comparing PRM with propranolol, the two drugs had comparable efficacy (5). Adverse effects occurred in about 20% to 30% of cases and led to discontinuance of treatment in a few patients. Adverse reactions consisted of somnolence, fatigue, vertigo, nausea, and unsteadiness, which subsided in many patients with continued use.

PB and phenylethylmalonamide (PEMA), the other active metabolite of PRM, showed little or no evidence of efficacy in essential tremor (8,10–13) (Table 54.1). PB was also compared with PRM (8) and with propranonol (12) and was found to be significantly less effective.

Based on published reports, the efficacy of propranolol and PRM in essential tremor is unequivocal, and both compounds can be used as drugs of first choice. To date, there are no guidelines to suggest a preference for one drug over the other. Propranonol is still the β-blocker of first choice. The starting dose is 20 mg twice daily. The optimal dose range is 240 to 320 mg/day. In the absence of a clear dose response, the minimal effective dose of PRM (250 mg/day) should be selected. To minimize acute adverse reactions, the daily dose of PRM may be titrated in 25- or 50-mg increments. In patients whose response to one drug is incomplete, the other drug may be added to increase treatment efficacy, although the increased efficacy of treatment combination awaits confirmation from well-designed randomized studies. PB and PEMA are not recommended for the treatment of essential tremor in clinical practice.

TABLE 54.1. RANDOMIZED CROSSOVER CLINICAL TRIALS OF PHENOBARBITAL, PRIMIDONE, AND PHENYLETHYLMALONAMIDE FOR ESSENTIAL TREMOR

Reference	No. Treated (age)	Treatment Duration (Double-Blind Period)	Daily Dose (mg) [Comparator]	Overall Results [No. Improved]	Adverse Events* [No. Withdrawals]
8	16 (60–78)	35 days	PRM, 750 PB, 150 [PLC]	Significant reduction of clinical measures with PRM compared with PB and PLC (PB ≈ PLC) [PRM, 8/13; PB, 1/13; PLC, 1/13]	PRM, 10/14; PB, 11/14; PLC, 5/14 [PRM, 1/16; PB, 1/16; PLC, 0/16]
10	18 (60–79)	35 days	PRM, 750 PB, 150 [PLC]	42% reduction of hand tremor with PRM (PB, 23%; PLC, 8%) [PRM, 12/15; PB, 8/15] Head tremor unaffected	PRM, 11/15; PB, 9/15; PLC, 5/15 [PRM, 1/18; PB, 1/18]
11	8 (28–69)	2 wk	PEMA, 400 [PLC]	No significant difference in any outcome measures	PEMA, 1/8; PLC, 0/8
12	17 (35–72)	1 mo	PB, 60–120 [PRP mean 1.7/kg; PLC]	PB ≈ PRP < PLC (subjective evaluation and reduction of tremor amplitude) PRP > PB ≈ PLC (clinical evaluation) PRP ≈ PB ≈ PLC (tremor frequency and performance tests) >50% tremor reduction: PB, 6/10; PRP, 6/10	PB, 5/12; PRP, 5/12; PLC, 1/12 [PRP, 1/12; PB, 0/12; PLC, 0/12]
13	12 (24–71)	5 wk	PB, 120 [PLC]	Reduction of tremor: PB, 11/11; PLC, 6/11 Clinical rating, but not performance or self-assessment, better with PB	PB, 8/11; PLC, 6/11 [PB, 1/12; PLC, 0/12]

PB, phenobarbital; PEMA, phenylethylmalonamide; PLC, placebo; PRM, primidone; PRP, propranolol.
*No. with any event or, if unavailable, with most common events.

NEONATAL CEREBRAL HEMORRHAGE

Premature infants weighing <1,500 g or having a gestational age <35 weeks are at a significantly higher risk of spontaneous cerebral hemorrhage (14). Neonatal cerebral hemorrhage can be effectively prevented with corticosteroids (15). Barbiturates have been repeatedly tested for the prevention of neonatal cerebral hemorrhage (Table 54.2). PB has been given to the mother in loading doses of ≤1,000 mg and in cumulative doses of 100 to 720 mg until delivery. Alternatively, PB has been given to the neonate at 10 to 20 mg/kg loading doses and at 2.5 to 5 mg/kg maintenance doses. The results of randomized clinical trials (16–30) (Table 54.2) are contradictory, and the apparent efficacy of barbiturates shown in the early studies can be interpreted on the basis of a less accurate diagnosis, selection bias, and an inconsistent use of steroids in both treatment groups. Rates of corticosteroid use were ~30% in the early studies and increased to 60% to 100% in more recent trials. A systematic review of some randomized studies on the preterm use of barbiturates confirms a reduction of treatment effect in more recent studies and the lack of significant trends toward a beneficial effect of barbiturates (31). In fact, although an initial analysis suggested a reduction in the risk of all grades of hemorrhages (relative risk [RR], 0.80; 95%

confidence interval [95% CI], 0.68 to 0.94) and severe hemorrhage (RR, 0.55; 95% CI, 0.35 to 0.87), after exclusion of trials with poor design and method, no significant effects were detected on the risk of infant mortality, all grades of periventricular hemorrhage, severe hemorrhage, neurodevelopmental abnormalities at 18 to 36 months of age, or combined outcomes (death and/or severe hemorrhage).

Despite its ability in suppressing motor activity, PB has been associated with an increased incidence of intraventricular hemorrhage in low-weight preterm infants with respiratory disease (32). On this basis, PB cannot be recommended to prevent intracranial hemorrhage in premature newborns.

INCREASED INTRACRANIAL PRESSURE

Increased intracranial pressure is an important complication of severe brain injury, with a high morbidity and mortality rate. Barbiturates may reduce intracranial pressure by reducing cerebral blood flow and metabolism (33). Treatment with barbiturates may thus diminish metabolic demand and may limit, if not prevent, neurologic injury. Randomized clinical trials provide conflict-

TABLE 54.2. RANDOMIZED CLINICAL TRIALS OF INTRAVENOUS PHENOBARBITAL TO PREVENT CEREBRAL HEMORRHAGE IN PRETERM NEWBORNS

Reference	No. Treated	Treatment Duration	Daily Dose (mg) (Comparator)	Significant Results (Neonatal Hemorrhage)	Adverse Events[a] (No. Withdrawals)
16	60 neonates	7 days	10/kg b.i.d. Maintenance: 2.5/kg b.i.d. [none]	PB, 4/30; CTR, 14/30 Mortality: PB, 6/30; CTR, 9/30	Hypoxia, hyperoxia, hypocapnia, hypercapnia, acidosis and hypotension in similar proportions
17	60 neonates	Single dose[b]	20/kg [PLC]	PB, 12/30; PLC, 11/30 Mortality: PB, 4/30; PLC, 6/30	Similar duration of acidosis with PB and PLC
18	42 neonates	6 days	10/kg b.i.d. (load) Maintenance: 2.5/kg b.i.d. [none]	PB, 10/21; CTR, 10/21 HEM in PB group significantly less severe	?
19	52 neonates	5 days	15/kg (load) 5/kg [i.v. glucose infusion]	PB, 8/25; CTR, 14/27 Severe HEM: PB, 3/25; CTR, 6/27 Mortality: PB, 2/25; CTR, 1/27	NR
20	101 neonates	5 days	15/kg at birth and 4 hours later Maintenance: 5/kg [i.v. glucose infusion]	PB, 15/47; CTR, 25/54 Severe HEM: PB, 4/47; CTR, 2/54 Severe neurodevelopmental impairment: PB, 5/47; CTR, 4/54	Hypoxia: PB, 11/47; CTR, 5/54
21	39 mothers	Until delivery	700 (load) maintenance: 500 (if not born within 24 h) [none]	Mortality: PB, 7/47; CTR, 3/54 PB, 2/21; CTR, 9/18 Severe HEM: PB, 0/21; CTR, 5/18	?
22	46 mothers	1–6 days	500 (load) 100 [none]	PB, 8/25; CTR, 13/23 Moderate to severe HEM: PB, 0/25; CTR, 5/23 Mortality: PB, 0/25; CTR, 4/23	NR [PB, 2/25]
23	280 neonates	4 days[b]	10/kg (load) 2.5 kg [PLC]	PB, 51/145; PLC, 26/135 Severe HEM: PB, 18/145; PLC, 8/135	NR
24	150 mothers and 150 neonates	1–6 days	390–780 (load) 2.5/kg (N) [2.5/kg only after birth (N)] [none]	PB, 16/75; CTR, 35/75 Severe HEM: PB, 4/75; CTR, 15/75 Mortality: PB, 3/75; CTR, 10/75	Sedation: PB, 75/75(?)
25	110 mothers	1 day[b]	500–700 (load) [PLC]	PB, 11/54; PLC, 19/67 Severe HEM: PB, 2/54; PLC, 10/67 Mortality: PB, 18%; PLC, 14%	No complications
26	139	0.06–31	720–780 (load) 240+ Vitamin K 10–20 + BMS 12 [PLC]	PB, 31/81; PLC, 40/83 Severe HEM: PB, 2/81; PLC, 5/83 Mortality: PB, 9/81; PLC, 5/83	Hypotension: PB, 10/83; PLC, 6/81 Acidosis: PB, 26/83; PLC, 17/81 Hyperglycemia, hypoglycemia and hypocalcemia in similar proportions
27	318 mothers	0.04–50 days[b]	As above	PB, 75/191; PLC, 84/181 Severe HEM: PB, 13/191; PLC, 15/181 Mortality: PB, 10%; PLC, 8%	Hypotension: PB, 20/181; PLC, 19/191 Acidosis: PB, 51/181; PLC, 44/191 Hyperglycemia, hypoglycemia and hypocalcemia in similar proportions
28	110 mothers	1–39 days	500–1,000 (load) 100 (27%)	PB, 14/62; CTR, 26/74 Severe HEM: PB, 1/62; CTR, 3/74 Mortality: PB, 5/62; CTR, 4/74	Hypotension: PB, 0/62; CTR, 0/74 Decrease of respiratory rate: PB, 0/62; CTR, 0/74
29	610 mothers	1–65 days[b]	10/kg (load) 100 [PLC]	PB, 70/344; PLC, 64/324 Severe HEM: PB, 12/344; PLC, 7/324 Periventricular leukomalacia: PB, 12/344; PLC, 9/324 Mortality (<72 h): PB, 14/344; PLC, 10/324	Sedation: PB, 253/290 PLC, 120/286
30	100 mothers	Single dose[b]	10/kg [PLC]	PB, 12/42; PLC, 29/46 Mild HEM: PB, 11/42; PLC, 26/46	?

b.i.d., twice daily; CTR, controls; HEM, hemorrhage; i.v., intravenous; N, neonate; NR, not reported; PB, phenobarbital; PLC, placebo.
[a]Number with any event or, if unavailable, with most common events.
[b]Double-blind trial.

TABLE 54.3. RANDOMIZED CLINICAL TRIALS OF INTRAVENOUS PENTOBARBITAL FOR ACUTE TRAUMATIC BRAIN INJURY AND INCREASED INTRACRANIAL PRESSURE

Reference	No. Evaluated (age)	Daily Dose (mg) [Comparator]	Significant Results	Adverse Events
34	26 (14–81 yr)	PTB loading 10/kg over 4 h; maintenance 1.6/kg/hr [none]	Mortality: PTB, 18/25; CTR, 36/43 (historical controls)	NR
35	59 (?)	PTB loading up to 10/kg; Maintenance 0.5–3/kg/h [MTL 20% 1,000/kg]	Mortality: PTB, 16/28; MTL, 15/31; PTB, 77%; MTL, 41% (ICP elevation); PTB, 40%; MTL 43% (evacuated hematomas)	(?)
36	53 (>12 yr)	PTB loading 5/10/kg to achieve burst suppression on EEG; maintenance 1–3/kg for at least 72 h [none]	Glasgow Outcome Scale: good outcome PTB, 11/27; CTR, 10/26 Mortality: PTB, 14/27; CTR, 13/26	Arterial hypotension: PTB, 14/27; CTR, 2/26 Acute respiratory disease: PTB, 7/27; CTR, 3/26 Sepsis: PTB, 9/27; CTR, 4/26 SIADH: PTB, 8/27; 5/26 CNS infection: PTB, 6/27; CTR, 2/26
37	73 (15–50 yr)	PTB loading 10/kg over 30 min; 5/kg q1 h × 3; Maintenance 1 kg/h repeated once if needed [none]	Fall of ICP < 20 mm Hg; (15 mm HG in skull opened) PTB, 32%; CTR, 17%; (no cardiovascular complications): PB, 40%; CTR, 9% Mortality: PTB, 23/37; CTR, 2/10	Arterial hypotension: PTB, 23/37; CTR 18/36
38	7 (14–68 yr)	PTB loading 2.5/kg every 15 min for 1 h, followed by 10/kg/h for 4 h; maintenance 1.5/kg/h [ETM induction 0.3/kg, followed by 0.02/kg/min for 24–72 h]	Mean ICP: PTB, 35 mm Hg (pretreatment); 26 mm Hg (posttreatment) ETM 33 mm Hg (pretreatment); 21 mm Hg (posttreatment)	Trial stopped because 3 patients receiving ETM developed renal failure. Mean systolic blood pressure: PTB, 106.5 mm Hg (pretreatment); PTB, 92.2 mm Hg (posttreatment)

CNS, central nervous system; CTR, controls; ETM, etomidate; ICP, intracranial pressure; MTL, mannitol; NR, not reported; PTB, pentobarbital; SIADH, syndrome of inappropriate antidiuretic hormone secretion.

ing results (Table 54.3) (34–38). Pentobarbital was no better than standard treatment and was less effective than mannitol in the control of increased intracranial pressure. A systematic review of randomized or quasirandomized studies of one or more barbiturate types administered for traumatic brain injury showed a pooled relative risk for death of 1.09 (95% CI, 0.81 to 1.47), a pooled risk of adverse neurologic outcome of 1.15 (95% CI, 0.81 to 1.64), and a pooled risk of uncontrolled intracranial pressure of 0.81 (95% CI, 0.62 to 1.06) (39). By contrast, barbiturates resulted in an increase in the occurrence of hypotension (pooled risk 1.80; 95% CI, 1.19 to 2.70). Mortality was similar in patients treated with barbiturates and in the controls (pooled risk 1.18; 95% CI, 0.73 to 1.92). Based on this review, it cannot be excluded that barbiturates reduce increased intracranial pressure, but they do not seem to affect the outcome of traumatic brain injury and may impair cerebral perfusion pressure by inducing hypotension. This adverse effect is likely to offset any benefit from reduction in intracranial pressure.

OTHER POTENTIAL INDICATIONS FOR NEUROPROTECTION

A single intravenous loading dose of thiopental (30 mg/kg) failed to ameliorate neurologic impairment in 262 comatose survivors of cardiac arrest who were enrolled in a multicenter randomized clinical trial (40). In this study, at the end of 1-year of follow-up, the proportion of deaths was 77% with thiopental and 80% with standard treatment; 17% of patients receiving thiopental and 14% of those receiving standard treatment recovered to their pre–cardiac arrest levels. Hypotension developed in 60% of the patients receiving experimental treatment and in 29% of those receiving standard treatment.

Along with traumatic brain injury and cardiac arrest, barbiturate coma was used in several clinical conditions, including Reye's syndrome, near drowning, bacterial meningitis, and hepatic encephalopathy (41). However, the negative results of randomized clinical trials and the controversial findings of open studies, coupled with the adverse hemodynamic effects of barbiturates, caution against the widespread use of these agents to prevent immediate and delayed complications of severe central nervous system insults with or without increased intracranial pressure.

NEONATAL HYPERBILIRUBINEMIA AND JAUNDICE

Neonatal kernicterus is an encephalopathy resulting from the disposition of unconjugated bilirubin in the central nervous system. The mainstays for the treatment of neonatal hyperbilirubinemia include phototherapy and exchange transfusions (42). Because barbiturates lower serum bilirubin levels by inducing hepatic conjugating enzymes, PB was used in the past to prevent or to treat neonatal hyperbilirubinemia. The effects on bilirubin disposition of different doses of PB (0, 4, 8, and 12 mg/kg in a single dose shortly after birth) were assessed in a randomized comparative trial in preterm infants (43). Only the highest dose was found to reduce serum bilirubin significantly. With this dose, the infants spent more time in quiet sleep than did the other groups. The absence of an effect when PB was given at <5 mg/kg was confirmed by other investigators (44,45).

OTHER CONDITIONS

Barbiturates were extensively used as sedative-hypnotic agents in the past. PB has been shown to produce significant dose-related reduction in sleep latency and number of awakenings, as well as an increase in total sleep time (46). However, the impairment of cognitive performance, the residual morning sedation, the significant potential for abuse (47), and the severe toxicity associated with overdose are reasons against the routine use of barbiturates as sedative-hypnotic agents. Barbiturates have also been used in drug withdrawal syndromes, although benzodiazepines are generally preferred for this indication.

PB, 15 to 150 mg/day, was compared with clonazepam, 1 to 10 mg/day, for the treatment of tardive dyskinesia (48). Both clonazepam and PB significantly reduced dyskinetic movements. Sleepiness and drowsiness were observed in about 50% of patients in both treatment groups. Neither drug was manifestly superior to the other, although clonazepam had a stronger effect on orofacial dyskinesia and PB for limb and axial movements.

Withdrawal symptoms in infants exposed to methadone *in utero* and born to drug-dependent women may require drug treatment. However, there is little evidence on the comparative value of different drug regimens used to treat neonatal abstinence syndrome (49). PB, paregoric (a preparation containing opiates, camphor, and alcohol), and diazepam have been all recommended for the treatment of neonatal abstinence syndrome. These three drugs were compared in a randomized trial and were found to be sim-

ilar (50). No difference was found in another randomized trial between PB and paregoric, with the exception of an increased blood level of partial pressure of carbon dioxide among PB-treated infants (51).

Bile acid dissolution therapy continues to be a safe and effective treatment for highly selected patients with cholesterol gallstone disease. Chenodeoxycholic acid (750 mg/day) and PB (90 or 180 mg/day) were compared in the treatment of gallstones. The effects of PB on the rate-limiting enzymes of liver cholesterol and bile acid synthesis were less than those of chenodeoxycholic acid, although a positive interaction was found when the two drugs were combined (52). PB alone seems ineffective in gallstone dissolution (53).

REFERENCES

1. Smith MC, Riskin BJ. The clinical use of barbiturates in neurological disorders. *Drugs* 1991;42:365–378.
2. Koller WC, Hristova A, Brin M. Pharmacologic treatment of essential tremor. *Neurology* 2000;54[Suppl 4]:S30–S38.
3. Findley LJ, Calzetti S. Double-blind controlled study of primidone in essential tremor: preliminary results. *BMJ* 1982;285:608.
4. Findley LJ, Cleeves L, Calzetti S. Primidone in essential tremor of the hands and head: a double blind controlled clinical study. *J Neurol Neurosurg Psychiatry* 1985;48:911–915.
5. Gorman WP, Cooper R, Pocock P, et al. A comparison of primidone, propranolol, and placebo in essential tremor, using quantitative analysis. *J Neurol Neurosurg Psychiatry* 1986;49:64–68.
6. Koller WC, Royse LV. Efficacy of primidone in essential tremor. *Neurology* 1986;36:121–124.
7. Dietrichson P, Espen E. Primidone and propranolol in essential tremor: a study based on quantitative tremor recording and plasma anticonvulsant levels. *Acta Neurol Scand* 1987;75:332–340.
8. Sasso E, Perucca E, Calzetti S. Double-blind comparison of primidone and phenobarbital in essential tremor. *Neurology* 1988;38:808–810.
9. Sasso E, Perucca E, Fava R, et al. Primidone in the long-term treatment of essential tremor: a prospective study with computerized quantitative analysis. *Clin Neuropharmacol* 1990;13:67–76.
10. Sasso E, Perucca E, Fava R, et al. Quantitative comparison of barbiturates in essential hand and head tremor. *Mov Disord* 1991;6:65–68.
11. Calzetti S, Findley LJ, Pisani F, et al. Phenylethylmalonamide in essential tremor: a double-blind controlled study. *J Neurol Neurosurg Psychiatry* 1981;44:932–934.
12. Baruzzi A, Procaccianti G, Martinelli P, et al. Phenobarbital and propranolol in essential tremor: a double-blind controlled clinical trial. *Neurology* 1983;33:296–300.
13. Findley LJ, Cleeves L. Phenobarbitone in essential tremor. *Neurology* 1985;35:1784–1787.
14. Ahmann PA, Lazzara A, Dykes FD, et al. Intraventricular hemorrhage in the high-risk preterm infant: incidence and outcome. *Ann Neurol* 1980;7:118–124.
15. Crowley P, Chalmers I, Keirse MJN. The effects of corticosteroid administration before preterm delivery: an overview of the evidence from controlled trials. *Br J Obstet Gynaecol* 1990;97:11–25.

16. Donn SM, Roloff DW, Goldstein GW. Prevention of intraventricular haemorrhage in preterm infants by phenobarbitone: a controlled trial. *Lancet* 1981;2:215–217.

17. Whitelaw A, Placzek M, Dubowitz L, et al. Phenobarbitone for prevention of periventricular haemorrhage in very low birthweight infants. *Lancet* 1983;2:1168–1170.

18. Bedard MP, Shankaran S, Slovis TL, et al. Effect of prophylactic phenobarbital on intraventricular hemorrhage in high-risk infants. *Pediatrics* 1984;73:435–439.

19. Ruth V. Brain protection by phenobarbitone in very low birthweight (VLBW) prematures: a controlled trial. *Klin Paediatr* 1985;197:170–171.

20. Ruth V, Virkola K, Paetau R, et al. Early high-dose phenobarbital treatment for prevention of hypoxic-ischemic brain damage in very low birth weight infants. *J Pediatr* 1988;112:81–86.

21. De Carolis S, De Carolis MP, Caruso A, et al. Antenatal phenobarbital in preventing intraventricular hemorrhage in premature newborns. *Fetal Ther* 1988;3:224–229.

22. Shankaran S, Cepeda EE, Ilagan N. Antenatal phenobarbital for the prevention of neonatal intracerebral hemorrhage. *Am J Obstet Gynecol* 1986;154:53–57.

23. Kuban KK, Leviton A, Krishnamoorthy KS. Neonatal intracranial hemorrhage and phenobarbital. *Pediatrics* 1986;77:443–450.

24. Morales WJ, Koerten J. Prevention of intraventricular hemorrhage in very low birth weight infants by maternally administered phenobarbital. *Obstet Gynecol* 1986;68:295–299.

25. Kaempf JW, Porreco R, Molina R, et al. Antenatal phenobarbital for the prevention of periventricular and intraventricular hemorrhage: a double-blind, randomized, placebo-controlled, multihospital trial. *J Pediatr* 1990;117:933–938.

26. Thorp JA, Parriott J, Ferrette-Smith D, et al. Antepartum vitamin K and phenobarbital for preventing intraventricular hemorrhage in the premature newborn: a randomized, double-blind, placebo-controlled trial. *Obstet Gynecol* 1994;83:70–76.

27. Thorp JA, Ferrette-Smith D, Gaston LA, et al. Combined antenatal vitamin K and phenobarbital therapy for preventing intracranial hemorrhage in newborns less than 34 weeks' gestation. *Obstet Gynecol* 1995;86:1–8.

28. Shankaran S, Cepeda E, Muran G, et al. Antenatal phenobarbital therapy and neonatal outcome. I. Effects on intracranial hemorrhage. *Pediatrics* 1996;97:644–648.

29. Shankaran S, Papile LA, Wright LL, et al. The effect of antenatal phenobarbital therapy on neonatal intracranial hemorrhage in preterm infants. *N Engl J Med* 1997;337:466–471.

30. Arroyo-Cabrales LM, Garza-Morales S, Hernandez-Pelaez G. Use of prenatal phenobarbital in the prevention of subependymal/intraventricular hemorrhage in premature infants. *Arch Med Res* 1998;29:247–251.

31. Crowther CA, Henderson-Smart DJ. Phenobarbital prior to preterm birth for preventing neonatal periventricular hemorrhage. In: *Cochrane database of systematic reviews,* 2000: CD000164.

32. Porter FL, Marshall RE, Moore JA, et al. Effect of phenobarbital on motor activity and intraventricular hemorrhage in preterm infants with respiratory disease weighing less than 1500 grams. *J Perinatol* 1985;2:63–66.

33. Trauner DA. Barbiturate therapy in acute brain injury. *J Pediatr* 1986;113:742–746.

34. Saul TG, Ducker TB. Effect of intracranial pressure monitoring and aggressive treatment on mortality in severe head injury. *J Neurosurg* 1982;56:498–503.

35. Schwartz ML, Tator CH, Rowed DW, et al. The University of Toronto Head Injury Treatment Study: a prospective randomized comparison of phenobarbital and mannitol. *Can J Neurol Sci* 1984;11:434–440.

36. Ward JD, Becker DP, Miller JD, et al. Failure of prophylactic barbiturate coma in the treatment of severe head injury. *J Neurosurg* 1985;62:383–388.

37. Eisenberg HM, Frankowski RF, Contant CF, et al. High dose barbiturate control of elevated intracranial pressure in patients with severe head injury. *J Neurosurg* 1988;69:15–23.

38. Levy ML, Aranda M, Zelman V, et al. Propylene glycol toxicity following continuous etomidate infusion in the control of refractory cerebral edema. *Neurosurgery* 1995;37:363–371.

39. Roberts I. Barbiturates for acute traumatic brain injury. In: *Cochrane database of systematic reviews,* 2000:CD000033.

40. Brain Resuscitation Clinical Trial I Study Group. Randomized clinical study of thiopental loading in comatose survivors of cardiac arrest. *N Engl J Med* 1986;314:397–403.

41. Rogers MC, Kirsch JR. Current concepts in brain resuscitation. *JAMA* 1989;261:3143–3147.

42. Rubaltelli FF. Current drug treatment options in neonatal hyperbilirubinemia and the prevention of kernicterus. *Drugs* 1998;56: 23–30.

43. Wallin A, Boreus LO. Phenobarbital prophylaxis for hyperbilirubinemia in preterm infants: a controlled study of bilirubin disappearance and infant behavior. *Acta Paediatr Scand* 1984;73: 488–497.

44. Ramboer C, Thompson RP, Williams R. Controlled trials of phenobarbitone therapy of neonatal jaundice. *Lancet* 1969;1: 966–968.

45. Del Castillo ED, Abdo-Bassol F, Jasso-Gutierrez L. Effect of minimal doses of phenobarbital on bilirubinemia in the newborn infant. *Bol Med Hosp Inf Mex* 1976;33:131–136.

46. Karacan I, Orr W, Roth T, et al. Dose-related effects of phenobarbitone on human sleep-waking patterns. *Br J Clin Pharmacol* 1981;12:303–313.

47. Miller NS, Gold MS. Sedative-hypnotics: pharmacology and use. *J Fam Pract* 1989;29:665–670.

48. Bobruff A, Gardos G, Tarsy D, et al. Clonazepam and phenobarbital in tardive dyskinesia. *Am J Psychiatry* 1981;138:189–193.

49. Theis JGW, Selby P, Ikizler Y, Koren G. Current management of the neonatal abstinence syndrome: a critical analysis of the evidence. *Biol Neonate* 1997;71:345–356.

50. Kaltenbach K, Finnegan LP. Neonatal abstinence syndrome, pharmacotherapy and developmental outcome. *Neurobehav Toxicol Teratol* 1986;8:353–355.

51. Carin I, Glass L, Parekh A, et al. Neonatal methadone withdrawal: effect of two treatment regimens. *Am J Dis Child* 1983; 137:1166–1169.

52. Coyne MJ, Bonorris GG, Goldstein LI, et al. Effect of chenodeoxycholic acid and phenobarbital on the rate-limiting enzymes of hepatic cholesterol and bile acid synthesis in patients with gallstones. *J Lab Clin Med* 1976;87:281–291.

53. Coyne MJ, Bonorris GG, Chung A, et al. Treatment of gallstones with chenodeoxycholic acid and phenobarbital. *N Engl J Med* 1975;292:604–607.

PHENOBARBITAL AND OTHER BARBITURATES

ADVERSE EFFECTS

MICHEL BAULAC
JOYCE A. CRAMER
RICHARD H. MATTSON

The safety and tolerability profiles of phenobarbital rest on a considerable background of knowledge owing to its worldwide use for almost a century. Phenobarbital has a reputation of safety because serious systemic side effects are very uncommon. Nonetheless, it presents a strong potential for inducing sedation, cognitive impairment, or behavioral disturbances, particularly in children. These types of neurologic adverse effects are not entirely specific to phenobarbital and also can be encountered with most of the other antiepileptic agents. Comparative studies, however, confirming the clinical experience, showed that many of these neurotoxic effects were more frequent and more pronounced with phenobarbital than with the other drugs. Because of this suboptimal tolerability, along with the increasing number of other therapeutic options, use of phenobarbital as long-term antiepileptic treatment continues to decrease in developed countries.

MOST COMMONLY OBSERVED ADVERSE EFFECTS

An overview of phenobarbital tolerability is given by the studies in which different antiepileptic drugs have been compared in monotherapy settings. The multicenter Veterans Administration (VA) study (1) has been pivotal from this point of view by showing that the rate of withdrawal for unacceptable adverse effects was 19% with phenobarbital, versus 16% with phenytoin, 12% with carbamazepine, and 33% with primidone. In this double-blind study, therapeutic blood concentrations had to be achieved very rapidly, and, in

case of seizure recurrence, daily dosages were increased up to maximum tolerated doses. These aspects of the design may have accounted for a globally high (20%) rate of withdrawal. Two recent, prospective, randomized, but unmasked studies have been conducted in newly diagnosed patients, with designs closer to clinical practice (2,3). These trials allowed a slow titration process and the maintenance of a relatively low dosage if seizures were controlled before therapeutic levels were reached. Globally, in adults (2), 10% of the patients were withdrawn owing to unacceptable adverse effects, with 22% of these subjects randomized to phenobarbital, versus 11%, 5%, and 3% to carbamazepine, sodium valproate, and phenytoin, respectively. A similar study was undertaken in children (3) to compare phenobarbital, carbamazepine, phenytoin, and sodium valproate. Of the 167 children with newly diagnosed epilepsy who were included, 6 of the first 10 children assigned to phenobarbital experienced unacceptable adverse effects, all cognitive or behavioral. No further children were assigned to this drug, leaving the phenobarbital arm of the study uncompleted. These data show that phenobarbital is among the less well tolerated of the conventional or old drugs. There are no comparative data between phenobarbital and any of the recent antiepileptic drugs, some of which are known for a favorable tolerability profile. Nearly all the adverse reactions leading to withdrawal of phenobarbital occurred in the domain of neurotoxicity.

Neurotoxicity

Various neurotoxic adverse effects can be encountered with the long-term use of phenobarbital, even at daily dosages maintaining serum concentrations of the drug in the broad therapeutic range of 15 to 40 µg/mL. Besides changes in affect, behavior, or cognitive function, high serum concentrations may cause neurologic signs of "drunkenness," including nystagmus, dysarthria, incoordination, and ataxia. Often, the neurotoxic side effects occur together in different degrees. Moreover, the terminologies used for their

Michel Baulac, MD: Hopital de la Salpetriere, Bat. P. Castaigne, Paris, France

Joyce A. Cramer, BS: Associate Research Scientist, Yale University School of Medicine, Veterans Affairs Connecticut Health Care System, West Haven, Connecticut

Richard H. Mattson, MD: Professor of Neurology and Director of Medical Studies, Department of Neurology, Yale University School of Medicine and Veterans Administration, West Haven, Connecticut

description are variable, making it difficult to separate one from the other. The occurrence and the magnitude of these neurotoxic symptoms can be reduced at the initial stages of the treatment by a slow titration process. All these neurologic adverse effects are dose dependent and reversible after dosage reduction, if a reduction is possible in terms of seizure control effectiveness. Treating physicians should be aware that patients or relatives might not report some of these symptoms because they can develop insidiously during long-term use.

Sedation

The hallmark of barbiturate toxicity in adults is sedation. In the VA study (1), two of three patients complained of sedation at one or more visits in the first year. Interestingly, phenobarbital produced no more acute sedation than the other drugs tested, probably because of cautious dose increases. Complaints of fatigue and tiredness are difficult to quantify and often are variable and subtle. The patient and family may describe listlessness or lack of spontaneity even when excessive sleeping time is not observed. As dosage is increased, overt sleepiness is observable and often manifests as difficulty with arousal in the morning and naps after school or work. An associated loss of interest, particularly in social activity or playing with friends, is common. Butler et al. (4) noted that patients complained of sedation at the onset of treatment when phenobarbital concentrations were only 5 µg/mL. Two weeks later, there were few complaints despite a fivefold increase in the serum levels. Others also have reported that sedation occurred primarily during the first few days of treatment and decreased rapidly as tolerance developed (5,6). Somnolence was even briefer if phenobarbital was restarted after a withdrawal period . It also was found that a dose that caused sedation during initiation of therapy in adults no longer caused sleepiness after 1 or 2 weeks of treatment (5). After tolerance was acquired, major adverse effects of phenobarbital were not observed when the serum concentration was less than 30 µg/mL. A subgroup of 58 patients taking phenobarbital in the VA study was examined at every visit for the first 3 months (1, 2, 4, 8, and 12 weeks) to assess the incidence of acute adverse effects and development of tolerance (7). Of the subgroup studied for tolerance, 33% of patients started on phenobarbital reported initial sedation, declining significantly to 24% by 12 weeks ($p < .04$). Development of tolerance was evidenced by decreasing symptoms despite increasing phenobarbital concentrations from 18 µg/mL at 2 weeks to 24 µg/mL at 12 weeks.

Mattson et al. (8), however, found many exceptions to the correlation between serum phenobarbital concentrations and complaints of tiredness. The variation among individuals was evident in that some patients were asymptomatic when serum phenobarbital levels were as high as 50 µg/mL, whereas others complained of feeling "drugged" when levels were as low as 15 µg/mL. The usual tolerable range of serum concentrations when phenobarbital is used as the sole drug is 15 to 30 µg/mL.

Neurologic Side Effects

Increasing the dosage of phenobarbital eventually leads to neurologic signs similar to those found with the use of other antiepileptic drugs. Dysarthria, incoordination, ataxia, dizziness, and nystagmus often appear as serum levels exceed 40 µg/mL. The VA study found that at lower levels and at initiation of therapy, these signs and symptoms were significantly less frequent with use of phenobarbital than with carbamazepine, phenytoin, or primidone ($p < .03$).

Behavior

Instead of the sedative effect of phenobarbital common in adults, paradoxical effects of the drug in children and, less commonly, in the elderly are insomnia and hyperactivity. Ounsted (9), in reviewing what he called "the hyperkinetic syndrome," found that many of the children receiving phenobarbital therapy were overactive. The pattern of behavior included signs of distractibility, shortened attention span, fluctuation of mood, and aggressive outbursts. Most of the children were boys. Wolf and Forsythe (10) also found a high incidence of behavioral disturbances. These problems developed in 42% of 109 children receiving daily phenobarbital therapy to prevent recurrence of febrile seizures. Surprisingly, 64% of the children exhibiting hyperactivity had serum phenobarbital concentrations of <15 µg/mL, indicating that such problems can be seen even in what would be considered the low or subtherapeutic range. The authors (10) also suggested that behavioral disturbances associated with phenobarbital use are more likely to become evident in children in the presence of organic brain disease or deficits.

In contrast, Camfield et al. (11) assessed 35 toddlers given phenobarbital and 30 given placebo and found no differences in hyperactivity between the groups after a year. Dose-related irritability and erratic sleep were common in the phenobarbital group, without frank hyperactivity. Reduction from 4 to 5 mg/kg/day to 2 to 3 mg/kg/day resolved these problems in four children. A randomized comparison of phenobarbital and phenytoin intended to detect behavioral side effects showed similar acceptability for the two drugs as monotherapy for childhood epilepsy in rural India (12), but the sensitivity of the procedures used for behavior assessment was limited (13). Another randomized trial comparing phenobarbital with phenytoin and valproate as initial treatment for epilepsy in India did not confirm that hyperactivity problems are more common with phenobarbital, and concluded that this drug should be considered as a possible first choice only for preschool children (14).

Elderly patients with organic brain disease also may become agitated rather than sedated with use of phenobarbital.

Mood and Affect

Phenobarbital therapy can produce alteration of affect, particularly depression. It is difficult to determine whether such mood changes are a reaction to the often newly diagnosed illness, the addition of another drug to treat severe seizures, or a direct neurotoxic effect of phenobarbital. Clinical observations in children suggest a direct effect of phenobarbital because changes to carbamazepine therapy have been associated with improved mood scores (15). In another study of children (16), phenobarbital (38%) was associated with a higher incidence of depression than was carbamazepine or no treatment (0%). Other studies in adults have not revealed statistically significant changes over time among patients on phenobarbital compared with other drugs (1). Early psychological problems with affect, mood, and cognition were reported by 13% of patients in the VA study at 1 month and by 12% at 3 months (7). This was not significantly different in phenobarbital-treated patients compared with carbamazepine, phenytoin, or primidone treatment. However, 40 of 56 patients treated for at least 1 year reported some psychological effect of phenobarbital during the first year. The risk for depression is increased in patients with a personal or family history of an affective disorder.

Cognition

A side effect of phenobarbital of considerable potential importance, especially in children, is a possible disturbance in cognitive function. Problems with memory or compromised work and school performance may develop independent of sedation and hyperactivity, although these factors may play a contributory role. Lennox (17) observed a marked impairment in affect and cognitive function in patients whose capacity had already been compromised: "Many physicians in attempting to extinguish seizures only succeed in drowning the finer intellectual processes of their patients." Such effects often are subtle and difficult to measure despite reports by patients, families, and teachers. Many reports and studies have dealt with this issue of cognitive changes induced by phenobarbital, in adults as in children, but their interpretation sometimes is difficult. Furthermore, some studies have been conducted in children with epilepsy whose persisting seizures or underlying brain damage may interfere with the results, whereas other studies have been done in children who do not have epilepsy who received phenobarbital for the prophylaxis of febrile seizures.

Changes in cognitive function have been measured by various standardized neuropsychological tests. Interestingly, in early reports, institutionalized epileptic patients showed some improvement in intelligence testing after treatment with antiepileptic drugs. Improved test scores could be attributed to decreased seizure frequency or a practice effect from repeated testing. Lennox (17) found 58% of his patients unchanged on subjective evaluation of mentality while using phenobarbital. He separated the improvement of patients because of diminished seizure frequency from the effect of the medication on mentality. A more detailed study by Somerfeld-Ziskind and Ziskind (18) showed no overall change in intelligence quotient (IQ) after phenobarbital therapy for 1 year. Twelve patients actually showed increased IQ scores, whereas 10 patients had lower scores (maximum change, 11 points); 79% had fewer seizures while receiving phenobarbital.

Stores (19) reviewed studies of the effect of phenobarbital on intellectual function in children. He commented that the educational problem for these children appears to be that their attainments fail to match their capacities as measured by standardized tests. Formal studies have not been able to assess this disparity. On careful testing, children treated with phenobarbital can perform at appropriate levels. It is difficult to assess subjective complaints unless the children are treated with a different medication and tested before and after the change from barbiturate therapy.

A double-blind, crossover comparison of psychological and behavioral effects of phenobarbital and valproate was performed in 21 epileptic children (aged 6 to 15 years) by Vining et al. (20). Cognitive function and behavior were significantly diminished during phenobarbital therapy ($p <$ .01), although differences were subtle. Overall intelligence assessed by the Wechsler Intelligence Scale for Children (Revised) (WISC-R) showed significantly lower performance and full-scale IQ scores for phenobarbital than for valproate treatment periods. Differences were seen both in verbal and nonverbal tasks, particularly for complex tests. The extensive neuropsychological testing showed important problems with epilepsy and developmental problems in children (20). The comparison with valproate, a drug not considered likely to cause cognitive impairments, provided information suggesting that phenobarbital can affect childhood learning and behavior.

In another study, children with epilepsy treated with phenobarbital (n = 32) or valproate (n = 32) were compared with healthy children (n = 66) for WISC scores. Total, verbal, and performance scores were lower for children receiving phenobarbital than for control subjects (21). Although valproate-treated and healthy children demonstrated a learning effect with improved scores on retest, the phenobarbital group did not improve, suggesting impaired ability to learn.

Camfield et al. (22) found a trend toward decreased memory and concentration scores in epileptic children taking phenobarbital compared with a placebo group ($p < .07$) that correlated well with serum levels ($p < .05$). They suggested caution in long-term exposure of children to phenobarbital, particularly at high dosage. In a careful study of children receiving an average daily dosage of 1.8 mg/kg of phenobarbital, however, Wapner et al. (23) compared learning behavior and intelligence before therapy and 6 weeks later and found that phenobarbital did not affect the function of the children in the classroom situation. Although seizure control was incomplete, there was no significant change in learning or intellect compared with a control group. It is possible that there is considerable variability in susceptibility to the adverse effects of barbiturates on learning and cognition. Recent case reports suggest that the manifestations of phenobarbital toxicity in children may even include regression of developmental milestones, mimicking a neurodegenerative disorder (24).

Schain et al. (15) found that when carbamazepine was substituted for phenobarbital in children, several mental functions were improved. In particular, they found a statistically significant difference in intelligence (as measured by WISC) and results of three problem-solving tests of attentiveness and impulse control. Parents and teachers also reported a significant improvement in alertness and attentiveness. These drug changes improved seizure control, but the psychological improvements were considered to be a function of removal of the sedating drug.

Other investigators (6) studied adults who had received phenobarbital for 2 weeks, allowing for the partial development of tolerance before performance testing. They found that phenobarbital did not diminish performance on simple tasks requiring attention but did affect tasks requiring sustained effort. Even the tasks requiring sustained effort showed improvement when patients were stimulated during the testing. Others also showed the difference between self-paced tests and tests in which sustained attention was necessary (25). Impaired vigilance and sensory perception during phenobarbital use have been noted in patients of average intelligence.

Hutt et al. (6) tested the effects of phenobarbital after tolerance had developed. Although sedation was less at the time of testing compared with the early acute effect, performance on perceptual-motor tests was significantly impaired in proportion to serum phenobarbital concentration. Tests requiring sustained vigilance were affected negatively. The author defined several factors that were significantly correlated with test performance: (a) serum phenobarbital concentration; (b) difficulty and duration of the task; and (c) tester interaction with the subject (i.e., external stimulation).

A closely related but separate issue is the question of memory impairment, which is a common complaint from epileptic patients and which unquestionably is related, in part, to the brain lesion (26). In detailed studies of patients tested when phenobarbital concentrations were at moderate and then high therapeutic levels, MacLeod et al. (27) compared short-term versus long-term memory storage. They found short-term memory scanning significantly impaired when phenobarbital levels were high, but retrieval of information stored in long-term memory was undiminished. Although this study was unfortunately brief in its 1-week trial at each dose, the data suggest that phenobarbital impairs access to information in short-term but not long-term memory. The authors suggested that impaired short-term memory might be an important influence in acquisition of new information because of impaired attention span. Oxley (28) indicated that a significant improvement in memory function could be achieved after a reduction in phenobarbital dose. This report was of interest because the patients experienced increased seizure frequency when the barbiturate level dropped, indicating that it is not seizure activity that impairs memory. In summary, the assessment indicated that phenobarbital has a deleterious effect on short-term memory, with test performance related to dose. Even when the serum concentration is within the therapeutic range, ability to concentrate and perform simple tasks is reduced.

Several studies have been done in children who received phenobarbital for the prevention of febrile seizures. Hirtz et al. (29) compared IQs of children receiving phenobarbital after a febrile seizure with an untreated group. IQs were significantly lower (7 points) in the phenobarbital-treated group, remaining 5 points lower even after medication was discontinued. The authors concluded that treatment with phenobarbital depressed cognitive performance in children. Farwell et al. (30) reported on the effect of phenobarbital on intelligence of children receiving the medication as prophylaxis for febrile seizures. Two years after randomization to phenobarbital therapy, children assigned to that group had Stanford-Binet IQ scores 8.4 points lower than children in the group assigned to placebo ($p < .006$). IQ scores remained 5.2 points lower for the group assigned to phenobarbital when tested 6 months after that group had treatment discontinued ($p < .05$). Only 64% of children continued to receive phenobarbital throughout the study, and only two-thirds of the phenobarbital blood levels were above 15 µg/mL during follow-up. These children were retested 3 to 5 years later, after they had entered school, to determine whether those effects persisted over the longer term and whether later school performance might be affected (31). On follow-up testing of 139 (of the original 217) children who had experienced febrile seizures, the phenobarbital group scored significantly lower than the placebo group on the Wide Range Achievement Test, and a nonsignificant mean difference of 3.71 IQ points was observed on the Stanford-Binet, with the phenobarbital-treated group scoring lower. The authors concluded that there might be a long-term adverse cognitive effect of phenobarbital on the developmental skills (language/verbal) being acquired during the period of treatment.

Another prospective study was performed to ascertain whether febrile convulsions in early childhood are associated with neurocognitive attention deficits in school-age children (32). A total of 103 children, confirmed to have febrile seizures by the age of 3 years, were followed up until at least the age of 6 years. An achievement test, behavioral ratings, and computerized neurocognitive battery assessing various subcomponents of attention were given to 87 children with febrile seizures and 87 randomly selected population-matched control subjects. Attention performance of the two groups was comparable, including the subgroup of children treated with phenobarbital.

Libido and Potency

A side effect of phenobarbital not documented in the literature and too little appreciated by treating physicians is decreased libido and impotence (1). In clinical practice, we have found that responses to specific questions reveal numerous complaints from men receiving phenobarbital. It is difficult to assess whether the problem is organic or related to psychological depression. Occasionally, dosage reduction improves the problem. Fifteen percent of the patients included in the VA study complained of decreased libido or potency, and this problem was found to be more common in patients treated with phenobarbital or primidone than in those receiving carbamazepine or phenytoin ($p < .06$) (1). Fourteen percent of 56 patients treated for 1 year with phenobarbital reported a transient or continuous decrease in sexual function. The reports increased over time, indicating that this is neither an acute problem nor one for which tolerance develops. Lowering the dosage allowed improvement in some instances, but the drug was discontinued for patients who did not improve.

Multiple mechanisms, including altered metabolism of testosterone (33,34) and psychosocial factors (35), may be responsible for these complaints. However, the problem usually disappeared when carbamazepine or phenytoin was substituted for phenobarbital, but not when phenobarbital was changed to another barbiturate. Psychosocial factors were comparable, testosterone levels (both total and free) were equal, and enzyme-inducing properties are similar for all drugs in the four treatment groups. Consequently, we concluded that the changes in sex behavior might be a direct neurogenic effect.

Precaution and Management

Many neurotoxic side effects improve with a simple reduction in dosage. Of course, improvement is gradual because of the slow elimination of phenobarbital. Such lowering of serum concentration provides less protection against seizures (36). In the past, when seizure control could be achieved only at the cost of neurotoxic side effects, sedation or hyperactivity sometimes were ameliorated with con-

comitant administration of amphetamines. Today, it is less necessary to subject patients to the additional complications attendant on the use of these stimulants. A change to treatment with an alternative antiepileptic drug may be equally effective and spare some side effects.

Dependence, Habituation, and Withdrawal

Phenobarbital shares the properties of other barbiturates in that prolonged use produces dependence, and abrupt discontinuation after high dosage produces abstinence symptoms. Such symptoms include anxiety, emotional lability, insomnia, tremors, diaphoresis, confusion, seizures, and possible status epilepticus (37,38). Reinstituting the drug can reverse these symptoms. It has been suggested that discontinuation of phenobarbital in epileptic patients may lead to exacerbation of seizures not only because of the underlying epilepsy but because of an additional barbiturate withdrawal mechanism (5). Even with abrupt discontinuation, the slow elimination of phenobarbital results in slowly decreasing plasma drug levels. Even so, gradual tapering may be advisable. In a study of the impact of withdrawal of different antiepileptic drugs on seizure recurrence (39), 1,013 patients, in remission of epilepsy for at least 2 years, were randomized to continued therapy or slow withdrawal over 6 months and were followed up for a median period of 5 years. No evidence was found that withdrawal of phenobarbital was associated with withdrawal seizures.

Because phenobarbital can cross the placenta and enter the fetal system, special care must be taken during the neonatal period of children born to mothers who received phenobarbital. The neonatal withdrawal syndrome was described by Desmond et al. (40) for infants born to epileptic mothers. The infants were allowed to withdraw from phenobarbital postpartum. Hyperexcitability, tremor, irritability, and gastrointestinal upset continued for several days to several months. Although the withdrawal syndrome is similar among infants born to heroin addicts, barbiturate addicts, and epileptic mothers, the infants of women on antiepileptic doses of phenobarbital have a milder and briefer withdrawal experience, with good results for all infants (41,42). There is no apparent residual damage after withdrawal. To calculate the probable length of withdrawal in neonates, it should be noted that the phenobarbital concentration in umbilical cord serum is approximately equal to the maternal serum concentration (43). The rate of elimination of phenobarbital in neonates often is slower than that in adults.

Systemic Toxicity

Megaloblastic Anemia

Megaloblastic anemia has been described during treatment with phenobarbital alone or, more commonly, when it is used with other antiepileptic drugs, particularly phenytoin.

Anticonvulsant megaloblastic anemia probably occurs in less than 1% of patients; the incidence was 0.15% to 0.75% in one report (44). The etiology and pathogenesis of macrocytosis and megaloblastic anemia during antiepileptic drug therapy are unknown, but these conditions usually respond to folate therapy.

Folate Deficiency

Frank serum and red blood cell folate deficiency is relatively common. Reynolds (45) surveyed 16 reports in which from 27% to as high as 91% of patients had subnormal serum folate levels, averaging 52%, in patients receiving long-term therapy with phenytoin, phenobarbital, or primidone. The significance of low folate levels is controversial.

Reynolds and Travers (46) reported improvement in psychiatric abnormalities in patients whose low serum folate concentrations were treated with folate therapy. However, such subjective observations are difficult to assess. Although controlled trials have not confirmed that replacement folate therapy in patients receiving phenobarbital or phenytoin either aggravates seizure susceptibility or improves patients' psychological status (47), it is possible that in some patients administration of folate therapy exacerbates seizures (45). Mattson et al. (48) found that serum phenobarbital and phenytoin concentrations decreased when folic acid was given in very high doses. It is possible that reports of seizure exacerbation resulted in part from the decrease in drug concentration rather than from an epileptogenic activity of folate, although the mechanism of this interaction is unknown. Although an inverse correlation exists between folate and phenobarbital levels in both serum and cerebrospinal fluid (CSF) (49), Mattson et al. (48) found no change in CSF folate concentration during folic acid therapy. In fact, animal studies (50) show clearly that even in severe folate deprivation, the brain maintains sufficient folate.

The significance of folate deficiency remains speculative. Other than in cases of obvious megaloblastic anemia, subnormal serum folate probably requires no therapeutic intervention. Except perhaps during pregnancy, proper nutritional balance is sufficient to maintain adequate folate levels during antiepileptic drug therapy. A clear exception exists for women of childbearing age. Supplementary folate reduces the risk of neural tube defects in the developing fetus and should be prescribed before conception (51).

Vitamin K

Another hematologic abnormality caused by antiepileptic drug therapy affects vitamin K. Phenobarbital and phenytoin, which enter the liver of the fetus, can interfere with vitamin K and decrease production of vitamin K–dependent clotting factors. This can occur even in the presence of normal clotting factors in mothers receiving drug therapy. Mountain et al. (52) reported 7 neonates with a severe coagulation defect in a series of 16 neonates whose mothers received various antiepileptic drugs (including 13 receiving barbiturates). The neonate can sustain intraperitoneal, intrathoracic, or intracranial bleeding if vitamin K–dependent coagulation factors are deficient. These signs occur within the first day or two postpartum. Vitamin K administered to mothers prepartum or to neonates at the time of birth prevents this coagulation deficiency (52,53).

Bone Disorders

Antiepileptic drug therapy may affect calcium and vitamin D metabolism, leading to hypocalcemia or, rarely, osteomalacia (54). Despite a high incidence of subnormal calcium levels, no more than 10% of epileptic patients were found to have osteomalacia, with the disorder developing only after many years of drug therapy (55). The incidence of this disorder may relate to climate and life-style (i.e., lack of exposure to sunlight) and diet. Bone mineral density measurements may help to detect subtle bone loss in children receiving phenobarbital over 24 months (56). Induction of liver enzymes leading to increased hydroxylation of vitamin D is a probable mechanism for altered calcium metabolism (57). Reversing signs of deficiency can be accomplished with less than 125 µg of vitamin D_3 per week (58).

Cardiovascular Risks

The potential effects of long-term phenobarbital therapy on the risk of atherosclerosis-related diseases have been differently addressed in the literature. Epidemiologic surveys suggest that antiepileptic drugs may have a protective effect against cardiovascular disease, with 29% less mortality due to ischemic heart disease than in respective control subjects (59). This also was supported by certain studies of serum lipoprotein patterns: through the activation of liver microsomal function, phenobarbital induces apolipoprotein A-1 and high-density lipoprotein synthesis and increases their serum levels, which would be expected to protect against atherosclerosis (60,61)

Other results suggest that, in contrast to the aforementioned finds, the effects on the serum lipid profile of long-term treatment with hepatic enzyme–inducing antiepileptic drugs (e.g., carbamazepine and phenobarbital) perhaps are not beneficial with regard to the risk of atherosclerosis-related disease: elevations of lipoprotein (1), an independent risk factor for atherosclerosis, have been observed in adults (62) and in children (63), and decreased levels of apolipoprotein A have been found in children (64). Finally, an elevated plasma concentration of homocysteine, another established risk factor for atherosclerosis, seems to be associated with antiepileptic drug treatments, including phenobarbital (65). Monitoring of serum cholesterol may be recommended in patients receiving long-term phenobarbital treatment, whatever their age.

Connective Tissue Disorders

A higher incidence of Dupuytren's contractures, palmar nodules, frozen shoulder, Ledderhose's syndrome (plantar fibromatosis), Peyronie's disease, heel and knuckle pads, and general joint pain has been noted in patients taking antiepileptic drugs than in the general population (66,67). These connective tissue disorders were first linked to patients with epilepsy in 1925, when Maillard and Renard (68) called attention to joint pain associated with the use of the newly introduced barbiturates, especially phenobarbital. Soon after, Beriel and Barbier (69) termed this disorder *rheumatism gardenalique.* Until recently, conflicting evidence was available to differentiate among probable etiologic agents. Data from another VA study (70) provided evidence of a statistically significant association between use of phenobarbital and primidone for at least 6 months and onset of all 10 cases of connective tissue disorders (71). None of the 107 patients receiving carbamazepine alone or the 121 on phenytoin experienced a problem ($p < .001$). Critchley et al. (71) were able to define phenobarbital as a common cause in contractures, and Janz and Piltz (72) associated primidone with frozen shoulder.

The incidence of barbiturate-related disorders ranges from 5% to 38%, depending on the population studied. Froscher and Hoffman (73) noted that their general outpatients with epilepsy had a 5% incidence of contractures, similar to that found in the VA study outpatients, but they noted a higher incidence (20%) in patients with severe epilepsy. Noble (74) reported a surgeon's point of view, having seen Dupuytren's contractures in 10% to 38% of institutionalized patients with epilepsy. Duration of treatment probably increases the incidence of disorders.

Reversibility has been seen during continued drug use (72), but improvement is most likely when the barbiturate is stopped early, particularly in patients with barbiturate-associated frozen shoulder and joint pain (67,75). Mattson et al. (70) also described clearing of signs and symptoms when carbamazepine, phenytoin, or valproate was substituted for the barbiturate.

Hepatic and Metabolic Disorders

Phenobarbital is a hepatotoxin only in unusually susceptible individuals. Liver disease induced by antiepileptic drugs, particularly phenobarbital or phenytoin, appears not to be dose dependent and has a low incidence. Most drugs are indirect hepatotoxins, selectively blocking metabolic pathways and producing structural changes by precise biochemical lesions (76). Idiosyncratic acute hepatic injury may be cytotoxic, cholestatic, or mixed. Cytotoxicity can lead to liver necrosis or cholestasis. These drugs probably produce hepatocellular injury—for example, liver necrosis or cholestasis (76) (see section on Hypersensitivity Reactions, later).

Enzymatic Effects

Antiepileptic drugs, particularly phenobarbital, are potent inducers of hepatic microsomal enzymes, which can lead to enhanced metabolism of other drugs or endogenous substances (77). Although some of these effects are considered drug interactions, the basis of these interactions must be considered a hepatic or metabolic side effect of phenobarbital therapy. When metabolism of other compounds is accelerated, the end effect of drugs or substances can be diminished or negated, or pathways can be modified to produce different, potentially effective or toxic metabolites. For example, the induction of microsomal valproate metabolism increases the concentration of the 4-en VPA hepatotoxic metabolite (78). Phenobarbital stimulates hydroxylation pathways related to numerous endogenous and exogenous substances, including thyroid hormones, sex hormones, and other steroids (79). Phenobarbital increases the excretion of 6β-hydroxycortisol, leading to decreased plasma cortisol half-life (80). It also has been shown to increase the rate of metabolism of dexamethasone and prednisone. The resulting lower serum concentrations of these drugs used by patients with bronchial asthma or rheumatoid arthritis disturbed the treatment of their underlying disorder (79). Withdrawal of phenobarbital allowed these changes to reverse (81). Enhanced hormone metabolism can cause failure of oral contraceptives, particularly with low-dose pills (33,82). Interference with the anticoagulation activity of coumarin drugs has been related to phenobarbital therapy (83). Erratic control of anticoagulation with decreased prothrombin time was noted during phenobarbital therapy, and increased dosage of the anticoagulant drug was necessary. However, if phenobarbital is withdrawn, allowing decreased enzyme stimulation, the other drug also requires dosage reduction, or bleeding may occur.

Patients treated with phenobarbital often show increased levels of serum alkaline phophatase and γ-glutamyl transferase. These abnormalities represent an epiphenomenon of enzyme induction and have no clinical significance (79).

Porphyria

Because phenobarbital can induce synthesis of liver enzymes, it has been shown to enhance the synthesis of γ-aminolevulinic acid (ALA) synthetase, which can aggravate porphyria. Granick (84) hypothesized that drugs such as barbiturates may interact with heme, thereby diminishing inhibition of enzymes controlling ALA synthase production. Hereditary acute porphyria can be exacerbated when barbiturates are used.

Hyperbilirubinemia

Bilirubin glucuronidation is induced by phenobarbital, and this has been used to treat neonatal hyperbilirubinemia (85).

Ethanol and Other Drugs

Cramer and Scheyer (86) reviewed the interactions between ethanol and antiepileptic drugs, noting several characteristics shared by phenobarbital and ethanol. Both compounds lead to hypertrophy of hepatic smooth endoplasmic reticulum, inducing nonspecific increases in numerous hepatic drug-metabolizing enzymes. Both compounds are oxidized by nicotinamide-adenine dinucleotide hydrogenase (NADH) microsomal systems (87,88). Barbiturate-hydroxylating enzymes are increased in men given alcohol (89). Enzyme induction allows for increased clearance of drugs in alcoholic patients as well as in those receiving barbiturates. Phenobarbital used with other drugs of abuse significantly affects their metabolism. In addition to altering ethanol metabolism, phenobarbital increases the rate of heroin deacetylation. This increase in detoxification is dose related, parallel to increased enzyme induction (90). Conversely, barbiturates can reduce alcohol dehydrogenase activity, allowing high levels of alcohol to occur when both compounds are used concurrently. The synergy of barbiturate and ethanol toxicity can cause respiratory depression, leading to unexpected death (91).

Gastrointestinal Disturbances

In the VA study (7), early gastrointestinal complaints occurred in 2% to 3% of patients, compared with 7% to 18% of patients on carbamazepine, phenytoin, or primidone (7). Although probably of central origin when nausea and vomiting occur acutely, as with primidone, some local gastrointestinal irritation is possible.

POTENTIALLY LIFE-THREATENING ADVERSE EFFECTS

Oncogenicity

Animal studies have shown liver tumors appearing with the use of phenobarbital and other drugs that activate liver enzymes. Although enzyme induction causes an increase in liver size, it also may protect against the carcinogenicity of other compounds (i.e., known chemical carcinogens) by enhancing their metabolism.

There is no evidence of an increased frequency of liver tumors in patients taking phenobarbital. In fact, Clemmensen et al. (92) found a decrease in tumor incidence in patients receiving anticonvulsants. White et al. (93) found an increase in cancer deaths for epileptic patients, but this was not statistically significant. A Danish study reviewed the incidence of cancer among 8,004 hospitalized patients with epilepsy. Their data suggest that exposure to phenobarbital did not correlate with brain tumor incidence, and that phenobarbital is not a carcinogen for humans (94).

Hypersensitivity Reactions

Phenobarbital causes various types of skin reactions. These usually are mild maculopapular, morbilliform, or scarlatini-

form rashes that fade rapidly when drug administration is stopped. The incidence has been reported to be as low as 1% to 3% of all patients receiving barbiturates (95). Overall, a hypersensitivity reaction to phenobarbital occurred in 9% of patients in the VA study (7), not significantly different from rate of the reaction to carbamazepine, phenytoin, or primidone. The rash was transient and did not require a change in treatment in 5 of 13 patients. None required hospitalization. Considering the universal usage of this drug, reports of exfoliative dermatitis, erythema multiforme, Stevens-Johnson syndrome, or toxic epidermal necrolysis are impressively rare. Welton (96) reported a case of exfoliative dermatitis with hepatitis caused by phenobarbital.

Hypersensitivity reactions are characterized by rash, eosinophilia, liver toxicity, lymphadenopathy, and fever, and may occur with phenobarbital as with other antiepileptic drugs (97). Histologic changes in the liver show eosinophilic or granulomatous inflammation (97). McGeachy and Bleemer (98) reviewed 17 instances of fatal sensitivity to phenobarbital. Another half-dozen cases of acute reaction to barbiturates and details of treatment were reported by Yatzidis (99). Corticosteroids may be of value in treatment (98,100), although their use in severe reactions affecting the skin has been questioned (101). Once sensitivity has been documented, only rarely should the patient be reexposed to the barbiturate (100).

Systemic lupus erythematosus (SLE) can develop with use of antiepileptic drugs. Alarcon-Segovia (102) suggests that the drugs elicit production of antinuclear antibodies by altering nuclear components. This may unmask SLE in predisposed individuals and can be reversed by prompt discontinuation of the drug.

SECOND-GENERATION EFFECTS

Long-Term Developmental Effects

Schain and Watanabe (103) reported that young rats showed retardation of brain growth and changes in behavior after long-term administration of phenobarbital. Hiilesmaa et al. (104) subsequently reported decreased fetal head growth associated with maternal use of antiepileptic drugs and suggested a phenobarbital effect. Several groups have found disturbed neuronal development in cultures containing phenobarbital comparable with or greater than what is found with other antiepileptic drugs (105–107). These findings may not be directly applicable to human use, but they raise special concerns because phenobarbital sometimes is used in pregnancy and in the treatment of neonates.

The neuropsychological consequences of antiepileptic treatment during pregnancy for school-age children and adolescents have been evaluated in 67 subjects (108). Maternal epilepsy and phenobarbital therapy during pregnancy appeared to have long-term effects on the offspring well into adolescence, as evidenced in electroencephalographic patterns, minor neurologic dysfunction, and intellectual performance. Severity of effects was most marked in the polytherapy group. Similar consequences were suggested in adults. A Danish study included 114 adult men born between 1959 and 1961 who were exposed to phenobarbital during gestation through maternal medical treatment and whose mothers had no history of a central nervous system disorder and no treatment during pregnancy with any other psychopharmacologic drug. Subjects exposed prenatally to phenobarbital had significantly lower verbal intelligence scores (approximately 0.5 standard deviation) than predicted (109). All these findings should be interpreted cautiously because of possible selection bias and influence of confounders. Moreover, detrimental environmental conditions may interact with prenatal biologic insults to magnify neuropsychological dysfunctions.

Teratogenicity

With the current awareness that most antiepileptic drugs have some teratogenic effects, counseling for the patient who wishes to become pregnant is indicated. It is difficult to correlate specific teratogenic effects with individual drug use in clinical studies of teratogenicity because of the frequent use of multiple drugs as well as other independent environmental and genetic risk factors. Animal studies suggest that most antiepileptic drugs have some potential for teratogenicity. However, when Chatot et al. (110) grew rat embryos in a medium containing human serum from patients taking antiepileptic drugs, malformed embryos were less common for phenobarbital than for carbamazepine, phenytoin, or valproate.

Speidel and Meadow (111) reported that a variety of malformations occurred in the offspring of six women who used only phenobarbital during their pregnancy: tracheoesophageal fistula, ileal atresia, diaphragmatic hernia with pulmonary hypoplasia, thumb and radius aplasia, congenital heart lesion with microcephaly, mental retardation, hypospadias, and meningomyelocele. In this report and in a similar retrospective survey by Nelson and Forfar (112), the lack of characteristic malformation associated with sole phenobarbital use suggests coincidence rather than causal relationship.

Fedrick (113) found phenytoin far more teratogenic than phenobarbital, but when the two drugs were used in combination, teratogenicity was even more pronounced. Only 4.9% of infants born to mothers who received only phenobarbital during the first trimester were known to have birth defects. This was much lower than incidence rates of 15.2% for sole phenytoin therapy and 22% for combined. Surprisingly, in the same study there was a 10.5% incidence of malformation when mothers with epilepsy took no drugs during pregnancy. A large cooperative study in the United States and Finland (114) implicated phenytoin as a possible

teratogen, but the question also was raised as to whether fetal damage was attributable to antiepileptic drugs or to epilepsy itself.

The Italian Multicenter Cohort Study (115) found reduced birth weight and head circumference in offspring of women treated with phenobarbital compared with other drugs. However, children of untreated epileptic women had the same outcome. The major drawback in all of these studies is the difficulty in obtaining precise information about maternal drug use. There is some evidence that higher drug dose and serum concentration correlate with increasing risk of malformation (116).

A prospective French study followed 156 pregnancies in women with epilepsy, 72 of whom were receiving phenobarbital alone (117). Valproate plus phenobarbital was the most common combination therapy. Microcephaly occurred in 18% of births in the valproate-only group and in 27% of the valproate plus phenobarbital group. The investigators also found a statistical association between cardiac defects and combined use of phenobarbital plus phenytoin, although phenytoin was the only significant variable in multivariate analyses.

The risk of major congenital abnormalities associated with specific antiepileptic drug regimens was assessed in a large retrospective cohort (118). The study included 1,411 children born between 1972 and 1992 in four provinces in The Netherlands who were born to mothers with epilepsy and using antiepileptic drugs during the first trimester of pregnancy, and 2,000 nonepileptic matched control subjects. Significantly increased risks of major congenital abnormalities for carbamazepine and valproate monotherapy were found, with evidence for a significant dose-response relationship for valproate. The risk of major congenital abnormalities was nonsignificantly increased for phenobarbital monotherapy when caffeine comedication was excluded, but a significant increase in risk was found when caffeine was included.

In a prospective, case–control cohort study of 174 pregnant women with epilepsy and their offspring (119), outcomes were compared with those of a control group of 355 healthy women and their offspring. Anomalies and fetal death were the primary outcome measures. Abnormal outcomes were associated with three major antiepileptic drugs (carbamazepine, phenytoin, and phenobarbital). In terms of abnormal outcome (death and anomalies), phenobarbital was associated with the highest relative risk, phenytoin with an intermediate relative risk, and carbamazepine with the lowest relative risk.

An analysis of pooled data from five prospective European studies found that prenatal exposure to either carbamazepine or valproate monotherapy was associated with a fivefold increase in risk of congenital malformations compared with the offspring of untreated nonepileptic mothers. Among 1,221 pregnancies exposed to antiepileptic drugs, the risk of malformations (relative to offspring exposed to phenytoin monotherapy) was increased for the combination of phenobarbital and ethosuximide (relative risk, 9.8), and the combination of phenytoin, phenobarbital, carbamazepine, and valproate (relative risk, 11.0).

A large, prospective, single-center study found that the rate of malformations in the offspring of 517 mothers exposed to antiepileptic drugs during pregnancy was 9.7%, without a significant difference in rates between exposure to polytherapy and exposure to monotherapy (9.6% versus 10.%, respectively). Among monotherapy exposures, structural abnormalities occurred in 15.9% of exposures for valproate (n = 44), compared with 8.6% for primidone (n = 35), 7.1% for carbamazepine (n = 113), 4.8% for phenobarbital (n = 83), and only 3.2% on phenytoin (n = 31). There were no malformations in the offspring of 25 untreated patients.

In another recent prospective analysis of 983 offspring of mothers with epilepsy (120), the incidence of congenital malformations in offspring without drug exposure was 3.1%, versus an incidence with drug exposure of 9.0%. The highest incidence in offspring exposed to a single antiepileptic drug occurred with primidone (14.3%), which was followed by valproate (11.1%), phenytoin (9.1%), carbamazepine (5.7%), and phenobarbital (5.1%).

In view of these data, which sometimes are contradictory, phenobarbital cannot be presented as a safe option for antiepileptic treatment during pregnancy. Drug selection may be influenced by the comparative risks carried by the other options on the one hand, and by other factors, including the need for using the agent that provides the best seizure control, on the other hand.

MANIFESTATIONS AND MANAGEMENT OF BARBITURATE OVERDOSE

Frank overdose of phenobarbital causing serum levels in excess of 50 to 60 µg/mL leads to progressive neurologic dysfunction and depression in levels of consciousness, sometimes even in patients on long-term therapy. Excessively high doses first produce ataxia, dysarthria, nystagmus, incoordination, and uncontrollable sleepiness. As the serum levels rise, these effects progress to stupor and coma. Ultimately, depression of cardiorespiratory function may lead to death. The severity of central nervous system depression is much greater in the drug-naive patient, in whom a level of 80 µg/mL is considered potentially lethal (121). Because of tolerance, the occasional individual on prolonged therapy may remain almost unaffected by serum levels that cause unconsciousness in the naive individual. Nonetheless, concentrations above 70 µg/mL can be expected to compromise levels of consciousness in almost all individuals.

In cases where reversing side effects and lowering serum concentration must be rapid, elimination can be accelerated by alkalinization and induction of forced diuresis (4).

Approximately one-third of an oral dose of phenobarbital is found in the urine unchanged. When necessary, administration of parenteral fluids up to 5 mg/kg/hr can increase excretion severalfold (122). If some of the fluid given is 1.25% sodium bicarbonate, the alkalinization of blood and urine further enhances elimination after overdose. At pH 7.4, 60% of phenobarbital is ionized and crosses cellular membranes poorly. Penetration into and out of tissue is possible for the 40% of the drug that is nonionized. When acidosis occurs, a higher percentage of phenobarbital is nonionized, allowing passage into the intercellular space. This effectively increases tissue concentrations without any change in total-body phenobarbital. Alkalosis has an opposite effect and leads to movement of phenobarbital out of brain and other tissues. Similarly, alkalinization of urine can appreciably increase elimination of phenobarbital from the body. Activated charcoal, by binding enterally secreted phenobarbital, also is effective in enhancing the elimination of the drug from the body, even when it is administered in the postabsorptive phase (123).

REFERENCES

1. Mattson RH, Cramer JA, Collins JF, et al. Comparison of carbamazepine, phenobarbital, phenytoin, and primidone in partial and secondary generalized tonic-clonic seizures. *N Engl J Med* 1985;313:145–151.
2. Heller AJ, Chesterman P, Elwes RD, et al. Phenobarbitone, phenytoin, carbamazepine, or sodium valproate for newly diagnosed adult epilepsy: a randomised comparative monotherapy trial. *J Neurol Neurosurg Psychiatry* 1995;58:44–50.
3. de Silva M, MacArdle B, McGowan M, et al. Randomised comparative monotherapy trial of phenobarbitone, phenytoin, carbamazepine, or sodium valproate for newly diagnosed childhood epilepsy. *Lancet* 1996;347:709–713.
4. Butler TC, Mahafee C, Waddell WJ. Studies of elimination accumulation, tolerance and dosage schedules. *J Pharmacol Exp Ther* 1954;111:425–435.
5. Buchthal F, Svensmark O, Simonsen H. Relation of EEG and seizures to phenobarbital in serum. *Arch Neurol* 1968;19: 567–572.
6. Hutt SJ, Jackson PM, Belsham A, et al. Perceptual motor behaviour in relation to blood phenobarbitone level: a preliminary report. *Dev Med Child Neurol* 1968;10:626–632.
7. Mattson RH, Cramer JA, Collins JF, and the VA Epilepsy Cooperative Study Group. Early tolerance to antiepileptic drug side effects: a controlled trial of 247 patients. *Recent Adv Epilepsy* 1986;149–156.
8. Mattson RH, Williamson PD, Hanahan E. Eterobarb therapy in epilepsy. *Neurology* 1976;26:1014–1017.
9. Ounsted C. The hyperkinetic syndrome in epileptic children. *Lancet* 1955;1:303–311.
10. Wolf SM, Forsythe A. Psychology, pharmacotherapy and new diagnostic approaches. *Adv Epileptol* 1977;124–127.
11. Camfield CS, Chaplin S, Doyle AB, et al. Side effects of phenobarbital in toddlers: behavioral and cognitive aspects. *J Pediatr* 1979;95:361–365.
12. Pal DK, Das T, Chaudhury G, et al. Randomised controlled trial to assess acceptability of phenobarbital for childhood epilepsy in rural India. *Lancet* 1998;351:19–23.

13. Trevathan E, Medina MT, Madrid A. Antiepileptic drugs in developing countries. *Lancet* 1998;351:1210–1211.
14. Thilothammal N, Banu K, Ratnam RS. Comparison of phenobarbitone, phenytoin with sodium valproate: randomized, double-blind study. *Indian Pediatr* 1996;33:549–555.
15. Schain RJ, Ward JW, Guthrie D. Carbamazepine as an anticonvulsant in children. *Neurology* 1977;27:476–480.
16. Brent DA, Crumrine PK, Varma R, et al. Phenobarbital treatment and major depressive disorder in children with epilepsy: a naturalistic follow-up. *Pediatrics* 1990;85:1086–1091.
17. Lennox WG. Brain injury, drugs and environment as causes of mental decay in epilepsy. *Am J Psychiatry* 1942;99:174–180.
18. Somerfeld-Ziskind E, Ziskind E. Effect of phenobarbital on the mentality of epileptic patients. *Arch Neurol Psychol* 1940;43:70–79.
19. Stores G. Behavioral effects of antiepileptic drugs. *Dev Med Child Neurol* 1975;17:647–658.
20. Vining EPG, Mellits ED, Dorsen MM, et al. Psychologic and behavioral effects of antiepileptic drugs in children: a double-blind comparison between phenobarbital and valproic acid. *Pediatrics* 1987;80:165–174.
21. Calandre EP, Dominguez-Granados R, Gomez-Rubio M, et al. Cognitive effects of long-term treatment with phenobarbital and valproic acid in school children. *Acta Neurol Scand* 1990;81:504–506.
22. Camfield CS, Chaplin S, Doyle AB, et al. Side effects of phenobarbital in toddlers: behavioral and cognitive aspects. *J Pediatr* 1979;95:361–365.
23. Wapner I, Thurston DL, Holowach J. Phenobarbital: its effect on learning in epileptic children. *JAMA* 1962;182:937.
24. Shinnar S, Kang H. Idiosyncratic phenobarbital toxicity mimicking a neurodegenerative disorder. *J Epilepsy* 1996;7:36–37.
25. Kornetsky C, Orzack MH. A research note on some of the critical factors on the dissimilar effects of chlorpromazine and secobarbital on the digit symbol substitution and continuous performance tests. *Psychopharmacology* 1964;6:79–86.
26. Delaney RC, Rosen AJ, Mattson RH, et al. Memory function in focal epilepsy: a comparison of nonsurgical, unilateral temporal lobe and frontal lobe samples. *Cortex* 1980;16:103–117.
27. MacLeod CM, Dekaban AS, Hunt E. Memory impairment in epileptic patients: selective effects of phenobarbital concentration. *Science* 1978;202:1102–1104.
28. Oxley J. The effect of antiepileptic drugs on psychological performance. *Epilepsy Int* 1979(abstr).
29. Hirtz DG, Lee YJ, Ellenberg JH, et al. Survey on the management of febrile seizures. *Am J Dis Child* 1986;140:909–914.
30. Farwell JR, Lee YJ, Hirtz DG, et al. Phenobarbital for febrile seizures: effects on intelligence and on seizure recurrence. *N Engl J Med* 1990;322:364–369.
31. Sulzbacher S, Farwell JR, Temkin N, et al. Late cognitive effects of early treatment with phenobarbital. *Clin Pediatr (Phila)* 1999;38:387–394.
32. Chang YC, Guo NW, Huang CC, et al. Neurocognitive attention and behavior outcome of school-age children with a history of febrile convulsions: a population study. *Epilepsia* 2000;41:412–420.
33. Levin W, Kuntzman R, Conney AH. Stimulatory effect of phenobarbital on the metabolism of the oral contraceptive 17-alpha-ethynylestradiol-3-methyl ether (Mestranol) by rat liver microsomes. *Pharmacology* 1979;19:255–294.
34. Toone BK, Wheeler M, Fenwick PBC. Sex hormone changes in male epileptics. *Clin Endocrinol* 1980;12:391–395.
35. Taylor DC. Sexual behavior and temporal lobe epilepsy. *Arch Neurol* 1969;21:510–516.
36. Svensmark O, Buchthal F. Accumulation of phenobarbital in man. *Epilepsia* 1963;4:199–206.
37. Hollister LE. Nervous system reactions to drugs. *Ann NY Acad Sci* 1965;123:342–353.
38. Isbell H, Fraser HF. Addiction to analgesics and barbiturates. *Pharmacol Rev* 1959;2:355–397.
39. Chadwick D. Does withdrawal of different antiepileptic drugs have different effects on seizure recurrence? Further results from the MRC Antiepileptic Drug Withdrawal Study. *Brain* 1999;122:441–448.
40. Desmond MM, Schwanecke RP, Wilson G, et al. Maternal barbiturate utilization and neonatal withdrawal symptomatology. *J Pediatr* 1972;80:190–197.
41. Bleyer WA, Marshall RE. Barbiturate withdrawal syndrome in a passively addicted infant. *JAMA* 1972;221:185–186.
42. Kuhnz W, Koch H, Helge H, et al. Primidone and phenobarbital during lactation period in epileptic women: total and free drug serum levels in the nursed infants and their effects on neonatal behavior. *Dev Pharmacol Ther* 1988;11:147–154.
43. Melchior JC, Svensmark O, Trolle D. Placental transfer of phenobarbitone in epileptic women, and elimination in newborns. *Lancet* 1967;2:860–861.
44. Hawkins CF, Meynell MJ. Macrocytosis and macrocytic anemia caused by anticonvulsant drugs. *Am J Med* 1958;27:45–63.
45. Reynolds EH. Chronic antiepileptic toxicity: a review. *Epilepsia* 1974;16:319–352.
46. Reynolds EH, Travers RD. Serum anticonvulsant concentrations in epileptic patients with mental symptoms: a preliminary report. *Br J Psychiatry* 1974;124:440–445.
47. Jensen ON, Olesen OV. Subnormal serum folate due to anticonvulsive therapy. *Arch Neurol* 1970;22:181–182.
48. Mattson RH, Gallagher BB, Reynolds EH, et al. Folate therapy in epilepsy: a controlled study. *Arch Neurol* 1973;29:78–81.
49. Reynolds EH, Mattson RH, Gallagher BB. Relationships between serum and cerebrospinal fluid anticonvulsant drug and folic acid concentrations in epileptic patients. *Neurology* 1972;22:841–844.
50. Klipstein FA. Subnormal serum folate and macrocytosis associated with anticonvulsant drug therapy. *Blood* 1964;23:68–86.
51. Yerby MS, Leavitt A, Erikson DM, et al. Antiepileptics and the development of congenital anomalies. *Neurology* 1992;42[Suppl 5]:132–140.
52. Mountain KR, Hirsh J, Gallus AS. Neonatal coagulation defect due to anticonvulsant drug treatment in pregnancy. *Lancet* 1970;1:265–268.
53. Renzulli P, Tuchschmid P, Eich G, et al. Early vitamin K deficiency bleeding after maternal phenobarbital intake: management of massive intracranial haemorrhage by minimal surgical intervention. *Eur J Pediatr* 1998;157:663–665.
54. Christiansen C, Rodbro P, Lund M. Incidence of anticonvulsant osteomalacia and effect of vitamin D: controlled therapeutic trial. *BMJ* 1973;4:695–701.
55. Stamp TCB. Effects of long-term anticonvulsant therapy on calcium and vitamin D metabolism. *Proc R Soc Med* 1974;67:64–68.
56. Chung S, Ahn C. Effects of anti-epileptic drug therapy on bone mineral density in ambulatory epileptic children. *Brain Dev* 1994;16:382–385.
57. Richens A, Rowe DJF. Disturbance of calcium metabolism by anticonvulsant drugs. *BMJ* 1970;4:73–76.
58. Offermann G, Pinto V, Kruse R. Antiepileptic drugs and vitamin D supplementation. *Epilepsia* 1979;20:3–15.
59. Muuronen A, Kaste M, Nikkila EA, et al. Mortality from

ischaemic heart disease among patients using anticonvulsive drugs: a case-control study. *BMJ* 1985;291:1481–1483.

60. Luoma PV. Microsomal enzyme induction, lipoproteins and atherosclerosis. *Pharmacol Toxicol* 1988;62:243–249.

61. Luoma PV. Gene activation, apolipoprotein A-1/high density lipoprotein, atherosclerosis prevention and longevity. *Pharmacol Toxicol* 1997;81:57–64.

62. Schwaninger M, Ringleb P, Annecke A, et al. Elevated plasma concentration of lipoprotein (a) in medicated epileptic patients. *J Neurol* 2000;247:687–690.

63. Aynaci FM, Orhan F, Orem A, et al. Effect of antiepileptic drugs on plasma lipoprotein (a) and other lipid levels in childhood. *J Child Neurol* 2001;16:367–369.

64. Eiris J, Novo-Rodriguez MI, Del Rio M, et al. The effects on lipid and apolipoprotein serum levels of long-term carbamazepine, valproic acid and phenobarbital therapy in children with epilepsy. *Epilepsy Res* 2000;41:1–7.

65. Schwaninger M, Ringleb P, Winter R, et al. Elevated plasma concentrations of homocysteine in antiepileptic drug treatment. *Epilepsia* 1999;40:345–350.

66. Battino D, Dukes G, Perucca E. Anticonvulsants. In: Dukes MNG, Aronson JK, eds. *Meyler's side effects of drugs.* Amsterdam: Elsevier Science BV, 2000:166–197.

67. Falasca GF, Toly TM, Reginato AJ, et al. Reflex sympathetic dystrophy associated with antiepileptic drugs. *Epilepsia* 1996; 35:396–399.

68. Maillard G, Renard G. Un nouveau traitement de l'epilepsie: la phenylethylmalonyturee. *Presse Med* 1925;33:315–317.

69. Beriel L, Barbier J. Le rhumatisme gardenalique. *Presse Med* 1934;42:67–69.

70. Mattson RH, Cramer JA, McCutchen CB, and the VA Epilepsy Cooperative Study Group. Barbiturate related connective tissue disorders. *Arch Intern Med* 1973;149:911–914.

71. Critchley EMR, Vakil SD, Hayward HW, et al. Dupuytren's disease in epilepsy: result of prolonged administration of anticonvulsants. *J Neurol Neurosurg Psychiatry* 1976;39: 498–503.

72. Janz D, Piltz U. Frozen shoulder induced by primidone. In: Oxley J, ed. *Antiepileptic therapy: chronic toxicity of antiepileptic drugs.* New York: Raven Press, 1983:155–159.

73. Froscher W, Hoffman F. Dupuytren's contracture in patients with epilepsy: follow-up study. In: Oxley J, ed. *Antiepileptic therapy: chronic toxicity of antiepileptic drugs.* New York: Raven Press, 1983:147–154.

74. Noble J. Connective tissue disorders: discussion. In: Oxley J, ed. *Antiepileptic therapy: chronic toxicity of antiepileptic drugs.* New York: Raven Press, 1983:169–173.

75. Horton P, Gerster JC. Reflex sympathetic dystrophy syndrome and barbiturates: a study of 25 cases treated with barbiturates compared with 124 cases treated without barbiturates. *Clin Rheumatol* 1984;3:493–500.

76. Zimmerman HJ. Drug-induced liver disease. *Drugs* 1978;16: 25–45.

77. Richens A. The clinical consequences of chronic hepatic enzyme induction by anticonvulsant drugs. *Br J Clin Pharmacol* 1974;1:185–187.

78. Baillie TA. Metabolic activation of valproic acid and drug-mediated hepatotoxicity: role of the terminal olefin, 2-n-propyl-4-pentenoic acid. *Chem Res Toxicol* 1988;1:195–199.

79. Perucca E. Clinical implications of hepatic microsomal enzyme induction by antiepileptic drugs. *Pharmacol Ther* 1987;33: 139–144.

80. Burstein S, Klaiber E. Phenobarbital induced increase in 6-beta-hydroxycortisol excretion: clue to its significance in human urine. *J Clin Endocrinol Metab* 1965;25:293–296.

81. Brooks SM, Werk EE, Ackerman SJ, et al. Adverse effects of phenobarbital on corticosteroid metabolism in patients with bronchial asthma. *N Engl J Med* 1972;286:1125–1128.

82. Janz D, Schmidt D. Antiepileptic drugs and failure of oral contraceptives. *Lancet* 1974;1:1113.

83. MacDonald MG, Robinson DS. Clinical observations of possible barbiturate interference with anticoagulation. *JAMA* 1968;204:95–100.

84. Granick S. Hepatic porphyria and drug-induced or chemical porphyria. *Ann NY Acad Sci* 1965;123:188–197.

85. Yeung CY, Tam LS, Chan A, et al. Phenobarbitone prophylaxis for neonatal hyperbilirubinemia poisoning. *Pediatrics* 1971;48: 372–376.

86. Cramer JA, Scheyer RD. The effect of alcohol use on antiepileptic drugs. In: Porter RJ, Mattson RH, Cramer JA, et al., eds. *Alcohol and seizures.* Philadelphia: FA Davis, 1990:241–250.

87. Conney AH, Jacobson M, Schneidman K, et al. Induction of liver microsomal cortisol 6β-hydroxylase by diphenylhydantoin or phenobarbital: an explanation for the increased excretion of 6-hydroxycortisol in humans treated with these drugs. *Life Sci* 1965;4:1091–1098.

88. Rubin E, Hutterer F, Lieber CS. Ethanol increases hepatic smooth endoplasmic reticulum and drug-metabolizing enzymes. *Science* 1968;159:1469–1470.

89. Rubin E, Lieber CS. Hepatic microsomal enzymes in man and rat: induction and inhibition by ethanol. *Science* 1968;162: 690–691.

90. Cramer JA, Cohn G, Meggs L. Effect of phenobarbital and heroin metabolism in the rat. *Fed Proc* 1975;34:814.

91. Hollister LE. Nervous system reactions to drugs. *Ann NY Acad Sci* 1965;123:342–353.

92. Clemmensen J, Fuglsang-Frederiksen V, Plum CM. Are anticonvulsants oncogenic? *Lancet* 1974;1:705–707.

93. White SJ, McLean AEM, Howland C. Anticonvulsant drugs and cancer: a cohort study in patients with severe epilepsy. *Lancet* 1979;2:458–461.

94. Olsen HH, Boice JD, Jensen JP, et al. Cancer among epileptic patients exposed to anticonvulsant drugs. *J Natl Cancer Inst* 1989;81:803–808.

95. Schmidt RP, Wilder BJ. *Epilepsy.* Philadelphia: FA Davis. 1968.

96. Welton DG. Exfoliative dermatitis and hepatitis due to phenobarbital. *JAMA* 1950;143:232–234.

97. Schlienger RG, Shear NH. Antiepileptic drug hypersensitivity syndrome. *Epilepsia* 1998;39[Suppl 7]:S3–S7.

98. McGeachy TE, Bleemer WE. The phenobarbital sensitivity syndrome. *Am J Med* 1953;14:600–604.

99. Yatzidis H. The use of ion exchange resins and charcoal in acute barbiturate poisoning. In: Matthew H, ed. *Acute barbiturate poisoning.* Amsterdam: Excerpta Medica, 1971:223–232.

100. Stuttgen G. Toxic epidermal necrolysis provoked by barbiturates. *Br J Dermatol* 1973;88:291–293.

101. Ruble J, Matsuo F. Anticonvulsant-induced cutaneous reactions. Incidence, mechanisms and management. *CNS Drugs* 1999;12:215–236.

102. Alarcon-Segovia D. Drug-induced lupus syndromes. *Mayo Clin Proc* 1966;44:664–681.

103. Schain RJ, Watanabe K. Origin of brain growth retardation in young rats treated with phenobarbital. *Exp Neurol* 1976;50: 806–809.

104. Hiilesmaa VK, Teramo K, Granstrom ML, et al. Fetal head growth retardation associated with maternal antiepileptic drugs. *Lancet* 1981;2:165–167.

105. Bergey GK, Swaiman KF, Schreir BK, et al. Adverse effects of

phenobarbital on morphological and biochemical development of fetal mouse spinal cord neurons in culture. *Ann Neurol* 1981; 9:584–589.

106. Neale EA, Sher PK, Graubard BI, et al. Differential toxicity of chronic exposure to phenytoin, phenobarbital, or carbamazepine in cerebral cortical cell cultures. *Pediatr Neurol* 1985;1:143–150.

107. Serrano EE, Kunis DM, Ransom BR. Effects of chronic phenobarbital exposure on cultured mouse spinal cord neurons. *Ann Neurol* 1988;24:429–438.

108. Koch S, Titze K, Zimmermann RB, et al. Long-term neuropsychological consequences of maternal epilepsy and anticonvulsant treatment during pregnancy for school-age children and adolescents. *Epilepsia* 1999;40:1237–1243.

109. Reinisch JM, Sanders SA, Mortensen EL, et al. In utero exposure to phenobarbital and intelligence deficits in adult men. *JAMA* 1995;274:1518–1825.

110. Chatot CL, Klein NW, Clapper ML, et al. Human serum teratogenicity studied by rat embryo culture: epilepsy, anticonvulsant drugs, and nutrition. *Epilepsia* 1984;25:205–216.

111. Speidel BD, Meadow SR. Maternal epilepsy and abnormalities of the fetus and newborn. *Lancet* 1972;2:839–843.

112. Nelson MM, Forfar JO. Associations between drugs administered during pregnancy and congenital abnormalities of the fetus. *BMJ* 1971;1:523–527.

113. Fedrick J. A report from the Oxford record linkage study. *BMJ* 1973;1:442–448.

114. Shapiro S, Hartz SC, Siskind V, et al. Anticonvulsants and parental epilepsy in the development of birth defects. *Lancet* 1976;1:272–275.

115. Mastroiacovo P, et al. Fetal growth in the offspring of epileptic women: results of an Italian multicentric cohort study. *Acta Neurol Scand* 1988;78:110–114.

116. Dansky L, Andermann NC, Sherwin A, et al. Maternal epilepsy and congenital malformation: a prospective study with monitoring of plasma anticonvulsant levels during pregnancy. *Neurology* 1980;30:438.

117. Dravet C, Julian C, Legras C, et al. Epilepsy, antiepileptic drugs, and malformations in children of women with epilepsy: a French prospective cohort study. *Neurology* 1992;42[Suppl 5]: 75–82.

118. Samren EB, van Duijn CM, Christiaens GC, et al. Antiepileptic drug regimens and major congenital abnormalities in the offspring. *Ann Neurol* 1999;46:739–746.

119. Waters CH, Belai Y, Gott PS, et al. Outcomes of pregnancy associated with antiepileptic drugs. *Arch Neurol* 1994;51:250–253.

120. Kaneko S, Battino D, Andermann E, et al. Congenital malformations due to antiepileptic drugs. *Epilepsy Res* 1999;33:145–158.

121. Berman LB, Jeghers HJ, Schreiner GE, et al. Hemodialysis, an effective therapy for acute barbiturate poisoning. *JAMA* 1956;161:820–827.

122. Mawer GE, Lee HA. Value of forced diuresis in acute barbiturate poisoning. *BMJ* 1968;2:790–792.

123. Goldberg MJ, Berlinger WG. Treatment of phenobarbital overdose with activated charcoal. *JAMA* 1982;247:2600–2601.

PHENOBARBITAL AND OTHER BARBITURATES

METHYLPHENOBARBITAL

MERVYN J. EADIE
WAYNE D. HOOPER

Two *N*-methyl barbituric acid derivatives were introduced as antiepileptic agents during the past 70 years, but only methylphenobarbital, which appeared in 1932 (1), remains in much use. Metharbital, first used in 1948, never became popular. It was discussed in earlier editions of this book (2), but is not considered further here. Methylphenobarbital is reputedly as effective as phenobarbital as an antiepileptic agent in humans, and is useful in the same types of epilepsy. There has been some interest in its pharmacokinetics and metabolism, especially their stereospecific aspects (3–5).

CHEMISTRY

Methylphenobarbital [mephobarbital, methylphenobarbitone, Mebaral (Sanofi Winthrop, New York, NY) Prominal], chemically 5-ethyl-1-methyl-5-phenylbarbituric acid, is the *N*-methylated analog of phenobarbital (Figure 56.1). It is a weakly acidic, white crystalline powder, pK_a 7.8, molecular weight 246.26, and is more lipid soluble than phenobarbital. It usually is supplied as a racemic mixture [i.e., as equal parts of the (*R*) (−)- and (*S*) (+)-enantiomers]. In what follows, *methylphenobarbital* should be taken to refer to the racemic substance, except where an individual enantiomer is specified; sometimes the prefix *rac-* is added to emphasize that the racemate is meant.

Mervyn J. Eadie, MD, PhD: Emeritus Professor, Department of Medicine, University of Queensland; and Honorary Consultant Neurologist, Royal Brisbane Hospital, Brisbane, Queensland, Australia

Wayne D. Hooper, PhD: Director, Center for Studies in Drug Disposition, University of Queensland, Royal Brisbane Hospital, Brisbane, Queensland, Australia

METHODS OF DETERMINATION

The earliest methods for measuring *N*-methylphenobarbital and its desmethylated derivative in biologic materials were ultraviolet spectrophotometric assays (6–8). Nitration, followed by thin-layer chromatography, was used to resolve methylphenobarbital from phenobarbital (9). Various gas–liquid chromatographic techniques were developed for measuring methylphenobarbital and phenobarbital (10) without derivatization (11), or as ethyl (12) or butyl derivatives (13). Gas chromatography–mass spectrometry provides specific measurement of methylphenobarbital and phenobarbital in the same sample of biologic material (14–17). Methylphenobarbital and phenobarbital can be measured at biologic concentrations without prior derivatization using high-performance liquid chromatography with ultraviolet detection (18). These chromatographic methods measure total methylphenobarbital—that is, the sum of the concentrations of the drug's two enantiomers. The value obtained is not correctly regarded as that of "racemic" methylphenobarbital; the concentrations of the two enantiomers in plasma rarely are equal (see later). In the following discussion, the result of such assays are expressed in terms of (*R*+*S*)-methylphenobarbital. Chiral separation chromatographic methods have been used for the measurement of the individual isomers of the drug (5,19,20).

ABSORPTION, DISTRIBUTION, AND ELIMINATION

Absorption

Clinicians have long known that the molar dose of *rac*-methylphenobarbital required to produce a given biologic effect is approximately twice that for phenobarbital. In urine from three humans, methylphenobarbital plus derived phenobarbital accounted for only 50% to 60% of the methylphenobarbital dose (6). It therefore sometimes was

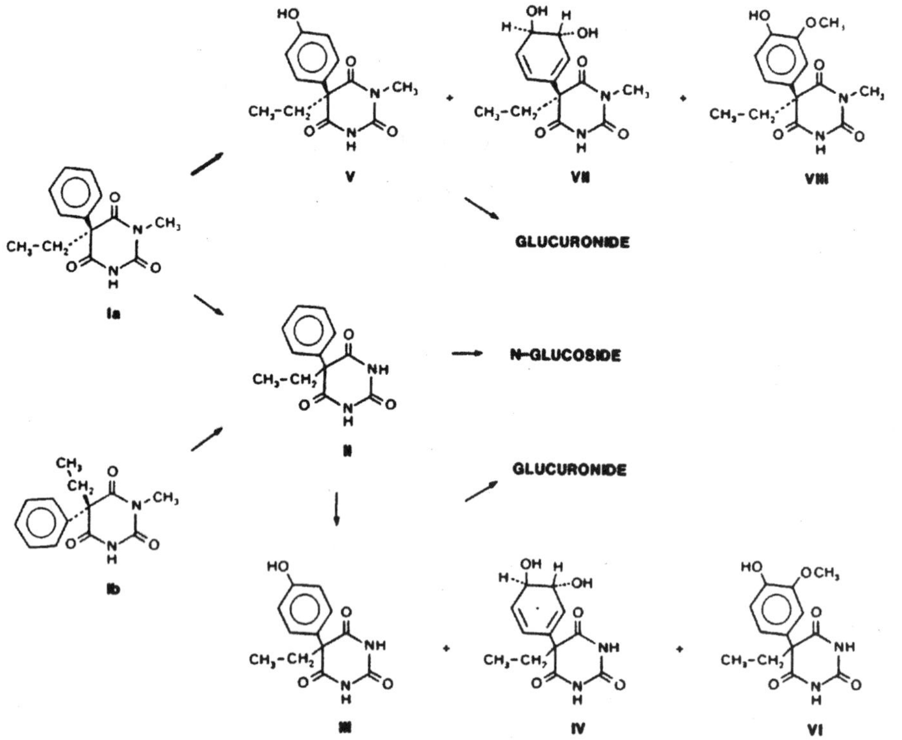

FIGURE 56.1. Metabolic pathways for (*R*)-methylphenobarbital (Ia) and (*S*)-methylphenobarbital (Ib). The (*R*)-enantiomer undergoes formation of phenolic (V), diol (VII), and *O*-methylcatechol (VIII) derivatives or may be demethylated to phenobarbital (II). The (*S*)-enantiomer is demethylated to phenobarbital, which may then undergo *N*-glucosidation or be oxidized to phenolic (III), diol (IV), or *O*-methylcatechol (VI) products. (From Hooper WD, Eadie MJ. Mephobarbital. In: Resor SJ Jr, Kutt H, eds. *The medical treatment of epilepsy*. New York: Marcel Dekker, 1992:363–370, with permission.)

assumed that only approximately 50% of an oral methylphenobarbital dose was absorbed. It is now known that in humans some 35% of a *rac*-methylphenobarbital dose is excreted in urine as the (*R*)- (predominantly) and (*S*)-enantiomers of a previously unidentified *p*-hydroxyphenyl glucuronide derivative (5,21). In two volunteers, the absolute bioavailability of oral methylphenobarbital was 75% (22). Hooper and Qing (23) pointed out that (*R*)-methylphenobarbital has a high oral clearance and is likely to undergo significant presystemic elimination, which may explain the incomplete oral bioavailability of the racemic drug.

The absorption half-time of (*R*+*S*)-methylphenobarbital after oral intake was 1.4 (24), 0.48, and 0.38 hour (22). Mean values (n = 6) of 0.20 hour and 0.94 hour were obtained for the (*R*)- and the (*S*)-enantiomers, respectively (5). Values for the time to maximum concentration (T_{max}) for plasma (*R*+*S*)-methylphenobarbital levels have been 2.5 to 7 hours (24), and for the (*R*)- and the (*S*)-enantiomers, 2.29 ± 1.03 hours (mean ± standard deviation) and 3.50 ± 1.52 hours, respectively (5). In young adult women and men and in elderly women and men, the T_{max} values for the (*R*)-enantiomer were 3.82 ± 1.67, 2.62 ± 1.48, 4.74 ± 1.56, and 4.17 ± 1.62 hours, respectively; the corresponding figures for the (*S*)-enantiomer were 5.96 ± 3.84, 17.3 ± 10.6, 9.18 ± 6.73, and 8.43 ± 3.24 hours (23).

Distribution

The calculated apparent volume of distribution (V_d) of *rac*-methylphenobarbital in humans (24) and dogs (25) exceeds that of total-body water. Such values and the known lipophilicity of the drug suggest that it may achieve higher concentrations in tissues (particularly adipose tissue and brain) than in plasma. In rats, brain methylphenobarbital levels were eight times those in blood (11). The (*R*)-isomer is more readily taken up than the (*S*)-isomer by the brains of Wistar rats, although the latter isomer has the more potent anesthetic effect (26). Values for the apparent V_d of (*R*+*S*)-methylphenobarbital have been 1.9 and 2.1 L/kg in two dogs (25), and in humans 153.5 and 188.3 L (22), and between 49 and 246 L (mean, 132 L) (24). The latter values assumed that the orally administered drug was fully bioavailable. In one human, the V_d of (*R*+*S*)-methylphenobarbital was 246 L and that of phenobarbital (administered separately on another occasion) 25.9 L (24). Assuming complete oral bioavailability, in healthy adults the V_d of (*R*)-methylphenobarbital averaged 5.32 ± 3.33 L/kg and the V_d of (*S*)-methylphenobarbital averaged 1.73 ± 0.31 L/kg (5). As mentioned previously, the (*R*)-enantiomer may not be fully bioavailable orally.

In vitro, 47% ± 2% of (*R*)-methylphenobarbital and 34% ± 2% of (*S*)-methylphenobarbital is bound to albumin (27). In human plasma, ~67% of the (*R*)-enantiomer and ~59% of the (*S*)-enantiomer were protein bound, with 41% and 29%, respectively, being bound to albumin (27). The percentage bound was slightly lower in young adults than in the elderly. The binding was not concentration dependent or influenced by plasma phenobarbital concentrations within the methylphenobarbital concentration range of 1 to 5 mg/L.

Elimination

Biotransformation

Methylphenobarbital undergoes biotransformation to phenobarbital (25), which might be metabolized further (e.g., to *p*-hydroxyphenobarbital and the dihydrodiol metabolite of phenobarbital) (28). Kunze et al. (18) and Hooper et al. (14) identified an additional major biotransformation pathway for the drug in humans, namely, aromatic hydroxylation. Both the *meta* and the *para* isomers of the hydroxylated product were identified in urine. The former appeared to be an artifact, probably formed from a postulated dihydrodiol derivative under conditions of acid hydrolysis of the glucuronide (and perhaps other conjugates). Treston et al. (29) identified small amounts of an *O*-methylcatechol derivative of methylphenobarbital in urine.

Kupfer and Branch (4) and Jacqz et al. (3) showed that methylphenobarbital undergoes a polymorphic pattern of metabolism that appears to be coregulated with that of mephenytoin (methoin). In subjects categorized either as extensive or as poor metabolizers of mephenytoin, Kupfer and Branch (4) showed that the extensive metabolizers excreted 2.5% to 48% of a racemic methylphenobarbital dose in urine as its *p*-hydroxyphenyl derivative over 8 hours, whereas the poor metabolizers excreted less than 1% of the dose in this form. Lim and Hooper (5) and Hooper and Qing (23) showed that (*R*)-methylphenobarbital is metabolized mainly by aromatic hydroxylation (the pathway that is coregulated with mephenytoin hydroxylation); the (*S*)-enantiomer is mainly oxidatively dealkylated to phenobarbital through cytochrome P450 (CYP) isoenzyme CYP2B6 activity (30), although a small amount of hydroxylation occurs (Figure 56.1). The metabolic products may undergo conjugations as well as further biotransformations. It is not clear whether methylphenobarbital, like phenobarbital (31), undergoes *N*-glucosidation.

Half-Life

Terminal half-life values for (*R*+*S*)-methylphenobarbital in individual subjects were 47.9 and 52.2 hours (22) and 34 and 47 hours (32). The first-dose mean half-life of (*R*+*S*)-methylphenobarbital was 49.0 ± 18.8 hours in four adults not receiving other drugs, but 19.6 ± 5.0 hours in five adults taking various drugs, mainly anticonvulsants (24). Lim and Hooper (5) showed that the mean half-life of the (*R*)-enantiomer was 7.50 ± 1.70 hours and that of the (*S*)-enantiomer was much longer (69.8 ± 14.8 hours). These (*R*+*S*)-methylphenobarbital half-life values represent the means of individual enantiomer values, and are potentially misleading (23). The derived phenobarbital had a half-life of 98.0 ± 19.7 hours.

Hooper and Qing (23) showed that the half-life of (*R*)-methylphenobarbital in young men (3.05 ± 1.68 hours) was shorter than in young women (6.94 ± 4.16 hours), elderly men (10.66 ± 7.70 hours), and elderly women (9.64 ± 5.07 hours). For (*S*)-methylphenobarbital, the half-life in young men again was shorter (50.5 ± 20.1 hours) than in the other groups (means of 85.4, 95.1, and 96.4 hours, respectively).

Clearance

The total-body clearance of orally administered (*R*+*S*)-methylphenobarbital averaged 1.85 ± 0.70 L/hr in noninduced subjects and 5.84 ± 2.70 L/hr in presumably induced subjects (24). After intravenous dosage of *rac*-methylphenobarbital, clearance values of 2.21 and 2.50 L/hr for the pooled enantiomers were obtained in two subjects (22). In six noninduced volunteers, the mean oral clearance was 0.47 ± 0.18 L/kg/hr for the (*R*)-isomer and 0.017 ± 0.001 L/kg/hr for the (*S*)-isomer (5). The former value is high enough to suggest that the (*R*)-enantiomer may undergo some presystemic elimination. The first-dose oral clearance of (*R*)-methylphenobarbital (169.9 ± 55.2 L/hr) was higher in young men than in healthy young women (45.1 ± 39.2), elderly men (35.0 ± 29.4), and elderly women (57.4 ± 57.7). Simultaneously measured oral clearances of (*S*)-methylphenobarbital (~1.1 to 1.6 L/hr) did not show appreciable differences related to age or sex (23).

Renal Excretion

Renal excretion of unmetabolized (*R*+*S*)-methylphenobarbital accounts for approximately 1.5% to 3.0% of an oral dose of the drug, with approximately 8% to 25% of the dose being excreted as phenobarbital (24). Possibly the urine collection may not have gone on long enough to determine the full amount of phenobarbital that ultimately would have been excreted by this route. *p*-Hydroxymethylphenobarbital accounts for 30% to 35% of the total dose and appears in human urine mainly as the phenolic glucuronide conjugate of the (*R*)-enantiomer (22). Lim and Hooper (5) found that 24.8% ± 2.3% of the oral dose of *rac*-methylphenobarbital was excreted in urine as (*R*)-*p*-hydroxymethylphenobarbital and 3.6% ± 2.0% as (*S*)-*p*-hydroxymethylphenobarbital. Again, the period of urine collection (at least 12 days) may not have been long enough to determine the full extent of the hydroxylation of the (*S*)-enantiomer.

INTERACTIONS WITH OTHER DRUGS

Any interaction that has been described for phenobarbital (Chapter 53) is likely to occur when methylphenobarbital provides the source of phenobarbital. Methylphenobarbital may contribute an additive sedative effect if coprescribed with other drugs with sedative properties. It probably possesses antiepileptic activity in its own right (see later), as well as by virtue of the phenobarbital it produces. When given with other appropriate antiepileptic drugs, it may produce additive antiepileptic effects. The degree of antiepileptic effect of the individual enantiomers of methylphenobarbital is not established.

Phenobarbital is a well known inducer of certain hepatic microsomal isoenzymes, namely, CYP2B1, CYP2B2, CYP2C6, and CYP3A (33). Methylphenobarbital intake might be expected to cause similar induction both by virtue of the phenobarbital to which it is biotransformed, and also directly (33). In patients, Lander et al. (34) found no interactions between methylphenobarbital and concurrently taken phenytoin or carbamazepine. Phenytoin, carbamazepine, and sulthiame dosage had no statistically significant effects on the relationship between plasma levels of parent methylphenobarbital or derived phenobarbital and methylphenobarbital dose (24). Valproate intake causes a progressive and sustained rise in plasma phenobarbital levels, and a lesser rise in plasma (R+S)-methylphenobarbital levels, in people taking methylphenobarbital (35).

RELATIONSHIP OF PLASMA CONCENTRATION TO SEIZURE CONTROL

Therapeutic Plasma Concentrations

When methylphenobarbital is taken on a long-term basis, steady-state plasma concentrations of phenobarbital become substantially higher than plasma methylphenobarbital levels. For clinical purposes, it usually is sufficient to use plasma phenobarbital levels as a guide to the therapeutic situation (Chapter 54) and to ignore simultaneous plasma methylphenobarbital levels.

Relationship of Dose to Plasma Concentration

Simultaneous steady-state plasma concentrations of both (R+S)-methylphenobarbital and derived phenobarbital are linearly related to the dose of methylphenobarbital (Figure 56.2). No comparable data are available for plasma levels of the individual enantiomers. A methylphenobarbital dosage of 3 to 4 mg/kg/day produces a mean steady-state plasma

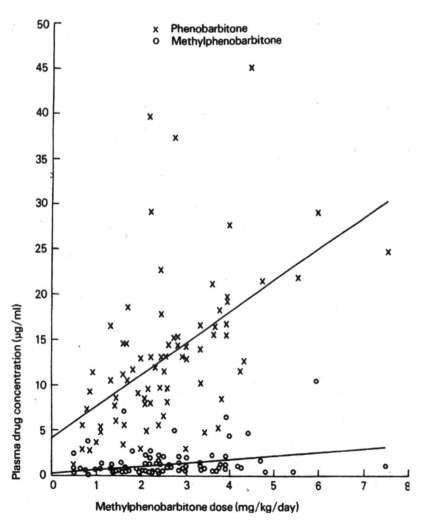

FIGURE 56.2. Relationship between steady-state plasma levels of (R + S)-methylphenobarbital and derived phenobarbital and dose of *rac*-methylphenobarbital in a group of treated epileptic patients. (From Eadie MJ, Bochner F, Hooper WD, et al. Preliminary observations on the pharmacokinetics of methylphenobarbitone. *Clin Exp Neurol* 1978;15:131–144, with permission.)

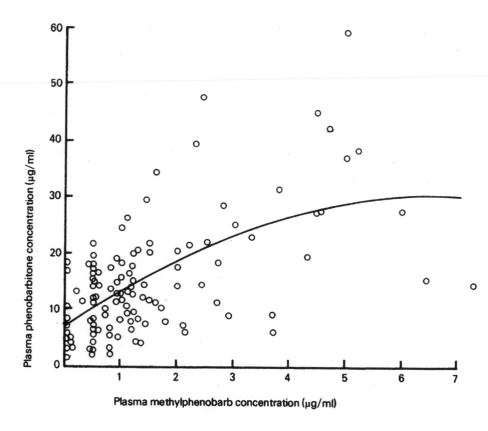

FIGURE 56.3. Relationship between simultaneous steady-state plasma levels of (*R* + *S*)-methylphenobarbital and derived phenobarbital in epileptic patients treated with *rac*-methylphenobarbital. (From Eadie MJ, Bochner F, Hooper WD, et al. Preliminary observations on the pharmacokinetics of methylphenobarbitone. *Clin Exp Neurol* 1978;15:131–144, with permission.)

phenobarbital level of 15 mg/L, and a dosage of 5 mg/kg/day a level of 20 mg/L. The relationship between simultaneous steady-state plasma phenobarbital and (*R+S*)-methylphenobarbital levels in the same patients is shown in Figure 56.3. Plasma phenobarbital levels between 10 and 20 mg/L (values commonly encountered in treating epilepsy) average 7 to 10 times simultaneous (*R+S*)-methylphenobarbital levels. However, at higher plasma methylphenobarbital levels, plasma phenobarbital levels tend to be proportionately less than at lower methylphenobarbital levels. Kupferberg and Longacre-Shaw (15) stated that plasma phenobarbital levels averaged 20 times those of (*R+S*)-methylphenobarbital.

In the individual, steady-state plasma phenobarbital levels up to at least 30 mg/L, and also (*R+S*)-methylphenobarbital plasma levels (36), appear linearly related to the methylphenobarbital dose (Figure 56.4). When phenobarbital itself is taken, the relationship in the individual between steady-state plasma phenobarbital level and phenobarbital dose appears curvilinear (37).

The methylphenobarbital dose (expressed relative to body weight) that produces a given plasma phenobarbital level decreases with age (37). To achieve a plasma phenobarbital level of 15 mg/L, a person younger than 15 years of age requires a mean daily methylphenobarbital dose of 4 mg/kg, and someone older than 40 years one of 2 mg/kg. For a given methylphenobarbital dose (corrected for body weight), men tend to have average plasma phenobarbital levels some 5 mg/L higher than women.

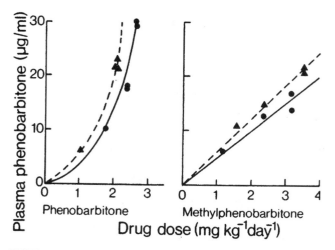

FIGURE 56.4. Relationship between steady-state plasma level of phenobarbital and phenobarbital dose (*left*) and between steady-state phenobarbital level and *rac*-methylphenobarbital dose (*right*), each in two subjects who took different doses of the drugs at different times. (From Eadie MJ, Lander CM, Hooper WD, et al. Factors influencing plasma phenobarbitone levels in epileptic patients. *Br J Clin Pharmacol* 1977;4:541–547, with permission.)

Relationship of Plasma Concentrations to Therapeutic and Toxic Effects

No data are available for the therapeutic range of plasma levels of (*R+S*)-methylphenobarbital or for the individual enantiomers. The conventional therapeutic range of plasma phenobarbital levels (15 to 30 or 10 to 40 mg/L) usually proves a reasonable guide to the antiepileptic effects of methylphenobarbital, although it probably underestimates the total antiepileptic activity present. Dose-determined toxic effects of methylphenobarbital correlate reasonably well with plasma phenobarbital levels. No information is available correlating plasma levels of the methylphenobarbital enantiomers with toxic effects of the drug.

Pharmacologic Aspects of Clinical Use

Steady-state plasma levels of (*R+S*)-methylphenobarbital (half-life approximately 2 days) should apply approximately 8 to 10 days after the most recent dosage change; steady-state conditions for the (*R*)-enantiomer would be expected after approximately 36 hours, and for the (*S*)-enantiomer after approximately 15 days. From the clinical point of view, the derived phenobarbital is likely to take approximately 2 to 3 weeks to attain steady-state after a methylphenobarbital dosage change.

Both (*S*)-methylphenobarbital and phenobarbital are rather slowly eliminated, and their steady-state plasma levels show relatively little fluctuation over 12-hour or even 24-hour dosage intervals, when the drug is taken only once a day (35). Plasma levels of the short half-life (*R*)-enantiomer might be expected to show appreciable interdosage fluctuation under "steady-state" conditions.

Pregnancy and Lactation

Plasma phenobarbital levels tend to fall during the course of pregnancy and to rise again in the puerperium at constant daily methylphenobarbital doses (38). Kaneko et al. (39) have obtained some evidence suggesting that methylphenobarbital is a teratogen in humans. Surprisingly, methylphenobarbital could not be found in the breast milk of women taking the drug (40).

Dose Required to Achieve a Given Plasma Concentration

Intravenous loading doses of methylphenobarbital (15 to 35 mg/kg) have been given to control convulsions in neonates (41), but the drug is better suited to long-term use than to single-dose intake.

Children require average oral methylphenobarbital doses of 5 mg/kg/day, young adults ones of 4 mg/kg/day, and adults older than 40 years of age, ones of 2 mg/kg/day to achieve a mean plasma phenobarbital level of 15 mg/L (24). If higher doses of methylphenobarbital are indicated, steady-state plasma phenobarbital levels can be expected to increase in proportion to the dose increment made.

Toxicity

It is difficult to distinguish between the toxicity of methylphenobarbital and that of its metabolite, phenobarbital (whose toxic manifestations are described in Chapter 56). Most of the toxic effects seen in patients taking methylphenobarbital involve depression of central nervous system function, usually manifested as drowsiness, intellectual blunting, decreased concentration, and irritability.

PHARMACODYNAMICS

Reinhard (42) tabulated the results of a number of studies in which methylphenobarbital appeared to protect against maximal electroshock seizures in the mouse, rat, and cat and against minimal electroshock seizures and pentylenetetrazol-induced seizures in the mouse and rat. Unfortunately, the investigators often have not determined whether phenobarbital had formed in the biologic systems in which they studied methylphenobarbital. After single doses of methylphenobarbital in rats, immediate protection against maximal electroshock seizures correlated better with brain (*R+S*)-methylphenobarbital than with levels of phenobarbital (13). Methylphenobarbital inhibits *N*-methyl-D-aspartate–mediated responses, but only at supratherapeutic concentrations (43).

With the exception of the work of Buch et al. (26), the biologic effects of the individual enantiomers of methylphenobarbital are still to be explored.

CONCLUSION

Methylphenobarbital often has been regarded as a more expensive and less completely absorbed but equally effective alternative to phenobarbital. However, accumulating pharmacokinetic and clinical pharmacologic data indicate that it is well absorbed after oral administration, may enter the brain more readily than phenobarbital, and possesses a useful antiepileptic effect in its own right. It has the advantage over phenobarbital that in the individual patient it produces plasma phenobarbital levels that vary in direct proportion to drug dose.

CONVERSIONS: METHYLPHENOBARBITAL

Conversion factor:

$$CF = 1,000/\text{mol. wt.} = 1,000/246.3 = 4.06$$

Conversion:

$$(\text{mg/L}) \text{ or } (\mu\text{g/mL}) \times 4.06 = \mu\text{mol/L}$$

$$(\mu\text{mol/L})/4.06 = \text{mg/L or } \mu\text{g/mL}$$

ACKNOWLEDGMENTS

The authors thank the editors and copyright owners of the *British Journal of Clinical Pharmacology* and *Clinical and Experimental Neurology* for permission to reproduce Figures 56.2 to 56.4 from previously published work; and Marcel Dekker, Inc. for permission to reproduce Figure 56.1.

REFERENCES

1. Blum E. Die Bekampfung epileptischer Anfalle und ihrer Forgeer scheinungen mit Prominal. *Dtsch Med Wochenschr* 1932;58:230–236.
2. Eadie MJ, Hooper WD. Other barbiturates: Methylphenobarbital and metharbital. In: Levy RH, Mattson RH, Meldrum BS, eds. *Antiepileptic drugs*, 4th ed. New York: Raven Press, 1995:421–437.
3. Jacqz E, Hall SD, Branch RA, et al. Polymorphic metabolism of mephenytoin in man: pharmacokinetic interaction with a coregulated substrate, mephobarbital. *Clin Pharmacol Ther* 1986;39:646–653.
4. Kupfer A, Branch RA. Stereoselective mephobarbital hydroxylation cosegregates with mephenytoin hydroxylation. *Clin Pharmacol Ther* 1985;38:414–418.
5. Lim W, Hooper WD. Stereoselective metabolism and pharmacokinetics of methylphenobarbitone in humans. *Drug Metab Dispos* 1989;17:212–217.
6. Butler TC, Waddell WJ. N-Methylated derivatives of barbituric acids, hydantoin and oxazolidine used in the treatment of epilepsy. *Neurology* 1958;8[Suppl 1]:106–112.
7. Butler TC, Waddell WJ, Poole DT. Demethylation of trimethadione and metharbital by rat liver microsomal enzymes: substrate concentration-yield relationships and competition between substrates. *Biochem Pharmacol* 1965;85:937–942.
8. Bush MT, Sanders-Bush E. Phenobarbital, mephobarbital and metharbital and their metabolites: chemistry and methods for determination. In: Woodbury DM, Penry JK, Schmidt RP, eds. *Antiepileptic drugs*. New York: Raven Press, 1972:293–302.
9. Huisman JW. The estimation of some important anticonvulsant drugs in serum. *Clin Chim Acta* 1966;13:323–328.
10. Rambeck B, Meijer JWA. Gas chromatographic methods for the determination of antiepileptic drugs: a systematic review. *Ther Drug Monit* 1980;2:385–396.
11. Craig CR, Shideman FE. Metabolism and anticonvulsant properties of mephobarbital and phenobarbital in rats. *J Pharmacol Exp Ther* 1971;176:35–41.
12. MacGee J. Rapid identification and quantitation of barbiturates and glutethimide in blood by gas-liquid chromatography. *Clin Chem* 1971;17:587–591.
13. Hooper WD, Dubetz DK, Eadie MJ, et al. Simultaneous assay of methylphenobarbitone and phenobarbitone using gas-liquid chromatography with on-column butylation. *J Chromatogr* 1975;110:206–209.
14. Hooper WD, Kunze HE, Eadie MJ. Simultaneous assay of methylphenobarbital and phenobarbital in plasma using GC-MS with selected ion monitoring. *J Chromatogr* 1981;223:426–431.
15. Kupferberg HJ, Longacre-Shaw J. Mephobarbital and phenobarbital plasma concentrations in epileptic patients treated with mephobarbital. *Ther Drug Monit* 1979;1:117–122.
16. Treston AM, Hooper WD. Metabolic studies with phenobarbitone, primidone and their N-alkyl derivatives: quantitation of substrates and metabolites using chemical ionization gas chromatography-mass spectrometry. *J Chromatogr B Biomed Appl* 1990;526:59–68.
17. Meatherall R. GC/MS confirmation of barbiturates in urine. *J Forensic Sci* 1997;42:1160–1170
18. Kunze HE, Hooper WD, Eadie MJ. High performance liquid chromatographic assay of methylphenobarbital and metabolites in urine. *Ther Drug Monit* 1981;3:45–49.
19. Ceccato A, Boulanger B, Chiap P, et al. Simultaneous determination of methylphenobarbital enantiomers in human plasma by on-line coupling of an achiral precolumn to a chiral liquid chromatographic column. *J Chromatogr A* 1998;819:143–153
20. Eto S, Noda H, Noda A. Simultaneous determination of antiepileptic drugs and their metabolites, including chiral compounds, via beta-cyclodextrin inclusion complexes by a column-switching chromatographic technique. *J Chromatogr B Biomed Appl* 1994;6658:385–390.
21. Hooper WD, Kunze HE, Eadie MJ. Qualitative and quantitative studies of methylphenobarbital metabolism in man. *Drug Metab Dispos* 1981;9:381–385.
22. Hooper WD, Kunze HE, Eadie MJ. Pharmacokinetics and bioavailability of methylphenobarbital in man. *Ther Drug Monit* 1981;3:39–44.
23. Hooper WD, Qing MS. The influence of age and gender on the stereoselective metabolism and pharmacokinetics of methylphenobarbital in humans. *Clin Pharmacol Ther* 1990;48:633–640.
24. Eadie MJ, Bochner F, Hooper WD, et al. Preliminary observations on the pharmacokinetics of methylphenobarbitone. *Clin Exp Neurol* 1978;15:131–144.
25. Butler TC. Quantitation studies of the metabolic fate of mephobarbital (N-methylphenobarbital). *J Pharmacol Exp Ther* 1952;106:235–245.
26. Buch H, Knabe J, Buzello W, et al. Stereospecificity of anaesthetic activity, distribution, inactivation and protein binding of the optical antipodes of two N-methylated barbiturates. *J Pharmacol Exp Ther* 1970;176:709–716.
27. O'Shea NJ, Hooper WD. Enantioselective binding of mephobarbital to plasma proteins. *Chirality* 1990;2:257–262.
28. Harvey DJ, Glazener L, Stratton C, et al. Detection of a 5-(3,4-dihydroxy-l,5-cyclohexadien-l-yl) metabolite of phenobarbital and mephobarbital in rat, guinea pig and human. *Res Commun Chem Pathol Pharmacol* 1972;3:557–566.
29. Treston AM, Philippides A, Jacobsen NW, et al. Identification and synthesis of O-methylcatechol metabolites of phenobarbital and some N-alkyl derivatives. *J Pharm Sci* 1987;76:496–501.
30. Kobayashi K, Abe S, Nakajima M, et al. Role of human CYP2B6 in S-mephobarbital N-demethylation. *Drug Metab Dispos* 1999;27:1429–1433
31. Tang BK, Kalow W, Grey AA. Metabolic fate of phenobarbital in man: N-glucoside formation. *Drug Metab Dispos* 1979;7:315–318.
32. Horning MG, Nowlin J, Butler CM, et al. Clinical applications of gas chromatograph/mass spectrometer/computer systems. *Clin Chem* 1975;21:1281–1287.
33. Murayama N, Shimada M, Yamazoe Y, et al. Distinct effects of phenobarbital and its N-methylated derivative on liver cytochrome P450 induction. *Arch Biochem Biophys* 1996;328:184–192
34. Lander CM, Eadie MJ, Tyrer JH. Interactions between anticonvulsants. *Proc Aust Assoc Neurol* 1975;12:111–116.
35. Eadie MJ, Tyrer JH. *Anticonvulsant therapy: pharmacological basis and practice*, 3rd ed. New York: Churchill Livingstone, 1989.
36. Eadie MJ. Plasma level monitoring of anticonvulsants. *Clin Pharmacokinet* 1976;1:52–66.
37. Eadie MJ, Lander CM, Hooper WD, et al. Factors influencing plasma phenobarbitone levels in epileptic patients. *Br J Clin Pharmacol* 1977;4:541–547.

38. Lander CM, Edwards VE, Eadie MJ, et al. Plasma anticonvulsant concentrations during pregnancy. *Neurology* 1977;27: 128–131.

39. Kaneko S, Otani K, Kondo T, et al. Malformations in infants of mothers with epilepsy receiving antiepileptic drugs. *Neurology* 1992;42[Suppl 5]:68–74.

40. Coradello H. Ueber die Ausscheidung von Antiepileptika in die Muttermilch. *Wien Klin Wochenschr* 1973;85:695–697.

41. Fischer K, Baarsma R [Treatment of convulsions in newborn infants.] *Ned Tijdschr Geneeskd* 1996;140:1557–1560

42. Reinhard JF, Reinhard JF Jr. Experimental evaluation of anti convulsants. In: Vida JA, ed. *Anticonvulsants*. New York: Academic Press, 1977:57–111.

43. Daniell LC. Effect of anesthetic and convulsant barbiturates on N-methyl-D-aspartate receptor-mediated calcium flux in brain membrane vehicles. *Pharmacology* 1994;49:296–307.

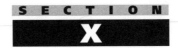

SECTION X

PHENYTOIN AND OTHER HYDANTOINS

PHENYTOIN AND OTHER HYDANTOINS

MECHANISMS OF ACTION

ROBERT J. DELORENZO
DAVID A. SUN

Phenytoin [diphenylhydantoin, Dilantin (Parke-Davis, Morris Plains, NJ); Figure 57.1], first synthesized in 1908 by Biltz (6), was introduced for the treatment of epilepsy in 1938 by Merritt and Putnam (87). The success of phenytoin as an anticonvulsant was one of the major pharmacologic advances in treating neurologic diseases and favorably altered the lives of many people with epilepsy worldwide. Phenytoin produces effective anticonvulsant action without troublesome sedation, and it is one of the most effective compounds for treating generalized tonic-clonic seizures (33,39) and status epilepticus (34,35).

As the first anticonvulsant drug without hypnotic effects (96,97), phenytoin had a major impact on patient care (33–37). Overdoses of phenytoin experimentally and clinically had excitatory rather than depressant effects (89). Because of its clinical importance, phenytoin has been extensively studied in both clinical and laboratory investigations (19,38,39,44). Phenytoin has been useful in studies elucidating the pathophysiology of epilepsy. Woodbury and coworkers (129–135) have contributed extensively to the understanding of the effects of phenytoin on nervous tissue and have written several reviews concerning the history, clinical uses, and mechanisms of action of this compound (2,32,57,80,82,104). More recently, Macdonald's group (78–82) and other laboratories (118,125) have provided evidence of a direct effect of phenytoin on the sodium channel.

Although limitations of space do not permit a complete review of the mechanisms of action of phenytoin, this chapter summarizes its major properties and effects on nervous tissue.

MULTIPLE ACTIONS OF PHENYTOIN

Early Phenytoin Research

Early research on phenytoin was directed at characterizing its metabolism, toxic effects, and clinical efficacy. This research is relevant to the basic mechanism of action of phenytoin because numerous aspects of its effect on the body indicated that it probably had multiple sites of action on physiologic function.

After oral or intravenous administration, phenytoin is widely distributed in the body with high plasma protein binding, giving maximum plasma solubility at 37°C of approximately 75 µg/mL (64). Phenytoin is not given by intramuscular injection. If the pH of the carrying vehicle is adjusted well below 7.8, phenytoin precipitates out of solution. Thus, with intravenous injection the high local concentration of the drug in a neutral pH environment around the injection site causes the drug to precipitate out of solution, with consequent slow absorption. For many years, it was thought that adequate phenytoin levels could be obtained only after several days of phenytoin loading to saturate all of the fat and other body stores for phenytoin. Loading with appropriate intravenous doses of phenytoin can produce adequate serum concentrations within 10 to 20 minutes. This allows phenytoin to be administered for the treatment of status epilepticus and other acute seizure problems. It also enables laboratory investigators to administer phenytoin in high concentrations quickly to various animals. The wide distribution of phenytoin in the brain

Robert J. DeLorenzo, MD, PhD, MPH: George B. Bliley III Professor of Neurology, Department of Neurology, Virginia Commonwealth University, Richmond, Virginia

David A. Sun, PhD: Research Scientist, Department of Neurology, Virginia Commonwealth University, Medical College of Virginia, Richmond, Virginia

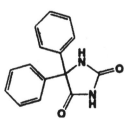

FIGURE 57.1. Structure of phenytoin.

and other body tissues has been studied extensively (91,135). Phenytoin clearly can have adverse effects on the skin, gastrointestinal system, and other major organ systems. The classic phenytoin facies is well documented and demonstrates that phenytoin affects other organ systems besides the central nervous system.

The toxic effects of phenytoin are numerous and have been extensively characterized. Fortunately, phenytoin has a very high therapeutic index, and therapeutic levels can be maintained without serious side effects. Consequently, clinical overdoses of phenytoin are easily recognized and usually not severe. Phenytoin can produce nystagmus, ataxia, and instability of gait at lower toxic levels. At higher toxic levels, dysarthria, incoordination, and unsteadiness often are seen. At very toxic levels, exceeding 30 µg/mL, phenytoin can produce drowsiness, lethargy, and coma. In addition, phenytoin at very high toxic levels can directly damage the cerebellar vermis, producing midline ataxia and a wide-based gait. Phenytoin at high toxic levels also can produce diplopia, hypotension, cardiac suppression, and even death. An important early finding indicated that phenytoin also can produce hyperexcitability, as well as irritability, hallucinations, and even psychotic reactions. These early clinical observations contributed to our understanding of the basic actions of phenytoin, indicating that it worked on multiple regulatory systems in the nervous system. Phenytoin, under certain conditions, clearly can act as an anticonvulsant and neuronal stabilizing compound. In other circumstances, however, it can be excitatory, and even cause psychotic phenomena.

Another hallmark of the multiple effects of phenytoin on the body is the gingival hypertrophy that can occur in patients younger than 21 years of age. This side effect has limited the use of phenytoin in children, although careful oral hygiene can minimize the problem, and research is being directed at inhibiting the effects of phenytoin on gingival cell growth. In adults, phenytoin does not produce much gingival hypertrophy. The developmental relationship of this side effect to the action of phenytoin and the specific cellular mechanisms by which phenytoin produces this effect are not clearly understood and could have important ramifications for developmental neurobiology. Phenytoin may cause mild hirsutism in some patients. It can have an adverse effect on the hematopoietic system and produce, in rare instances, megaloblastic anemia. Phenytoin rarely may produce lupus erythematosus, and is well known to exacerbate this condition.

These early clinical investigations demonstrated that phenytoin affected multiple organ systems and several physiologic and biochemical processes in the body. Much of the research directed at understanding the mechanisms of action of phenytoin was initiated to explain the many effects of this compound in clinical and laboratory settings.

Major Sites of Actions

Phenytoin is probably the most widely studied anticonvulsant. The numerous effects of phenytoin on electrophysiologic and biochemical systems in brain and other tissues have been extensively reviewed by Woodbury and coworkers (129–135) and others (32,39,78–82,104,107). These studies have shown that phenytoin acts on ion conductances, sodium–potassium adenosine triphosphatase (ATPase) activity, various enzyme systems, synaptic transmission, posttetanic potentiation (PTP), neurotransmitter release, and cyclic nucleotide metabolism. These findings suggest that phenytoin has many sites of action in the central nervous system and that it most likely interacts with numerous biochemical processes that regulate neuronal function.

A different point of view from this original theory is that phenytoin may interact with a few important major regulatory systems in the nervous system that could then regulate numerous other cellular processes controlled by these regulators (26–31). Phenytoin has been shown to regulate sodium–potassium ATPase and sodium ion channels. This could have widespread regulatory effects on numerous excitatory and inhibitory systems. Phenytoin also has been shown to regulate calcium–calmodulin-dependent enzyme systems, which also may provide insight into the multiple effects of phenytoin. The effects of phenytoin on cyclic nucleotide metabolism levels also could provide a focal point for multiple effects on cell function. Thus, the effects of phenytoin on several second messenger systems, such as the cyclic nucleotides and calcium systems, might explain the widespread action of this compound on numerous cells and physiologic functions. However, no single action of phenytoin is likely to explain all of its diverse effects on the nervous system.

Whether phenytoin has few or numerous sites of action is still a matter of debate. Although the precise anticonvulsant effect or effects of this compound on neuronal tissue need to be elucidated, the effect of phenytoin on the sodium channel is becoming widely accepted as a major mechanism of action. The following topics represent those areas of research that scientists generally agree have some importance in the action of phenytoin.

EFFECTS OF PHENYTOIN ON NEURONAL EXCITABILITY

Phenytoin limits the development of maximal seizure activity and reduces the spread of seizure discharge from a seizure focus. Both of these experimental observations are pertinent to the clinical effects of phenytoin on generalized tonic-clonic seizures and focal epilepsy. A major anticonvulsant effect of phenytoin is believed to be its ability to block the epileptogenic focus from recruiting surrounding neurons, preventing the spread of seizure discharge.

In contrast to phenobarbital, phenytoin does not significantly elevate the threshold for seizures induced by electrical stimulation with 60-Hz alternating current or by pentylenetetrazol, strychnine, or picrotoxin. In fact, phenytoin actually can potentiate the convulsant effect of pentylenetetrazol and picrotoxin. Thus, studies currently indicate that, although there are some similarities between anticonvulsant drugs, there are important differences in their mechanism of action and the way they produce control of seizure activity.

Despite its inability to elevate the seizure threshold of electrical stimulation of the brain with 60-Hz alternating current, phenytoin does slightly elevate the threshold for seizures induced by 6-Hz stimulation of the brain. Phenytoin's effect is not as dramatic as the effect of phenobarbital in this system, but is clearly distinct from its effect on high-frequency stimulation. Recent evidence, described later, on the effects of phenytoin on use-dependent inhibition of sodium channel function might be related to this interesting physiologic phenomenon.

Phenytoin blocks the tonic phase of tonic-clonic seizures induced by supramaximal electroshock (5,55,123,124). This effect of phenytoin in animals also has been documented in humans undergoing electroconvulsive therapy (123). Phenytoin also blocks the tonic phase of seizures induced by picrotoxin, pentylenetetrazol, and fluorothyl. In spinal preparations, phenytoin abolishes the tonic phase of seizures elicited by supramaximal electroshock (53–55). However, this effect requires higher doses than those that are able to block the tonic phase of seizures in the cerebral cortex.

Phenytoin reduces the prolonged increase in excitability and independent repetitive firing that occurs in the peripheral nerve after supramaximal rapid stimulation (118,121). The hyperexcitability of the peripheral nerve induced by low calcium or a combination of low calcium and low magnesium in the bathing medium also is reduced by phenytoin (73,104,105). These effects on the peripheral nerve suggest that phenytoin has an overall stabilizing effect on the neuronal membrane that may be related in some way to the effects of calcium or sodium on neuronal excitability.

Phenytoin prevents the spread of seizure activity in most areas of the central nervous system. However, its effects on seizure threshold are directed somewhat more toward the cerebral cortex. In several species, phenytoin has been shown to elevate seizure threshold in the hippocampus, amygdala, and anterior dorsal nucleus of the thalamus (1,21), but does not significantly affect the threshold in the reticular activating system and does not influence the sensory relay path to the pyramidal tract (7). Some of these results indicate that phenytoin is most effective in reducing seizure threshold in anatomic regions that contain numerous synaptic connections. Gangloff and Monnier (62)

showed that phenytoin elevated the seizure threshold of the diencephalon, but Morell et al. (90) could not confirm this result. This effect was in contradiction to the effects of phenobarbital and trimethadione on this region of the nervous system. Morell et al. (90) felt that the inability of phenytoin to affect the diencephalon is consistent with some of its clinical effects. Phenytoin can block generalized tonic-clonic seizures but may not block tonic-clonic seizures of cortical origin. Phenytoin does not completely block the sensory or other prodromal signs associated with some partial complex seizures. These authors argued that some of these other effects might result from the inability of phenytoin to alter the seizure threshold in the diencephalon. However, at high concentrations, phenytoin may have marked effects on this structure, and the discrepancy in the findings may relate to the concentrations of the drug used in each experimental system.

The studies described in the foregoing paragraphs pioneered the research efforts into the mechanisms of action of phenytoin on the central nervous system. Phenytoin clearly produces dramatic and clinically useful suppression of the spread of seizure activity in the cortex and other regions of the brain. This effect is not universal, however, and is somewhat selective for specific types of seizures initiated by maximal electroshock but not by several chemical convulsants. In addition, phenytoin appears to be somewhat selective in seizure phase in that it inhibits the tonic phase more potently than the clonic phase of tonic-clonic seizures.

PHYSIOLOGIC EFFECTS OF PHENYTOIN

The well documented effects of phenytoin on seizure discharge and the spread of neuronal excitability set the stage for studying the physiologic mechanisms underlying these effects. Rapid advances in molecular neurobiology, with sophisticated intracellular and extracellular recording techniques, have greatly facilitated this research since the early 1980s. Phenytoin has been shown to modify several important physiologic processes, including PTP and sustained repetitive firing (2,80).

Effects of Phenytoin on Posttetanic Potentiation

PTP is a physiologic phenomenon that has been implicated in the development of hyperexcitable areas in the brain during seizure activity (122). PTP also is thought to be an important mechanism leading to high-frequency trains of impulses in excitatory brain circuits and to the spread of this activity to adjoining neurons, as well as to their propagation to distant neuronal aggregates, resulting in uncontrolled spread of excitation to the whole brain in the maximal tonic seizure discharge (101,107). Thus, PTP is considered an important physiologic process inherent in normal neuronal circuitry that could regulate the spread of neuronal excitability.

PTP specifically refers to the augmentation of the postsynaptic compound action potential elicited by presynaptic stimulation after a repetitive stimulus (100,101,106). Thus, stimulating a neuronal circuit, after a number of intense repetitive stimulations (tetanus) of the same circuit, results in a more dramatic response than before tetanus. This tetanus, or intense stimulation, somehow alters the normal resting levels of excitability of the system and produces a hyperexcitable state. This phenomenon suggests that repetitive use of a neuronal pathway sensitizes it for a given time to enhanced discharge. These types of phenomena could develop a reverberating or "building" hyperexcitability in the neuronal circuitry and implicate normal neuronal mechanisms in the development and spread of the epileptogenic focus. Although this model is appealing, the question of whether PTP is a major mechanism for producing spread of the seizure focus in humans remains unanswered.

Phenytoin effectively blocks PTP (100,101), and this effect may represent one of its major sites of action in preventing the spread of seizures. Phenytoin inhibits PTP in spinal cord preparations as well as in preparations of stellate ganglion in the cat (50,101). In addition, phenytoin blocks PTP at intramedullary terminals and the neuromuscular junction (100). Not all anticonvulsants are effective in blocking PTP. Phenobarbital, trimethadione, and valproic acid have little or no effect on PTP. However, carbamazepine and the anticonvulsant benzodiazepines are effective in blocking PTP.

The mechanism by which phenytoin regulates PTP has not been clearly established. Both the accumulation of calcium in the nerve terminal during the tetanus and the ability of phenytoin to block sodium channels in a use-dependent fashion may contribute as mechanisms for phenytoin's action in blocking PTP (30,31,106).

Effects of Phenytoin on Sustained Repetitive Firing

A growing body of evidence (81–86) indicates that sustained high-frequency repetitive firing (SRF) is an important property of vertebrate and invertebrate neurons and plays a role in regulating the excitability of the cell. SRF is manifested in several types of central nervous system neurons and may be involved in anticonvulsant drug action and epileptogenesis. Although no direct evidence has demonstrated the link between SRF and epilepsy, information obtained from *in vitro* studies on isolated neurons concerning SRF may have some bearing on altered neuronal excitability and anticonvulsant drug action.

Phenytoin is effective in regulating SRF (78–86) (Chapter 4). The correlation of specific anticonvulsant drug activity with actions on SRF has indicated that the SRF model is useful for studying drug effects against generalized tonic-clonic and maximal electroshock–induced seizures (78–80). Anticonvulsants effective against generalized absence seizures, such as ethosuximide and trimethadione, are not effective against SRF. Therapeutic cerebrospinal fluid levels of phenytoin in humans are within the concentration range that inhibits SRF in isolated cultured neurons (80).

The ability of phenytoin to limit SRF has been shown in a wide variety of neurons maintained in culture and several invertebrate preparations (78–86). Phenytoin's ability to limit SRF is an attractive hypothesis for some of the neuronal stabilizing effects of this drug. Evidence is now accumulating that the effects of phenytoin on SRF are mediated by the use-dependent blockage of sodium channels produced by phenytoin (Chapter 4).

EFFECTS OF PHENYTOIN ON SODIUM–POTASSIUM TRANSPORT AND SODIUM ION MOVEMENTS

In 1955, Woodbury (129) provided evidence that phenytoin played a major role in altering sodium ion movements across nerve cell membranes. This work set the stage for much of the following research over the next 30 years with regard to the effects of phenytoin on ion conductances in neuronal membranes. On the basis of calculated intracellular sodium concentrations, Woodbury suggested that phenytoin might regulate sodium transport in the brain by affecting sodium–potassium ATPase (22,130–134). The more recent electrophysiologic studies of Macdonald's group (78–80) have clearly established that concentration ranges of phenytoin that are consistent with anticonvulsant levels in humans produce a use-dependent blockage of the voltage-gated sodium channel.

Sodium–Potassium ATPase

Sodium–potassium ATPase and its regulation by phenytoin have been extensively studied and reviewed (22,23). The early research studies showed that phenytoin, under some conditions, increased the activity of the sodium–potassium ATPase. In brain synaptosomes, phenytoin increased sodium–potassium ATPase activity after systemic administration to animals (63,75) and after administration *in vitro* (60,128). Phenytoin also increased the activity of sodium–potassium ATPase in the adrenal medulla (65). Some conflict developed in this field when it was found that under some experimental conditions phenytoin did not affect sodium–potassium ATPase in *in vitro* brain synaptosome experiments. These results have been carefully examined by numerous investigators (22), and it now appears that the difference in experimental results relates to the ratio of sodium to potassium in the experimental systems.

Deupree (48,49) concluded that phenytoin, under certain conditions, does not affect sodium–potassium ATPase and that earlier studies may be explained by the contamination of phenytoin with potassium, which would increase the potassium ratio. However, Delgado-Escueta and Horan (22) reviewed these data and found that the effects of phenytoin on active transport of potassium in synaptosomes occur under conditions in which the potassium content of the cell is lowered and the sodium concentration is increased. This latter condition is thought to be more closely analogous to the environment of the epileptogenic focus.

These results may explain why phenytoin lacks toxic effects on normal neuronal function, but can have a marked neuronal stabilizing effect during an excitable discharge. Under normal conditions, phenytoin may not play a role in regulating sodium–potassium ATPase activity. However, in an epileptogenic focus, where the ratio of sodium to potassium across the membrane may be altered, phenytoin may regulate the activity of this important membrane enzyme system. These studies on sodium and sodium–potassium ATPase represented a major advance in understanding the mechanism of action of anticonvulsant drugs. This research represents one of the first neurochemical insights into the mechanism of action of phenytoin and serves as a model for its testing in numerous other biochemical systems.

Phenytoin Effects on Sodium Conductances

After the initial observations by Woodbury that phenytoin may regulate neuronal excitability by affecting sodium permeability across the cell membrane, several relevant investigations over the next 30 years used new techniques for studying the action of phenytoin on neuronal tissue. The membrane "stabilizer" effect of phenytoin and its ability to prevent repetitive electrical activity (13,59,71,73,121) indicated that phenytoin's action on sodium conductance might be an important area for further research. Lipicky et al. (76) observed that phenytoin decreased the early sodium current in the voltage-clamped squid axon, suggesting that the drug decreased the number of open channels in the early phase of the action potential. Johnson and Ayala (70) also observed in *Aplysia* that phenytoin decreased sodium influx. Further evidence for an effect of phenytoin on sodium influx was provided by Swanson and Crane (115) using guinea pig cerebral cortical slices, and by Schwarz and Vogel (109) in voltage-clamp experiments on single myelinated neurofibers. These studies also suggested that phenytoin decreased the action potential amplitude and increased the threshold to fire. These results led to the hypothesis that phenytoin might reduce the conduction velocity by affecting sodium currents.

More recent observations by DeWeer (50) and Perry et al. (94) on the isolated squid axon provided additional evidence that phenytoin affects sodium influx. These investigators postulated that phenytoin behaved like tetrodotoxin in blocking sodium channels. Their studies also confirmed the observations of Schwarz and Vogel (109) that phenytoin induced membrane hyperpolarization. Thus, numerous studies have demonstrated that phenytoin has a significant effect on sodium influx in neuronal membranes (20,105). The results are consistent with the original observations of Woodbury and may explain some of the neuronal stabilizing effects of this anticonvulsant.

Use-Dependent Inhibition of Sodium Channels

A major contribution of Macdonald's laboratory (78–80) has been to demonstrate, using electrophysiologic techniques and kinetic analysis, that phenytoin interacts with sodium channels at concentrations found in the plasma of patients treated for epilepsy. Phenytoin directly reduces the frequency of SRF of action potentials in isolated neurons maintained in culture (78–86). An important aspect of this effect of phenytoin on the action potential was that it did not reduce the amplitude or duration of a single action potential but reduced only the ability of the neuron to fire trains of action potentials at high frequency. Outside-out patch recordings in hippocampal neuronal cultures demonstrated that phenytoin more effectively inhibited late sodium channel openings, believed to underlie ictal epileptiform activity, than the transient sodium channel openings that comprise the peak sodium current (110). This ability of phenytoin to limit high-frequency repetitive firing was voltage dependent, increased after depolarization, and reduced by hyperpolarization. The limitation of firing was prolonged enough to last for several hundred milliseconds.

It was postulated from these studies that one of phenytoin's anticonvulsant actions may be to shift the sodium channel to an inactive state similar to the normally occurring inactive state of the channel, but from which recovery was delayed (80). The ability of phenytoin to limit SRF implies an action that occurs only under abnormal conditions, where neurons are firing repetitively at high frequencies. Thus, phenytoin can decrease the high-frequency spread of seizure discharge during the development of seizure activity without inhibiting the normal, less frequent firing of the neuron under background conditions. This experimental finding, along with the finding that phenytoin preferentially inhibits late sodium channel openings (110), is attractive because it seems to explain why phenytoin has so few sedative or cognitive effects relative to its potent anticonvulsant action. Other studies have supported the findings of Macdonald's group and further substantiated the effect of phenytoin on sodium channels using electrophysiologic techniques. Schwarz and Vogel (109) showed that phenytoin produced a voltage-dependent block of sodium channels that could be removed by hyperpolarization in mammalian myelinated nerve fibers. Phenytoin caused a shift of the steady-state sodium channel inactivation curve to the more negative voltages in these experiments. Also, phenytoin reduced the rate of recovery of sodium channels from inactivation. These studies showed that under normal conditions, sodium channels recovered from the inactivation state in a few milliseconds after a 500-millisecond depolarization to 25 mV. In the presence of phenytoin, however, recovery from the inactive state took greater than 90 milliseconds. In addition, phenytoin was shown in this preparation to produce a frequency-dependent block of action potentials. The advantage of this experimental model was that it could be used to apply more sophisticated kinetic analysis. These studies suggested that the effect of phenytoin on sodium channel inhibition assumed first-order kinetics, indicating that the anticonvulsant was binding at one site near or at the sodium channel.

Similar studies were performed on isolated mammalian neurons by Wakamori et al. (127). These studies investigated the effect of phenytoin on hippocampal pyramidal neurons isolated from CA1 regions from 1- to 2-week-old rats. Phenytoin produced a negative shift in the steady-state inactivation curve for sodium channels in these cells and also produced frequency-dependent block of sodium channels. Thus, phenytoin has been shown to inactivate sodium channels in a use-dependent manner in both mammalian myelinated nerve fibers as well as isolated neurons in culture.

Phenytoin also has been shown to affect human sodium channels (125). Electrophysiologic studies of the human brain sodium channels expressed in the oocytes were blocked by phenytoin in a voltage-, frequency-, and time-dependent fashion. The authors (125) concluded that the effects of phenytoin on human sodium channels were similar to those in cultured neurons, rat myelinated nerve, and rat hippocampal pyramidal neurons (80).

More recent studies have investigated the specific kinetics and binding actions of phenytoin to sodium channels (80,118,125). Phenytoin appears to stabilize the inactive form of the sodium channel in a voltage-dependent fashion. Kinetic data suggest that opening of the sodium channel allows the phenytoin molecule to diffuse through the channel and bind to a receptor site on the inside of the membrane surface. Thus, the effect occurs in a voltage-dependent manner. The affinity of phenytoin for the sodium channel is short-lived, and the channel returns to normal activity within milliseconds. Therefore, the sodium channel can quickly recover from this use dependent block.

The characteristics of this binding and the elucidation of the possible site of the phenytoin sodium channel have been actively pursued (14,69,99,118). Site-directed mutagenesis studies have shown that three amino acids in the S6 transmembrane α helix of domain IV of the pore-forming α subunit glycoprotein of the sodium channel are critical for phenytoin binding. Mutation of these three amino acids has been found to reduce phenytoin binding to the inactivated state of the sodium channel (14). The anticonvulsants carbamazepine and lamotrigine, and local anesthetics, share this common receptor site, as well as the mechanism of stabilizing the inactivated state of the channel (14). A two–phenyl-ring structure also is common to these drugs and has been implicated in forming the ligand for the binding interaction (69).

The effect of phenytoin on limiting sustained repetitive firing through use-dependent blockage of the sodium channel provides a biochemical mechanism for preventing rapid neuronal discharge from spreading from one neuron to another without interfering with normal action potential communication between neurons.

EFFECTS OF PHENYTOIN ON NEUROTRANSMISSION

Phenytoin has long been known to depress synaptic transmission. Since the early 1970s, new electrophysiologic techniques have allowed the inhibitory effects of phenytoin to be studied in more detail. It appears that phenytoin can inhibit depolarization-dependent synaptic transmission but can increase the frequency of miniature end-plate potentials (MEEPs) at rest in the synapse (136). These mechanisms provide insight into the ability of phenytoin to be both excitatory and inhibitory in the nervous system.

It has been shown in *in vitro* synaptosome preparations that phenytoin inhibits norepinephrine and acetylcholine release (27–29). Studies (27–31) have shown that phenytoin can inhibit neurotransmitter release from synaptosomes by blocking calcium entry during depolarization. In addition, under conditions where calcium enters the synaptosomes through an ionophore, phenytoin still could inhibit neurotransmitter release by direct inhibition of intracellular synaptosomal biochemical processes, such as protein phosphorylation and other calmodulin-regulated events. These studies provide the first evidence that at least two mechanisms exist for explaining the effects of phenytoin on synaptic transmitter release. Phenytoin most likely blocks transmitter release during an action potential by minimizing or limiting calcium entry and by having a specific effect on other molecular processes in the nerve terminal that modulate transmitter release. The effects of phenytoin on MEEPs are postulated to be the result of increased intracellular calcium concentrations induced by the drug. Phenytoin not only inhibits calcium uptake into synaptosomes but can block calcium uptake into mitochondria. As an important intracellular calcium buffering system, the mitochondria keep the calcium concentration in the nerve terminal at a low level. By inhibiting this process, phenytoin can slightly elevate intrasynaptosomal calcium, causing hyperexcitability manifested as a significant increase in MEEPs.

EFFECTS OF PHENYTOIN ON CALCIUM CHANNELS AND CALCIUM SYSTEMS

Phenytoin has been shown to inhibit calcium influx in numerous preparations. The mechanisms by which phenytoin inhibits calcium influx are not completely understood. However, several studies have provided convincing evidence that this drug regulates the calcium conductances in nerve preparations as well as in other tissues (92).

Effects of Phenytoin on Calcium Channels and Sequestration Mechanisms

Studies by Ferrendelli and coworkers (57,58,111,112) elegantly demonstrated that phenytoin inhibits depolarization-dependent calcium influx in preparations of presynaptic nerve terminals *in vitro*. This work provided the initial evidence that phenytoin inhibits both sodium and calcium influx during depolarization and suggests that these conductances are affected independently of each other. Phenytoin has been shown moderately to inhibit L-type calcium channels in neuronal (68,108) and nonneuronal preparations (88,103). Phenytoin also inhibits T-type calcium currents (68,119). Recent studies have demonstrated that phenytoin inhibition of T-type currents may be subject to subunit variation of the T-type calcium channel (74,120). Phenytoin caused a moderate blockade of native dorsal root ganglia T-currents, but a complete, although lower-affinity, blockade of currents from transfected α1G subunits in HEK293 cells. Interestingly, a complete, lower-affinity block similar to that of α1G T-currents was seen in some α1H currents, whereas other α1H T-currents demonstrated a partial, higher-affinity blockade similar to the native DRG neurons (120). The investigators suggested that there could be an as yet unknown regulatory factor present in DRG neurons, and some HEK293 cells, that selectively regulates α1H subunit T-currents (120). Further investigation is required to elucidate the complete role of phenytoin on depolarization-dependent calcium influx and the potential for anticonvulsant action.

Phenytoin also blocks calcium sequestration in a number of different preparations. Calcium uptake is inhibited in the intact neuromuscular junction preparations as well as in the synaptosome preparation (102,135). Several other studies on the effects of phenytoin on calcium uptake and metabolism have been extensively reviewed (117,131). Cytosolic calcium levels in gingival fibroblasts are modulated by phenytoin (89), possibly providing mechanistic insight into the gingival hyperplasia associated with phenytoin use in children.

An overwhelming body of evidence suggests that phenytoin can inhibit calcium influx during depolarization and also inhibit the uptake and sequestration of calcium in the nerve terminal after its entry. Thus, phenytoin has both a depressive effect by blocking calcium uptake and a poten-

tially excitatory effect by blocking the uptake and sequestration of calcium in the nerve terminal. This latter effect could result in prolonged elevated calcium concentrations in the nerve terminal after tetanic stimulation or the spread of repetitive firing. This molecular insight might have some bearing on the clinical observations that phenytoin can have both neuronal stabilizing and anticonvulsant properties, as well as cause hyperexcitability in the nervous system. Depending on the balance in the system, phenytoin could either suppress neuronal activity by decreasing calcium entry or cause hyperexcitability of the nervous system by delaying the recovery of resting intracellular calcium in the nerve terminal after repetitive discharge. These results have led several investigators (30,31) to suggest that the effect of phenytoin on calcium metabolism may explain some of its anticonvulsant activity and effects on hyperexcitable nervous tissue.

Effects of Phenytoin on Calmodulin Target Enzymes

Calmodulin is a major calcium-binding protein that mediates some of the second messenger effects of calcium on cell function (16,17,72). Calmodulin binds calcium, and this calcium–calmodulin complex can regulate several enzyme systems in the cell (17). Major enzymes regulated by calcium and calmodulin are the calcium- and calmodulin-dependent protein kinases such as calmodulin kinase II. Phenytoin inhibits calcium–calmodulin-regulated protein phosphorylation in neuronal preparations and in preparations of presynaptic nerve terminals (24–46). The ability of phenytoin to regulate this major calcium-dependent enzyme system suggests that phenytoin modulates many of the second messenger effects of calcium in the nervous system, which may provide a major pathway by which phenytoin can regulate many cellular processes. The effect of phenytoin on calmodulin-regulated systems may occur at higher-than-physiologic concentrations, and thus may account for some of the toxic effects of phenytoin on neuronal tissue. The precise role of phenytoin inhibition of calcium–calmodulin-regulated enzyme systems is an important area for further investigation.

Because calcium has been implicated in regulating many physiologic processes in the brain, the influence of phenytoin on some of these processes by blocking calcium entry, regulating intracellular calcium levels, or affecting one or more major calcium–calmodulin-regulated enzyme system could account for some of the broad anticonvulsant and toxic effects of phenytoin on the central nervous system.

EFFECTS OF PHENYTOIN ON CHLORIDE PERMEABILITY

Phenytoin increases chloride conductance in mammalian cortical neurons as well as in crayfish stretch receptor neurons (3). This chloride conductance is associated with the γ-aminobutyric acid A (GABA$_A$) receptor. At nanomolar concentrations, phenytoin postsynaptically modifies the gating mechanism, thereby decreasing the rate of closing of the chloride channel. Phenytoin apparently enhances the chloride conductance of the GABA$_A$ receptor, which underlies the inhibitory postsynaptic potential, leading to increased hyperpolarization of the neuronal membrane. Therefore, similar to benzodiazepines and barbiturates, phenytoin apparently enhances the effect of the GABA$_A$ receptor.

Although phenytoin-enhanced GABA$_A$ receptor chloride currents are an attractive anticonvulsant mechanism, phenytoin's inability effectively to inhibit pentylenetetrazol-induced seizures in animals somewhat discredits this hypothesis. Pentylenetetrazol-induced seizures are very sensitive to benzodiazepines, working through the GABA$_A$–benzodiazepine complex. This anticonvulsant complex functions to increase the GABA$_A$ receptor chloride current. If phenytoin's anticonvulsant properties are similarly mediated through increased chloride conductances, then phenytoin should inhibit pentylenetetrazol-induced seizures. Because phenytoin is ineffective in this model, the significance of phenytoin's action on chloride currents requires further investigation.

EFFECTS OF PHENYTOIN ON BIOCHEMICAL SYSTEMS

Phenytoin, particularly at toxic concentrations, affects numerous biochemical systems and processes, as noted in the reviews by Woodbury (131–133). A complete discussion of all of these effects goes beyond the scope of this chapter. However, several effects of phenytoin on major second messenger and biochemical systems are worth discussing in some detail because they may have an important contribution to some of the anticonvulsant or toxic effects of this drug.

Effects of Phenytoin on Cyclic Nucleotide Metabolism

Phenytoin regulates the metabolism of adenosine 3',5'-monophosphate (cyclic AMP) and guanosine 3',5'-monophosphate (cyclic GMP). Both of these cyclic nucleotides have been implicated as major second messengers in cell function. The effects of phenytoin on cyclic nucleotide metabolism have been studied and reviewed by Ferrendelli (56,58). Phenytoin depresses the basal levels of cyclic GMP in the cerebellum *in vivo*. Phenytoin also prevents electroshock convulsion–induced elevation of brain cyclic AMP and cyclic GMP levels in the cerebral cortex. Phenytoin also inhibits the elevation of brain cyclic nucleotides caused by depolarizing agents that increase sodium influx in synaptosome fractions.

These studies suggest that phenytoin may act directly on nucleotide metabolism or that the effects may be secondary to some neuronal stabilizing effects of phenytoin that block depolarization-induced production or metabolism of cyclic nucleotides. The possible relationship of these effects of phenytoin to its anticonvulsant action or toxic effects is an important area for further research.

Effects of Phenytoin on Neurotransmitter Systems

As discussed earlier, phenytoin affects neurotransmitter release and metabolism in numerous preparations [see review by Woodbury (131)]. Phenytoin inhibits the release of norepinephrine and other neurotransmitters *in vivo* and from intact nerve terminal preparations *in vitro*. Phenytoin also inhibits neurotransmitter reuptake. These effects are dose dependent because different effects are attained at different concentrations of phenytoin. These results suggest that phenytoin may act at different sites in regulating transmitter release and uptake.

Phenytoin also decreases the concentration of glutamic acid in the brain and increases the concentration of glutamine and GABA. The effect of phenytoin on GABA systems has been observed in different preparations and in different species. Thus, phenytoin may play a role in regulating the level and metabolism of this major inhibitory neurotransmitter. Furthermore, phenytoin affects the metabolism and activity of acetylcholine. These examples indicate that phenytoin may play an important role in regulating neurotransmitter systems in the brain by affecting the metabolism, storage, release, or uptake of these compounds, possibly through its effects on calcium and cyclic nucleotide second messenger systems.

Effects of Phenytoin on Calmodulin Systems

Phenytoin inhibits calcium–calmodulin-dependent protein kinase in neuronal preparations (4,24,31,43). Phenytoin's ability to regulate protein phosphorylation may play an important role in regulating the anticonvulsant or side effects of this compound on neuronal and nonneuronal tissue. Because calcium-dependent protein phosphorylation may play a major role in regulating numerous cellular processes, the ability of phenytoin to inhibit this system could account for many of its effects on cellular metabolism and, ultimately, on numerous cells in the body. The role of phenytoin in regulating other calmodulin-controlled enzyme systems needs further investigation.

NEUROPROTECTIVE EFFECTS OF PHENYTOIN

Phenytoin's ability to block calcium entry suggests that it may be a potent neuroprotective agent in ischemia or anoxia. Studies from Taft et al. (116) demonstrate that phenytoin protects against ischemia-induced neuronal cell death in a well characterized gerbil forebrain ischemia model. This model entails brief bilateral carotid occlusion that results in complete forebrain ischemia. After 5 minutes of carotid occlusion, almost complete neuronal destruction in the CA1 sector of the hippocampus is observed, with preservation of other hippocampal neuronal structures. This is a very controllable experimental model for studying effects of neuroprotective agents. Phenytoin treatment (200 mg/kg) blocked the ischemia-induced neuronal cell death. Phenytoin was also neuroprotective with longer durations of ischemia and was more effective at higher concentrations.

These studies indicate that phenytoin may be a useful neuroprotective agent for the treatment of brain injury or cerebrovascular disease. The precise mechanism by which phenytoin accomplishes its neuroprotective effects has not been clearly established (66). The ability of phenytoin to inhibit calcium entry or calcium-dependent enzymes may play an important role in this neuroprotective effect. However, the possibility of reducing depolarization through block of the sodium channel or subsequent seizure activity associated with neuronal injury also must be considered. Phenytoin also inhibits spreading depression in retinal preparations (15). Phenytoin therefore may have an important role in the future as a neuroprotective or adjunct neuroprotective agent.

PHENYTOIN RECEPTOR MOLECULES

Receptor neuropharmacology has played a major role in the development of many drugs since the early 1980s. Specific receptors for the benzodiazepines, steroids, catecholamines, and other neuroleptic compounds have provided important mechanisms of action for several of these neuropharmacologic agents. However, at present, except for the high-affinity benzodiazepine receptor (10), there is no evidence for a specific anticonvulsant binding site. Recent studies (8,9) have identified a novel class of benzodiazepine-binding proteins that bind benzodiazepines with a potency series and a therapeutic concentration range that are consistent with the effects of the benzodiazepines on SRF and effects on maximal electroshock–induced seizures in animals. Studies also have indicated that phenytoin effectively competes in therapeutic concentrations with the benzodiazepines for this low-affinity receptor. These results suggest that these novel benzodiazepine receptors also may bind phenytoin in therapeutic concentrations and provide evidence of a specific binding protein for phenytoin in the central nervous system. Further investigations must be conducted to determine the significance and relevance of this phenytoin-binding protein to its actions as a stabilizer of neuronal membranes. It is clear that research directed at identifying anticonvulsant receptors would have important implications in developing new therapeutic agents to regulate seizures and in understanding mechanisms of action of anticonvulsant drugs. This is an area that needs further research.

FOSPHENYTOIN

Fosphenytoin [ACC-9653; CI 982; Cerebyx (Parke-Davis)], first synthesized in 1973 by Stella and Higuchi (114), is a disodium phosphate ester of phenytoin. As a highly water-soluble prodrug of phenytoin, fosphenytoin offers an alternative composition of this anticonvulsant that lacks many of the adverse effects of phenytoin administration. As discussed earlier, intramuscular phenytoin administration is painful and ineffective owing to drug precipitation induced by the lower pH effect of phenytoin injection in tissue (93). Intravenous administration of phenytoin also is painful and can cause vascular tissue damage (113) and phlebitis (95). Rapid intravenous administration of phenytoin can cause cardiovascular collapse, presumably because of the 40% propylene glycol vehicle (77). Fosphenytoin, because of its high water solubility [over 4,000 times greater than phenytoin (126)], is an excellent alternative to phenytoin for parenteral administration. Fosphenytoin does not produce the vascular and cardiac toxicities of phenytoin preparations and therefore is safer and can be administered more rapidly.

Fosphenytoin has no known intrinsic activity. Fosphenytoin's anticonvulsant effects only become apparent after its rapid and complete metabolism to phenytoin by phosphatases (Figure 57.2) in the heart, lungs, liver, spleen, kid-

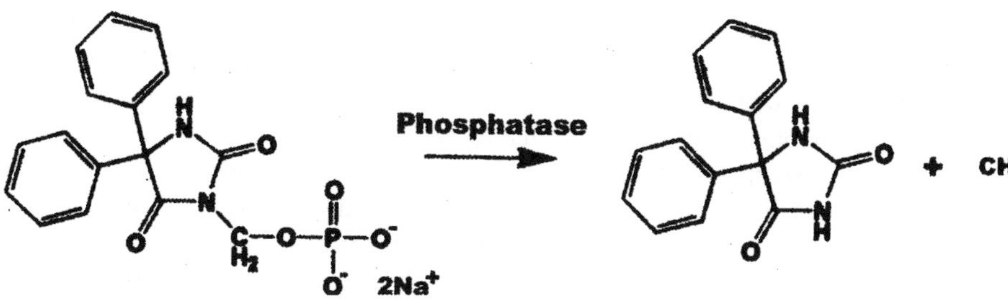

FIGURE 57.2. Enzymatic conversion of fosphenytoin to phenytoin, formate, and phosphate by phosphatases.

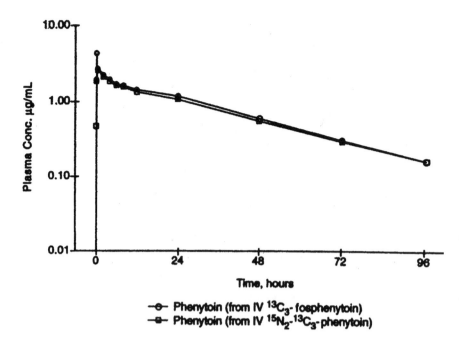

FIGURE 57.3. Plasma total phenytoin concentrations derived from fosphenytoin (*circles*) and from phenytoin (*squares*) after simultaneous intravenous infusion of 150 mg phenytoin equivalents are virtually identical over time. (From Browne TR, Szabo GK, McEntegart C, et al. Bioavailability studies of drugs with nonlinear pharmacokinetics: II. absolute bioavailability of intravenous phenytoin prodrug at therapeutic phenytoin serum concentrations determined by double-stable isotope technique. *J Clin Pharmacol* 1993;33:89–94, with permission.)

neys, and small intestine, (98). At this time, no drugs are known to alter the conversion of fosphenytoin to phenytoin (18). The bioavailability of phenytoin derived from intravenous fosphenytoin administration is rapid and virtually identical to that of intravenous phenytoin (12) (Figure 57.3). Like phenytoin, protein binding of fosphenytoin to plasma proteins like albumin is high (95% to 99%) (67). However, in contrast to phenytoin, this binding is nonlinear (67). This extensive binding displaces phenytoin from albumin and increases the plasma free fraction of phenytoin (51,52). Direct renal excretion of fosphenytoin is minimal and clinically insignificant (12).

Fosphenytoin has fewer local adverse effects at the administration site than phenytoin. Adverse effects of fosphenytoin in the central nervous system (nystagmus, headache, ataxia, and somnolence) are attributed to the phenytoin derived from fosphenytoin metabolism, rather than the prodrug itself. Electrocardiographic changes and hypotension sometimes seen with rapid phenytoin administration are not seen with fosphenytoin (52). Transient paresthesias that resolve without further consequence have been reported with intravenous administration of fosphenytoin (11,61). These paresthesias have not been associated with phenytoin use, but are not associated with permanent symptoms.

Fosphenytoin is a better preparation for rapid administration and for parenteral indications of phenytoin (47). The U.S. Food and Drug Administration has approved fosphenytoin for intramuscular loading and maintenance dosing in adults and children older than 5 years of age and for the intravenous treatment of status epilepticus. Fosphenytoin shares the same contraindications as phenytoin. Although fosphenytoin is more expensive than phenytoin,

economic savings can be realized with this drug over phenytoin because of the savings associated with decreased adverse effects at the site of administration, decreased time and supplies associated with restarted and new intravenous lines, and decreased risk of cardiovascular complications.

UNIFYING MECHANISMS OF ACTION—SUMMARY

There is no single action of phenytoin that can completely account for its numerous effects on neuronal and nonneuronal tissue. The preponderance of evidence suggests that phenytoin may produce its numerous effects by regulating several important aspects of cellular function. Phenytoin's ability to regulate sodium transport across neuronal membrane is a major mechanism of action that almost certainly underlies some of its clinical effects on neuronal tissue. The use-dependent inhibition of sodium channels characteristic of phenytoin provides an important potential mechanism allowing phenytoin to regulate excitability ictally, but not interictally, during normal neuronal activity. Further research on the effect of phenytoin on sodium channels potentially will elucidate how its molecular effect might underlie its specific clinical effects. The ability of phenytoin to modulate sustained repetitive firing may underlie its ability to inhibit the tonic phase of generalized tonic-clonic seizures. The ability of phenytoin to regulate calmodulin and cyclic nucleotide second messenger systems could account for some of its widespread effects on cellular processes. It is difficult to find a biochemical or physiologic process that is not in some way regulated by cyclic nucleotides or calcium. Thus, the effects of phenytoin on these second messenger systems would be dramatically amplified in terms of the diverse clinical and toxic effects that might result from its use. These effects may account for the wide diversity of phenytoin's actions. The ability of phenytoin to regulate and inhibit voltage-dependent neurotransmitter release at the synapse also may play an important role in its anticonvulsant action. Although the precise mechanisms of this effect are not known, it is clear that inhibition of calcium channels and calcium sequestration by phenytoin in the nerve terminal plays an important role in the excitatory and inhibitory actions of this anticonvulsant. The effect of phenytoin on PTP also may underlie some of its important anticonvulsant properties. Some of the effects of phenytoin on PTP may be mediated at the molecular level by its effect on calcium and sodium systems. Advances in molecular neurobiology and neuroscience have increased our understanding of the mechanisms of action of phenytoin. Major advances described in this chapter shed light on how phenytoin may mediate neuronal stabilizing and excitatory phenomena. More recent advances have lead to the synthesis and characterization of fosphenytoin, which shares the anticonvulsant mechanisms of action of phenytoin while reducing some of the adverse effects associated with parenteral administration.

REFERENCES

1. Aston R, Domino EF. Differential effects of phenobarbital, pentobarbital and diphenylhydantoin on motor cortical and reticular thresholds in the rhesus monkey. *Psychopharmacologia* 1961; 2:304–317.
2. Ayala GF, Johnston D. The influences of phenytoin on the fundamental electrical properties of simple neural systems. *Epilepsia* 1977;18:299–307.
3. Ayala GF, Lin S, Johnston D. The mechanism of action of diphenylhydantoin on invertebrate neurons: I. effects on basic membrane properties. *Brain Res* 1977;121:245–258.
4. Babcock Atkinson E, Norenberg LO, et al. Diazepam inhibits calcium, calmodulin-dependent protein kinase in primary astrocyte cultures. *Brain Res* 1989;484:399–403.
5. Barany EH, Stein-Jensen E. The mode of action of anticonvulsant drugs on electrically-induced convulsions in the rabbit. *Arch Int Pharmacodyn Ther* 1946;73:1–47.
6. Biltz H. Uber die Konstitution der Einwirkungsprodukte von substituierten Harnstoffen auf Benzil und uber einige neue Methoden zur Darstellung der 5,5 Diphenylhydantoin. *Berl Dtsch Chem Ges* 1908;41:1379.
7. Blum B. A differential action of diphenylhydantoin on the motor cortex of the cat. *Arch Int Pharmacodyn Ther* 1964;149: 45–55.
8. Bowling AC, DeLorenzo RJ. Micromolar benzodiazepine receptors: identification and characterization in central nervous system. *Science* 1982;216:1247–1250.
9. Bowling AC, DeLorenzo RJ. Photoaffinity labeling of a novel benzodiazepine binding protein in rat brain. *Eur J Pharmacol* 1987;135:97–100.
10. Braestrup C, Squires RF. Pharmacological characterization of benzodiazepine receptors. *Eur J Pharmacol* 1978;48:263–270.
11. Broumer K, Matier WL, Quon CY. Absolute bioavailability of phenytoin after IV 3-phosphoryloxymethyl phenytoin disodium. *Clin Pharmacol Ther* 1988;43:178(abstr).
12. Browne TR, Szabo GK, McEntegart C, et al. Bioavailability studies of drugs with nonlinear pharmacokinetics: II. absolute bioavailability of intravenous phenytoin prodrug at therapeutic phenytoin serum concentrations determined by double-stable isotope technique. *J Clin Pharmacol* 1993;33:89–94.
13. Carnay L, Grundfest S. Excitable membrane stabilization by diphenylhydantoin and calcium. *Neuropharmacology* 1974;13: 1097–1108.
14. Catterall WA. Molecular properties of brain sodium channels: an important target for anticonvulsant drugs. *Adv Neurol* 1999; 79:441–456.
15. Chebabo SR, DoCarmo RJ. Phenytoin and retinal spreading depression. *Brain Res* 1991;551:16–19.
16. Cheung WY. Cyclic 3′,5′-nucleotide phosphodiesterase: demonstration of an activator. *Biochem Biophys Res Commun* 1970;38:533–538.
17. Cheung WY. Calmodulin role in cellular regulation. *Science* 1980;207:19–27.
18. Cerebyx (fosphenytoin sodium injection) package insert. Morris Plains, NJ: Parke–Davis, 1996.
19. Czuczwar S, Frey H, Loscher W. *N*-methyl-*d*,*l*-aspartic acid-induced convulsions in mice and their blockade by antiepileptic drugs and other agents. In: Nistico G, Morselli P, Lloyd K, et al., eds. *Neurotransmitters, seizures and epilepsy III*. New York: Raven Press, 1986, 235–246.
20. Davies JA. Mechanisms of action of antiepileptic drugs. *Seizure* 1995;4:267–271.
21. Delgado JMR, Mihailovic L. Use of intracerebral electrodes to evaluate drugs that act on the central nervous system. *Ann NY Acad Sci* 1956;64:644–666.
22. Delgado-Escueta AV, Horan MP. Phenytoin: biochemical membrane studies. *Adv Neurol* 1980;27:377–398.
23. Delgado-Escueta AV, Ward AA, Woodbury DM, et al., eds. Basic mechanisms of the epilepsies: molecular and cellular approaches. *Adv Neurol* 1986;44:3–55.
24. DeLorenzo RJ. Antagonistic action of diphenylhydantoin and calcium on the endogenous phosphorylation of specific brain proteins. *Neurology* 1976;26:386.
25. DeLorenzo RJ. Antagonistic action of diphenylhydantoin and calcium on the level of phosphorylation of particular rat and human brain proteins. *Brain Res* 1977;134:125–138.
26. DeLorenzo RJ. Phenytoin: calcium- and calmodulin-dependent protein phosphorylation and neurotransmitter release. In: Glaser GH, Penry JK, Woodbury DM, eds. *Antiepileptic drugs: mechanisms of action*. New York: Raven Press, 1980: 399–414.
27. DeLorenzo RJ. Role of calmodulin in neurotransmitter release and synaptic function. *Ann NY Acad Sci* 1980;356:92–109.
28. DeLorenzo RJ. The calmodulin hypothesis of neurotransmission. *Cell Calcium* 1981;2:365–385.
29. DeLorenzo RJ. Calmodulin in neurotransmitter release and synaptic function. *Fed Proc* 1982;41:2275.
30. DeLorenzo RJ. Calcium-calmodulin protein phosphorylation in neuronal transmission: a molecular approach to neuronal excitability and anticonvulsant drug action. *Adv Neurol* 1983; 34:325–338.
31. DeLorenzo RJ. A molecular approach to the calcium signal in brain: relationship to synaptic modulation and seizure discharge. *Adv Neurol* 1986;44:325–338.
32. DeLorenzo RJ. Mechanisms of action in anticonvulsant drugs. *Epilepsia* 1988;29[Suppl 2]:S35–S47.
33. DeLorenzo RJ. The epilepsies. In: Bradley WG, Daroff RB, Fenichel GM, et al., eds. *Neurology in clinical practice*. Stoneham, MA: Butterworth Publishers, 1989:1443–1478.

34. DeLorenzo RJ. Status epilepticus. *Curr Ther Neurol Dis* 1990; 3:47–53.

35. DeLorenzo RJ. Management of status epilepticus. *Virginia Medical Q* 1996;123:103–111.

36. DeLorenzo RJ. Regulation of neuronal excitability: molecular foundations for the study of alcohol withdrawal. In: Porter RJ, Mattson RH, Cramer JA, et al., eds. *Alcohol and seizures: basic mechanisms and clinical concepts.* Philadelphia: FA Davis, 1990.

37. DeLorenzo RJ. Status epilepticus: concepts in diagnosis and treatment. *Semin Neurol* 1990;10:396–405.

38. DeLorenzo RJ, Bowling AC, Taft WC. A molecular approach to the development of anticonvulsants. *Ann NY Acad Sci* 1986; 477:238–246.

39. DeLorenzo RJ, Dashefsky L. Anticonvulsants. *Hand Neurochem* 1985;9:363–403.

40. DeLorenzo RJ, Emple GP, Glaser GH. Regulation of the level of endogenous phosphorylation of specific brain proteins by diphenylhydantoin. *J Neurochem* 1976;28:21–30.

41. DeLorenzo RJ, Freedman SD. Possible role of calcium-dependent protein phosphorylation in mediating neurotransmitter release and anticonvulsant action. *Epilepsia* 1977;18:357–365.

42. DeLorenzo RJ, Freedman SD, Yohe WB, et al. Stimulation of Ca^{2+}-dependent neurotransmitter release and presynaptic nerve terminal protein phosphorylation by calmodulin and a calmodulin-like protein isolated from synaptic vesicles. *Proc Natl Acad Sci U S A* 1979;76:1838–1842.

43. DeLorenzo RJ, Glaser GH. Effect of diphenylhydantoin on the endogenous phosphorylation of brain protein. *Brain Res* 1976;105:381–386.

44. DeLorenzo RJ, Sgro JA. Basic mechanisms of neuronal excitability and anticonvulsant action. In: Suzuki J, Seino M, eds. *Art and science of epilepsy.* New York: Elsevier, 1989:39–45.

45. DeLorenzo RJ, Taft WC. Regulation of depolarization-induced calcium uptake. In: *Advances in epileptology: The XVth epilepsy international symposium.* 1984;37–42.

46. DeLorenzo RJ, Taft WC, Andrews WT. Regulation of voltage-sensitive calcium channels in brain by micromolar affinity benzodiazepine receptors. In: Katz B, Rahamimoff R, eds. *Calcium, neuronal function and neurotransmitter release.* Boston: Martinus Nijhoff, 1985:375–394.

47. DeToledo JC, Ramsay RE. Fosphenytoin and phenytoin in patients with status epilepticus: improved tolerability versus increased costs. *Drug Saf* 2000;22:459–466.

48. Deupree JD. Evidence that diphenylhydantoin does not affect adenosine triphosphatase from brain. *Neuropharmacology* 1976;15:187–195.

49. Deupree JD. The role or non-role of ATPase activation by phenytoin in the stabilization of excitable membranes. *Epilepsia* 1977;18:309–315.

50. De Weer P. Phenytoin: blockage of resting sodium channels. *Adv Neurol* 1980;27:353–361.

51. Eldon MA, Loewen GR, Voightman RE, et al. Pharmacokinetics and tolerance of fosphenytoin and phenytoin administration intravenously to healthy subjects. *Can J Neurol Sci* 1993;20[Suppl 4]:S180(abstr).

52. Eldon MA, Loewen GR, Voightman RE, et al. Safety, tolerance, and pharmacokinetics of intravenous fosphenytoin. *Clin Pharmacol Ther* 1993;53:212(abstr).

53. Esplin DW. Effects of diphenylhydantoin on synaptic transmission in cat spinal cord and stellate ganglion. *J Pharmacol Exp Ther* 1957;120:301–323.

54. Esplin DW, Freston JW. Physiological and pharmacological analysis of spinal cord convulsions. *J Pharmacol Exp Ther* 1960;130:68–80.

55. Esplin DW, Laffan RJ. Determinants of flexor and extensor components of maximal seizures in cats. *Arch Int Pharmacodyn Ther* 1957;113:189–202.

56. Ferrendelli JA. Phenytoin: cyclic nucleotide regulation in the brain. *Adv Neurol* 1980;27:429–433.

57. Ferrendelli JA. Pharmacology of antiepileptic drugs. *Epilepsia* 1987;28[Suppl 3]:S14–S16.

58. Ferrendelli JA, Kinscherf DA. Phenytoin: effects on calcium flux and cyclic nucleotides. *Epilepsia* 1977;18:331–348.

59. Fertziger AP, Liuzzi SE, Dunham PB. Diphenylhydantoin (Dilantin): stimulation of potassium influx in lobster axons. *Brain Res* 1971;33:592–596.

60. Festoff BW, Appel SH. Effect of diphenylhydantoin on synaptosome sodium-potassium ATPase. *J Clin Invest* 1968;47: 2752–2758.

61. Fischer PA, Sloan EP, Turnbull TL, et al. Safety and pharmacokinetics of intravenous loading doses of fosphenytoin for the acute treatment of seizures. *Epilepsia* 1995;36[Suppl 3]:S160 (abstr).

62. Gangloff H, Monnier M. The action of anticonvulsant drugs tested by electrical stimulation of the rabbit cortex, diencephalon and rhinencephalon in the unanesthetized rabbit. *Electroencephalogr Clin Neurophysiol* 1957;9:43–58.

63. Gibbs MK, Ng KT. Diphenylhydantoin facilitation of labile protein-independent memory. *Brain Res Bull* 1976;1:203–208.

64. Glazko AJ. Diphenylhydantoin: chemistry and methods for determination. In: Woodbury DM, Penry JK, Schmidt RP, eds. *Antiepileptic drugs.* New York: Raven Press, 1972:103–112.

65. Gutman Y, Boonyaviroj P. Mechanism of inhibition of catecholamine release form adrenal medulla by diphenylhydantoin and by low concentration of ouabain (10^{-10} M). *Naunyn Schmiedebergs Arch Pharmacol* 1977;296:293–296.

66. Hall R, Murdoch J. Brain protection: physiological and pharmacological considerations: Part II. the pharmacology of brain protection. *Can J Anaesth* 1990;37:762–777.

67. Hussey EK, Dukes GE, Messenheimer JA, et al. Evaluation of the pharmacokinetic interaction between diazepam and ACC-9653 (a phenytoin prodrug) in healthy male volunteers. *Pharm Res* 1990;7:1172–1176.

68. Kito M, Maehara M, Watanabe K. Antiepileptic drugs: calcium current interaction in cultured human neuroblastoma cells. *Seizure* 1994;3:141–149.

69. Kuo CC, Huang RC, Lou BS. Inhibition of Na(+) current by diphenhydramine and other diphenyl compounds: molecular determinants of selective binding to the inactivated channels. *Mol Pharmacol* 2000;57:135–143.

70. Johnston D, Ayala GF. Diphenylhydantoin: the action of a common anticonvulsant on bursting pacemaker cells in *Aplysia Sci* 1975;189:1009–1011.

71. Julien RM, Halpern LM. Effects of diphenylhydantoin and other antiepileptic drugs on epileptiform activity and Purkinje cell discharge rates. *Epilepsia* 1972;13:387–400.

72. Klee CB, Crouch TH, Richmand PG. Calmodulin. *Annu Rev Biochem* 1980;49:489–515.

73. Korey SR. Effect of Dilantin and Mesantoin on the giant axon of the squid. *Proc Soc Exp Biol Med* 1951;79:297–299.

74. Lacinova L, Klugbauer N, Hofmann F. Regulation of the calcium channel alpha(1G) subunit by divalent cations and organic blockers. *Neuropharmacology* 2000;39:1254–1266.

75. Lewin E, Bleck V. The effect of diphenylhydantoin administration on cortex potassium-activated phosphatase. *Neurology* 1971;21:417–418.

76. Lipicky RJ, Gilbert DL, Stillman IM. Diphenylhydantoin inhibition of sodium conductance in squid giant axon. *Proc Natl Acad Sci U S A* 1972;69:1758–1760.

77. Louis S, Kutt H, McDowell F. The cardiocirculatory changes

caused by intravenous Dilantin and its solvent. *Am Heart J* 1967;74:523–529.

78. Macdonald RL. Anticonvulsant drug actions on neurons in cell culture. *J Neural Transm* 1988;72:173–183.

79. Macdonald RL. Antiepileptic drug actions. *Epilepsia* 1989;30 [Suppl 1]:S19–S28.

80. Macdonald RL, Kelly KM. Antiepileptic drug mechanisms of action. *Epilepsia* 1995;36[Suppl 2]:S2–S12.

81. Macdonald RL, McLean MJ. Cellular bases of barbiturate and phenytoin anticonvulsant drug action. *Epilepsia* 1982;23: S7–S18.

82. Macdonald RL, McLean MJ. Anticonvulsant drugs: mechanisms of action. *Adv Neurol* 1986;44:713–736.

83. Macdonald RL, McLean MJ. Mechanisms of anticonvulsant drug action. *Electroencephalogr Clin Neurophysiol Suppl* 1987. 39: 200–208.

84. McLean MJ, Macdonald RL. Multiple actions of phenytoin on mouse spinal cord neurons in cell culture. *J Pharmacol Exp Ther* 1983;227:779–789.

85. McLean MJ, Macdonald RL. Limitation of high frequency repetitive firing of cultured mouse neurons by anticonvulsant drugs. *Neurology* 1984;34[Suppl 1]:288.

86. McLean MJ, Macdonald RL. Sodium valproate, but not ethosuximide, produces use- and voltage-dependent limitation of high frequency repetitive firing of action potential of mouse central neurons in cell culture. *J Pharmacol Exp Ther* 1986. 237:1001–1011.

87. Merritt HH, Putnam TJ. A new series of anticonvulsant drugs tested by experiments on animals. *Arch Neurol Psychiatry* 1938; 39:1003–1015.

88. Miyazaki T, Hashiguchi T, Hashiguchi M, et al. Phenytoin partially antagonized L-type Ca^{2+} current in glucagon-secreting tumor cells (ITC-1). *Naunyn Schmiedebergs Arch Pharmacol* 1992;345:78–84.

89. Modeer T, Brunius G, Mendez C, et al. Influence of phenytoin on cytoplasmic free Ca^{2+} level in human gingival fibroblasts. *Scand J Dent Res* 1991;99:310–315.

90. Morell F, Bradley W, Ptashne M. Effect of diphenylhydantoin on peripheral nerve. *Neurology* 1958;8:140–144.

91. Noach EL, Woodbury DM, Goodman LS. Studies on the absorption, distribution, fate and excretion of 4-^{14}C-labeled diphenylhydantoin. *J Pharmacol Exp Ther* 1958;122:301–314.

92. Perlin JB, DeLorenzo RJ. Calcium and epilepsy. In: Pedley TA, Meldrum BS, eds. *Recent advances in epilepsy.* New York: Churchill Livingstone, 1992:15–36.

93. Perrier D, Rapp R, Young B, et al. Maintenance of therapeutic phenytoin plasma levels via intramuscular administration. *Ann Intern Med* 1976;85:318–321.

94. Perry JG, McKinney L, DeWeer P. The cellular mode of action of antiepileptic drug 5,5-diphenylhydantoin. *Nature* 1978;272: 271–273.

95. Pfeifle CE, Adler DS, Gannaway WL. Phenytoin sodium solubility in three intravenous solutions. *Am J Hosp Pharm* 1981;38: 358–362.

96. Putnam TJ, Merritt HH. Experimental determination of anticonvulsant properties of some phenyl derivatives. *Science* 1937; 85:525–526.

97. Putnam TJ, Merritt HH. Chemistry of anticonvulsant drugs. *Arch Neurol* 1941;45:505–516.

98. Quon CY, Stampfli HE. In vitro hydrolysis of ACC-9653 (phosphate ester prodrug of phenytoin) by human, dog, rat, blood, and tissues. *Pharm Res* 1986;3[Suppl 5]:134S(abstr).

99. Ragsdale DS, McPhee JC, Scheuer T, et al. Common molecular determinants of local anesthetic, antiarrhythmic, and anticonvulsant block of voltage-gated Na+ channels. *Proc Natl Acad Sci U S A* 1996;93:9270–9275.

100. Raines A, Standaert FG. Pre- and post-junctional effects of diphenylhydantoin at the soleus neuromuscular junction. *J Pharmacol Exp Ther* 1966;153:361–366.

101. Raines A, Standaert FG. An effect of diphenylhydantoin on post-tetanic hyperpolarization of intramedullary nerve terminals. *J Pharmacol Exp Ther* 1967;156:591–597.

102. Rampe D, Ferrante J, Triggle DJ. The actions of diazepam and diphenylhydantoin on fast and slow Ca^{2+} uptake processes in guinea pig cerebral cortex synaptosomes. *Can J Physiol Pharmacol* 1987;65:538–543.

103. Rivet M, Bois P, Cognard C, et al. Phenytoin preferentially inhibits L-type calcium currents in whole-cell patch-clamped cardiac and skeletal muscle cells. *Cell Calcium* 1990;11: 581–588.

104. Rogawski MA, Porter RJ. Antiepileptic drugs: pharmacological mechanisms and clinical efficacy with consideration of promising developmental stage compounds. *Pharmacol Rev* 1990;42: 223–286.

105. Rosenberg P, Bartels E. Drug effects on the spontaneous electrical activity of the squid giant axon. *J Pharmacol* 1967;155: 532–544.

106. Rosenthal J. Post-tetanic potentiation at the neuromuscular junction of the frog. *J Physiol (Lond)* 1969;203:121–133.

107. Schmidt RP, Wilder J. *Epilepsy.* Contemporary neurology series. Philadelphia: FA Davis, 1968.

108. Schumacher TB, Beck H, Steinhauser C, et al. Effects of phenytoin, carbamazepine, and gabapentin on calcium channels in hippocampal granule cells from patients with temporal lobe epilepsy. *Epilepsia* 1998;39:355–363.

109. Schwarz JR, Vogel W. Diphenylhydantoin: excitability reducing action in single myelinated nerve fibers. *Eur J Pharmacol* 1977; 44:241–249.

110. Segal MM, Douglas AF. Late sodium channel openings underlying epileptiform activity are preferentially diminished by the anticonvulsant phenytoin. *J Neurophysiol* 1997;77:3021–3034.

111. Sohn RS, Ferrendelli JA. Inhibition of Ca^{++} transport into rat brain synaptosomes by diphenylhydantoin (DPH). *J Pharmacol Exp Ther* 1973;185:272–275.

112. Sohn RS, Ferrendelli JA. Anticonvulsant drug mechanisms. *Arch Neurol* 1976;33:626–629.

113. Spengler RF, Arrowsmith JB, Kilarski DJ, et al. Severe soft-tissue injury following intravenous infusion of phenytoin: patient and drug administration risk factors. *Arch Intern Med* 1988; 148:1329–1333.

114. Stella V, Higuchi T. Esters of hydantoic acids as prodrugs of hydantoins. *J Pharm Sci* 1973;62:962–967.

115. Swanson PD, Crane PO. Diphenylhydantoin and movement of radioactive sodium into electrically stimulated cerebral slices. *Biochem Pharmacol* 1972;21:2899–2905.

116. Taft WC, Clifton GL, Blair RE, et al. Phenytoin protects against ischemia-produced neuronal cell death. *Brain Res* 1988; 483:143–148.

117. Taft WC, DeLorenzo RJ. Regulation of calcium channels in brain: implications for the clinical neurosciences. *Yale J Biol Med* 1987;60:99–106.

118. Thomsen W, Hays SJ, Hicks JL, et al. Specific binding of the novel Na+ channel blocker PD85,639 to the alpha subunit of rat brain Na+ channels. *Mol Pharmacol* 1993;43:955–964.

119. Todorovic SM, Lingle CJ. Pharmacological properties of T-type Ca^{2+} current in adult rat sensory neurons: effects of anticonvulsant and anesthetic agents. *J Neurophysiol* 1998;79:240–252.

120. Todorovic SM, Perez-Reyes E, Lingle CJ. Anticonvulsants but not general anesthetics have differential blocking effects on different T-type current variants. *Mol Pharmacol* 2000;58: 98–108.

121. Toman JEP. Neuropharmacology of peripheral nerve. *Pharmacol Rev* 1952;4:168–218.
122. Toman JEP. Further observations on diphenylhydautoin. In: Jasper HH, Ward AA Jr, Pope A, eds. *Basic mechanisms of the epilepsies*. Boston: Little, Brown & Co, 1969:682–688.
123. Toman JEP, Loewe S, Goodman LS. Physiology and therapy of convulsive disorders: I. effect of anticonvulsant drugs on electroshock seizures in man. *Arch Neurol* 1947;58:312–324.
124. Toman JEP, Swinyard EA, Goodman LS. Properties of maximal seizures and their alterations by anticonvulsant drugs and other agents. *J Neurophysiol* 1946;9:231–240.
125. Tomaselli GF, Marban E, Yellen G. Sodium channels from human brain RNA expressed in *Xenopus* oocytes: brain electrophysiologic characteristics and their modification by diphenylhydantoin. *J Clin Invest* 1989;83:1724–1732.
126. Varia SA, Stella VJ. Phenytoin prodrugs: V. in vivo evaluation of some water-soluble phenytoin prodrugs in dogs. *J Pharm Sci* 1984;73:1080–1087.
127. Wakamori M, Kaneda M, Oyama Y, et al. Effects of chlordiazepoxide and haloperidol on the voltage-dependent sodium current of isolated mammalian brain neurons. *Brain Res* 1989;494:374–378.
128. Wilensky AJ, Lowden JA. The inhibitory effect of diphenylhydantoin and microsomal ATPases. *Life Sci* 1972;11:319–327.
129. Woodbury DM. Effect of diphenylhydantoin on electrolytes and on sodium turnover in brain and other tissues of normal, hypernatremic and postictal rats. *J Pharmacol Exp Ther* 1955;115:74–95.
130. Woodbury DM. Mechanisms of action of anticonvulsants. In: Jasper HH, Ward AA Jr, Pope A, eds. *Basic mechanisms of the epilepsies*. Boston: Little, Brown & Co, 1969:647–681.
131. Woodbury DM. Phenytoin: proposed mechanisms of anticonvulsant action. *Adv Neurol* 1980;27:447–471.
132. Woodbury DM. Phenytoin: mechanisms of action. In: Woodbury DM, Penry JK, Pippenger CE, eds. *Antiepileptic drugs*, 2nd ed. New York: Raven Press, 1982:269–282.
133. Woodbury DM, Esplin DW. Neuropharmacology and neurochemistry of anticonvulsant drugs. *Res Publ Assoc Res Nerv Ment Dis* 1959;37:24–56.
134. Woodbury DM, Kemp JW. Pharmacology and mechanisms of action of diphenylhydantoin. *Psychiatr Neurol Neurochir* 1971;74:91–117.
135. Woodbury DM, Swinyard EA. Diphenylhydantoin: absorption, distribution and excretion. In: Woodbury DM, Penry JD, Schmidt RP, eds. *Antiepileptic drugs*. New York: Raven Press, 1972:113–123.
136. Yaari Y, Pincus JH, Argov Z. Depression of synaptic transmission by diphenylhydantoin. *Ann Neurol* 1977;1:334–338.

Antiepileptic Drugs, 5th Edition. Edited by R.H. Levy, R.H. Mattson, B.S. Meldrum, and E. Perucca. Lippincott Williams & Wilkins, Philadelphia © 2002.

PHENYTOIN AND OTHER HYDANTOINS

CHEMISTRY AND BIOTRANSFORMATION

THOMAS R. BROWNE
BARBARA LEDUC

CHEMISTRY

Phenytoin is the generic name for 5,5-diphenylhydantoin (acid form). The *Chemical Abstracts* name is 5,5-diphenyl-2,4-imidazolidinedione. It has the chemical structure shown in Figure 58.1. The free acid has a molecular weight of 252.26; the sodium salt has a molecular weight of 274.25, equivalent to acid content of 91.98%. The acid form is used in formulations of aqueous suspensions (Pediatric Dilantin-30 Suspension and Dilantin-125 Suspension; Pfizer, New York, NY) containing 30 mg or 125 mg of phenytoin acid per 5 mL. The free acid also is used in formulating chewable tablets (Dilantin Infatabs; Pfizer) containing 50 mg phenytoin acid per tablet. However, other products are formulated with the sodium salt of phenytoin (phenytoin sodium; acid equivalents = 91.98%). With these preparations, the drug content is expressed in terms of the sodium salt rather than the free acid. Thus, the gelatin capsules (Dilantin Sodium Kapseals; Pfizer) are formulated to contain either 30 mg or 100 mg of phenytoin sodium (= 27.6 mg or 92.0 mg of phenytoin acid equivalents) per capsule. The Mylan extended-release 100-mg capsules also are formulated with sodium phenytoin. This 8% difference in drug content should be taken into account when changing from one product to another. The sodium salt also is used in parenteral formulations [Parenteral Dilantin (Pfizer); phenytoin sodium injection (generic)]. The drug content is given in terms of the sodium salt.

Phenytoin is a weak organic acid that is poorly soluble in water. The apparent dissociation constant (pKN_a), representing the pH at which half the drug is ionized, is in the range of 8.1 to 9.2. The acid essentially is nonionized at pH 5.4 (solubility approximately 19.4 μg/g at 25.4°C), whereas at pH 7.4 (approximately 80% nonionized), the acid has a

water solubility of 20.5 μg/g (25.2°C). Higher concentrations of phenytoin required strongly alkaline solutions, with solubility measurements of 165 μg/mL at pH 9.1 and 1,520 μg/mL at pH 10. Parenteral phenytoin sodium is made up in an aqueous vehicle containing propylene glycol, ethanol, and sodium hydroxide. It contains 50 mg phenytoin sodium per mL (= 46 mg phenytoin acid per mL). The solubility of phenytoin in blood plasma is approximately 75 μg/mL (37°C), at least in part because of binding of the drug on the plasma proteins.

Phenytoin sodium is not recommended as an analytical standard because of its variable water content (hydrate formation) and partial conversion to the free acid on exposure to carbon dioxide.

This section was based on Glazko (61), which should be consulted for details and references.

BIOTRANSFORMATION

Phenytoin (5,5-diphenylhydantoin; Dilantin) is eliminated almost entirely by metabolic transformation before excretion in the form of metabolites. Less than 5% of an administered dose is excreted unchanged in the urine (45,62, 114,121). The principal metabolic pathway of phenytoin in humans is the 5-(4-hydroxyphenyl)-5-phenylhydantoin (*p*-HPPH) and dihydrodiol pathway, accounting for 70% to 90% of administered phenytoin (Figure 58.2). The first

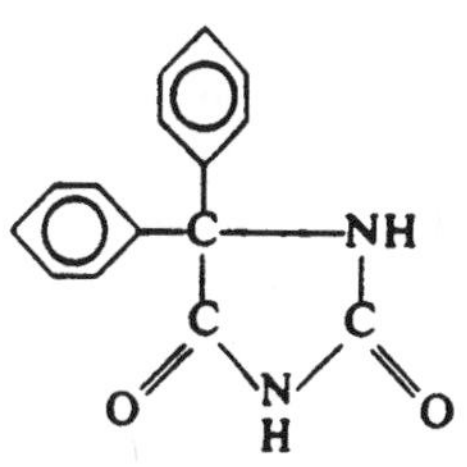

Thomas R. Browne, MD: Professor of Neurology, Department of Neurology, Boston University School of Medicine, Boston, Massachusetts

Barbara LeDuc, PhD: Massachusetts College of Pharmacy and Allied Sciences, Boston, Massachusetts

FIGURE 58.1. Structure of phenytoin.

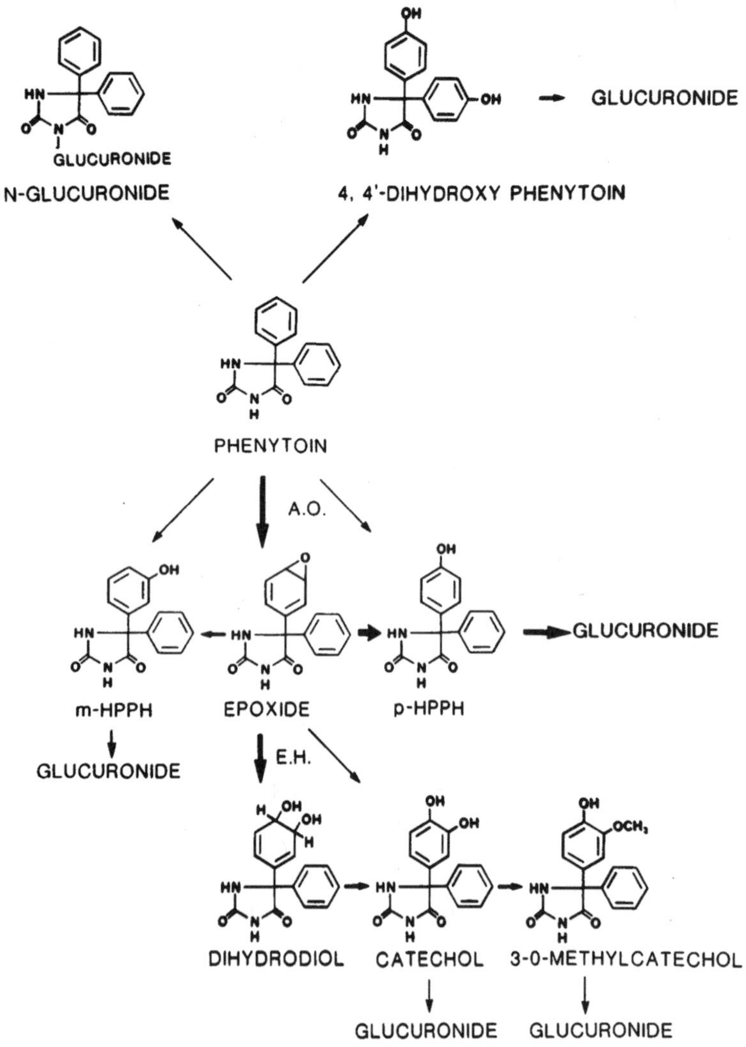

FIGURE 58.2. Pathways of phenytoin metabolism.

step of this pathway [involving the cytochrome P450 (CYP) enzymes CYP2C9 and CYP2C19] exhibits nonlinear enzyme kinetics, which has significant effects on phenytoin's clinical pharmacokinetics. A number of minor metabolic pathways for phenytoin also have been described, some of which involve the CYP enzymes CYP2C9, CYP2C19, and CYP3A4 (Figure 58.2). Species differences in the biotransformation of phenytoin have been reported.

The *Para*-HPPH and Dihydrodiol Pathways

Para-HPPH accounts for 67% to 88%, and dihydrodiol accounts for 7% to 11% of human urinary metabolites of phenytoin (23,24,32,43,75,90). The first step in this pathway is the formation of an arene oxide intermediate through the enzymes CYP2C9 and CYP2C19 (Figure 58.2). The arene oxide is converted spontaneously to *p*-HPPH and is converted by the enzyme epoxide hydrolase to dihydrodiol (Figure 58.2).

Cytochrome P450 Enzymes Active in Phenytoin Metabolism and Their Genetic Variants

Enzymes belonging to the CYP2C subfamily and the CYP3A family have been implicated in the biotransformation of phenytoin and its metabolites (40,95). A substantial number of human allelic variants of these enzymes have been identified.

Four members of the CYP2C subfamily, CYP2C8, CYP2C9, CYP2C18, and CYP2C19, have been identified in humans (64,110). The CYP2C enzymes, which constitute approximately 20% of total hepatic CYP content, are encoded by a cluster of four genes at chromosomal location 10q24 (85,138). Both the CYP2C9 and CYP2C19 enzymes are active in phenytoin hydroxylation, with CYP2C9 being the more vigorous catalyst (10,51,82,154, 167). Although earlier *in vitro* studies suggested a role for CYP2C8 and CYP2C18, their contribution to phenytoin metabolism *in vivo* has been questioned, and studies have indicated that only negligible amounts of CYP2C18 are expressed in human liver (130). CYP2C9 catalyzes the formation of both (*R*)- and (*S*)-HPPH [5-(4′-hydroxyphenyl)-,5-phenylhydantoin] but is highly stereoselective for (*S*)-HPPH, whereas CYP2C19 exhibits little stereoselectivity and thus contributes more to the formation of the (*R*)-enantiomer (82,110,167). In addition, studies have identified CYP2C19, CYP2C9, and several CYP3A forms as the catalysts for the further hydroxylation of 3′- and 4′-HPPH to the catechol 3′,4′-diHPPH [5-(3′,4′-dihydroxyphenyl)-,5-phenylhydantoin] (40,95).

Four alleles of CYP2C9 have been identified. The wild-type enzyme, CYP2C9*1, contains arginine at position 144 and isoleucine at position 359 (132). The variant CYP2C9*2 contains a single amino acid substitution at position 144 (Arg144Cys), whereas in CYP2C9*3, leucine is substituted at position 359 (Ile359Leu) (39,69,122,128,141). Another mutation generating an amino acid substitution at position 359 has been identified in CYP2C9*4 (Ile359Thr) (84). (For a current listing of human CYP450 alleles, see www.imm.ki.sec/CYPalleles). Although the activity of CYP2C9*2 for HPPH formation is reported to be only moderately diminished compared with that of CYP2C9*1, CYP2C9*3 shows markedly decreased catalytic activity both *in vitro* and *in vivo* (9,40,52,72,110,122,128,143,154). Interestingly, a white patient with epilepsy displaying a very low clearance of phenytoin was found to be homozygous for CYP2C9*3 (91). The CYP2C9*4 mutation (Ile359Thr) is extremely rare, but was associated also with a diminished rate of phenytoin hydroxylation *in vivo* (83). It has been suggested that amino acid 359 is located in the enzyme's substrate recognition site; this would explain the large detrimental effect of substitutions at this position (67). To date, poor metabolizers of phenytoin have been shown to have mutations of either CYP2C9 or CYP2C19. Although CYP2C9*3 is the primary determinant of slow phenytoin metabolism, defective CYP2C19 alleles also contribute, especially at high doses (120).

The incidence of allelic variants of CYP2C9 varies significantly between different racial groups. The gene frequency of CYP2C9*2 has been estimated as 0.08 to 0.125 in whites, 0.01 in Africans, and zero in East Asians (9,122,140,141). The predicted frequency of CYP2C9*3 in whites is 0.06 to 0.10, in East Asians, 0.017 to 0.026, and in Africans, 0.005 (9,92,122,140,141,157).

In contrast to CYP2C9, most variant alleles of CYP2C19 identified thus far appear to result in nonfunctional or absent enzymes. The CYP2C19 polymorphism is responsible for the variation in human 4′-hydroxylation of (*S*)-mephenytoin (41,42). Poor metabolizers of (*S*)-mephenytoin constitute approximately 2% to 6% of white or African, and 18% to 23% of East Asian populations (92,119,164–166). Two wild-type and seven defective alleles of CYP2C19 have been

identified thus far (87). As with CYP2C9, the incidence of specific alleles varies significantly among different ethnic groups. CYP2C19*1A and CYP2C19*1B are the wild-type forms (129,132). The allelic variants CYP2C19*2 (CYP2C19m1), CYP2C19*3 (CYP2C19 m2), and CYP2C19*5 account for approximately 99% of East Asian, but only 75% to 85% of white poor metabolizers of (*S*)-mephenytoin (54,87). CYP2C19*2B, CYP2C19*4, CYP2C19*5B, and CYP2C19*6 account for the remainder of slow metabolism in whites (54). The mutations found in CYP2C19*2A and CYP2C19*2B are due to G6A point mutations in exon 5, leading to aberrant splice sites (41,42,80). CYP2C19*3 is due to a G6A point mutation in exon 4, causing premature termination (41,42). In CYP2C19*4, an A→G mutation disrupts the initiation codon (50). CYP2C19*5A contains an amino acid substitution (Arg433Trp), and CYP2C19*5B contains this, plus an additional substitution (Arg433Trp; Ile331Val); both enzymes appear to lack activity (79,80,163). CYP2C19*6 (Arg132Gln; Ile331Val), CYP2C19*7 (splicing defect), and CYP2C19*8 (Trp120Arg) apparently are absent or inactive as well (80,81).

Although CYP2C9 is the primary determinant, a number of studies have confirmed that the activity of CYP2C19 is clinically significant to overall phenytoin metabolism. Diminished renal elimination of (*R*)-HPPH and total HPPH, a substantially decreased urinary (*R*)-HPPH/phenytoin ratio, elevated serum phenytoin concentrations, and an elevated Michaelis constant (K_m) for phenytoin have been demonstrated in Japanese subjects who were either heterozygous or homozygous for mutant CYP2C19 alleles (82,110,116,120,122,157,158). Furthermore, ticlopidine, a potent inhibitor of CYP2C19, has been implicated in drug interactions resulting in phenytoin toxicity (47).

The gene frequency of CYP2C19*2 has been estimated as 0.11 to 0.13 in whites and in Africans, but 0.27 to 0.37 in East Asians (16,30,92,112,133,142,163). In contrast, the CYP2C19*3 allele is rare or absent in whites, whereas its frequency is approximately 0.5 to 0.11 in East Asians (92,133,163). Interestingly, in Japanese but not whites, mutations of CYP2C18 and CYP2C19 appear to be completely linked, that is, the occurrence of CYP2C18m2 coincides with that of CYP2C19*32, and CYP2C18m1 occurs with CYP2C19*3 (96,109,116). The CYP2C9 mutations were found to be independent of either CYP2C18 and CYP2C19 alleles (86).

Collectively, the CYP3A enzymes constitute most of the total hepatic CYP. Four genes have been described: CYP3A4, CYP3A5, CYP3A7, and a newly identified form, CYP3A43 (56,147). cDNA analysis of CYP3A4, CYP3A5, and CYP3A7 sequences confirms at least 90% homology between them (71,160). CYP3A43 is predicted to be at least 71% homologous with other CYP3A forms (56). The CYP3A forms display broad and overlapping substrate specificities, and are thought to participate in the metabolism of at least 50% of all drugs (49,103). Although CYP3A4 exhibited the greatest activity, recombinant CYP3A4, CYP3A5, and CYP3A7 isoforms were shown to be capable of catalyzing the conversion of 3′- and 4′-HPPH to the catechol diHPPH *in vitro* (40,93). In humans, total CYP3A activity displays large interindividual and interethnic variations that might be due to differences in induction, inhibition, or regulation of expression (97,138). To facilitate study of the control of CYP3A gene expression, the human CYP3A gene locus at 7q21.1 has been sequenced (56).

CYP3A4 is the most common form of CYP450 in liver and intestine. CYP3A4*1A is the wild-type form (65). Although CYP3A4*1B contains an A→G point mutation in the 5′-flanking region, there appears to be no difference in the level of hepatic expression of the enzyme compared with the wild-type form (89,161). The frequency of this mutation is 4.2% to 9% in whites, 53% to 66% in African Americans, and 0% in Taiwanese subjects (134,156). CYP3A4*2 contains a Ser222Pro substitution, resulting in lower *in vitro* nifedipine metabolism but, curiously, no difference in testosterone β-hydroxylation (134). This variant was found in 2.7% of white subjects, but was absent in both East Asians and African Americans (134). A CYP3A4*3 variant, containing a Met445Thr substitution, was found in only one Chinese subject (132). Recently, Hsieh et al. identified three rare variants in Chinese subjects, CYP3A4*4 (Ile118Val), CYP3A4*4 (Pro102Arg), and CYP3A4*6 (frameshift), which were associated with decreased β-hydroxycortisol formation (77).

CYP3A5 appears to be expressed considerably more frequently than previously thought (13,97). The isoform constitutes up to 50% of total CYP3A in subjects who express the gene, and may be an important contributor to interindividual and interracial differences in CYP3A-dependent drug disposition (97). Only subjects having at least one copy of CYP3A5*1 express large amounts of the enzyme (95). The CYP3A5*1B and CYP3A5*1C variants differ from the wild-type gene (CYP3A5*1A) by having nucleotide substitutions in the promoter region, although these mutations are not associated with differences in enzyme activity *in vivo* (1,97). The CYP3A5*2, CYP3A5*3, and CYP3A5*6 variants appear to result in absence of the hepatic enzyme (89,97). Hepatic CYP3A5 is expressed much more frequently in African Americans (66%) than in whites (33%) (97).

CYP3A7 is the fetal form of the enzyme, although expression has been known to persist into adulthood in some people (70,135). A partial explanation for this continued expression may be the discovery of the CYP3A7*1C variant, in which a segment of the CYP3A4 promoter is substituted into the equivalent CYP3A7 promoter region. Interestingly, this CYP3A7*1C allele is three times more common in African Americans than in whites (97).

Arene Oxide

The arene oxide of phenytoin has never been isolated from plasma or urine, presumably because it is rapidly converted to further metabolic products. The existence of an arene oxide intermediate in the formation of *p*-HPPH was suggested by early kinetic experiments (148) and was established using the "NIH shift" technique (38,117).

The NIH shift technique depends on the observation that arene oxides spontaneously break down to form a hydroxylated metabolite, and that when this happens the hydrogen molecule at the site of the hydroxyl group is lost 50% of the time and is shifted (NIH shift) to the adjacent carbon, where the oxygen molecule had been attached 50% of the time. The NIH shift experiment of Claesen et al. (38) is shown in Figure 58.3. Racemic 5-(4-deuteriophenyl)-5-phenylhydantoin (p-[^{2}H]-DPH) was administered to volunteers, and urine was collected. After enzymatic hydrolysis of the urine, deuterium retention by *p*-HPPH metabolites was determined. The expected percentage of deuterium retention by *p*-HPPH in the presence of an arene oxide/NIH shift pathway was 75%, and the measured values were 65% to 75% in four volunteers.

Phenytoin is known to exhibit nonlinear pharmacokinetics in humans (see later), implying that substrate saturation must be occurring in one or more of the enzymes metabolizing phenytoin. The CYP2C9 and CYP2C19 enzymes appear to be the site of substrate saturation resulting in nonlinear pharmacokinetics in humans based on the following observations: (a) Browne et al. (18) demonstrated that the rate of urinary excretion of *p*-HPPH varies inversely with phenytoin plasma concentration in humans ($r = -0.640$, $p < 0.005$) (9); (b) Tsuru et al. (149) demonstrated that the rate of formation of *p*-HPPH from rat hepatocytes and rat hepatic microsomes varies inversely with phenytoin concentration in the medium. Phenytoin is the probable substance causing competitive inhibition of the arene oxidase enzyme (25). There is some evidence that high concentrations of *p*-HPPH competitively inhibit hydroxylation of phenytoin in animals (76), but this phenomenon has not been demonstrated *in vivo* in humans (25,32). Arene oxides have attracted considerable attention because of their reactivity and possible role in toxicity and teratogenicity mechanisms.

Para-HPPH and Meta-HPPH

The principal urinary metabolite of phenytoin is *p*-HPPH in humans (27,28,146). Most *p*-HPPH is excreted as a glucuronide, and only small amounts of free *p*-HPPH are found in human urine (31,114). Very small amounts of *m*-HPPH also are found in human urine (5,29,63). Species differences in the patterns of *p*-HPPH and *m*-HPPH exist (5,28,73,121). The details of these differences have been reviewed previously (17).

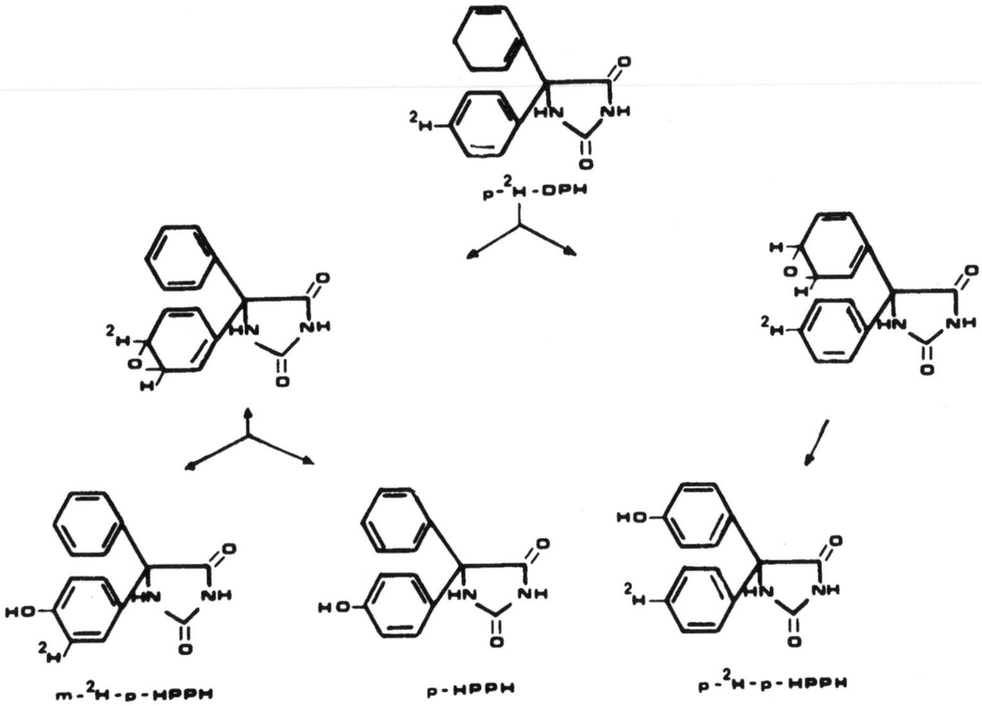

FIGURE 58.3. Arene oxide–NIH shift pathway for *para*-hydroxylation of phenytoin. (From Claesen M, Moustafa MAA, Adline J, et al. Evidence for an arene oxide–NIH shift pathway in the metabolic conversion of phenytoin to 5-(4-hydroxyphenyl)-5-phenylhydantoin in the rat and in man. *Drug Metab Dispos* 1982;10:667–671, with permission.)

Mechanism of Formation

NIH shift experiments indicate that most *p*-HPPH in humans is produced through an arene oxide intermediate (see earlier). CYP2C9 and CYP2C19 are the enzymes responsible for the formation of arene oxide (see earlier).

A minority of patients are "slow metabolizers" of phenytoin (32,63,98,99,152,153). In these individuals, toxic phenytoin plasma concentrations develop at average dosing rates of phenytoin. Mutations of CYP2C9 or CYP2C19 are the causes of slowed metabolism (see earlier).

Dihydrodiol

We (17) have reviewed the key papers on phenytoin dihydrodiol.

Mechanism of Formation

Phenytoin dihydrodiol is believed to be formed from phenytoin arene oxide through the enzyme epoxide hydrolase (Figures 58.2 and 58.4). This belief is supported by several lines of evidence. First, the usual metabolic pathway leading to formation of dihydrodiols is conversion of an epoxide intermediate to a dihydrodiol by the enzyme epoxide hydrolase (32,68,88,123). Second, administration of an epoxide hydrolase inhibitor (1,2-epoxy-3,3,3-trichlorophropane) to pregnant Swiss mice reduced the incidence of phenytoin-related teratogenesis and the covalent binding of ^{14}C radioactivity in

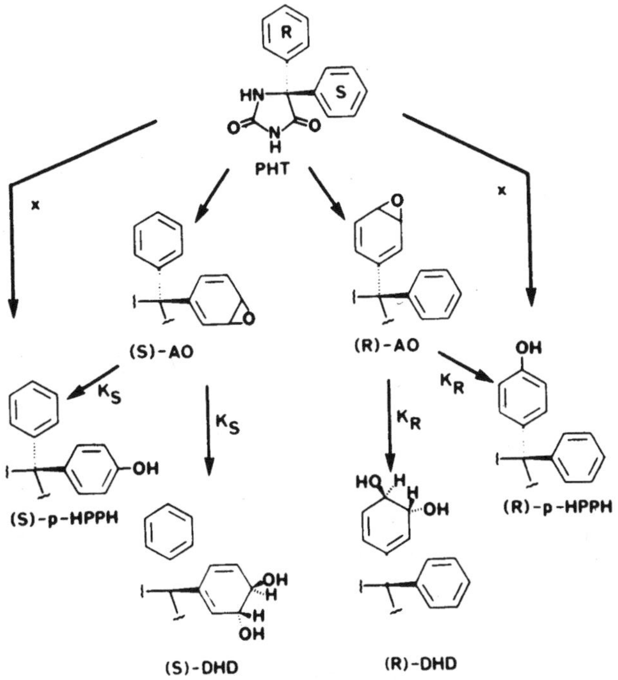

FIGURE 58.4. Scheme depicting stereoselective metabolic pathways involved in the production of 5-(4-hydroxyphenyl)-5-phenylhydantoin (*p*-HPPH) and dihydrodiol (DHD). Possible stereoselective direct hydroxylation pathways are indicated with an "X." [From Maguire JH, Butler TC, Dudley KH. Absolute configuration of (+)-5-(3-hydroxyphenyl)-5-phenylhydantoin, the major metabolite of 5,5-diphenylhydantoin in the dog. *J Med Chem* 1978;21:1194–1297, with permission.]

the fetus after administration of ^{14}C-labeled phenytoin, while maternal phenytoin serum concentrations remained unchanged (111). This implies that the initial step of phenytoin metabolism (presumably the arene oxide formation) is unaffected by epoxide hydrolase inhibition and that a metabolic intermediate with teratogenic and covalent binding properties (presumably arene oxide) accumulates in greater-than-usual amounts when epoxide hydrolase is inhibited. Third, incubation of phenytoin with human liver fractions known to contain epoxide hydrolase results in the formation of phenytoin dihydrodiol (127). There is evidence that chronic administration of phenytoin may induce epoxide hydrolase activity in humans (18,127).

Stereoselective Formation of HPPH and Dihydrodiol

Phenytoin is a prochiral compound. Introduction of a hydroxyl group in one of the phenyl rings leads to the creation of a chiral center and results in the formation of enantiomeric phenolic metabolites (Figure 58.4). CYP2C19 catalyzes the formation of both (R)-HPPH and (S)-HPPH, whereas CYP2C9 is more stereoselective in the formation of (S)-HPPH (82,110,167). The p-HPPH from human urine consists of a 10:1 mixture of levorotatory and dextrorotatory isomers (29,51,108). The amount of m-HPPH in human urine is too low to permit isolation and measurement of optical rotation. Most dihydrodiol in human urine is in the (S) configuration [3:1 ratio of (S):(R)] (105,107,108,124). Although an arene oxide of phenytoin has not been directly isolated and characterized, a large body of evidence has accumulated in support of the existence of (S) and (R) arene oxide intermediates. The proposed pathway is depicted in Figure 58.4. There are species differences in the chirality of p-HPPH, m-HPPH, and dihydrodiol excreted in the urine (29,51,105,107,108).

Effects of Head Trauma and Pregnancy

After head trauma, there is decrease in plasma albumin concentration that begins immediately, reaches a minimum at 5 to 7 days, and does not return to normal for 3 to 4 weeks (2). After head trauma, there also is an increase in phenytoin metabolism (3,15). These changes are accompanied by a decrease in free and total phenytoin plasma concentration and an increase in free fraction of phenytoin (2,4,15). Frequent monitoring of free phenytoin plasma concentration and frequent adjustment of phenytoin dosage often are necessary after head injury.

Phenytoin does not appear to be metabolized to p-HPPH or derivatives by the human placenta (94).

Minor Metabolic Pathways

Catechol and 3-O-Methylcatechol Metabolites

Relatively small amounts of a 3,4-catechol metabolite, -(3,4-dihydroxyphenyl)-5-phenylhydantoin, and a 3-O-methylcatechol metabolite, 5-(4-hydroxy-3-methoxyphenyl)-5-phenylhydantoin, have been identified in the urine of humans and other species (12,14,33,34,115). The same metabolites also have been identified as glucuronides in the bile from isolated, perfused rat liver (60).

The catechol could be formed through dehydrogenation of the dihydrodiol metabolite by a mechanism similar to those described by Ayengar et al. (8). In a preliminary experiment, ^{14}C-labeled dihydrodiol metabolite isolated from rat urine was administered perorally to rats. It did not result in the appearance of the catechol metabolite in urine (33). The catechol metabolite could be formed by further hydroxylation of m-HPPH or p-HPPH. Gerber and Thompson (57) identified small amounts of the catechol and 3-O-methylcatechol in rat bile by gas chromatography/mass spectrometry (GC/MS) techniques after administration of m-HPPH or p-HPPH to rats or by addition of these compounds to an isolated, perfused rat liver preparation. More recently, Billings and Fischer (12) and Chow and Fischer (36) provided evidence that the catechol metabolite of phenytoin was formed from both dihydrodiol and p-HPPH in rats and mice. However, the predominant route was through p-HPPH (36).

In rat urine, the concentration of the 3-O-methylcatechol metabolite was approximately fivefold greater than that of the catechol, indicating extensive O-methylation in this species (33). Evidence obtained by Chang et al. (34) indicates that the 3-O-methylcatechol metabolite of phenytoin is formed from the catechol. Administration of the synthetic 3,4-dihydroxycatechol to rats resulted in the prompt appearance of 3-O-methylcatechol in the urine (33). It is reasonable to assume that the enzyme catechol-O-methyltransferase is involved in the formation of this metabolite because it is known to methylate other catechols, including catecholamines (7).

4,4N-Dihydroxy Metabolite and N-Glucuronide of Phenytoin

Two minor metabolites of phenytoin—namely, 5,5-bis(4-hydroxyphenyl) hydantoin (145) and an N-glucuronide of phenytoin (139)—were identified in rats and in humans (Figure 58.2). The 4,4N-dihydroxy metabolite was excreted as a glucuronide and accounted for approximately 1% of the total hydroxylated metabolites. The pathway that leads to the formation of this metabolite is not known. When p-HPPH was added to the perfusate of an isolated rat liver preparation, there was no evidence of the formation of the 4,4N-dihydroxy metabolite (145). However, addition of the synthetic 4,4N-dihydroxy compound to the same *in vitro* preparation (145) resulted in the formation of a monoglucuronide, a trihydroxyphenytoin glucuronide, and a dihydroxymethoxyphenytoin glucuronide, indicating further hydroxylation of the dihydroxy metabolite. Whether the trihydroxylated product represents normal phenytoin metabolites in intact animals is not known.

The glucuronide of phenytoin was isolated from a patient receiving phenytoin and was characterized as the *N*-3 glucuronide by GC/MS. The same metabolite also was present in the bile of an isolated, perfused rat liver preparation. The structure assignment was based on the mass spectra of various permethylated derivatives and a comparison of the reaction of the metabolite and 5,5-diphenyl-3-methylhydantoin with diazomethane (139). Subsequently, Hassell et al. (73) reported that phenytoin *N*-glucuronide was the major metabolite in cat urine.

A number of other minor metabolites of phenytoin, some not yet identified, are known to exist (31,32).

The metabolite distribution patterns in human urine were reported by Chang and coworkers (32,35): 68% to 81% *p*-HPPH, 7% to 11% dihydrodiol, 2.5% 3-*O*-methylcatechol, 1% unchanged phenytoin, and approximately 1% catechol. Metabolites in human feces (1% of fecal radioactivity) were identified as *p*-HPPH (50% to 80%), dihydrodiol (15% to 35%), and catechol (5% to 10%). Later studies have confirmed these values (43).

SPECIES DIFFERENCES IN METABOLISM

With the exception of the dog and cat, the major metabolic product of phenytoin in all species, including humans, is a glucuronide conjugate of *p*-HPPH (17,66,106). Significant amounts of free *p*-HPPH were observed in the urine of mice and rats (32). The dihydrodiol metabolite was found in higher concentrations in urine of rats and monkeys than in that of mice, dogs, or cats. The catechol and 3-*O*-methylcatechol metabolites were detected in rat urine after repeated administration of phenytoin in the diet and accounted for 2% and 20%, respectively, of the total metabolite present (34). In dog urine, the major metabolite was the glucuronide conjugate of *m*-HPPH, whereas phenytoin *N*-glucuronide was the major urinary product in cat.

Species differences in the formation of glucuronide conjugates of *m*-HPPH or *p*-HPPH in rat or dog liver supernatant were reported by Gabler (53). Conjugation of *m*-HPPH was greater than that of *p*-HPPH in the dog liver, whereas the opposite effect was found with rat liver supernatant.

NONLINEAR PHARMACOKINETIC PROPERTIES OF PHENYTOIN

The rate of change of plasma concentration (C) of a drug by an enzyme system can be expressed by the Michaelis-Menten equation:

$$\frac{dC}{dt} = \frac{V_{max}}{K_m + C}\, C \qquad [1]$$

where t is time, V_{max} is the maximum velocity of the enzyme system, and K_m is the Michaelis constant of the enzyme system (plasma concentration at which half of the maximum velocity of the enzyme system is attained). Mean steady-state plasma drug concentration (C_{ss}) can be expressed as

$$C_{ss} = \frac{RK_m}{V_{max} - R} \qquad [2]$$

where R is dosing rate (102). When C is similar to or greater than K_m, dC/dt varies in a nonlinear fashion with C; when R is equal to or greater than 0.1 V_{max}, C_{ss} will vary in a nonlinear fashion with R. These observations are the basis of nonlinear pharmacokinetics.

The mean apparent value for phenytoin K_m in adults is 6.2 µg/mL, with a range of 1.5 to 30.7 µg/mL based on 55 reported determinations; the mean apparent value for phenytoin V_{max} in adults is 0.45 µg/mL/hr, with a range of 0.14 to 1.36 µg/mL/hr based on 54 reported determinations (6,19,48,55,59,74,113,126). These values appear to be determined principally by CYP2C9 and CYP2C19 K_m and V_{max} values. The other pathways shown in Figure 58.2 potentially could have modifying effects on the apparent values of K_m and V_{max} for phenytoin in humans (104). However, attempts to demonstrate an effect of these other pathways on phenytoin pharmacokinetic parameters in humans have been negative (23).

The apparent K_m values computed for humans are based on total (protein-bound and non–protein-bound) phenytoin plasma concentration. Because only non–protein-bound phenytoin can be acted on by the metabolizing enzyme system and the non–protein-bound fraction for phenytoin is approximately 10% in humans (162), the K_m of the enzyme responsible for parahydroxylation of phenytoin actually should be approximately 0.6 µg/mL. This prediction has been verified in rat liver microsomes (149).

Eadie et al. (48) performed the largest comprehensive comparison of phenytoin K_m and V_{max} values in children and adults. The K_m values from 21 adults (mean = 5.8 µg/mL) and 15 children (mean = 5.3 µg/mL) were not significantly different. The V_{max} values from 21 adults (mean = 0.48 µg/mL/hr, assuming phenytoin volume of distribution = 0.7 L/kg) were significantly (*p* < .025) less than the V_{max} values from 15 children (mean = 0.74 µg/mL/hr, assuming phenytoin volume of distribution = 0.7 L/kg). These observations predict that the clearance (V_{max}/[K_m + C]) of phenytoin should be greater in children than in adults. This prediction is confirmed by the observations that the elimination half-life of phenytoin is shorter in children than in adults and that the average dosing rate of phenytoin (in milligrams per kilogram per day) required to achieve a given plasma concentration is greater in children than in adults (46,98).

The V_{max} for phenytoin increases significantly during pregnancy (44). This explains part or all of the observed decreases in phenytoin steady-state plasma concentration during pregnancy (equation [2]).

Phenytoin exhibits nonlinear pharmacokinetic properties in most patients because the usual therapeutic plasma concentration values (10 to 20 μg/mL; Chapter 60) exceed the usual K_m (6.2 μg/mL), and the usual dosing rate (0.15 to 0.45 μg/mL/hr) is greater than 0.1 times the usual value of V_{max} (0.45 μg/mL/hr). Note that the metabolism of phenytoin is linear at low plasma concentrations and nonlinear at therapeutic and higher plasma concentrations (151). The consequences of nonlinear pharmacokinetics are discussed later.

Steady-State Plasma Concentration Varies in a Nonlinear Fashion with Dosing Rate

For drugs with nonlinear pharmacokinetics, steady-state plasma concentration increases faster than dosing rate when dosing rate is increased, and plasma concentration decreases faster than dosing rate when dosing rate is decreased (equation 2) (27,44,131) (Figure 58.5). Thus, the steady-state plasma concentration of a drug with nonlinear pharmacokinetic properties at one dosing rate does not directly pre-

dict the steady-state plasma concentration of the drug at another dosing rate.

If the clinician attempts to increase or decrease the phenytoin steady-state plasma concentration by simple linear extrapolation from a known plasma concentration versus dosing rate point, the result often is an unexpectedly high or low plasma concentration when the new steady-state value is attained (Figure 58.5). Numerous mathematical and tabular methods have been published that claim to be able to predict the phenytoin dosing rate necessary to produce a given steady-state plasma concentration from a single steady-state plasma concentration versus dose point, and these methods have been critically reviewed elsewhere (7,19,27,37,78,118,126,136,137). A useful rule of thumb in titrating phenytoin dosage upward in adults is to increase dosing rate in increments of 100 mg/day at monthly intervals (see later) until a steady-state phenytoin plasma concentration of 5 to 10 μg/mL (a value approximately equal to K_m) is attained; later increases should not exceed 50 mg/day at monthly intervals.

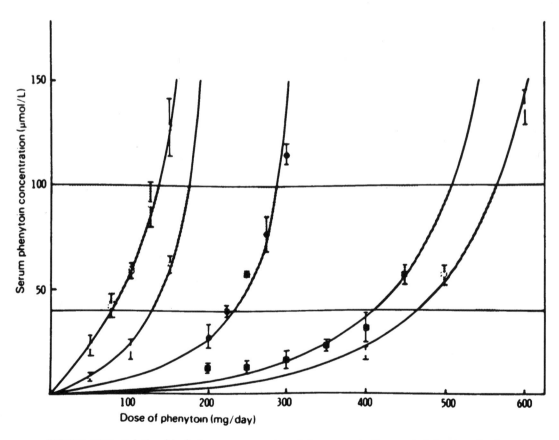

FIGURE 58.5. Relationship between serum phenytoin concentration and daily dose in five patients. Each point represents the mean (± standard deviation) of three to eight measurements of serum phenytoin concentration at steady state. The curves were fitted by computer using the Michaelis-Menten equation. (From Richens A, Dunlop A. Serum phenytoin levels in the management of epilepsy. *Lancet* 1975;2:247–248, with permission.)

Generic Equivalence

Nonlinear pharmacokinetics complicate the issue of generic equivalence of phenytoin products. The weighted mean value for absolute bioavailability of brand-name (Dilantin Kapseals, 100 mg) phenytoin was 86% in three studies (18). Less-than-complete absorption of brand-name phenytoin is, at least in part, a consequence of the use of a sustained-release preparation (Chapter 13). Different generic preparations of phenytoin thus have the potential to differ in absolute bioavailability from the brand-name preparation by +14% and −14% or more. Because of phenytoin's nonlinear pharmacokinetics, a 14% difference in bioavailability would result in a >14% increase or decrease in steady-state plasma concentration. A national epidemic of phenytoin intoxication occurred in Australia when a more bioavailable formulation was substituted for an older formulation (125,150). Ludden et al. (104) and Browne et al. (26) have reviewed the effect of nonlinear pharmacokinetics on bioavailability studies in more detail.

Clearance Varies Inversely, and Elimination Half-Life Directly, with Plasma Concentration

Drug clearance is equal to $V_{max}/(K_m + C)$. Drug elimination half-life is equal to $0.693 \times$ volume of distribution/clearance. Thus, phenytoin clearance varies inversely with plasma concentration, and phenytoin elimination half-life varies directly with plasma concentration (18,20,27) (Figure 58.6). Browne et al. (20,27) described and validated a method for calculating phenytoin elimination half-life at any given phenytoin plasma concentration if the patient's K_m and V_{max} values for phenytoin are known. The results were as follows for a group of six adult men on phenytoin monotherapy (plasma concentration − mean calculated elimination half-life): 1 µg/mL—12.8 hours; 10 µg/mL—25.8 hours; 20 µg/mL—40.2 hours; 40 µg/mL—69.1 hours. Note that the often-quoted elimination half-life of 24 hours for phenytoin applies principally to plasma concentration values in the low therapeutic range (10 µg/mL) and that the elimination half-life often is longer at higher plasma concentrations (Figure 58.6). The range of elimination half-life values at phenytoin plasma concentration 40 µg/mL was 37.1 to 96.8 hours. Because of phenytoin's long and variable elimination half-life values at toxic plasma concentration values, the time required for phenytoin plasma concentration to fall from a toxic value to a therapeutic value cannot be predicted in a given individual . In such circumstances, the clinician must withhold phenytoin and obtain daily plasma concentration determination values until the plasma concentration has fallen back into the therapeutic range.

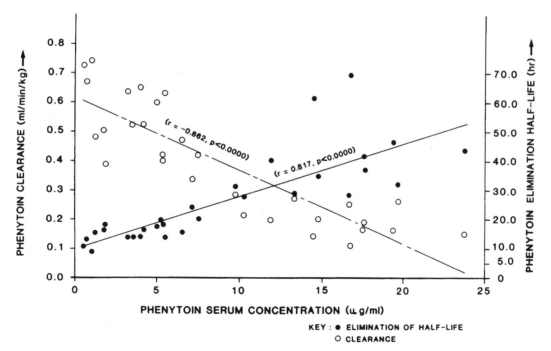

FIGURE 58.6. Phenytoin clearance and elimination half-life values determined by stable isotope tracer techniques at 30 different serum concentration values in 18 adult men on phenytoin monotherapy. (Based in part on data from references 18, 21, and 23, with permission.)

Time to Reach Steady-State Plasma Concentration Varies Nonlinearly with Dosing Rate and Linearly with Plasma Concentration

As phenytoin plasma concentration rises, phenytoin clearance decreases (see earlier). This results in a further rise in phenytoin plasma concentration and a further decrease in phenytoin clearance. This self-propagating cycle can require a long period to go to completion. The time (t) required to attain a given plasma concentration can be computed by the equation

$$t = \frac{V_d(C_{s,t} - C_{s,0})}{R - V_{max}} - \frac{V_d K_m V_{max}}{(R - V_{max})^2}$$

$$\ln \frac{(R - V_{max})C_{s,t} + RK_m}{(R - V_{max})C_{s,0} + RK_m} \quad [3]$$

where V_d is the volume of distribution, $C_{s,t}$ is the plasma concentration at time t, and $C_{s,0}$ is the plasma concentration at time 0 (89). Assuming average values for K_m and V_{max}, it is possible to compute an accumulation ½half-life (t½A) for phenytoin as follows:

$$t_{½A} = 0.270 C_{ss} \quad [4]$$

where $t_{1/2,A}$ has units of days, and C_{ss} has units of μg/mL (100). Equations [3] and [4] predict, and empirical data confirm, the following: (a) the time to reach steady-state plasma concentration varies nonlinearly with dosing rate; (b)

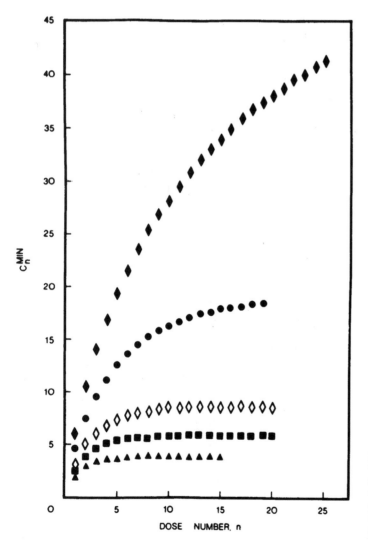

FIGURE 58.7. Plot of minimum serum concentration after the Nth dose, C^{min}, versus dose number *n*. Symbols and dosing rates (g/day) are: ◆, 0.50; ●, 0.40; ◇, 0.30; ■, 0.25; and ▲, 0.20. (From Wagner JG. Time to reach steady state and prediction of steady state concentration for drugs obeying Michaelis-Menten elimination kinetics. *J Pharmacokinet Biopharm* 1978;6:209–225, with permission.)

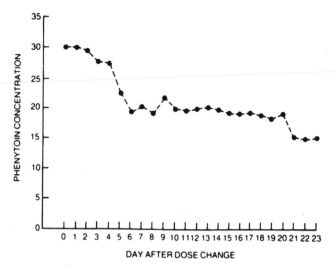

FIGURE 58.8. Changes in serum phenytoin concentration after reduction in phenytoin dosing rate from 250 to 200 mg/day. Serum phenytoin concentration stabilized after day 23. (From Theodore WH, Qu P, Tsay JY, et al. Phenytoin: the pseudosteady-state phenomenon. *Clin Pharmacol Ther* 1984;25:822–825, with permission.)

Typical Changes in Phenytoin Pharmacokinetics during Chronic Administration

When a patient starts phenytoin monotherapy, his or her plasma phenytoin concentration progressively rises. This has the following effects on phenytoin biotransformation and pharmacokinetic values (18): Rate of formation of *p*-HPPH decreases, clearance decreases, and elimination half-life increases (Figure 58.6). Table 58.1 illustrates typical values for these changes in a group of six patients started on phenytoin monotherapy.

ACKNOWLEDGMENT

This work was supported in part by the Department of Veterans Affairs.

CONVERSION

Conversion Factor:

$$CF = \frac{1,000}{mol.\ wt.} = \frac{1,000}{252.3} = 3.96$$

Conversion:

$$(\mu g/m) \times 3.96 = \mu mol/L \div 3.96 = \mu g/mL$$

$$(\mu mol/L) \div 3.96 = \mu g/mL$$

the time to reach steady-state plasma concentration varies linearly with plasma concentration; and (c) the time required to attain new steady-state plasma concentration values after starting phenytoin therapy or increasing or decreasing phenytoin dosing rate may be as long as 28 days (19,27, 101,144,155) (Figures 58.7 and 58.8). Therefore, a plasma phenytoin concentration value measured less than 28 days after a change in phenytoin dosing rate may not be an accurate indication of the ultimate new steady-state plasma concentration that will result from the change in dosing rate.

TABLE 58.1. PHENYTOIN BIOTRANSFORMATION AND PHARMACOKINETIC VALUES FOR SIX PATIENTS AT THREE TIMES DURING MONOTHERAPY DETERMINED WITH 150-MG TRACER DOSES OF STABLE ISOTOPE–LABELED PHENYTOIN[a]

	Week 0[b]	Week 4[c]	Week 12[d]	Significance[e]
Rate of formation of *p*-HPPH (mg labeled *p*-HPPH excreted per 48 hr):	98.5 ± 31.45[f]	82.2 ± 20.1	69.2 ± 31.9	$p < .01$
Clearance (mL/min/kg)[g]:	0.587 ± 0.149	0.456 ± 0.147	0.387 ± 0.187	$p < .05$
Elimination half-life (hr)[g]:	13.2 ± 3.6	18.4 ± 5.0	25.9 ± 9.7	$p < .01$

p-HPPH, 5-(*p*-hydroxyphenyl)-5-phenylhydantoin [a]From Browne TR, Evans JE, Szabo GK, et al. Studies with stable isotopes: I. changes in phenytoin pharmacokinetics and biotransformation during monotherapy. *J Clin Pharmacol* 1985;25:43–50, with permission.)
[b]Week 0 = value from single-dose (150 mg) study performed before monotherapy.
[c]Week 4 = value after 4 weeks on monotherapy (300 mg/day).
[d]Week 12 = value after 12 weeks on monotherapy (300–500 mg/day).
[e]Difference among values for weeks 0, 4, and 12 by analysis of variance for one group with repeated measures.
[f]Mean ± standard deviation, here and throughout table.
[g]Value for tracer dose of phenytoin.

REFERENCES

1. Aoyama T, Yamano S, Waxman DJ, et al. Cytochrome P450-hPCN3, a novel cytochrome P-450IIIA gene product that is differentially expressed in adult human liver: cDNA and deduced amino acid sequence in distinct specificities of cDNA-expressed hpCN1 and hpCN3 for the metabolism of steroid hormones and cyclosporine. *J Biol Chem* 1989;264:100388–100395.
2. Anderson GD, Gidal BE, Hendryx RJ, et al. Decreased plasma protein binding of valproate in patients with acute head trauma. *Br J Clin Pharmacol* 1994;37:559–562.
3. Anderson GD, Kaines KB, Kobayashi KA, et al. Phenytoin pharmacokinetics in post-traumatic head injury patients. *Epilepsia* 1991;32[Suppl 3]:9(abstr).
4. Anderson GD, Pak C, Doane KW, et al. Revised Winter-Tozer equation for normalized phenytoin concentrations in trauma and elderly patients with hypoalbuminemia. *Ann Pharmacother* 1997;31:279–284.
5. Atkinson AJ Jr, MacGee J, Strong J, et al. Identification of 5-methohydroxyphenyl-5-phenyl hydantoin as a metabolite of diphenylhydantoin. *Biochem Pharmacol* 1970;19:2483–2491.
6. Atkinson AJ, Shaw JM. Pharmacokinetic study of a patient with diphenylhydantoin toxicity. *Clin Pharmacol Ther* 1973;14:521–528.
7. Axelrod J, Tomachick R. Enzymatic O-methylation of epinephrine and other catechols. *J Biol Chem* 1950;233:702–705.
8. Ayengar PK, Hayaisnio M, Nakajima M, et al. Enzymatic aromatization of 3,5-cyclohexadiene-1,2-diol. *Biochim Biophys Acta* 1959;33:111–119.
9. Aynacioglu AS, Brockmoller J, Bauer S, et al. Frequency of cytochrome P450 CYP2C9 variants in a Turkish population and functional relevance for phenytoin. *Br J Clin Pharmacol* 1999;48:409–15.
10. Bajpai M, Roskos LK, Shen DD, et al. Roles of cytochrome P4502C9 and cytochrome P4502C19 in the stereoselective metabolism of phenytoin to its major metabolite. *Drug Metab Dispos* 1996;24:1401–1403.
11. Billings RE. Sex differences in rats in the metabolism of phenytoin to 5-(3,4-dihydroxyphenyl)-5-phenyl hydantoin. *J Pharmacol Exp Ther* 1983;225:630–636.
12. Billings RE, Fischer LJ. Oxygen-18 incorporation studies of the metabolism of phenytoin to the catechol. *Drug Metab Dispos* 1985;13:312–317.
13. Boobis AR, Edwards RJ, Adams DA, et al. Dissecting the function of cytochrome P450. *Br J Clin Pharmacol* 1996;42:81–89.
14. Borga O, Garle M, Gutova M. Identification of 5-(3,4-dihydroxyphenyl)-5-phenylhydantoin as a metabolite of 5,5-diphenylhydantoin (phenytoin) in rats and man. *Pharmacology* 1972;7:129–137.
15. Boucher BA, Rodman JH, Jaresko GS, et al. Phenytoin pharmacokinetics in critically ill trauma patients. *Clin Pharmacol Ther* 1988;44:675–683.
16. Brockmoller J, Rost KL, Gross D, et al. Phenotyping of CYP2C19 with enantiospecific HPLC-quantification of R- and S-mephenytoin and comparison with the intron4/exon5 G—A-splice site mutation. *Pharmacogenetics* 1995;5:80–88.
17. Browne TR, Chang T. Phenytoin: biotransformation. In: Levy RH, Dreifuss FE, Mattson RH, et al., eds. *Antiepileptic drugs*, 3rd ed. New York: Raven Press, 1989:197–213.
18. Browne TR, Evans JE, Szabo GK, et al. Studies with stable isotopes: I. changes in phenytoin pharmacokinetics and biotransformation during monotherapy. *J Clin Pharmacol* 1985;25:43–50.
19. Browne TR, Greenblatt DJ, Evans JE, et al. Determination of the in vivo K_m and V_{max} of a drug with tracer studies. *J Clin Pharmacol* 1987;27:321–324.
20. Browne TR, Greenblatt DJ, Evans JE, et al. Estimation of a drug's elimination half-life at any serum concentration when the drug's K_m and V_{max} are known: calculation and validation with phenytoin. *J Clin Pharmacol* 1987;27:318–320.
21. Browne TR, Szabo GK, Evans JE, et al. Phenobarbital does not alter phenytoin steady-state serum concentration or pharmacokinetics. *Neurology* 1988;38:639–642.
22. Browne TR, Szabo GK, Evans JE, et al. Carbamazepine increases phenytoin serum concentration and reduces phenytoin clearance. *Neurology* 1988;38:1146–1150.
23. Browne TR, Davondi H, Donn KH, et al. Bioavailability of ACC-9653 (phenytoin prodrug). *Epilepsia* 1989;30[Suppl 2]:527–532.
24. Browne TR, Szabo GK, Schumacher GE, et al. Effects of epoxide hydrolase and other minor metabolic pathways on phenytoin's non-linear pharmacokinetics. *J Clin Pharmacol* 1989;29:857.
25. Browne TR, Szabo GK, Walsh CT, et al. New pharmacokinetic methods: II. determination of presence or absence of product inhibition in drugs with non-linear pharmacokinetics. *J Clin Pharmacol* 1990;30:578–584.
26. Browne TR, Szabo GK, Schumacher GE, et al. Bioavailability studies of drugs with non-linear pharmacokinetics: I. tracer dose A.U.C. varies directly with serum concentration. *J Clin Pharmacol* 1992;32:1141–1145.
27. Browne TR, Szabo GK, Evans JE, et al. Studies of nonlinear pharmacokinetics with stable isotope labeled phenytoin. In: Baillie TA, Jones JP, eds. *Synthesis and applications of isotopically labeled compounds.* Amsterdam: Elsevier, 1994:157–162.
28. Butler TC. The metabolic conversion of 5,5-diphenylhydantoin to 5-(p-hydroxyphenyl)-5-phenylhydantoin. *J Pharmacol Exp Ther* 1957;199:1–11.
29. Butler TC, Dudley KH, Johnson D, et al. Studies of the metabolism of 5,5-diphenylhydantoin relating principally to the stereoselectivity of the hydroxylation reactions in man and the dog. *J Pharmacol Exp Ther* 1976;199:82–92.
30. Chang M, Dahl ML, Tybring G, et al. Use of omeprazole as a probe for CYP2C19 phenotype in Swedish Caucasians: comparison with S-mephenytoin hydroxylation phenotype and CYP2C19 genotype. *Pharmacogenetics* 1995;5:358–363.
31. Chang T, Glazko AJ. Diphenylhydantoin: biotransformation. In: Woodbury DM, Penry JK, Schmidt RP, eds. *Antiepileptic drugs.* New York: Raven Press, 1972:149–162.
32. Chang T, Glazko AJ. Phenytoin: biotransformation. In: Woodbury DM, Penry JK, Pippenger CE, eds. *Antiepileptic drugs*, 2nd ed. New York: Raven Press, 1982:204–226.
33. Chang T, Okerholm RA, Glazko AJ. Identification of 5-(3,4-dihydroxyphenyl)-5-phenylhydantoin: a metabolite of 5,5-diphenylhydantoin (Dilantin) in rat urine. *Anal Lett* 1972;5:195–202.
34. Chang T, Okerholm RA, Glazko AJ. A 3-O-methylated catechol metabolite of diphenylhydantoin (Dilantin) in rat urine. *Res Commun Chem Pathol Pharmacol* 1972;4:13–23.
35. Chang T, Young R, Maschewske E, et al. Metabolite studies with 13C-14C doubly labeled phenytoin in human subjects. *Epilepsia* 1977;18:191.
36. Chow SA, Fischer LJ. Phenytoin metabolism in mice. *Drug Metab Dispos* 1982;10:156–160.
37. Choy M, Winter ME. Comparing a mass balance algorithm with a Baysian regression analysis computer program for predicting serum phenytoin concentrations. *Am J Health Syst Pharm* 1998; 55:2392–2396.

38. Claesen M, Moustafa MAA, Adline J, et al. Evidence for an arene oxide–NIH shift pathway in the metabolic conversion of phenytoin to 5-(4-hydroxyphenyl)-5-phenylhydantoin in the rat and in man. *Drug Metab Dispos* 1982;10:667–671.

39. Crespi CL, Miller VP. The R144C change in the CYP2C9*2 allele alters interaction of the cytochrome P450 with NADPH: cytochrome P450 oxidoreductase. *Pharmacogenetics* 1997;7: 203–210.

40. Cuttle L, Munns A, Hogg NA, et al. Phenytoin metabolism by human cytochrome P450: involvement of P450 3A and 2C forms in secondary metabolism and drug-protein adduct formation. *Drug Metab Dispos* 2000;28:945–950.

41. deMorais SMF, Wilkinson GR, Blaisdell J, et al. The major defect responsible for the polymorphism of S-mephenytoin metabolism in humans. *J Biol Chem* 1994;269:15419–15422.

42. deMorais SM, Wilkinson GR, Blaisdell J, et al. Identification of a new genetic defect responsible for the polymorphism of (S)-mephenytoin metabolism in Japanese. *Mol Pharmacol* 1994;46: 594–598.

43. Dickinson RG, Hooper WD, Patterson M, et al. Extent of urinary excretion of p-hydroxyphenytoin in healthy subjects given phenytoin. *Ther Drug Monit* 1985;7:283–289.

44. Dickinson RG, Hooper WD, Wood B, et al. The effect of pregnancy in humans on the pharmacokinetics of stable isotope labeled phenytoin. *Br J Clin Pharmacol* 1989;28:17–27.

45. Dill WA, Kazenko A, Wold LM, et al. Studies on 5,5-diphenylhydantoin (Dilantin) in animals and man. *J Pharmacol Exp Ther* 1956;118:270–279.

46. Dodson WE. Phenytoin elimination in childhood: effect of concentration-dependent kinetics. *Neurology* 1980;30:196–199.

47. Donahue SR, Flockhart DA, Abernethy DR, et al. Ticlopidine inhibition of phenytoin metabolism mediated by potent inhibition of 2C19. *Clin Pharmacol Ther* 1997;62:572–577.

48. Eadie MJ, Tyrer JH, Bochner F, et al. The elimination of phenytoin in man. *Clin Exp Pharmacol Physiol* 1976;3:217–224.

49. Evans WE, Relling MV. Pharmacogenetics: translating functional genomics into rational therapeutics. *Science* 1999;286: 487–491.

50. Ferguson RJ, deMorais SM, Benhamou S, et al. A new genetic defect in human CYP2C19: mutation of the initiation codon is responsible for poor metabolism of S-mephenytoin. *J Pharmacol Exp Ther* 1998;284:356–361.

51. Fritz S, Linder W, Roots I, et al. Stereochemistry of aromatic phenytoin hydroxylation in humans. *J Pharmacol Exp Ther* 1987;241:615–622.

52. Furuya H, Fernandez-Salguero P, Gregory W, et al. Genetic polymorphism of CYP2C9 and its effect on warfarin maintenance dose requirement in patients undergoing anticoagulation therapy. *Pharmacogenetics* 1995;5:389–392.

53. Gabler WL. A method for assaying conjugation of diphenylhydantoin metabolites. *Fed Proc* 1974;33:525.

54. Garcia-Barcelo M, Chow LY, Kum Chiu HF, et al. Frequencies of defective CYP2C19 alleles in a Hong Kong Chinese population: detection of the rare allele CYP2C19*4. *Clin Chem* 1999; 45:2273–2274.

55. Garrettson LK, Jusko WJ. Diphenylhydantoin elimination kinetics in overdosed children. *Clin Pharmacol Ther* 1975;17: 481–491.

56. Gellner K, Eiselt R, Hustert E, et al. Genomic organization of the human CYP3A locus: identification of a new, inducible CYP3A gene. *Pharmacogenetics* 2001;11:111–121.

57. Gerber N, Thompson RM. Identification of catechol glucuronide metabolites of hydroxydiphenylhydantoins (m-HPPH, p-HPPH) in rat bile. *Fed Proc* 1974;33:525.25.

58. Gerber N, Wagner JG. Explanation of dose-dependent decline of diphenylhydantoin levels by fitting to the integrated form of the Michaelis-Menten equation. *Res Commun Chem Pathol Pharmacol* 1972;3:455–466.

59. Gerber N, Lynn R, Oates J. Acute intoxication with 5,5-diphenylhydantoin (Dilantin) associated with impairment of biotransformation: plasma levels urinary metabolites; and studies in healthy volunteers. *Ann Intern Med* 1972;77:756–771.

60. Gerber N, Seibert RA, Thompson RM. Identification of a catechol glucuronide metabolite of 5,5-diphenylhydantoin (DPH) in rat bile by gas chromatography (GC) and mass spectrometry (MS). *Res Commun Chem Path Pharmacol* 1973; 6:499–511.

61. Glazko AJ. Phenytoin: chemistry and methods of determination. In: Levy RH, Mattson RH, Meldrum B, et al., eds. *Antiepileptic drugs*, 3rd ed. New York: Raven Press, 1989:159–160.

62. Glazko AJ, Chang T, Baukema J, et al. Metabolic disposition of diphenylhydantoin in normal human subjects following intravenous administration. *Clin Pharmacol Ther* 1969;10:498–504.

63. Glazko AJ, Peterson FE, Smith TC, et al. Phenytoin metabolism in subjects with long and short plasma half-lives. *Ther Drug Monit* 1982;4:281–292.

64. Goldstein JA, deMorais SMF. Biochemistry and molecular biology of the human CYP2C subfamily. *Pharmacogenetics* 1994;4: 285–289.

65. Gonzalez FJ, Schmid BJ, Umeno M, et al. Human P450PCN1: sequence, chromosome localization, and direct evidence through cDNA expression that P450PCN1 is nifedipine oxidase. *DNA* 1988;7:79–86.

66. Gorvin JH, Brownlee G. Metabolism of 5,5-diphenylhydantoin in the rabbit. *Nature* 1957;179:1248.

67. Gotoh O. Substrate recognition sites in cytochrome P450 family 2 (CYP2) proteins inferred from comparative analyses of amino acid and coding nucleotide sequences. *J Biol Chem* 1992; 267:83–90.

68. Grover PL, Hewer A, Sims P. Epoxides as microsomal metabolites of polycyclic hydrocarbons. *FEBS Lett* 1971;18:76–80.

69. Haining RL, Hunter AP, Veronese ME, et al. Allelic variants of human cytochrome P450 2C9: baculovirus-mediated expression, purification, structural characterization, substrate stereospecificity, and prochiral selectivity of the wild-type and I359L mutant forms. *Arch Biochem Biophys* 1996;333:447–458.

70. Hakkola J, Tanaka E, Pelkonen O. Developmental expression of cytochrome P450 enzymes in human liver. *Pharmacol Toxicol* 1998;82:209–217.

71. Hashimoto H, Toide K, Katamura R, et al. Gene structure of CYP3A4, an adult-specific form of cytochrome P450 in human livers, and its transcriptional control. *Eur J Biochem* 1993;218: 585–595.

72. Hashimoto Y, Otsuki Y, Odani A, et al. Effect of CYP2C polymorphisms on the pharmacokinetics of phenytoin in Japanese patients with epilepsy. *Biol Pharm Bull* 1996;19:1103–1105.

73. Hassell TM, Maguire JH, Cooper CG, et al. Phenytoin administered in the cat after long-term administration. *Epilepsia* 1984; 25:556–563.

74. Holcomb R, Lynn R, Harvey B, et al. Intoxication with 5,5-diphenylhydantoin (Dilantin): clinical features, blood levels, urinary metabolites and metabolic changes in a child. *J Pediatr* 1972;80:627–632.

75. Horning MG, Lertratanangkoon K. Effect of chronic administration on urinary profiles of phenytoin metabolites. *Fed Proc* 1977;36:966.

76. Horning MG, Stratton C, Wilson A, et al. Detection of 5-(3,4-di-p-phdroxy-1,5-cyclohexadien-1-yl)-5-phenyl-hydantoin as a major metabolite of 5,5-diphenylhydantoin (Dilantin) in newborn human. *Anal Lett* 1971;4:537–545.

77. Hsieh KP, Lin YY, Cheng CL, et al. Novel mutations of CYP3A4 in Chinese. *Drug Metab Dispos* 2001;29:268–273.

78. Hudson SA, Farqyhar DL, Thompson P, et al. Phenytoin dosage individualization: five methods compared in the elderly. *J Clin Pharmacol Ther* 1990;15:25–34.

79. Ibeanu GC, Blaisdell J, Ghanayem BI, et al. An additional defective allele, CYP2C19*5, contributes to the S-mephenytoin poor metabolizer phenotype in Caucasians. *Pharmacogenetics* 1998;8:129–135.

80. Ibeanu GC, Goldstein JA, Meyer U, et al. Identification of new human CYP2C19 alleles (CYP2C19*6 and CYP2C19*2B) in a Caucasian poor metabolizer of mephenytoin. *J Pharmacol Exp Ther* 1998;286:1490–1495.

81. Ibeanu GC, Blaisdell J, Ferguson RJ, et al. A novel transversion in the intron 5 donor splice junction of CYP2C19 and a sequence polymorphism in exon 3 contribute to the poor metabolizer phenotype for the anticonvulsant drug S-mephenytoin. *J Pharmacol Exp Ther* 1999;290:635–640.

82. Ieiri I, Mamiya K, Urae A, et al. Stereoselective 4′-hydroxylation of phenytoin: relationship to (S)-mephenytoin polymorphism in Japanese. *Br J Clin Pharmacol* 1997;43:441–445.

83. Ieiri I, Tainaka H, Morita T, et al. Polymorphism of the cytochrome P450 (CYP) 2C9 gene in Japanese epileptic patients: genetic analysis of the CYP2C9 locus. *Pharmacogenetics* 2000;10:85–89.

84. Imai J, Ieiri I, Mamiya K, et al. Polymorphism of cytochrome P450 (CYP) 2C9 gene in Japanese epileptic patients: genetic analysis of the CYP2C9 locus. *Pharmacogenetics* 2000;10:85–89.

85. Inoue K, Yamazaki H, Imiya K, et al. Relationship between CYP2C9 and CYP2C19 genotypes and tolbutamide methyl hydroxylation and S-mephenytoin 4′-hydroxylation activities in livers of Japanese and Caucasian populations. *Pharmacogenetics* 1997;7:103–113.

86. Inoue K, Yamazaki H, Shimada T. Linkage between the distribution of mutations in the CYP2C18 and CYP2C19 genes in the Japanese and Caucasian. *Xenobiotica* 1998; 28:403–411.

87. Itoh K, Inoue K, Nakao H, et al. Polymerase chain reaction-single-strand conformation polymorphism based determination of two major genetic defects responsible for a phenotypic polymorphism of cytochrome P450 (CYP) 2C19 in the Japanese population. *Anal Biochem* 2000;284:160–162.

88. Jerina DM, Daly JW, Witkop B, et al. 1,2-Naphthalene oxide as an intermediate in the microsomal hydroxylation of naphthalene. *Biochemistry* 1970;9:147–155.

89. Jounadi Y, Hyrailles V, Gervot L, et al. Detection of CYP3A5 allelic variant: a candidate for the polymorphic expression of the protein? *Biochem Biophys Res Commun* 1996;221:466–470.

90. Jusko WJ. Bioavailability and disposition kinetics of phenytoin in man. In: Kellaway P, Petersen I, eds. *Quantitative analytic studies in epilepsy*. New York: Raven Press, 1976:115–136.

91. Kidd RS, Straughn AB, Meyer MC, et al. Pharmacokinetics of chlorpheniramine, phenytoin, glipizide, and nifedipine in an individual homozygous for the CYP2C9*3 allele. *Pharmacogenetics* 1999;9:71–80.

92. Kimura M, Ieire I, Mamiya K, et al. Genetic polymorphisms of the cytochrome P450s, CYP2C19 and CCP2C9 in Japanese population. *Ther Drug Monit* 1998;20:243–247.

93. Kimura SJ, Pastewka J, Gelboin HV, et al. cDNA and amino acid sequences of two members of the human P450 IIC gene subfamily. *Nucleic Acids Res* 1987;15:10053–10054.

94. Kluck RM, Cannell GR, Hooper WD, et al. Disposition of phenytoin and phenybarbitone in isolated perfused human placenta. *Clin Pharmacol Physiol* 1988;15:827–836.

95. Komatsu T, Yamazaki H, Asahi S, et al. Formation of a dihydroxy metabolite of phenytoin in human liver microsomes /

cytosol: roles of cytochromes P450 2C9, 2C19, and 3A4. *Drug Metab Dispos* 2000;28:1361–1368.

96. Kubota T, Hibi N, Chiba K. Linkage of mutant alleles of CYP2C18 and CYP2C19 in a Japanese population. *Biochem Pharmacol* 1998;55:2039–2042.

97. Kuehl P, Zhang J, Lin Y, et al. Sequence diversity in CYP3A promoters and characterization of the genetic basis of polymorphic CYP3A5 expression. *Nat Genet* 2001;27:383–391.

98. Kutt H. Phenytoin: relation of plasma concentration to seizure control. In: Woodbury DM, Penry JK, Pippenger CE, eds. *Antiepileptic drugs*, 2nd ed. New York: Raven Press, 1982: 241–246.

99. Kutt H, Wolk M, Scherman R, et al. Insufficient parahydroxylation as a cause of diphenylhydantoin toxicity. *Neurology* 1964; 14:542–548.

100. Lai C, Moore P, Matier WL, et al. Bioequivalence of ACC-9653, a phosphate ester prodrug of phenytoin, to phenytoin sodium after i.v. administration in dogs. *Pharmacologist* 1987; 29:143.

101. Lam G, Chiou WL. Integrated equation to evaluate accumulation profiles of drugs eliminated by Michaelis-Menten kinetics. *J Pharmacokinet Biopharm* 1979;7:227–232.

102. Levy RH. General principles: drug absorption, distribution and elimination. In: Woodbury DM, Penry JK, Pippenger CE, eds. *Antiepileptic drugs*, 2nd ed. New York: Raven Press, 1982:11–24.

103. Li AP, Kaminski DL, Rasmussen A. Substrates of human hepatic cytochrome P450 3A4. *Toxicology* 1995;104:1–8.

104. Ludden TM, Allerheiligen SR, Browne TR, et al. Sensitivity analysis of the effect of bioavailability or dosage form content on mean steady state phenytoin concentration. *Ther Drug Monit* 1991;13:120–125.

105. Maguire JH, Wilson DC. Urinary dihydrodiol metabolites of phenytoin: high performance liquid chromatography assay of diastereometric composition. *J Chromatogr* 1985;342:323–332.

106. Maguire JH, Butler TC, Dudley KH. Absolute configuration of (+)-5-(3-hydroxyphenyl)-5-phenylhydantoin, the major metabolite of 5,5-diphenylhydantoin in the dog. *J Med Chem* 1978; 21:1194–1297.

107. Maguire JH, Butler TC, Dudley KH. Absolute configurations of the dihydrodiol metabolites of 5,5-diphenylhydantoin (phenytoin) from rat, dog, and human urine. *Drug Metab Dispos* 1980;8:325–331.

108. Maguire JH, McClanahan JS. Evidence for stereoselective production of phenytoin (5,5-diphenylhydantoin) arene oxides in man. *Life Sci* 1983;897–902.

109. Mamiya K, Ieiri I, Miyahara S, et al. Association of polymorphisms in the cytochrome P450 (CYP) 2C19 and 2C18 genes in Japanese epileptic patients. *Pharmacogenetics* 1998;8:87–90.

110. Mamiya K, Ieieri I, Shimamoto J, et al. The effects of genetic polymorphisms of CYP2C9 and CYP2C19 on phenytoin metabolism in Japanese adult patients with epilepsy: studies with stereoselective hydroxylation and population pharmacokinetics. *Epilepsia* 1998; 39:1317–1323.

111. Martz F, Failinger C III, Blake D. Phenytoin teratogenesis: correlation between embryopathic effects and covalent binding of putative arene oxide metabolite in gestational tissue. *J Pharmacol Exp Ther* 1977;203:231–239.

112. Masimirembwa C, Bertilsson L, Johansson I, et al. Phenotyping and genotyping of S-mephenytoin hydroxylase (cytochrome P450 2C19) in a Shona population of Zimbabwe. *Clin Pharmacol Ther* 1995;57:656–661.

113. Mawer GE, Mullen PW, Rodgers M, et al. Phenytoin dose adjustment in epileptic patients. *Br J Clin Pharmacol* 1974;1: 163–168.

114. Maynert EW. The metabolic fate of diphenylhydantoin in the dog, rat, and man. *J Pharmacol Exp Ther* 1960;130:275–284.

115. Midha KK, Hindmarsh KW, McGilvrary IJ, et al. Identification of urinary catechol and methylated catechol metabolites of phenytoin in human, monkeys, and dogs by GLC and GLC-mass spectrometry. *J Pharm Sci* 1977;66:1596–1602.

116. Mizugaki M, Hiratsuka M, Agatsuma Y, et al. Rapid detection of CYP2C18 genotypes by real-time fluorescence polymerase chain reaction. *J Pharm Pharmacol* 2000;52:199–205.

117. Moustafa MAA, Claesen M, Adline J, et al. Evidence for an arene-3,4-oxide as metabolic intermediate in the meta- and para-hydroxylation of phenytoin in the dog. *Drug Metab Dispos* 1983;11:574–580.

118. Mullen PW, Foster RW. Comparative evaluation of six techniques for determining the Michaelis-Menten parameters relating phenytoin dose and steady state serum concentrations. *J Pharm Pharmacol* 1979;31:100–104.

119. Nakamura K, Goto F, Ray WA, et al. Interethnic differences in genetic polymorphism of debrisoquine and mephenytoin hydroxylation between Japanese and Caucasian populations. *Clin Pharmacol Ther* 1985;38:402–408.

120. Ninomiya H, Mamiya K, Matsuo S, et al. Genetic polymorphism of the CYP2C subfamily and excessive serum phenytoin concentration with central nervous system intoxication. *Ther Drug Monit* 2000;22:230–232.

121. Noach EL, Woodbury DM, Goodman LS. Studies on the absorption, distribution, fate and excretion of 4-14C-labeled diphenylhydantoin. *J Pharmacol Exp Ther* 1958;122:301–314.

122. Odani A, Hashimoto Y, Otsuki Y, et al. Genetic polymorphism of the CYP2C subfamily and its effect on the pharmacokinetics of phenytoin in Japanese patients with epilepsy. *Clin Pharmacol Ther* 1997;62:287–292.

123. Oesch F, Kaubisch N, Jerina DM, et al. Hepatic epoxide hydrase: structure–activity relationships for substrates and inhibitors. *Biochemistry* 1971;10:4858–4866.

124. Poupaert JH, Cavalier R, Claesen MH, et al. Absolute configuration of the major metabolite of 5,5-diphenylhydantoin, 5-(4-hydroxyphenyl)-5-phenylhydantoin. *J Med Chem* 1975;18:1268–1271.

125. Rail L. Dilantin overdosage. *Med J Aust* 1968;2:339.

126. Rambeck B, Boenigk HE, Dunlop A, et al. Predicting phenytoin dose: A revised monogram. *Ther Drug Monit* 1979;1:325–333.

127. Rane A, Peug D. Phenytoin enhances epoxide metabolism in human fetal liver cultures. *Drug Metab Dispos* 1985;13:382–385.

128. Rettie AE, Haining RL, Bajpai M, et al. A common genetic basis for idiosyncratic toxicity of warfarin and phenytoin. *Epilepsy Res* 1999;35:253–255.

129. Richardson TH, Jung F, Griffin KJ, et al. A universal approach to the expression of human and rabbit cytochrome P450s of the 2C subfamily in *Escherichia coli*. *Arch Biochem Biophys* 1995;323:87–96.

130. Richardson TH, Griffin KJ, Jung F, et al. Targeted antipeptide antibodies to cytochrome P450 2C18 based on epitope mapping of an inhibitory monoclonal antibody to P450 2C51. *Arch Biochem Biophys* 1997;338:157–162.

131. Richens A, Dunlop A. Serum phenytoin levels in the management of epilepsy. *Lancet* 1975;2:247–248.

132. Romkes M, Faletto MB, Blaisdell JA, et al. Cloning and expression of complementary DNAs for multiple members of the human cytochrome P450IIC subfamily. *Biochemistry* 1991;30:3247–3255.

133. Ruas JL, Lechner MC. Allele frequency of CYP2C19 in a Portuguese population. *Pharmacogenetics* 1997;7:333–335.

134. Sata F, Sapone A, Elizondo G, et al. CYP3A4 allelic variants with amino acid substitutions in exons 7 and 12: evidence for an allelic variant with altered catalytic activity. *Clin Pharmacol Ther* 2000;67:48–56.

135. Schuetz J, Beach P, Guzelian PS. Selective expression of cytochrome P450 CYP3A mRNAs in embryonic and adult human liver. *Pharmacogenetics* 1994;4:11–20.

136. Schumacher GE. Using pharmacokinetics in drug therapy: VI. comparing methods for dealing with nonlinear drugs like phenytoin. *Am J Hosp Pharm* 1980;37:128–132.

137. Sheiner LB, Beal SL. Evaluation of population methods for estimating pharmacokinetic parameters: I. Michaelis-Menten model: routine pharmacokinetic data. *J Pharmacokinet Biopharm* 1980;8:553–571.

138. Shimada T, Yamazaki H, Mimura M, et al. Interindividual variations in human liver cytochrome P-450 enzymes involved in the oxidation of drugs, carcinogens, and toxic chemicals: studies with liver microsomes of 30 Japanese and 30 Caucasians. *J Pharmacol Exp Ther* 1994;270:414–423.

139. Smith RG, Daves GD Jr, Lynn RK, et al. Hydantoin ring glucuronidation: characterization of a new metabolite of 5,5-diphenylhydantoin in man and the rat. *Biomed Mass Spectrom* 1977;4:275–279.

140. Stubbins MJ, Haries LW, Smith G, et al. Genetic analysis of the human cytochrome P450 CYP2C9 locus. *Pharmacogenetics* 1996;6:429–439.

141. Sullivan-Klose TH, Ghanayem BI, Bell DA, et al. The role of the CYP2C9-Leu359 allelic variant in the tolbutamide polymorphism. *Pharmacogenetics* 1996;6:341–349.

142. Takakubo F, Kuwano A, Kondo I. Evidence that poor metabolizers of (S)-mephenytoin could be identified by haplotypes of CYP2C19 in Japanese. *Pharmacogenetics* 1996;6:265–267.

143. Takanashi K, Tainaka H, Kobayashi K, et al. CYP2C9Ile359 and Leu359 variants: enzyme kinetic study with seven substrates. *Pharmacogenetics* 2000;10:95–104.

144. Theodore WH, Qu P, Tsay JY, et al. Phenytoin: the pseudosteady-state phenomenon. *Clin Pharmacol Ther* 1984;25:822–825.

145. Thompson RM, Beghin J, Fife WK, et al. 5,5-Bis(4-hydroxyphenyl)hydantoin, a minor metabolite of diphenylhydantoin (Dilantin) in the rat and human. *Drug Metab Dispos* 1976;4:349–356.

146. Thompson RM, Gerber N, Seibert RA, et al. A rapid method for the mass spectrometric identification of glucuronides and other polar drug metabolites in permethylated rat bile. *Drug Metab Dispos* 1973;1:489–505.

147. Thummel KE, Wilkinson GR. In vitro and in vivo drug interactions involving human CYP3A. *Annu Rev Pharmacol Toxicol* 1998;38:389–430.

148. Tomaszewski JE, Jerina DM, Daly JW. Deuterium isotope effect during formation of phenols by hepatic monoxygenases: evidence for an alternative to the arene oxide pathway. *Biochemistry* 1975;14:2024–2031.

149. Tsuru M, Erickerson RR, Holtzman JL. The metabolism of phenytoin by isolated hepatocytes and hepatic microsomes from male rats. *J Pharmacol Exp Ther* 1982;222:658–661.

150. Tyrer JH, Eadie MJ, Sutherland JM. Outbreak of anticonvulsant intoxication in an Australian city. *BMJ* 1970;4:271–273.

151. Valodia PN, Seymour SA, McFayden ML, et al. Validation of population pharmacokinetic parameters of phenytoin using a parallel Michaelis-Menten and first-order elimination model. *Ther Drug Monit* 2000;22:313–319.

152. Vasko MR, Bell RD, Daly DD, et al. Inheritance of phenytoin hypometabolism: a kinetic study in one family. *Clin Pharmacol Ther* 1979;27:96–103.

153. Vermeij P, Ferrari MD, Buruma PJ, et al. Inheritance of poor phenytoin parahydroxylation capacity in a Dutch family. *Clin Pharmacol Ther* 1988;44:588–593.

154. Veronese ME, Doecke CJ, Mackenzie PI, et al. Site-directed mutation studies of human liver cytochrome P-450 isoenzymes in the 2C subfamily. *Biochem J* 1993;289:533–538.

155. Wagner JG. Time to reach steady state and prediction of steady state concentration for drugs obeying Michaelis-Menten elimination kinetics. *J Pharmacokinet Biopharm* 1978;6:209–225

156. Walker AH, Jaffe JM, Gunasegaram S, et al. Characterization of an allelic variant in the nifedipine-specific element of CYP3A4: ethnic distribution and implications for prostate cancer risk. *Hum Mutat* 1998;12:289–293.

157. Wang SL, Huang JD, Lai MD, et al. Detection of CYP2C9 polymorphism based on the polymerase chain reaction in Chinese. *Pharmacogenetics* 1995;5:37–42.

158. Watanabe M, Iwahashi K, Kugoh T, et al. The relationship between phenytoin pharmacokinetics and the CYP2C19 genotype in Japanese epileptic patients. *Clin Neuropharmacol* 1998; 21:122–126.

159. Weber BL, Rebbeck TR. Characterization of an allelic variant in the nifedipine-specific element of CYP3A4: ethnic distribution and implications for prostate cancer risk. *Hum Mutat* 1998;12:289–293.

160. Watkins PB. Noninvasive tests of CYP3A enzymes. *Pharmacogenetics* 1994;4:171–184.

161. Westlind A, Lofberg L, Tindberg N, et al. Interindividual differences in hepatic expression of CYP3A4: relationship to genetic polymorphism in the 5′-upstream regulatory region. *Biochem Biophys Res Commun* 1999;259:201–205.

162. Woodbury DM. Phenytoin: absorption, distribution, and excretion. In: Woodbury DM, Penry JK, Pippenger CE, eds. *Antiepileptic drugs*, 2nd ed. New York: Raven Press, 1982: 191–207.

163. Xiao ZS, Goldstein JA, Xie HG, et al. Differences in the incidence of the CYP2C19 polymorphism affecting the S-mephenytoin phenotype in Chinese Han and Bai populations and identification of a new rare CYP2C19 mutant allele. *J Pharmacol Exp Ther* 1997;281:604–609.

164. Xie HG, Kim RB, Stein CM, et al. Genetic polymorphism of (S)-mephenytoin 4′-hydroxylation in populations of African descent. *Br J Clin Pharmacol* 1999;48:402–408.

165. Xie HG, Stein CM, Kim RB, et al. Allelic, genotypic and phenotypic distributions of S-mephenytoin 4′-hydroxylase (CYP2C19) in healthy Caucasian populations of European descent throughout the world. *Pharmacogenetics* 1999;9: 539–549.

166. Xie HG. Genetic variations of S-mephenytoin 4′-hydroxylase (CYP2C19) in the Chinese population. *Life Sci* 2000;66: PL175–PL181.

167. Yasumori T, Chen LS, Li QH, et al. Human CYP2C-mediated stereoselective phenytoin hydroxylation in Japanese: difference in chiral preference of CYP2C9 and CYP2C19. *Biochem Pharmacol* 1999;57:1297–1303.

Antiepileptic Drugs, 5ᵗʰ Edition. Edited by R.H. Levy, R.H. Mattson, B.S. Meldrum, and E. Perucca. Lippincott Williams & Wilkins, Philadelphia © 2002.

PHENYTOIN AND OTHER HYDANTOINS

INTERACTIONS WITH OTHER DRUGS

ISABELLE RAGUENEAU-MAJLESSI
MANOJ BAJPAI
RENÉ H. LEVY

Numerous interactions between phenytoin (PHT) and other drugs have been reported, involving different therapeutic classes, and resulting in signs of intoxication or lack of effectiveness of PHT or the other drug(s). Most of the drug interactions observed with PHT involve inhibition of its biotransformation or alteration of its protein binding. In addition, PHT is a potent inducer of the metabolism of various compounds.

This chapter is divided as follows: Alteration of PHT Kinetics by Antiepileptic Drugs (AEDs); Alteration of PHT Kinetics by Other Drugs; Effects of PHT on Kinetics of Other AEDs; and Effects of PHT on Kinetics of Other Drugs. In each section, drugs or drug classes are presented in alphabetical order.

MECHANISMS OF PHARMACOKINETIC INTERACTIONS

Absorption

PHT is slowly but almost completely absorbed. In clinical studies using low dosages of antacids (10 mL every 6 hours), little or no effect was seen (70). Higher doses (15 to 45 mL), however, were found to reduce PHT bioavailability (14,19). The effect usually is more noticeable if the antacid is given at the same (or nearly the same) time as PHT; therefore, it is advisable to keep a minimum interval of about 2 hours between the administration of PHT and the ingestion of antacids.

Isabelle Ragueneau-Majlessi, MD: Research Associate, Department of Pharmaceutics, University of Washington, Seattle, Washington

Manoj Bajpai, PhD: Department of Pharmaceutics and Drug Metabolism, Amgen Incorporated, Thousand Oaks, California

René H. Levy, PhD: Professor and Chair, Department of Pharmaceutics, Professor of Neurological Surgery, University of Washington School of Pharmacy and Medicine, Seattle, Washington

Food has been found to have variable but modest, usually enhancing, effects on PHT absorption (14). Lipid meals were found to increase PHT bioavailability (101). A protein-rich diet had the same effect on PHT acid but not on the sodium salt (41). A constant relationship in time between food intake and ingestion of PHT is recommended (41,59). Low levels of PHT have been found in some patients receiving liquid food concentrates given either by nasogastric tube or orally (108).

Activated charcoal delays and reduces absorption of PHT and influences the enterohepatic recirculation; therefore, it is beneficial to give large doses of charcoal in the early phases of massive PHT overdose (115).

Protein Binding

Approximately 90% of the total PHT in the plasma is protein bound. Other strongly bound drugs, such as tolbutamide (116), salicylates (27), valproate (63), and phenylbutazone (104), can displace PHT from its binding sites. Plasma protein binding interactions *per se* are not expected to modify the pharmacologic effect of PHT, but they should be taken into account when interpreting total serum PHT concentrations. In fact, in the presence of a displacing agent, therapeutic and toxic effects are expected to occur at total serum PHT concentrations lower than usual.

Biotransformation

PHT undergoes extensive metabolism, with less than 5% of the dose excreted unchanged in urine. PHT is metabolized by cytochrome P450 (CYP) isoforms CYP2C9 and CYP2C19 to the two enantiomers of its primary metabolite, *p*-HPPH [5-(4-hydroxyphenyl)-5-phenylhydantoin] (6). CYP2C9 is the major contributor in the formation of the (*S*)-enantiomer of *p*-HPPH. Both CYP2C9 and

CYP2C19 are expressed polymorphically in the human population, with two functionally defective alleles of CYP2C9 and four null alleles of CYP2C19 currently recognized. Genetically determined defects in the expression of CYP2C9 and CYP2C19 could explain the occurrence of high serum PHT concentrations in some patients treated with normal doses of PHT.

ALTERATION OF PHENYTOIN KINETICS BY ANTIEPILEPTIC DRUGS

Carbamazepine. The effect of carbamazepine on the plasma PHT level varies among patients. A lowering effect (120), no significant changes, and an upward trend has been observed (25,79,124). Prolongation of PHT half-life by carbamazepine in several but not all patients was seen using a stable isotope–labeled PHT test dose (13). What to expect in an individual patient is largely unpredictable and concurrent use should be monitored.

Chlordiazepoxide. Chlordiazepoxide has caused elevated PHT concentrations in some patients (47,112).

Clobazam. Clobazam may have no marked effect on plasma PHT level in many patients (102), but it has caused an increase in PHT concentration and intoxication in some (125).

Clonazepam. Clonazepam has been reported to lower the plasma PHT level in some patients (95), but in other studies, clonazepam has caused a rise in the PHT level (120) or no significant changes (35,38).

Diazepam. The effect of diazepam on the plasma PHT level varies among patients, with elevations (112) or decreases (35) of PHT levels. In most patients, the commonly used diazepam doses do not seem to cause significant changes in PHT level.

Felbamate. Felbamate has been shown to inhibit CYP2C19 in vitro with an inhibition constant in the therapeutic range (K_i, 225 μmol/L) (29). Recently, Sachdeo et al. showed that when 10 patients on PHT monotherapy received increasing dosages of felbamate (1,200, 1,800, 2,400 to 3,600 mg/day), PHT plasma concentrations increased and PHT dose reductions of at least 20% were required (96).

Flunarizine. In several studies, the addition of flunarizine caused little change in PHT levels (111).

Gabapentin. Gabapentin usually is not found to alter PHT levels (88).

Lamotrigine. Single and repeated doses of lamotrigine do not alter PHT kinetics significantly (74).

Levetiracetam. Levetiracetam has no effect *in vitro* on PHT metabolism (68). In most studies, levetiracetam did not modify plasma PHT levels in epileptic patients (72).

Methsuximide. Comedication of epileptic patients with PHT and methsuximide caused varying degrees of elevation in the plasma PHT level (86).

Oxcarbazepine. Oxcarbazepine is an inhibitor of CYP2C19 and therefore may cause a moderate increase in plasma PHT concentration (7).

Phenobarbital. Phenobarbital induces CYP2C enzymes (46), but is also is a substrate for those enzymes (73). This dual effect leads to variable results in patients taking PHT and phenobarbital together, with an increase, a decrease, or no change in PHT levels having been reported.

Progabide. Progabide given as add-on medication caused elevation of PHT levels to varying extents in most patients (52).

Stiripentol. Stiripentol reduced the clearance of PHT in a dose-dependent manner up to 40% (51).

Tiagabine. Tiagabine (90,91) does not cause significant alterations of plasma PHT levels.

Topiramate. Topiramate occasionally may cause an increase in plasma PHT concentration (76), probably by inhibiting CYP2C19.

Valproate. The effect of valproate on PHT plasma level varies among patients and may vary in the same patient during the course of therapy. Thus, a persistent fall (54) or a transient fall (63) or even a rise (120) within days after the addition of valproate occurs in some patients. When a fall in plasma PHT concentration occurs, this can be ascribed to displacement of PHT from plasma protein binding sites (66), and the free plasma concentration is not reduced or even may be increased (54,75). Clinically, the need to adjust PHT dose is rare.

Vigabatrin. Vigabatrin may cause up to a 40% decline in PHT levels in some patients, sometimes as late as a few weeks after starting combined therapy (92). Comparing groups of patients taking PHT with and without vigabatrin revealed only small differences in PHT plasma levels (58).

Zonisamide. The effect of zonisamide on blood PHT levels is modest and variable, and there was no need to adjust the PHT dose because of the interaction (34).

ALTERATION OF PHENYTOIN KINETICS BY OTHER DRUGS

Activated Charcoal. As discussed previously, activated charcoal effectively inhibits the absorption of PHT from the gastrointestinal tract (115).

Analgesics, Antipyretics, and Nonsteroidal Antiinflammatory Drugs

Phenylbutazone. Prolongation of PHT half-life and PHT intoxication has occurred in some epileptic patients taking phenylbutazone (104). The major factors in this interaction are displacement of PHT from plasma binding sites and inhibition of PHT metabolism (inhibition of CYP2C9). Thus, an increase in the plasma concentration of free, pharmacologically active PHT also may occur in the absence of any change in total plasma PHT concentration. It may be necessary to adjust PHT dosage in some patients.

Propoxyphene. The PHT plasma level increased slightly in five patients after they received 65 mg of propoxyphene three times daily for 6 days (18). In another patient who took large amounts (650 mg/day) of propoxyphene for several days (47), PHT accumulated to the toxic range. These effects are consistent with inhibition of CYP2C9.

Salicylates. Salicylates can displace PHT from plasma protein binding sites *in vitro* and *in vivo*. In clinical studies, an increase in the unbound fraction of PHT from the usual 10% to near 16% and an increase in PHT clearance by acetylsalicylic acid was observed (27). This interaction is unlikely to be clinically relevant.

Anticoagulants and Inhibitors of Platelet Aggregation

Bishydroxycoumarin. Bishydroxycoumarin (104) and, to a lesser extent, phenprocoumon have been reported to cause elevations of PHT plasma levels in some patients.

Ticlopidine. Several cases of PHT toxicity during concomitant ticlopidine therapy have been reported (43,83). In a clinical study performed in six patients treated with PHT, 250 mg ticlopidine twice daily inhibited the clearance of PHT (20). These interactions are consistent with in vitro findings that ticlopidine is a potent inhibitor of CYP2C19.

Antidepressants

Fluoxetine. Two case reports have described signs of PHT toxicity resulting from combined administration of fluoxetine and PHT (37). In both cases, PHT plasma levels increased significantly when fluoxetine was coadministered, and removal or gradual reduction of fluoxetine resulted in complete recovery. This interaction with PHT can be explained by inhibition of CYP2C19 by fluoxetine.

Fluvoxamine. A recent report described the case of a patient with PHT plasma concentrations that increased from 16.6 to 49.1 µg/mL when fluvoxamine was coadministered, associated with clinical symptoms of PHT toxicity (53).

Imipramine. Imipramine caused an increase in PHT levels in some studies, but in other studies no significant alteration of PHT kinetics was seen. It appears that the tricyclic antidepressants rarely necessitate PHT dosage adjustments.

Sertraline. Sertraline, a known inhibitor of the CYP2C family, increased PHT plasma levels in two elderly patients, without symptoms of toxicity (32).

Trazodone. The PHT level increased from 17 to 46 µg/mL in a patient within a few weeks after trazodone administration. Clinical intoxication occurred and the PHT dose had to be reduced (23).

Viloxazine. Viloxazine increased plasma PHT levels by 7% to 94% and caused intoxication in 4 of 10 epileptic patients (78).

Antifungal Agents

Fluconazole. Several case reports have been published describing PHT toxicity in the presence of fluconazole (15,36,61), with significant increases in PHT plasma levels. In addition to these clinical reports, several controlled trials in healthy subjects have shown that fluconazole increases the serum concentration of PHT (10,49,110). Based on in vitro studies, the interaction between PHT and fluconazole can be attributed to inhibition of CYP2C9 and CYP2C19.

Miconazole. In one patient well controlled by PHT, miconazole in combination with flucytosine caused an elevation of PHT levels associated with symptoms of PHT toxicity (94). Miconazole is an inhibitor of CYP2C9.

Antihistaminics

Chlorpheniramine. A modest elevation of plasma PHT levels has occurred in some patients after the addition of chlorpheniramine, but without the need to change dosages (84).

Terfenadine. Terfenadine caused essentially no changes in PHT pharmacokinetics (17).

Antimicrobial Agents

Chloramphenicol. Chloramphenicol has caused modest elevations of PHT plasma levels in some patients and marked elevations in others (44,66). The need to reduce the PHT dose has varied.

Isoniazid. Isoniazid noncompetitively inhibits PHT metabolism *in vitro* and *in vivo* (46,121). In patients taking PHT and isoniazid, significant PHT accumulation and intoxication have been reported in 10% to 15% of the subjects (21,121), some of whom were identified as very slow acetylators (12,114).

Rifampin. Rifampin can lower PHT levels and increase its clearance by a factor of two. Furthermore, rifampin comedication minimizes the inhibitory effect of isoniazid even in the slow isoniazid acetylators (40).

Sulfonamides. A number of bacteriostatic sulfonamides, including sulfadiazine, sulfamethizole, sulfamethoxazole, and sulfaphenazole, can reduce PHT clearance and prolong its half-life (62). The mechanism appears to be inhibition of CYP2C enzymes, and sulfaphenazole is the strongest inhibitor (22,62) of PHT metabolism. Some sulfonamides also may displace PHT from plasma binding sites. Adjustment of PHT dosage may become necessary during sulfonamide therapy.

Antineoplastic Agents

Low PHT levels have been observed in several patients undergoing antineoplastic therapy with vinblastine, cisplatinum, or bleomycin and adriamycin (11,107).

Tamoxifen. High-dose tamoxifen therapy was associated with clinical signs of PHT toxicity and increased serum PHT levels (85).

Antipsychotics

Thioridazine. Two case reports described PHT intoxication during concurrent administration of thioridazine (113). However, a retrospective study (99) in 27 adult patients treated with PHT showed no clinically important alterations in PHT serum concentration with thioridazine.

Antiulcer Agents

Antacids. Antacids such as aluminum and magnesium hydroxides and calcium carbonate have been found to reduce or maintain low blood PHT levels in some patients but not in others. It appears that the total dose of antacid and the time of administration are determining factors.

Cimetidine. Cimetidine has been found to increase PHT concentrations (50,77) by inhibition of metabolism (inhibition of CYP2C19). In one study (77), 300 mg of cimetidine given four times a day caused elevation of blood PHT levels in a few days in five of nine subjects. In another study (97), PHT levels increased in six patients, causing intoxication in two, after addition of cimetidine.

Omeprazole. Gugler and Jensen (30) have shown that omeprazole, a weak inhibitor of CYP2C19, causes a small but consistent elevation of PHT levels in healthy subjects. Prichard et al. (82) also have shown significant increases in the plasma levels of PHT in healthy subjects receiving omeprazole.

Cardiovascular Agents

Amiodarone. Amiodarone caused a twofold to threefold increase in PHT plasma levels in three patients (57) and increased the PHT half-life severalfold in healthy volunteers (69) by inhibition of PHT metabolism (inhibition of CYP2C9).

Calcium Channel Blockers. Among calcium channel blockers, verapamil and nifedipine had little or no effect on PHT concentration, but diltiazem caused elevations and intoxication in 3 of 14 patients (5).

Diazoxide. Diazoxide reduced the protein binding of PHT, with a consequent increase in the free fraction and a slight decrease in the total plasma PHT concentration (93).

Hypoglycemic Agents

Tolbutamide. Tolbutamide was found to displace PHT from plasma binding sites and to lower plasma PHT levels in patients (116).

Other Agents

Disulfiram. Disulfiram noncompetitively inhibits PHT metabolism and causes an increase in plasma PHT concentrations and signs of PHT intoxication in most patients (71). A study by Svendsen et al. (106) with healthy volunteers demonstrated that disulfiram reduced PHT clearance from approximately 50 to 34 mL/min. Dosage adjustment of PHT is necessary when these two drugs are administered together.

Ethanol. Prolonged use of ethanol can reduce PHT plasma level (98), perhaps through enzyme induction. Elevation of the PHT plasma level, on the other hand, has been observed during occasional moderate or heavy intake of ethanol (47).

EFFECTS OF PHENYTOIN ON KINETICS OF ANTIEPILEPTIC DRUGS

Carbamazepine. PHT is a potent inducer of carbamazepine biotransformation (25,48), probably through induction of CYP3A4. The plasma concentration of 10,11-carbamazepine epoxide, which usually equals 10% to 20% of the parent compound in patients on monotherapy, may remain unchanged after the addition of PHT, or may undergo a small rise or fall (89).

Clobazam. PHT induces clobazam metabolism. The plasma levels of clobazam were lower, whereas those of the active metabolite norclobazam were higher during comedication (102).

Clonazepam. PHT increased clonazepam clearance by 46% to 58% in healthy subjects (42).

Flunarizine. Flunarizine levels were lower in patients receiving combined medication with enzyme inducers, including PHT (111).

Lamotrigine. Lamotrigine clearance is increased and plasma levels are lowered by comedication with PHT, suggesting induction of glucuronidation (74).

Levetiracetam. PHT does not appear to modify the plasma levels of levetiracetam to any significant extent (72).

Methsuximide. PHT was found to increase the levels of the pharmacologically active metabolite N-desmethylmethsuximide in epileptic patients (86).

Phenobarbital. PHT has been reported to cause an elevation of plasma phenobarbital levels in some patients (64,120). Also, in some patients stabilized on combination therapy, a decrease in phenobarbital plasma levels was noted after PHT was discontinued (25,64). In most patients, however, PHT does not cause significant changes in plasma phenobarbital levels, and the need to adjust dosages because of this interaction is expected to be rare.

Primidone. PHT induces primidone biotransformation, but this interaction rarely leads to a need for dosage adjustments.

Oxazepam. Induction of oxazepam metabolism has been demonstrated in epileptic patients treated with PHT alone or in combination with phenobarbitone (100).

Oxcarbazepine. PHT reduces to a moderate extent the plasma levels of 10-hydroxycarbazepine, the active metabolite of oxcarbazepine (4).

Tiagabine. The plasma levels of tiagabine are reduced markedly by PHT (91).

Topiramate. PHT induces the metabolism of topiramate and reduces its concentration in plasma (76).

Valproate. There is extensive evidence that plasma valproic acid levels are lower in patients who receive polytherapy with enzyme inducers. In particular, PHT was shown to have the strongest reducing effect (up to 50%) on plasma valproic acid levels (56).

Zonisamide. PHT is a more effective inducer of zonisamide metabolism than is carbamazepine, and reduces plasma zonisamide levels to a considerable extent (34).

EFFECTS OF PHENYTOIN ON KINETICS OF OTHER DRUGS

Analgesics and Antipyretics

Acetaminophen (Paracetamol). The elimination of acetaminophen is accelerated by PHT, perhaps through induction of its biotransformation (66).

Meperidine (Pethidine). Meperidine half-life declined from 6.4 to 4.3 hours, and the area under the concentration–time curve (AUC) of the primary metabolite of meperidine increased after the addition of PHT (81). Patients given PHT may need higher doses of meperidine.

Methadone. Plasma methadone levels decreased by 50% in five patients on methadone maintenance who had received PHT for 3 weeks (109). Several of these patients started to have withdrawal signs and symptoms while receiving a previously adequate methadone maintenance dose.

Antiasthmatics

Theophylline. Daily doses of 300 to 400 mg of PHT, producing blood levels of 10 to 20 μg/mL, reduced the half-life of intravenously administered theophylline by 40% and increased its clearance in 10 volunteers. It was suggested that patients receiving PHT may need higher or more frequent doses of theophylline (39,103).

Anticoagulants

Acenocoumarol. A case was reported of an interaction between PHT and acenocoumarol, possibly potentiated by concomitant treatment with paroxetine, leading to a retroperitoneal hematoma (1). Monitoring of anticoagulant response is recommended in patients started on the combination of PHT and acenocoumarol, or when PHT is removed from combination therapy.

Dicoumarol. PHT can reduce the blood level of dicoumarol, leading to a need for increased dosage of that anticoagulant (31).

Warfarin. The effect of PHT on warfarin is variable. Although PHT is expected to reduce the effect of warfarin through enzyme induction, an increased anticoagulant effect has been reported in some patients given this combination (65). Close monitoring of anticoagulant effect is recommended whenever PHT is added or removed from the therapeutic regimen of patients stabilized on warfarin.

Antifungals

Itraconazole. In healthy volunteers given itraconazole (single dose of 200 mg orally) alone and after 15 days of 300 mg PHT once daily (24), PHT decreased the itraconazole AUC by more than 90%, from 3,203 to 224 ng/hr/mL, with a decrease in the itraconazole half-life from 22.3 to 3.8 hours. Similar changes were observed for hydroxyitraconazole. Given this marked reduction in itraconazole serum concentrations, it would be prudent to use an alternative antifungal agent in patients receiving PHT.

Antimicrobials

Chloramphenicol. PHT was found to reduce chloramphenicol levels in patients (45).

Doxycycline. The elimination of doxycycline was increased in patients receiving PHT (67).

Praziquantel. The plasma levels of the anthelmintic praziquantel were reduced twofold to threefold during comedication with PHT, probably because of enzyme induction. Higher-than-average doses of praziquantel were recommended for comedicated patients with poor response in the treatment of neurocysticercosis (9).

Antineoplasic Agents

Cyclophosphamide. PHT increased the clearance of (R)- and (S)-cyclophosphamide by 100% and 150%, respectively, in three bone marrow transplant recipients (118).

Antipsychotics

Quetiapine. PHT induced the metabolism of quetiapine, a newly introduced antipsychotic, in schizophrenic patients, resulting in a fivefold increase in quetiapine clearance (123). Dosage adjustment of quetiapine may be necessary when the two drugs are given concurrently.

Cardiovascular Agents

Digitoxin. In some patients receiving PHT, digitoxin levels were reduced to a modest extent (105).

Digoxin. Coadministration of PHT caused a significant reduction in digoxin half-life and a 27% increase in its clearance in healthy subjects (87).

Disopyramide. PHT can induce disopyramide metabolism but, because the dealkylated metabolite also is pharmacologically active, a loss of effectiveness may not occur (3).

Furosemide. The diuretic effect of furosemide is reduced by PHT to some degree. There is evidence that PHT reduces furosemide absorption, but interference with furosemide action in the kidney may occur as well (2,119).

Mexiletine. PHT has been shown to enhance the metabolism of mexiletine and to reduce the AUC of mexiletine by 55% in healthy subjects (8). This interaction is likely to be clinically significant.

Nisoldipine. PHT increased the metabolism of nisoldipine to a clinically important extent in 12 epileptic patients (60), with a mean decrease in the nisoldipine AUC of 90%.

Quinidine. PHT has been found to reduce the half-life of quinidine by 50%. An increase in the dosage of quinidine may be required to maintain effective plasma quinidine levels. Conversely, if PHT is discontinued, the quinidine dosage may need to be reduced (66).

Immunosuppressants

Cyclosporine. PHT reduced the maximal concentration, AUC, and half-life of cyclosporine. This may lead to a reduction in the clinical efficacy of cyclosporine (28).

Miscellaneous

Misonidazole. PHT has been found to reduce the half-life of misonidazole and to accelerate its demethylation. This may diminish the toxicity of misonidazole while not reducing its effectiveness as an enhancer in radiation therapy (117).

Vecuronium. Patients treated chronically with PHT needed higher and more frequent doses of vecuronium than average to obtain and maintain required muscle relaxation during neurosurgical procedures. This is likely to be induction related because newly started PHT had much smaller effect on vecuronium (80).

Tirilazad. Repeated administration of PHT (100 to 200 mg three times daily for 7 days) increased the clearance of the antioxidant tirilazad (1.5 mg/kg intravenously every 6 hours) by 91.8% in healthy volunteers (26).

Steroids

Dexamethasone. PHT induces the metabolism of dexamethasone considerably. The elimination half-life of the steroid was reduced from 3.5 to 1.8 hours after the addition of PHT (16). In six patients, dexamethasone levels dropped by 50% with PHT comedication (122).

Oral Contraceptives. Failure of oral contraceptives has been reported in some epileptic patients taking enzyme-inducing AEDs, including PHT (33). Higher-dose contraceptive pills may need to be given in patients comedicated with PHT (55).

Prednisone/Prednisolone. Effectiveness of prednisone and prednisolone is reduced in patients taking enzyme-inducing AEDs, including PHT (66). Higher dosages of these steroids are needed in patients comedicated with PHT.

CONCLUSION

PHT is associated with a wide range of drug interactions, including enzyme induction and inhibition and protein binding displacement. PHT induction of extensively metabolized drugs (e.g., itraconazole, quetiapine, nisoldipine) or drugs with narrow therapeutic indices (e.g., theophylline) results in patient exposure to suboptimal levels of concurrent therapy if dosages are not adjusted by clinical or laboratory monitoring. On the other hand, interactions involving inhibition of PHT metabolism can result in clinical signs of PHT toxicity, and coprescription of known inhibitors of CYP2C9 and CYP2C19, the isoenzymes involved in PHT metabolism (e.g., amiodarone, ticlopidine, fluoxetine), requires careful monitoring. Interactions involving displacement from plasma protein binding sites need to be taken into account when interpreting total plasma PHT concentrations, but they are unlikely to be clinically significant unless additional mechanisms such as enzyme induction or inhibition also are present.

By understanding the different mechanisms involved in PHT interactions, clinicians can predict potential interactions and avoid clinical toxicity with careful monitoring and dosage adjustments.

REFERENCES

1. Abad-Santos F, Carcas AJ, Capitan C, et al. Retroperitoneal haematoma in a patient treated with acenocoumarol, PHT and paroxetine. *Clin Lab Haematol* 1995;17:195–197.
2. Ahmad S. Renal insensitivity to furosemide caused by chronic anticonvulsant therapy. *BMJ* 1974;3:657–659.
3. Aitio ML, Mansbury L, Tala E, et al. The effect of enzyme induction on the metabolism of disopyramide in man. *Br J Clin Pharmacol* 1981;11:279–286.
4. Arnoldussen W, Rentmeester T. Interaction between oxcarbazepine and PHT. *Epilepsia* 1993;34[Suppl 6]:37.
5. Bahls FH, Ozuma J, Ritchie DE. Interactions between calcium channel blockers and anticonvulsants carbamazepine and PHT. *Neurology* 1991;41:470–472.
6. Bajpai M, Roskos LK, Shen DD, et al. Roles of cytochrome P4502C9 and cytochrome P4502C19 in the stereoselective metabolism of PHT to its major metabolite. *Drug Metab Dispos* 1996;24:1401–1403.
7. Barcs G, Walker EB, Elger CE, et al. Oxcarbazepine placebo-controlled, dose ranging trial in refractory partial epilepsy. *Epilepsia* 2000;41:1597–1607.
8. Begg EJ, Chinwah PM, Webb C, et al. Enhanced metabolism of mexiletine after PHT administration. *Br J Clin Pharmacol* 1982;14:219–223.
9. Bittencourt PRM, Gracia CM, Martins R, et al. PHT and carbamazepine decrease oral bioavailability of praziquantel. *Neurology* 1992;42:492–496.
10. Blum RA, Wilton JH, Hilligross DM, et al. Effect of fluconazole on disposition of PHT. *Clin Pharmacol Ther* 1990;47:182.
11. Bollini P, Riva R, Albani F, et al. Decreased PHT level during antineoplastic therapy: a case report. *Epilepsia* 1983;24:75–78.
12. Brennan RW, Deheija H, Kutt H, et al. Diphenylhydantoin intoxication attendant to slow inactivation of isoniazid. *Neurology (Minneap)* 1970;21:383–385.
13. Browne TR, Szabo GK, Evans JE, et al. Carbamazepine increases PHT concentration and decreases PHT clearance. *Neurology* 1988;38:1146–1150.
14. Cacek AJ. Review of alterations in oral PHT bioavailability associated with formulation, antacids and food. *Ther Drug Monit* 1986;8:166–171.
15. Cadle RM, Zenon GJ III, Rodriguez-Barradas MC, et al. Fluconazole-induced symptomatic phenytoin toxicity. *Ann Pharmacother* 1994;28:191–195.
16. Chalk JB, Ridgeway K, Brophy T, et al. PHT impairs the bioavailability of dexamethasone in neurological and neurosurgical patients. *J Neurol Neurosurg Psychiatry* 1984;47:1087–1090.
17. Coniglia AA, Garnett WR, Pellock JH, et al. Effect of acute and chronic terfenadine on free and total serum concentration in epileptic patients. *Epilepsia* 1989;30:611–615.
18. Dam M, Christensen JM, Brandt J, et al. Antiepileptic drugs: interaction with dextropropoxyphene. In: Johannessen SI, Morselli PL, Pippenger CE, et al., eds. *Antiepileptic therapy: advances in drug monitoring.* New York: Raven Press, 1980:299–304.
19. D'Arcy PF, McElnay JC. Drug and antacid interactions of clinical importance. *Drug Intell Clin Pharm* 1987;21:607–617.
20. Denahue S, Flockart DA, Albernethy DR. Ticlopidine inhibits PHT clearance. *Clin Pharmacol Ther* 1999;66:563–568.
21. de Wolff F, Vermeij P, Ferrari MD, et al. Impairment of PHT parahydroxylation as a cause of severe intoxication. *Ther Drug Monit* 1983;5:213–215.
22. Doecke CJ, Veronese ME, Pond SM, et al. Relationship between PHT and tolbutamide hydroxylation in human microsomes. *Br J Clin Pharmacol* 1991;34:125–130.
23. Dorn JM. A case of PHT toxicity possibly precipitated by trazodone. *J Clin Psychiatry* 1986;47:89–90.
24. Ducharme MP, Slaughter RL, Warbasse LH. Itraconazole and hydroxyitraconazole serum concentrations are reduced more than tenfold by PHT. *Clin Pharmacol Ther* 1995;58:617–624.
25. Duncan JS, Patsalos PN, Shovron SD. Effects of discontinuation of PHT, carbamazepine and valproate on concomitant antiepileptic medication. *Epilepsia* 1991;32:101–115.
26. Fleishaker JC, Pearson LK, Peters GR. Induction of tirilazad clearance by PHT. *Biopharm Drug Dispos* 1998;19:91–96.
27. Fraser DG, Ludden TM, Evens RP, et al. Displacement of PHT from plasma binding sites by salicylate. *Clin Pharmacol Ther* 1980;27:165–169.
28. Freeman DJ, Laupacis A, Keown A, et al. Evaluation of cyclo-

sporin and PHT interaction with observations on cyclosporin metabolites. *Br J Clin Pharmacol* 1984;18:887–893.

29. Glue P, Banfield CR, Perhach JL, et al. Pharmacokinetic interactions with felbamate: in vitro–in vivo correlation. *Clin Pharmacokinet* 1997;33:214–224.

30. Gugler R, Jensen JC. Omeprazole inhibits oxidative drug metabolism. *Gastroenterology* 1985;89:1235–1241.

31. Hansen JJM, Siersbaek-Nielsen K, Kristensen M, et al. Effect of diphenylhydantoin on the metabolism of dicoumarol in man. *Acta Med Scand* 1971;189:15–19.

32. Haselberger MB, Freedman LS, Tolbert S. Elevated serum PHT concentrations associated with coadministration of sertraline. *J Clin Psychopharmacol* 1997;17:107–109.

33. Hempel E, Klinger W. Drug stimulated biotransformation of hormonal steroid contraceptives: clinical implications. *Drugs* 1976;12:442–448.

34. Henry TR, Sackellares JC. Zonisamide. In: Resor SR Jr, Kutt H. eds. *The medical treatment of epilepsy.* New York: Marcel Dekker, 1992:423–427.

35. Houghton GW, Richens A. The effect of benzodiazepines and pheneturide on PHT metabolism in man. *Br J Clin Pharmacol* 1974;1:344–345.

36. Howitt KM, Oziemski MA. PHT toxicity induced by fluconazole. *Med J Aust* 1989;151:603–604.

37. Jalil P. Toxic reaction following the combined administration of fluoxetine and PHT: two case reports. *J Neurol Neurosurg Psychiatry* 1992;55:412–413.

38. Johannessen SI, Strandjord RE, Munthekaas AW. Lack of effect of clonazepam on serum levels of diphenylhydantoin, phenobarbital and carbamazepine. *Acta Neurol Scand* 1977;55:506–512.

39. Jonkman JHG, Upton RA. Pharmacokinetic drug interactions with theophylline. *Clin Pharmacokinet* 1984;9:309–334.

40. Kay L, Kampmann JP, Svendsen TL, et al. Influence of rifampin and isoniazid on the kinetics of PHT. *Br J Clin Pharmacol* 1985;20:323–326.

41. Kennedy MC, Wade DN. The effect of food on the absorption of PHT. *Aust N Z J Med* 1982;12:258–261.

42. Khoo KC, Mendels J, Rothbart M. Influence of PHT and phenobarbital on the disposition of a single oral dose of clonazepam. *Clin Pharmacol Ther* 1980;28:368–75.

43. Klaassen SL. Ticlopidine-induced PHT toxicity. *Ann Pharmacother* 1998;32:1295–1298.

44. Koup JR. Interaction of chloramphenicol with PHT and phenobarbital: a case report. *Clin Pharmacol Ther* 1978;24:571–575.

45. Krasinski K, Kusmiesz M, Nelson JD. Pharmacologic interactions among chloramphenicol, PHT and phenobarbital. *Pediatr Infect Dis* 1982;1:232–235.

46. Kutt H. Interactions with antiepileptic drugs involving multiple mechanisms. In: Morselli PL, Garattini S, Cohen SN, eds. *Drug interactions.* New York: Raven Press, 1974;211–222.

47. Kutt H. Interactions between anticonvulsants and other commonly prescribed drugs. *Epilepsia* 1984;25[Suppl 2]:S118–S131.

48. Lander CM, Eadie MJ, Tyrer JH. Interactions between anticonvulsants. *Proc Aust Assoc Neurol* 1975;12:111–116.

49. Lazar JD, Wilner KD. Drug interactions with fluconazole. *Rev Infect Dis* 1990;12:S327–S333.

50. Levine M, Jones MW, Sheppard I. Differential effect of cimetidine on serum concentrations of carbamazepine and PHT. *Neurology* 1985;35:562–565.

51. Levy RH, Loiseau P, Guyot M, et al. Stiripentol kinetics in epilepsy: nonlinearity and interactions. *Clin Pharmacol Ther* 1984;36:661–669.

52. Loiseau P, Duche B. Progabide. In: Resor SR Jr, Kutt H. eds. *The medical treatment of epilepsy.* New York: Marcel Dekker, 1992:393–398.

53. Mamiya K, Kojima K, Yukawa E, et al. PHT intoxication induced by fluvoxamine. *Ther Drug Monit* 2001;23:75–77.

54. Mattson RH, Cramer JA, Williamson PC, et al. Valproic acid in epilepsy: clinical and pharmacological effects. *Ann Neurol* 1978;3:20–25.

55. Mattson RH, Cramer JA. Epilepsy, sex hormones and antiepileptic drugs. *Epilepsia* 1985;26[Suppl]:S40–S55.

56. May T, Rambeck B. Serum concentrations of valproic acid: influence of dose and co-medication. *Ther Drug Monit* 1985;7:387–390.

57. McGovern B, Geer VR, Laraia PJ, et al. Possible interaction between amiodarone and PHT. *Ann Intern Med* 1984;101:650–651.

58. McKee PJW, Blacklaw J, Friel E, et al. Adjuvant vigabatrin in refractory epilepsy: a ceiling to effective dosage. *Epilepsia* 1993;34:937–943.

59. Melander A, Brante G, Johansson O, et al. Influence of food on the absorption of PHT in man. *Eur J Clin Pharmacol* 1979;15:269–274.

60. Michelucci R, Cipolla G, Passarelli D. Reduced plasma nisoldipine concentrations in phenytoin-treated patients with epilepsy. *Epilepsia* 1996;37:1107–1110.

61. Mitchell AS, Holland JT. Fluconazole and phenytoin: a predictable interaction. *BMJ* 1989;298:1315.

62. Molholm Hansen J, Kampmann JP, Siersbaek-Nielsen K, et al. The effect of different sulfonamides on PHT metabolism in man. *Acta Med Scand Suppl* 1979;624:106–110.

63. Monks A, Richens A. Effects of single doses of sodium valproate on serum PHT levels and protein binding in epileptic patients. *Clin Pharmacol Ther* 1980;27:89–95.

64. Morselli PL, Rizzo M, Garattini S. Interaction between phenobarbital and diphenylhydantoin in animals and in epileptic patients. *Ann NY Acad Sci* 1971;179:88–107.

65. Nappi J. Warfarin and PHT interaction. *Ann Intern Med* 1979;90:852.

66. Nation RL, Evans AM, Milne RW. Pharmacokinetic interactions with PHT. *Clin Pharmacokinet* 1990;18:37–60.

67. Neuvonen PJ, Penttila O, Lehtovaara R, et al. Effects of antiepileptic drugs on the elimination of various tetracycline derivatives. *Eur J Clin Pharmacol* 1975;9:147–154.

68. Nicolas JM, Collart P, Gerin B, et al. In vitro evaluation of potential drug interactions with levetiracetam, a new antiepileptic agent. *Drug Metab Dispos* 1999;27:250–254.

69. Nolan PE, Marcus FI, Hoyer GL, et al. Pharmacokinetic interaction between intravenous PHT and amiodarone in healthy volunteers. *Clin Pharmacol Ther* 1989;46:43–50.

70. O'Brien LS. Failure of antacids to alter pharmacokinetics of PHT. *Br J Pharmacol* 1978;6:176–177.

71. Olesen OV. The influence of disulfiram and calcium carbamide on the serum diphenylhydantoin. *Arch Neurol* 1967;16:642–644.

72. Patsalos PN. Pharmacokinetic profile of levetiracetam: toward ideal characteristics. *Pharmacol Ther* 2000;85:77–85.

73. Patsalos PN, Lascelles PT. In vitro hydroxylation of diphenylhydantoin and its inhibition by other commonly used anticonvulsant drugs. *Biochem Pharmacol* 1977;266:1929–1933.

74. Peck AW. Clinical pharmacology of lamotrigine. *Epilepsia* 1991;32[Suppl 2]:S2–S12.

75. Perucca E, Hebdige S, Frigo GM, et al. Interaction between PHT and valproic acid: plasma protein binding and metabolic effects. *Clin Pharmacol Ther* 1980;28:779–789.

76. Perucca E, Bialer M. The clinical pharmacokinetics of the newer

antiepileptic drugs: focus on topiramate, zonisamide and tiagabine. *Clin Pharmacokinet* 1996;31:29–46.

77. Phillips P, Hansky J. PHT toxicity secondary to cimetidine administration. *Med J Aust* 1984;141:602.

78. Pisani F, Fazio A, Artesi I, et al. Elevation of plasma PHT by viloxazine in epileptic patients: a clinically significant drug interaction. *J Neurol Neurosurg Psychiatry* 1992;55:126–127.

79. Pitlick WH, Levy RH. Carbamazepine: interactions with other drugs. In: Levy RH, Dreifuss FE, Mattson RH, Meldrum BS, et al., eds. *Antiepileptic drugs*, 3rd ed. New York: Raven Press, 1989:521–531.

80. Platt PR, Thackery NM. PHT-induced resistance to vecuronium. *Anesth Intensive Care* 1993;21:185–191.

81. Pond SM, Kretschzmar KM. Effect of PHT on meperidine clearance and normeperidine formation. *Clin Pharmacol Ther* 1981;30:680–686.

82. Prichard PJ, Walt RP, Kitchingman GK, et al. Oral PHT pharmacokinetics during omeprazole therapy. *Br J Clin Pharmacol* 1987;24:543–545.

83. Privitera M, Welty TE. Acute PHT toxicity followed by seizure breakthrough from a ticlopidine-PHT interaction. *Arch Neurol* 1996;53:1191–1192.

84. Pugh RNH, Geddes AM, Yeoman WB. Interaction of PHT and chlorpheniramine. *Br J Clin Pharmacol* 1975;2:173–174.

85. Rabinowicz AL, Hinton DR, Dyck P, et al. High-dose tamoxifen in treatment of brain tumors: interaction with antiepileptic drugs. *Epilepsia* 1995;36:513–515.

86. Rambeck B. Pharmacological interactions of methsuximide with phenobarbital and PHT in hospitalized epileptic patients. *Epilepsia* 1979;20:147–156.

87. Rameis H. On the interaction between PHT and digoxin. *Eur J Clin Pharmacol* 1985;29:49–53.

88. Ramsay RE. Advances in the chemotherapy of epilepsy. *Epilepsia* 1993;34[Suppl 5]:S9–S16.

89. Ramsay RE, McManus DQ, Guterman A, et al. Carbamazepine metabolism in humans: effect of concurrent anticonvulsant therapy. *Ther Drug Monit* 1990;12:235–241.

90. Ramsay RE, Slater JD, Brown MC, et al. Double-blind three dose parallel placebo-controlled efficacy of tiagabine in partial seizures. *Epilepsia* 1993;34[Suppl 6]:103–104.

91. Richens A, Gustavson LE, McKelvy JF, et al. Pharmacokinetics and safety of single-dose tiagabine-HCl in epileptic patients chronically treated with four other antiepileptic drug regimens. *Epilepsia* 1991;32[Suppl 3]:12.

92. Rimmer EM, Richens A. Interaction between vigabatrin and PHT. *Br J Clin Pharmacol* 1989;27[Suppl 1]:S27–S33.

93. Roe TF, Podosin RL, Blaskovics ME. Drug interaction: diazoxide and diphenylhydantoin. *J Pediatr* 1975;87:480–484.

94. Rolan PE, Somogy AA, Drew MR, et al. PHT intoxication during treatment with parenteral miconazole. *BMJ* 1983;287:1760.

95. Saavedra IN, Aguilera LI, Galdames DG. PHT/clonazepam interaction. *Ther Drug Monit* 1985;7:481–484.

96. Sachdeo R, Wagner ML, Sachdeo S, et al. Coadministration of PHT and felbamate: evidence of additional PHT dose-reduction requirements based on pharmacokinetics and tolerability with increasing doses of felbamate. *Epilepsia* 1999;40:1122–1228.

97. Salem RB, Breland BD, Mishra SK, et al. Effect of cimetidine on PHT serum level. *Epilepsia* 1983;24:284–288.

98. Sandor P, Sellers EM, Dumbell M, et al. Effect of long and short term alcohol on PHT kinetics in chronic alcoholics. *Clin Pharmacol Ther* 1981;30:390–397.

99. Sands CD, Robinson JD, Salem RB, et al. Effect of thioridazine on PHT serum concentration: a retrospective study. *Drug Intell Clin Pharm* 1987;21:267–272.

100. Scott AK, Khir AS, Steele WH, et al. Oxazepam pharmacokinetics in patients with epilepsy treated long-term with PHT alone or in combination with phenobarbitone. *Br J Clin Pharmacol* 1983;16:441–444.

101. Sekikawa H, Nakano M, Takada M, et al. Influence of dietary components on the bioavailability of PHT. *Chem Pharm Bull* 1980;22:2443–2449.

102. Sennoune S, Mesdjian E, Bonneton J, et al. Interaction between clobazam and standard antiepileptic drugs in patients with epilepsy. *Ther Drug Monit* 1992;14:269–274.

103. Sklar SJ, Wagner JC. Enhanced theophylline clearance secondary to PHT therapy. *Drug Intell Clin Pharm* 1985;19:34–36.

104. Skovsted L, Hansen JM, Kristensen M, et al. Inhibition of drug metabolism in man. In: Morselli PL, Garattini S, Cohen SN, eds. *Drug interactions*. New York: Raven Press, 1974:81–90.

105. Solomon HM, Reich S, Spirt N, et al. Interaction between digitoxin and other drugs *in vitro* and *in vivo*. *Ann NY Acad Sci* 1971;79:362–369.

106. Svendsen TL, Kristensen M, Hansen JM, et al. The influence of disulfiram on the half-life and metabolic clearance rate of diphenylhydantoin and tolbutamide in man. *Eur J Clin Pharmacol* 1976;9:439–441.

107. Sylvester RK, Lewis FB, Caldwell KC, et al. Impaired PHT bioavailability secondary to cisplatinum, vinblastin and bleomycine. *Ther Drug Monit* 1984;6:302–305.

108. Taylor DM, Massay CA, Wilson WG, et al. Lowered serum PHT concentrations during therapy with liquid food concentrates. *Ann Pharmacother* 1992;27:369.

109. Tong TG, Pond SM, Kreek MJ, et al. PHT-induced methadone withdrawal. *Ann Intern Med* 1981;94:349–351.

110. Touchette MA, Chandrasekar PH, Milad MA, et al. Contrasting effects of fluconazole and ketoconazole on phenytoin and testosterone disposition in man. *Br J Clin Pharmacol* 1992;34:75–78.

111. Treiman DM, Pledger GW, DeGiorgio C, et al. Increasing plasma concentration tolerability study of flunarizine in comedicated epileptic patients. *Epilepsia* 1993;34:944–953.

112. Vaijda FJE, Prineas RJ, Lowell RRH. Interaction between PHT and the benzodiazepines. *BMJ* 1971;1:346.

113. Vincent FM. Phenothiazine-induced phenytoin intoxication. *Ann Intern Med* 1980;93:56–57.

114. Walubo A, Aboo A. PHT toxicity due to concomitant antituberculosis therapy. *S Afr Med J* 1995;85:1175–1176.

115. Welling PG. Interactions affecting drug absorption. *Clin Pharmacokinet* 1984;9:404–434.

116. Wesseling H, Molsthurkow I. Interaction of diphenylhydantoin (DPH) and tolbutamide in man. *Eur J Clin Pharmacol* 1975;8:75–78.

117. Williams K, Begg E, Wade D, et al. Effects of PHT, phenobarbital and ascorbic acid on misonidazole elimination. *Clin Pharmacol Ther* 1983;33:314–321.

118. Williams ML, Wainer IW, Embree L, et al. Enantioselective induction of cyclophosphamide metabolism by phenytoin. *Chirality* 1999;11:569–574.

119. Williamson HE. Interaction of furosemide and PHT in the rat. *Proc Soc Exp Biol Med* 1986;182:322–324.

120. Windorfer A Jr, Sauer W. Drug interactions during anticonvulsant therapy in childhood: diphenylhydantoin, primidone, phenobarbitone, clonazepam, nitrazepam, carbamazepine, and dipropylacetate. *Neuropaediatrie* 1977;8:29–41.

121. Witmer DR, Ritschel WA. PHT and isoniazid interaction: a kinetic approach to management. *Drug Intell Clin Pharm* 1984;18:483–486.

122. Wong DD, Longenecker RG, Liepman M, et al. PHT-dexamethasone: a possible drug–drug interaction. *JAMA* 1985;254: 2062–2063.

123. Wong YW, Yeh C, Thyrum PT. The effects of concomitant PHT administration on the steady-state pharmacokinetics of quetiapine. *J Clin Psychopharmacol* 2001;21:89–93.

124. Zielinski J, Haydukewych D, Leheta BJ. Carbamazepine–PHT interaction: elevation of plasma PHT concentrations due to carbamazepine co-medication. *Ther Drug Monit* 1985;7: 51–53.

125. Zifkin B, Sherwin A, Andermann F. PHT toxicity due to interaction with clobazam. *Neurology* 1991;41:313–314.

PHENYTOIN AND OTHER HYDANTOINS
CLINICAL EFFICACY AND USE IN EPILEPSY

B. JOE WILDER
JOSEPH BRUNI

Discovery of the anticonvulsant properties of phenytoin (PHT) by Merritt and Putnam (1) in 1938 created a revolution in the treatment of epilepsy and anticonvulsant drug research. Their questioning of the traditional idea that sedation was requisite for anticonvulsant activity opened a new era of drug development and patient management. PHT was the first drug to control seizures without producing sedation, and its efficacy against seizures induced in animals by the maximal electroshock test (2) indicated its efficacy in tonic-clonic and partial seizures. For the first time, an antiepileptic drug (AED) that was effective clinically had been tested experimentally in pioneering work in animal models.

Since the introduction of PHT, many drugs have been licensed in the United States for the treatment of epilepsy. Almost all of these are recommended for the treatment of partial and tonic-clonic seizures. Since the mid-1980s, controlled, randomized clinical trials and double-blind studies comparing other AEDs with PHT (3–12) have shown that PHT remains one of the most effective drugs for the treatment of partial and generalized tonic-clonic seizures. When compared with newer AEDs, PHT is equally effective as lamotrigine and oxcarbazepine as monotherapy in the treatment of localization-related epilepsy (13).

FORMULATIONS

Oral preparations of PHT are either the sodium salt of PHT or PHT acid. The sodium salt is a crystalline preparation that is absorbed slowly from the gastrointestinal tract and has relatively slow clearance, which in adolescents and adults usually permits single or twice-daily dosing. Dosing twice a day is preferable in children. PHT sodium is marketed as 30- and 100-mg capsules. PHT acid is absorbed more rapidly and is available as a 50-mg chewable tablet and as 30-mg/5-mL and 125-mg/5-mL oral suspensions for children and adults.

PHT is also available in a parenteral formulation dissolved in propylene glycol at pH 10 that can be diluted in normal saline or half-normal saline (2 to 10 μg/mL) to avoid tissue reactions and to facilitate administration with routine intravenous (i.v.) techniques (14,15). This parenteral form of PHT should not be administered by the intramuscular route. Crystalline precipitation in the muscle after intramuscular PHT injection results in a marked delay in absorption and tissue necrosis (16). The prodrug, fosphenytoin, is water soluble and is much less irritating to tissue, so it is a clinically preferable formulation.

INDICATIONS FOR USE

In North America, PHT remains the most commonly used AED. PHT is a drug of choice in patients with simple and complex partial seizures and in those with generalized tonic and tonic-clonic seizures. It is ineffective in absence seizures and is of limited value in clonic, myoclonic, and atonic or akinetic seizures. In the epilepsy syndromes, PHT is most effective in symptomatic or secondary epilepsy manifested by partial and secondary generalized seizures. Its role in primary or genetic epilepsy characterized by generalized tonic-clonic convulsions has not been studied in randomized clinical tests.

In patients with absence, myoclonus, and tonic-clonic seizures, PHT is of value as adjunctive therapy if other drugs fail to control the tonic-clonic seizures. PHT also is effective in young adults with primary epilepsy and tonic-clonic seizures only (9). Ramsay et al. (17) reported both

B. Joe Wilder, MD: Associate Professor, Department of Medicine, University of Toronto, Toronto, Ontario, Canada

Joseph Bruni, MD, FRCP(C): Associate Professor, Department of Medicine, University of Toronto; and Consultant Neurologist, Department of Medicine, St. Michael's Hospital, Toronto, Ontario, Canada

valproic acid (VPA) and PHT to be efficacious in patients with primary epilepsy with spike-and-wave electroencephalographic discharge and tonic-clonic seizures.

PHT is usually not effective in infantile spasms and is of limited value in the Lennox-Gastaut syndrome; it is effective only in the tonic-clonic component of the syndrome. It is not effective as a monotherapeutic agent in the progressive myoclonic epilepsies and has been reported to worsen Baltic myoclonic epilepsy (18,19).

The use of PHT is often recommended after head trauma, intracranial neurosurgical procedures, and hemorrhagic stroke. However, double-blind studies do not demonstrate the efficacy of PHT in preventing epilepsy after stroke or supratentorial neurosurgical procedures. PHT does prevent early seizures after severe head trauma (20), nor is it useful in the prevention of alcohol withdrawal seizures (21).

After phenobarbital, PHT is the drug of choice in neonatal seizures when the drug is administered by the i.v. route (22). Fosphenytoin is the clear choice of formulations because of difficult parenteral accessibility and tissue toxicity of PHT. Therapeutic plasma PHT levels are difficult to maintain after oral administration in neonates because of erratic and sometimes incomplete absorption. PHT is generally well tolerated in children, adolescents, adults, and the elderly. However, elderly patients often are receiving multiple drugs, and PHT enhances the metabolism of these drugs. The doses of theophylline, warfarin, digoxin, steroids, and other drugs commonly used by adults and the elderly must be increased when PHT is concurrently administered. Because of the nonlinear kinetics of PHT, careful monitoring after an increase in dose in elderly patients is especially important.

PHT (as PHT or the prodrug fosphenytoin) is considered by many epilepsy specialists in the United States to be a drug of choice in the treatment of status epilepticus, as well as in acute and serial seizures (23–28). In conjunction with a rapid-acting benzodiazepine, PHT is valuable for treating status epilepticus or other acute seizures because it is available in an easily administered i.v. solution. It relatively rapidly penetrates the blood–brain barrier to achieve therapeutic concentrations at the site of action. PHT controls seizures in most cases, and it has a time span of action that permits follow-up oral administration to maintain a therapeutic response. Respiratory or cardiac depression does not occur with careful administration (usually 50 mg/min for normal adults), and no major changes are observed in the neurologic examination. PHT does not potentiate central nervous system depression produced by previously administered agents (e.g., benzodiazepines or barbiturates). The delay in action resulting from the slow rate of administration is reason to coadminister a benzodiazepine when rapid control of seizures is needed.

DOSAGE AND ADMINISTRATION

In patients with newly diagnosed epilepsy, PHT therapy can be initiated at a dose of 4 to 7 mg/kg given once or twice daily. Children require higher doses (mg/kg/day) than do adults, and it is usually preferable to give the drug at 12-hour intervals. Most adults can take PHT once daily, either in the morning or in the evening. Our practice with adults is to give PHT once a day if the dose is 400 mg/day or less and twice a day if it is >400 mg/day. A survey of 220 adults receiving stable PHT doses showed an average daily dose of 342 mg/day (B. Joe Wilder and J. R. McLean, *unpublished data*). After initiation of therapy, steady state is achieved in 1 to 3 weeks because of the wide variation in metabolism among individual patients and the nonlinear kinetics of PHT. Therefore, monitoring for PHT–dose–plasma level relationships should be delayed for 2 to 3 weeks. When PHT levels are in the low to intermediate target range (8 to 15 µg/mL), increases in the dose should be made, aided by follow-up blood level monitoring. Our practice is to use the 30-mg capsules for dose increases. In general, an increase in the PHT dose of 10 mg/day will result in an approximately 1 µg/mL increase in the plasma PHT level of a patient with a level of 10 µg/mL and in a 3 µg/mL increase in a patient with a 20 µg/mL level because of saturating kinetics. This should be kept in mind when one changes the daily dose of PHT.

If seizure frequency makes a more rapid achievement of therapeutic levels desirable, PHT can be loaded orally or by the i.v. route. Oral loading can be achieved by giving 15 mg/kg in three doses at 1-hour intervals. A maintenance dose of 4 to 7 mg/kg can be given daily thereafter. The low target range of the plasma PHT level is achieved 8 to 12 hours after the loading dose (29). An i.v. loading dosage of 15 mg/kg gives immediate therapeutic levels. Our practice is to mix PHT 50 mg/mL in normal saline to a dilution of approximately 5 mg/mL and to administer it slowly over 1 to 2 hours (14,15). After oral or i.v. loading doses, transient vertigo and nausea may rarely occur.

The i.v. administration of PHT should not exceed a rate of 50 mg/min. PHT depresses the Purkinje conduction system of the heart, and slowing of the pulse rate and a drop in blood pressure may occur with rapid administration. Rarely, transient diastolic pauses may occur. The i.v. administration of PHT should be done with care in patients with heart block. The propylene glycol, alcohol, and a pH adjusted to 12, used to bring PHT into solution, may be responsible for some of the toxicity observed during rapid i.v. administration.

In young children, PHT suspension (30 mg/5 mL and 125 mg/5 mL) in individually packaged doses should be used. PHT is poorly soluble, and in large bottles, dosing errors are made because of too little or too much PHT in an individual teaspoon or tablespoon dose.

Older children can be treated with 50-mg chewable tablets. Twice-a-day administration is preferable in children. Metabolism is faster in children than in adults, and the sodium PHT in the suspension and in chewable tablets is absorbed faster. Thus, peaking of plasma PHT levels after large single daily doses may cause transient toxicity.

The accepted therapeutic plasma PHT level ranges from 10 to 30 μg/mL (40 to 80 μmol/L) (30). However, this range should only be viewed as a guide; proper management depends on the clinical response (31). Patients with partial seizures require a higher dose and higher serum PHT levels to achieve seizure control than do patients with generalized tonic-clonic seizures (32).

Any factors or substances that interfere with the solubility of PHT in the intestinal tract will retard or prevent its complete absorption. Anecdotal reports of altered absorption of PHT with the concurrent administration of antacids and other drugs are probably reliable. In some patients, absorption may be defective (33), particularly under certain conditions. For example, a marked absorption defect was observed in a pregnant woman during her second and third trimesters (B. Joe Wilder and E. Ramsay, *unpublished data*). Dosage requirements of PHT increased from 400 to 1,300 mg/day, with large quantities of drug excreted in the feces.

Status Epilepticus and Acute Seizures

PHT is commonly used in acute treatment of serial seizures to achieve prompt control and with a benzodiazepine to treat status epilepticus (Treiman et al.) For the treatment of status epilepticus and other acute seizures, concentrations of 5 to 20 mg of PHT per milliliter of normal saline can be administered at a rate of 50 mg/min without producing significant adverse clinical effects. Care must be taken to prevent extravasation from the vein, because severe tissue reaction may occur (34,35). A mild decrease in blood pressure or slowing of the pulse occasionally occurs, and this can be controlled by decreasing the rate of administration (25,27). An infusion rate exceeding 50 mg/min may produce a decrease in blood pressure and slowing of the pulse rate (23). Respiratory depression does not occur in patients receiving i.v. loading doses of 10 to 20 mg/kg of PHT. Asystole may occur after bolus i.v. injection. Subjective side effects resulting from i.v. loading are rare. Vertigo and nausea may occur. Except for nystagmus, the neurologic examination is unchanged.

PHT rapidly penetrates the brain during i.v. infusion (27,36) and is concentrated by brain phospholipids. One hour after i.v. infusion, the brain:plasma ratio is greater than 1.5 in both experimental animals and humans (26,36).

Patients in status epilepticus or experiencing serial epileptic seizures, alcohol or drug withdrawal seizures, or seizures of undetermined origin respond promptly to i.v. PHT. Wilder (26) and Leppik et al. (25) reported that 60%

to 80% of patients responded within 20 minutes after the initiation of PHT infusion. Plasma PHT levels were ≥10 μg/mL 12 hours after a mean i.v. dose of 13 mg/kg in eight of 14 patients (26). Higher levels were reached after an initial higher i.v. dose (25). Fosphenytoin, a water-soluble prodrug formulation, is preferred because of improved tolerability to tissue irritability.

Monotherapy versus Polytherapy

PHT, like other AEDs, is easier to use in a monotherapy regimen. Unfortunately, some 30% of epileptic patients are refractory to monotherapy and require polytherapy with other AEDs. PHT has been used with virtually every other AED, but there appear to be favorable combinations. The selection of a drug combination should be based on certain basic principles: Select combinations of drugs with different mechanisms of action, avoid drugs that have adverse additive effects, and avoid drugs with the potential for drug interactions. The last principle is difficult to follow with PHT, because it is an enzyme inducer of the cytochrome P450 mixed oxidase system and therefore increases the metabolic rate of other drugs also metabolized by this route.

Mirza et al. (37) showed that PHT with VPA is a favorable combination for enhancing seizure control in refractory patients. Bates et al. (38) reported that PHT and low doses of phenobarbital were efficacious in a large cohort of mentally retarded patients with refractory seizures that did not respond to monotherapy. Ultimately, the combination of drugs that works is the best. Whenever PHT is used with other AEDs, interactions may occur. With the development of newer AEDs drugs such as gabapentin, vigabatrin, lamotrigine, topiramate, levetiracetam, zonisamide, and oxcarbazepine a rational algorithm has to be developed to optimize combination therapy (39–42).

DRUG INTERACTIONS

Although felbamate, carbamazepine, sulfonamides, clobazam, chloramphenicol, diltiazem, cimetidine, disulfiram, isoniazid, methsuximide, and antimetabolites used in cancer chemotherapy may increase PHT levels by inhibition of metabolism. Only a few drugs interact sufficiently with PHT to necessitate a change in the dose of PHT. Antacids, large doses of salicylates, tolbutamide, and phenylbutazone may alter PHT total and free levels by altering absorption and protein binding (31,43). Felbamate increases PHT levels, and careful monitoring of PHT levels is required. With the addition of felbamate to PHT, the guiding principle should be clinical changes rather than an automatic reduction in the PHT dose. Seizures and possible status epilepticus may be precipitated by an abrupt decrease in PHT dosage (44).

The effect of PHT on other drugs may be clinically significant (33,43). Doses of dicumarol, tiagabine, zonisamide, lamotrigine, topiramate, theophylline, chloramphenicol, doxycycline, digitoxin, quinidine, dexamethasone, oral contraceptives, or folic acid may have to be increased because of enzyme induction by PHT.

Interactions are usually not seen when PHT is used in combination with phenobarbital, diazepam, or clonazepam (31). The interaction of PHT with vigabatrin is generally not clinically significant.

VPA transiently lowers PHT levels in patients whose PHT levels are less than the saturation point of the metabolizing enzymes (45), but by displacing PHT from protein binding sites, VPA increases levels of free PHT so no change in the dose of PHT is generally required. However, the increase in free PHT levels resulting from VPA displacement of PHT from protein binding sites may be sufficient to produce signs of PHT toxicity without a significant change in the total level of PHT (46). Patients should be warned that this interaction may occur; and if signs of PHT intoxication develop after the dose of VPA, free levels of PHT should be determined, and dosage adjustments of VPA should be made. Reducing the peak plasma levels of VPA by giving lower doses more frequently, giving the drug with meals to slow absorption, or use of the slow-release form will generally relieve the problem. No interactions occur when PHT is used in combination with gabapentin (44).

PHT induces the metabolism of VPA, and it markedly increases the dose of VPA needed to achieve a therapeutic serum level (47). When VPA is given with PHT or carbamazepine, the dose of VPA required to maintain therapeutic serum levels may be 50% to 100% greater than that needed with VPA monotherapy (46). PHT increases the metabolism of lamotrigine and felbamate and lowers plasma concentrations (48).

When PHT is combined with primidone, the plasma primidone level falls and the level of phenobarbital rises, giving a marked increase in the ratio of phenobarbital to primidone (46,49). This combination should generally be avoided because of resulting phenobarbital toxicity.

PHT induces the metabolism of carbamazepine; and when the two drugs are used in combination, the dose of carbamazepine required is higher than when carbamazepine is given alone. Carbamazepine inhibits the metabolism of PHT (46,50) and increases plasma PHT levels. An extensive review of PHT interactions is given in Chapter 59.

ADVERSE EFFECTS

Dysfunction of the ocular and cerebellovestibular systems may occur at plasma PHT levels higher than the usual therapeutic range of 10 to 30 μg/mL. Nystagmus and ataxia appear at plasma PHT levels >30 μg/mL; dysarthria, lethargy, and mental changes occur at levels >30 to 40 μg/mL; and stupor occurs at levels >40 to 60 μg/mL (30,31). Because the neurologic effects of PHT are usually dose related, reduction of the dose should eliminate them.

Other adverse effects of PHT may be hypersensitivity reactions, such as rash, fever, abnormal liver function, lymphadenopathy, eosinophilia, blood dyscrasias, renal failure, and serum sickness–like illness (51). Other systemic adverse effects include the following: gingival hyperplasia (19,52, 53); hirsutism; hematologic reactions and folate deficiency including megaloblastic anemia (53), neonatal coagulation defects (54), aplastic anemia, granulocytosis, and thrombopenia; thyroid dysfunction (55,56); and decrease in serum immunoglobulin A (57–59). An extensive review of the toxicity of PHT, as well as its cognitive effects and teratogenicity, is given in Chapter 63.

CLINICAL USE: OTHER HYDANTOINS

With the availability of newer-generation AEDs, the use of other hydantoins such as ethotoin and mephenytoin is only of historical interest. There is probably a very limited role in the use of other drugs in the treatment of epilepsy because of better efficacy and tolerance of the newer agents.

Ethotoin

Ethotoin is an approved drug by the United States Food and Drug Administration for the treatment of complex partial and tonic-clonic seizures. It is ineffective against other seizure types. Clinical efficacy has been determined through uncontrolled clinical trials (60,61).

In a study of 17 patients with refractory seizures, 16 patients responded favorably to adjunctive therapy with ethotoin (60). Control, however, was not defined. The number of patients was small and represented a very heterogeneous population. No adverse effects were reported.

A retrospective study of 46 patients with intractable seizures reported a >50% seizure reduction in approximately 51% of the patients (61). This was reduced to about 25% for the last 3 months of the study. Ten patients experienced side effects including allergy, gastrointestinal effects, weight loss, psychiatric effects, tremors, and ataxia. Gingival hyperplasia was not observed. Other side effects observed in six patients included leukopenia, pseudolymphoma, elevated liver enzymes, and, in one patient, choreoathetosis. Although the clinical experience is limited, it is generally believed that the risk of congenital anomalies and malformations is similar to the incidences associated with PHT (62).

Therapy should be initiated with doses ≤1,000 mg. The optimal dose is in the range of 3,000 to 4,000 mg and initially should be administered in four to six divided doses. Once steady-state levels are achieved, administration can be reduced to three daily doses.

SUMMARY

After many decades of use, PHT remains a drug of choice for the treatment of partial (simple and complex) and generalized tonic-clonic seizures. It is not effective in absence or myoclonic seizures or infantile spasms. PHT is effective in neonatal seizures, but adequate blood levels may be difficult to maintain with the oral preparation. PHT is considered by many clinicians to be a drug of choice for the treatment of acute seizures and status epilepticus. In this case, its action is enhanced by the simultaneous use of diazepam or lorazepam.

Drug interactions may occur when PHT is used concurrently with other drugs, including some AEDs. Generally, PHT induces the metabolism and increases the dose requirements of other drugs, and caution is indicated when PHT is used in combination with other drugs.

The acute toxic effects of PHT (e.g., nystagmus, ataxia, and incoordination) are dose related. Individual variation can result in adverse effects over a wide range of blood PHT levels. Thus, the response to therapy must be judged clinically, with "therapeutic" or "toxic" blood PHT levels used as general guidelines to treatment. The clinical uses of ethotoin and mephenytoin in the treatment of epilepsy are limited.

REFERENCES

1. Merritt HH, Putnam TJ. Sodium diphenyl hydantoinate in the treatment of convulsive disorders. *JAMA* 1938;111: 1068–1073.
2. Merritt HH, Putnam TJ. A new series of anticonvulsant drugs tested by experiments in animals. *Arch Neurol Psychiatry* 1938; 39:1003–1015.
3. Callaghan N, Kenny RA, O'Neill B, et al. A prospective study between carbamazepine, phenytoin and sodium valproate as monotherapy in previously untreated and recently diagnosed patients with epilepsy. *J Neurol Neurosurg Psychiatry* 1985;48: 639–644.
4. Heller AJ, Chesterman P, Elwes RDC, et al. Monotherapy for newly diagnosed adult epilepsy: a comparative trial and prognostic evaluation. *Epilepsia* 1989;30:648.
5. Mattson RH, Cramer JA, Collins JF, et al. Comparison of carbamazepine, phenobarbital, phenytoin, and primidone in partial and secondarily generalized tonic-clonic seizures. *N Engl J Med* 1985;313:145–151.
6. Pellock JM, for the Collaborative Study Group at the Medical College of Virginia. Use of carbamazepine and phenytoin in the treatment of epilepsy in children under six years of age. Paper presented at the Child Neurology Society, Nova Scotia, September, 1988.
7. Ramsay RE, Wilder BJ, Berger JR, et al. A double-blind study comparing carbamazepine with phenytoin as initial seizure therapy in adults. *Neurology* 1983;33:904–910.
8. Turnbull DM, Howel D, Rawlins MD, et al. Which drug for the adult epileptic patient: phenytoin or valproate. *BMJ* 1985; 290:815–819.
9. Wilder BJ, Ramsay RE, Murphy JV, et al. Comparison of valproic acid and phenytoin in newly diagnosed tonic-clonic seizures. *Neurology* 1983;33:1474–1476.
10. DeSilva M, McArdle B, McGowan M, et al. Randomized comparative monotherapy trial of phenobarbitone, phenytoin, carbamazepine or sodium valproate for newly diagnosed childhood epilepsy. *Lancet* 1996;347:709–713.
11. Brodie MJ, Dichter MA. Antiepileptic drugs. *N Engl J Med* 1996;334:168–175.
12. Heller AJ, Chesterman P, Elwes RDC, et al. Phenobarbitone, phenytoin, carbamazepine or sodium valproate for newly diagnosed adult epilepsy: a randomized comparative monotherapy trial. *J Neurol Neurosurg Psychiatry* 1995;58:44–50.
13. Brodie MJ, Clifford YS, Yuen AWC, et al. Open multicenter trial of Lamictal (lamotrigine) in patients with treatment-resistant epilepsy withdrawing from a add-on to Lamictal monotherapy. *Epilepsia* 1995;35[Suppl 7]:69–70.
13a. Steiner TJ, Dellaportes CI, Findley LJ, et al. Lamotrigine monotherapy in newly diagnosed untreated epilepsy: a double-blind randomized comparison with phenytoin. *Epilepsia* 1999; 40:601–607.
13b. Bill PA, Vigonius W, Pohlman H, et al. A double-blind clinical treal of oxcarbazepine versus phenytoin in adults with previously untreated epilepsy. *Epilepsy Res* 1997;27:195–204.
14. Salem RB, Yost RL, Torosian G, Davis FT. Investigation of the crystallization of phenytoin in normal saline. *Drug Intell Clin Pharm* 1980;14:605–608.
15. Salem RB, Wilder BJ, Yost RL, et al. Rapid infusion of phenytoin sodium loading doses. *Am J Hosp Pharm* 1981;38: 354–357.
16. Serrano EE, Wilder BJ. Intramuscular administration of diphenylhydantoin. *Arch Neurol* 1974;31:276–278.
17. Ramsay RE, Wilder BJ, Murphy JV, et al. Efficacy and safety of valproic acid versus phenytoin as sole therapy in newly diagnosed primary tonic-clonic seizures. *J Epilepsy* 1992;5:55–60.
18. Ethridge R, Iivanien M, Stern R, et al. "Baltic" myoclonus epilepsy: hereditary disorder of childhood made worse by phenytoin. *Lancet* 1983;2:838–842.
19. Hurd RW, Perchalski RJ, Wilder BJ, et al. The role of copper in the differing effects of valproic acid (VPA) and phenytoin (PHT) in progressive myoclonus epilepsy of the Unverricht-Lundborg type (PME-UL). *Neurology* 1994;44[Suppl 2]:A295.
20. Temkin NR, Dikmen SS, Wilensky AJ, et al. A randomized, double-blind study of phenytoin for the prevention of post-traumatic seizures. *N Engl J Med* 1990;323:497–502.
21. Rathlev NK, D'Onofrio G, Fish SS, et al. The lack of efficacy of phenytoin in the prevention of recurrent alcohol-related seizures. *Ann Emerg Med* 1994;23:513–518.
22. Painter MJ, Stein AD, et al. Phenobarbital compares with phenytoin for the treatment of neonatal seizures. *N Engl J Med* 1999;341:485–489.
23. Cranford RE, Leppik IE, Patrick B, et al. Intravenous phenytoin: clinical and pharmacokinetic aspects. *Neurology* 1978;28: 874–880.
24. Delgado-Escueta AV, Wasterlain C, Treiman DM, et al. Management of status epilepticus. *N Engl J Med* 1982;306: 1337–1340.
25. Leppik IE, Patrick BK, Cranford RE. Treatment of acute seizures and status epilepticus with intravenous phenytoin. *Adv Neurol* 1983;34:447–451.
26. Wilder BJ. Efficacy of phenytoin in the treatment of status epilepticus. *Adv Neurol* 1983;34:441–446.
27. Wilder BJ, Ramsay RE, Willmore LJ, et al. Efficacy of intravenous phenytoin in the treatment of status epilepticus: kinetics of central nervous system penetration. *Ann Neurol* 1977;1: 511–518.
28. Lowenstein DH, Alldredge BK. Status epilepticus. *N Engl J Med* 1998;338:970–976.
29. Wilder BJ, Streiff RR, Hammer RH. Diphenylhydantoin:

absorption, distribution, and excretion: clinical studies. In: Woodbury DM, Penry JK, Schmidt RP, eds. *Antiepileptic drugs.* New York: Raven Press, 1972:137–148.

30. Davis JA, Barnes DW, Wilder BJ, et al. The use of free serum phenytoin concentrations, albumin and neurologic assessment to improve dosing of phenytoin. *Epilepsia* 1992;33[Suppl 3]:107.

31. Wilder BJ, Bruni J. Medical management of seizure disorders. In: *Seizure disorders: a pharmacological approach to treatment.* New York: Raven Press, 1981:35–39.

32. Schmidt D, Einicke I, Haenel F. The influence of seizure type on the efficacy of plasma concentrations of phenytoin, phenobarbital and carbamazepine. *Arch Neurol* 1986;43:263–265.

33. Kutt H, Haynes J, McDowell F. Some causes of ineffectiveness of diphenylhydantoin. *Arch Neurol* 1966;14:489–492.

34. Kilarski DJ, Buchanan C, Von Behren L. Soft-tissue damage associated with intravenous phenytoin. *N Engl J Med* 1984; 311:1186–1187.

35. Rao VK, Feldman PD, Dibbell DG. Extravasation injury to the hand by intravenous phenytoin: report of three cases. *J Neurosurg* 1988;68:967–969.

36. Ramsay RE, Hammond EJ, Perchalski RJ, et al. Brain uptake of phenytoin, phenobarbital, and diazepam. *Arch Neurol* 1979;36: 535–539.

37. Mirza W, Credeur LJ, Penry JK. Results of antiepileptic drug reduction in patients with multiple handicaps and epilepsy. *Drug Invest* 1993;5:320–326.

38. Bates ER, Wilder BJ, Dubay C, et al. Antiepileptic drug reduction program revisited at a center for the developmentally disabled. *Epilepsia* 1993;34[Suppl 6]:108.

39. Schneiderman JH. Monotherapy versus polytherapy in epilepsy: a framework for patient management. *Can J Neurol Sci* 1998;25[Suppl 4]:S9–S13.

40. Ferrendelli JA. Pharmacology of antiepileptic drug polypharmacy. *Epilepsia* 1999;40[Suppl 5]:S81–S83.

41. Leppik IE. Monotherapy and polytherapy. *Neurology* 2000:55 [Suppl 3]:S25–S29.

42. Deckers CLP, Czuczwar SJ, Hekster YA, et al. Selection of antiepileptic drug polytherapy based on mechanisms of action: the evidence reviewed. *Epilepsia* 2000;41:1364–1374.

43. Kutt H. Phenytoin: interactions with other drugs. In: Levy R, Mattson R, Meldrum B, et al., eds. *Antiepileptic drugs,* 4th ed. New York: Raven Press, 1995:315–328.

43a. Treiman DM, Meier PD, et al. Treatment of status epilepticus. *N Engl J Med* 1998;339:792–798.

44. Wilder BJ. How about the new antiepileptic drugs? *Can J Neurol Sci* 1994;21[Suppl 3]:S3–S6.

45. Bruni J, Wilder BJ, Willmore LJ, et al. Valproic acid and plasma levels of phenytoin. *Neurology* 1979;29:904–905.

46. Wilder BJ, Rangel RJ. Clinically relevant antiepileptic drug

interactions. In: Pitlick WH, ed. *Antiepileptic drug interactions.* New York: Demos, 1989:65–75.

47. May T, Rambeck B. Serum concentration of valproic acid: influence of dose and comedication. *Ther Drug Monit* 1985;7: 387–390.

48. Harden CL. New antiepileptic drugs. *Neurology* 1994;44: 787–795.

49. Fincham RW, Schottelius DD. Primidone: interactions with oher drugs. In: Levy R, Mattson R, Meldrum B, et al., eds. *Antiepileptic drugs,* 3rd ed. New York: Raven Press, 1989: 413–422.

50. Browne TR, Szabo MT, Evans JE, et al. Carbamazepine increases phenytoin serum concentration and reduces phenytoin clearance. *Neurology* 1988;38:1146–1150.

51. Haruda F. Phenytoin hypersensitivity: 38 cases. *Neurology* 1979; 29:1480–1485.

52. Angelopoulos AP, Goaz PW. Incidence of diphenylhydantoin gingival hyperplasia. *Oral Surg Oral Med Oral Oncol* 1972;34: 898.

53. Reynolds EH. Chronic antiepileptic toxicity: a review. *Epilepsia* 1975;16:319–352.

54. Solomon GE, Hilgartner MW, Kutt H. Coagulation defects caused by diphenylhydantoin. *Neurology* 1972;22:1165–1171.

55. Cantu RC, Schwab RS. Ceruloplasmin rise and protein bound fall in human serum during diphenylhydantoin (Dilantin) administration. *Trans Am Neurol Assoc* 1966;91:201–203.

56. Yeo PPB, Bates D, Howe JG, et al. Anticonvulsants and thyroid function. *BMJ* 1978;1:1581.

57. Bardana EJ, Gabourel JD, Davies GH, et al. Effect of phenytoin on man's immunity: evaluation of changes in serum immunoglobulin complement, and antinuclear antibody. *Am J Med* 1983;74:289–296.

58. Burks AW, Charlton R, Casey P, et al. Immune function in patients treated with phenytoin. *J Child Neurol* 1989;4:25.

59. Ruff ME, Pincus LG, Sampson HA. Phenytoin-induced IgA depression. *Am J Dis Child* 1987;141:858.

60. Carter CA, Helms RA, Boechm R. Ethotoin in seizures of childhood and adolescence. *Neurology* 1984;34:791–795.

61. Biton V, Gates J, Ritter FS, et al. Adjunctive therapy for intractable epilepsy with ethotoin. *Epilepsia* 1990;31:433–437.

62. Finnell RH, Di Liberti JH. Hydantoin-induced teratogenesis: are arene oxide intermediates really responsible? *H Paediatr Acta* 1983;38:171–177.

63. Kupferberg HJ. Other hydantoins: mephenytoin and ethotoin. In: Levy R, Mattson R, Meldrum B, et al., eds. *Antiepileptic drugs,* 4th ed. New York. Raven Press, 1995:351–357.

64. Troupin A. Mephenytoin. In: Resor SR Jr, Kutt H, eds. *The medical treatment of epilepsy.* New York: Marcel Dekker, 1992: 399–404.

PHENYTOIN AND OTHER HYDANTOINS

CLINICAL EFFICACY AND USE IN OTHER NEUROLOGICAL DISORDERS

ETTORE BEGHI

Phenytoin (PHT) reduces the frequency of sustained repetitive firing of action potentials in neurons through a use-dependent inhibition of sodium channels. The drug also exerts an action on calcium or sodium ions that regulate voltage-dependent neurotransmitter release at the synaptic cleft (1). These actions on neurotransmitter receptors and ion channels tend to explain the use of PHT and other anticonvulsants in neurologic conditions other than epilepsy. These mechanisms of action may explain the postulated efficacy of PHT in conditions such as neuropathic pain and pain syndromes, spasticity, myotonia, and other muscle disorders. Although several reports have been published on the use of PHT for the treatment of these and other nonepileptic conditions, evidence of efficacy from randomized clinical trials is scant.

NEUROPATHIC PAIN

Neuropathic pain is a spectrum of neuralgic pain syndromes including trigeminal neuralgia and neuralgias affecting other cranial or peripheral nerves (glossopharyngeal, superior-laryngeal, postherpetic), diabetic neuropathy, thalamic syndrome, phantom limb pain, tabetic pain, and cancer pain, among others.

Trigeminal and Other Cranial Neuralgias

Trigeminal neuralgia is a paroxysmal form of facial pain commonly affecting the second and third divisions of the trigeminal nerve. Unlike with carbamazepine (Chapter 24),

Ettore Beghi, MD: Chief, Neurophysiological Unit, "San Gerardo" Hospital, Monza, Italy; and Head, Neurological Disorders Laboratory, Institute for Pharmacological Research "Mario Negri," Milan, Italy

evidence of efficacy of PHT in trigeminal neuralgia and similar conditions is based only on uncontrolled studies. In his extensive review of the neurophysiology of the main pain syndromes and the presumed mechanisms of actions of PHT and other anticonvulsants, Swerdlow (2) reported that PHT was effective as first-aid treatment in ≤80% of patients with trigeminal neuralgia. The drug was used in daily doses ranging from 300 to 600 mg/day. Because trigeminal neuralgia responds to carbamazepine, this is the drug of choice; if symptoms persist with carbamazepine, PHT should be added to the regimen. In contrast to trigeminal neuralgia, the response of glossopharyngeal neuralgia to PHT has been varied. Information on the safety and tolerability of PHT in these cases was insufficient. For these reasons, PHT can be considered an alternative to other treatments in patients with neuralgia, but other drugs such as carbamazepine are preferred.

Other Pain Syndromes

The results of five randomized clinical trials on the use of PHT in pain syndromes other than cranial nerve neuralgias are given in Table 61.1. The neuropathic conditions in these studies included diabetic neuropathy, Fabry's disease, and cold-induced pain. The drug was administered orally (average daily dose 300 mg/day) (3–6) or as intravenous infusion (15 mg/kg) (7). The results of the two placebo-controlled studies in patients with diabetic neuropathy treated for 2 and 23 weeks were contradictory (PHT was superior to placebo in one study and was similar to placebo in the other study). The number needed to treat for effectiveness of PHT compared to placebo is 2.1 (95% confidence interval, 1.5 to 3.6) (8). In patients with Fabry's disease, PHT given for 3 weeks was better than aspirin 1,700 mg/day and placebo in reducing the intensity of pain (3). In diabetic neuropathy, the efficacy of PHT 300 mg/day was at best modest (4–5). The anal-

TABLE 61.1. RANDOMIZED CLINICAL TRIALS OF PHENYTOIN FOR NEUROPATHIC PAIN OTHER THAN TRIGEMINAL NEURALGIA

Reference	No. Treated (age) (Disease)	Treatment Duration (Double-Blind Period)	Daily Dose (mg) [Comparator]	Significant Results [No. Improved]	Adverse Events[a] [No. Withdrawals]
3	8 (13–32) [Fabry's disease]	3 wk	≤300 or 4–6/kg [ASP 1,700]	Mean subjective pain relief (score = 0–3) PHT, 2.7; ASP, 0.5; PLC, 0.9	PHT, 1/8
4	12 (39–75) [Diabetic neuropathy]	23 wk	300 [PLC]	Mean pain score (distance in mm from "none") PHT, 7.2 mm (PL, <5 mg/L), PLC, 8 mm; PHT, 19.1 mm (PL <5 mg/l), PLC, 20 mm	PHT, 10/12; PLC, 4/12 [PHT, 2/12; PLC, 0/12]
5	40 (?) [Diabetic neuropathy]	2 wk	300 [PLC]	[PHT, 28/38; PLC, 10/38]	Ataxia: PHT, 4/38; PLC, 0/38
6	12 (20–26) [Cold-induced pain]	Single	300 [LTG, 300; DHC, 90; PLC]	Main pain AUC changes[b]: PHT, +65; LTG, +37; DHC, +91; PLC, −17	PHT, 2/15; LTG, 1/15; DHC, 5/15: PLC, 0/15
7	20 (25–60) [Radiculopathy, 10; neuritis, 5; diabetic neuropathy, 3; digital neuroma 2]	2 h	15/kg infusion [PLC]	During PHT infusion: significant decrease of burning, shooting, and overall pain, sensitivity, and numbness. After infusion: significant decrease of overall pain (day 1), shooting pain (day 5), and sensitivity (day 3). No change with PLC [PHT, 14/20; PLC, 0/20]	?

AMT, amitriptyline; ASP, aspirin; AUC, area under the drug plasma concentration; DHC, dihydrocodeine; LTG, lamotrigine; PHT, phenytoin; PL, plasma level; PLC, placebo; VAS, visual analog scale.
[a]No. with any event or, if unavailable, with commonest events.
[b]Positive value means pain decrease.

gesic activity of PHT on cold-induced pain in healthy volunteers was compared with that of lamotrigine and dihydrocodeine and was found to be similar (6). The three drugs did not show significant differences in sedation compared with placebo. In a double-blind placebo-controlled crossover study, intravenous infusion of PHT showed a significant analgesic effect in acute exacerbations of neuropathic pain, which outlived the infusion time and the plasma half-life of the drug. Based on the available findings, the evidence of efficacy of PHT ≤300 mg/day for the treatment of neuropathic pain is at best modest, even though the drug is thought to potentiate other analgesic agents (2), and it seems able to control acute exacerbations of neuropathic pain when it is given in intravenous infusion. PHT is well tolerated and does not seem to provoke sedation and cognitive impairment.

MYOTONIA

Myotonia is a clinical manifestation of different muscle disorders and is characterized by altered muscle membrane physiology. Treatment of myotonia with PHT 200 to 400 mg/day orally was investigated in two small double-blind comparative studies (Table 61.2) (9,10). The drug showed an efficacy similar to that of the two comparators (procainamide and carbamazepine) and was superior to placebo, as shown by the improvement of myotonic symptoms and the delay in muscle relaxation, documented ergographically. Based on the results of these studies, PHT and carbamazepine can be used interchangeably for the treatment of myotonia. Specific attention should be paid to adverse treatment events, which were not sufficiently documented in the randomized studies.

MOTION SICKNESS

PHT may be effective in motion sickness by acting on the central and peripheral vestibular pathways (11). The prophylactic action of PHT in 35 patients susceptible to motion sickness was tested in a double-blind trial (12). The patients received 200 mg of PHT or placebo in single dose. Based on clinical and electrophysiologic tests, PHT prevented gastric tachyarrhythmia and reduced the intensity of motion sickness symptoms.

TABLE 61.2. RANDOMIZED CLINICAL TRIALS OF PHENYTOIN FOR MYOTONIA

Reference	No. Treated (age) (Disease)	Treatment Duration (Double-Blind Period)	Daily Dose (mg) [Comparator]	Significant Results [No. Improved]	Adverse Events[a] [No. Withdrawals]
9	9 (?) [Myotonic dystrophy 7; myotonia congenita 2]	3 wk	300–400 [PCN, 2,000–4,000; PLC]	Grasp phase showed by PLC and PCN, not by PHT; relaxation affected by PHT and PCN (no difference), not by PLC PHT and PCN both relieved myotonia [PHT, 5/9; PCN, 5/9; PLC, 2/9]	PCN, 6/9; PHT, 1?/9
10	6 (?) [Myotonic dystrophy]	Two 15-day periods	200, 300 [CBZ, 600, 800; PLC]	Decrease in time of myotonic after-discharge (CBZ ≈PHT>PLC) with moderate effect of dose Improved score of myotonic symptoms (CBZ ≈PHT>PLC) with no effect of dose	Asthenia and somnolence: PHT, 2/6; CBZ, 2/6 Increase of P-Q interval: CBZ, 1/6 [CBZ,0/6; PHT, 1/6]

PLC, placebo; PCN, procainamide.
[a]No. with any event or, if unavailable, with commonest events.

REFERENCES

1. DeLorenzo RJ. Phenytoin: mechanisms of action. In: Levy RH, Mattson RH, Meldrum BS, eds. *Antiepileptic drugs,* 4th ed. New York: Raven Press, 1995:271–282.
2. Swerdlow M. Anticonvulsant drugs and chronic pain. *Clin Neuropharmacol* 1984;7:51–82.
3. Lockman LA, Hunningghake DB, Krivit W, et al. Relief of pain of Fabry's disease by diphenylhydantoin. *Neurology* 1973;23:871–875.
4. Saudek CD, Werns S, Reidenberg MM. Phenytoin in the treatment of diabetic symmetrical polyneuropathy. *Clin Pharmacol Ther* 1977;22:196–199.
5. Chadda VS, Mathur MS. Double blind study of the effects of diphenylhydantoin sodium on diabetic neuropathy. *J Assoc Physicians India* 1978;26:403–406.
6. Webb J, Kamali F. Analgesic effects of lamotrigine and phenytoin on cold-induced pain: a crossover placebo-controlled study in healthy volunteers. *Pain* 1998;76:357–363.
7. McCleane GJ. Intravenous infusion of phenytoin relieves neuropathic pain: a randomized, double-blinded, placebo-controlled, crossover study. *Anesth Analg* 1999;89:985–988.
8. Wiffen P, Collins S, McQuay H, et al. Anticonvulsant drugs for acute and chronic pain. In: *Cochrane database of systematic reviews,* 2000:CD001133.
9. Munsat TL. Therapy of myotonia: a double-blind evaluation of diphenylhydantoin, procainamide, and placebo. *Neurology* 1967;17:359–367.
10. Sechi GP, Traccis S, Durelli L, et al. Carbamazepine versus diphenylhydantoin in the treatment of myotonia. *Eur Neurol* 1983;22:113–118.
11. Knox GW, Woodard D, Chelen W, et al. Phenytoin for motion sickness: clinical evaluation. *Laryngoscope* 1994;104:935–939.
12. Stern RM, Uijtdehaage SH, Muth ER, et al. Effects of phenytoin on vection-induced motion sickness and gastric myoelectric activity. *Aviat Space Environ Med* 1994;65:518–521.

SUGGESTED READING

Beghi E. The use of anticonvulsants in neurological conditions other than epilepsy: a review of the evidence from randomized controlled trials. *CNS Drugs* 1999;11:61–82.

Antiepileptic Drugs, 5th Edition. Edited by R.H. Levy, R.H. Mattson, B.S. Meldrum, and E. Perucca. Lippincott Williams & Wilkins, Philadelphia © 2002.

PHENYTOIN AND OTHER HYDANTOINS

CLINICAL EFFICACY AND USE IN PSYCHIATRIC DISORDERS

FRANCESCO MONACO
MARCO MULA

The use of antiepileptic drugs (AEDs) in the treatment of psychiatric disorders has reached a new phase of clinical and theoretical interest (1). Initially, as various became available, anecdotal observations and clinical studies suggested that they could be associated with either improvement or worsening of mood and psychosis in patients with epilepsy (2). Later assessments of the behavioral effects of AEDs yielded a series of clinical trials on psychiatric patients who had no evidence of seizure disorders (3). Phenytoin (PHT) (Chapter 58) was one of the first AEDs to be used in psychiatric disorders (4). Conversely, to our knowledge, the other hydantoins (mephenytoin and ethotoin) were very seldom employed for this use (5), and no significant data are available in the literature.

SPECTRUM OF EFFICACY IN PSYCHIATRIC DISORDERS

Psychoses

In 1943, Kalinowsky and Putnam (4) treated 41 patients with schizophrenia with an oral dose of 700 mg/day of diphenylhydantoin (the older term for PHT) sodium, and these investigators reported substantial improvement in excitement, agitation, hyperactivity, and aggression in these patients. In 1945, Freyhan (6) treated 25 patients with schizophrenia with 300 to 600 mg of PHT daily and observed encouraging results, mainly in the alleviation of catatonic excitement. In 1946, Kubanek and Rowell (7) administered PHT (300 to 700 mg/day) to 35 chronically psychotic hospitalized patients, eight of whom showed marked improvement in their behavior. Taking into account all the patients studied in the three (uncontrolled)

Francesco Monaco, MD: Chief and Professor of Neurology, Department of Neurology, University of Piemonte Orientale "Amedeo Avogadro," Novara, Italy

Marco Mula, MD: Research Fellow, Department of Neurology, University of Piemonte Orientale "Amedeo Avogadro," Novara, Italy

studies, there was an overall improvement rate of 45%, a rather impressive figure considering the severe and long-term nature of the disturbances shown by most of these patients. In 1969, Haward (8), in the first double-blind, placebo-controlled study performed for the use of PHT in the treatment of chronic schizophrenia, reported that both aggressive behavior and assaultive ward behavior were reduced in the 20 patients studied when PHT ($\leq$200 mg/day) was administered.

In 1974, Simopoulos et al. (9) conducted a double-blind, placebo-controlled trial to clarify the effect of PHT in patients with chronic schizophrenia, with particular interest on the effect of the drug on hostility. In this study, 26 men and 50 women (age range, 20 to 59 years) with a primary diagnosis of schizophrenia, who had been hospitalized and had been taking continuous phenothiazine medication for at least 6 months, were selected. PHT was administered according to the following dosage: 375 mg/day for the first 2 weeks, 500 mg for the third and fourth weeks, and 625 for the remaining 4 weeks. Measures used were the Brief Psychiatric Rating Scale, the Nurses Observation Scale for Inpatient Evaluation, and the Crownsville Psychiatric Scale (parts I and II). Patients receiving both PHT and placebo worsened on both measures (in this study, all phenothiazines were discontinued on the first day of PHT administration); differences in favor of PHT were found for the Brief Psychiatric Rating Scale variables of hostility and thought content. The optimal dosage appeared to be <500 mg/day (because retardation and blunted affect were more predominant at the highest dose levels), and the indication seemed to be a high initial disorder score, especially for hostility. The therapeutic effects of PHT were of short duration and occurred in the early phases of treatment. These effects did not continue into the later period of treatment, when doses were >525 mg/day. The same authors (10) conducted a double-blind study to evaluate the response of patients with chronic schizophrenia to a combination of PHT and neuroleptics, and results were the same as those of the previous study.

Mood Disorders

The early studies, particularly in the 1940s, were largely based on uncontrolled clinical observations. In 1943, Kalinowsky and Putnam (4) reported that eight of nine patients with mania improved during treatment with PHT, as did three of five patients in the depressed phase. In 1945, Freyhan (6) reported that five of six patients were doubtful responders to treatment with PHT. However, he reported one patient who appeared to be an unequivocal responder. This patient's severe manic illness improved on four occasions in response to PHT and showed repeated exacerbations when the drug was discontinued. In 1967, both Jonas (11) and Turner (12) studied the effects of PHT in less severely ill outpatients with mood disturbances who could be classified as having neurotic or nonendogenous depressive illness. In 1983, Post and Uhde (2), in a double-blind, placebo-controlled trial with three different AEDs (carbamazepine, PHT, and valproic acid) in patients with recurrent manic illness, showed a notable response to carbamazepine but showed no evidence of response to treatment with the PHT or valproic acid. From this finding, these investigators theorized a different biochemical mechanism of action and neural substrate for carbamazepine and PHT, in spite of the similar clinical and experimental spectrum of clinical efficacy. Compared with PHT, carbamazepine is actually more effective in inhibiting amygdala-kindled afterdischarges and seizures and in raising the threshold for amygdala seizures (13–17).

As a new phase of interest in the use of PHT for mania has begun (1,18,19), and the cognitive side effects of PHT have been reassessed favorably (20,21), it may be of clinical value to add PHT to the therapeutic regimen in some patients with bipolar illness. Mishory et al. (19) conducted a controlled study on the use of PHT for mania and used an add-on design with ongoing neuroleptic treatment; 39 patients with either bipolar I disorder, manic type, or schizoaffective disorder, manic type, entered a 5-week, double-blind, placebo-controlled trial of haloperidol plus PHT versus haloperidol plus placebo. PHT or placebo was begun at a dose of 300 mg/day, and the dose was increased to 400 mg after 4 days. Of 39 patients, 30 completed at least 3 weeks, and 25 completed 5 weeks of treatment. Improvement with PHT was observed on the Brief Psychiatric Rating Scale and Clinical Global Impression scores in patients with bipolar mania but not with schizoaffective mania. This conclusion should be interpreted cautiously, because the Young Mania Rating Scale scoring did not show significant improvement. The study, as underlined by the authors themselves, is limited by the small sample size, by the finding that the schizoaffective group included more patients nonresponsive to previous treatment, and by the situation that all patients received haloperidol, the plasma levels of which have been demonstrated to be reduced by PHT (22).

Aggression and Behavior Disorders

Many different drugs have been advocated to be useful in treating aggressive patients (23). Aggression is a symptom, and it is important for the clinician to clarify underlying causal agents or psychological factors before treating the patient. For example, violence can exist in association with a psychotic condition such as catatonic excitement or an acute toxic psychotic state. Organic factors such as latent epilepsy or, in rare instances, overt partial temporal lobe epilepsy, with complex symptoms, may or may not underlie such conditions. Episodic rage, fear attacks, memory disturbances, fugues, and impulsive actions are typical of partial epilepsy and are strongly reminiscent of various aspects of other illnesses such as character disorders of hysterical and emotionally unstable type (2,24,25). Because of the similarity in clinical features, investigators have suggested that AEDs be used in treating such patients (26).

PHT has long been advocated to reduce aggressiveness in psychiatric patients (27,28). In 1945, Freyhan (29) reported good results using PHT in adult patients with agitated depression. In 1967, Klein and Greenberg (26) studied the efficacy of PHT in hospitalized older adolescents and adult psychiatric patients with a main diagnosis of agitated depression and behavior characterized by impulsive actions and rage attacks unrelated to appropriate stimuli; 13 patients were treated with PHT as the sole psychotropic agent, and 15 others were treated with PHT added as an adjunctive medication to another psychotropic agent. All patients received 100 mg of PHT three times a day for at least 2 weeks; control measures were not taken, nor there was any attempt to mask the identification of the drug. This study showed no beneficial effect of PHT, whether administered alone or in association with phenothiazines or imipramine. The only patient who had a maximum clinical response to PHT had a previous diagnosis of "psychomotor" epilepsy. Several controlled studies have shown that the drug is no more effective than placebo or other medications (30–32).

In 1968, Boelhouwer et al. (33), in a double-blind study, showed that a combination of benzodiazepines and PHT was useful in aggressive patients, and another controlled study showed that PHT alone was useful for treating anxiety, irritability, and anger in neurotic patients (34). The complexities of clinical diagnosis and evaluation are further emphasized by isolated reports of worsening of episodic disorders by PHT and chlordiazepoxide (35). Many of these studies were carried out on criminals, in whom the degree of aggressiveness was not specified and was not associated with a well-defined psychiatric disorder (31).

To date, there is more negative than positive evidence in the literature on this topic. For example, in a controlled trial, Yudofsky et al. (36) demonstrated no efficacy for PHT in aggression. More recently, Barratt (37) theorized that the equivocal findings in the early studies resulted from poor criterion measures, inappropriate inclusion and exclusion criteria for patients, and a different nosologic basis for classifying various types of aggression. He therefore proposed that aggression could be divided into three broad categories: (a) medically related (aggression is a symptom related to a psychiatric, neurologic, or other medical disorder); (b) premeditated or planned (the aggressive act is an instrumental response); and (c) impulsive. Barratt hypothesized that selected anticonvulsants (e.g., PHT) would have a therapeutic effect on impulsive aggression. For these reason, Barratt et al. conducted a double-blind, placebo-controlled, crossover study (38). Sixty inmates were divided into two groups on the basis of committing impulsive aggressive acts or premeditated aggressive acts committed while the inmates were in prison; medical aggression was ruled out by subject selection. As hypothesized, PHT (300 mg/day) significantly reduced impulsive aggressive acts but not premeditated aggressive acts. However because aggression is a complex phenomenon that is undoubtedly multifactorially determined, it appears very difficult to evaluate a specific antiaggressive pharmacotherapeutic agent.

Eating Disorders

The pharmacotherapy of anorexia nervosa and bulimia is mainly based on antidepressant drugs (39,40); alternative drugs therapies include anticonvulsants (PHT and carbamazepine) and lithium (41). Evidence for the use of AEDs in eating disorders is based on the early observations of Lundberg and Walinder (42) who, in 1967, reported on five patients with anorexia nervosa who showed clear clinical signs of underlying neurologic disease. In 1974, Green and Rau (5) speculated that some patients with disturbances in eating behavior could suffer from hypothalamic neurologic dysfunction. Whether such dysfunction could be directly caused by lesions in the hypothalamus or from the feedback effects of cortical lesions was unknown. Furthermore, persons with severe eating disorders resulting from cerebral lesions could be expected to have abnormal electroencephalographic (EEG) patterns, and these patients could be responsive to AEDs. In the study by Green and Rau (5), 10 patients with symptoms of compulsive eating were treated pharmacologically with PHT at doses ranging from 200 to 400 mg/day. Nine of these patients were treated successfully, with normalization of eating behavior and weight loss in the overweight group. Two patients developed allergic reactions; one dropped out of the study, and the second patient was less successfully treated with mephenytoin (300 mg/day). For these two patients, interruption of medication was shortly followed by a recurrence of symptoms. In the patient who could resume PHT treatment, the compulsive eating behavior decreased significantly. All these patients had abnormal EEGs (six of them showed 14- and six-per-second positive spiking in the temporal and occipital areas, and four of them showed spiking in temporal and occipital areas), indicating that a neurologic dysregulation may have been an etiologic factor.

The foregoing study stimulated Wermuth et al. (43) to test the efficacy of PHT treatment in a controlled clinical trial. Nineteen subjects completed a 12-week, double-blind, crossover study comparing PHT (300 mg/day) with placebo. The data were first analyzed by comparing the mean number of binges per week estimated by subjects (historical control) and those during both experimental periods (placebo-PHT and PHT-placebo sequence). In the placebo-PHT sequence, the number of binges per week during the placebo period was not significantly different from the historical control. However, there was a significant decrease during PHT treatment. Nevertheless, the efficacy of PHT was considerably less in this study than in the previous one, in which 90% of the subjects returned to normal eating habits. As suggested by the authors, this discrepancy could have resulted from the inclusion of more seriously affected subjects (in this study, patients who had frequent binges were intentionally selected; those with milder forms were therefore excluded) and the shorter duration of treatment. Results were further confounded by the effect of treatment sequence, in which there was an unexpected persistence of treatment effect in the placebo period for subjects in the PHT-placebo sequence. The action of PHT ended soon after the drug was discontinued, and during placebo period, virtually all subjects had no detectable plasma drug concentrations. Thus, a prolonged drug effects was most unlikely, so it could be speculated that a learning effect was created once the pattern of binge eating was interrupted.

MODE OF USE

The previously described data provide the tempting suggestion that PHT, in carefully adjusted doses, may be of therapeutic value at least in some psychiatric disorders, particularly for its lack of sedative action. An initial dose of 300 mg/day seems to be useful in mood disorders and aggressive behavior. In some patients, such as those with schizophrenia, particularly those with high levels of hostility, the initial dose of 300 mg/day of PHT must be raised 100 mg/wk until a good clinical response is obtained; the optimal dose appears to be 500 mg/day. However, a good clinical response has been described mainly for patients with EEG abnormalities (34).

Long-term prophylactic studies of PHT in patients with bipolar disorder and with schizophrenia will need to take into account the danger of gingival hyperplasia, leukopenia, or anemia and the risks of toxicity resulting from nonlinear kinetic and pharmacokinetic and pharmacodynamic interactions with other drugs in such combined therapies. Moreover, patients with organic mania induced by PHT are described in the literature (44–46). For clinicians managing psychiatric disorders, PHT pharmacokinetic interactions with psychotropic drugs are quite relevant (47). PHT is 90% metabolized by the cytochrome P450 enzyme system, mainly by the subfamily CYP2C9 and to a lesser extent also by CYP2C19 (Chapter 52), and it is a potent inducer of the CYP3A4, epoxide hydrolase, and the uridine diphosphate glucuronosyltransferase enzyme system (48). Chapter 59 deals with the pharmacologic interactions of PHT, so here we simply mention some aspects of the problem.

As far as antipsychotic drugs are concerned, an increase in PHT plasma concentrations and neurotoxicity was reported after the addition of typical phenothiazines (thioridazine, chlorpromazine, and prochlorperazine) (49,50), whereas plasma concentrations of butyrophenone (as haloperidol) have been demonstrated to be reduced by PHT (21). For atypical antipsychotic drugs, anecdotal reports have described a reduction of clozapine plasma levels in patients treated with PHT (51), as well as the appearance of extrapyramidal symptoms during the coadministration of PHT and risperidone (52). Among antidepressant drugs, fluoxetine (53), viloxazine (54), trazodone, and tricyclic antidepressants (55) demonstrated an increase in PHT plasma levels, whereas PHT was shown to induce paroxetine metabolism and to decrease its plasma concentrations by about 50% (56). In conclusion, PHT, a powerful AED of the first generation, shows many properties, other than its anticonvulsant action, that could have relative efficacy in some psychiatric disorders.

REFERENCES

1. Dunn RT, Frye MS, Kimbrell TA, et al. The efficacy and use of anticonvulsant in mood disorders. *Clin Neuropharmacol* 1998; 21:215–235.
2. Post RM, Uhde TW. Treatment of mood disorders with antiepileptic medications: clinical and theoretical implications. *Epilepsia* 1983;24[Suppl 2]:S97–S108.
3. Post RM, Ballenger JC, Uhde TW, et al. Efficacy of carbamazepine in manic-depressive illness: implications for underlying mechanisms. In: Post RM, Ballenger JC, eds. *Neurobiology of mood disorders.* Baltimore: William & Wilkins, 1983:777–816.
4. Kalinowsky LB, Putnam TJ. Attempts at treatment of schizophrenia and other nonepileptic psychoses with Dilantin. *Arch Neurol Psychiatry* 1943;49:414–420.
5. Green RS, Rau JH. Treatment of compulsive eating disturbances with anticonvulsant medication. *Am J Psychiatry* 1974;131: 428–431.
6. Freyhan FA. Effectiveness of diphenylhydantoin in management of nonepileptic psychomotor excitement states. *Arch Neurol Psychiatry* 1945;53:370–374.
7. Kubanek JL, Rowell RC. The use of Dilantin on the treatment of psychotic patients unresponsive to other treatment. *Dis Nerv Syst* 1946;7:47–750.
8. Haward LRC. Differential modifications of verbal aggression by psychotropic drugs. In: Carattini S, Sigg EB, eds. *Aggressive behaviour: proceeding of the International Symposium on the biology of aggressive behaviour.* Amsterdam: Excerpta Medica, 1969:317–321.
9. Simopoulos AM, Pinto A, Uhlenhuth EH, et al. Diphenylhydantoin effectiveness in the treatment of chronic schizophrenics. *Arch Gen Psychiatry* 1974;30:106–111.
10. Pinto A, Simopoulos AM, Uhlenhuth EH, et al. Responses of chronic schizophrenic females to a combination of diphenylhydantoin and neuroleptics: a double-blind study. *Compr Psychiatry* 1975;16:529–536.
11. Jonas AD. The diagnostic and therapeutic use of diphenylhydantoin in the subictal state and nonepileptic dysphoria. *Int J Neuropsychiatry* 1967;3:S21–S29.
12. Turner WJ. The usefulness of diphenylhydantoin in treatment of non-epileptic emotional disorders. *Int J Neuropsychiatry* 1967;3: S8–S20.
13. Wada JA, Sato M, Wake A, et al. Prophylactic effects of phenytoin, phenobarbital, and carbamazepine examined in kindled cat preparations. *Arch Neurol* 1976;33:426–434.
14. Babington RG. The pharmacology of kindling. In: Hanin I, Usdin E, eds. *Animal models of psychiatry and neurology.* Oxford: Pergamon Press, 1977:141–149.
15. Wada JA. Pharmacological prophylaxis in the kindling model of epilepsy. *Arch Neurol* 1977;34:389–395.
16. Albright PS, Burnham WM. Development of a new pharmacological seizure model: effects of anticonvulsants on cortical- and amygdala-kindled seizures in rat. *Epilepsia* 1980;21:681–689.
17. Albright PS. Effects of carbamazepine, clonazepam and phenytoin on seizure threshold in amygdala and cortex. *Exp Neurol* 1983;79:11–17.
18. Kecke PE, McElroy SL. Anticonvulsants in the treatment of rapid-cycling bipolar disorder. In: McElroy SL, Pope HG eds. *Uses of anticonvulsants in psychiatry.* Clifton, NJ: Oxford Health Care, 1988:115–125.
19. Mishory A, Yaroslavsky Y, Bersudsky Y, et al. Phenytoin as an antimanic anticonvulsant: a controlled study. *Am J Psychiatry* 2000;157:463–465.
20. Devinsky O. Cognitive and behavioral effects of antiepileptic drugs. *Epilepsia* 1995;36[Suppl 2]:S46–S65.
21. Fenwick PB. Antiepileptic drugs and their psychotropic effects. *Epilepsia* 1992;33[Suppl 6]:S33–S36.
22. Linnoila M, Viukari M, Vaisanen K, et al. Effect of anticonvulsants on plasma haloperidol and thioridazine levels. *Am J Psychiatry* 1980;137:819–821.
23. Cherkasy S, Hollander E. Neuropsychiatric aspects of impulsivity and aggression. In: Yudofsky SC, Hales RE, eds. *Textbook of neuropsychiatry.* Washington, DC: American Psychiatric Press, 1997:485–499.
24. Wiegartz P, Seidenberg M, Woodard A, et al. Co-morbid psychiatric disorder in chronic epilepsy: recognition and aetiology of depression. *Neurology* 1999;53[Suppl 2]:S3–S8.
25. Lancman M. Psychosis and peri-ictal confusional states. *Neurology* 1999;53[Suppl 2]:S33–S38.
26. Klein FD, Greenberg IM. Behavioral effects of diphenylhydantoin in severe psychiatric disorders. *Am J Psychiatry* 1967;124: 155–157.
27. Goldstein M. Brain research and violent behavior. *Arch Neurol* 1974;30: 1-35.
28. Lion JR. Conceptual issues in the use of drugs for the treatment of aggression in man. *J Nerv Ment Dis* 1975;160:76–82.
29. Freyhan F. Dilantin in agitated depression. *Arch Neurol Psychiatry* 1945;53:370–374.
30. Conners CK, Kramer R, Rothschild GH, et al. Treatment of young delinquent boys with diphenylhydantoin sodium and methylphenidate. *Arch Gen Psychiatry* 1971;24:156–160.
31. Gottschalk LA, Covi L, Uliana R, et al. Effects of diphenylhydantoin on anxiety and hostility in institutionalised prisoners. *Compr Psychiatry* 1973;14:503–511.
32. Lefkowitz MM. Effects of diphenylhydantoin in disruptive behaviour;study of male delinquent. *Arch Gen Psychiatry* 1969; 29:643–651.
33. Boelhouwer C, Henry CE, Gleck BC. Positive spiking;a double blind study on its significance in behavior disorders, both diagnostically and therapeutically. *Am J Psychiatry* 1968;125: 473–481.
34. Stephens JH, Shaffer JW. A controlled study of the effects of

diphenylhydantoin on anxiety, irritability and anger in neurotic outpatients. *Psychopharmacology (Berl)* 1970;17:169–181.

35. Monroe RR. Anticonvulsants in the treatment of aggression. *J Nerv Ment Dis* 1975;160:119–126.

36. Yudofsky SC, Silver JM, Schneider SE. Pharmacologic treatment of aggression. *Psychiatr Ann* 1987;17:397–407.

37. Barratt ES. The use of anticonvulsants in aggression and violence. *Psychopharmacol Bull* 1993;29:75–81.

38. Barratt ES, Stanford MS, Felthous AR, et al. The effects of phenytoin on impulsive and premeditated aggression: a controlled study. *J Clin Psychopharmacol* 1997;17:341–349.

39. Mitchell JE. Psychopharmacology of anorexia nervosa. In: Meltzer HY, ed. *Psychopharmacology: the third generation of progress.* New York: Raven Press, 1987:1273–1276.

40. Trygstat O. Drugs in the treatment of bulimia nervosa. *Acta Psychiatr Scand* 1990;82:34–37.

41. Steinhausen HC. Anorexia and bulimia nervosa. In: Rutter M, Taylor E, Hersoy L, eds. *Child and adolescent psychiatry.* Oxford: Blackwell Scientific, 1994:425–440.

42. Lundberg O, Walinder J. Anorexia nervosa and signs of brain damage. *Int J Neuropsychiatry* 1967;3:165–173.

43. Wermuth BM, Davis KL, Hollister LE, et al. Phenytoin treatment of binge-eating syndrome. *Am J Psychiatry* 1977;134:1249–1253.

44. Franks RD, Richter AJ. Schizophrenia-like psychosis associated with anticonvulsant toxicity. *Am J Psychiatry* 1979;136:973–974.

45. Kato H. Antiepileptic drugs and psychiatric disorders: mechanism involved in manifestation of psychotic symptoms of high blood level of antiepileptics. *Folia Psychiatr Neurol Jpn* 1983;37:283–289.

46. Pattern SB, Klein GM, Lussier C, et al. Organic mania induced by phenytoin: a case report. *Can J Psychiatry* 1989;34:827–828.

47. Monaco F, Cicolin A. Interactions between anticonvulsant and psychoactive drugs. *Epilepsia* 1999;40[Suppl 10]:S71–S76.

48. Riva R, Albani F, Conin M et al. Pharmacokinetic interactions between antiepileptic drugs: clinical considerations. *Clin Pharmacokinet* 1996;31:470–493.

49. Vincent FM. Phenothiazine-induced phenytoin intoxication. *Ann Intern Med* 1980;93:56–57.

50. Gay PE, Madsen JA. Interaction between phenobarbital and thioridazine on phenytoin serum concentration. *Neurology* 1983;33:1631–1632.

51. Miller DD. Effect of phenytoin on plasma clozapine concentrations in two patients. *J Clin Psychiatry* 1991;52:23–25.

52. Sanderson DR. Drug interaction between risperidone and phenytoin resulting in extrapyramidal symptoms. *J Clin Psychiatry* 1996;57:177.

53. Darley J. Interaction between phenytoin and fluoxetine. *Seizure* 1994;3:151–152.

54. Pisani F, Fazio A, Artesi C, et al. Elevation of plasma phenytoin by viloxazine in epileptic patients: a clinically significant drug interaction. *J Neurol Neurosurg Psychiatry* 1992;55:126–127.

55. Perucca E, Richens A. Interaction between phenytoin and imipramine. *Br J Clin Pharmacol* 1977;4:485–486.

56. Nemeroff C, De Vane C, Pollock B. Newer antidepressants and the cytochrome P450 system. *Am J Psychiatry* 1996;153:311–320.

Antiepileptic Drugs, 5th Edition. Edited by R.H. Levy, R.H. Mattson, B.S. Meldrum, and E. Perucca. Lippincott Williams & Wilkins, Philadelphia © 2002.

PHENYTOIN AND OTHER HYDANTOINS
ADVERSE EFFECTS

JOSEPH BRUNI

PHENYTOIN

Toxicity

The toxicity of antiepileptic drugs can be a limiting factor in the long-term management of the patient with epilepsy. The physician should be aware of the potential acute, idiosyncratic, chronic, and teratogenic side effects of these agents.

Central nervous system (CNS) toxicity is usually dose related; however, significant toxicity and adverse effects may involve other systems: hematopoietic, gastrointestinal, immune, endocrine, skeletal, and skin. The intravenous administration of phenytoin may also precipitate cardiac arrhythmias.

Since its introduction in 1938, phenytoin has remained one of the most widely used antiepileptic drugs, and because of its widespread use, a large literature on the adverse effects of phenytoin has accumulated. This summary is based on reviews in previous editions of this book (1–3) as well as on several other reviews (4–8).

Acute Toxicity

Acute toxicity from antiepileptic drugs is usually the result of overdosage and is less often secondary to an allergic or idiosyncratic reaction. The CNS signs of acute toxicity can usually be predicted on the basis of drug dose–weight or drug dose–plasma concentration relationships. This toxicity occurs as a result of direct drug action on receptor sites as therapeutic concentrations are exceeded. The cerebellovestibular, pyramidal, and higher integrative functions may be involved separately or in various combinations with phenytoin therapy. Initially, cerebellovestibular dysfunction (nystagmus, ataxia, incoordination, dysarthria, and hand tremor) may be observed. As toxicity increases, higher cortical functions (judgment, concentration, behavior, speech,

and mood) are altered. With more severe toxicity, pyramidal and extrapyramidal signs of dystonic posturing, asterixis, athetoid and choreiform movements, and (rarely) myoclonic jerks develop. Epileptic seizures may be exacerbated. With prolonged toxicity, autonomic dysfunction and altered level of consciousness may occur. Phenytoin intoxication is not always easy to recognize clinically, and antiepileptic drug plasma level monitoring can be invaluable in detecting subtle toxicity.

Cerebellar Syndrome

Cerebellovestibular dysfunction with nystagmus and ataxia is well recognized as a manifestation of acute phenytoin toxicity, and it is usually dose related (9). Often, one sees a stepwise effect of nystagmus, ataxia, and mental changes, but this is not universally so. Some patients may demonstrate only one of the symptoms or signs. Neurologically handicapped patients and patients receiving polytherapy generally experience adverse effects at lower plasma concentrations, and a wide interindividual difference exists regarding what plasma concentrations will be associated with toxicity.

Prolonged treatment with phenytoin, especially at high doses, may lead to irreversible cerebellar deficits, and the distinction between reversible cerebellar syndrome and chronic ataxia may be difficult to make on clinical grounds (10). Cerebellar degeneration has been attributed to large doses of phenytoin or prolonged phenytoin therapy (9,11,12). Dam (13) noted Purkinje cell degeneration and astrocytic changes in patients receiving long-term phenytoin therapy. The relative contribution of phenytoin toxicity and repeated episodes of seizures is not uniformly agreed on, however, although phenytoin-related cerebellar degeneration has been reported in nonepileptic patients (14) and after acute intoxication (15). Considering the number of patients treated with prolonged phenytoin therapy, clinically significant permanent cerebellar deficits are uncommon. The long-term effects of high phenytoin levels in patients who do not demonstrate clinical signs of toxicity are unknown.

Joseph Bruni, MD, FRCP(C): Associate Professor, Department of Medicine, University of Toronto; and Consultant Neurologist, Department of Medicine, St. Michael's Hospital, Toronto, Ontario, Canada

Extrapyramidal and Pyramidal Signs

Anticonvulsant-induced dyskinesia, chorea, ballismus, and dystonia are clinically similar to those conditions induced by neuroleptic drugs (16). The dyskinetic movements may involve the extremities, trunk, and face and generally occur early in the course of therapy. The dyskinesias are more frequently observed with high phenytoin concentrations, but some patients may demonstrate similar adventitious movements with concentrations that generally are within the usually accepted therapeutic range. With reduction in the phenytoin dosage, these symptoms often improve.

Spasticity and transient hemiparesis have been observed with high phenytoin concentrations (17,18). Choreoathetosis is an uncommonly observed movement disorder (19). Anterior horn cell dysfunction resulting in muscle fasciculations was observed in one patient (20). Occasionally, a parkinsonian syndrome or aggravation of Parkinson's disease can occur. These are isolated case reports, and their relationship with antiepileptic drug therapy is not definitely established. Considering the large number of patients treated with phenytoin, these are extremely rare occurrences.

Acute Encephalopathy

It is well recognized that phenytoin can cause encephalopathy that can exacerbate seizures (21,22). This usually occurs in association with a high phenytoin concentration and may lead to stupor and coma. Dyskinetic movements may be observed concurrently, and ophthalmoplegia may be observed (23).

A syndrome of chronic phenytoin encephalopathy characterized by the insidious deterioration of intellect and behavior with or without seizure exacerbation, mild cerebrospinal fluid pleocytosis, and moderate increase in protein has also been observed. This encephalopathy is more common in children, and preexisting brain damage may be a risk factor (24).

Allergic and Idiosyncratic Reactions

Phenytoin hypersensitivity reactions are well documented. Idiosyncratic drug reactions are rare but are potentially serious. Idiosyncratic reactions generally occur early in the course of therapy and represent genetically determined abnormal responses to drugs. Skin rashes, mostly morbilliform, represent the most frequently observed reactions. Less frequently, exfoliative dermatitis with systemic symptoms or toxic epidermal necrolysis (Lyell's syndrome) may be observed. These conditions are potentially lethal. Cutaneous vasculitis, a lupuslike syndrome, lichenoid eruptions, and purpuric rashes are less frequently observed manifestations (25). Less common reactions include pancytopenia, thrombocytopenia, erythema multiforme, pseudolymphoma, interstitial nephritis, myositis, polyarteritis nodosa, disseminated intravascular coagulation, and red cell aplasia (2,7,26,27). With intravenous phenytoin, extravasation of the drug into interstitial tissues can cause limb ischemia and skin necrosis. Rarely, hepatic necrosis, with a 25% mortality rate, can occur (28). Mild elevation of hepatic enzymes may be seen in 10% to 15% of patients.

Lymphadenopathy may be associated with systemic symptoms such as fever, rash, arthralgias, and hepatosplenomegaly. Most frequently, this is a benign condition and is reversible with discontinuation of phenytoin therapy, but it may be confused with Hodgkin's lymphoma. This syndrome may be secondary to decreased immunologic surveillance, and depressed cellular and humoral immunity may be found in phenytoin-treated patients. Immunoglobulin A (IgA) production is reduced, and IgG and IgM production may be altered (29).

Chronic Toxicity

Chronic toxicity of phenytoin may involve the following systems or may cause certain deficiency states: neurologic toxicity, connective tissue and dermatologic effects, endocrine disturbances and metabolic effects, hematologic effects and deficiency states, and immunologic effects.

Neurologic Toxicity

Peripheral Neuropathy. Although electrophysiologic abnormalities are common in patients maintained on long-term phenytoin therapy, clinically significant neuropathy is rare. In one report, lower limb areflexia was observed in 15% of patients after ≥5 years of treatment (30). In >50% of those tested, nerve conduction velocities were slow. Transient dysfunction associated with acute toxicity and high phenytoin levels may also occur.

Although phenytoin has been implicated in the neuropathy after long-term therapy, many patients reported that they were concurrently receiving other antiepileptic drugs. Folate deficiency and vitamin B_{12} deficiency are not significant factors. Whether phenytoin monotherapy results in neuropathy after prolonged use is uncertain. One study (31) failed to show evidence of neuropathy in patients treated with phenytoin for ≤5 years.

Disturbances of Higher Cortical Functions. Cognitive and behavioral side effects of antiepileptic drugs have received wide attention (24,32–35). The barbiturate drugs have the greatest importance. However, other antiepileptic drugs such as phenytoin may impair motor speed, concentration, and memory. These disturbances appear to be dose related (33,36). Meador et al. (34) assessed the neuropsychological effects of phenytoin and carbamazepine in 21 healthy adults with various cognitive measures and found that the differences in cognitive effects of carbamazepine and phenytoin were not clinically significant. Both drugs, however, impaired subjects on certain tests as compared with non–drug-related conditions. Dodrill and Troupin (33) also found no significant differences between phenytoin and carbamazepine when adjustments were made for serum plasma levels. Most studies support the absence of a clinically significant effect in most patients, although subtle defects may be identified on formal neuropsychological evaluations.

Connective Tissue Effects

Thickening of subcutaneous tissue, enlargement of lips and nose, coarsening of facial features, and subcutaneous fibrous deposits are often recognized in epileptic patients who receive long-term phenytoin therapy. The term *hydantoin facies* has been used to describe these features, which are common in institutionalized patients (37). These changes may be related to long-term therapy with multiple drugs and high phenytoin levels. Dermatologic changes of hirsutism, acne, and hyperpigmentation may also contribute to the characteristic facies.

There appears to be an association between Dupuytren's contracture and antiepileptic drug therapy, most frequently phenobarbital. Phenytoin may increase the risk of this condition by its influence on collagen synthesis and fibroblast proliferation (38).

Gingival hyperplasia may occur in ≤50% of patients receiving phenytoin therapy. This disorder is more frequently observed in children and in institutionalized patients. Poor oral hygiene (39) and a deficiency in saliva IgA may play a role (40). Genetic factors and high phenytoin concentrations may also be contributory. Gingival hyperplasia usually becomes apparent in the first few months of therapy. Alveolar bone loss is not increased (1). Pulmonary fibrosis secondary to phenytoin-induced pulmonary toxicity rarely has been described, and investigators have suggested that it may represent an immune-complex injury (41).

Endocrine Disturbances and Metabolic Effects

At least four endocrine systems and processes are targets for antiepileptic drug effects: bone metabolism, thyroid gland, pancreatic β cells, and the pituitary-adrenal-gonadal axis. Such effects are found by laboratory tests, but occasionally they result in clinical changes.

Metabolic Bone Disease. Although biochemical abnormalities such as elevated alkaline phosphatase, reduced serum calcium, and decreased serum 2-hydroxycholecalciferol are seen in many patients, clinically significant metabolic bone disease with osteomalacia and rickets is uncommon. It is more prominent in institutionalized patients and in patients receiving multiple drug therapy. Dietary factors and the amount of sunlight exposure may be contributory factors. In a bone biopsy study (42), osteomalacia was found in 53% of patients along with evidence of increased bone resorption (secondary hyperparathyroidism). In another bone biopsy study (43), bone mineral mass was decreased in 44%, but no clinical evidence of metabolic bone disease was found in any of the patients.

Metabolic bone disease may be secondary to decreased intestinal absorption of calcium, altered hepatic vitamin D hydroxylation, and inhibition of parathyroid hormone–induced release of calcium from bone. Metabolic bone disease may lead to fractures, postural changes, and muscle weakness, including a specific myopathy. In populations at risk, long-term treatment with vitamin D should be considered in patients with elevated serum alkaline phosphatase and decreases in serum 25-hydroxycholecalciferol or bone mineral mass.

Thyroid Function. The decline of serum protein iodine sometimes induced by phenytoin is related to changes in protein binding of the thyroid hormones and increased clearance (44). Uptake of triiodothyronine and radioactive iodine by red blood cells is not altered, and most patients are clinically euthyroid. Triiodothyronine and thyroid-stimulating hormone levels are usually normal. The symptoms of phenytoin toxicity may mimic those of hypothyroidism.

Pancreatic β Cells. Most patients receiving long-term phenytoin therapy have normal carbohydrate metabolism, but insulin secretion may be impaired in some patients, especially those with prediabetes or diabetes. This effect may be manifested by an abnormal glucose tolerance test, and acute phenytoin intoxication may be associated with high blood glucose levels. Experimentally, phenytoin can cause hyperglycemia (45).

Pituitary-Adrenal-Gonadal Axis. Phenytoin can influence the pituitary-adrenal-gonadal axis. Short-term administration of large doses may initially increase circulating adrenocorticotropic hormone and cortisol levels. Long-term administration may lead to a shift in steroid metabolism, with an increase in urinary exertion of 6-hydroxycortisol. Phenytoin administration can result in erroneous results on metyrapone and 2-mg dexamethasone suppression tests (46). Phenytoin may also depress the release of antidiuretic hormone.

Testosterone and estradiol metabolism may also be enhanced by phenytoin. Long-term therapy may be associated with elevated plasma concentrations of sex hormone–binding globulin in male and female patients (47). The effect on sexual function of increased testosterone binding to the excess globulin and lower free testosterone levels is uncertain. In male rats, phenytoin treatment for 2 months did not affect fertility (48).

In men with epilepsy, a higher incidence of hyposexuality and sperm abnormalities has been observed (49,50). This may be as a result of altered pituitary hormones, or it may be a direct result of an effect on the testes. In epileptic patients, phenytoin has been reported to stimulate secretion of luteinizing hormone, follicle-stimulating hormone, and prolactin.

Hematologic Effects and Deficiency States

The effects of phenytoin on the hematopoietic system can be classified under neonatal coagulation defects, bone marrow suppression, and folate deficiency.

Neonatal Coagulation Defects. Neonatal coagulation defects have been associated with both phenytoin and phenobarbital (51). Although coagulation disturbances are common, clinical hemorrhage that may become apparent in the first 24 hours is uncommon. Bleeding is caused by a deficiency of vitamin K–dependent clotting factors (II, VII, IX, X). Vitamin K administered to the mother before delivery and to the infant at delivery will prevent this coagulopathy.

Bone Marrow Suppression. Agranulocytosis, pancytopenia, neutropenia, leukopenia, thrombocytopenia, and aplastic anemia occur very rarely with phenytoin use (52). Selective red cell aplasia has been reported with phenytoin, and this may be secondary to inhibition of the incorporation of uridine into normoblasts (53). Mild leukopenia is commonly observed in patients treated with standard antiepileptic drugs. This generally does not require discontinuation of therapy.

Megaloblastic Anemia and Folate Deficiency. Folate deficiency is common in patients with epilepsy who receive long-term treatment. The incidence varies from 27% to 41% (7). The clinical significance is uncertain, except in the case of the megaloblastic anemia induced by phenytoin, which is unassociated with vitamin B_{12} deficiency. This anemia always responds to folate therapy. Folic acid deficiency can be confirmed by low red cell and serum folate levels.

Although megaloblastic anemia is rare, mild macrocytosis can be observed in ≤50% of patients. Other indicators of folate deficiency include decreased folate concentrations in cerebrospinal fluid, marrow megaloblastosis, decreased serum lactic dehydrogenase, and hypersegmentation of peripheral neutrophils. Theoretically, widespread CNS damage, such as Purkinje cell loss, chronic encephalopathy and other neuropsychiatric symptoms, and peripheral neuropathy, could result from severe folic acid deficiency. Such changes, however, have not been commonly reported.

The mechanism by which phenytoin produces folate deficiency is not clear, although several mechanisms are possible. Folate absorption (54,55), folate coenzyme metabolism, and tissue use of folate (53) may be altered. Investigators have suggested a possible relationship between the antifolate effects of antiepileptic drugs and seizure control, although the major mechanisms of action of the standard drugs are not related to folate.

Immunologic Effects

Some phenytoin-treated patients have depressed cellular and humoral immunity (56). The reduced production of IgA in some patients has been confirmed (29,57,58). It has been suggested that IgA deficiency is more likely to develop in phenytoin-treated patients possessing the HLA-A$_2$ histocompatibility antigen (59). Antinuclear antibodies and lymphocytotoxins of the IgM class have been found in epileptic patients receiving phenytoin (60). These findings may have importance in the genesis of an altered immune state in epileptic patients receiving phenytoin.

Teratogenicity

The incidence of congenital anomalies and major malformations in children born of epileptic mothers is about three times that in children of nonepileptic mothers. The role of antiepileptic drugs, nutritional factors, and genetic factors has to be considered. Most epileptic patients receive multiple drug therapy, and interpretation of potential individual drug teratogenesis is difficult. A higher incidence of anomalies has been found in infants born to mothers receiving multiple drugs than in those born to mothers receiving monotherapy. Teratogenesis in pregnancy has been reviewed (61–65).

Malformation and abnormalities described with an increase incidence include cleft lip and palate, cardiac defects, skeletal and CNS defects, hypospadias, intestinal atresia, and hypoplastic phalanges and nails. A fetal hydantoin syndrome was described by Hanson and Smith (66), but whether a true anticonvulsant drug syndrome exists has been questioned. This syndrome has been reported to be associated with cranial anomalies, limb anomalies, and growth and mental deficiency; however, the significance of the dysmorphic features remains unclear. In a prospective study of 121 children, none had the fetal hydantoin syndrome, and the only dysmorphic features attributable to hydantoin exposure were hypertelorism and digital hypoplasia (67). Several studies on the incidence and types of major and minor anomalies have been reported (68–70).

The pharmacologic mechanisms of teratogenesis are poorly understood, and the precise molecular mechanisms are unknown. Folate deficiency, altered oxidative metabolism, and chromosomal abnormalities may be contributing factors (71–73). Certain drug combinations may carry a greater risk because of changes in enzymatic metabolism with inhibition or induction of enzymes (74). Consensus guidelines for the management of the pregnant woman with epilepsy have been developed (75–77).

Summary

Many decades of clinical use of phenytoin have allowed extensive experience with adverse effects. Acute and excessive dose effects are most frequent, and they are characterized by cerebellovestibular signs and symptoms. With increasing dose, cognitive and sedative effects are observed. Acute idiosyncratic systemic toxicity is characterized by a rash, which occasionally may be quite serious and may involve many organs.

Chronic neurologic effects include gingival hyperplasia, hirsutism, and coarsening of the facies. Other systemic dysfunction is uncommon. Neuropathy and cerebellar degeneration may occur with long-term use. Despite the extensive number of adverse effects reported, most patients receiving the drug have little or no toxicity.

ETHOTOIN

Ethotoin is a drug approved by the United States Food and Drug Administration for the treatment of complex partial and tonic-clonic seizures, although it is uncommonly used. Adverse effects include allergic skin reactions, gastrointestinal side effects, sedation, and lymphadenopathy. These adverse effects are uncommon (78). With toxic doses, a cerebellar ataxic syndrome can occur. Hallucinations, memory impairment, and aggression have also been described. Gingival hyperplasia has not been observed (78). Congenital malformations have been reported (79,80).

MEPHENYTOIN

Mephenytoin is uncommonly used in the treatment of partial and tonic-clinic seizures because of its greater incidence of serious toxicity. Gingival hyperplasia, hirsutism, gastrointestinal side effects, and ataxia are less common than with phenytoin. Drowsiness, serious allergic reactions, hepatitis, and hematologic toxicity are more common than with phenytoin (81). Patients with deficiency in the hydroxylation of (S)-mephenytoin may be predisposed to greater toxicity because of drug accumulation. Approximately 4% of white persons and 20% of Japanese persons are poor hydroxylators and are particularly prone to mephenytoin toxicity (82).

REFERENCES

1. Dam M. Phenytoin toxicity. In: Woodbury DM, Penry JK, Pippenger CE, eds. *Antiepileptic drugs,* 2nd ed. New York: Raven Press, 1982:247–256.
2. Reynolds EH. Phenytoin: toxicity. In: Levy R, Mattson RH, Meldrum B, et al., eds. *Antiepileptic drugs,* 3rd ed. New York; Raven Press, 1989:241–255.
3. Bruni J. Phenytoin toxicity. In: Levy RH, Mattson RT, Meldrum BS, eds. *Antiepileptic drugs,* 4th ed. New York: Raven Press, 1995: 345–350.
4. Bruni J, Wilder BJ. The toxicity of antiepileptic drugs. In: Vinken PJ, Bruyn G, eds. *Handbook of clinical neurology,* vol 37: *Intoxications of the nervous system,* part 20. New York: North-Holland Publishing, 1979:199–222.
5. Plaa GL. Acute toxicity of antiepileptic drugs. *Epilepsia* 1975;16: 183–191.
6. Pugh CB, Garnett WR. Current issues in the treatment of epilepsy. *Clin Pharm* 1991;10:335–358.
7. Reynolds EH. Chronic antiepileptic drug toxicity: a review. *Epilepsia* 1975;16:319–352.
8. Schmidt D, ed. *Adverse effects of antiepileptic drugs.* New York: Raven Press, 1982.
9. Ghatak NR, Santoso RA, McKinney WM. Cerebellar degeneration following long term phenytoin therapy. *Neurology* 1976;26: 818–820.
10. Munoz-Garcia D, Delser T, Bermejo F, et al. Truncal ataxia in chronic anticonvulsant treatment: association with drug-induced folate deficiency. *J Neurol Sci* 1982;55:305–311.
11. Haberland C. Cerebellar degeneration with clinical manifestation in chronic epileptic patients. *Psychiatr Neurol* 1962;143:29–44.
12. Hoffbrand AV, Necheles TH. Mechanism of folate deficiency in patients receiving phenytoin. *Lancet* 1968;2:528–530.
13. Dam M. *The density and ultrastructure of the Purkinje cells following diphenylhydantoin treatment in animals and man.* Copenhagen: Bogtrykkeriet Forum, 1972.
14. Rapport RL, Shaw C-M. Phenytoin-related cerebellar degeneration without seizures. *Ann Neurol* 1977;2:437–439.
15. Masur H. Cerebellar atrophy following acute intoxication with phenytoin. *Neurology* 1990;40:1800.
16. Chadwick DD, Reynolds EH, Marsden CD. Anticonvulsant-induced dyskinesia: a comparison with dyskinesia induced by neuroleptics. *J Neurol Neurosurg Psychiatry* 1976;39:1210–1218.
17. Findler G, Lavy S. Transient hemiparesis: a rare manifestation of diphenylhydantoin toxicity. *J Neurosurg* 1979;50:685–687.
18. Stark RJ. Spasticity due to phenytoin toxicity. *Med J Aust* 1979; 1:156.
19. Rasmussen S, Kristensen M. Choreo-athetosis during phenytoin treatment. *Acta Med Scand* 1977;201:239–244.
20. Direkze M, Fernando PSL. Transient anterior horn cell dysfunction in diphenylhydatoin therapy. *Eur Neurol* 1977;15:131–134.
21. Glaser GH. Diphenylhydantoin: toxicity. In: Woodbbury DM, Penry JK, Schmidt RP, eds. *Antiepileptic drugs.* New York: Raven Press, 1972:219–226.
22. Levy LL, Fenichel GM. Diphenylhydantoin-activated seizures. *Neurology* 1965;15:716–722.
23. Spector RH, Davidoff RA, Schwartzman J. Phenytoin-induced ophthalmoplegia. *Neurology* 1976;26:1031–1034.
24. Reynolds EH, Travers RD. Serum antconvulsant concentration in epileptic patients with mental symptoms. *Br J Psychiatry* 1974; 124:440–445.
25. Chang DKM, Shear NH. Cutaneous reactions to anticonvulsants. *Semin Neurol* 1991;12:329–336.
26. Haruda F. Phenytoin hypersensitivity: 38 cases. *Neurology* 1979; 29:1480–1485.
27. Pelekanos J, Camfield P, Camfield C, et al. Allergic rash due to anti-epileptic drugs: clinical features and management. *Epilepsia* 1991;32:554–559.
28. Parker WA, Shearer CA. Phenytoin hepatotoxicity: a case report and review. *Neurology* 1979;29:175–178.
29. Slavin BN, Fenton GM, Laundy M, et al. Serum immunoglobulins in epilepsy. *J Neurol Sci* 1974;23:353–357.
30. Lovelace RE, Horwitz SJ. Peripheral neuropathy in long-term diphenylhydantoin therapy. *Arch Neurol* 1968;18:69–77.
31. Shorvon SD, Reynolds EH. Anticonvulsant peripheral neuropathy: a clinical and electrophysiological study of patients on single drug treatment with phenytoin, carbamazepine or barbiturates. *J Neurol Neurosur Psychiatry* 1982;45:620–626.
32. Dodrill CB. Effects of antiepileptic drugs on abilities. *J Clin Psychiatry* 1988;49:31–34.
33. Dodrill CB, Troupin AS. Neuropsychological effects of carbamazepine and phenytoin: a reanalysis. *Neurology* 1991;41:141–143.
34. Meador KJ, Loring DW, Allen ME, et al. Comparative cognitive effects of carbamazepine and phenytoin in health adults. *Neurology* 1991;41:1537–1540.
35. Trimble MR. Neurobehavioural effects of anticonvulsants. *JAMA* 1991;265:1307–1308.

36. Aman MG, Werry JS, Paxton JW, et al. Effects of phenytoin on cognitive-motor performance in children as a function of drug concentration, seizure type, and time of medication. *Epilepsia* 1994;35:172–180.

37. Falconer MA, Davidson S. Coarse features in epilepsy as a consequence of anti-convulsant therapy. *Lancet* 1973;2:1112–1114.

38. Houck TC, Cheng RF, Waters MD. In: Woodbury DM, Penry JK, Schmidt RP, eds. *Antiepileptic drugs.* New York: Raven Press, 1972:267–274.

39. Angelopoulos AP, Goaz PW. Incidence of diphenylhydantoin gingival hyperplasia. *Oral Surg* 1972;34:898–906.

40. Aarli J A. Phenytoin-induced depression of salivary IgA and gingival hyperplasia. *Epilepsia* 1976;17:283–291.

41. Bayer AS, Targan SR, Pitchon HE, et al. Dilantin toxicity: miliary pulmonary infiltrates and hypoxemia. *Ann Intern Med* 1976;85:475–476.

42. Bell RD, Paky C, Zerwkh J, et al. Effect of phenytoin on bone and vitamin D metabolism. *Ann Neurol* 1979;5:374–378.

43. Polypchuk G, Oreopoulos DG, Wilson DR, et al. Calcium metabolism in adult outpatients with epilepsy receiving long-term anticonvulsant therapy. *Can Med Assoc J* 1978;118:635–638.

44. Yeo PPB, Bates D, Howe JG, et al. Anticonvulsants and thyroid function. *BMJ* 1989;1:1581–1583.

45. Kiser JS, Vargas-Cordon M, Brendel K, et al. The *in vitro* inhibition of insulin secretion by diphenylhydantoin. *J Clin Invest* 1979;49:1942–1948.

46. Gharib H, Munoz JM. Endocrine-manifestations of diphenylhydantoin therapy. *Metabolism* 194;23:515–524.

47. Cramer JA, Jones EE. Reproductive function in epilepsy. *Epilepsia* 1991;32[Suppl 6]:S19–S26.

48. Cohn DF, Axelrod T, Hommonnai ZT, et al. Effect of diphenylhydantoin on the reproductive functionof the male rat. *J Neurol Neurosurg Psychiatry* 1978;41:858–860.

49. Herzog AG, Levesque LA, Drislane FW, et al. Phenytoin-induced elevation of serum estradol and reproductive dysfunction in men with epilepsy. *Epilepsia* 1991;32:550–553.

50. Taneja N, Kucheria K, Jain S, et al. Effect of phenytoin on semen. *Epilepsia* 1994;35:136–140.

51. Solomon GE, Hilgartner MW, Kutt H. Coagulation defects caused by diphenylhydantoin. *Neurology* 1972;22:1165–1171.

52. Pisciotta AV. Phenytoin: hematological toxicity. In: Woodbury DM, Penry JK, Schmidt RP, eds. *Antiepileptic drugs.* New York: Raven Press, 1972:257–268.

53. Yunis AA, Arimura BK, Lutcher CL, et al. Biochemical lesion in Dilantin-induced erythroid aplasia. *Blood* 1967;30:587–600.

54. Hofman WW. Cerebellar lesions after parenteral dilantin administration. *Neurology* 1958;9:210–214.

55. Rosenberg IH, Streiff RR, Goodwin HA, et al. Impairment of intestinal deconjugation of dietary folate: a possible explanation of megaloblastic anemia associated with phenytoin therapy. *Lancet* 1968;2:530–532.

56. Sorel TC, Forbes IJ, Burness FR, et al. Depression of immunologic function in patients treated with phenytoin sodium (sodium diphenylhydantoin) *Lancet* 1971;2:1233–1235.

57. Bardana EJ, Gaboourel JD, Davies GH, et al. Effect of phenytoin on man's immunity. *Am J Med* 1983;74:289–296.

58. Ruff ME, Pincus LG, Sampson PA. Phenytoin-induced IgA depression. *Am J Dis Child* 1987;141:858–861.

59. Shakir RA, Behan PO, Dick H, et al. Metabolism of immunoglobulin A_1 lymphocyte function and histocompatability antigens in patients on anticonvulsants. *J Neurol Neurosurg Psychiatry* 1978;41:307–311.

60. Ooi BS, Kant KS, Hanenson IB, et al. Lymphocytotoxins in epileptic patients receiving phenytoin. *Clin Exp Immunol* 1977;30:56–61.

61. Delgado-Escueta AV, Janz D, Beck-Mannagetta G. Pregnancy and teratogenesis in epilepsy. *Neurology* 1992;42[Suppl 5]:S8–S16.

62. Waters CH, Belai Y, Gott PS, et al. Outcomes of pregnancy associated with antiepileptic drugs. *Arch Neurol* 1994;51[Suppl 3]:250–253.

63. Jick SS, Terris B. Anticonvulsants and congenital malformations. *Pharmacotherapy* 1997;17:561-00564.

64. Olafsson E, Halgrimsson JT, Hauser WA, et a. Pregnacies of women with epilepsy: a population-based study in Iceland. *Epilepsia* 1998;39:88700-892.

65. Canger B, Battino D, Canevini MP, et al. Malformations in offspring of women with epilepsy: a prospective study. *Epilepsia* 1999;40:1231-001236.

66. Hanson JH, Smith DW. Fetal hydantoin syndrome. *J Pediatr* 1975;87:28500-290.

67. Dravet C, Julian C, Legras C, et al. Epilepsy, antiepileptic drugs, and malformations in children of women with epilepsy: a French prospective cohort study. *Neurology* 1992;42[Suppl 5]:7500-82.

68. Gailey E, Granstrom M-L. Minor anomalies in children of mothers with epilepsy. *Neurology* 1992;42[Suppl 5]:128-00131.

69. Tanganelli P, Regesta G. Epilepsy, pregnancy, and major birth anomalies: an Italian prospective controlled study. *Neurology* 1992;42[Suppl 5]:89–93.

70. Yerby MS, Leavitt A, Erickson DM, et al. Antiepileptics and the development of congenital anomalies. *Neurology* 1992;42[Suppl 5]:132–140.

71. Buehler BA, Delimont D, Van Waes M, et al. Prenatal prediction of risk of the fetal hydantoin syndrome. *N Engl J Med* 1990;332:1567–1572.

72. Dansky LV, Rosenblatt DS, Andermann E. Mechanisms of teratogenesis: folic acid and antiepileptic therapy. *Neurology* 1992;42[Suppl 5]:32–42.

73. Finnell RH, Kerr BM, Van Waes, et al. Protection from phenytoin-induced congenital malformations by coadministration of the antiepileptic drug stiripentol in a mouse model. *Epilepsia* 1994;35:141–147.

74. Lindhout D. Pharmacogenetics and drug interactions: role in antiepileptic drugs induced teratogenesis. *Neurology* 1992;42[Suppl 5]:43—47.

75. Delgado-Escueta AV, Janz D. Consensus guidelines: preconception counselling, management, and care of the pregnant woman with epilepsy. *Neurology* 1992;42[Suppl 5]:149–160.

76. Zahn C. Neurologic care of pregnant women with epilepsy. *Epilepsia* 1998;39[Suppl 8]:S26–S31.

77. Report on the Quality Standards Committee of the American Academy of Neyrology. Practice parameters: management issue for women with epilepsy. *Neurology* 1998;51;944–948.

78. Biton V, Gates JR, Her FJ, et al. Adjunctive therapy for intractable epilepsy with ethotoin. *Epilepsia* 1990;31:433–437.

79. Finnell RH, Diliberti JH. Hydantoin-induced teratogenesis: are arene oxide intermediates really responsible? *Helv Paediatr Acta* 1983;38:171–177.

80. Zablen M, Brand N. Cleft lip and cleft palate with the anticonvulsant ethotoin. *N Engl J Med* 1977;297:1404.

81. Troupin AS. Mephenytoin. In: Resor SD Jr, Kutt H, eds. *The medical treatment of epilepsy.* New York: Marcel Dekker, 1992:399–404.

82. Nakamura E, Goto F, Ray WA, et al. Interethnic differences in genetic polymorphism of debrisoquin and mephenytoin hydroxylation between Japanese and Caucasian populations. *Chin Pharmacol Ther* 1985;38:402–408.

PHENYTOIN AND OTHER HYDANTOINS

FOSPHENYTOIN

FLAVIA M. PRYOR
R. EUGENE RAMSAY

BACKGROUND

Fosphenytoin sodium (Cerebyx, Parke-Davis) is the disodium phosphate ester of 3-hydroxymethyl-5,5-diphenylhydantoin (Figure 64.1). It was originally formulated in the early 1970s and was subsequently marketed as a replacement for parenteral phenytoin (PHT; Dilantin) (2).

Fosphenytoin is a phosphate ester prodrug of PHT. The phosphate moiety is rapidly and completely (conversion half-life of ~8 to 15 minutes) hydrolyzed by phosphatases found in blood and vascularized tissue such as muscle (Figure 64.2). There is little interindividual variability (2–11), and it is not dependent on plasma fosphenytoin or PHT concentrations (2,4,9,12,13). The conversion of fosphenytoin to PHT is not influenced by age, race, or gender (14). Administration of fosphenytoin by the intravenous (i.v.) route appears to be better tolerated than PHT administered parenterally (15).

PHYSICAL AND CHEMICAL PROPERTIES

Fosphenytoin has a molecular weight of 406.24 and consists of an off-white congregated powder. Its water solubility at 37°C is 7.5×10^4 µg/mL (compared with 20.5 µg/mL for PHT) (2). Dosages of fosphenytoin are expressed as PHT equivalents (PE), a term that refers to the mg of active PHT delivered as fosphenytoin. Thus, 150 mg of fosphenytoin is equivalent to 100 mg PE, which is equivalent to 100 mg of parenteral PHT. Fosphenytoin is available as a ready-mixed solution of 50 mg PE/mL in water for injection USP, tromethamine USP (TRIS), buffer adjusted to

pH 8.6 to 9.0 with either hydrochloric acid NF or sodium hydroxide NF (16). In contrast to fosphenytoin, parenteral PHT requires a chemical vehicle consisting of 40% propylene glycol and 10% ethanol in water adjusted to pH 12 with sodium hydroxide. Local and systemic adverse effects of parenteral PHT have been attributed to the relatively high pH of its chemical vehicle (14,15,17).

Fosphenytoin is a disodium phosphate ester of PHT. The attachment of a large phosphate ester to the central five-membered ring of PHT changes its physical chemical properties and renders it water soluble (18). It has a pH of 8.6 to 9.0 and does not require excipients such as propylene glycol or alcohol to remain in solution (18). The increased water solubility of fosphenytoin obviates the need for the propylene glycol and alcohol, which are required to make PHT water soluble. On entry into the vascular compartment, the phosphate molecule is removed by nonspecific tissue phosphatases, thus converting fosphenytoin into active PHT. The half-life of conversion is 8 to 15 minutes and is the same regardless of dose or fosphenytoin concentration range achieved (4,19). The plasma clearance of fosphenytoin is not dependent on dose administration and is 19.8±1.6 L/hr. The conversion is rapid after an i.v. infusion and is essentially completed within 30 to 45 minutes (4).

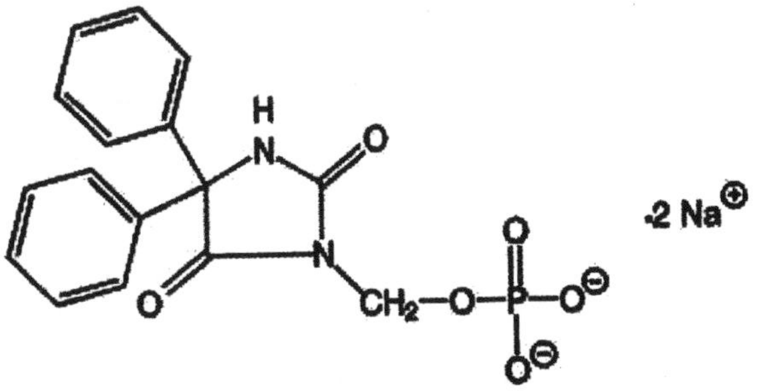

FIGURE 64.1. Structure of fosphenytoin (5,5-diphenyl-3-[(phosphonooxy)methyl]-2,4-imidazolidinedione disodium salt.

R. Eugene Ramsay, MD: Professor of Neurology and Psychiatry, Department of Neurology, University of Miami School of Medicine, Miami, Florida

Flavia M. Pryor, RN, BSN: Nurse Researcher, Department of Neurology Service, Miami Veterans Affairs Medical Center, Miami, Florida

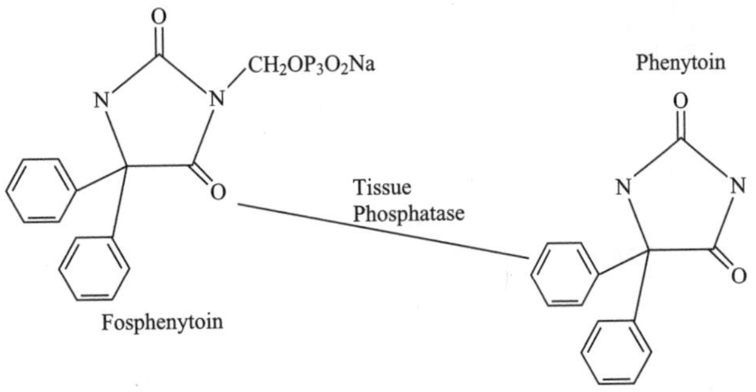

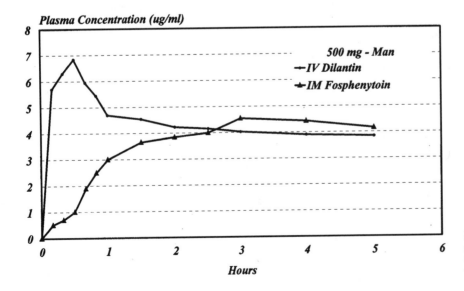

FIGURE 64.2. Conversion of fosphenytoin to phenytoin.

CLINICAL PHARMACOLOGY

Bioavailability

The bioavailability of PHT from fosphenytoin as compared with i.v. PHT sodium was determined in healthy volunteers after i.v. and intramuscular (i.m.) administration of fosphenytoin (12). The mean absolute bioavailability of fosphenytoin was 0.992 after i.v. administration and 1.012 after i.m. injection, a finding demonstrating complete bioavailability irrespective of route of administration. Twelve healthy volunteers were randomized, in a double-blind, crossover fashion to receive PHT sodium and fosphenytoin i.v. in 30 minutes (15). The conversion half-life of fosphenytoin to PHT was 9.3±2.7 minutes. Greater than 99% of fosphenytoin was converted to PHT, and no fosphenytoin was detected in the urine. Fosphenytoin was shown to be bioequivalent to PHT and produced less irritation at the injection site than PHT.

Fosphenytoin is undetectable 4 hours after i.m. injection. Fosphenytoin bioavailability studies have demonstrated i.m. fosphenytoin to be 100% bioavailable (2). Two

hours after administration, the plasma PHT level is essentially the same after equivalent doses of i.v. PHT and i.m. fosphenytoin. Levels >10 μg/mL can be achieved within 45 minutes of i.m. administration of a 20 mg/kg loading dose of fosphenytoin (Figure 64.3). Leppik et al compared the maximum concentration and time to maximum concentration of fosphenytoin administered i.m. on a single site versus two sites (4). For the single injection, the time to maximum concentration was 0.97±1.8 hours compared with 0.32±0.4 hours. The maximum concentration for a single site injection was 8.9 mg/L compared with 16.8 mg/L for two injection sites. Thus, faster and higher peaks are attained after injections at two sites. The tissue phosphatases responsible for the conversion of fosphenytoin to PHT are ubiquitous. Phosphatase activity is present at all ages and the activity is not altered by age, disease states, or medications. Thus, the conversion should be similar in all patients.

Protein Binding

The protein binding and pharmacokinetics of fosphenytoin, diazepam, and PHT were evaluated in nine healthy male volunteers (20). PHT free fraction increased significantly with rising fosphenytoin concentrations, a finding suggesting PHT displacement from its binding sites by fosphenytoin. Fosphenytoin is highly bound (95.7±0.48%) to serum proteins, predominantly albumin. Increased clearance of fosphenytoin may occur in hypoalbuminemia (21). Fosphenytoin competes with PHT for binding sites. Rapid infusion rates (50 to 150 mg/min) of fosphenytoin at relatively high doses (≥15 mg/kg) will result in increased PHT unbound fraction (22). However, PHT binding stabilizes as plasma fosphenytoin concentrations decline (30 to 60 minutes after infusion).

FIGURE 64.3. Plasma phenytoin levels after administration of 500 mg phenytoin (Dilantin) intravenously *(filled boxes)* or 500 mg fosphenytoin intramuscularly *(filled wedges)*.

Distribution

The volume of distribution of fosphenytoin was evaluated in two pharmacokinetic studies. Fosphenytoin was administered by the i.v. route over 30 minutes using doses of 150, 300, 600, and 1,200 mg to four different groups of volunteers (3). The area under the curve (AUC) was 10, 19, 43, and 55 mg/hr/L respectively, and it was proportional to dose. Total clearance was 14 L/hr and was independent of dose. The volume of distribution was approximately 2.6 L, a finding suggesting the most of the dose remained in plasma. Ten patients (one female and nine male patients) received a single i.v. dose of 100 to 200 mg PE, and an equivalent i.m. dose was administered 1 week later (6). The volume of distribution for the i.v. dose was 0.040±0.0084 L/kg, with a conversion half-life of 8.0±2.9 minutes. Mean clearance overall was 0.24±0.080 L/kg/hr in the 10 patients. The volume of distribution was 2.8 L in this group of patients, similar to that previously reported in healthy volunteers.

Chemical Stability

Admixtures of fosphenytoin 1, 8, and 20 mg with sodium chloride 0.9% injection, dextrose 5%, and 11 other i.v. solutions were prepared and stored at −20°C in glass or polyvinyl chloride containers for 7 days (23). Additionally, 63 syringes were filled with fosphenytoin sodium 50 mg PE/mL (undiluted) and were stored at 25°, 4°, or −20°C. There were no discernible changes in color or clarity in any of the fosphenytoin solutions throughout the study. No visible precipitation was observed. Fosphenytoin concentrations remained stable at each sampling, regardless of container, concentration, i.v. solution, or storage temperature. Fosphenytoin remains stable for at least 30 days at room temperature, under refrigeration, or frozen. Furthermore, solutions of fosphenytoin in numerous different i.v. fluids were stable for at least 7 days at room temperature. Findings from a subsequent study indicate that fosphenytoin remains physically stable from at least 2 years at 25°C in pH ranging from 7.4 to 8.0 (24).

Intramuscular Clinical Trials

Of 882 patients and subjects involved in the clinical trials with fosphenytoin, 411 received i.m. injections. These include pharmacokinetics, dosage maintenance, and loading dose studies. In a double-blind parallel study, 240 patients were randomized to receive either oral PHT and i.m. placebo (n = 61) or oral placebo and i.m. fosphenytoin (n = 179) (25). This study was conducted in patients receiving oral PHT once a day for the treatment of epilepsy or seizure prophylaxis after neurosurgery. The dose given to each patient remained constant throughout the study. The fosphenytoin dose for each patient provided an equivalent amount of PHT as the dose of PHT taken during the baseline period. The trough plasma levels remained the same during open baseline and the double-blind treatment phase. The injection sites were evaluated for pain, burning, and itching after the loading and maintenance doses. The rating scale was none (score = 0), mild (score = l), moderate (score = 2), and severe (score = 3). No severe reactions were reported. The average score 5 minutes after injection was less than 0.3 for all measures, except pain in the i.m. placebo group, which was 0.51. There was no difference in the scores for i.m. fosphenytoin and placebo for burning or itching. In a subset of 13 of the patients participating in this trial, serial timed plasma levels were drawn after oral PHT during baseline and on the last day of i.m. fosphenytoin administration during the blinded treatment period (11). The average plasma level as measured by the AUC of the plasma level versus time was higher with i.m. fosphenytoin (AUC = 418) than with oral PHT (AUC = 400), but this difference was not clinically significant. The trough plasma level at 24 hours was the same for both groups.

A prospective open-label study on the safety, tolerance, and pharmacokinetics was conducted in 118 patients (26). Neurosurgical patients ≥12 years old who were to be treated with PHT were included. Patients were given an i.m. loading dose of fosphenytoin (8 to 12 mg/kg), after which timed plasma samples were obtained for total and free fosphenytoin and PHT concentrations. The initial dose administered ranged from 480 to 1,500 mg (8 to 22 mg/kg). By the time the first PHT sample was drawn at 1 hour after administration, the total level was 11 μg/mL and the free PHT level was ~1.5 μg/mL. Over the next 2 to 14 days, these patients were given maintenance doses of fosphenytoin that ranged from 130 to 1,250 mg/day (1.7 to 17.2 mg/kg/day). The duration of maintenance treatment varies: 98.8% (n = 116) of the patients received 2 days and 14.4% (n = 17) received 7 days of i.m. fosphenytoin. Trough plasma levels were obtained and remained stable. The injection sites were evaluated daily, with 96% of the patients reporting no discomfort or pain after the loading dose. At the end of the maintenance period, 98% of the patients reported no injection site discomfort. No adverse reactions were noted from the i.m. administration of fosphenytoin. These authors demonstrated the rapid and consistent attainment of therapeutic plasma total and free PHT after i.m. fosphenytoin.

The experiences derived from these studies indicate that dosage adjustments are not usually necessary when one converts from oral PHT to i.m. fosphenytoin for 1 to 2 weeks. The plasma total and free PHT concentrations were maintained in the therapeutic range after conversion from oral PHT to equimolar i.m. fosphenytoin. A 100-mg PHT (Dilantin) capsule actually contains 92 mg PHT, whereas the i.v. preparation actually contains 100 mg PHT per 1.0 mL of solution. Longer-term maintenance on fosphenytoin could result in some increase in the plasma level. The plasma level should be checked after 2 or more weeks of i.m. or i.v. fosphenytoin therapy.

The safety and tolerance of i.m. fosphenytoin were tested in 60 patients (35 male and 25 female patients) requiring a loading dose of PHT (27). The mean age of patients was 43 years (range, 16 to 80 years); their mean weight was 79 kg (range, 40 to 146 kg). Reasons justifying the use of a loading dose included the following: noncompliance, 18%; first-time PHT treatment, 30%; decreased phenytoin serum levels, 37%; other factors, 15%. A dose of 20 mg/kg of PHT was given to patients with nondetectable plasma levels. Those with a plasma level <7.1 μg/mL were included in the study and were given a loading dose of 15 mg/kg. The mean loading dose administered was 17.7 mg/kg (range, 5.4 to 30.3 mg/kg) for a mean total dose of 1,359.8 mg (range, 525 to 2,250 mg). Most loading doses required 15 to 20 mL of fosphenytoin solution. Fosphenytoin was given as a single site injection in 29 cases, and multiple injection sites were used in the remaining 31 cases. Site of administration was the gluteus in 58 cases and the deltoid in two cases. Despite the relatively large volume of the i.m. injection, patients had no unusual discomfort or side effects with gluteal or deltoid injections. Local irritation at the site of injection occurred in 5% of patients and was considered mild in each case. No serious local adverse reactions were noted. The largest volume injected was 30 mL, which was given into a single muscle site. This patient reported no pain, burning, or discomfort, and this finding attests to how well i.m. fosphenytoin is tolerated. Forty patients reported experiencing some adverse events after the i.m. injection, with the most frequent being nystagmus (47%), dizziness (17%), and ataxia (13%).

Eighty-two percent of the adverse events reported were considered mild. The nature and frequency of side effects reported after i.m. loading of fosphenytoin were similar to those experienced after i.v. PHT.

The rate and extent of absorption and the tolerability of i.m. fosphenytoin were evaluated in an open-label, double-blind study (28). Twenty-four patients, 12 male and 12 female, were enrolled. Patients selected required a loading dose of PHT for the treatment of epilepsy or for seizure prophylaxis, or they volunteered to participate in the study. Each patient received 10 mg/kg of fosphenytoin i.m. and a saline injection to compare tolerability. Half of the patients received a volume of saline equal to that of the fosphenytoin, whereas the other half received only 2 mL of saline. The group ranged in age from 19 to 60 years (mean, 35±10 standard deviation years). Weight ranged from 49.1 to 97.3 kg (mean, 79.4±13.9 standard deviation kg). Doses of fosphenytoin ranged from 491 to 973 mg PE, which corresponded to injection volumes ranging from 9.8 to 19.5 mL. The accepted loading dose of fosphenytoin is 20 mg PE/kg, which corresponds to injection volumes ranging from 20 to 40 mL. Typically, this full loading dose is divided into two injection of 10 mg/kg each. Because study participants would be receiving saline injections on the opposite side for tolerability comparison, we used a loading dose of 10 mg/kg to abide by standard clinical practice and to avoid multiple injections of fosphenytoin. Therapeutic serum concentrations of PHT were achieved as early as 5 minutes after the i.m. administration of fosphenytoin in 14.3% of patients and in 26.3% after 10 minutes. By 20 minutes, 37% of the patients had achieved PHT serum concentra-

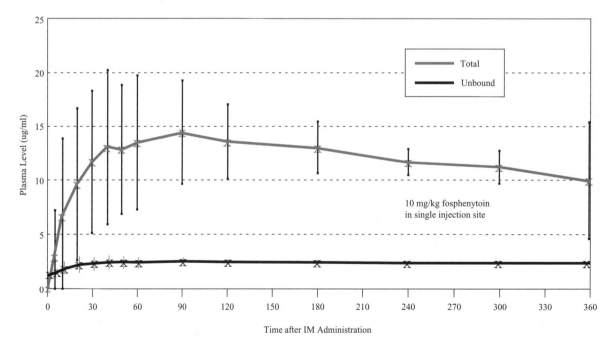

FIGURE 64.4. Intramuscular fosphenytoin total and free levels.

tions >10 μ/mL. More than half the patients had therapeutic serum concentrations at 30 minutes. Nearly 40% of patients had a free PHT level of 1.0 μg/mL by 40 minutes. At 50 minutes, 14 of 18 patients had achieved unbound PHT levels of ≥1.0 μg/mL (Figure 64.4). There was a statistically significant difference in pain between the fosphenytoin and saline sides immediately after injection and at 30 minutes (X^2 = .0386 and X^2 = .0386, respectively). However, there was no significant difference in pain at 60 minutes and thereafter. Fosphenytoin injections were slightly more uncomfortable than saline injections; however, volume did not appear to be the determining factor. These investigators demonstrated that i.m. administration of fosphenytoin produces therapeutic PHT serum concentrations very rapidly (as early as 5 to 20 minutes), and it is well tolerated by most patients irrespective of injection volume.

POTENTIAL CLINICAL USES FOR INTRAMUSCULAR FOSPHENYTOIN

Despite the efficacy of i.v. PHT in the treatment of status epilepticus and acute seizures, the potential side effects of the i.v. formulation have limited its use to situations in which adequate venous access is secured and appropriate monitoring systems are available. Fosphenytoin can be safely given i.m. by rescue squads in the field or at home by family members. It is rapidly absorbed and has a sustained serum half-life. The availability of fosphenytoin has the potential to revolutionize the way we treat serial seizures and tonic-clonic status epilepticus.

INTRAVENOUS CLINICAL TRIALS

The pharmacokinetics, safety, and tolerance of i.v. fosphenytoin were investigated in 17 clinical studies. Of 925 patients and subjects involved in fosphenytoin clinical trials, 514 received i.v. injections. Nine clinical trials involving 136 healthy subjects were completed using doses of 100 to 1,200 mg and infusion rates of 3.3 to 150 mg/min. Fosphenytoin, total PHT, and free PHT concentrations and pharmacokinetic parameters were similar in patients and in healthy subjects. Plasma fosphenytoin concentration increases with increasing dose and infusion rate, peaks at the end of infusion, and then declines with a half-life of ~0.25 hour. The half-life is independent of dose and infusion rate (19). With the addition of the phosphate moiety to the PHT molecule, fosphenytoin weighs more than PHT. A dose of 150 mg of fosphenytoin is equivalent to 100 mg of PHT, and both are described as being equal in molar quantities of PHT. Dosing can be reported in actual weight of fosphenytoin or as PE, which refers on a one-to-one basis to a dose of PHT.

A total of 378 patients received fosphenytoin in doses ranging from 205 to 2,280 mg (2.7 to 20.3 mg/kg) of PE and infusion rates of 3.3 to 167 mg PE/min. To investigate bioequivalence, 43 patients with chronic epilepsy were entered into an open-labeled, single-dose safety and pharmacokinetic study (4). These patients had been treated with PHT with documented stable levels. Mean trough PHT levels were the same after oral PHT, i.v. fosphenytoin, and i.m. fosphenytoin. Analysis of electrocardiograms revealed no significant change in RR, PR, QRS, and QT intervals and no disturbances of cardiac rhythms after i.v. administration of fosphenytoin. Minor and transient discomfort was reported with i.v. infusion (17%) and i.m. injection (14%).

To compare the safety and tolerance of i.v. fosphenytoin, a single-dose, double-blind study was conducted in patients requiring a loading dose of PHT (29). Fifty-two patients were randomized to receive either i.v. fosphenytoin (n = 39) or i.v. PHT (n = 13). Patients in the treatment group received similar doses of study drug (899 mg PE; 12.7 mg/kg) or PHT (879 mg; 11.3 mg/kg). However, the fosphenytoin was infused at nearly twice the rate of administration (82 mg PE/min; range, 40 to 103 mg PE/min) compared with patients in the PHT group (42.4 mg/min). Despite the higher rate of infusion, fosphenytoin was well tolerated and produced no significant cardiac arrhythmias or changes in heart rate, respiration, or diastolic blood pressure. A decline in systolic blood pressure occurred and was reported to be statistically but not clinically significant. A similar study was subsequently conducted, but patients were given maintenance doses of i.v. fosphenytoin or i.v. PHT for 3 to 14 days after receiving a loading dose (30). Patients were randomized to receive i.v. fosphenytoin (n = 88; mean dose, 1,088 mg PE or 15.3 mg PE/kg) or i.v. PHT (n = 28; mean dose, 1,082 mg or l5.0 mg/kg). Maintenance therapy was given for >4 days (fosphenytoin for 4.3 days; PHT for 4.7 days). Similar infusion rates were used (fosphenytoin, 37 mg PE/min; PHT, 33 mg/min). A significantly greater number of patients reported pain in the infusion site with PHT (17%) compared with fosphenytoin (2%). No electrocardiographic changes were found. Reduction in systolic and diastolic blood pressure was reported in five patients in both groups. However, symptomatic hypotension requiring reduction in infusion rates occurred four times more often with i.v. PHT (n = 4; 17.9%). A subset of 10 patients had serial timed total and free plasma fosphenytoin and PHT levels drawn after the loading dose. At the first sample drawn at 1 hour after infusion, all patients had total PHT levels >10 μg/mL, and the mean concentrations were essentially the same for the two groups.

PEDIATRIC POPULATIONS

In a retrospective study, 52 pediatric patients who received fosphenytoin i.v. therapy for seizures were evaluated (31). Age ranged from 4 days to 16 years of age. PHT serum levels were maintained within the therapeutic range (10 to 20 µg/mL). No infusion site complications were reported in any of the patients. Only one patient experienced cardiac arrhythmia from an accidental overdose. Eight neonates (1 to 146 days old) received i.v. fosphenytoin for the treatment of status epilepticus (32). In six patients, treatment with phenobarbital had failed. Of these six patients, two had received lorazepam as well. Loading doses of fosphenytoin PE ranged from 14.5 to 24.3 mg/kg. Seven of the eight patients achieved therapeutic PHT levels. Complete seizure control was obtained in 50%. No side effects were observed in any of the patients.

CLINICAL EFFICACY

Status Epilepticus

PHT given by the i.v. route has been the mainstay of the treatment of status epilepticus. The previously described studies used fosphenytoin infusion rates of approximately 100 mg PE/min. At this rate, the free PHT levels reached were less than that those achieved with 50 mg/min of PHT, a rate commonly employed in the treatment of status epilepticus. Fosphenytoin must be given at 150 mg PE/min to produce a free PHT level bioequivalent to that produced by 50 mg/min of PHT. Thus, additional clinical experience was needed in the area of status epilepticus with faster rates of infusion.

The treatment of overt status epilepticus was evaluated in a Veterans Affairs Cooperative Study (33). The highest treatment success rate was obtained with parenteral lorazepam (64.9%), followed by phenobarbital (58.2%), diazepam/PHT (55.8%), and PHT alone (43.6%). Based on these findings, the recommended first-line treatment for generalized convulsive status epilepticus is i.v. lorazepam. Fosphenytoin or PHT is still recommended as a second-line agent if status epilepticus is not controlled within 5 to 7 minutes (34).

A double-blind parallel safety and tolerance study was conducted comparing i.v. fosphenytoin given at 150 mg PE/min versus PHT at 50 mg/min (27). Patients were randomized on a 4:1 basis to receive i.v. fosphenytoin (n = 90) or PHT (n = 22). The loading dose was either 20 mg/kg (patients with no detectable PHT in the plasma) or 15 mg/kg if the plasma PHT level was ≤7µg/mL. The most common reasons for patient inclusion were treatment of acute seizures, low PHT levels in patients with epilepsy, or seizure prophylaxis in neurosurgical patients. Patient demographics were similar between the fosphenytoin and PHT groups. Infusions had to be slowed or discontinued significantly more often with i.v. PHT than with fosphenytoin. Adverse events with the two drugs were different, with pruritus, at times very uncomfortable, more common with fosphenytoin (48.9%) and pain at the site of infusion more frequently reported with PHT (63.6%). The other side

effects of dizziness, somnolence, and ataxia are typical of PHT and were the same for both drugs. The pruritus associated with fosphenytoin typically occurred in the trunk, especially in the groin region, or at the back of the head. Pruritus, when reported, presented soon after initiation of the infusion and abated rapidly when the infusion was discontinued. The occurrence and severity of the pruritus were rate-dependent phenomena because lowering the rate reduced or abolished the symptom. Changes in blood pressure were noted in both groups, with a mean decline in systolic pressure of 13.7 mm Hg with fosphenytoin and 5.9 mm Hg with PHT. By this one measure, the decrease was statistically more common with fosphenytoin, but it was not believed to be clinically significant. Direct cardiovascular effects in this study were difficult to compare because the duration of infusions were different (fosphenytoin, 13 minutes; PHT, 44 minutes). Blood pressure changes occurred 10 to 20 minutes after the initiation of the i.v. infusion. The decrease in systolic blood pressure was gradual and lasted for 10 to 15 minutes. Patients with preexisting hypertension and who were being treated with antihypertensives were at increased risk (13 of 16) of a systolic blood pressure decline of 20 mm Hg or more. There was no association between specific antihypertensive medication and a drop in systolic blood pressure. Patients with underlying ischemic heart disease also seemed to be at increased risk of a mild decline in blood pressure (9 of 13). In no case was the hypotension judged severe enough to justify discontinuation of treatment, although the i.v. infusion rate was reduced in a total of six patients (fosphenytoin, four patients or 4.7%; PHT, two patients or 9. 1%). Several clinically unstable ICU patients with neurosurgical, neurologic, or cardiac problems were included in the protocol. These patients tolerated the rapid infusions of i.v. fosphenytoin without clinically significant changes in blood pressure or cardiac arrhythmias.

An open-label, single-dose, safety, tolerance, and pharmacokinetic trial of fosphenytoin was completed in 85 patients in convulsive status epilepticus (35). Infusion rates of 100 mg/min were used in the first 10 patients, and rates of 150 mg/min were used in the remaining 75 patients. Patients ≥5 years old who had two or more generalized convulsions without regaining consciousness between seizures were included. The study included 10 patients <16 years of age (mean, 7.6 years) and 75 patients ranging from 18 to 82 years of age (mean, 43.7 years). Applying the same criteria used in the Veterans Affairs Cooperative Study 265 on status epilepticus (33), seizures were controlled in 79 (92.3%) patients with fosphenytoin. Only two patients experienced seizure recurrence within the next 24 hours. Three patients did not have their seizures controlled, and one was not evaluated because of the inadequate dose given (2 mg PE/kg). The mean dose administered was 967 mg PE (16.4 mg PE/kg) and ranged from 216 to 2,000 mg PE (8.2 to 26.1 mg PE/kg). The mean rate of infusion was 2.6 mg/kg/min in children and 135 mg

PE/min (36.4 to 218 mg PE/min) in adults. The mean duration of the i.v. infusion was 11 minutes. The infusion rate was not reduced in any patient. Hypotension, which has been a concern with high-dose high-rate infusion of i.v. PHT, was not encountered. Significantly higher free PHT levels were obtained in patients receiving fosphenytoin 20 mg/kg at 150 mg/min, with more than half having free levels ranging from 5 to 20 μg/mL. These levels are much higher than achieved using the same loading dose of parenteral PHT and may explain the better rate of control of status epilepticus. Blood samples were drawn at the conclusion of the infusion. Free levels >5 μg/mL were achieved in the majority of the patients, and this is likely the reason for the greater efficacy found in this study. No cardiac arrhythmias were observed, and no adjustments in infusion rates were required because of changes in vital signs. Some decline in blood pressure was observed during or after the infusion but was not judged to be clinically significant. At follow-up evaluation 24 hours later, only 3% of the patients reported tenderness at the infusion site, and no inflammation or phlebitis was found.

COST CONSIDERATIONS

The cost effectiveness of using parenteral fosphenytoin versus PHT for the treatment of acute seizures and status epilepticus remains a controversial issue. The cost per package for fosphenytoin is approximately 26 times greater than that for parenteral PHT (based on Parke-Davis catalog prices) (36). However, other factors must be considered in determining cost effectiveness of a prescription. Marchetti et al. (1996) conducted a multicenter, double-blind, parallel group study to evaluate costs of administering i.v. fosphenytoin versus i.v. PHT in emergency departments (37). Fifty-two patients were enrolled; 39 were randomized to the i.v. fosphenytoin group and 13 to the i.v. PHT group. The acquisition cost per loading dose was significantly higher for fosphenytoin ($90.00) compared with PHT ($6.72). The average wholesale price for PHT was $1.68 per package, and it was $45.00 per package for fosphenytoin (500-mg equivalent of phenytoin). Total adverse event monitoring costs were $536.86 for i.v. PHT versus $66.20 for i.v. fosphenytoin. The most common side effects reported with the use of PHT were significant neurologic toxicity (moderate to severe ataxia or vertigo), severe i.v. site reaction, and symptomatic decrease in blood pressure (>20 mm Hg systolic). Only the last side effect was reported with fosphenytoin. The adverse events resulted in higher use of resources. There was a significant cost savings of $386.89 (11%) with i.v. fosphenytoin compared with i.v. PHT, primarily based on the less favorable side effect profile of PHT.

Armstrong et al. (1999) developed a model of cost and clinical outcomes to compare the cost effectiveness of parenteral PHT versus fosphenytoin (38). The data were collected using a questionnaire. This model assumed that 50%

of PHT would be replaced by fosphenytoin. They calculated mean cost-effectiveness ratios (defined as the cost to achieve the desired goal of administering a loading dose without complication) for PHT alone, for fosphenytoin plus PHT (50% fosphenytoin and 50% PHT), and for fosphenytoin alone. The average cost of a loading dose of PHT ($58) was less than the average cost of both 50%-50% fosphenytoin-PHT ($94) and fosphenytoin alone ($130). However, the average cost-effectiveness ratios were $225 for PHT, $149 for the 50%-50% option, and $130 for fosphenytoin alone. PHT-induced peripheral vascular failure (phlebitis-type effects) frequently required central line placement. In the PHT group, 62.3±43.4% of patients receiving loading doses and 74.0±32.9% receiving maintenance doses experienced venous irritation. In the fosphenytoin group, side effects were uncommon (0.3±1.0%). These investigators concluded that institutions with comparable drug costs should consider replacing PHT with fosphenytoin for loading and maintenance doses, primarily based on the reduction of side effects. Further pharmacoeconomic studies are needed to define more precisely the cost effectiveness of replacing parenteral PHT with fosphenytoin. However, present information indicates that fosphenytoin is most cost effective.

CONCLUSION

PHT is a very effective anticonvulsant, and despite significant problems with its parenteral formulation, it has been the mainstay of the treatment of various forms of acute seizures for many decades. In contrast to parenteral PHT, fosphenytoin does not need propylene glycol and alcohol vehicles for water solubility, so it is a much safer and better-tolerated preparation. PHT and fosphenytoin have identical therapeutic profiles. However, because much higher unbound PHT can be achieved when a loading dose of fosphenytoin is infused at the maximal approved rate, fosphenytoin appears to be more effective in status epilepticus. Given the risks associated with the use of parenteral PHT, fosphenytoin should entirely replace PHT in all its present i.v. indications. Moreover, the safety and tolerability of i.m. fosphenytoin extend its use to other clinical situations in which prompt administration of a nondepressing anticonvulsant is indicated but secure i.v. access and cardiac monitoring are not available such as in the following situations: (a) in the treatment of tonic-clonic status epilepticus by rescue workers in the field; (b) in the management of serial seizures in patients with intractable epilepsy; and (c) possibly in the treatment of acute ischemic stroke.

REFERENCES

1. Stella VJ, Higuchi T. Esters of hydantoic acid as prodrugs of hydantoins. *J Pharmacol Sci* 1973;62:962–962.

2. Browne TR, Szabo GK, McGovern J. Bioavailability studies of drugs with nonlinear pharmacokinetics. II. Absolute bioavailability of intravenous phenytoin prodrug at therapeutic phenytoin serum concentration determined by double stable isotope technique. *J Pharmacol Sci* 1993;33:89–94.

3. Gerber N, Mays DC, Donn KH. Safety, tolerance, and pharmacokinetics of intravenous doses of phosphate ester of 3-hydroxymethyl-5-diphenyl hydantoin: a new prodrug of phenytoin. *J Clin Pharmacol* 1988;28:1023–1032.

4. Leppik IE, Boucher BA, Wilder BJ, et al. Pharmacokinetics and safety of a phenytoin prodrug given IV in patients. *Neurology* 1990;40:456–460.

5. Browne TR, Le Duc B. Phenytoin and fosphenytoin: biotransformation. In: Levy RY, Mattson R, Meldrum BS, eds. *Antiepileptic drugs,* 4th ed. New York: Raven Press, 1995:283–300.

6. Boucher BA, Bombassaro A, Rasmussen SN, et al. Phenytoin prodrug 3-phosphoryloxy-methyl phenytoin (ACC-9653): pharmacokinetics in patients following intravenous and intramuscular administration. *J Pharmacol Sci* 1989;78:929–932.

7. Eldon MA, Loewen GR, Voigtman RE, et al. Safety, tolerance, and pharmacokinetics of intravenous fosphenytoin. Clinical Pharmacological Therapy 1993;53:212–212.

8. Aweeka F, Alldredge B, Boyer T, et al. Conversion of ACC-9653 to phenytoin in patients with renal or hepatic diseases. *Clin Pharmacol Ther* 1989;45:152–152.

9. Broumer K, Matier WL, Quon CY. Absolute bioavailability of phenytoin after IV 3-phosphoryloxymethyl phenytoin disodium. *Clin Pharmacol Ther* 1988;43:178–178.

10. Boucher BA, Kugler AR, Hess MM, et al. Pharmacokinetics of fosphenytoin, a phenytoin prodrug, following intramuscular administration in critically ill neurosurgery patients. *Crit Care Med* 1995;23:A78–A78.

11. Garnett WR, Kugler AR, O'Hara KA, et al. Pharmacokinetics of fosphenytoin following intramuscular administration of fosphenytoin substituted for oral phenytoin in epileptic patients. *Neurology* 1995;45:A248.

12. Browne TR, Davoudi H, Donn KH, et al. Bioavailability of ACC-9653 (phenytoin prodrug). *Epilepsia* 1989;30:S27–S32.

13. Eldon MA, Loewen GR, Voigtman RE, et al. Pharmacokinetics and tolerance of fosphenytoin and phenytoin administered intravenously to healthy subjects. *Can J Neurol Sci* 1993;20:S180–S180.

14. Kugler AR, Knapp LE, Eldon MA. Intravenous administration of fosphenytoin: pharmacokinetics and dosing considerations in special populations. *Epilepsia* 1996;37:156.

15. Jamerson B. Venous irritation related to intravenous administration of phenytoin versus fosphenytoin. *Pharmacotherapy* 1994;14:47–52.

16. Parke-Davis. *Cerebyx injection.* Package insert. Parke-Davis, 1998.

17. Hanna DR. Purple glove syndrome: a complication of intravenous phenytoin. *J Neurosci Nurs* 1992;24:340–345.

18. Smith RD, Brown BS, Maher RW, et al. Pharmacology of ACC-9653 (phenytoin prodrug)). *Epilepsia* 1989;30[Suppl 2]:S15–S21.

19. Besserer J, Cook J, Eldon M. A randomized, double blind, placebo controlled, rising single dose study of the pharmacokinetic and tolerance profiles of intravenous fosphenytoin sodium (CI-982) administered at five different infusion rates to healthy subjects. Unpublished data, 1994.

20. Hussey EK, Dukes GE, Messenheimer JA, et al. Evaluation of the pharmacokinetic interaction between diasepam and ACC-9653 (a phenytoin prodrug) in healthy male volunteers. *Pharm Res* 1990;7:1172–1176.

21. Lai CM, Moore P, Quon CY. Binding of fosphenytoin, phosphate ester pro drug of phenytoin, to human serum proteins and competitive binding with carbamazepine, diazepam, phenobarbital, phenylbutazone, phenytoin, valproic acid or warfarin. *Res Commun Mol Pathol Pharmacol* 1995;88:51–62.

22. Dow M, Barry E, Bell W, et al. A double-blind, placebo-controlledstudy of vigabatrin 3 g/day in patients with uncontrolled complex partial seizures. Pfizer Inc. Data on file, 1995 and 2002.

23. Fischer J, Cwik MJ, Luer MS, et al. Stability of fosphenytoin sodium with intravenous solutions in glass bottles, polyvinyl chloride bags, and polypropylene syringes. *Ann Pharmacother* 1997;31:553–559.

24. Narisawa S, Stella VJ. Increased shelf-life of fosphenytoin: solubilization of a degradant, phenytoin, through complexation with (SBE)7m-beta-CD. *J Pharm Sci* 1998;87:926–930.

25. Wilder BJ, Ramsay RE, Serrano EE, et al. A method for shifting from oral to intramuscular diphenylhydantoin administration. *Clin Pharmacol Ther* 1974;16:507–513.

26. Dean JC, Smith KR, Boucher BA, et al. Safety, tolerance and pharmacokinetics of intramuscular (IM) fosphenytoin, a phenytoin prodrug, in neurosurgery patients. *Epilepsia* 1993;34:111.

27. Ramsay RE, Philbrook B, Martinez OA, et al. A double-blinded, randomized safety comparison of rapidly infused intravenous loading doses of fosphenytoin vs. phenytoin. *Epilepsia* 1995;36 [Suppl 4]:52.

28. Pryor FM, Ramsay RE, Gidal BE, et al. Fosphenytoin: pharmacokinetics and tolerance of intramuscular loading doses. *Epilepsia* 2001;42:245–250.

29. Fischer J, Turnbull T, Uthman BM, et al. Safety, tolerance, pharmacokinetics of intravenous loading doses of fosphenytoin versus Dilantin. *Neurology* 1995;45:A202.

30. Baron BA, Hankin S, Knapp LE. Advantages of intravenous fosphenytoin (Cerebyx) compared with IV phenytoin (Dilantin). *Neurology* 1995;45:248–249.

31. Morton LD, O'Hara KA, Meloche NM, et al. Fosphenytoin experience in pediatric patients. *Epilepsia* 1999;40:131–131.

32. Gustafson MC, Ritter FJ, Minnesota Epilepsy Group PA. Fosphenytoin loading for status epilepticus in the neonate. *Epilepsia* 1999;40:124–124.

33. Treiman DM, Meyers PD, Walton NY, et al. Treatment of generalized convulsive status epilepticus: a randomized double-blind comparison of four intravenous regimens. *N Engl J Med* 1998; 339:792–798.

34. Bleck TP. Management approaches to prolonged seizures and status epilepticus. *Epilepsia* 1999;40[Suppl 1]:S59–S63.

35. Allen FH, Bunge JW, Legarda S, et al. Safety, tolerance and pharmacokinetics of intravenous fosphenytoin (Cerebyx) in status epilepticus. *Epilepsia* 1995;36[Suppl 4]:90.

36. Fierro L, Hudak J. Cost of fosphenytoin. *Ann Emerg Med* 1998; 31:137–138.

37. Marchetti A, Magar R, Fischer J, et al. A pharmacoeconomic evaluation of intravenous fosphenytoin (Cerebyx) versus intravenous phenytoin (Dilantin) in hospital emergency departments. *Clin Ther* 1996;18:953–966.

38. Armstrong EP, Sauer KA, Downey MJ. Phenytoin and fosphenytoin: a model of cost and clinical outcomes. *Pharmacotherapy* 1999;19:844–853.

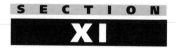

SECTION XI

PRIMIDONE

65

PRIMIDONE

RICHARD W. FINCHAM
DOROTHY D. SCHOTTELIUS

Primidone (PRM) can provide effective treatment for partial or tonic-clonic seizures, singly or as adjunctive therapy. Its clinical use began in 1952 (1), although controlled testing for efficacy waited more than a decade (2–5). Clinical efficacy and toxicity were most extensively evaluated in a double-blind, controlled study published in 1985, with comparison made among phenytoin (PHT), carbamazepine (CBZ), valproic acid (VPA), and PRM in treatment of secondarily generalized seizures (6). PRM was identified as less effective for partial seizures compared with CBZ and possessed the greatest potential for poor tolerability at initiation. It has since been regarded as a drug of second choice in the treatment of epilepsy.

Extensive testing in animal models of epilepsy, such as are required today, did not precede the first use of PRM in treatment of epilepsy in humans (7). Excellent reviews of these studies of PRM are available in Chapters 33 and 34 of the fourth edition of this text, *Antiepileptic Drugs* (8,9). A variant of the standard maximal electroshock seizures (MES) model established pharmacologic and toxic properties of PRM (10). The drug was found to lack potency in chemoconvulsant models of epilepsy such as determined by pentylenetetrazole. This dichotomy in response to two standard animal models of epilepsy indicated a pharmacodynamic effect of PRM leading to inhibition of the spread of seizures, rather than one raising the threshold for their development.

CHEMISTRY AND METABOLISM

PRM (5-ethyldihydro-5 phenyl-4,6-(1H, 5H)-pyrimidedione) was first synthesized and used as an anticonvulsant in 1952 (11). It is a desoxyphenobarbital differing from phenobarbital (PB) by the absence of the carbonyl group in position 2 of the pyrimidine ring (Figure 65.1). Because it contains only two carbonyl groups and not three, PRM is not, *per se,* a barbiturate but is considered clinically in that group.

PRM (molecular weight, 218.25) is an odorless crystalline white powder with a slightly bitter taste and a melting point of 279° to 282°C. Pharmacokinetic properties of PRM are influenced by its physicochemical characteristics, namely, its low solubility in water (600 μg/mL), weak acidity (negative log of dissociation constant, 13), and low lipophilic partition coefficients compared with PB. Quantitative discussions of serum concentrations may involve either micrograms per milliliter or micromoles per liter; therefore, a conversion factor of 4.58 may be used (μg/mL × 4.58 = μmol/L; μmol/L ÷ 4.58 = μg/mL).

The clinical use of PRM requires an understanding of its pharmacokinetics, which is complicated by the presence of two active metabolites: PB and phenylethylmalonamide (PEMA). Figure 65.1 illustrates the primary and most relevant metabolic pathways of PRM. The transformation of PRM to PEMA and PB was not recognized until after the clinical introduction of PRM. Bogue and Carrington (12) identified PEMA as a metabolite in rats, and Butler and Waddell (13) found PB as well as *p*-hydoxyphenobarbital in urine and in the plasma of a dog and a patient receiving PRM. Later, both PEMA and PB were shown to have anticonvulsant properties. Minor metabolites identified include α-phenylbutyramide (14), *p*-hydoxyprimidone (15,16), and α-phenyl-γ-butyrolactone (17), but no evidence indicates that these metabolites have any importance during therapy with PRM. The biotransformation of PRM has been shown to take place in all animals tested, although with variable rates and extent. It is necessary to consider the pharmacokinetics of the two active metabolites along with PRM. PB is discussed in Chapter 51 and is considered only with regard to its influence on PRM; PEMA is considered concurrently.

The rate and extent of absorption of PRM have been studied indirectly in humans because only oral preparations (tablets and syrup) are available. Such studies have indi-

Richard W. Fincham, MD: Deceased, November 11, 2000.
Dorothy D. Schottelius, PhD: Research Scientist, Department of Neurology, University of Iowa, Iowa City, Iowa

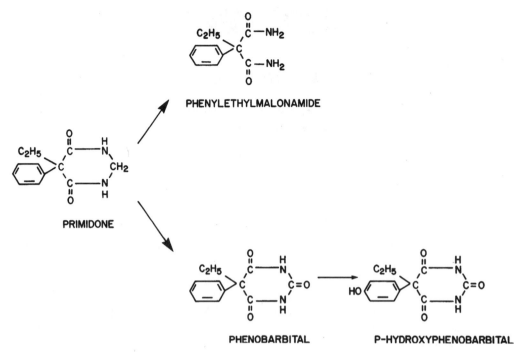

FIGURE 65.1. The main biotransformation pathways of primidone consist of formation of phenylethylmalonamide by ring scission and oxidation to phenobarbital, which is then parahydroxylated.

cated average peak absorption time between 2.7 and 4.2 hours after single-dose administration in adult patients (18,19). In one case, we gave a single 125-mg dose to a woman and found that 60% of the dose was absorbed in 0.5 hour, and the patient complained of minor side effects. A study of ^{14}C-labeled PRM in 10 patients receiving combination therapy indicated that almost 100% of PRM is rapidly absorbed (20). Kauffman et al. (21) studied absorption of PRM in children; an average of 92% of dose was absorbed, with a peak plasma concentration at 4 to 6 hours. All these studies suggest a great deal of variability in the rate and extent of absorption of PRM. Toxicity symptoms associated with the initial dose of PRM are discussed later, in relation to determining dosage schedules for treatment with this drug.

Differences in formulation of PRM may have an influence on rate and extent of absorption, as observed in two instances (22,23). Few studies have been reported on the influence of age, pregnancy, and other diseases or conditions on the rate and extent of absorption of PRM. The bioavailability and peak absorption time for PEMA determined in adult volunteers averaged 91% and 3 hours (24).

The distribution of PRM throughout body tissues and fluids is apparently similar to that of PB (25). Several animal studies (10,26,27) have indicated that PRM enters the brain rapidly, with the brain:plasma ratio remaining constant for ≤2 hours. The distribution of PEMA and PB involves the rate of biotransformation from PRM as well as

their physiochemical properties, with both reaching maximum plasma and brain concentrations 6 to 8 hours after orally administered PRM (27–29). Houghton et al. (30) reported an average brain: serum ratio of 0.87 in humans. PRM was present in muscle, skin, and bone, but this distribution correlated poorly with concentration in plasma.

PRM does not bind significantly to plasma proteins, and several studies using either equilibrium dialysis or ultrafiltration show a range of 9% to 20%. (18,23,27,31–42). Saliva values equal 70% to 80% of total plasma concentrations (21,42–44). PRM concentration in the cerebrospinal fluid (CSF) averages 70% to 100% of that in plasma (31,32,36–41,45); the variance may result from time required for PRM to equilibrate between these fluids. Our data indicated a CSF:serum ratio of 0.6 at a dose-sample interval of 2.6 hours when patients were taking PRM alone or PRM plus PHT (46). When samples were obtained approximately 7.2 hours after administration, the ratio was approximately 0.997. The relatively low penetration of PRM across lipid membranes could account for the time- and flow-related differences in CSF or saliva and plasma ratios. Distribution volumes of PRM have been characterized in patients with means of 0.72 L/kg (20) and 0.65 kg/L (47). The distribution volume for PEMA is similar to that of PRM (37).

Elimination of PRM is highly variable (half-life range, 3.3 to 22.4 hours) because of factors such as age and concomitant therapy (18,19,21,24,47,48). Studies indicate that PRM half-life after a single dose is independent of dose or plasma concentration, a finding consistent with a first-order, linear pharmacokinetic model. Long-term PRM therapy could decrease its half-life for various, such as microsomal enzyme induction, structural similarity of PB and PRM, and the presence of other antiepileptic drugs (AEDs) (18,20,21,40,47,48). When PEMA is administered directly to humans, its half-life ranges from 10 to 25 hours (22,37).

Correlation between PRM daily dose and steady-state concentrations results in large measure from a wide range of clearance found in patients. Clearance is not affected by the size of dose but is altered by concomitant AED therapy with an increase of approximately 50% (28,47). Changes in clearances may also be time dependent, with increases of 30% to 200%, which may be a result of PB-mediated enzyme induction.

The liver appears to be responsible for most of the biotransformation of PRM, although the kidney may also play a role (27,49–52). PRM and its metabolites are primarily eliminated by renal excretion (20), with 75% to 77% of a dose recovered during a 5-day collection period. Patients receiving monotherapy excreted 64% as PRM, whereas those receiving concomitant AED therapy excreted 40% of PRM. Advanced age, pregnancy, lactation, and liver disease may all have an influence on PRM pharmacokinetics, and care must be taken in clinical situations when PRM is used in anticonvulsant therapy.

Biotransformation of PRM to two active metabolites (PB and PEMA; Figure 65.1) illustrates the complexities involved when a drug with pharmacologic activity of its own is converted into active metabolites. The attempts to ascertain the basis of mechanisms of action of PRM were complicated by the uncertainty regarding whether it has independent antiepileptic activity. In long-term therapy with PRM in humans, in all but a few instances (5), PB is present.

In a clinical study of epileptic patients, PRM was found to be more effective than PB against generalized tonic-clonic seizures. Several experiments in animals have shown independent anticonvulsant activity of PRM; dogs were found to be protected against chemically induced seizures at a lower concentration of PB when PRM was also present (53). Rats were protected against induced seizures after a single dose of PRM before the active metabolites were detectable (10); similar seizure protection was achieved in mice and fowl when pretreatment of a liver enzyme inhibitor SKF 52A was used (27,51,52). Some evidence suggests that the anticonvulsant spectra of PRM and PB differ, that is, PRM and PB are equally potent against seizures induced by MES, but against seizures produced chemically, PB is effective but PRM is totally ineffective. Therefore, the two compounds may have different mechanisms of action. PRM has an anticonvulsant spectrum similar to that of CBZ and PHT. A relatively weak anticonvul-

sant activity was found for PEMA in rats (48) as well as in mice (27,51). These experimental results, together with blood levels in patients receiving long-term therapy with PRM, suggest that PEMA contributes little or not at all to the antiepileptic effect or clinical toxicity of PRM in patients.

The question of the relative amounts of PRM converted to its metabolites after single or multiple doses has been the subject of several studies. Rabbits were given single or multiple oral doses of PRM (50), and the amount of PRM excreted unchanged in urine was calculated to be about 20% of a single dose, whereas 48% was excreted as PEMA and 10% as PB and *p*-hydroxyphenobarbital. The conversion to PEMA occurred earlier and more rapidly than conversion to PB. In another study (35) in which PRM was given intravenously, 20% of the dose was excreted as unchanged PRM, 40% was metabolized to PEMA, and 40% was metabolized to PB. PHT pretreatment increased the total body clearance of PRM, PEMA, and PB and accelerated the rate of formation of the metabolites.

Studies of quantitative aspects of PRM transformation in humans have been assessed. One study (2) concluded that 24.5% of PRM was converted to PB. Another study (55a) found that, to achieve the same PB levels, the PRM dose had to be five times higher than a corresponding dose of PB.

Two groups of patients with epilepsy (group I with no previous exposure to anticonvulsants and group II taking over anticonvulsants) were studied using an intravenous infusion of ^{14}C PRM (20). The mean plasma half-life was 50% shorter in group I, although the total amount of PRM was approximately equal. The relative amounts of the compounds excreted were different in the two groups: PRM, 42% unchanged, 2% PEMA, 1.2% PB, and 1.5% unidentified products in group I; in group II, 31% unchanged PRM, 10% PEMA, 1.3% PB, and 1.5% unidentified products (considered to be free and conjugated *p*-hydroxyphenobarbital). The profile of PRM and the rate of production of its two main metabolites were studied in a group of 12 children (21), with a pronounced interpatient variability.

The quantitative assessment of PRM biotransformation has also been evaluated using steady-state blood concentrations between PRM and its two main metabolites. The levels of PRM fluctuate more than the levels of the metabolites because of the drug's short half-life, and the concentration ratios are therefore not constant. If comparisons are made between the PB:PRM ratio in patients receiving monotherapy and that in patients receiving combination therapy, there is a threefold increase in this ratio. The :PRM ratio approximately doubles (5,40,47,55b).

Several factors can cause change in these ratios, such as age (49,56), pregnancy (57), and disease, that is, viral hepatitis (28). From all the current information, PRM is both a drug in itself and a PB prodrug that has implications for the clinical use of this drug.

DRUG INTERACTIONS

The many interactions reported between PRM and other drugs can be beneficial as well as potentially damaging. PRM biotransformation creates a kind of polypharmacy in a setting of monotherapy, and the use of other drugs enhances the complexity of these biotransformations. Because PRM and PB appear to induce enzyme activity, their influence on other drugs is important (58).

Drugs that can affect the gastrointestinal tract and can produce changes such as alteration in pH, motility of the tract, and possible formation of insoluble complexes can delay or prevent absorption of PRM. Conversely, PRM may affect the transport system of the brush border of the enterocyte (59). Acetazolamide may impair the absorption of PRM (60). PRM has been shown to impair biotransport in human intestine in a concentration-dependent manner (59). Folate metabolism or absorption has been shown to be affected by anticonvulsants including PRM (61). Distribution, including protein binding of either PRM or its main metabolites, does not seem to be altered by biotransformation.

Because PRM is a weak organic acid, excretion may be altered by changes in the pH of the urine. Patients receiving only PRM eliminated it more slowly than those patients taking PRM in combination with other AEDs, particularly PHT (47,62), and CBZ (63).

The main pharmacokinetic interactions concern the biotransformation or metabolism of PRM and its metabolites. The biotransformation of PRM to PB and PEMA can be both markedly induced and markedly inhibited by other drugs, and this inducibility is influenced by various factors, including genetics, age, and disease processes. The effect of induction was studied extensively in adults and children, and findings clearly indicated that the presence of other drugs decreased the amount of unchanged PRM approximately 20% (5,10,20,64).

Clinical studies also indicate the possibility of substance interaction. The delayed appearance of PEMA and PB in plasma (18,47,48) and the influence of repeated administration on that delay (5,10,64) suggest that the enzyme systems responsible for the biotransformation of PRM may be altered by interactions among all three of these compounds (40,58).

The combination of PHT and PRM results in a pronounced acceleration of the enzymatic transformation (5, 32,47,65) and in a marked increase in the PB:PRM ratio (5,32,66; Table 65.1). Determining the exact mechanism responsible for this enzyme induction and/or inhibition of hydroxylation of PB (47,67) is not critical before one decides that this is a clinically significant finding.

CBZ also increases the metabolism of PRM to its metabolites in both animals (47) and humans (20,63, 68–70). An apparent opposite effect was found in one study (71). It has been reported that PRM lowers the serum level

TABLE 65.1. EFFECT OF PHENYTOIN ON PRIMIDONE BIOTRANSFORMATION[a]

	Primidone Only (n = 80)	Primidone and Phenytoin (n = 127)
PRM dose (mg/kg)	9.7 ± 0.2	10.6 ± 0.4
PHT dose (mg/kg)	—	4.8 ± 0.1
Serum PHT level (µg/mL)	—	12.1 ± 0.1
Serum PRM level (µg/mL)	11.3 ± 0.2	8.1 ± 0.4
Serum PB level (µg/mL)	15.0 ± 0.4	27.2 ± 1.4
PB/PRM	1.45 ± 0.10	3.82 ± 0.24

PRM, primidone; PHT, phenytoin; PB, placebo.
[a]Values are expressed as mean ± standard error.

of CBZ (70–73) and decreases the CBZ:CBZ-epoxide ratio (69).

VPA has been reported to alter the serum levels of PRM (74–77) and to change the PRM:PB ratio. Our results, in 16 patients, did not show an average change when VPA was added to the regimen, although there was marked interindividual variability (58).

Clonazepam apparently causes a significant increase in PRM concentration (78), in contrast to other AEDs. Two drugs, isoniazid and nicotinamide (51,79–81), decrease the conversion of PRM to PB, and it has been postulated that this action results from inhibition of the cytochrome P450 enzyme system. Interaction of PRM with several other drugs has been investigated (66,82–85).

Table 65.1 summarizes most of the reported interactions of PRM and its metabolites. As with all drug interactions, individual variability is of marked concern and points out the necessity and benefits of using serum drug levels to gain maximum therapeutic effect of all drugs.

PRIMIDONE AS AN ANTICONVULSANT

Animal Studies

Initial support for an independent anticonvulsant effect of PRM was provided by Frey and Hahn (53), with their demonstration of protection against pentylenetetrazole-induced seizures in dogs with lower concentrations of PB in the presence of PRM. Studies in rats by Baumel et al. (10) indicated an independent anticonvulsant effect for PRM, with protection of 50% of the rats from MES in the first 6 hours after administration and before the appearance of its metabolites PB and PEMA in the brain. This was accomplished with 3.9 mg/kg compared with a median effective dose of 5 mg/kg for PB and of 62.5 mg/kg for PEMA. PRM did not show protection against pentylenetetrazole- or hexafluorodiethyl ether–induced seizures at this low concentration. Protection against these two systemic chemoconvulsants required time for PRM's biotransformations to

PB and PEMA. Thus, different pharmacodynamic effects for PRM and PB were indicated by this study.

PRM was shown to have an independent anticonvulsant effect in seizures induced in epileptic fowl by intermittent photic stimulation (52). The metabolic inhibitor SKF 525A prevented PRM's conversion to PEMA and PB in this study. Leal et al. (27), using SKF 525A, showed similar independent effectiveness of PRM against MES in mice. Further comparison of protection against seizures, by using brain concentrations of PRM, PB, and PEMA after single doses of PRM without SKF 525A, led these investigators to conclude that PB probably gave the greatest anticonvulsant effect in that circumstance.

Another study of PRM and its two major metabolites PB and PEMA in mice, showed PRM to raise the electroconvulsant threshold, but with 1.7 times less potency than PB (33). Eighty percent of the anticonvulsant effect in this study was attributed to PRM when brain concentrations of PRM, PB, and PEMA were measured at the time of the test. Seizures were produced in gerbils using a blast of compressed air, and PRM was responsible for the main anticonvulsant effect in the first hours after administration using measures of serum and brain concentrations (86). In a long-term, study only one of 15 dogs was shown to have improved control of seizures when PRM was substituted for PB at comparable serum concentrations of PB (87).

Bourgeois et al. (51,80) performed a series of experiments in mice to assess neurotoxicity of PRM and its metabolites and to view the pharmacodynamic interactions of PRM, PB, and PEMA with regard to their anticonvulsant potency and neurotoxicity. Seizure protection was quantitated as median effective brain concentration (EC_{50}) against MES and pentylenetetrazole-induced seizures. Neurotoxicity was measured as median toxic brain concentration (TC_{50}) with employment of the rotorod test. Therapeutic indices (TI = TC_{50}/EC_{50}) were also individually assessed for PRM, PB, and PEMA. Brain concentrations were used to eliminate any possible pharmacokinetic interactions from the test. The median neurotoxic concentration for PRM was much higher than that for PB, a finding indicating PRM to be 2.5 times less neurotoxic in this model than PB. PRM was as potent as PB in controlling MES seizures, with a resultant higher therapeutic index because of its lesser neurotoxicity. PRM showed no effectiveness against the chemoconvulsant models employing pentylenetetrazole (with brain concentrations of 81.7 μg/mL) and bicuculline (with brain concentrations of 103.3 μg/mL). PB, however, showed similar potency against MES and chemoconvulsant seizures. PEMA showed an anticonvulsant spectrum similar to that of PB for both the MES and chemoconvulsant models, but it was 16 times less potent for each.

PRM's differential effectiveness against MES seizures and its inability to influence chemoconvulsant seizures reconfirmed the finding of Baumel et al. (10). As indicated earlier, PB and PRM are different anticonvulsants with two different mechanisms of action; PRM has a spectrum of effectiveness similar to that of CBZ and PHT (88).

Bourgois et al., acknowledging the eventual obligatory presence of PB and PEMA with use of PRM, addressed the potential for toxicity as well as effectiveness in this mouse model (89). Bourgeois et al. hypothesized that if neurotoxicity is lower for PRM than PB, as in this mouse model, then an upper therapeutic limit for serum PRM concentrations is meaningless in naturally occurring PB:PRM ratios. Animal studies have provided a preponderance of evidence that PRM has antiepileptic effects independent of metabolically derived PB.

Results of clinical studies have demonstrated arguments both for and against the independence of PRM as an AED. Most early studies were not prospective or controlled and used PRM as add-on therapy. Early double-blind studies, such as that of White et al. (90), found no significant difference in the anticonvulsant efficacy of PRM, PB, or PHT, and toxicity was comparable among the three drugs. Booker et al. (18) studied 30 patients taking only PRM and showed effectiveness with a PB:PRM ratio of 3:1. Several comparative clinical studies of PRM have been performed since the 1960s (91–95), and only one showed that PRM was superior in efficacy (96). Other clinical studies (58,91,95) have demonstrated seizure control with PRM when PB was not within therapeutic range.

Clinical Observations

PRM was first used in the treatment of patients before its metabolic transformations were understood and before any controlled trials had been undertaken. Initial enthusiasm for treatment of epilepsy in humans with PRM (1,50, 90,98–103) was tempered by the discovery that PB was a major metabolite. Clear evidence for the effectiveness of PRM beyond that provided by PB was not established in numerous clinical investigations (6,19,92,104–107).

An add-on study by Rodin et al. (94) is of interest with regard to seizure control with and side effects of PRM in comparison with those of CBZ when both drugs were used as adjunctive therapy. Forty-five patients with partial or tonic-clonic seizures occurring at least twice monthly completed a 6-month study, with each patient serving as his or her own control. Either PRM or CBZ was added to a stable regimen of PHT after all other drugs had been withdrawn. One adjunctive drug (either CBZ or PRM) was given for 3 months, after which the other was substituted for the next 3 months. Single-blind observations by the treating neurologist and double-blind observations by the electroencephalographer and psychologists indicated no difference between the two drugs in their effectiveness in controlling seizures and noted "somewhat more side effects— nonserious—with CBZ than with PRM." However, they did find more severe impairment on a repeatable neuropsychological test battery and an increase on the psychopathic deviation scale of the Minnesota Multiphasic Personality Inventory with use of PRM. They also reported that CBZ led to lessened depressive feelings, if that mood change was present, in contrast to PRM. These investigators speculated that an intellectually and emotionally intact patient could do better with PRM, but they favored CBZ for patients with a history of emotional or intellectual deficits.

The double-blind prospective study of treatment of patients with partial or secondarily generalized seizures in the nationwide Veterans Administration (VA) Cooperative Study was completed in 1985 and provides the most definitive clinical insights available regarding therapy with the four studied anticonvulsant drugs: PB, PRM, PHT, and CBZ (6,107). Patients were randomized to therapy with one of the four drugs. CBZ and PHT showed the best success with treatment, followed by PB and, finally, by PRM. The length of time that the patient received treatment (patient retention time) constituted one of the end point measures of efficacy. This retention rate was poorest for PRM despite limiting initial dosing to 125 mg. The common appearance of acute side effects of nausea, vomiting, dizziness, and sedation led to early discontinuation of PRM in this study. When this problem was not encountered or was manageable, the patients usually completed the study. Similar side effects have been observed during induction of PRM when it is used in treating essential tremor (108).

Another end point in a later VA study (96) compared the percentage of patients who were free of tonic-clonic seizures while taking each of the drugs. No significant differences were found in this measure, with 63% of patients receiving PRM, 58% receiving PB, 55% receiving CBZ, and 48% receiving PHT being free of tonic-clonic seizures at the end of 1 year, but CBZ was more effective than PB and PRM for partial seizures. PRM showed fewer adverse behavioral effects as measured by the total behavioral toxicity battery than either PHT or PB (95). PRM showed a definitely different behavioral profile on the subtests of the behavioral toxicity battery and on the total behavioral toxicity battery score than was shown by PB. This difference in toxicity between PRM and PB pointed to PRM's effects being independent of those related to PB. These behavioral differences as measured by this psychological test battery are of interest to consider in relation to the differential action and inaction of PB and PRM in the chemoconvulsant animal models of epilepsy. Relatively subtle structural differences in chemical makeup appear capable of bringing about noteworthy differences in anticonvulsant and behavioral changes.

PB's obligatory appearance with biotransformation of PRM led Bourgeois et al. (80) to look for an optimal PB:PRM ratio for treating seizures in their experiments with mice. These researchers found brain concentrations of PB and PRM to be optimal at 1:1, with resultant effect of potentiation of both drugs against electroshock seizures. Leal et al. (27) showed that brain penetration is better for PB than for PRM and that PB concentrations in the brain were twice that of PRM with equal plasma concentrations in the mouse model. The plasma PB:PRM ratio would, in this way, underestimate the cerebral ratio. Data from the VA study (95) indicated minimal plasma levels of PB in the first week of therapy that climbed to a higher and relatively stable concentration in 1 month. Additional data indicated a poor correlation between dose and serum concentration of PRM and between serum PRM and serum PB concentrations, except for a tendency of higher serum PB concentrations to correlate with higher serum PRM levels. The mean serum PB:PRM ratio for the first year was 1.2:1, close to the ratio favored by Bourgeois et al. (80), although their ratio used brain and not serum concentrations. Our conclusions that PRM itself was an effective antiseizure drug were based on our study of 80 patients who had received only PRM for at least 12 months (5). Twenty-nine patients with excellent control of seizures had plasma PB concentrations of <15 µg/mL (mean derived PB concentrations at 12 months, 13.4 µg/mL; range, 12.1 to 15.4 µg/mL at 12 months) and led us to the conclusion that PRM, *per se,* possessed anticonvulsive potency. If brain concentrations had been measured, PB could have been present at much higher concentration, and this, with a consideration of PRM's half-life, would lessen the strength of our conclusion. Bourgeois et al. noted that the mouse model (80), which showed lesser neurotoxicity for PRM than PB (rotorod test) and higher brain concentrations of PB than PRM, would render an upper therapeutic limit for serum PRM concentrations without meaning.

Oxley et al. (109) provided clinical evidence that PRM was superior to PB in treating certain seizures. Twenty-one residents of the Chalfont Centre for Epilepsy who were taking either PRM or PB for at least 1 year along with several other AEDs were included in this study. Doses of the concomitant AEDs were held constant, whereas doses of PRM and PB were adjusted to obtain comparable levels of PB for those receiving PRM and those receiving PB. One year of observation was followed by interchanging PRM and PB and readjusting plasma PB to similar levels for each group and another year of observation. Mean serum PB during treatment was 30.1 + 12.8 µg/mL with concurrent PRM values of 29.9 + 11.6 µg/mL. Fourteen of 21 patients experienced better control of generalized tonic-clonic seizures when they were taking PRM, and four had more frequent seizures. Patients with complex partial and generalized absence seizures did not show a difference in response to the two drugs.

A study using 24-hour video electroencephalographic (EEG) monitoring correlating EEG paroxysms, seizure frequency, and plasma PRM and PB levels demonstrated that peak plasma levels were associated with periods of decreased clinical seizures and fewer EEG paroxysms. Dosing intervals of PRM were closer (8 hours), and there was little fluctuation in drug level in a patient receiving PRM monotherapy. These data indicated a better correlation with EEG and clinical changes with PRM levels than PB (110)

These clinical observations present strong but not conclusive evidence for the independent antiepileptic activity of PRM. Before discussing the clinical use of this drug, we should discuss the adverse effects associated with its use.

ADVERSE EFFECTS

Assessment of PRM for adverse effects necessarily includes attention to its metabolic derivative PB (13), except for a singular initial interval after its first dosage, before conversion to PB has taken place. Booker et al. (18) showed that this interval may last up to 48 hours in testing serum of normal volunteers given their first dose of PRM. Two of these six volunteers experienced this noteworthy acute initial toxicity of PRM defined by marked dizziness, slurred speech, giddiness, and altered mental status (difficulty with concentration) when only PRM is present. PB is almost always present with PRM, thus rendering it impossible to separate its adverse effects from those of PRM.

Clinicians must consider potential adverse events as well as therapeutic efficacy in their choice of available AEDs. Classification systems for adverse events have been designed to help recognize, prevent, and treat potential adverse events of AEDs (111). PRM's clinical usage since 1952 must have allowed for recognition of most of its adverse events. This discussion employs an approach using involvement of organ systems with some consideration of mechanistic processes (teratogenicity and hypersensitivity reaction). Attention is focused on adverse effects involving the central nervous system (CNS) with recognition that those undesired effects that can be unequivocally attributed to PRM can only be identified in one interval, not exceeding 48 hours, after its initial dosage. Long-term use of PRM, with its obligatory metabolite PB, is necessarily associated with adverse events relatable to PB (Chapter 55).

Adverse Events Viewed in Organ Systems

It is not surprising that therapeutic intervention with AEDs designed to prevent clinical seizures may affect these other neuronal activities. Lennox expressed concern about this ability of AEDs to impair other neurologic functions in 1942 (112) with the observation that "many physicians in attempting to extinguish seizures only succeed in drowning the finer intellectual processes of their patients."

Consistent interest in and studies of possible cognitive side effects of AEDs appeared in the 1970s (113,114). All established AEDs were recognized to possess cognitive side effects (115), with PB, the obligate metabolite of PRM, showing the least favorable cognitive profile of all (116).

Acute initial toxicity appears as PRM's unique contribution to CNS toxicity, apart from those engendered by its usual companion, PB. Goldin (117) and Timberlake et al. (102) commented about this in early reports of clinical use of PRM. Other reports of toxicity followed (92,106). Mattson et al. (91) listed clinical identifiers for this state of acute CNS toxicity similar to those noted by Booker et al. (18): drowsiness, dizziness, ataxia, nausea, and vomiting, with observation that these untoward effects of PRM often resulted in its therapeutic discontinuation. Although intensely disabling, these acutely altered mental states usually end within hours of discontinuation of PRM. The appearance of this state of toxicity follows ingestion of PRM by an hour or so and before the appearance of serum PB, a finding thereby indicating PRM to have causal importance for this state of toxicity. PEMA serum levels may equal those of PRM, but PEMA has been believed to play a small role if any, in the appearance of this toxicity on the basis of animal studies (51).

This acute state of toxicity may appear with even a limited first dose of 50 mg of PRM, although it is much more likely to develop after higher doses. Serum concentrations of PRM near 10 μg/mL after 500-mg doses were found in normal volunteers (18). Other investigators noted this acute state of toxicity with lower serum concentrations (118). Some patients decide at this point to discontinue trial use of PRM, whereas others, perhaps with less severe acute toxicity, persevere and are able to tolerate the drug and eventually live comfortably with much larger doses in long-term therapy. Leppik et al. (118) explored this development of tolerance to PRM, which can occur in hours or days, by comparing clinical toxicity scores with serum concentrations of PRM. Toxicity scores were seen to decline with time, despite identical and even higher serum concentrations of PRM. The possibility that PB could produce a cross-tolerance to acute PRM toxicity had been suggested after noting that patients receiving long-term PB therapy were less likely to experience this severe toxicity on their first exposure to PRM (106).

Bourgeois et al. (80), noting the obligatory appearance of both PB and PEMA with ingestion of PRM, studied the potential of these metabolites with regard to neurotoxicity and efficacy in controlling electroshock and chemoconvulsant seizures in a mouse model. Combined brain concentrations of PRM and PB near a ratio of 1:1 provided maximal protection against MES with minimal neurotoxicity (rotorod test). Brain concentrations of PB were found to be twice those of PRM (80,119), a finding confirming that of Leal et al. (27) that brain penetration is better for PB than for PRM. Observation of variable PB:PRM ratios in clinical settings indicate that the 1:1 ratio is approached in settings of monotherapy with PRM, with enhancement of PB concentrations by a factor of more than 3 in the presence of enzyme-inducing comedications such as CBZ and PHT (120). Bourgeois (9) believed that these data indicated that it would be meaningless to set an upper therapeutic limit for serum PRM concentrations with naturally occurring PB:PRM ratios.

Symptoms of CNS toxicity beyond those of acute initial toxicity include personality changes (99,121). Rodin et al. (94) stabilized 45 patients with partial and tonic-clonic seizures on PHT therapy. CBZ was added to this regimen for half of the group, with the others given PRM for 3 months. These comedications were then interchanged for the next 3 months. Patients receiving PRM showed a significantly higher psychopathic deviate scale on testing with the Minnesota Multiphasic Inventory in comparison with those receiving CBZ. Depressive feelings, when present, lessened when CBZ was substituted for PRM in this study.

PB, PRM's companion in long-term therapy, has been associated with behavioral changes and depression in adults (122,123) and in adults and children (124). Dodrill's review of 90 studies (125) emphasized negative behavioral changes, including depression, with the use of PB in comparison with PHT, CBZ, and VPA in the treatment of epilepsy.

Cognitive impairments in memory functions and psychological development have been related to use of PB, without dosage data, in comparison with no treatment (126–129). Psychotic symptoms have been observed with PRM in combination with PHT (130).

The best documentation of the role of PRM in the development of sexual impotence comes from Mattson et al. (6). Three patients intoxicated with PRM and PHT were reported with partial or complete external ophthalmoplegia (131).

Integumentary System

Rare benign maculopapular rash may appear within 2 months of starting PRM. The role of derived PB in this setting is not clear. Disappearance of the rash is anticipated within 2 weeks of PRM's discontinuation. Association of rashes with systemic reactions is even more uncommon, but those rashes are much more serious.

Hematologic and Lymphatic Systems

Several instances of megaloblastic anemia have been reported (132). Severe megaloblastic anemia was reported to follow PRM's substitution for PHT in a regimen of PHT and PB that had been given for the 4 years preceding the anemia (133). PRM's substitution for PB was followed in 4 months by megaloblastic anemia in one patient and appeared after 2 years of monotherapy with PRM in another (134). The macrocytic anemias associated with use of PRM have been reported to respond to folic acid in some patients and to vitamin B_{12} in others (135,136).

An instance of a neonatal coagulation defect was related to maternal use of PRM and was suspected in others (137). Prophylactic use of vitamin K is indicated in the treatment of women receiving PRM during pregnancy.

Thrombocytopenia appeared in one patient who was given PRM to replace PHT after the latter had caused bone marrow depression (138). Another instance of thrombocytopenia was also reported with PRM therapy (139). Unusually transient leukopenias (140) have also been noted. Lymphadenopathy has been observed in association with folate-deficient anemias in patients taking PRM (141).

Hepatic Toxicity

Induction of liver enzymes with asymptomatic slight elevations of liver enzymes has been noted as with other AEDs (142). There is no report linking PRM to the appearance of hepatitis (143). PRM's derived metabolite, PB, could be of causal import in serious hepatotoxicity in the very rare AED hypersensitivity syndrome (144). Granick (145) hypothesized that drugs such as PB could interact with heme and so could diminish inhibition of enzymes controlling γ-aminolevulinic acid synthetase production, thereby allowing the appearance of hereditary acute porphyria. Potential metabolic effects of PB's potent ability to induce hepatic microsomal enzymes are worthy of consideration (142).

Renal Effects

Crystalluria has been recognized as a sign of PRM intoxication in humans (119,131,146,147). The identified urinary crystals have been found to be mostly PRM (148). Renal problems, however, such as hematuria and acute or chronic renal failure have not appeared even after massive overdoses (146).

Skeletal Disorders

Enzyme-inducing AEDs may affect bone metabolism by increased conversion of active metabolites of vitamin D to inactive forms (149). Studies have shown reduced bone mineral density and impaired calcium metabolism in patients being treated with enzyme-inducing AEDs, and this list would include metabolically derived PB as well as PRM. Clinical incidence of osteomalacia is rare (150), and it is perhaps most reflective of the patient's diet and exposure to the sun (151). Calcium and vitamin D supplementation can be helpful in high-risk patients (152).

Connective Tissue Disorders

Dupuytren's contractures, various nodules, and other connective tissue changes may be included in this grouping of possible side effects. The VA study data (153) indicated statistically significant associations between use of PB and PRM for at least 6 months and the development of 10 instances of connective tissue disorders. PB had previously been identified as having causal importance in the development of contractures (154). PRM had been associated with appearance of the frozen shoulder syndrome (155). The frozen shoulder syndrome was reported to be reversible with continued therapy, although Mattson et al. (153) reported clearing of these changes when PHT, CBZ, and VPA were substituted for PRM.

Teratogenicity

A significant increase in cleft palates was demonstrated in mice given 100 to 250 mg/kg during 6 to 16 days of their pregnancies, with peak PRM concentrations of 43 µg/mL in comparison with untreated controls (156,157). Sprague-Dawley rats were given PRM (0 or 120 mg/kg) by gavage on gestational days 8 to 20, with PRM proving to be embryolethal for 57% of the dams (100% of the pregnant controls produced offspring) and with evidence of a specific learning deficit in the PRM-treated offspring (158).

A human syndrome of hirsute forehead, thick nasal root, anteverted nostrils, long philtra, and thin upper lips with distal digital hypoplasia and increased risks of heart defects and psychomotor retardation has been reported (159). These features have also been reported with many other AEDs. Aqueductal stenosis and enteroencephalocele have been observed with the use of PRM in pregnancy (119,134,158,160). The linkage of PRM to human malformations was complicated by the rarity of use of PRM as the sole agent (160). A survey of 983 births to epileptic mothers treated with AEDs in Japan, Italy, and Canada indicated PRM to be associated with the highest incidence of congenital malformations related to use of a single drug (161). A complex study of antiepileptic therapy during pregnancy suggested long-term effects on intellectual performance of children into adolescence in those instances of treatment with PRM (162).

Antiepileptic Drug Hypersensitive Syndrome

Various types of skin reactions can occur with the use of PRM and PB; the incidence is low (1% to 3%) (163) and usually occurs at the onset of therapy. A fatal case of dermatitis bullosa was reported (164). A patient taking PRM developed eosinophilia, edema, and a rash during the first month of pregnancy, and the rash cleared when PH was substituted (165). Systemic lupus erythematosus was associated with PRM in one case that cleared when PHT was substituted (166). It has been suggested that AEDs elicit the production of antinuclear antibodies by altering nuclear components that may unmask systemic lupus erythematosus in predisposed persons (167). This AED hypersensitivity syndrome has been reviewed (168).

CLINICAL USE

The choice of PRM as a single drug for treatment of partial or secondarily generalized seizures is valid during its first usage and for up to the next 48 hours, but the appearance of its metabolic derivative PB thereafter creates a more complex state of polypharmacy. This situation has led some investigators to view PRM as only a prodrug for PB, with PB regarded as providing the major or perhaps only antiepileptic effect (169). Eadie recognized antiepileptic effectiveness with both PRM and PB but believed that PB probably provided the major anticonvulsant effect (170). PRM's other major metabolic derivative, PEMA, has not been believed to contribute notably to either therapy or toxicity in humans. Our observation that 29 of 80 patients receiving PRM monotherapy for 12 months had excellent control of their seizures with derived serum concentrations of <15 µg/mL provided evidence of the efficacy of this drug (5). Wylie et al. (23) presented evidence in a case report that indicated that PRM possesses antiepileptic potency and pointed out an instance in which its generic substitution was followed by low serum concentrations of PRM. A 16-year-old girl with two tonic-clonic and atonic seizures weekly suddenly experienced a dramatic rise in frequency of seizures after generic substitution of PRM. Reinstitution of treatment with the brand name Mysoline was followed by return of her seizures to their baseline frequency. Generic PRM was again administered 3 months later during hospitalization, and, again, there was an increase in seizures. At this time, plasma PRM concentration had decreased by 53%, and plasma PB concentration had decreased by 16%. It was viewed as unlikely that the relatively small decline in plasma PB from 19.1 to 15.9 µg/mL was of importance in the patient's increasingly frequent seizures. Return to the brand name drug resulted in decreasing frequency of seizures to baseline values and return of plasma PRM levels.

Initiation of Therapy

Administration of large initial doses of PRM followed by rapid escalation to a desired final regimen is not possible without high likelihood of a very unpleasant experience in drug toxicity for the patient. This will almost certainly lead to discontinuation of its use. First-time users of AEDs are at the greatest risk. This potential ordeal for the patient has been noted for some time (18,171), and it has been correlated with the appearance of PRM in serum and presumably brain (48) before the appearance of either of its metabolites PB or PEMA. Discontinuation of PRM is followed by clearance of this state of toxicity in hours or sometimes days, but it will leave the patient with a distressing recollection. Patients who have been receiving AEDs, particularly drugs that induce activity of the cytochrome P450 system, usually tolerate the addition of PRM to their drug regimen with less difficulty, and that allows a higher initial dose and a more rapid upward titration of PRM. It is reasonable to recall here that experimentally shown cross-tolerance to neurotoxic effects of PRM by pretreatment with

PB in mice (118) and rats (172) supports the clinical observations that individuals previously treated with PB have fewer side effects on first exposure to PRM (19,106).

How should PRM be started? It should begin with a discussion with the patient about potential acute side effects (dizziness, nausea, unsteadiness, sedation), followed by noting possible long-term effects. If a decision to use PRM is made, and the patient has not previously taken AEDs, an initial dose of 25 or 50 mg at bedtime may be given for several days. This should be followed by an increase to 50 mg twice daily (b.i.d.) for several more days, followed by an increase to 125 mg b.i.d. for 4 days, with a final increase to 250 mg b.i.d. as the initial goal. Some patients who have tolerated other AEDs, including those that induce hepatic cytochrome enzyme systems, may also benefit from this conservative approach, whereas others may tolerate an initial dose of 125 mg daily with a more rapid increase to a 125- and 250-mg b.i.d. schedule. At this point, a trough PRM value of ≥ 6 μg/mL is often achieved. It may be necessary to increase the dose to 250 mg three times daily or more to achieve satisfactory seizure control. If satisfactory control of seizures has not been achieved with serum PRM levels in the 15 μg/mL range, success is not likely with this drug in monotherapy, and other therapeutic regimens will need to be considered, although clinically unacceptable side effects are the ultimate measure of AED failure.

Serum Concentrations and Control of Seizures

A poor correlation has been noted between dose of PRM and plasma PB and plasma PRM concentrations in several studies (5,95), as is true for other AEDs. Plasma PRM concentrations do correlate with brain concentrations, and therefore dosing decisions in each patient can be guided by plasma PRM values. Plasma PB levels do not predict plasma PRM concentrations, but they do give information about the PRM:PB ratio, which may be the most important factor in determining clinical success; it is important to adjust the dose of PRM on the basis of both levels. The cooperative VA study suggests that the optimal mean plasma PRM level is 12 μg/mL, with an associated mean derived PB level of 15 μg/mL, resulting in a PRM:PB ratio of 0.8. There is great interpatient variability. Toxicity in long-term PRM therapy appears to be associated with low ratios, such as found when PRM is coadministered with PHT. Investigators have suggested that autoinduction on monotherapy with PRM does not occur to any clinically significant degree (173), and in rare patients it does not occur at all (5).

The half-life of PRM in humans ranges from 3 to >20 hours (18,19,47,174), and this range makes the assessment of PRM levels alone difficult. Without a detailed pharmacokinetic study in each patient, the timing of a trough level is complex and leads to inaccuracies (58).

Drug interactions have a significant effect on plasma PRM levels, as previously noted, and the variability in the PRM:PB ratio may be markedly altered. Measurement of plasma levels is necessary whenever PRM is used in conjunction with other drugs and especially other AEDs. Any instance of abrupt change in seizure control should alert one to the possibility of drug interaction, and one should treat the patient and not the plasma drug level.

The effect of age, both young and old, with concomitant changes in metabolism may influence the clinical effectiveness of PRM, and the variability of the PRM:PB ratio may be enhanced. Steady-state PRM concentrations are even more variable in children than in adults (175). In elderly patients, the half-life of PRM may be somewhat prolonged, but PB still accumulates (176). This population may be more sensitive to the hypnotic effects of PB and may not tolerate the usual doses of PRM. It would seem wise to monitor the plasma PRM and PB levels in children, adolescents, and the elderly more frequently, probably as often as every 3 months.

The usefulness of PRM in patients with psychiatric problems has been the subject of few investigations. One investigation demonstrated a persistent positive therapeutic effect of PRM as an adjunctive therapy in 31% of patients with refractory bipolar disorders (177).

Treatment of the developmentally delayed patient is one of the most challenging problems presented to the physician. The use of barbiturates in these patients has fallen into disfavor, but one study indicates the usefulness of PRM in retarded patients with mixed seizure types (178–180).

The metabolism of most AEDs changes during pregnancy, and PRM is no exception. The levels of PB and PEMA tend to decrease during the first trimester, although the plasma levels of PRM tend to remain fairly stable (181) or may even increase (57,182). The large decrease in PB during pregnancy is often followed by a rapid increase after delivery. Increased seizure activity is not associated with these changes. Transplacental passage of PRM is well documented (157,183,184) and has been associated with a syndrome of tremulousness, jitteriness, disturbance of sleep rhythm, and unmotivated crying in neonates. No PRM levels are detectable, although PEMA and PB concentrations are still considerable (185,186), thus providing evidence of PRM withdrawal as the significant feature. The possibility of specific PRM teratogenicity has been raised in several reports (157,159,186–188), but the data are still insufficient to allow meaningful assessment of PRM teratogenicity independent of its derived PB.

Discontinuing PRM therapy, unless there is a specific reason to proceed more quickly, should be tapered in a linear fashion during 3 to 6 months, with dosage reductions at monthly intervals. Withdrawal of barbiturates seems to be associated with a higher overall risk of withdrawal seizures, and, therefore, because of its metabolite PB, PRM should be gradually tapered.

Other Uses

Although the use of PRM for epilepsy therapy has decreased, especially with the introduction of newer AEDs, a major role has evolved in the treatment of essential postural tremor. Eight double-blind, placebo-controlled trials were reviewed by Koller et al. (189) and indicated consistent evidence of efficacy comparable to results from β-adrenergic blockers. Doses ranged from 50 to 1000 mg/day. Adverse effects were often experienced at initiation of treatment unless low doses (25 to 50 mg) were used and were titrated slowly. Koller and Veter-Olderfiled (108) showed that the effect on tremor was the result of PRM rather than metabolically derived PB. Tremor subsided acutely after PRM initiation before clinically significant blood levels of PB had appeared, and substitution of PB for PRM resulted in recurrence of the tremor.

SUMMARY

PRM has been demonstrated to be an effective drug in the treatment of partial and secondarily generalized epilepsy and is still widely used in the treatment of epilepsy. It has also become a drug of choice for treatment of essential tremor. It is an intriguing drug because of the unique quantitative and qualitative aspects of its metabolism. PRM is both a drug in itself and, under certain circumstances, a prodrug for PB.

The liver metabolism of PRM results in the production of two metabolites with antiepileptic activity, and this has led to the confusion about whether its activity is a result of the parent compound or its PB metabolite. The other metabolites of PRM have little clinical efficacy. Numerous clinical investigations have not provided a completely clear answer to this question, although various animal studies have demonstrated the independent activity of PRM. PRM is infrequently used as a drug of first choice because of the unpleasant side effects occurring on initiation of therapy. When PRM is used as adjunctive therapy, especially with PHT, there is increased metabolism to PB that can lead to adverse effects. The clinical use of PRM represents an obligatory combination between a drug with a short elimination half-life and a drug with a long elimination half-life. The PRM:PB serum concentration ratio should be maintained as high as possible. Thus, the combination of PRM with enzyme-inducing drugs should be avoided, and it makes no sense to prescribe PB in combination with PRM. Side effects, except those appearing on initiation of therapy, are relatively uncommon, and, aside from connective tissue changes, they disappear readily on discontinuing use of PRM. Despite the introduction of several newer drugs for the treatment of epilepsy, PRM is still a drug that should be considered in certain patients.

ACKNOWLEDGMENTS

Richard Fincham died unexpectedly on November 11, 2000 without completing those sections he was writing, and I, Dorothy Schottelius, assume full responsibility for the entire chapter. Completion of this chapter would not have been possible without the assistance of Carol Devore.

REFERENCES

1. Handley R, Stewart ASR. Mysoline: a new drug in the treatment of epilepsy. *Lancet* 1952;1:742–744.
2. Olesen OV, Dam M. The metabolic conversion of primidone (Mysoline) to phenobarbital in patients under long-term treatment. *Acta Neurol Scand* 1967;43:348–356.
3. Booker HE. Primidone: relation of plasma levels to conical control. In: Woodbury D, Penry K, Schmidt R, eds. *Antiepileptic drugs.* New York: Raven Press, 1972:373–376.
4. Sapin JI, Riviello JJ Jr, Grover WD. Efficacy of primidone for seizure control in neonates and young infants. *Pediatr Neurol* 1988;4:292–295.
5. Fincham RW, Schottelius DD, Sahs AL. The influence of diphenylhydantoin on primidone metabolism. *Arch Neurol* 1974;30:259–262.
6. Mattson RH, Cramer JA, Collins JF, et al. Comparison of carbamazepine, phenobarbital, phenytoin, and primidone in partial and secondarily generalized tonic-clonic seizures. *N Engl J Med* 1985;313:145–151.
7. Levy RH, Mattson RH, Meldrum BS, eds. *Antiepileptic drugs,* 4th ed. New York: Raven Press, 1995:439–449.
8. Frey HH. Primidone. In: Levy RH, Mattson RH, Medrum BS, eds. *Antiepileptic drugs,* 4th ed. New York: Raven Press, 1995: 439–449.
9. Bourgeois BFD. Primidone: chemistry and biotransformation. In: Levy RH, Mattson RH, Meldrum, eds. *Antiepileptic drugs,* 4th ed. New York: Raven Press, 1995:449–457.
10. Baumel IP, Gallagher BB, Di Micco D, et al. Metabolism and anticonvulsant properties of primidone in the rat. *J Pharmacol Exp Ther* 1973;186:305–314.
11. Bogue JY, Carrington HC. Personal communication (1952). Cited by Goodman LS, Swinyard EA, Brown WC, et al. Anticonvulsant properties of 5-phenyl-ethylhexahydropyrimidine-4,6-dione (Mysoline), a new antiepileptic. *J Pharmacol Exp Ther* 1953;108:428–436.
12. Bogue JY, Carrington HC. The evaluation of Mysoline: a new anticonvulsant drug. *Br J Pharmacol* 1953;8:230–235.
13. Butler TC, Waddell WJ. Metabolic conversion of primidone (Mysoline) to phenobarbital. *Proc Soc Exp Biol Med* 1956;93: 544–546.
14. Foltz RL, Couch MW, Greer M, et al. Chemical ionization mass spectrometry in the identification of drug metabolites. *Biochem Med* 1972;6:294–298.
15. Hooper WD, Treston AM, Jacobsen NW, et al. Identification of *p*-hydroxyprimidone as a minor metabolite of primidone in rat and man. *Drug Metab Dispos* 1983;11:607–610.
16. Horning MG, Nowlin J, Buller CM, et al. Clinical applications of gas chromatograph/mass spectrometer/computer systems. *Clin Chem* 1975;21:1282–1287.
17. Andresen BD, Davis FT, Templeton JL, et al. Synthesis and characterization of alpha-phenyl-gamma-butyrolactone, a metabolite of gluthetimide, phenobarbital and primidone in human urine. *Res Commun Chem Pathol Pharmacol* 1976;15:21–30.

18. Booker H, Hosokowa K, Burdette R, et al. A clinical study of serum primidone levels. *Epilepsia* 1970;11:395–402.

19. Gallagher BB, Baumel IP, Mattson RH. Metabolic disposition of primidone and its metabolites in epileptic subjects after single and repeated administration. *Neurology* 1972;22:1186–1192.

20. Zavadil P, Gallagher B. Metabolism and excretion of ^{14}C-primidone in epileptic patients. In: Janz D, ed. *Epileptology.* Stuttgart: Georg Thieme-Verlag, 1976;129–138.

21. Kauffman RE, Habersang R, Lansky L. Kinetics of primidone metabolism and excretion in children. *Clin Pharmacol Ther* 1977;22:200–205.

22. Bielmann P, Levac T, Langlois Y, et al. Bioavailability of primidone in epileptic patients. *Int J Clin Pharmacol* 1979;9:132–137.

23. Wylie E, Pippenger CE, Rothner AD. Increased seizure frequency with generic primidone. *JAMA* 1987;258:1216–1217.

24. Pisani F, Richens A. Pharmacokinetics of phenylethylmalonamide (PEMA) after oral and intravenous administration. *Clin Pharmacokinet* 1983;8:272–276.

25. Guelen PHM, van der Kleijn E. *Rational antiepileptic drug therapy.* Amsterdam: Elsevier, 1978.

26. Lagenstein I, Sternowsky HJ, Iffland E, et al. Intoxication with primidone: continuous monitoring of serum primidone and its metabolites during forced diuresis. *Neuropaediatrie* 1977;8:190–195.

27. Leal KW, Rapport RL, Wilensky AJ, et al. Single-dose pharmacokinetics and anticonvulsant efficacy of primidone in mice. *Ann Neurol* 1979;5:470–474.

28. Pisani F, Perucca E, Primerano G, et al. Single-dose kinetics of primidone in acute viral hepatitis. *Eur J Clin Pharmacol* 1984;27:465–469.

29. El-Masri HA, Portier CJ. Physiologically based pharmacokinetics model of primidone and its metabolites phenobarbital and phenylethylmalonamide in humans, rats, and mice. *Drug Metab Dispos* 1998;26:585–594.

30. Houghton G, Richens A, Toseland P, et al. Brain concentrations of phenytoin, phenobarbitone and primidone in epileptic patients. *Eur J Clin Pharmacol* 1975;9:73–78.

31. Bartels H, Gunther E, Wallis S. Flow-dependent salivary primidone levels in epileptic children. *Epilepsia* 1979;20:431–436.

32. Battino D, Avanzini G, Bossi L, et al. Plasma levels of primidone and its metabolite phenobarbital: effect of age and associated therapy. *Ther Drug Monit* 1983;5:73–79.

33. Frey H, Gobel W, Löscher W. Pharmacokinetics of primidone and its active metabolites in the dog. *Arch Int Pharmacodyn* 1979;242:14–30.

34. Goldsmith RF, Ouvrier RA. Salivary anticonvulsant levels in children: a comparison of methods. *Ther Drug Monit* 1981;3:151–157.

35. Hunt RJ, Miller KW. Disposition of primidone, phenylethylmalonamide, and phenobarbital in the rabbit. *Drug Metab Dispos* 1978;6:75–81.

36. Knott C, Reynolds F. The place of saliva in antiepileptic drug monitoring. *Ther Drug Monit* 1984;6:35–41.

37. MacAulife JJ, Sherwin AL, Leppik IE, et al. Salivary levels of anticonvulsants: a practical approach to drug monitoring. *Neurology* 1977;27:409–413.

38. Schmidt D, Kupferberg HJ. Diphenylhydantoin, phenobarbital and primidone in saliva, plasma and cerebralspinal fluid. *Epilepsia* 1975;16:735–741.

39. Schottelius DD. Primidone: absorption, distribution and excretion. In: Woodbury DM, Penry JL, Pippenger CE, eds. *Antiepileptic drugs,* 2nd ed. New York: Raven Press, 1982:405–413.

40. Streete J, Berry D, Pettit L, et al. Phenylethylmalonamide serum levels in patients treated with primidone and the affects of other antiepileptic drugs. *Ther Drug Monit* 1986;8:161–165.

41. Troupin AS, Friel P. Anticonvulsant level in saliva, serum and cerebralspinal fluid. *Epilepsia* 1975;16:223–227.

42. Van der Klein E, Guelen PMJ, Van Wijk C, Baars I. Clinical pharmacokinetics in monitoring chronic medication with antiepileptic drugs. In: Schnieder H, Janz D, Gardner-Thorpe C, et al., eds. *Clinical pharmacology of antiepileptic drugs.* Berlin: Springer-Verlag, 1975.

43. Bardy A, Teramo K, Hiilesmaa V. Apparent plasma clearances of phenytoin, phenobarbitone, primidone, and carbamazepine during pregnancy: results of the prospective Helsinki study. In: Janz D, et al., eds. *Epilepsy, pregnancy, and the child.* New York: Raven Press, 1982:141–145.

44. Van Heijst A, de Jong W, Seldenrijk R, et al. Coma and crystalluria: a massive primidone intoxication treated with haemoperfusion. *J Toxicol Clin Toxicol* 1983;20:307–318.

45. Nagaki, S, Ratnaraj N, Patsalos PN. Blood and cerebrospinal fluid pharmacokinetics of primidone and its primary pharmacologically actives metabolites, phenobarbital and phenylethylmalonamide in the rat. *Eur J Drug Metab Pharmacokinet* 1999;24:255–264.

46. Schottelius DD, Fincham RW. Cerebrospinal fluid/serum ratios of primidone: inferences to protein binding. *Epilepsia* 1977;18:291.

47. Cloyd J, Miller K, Leppik IE. Primidone kinetics: effects of concurrent drugs and duration of therapy. *Clin Pharmacol Ther* 1981;29:402–407.

48. Baumel IP, Gallagher BB, Mattson RH. Phenylethylmalonamide (PEMA): an important metabolite of primidone. *Arch Neurol* 1972;27:34–41.

49. Alvin J, Gohr E, Bush MT. Study of the hepatic metabolism of primidone by improved technology. *J Pharmacol Exp Ther* 1975;194:117–125.

50. Swinyard EA, Tedeschi DH, Goodman LS. Effects of liver damage and nephrectomy on anticonvulsant activity of Mysoline and phenobarbital. *J Am Pharm Assoc* 1954;43:114–116.

51. Bourgeois BFD, Dodson WE, Ferrendelli JA. Primidone, phenobarbital and PEMA. I. Seizure protection, neurotoxicity and therapeutic index of individual compounds in mice. *Neurology* 1983;33:283–290.

52. Johnson DD, Davis HL, Crawford RD. Epileptiform seizures in domestic fowl. VIII. Anti-convulsant activity of primidone and its metabolites, phenobarbital and phenylethylmalonamide. *Can J Physiol Pharmacol* 1978;56:630–633.

53. Frey HH, Hahn I. Untersuchungen über die Bedeutung des durch Biotransformation gebildeten Phenobarbital für die antikonvulsive Wirkung von Primidon. *Arch Int Pharmacodyn Ther* 1960;128:281–290.

54. Fujimoto JM, Mason WH, Murphy M. Urinary excretion of primidone and its metabolites in rabbits. *J Pharmacol Exp Ther* 1968;159:379–388.

55a. Bogan J, Smith H. The relation between primidone and phenobarbitone blood levels. *J Pharm Pharmacol* 1968;20:64–67.

55b. Haidukewych D, Rodin EA. Monitoring 2-ethyl-2-phenylmalonamide in serum by gas-liquid chromatography: application to retrospective study in epilepsy patients dosed with primidone. *Clin Chem* 1980;26:1537–1539.

56. Powell C, Painter MJ, Pippenger CE. Primidone therapy in refractory neonatal seizures. *J Pediatr* 1984;105:651–654.

57. Battino D, Binelli S, Bossi L, et al. Changes in primidone/phenobarbitone ratio during pregnancy and the puerperium. *Clin Pharmacokinet* 1984;9:252–260.

58. Schottelius DD, Fincham RW. Clinical application of serum primidone levels. In: Pippenger CE, Penry JK, Jutt H, eds. *Antiepileptic drugs: quantitative analysis and interpretation.* New York: Raven Press, 1978:273–282.

59. Redho R, Nylander W. Biotin transport in the human intestine: inhibition by anticonvulsant drugs. *Am J Clin Nutr* 1989;49: 127–131.

60. Syverson GB, Morgan JP, Weintraub M, et al. Acetazolamide-induced interference with primidone absorption. *Arch Neurol* 1977;34:80–84.

61. Reynolds EH, Mattson RH, Gallagher BB. Relationship between serum and cerebrospinal fluid anticonvulsant drug and folic acid concentrations in epileptic patients. *Neurology* 1972; 22:841–844.

62. Morselli PL, Rizzo M, Garratin S. Interaction between phenobarbital and diphenylhdantoin in animals and in epileptic patients. *Ann NY Acad Sci* 1971;179:88–107.

63. Callaghan N, Duggan B, O'Hare J, et al. Serum levels of phenobarbitone and phenylethylmalonamide with primidone used as a single drug and in combination with carbamazepine or phenytoin. In: Johannessen SL, Morrelli PL, Pippenger CE, et al., eds. *Antiepileptic therapy: advances in drug monitoring.* New York: Raven Press, 1980:307–313.

64. Huisman JW. Disposition of primidone in man: an example of autoinduction of a human enzyme system? *Pharm Weekbl* 1969; 104:799–802.

65. Reynolds EH, Fenton G, Fenwick P, et al. Interaction of phenytoin and primidone. *BMJ* 1975;2:594–595.

66. Schmidt D. The effect of phenytoin and ethosuximide on primidone metabolism in patients with epilepsy. *J Neurol* 1975;209: 115–123.

67. Porro MG, Kupferberg HG, Porter RJ, et al. Phenytoin: an inhibitor and inducer of primidone metabolism in an epileptic patient. *Br J Clin Pharmacol* 1982;14:294–297.

68. Baciewicz AM. Carbamazepine drug interactions. *Ther Drug Monit* 1986;8:305–317.

69. Brodie MJ, Forrest G. Rapaport WG. Carbamazepine 10,11 epoxide concentrations in epileptics on carbamazepine alone and in combination with other anticonvulsants. *Br J Clin Pharmacol* 1983;16:747–749.

70. Callaghan N. Feeley M, Duggan F, et al. The effect of anticonvulsant drugs which induce liver microsomal enzymes on derived and ingested phenobarbital levels. *Acta Neurol Scand* 1977;56:1–6.

71. Cereghino JJ, Van Meter JC, Brock JT, et al. Preliminary obsrevations of serum carbamazepine concentration in epileptic patients. *Neurology* 1973;23:356–366.

72. Rambeck R, May T, Jurgens V. Serum concentration of carbamazepine and its epoxide and diol metabolites in epileptic patients: the influence of dose and comedications. *Ther Drug Monit* 1987;9:298–303.

73. Schneider H. Carbamazepine: the influence of other antiepileptic drugs on its serum level. In: Schneider H., Janz D, Gardner-Thorpe C, et al., eds. *Clinical pharmacology of antiepileptic drugs.* New York: Springer-Verlag, 1975:189–196.

74. Windorfer A, Sauer W, Gadeke R. Elevation of diphenylhydantoin and primidone serum concentrations by addition of dipropylacetate,, a new anticonvulsant drug. *Acta Paediatr Scand* 1975;64:771–772.

75. Adams DJ, Luder H, Pippenger CE. Sodium valproate in the treatment of intractable seizure disorders: a clinical and electroencephalographic study. *Neurology* 1978;28:152–157.

76. Richens A, Ahmad S. Controlled trial of sodium valproate. *BMJ* 1975;4:255–256.

77. Varma R, Hoshino A. Simultaneous gas-chromatographic measurement of valproic acid in psychiatric patients: effects on levels of other simultaneously administered anticonvulsants. *Neurosci Lett* 1979;11:353–356.

78. Windorfer A, Sauer W. Drug intereactions during anticonvulsant therapy in childhood: diphenylhydantoin, primidone, phenobarbitone, clonazepam, nitrazepam, carbamazepine and dipropylacetate. *Neuropaediatrie* 1977;8:29–41.

79. Bourgeois BFD, Dodson WE, Ferrendelli JA. Interactions between primidone, carbamazepine and nicotinamide. *Neurology* 1982;32:1122–1126.

80. Bourgeois BFD, Dodson WE, Ferrendelli JA. Primidone, phenobarbital and PEMA. II. Seizure protection, neurotoxicity, and therapeutic index of varying combinations in mice. *Neurology* 1983;33:291–295.

81. Sutton G, Kupferberg HJ. Isoniazid as an inhibitor of primidone metabolism. *Neurology* 1975;25:1179–1181.

82. Browne TR, Feldman RG, Buchanan RA, et al. Methsuximide for complex partial seizures: efficacy, toxicity, clinical pharmacology, and drug interactions. *Neurology* 1983;33:414–418.

83. Young MC, Hughes IA. Loss of therapeutic control in congenital adrenal hyperplasia due to interaction between dexamethasone and primidone. *Acta Paediatr Scand* 1991;80:120–124.

84. Huisman JW, van Heycopten H, van Zihl CH. Influence of ethylphenacemide on serum levels of other antiepileptic drugs. *Epilepsia* 1970;11:207–215.

85. Garrettson LK, Perel JM, Dayton PG. Methylphenidate interaction with both anticonvulsants and ethyl biscoumacetate. *JAMA* 1969;207:2053–2056.

86. Frey HH, Löscher W, Reiche R, et al. Anticonvulsant effect of primidone in the gerbil: time course and significance of the active metabolites. *Pharmacology* 984;28:329–335.

87. Farnbach GC. Efficacy of primidone in dogs with seizures unresponsive to phenobarbital. *J Am Vet Med Assoc* 1984;195: 867–868.

88. Boer HE, Hosokowa K, Burdette RD, et al. A clinical study of serum primidone levels. *Epilepsia* 1970;11:395–402.

89. Bourgeois BFD. Individual and crossed tolerance to the anticonvulsant effect and neurotoxicity of phenobarbital and primidone in mice. In: Frey HH. Fröscher W, Koella WP, et al., eds. *Tolerance to beneficial and adverse effects of antiepileptic drugs.* New York: Raven Press, 1986:17–24.

90. White PT, Plott D, Norton J. Relative anticonvulsant potency of primidone: a double blind comparison. *Arch Neurol* 1966;14: 31–35.

91. Smith DB, Craft BR, Collins J, et al. Behavioral characteristics of epilepsy patients compared with normal controls. *Epilepsia* 1986;27:760–768.

92. Millichap JC, Aymat F. Controlled evaluation of primidone and diphenylhydantoin sodium. Comparative anticonvulsant efficacy and toxicity in children. *JAMA* 1968;204:738–739.

93. Oxley H, Hebdige S, Richens A. A comparison of phenobarbitone and primidone in the control of seizures in chronic epilepsy. *Br J Clin Pharmacol* 1979;7:414P.

94. Rodin EA, Choo SR, Hideki K, et al. A comparison of the effectiveness of primidone versus carbamazepine in epileptic outpatients. *J Nerv Ment Dis* 1976;163:41–46.

95. Smith DB, Mattson RH, Cramer JA, et al. Results of a nationwide Veterans Administration cooperative study comparing the efficacy and toxicity of carbamazepine, phenobarbital, phenytoin, and primidone. *Epilepsia* 1987;28[Suppl 3]:S50–S58.

96. Oxley J, Hebdige S, Laidlaw J, et al. A comparative study of phenobarbitone and primidone in patients under long-term treatment. *Acta Neurol Scandinav* 1967;43:348–356.

97. Calnan WL, Borrell YM. Mysoline in the treatment of epilepsy. *Lancet* 1953;2:42–43.

98. Doyle PJ, Livingston S. Use of Mysoline in treatment of epilepsy. *J Pediatr* 1953;43:413–416.

99. Livingston S, Petersen D. Primidone (Mysoline) in the treatment of epilepsy. *N Engl J Med* 1956;254:327–329.

100. Smith B, Forster FM. Mysoline and Milontin: two new medicines for epilepsy. *Neurology* 1954;4:137–142.

101. Smith BH, McNaughton FL. Mysoline, new anticonvulsant drug: its value in refractory cases of epilepsy. *Can Med Assoc J* 1953;68:464–467.

102. Timberlake WH, Abbott HA, Schwab RS. Mysoline: an effective anticonvulsant with initial problems of adjustment. *N Engl J Med* 1955;252:304–307.

103. Travers RD, Reynolds EH, Gallagher BB. Variation in response to anticonvulsants in a group of epileptic patients. *Arch Neurol* 1972;27:29–33.

104. Bogue JY, Carrington HC, Bentley S. L'activité anticonvulsive de la Mysoline. *Acta Neurol Psychiatr Belg* 1956;56:640–650.

105. Gallagher BB, Baumel IP. Primidone: interaction with other drugs. In: Woodbury D, Penry K, Schmidt R, eds. *Antiepileptic drugs.* New York: Raven Press, 1972:367–371.

106. Gallagher BB, Baumel IP, Mattson RH, et al. Primidone, diphenylhydantoin and phenobarbital: aspects of acute and chronic toxicity. *Neurology* 1973;23:145–149.

107. Smith DB. Unpublished data from VA Cooperative Study Group 118, 1986.

108. Koller WC, Vetere-Overfield B. Acute and chronic effects of propranolol and primidone in essential tremor. *Neurology* 1989; 39:1587–1588.

109. Oxley J, Hebdige S, Laidlaw J, et al. A comparative study of phenobarbitone and primidone in the treatment of epilepsy. In: Johannessen SI, et al., eds. *Antiepileptic therapy: advances in drug monitoring.* New York: Raven Press, 1980:237–245.

110. Rowan AJ, Pippenger CE, McGregor PA, et al. Seizure activity and anticonvulsant drug concentration: 24 hour sleep waking studies. *Arch Neurol* 1975;32:281–288.

111. Greenwood RS. Adverse effects of antiepileptic drugs. *Epilepsia* 2000;41[Suppl 2]:S42–S52.

112. Lennox WG. *Epilepsy and related disorders.* Boston: Little, Brown, 1960.

113. Ideström CM, Schalling D, Carlquist U, et al. Behavioral and psychological studies: acute effects of diphenylhydantoin in relation to plasma levels. *Psychiatr Med* 1972;2:111–120.

114. Dodrill CB, Troupin AS. Psychotropic effects of carbamazepine in epilepsy: a double-blind comparison with phenytoin. *Neurology* 1977;27:1023–1028.

115. Vermeulen J, Aldenkamp AP. Cognitive side effects of chronic antiepileptic drug treatment: a review of 25 years of research. *Epilepsy Res* 1995;22:65–95.

116. Meador KJM, Loring DW, Huh K, et al. Comparative cognitive effects of anticonvulsants. *Neurology* 1990;40:391–394.

117. Goldin S. Toxic effects of primidone. *Lancet* 1954;1:102–103.

118. Leppik IE, Cloyd JC, Miller K. Development of tolerance to the side effects of primidone. *Ther Drug Monit* 1984;6: 189–191.

119. Brillman J, Gallagher BB, Mattson RH. Acute primidone intoxication. *Arch Neurol* 1974;30:255–258.

120. Schottelius DD. Primidone: biotransformation. In: Woodbury DM, Penry JK, Pippenger CE, eds. *Antiepileptic drugs,* 2nd ed. New York: Raven Press, 1982:415–420.

121. Nathan PW. Primidone in treatment of non-idiopathic epilepsy. *Lancet* 1954;1:21.

122. Hermann BP, Whitman S. Psychological predictors of interictal depression. *J Epilepsy* 1989;2:231–237.

123. Smith DB, Collins JB. Behavioral effects of carbamazepine, phenobarbital, phenytoin and primidone. *Epilepsia* 1987;28: 598(abst).

124. Brent DA, Crumrine PK, Varma RR, et al. Phenobarbital treatment and major depressive disorder in children with epilepsy. *Paediatrics* 1987;80:909–917.

125. Dodrill CB. Behavioral effects of antiepileptic drugs. *Adv Neurol* 1991;55:213–224.

126. MacLeod CM, Dekaban AS, Hunt E. Memory impairment in epileptic patients: selective effects of phenobarbital concentration. *Science* 1978;202:1102–1104.

127. Vining EP, Mellitis ED, Dorsen MM, et al. Psychologic and behavioral effects of antiepileptic drugs in children: a double-blind comparison between phenobarbital and valproic acid. *Pediatrics* 1987;80.

128. Calandre EP, Dominguez-Granados R, Gomez-Rubio M, et al. Cognitive effects of long-term treatment with phenobarbital and valproic acid in school children. *Acta Neurol Scand* 1990; 81:504–506.

129. Gallassi R, Morreale A, Di Sarro R, et al. Cognitive effects of antiepileptic drug discontinuation. *Epilepsia* 1992;33[Suppl 6]: 41–44.

130. Franks RD, Richter AJ. Schizophrenia-like psychosis associated with anticonvulsant toxicity. *Am J Psychiatry* 1979;136: 973–974.

131. Bailey DN, Jatlow PI. Chemical analysis of massive crystalluria following primidone overdose. *Am J Clin Pathol* 1972;58: 583–589.

132. Flexner JM, Hartmann RC. Megaloblastic anemia associated with anticonvulsant drugs. *Am J Med* 1960;28:386–396.

133. Chalmers JNM, Boheimer K. Megaloblastic anemia and anticonvulsant therapy. *Lancet* 1954;2:920–921.

134. Fuld H, Moorhouse EH. Observations on megaloblastic anemias after primidone. *BMJ* 1957;1:344.

135. Montgomery D, Craig J. Megaloblastic anemia during primidone therapy: report of a case responding to vitamin B$_{12}$. *Scott Med J* 1958;3:460.

136. Newman MJD, Sumner DW. Megaloblastic anemia following the use of primidone. *Blood* 1957;12:183–188.

137. Mountain KR, Hirsh J, Gallus AS. Neonatal coagulation defects due to anticonvulsant drug treatment in pregnancy. *Lancet* 1970;1:265–268.

138. Parker WA. Primidone thrombocytopenia. *Ann Intern Med* 1974;81:559–560.

139. Livingston S. *Drug therapy for epilepsy.* Springfield, IL: Charles C Thomas, 1966.

140. Langlands AO, MacLean N, Pearson JG, et al. Lymphadenopathy and megaloblastic anemia in patients receiving primidone. *BMJ* 1967;1:215–217.

141. Hartlage LC, Stovall K, Kocack B. Behavioral correlates of anticonvulsant blood levels. *Epilepsia* 1980;21:185.

142. Richens A. The clinical consequences of chronic hepatic enzyme induction by anticonvulsant drugs. *Br J Clin Pharmacol* 1974;1:185–187.

143. Fincham RW, Schottelius DD. Primidone interactions with other drugs. In: Woodbury JDM, Penry JK, Pippenger CE. *Antiepileptic drugs,* 2nd ed. New York: Raven Press, 1982.

144. McGeachy TE, Bleemer WE. The phenobarbital sensitivity syndrome. *Am J Med* 1953;14:600–604.

145. Granick S. Hepatic porphyria and drug-induced or chemical porphyria. *Ann NY Acad Sci* 1965;123:188–197.

146. Matzke GR, Cloyd JC, Sawchuk RJ. Acute phenytoin and primidone intoxication: a pharmacokinetic analysis. *J Clin Pharmacol* 1981;21:92–99.

147. Morley D, Wynne NA. Acute primidone poisoning in a child. *BMJ* 1957;1:90.

148. Lehman DF. Primidone crystalluria following overdose: a report of a case and an analysis of the literature. *Med Toxicol Adverse Drug Exp* 1987;2:383–387.

149. Richens A, Rowe DJF. Disturbance of calcium metabolism by anticonvulsant drugs. *BMJ* 1970;4:73–76.

150. Christiansen C, Rodbro P, Lund M. Incidence of anticonvulsant osteomalacia and effect of vitamin D: controlled therapeutic trial. *BMJ* 1973;4:695–701.

151. Stamp TCB. Effects of long-term anticonvulsant therapy on cal-

cium and vitamin D metabolism. *Proc R Soc Med* 1974;67:
64–68.

152. Offermann G, Pinto V, Kruse R. Antiepileptic drugs and vitamin D supplementation. *Epilepsia* 1979;20:3–15.

153. Mattson RH, Cramer JA, McCutchen CB, et al. Barbiturate related connective tissue disorders. *Arch Intern Med* 1973;149:911–914.

154. Critchley EMR, Vakil SD, Hayward HW, et al. Dupuytren's disease in epilepsy: result of prolonged administration of anticonvulsants. *J Neurol Neurosurg Psychiatry* 1976;39:498–503.

155. Janz D, Piltz U. Frozen shoulder induced by primidone. In: Oxley J, ed. *Antiepileptic therapy: chronic toxicity of antiepileptic drugs.* New York: Raven Press, 1983:155–159.

156. McElhatton PR, Sullivan FM. Teratogenic effects of primidone in mice. *Br J Pharmacol* 1975;54:267P–268P.

157. McElhatton PR, Sullivan FM, Toseland PA. Teratogenic activity and metabolism of primidone in the mouse. *Epilepsia* 1977;18:1–11.

158. Gustavson EE, Chen H. Goldenhar syndrome: enteroencephalocele and aqueductal stenosis following fetal primidone exposure. *Teratology* 1985;32:13–17.

159. Rudd NL, Freedom RM. A possible primidone embryopathy. *J Pediatr* 1979;94:835–837.

160. Fredrick J. Epilepsy and pregnancy: a report from the Oxford record linkage study. *BMJ* 1973;1:442–448.

161. Kaneko S, Battino D, Andermann E, et al. Congenital malformations due to antiepileptic drugs. *Epilepsy Res* 1999;33:145–158.

162. Koch S, Titze K, Zimmermann RB, et al. Long-term neuropsychological consequences of maternal epilepsy and anticonvulsant treatment during pregnancy for school-age children and adolescents. *Epilepsia* 1999;40:1237–1243.

163. Schmidt RP, Wilder BJ. *Epilepsy.* Philadelphia: FA Davis, 1968.

164. Rodriguez VLE, Ovideo SGV. Dermatitis ampollosa mortal desencadenada por la primidona (Mysoline). *Rev Esp Pediatr* 1957;13:737–747.

165. Gabriel RM. Delayed reaction to PRM in pregnancy. *BMJ* 1957;1:344.

166. Ahuja GK, Schumacher GA. Drug induced systematic lupus erythematosus: primidone as a possible cause. *JAMA* 1966;198:669–671.

167. Alarcon-Segovia D. Drug-induced lupus syndromes. *Mayo Clin Proc* 1966;44:664–681.

168. Hamer HM, Morris HH. Hypersensitivity syndrome to antiepileptic drugs: a review including new anticonvulsants. *Cleve Clin J Med* 1999;66:239–245.

169. Shorvon S. The treatment of epilepsy by drugs. In: Hopkins A, ed. *Epilepsy.* New York: Demos Publications, 1987:229–282.

170. Eadie MJ. Formation of active metabolites of anticonvulsant drugs: a review of their pharmacokinetic and therapeutic significance. *Clin Pharmacokinet* 1991;21:27–41.

171. Booker HE. Primidone toxicity. In: Woodbury DM, Penry JK, Schmidt RP, eds. *Antiepileptic drugs,* New York: Raven Press, 1972:377–383.

172. Leppik IE, Cloyd JC. Primidone toxicity. In: Levy R, Mattson R, Meldrum B, et al., eds. *Antiepileptic drugs,* 3rd ed. New York: Raven Press, 1989:439–445.

173. Cornaggia CM, Altamura AC, Bianchi M, et al. PB: PRM ratio in patients with epilepsy treated with primidone. *Int J Clin Pharmacol Res* 1983;3:185–193.

174. Fincham RW, Schottelius DD. Primidone: relation of plasma concentration to seizure control. In: Woodbury DM, Penry JK, Pippenger CE, eds. *Antiepileptic drugs,* 2nd ed. New York: Raven Press, 1982:429–440.

175. Armijo JA, Herranz JL, Arteaga R, et al. Poor correlation between single-dose data and steady-state kinetics for phenobarbitone, primidone, carbamazepine and sodium valproate in children during monotherapy: possible reasons for the lack of correlation. *Clin Pharmacokinet* 1986;11:323–335.

176. Bruni J, Albright PS. The clinical pharmacology of antiepileptic drugs. *Clin Neuropharmacol* 1984;7:1–34.

177. Schaffer LC, Schaffer CB, Caretto J. The use of primidone in the treatment of refractory bipolar disorder. *Ann Clin Psychiatry* 1999;11:61–66.

178. DeToledo JC, Smith DB, Haddad H, et al. Phenobarbital revisited in the institutionalized mentally retarded. *Epilepsia* 1990;31:614.

179. DeToledo JC, Haddad H, Smith DB. Pseudotoxicity of antiepileptic drugs in the mentally retarded. *Electroencephalogr Clin Neurophysiol* 1991;79:59P.

180. DeToledo JC, Haddad H, Smith DB. Behaviors mimicking epilepsy in the mentally retarded. *Electroencephalogr Clin Neurophysiol* 1991;79:58P.

181. Rating D, Jager-Roman E, Gopfert-Geyer I, et al. Teratogenic and pharmacokinetic studies of primidone during pregnancy and in the offspring of epileptic women. *Acta Paediatr Scand* 1982;71:301–311.

182. Levy RH, Yerby MS. Effects of pregnancy on antiepileptic drug utilization. *Epilepsia* 1985;26[Suppl 1]:S52–S57.

183. Martinez G, Snyder RD. Transplacental passage of primidone. *Neurology* 1973;23:381–383.

184. Nau H, Schmidt D, Beck-Mannagetta G, et al. Anticonvulsants during pregnancy and lactation: transplacental, maternal and neonatal pharmacokinetics. *Clin Pharmacokinet* 1982;7:508–543.

185. Nau H, Schmidt D, Beck-Mannagetta G, et al. Pharmacokinetics of primidone and metabolites during human pregnancy. In: Janz D, Dam M, Richens A, et al., eds. *Epilepsy, pregnancy and the child.* New York: Raven Press, 1981:349–355.

186. Rating D, Jager-Roman E, Koch S, et al. Enzyme induction in neonates due to antiepileptic therapy during pregnancy. In: Janz D, Dam M, Richens A, et al., eds. *Epilepsy, pregnancy and the child.* New York: Raven Press, 1981:349–355.

187. Krauss CM, Holmes LB, VanLang QN, et al. Four siblings with similar malformations after exposure to phenytoin and primidone. *J Pediatr* 1984;105:750.

188. Myhre SA, Williams R. Teratogenic effects associated with maternal primidone therapy. *J Pediatr* 1981;99:160–162.

189. Koller, WC, Kristova, A, Brin, M. Pharmacological treatment of essential tremor. *Neurology* 2000;54[Suppl 4]:S30–S38.

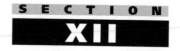

SUCCINIMIDES

SUCCINIMIDES

MECHANISMS OF ACTION

KATHERINE D. HOLLAND
JAMES A. FERRENDELLI

Succinimides, especially ethosuximide (ESM), α-ethyl-α-methyl succinimide, have been used extensively for the treatment of absence *(petit mal)* seizures. Despite the frequent use of these agents, the sites and mechanisms of action of succinimides are still poorly defined. In this chapter, the available published data on basic pharmacologic actions of succinimides are reviewed. Most of the available literature has focused on ESM; therefore, the main emphasis of this chapter is the mechanism of action of this succinimide. After reviewing its effects on clinical and experimental seizures, its molecular and cellular actions, and its neuronal systems effects, we present a hypothesis explaining its probable mechanism of action.

EFFECTS ON EPILEPTIFORM DISCHARGES

One of the most intriguing facts about ESM is its highly selective effect on clinical and experimental seizures. It completely, or almost completely, controls absence seizures in ~50% of patients with absence epilepsy and reduces the frequency of these seizures in another 40% to 45% of patients (1). The electroencephalographic (EEG) hallmark of absence seizures is generalized 3-Hz spike-and-wave complexes. Succinimides are able to eliminate these discharges in most patients (2,3). ESM is also highly effective at controlling epileptic negative myoclonus (4,5). In contrast, it has no apparent effect against generalized tonic-clonic convulsions or partial seizures. Methsuximide has a broader spectrum of action. It has been reported to be effective in some patients with partial seizures and in children with atypical absence seizures (6,7).

The high degree of therapeutic specificity of ESM in human seizure disorders is reflected by its selective anticon-

vulsant action against experimental seizures. It is well known that ESM prevents pentylenetetrazol (PTZ; Metrazol) seizures at nontoxic doses in experimental animals. However, it has no effect on maximal electroshock seizures, except at very high, toxic concentrations (8). ESM blocks spontaneous absencelike seizures, which occur in some genetically epilepsy-prone mice (9). It also has been reported to have an anticonvulsant effect on seizures induced by implantation of cobalt into the cerebral cortex (10–12), systemic administration of γ-hydroxybutyric acid (GHB) (13–15), application of conjugated estrogen to the brain (16), inhalation of fluorothyl (17) or enflurane (18), barbiturate withdrawal (19), and systemic administration of penicillin, picrotoxin, and a benzodiazepine receptor inverse agonist (20,21). However, it seems to be inactive against allylglycine seizures in photosensitive baboons (22), stroboscopic seizures in epileptic fowl (23), seizures produced by application of aluminum hydroxide (24) to the cerebral cortex, and seizures produced by the systemic administration of bicuculline, N-methyl-D-aspartate, strychnine, or aminophylline (20).

It has become increasingly clear that subcortical brain regions play a crucial role in the propagation of generalized seizures. An important characteristic of anticonvulsant compounds is their ability to depress repetitive impulses in the reticular core. Antiabsence drugs such as ESM have been shown to depress descending reticular inhibitory pathways (25). In addition, there is selective enrichment of ^{14}C-2-deoxyglucose uptake into the mammillary bodies and their connections during ESM-induced suppression of PTZ seizures (26). The ability of ESM to block PTZ-induced EEG phenomena in rats requires an intact hindbrain (27). This is not required for the action of other antiabsence agents such as valproate. These findings suggest a unique neurosystemic action of ESM that is important for its anti-PTZ, and perhaps antiabsence, activity. However, these observations do not clearly establish the functional anatomy of ESM action, and additional research on this question is needed.

Fromm and coworkers showed that antiabsence drugs preferentially depress central nervous system inhibitory

Katherine D. Holland, MD, PhD: Staff Physician, Department of Neurology, Cleveland Clinic Foundation, Cleveland, Ohio

James A. Ferrendelli, MD: Professor and Chairman, Department of Neurology, University of Texas, Houston Medical School; and Chief, Department of Neurology Service, Hermann Hospital, Houston, Texas

pathways that require considerable repetitive stimulation for activation (25,28–30). These investigators suggest that this accounts for the therapeutic specificity of ESM. In addition, they believe that absence seizures involve paroxysmal activity in inhibitory pathways (25,31). If this is the case, the observation that γ-aminobutyric acid (GABA) responses are reduced by ESM could provide a basis for the antiabsence properties of this drug. However, this theory cannot account for the ability of ESM to protect animals from seizures caused by picrotoxin, whose convulsant actions are thought to result from its ability to antagonize GABA-mediated inhibition noncompetitively.

In cultured neurons, ESM has no effect on the use-dependent firing of action potentials (32); however, *in vivo*, ESM is able to depress specific types of repetitive activation. ESM significantly reduces PTZ-induced photic recruitment and photic afterdischarges, and it completely suppresses PTZ-induced spindle activity (33). These rhythmic activities are thought to be an expression of synchronous afterdischarges of the thalamocortical system.

Investigators have suggested that the effect of ESM is mediated either by direct influences on inhibitory cells in the thalamic relay or by actions on ascending reticular activation. The lateral geniculate body has been discounted as the site of action because injections of ESM into the lateral geniculate could not abolish these photic afterdischarges (34). The actions of anticonvulsants on thalamocortical excitability have been examined by recording the cortical response elicited by a pair of stimuli given to the ventral lateral thalamus (31,35,36). These reports show that phenytoin, carbamazepine, and diazepam depressed evoked responses at all frequencies, and ESM and valproate decreased evoked responses at 3 Hz. This provides a basis for the effectiveness of ESM and valproate in controlling absence seizures characterized by 3-Hz spike-and-wave activity. Additionally, Pelligrini and associates (37) studied the effect of ESM on thalamic and cortical neuronal activity in cats. They concluded that ESM acts by disruption of spontaneous intrathalamic synchronizing mechanisms resulting in less efficient thalamocortical impulses necessary for cortical spike-and-wave discharges.

Studies of thalamic neurons reveal that they have tonic and burst-firing properties (38,39). This burst firing may underlie spike-and-wave discharges associated with generalized epilepsy (40). ESM decreases the probability that thalamic neurons will fire in a burst (39,41).

PHYSIOLOGIC EFFECTS

Effects on Excitability or Inhibition

A relationship between ESM and GABA has been suggested by several studies (42,43). Because anticonvulsants such as valproate, phenobarbital, and benzodiazepines potentiate GABA function, several laboratories have examined the possibility

that ESM may modify GABAergic neurotransmission. These studies reveal that ESM decreases GABA responses in cultured cortical, hippocampal, thalamic, and spinal cord neurons (32,44–46). Barnes and Dichter (44) report that 500 µmol/L ESM decreased the mean GABA response by 30%. The GABA receptor–chloride ionophore complex contains at least three distinct binding sites: the GABA site, the benzodiazepine site, and the picrotoxin site. In radioligand binding studies, ESM has no effect on diazepam and GABA binding to rat brain membranes at concentrations <1 mmol/L (47,48). At higher concentrations, ESM substantially inhibits GABA, but not benzodiazepine binding (47). In contrast, the binding of ^{35}S-t-butylbicyclophosphorothionate, the radioligand used to study the picrotoxin receptor, is decreased competitively at concentrations comparable to those used by Barnes and Dichter (47,49). This finding suggests that ESM-induced antagonism of GABA responses results from its action at the picrotoxin site and also implies that the anticonvulsant actions of ESM are not mediated by a postsynaptic enhancement of GABAergic responses.

The role of excitatory amino acids in the pathogenesis of epilepsy is the subject of intense research. Although the relationship between ESM and excitatory amino acids has yet to be fully investigated, some evidence suggests ESM does not work by a blockade of excitatory pathways. For example, ESM does not prevent seizures induced by either kainic acid or N-methyl-D-aspartate, but nonspecific excitatory amino acid antagonists are very potent blockers of these seizure types (50,51). In addition, the anticonvulsant profiles of ESM and certain excitatory amino acid antagonists differ substantially. These data are certainly not conclusive, but they do suggest that ESM does not alter excitatory amino acid function, at least by postsynaptic mechanisms.

Effects on Ion Channels and Transport

Investigators have shown that ESM has no effect on the basal level of calcium ion (Ca^{2+}) uptake into synaptosomes (52). Unlike phenytoin and carbamazepine, which inhibit Ca^{2+} accumulation into veratridine-depolarized synaptosomes at therapeutic concentrations, ESM is ineffective except at concentrations exceeding 10 mmol/L. Crowder and Bradford (53) confirmed this and additionally showed that ESM has no effect on veratridine-stimulated amino acid neurotransmitter release.

Calcium channels play an important role in neuronal excitability. Originally, three classes of channels that mediate calcium entry into neurons were identified: L (large), T (tiny), and N (neither) channels (54). These channels differ in their magnitude, voltage dependence, activation properties, and pharmacologic profiles. The low-threshold calcium channel (LTCC) is analogous to the T channel and is a transient, low-conductance channel present in thalamic neurons. Experiments by Coulter, Huguenard, and Prince (39,55–57) showed that therapeutic concentrations of ESM reduce the LTCC in thalamic neurons. ESM did not affect the gating properties of the channel; it reduced either the number of LTCC channels or the single-channel conductance. Dimethadione, another antiabsence drug, had the same action. Carbamazepine, phenytoin, and valproate had no effect on the LTCC at clinically relevant concentrations. Convulsant succinimide compounds, such as tetramethylsuccinimide, do not alter thalamic LTCCs. ESM also inhibited high-threshold calcium channels, but to a lesser extent than its effect on the LTCC, and at concentrations significantly higher than the therapeutic range of ESM. Similar effects of ESM on T currents have been demonstrated in sensory neurons (58), but other researchers have failed to find any effects of ESM on T-type calcium currents in numerous other types of neurons (59–61).

More recently, Leresche and colleagues (41) studied the action of ESM in thalamic neurons. They found that ESM decreased noninactivating sodium ion (Na^+) currents in thalamocortical neurons at clinically relevant concentrations. It did not alter transient Na^+ currents. ESM also blocked Ca^{2+}-dependent potassium ion (K^+) channels. In contrast to the work by Coulter et al. (45,53,55–57), Leresche did not find any effect on the LTCC despite studying various types of thalamic neurons in various strains of rats. The reason for this discrepancy is unclear.

Effects on Voltage Sensitive Receptors

Fohlmeister, Aldelman, and Brennan (62) examined the effects of ESM and valproate on excitable Na^+- and K^+-channels in voltage-clamped squid giant axons. These researchers reported that ESM applied to the external surface of the axon reduced Na^+-current in a voltage-independent manner, reduced maximal K^+ conductance, and slowed K^+ channel gating. Internally applied ESM slowed Na^+ and K^+ channel gating and reduced the peak conductance of the Na^+ channel in a voltage-dependent fashion. The significance of these observations in invertebrate neurons as related to the anticonvulsant mechanism of ESM is unclear because of both the species difference and the heroic concentrations of ESM used (60 mmol/L). Other investigators have reported that ESM is unable to inhibit ^{2}H-batrachotoxinin A 20-α-benzoate binding to sodium channels and batrachotoxinin-induced Na^+ flux in neuroblastoma cells and rat brain synaptosomes at concentrations up to 1 mmol/L (63,64). These data suggest that this sodium channel is not ESM's site of anticonvulsant action.

BIOCHEMICAL EFFECTS

The molecular bases for changes in neuronal excitability involve actions on brain enzyme activity, neuron transmitter processes, and ion channels. The effects of ESM on each of these are discussed.

Effects on Biochemical Systems

Two laboratories have reported that ESM inhibits (Na^+, K^+)–adenosine triphosphatase (ATPase) activity but not magnesium ion–ATPase activity in subcellular fractions of cortical tissue (21,65–67). The data of Gilbert and colleagues suggest that the site of (Na^+, K^+)-ATPase inhibition may be restricted to the nerve terminal plasma membrane (21). Unfortunately, these effects were found at ESM concentrations (2.5 and 25 mmol/L) considerably greater than those producing anticonvulsant effects. In addition, although Leznicki and Dymecki (67) reported that ESM inhibits (Na^+, K^+-ATPase in brain homogenates, they also found that long-term treatment of animals resulted in an increase in (Na^+, K^+)-ATPase activity.

Although ESM has been reported to have little or no direct effect on the GABA- synthesizing enzyme glutamic acid decarboxylase (67), it antagonizes isoniazid-induced inhibition of this enzyme (68). However, single-dose administration of ESM in anticonvulsant doses has no effect on brain GABA concentration (69). Thus, alterations in brain GABA do not contribute to the anticonvulsant effects of ESM. ESM has no effect on the activities of various enzymes involved in the breakdown of neurotransmitters including GABA transaminase, monoamine oxidase, acetylcholinesterase, and arylsulfatase (67).

ESM inhibits NADPH (reduced form of nicotinamideadenine dinucleotide phosphate)–linked aldehyde reductase in bovine brain (70). This enzyme can convert succinic semialdehyde to GHB and may be the mechanism by which long-term ESM treatment decreases brain GHB levels (71,72). In light of the behavioral and EEG similarities between human absence seizures and administration of exogenous GHB, alterations in endogenous GHB levels could be relevant to the antiabsence actions of ESM (13,14,73). However, this is unable to account for either the anti-PTZ actions of ESM or the ability of ESM to block seizures caused by exogenous GHB. In addition, single-dose administration of ESM produces an increase in brain GHB, possibly by inhibition of GHB dehydrogenase (74), and that this increase coincides with the onset of anticonvulsant effects (72).

Studies in genetic absence epilepsy in rats from Strasbourg (GAERS) have shown that endogenously released nitric oxide can suppress generalized spike-and-wave discharges (75). ESM has been shown to promote nitric oxide release in GAERS animals and also to suppress the epileptiform discharges in these animals. The molecular biochemical basis for this increase in nitric oxide release is unknown.

Neuroprotective Effects

Potential neuroprotective effects of ESM have not been studied. However, from information about its lack of action at excitatory amino acid receptors (50,51), and a study showing that ESM can release nitric oxide (75), a compound associated with neuronal injury, it is unlikely that ESM has significant neuroprotective properties (76).

Effects at Synapse–Drug Receptor Interactions

Several laboratories have demonstrated that GHB produces seizures in experimental animals. These seizures resemble human absence seizures behaviorally, electrically, and pharmacologically (13–15,72). Although the mechanism by which GHB produces seizures remains obscure, specific high-affinity GHB binding sites associated with the GABA-mediated chloride ionophore have been identified (77,78). It has also been established that GHB is capable of blocking flow through dopaminergic neurotransmitter systems (19). ESM is highly effective in preventing GHB-induced seizures. However, ESM is not able to compete with ^{3}H-GHB for binding to rat brain (77). This finding suggests that the anti-GHB and antiabsence effects of this drug are not the result of direct action at the putative GHB binding site. ESM inhibits depolarization-evoked release of GHB from hippocampal slices (79). Although this may explain the rise in brain GHB concentration after single-dose ESM administration, it cannot account for the ability of ESM to block seizures produced by exogenously supplied GHB.

Fluphenazine, a dopamine receptor antagonist, and α-methylparatyrosine, an inhibitor of dopamine synthesis, can block the protective effects of ESM in the GHB seizure model (80). This finding indicates that the anticonvulsant action of ESM, at least in the GHB model, may be related to some effect on dopaminergic neurotransmission, possibly by augmentation of dopamine-mediated inhibition in the central nervous system. The involvement of dopaminergic systems in the action of ESM is supported by the following observations. First, L-DOPA, a dopamine precursor, prevents cobalt-induced seizures that are also prevented by ESM (12). Second, cortical spikes produced by the topical application of penicillin are prevented by systemic L-DOPA and by topical dopamine but not by topical norepinephrine (81). As mentioned earlier, ESM prevents seizures produced by systemic administration of penicillin (82). Finally, dopamine receptor agonists decrease the duration of spike-and-wave discharges in rats with spontaneous absencelike seizures (83). ESM is also able to abolish seizures in this form of epilepsy (84). However, these results must be interpreted cautiously because, at present, ESM has not been shown directly to alter dopamine-mediated processes either *in vivo* or *in vitro*.

SUMMARY OF "UNIFIED MECHANISM"

Any complete description of the mechanisms of action of an antiepileptic drug would require a full understanding of the pathophysiologic mechanisms of epilepsy and an explanation of how the drug modifies these to prevent seizures. Because the pathophysiologic mechanisms of epilepsy are still incompletely understood, one can only speculate about the mechanisms of action of most antiepileptic drugs.

Anticonvulsant drugs are widely believed to act by (a) direct modification of membrane function in excitable cells, (b) alteration of chemically mediated neurotransmission, and/or (c) alteration in the activity of ion channels. There is no evidence that ESM indirectly and nonspecifically alters membrane structure, thereby disrupting ionic channels. ESM is highly water soluble, so it is unlikely that much of it inserts into cellular membranes that have a high lipid content. Furthermore, it has none of the properties of general anesthetics that are thought to exert their effects by a direct action on cellular membranes.

The action of ESM does not appear to be directly related to its known actions on neurotransmitter processes. Indirect evidence indicates that it may deplete excitatory neurotransmitter stores mediating the spinal monosynaptic reflex. This is thought to occur by an increase in fractional release per stimulus without resultant increase in synthesis. Although a similar effect in brain could selectively depress repetitive impulses, thereby preventing seizures, it is not likely because the increased release of excitatory neurotransmitters on initial impulses could be enough to potentiate seizure activity. In addition, direct measurements of neurotransmitters indicate that, in many systems, synthesis can more than compensate for increased release even at the highest firing rates attainable. A more tenable explanation would be that ESM may increase the influence of inhibitory neurotransmitters. The suggested depressant effects on corticofugal inhibition of the spinal trigeminal nucleus may well be a result of some action on neuronal pathways subserved by inhibitory neurotransmitters. However, present evidence suggests that ESM does not significantly increase, but rather diminishes, GABA-mediated inhibitory processes. Possibly the anticonvulsant effect of ESM may involve dopamine-mediated neurotransmission, but this is also uncertain. Other still unidentified, inhibitory neurotransmitter systems may be responsible for or may have a role in ESM mechanisms of action.

Experimental models suggest that thalamic neurons play an important role in the generation of thalamocortical rhythmicity that underlies the 3-Hz spike-and-wave discharges seen during absence seizures (85), and calcium currents are involved in the production of low-threshold calcium spikes involved in the generation of sleep spindles. Studies on the kinetic properties of calcium currents in thalamocortical relay neurons suggest that the T current or LTCC is necessary and sufficient to generate the low-threshold calcium spikes produced in thalamic relay neurons. Although multiple studies have shown that ESM can decrease the bursting of these thalamocortical neurons, the molecular mechanism is unclear. Some researchers have shown that ESM can effect T currents, whereas others have not been able to reproduce this finding. An alternative hypothesis is that ESM blocks spike-and-wave discharges and burst firing in thalamocortical neurons by inhibition of a noninactivating sodium current in thalamic neurons.

REFERENCES

1. Browne TR, Dreifuss FE, Dyken PR, et al. Ethosuximide in the treatment of absence (petit mal) seizures. *Neurology* 1975;25: 515–524.
2. Browne TR, Dreifuss FE, Penry JK, et al. Clinical and EEG estimates of absence seizure frequency. *Arch Neurol* 1983;40: 469–472.
3. Blomquist HK, Zetterlaund B. Evaluation of treatment in typical absence seizures: the roles of long-term EEG monitoring and ethosuximide. *Acta Paediatr Scand* 1985;74:409–415.
4. Oguni H, Uehara T, Tanaka T, et al. Dramatic effect of ethosuximide on epileptic negative myoclonus: implications for the neurophysiological mechanism. *Neuropediatrics* 1998;29:29–34.
5. Capovilla G, Beccaria F, Veggiotti P, et al. Ethosuximide is effective in the treatment of epileptic negative myoclonus in childhood partial epilepsy. *J Child Neurol* 1999;14:395–400.
6. Wilder BJ, Buchanan RB. Methsuximide for refractory complex partial seizures. *Neurology* 1981;31:741–744.
7. Tennison MB, Greenwood RS, Miles MV. Methsuximide for intractable childhood seizures. *Pediatrics* 1991;87:186–189.
8. Chen A, Weston JK, Bratton AC Jr. Anticonvulsant activity and ethosuximide. *Epilepsia* 1963;XX:66–76.
9. Heller AH, Dichter MA, Sidman RL. Anticonvulsant sensitivity of absence seizures in the tottering mutant mouse. *Epilepsia* 1983;25:25–34.
10. Dow RC, Forfar JC, McQueen JK. The effects of some anticonvulsant activity on cobalt-induced epilepsy. *Epilepsia* 1973;14: 203–212.
11. Kastner I, Klingberg F, Muller M. Zur Wirkung des Ethosuximids auf die Kobalt-in-duzierte "Epilepsie" der Ratte. *Arch Int Pharmacodyn Ther* 1970;186:220–226.
12. Scuvee-Moreau J, Lepot M, Brotchi J, et al. Action of phenytoin, ethosuximide, and of the carbidopa–L-dopa association in semichronic cobalt-induced epilepsy in the rat. *Arch Int Pharmacodyn Ther* 1977;230:92–99.
13. Godschalk M, Dzoljíc MR, Bonta IL. Antagonism of gamma-hydroxybutyrate-induced hypersynchronization in the ECoG of the rat by anti-petit mal drugs. *Neurosci Lett* 1976;3:145–150.
14. Snead OC. Gammahydroxybutyrate in the monkey. II. Effect of chronic oral anticonvulsant drugs. *Neurology* 1978;28:643–648.
15. Snead OC. Gammahydroxybutyrate in the monkey. III. Effect of intravenous anticonvulsant drugs. *Neurology* 1978;28: 1173–1178.
16. Julien RM, Fowler GW, Danielson MG. The effect of antiepileptic drugs on estrogen-induced electrographic spike–wave discharges. *J Pharm Exp Ther* 1975;193:647–656.
17. Adler MW. The effect of single and multiple lesions of limbic system on cerebral excitability. *Psychopharmacologia* 1972;24: 218–230.
18. Schettine A, Wilder BJ. Effects of anticonvulsant drugs on enflurane cortical dysrhythmias. *Anesth Analg* 1974;53:951–962.
19. Roth RH, Walters JR, Aghajanian GK. Effect of impulse flow on the release and synthesis of dopamine in the rat striatum. In: Udsin E, Snyder SH, eds. *Frontiers in catecholamine research.* Oxford: Pergamon Press, 1973:567–574.
20. Ferrendelli JA, Holland KD, McKeon AC, et al. Comparison of the anticonvulsant activities of ethosuximide, valproate, and a new anticonvulsant, thiobutyrolactone. *Epilepsia* 1989;30: 617–622.
21. Gilbert JC, Wyllie MG. The effects of the anticonvulsant ethosuximide on adenosine triphosphatase activities of synaptosomes prepared from rat cerebral cortex. *Br J Pharmacol* 1974;52: 139P–140P.
22. Meldrum BS, Horton RW, Toseland PA. A primate model for testing anticonvulsant agents. *Mol Pharmacol* 1975;14:347–356.
23. Davis HL, Johnson DD, Crawford RD. Epileptiform seizures in domestic fowl. IX. Implication of the absence of anticonvulsant activity on ethosuximide in a pharmacological model of epilepsy. *Can J Physiol Pharmacol* 1978;56:893–896.
24. Lockard JS, Levy RH, Congdon WC, et al. Efficacy testing of valproic acid compared to ethosuximide in monkey model. II. Seizure, EEG, and diurnal variation. *Epilepsia* 1977;18:205–224.
25. Fromm GH, Terrence CF. Effect of antiepileptic drugs on the brainstem. In: Fromm GH, Faingold DL, Browning RA, et al., eds. *Epilepsy and the reticular formation: the role of the reticular core in convulsive seizures.* New York: Alan R. Liss, 1987: 119–136.
26. Mirski MA, Ferrendelli JA. Selective metabolic activation of the mammillary bodies and their connections during ethosuximide induced suppression of pentylenetetrazol seizures. *Epilepsia* 1986; 27:194–203.
27. Mares P, Pohl M, Kubova H, et al. Is the site of action of ethosuximide in the hindbrain? *Physiol Res* 1994;43:51–56.
28. Fromm GH, Glass JD, Chattha AS, et al.. Effect of anticonvulsant drugs on inhibitory and excitatory pathways. *Epilepsia* 1981; 22:65–73.
29. Fromm GH, Glass JD, Chattha AS, et al. Antiabsence drugs and inhibitory pathways. *Neurology* 1980;30:126–131.
30. Shibuya T, Fromm GH, Terrence CF. Differential effect of ethosuximide and of electrical stimulation on inhibitory and excitatory mechanisms. *Epilepsy Res* 1987;1:35–39.
31. Englander RN, Johnson RN, Brickley JJ, et al. Ethosuximide and bicuculline inhibition in petit mal epilepsy. *Neurol Neurochir Psychiatr* 1977;18:265–275.
32. McLean MJ, MacDonald RL. Sodium valproate, but not ethosuximide, produces use- and voltage-dependent limitation of high frequency repetitive firing of action potentials of mouse central neurons in cell culture. *J Pharmacol Exp Ther* 1986;237: 1001–1011.
33. Wenzel J, Krueger E, Mueller M. Hemmung pentylenetetrazol-induzierter hypersynchroner Aktivität im thalamokortikalen System durch Ethosuximid. *Acta Biol Med Germ* 1971;26:567–572.
34. Kastner I, Rougerie A. Photisch Ausgelöste potentialfolgen nach lokaler Aplikation von Ethosuximid ins Corpus geniculatum laterale. *Acta Biol Med Germ* 1978;37:677–679.
35. Englander RN, Johnson RN, Brickley JJ, et al. Effects of antiepileptic drugs on thalamocortical excitability. *Neurology* 1977;27:1134–1139.
36. Nowack WJ, Johnson RN, Englander RN, et al. Effects of valproate and ethosuximide on thalamocortical excitability. *Neurology* 1979;29:96–99.
37. Pelligrini A, Dossi RC, Dal Pos F, et al. Ethosuximide alters intrathalamic and thalamocortical synchronizing mechanisms: a possible explanation of its antiabsence effect. *Brain Res* 1989;497: 344–360.
38. Huguenard JR, Prince DA. A novel type of T-current underlies prolonged Ca^{2+} dependent burst firing in GABAergic neurons of rat thalamic reticular nucleus. *J Neurosci* 1992;12:3804–3817.
39. Huguenard JR, Prince DA. Intrathalmic rhythmicity studied *in vitro*: nominal T-current modulation causes robust antioscillatory effects. *J Neurosci* 1994;14:5485–5502.
40. Inoue M, Duysens J, Vossen JMH, et al. Thalamic multiple-unit

activity underlying spike-wave discarges in anesthetized rats. *Brain Res* 1993;612:35–40.

41. Leresche N, Parri H, Erdemli G, et al. On the action of the anti-absence drug ethosuximide in the rat and cat thalamus. *J Neurosci* 1998;18:4842–4845.

42. Klunk WE, Covey DF, Ferrendelli JA. Structure-activity relationships of alkyl substituted γ-butyrolactones and succinimides. *Mol Pharmacol* 1982;22:444–450.

43. Klunk WE, Kalman BL, Ferrendelli JA, et al. Computer-assisted modeling of the picrotoxinin and γ-butyrolactone receptor site. *Mol Pharmacol* 1983;23:511–518.

44. Barnes DM, Dichter MA. Effects of ethosuximide and tetramethylsuccinimide on cultured cortical neurons. *Neurology* 1984; 34:620–625.

45. Coulter, DA, Huguenard JR, Price DA. Differential effects of petit mal anticonvulsants and convulsants on thalamic neurones: GABA current blockade. *Br J Pharmacol* 1990;100:807–813.

46. Holland KD, Ferrendelli JA, Covey DF, et al. Physiological regulation of the picrotoxin receptor by γ-butyrolactones and γ-thiobutyrolactones in cultured hippocampal neurons. *J Neurosci* 1990;10:1719–1727.

47. Holland KD, McKeon AC, Covey DF, et al. Binding interactions of convulsant and anticonvulsant γ-butyrolactones and γ-thiobutyrolactones with the picrotoxin receptor. *J Pharmacol Exp Ther* 1990;254:578–583.

48. Skerritt JH, Johnston GAR. Interactions of some anesthetic, convulsant, and anticonvulsant drugs at GABA-benzodiazepine receptor-ionophore complexes in rat brain synaptosomal membranes. *Neurochem Res* 1983;8:1351–1362.

49. Pitkänen A, Saano V, Tuomisto L, et al. Effect of anticonvulsant drugs on (^{35}S)t-butylbicyclophosphorothionate binding *in vitro* and *ex vivo*. *Pharmacol Toxicol* 1987;61:103–106.

50. Clifford DB, Lothman EW, Dodson WE, et al. Effect of anticonvulsant drugs on kainic acid-induced epileptiform activity. *Exp Neurol* 1982;76:156–167.

51. Czuczwar SJ, Frey H-H, Löscher W. N-Methyl-D,L-aspartic acid-induced convulsions in mice and their blockade by antiepileptic drugs and other agents. In: Nisticô G, Morselli PL, Lloyd KG, et al., eds. *Neurotransmitters, seizures, and epilepsy III*. New York: Raven Press, 1986:235–246.

52. Sohn RS, Ferrendelli JA. Anticonvulsant drug mechanisms phenytoin, phenobarbital, and ethosuximide and Ca^{2+} flux in isolated presynaptic endings. *Arch Neurol* 1976;33:626–629.

53. Crowder JM, Bradford HF. Common anticonvulsants inhibit Ca^{2+} uptake and amino acid neurotransmitter release *in vitro*. *Epilepsia* 1987;28:378–382.

54. Nowycky MC, Fox AP, Tsien RW. More types of neuronal calcium channels with different agonist sensitivity. *Nature* 1985; 316:440–443.

55. Coulter, DA, Huguenard JR, Price DA. Characterization of ethosuximide reduction of low-threshold calcium current in thalamic neurons. *Ann Neurol* 1989;25:582–593.

56. Coulter, DA, Huguenard JR, Price DA. Specific petit mal anticonvulsants reduce calcium currents in thalamic neurons. *Neurosci Lett* 1989;98:74–78.

57. Coulter, DA, Huguenard JR, Price DA. Differential effects of petit mal anticonvulsants and convulsants on thalamic neurones: calcium current blockade. *Br J Pharmacol* 1990;100:800–806.

58. Kostyuk PG, Molokanova EA, Pronchuck NF, et al. Different action of ethosuximide on low- and high-threshold calcium currents in rat sensory neurons. *Neuroscience* 1992;51:755–758.

59. Pfrieger FW, Veselovsky NS, Gottmann K, et al. Pharmacological characterization of calcium currents and synaptic transmission between thalamic neurons *in vitro*. *J Neurosci* 1992;12: 4347–4357.

60. Sayer RJ, Brown AM, Schwindt PC. Calcium currents in acutely isolated human neocortical neurons. *J Neurophysiol* 1993;69: 1596–1606.

61. Thompson SM, Wong RS. Development of calcium current subtypes in isolated rat hippocampal pyramidal cells. *J Physiol (Lond)* 1991;439:671–689.

62. Fohlmeister JF, Adelman WJ, Brennan JJ. Excitable channel currents and gating times in the presence of anticonvulsant ethosuximide and valproate. *J Pharmacol Exp Ther* 1984;230:75–81.

63. Willow M, Catterall WA. Inhibition of binding of [^{3}H]batrachotoxinin A 20-α-benzoate to sodium channels by the anticonvulsant drugs diphenylhydantoin and carbamazepine. *Mol Pharmacol* 1982;22:267–635.

64. Willow M, Kuenzel EA, Catterall WA. Inhibition of voltage-sensitive sodium channels in neuroblastoma cells and synaptosomes by the anticonvulsant drugs diphenylhydantoin and carbamazepine. *Mol Pharmacol* 1984;25:228–234.

65. Gilbert JC, Buchan P, Scott AK. Effects of anticonvulsant drugs on monosaccharide transport and membrane ATPase activities of cerebral cortex. In: Harris P, Mawdsley C, eds. *Epilepsy*. Edinburgh: Churchill Livingstone, 1974:98–104.

66. Gilbert JC, Scott AK, Wyllie MG. Effects of ethosuximide on adenosine triphosphatase activities of some subcellular fractions prepared from rat cerebral cortex. *Br J Pharmacol* 1974;50: 452P–453P.

67. Leznicki A, Dymecki J. The effect of certain anticonvulsants *in vitro* and *in vivo* on enzyme activities in rat brain. *Neurol Neurochir Pol* 1974;24:413–419.

68. Löscher W, Frey H-H. Effects of convulsant and anticonvulsant agents on level and metabolism of γ-aminobutyric acid in mouse brain. *Naunyn Schmiedebergs Arch Pharmacol* 1977;296; 263–269.

69. Lin-Mitchell E, Chweh AY, Swinyard EA. Effect of ethosuximide alone and in combination with γ-aminobutyric acid receptor agonists on brain γ-aminobutyric acid concentration, anticonvulsant activity and neurotoxicity in mice. *J Pharmacol Exp Ther* 1986;237:486–489.

70. Erwin VG, Deitrich RA. Inhibition of bovine brain aldehyde reductase by anticonvulsant compounds. *Biochem Pharmacol* 1973;2:2615–2624.

71. Snead OC, Bearden LJ, Pergram V. Effect of acute and chronic anticonvulsant administration on endogenous γ-hydroxybutyrate in rat brain. *Neuropharmacology* 1980;19:47–52.

72. Tabakoff B, von Wartburg JP. Separation of aldehyde reductases and alcohol dehydrogenase from brain by affinity chromatography: metabolism of succinic semialdehyde and ethanol. *Biochem Biophys Res Commun* 1975;63:957–966.

73. Winters WD, Spooner CE. A neurophysiological comparison of gamma-hydroxybutyrate with pentobarbital in cats. *Electroencephalogr Clin Neurophysiol* 1965;18:287–296.

74. Hechler V, Ratomponirina C, Maitre M. Gamma-hydroxbutyrate conversion into GABA induces displacement of GABAB binding that is blocked by valproate and ethosuximide. *J Pharmacol Exp Ther* 1996;281:753–760.

75. Faradji H, Rousset C, Deilly G, et al. Sleep and epilepsy: a key role for nitric oxide? *Epilepsia* 2000;41:794–801.

76. Matsui T, Nagafuji T, Kumanishi T, et al. Role of nitric oxide in pathogenesis underlying ischemic cerebral damage. *Cell Mol Neurobiol* 1999;19:177–189.

77. Snead OC, Liu C-C. Gamma-hydroxybutyric acid binding sites in rat and human brain synaptosomal membranes. *Biochem Pharmacol* 1984;33:2587–2590.

78. Snead OC, Nichols AC. γ-Hydroxybutyric acid binding sites: evidence for coupling to a chloride anion channel. *Neuropharmacology* 1987;26:1519–1523.

79. Vayer P, Charlie B, Mandel P, et al. Effect of anticonvulsant drugs on γ-hydroxybutyrate release from hippocampal slices: inhibition by valproate and ethosuximide. *J Neurochem* 1987;49:1022–1024.

80. Klunk WE, Ferrendelli JA. Reversal of the anticonvulsant action of ethosuximide by drugs that diminish CNS dopaminergic neurotransmission. *Neurology* 1980;30:421.

81. Kobayashi K, Shirakabe T, Kishikawa H, et al. Catecholamine levels in penicillin-induced epileptic focus of the cat cerebral cortex. *Acta Neurochir Suppl (Wien)* 1976;23:93–100.

82. Guberman AG, Gloor P, Sherwin AL. Response of generalized penicillin epilepsy in the cat to ethosuximide and diphenylhdantoin. *Neurology* 1975;25:758–764.

83. Warter J-M, Vergnes M, Depaulis A, et al. Effects of drugs affecting dopaminergic neurotransmission in rats with spontaneous *petit mal*-like seizures. *Neuropharmacology* 1988;27:269–274.

84. Micheletti G, Vergnes M, Marescaux C, et al. Antiepileptic drug evaluation in a new animal model: spontaneous *petit mal* epilepsy in the rat. *Arzneimittelforschung* 1985;35:473–475.

85. Gloor P, Fariello RG. Generalized epilepsy: some of its cellular mechanisms differ from those of focal epilepsy. *Trends Neurosci* 1988;11:63–68.

SUCCINIMIDES

ETHOSUXIMIDE: CHEMISTRY, BIOTRANSFORMATION, PHARMACOKINETICS, AND DRUG INTERACTIONS

FRANCESCO PISANI
EMILIO PERUCCA
MEIR BIALER

Ethosuximide was discovered at Parke-Davis Laboratories in the early 1950s. After many decades of clinical use (1), it remains a major therapeutic tool for the management of absence seizures.

CHEMISTRY

Ethosuximide, or 2-ethyl-2-methylsuccinimide ($C_7H_{11}NO_2$), a weak acid (negative log of dissociation constant, 9.3), is a white crystalline powder with a molecular weight of 141.17, a melting point of 64° to 65°C, a chloroform/water partition coefficient of 9 at pH 7, and a water solubility of 190 mg/mL.

Its structure (Figure 67.1) includes a five-membered ring with two negatively charged carbonyl oxygen atoms separated by a distance of about 4.5 A. A ring nitrogen is situated between the two groups, and this feature has been suggested to be required for the anticonvulsant effect (2). Because of the occurrence of a chiral carbon at the 2 position of the succinimide ring, ethosuximide exists as a racemic mixture of two separate enantiomers.

Francesco Pisani, MD: Associate Professor of Neurology, Department of Neurosciences, Psychiatric and Anaesthesiological Sciences, University of Messina, Messina, Italy

Emilio Perucca, MD, PhD, FRCP (Edin): Professor of Medical Pharmacology, Clinical Pharmacology Unit, Department of Internal Medicine and Therapeutics, University of Pavia; and Consultant Clinical Pharmacologist, Institute of Neurology, C. Mondino Foundation, Pavia, Italy

Meir Bialer, PhD, MBA: David H. Eisenberg Professor of Pharmacy, Department of Pharmaceutics, School of Pharmacy, Faculty of Medicine, The Hebrew University of Jerusalem, Jerusalem, Israel

BIOTRANSFORMATION

Both in animals and in humans, only a relatively small proportion (about 20%) of an administered dose of ethosuximide is excreted unchanged in urine (3–6). Ethosuximide is eliminated primarily by metabolism, and the most important pathways are summarized in Figure 67.1. In humans, 30% to 60% of the administered dose is recovered in urine as the isomers of 2-(1-hydroxyethyl)-2-methylsuccinimide, and at least 40% of these are excreted as glucuronide conjugates (3,7–11). The 2- and 3-hydroxy derivatives and 2-carboxymethyl-2-methylsuccinimide represent less important metabolites (3,12,13). There is no evidence that the metabolites of ethosuximide possess significant anticonvulsant activity, except for a report suggesting weak protective effects of 2-(1-hydroxyethyl)-2-methylsuccinimide against pentylenetetrazol-induced seizures in mice (3). In any case, the finding that the unchanged drug is the predominant plasma component in all species including humans argues against an important pharmacodynamic contribution of ethosuximide metabolites.

Studies in rats suggest that ethosuximide metabolism is mediated primarily by cytochrome P450 (CYP) isozymes, with a major contribution from CYP3A and, to a lesser extent, CYP2E and CYP2B/C (10,14,15). In humans, ethosuximide metabolism is stimulated by concomitant administration of rifampicin (16), phenobarbital, phenytoin, and carbamazepine (17,18), all of which are known inducers of cytochrome CYP3A/4.

Although ethosuximide is an enantiomeric drug, potential stereoselectivity in its disposition has been minimally investigated. In one study, the ratio between the two enantiomers measured by chiral gas chromatography in plasma samples from 33 patients receiving long-term treatment was close to unity (19). This finding is consistent with a similar disposition rate for the two enantiomers.

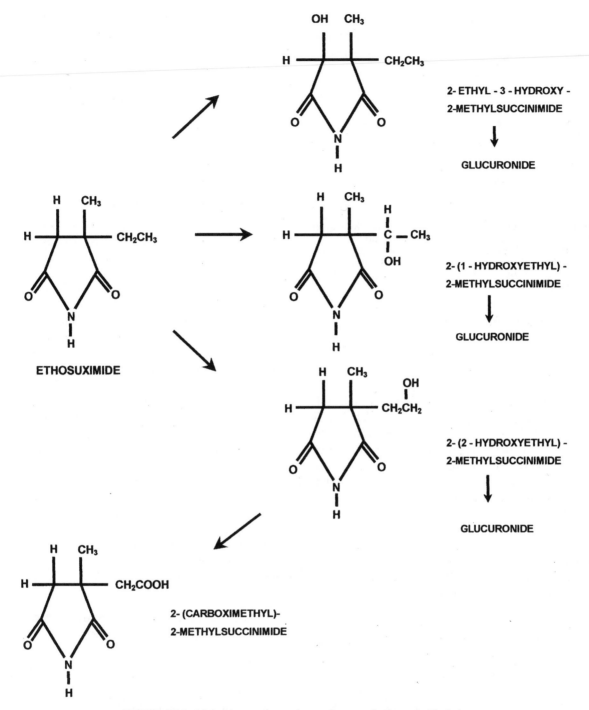

FIGURE 67.1. Main biotransformation pathways of ethosuximide in humans.

PHARMACOKINETICS

Absorption

Ethosuximide is available clinically only in oral dosage forms. After intake of single doses (two 250-mg capsules), the drug is absorbed relatively rapidly and reaches peak plasma concentrations within 3 to 5 hours in both children and adults (4,20,21). The bioavailability of syrup and cap-sules is equivalent, but absorption occurs at a faster rate with the syrup (4) (Figure 67.2).

Being a low-clearance drug, ethosuximide does not undergo significant liver first-pass metabolism, and its gastrointestinal absorption is generally assumed to be complete, even though bioavailability studies using an intravenous reference standard in humans have not been reported. Studies in dogs (22) and monkeys (23,24)

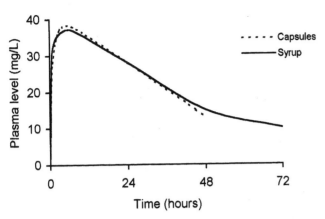

FIGURE 67.2. Mean plasma ethosuximide concentrations after single oral doses of ethosuximide (500 mg) as a syrup *(solid line)* or as capsules *(dotted line)* in children. (From Buchanan RA, Fernandez L, Kinkel AW. Absorption of elimination of ethosuximide in children. *J Clin Pharmacol* 1969;7:213–218, with permission.)

found that the absolute oral bioavailability is virtually complete.

Distribution

The apparent volume of distribution of ethosuximide, calculated by assuming complete oral bioavailability, is approximately 0.7 L/kg in both children and adults (4,17,21), a finding suggesting that the drug is distributed through total body water. Ethosuximide is not bound to plasma proteins, and it is present in cerebrospinal fluid, saliva, and tears at concentrations similar to those found in plasma (5,25–28).

Ethosuximide penetrates rapidly the blood–brain barrier. In dogs, the half-life of entry of unchanged drug into the cerebrospinal fluid has been estimated at about 4 to 5 minutes, and this implies that after 20 to 30 minutes, the concentration in the cerebrospinal fluid reaches values identical to those found in plasma (22,29). By comparison, half-lives of entry into the cerebrospinal fluid have been found to be in the order of 3 minutes for diazepam, 12 minutes for valproic acid, 16 minutes for phenobarbital, 17 minutes for phenytoin, 18 minutes for carbamazepine, and 43 minutes for primidone (29).

Studies using unlabeled ethosuximide in rats indicate even distribution throughout the body, except for the adipose tissue, in which concentrations are only about one-third of those reached in plasma, brain, and other tissues (30). Ethosuximide also shows a uniform distribution in discrete brain regions, without significant differences in concentration among the cerebral cortex, the midbrain, the cerebellum, and the pons medulla (31).

Ethosuximide crosses the human placenta and is found in neonatal plasma at concentrations similar to those observed in the mother (45). Ratios of breast milk to plasma concentration are in the order of 0.8 to 0.9 (32–36).

Koup et al. (32) estimated that if a nursing infant receives 200 to 600 mL of milk from a mother who has a plasma ethosuximide concentration of 64 μg/mL, the daily dose of ethosuximide ingested by the infant would be 13 to 38 mg. Rane and Tunell (48) reported that the plasma ethosuximide concentration in a suckling infant during the first 5 months of age was about 30% of the maternal plasma concentration. In a separate study, nursed infants had serum ethosuximide concentrations of 15 to 40 μg/mL, that is, ~50% of the value found in their mothers (34).

Elimination and Excretion

After single oral doses in adults, ethosuximide is eliminated with mean plasma half-lives of 40 to 60 hours (6,20,21,30). Total body clearance, which is about 0.01 l/kg^{-1}/hr (11,20), is considerably lower than liver blood flow, a finding indicating that ethosuximide does not undergo a significant first-pass effect and follows restrictive, flow-independent elimination. Plasma ethosuximide half-lives determined after discontinuation of a multiple-dose regimen are similar to those recorded after a single dose (8), whereas total body clearance may decrease slightly during repeated doses, probably because of a reduction in biotransformation rate (6). Although ethosuximide may induce microsomal enzyme activity in rodents (37,38), there is no evidence that enzyme induction occurs in patients receiving long-term treatment (11). Autoinduction of ethosuximide metabolism has been described in rats (14), but it does not seem to occur in humans (6,7).

The half-life of ethosuximide is generally shorter and clearance is generally higher in children than in adults. Mean half-lives of 29 to 39 hours (range, 15 to 68 hours) have been reported in children aged 5 to 15 years (3,4,39). Preliminary data suggest that half-lives in newborns are within the range reported for children (32,33).

Steady-State Plasma Concentrations and Relationship with Dosage

An interval of 7 to 12 days is required for plasma ethosuximide concentrations to reach steady-state conditions after a dosage adjustment (5,8,40). Because of the slow rate of elimination, daily fluctuations in plasma ethosuximide concentration during repeated doses are relatively minor. Therapeutic levels can be maintained throughout a 24-hour period even with once-daily administration (5,8,41,42), but a twice-daily regimen is more frequently used to minimize gastrointestinal side effects potentially associated with large individual doses (42).

In most patients, daily doses of 15 to 40 mg/kg are required to achieve steady-state plasma ethosuximide concentrations within the commonly quoted optimal range of 280 to 700 μmol/L (40 to 100 μg/mL), but the interindividual variation in plasma levels among patients receiving

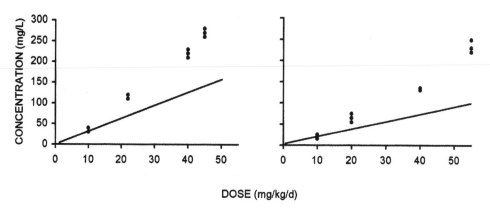

FIGURE 67.3. Relationship between steady-state serum ethosuximide concentration and dosage in two patients with absence seizures. The *solid line* shows the relationship anticipated from the lowest concentration–dose data pair if one assumes linear kinetics. The concentration increases disproportionately with increasing daily dosage. (From Bauer LA, Harris C, Wilensky AJ, et al. Ethosuximide kinetics: possible interaction with valproic acid. *Clin Pharmacol Ther* 1982;31:741–745, with permission.)

the same dose is considerable, and dosage needs to be titrated to meet individual needs (40,43–44).

Information on the relationship between plasma ethosuximide concentration and daily dosage is somewhat controversial. In a carefully controlled study in 20 adult volunteers, Goulet et al. (8) found that a dosage increase from 500 to 750 mg/day produced a 50% increment in plasma concentration, a finding suggesting a linear relationship between plasma levels and dose. Smith et al. (44), however, reported that in some patients increments in ethosuximide dosage resulted in a disproportionate increase in plasma drug concentration. In a retrospective survey, Bauer et al. (6) also found similar evidence of nonlinear (saturation) kinetics in seven of 10 patients studied at different dosage levels (Figure 67.3). Overall, these data suggest that in individual patients the metabolism of ethosuximide may become saturated within the therapeutic dosage range. This can result in a disproportionately large rise in plasma ethosuximide concentration when dosage is increased, but this phenomenon appears to be less consistent and less important clinically compared with that observed with phenytoin.

Influence of Developmental Factors, Pregnancy, and Disease States on Plasma Ethosuximide Concentrations

Plasma ethosuximide concentrations tend to be lower in children than in adults receiving comparable weight-adjusted doses (40,43,45). In a large epidemiologic study, the ratio between ethosuximide concentrations (µg/mL) and daily dosage (mg/kg/day) was found to be 2.23±0.15 in children aged 2.5 to 10 years (n = 48) compared with 3.14±0.15 in older children (≤15 years of age, n = 79) and 3.34±0.l5 in patients aged l6 to 34 years (n = 71) (45). There is also some evidence that plasma ethosuximide concentrations decrease during pregnancy and return to baseline after delivery (32,34,35,46), but this requires confirmation.

Because ethosuximide is eliminated largely by hepatic metabolism, its elimination would be expected to be impaired in patients with liver disease, although this has not been formally investigated. Patients with impaired renal

function may also exhibit some decrease in ethosuximide clearance, but the effect of renal disease is not anticipated to be marked.

Ethosuximide is not bound to plasma proteins, and it is removed relatively efficiently by hemodialysis. It has been estimated that the half-life of ethosuximide drops to about 3 to 4 hours during dialysis, and ~50% of the drug in the body can be removed during a 6-hour dialysis interval (47). In an epileptic girl undergoing peritoneal dialysis, increasing the daily duration of dialysis caused a decrease in plasma ethosuximide and phenobarbital concentrations that may have contributed to precipitating seizure activity (48). Patients receiving dialysis and who are treated with ethosuximide may need supplemental doses at the beginning or at the end of the dialytic procedure, and hemodialysis could be useful in cases of drug overdose.

Pharmacokinetic Drug Interactions
Effect of Other Drugs on the Kinetics of Ethosuximide

Because valproic acid is frequently combined with ethosuximide, the possibility of a pharmacokinetic interaction between these drugs has been repeatedly investigated. In rats, valproic acid may increase the brain concentration of concurrently administered ethosuximide, possibly by inhibiting its metabolism (49). In epileptic patients, one report indicated that valproic acid may increase plasma ethosuximide levels (50), but the opposite effect has also been described (45,51). Of two studies that formally evaluated this interaction in normal volunteers, one reported no change in ethosuximide kinetics after addition of valproic acid at a dose of 500 mg daily (6), whereas the other documented a small but statistically significant increase in plasma ethosuximide concentration after administration of a larger dose of valproate (800 to 1,600 mg/day) (21). In practice, the combination of valproic acid and ethosuximide is often clinically beneficial. Rowan et al. (52) found that absence seizures refractory to either drug may respond remarkably well to the combination: the mechanism underlying this favorable response does not appear to involve major pharmacokinetic changes, and it is probably pharmacodynamic (49).

Because ethosuximide is eliminated primarily by oxidative biotransformation, it is not surprising that its rate of metabolism is accelerated by enzyme-inducing anticonvulsants, such as phenobarbital, primidone, phenytoin, and carbamazepine (11,16–18). In one study, Giaccone et al. (18) found that ethosuximide clearance in 10 epileptic patients receiving long-term therapy with phenobarbital, phenytoin, or carbamazepine was about 65% higher than that observed in 12 study subjects who did not receive comedication. In an earlier study in six healthy volunteers, a carbamazepine dose as low as 200 mg daily was sufficient to decrease plasma ethosuximide concentrations by 17% and to shorten its half-life from 54 to 45 hours (17).

Information about the effect of nonanticonvulsants on ethosuximide kinetics is scant. Coadministration of rifampicin increases ethosuximide clearance in normal volunteers, presumably because of enzyme induction (16). Another drug used for the treatment of tuberculosis, isoniazid, may cause ethosuximide intoxication by inhibiting its metabolism (53), but evidence for this interaction is inconclusive. In rats, ethosuximide clearance can be markedly reduced by certain enzyme inhibitors, including relatively selective inhibitors of cytochrome CYP3A such as triacetyloleandomycin (15,54). If ethosuximide is metabolized by the same cytochrome in humans, similar interactions would be expected to occur in a clinical setting.

Effect of Ethosuximide on the Kinetics of Other Drugs

Contrary to findings obtained in rodents (14,37–38), no evidence indicates that therapeutic doses of ethosuximide cause enzyme induction in humans (11,55). Ethosuximide is not bound to plasma proteins, and therefore competition with other drugs at plasma protein binding sites cannot occur. Because of these properties, ethosuximide has a lower interaction potential than many other anticonvulsants.

In rats, ethosuximide was found to increase the brain concentration of concurrently administered valproic acid, but this effect was observed only at neurotoxic doses (49). In epileptic patients, sporadic reports suggest that ethosuximide may increase the concentration of phenytoin (56,57) and phenobarbital derived from primidone (58), but the clinical significance of these potential interactions is unclear.

REFERENCES

1. Zimmerman FT, Burgmeister BB. A new drug for petit mal epilepsy. *Neurology* 1958;8:769–775.
2. Edwardson JM, Dean PM. Inhibition of alloxan-induced hypercalcemia by compounds of similar molecular structure. *Biochem Pharmacol* 1992;44:2111–2115.
3. Chang T. Ethosuximide: biotransformation. In: Levy R, Mattson R, Meldrum B, Penry JR, et al., eds. *Antiepileptic drugs,* 3rd ed. New York: Raven Press, 1989:679–683.
4. Buchanan RA, Fernandez L, Kinkel AW. Absorption of elimination of ethosuximide in children. *J Clin Pharmacol* 1969;7:213–218.
5. Buchanan RA, Kinkel AW, Smith TC. The absorption and excretion of ethosuximide. *Int J Clin Pharmacol* 1973;7:213–218.
6. Bauer LA, Harris C, Wilensky AJ, et al. Ethosuximide kinetics: possible interaction with valproic acid. *Clin Pharmacol Ther* 1982;31:741–745.
7. Glazko AJ. Antiepileptic drugs: biotransformation. metabolism, and serum half-life. *Epilepsia* 1975;16:367–391.
8. Goulet GR, Kinkel AW, Smith TC. Metabolism of ethosuximide. *Clin Pharmacol Ther* 1976;20:213–218.
9. Millership JS, Mifsud J, Collier PS. The metabolism of ethosuximide. *Eur J Drug Metab Pharmacokinet* 1993;18:349–353.
10. Pisani F, Bialer M. Chemistry and biotransformation. In: Levy RH, Mattson RH, Meldrum BS, eds. *Antiepileptic drugs,* 4th ed. New York: Raven Press, 1995:655–658.
11. Eadie MJ, Vajda FJE. Older anticonvulsants continuing in use but with limited advances in knowledge. In: Eadie MJ, Vajda FJE, eds. *Handbook of experimental pharmacology,* vol 13: *Antiepileptic drugs, pharmacology and therapeutics,* Berlin: Springer-Verlag, 1999:189-228.
12. Horning MO, Stratton J, Nowlin DJ, et al. Metabolism of 2-ethyl-2-methyl succinimide (ethosuximide) in the rat and human. *Drug Metab Dispos* 1973;3:569–576.
13. Pettersen JE. Urine metabolites of 2-ethyl-2 methyl-succinimide (ethosuximide) studied by combined gas chromatography mass spectrometry. *Biomed Mass Spect* 1978;5:601–603.
14. Bachmann KA, Jahn D, Yang C, et al. Ethosuximide disposition kinetics in rats. *Xenobiotica* 1988;18:373–380.
15. Bachmann KA, Chu CA, Grear V. *In vivo* evidence that ethosuximide is a substrate for cytochrome P450IIIA. *Pharmacology* 1992;45:121–128.
16. Bachmann KA, Jauregui L. Use of single sample clearance estimates of cytochrome P450 substrates to characterize human hepatic CYP status *in vivo. Xenobiotica* 1993;3:307–315.
17. Warren JW, Benmaman JD, Wannamaker BB, et al. Kinetics of a carbamazepine-ethosuximide interaction. *Clin Pharmacol Ther* 1980;28:646–651.
18. Giaccone M, Bartoli A, Gatti G, et al. Effects of enzyme inducing anticonvulsants on ethosuximide pharmacokinetics in epileptic patients. *Br J Clin Pharmacol* 1996;41:575–579.
19. Villen T, Bertilsson L, Sjoqvist F. Nonstereoselective disposition of ethosuximide in humans. *Ther Drug Monit* 1990;l2:514–316.
20. Eadie MJ, Tyrer JH, Smith JA, et al. Pharmacokinetics of drugs used for petit mal absence epilepsy. *Clin Exp Neurol* 1977;14:172–183.
21. Pisani P, Narbone MC, Trunfio C, et al. Valproic acid-ethosuximide interaction: a pharmacokinetic study. *Epilepsia* 1984;25:229–233.
22. El Sayed MA, Loscher W, Frey HH. Pharmacokinetics of ethosuximide in the dog. *Arch Int Pharmacodyn Ther* 1976;234:180–192.
23. Patel IH, Levy RH. Pharmacokinetic properties of ethosuximide in monkeys. II. Chronic intravenous and oral administration. *Epilepsia* 1975;16:717–730.
24. Patel IH, Levy RH. Bauer TG. Pharmacokinetic properties of ethosuximide in monkeys. I. Single dose intravenous and oral administration. *Epilepsia* 1975;16:705–716.
25. Horning MG, Brown L, Nowlin J, et al. Use of saliva in therapeutic drug monitoring. *Clin Chem* 1977;23:157–164.
26. McAuliffe JJ, Sherwin AL, Leppik IE, et al. Salivary levels of anticonvulsant: a practical approach to drug monitoring. *Neurology* 1977;27:409–413.

27. Piredda S, Monaco F. Ethosuximide in tears, saliva and cerebral fluid. *Ther Drug Monit* 1981;3:321–323.
28. Loscher W. A comparative study of the protein binding of anticonvulsant drugs in serum of dog and man. *J Pharmacol Exp Ther* 1979;208:429–435.
29. Loscher W, Frey HH. Kinetics of penetration of common antiepileptic drugs into cerebrospinal fluid. *Epilepsia* 1984;25:346–352.
30. Dill WA, Peterson L, Chang T, et al. Physiologic disposition of alpha-methyl-alpha- ethylsuccinimide (ethosuximide; Zarontin) in animals and in man. In: *Abstracts of papers, 149th national meeting, American Chemical Society, Detroit, Michigan.* Washington, DC: American Chemical Society, 1965:30N.
31. Patel IH, Levy RH, Rapport RL. Distribution characteristics of ethosuximide in discrete areas of rat brain. *Epilepsia* 1977;18:533–541.
32. Koup JR, Rose JQ, Cohen ME. Ethosuximide pharmacokinetics in a pregnant patient and her newborn. *Epilepsia* 1978;19:535–539.
33. Kaneko S, Sato T, Suzuki K. The levels of anticonvulsant in breast milk. *Br J Clin Pharmacol* 1979;7:624–627.
34. Kuhnz W, Koch S, Jacob S, et al. Epileptic women during pregnancy and lactation: placental transfer, serum concentration in nursed infants and clinical status. *Br J Clin Pharmacol* 1984;18:671–677.
35. Rane A, Tunell R. Ethosuximide in human milk and in plasma of a mother and her nursed infant. *Br J Clin Pharmacol* 1981;12:855–858.
36. Hagg S, Spigset O. Anticonvulsant use during lactation. *Drug Saf* 2000;22:425–440.
37. Orton TC. Nicholls PJ, Effect in rats of subacute administration of ethosuximide, methsuximide ad phensuximide on hepatic microsomal enzymes of porphyrin turnover. *Biochem Pharmacol* 1972;21:2253–2261.
38. Stevenson IH, O'Malley K, Shepherd AMM. Relative induction potency of anticonvulsant drugs. In: Richens A, Woodford FP, eds. *Anticonvulsant drugs and enzyme induction.* Oxford: Elsevier, 1976:37–46.
39. Buchanan RA, Kinkel AW, Turner JL, et al.. Ethosuximide dosage regimens. *Clin Pharmacol Ther* 1976;19:143–147.
40. Browne TR, Dreifuss FE, Dyken PR, et al. Ethosuximide in the treatment of absence (petit mal) seizures. *Neurology* 1975;25:515–524.
41. Colburn WA, Gibaldi M. Use of MULTIDOS for pharmacokinetic analysis of ethosuximide data during repeated administration of single or divided daily doses. *J Pharm Sci* 1978;67:574–573.
42. Dooley JM, Camfield PR, Camfield CS, et al. Once daily ethosuximide in the treatment of absence epilepsy. *Pediatr Neurol* 1990;6:38–39.
43. Sherwin AL. Ethosuximide: clinical use. In: Levy RH, Dreifuss FE, Mattson RH, et al., eds. *Antiepileptic drugs,* 3rd ed. New York: Raven Press, 1989:679–698.
44. Smith GA, McKauge L, Dubety D, et al. Factors influencing plasma concentrations of ethosuximide. *Clin Pharmacokinet* 1979;4:38–52.
45. Battino D, Cusi C, Franceschetti S, et al. Ethosuximide plasma concentrations: influence of age and associated concomitant therapy. *Clin Pharmacokinet* 1982;7:176–180.
46. Eadie MJ, Lander CM, Tyrer JH. Plasma drug level monitoring in pregnancy. *Clin Pharmacokinet* 1977;2:427–436.
47. Marbury TC, Lee CC, Perchalski RJ. Hemodialysis clearance of ethosuximide in patients with chronic renal failure. *Am J Hosp Pharmacol* 1981;38:1757–1760.
48. Marquardt ED, Ishisaka DY, Batra KK, et al. Removal of ethosuximide and phenobarbital by peritoneal dialysis in a child. *Clin Pharmacol* 1992;11:1030–1031.
49. Bourgeois BFD. Combination of valproate and ethosuximide: antiepileptic and neurotoxic interaction. *J Pharmacol Exp Ther* 1988;247:1128–1132.
50. Mattson RH, Cramer JA. Valproic acid and ethosuximide interaction. *Ann Neurol* 1980: 583–584.
51. Flachs H, Wurtz-Iorgensen A, Gram L, et al. Sodium di-*n*-propylacetate: its interaction with other antiepileptic drugs. In: Schneider H, Janz D, Gardner-Thorpe C, et al., eds. *Clinical pharmacology of antiepileptic drugs.* Berlin: Springer-Verlag, 1975:163–172.
52. Rowan AJ, Meijer JWA, de Beer-Pawlikowski N, et al. Valproate ethosuximide combination therapy for refractory absence seizures. *Arch Neurol* 1983;40:797–802.
53. Van Wieringen A, Vrijlandt CM. Ethosuximide intoxication caused by interaction with isoniazid. *Neurology* 1983;33:1227–1228.
54. Bachmann KA, Madhira MS, Rankin GO. The effect of cobalt chloride, SKF-525A, and N- (3,5-dichlorophenyl) succinimide on *in vivo* hepatic mixed function oxidase activity as determined by single-sample plasma clearances. *Xenobiotica* 1992;22:27–31.
55. Gilbert JC, Scott AK. Galloway DB, et al. Ethosuximide: liver enzyme induction of D-glucaric acid excretion. *Br J Clin Pharmacol* 1974;1:249–252.
56. Dawson GW, Brown HW, Clark BG. Serum phenytoin after ethosuximide. *Ann Neurol* 1978;4:583–584.
57. Lander CM, Eadie MJ, Tyrer J. Interactions between anticonvulsants. *Proc Aust Assoc Neurol* 1975;12:111–116.
58. Schmidt D. *J Neurol* 1975;209:115–123.

SUCCINIMIDES

CLINICAL EFFICACY AND USE IN EPILEPSY

ALLAN L. SHERWIN

SPECTRUM OF EFFICACY

Ethosuximide, a succinimide derivative, was initially used for the treatment of generalized absence seizures, but it also proved effective in certain other seizure types including atypical absence attacks and myoclonic seizures (1). This agent has also been reported to prevent epileptic negative myoclonus (2,3), which is a seizure type observed in certain childhood epileptic syndromes.

Typical Absence Seizures

Absence seizures are an age-related manifestation of generalized epilepsy with onset between 4 and 8 years of age (4). Absence seizures are accompanied by very characteristic bilateral spike-and-wave discharges in the electroencephalogram (EEG), as shown in Figure 68.1. This disorder is rare, with an annual incidence of newly diagnosed cases of 1 in 100,000 (5). It occurs in 8% of children with epilepsy between the ages of 5 and 14 years (6), and it is more common in girls (60% to 70%) than in boys. Epidemiologic studies indicate that a family history of epilepsy is present in 15% to 44% of cases.

Despite their brevity, frequent absence seizures require treatment because of their disruptive effect on the child's normal activities (7). Often they lead to embarrassment at school or interference with work, and the possibility of accidental injury is always present. There is also evidence that the generalized 3-Hz spike-and-wave epileptic discharge (Figure 68.1), the hallmark of this seizure pattern, causes impairment in sustained attention (8,9).

Browne et al. (10) and Penry et al. (9) were the first to carry out a prospective study of the efficacy of ethosuximide in controlling absence attacks. These investigators reported

Allan L. Sherwin, MD, FRCP(C): Professor of Neurology, Department of Neurology and Neurosurgery, McGill University; and Emeritus Neurologist, Montreal Neurological Hospital and Institute, Montreal, Quebec, Canada

that 18 of 37 patients (49%) had a ≥90% reduction, and 35 (95%) had a ≥50% reduction in seizures. My colleagues and I carried out a prospective study of 70 patients with absence seizures treated with ethosuximide. The group comprised 38 female and 32 male patients ranging in age from 4 to 28 years (median, 12 years). Absence attacks were the sole manifestation of epilepsy in 38 of the patients (54%). Tonic-clonic seizures were also present in 21 patients (30%), and additional 11 patients (16%) had a history of one or more other generalized seizures before they entered the study. The dosage of ethosuximide employed

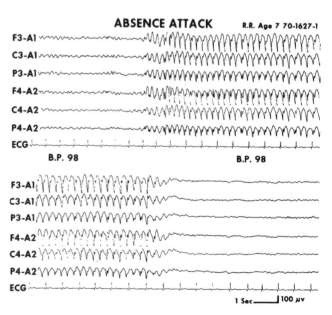

FIGURE 68.1. Electroencephalogram recorded from a 7-year-old boy before and during an absence seizure that lasted approximately 9 seconds. The generalized and bilaterally synchronous spike-and-wave activity at 2.5 to 3 Hz emerges abruptly from normal background activity. Complete seizure control was achieved with ethosuximide monotherapy (30 mg/kg, plasma concentration 85 µg/mL). Epilepsy remitted at 13 years; the child had no history of tonic-clonic seizures.

ranged from 0.5 to 1.75 g/day (9.4 to 73.5 mg/kg). Medications administered to prevent tonic-clonic seizures were phenytoin (30 patients) and phenobarbital (six patients). In the group of 33 patients who had completely seizures, only 9% were found to have serum ethosuximide levels <40 μg/mL, with none <30 μg/mL. Thus, efforts were directed toward achieving levels >40 μg/mL in patients with uncontrolled seizures. A significant improvement in the clinical control of absence seizures was observed within the first 2½ years (Figure 68.2).

Patients with absence seizures tend to cease having attacks with advancing age (11), although some studies have reported a more guarded prognosis (12). Janz (13) observed that the rate of spontaneous remission of absence seizures over 2-year periods was 3%. This gradual rate of improvement could not account for the observed increase in the number of patients with controlled seizures in the study conducted by my colleagues and I (1); however, patients who continued to have tonic-clonic seizures were less likely to have attained control of absence seizures. There is no clear evidence that ethosuximide influences the remission rate of absence seizures (14).

Controlled trials in which ethosuximide and valproate were compared indicate that both drugs are equally effective in controlling absence seizures (15,16). In clinical practice, individual patients may respond to one or the other drug in monotherapy. Rowan et al. (17) carefully studied five patients with absence seizures refractory to treatment with either ethosuximide or valproate monotherapy whose seizures became controlled when the two agents were combined.

If absence attacks are the sole seizure pattern, ethosuximide provides a relatively safe and effective form of monotherapy. If tonic-clonic seizures are also present, ethosuximide can be readily combined with another antiepileptic agent, because clinically significant drug interactions are rare. Alternatively, monotherapy with valproate, lamotrigine, zonisamide, or another antiepileptic drug that protects against both absence and tonic-clonic seizures is a more direct approach (7,18,19). Children ≥7 years old with generalized childhood absence epilepsy have a high incidence (~40%) of new-onset tonic-clonic seizures.

Atypical Absence Seizures

Patients with atypical absence seizures, in whom the attacks usually have a more gradual onset and cessation, more pronounced alteration of tone, and more heterogeneous EEG findings, also respond to ethosuximide. These patients often exhibit other types of seizures including myoclonus, tonic-clonic seizures, and drop attacks.

Absence Status

Absence status, an almost continuous state of abnormal behavior and responses ranging from mild confusion to stupor (20,21), can often be prevented or controlled by ethosuximide, especially when plasma ethosuximide levels are >120 μg/mL.

Epileptic Negative Myoclonus

Ethosuximide is also very efficacious in epileptic negative myoclonus, a rare form of partial seizures seen in various epileptic syndromes of childhood. This seizure type has been defined as a brief and involuntary loss of postural tone, which is time related to spike-and-wave complexes in the contralateral cerebral hemisphere. Negative myoclonus is caused by muscular inhibition with a brief loss of postural tone, in contrast to the more frequently observed brisk jerks of positive myoclonus. Epileptic negative myoclonus in a lower limb may result in an unexpected fall, but the attacks are usually more subtle and must be documented by simultaneous EEG and electromyography (EMG) recordings (Figure 68.3).

The localization and morphology of paroxysmal abnormalities, such as high-amplitude spikes followed by large slow waves over the contralateral motor area, suggest this disorder. Ethosuximide may prevent this negative motor seizure phenomenon by selectively blocking T-type calcium channels in the thalamus (22). Oguni et al. (2) reported that ethosuximide achieved complete control of epileptic negative myoclonus in six patients, in contrast to their findings with carbamazepine, which was ineffective in eight patients. Capovilla et al. (3) carried out a detailed prospective study of epileptic myoclonus in nine patients with partial epilepsy of varying causes including benign epilepsy with centrotemporal spikes, cryptogenic partial epilepsy, cortical dysplasia, and tuberous sclerosis. Epileptic negative myoclonus appeared as brief interruptions of the tonic EMG activity related to a contralateral focal or diffuse spike-and-wave complex. Back averaging of EEG activity revealed that the onset of the slow wave followed the onset

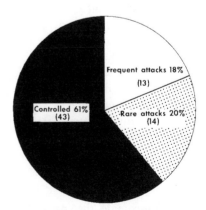

FIGURE 68.2. Control of absence attacks in a study performed when ethosuximide was the only safe antiepileptic drug available for this seizure type. Approximately two-thirds of the patients received ethosuximide monotherapy.

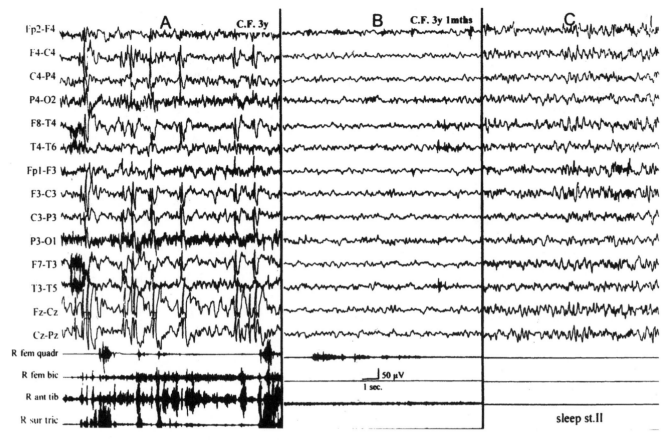

FIGURE 68.3. A: Waking electroencephalogram (EEG) before ethosuximide introduction showing triphasic vertex spikes diffusing mainly to left parasagittal regions associated with epileptic negative myoclonus in both right tibialis anterior and triceps surae. **B:** Waking EEG after ethosuximide monotherapy showing complete disappearance of paroxysms. **C:** Confirmation of this finding by means of a sleep EEG. (From Capovilla G, Beccaria F, Veggiotti P, et al. Ethosuximide is effective in the treatment of epileptic negative myoclonus in childhood partial epilepsy. *J Child Neurol* 1999;14:395–400, with permission.)

of the EMG silent period. Ethosuximide was added to pre-existing antiepileptic medications, which were maintained unchanged for the next 6 months. Epileptic negative myoclonus disappeared in all patients when an effective therapeutic dose was attained, usually within 15 to 30 days. Plasma ethosuximide levels in patients with controlled seizures ranged from 55 to 89 µg/mL.

The EEG and EMG findings in a child studied before and after the start of ethosuximide monotherapy are shown in Figure 68.3. The clinical responses observed in these patients did not appear to be influenced by the nature of the preexisting treatment, and various more modern antiepileptic drugs had been ineffective. Shirasaka et al. (23) also reported a patient with epileptic negative myoclonus in whom active unilateral interictal focal epileptic discharges were recorded from the centrotemporal region. Carbamazepine, zonisamide, and valproate exacerbated the negative myoclonus, but complete control of this seizure type was achieved after the addition of ethosuximide to the preexisting medication.

Myoclonic and Miscellaneous Seizure Types

Ethosuximide is also useful as an adjunctive agent in patients with myoclonic epilepsy in infancy, juvenile myoclonic epilepsy (18,19), and Lennox-Gastaut syndrome (24). Likely because of its inhibitory effects on thalamic oscillatory discharges, ethosuximide has been helpful in epilepsy with continuous spikes and waves during slow-wave sleep. Anecdotal reports indicate that ethosuximide is efficacious in some patients with photosensitive seizures (25).

MODE OF USE

Guidelines for ethosuximide therapy are summarized in Table 68.1. Treatment should be started with a small dose to minimize side effects, but care should be taken to prescribe an adequate final dose based on the weight of the patient.

TABLE 68.1. GUIDELINES FOR ETHOSUXIMIDE THERAPY

Indications: Absence seizures, both typical and atypical; adjunctive therapy of myoclonic epilepsy and epileptic negative myoclonus
Maintenance dosage: 15–40 mg/kg/day, once daily or with meals
Peak levels: Children, 3–7 h; adults, 2–4 h
Dose-related effects: Gastric distress, nausea, vomiting, anorexia, fatigue, lethargy, headache, dizziness, hiccups, and behavioral changes
Plasma concentrations: Effective levels 40–100 µg/mL (300–700 µmol/L); but levels of up to 150 µg/mL (1,000 µmol/L) may be required and well tolerated
Time to reach steady state: Children, 6 days; adults, 12 days
Interactions: Minimal with other antiepileptic drugs; negligible binding by plasma proteins; levels increased by valproate alone or in combination
Indications for plasma level monitoring: Poor response, poor compliance, suspected toxicity, maintenance of optimal concentrations following addition or withdrawal of potentially interacting drugs

Daily administration of 20 mg/kg ethosuximide in children ≤11 years of age will result in mean plasma levels of 50 µg/mL, whereas in older patients, the administration of approximately 15 mg/kg will result in similar levels (Figure 68.4). The generally accepted maximum daily dosage is 30 mg/kg for adults and 40 mg/kg for children. The daily dose may be increased every 4 to 7 days until seizure control is achieved.

Although ethosuximide therapy can usually be individualized empirically based on clinical and EEG monitoring of drug response, measurement of plasma ethosuximide levels can be helpful when good seizure control is not easily achieved, such as because of to noncompliance, but frequent measurements are not necessary as long as the dosage is adjusted to account for weight gain (Figure 68.4). Plasma ethosuximide levels ranging from 40 to 100 µg/mL have been associated with practical seizure control in 80% of patients, with 60% becoming seizure free (Figure 68.2). Overall, concentrations ranging from 40 to 100 µg/mL are considered optimal for effective seizure control, but concentrations ≤150 µg/mL may be required and tolerated if achieved by slow titration (1).

Plasma ethosuximide levels remain extremely stable on successive examination of patients when the medication is taken regularly. Although trough levels are theoretically more accurate, it appears that the time of day that the blood sample is obtained is not likely to change the therapeutic implications of the plasma level significantly. Saliva and plasma ethosuximide levels are very similar, and salivary levels can be used to monitor therapy (26).

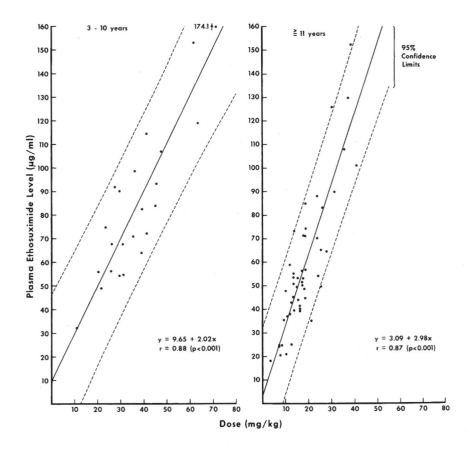

FIGURE 68.4. Relation of plasma ethosuximide concentration to dosage at steady state. The slope of the regression line for patients ranging in age from 2 to 10 years (n = 23) is significantly less than that for patients ≥11 years of age (n = 49) (p < .01). The regression lines are useful as guidelines for selecting the appropriate dosage. Significant differences between boys and girls were not observed.

USE DURING PREGNANCY AND BREAST-FEEDING

Fortunately, typical absence seizures have often ceased to be a major problem by the time many patients reach child-bearing age. If so, it may be possible to discontinue therapy before conception, although therapy with other agents must be maintained if tonic-clonic seizures are also present (27). Preliminary findings suggest that plasma ethosuximide levels tend to decrease somewhat during pregnancy, with modest increases in maternal levels reported after delivery (28). The mean fetal:maternal plasma concentration ratio was 0.97 at birth, a finding indicating that the fetus is exposed to similar drug concentrations as the mother. There are insufficient data on ethosuximide monotherapy in pregnancy to predict the precise risk of fetal malformations. Congenital malformations have been described in some patients taking ethosuximide therapy during pregnancy, but these patients were also taking at the same time other anticonvulsants known to be teratogenic (29). Dansky et al. (30) monitored ethosuximide in five patients, one of whom had a malformed child. Her mean dosage (17 mg/kg) and mean plasma level (42 µg/mL), although within the therapeutic range, were about twice the corresponding mean values for the four mothers with normally formed children (10 mg/kg, 27 µg/mL). Because uncontrolled absence seizures, unlike tonic-clonic seizures, are unlikely to cause any harm to the fetus, it would seem prudent to minimize fetal exposure to ethosuximide by keeping plasma drug levels as low as possible during the first trimester of pregnancy and in women who are planning to become pregnant.

Breast milk ethosuximide concentrations are approximately 90% of the mother's steady-state plasma levels. Kuhnz et al. (31) reported hyperexcitability during the first 2 weeks in a newborn who had been breast-fed for 10 days, during which time the mother received ethosuximide monotherapy. In a group of five infants exposed to ethosuximide through breast milk, plasma levels ranged between 15 and 40 µg/mL, whereas the corresponding maternal plasma concentrations ranged between 28 and 84 µg/mL. Based on the high ethosuximide plasma levels found in suckling infants and the reports of behavioral effects, infants breast-fed by mothers taking ethosuximide should be carefully monitored for potential adverse effects (32).

CONCLUSION

Ethosuximide is particularly effective as monotherapy in patients with absence seizures as the sole seizure type when both the intelligence quotient and the EEG background activity are within the normal range. However, ethosuximide is also highly effective in atypical absence seizures, and it can be valuable in patients with myoclonic seizures and epileptic negative myoclonus. If seizure control is not attained with ethosuximide, the patient should be gradually switched to monotherapy with another medication. If seizures remain uncontrolled, then combination therapy, particularly with ethosuximide and valproate, is frequently successful, especially in patients with myoclonic absences (19) or partial seizures with epileptic negative myoclonus (2,3,23). In patients with a history of tonic-clonic seizures, ethosuximide should also be associated with another antiepileptic drug.

When absence seizures have been controlled for 2 years, consideration may be given to discontinuing therapy, particularly if the EEG examination, including 3 minutes of forceful hyperventilation, fails to reveal evidence of 3-Hz spike-and-wave discharges. Ethosuximide therapy can be discontinued, but the patient should be reexamined 1 month later, and the EEG with hyperventilation should be repeated (33). Ambulatory EEG monitoring has been demonstrated to be an effective technique to identify those patients in whom ethosuximide therapy can be discontinued (34). A similar approach applies when ethosuximide is administered for the control of epileptic negative myoclonus. If behavioral seizures or epileptogenic discharges are recorded, continuation of drug therapy for an additional period should be considered.

REFERENCES

1. Sherwin AL, Robb JP, Lechter M. Improved control of epilepsy by monitoring plasma ethosuximide. *Arch Neurol* 1973;28:178–181.
2. Oguni H, Uehara T, Tanaka T, et al. Dramatic effect of ethosuximide on epileptic negative myoclonus: implications for the neurophysiological mechanism. *Neuropediatrics* 1998;29:29–34.
3. Capovilla G, Beccaria F, Veggiotti P, et al. Ethosuximide is effective in the treatment of epileptic negative myoclonus in childhood partial epilepsy. *J Child Neurol* 1999;14:395–400.
4. Berkovic SF, Andermann F, Andermann E, et al. Concepts of absence epilepsies: discrete syndromes or biological continuum. *Neurology* 1987;37:993–1000.
5. Loiseau J, Loiseau P, Guyot M, et al. A survey of epileptic disorders in Southwest France: seizures in elderly patients. *Ann Neurol* 1990;27:232–237.
6. Cavazzuti GB. Epidemiology of different types of epilepsy in school age children of Modena, Italy. *Epilepsia* 1980;22:57–62.
7. Pellock JM. Treatment of epilepsy in the new millenium. *Pharmacotherapy* 2000;20[Suppl S]:129S –138S.
8. Browne TR, Penry JK, Porter RJ, et al. Responsiveness before, during and after spike-wave paroxysms. *Neurology* 1974;24:659–665.
9. Penry JK, Porter RJ, Dreifuss FE. Simultaneous recording of absence seizures with video tape and electroencephalography: a study of 374 seizures in 48 patients. *Brain* 1975;98;427–440.
10. Browne TR, Dreifuss FE, Dyken PR, et al. Ethosuximide in the treatment of absence (petit mal) seizures. *Neurology* 1975;25:515–524.
11. Dalby MA. Epilepsy and 3 per second spike-and-wave rhythms. *Acta Neurol Scand* 1969;45[Suppl 40]:1–83.
12. Rodin EA. *The prognosis of patients with epilepsy.* Springfield, IL: Charles C Thomas, 1968.

13. Janz D. *Die Epilepsien-Spezielle Pathologie und Therapie.* Stuttgart: Georg Thieme, 1969:94.

14. Okuma T, Kumashiro H. Natural history and prognosis of epilepsy: report of a multi-institutional study in Japan. *Epilepsia* 1981;22:35–53.

15. Sato S, White BG, Penry JK. Valproic acid versus ethosuximide in the treatment of absence seizures. *Neurology* 1982;32:157–163.

16. Callaghan N, O'Hare J, O'Driscoll D, et al. Comparative study of ethosuximide and sodium valproate in the treatment of typical absence seizures (petit mal). *Dev Med Child Neurol* 1982;24:830–836.

17. Rowan AJ, Meijer JW, de Beer-Pawlikowski N, et al. Valproate-ethosuximide combination therapy for refractory absence seizures. *Arch Neurol* 1983;40:797–802.

18. Brodie MJ, Dichter MA. Established antiepileptic drugs. *Seizure* 1997;6:159–174.

19. Wallace SJ. Myoclonus and epilepsy in childhood: a review of treatment with valproate, ethosuximide, lamotrigine and zonisamide. *Epilepsy Res* 1998;29:147–154.

20. Andermann F, Robb JP. Absence status: a reappraisal following a review of 38 patients. *Epilepsia* 1972;13:177–187.

21. Porter RJ, Penry JK. Petit mal status. *Adv Neurol* 1983;34:61–67.

22. Huguenard JR. Neuronal circuitry of thalamortical epilepsy and mechanisms of antiabsence drug action. *Adv Neurol* 1999;79:991–999.

23. Shirasaka Y, Mitsuyshi I. A case of epileptic negative myoclonus: therapeutic considerations. *Brain Dev* 1999;21:209–212.

24. Schmidt D, Bourgeois B. A risk-benefit assessment of therapies for Lennox-Gastaut syndrome. *Drug Saf* 2000,22:467–477.

25. Zifkin B, Andermann F. Epilepsy with reflex seizures. In: Wyllie E, ed. *The treatment of epilepsy: principles and practices,* 3rd ed. Philadelphia: Lea & Febiger, 1993;614–623.

26. Liu H, Delgado MR. Therapeutic drug concentration monitoring using saliva samples. *Clin Pharmacokinet* 1999;36:453–470.

27. Schmidt D, Beck-Mannagetta G, Janz D, et al. The effect of pregnancy on the course of epilepsy: a prospective study. In: Janz D, Dan M, Pickens A, et al., eds. *Epilepsy, pregnancy and the child.* New York: Raven Press; 1982:39–49.

28. Koup JR, Rose JQ, Cohen ME. Ethosuximide pharmacokinetics in a pregnant patient and her newborn. *Epilepsia* 1978;19:535–539.

29. Samren EB, van Duijn CM, Koch S, et al. Maternal use of antiepileptic drugs and the risk of major congenital malformations: a joint European prospective study of human tetragenesis associated with maternal epilepsy. *Epilepsia* 1997;38:981–990.

30. Dansky L, Andermann E, Sherwin AL. Maternal epilepsy and birth defects: a prospective study with monitoring of plasma anticonvulsant levels during pregnancy. In: Dam M, Gram L, Penry JK, eds. *Advances in epileptology: XIIth Epilepsy International Symposium.* New York: Raven Press, 1981:607–612.

31. Kuhnz W, Koch S, Jakob S, et al. Ethosuximide in epileptic women during pregnancy and lactation period: placental transfer, serum concentrations in nursed infants and clinical status. *Br J Clin Pharmacol* 1984;18:671–677.

32. Häag S, Spigset O. Anticonvulsant use during lactation. *Drug Saf* 2000;6:425–440.

33. Dreifuss FE. Treatment of the nonconvulsive epilepsies. *Epilepsia* 1983;24[Suppl 1]:S45–S54.

34. Amit R, Vitale S, Maytal J. How long to treat childhood onset absence epilepsy. *Clin Electroencephalogr* 1995;26:163–165.

SUCCINIMIDES

ADVERSE EFFECTS

TRACY A. GLAUSER

The first anticonvulsants to demonstrate efficacy against absence seizures, trimethadione and its analog paramethadione, were introduced in the 1940s but displayed significant toxicity (1–4). These toxicity issues spurred the discovery and testing in the 1950s of the succinimide family of anticonvulsants (ethosuximide, methsuximide, and phensuximide), in the hope of finding more effective, safer, and better-tolerated anticonvulsants for patients with absence seizures (4,5). Among the succinimide family, ethosuximide has the greatest efficacy against absence seizures with the least toxicity and has been considered as possible first-line therapy for absence seizures since its introduction in 1958 (4,6,7). Methsuximide and phensuximide are used as later treatment options because they exhibit less favorable efficacy and side effects profiles compared with ethosuximide.

The adverse event profile of the succinimide class of anticonvulsants can be separated into four categories: (a) most commonly observed adverse effects; (b) less common, but clinically relevant adverse effects; (c) potentially life-threatening adverse effects; and (d) manifestations of overdose. As with most drugs (8,9), the most commonly observed adverse effects of drugs of the succinimide class are usually predictable, dose dependent, and host independent, and they resolve with dose reduction. The less common but clinically relevant adverse effects may result from multiple mechanisms, including (a) dose-dependent side effects, (b) effects of long-term therapy, effects of the cumulative dose, and (c) delayed effects (e.g., teratogenicity and carcinogenicity) that are host dependent but not necessarily dose dependent (8,9). The potentially life-threatening adverse events, frequently called idiosyncratic drug reactions, cannot be predicted based on the known pharmacologic effect of the drug. These side effects do not demonstrate a simple dose–response relationship, they are host dependent, and they can be serious and life-threatening (10). Preclinical animal toxicology testing may not detect these reactions, and often these reactions cannot be reproduced in animal models (8,9). Although

rare, the symptoms of succinimide (especially methsuximide) overdose are important to recognize so appropriate therapy can be initiated as soon as possible.

MOST COMMONLY OBSERVED ADVERSE EFFECTS

Ethosuximide

During the first 8 years after ethosuximide's release, the results of 12 large clinical trials (each involving >50 patients) were published, detailing the spectrum of ethosuximide's adverse effects. Browne summarized these studies and found that the overall incidence of ethosuximide-related adverse effects ranged from 26% to 46% (Table 69.1) (11–23). In half of these large trials, ≥37% of the subjects experienced adverse effects (11).

The most common ethosuximide concentration-dependent adverse effects involve the gastrointestinal system. These gastrointestinal symptoms include nausea (the most common), abdominal discomfort, anorexia, vomiting, and diarrhea (5,7,24–27). Symptoms usually occur at the onset of therapy, they affect 20% to 33% of children, are they considered mild and resolve promptly to dose reduction (24–27). In some patients, the adverse effect is transient, and no dose reduction is needed, whereas for other patients, dividing the total daily dosage and administering the smaller doses at mealtime is another technique to lessen the symptoms (6,11). Gastrointestinal symptoms are seldom severe enough to cause discontinuation of ethosuximide (11).

Central nervous system–related adverse events, such as drowsiness, are the second most common form of ethosuximide concentration-dependent adverse events (11). Similar to the gastrointestinal side effects, drowsiness usually occurs at the onset of therapy and resolves promptly when the ethosuximide dose is reduced (6,24,25,27).

Additional commonly observed central nervous system–related adverse events include dizziness, hiccups, lethargy, fatigue, ataxia, insomnia, and behavior changes (e.g., aggression, euphoria, irritability, hyperactivity) (7,27). Nervousness is reported in 12% of children (7,27). A direct

Tracy A. Glauser, MD: Division of Neurology, Children's Hospital Medical Center, Cincinnati, Ohio

TABLE 69.1. SUMMARY OF ADVERSE EFFECT PROFILES NOTED IN EARLY STUDIES INVOLVING 50 OR MORE SUBJECTS RECEIVING EITHER ETHOSUXIMIDE (12 REPORTS, 1958–1966)[a] OR METHSUXIMIDE (EIGHT REPORTS, 1957–1977)[b]

Adverse Effect	Ethosuximide Range (Median, Both in %)	Methsuximide Range (Median, Both in %)
Any adverse effect	26–46 (37)	11–57 (35)
Gastrointestinal disturbances (nausea, abdominal discomfort, anorexia, vomiting and diarrhea)	4–29 (13)	2–30 (6)
Drowsiness	0–16 (7)	0–28 (16)
Rash	0–6 (0)	0–17 (6)
Ataxia	0–1 (0)	0–13 (6)
Dizziness	0–4 (1)	0–13 (0)
Hiccups	0–5 (0)	0–6 (0)
Irritability	0 (0)	0–6 (0)

[a]Ethosuximide references 12–23.
[b]Methsuximide references 33–40.
Modified from Lennox W. The peritoneal epilepsies: their treatment with tridione. *JAMA* 1945;129:1069–1074, with permission.

relationship between ethosuximide therapy and reported behavioral changes is not certain because poor methodology (e.g., the lack of reliable methods for objectively measuring behavior changes, the confounding variable of polypharmacy, and the lack of serum antiepileptic drug concentrations) make analysis of existing reports difficult at best (24,25).

Approximately 14% of children taking ethosuximide develop headaches. In contrast to the other central nervous system side effects described earlier, these headaches do not appear to be concentration dependent, they may not respond to dose reduction, and they may be persistent (6,24,25,27,28).

Assessing ethosuximide's effects on cognition is difficult because few trials have examined the issue in a controlled fashion accounting for confounding variables such as plasma concentrations, underlying mental retardation, concomitant antiepileptic drug use, or seizure type. Memory, speech, and emotional disturbances were noted on psychometric testing in 25 children receiving ethosuximide for various seizure types in one early report (29). Confounding these results are multiple methodologic issues including the finding that all the patients were also taking barbiturates, 60% of the cohort had intelligence quotient (IQ) scores <83, no ethosuximide plasma concentrations were measured, and no matched control group was used (29). In contrast, ethosuximide therapy resulted in a significant improvement in verbal and full-scale IQ scores without change in motor performance or personality test scores in a cohort of children without epilepsy but with learning disorders and 14 and six per second positive spikes on the electroencephalogram (30). Similarly, psychometric performance improved significantly over 8 weeks of ethosuximide therapy in 17 of 37 (46%) children with absence seizures in a well-designed study by Browne et al. (31). This improvement was significantly different compared with a control group of patients tested in the same fashion over the same interval (31). Only 25% of the study group had IQ scores <83, and only 32% were taking other antiepileptic drugs (31).

Methsuximide

Although methsuximide's adverse effect profile is qualitatively similar to that of ethosuximide, overall its adverse effects occur with higher incidence, have greater severity, and persist long than ethosuximide's (6,7,11,32). Browne noted that drowsiness and gastrointestinal symptoms (e.g., nausea, vomiting, anorexia, constipation, diarrhea, and abdominal pain) were the most commonly reported side effects in eight large methsuximide clinical trials performed from 1957 to 1977 (Table 69.1) (11,33–40).

In comparison with ethosuximide, methsuximide's adverse effects were less likely to resolve spontaneously without a dosage adjustment and were more likely to lead to the need to discontinue the medication (11,32). Multiple authors propose that some of the central nervous system symptoms (e.g., drowsiness, ataxia, irritability) observed during methsuximide therapy could be related to a pharmacokinetic interaction between methsuximide and other anticonvulsants such as phenobarbital and phenytoin, rather a direct effect of methsuximide (11,32,34,41).

Commonly noted methsuximide-associated central nervous system adverse effects include dizziness, ataxia, confusion, somnolence, lethargy, irritability, hiccups, personality change, fearfulness, irritability, photophobia, nervousness, and headaches. Methsuximide therapy has also been associated with vertigo, diplopia, blurred vision, increased seizures, inattention, dysarthria, incoordination, slurred speech, and adventitious movements (7,34,35,42–46). In one study, two patients experienced psychic changes, including "depression, withdrawal, weepiness and impulsive behavior" (43).

Phensuximide

The most common adverse effects noted with phensuximide usage involve gastrointestinal symptoms (nausea and vomiting) and central nervous system symptoms (drowsiness and dizziness) (11). Other commonly noted phensuximide-associated central nervous system adverse effects include headaches and hiccups (45). The actual rate of these adverse effects is unknown; some authors propose the incidence to be at least the rate of other succinimides (11,47). High doses of phensuximide can produce a dreamlike state, unlike with other succinimides (11,47). Long-term phensuximide use has been reported to be associated with urinary frequency, burning, hematuria, proteinuria, hemorrhagic cystitis, and mild nephrotoxicity (45,47–49).

LESS COMMON, BUT CLINICALLY RELEVANT ADVERSE EFFECTS

Ethosuximide

Episodes of psychotic behavior (anxiety, depression, visual hallucinations, auditory hallucinations, and intermittent impairment of consciousness) have been noted in patients taking ethosuximide (12,14,24,50,51). Risk factors for this adverse effect include age (young adults in their teens or twenties) and a history of mental illness (6,11,24). Reported acute psychotic episodes appeared after ethosuximide-induced seizure control with associated electroencephalographic improvement; the episodes resolved when ethosuximide was stopped and the seizures returned, a finding illustrating the phenomenon of *forced normalization* (6,24). Psychotic symptoms have recurred when ethosuximide therapy is resumed in patients with previous ethosuximide-related psychotic episodes (24). This forced normalization reaction is not dose dependent and, among all antiabsence antiepileptic drugs, occurs with highest frequency with ethosuximide (6,52). This type of side effect seldom occurs in young children with no previous history of psychiatric disease who are receiving ethosuximide for typical absence seizures (11).

Most studies find no evidence of ethosuximide-associated seizure exacerbation (16,21,23,24,31,53). There are scattered reports of exacerbation of myoclonic and absence seizures and transformation of absence into grand mal seizures in patients receiving ethosuximide (24,54,55). Dreifuss considered that the appearance of grand mal seizures is simply a consequence of the high incidence of generalized tonic-clonic seizures in patients with absences seizures coupled with ethosuximide's lack of efficacy against generalized tonic-clonic seizures (24).

In early studies, the incidence of ethosuximide-related granulocytopenia ranged from 0% to 7% (11). Dreifuss considered this symptom to be probable dose-dependent granulocytopenia that often resolved with dose reduction

without requiring termination of ethosuximide therapy (24,25). It is critical to distinguish between this probable dose-dependent adverse event and ethosuximide-associated idiosyncratic bone marrow depression (see later). Careful clinical and laboratory monitoring is essential in making this decision. Ethosuximide therapy is not reported to cause hepatotoxicity or serious endocrine adverse effects (11). Ethosuximide can precipitate an attack of acute intermittent porphyria (27,56).

Long-term cumulative dose ethosuximide side effects are infrequent. Extrapyramidal reactions (e.g., severe bradykinesia, akathisias, dyskinesias, and parkinsonian syndrome) have been reported after several years of ethosuximide treatment (15,57).

In mice, ethosuximide exhibits considerably less teratogenic effect than carbamazepine, phenytoin, phenobarbital, or primidone (58). However, in one report of 10 women with epilepsy who were taking ethosuximide, two of 13 newborns had major malformations (bilateral clefting, hare lip), and the cohort had a higher rate of minor abnormalities compared with a pair-matched control group of newborns of women without epilepsy (59). The mothers of these two seriously affected newborns were taking ethosuximide in combination with phenobarbital in one mother and primidone in the other mother (59). In another small series, one of five infants born to a mother taking ethosuximide was malformed (60). Little information is available about the overall risks maternal ethosuximide use poses to the fetus (24). Data are currently insufficient to assess the teratogenic effect of ethosuximide accurately in humans.

Methsuximide

Restless legs syndrome was described in two patients taking methsuximide and phenytoin (61). Methsuximide can precipitate an attack of acute intermittent porphyria (56,62). Periorbital edema, proteinuria, microscopic hematuria, and hyperemia have been seen (32). One article proposed that methsuximide therapy caused or aggravated irreversible cerebellar damage in two patients (63).

Phensuximide

Phensuximide can precipitate an attack of acute intermittent porphyria (56).

POTENTIALLY LIFE-THREATENING ADVERSE EFFECTS

Overview

Idiosyncratic drug reactions are unpredictable, at times dose-independent, host-dependent reactions that cannot be predicted based on the known pharmacologic effect of the drug, and they can be serious and life-threatening (8,9). In general, the skin is the most commonly affected site, followed by the formed elements of the blood and the liver and, to a lesser extent, the nervous system and kidneys (8,64). These reactions can be very organ specific, or they may present with generalized nonspecific symptoms, such as lymphadenopathy, arthralgias, eosinophilia, and fever (8,65). Idiosyncratic reactions are proposed to result from toxic metabolites that either directly or indirectly (by way of an immunologic response or free radical mediated process) cause injury (10).

Ethosuximide

Ethosuximide has been associated (to varying degrees) with many different idiosyncratic reactions (24,25,27,66), including allergic dermatitis, rash, erythema multiforme, Stevens-Johnson syndrome (67), systemic lupus erythematosus (68–70), a lupuslike syndrome (24,71–73), blood dyscrasias (aplastic anemia, agranulocytosis) (17,22,31,53, 74–79), dyskinesia (80,81), akathisia (80), autoimmune thyroiditis (82), and diminished renal allograft survival (83).

The mild cutaneous reactions, allergic dermatitis and rash, are the most common ethosuximide-associated idiosyncratic reaction. These reactions frequently resolve with withdrawal of ethosuximide, but some patients may require steroid therapy. Patients developing Stevens-Johnson syndrome, a potentially life-threatening condition, require more aggressive therapy in the hospital.

The symptoms of the lupuslike syndrome are described as "fever, malar rash, arthritis, lymphadenopathy, and, on occasion, pleural effusions, myocarditis, and pericarditis" (24). After ethosuximide discontinuation, patients with the lupuslike syndrome usually fully recover, but recovery may be prolonged (24).

The manifestations of ethosuximide-associated blood dyscrasias range from thrombocytopenia to pancytopenia and aplastic anemia (17,22,31,53,74–78). Between 1958 and 1994, only eight cases of ethosuximide-associated aplastic anemia were reported, with an onset 6 weeks to 8 months after ethosuximide was initiated (77). Six patients were receiving polypharmacy, and five were taking either phenytoin or ethotoin in combination with ethosuximide (77). Despite therapy, five of the eight patients died (17,22, 31,53,74–78).

There is no evidence that laboratory monitoring of blood counts during ethosuximide therapy anticipates ethosuximide's idiosyncratic hematologic reactions. Patients need to be educated to watch for fever, sore throat, and cutaneous or other hemorrhages and to alert their physician immediately if these symptoms occur (24). However, one recommendation for blood monitoring has been "that periodic blood counts be performed at no greater than monthly intervals for the duration of treatment with ethosuximide and that the dosage be reduced or the drug discontinued should the total white-blood-cell count fall below 3,500 or the proportion of granulocytes below 25% of the total white-blood-cell count" (24).

Methsuximide

Similar to ethosuximide, methsuximide therapy has been associated with various idiosyncratic reactions including rashes and hypersensitivity reactions (11). Some reports describe patients who experienced cross-sensitivity between phenytoin and methsuximide; these patients had a history of a hypersensitivity reaction to phenytoin and then developed a hypersensitivity reaction to methsuximide (84,85). Other idiosyncratic reactions have included isolated cases of Stevens-Johnson syndrome, two cases of transient nonfatal leukopenia, a single case of fatal pancytopenia, a single case of fatal aplastic anemia, and one patient with reversible osteomalacia (11,45,86). Methsuximide therapy is not associated with hepatotoxicity (11).

Phensuximide

Phensuximide is associated with a higher rate of idiosyncratic reactions than other succinimides (11). These reactions include fever, rash, erythema multiforme, leukopenia, and renal damage manifested by proteinuria, microscopic hematuria, and granular casts (11,47). There is one report of megaloblastic anemia in a patient taking phensuximide and phenobarbital (87).

MANIFESTATIONS AND MANAGEMENT OF OVERDOSE

Manifestations of Overdose

The manifestations of acute ethosuximide overdose include nausea, vomiting, and symptoms of central nervous system depression including stupor and coma leading to respiratory depression. At least five cases of methsuximide overdose have been reported; four patients survived without sequelae, and one died after an overdose of methsuximide and primidone (88–92). The major symptoms associated with methsuximide overdose are stupor and coma, although respiratory depression, central neurogenic hyperventilation, increased or decreased reflexes, coffee ground emesis, second-degree heart block, and myoclonus have also been reported (32,93).

Development of stupor and coma after methsuximide overdose may occur in a monophasic or biphasic fashion. The biphasic course can present with initial ataxia, dizziness, loss of consciousness, or stupor, followed by a period of improved alertness or arousal, then followed by a lapse into a coma within 24 hours (90,92,93). Three proposed explanations for the biphasic course include (a) methsuximide's conversion into the *N*-desmethylmethsuximide (normethsuximide) metabolite with subsequent accumulation, (b) methsuximide's interference with the metabolism of other antiepileptic medications (32), and (c) delayed absorption (45). There have not been any published reports of phensuximide overdose (45).

Management of Overdose

The management of a succinimide overdose involves life-support measures, symptomatic treatment, procedures to decrease drug absorption, and procedures to enhance drug elimination. Life-support measures involve initial and immediate evaluation and stabilization of the patient's airway, breathing, and circulation. Symptomatic treatment involves the subsequent care for each of the patient's overdose symptoms as they occur. No specific antidote exists for a succinimide overdose.

Three potentially useful methods to decrease drug absorption after any overdose include the following: induction of emesis, use of activated charcoal, and use of gastric lavage. Because succinimide overdose can rapidly lead to significant alteration of consciousness, induction of emesis is not recommended (93). In conscious patients who are able to protect their airway, administration of activated charcoal as an aqueous slurry may reduce absorption; effectiveness is greatest if it is given within 1 hour of succinimide overdose (93). If emesis or rapid deterioration of consciousness occurs or is impending, only personnel skilled in airway management should administer activated charcoal to minimize the potential for aspiration. Contraindications for the use of activated charcoal include a patient with an unprotected airway or a situation in which the therapy increases the risk or severity of aspiration (94). The recommended dose of activated charcoal is 1 g/kg of weight for infants ≤1 year old, 25 to 50 g in children between 1 and 12 years old, and 25 to 100 g in adults. The optimal dose has not been established (94).

Gastric lavage with a large-bore orogastric tube may be considered if a potentially life-threatening amount of succinimide has been ingested and the procedure can be performed within 1 hour of the ingestion (95). Because of the risk of significant morbidity associated with the procedure, gastric lavage should not be employed routinely in the management of patients after an overdose of succinimides (95).

Four potentially useful methods to decrease absorption after a drug overdose include hemodialysis, hemoperfusion, exchange transfusion, and forced diuresis. Hemodialysis may be useful in the treatment of ethosuximide overdose, based on an observed extraction efficiency of 61% to 100% in one study of four patients with chronic renal disease who were supported by hemodialysis and who received a single dose of 500 mg of ethosuximide 4 hours before dialysis. In this study, the elimination half-life of ethosuximide was reduced by dialysis to an average of 3.5 hours (96).

Hemoperfusion with a cellulose-activated charcoal hemoperfusion column led to rapid improvement in one patient after a methsuximide overdose through rapid clearance of methsuximide's primary metabolite, *N*-desmethyl-methsuximide (88). Both exchange transfusion and forced diuresis have little use in the treatment of succinimide overdose because succinimides have low protein binding, and little of the parent succinimide compound is excreted unchanged in the urine.

REFERENCES

1. Lennox W. The petit mal epilepsies: their treatment with tridione. *JAMA* 1945;129:1069–1074.
2. Lennox W. Tridione in the treatment of epilepsy. *JAMA* 1947; 134:138–143.
3. Mattson RH. Efficacy and adverse effects of established and new antiepileptic drugs. *Epilepsia* 1995;36:S13–S26.
4. Rogawski M, Porter R. Antiepileptic drugs: pharmacological mechanisms and clinical efficacy with consideration of promising developmental state compounds. *Pharmacol Rev* 1990;42: 223–286.
5. Brodie M, Dichter M. Established antiepileptic drugs. *Seizure* 1997;6:159–174.
6. Sabers A, Dam M. Ethosuximide and methsuximide. In: Shorvon S, Dreifuss F, Fish D, et al., eds. *The treatment of epilepsy.* London: Blackwell Science, 1996:414–420.
7. Bromfield E. Ethosuximide and other succinimides. In: Engel J, Pedley T, eds. *Epilepsy: a comprehensive textbook.* Philadelphia: Lippincott–Raven, 1997:1503–1508.
8. Park BK, Pirmohamed M, Kitteringham NR. Idiosyncratic drug reactions: a mechanistic evaluation of risk factors. *Br J Clin Pharmacol* 1992;34:377–395.
9. Pirmohamed M, Kitteringham NR, Park BK. The role of active metabolites in drug toxicity. *Drug Saf* 1994;11:114–144.
10. Glauser TA. Idiosyncratic reactions: new methods of identifying high-risk patients. *Epilepsia* 2000;41:S16–S29.
11. Browne T. Ethosuximide (Zarontin) and other succinimides. In: Browne T, Feldman R, eds. *Epilepsy: diagnosis and management.* Boston: Little, Brown, 1983:215–224.
12. Cohardon R, Loiseau P, Cohardon S. Results of treatment of certain forms of epilepsy of the petit mal type by ethosuximide. *Rev Neurol* 1964;110:201.
13. Dongier MS, Gastaut H, Roger J. Essai d'un nouvel anti-épileptique (PM671, alpha-ethyl-alpha-methyl-succinimide) chez l'enfant. *Rev Neurol (Paris)* 1961;104:441.
14. Fischer M, Korskjaer G, Pedersen E. Psychotic episodes in Zarontin treatment: effects and side-effects in 105 patients. *Epilepsia* 1965;6:325–334.
15. Goldensohn E, Hardie J, Borea E. Ethosuximide in the treatment of epilepsy. *JAMA* 1962;180:840–842.
16. Heathfield K, Jewesbury E. Treatment of petit mal with ethosuximide. *BMJ* 1961;2:565.
17. Kiorboe E, Paludan J, Trolle E, et al. Zarontin (ethosuximide) in the treatment of petit mal and related disorders. *Epilepsia* 1964; 5:83–89.
18. Lorentz de Haas AM, Stoel LMK. Experiences with alpha-ethyl-alpha-methyl succinimide in the treatment of epilepsy. *Epilepsia* 1960;1:501.
19. Matthes A, Mallman-Muhlberger E. Erfahrungen bei der Behandlung kleiner epileptische Anfalle in Kindersalter mit Methyl-athyl-succinimid (MAS). *Munch Med Wochenschr* 1962; 104:1095.
20. Spinner A. Indikation und Wirkung von Suxinutin bei Petit-mal-Epilepsien. *Munch Med Wochenschr* 1961;103:1110.

21. Vossen R. Uber die antikonvulsive Wirkung von Succinimiden. *Dtsch Med Wochenschr* 1958;29:1227–1230.

22. Weinstein A, Allen R. Ethosuximide treatment of petit mal seizures: a study of 87 pediatric patients. *Am J Dis Child* 1966; 111:63–67.

23. Zimmerman F, Bergemeister B. A new drug for petit mal epilepsy. *Neurology* 1958;8:769–776.

24. Dreifuss F. Ethosuximide: toxicity. In: Levy R, Mattson R, Meldrum B, eds. *Antiepileptic drugs,* 4th ed. New York: Raven Press, 1995:675–679.

25. Dreifuss F. Ethosuximide: toxicity. In: Levy R, Mattson R, Meldrum B, et al., eds. *Antiepileptic drugs,* 3rd ed. New York: Raven Press, 1989:699–705.

26. Wallace SJ. Use of ethosuximide and valproate in the treatment of epilepsy. *Neurol Clin* 1986;4:601–616.

27. Wallace SJ. A comparative review of the adverse effects of anticonvulsants in children with epilepsy. *Drug Saf* 1996;15: 378–393.

28. Abu-Arafeh I, Wallace S. Unwanted effects of antiepileptic drugs. *Dev Med Child Neurol* 1988;30:117–121.

29. Guey J, Charles C, Coquery C, et al. Study of psychological effects of ethosuximide (Zarontin) on 25 children suffering from petit mal epilepsy. *Epilepsia* 1967;8:129–141.

30. Smith L, Phillips M, Guard H. Psychometric study of children with learning problems and 14-6 positive spike EEG patterns, treated with ethosuximide (Zarontin) and placebo. *Arch Dis Child* 1968;43:616–619.

31. Browne TR, Dreifuss FE, Dyken PR, et al. Ethosuximide in the treatment of absence (petit mal) seizures. *Neurology* 1975;25: 515–524.

32. Browne T. Other succinimides: methsuximide. In: Levy R, Mattson R, Meldrum B, eds. *Antiepileptic drugs,* 4th ed. New York: Raven Press, 1995:681–687.

33. Dow RS, McFarlane JP, Stevens JR. Celontin in patients with refractory epilepsy. *Neurology* 1958;8:201.

34. French EG, Rey-Bellet J, Lennox WG. Methsuximide in psychomotor and petit-mal seizures. *N Engl J Med* 1958;258:892.

35. Livingston S, Pauli L. Celontin in the treatment of epilepsy. *Pediatrics* 1957;19:614.

36. Stenzel E, Boenigk HE, Rambeck B. Methsuximide in the treatment of epilepsies. *Nervenarzt* 1977;48:377–382.

37. Rabe F. Celontin (Petinutin): Ein Beitrag zur differenzierten Epilepsiebehandlung. *Nervenarzt* 1960;31:306.

38. Scholl ML, Abbott JA, Schwab RS. Celontin: a new anticonvulsant. *Epilepsia* 1960;1:105.

39. Trolle E, Kiorboe E. Treatment of petit-mal epilepsy with new succinimides: PM60 and Celontin (a clinical comparative study). *Epilepsia* 1960;1:587–597.

40. Zimmerman FT. Evaluation of *N*-methyl-alpha,alpha-methyl-phenylsuccinimide in the treatment of petit mal epilepsy. *NY State J Med* 1956;56:1460.

41. Rambeck B. Pharmacological interactions of methsuximide with phenobarbital and phenytoin in hospitalized epileptic patients. *Epilepsia* 1979;20:147–156.

42. Wilder BJ, Buchanan RA. Methsuximide for refractory complex partial seizures. *Neurology* 1981;31:741–744.

43. Browne T, Feldman R, Buchanan R. Methsuximide for complex seizures: efficacy, toxicity, clinical pharmacology, and drug interactions. *Neurology* 1983;33:414–418.

44. Dasheiff RM, McNamara D, Dickinson L. Efficacy of second line antiepileptic drugs in the treatment of patients with medically refractive complex partial seizures. *Epilepsia* 1986;27: 124–127.

45. Porter R, Kupferberg H. Other succinimides: methsuximide and phensuximide. In: Woodbury D, Penry J, Pippenger C, eds. *Antiepileptic drugs,* 2nd ed. New York: Raven Press, 1982:663–671.

46. Dooley J, Camfield P, Buckley D, et al. Methsuximide-induced movement disorder. *Pediatrics* 1991;88:1291–1292.

47. Millichap JG. Milontin: a new drug in the treatment of petit mal. *Lancet* 1952;2:907.

48. Rankin GO, Beers KW, Nicoll DW, et al. Role of *para*-hydroxylation in phensuximide-induced urotoxicity in the Fischer 344 rat. *Toxicology* 1992;74:77–88.

49. Newmark ME. Phensuximide. In: Resor SR, Kutt H, eds. *The medical treatment of epilepsy,* vol 10. New York: Marcel Dekker, 1992:385–387.

50. Lairy C. Psychotic signs in epileptics during treatment with ethosuximide. *Rev Neurol* 1964;110:225–226.

51. Sato T, Kondo Y, Matsuo T, et al. Clinical experiences of ethosuximide (Zarontin) in therapy-resistant epileptics. *Brain Nerve (Toyko)* 1965;17:958–964.

52. Wolf P, Inoue Y, Roder-Wanner U-U, et al. Psychiatric complications of absence therapy and their relation to alteration of sleep. *Epilepsia* 1984;25[Suppl 1]:S56–S59.

53. Buchanan R. Ethosuximide: toxicity. In: Woodbury D, Penry J, Schmidt R, eds. *Antiepileptic drugs.* New York: Raven Press, 1972:449–454.

54. Gordon N. Treatment of epilepsy with *O*-ethyl-*o*-methylsuccinimide (P.M. 671). *Neurology* 1961;11:266–268.

55. Todorov A, Lenn N, Gabor A. Exacerbation of generalized nonconvulsive seizures with ethosuximide therapy. *Arch Neurol* 1978; 35:389–391.

56. Reynolds NC Jr, Miska RM. Safety of anticonvulsants in hepatic porphyrias. *Neurology* 1981;31:480–484.

57. Porter R, Penry J, Dreifuss F. Responsiveness at the onset of spike-wave bursts. *Electroencephalogr Clin Neurophysiol* 1973;34: 239–245.

58. Sullivan F, McElhatton P. A comparison of the teratogenic activity of the antiepileptic drugs carbamazepine, clonazepam, ethosuximide, phenobarbital, phenytoin, and primidone in mice. *Toxicol Appl Pharmacol* 1977;40:365–378.

59. Kuhnz W, Koch S, Hartmann A, et al. Ethosuximide in epileptic women during pregnancy and lactation period: placental transfer, serum concentrations in nursed infants and clinical status. *Br J Clin Pharmacol* 1984;18:671–677.

60. Dansky L, Andermann E, Sherwin A. Maternal epilepsy and birth defects: a prospective study with monitoring of plasma anticonvulsant levels during pregnancy. In: Dam M, Gram L, Penry J, eds. *Advances in Epileptology: XIIth Epilepsy International Symposium.* New York: Raven Press, 1981:607–612.

61. Drake ME. Restless legs with antiepileptic drug therapy. *Clin Neurol Neurosurg* 1988;90:151–154.

62. Birchfield R, Cowger M. Acute intermittent porphyria with seizures. *Am J Dis Child* 1966;112:561–565.

63. Hammers R, Zehner J. Irreversible cerebellar damage by methsuximide? Two case reports. *Epilepsia* 1988;29:344.

64. Uetrecht JP. The role of leukocyte-generated reactive metabolites in the pathogenesis of idiosyncratic drug reactions. *Drug Metab Rev* 1992;24:299–366.

65. Gibaldi M. Adverse drug effect: reactive metabolites and idiosyncratic drug reactions. I. *Ann Pharmacother* 1992;26: 416–421.

66. Pellock JM. Standard approach to antiepileptic drug treatment in the United States. *Epilepsia* 1994;35:S11–S18.

67. Taaffe A, O'Brien C. A case of Stevens-Johnson syndrome associated with the anti-convulsants sulthiame and ethosuximide. *Br Dent J* 1975;138:172–174.

68. Dabbous IA, Idriss HM. Occurrence of systemic lupus erythematosus in association with ethosuccimide therapy: case report. *J Pediatr* 1970;76:617–620.

69. Alter BP. Systemic lupus erythematosus and ethosuccimide. *J Pediatr* 1970;77:1093–1095.

70. Ansell BM. Drug-induced systemic lupus erythematosus in a nine-year-old boy. *Lupus* 1993;2:193–194.

71. Singsen B, Fishman L, Hanson V. Antinuclear antibodies and lupus-like syndromes in children receiving anticonvulsants. *Pediatrics* 1976;57:529–534.

72. Teoh PC, Chan HL. Lupus-scleroderma syndrome induced by ethosuximide. *Arch Dis Child* 1975;50:658–661.

73. Takeda S, Koizumi F, Takazakura E. Ethosuximide-induced lupus-like syndrome with renal involvement. *Intern Med* 1996;35:587–591.

74. Cohn R. A neuropathological study of a case of petit mal epilepsy. *Electroencephalogr Clin Neurophysiol* 1968;24:282.

75. Kousoulieris E. Granulopenia and thrombocytopenia after ethosuximide. *Lancet* 1967;2:310–311.

76. Spittler J. Agranulocytosis due to ethosuximide with a fatal outcome. *Klin Paediatr* 1974;186:364–366.

77. Massey GV, Dunn NL, Heckel JL, et al. Aplastic anemia following therapy for absence seizures with ethosuximide. *Pediatr Neurol* 1994;11:59–61.

78. Mann L, Habenicht H. Fatal bone marrow aplasia associated with administration of ethosuximide (Zarontin) for petit mal epilepsy. *Bull Los Angeles Neurol Soc* 1962;27:173–176.

79. Seip M. Aplastic anemia during ethosuximide medication: treatment with bolus-methylprednisolone. *Acta Paediatr Scand* 1983;72:927–929.

80. Ehyai A, Kilroy A, Fenicheal G. Dyskinesia and akathisia induced by ethosuximide. *Am J Dis Child* 1978;132:527–528.

81. Kirschberg G. Dyskinesia: an unusual reaction to ethosuximide. *Arch Neurol* 1975;32:137–138.

82. Nishiyama J, Matsukura M, Fugimoto S, et al. Reports of 2 cases of autoimmune thyroiditis while receiving anticonvulsant therapy. *Eur J Pediatr* 1983;140:116–117.

83. Wassner S, Pennisi A, Malekzadeh M, et al. The adverse effect of anticonvulsant therapy on renal allograft survival: a preliminary report. *J Pediatr* 1976;88:134–137.

84. Stein S, Pembrook R. Cross-sensitivity to Dilantin (diphenylhydantoin) and Celontin (methsuximide). 1965;66:799–801.

85. Tennison MB, Greenwood RS, Miles MV. Methsuximide for intractable childhood seizures. *Pediatrics* 1991;87:186–189.

86. Green R, Gilbert M. Fatal bone marrow aplasia associated with Celontin therapy. *Minn Med* 1959; 42.

87. Doig A, Stanton J. Megaloblastic anemia during combined phensuximide and phenobarbital therapy. *BMJ* 1961;2:998–999.

88. Baehler RW, Work J, Smith W, et al. Charcoal hemoperfusion in the therapy for methsuximide and phenytoin overdose. *Arch Intern Med* 1980;140:1466–1468.

89. Johnson GF, Least CJ Jr, Serum JW, et al. Monitoring drug concentrations in a case of combined overdosage with primidone and methsuximide. *Clin Chem* 1976;22:915–921.

90. Karch SB. Methsuximide overdose: delayed onset of profound coma. *JAMA* 1973;223:1463–1465.

91. Gellman V. A case of accidental methsuximide (Celontin) ingestion. *Manitoba Med Rev* 1956;45:141–143.

92. Schulte C, Good T. Acute intoxication due to methsuximide and diphenylhydantoin. *J Pediatr* 1966;68:635–637.

93. Toll L, Hurlbut K, eds. Succinimides: anticonvulsants. In: *POISINDEX system: Healthcare series,* vol 108. Greenwood Village, CO: MICROMEDEX, 2001.

94. Chyka PA, Seger D. Position statement: single-dose activated charcoal. American Academy of Clinical Toxicology, European Association of Poisons Centres and Clinical Toxicologists. *J Toxicol Clin Toxicol* 1997;35:721–741.

95. Vale JA. Position statement: gastric lavage. American Academy of Clinical Toxicology, European Association of Poisons Centres and Clinical Toxicologists. *J Toxicol Clin Toxicol* 1997;35:711–719.

96. Marbury TC, Lee CS, Perchalski RJ, et al. Hemodialysis clearance of ethosuximide in patients with chronic renal disease. *Am J Hosp Pharm* 1981;38:1757–1760.

SUCCINIMIDES

METHSUXIMIDE

THOMAS R. BROWNE

The three marketed succinimide antiepileptic drugs are ethosuximide (Zarontin), methsuximide (Celontin), and phensuximide (Milontin). These drugs are all derivatives of a five-membered succinimide ring (6) (Table 70.1).

Numerous succinimide derivatives have undergone animal screening tests for antiepileptic activity (11,12,38). The results show that methyl and ethyl substitutions at the 2 and 3 positions produce drugs that are more effective against pentylenetetrazol-induced seizures than against maximal electroshock seizures, methylation at the 5 position results in increased activity against pentylenetetrazol-induced seizures, activity against pentylenetetrazol-induced seizures decreases with increasing length of alkyl chain substitutions at the 2, 3, and 5 positions, and phenyl substitution at the 2 and 3 positions decreases activity against pentylenetetrazol-induced seizures and increases activity against maximal electroshock seizures.

Effectiveness against pentylenetetrazol-induced seizures in animals is thought to correlate with clinical efficacy against absence seizures in humans, and activity against maximal electroshock seizures in animals is thought to correlate with activity against tonic-clonic and complex partial seizures in humans (Chapter 3). The rank order of the therapeutic index of succinimides against pentylenetetrazol-induced seizures in animals is (from most to least effective) ethosuximide, methsuximide, and phensuximide (10). Clinical experience indicates that ethosuximide is the most effective succinimide against absence seizures. The rank order of the therapeutic index of succinimides against maximal electroshock seizures in animals is (from most to least effective) methsuximide, phensuximide, and ethosuximide (12). Clinical experience indicates that methsuximide has some efficacy against complex partial seizures, whereas ethosuximide has almost none.

In more recent work, N-desmethylmethsuximide (active metabolite of methsuximide) has been shown to be effective in the spontaneous generalized low-magnesium ion thalam-ocortical slice model of epilepsy (56). This work predicts efficacy for absence and primarily generalized tonic-clonic seizures (56).

CHEMISTRY

Methsuximide has the structure shown in Figure 70.1. It has the following physical characteristics: molecular weight of 203.23, melting point of 52°C, and water solubility at pH 7.0 (25°C) of mg/mL (24). Methsuximide is prepared by the action of methylamine on methylphenylsuccinic acid (39). Methsuximide is marketed in the United States as 150-mg and 300-mg capsules.

METHODS OF ANALYSIS

Methsuximide is rapidly demethylated to form 2-methyl-2-phenylsuccinimide (N-desmethylmethsuximide) (Table 70.1) (18,24,32,48,49). Only N-desmethylmethsuximide accumulates in the plasma in detectable quantities during long-term methsuximide administration in children or adults (8,23,24,37,40,48). Gibbs et al. (23) reported no plasma methsuximide concentrations >1 μg/mL in >100 patients receiving long-term methsuximide therapy.

TABLE 70.1. SUCCINIMIDES

Substituents				
R1	R2	R3	Generic Name	Trade Name
C_2H_5	CH_3	H	Ethosuximide	Zarontin
C_6H_5[a]	CH_3	CH_3	Methsuximide	Celontin
C_6H_5[a]	CH_3	H	N-desmethyl-methsuximide[b]	None
C_6H_5[a]	H	CH_3	Phensuximide	Milontin

[a]Phenyl ring.
[b]Active metabolite of methsuximide.
From Browne TR. Ethosuximide and other succinimides. In: Browne TR, Feldman RG, eds. *Epilepsy: diagnosis and management*. Boston: Little, Brown, 1983:215–224, with permission.

Thomas R. Browne, MD: Professor of Neurology, Department of Neurology, Boston University School of Medicine, Boston, Massachusetts

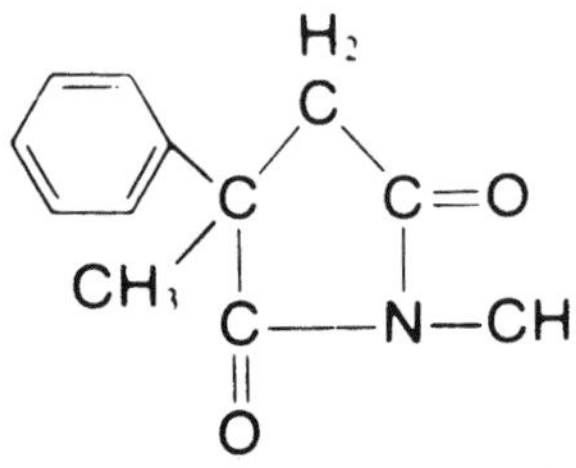

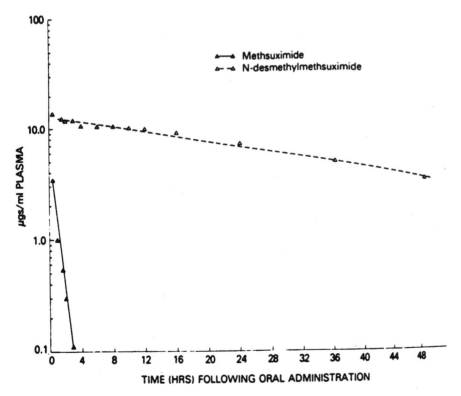

FIGURE 70.1. Structure of methsuximide.

Colorimetric and gas–liquid chromatographic methods have been reported for the determination of methsuximide in biologic fluids (18,24,53). However, the sensitivity of these methods is not sufficient to detect the low concentrations of methsuximide present in plasma after administration of methsuximide at typical dosing rates (Figure 70.2) (40,48). Two gas chromatographic–mass spectrometric methods with sufficient sensitivity (0.1 μg/mL) to detect the usual plasma concentrations of methsuximide and *N*-desmethylmethsuximide have been reported (40,48).

For routine therapeutic drug monitoring, only the plasma concentration of *N*-desmethylmethsuximide needs to be followed (8,23,37,30,48,52). High-performance liquid chromatographic (24,25,36,49), capillary gas chromatography (10), enzyme-multiplied immunoassay (36), and fluorescence polarization immunoassay (36) techniques have been reported.

ABSORPTION, DISTRIBUTION, AND EXCRETION

The absorption, distribution, and excretion of methsuximide in animals were reviewed by Porter and Kupferberg (39). Maximal plasma concentration of *N*-desmethylmethsuximide occurs 1 to 4 hours after an oral dose in humans of all ages (24,37). The protein binding of *N*-desmethylmethsuximide is 45% to 60% in human plasma (52). Animal research indicates that methsuximide crosses the blood–brain barrier (24,39). Less than 1% methsuximide is excreted unchanged in humans (24).

Biotransformation and Clinical Pharmacokinetics

Methsuximide is rapidly converted to *N*-desmethylmethsuximide, with an elimination half-life of 1.0 to 2.6 hours (Table 70.2 and Figure 70.2) (24,40,48). *N*-desmethylmethsuximide is then slowly metabolized, with an elimination half-life of 34 to 80 hours in adults (Figure 70.2) (8,23,40) and 16 to 45 hours in children (37). *N*-desmethylmethsuximide accumulates to steady-state plasma concentrations that are, on the average, about 600 to 800 times higher than the concentration of the parent drug methsuximide (39,40,48). Based on the following observations, *N*-desmethylmethsuximide is probably the major antiepileptic substance in the plasma of patients receiving methsuximide: (a) *N*-desmethylmethsuximide plasma levels

FIGURE 70.2. Serum concentration versus time course for methsuximide and *N*-desmethylmethsuximide after a single 1,200-mg dose of methsuximide. (From Porter RJ, Penry JK, Lacey JR, et al. Plasma concentrations of phensuximide, methsuximide, and their metabolites in relation to clinical efficacy. *Neurology* 1979; 29:1509–1513, with permission.)

TABLE 70.2. PHARMACOKINETIC VALUES FOR METHSUXIMIDE AND N-DESMETHYLMETHSUXIMIDE

Pharmacokinetic Parameter	Range of Values	References
MSM time to reach maximal serum concentration (hr)[a]	1–4	24,37
MSM elimination half-life (hr)[b]	1.0–2.6	23,36,42
NDM accumulation half-life (hr)[c]	39–81	7
NDM elimination half-life (hr)[b]	34–48	22,23,36,42
NDM elimination half-life (hr)[d]	52–80	7
NDM elimination half-life (hr)[e]	16–45	33
Therapeutic range of NDM plasma concentration (µg/mL)	10–40	17,40,46, 48,54

MSM, methsuximide; NDM, *N*-desmethylmethsuximide.
[a]Adults and children.
[b]Values for low plasma concentrations of NDM in adults on MSM monotherapy.
[c]Values for low plasma concentration of NDM in adults taking other antiepileptic drugs.
[d]Children.

are much higher than methsuximide serum levels; (b) methsuximide and *N*-desmethylmethsuximide have similar effectiveness against pentylenetetrazol and maximal electroshock seizures in animals (11); and (c) a small clinical trial has shown that methsuximide and *N*-desmethylmethsuximide have similar clinical effectiveness against absence seizures (57).

The major urinary metabolites of methsuximide are hydroxylated at the 3 and 4 positions of the phenyl ring by an epoxide-diol pathway (27). This pathway uses the cytochrome P450 enzyme CYP2C19 (26,56). CYP2C19 is discussed in detail in Chapter 58. The following substances are lesser urinary metabolites of methsuximide: unmetabolized methsuximide; *N*-desmethyl-2-hydroxy-methyl-2-phenylsuccinimide; *N*,2-dimethyl-3-hydroxy-2-phenylsuccinimide; and a dihydrodiol derivative (24,37,39).

The CYP2C19 pathway exhibits nonlinear (concentration-dependent) pharmacokinetics for phenytoin at therapeutic plasma concentrations in humans (Chapter 58). This raises the possibility that *N*-desmethylmethsuximide may exhibit nonlinear pharmacokinetics at therapeutic plasma concentrations in humans, and my colleagues and I (8) presented indirect evidence of this possibility. If *N*-desmethylmethsuximide has nonlinear pharmacokinetics, then the elimination half-life of *N*-desmethylmethsuximide would be longer at steady-state serum concentrations than in single-dose studies (7–9).

The package insert states that increases in methsuximide dosing rate may be made at weekly intervals. However, increases in methsuximide dosing rate should only be made at intervals of 14 days or longer in adults because (a) a drug's accumulation half-life should be similar to its elimination half-life, and five half-lives are required to attain a steady-state plasma concentration (8); and (b) the elimina-

tion half-life of *N*-desmethylmethsuximide at low plasma concentrations is 34 to 80 hours in adults and may be longer at steady-state plasma concentrations. If methsuximide dosage is increased at weekly intervals, then the plasma concentration of *N*-desmethylmethsuximide will rise rapidly because of the combined effects of the continuing rise in plasma concentration from the previous dosing rate (which had not risen to steady-state value) and the new increase in dosing rate. This may lead to toxic plasma concentrations of *N*-desmethylmethsuximide (8).

RELATIONSHIP OF PLASMA CONCENTRATION TO SEIZURE CONTROL

The plasma concentration of methsuximide in patients taking the usual doses of the drug is so small that it can be measured accurately only by gas chromatography–mass spectroscopy (8,40,48). There is no apparent correlation between the administered dose of methsuximide and the antiepileptic effect or the plasma concentration of methsuximide, presumably because methsuximide is converted to *N*-desmethylmethsuximide so rapidly (8).

There is a significant correlation between the administered dose of methsuximide and the plasma concentration of *N*-desmethylmethsuximide (4,48). On average, the plasma concentration of *N*-desmethylmethsuximide in micrograms per milliliter is 1.6 to 2.0 times the daily dose of methsuximide in milligrams per kilogram (8,48). Several studies indicate that the range of therapeutic plasma concentration of *N*-desmethylmethsuximide is 10 to 40 µg/mL (8,16,40,46,48,54) in adults. Children appear to tolerate higher plasma concentrations of *N*-desmethylmethsuximide, and the upper value for the therapeutic range may be 50 µg/mL in children (37,46).

DRUG INTERACTIONS

Patients taking methsuximide in addition to phenytoin or phenobarbital have higher values for *N*-desmethylmethsuximide plasma concentration than patients taking methsuximide alone (41). The addition of methsuximide to a regimen of phenytoin or phenobarbital results in an appreciable increase in the plasma concentration of the latter two drugs in many patients (8,41,47). These observed interactions among phenytoin, phenobarbital, and *N*-desmethylmethsuximide probably occur as a result of competition for a common arene oxidase metabolic pathway, probably cytochrome P450 CYP2C isoforms shared by all three drugs.

My colleagues and I (8) reported that the addition of methsuximide to primidone was accompanied by a significant (17%, *p* < .05) increase in the serum concentration of phenobarbital derived from primidone. The addition of methsuximide to carbamazepine was accompanied by a

23% decrease in carbamazepine plasma concentration in six adult patients (p = .08) (8). Similarly, Tennison et al. (50) reported decreases of 26% to 44% in carbamazepine plasma concentration when methsuximide was added to carbamazepine in five children (p = .01). These observations suggest that methsuximide may induce CYP3A4.

The addition of methsuximide to lamotrigine results in a drop in lamotrigine plasma concentration of 36% to 72% (4,34). The addition of methsuximide to combination therapy of lamotrigine and valproic acid also results in a decrease in lamotrigine plasma concentration, but not as great a decrease as when methsuximide is added to lamotrigine monotherapy (34).

DOSE-RELATED SIDE EFFECTS

Common Side Effects

Large series report side effects of methsuximide in 11% to 57% (median, 35%) of patients taking the drug. The frequency of common side effects of methsuximide is shown in Table 70.3. Because patients are less apt to develop tolerance to the common side effects of methsuximide than with ethosuximide, methsuximide has to be discontinued because of side effects more often than ethosuximide. Some of the drowsiness, irritability, and ataxia reported in association with methsuximide therapy may result from interference with the elimination of phenobarbital or phenytoin caused by methsuximide drug interactions, rather than from a direct toxic effect of methsuximide or its metabolites.

Overdosage

Four reported patients with methsuximide overdose all recovered without sequelae (4,22,30,45). Methsuximide overdose is characterized by stupor and coma, which may develop slowly or may have a biphasic (coma–more alert–

coma) course. The late worsening may be the result of conversion of methsuximide to *N*-desmethylmethsuximide or interference with metabolism of other antiepileptic drugs caused by methsuximide. Other clinical features reported with methsuximide overdosage include respiratory depression, central neurogenic hyperventilation, increased reflexes, decreased reflexes, myoclonus, and second-degree heart block. Charcoal hemoperfusion was employed in one case and was reported to result in a high rate of *N*-desmethylmethsuximide clearance and rapid clinical improvement (32). A single case of massive combined overdosage of methsuximide and primidone resulted in flaccid coma, respiratory arrest, hypotension, and death (29).

IDIOSYNCRATIC SIDE EFFECTS

Extensive toxicity testing of methsuximide in animals showed no abnormalities on hematologic and chemical tests of blood (12). Autopsy studies of mice, rats, dogs, and monkeys showed no abnormalities except for "mild centrilobular hepatic necrosis" in rats receiving 600 mg/kg/day of the drug (12). These changes were believed to be reversible and of no functional consequence (12).

No serious hepatic damage has ever been attributed to methsuximide. Dow et al. (19) reported an increase in cephalin flocculation in two of 62 patients taking methsuximide. Both patients were taking other antiepileptic drugs as well.

Trolle and Kiorboe (51) reported one case of transient leukopenia in which blood cell counts returned to normal while the patient was still taking methsuximide. Stenzel et al. (47) reported another case of apparently transient leukopenia. Trolle and Kiorboe (51) reported one patient with multiple small bruises in whom a platelet count was not performed.

The only reported fatal blood dyscrasia associated with methsuximide was a case of pancytopenia occurring in a

TABLE 70.3. REPORTED INCIDENCE OF SIDE EFFECTS OF ETHOSUXIMIDE AND METHSUXIMIDE IN SERIES WITH 50 OR MORE PATIENTS

Side Effect	Ethosuximide[a]		Methsuximide[b]	
	Range (%)	Median (%)	Range (%)	Median (%)
Drowsiness	0–16	7	0–28	16
Gastrointestinal disturbances (anorexia, nausea, vomiting, or abdominal pain)	4–29	13	2–30	6
Hiccoughs	0–5	0	0–6	0
Ataxia	0–1	0	0–13	6
Dizziness	0–4	1	0–13	0
Irritability	0	0	0–6	0
Rash	0–6	0	0–17	6
Leukopenia	0–7	0	0–2	0
Any side effect	26–46	37	11–57	35

[a]Based on 12 published reports. See Browne (6) for original references.
[b]Based on 8 published reports. See Browne (6) for original references.
From Browne TR. Ethosuximide and other succinimides. In: Browne TR, Feldman RG, eds. *Epilepsy: diagnosis and management.* Boston: Little, Brown, 1983:215–224, with permission.

middle-aged woman 3 months after beginning methsuximide (25). It is not certain that methsuximide was the cause of the pancytopenia because the woman had breast carcinoma and was taking four other medications.

There is a reported case of neonatal hemorrhage after combined maternal therapy with methsuximide and metharbital (5). Other rare reported complications with methsuximide are behavioral changes, confusion, diplopia, headache, periorbital edema, extrapyramidal reactions, Stevens-Johnson syndrome, restless legs syndrome, and reversible osteomalacia (3,17,20,24,39). Methsuximide may precipitate attacks of hepatic porphyria in susceptible patients (42). Rashes can occur with methsuximide (Table 70.3).

MECHANISM OF ACTION

Methsuximide possesses activity against both absence and partial seizures. There is considerable experimental evidence that the antiabsence activity of succinimides in general (14,15,31,56), and of *N*-desmethylmethsuximide in particular (16) (Figure 70.3), is the result of blockage of low-

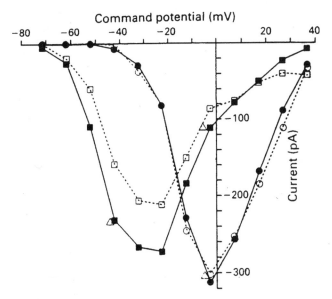

FIGURE 70.3. Effects of *N*-desmethylmethsuximide (NDM, 200 μmol/L) on calcium currents in a thalamic neuron. Plot of voltage command potential versus transient and sustained calcium current amplitude under control, NDM-exposed, and wash conditions. Transient current was defined as the portion of current that decayed during the 200-millisecond duration of the step command, and the sustained current was defined as the portion of the current that remained at the end of the 200-millisecond step command. NDM specifically reduced the transient, low-threshold calcium current, and this effect was fully reversible. *Solid box,* control transient current; *open box,* transient current in the presence of NDM; *solid circle,* control sustained current; *open circle,* sustained current in the presence of NDM; *solid triangle,* recovery. (From Coulter DA, Huguenard JR, Prince DA. Differential effects of petit-mal anticonvulsants and convulsants on thalamic neurones: calcium current reduction. *Br J Pharmacol* 1990;100:800–806, with permission.)

threshold calcium currents (T-calcium currents) of thalamic neurons (Chapter 66). Blockage of T-calcium channels may also inhibit primarily generalized tonic-clonic seizures (56). Because of the structural and functional similarities of methsuximide and *N*-desmethylmethsuximide with phenytoin, it has been presumed that the antiepileptic activity of methsuximide against partial seizures results from sodium channel inactivation similar to that induced by phenytoin (Chapter 57).

THERAPEUTIC USE

Absence Seizures

Treatment of absence seizures is the only indication for methsuximide approved by the United States Food and Drug Administration. In four reported series with 20 or more patients in whom methsuximide was used as an adjunctive drug for absence seizures, the seizures were completely controlled in 0% to 31% of cases, and the frequency of absence seizures was reduced by ≥50% in 13% to 66% of cases (19,21,33,58). In the one reported study in which methsuximide was used as the first drug for previously untreated absence seizures, only 20% of patients had a ≥50% reduction in frequency of seizures, and none had complete seizure control (33).

Ethosuximide offers the following advantages over methsuximide for treatment of absence seizures: (a) ethosuximide controls absence seizures in a higher percentage of cases (Chapter 68); (b) the common side effects of succinimides (drowsiness, gastrointestinal upset) are less severe and less persistent with ethosuximide (Table 70.3); (c) ethosuximide plasma concentration determinations are more generally available; and (d) ethosuximide has fewer drug interactions with other antiepileptic drugs (Chapter 67). Methsuximide is indicated for absence seizures only when less toxic drugs fail to control seizures adequately.

Complex Partial Seizures

In eight reported series with 18 or more patients in whom methsuximide was used as an adjunctive antiepileptic drug for complex partial seizures, complete seizure control was obtained in 4% to 30% of patients, and a ≥50% reduction in seizure frequency was obtained in 25% to 80% of patients (1,8,13,17,21,44,54,59). The four most recent series (1,8,17,54) are most applicable to current-day practice and indicate the following: (a) many patients in whom a trial of phenytoin and phenobarbital has failed will have a ≥50% reduction in seizure frequency immediately after the addition of methsuximide; (b) most patients in whom a trial of phenytoin, phenobarbital, and carbamazepine has failed will not have a ≥50% reduction in seizure frequency after the addition of methsuximide; (c) some patients will develop tolerance to the antiepileptic effect of methsuximide after 4 to 7 months of maximal therapy; (d) the response rate may be higher in patients with focal spike–wave electroencephalographic patterns (complexes consisting of a spike, often blunt, followed by a slow wave at a frequency of 1 to 2 Hz occurring predominantly in one temporal region). In the one reported study in which methsuximide was used as the first antiepileptic drug in previously untreated patients with complex partial seizures, a ≥50% reduction in seizure frequency occurred in 27% of patients, and 18% of patients experienced complete control of seizures (33).

Other Seizure Types

Stenzel et al. (47) reported some success with methsuximide in patients with "complex atypical absences" and "slow spike–wave, or sharp and slow." Tennison et al. (50) reported some success with methsuximide in children with tonic, "astatic/myoclonic," and atypical absence seizures. In a review, Schmidt and Bourgeois (43) recommended methsuximide as a fourth-line drug for Lennox-Gastaut syndrome. An open-label study reported good results with methsuximide in the treatment of juvenile myoclonic epilepsy (28). Trials of methsuximide for tonic-clonic and simple partial seizures generally have been discouraging.

Dosage and Administration

The usual starting dose of methsuximide is 300 mg/day. The daily dosage of methsuximide may be increased in increments of 150 mg or 300 mg/day at intervals of at least 2 weeks. The smaller increment is preferred in small children and persons of any age who are taking other antiepileptic drugs because of the longer elimination half-life and, therefore, reduced clearance of N-desmethylmethsuximide in patients receiving polytherapy. Dosage is increased until seizures are controlled, toxicity develops, or a maximal dosing rate of 1,200 mg/day is reached. Because N-desmethylsuccinimide elimination half-life is shorter in children than in adults, children will require a larger dose (mg/kg/day) of methsuximide to attain a given plasma concentration than adults (37).

CONVERSION

Conversion factor:

$$CF = \frac{1,000}{mol\ wt} = \frac{1,000}{203.23} = 4.92$$

Conversion:

$$(\mu g/mL) \times 4.92 = \mu mol/L$$

$$(\mu mol/L) \div 4.92 = \mu g/mL$$

REFERENCES

1. Ali A, Harden CL, Milrod L, et al. Antiepileptic drugs of last resort: recent clinical experience. *Epilepsia* 1993;34[Suppl 6]: 103.
2. Aponte CJ, Petrelli MP. Anticonvulsants and vitamin D metabolism. *JAMA* 1973;225:1248.
3. Baehler RW, Work J, Smith W, et al. Charcoal hemoperfusion in therapy of methsuximide and phenytoin overdose. *Arch Intern Med* 1980;140:1466–1468.
4. Besag FM, Berry DJ, Pool F. Methsuximide lowers lamotrigine blood levels: a pharmacokinetic antiepileptic drug interaction. *Epilepsia* 2000;41:624–627.
5. Bleyer WA, Skinner AL. Fatal neonatal hemorrhage after maternal anticonvulsant therapy. *JAMA* 1976;235:626-627.
6. Browne TR. Ethosuximide and other succinimides. In: Browne TR, Feldman RG, eds. *Epilepsy: diagnosis and management.* Boston: Little, Brown, 1983:215–224.
7. Browne TR, Evans JE, Szabo GK, et al. Studies with stable isotopes. I. Changes in phenytoin pharmacokinetics and biotransformation during monotherapy. *J Clin Pharmacol* 1985; 25:43–50.
8. Browne TR, Feldman RG, Buchanan RA, et al. Methsuximide for complex partial seizures: efficacy, toxicity, clinical pharmacology, and drug interactions. *Neurology* 1983;33:414–418.
9. Browne TR, Greenblatt DJ, Evans JE, et al. Estimation of a drug's elimination half-life at any serum concentration when the drug's K_m and V_{max} are known: calculations and validation with phenytoin. *J Clin Pharmacol* 1987;27:318–320.
10. Cardella DS, Leutzow CB, Rafai N, et al. Measurement of methsuximide and N-desmethylmethsuximide using solid phase extraction and wide-bore capillary gas chromatography. *Clin Biochem* 1988;21:329–331.
11. Chen G, Portman R, Ensor CR, et al. The anticonvulsant activity of ?[SC]-phenyl succinimides. *J Pharmacol Exp Ther* 1951; 103:54–61.
12 Chen G, Weston JK, Bratton AC Jr. Anticonvulsant activity and toxicity of phensuximide, methsuximide and ethosuximide. *Epilepsia* 1963;4:66–76.
13. Cardoba EF, Strobos RRJ. N-methyl-?[SC]-?[SC] methylphenyl-succinimide in psychomotor epilepsy. *Dis Nerv Syst* 1956;17: 383–385.
14. Coulter DA, Huguenard JR, Prince DA. Specific petit-mal anticonvulsants reduce calcium currents in thalamic neurones. *Neurosci Lett* 1989;98:74–78.
15. Coulter DA, Huguenard JR, Prince DA. Characterization of ethosuximide reduction of low-threshold calcium current in thalamic neurones. *Ann Neurol* 1989;25:582–593.
16. Coulter DA, Huguenard JR, Prince DA. Differential effects of petit-mal anticonvulsants and convulsants on thalamic neurones: calcium current reduction. *Br J Pharmacol* 1990;100:800–806.
17. Dasheiff RM, McNamara D, Dickson LV. Efficacy of second line antiepileptic drugs in the treatment of patients with medically refractive complex partial seizures. *Epilepsia* 1986;27:124–127.
18. Dobrinska MR, Welling PG. Pharmacokinetics of methsuximide and a major metabolite in dog. *J Pharm Sci* 1977;66:688–692.
19. Dow RS, Macfarlane JP, Stevens JR. Celontin in patients with refractory epilepsy. *Neurology* 1958;8:201–207.
20. Drake ME. Restless legs with antiepileptic drug therapy. *Clin Neurol Neurosurg* 1988;90:151–154.
21. French EG, Rey-Bellet J, Lennox WG. Methsuximide in psychomotor and petit-mal seizures. *N Engl J Med* 1958;258: 892–894.
22. Gellman V. A case of accidental methsuximide (Celontin) ingestion. *Manitoba Med Rev* 1956;45:141–143.

23. Gibbs EL, Gibbs TJ, Appell MR. Subtle side effects caused by Dilantin and Celontin: a report of two pilot volunteer studies. *Clin Electroencephalogr* 1974;5:192–198.

24. Glazko AJ, Dill WA. Other succinimides. Methsuximide and phensuximide. In: Woodbury DM, Penry JK, Schmidt RP, eds. *Antiepileptic drugs.* New York: Raven Press, 1972:455–464.

25. Green RA, Gilbert MG. Fatal bone marrow aplasia associated with Celontin therapy. *Minn Med* 1959;42:130.

26. Hall SD, Guengerich FP, Branch RA, et al. Characterization and inhibition of mephenytoin 4-hydroxylase activity in human liver microsomes. *J Pharmacol Exp Ther* 1987;240:216–222.

27. Horning MG. Metabolism of *N*,2-dimethyl-2-phenylsuccinimide (methsuximide) by epoxide-diol pathway in rat, guinea pig, and human. *Res Commun Chem Pathol Pharmacol* 1973;6:565–578.

28. Hurst DL. Methsuximide therapy of juvenile myoclonic epilepsy. *Seizure* 1996;5:47–50.

29. Johnson GF, Least CJ Jr, Serum JW, et al. Monitoring drug concentration in a case of combined overdosage with primidone and methsuximide. *Clin Chem* 1976;22:915–921.

30. Karch SB. Methsuximide overdose: delayed onset of profound coma. *JAMA* 1973;223:1463–1465.

31. Klunk WE, Convey DF, Ferendelli JF. Structure activity relationships of alky-substituted ?[SC]-butyrolactones and succinimides. *Mol Pharmacol* 1982;27:444–450.

32. Kupferberg HJ, Yonekawa WD, Lacy JR, et al. Comparison of methsuximide and phensuximide metabolism in epileptic patients. In: Gardner-Thrope C, Janz D, Meinardi H, et al., eds. *Antiepileptic drug monitoring.* Tunbridge Wells, UK: Pitman Medical, 1977:173–180.

33. Livingston S, Pauli L. Celonin in the treatment of epilepsy. *Pediatrics* 1957;19:614–617.

34. May TW, Rambeck B, Jurgens U. Influence of oxcarbazepine and methsuximide on lamotrigine concentrations in epileptic patients with and without valproic acid comedication: results of a retrospective study. *Ther Drug Monit* 1999;21:175–181.

35. Meatherall R, Ford D. Isocratic liquid chromatographic determination of theophylline, acetaminophen, chloramphenicol, caffeine, anticonvulsants, and barbiturates in serum. *Ther Drug Monit* 1988;10:101–115.

36. Miles MV, Howlett CM, Tennison MB. Determination of *N*-desmethylmethsuximide serum concentrations using enzyme-multiplied and fluorescence polarization immunoassays. *Ther Drug Monit* 1989;11:337–342.

37. Miles MV, Tennison MB, Greenwood RS. Pharmacokinetics of *N*-desmethylmethsuximide in pediatric patients. *J Pediatrics* 1989;114:647–650.

38. Miller CA, Long LM. Anticonvulsants: an investigation of *N-R*-?[SC]-R₁-?[SC]-phenylsuccinimides. *J Am Chem Soc* 1951;73:4895–4898.

39. Porter RJ, Kupferberg HJ. Other succinimides: methsuximide and phensuximide. In: Woodbury DM, Penry JK, Pippenger CE, eds. *Antiepileptic drugs,* 2nd ed. New York: Raven Press, 1982:663–671.

40. Porter RJ, Penry JK, Lacey JR, et al. Plasma concentrations of phensuximide, methsuximide, and their metabolites in relation to clinical efficacy. *Neurology* 1979;29:1509–1513.

41. Rambeck B. Pharmacological interactions of methsuximide with phenobarbital and phenytoin in hospitalized epileptic patients. *Epilepsia* 1979;20:147–156.

42. Reynolds NC, Miska RM. Safety of anticonvulsants in hepatic porphyrias. *Neurology* 1981;31:480–484.

43. Schmidt D, Bourgeois B. A risk-benefit assessment of therapies for Lennox-Gastaut syndrome. *Drug Saf* 2000;22:467–477.

44. Scholl ML, Abbot JA, Schwab RS. Celontin: a new anticonvulsant. *Epilepsia* 1959;1:105–109.

45. Schulte CJA, Good TA. Acute intoxication due to methsuximide and diphenylhydantoin. *J Pediatr* 1966;68:635–637.

46. Sigler M, Strassburg HM, Boenigk HE. Effective and safe but forgotten: methsuximide in intractable epilepsies in childhood. *Seizure* 2001;10:120–124.

47. Stenzel E, Boenigk HE, Rambeck B. Methsuximide in der Epilepsiebenhandlung. *Nervenarzt* 1977;48:377–384.

48. Strong JM, Abe T, Gibbs EL, et al. Plasma levels of methsuximide and *N*-desmethylmethsuximide during methsuximide therapy. *Neurology* 1974;24:250–255.

49. Szabo GK, Browne TR. Improved isocratic liquid-chromatographic simultaneous measurement of phenytoin, phenobarbital, primidone, carbamazepine, ethosuximide, and *N*-desmethylsuximide in serum. *Clin Chem* 1982;28:100–104.

50. Tennison MB, Greenwood RS, Miles MV. Methsuximide for intractable childhood seizures. *Pediatrics* 1991;87:186–189.

51. Trolle R, Kiorboe E. Treatment of petit-mal epilepsy with new succinimides: PM60 and Celontin (a clinical comparative study). *Epilepsia* 1960;1:587–697.

52. Wad N, Bourgeois B, Kramer G. Serum protein binding of desmethyl-methsuximide. *Clin Neuropharmacol* 1999;22:239–240.

53. Watson JR, Lawrence RC, Lovering EB. Simple GLC analysis of anticonvulsant drugs in commercial dosage forms. *J Pharm Sci* 1978;67:950–953.

54. Wilder BJ, Buchanan RB. Methsuximide for refractory complex partial seizures. *Neurology* 1981;31:741-744.

55. Wright JD, Helsby NA, Ward SA. The role of S-mephenytoin hydroxylase (CYP2C19) in the metabolism of the antimalarial biguanides. *Br J Clin Pharmacol* 1995; 39:441–444.

56. Zhang YF, Gibbs JW, Coulter DA. Anticonvulsant drug effects spontaneous thalamocortical rhythms in vitro:valproic acid, clonazepam, and alpha-methyl-alpha-phenylsuccinimide. *Epilepsy Res* 1996;5:37–53.

57. Zimmerman FT. New drugs in the treatment of petit-mal epilepsy. *Am J Psychiatry* 1953;109:767–773.

58. Zimmerman FT. Milontin in the treatment of epilepsy. *NY State J Med* 1955;56:1460–1465.

59. Zimmerman FT. *N*-methyl-?[SC]-?[SC]-methylphenylsuccinimide in psychomotor epilepsy therapy. *Arch Neurol Psychiatry* 1956;76:65–71.

Antiepileptic Drugs, 5th Edition. Edited by R.H. Levy, R.H. Mattson, B.S. Meldrum, and E. Perucca. Lippincott Williams & Wilkins, Philadelphia © 2002.

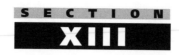

TIAGABINE

TIAGABINE

MECHANISMS OF ACTION

WILLIAM J. GIARDINA

Tiagabine HCl (*R*-*N*-(4,4-di-(3-methyl-2-thienyl)-3-butenyl)nipecotic acid, hydrochloride) (Figure 71.1) is a potent blocker of γ-aminobutyric acid (GABA) uptake by neurons and glia. Novo-Nordisk scientists discovered tiagabine HCl in 1987 in Denmark. GABA is the major inhibitory neurotransmitter in the central nervous system, and a reduction in GABA-mediated inhibition has been implicated in the origin of epilepsy and other neurologic disorders (1,2). Two important observations formed the basis of the Novo-Nordisk drug discovery program. First, nipecotic acid and several other cyclic amino acids, such as guvacine, hydroxynipecotic acid, and homo-β-proline, block GABA uptake into glia and neurons *in vitro*, and second, nipecotic acid protects mice against sound-induced seizures after intracerebroventricular injection (2,3). Nipecotic acid does not cross the blood–brain barrier after systemic administration. Novo-Nordisk scientists synthesized and evaluated a series of compounds in which nipecotic acid was linked by an aliphatic chain to different lipophilic groups. These compounds were designed to be orally active blockers of GABA uptake that would readily cross the blood–brain barrier. Tiagabine HCl emerged from this program as the best of these compounds to become a candidate for clinical study in epilepsy. Tiagabine HCl has received regulatory approval in the United States and in many countries around the world for use as adjunctive therapy in the treatment of partial seizures with and without generalization.

The anticonvulsant profile of tiagabine HCl in animal seizure models is summarized in Table 71.1. Tiagabine HCl blocks seizures induced by pentylenetetrazol (PTZ) and DMCM (6,7-dimethoxy-4-ethyl-β-carboline-3-carboxylate), but it only weakly inhibits maximal electroshock seizures (4,5). It blocks the kindling process and the expression of amygdala-kindled seizures in rats (6,7). Thus, the screening profile of tiagabine HCl is unique among the older, first-generation, and the newer, second-generation, anticonvul-

sants. Tiagabine HCl provides maximal protection of only 50% to 60% against PTZ and DMCM clonic seizures at doses in the range of 1 to 10 mg/kg intraperitoneally (i.p.), and a dose of 30 mg/kg i.p., it fails altogether to block clonic seizures. In contrast, tiagabine HCl blocks PTZ tonic seizures and death in a dose-related manner (4,5). Tiagabine HCl is effective in three animal models of reflex epilepsy: sound-induced seizures in the epilepsy-prone rat and the DBA/2 mouse and photic-induced seizures in the baboon (5,8,9). Tiagabine HCl is also effective in controlling status epilepticus in cobalt-lesioned rats (10). Anticonvulsant tolerance, an activity-dependent liability of benzodiazepine anticonvulsants and of other GABAergic compounds, does not develop after repeated doses of tiagabine HCl in the mouse (11). In rodents, tiagabine HCl produces sedation at doses 10 to 14 times higher than anticonvulsant doses and impairs motor coordination at doses four to six times higher than anticonvulsant doses (5). With long-term administration, a substantial tolerance develops to the sedative and motor-impairing effects of tiagabine HCl in rodents. In addition to its well-characterized anticonvulsant activity, tiagabine HCl has also been shown to have antiallodynic pharmacology in a rodent model of neuropathic pain and antinociceptive and anxiolytic pharmacology in rodent behavioral models (12–14).

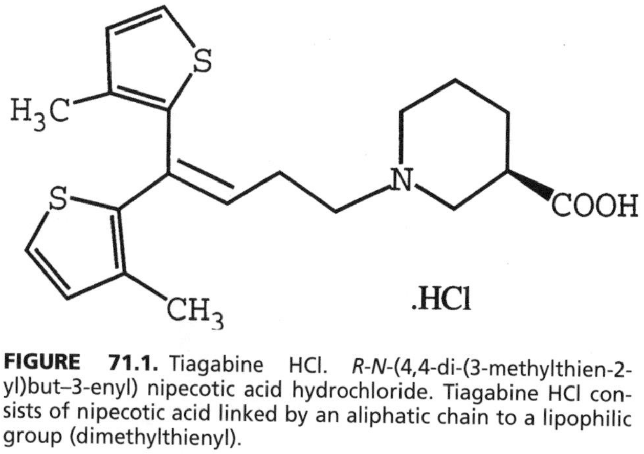

FIGURE 71.1. Tiagabine HCl. *R*-*N*-(4,4-di-(3-methylthien-2-yl)but–3-enyl) nipecotic acid hydrochloride. Tiagabine HCl consists of nipecotic acid linked by an aliphatic chain to a lipophilic group (dimethylthienyl).

William J. Giardina, PhD: Associate Research Fellow, Central Nervous System Diseases Research, Abbott Laboratories, Abbott Park, Illinois

TABLE 71.1. ANTICONVULSIVE ACTIVITY OF TIAGABINE HYDROCHLORIDE IN ANIMAL MODELS OF EPILEPSY

Seizure Model (Reference)	Effects of Tiagabine Hydrochloride
Pentylenetetrazol-induced tonic and clonic seizures in mice (5)	Blocks tonic seizures, ED_{50} = 0.8 mg/kg, i.p.
	Blocks clonic seizures, ED_{50} = 2 mg/kg i.p., ineffective at 30 mg/kg, i.p.
DMCM (6,7-dimethoxy-4-ethyl-β-carboline-3-carboxylate)-induced tonic and clonic seizures in mice (4,5)	Blocks tonic seizures, ED_{50} = 0.8 mg/kg, i.p.
	Blocks clonic seizures ED_{50} = 0.8 mg/kg, i.p., ineffective at 100 mg/kg, i.p.
Maximal electroshock seizures in mice (5)	Ineffective up to 30 mg/kg, i.p.
Bicuculline-induced seizures in mice (4)	40% antagonism at 8 mg/kg, i.p., ineffective at higher doses
Amygdala-kindled seizures in rats (6)	Suppresses the kindling process and expression of kindled seizures at 10 mg/kg, i.p.
Sound-induced tonic and clonic seizures in DBA/2 mice (5)	Blocks clonic seizures, ED_{50} = 0.4 mg/kg, i.p.
	Blocks tonic seizures, ED_{50} = 0.4 mg/kg, i.p.
Sound-induced clonic seizures in genetically epilepsy-prone rats (8)	Blocks clonic seizures, ED_{50} = 10 mg/kg, i.p. at 30 min after dosing
Photically induced myoclonic seizures in *Papio papio* (9)	Reduces myoclonus at 0.2–1 mg/kg, i.v.
	Approximate ED_{50} of 0.6 mg/kg, i.v.
Homocysteine thiolactone-induced status epilepticus in cobalt-lesioned rats (10)	Controls generalized tonic-clonic seizures at 8.3 mg/kg, i.p.

ED_{50}, dose protecting 50% of animals; i.p., intraperitoneally; i.v., intravenously.

EFFECTS ON GABA UPTAKE

After release into the synapse from presynaptic nerve terminal vesicles, GABA binds to certain functional sites: $GABA_A$ and $GABA_B$ receptors and a family of GABA uptake transporters. The $GABA_A$ receptor, the more prevalent of the two GABA receptors in the central nervous system, is a postsynaptic, multisubunit, receptor–chloride ion channel complex that, when activated by GABA, increases chloride permeability (Figure 71.2). The increase in chloride permeability results in the hyperpolarization of the nerve membrane potential and thus a decrease in nerve excitability. Experimental evidence suggests that alterations in $GABA_A$ receptor activity are involved in the initiation and spread of seizure activity (1). The $GABA_B$ receptor is coupled to cellular membrane calcium and potassium ion channels

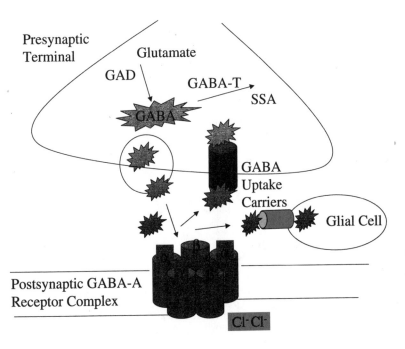

FIGURE 71.2. The $GABA_A$ synapse. Glutamate is metabolized by glutamic acid decarboxylase (GAD) to form GABA. After release from synaptic vesicles, GABA is inactivated by uptake in glia and presynaptic endings. GABA is metabolized by GABA transaminase ($GABA_T$) in mitochondria to form succinic semialdehyde (SSA).

through intracellular second messenger systems. $GABA_B$ receptors are found on presynaptic terminals, where they function to decrease neurotransmitter release through depolarization, and on postsynaptic sites, where they serve to hyperpolarize cells. After release into the synapse, unbound GABA is removed from the synapse into presynaptic nerve endings and astroglia by high-affinity, sodium-dependent membrane transporter proteins. Molecular cloning has revealed four such GABA transporters in the central nervous system: GAT-1, GAT-2, GAT-3, and BGT-1 (15,16). Tiagabine HCl is a highly selective blocker of the GAT-1 transporter, which is the predominant transporter in rat forebrain (cortex, striatum, and hippocampus (15,16).

Braestrup and colleagues did the pioneering work that characterized the biochemistry and pharmacology of tiagabine HCl (17). Tiagabine HCl inhibits the uptake of [^{3}H]-GABA into rat forebrain-derived synaptosomes with an IC_{50} value, which is the concentration that inhibits the uptake of [^{3}H]-GABA by 50%, of 67 nmol/L, and in primary cultures of neurons and astrocytes with IC_{50} values of 466 and 182, respectively. Tiagabine HCl produces a mixed competitive-noncompetitive type of inhibition of [^{3}H]-GABA uptake. In the same assays, tiagabine HCl is more potent than nipecotic acid (IC_{50} values of 3,790, 16,800, and 33,000 in synaptosomes, neurons, and astrocytes, respectively), and it is more potent than a guvacine-derived uptake inhibitor SKF-100330A (IC_{50} values of 331, 1,772, and 559 in synaptosomes, neurons, and astrocytes, respectively). Tiagabine HCl (200 nmol/L) significantly reduces the uptake of GABA into human astrocytes cultured from human adult brain tissue (18). Tiagabine HCl, the *(R)*-(−)-enantiomer of the racemic compound, is more potent than the corresponding *(S)*-(+)-enantiomer in these assays, a finding indicating a stereospecific interaction at the GAT-1 transporter. Tiagabine HCl is a specific inhibitor of the GAT-1 transporter, as indicated by the finding that it has no significant binding affinity for catecholamine, serotonin, or glutamate transporters. It also does not bind to catecholamine, acetylcholine, adenosine, serotonin, histamine, opiate, glycine, or glutamate receptors, and it has no affinity for voltage-gated calcium or sodium ion channels.

Tiagabine HCl (100 to 300 nmol/L) and vigabatrin (100 µmol/L), an inhibitor of GABA transaminase, or the combination of both, reduce [^{14}C]GABA uptake in primary cultures of rat cortical astrocyte (19). In these experiments, the inhibition of GABA uptake in cultures exposed to both compounds was greater than that observed for each drug alone, but the combined effect was infraadditive, a finding suggesting a common site of action for both compounds. Vigabatrin may affect GABA transport in these cultures by acting as a substrate for the GABA transporter (19). Tiagabine HCl is not a substrate for the GAT-1 transporter and is not transported into neurons (17). Because it is not transported into neurons, tiagabine HCl does not stimulate the release of GABA or act as a false neurotransmitter.

Several experiments show that the oral and parenteral administration of tiagabine HCl, at pharmacologically relevant doses, increases the extracellular levels of GABA. The ED_{50} (11.5 mg/kg i.p., the dose blocking seizures in 50% of animals) and ED_{85} (21 mg/kg i.p.) doses of tiagabine HCl for inhibiting PTZ-induced seizures in rats produce dose-related increases in the extracellular levels of GABA in rat brain (20). In these experiments, in which extracellular GABA was measured by *in vivo* microdialysis technique, GABA levels increased 250% and 350% over basal levels in the globus pallidus and ventral tegmentum. The time course of the increase in brain GABA levels coincides with peak anticonvulsant activity in the rat. In kindled rats in which the baseline extracellular GABA levels in rat frontal cortex are increased 100% over control animals, tiagabine HCl (10 mg/kg intravenously) causes a further increase in extracellular GABA levels (21). A delay between the rise in plasma concentrations of tiagabine HCl and the increase in GABA levels was observed in these kindled rats. Tiagabine HCl has also been reported to increase GABA levels in the hippocampus of human patients after oral administration (22). The antinociceptive and neuroprotective effects of tiagabine HCl in the rat and gerbil, respectively, are also correlated with increases in extracellular brain GABA levels (13,23).

EFFECTS ON NERVE EXCITABILITY

GABA produces a fast inhibitory postsynaptic potential (IPSP) in neurons by increasing chloride conductance at the $GABA_A$ receptor–chloride ion channel complex. Tiagabine HCl enhances the GABA-induced increase in membrane conductance in CA1 pyramidal cells (24). In these experiments, GABA was applied iontophoretically to the dendritic or somatic regions of pyramidal neurons during the perfusion of the slice with tiagabine HCl. The decay time of the conductance increase was prolonged by tiagabine HCl, and tiagabine HCl did not affect resting membrane potential. Tiagabine HCl also increases endogenous GABA-mediated IPSPs that are evoked antidromically in the hippocampal slice by electrical stimulation of the axons of the pyramidal cells (24).

The effects of tiagabine HCl on IPSPs were also tested in rat hippocampal slice cultures, which contain large numbers of GABAergic interneurons that form correct axosomatic and axodendritic synapses with pyramidal cells (25). In this preparation, tiagabine HCl prolongs the duration of both $GABA_A$ and $GABA_B$ receptor-mediated monosynaptic IPSPs produced by excitatory amino acid antagonists. In the presence of tiagabine HCl, the mean decay time constant increased from 16 to 250 milliseconds. Tiagabine HCl also reduces the spontaneous and evoked epileptiform bursting induced by increasing extracellular potassium ion concentration. Tiagabine HCl (20 µmol/L) increases the rise time and duration of IPSPs of CA1 pyramidal cells of genetically epileptic mice until they resemble those of control mice (26). A study comparing the effects of tiagabine, vigabatrin, gabapentin, and valproate on the function of the mouse brain GAT-1 transporter expressed in *Xenopus* oocytes found that all these anticonvulsant compounds inhibit the uptake of GABA at clinically relevant concentrations in this preparation, but only tiagabine HCl (20 μmol/L) blocks the GAT-1–mediated steady-state current and transient charge movement at clinically relevant concentrations (27).

HYPERSYNCHRONOUS ELECTROENCEPHALOGRAPHIC EFFECTS

Tiagabine HCl produces hypersynchronous electroencephalograms (EEGs) at anticonvulsive doses in several different behavioral models in the rat and mouse. Repetitive 1- to 10-second episodes of hypersynchronous EEG waves in the frequency range of 4 to 7 Hz occur in the normal EEG of the rat after a dose of 10 mg/kg i.p. of tiagabine HCl and, to a lesser extent, after a dose of 2 mg/kg i.p. (28). The hypersynchronous EEG episodes appear only during wakefulness and are accompanied by low muscle activity, generally within 15 minutes of a dose of tiagabine HCl. Apart from the hypersynchronous activity, tiagabine HCl has no other effect on EEG of the awake rat. In the sleeping rat, a dose of 10 mg/kg i.p. of tiagabine HCl significantly increases the latency to rapid eye movement sleep, but it does not affect the latency to non–rapid eye movement sleep or the number or average duration of the non–rapid eye movement sleep episodes (28). This dose of tiagabine HCl tends to elevate the EEG power density in the frequencies between 1 and 8 Hz during non–rapid eye movement sleep.

Tiagabine HCl produces a nonconvulsive type epilepsy in the WAG/Rij rats, an animal model of generalized nonconvulsive epilepsy (29). In these animals, tiagabine HCl increases the number and duration of spike–wave discharges in cortical EEG in a dose-related manner over the dose range of 1 to 10 mg/kg i.p., without causing behavioral effects and with little effect on the spectral EEG, except to increase the power in the β band of 25 to 39 Hz at doses of 3 and 10 mg/kg i.p. Tiagabine HCl produces a dose-dependent increase in the frequency and duration of absence seizures at doses greater than 1 mg/kg i.p., and absence status epilepticus at 11 mg/kg i.p., in the lethargic (lh/lh) mouse model of absence seizures (30). In nonepileptic rats, a very high dose of tiagabine HCl (100 mg/kg i.p.) produces an abnormal, hyporeactive behavioral state that is accompanied by an EEG pattern of high-amplitude, frontally dominant, rhythmic, 3- to 5-Hz spike–wave activity (10).

The effects of tiagabine HCl in normal and epileptic rodents suggest a potential association of tiagabine HCl with generalized spike–wave discharge of nonconvulsive status epilepticus. Such absencelike seizures may be mediated by GABA_B receptor stimulation. Experimental absence seizures in rats are prolonged by baclofen, a GABA_B agonist, and are attenuated by CGP35348, a GABA_B antagonist (31). There have been case reports of possible nonconvulsive absence seizures associated with tiagabine HCl therapy (32–35). However, the results of a clinical study of tiagabine HCl as initial treatment of adult-onset partial epilepsy did not find any confusional states or nonconvulsive status epilepticus associated with tiagabine HCl treatment, and tiagabine HCl was not associated with new interictal slow-wave discharges (36). An analysis of data on status epilepticus and tiagabine HCl that included an expert review of the EEGs of patients showing slow-wave discharge and a comparison of tiagabine HCl treated patients with placebo-treated patients showed that tiagabine HCl toxicity may be associated with spike–wave discharges, especially in patients with a history of spike–wave discharge, and the incidence of complex partial status epilepticus is not higher in patients taking tiagabine HCl (37).

Tiagabine HCl has been reported to cause an activity-dependent enhancement of hyperpolarizing as well as depolarizing GABA-mediated responses in CA1 pyramidal cells of an *in vitro* rat hippocampal slice preparation (38). In contrast to the well-known inhibitory effects of GABA, the high-frequency stimulation (100 Hz) of inhibitory pathways in the hippocampal slice evokes GABA-mediated depolarization responses capable of triggering seizurelike bursts of action potentials in hippocampal pyramidal cells (39). The bath application of tiagabine HCl (20 μmol/L) prolongs the duration of hyperpolarizing IPSPs in CA1 pyramidal cells evoked by a single, high- or low-intensity electrical stimulation of inhibitory interneurons. In contrast, tiagabine HCl greatly increases the GABA-mediated depolarizing responses in the hippocampus evoked by low- or high-intensity, high-frequency stimulation of the same inhibitory interneurons (38). Tiagabine HCl (50 μmol/L) evokes large, slow depolarizations in cortical wedges prepared from audiogenic seizure-prone mice (40). The depolarizing and desensitizing effects of tiagabine HCl may be the mechanisms by which large doses of tiagabine HCl cause tremor and seizurelike movements of the forelimbs in animals (4). Such proconvulsant effects of tiagabine HCl are in line with the convulsant effects of direct-acting GABA_A receptor agonists, which cause GABA receptor depolarization and desensitization (41).

NEUROPROTECTIVE EFFECTS

A dose of 50 mg/kg/day of tiagabine HCl delivered by subcutaneous osmotic pump blocks generalized clonic seizures, prevents seizure-induced damage in the CA1 and CA3 areas of the hippocampus, and reduces impairment of spatial learning and memory on the Morris water maze in the perforant pathway stimulation model of status epilepticus in the rat (42). In this study, the protective effects of tiagabine HCl were greater in the pyramidal cell layer than in the hilus of the dentate gyrus or in the extrahippocampal areas. A dose of 50 mg/kg i.p. of tiagabine HCl administered immediately before and 1, 24, and 48 hours after transient global ischemia reduces ischemic cell loss of CA1 pyramidal cells in the rat four-vessel occlusion model (43). Tiagabine HCl (45 mg/kg i.p.) also slows pyramidal cell loss in the gerbil hippocampus after global ischemia (23). The neuroprotective effect of this dose of tiagabine HCl in gerbils is associated with an elevation of extracellular GABA levels and the induction of mild hypothermia. A dose of 20 mg/kg i.p. of tiagabine HCl administered to rats 1 hour after occlusion of the middle cerebral artery significantly reduces infarction volume after focal ischemic injury (44). There is no neuroprotective effect when tiagabine HCl is administered either 15 minutes before or 3 or 6 hours after focal ischemic injury. Taken together, the results of these studies indicate that tiagabine HCl is neuroprotective in animals. It can be postulated that this protection is the result of a GABA-mediated decrease in nerve excitation that ultimately prevents calcium-induced neurotoxicity.

SUMMARY OF UNIFIED MECHANISM

Tiagabine HCl evolved from a discovery program that was designed to identify potent and specific GABA uptake inhibitors as anticonvulsants for the treatment of epilepsy. Impairment of GABA inhibitory function may play a role in the pathogenesis of epilepsy and other neurologic disorders. The results of *in vitro* neuropharmacology studies show the specificity and potency of tiagabine HCl as a GABA uptake inhibitor and demonstrate that tiagabine HCl can strengthen the inhibitory neuropharmacologic actions of GABA at both GABA$_A$ and GABA$_B$ receptors. In animal seizure models, the anticonvulsive pharmacology of tiagabine HCl is correlated with increases in extracellular GABA brain levels. Presumably, the increase in extracellular GABA levels results in a greater distribution and prolonged action of GABA. The ability of tiagabine HCl to block DMCM clonic seizures in mice suggests that it acts *in vivo* to block seizures at the GABA$_A$ receptor. DMCM, an inverse agonist at the benzodiazepine receptor on the GABA$_A$ receptor–ion channel complex, produces convulsions by impairing GABAergic neurotransmission (5). The anticonvulsant and antinociceptive effects of tiagabine HCl occur in the same dose range of 1 to 30 mg/kg i.p. Whereas the anticonvulsant effects of tiagabine HCl appear to be mediated by GABA$_A$ receptors, GABA$_B$ receptors appear to modulate the antinociceptive effects of tiagabine HCl in the mouse and rat because these effects are blocked by a GABA$_B$ receptor blocker (13). Taken together, the results of bio-

chemical and pharmacologic mechanism of action studies support the hypothesis that the primary antiepilepsy effect of tiagabine HCl is achieved through inhibition of GABA uptake by nerves and glia that results in an increase in GABA-mediated inhibitory events.

REFERENCES

1. Olsen RW, Avoli M. GABA and epileptogenesis. *Epilepsia* 1997; 38:399–407.
2. Krogsgaard-Larsen P, Falch E, Larsson OM, et al. GABA uptake inhibitors: relevance to antiepileptic drug research. *Epilepsy Res* 1987;1:77–93.
3. Horton RW, Collins JF, Anlezark BM, et al. Convulsant and anticonvulsant actions in DBA/2 mice of compounds blocking the reuptake of GABA. *Eur J Pharmacol* 1979;59:75–83.
4. Nielsen EB, Suzdak PD, Andersen KE, et al. Charterization of tiagabine (NO-328), a new potent and selective GABA uptake inhibitor. *Eur J Pharmacol* 1991;196:257–266.
5. Dalby NO, Nielsen EB. Comparison of the preclinical anticonvulsant profiles of tiagabine, lamotrigine, gabapentin and vigabatrin. *Epilepsy Res* 1997;28:63–72.
6. Dalby NO, Nielsen EB. Tiagabine exerts an anti-epileptogenic effect in amygdala kindling epileptogenesis in the rat. *Neurosci Lett* 1997;229:135–137.
7. Morimoto K, Sato H, Yamamoto Y, et al. Antiepileptic effects of tiagabine, a selective GABA uptake inhibitor, in the rat kindling model of temporal lobe epilepsy. *Epilepsia* 1997;38:966–974.
8. Faingold CL, Randall ME, Boersma Anderseon CA. Blockade of GABA uptake with tiagabine inhibits audiogenic seizures and reduces neuronal firing in the inferior colliculus of the genetically epilepsy-prone rat. *Exp Neurol* 1994;126:225–232.
9. Smith SE, Parvez NS, Chapman AG, et al. The γ-aminobutryic acid uptake inhibitor, tiagabine, is anticonvulsant in two animal models of reflex epilepsy. *Eur J Pharmacol* 1995;273:259–265.
10. Walton NY, Gunawan S, Trieman DM. Treatment of experimental status epilepticus with the GABA uptake inhibitor, tiagabine. *Epilepsy Res* 1994;19:237–244.
11. Suzdak PD. Lack of tolerance to the anticonvulsant effects of tiagabine following chronic (21 day) treatment. *Epilepsy Res* 1994;19:205–213.
12. Giardina WJ, Decker MW, Porsolt RD, et al. An evaluation of the GABA uptake blocker tiagabine in animal models of neuropathic and nociceptive pain. *Drug Dev Res* 1998;44:106–113.
13. Ippioni A, Lamberi C, Medica A, et al. Tiagabine antinociception in rodents depends on GABA$_B$ receptor activation: parallel antinociception testing and medial thalamus GABA microdialysis. *Eur J Pharmacol* 1999;368:205–211.
14. Schmitt U, Hiemke C. Effects of GABA-transporter (GAT) inhibitors on rat behavior in open-field and elevated plus-maze. *Behav Pharmacol* 1999;10:131–137.
15. Borden LA, Murali Dhar TG, Smith KE, et al. Tiagabine, SK&F 89976, CI-966, and NNC-711 are selective for the cloned GABA transporter GAT-1. *Eur J Pharmacol* 1994;269:219–234.
16. Borden LA. GABA transporter heterogeneity: pharmacology and cellular localization. *Neurochem Int* 1996;29:335–356.
17. Braestrup C, Nielsen EB, Sonnewald, et al. R-N-[4,4-bis(3-methyl-2-thienyl)but-3-3n-1-yl]nipecotic acid binds with high affinity to the brain γ-aminobutyric acid uptake carrier. *J Neurochem* 1990;54:639–647.
18. Fraser CM, Sills GJ, Butler E, et al. Effects of valproate, vigabatrin and tiagabine on GABA uptake into human astrocytes cultures from foetal and adult brain tissue. *Epileptic Disord* 1999;1: 153–157.

19. Leach JP, Sills GJ, Majid A, et al. Effects of tiagabine and vigabatrin on GABA uptake into primary cultures of rat cortical astrocytes. *Seizure* 1996;5:229–234.

20. Fink-Jensen A, SuzdakPD, Swedberg ME, et al. The γ-aminobutyric acid (GABA) uptake inhibitor, tiagabine, increase extracellular brain levels of GABA in awake ras. *Eur J Pharmacol* 1992; 220:197–201.

21. Cleton A, Altorf BA, Voskuyl RA, et al. Effect of amygdala kindling on the central nervous system effects of tiagabine: EEG effects versus brain GABA levels. *Br J Pharmacol* 2000;130: 1037–1044.

22. During M, Mattson R, Scheyer R, et al. The effect of tiagabine hydrochloride on extracellular GABA levels in the human hippocampus. *Epilepsia* 1992;33[Suppl 3]:83.

23. Inglefield JR, Perry JM, Schwartz RD. Postischemic inhibition of GABA reuptake by tiagabine slows neuronal death in the gerbil hippocampus. *Hippocampus* 1995;5:460–468.

24. Rekling JC, Jahnsen H, Laursen AM. The effect of two lipophilic γ-aminobutyric acid uptake blockers in CA1 of the rat hippocampal slice. *Br J Pharmacol* 1990;99:103–106.

25. Thompson SM, Gahwiler BH. Effects of the GABA uptake inhibitor tiagabine on inhibitory synaptic potentials in rat hippocampal slice cultures. *J Neurophysiol* 1992;67:1698–1701.

26. Lambert JDC, Fueta Y, Roepstorff A, et al. Analysis of the kinetics of synaptic inhibition points to a reduction in GABA release in area CA1 of the genetically epileptic mouse, EL. *Epilepsy Res* 1996;26:15–23.

27. Eckstein-Ludwig U, Fei J, Schwarz W. Inhibition of uptake, steady-state currents, and transient charge movements generated by the neuronal GABA transporter by various anticonvulsant drugs. *Br J Pharmacol* 1999;128:92–102.

28. Lancel M, Faulhaber J, Deisz RA. Effect of the GABA uptake inhibitor tiagabine on sleep and EEG power spectra in the rat. *Br J Pharmacol* 1998;123:1471–1477.

29. Coenen AML, Blezer EHM, van Luijtelaar ELJM. Effects of the GABA-uptake inhibitor tiagabine on electroencephalogram, spike–wave discharges and behaviour of rats. *Epilepsy Res* 1995;21:89–94.

30. Hosford DA, Wang Y. Utility of the lethargic (lh/lh) mouse model of absence seizures in predicting the effects of lamotrigine, vigabatrin, tiagabine, gabapentin, and topiramate against human absence seizures. *Epilepsia* 1997; 38:408–414.

31. Snead OC. Evidence for GABA-B-mediated mechanism in experimental generalized absence seizures. *Eur J Pharmacol* 1992; 213:343–349.

32. Schapel G, Chadwick D. Tiagabine and non-convulsive status epilepticus. *Seizure* 1996;5:153–156.

33. Eckardt KM, Steinhoff BJ. Non-convulsive status epilepticus in two patients receiving tiagabine treatment. *Epilepsia* 1998;39: 671–674.

34. Ettinger AB, Bernal OG, Andriola MR, et al. Two cases of nonconvulsive status epilepticus in association with tiagabine therapy. *Epilepsia* 1999;40:1159–1162.

35. Knake S, Hamer HM, Schomburg U, et al. Tiagabine-induced absence status in idiopathic generalized epilepsy. *Seizure* 1999;8: 314–317.

36. Kalviainen R, Leena J, Salmanpera T, et al. The EEG effects of initial tiagabine monotherapy. *Epilepsia* 2000;41[Suppl 7]:224 (abst).

37. Shinnar S, Berg AT, Treiman D, et al. Status epilepticus and tiagabine therapy: review of safety data and epidemiological comparisons. *Epilepsia* 2001;42:372–379.

38. Jackson MF, Esplin B, Capek R. Activity-dependent enhancement of hyperpolarizing and depolarizing γ-aminobutyric acid (GABA) synaptic responses following inhibition of GABA uptake by tiagabine. *Epilepsy Res* 1999;37:25–36.

39. Grover LM, Lambert NA, Schwartzkroin PA, et al. Role of HCO3-ions in depolarizing GABA-A receptor mediated responses in pyramidal cells of rat hippocampus. *J Neurophysiol* 1993;69:1541–1555.

40. Hu RQ, Davies JA. Tiagabine hydrochloride, a inhibitor of gamma-aminobutyric acid (GABA) uptake, induces cortical depolarizations *in vitro*. *Brain Res* 1997;753:260–268.

41. Meldrum BS. GABAergic mechanism in the pathogenesis and treatment of epilepsy. *Br J Clin Pharmacol* 1989;27[Suppl]:3–11.

42. Halonen T, Nissinen J, Jansen JA et al. Tiagabine prevents seizures, neuronal damage and memory impairment in experimental status epilepticus. *Eur J Pharmacol* 1996;299:69–81.

43. Johansen FF, Diemer NH. Enhancement of GABA neurotransmission after cerebral ischemia in the rat reduces loss of hippocampal CA1 pyramidal cells. *Acta Neurol Scand* 1991;84:1–6.

44. Xu WC, Yi YY, Qiu L, et al. Neuroprotective activity of tiagabine in a focal embolic model of cerebral ischemia. *Brain Res* 2000; 874:57–77.

TIAGABINE

CHEMISTRY, BIOTRANSFORMATION, AND PHARMACOKINETICS

KENNETH W. SOMMERVILLE
STEPHEN D. COLLINS

Tiagabine (Gabitril) is a nipecotic acid derivative developed specifically for the treatment of epilepsy. The synthesis and development of tiagabine were motivated by the therapeutic goal of preventing or reducing the uptake of γ-aminobutyric acid (GABA) by presynaptic neurons and glial cells.

GABA is extensively distributed in the mammalian brain, and as a major inhibitory transmitter it is thought to be an important part of most integrative central nervous system functions (1). Reduced GABAergic neurotransmission activity has been implicated in numerous neurologic disorders, including anxiety, pain, and epilepsy (2). The pharmacologic enhancement of GABAergic function is a possible therapeutic approach to alleviating these disorders. Enhancement of GABAergic function could conceivably be effected through direct receptor agonism, inhibition of the enzymatic breakdown of GABA, or action on GABA-coupled ion channels. However, inhibition of the uptake of synaptic GABA by neurons and glial cells offers the advantage of enhancing natural physiologic mechanisms (3).

Nipecotic acid and related cyclic amino acids exhibit anticonvulsant activity in mice, through inhibition of GABA uptake (4); however, the inability of these compounds to cross the blood–brain barrier renders them unsuitable for therapeutic use. Tiagabine, originally synthesized by scientists at Novo-Nordisk in Denmark, has a lipophilic anchor attached via an aliphatic chain to the amino acid nitrogen of nipecotic acid, and readily crosses the blood–brain barrier (5). Tiagabine has demonstrated clinical efficacy against a range of partial seizure types, both as adjunctive therapy (6) and as monotherapy (7–9).

CHEMISTRY

Tiagabine HCl (hereafter referred to as tiagabine) is a whitish, odorless, crystalline powder, with the chemical name (−) - (R)-1-[4,4-bis(3-methyl-2-thienyl)-3-butenyl]-3-nipecotic acid hydrochloride, and the empiric formula $C_{20}H_{25}NO_2S_2HCl$; its structure is shown in Figure 72.1. Tiagabine has a molecular weight of 412.0 and a melting point between 193°C and 195°C. Tiagabine is soluble in water to 3% and is insoluble in heptane. The negative log of dissociation constant (pKa) of the −COOH group is 3.3, and the pKa of the −NH₂ moiety is 9.4. Tiagabine has a partition coefficient of 39.3 in octanol and water at pH 7.4. The nipecotic acid moiety has an asymmetric carbon atom; the (R)-(−)-enantiomer is four times more potent than the (S)-(+)-enantiomer, and the name *tiagabine* refers to the (R)-(−)-enantiomer.

Tiagabine can be quantified in samples of human plasma through the use of a sensitive and precise high-performance liquid chromatography procedure developed at Abbott Laboratories in Illinois. The procedure involves separation on a C18 column using a mobile phase containing the ion-pairing reagent sodium octane sulfonate; the limit of detection is 2 ng/mL. Tiagabine is stable in plasma samples; no evidence of degradation is observed after 23 hours at room temperature or after 2 months at −20°C (10).

ABSORPTION

Tiagabine is rapidly absorbed, with the time to maximal plasma concentration (T_{max}) <2 hours in healthy volunteers

Kenneth W. Sommerville, MD: Medical Director, Neuroscience, Department of Marketed Products, Clinical Research, Abbott Laboratories, Abbott Park, Illinois

Stephen D. Collins, MD, PhD: Associate Medical Director, Department of Marketed Products, Abbott Laboratories, Abbott Park, Illinois

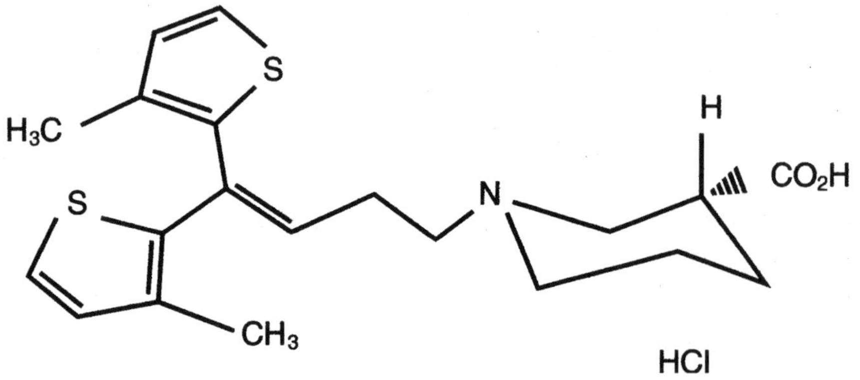

FIGURE 72.1. Chemical structure of tiagabine.

under fasting conditions. The elimination half-life ($t\frac{1}{2}$) ranges from 4 to 9 hours, regardless of dose. Absorption and elimination of tiagabine are linear processes across the therapeutic range of tiagabine doses, in both single-dose and steady-state studies (11).

Tiagabine absorption was examined after single doses (dose range, 2 to 24 mg) administered to 58 healthy male subjects (11) in three phase I studies. Tiagabine was rapidly absorbed across all doses; T_{max} occurred ≤1 hour after administration in most subjects. The maximum plasma concentration (C_{max}) was proportional to the dose; no evidence of nonlinearity was found throughout the dose ranges studied (study I, 2 to 24 mg; study II, 2 to 10 mg; study III, 6 or 12 mg). Both the dose-adjusted area under the plasma concentration–time curve (AUC_∞) and C_{max} were independent of the administered dose; the dose-adjusted AUC_∞ averaged 105 ng·hr/mL/mg, and the dose-adjusted C_{max} averaged 20.8 ng/mL/mg in study I. In most subjects, plasma concentration–time curves were biphasic and indicated possible enterohepatic recirculation. The recirculation created some uncertainty regarding the estimation of elimination $t\frac{1}{2}$; the harmonic mean $t\frac{1}{2}$ was 6.7 hours. The single-dose pharmacokinetic properties of tiagabine are summarized in Table 72.1.

Tiagabine pharmacokinetics at steady state also demonstrate dose-proportional behavior. In a study of healthy male subjects receiving once-daily doses of tiagabine (dose range, 2 to 10 mg/day) for 5 days, dose-adjusted C_{max} values (range, 16.0 to 26.5 ng/mL/mg) were generally independent of the dose administered (11). The dose-adjusted AUC also appeared to be independent of dose at day 1 and day 5, with accumulation ratios throughout the 5-day regimen clustered near 1.0. As in the single-dose study, tiagabine was rapidly absorbed: T_{max} was reached 0.5 to 1.5 hours after administration under fasting conditions. T_{max} values were independent of both the size of the dose and the number of doses administered (Table 72.2).

BIOAVAILABILITY

Tiagabine exhibits high bioavailability regardless of the formulation. The mean absolute bioavailability was 89.9±9.7% in a study comparing oral tablets and intravenous infusions in healthy subjects (12). The bioavailability of tiagabine administered as tablets, capsules, and oral solution is essentially identical (13).

TABLE 72.1. PHARMACOKINETICS OF TIAGABINE FOLLOWING A SINGLE DOSE

Dose (mg)	n	T_{max} (h)	C_{max} (ng/mL)	$T_{1/2}$ (h)[a]	AUC_∞ (ng · h/mL)
2	5	0.8 ± 0.5	43.4 ± 14.7	6.9	228 ± 71.4
8	5	1.0 ± 0.0	150 ± 26.2	5.4	727 ± 165
12	5	1.3 ± 1.0	241 ± 78.7	8.0	1450 ± 420
24	4	1.1 ± 0.8	552 ± 189	7.3	2190 ± 597

AUC_∞, C_{max}, and T_{max} are reported as mean ± standard deviation; $T_{1/2}$, half-life.
[a]Harmonic mean.
Adapted from Gustavson LE, Mengel HB. Pharmacokinetics of Tiagabine, a γ-aminobutyric acid-uptake inhibitor, in healthy subjects after single and multiple doses. *Epilepsia* 1995;36:605–611, with permission.

TABLE 72.2. SUMMARY OF TIAGABINE PHARMACOKINETICS IN THREE STUDIES OF HEALTHY VOLUNTEERS

Study	T_{max} (hr)	Dose-adjusted C_{max} (ng/mL/mg)	$T_{1/2}$ (hr)	Dose-adjusted AUC (ng · hr/mL/mg)
I				
Day 1	0.8–1.3	18.8–23.0	5.4–8.0	91.2–121
II				
Day 1	0.8–2.2	16.0–26.5	5.5–7.2	82.7–105
Day 5	0.8–1.5	16.2–21.5	4.5–8.1	92.3–135
III				
Day 1	1.2–1.5	15.5–20.1	5.5–8.5	75.7–107
Day 9	1.5–1.7	15.2–25.0	5.5–6.2	94.2–124
Day 14	1.0–1.5	18.8–21.8	4.6–5.0	92.3–117

AUC, area under the plasma concentration-time curve, a measure of drug exposure; C_{max}, maximum plasma concentration after a dose; T_{max}, time to maximum plasma concentration after a dose; $T_{1/2}$, half-life.

The intake of food concomitant with tiagabine administration appears to reduce the rate of tiagabine absorption, but not its extent. Whereas T_{max} is extended more than twofold and the peak plasma concentration is lower in the fed state than in the fasting state, the AUC_∞ is similar (14). Clinical efficacy trials of tiagabine were conducted using administration in the fed state, to reduce variations in plasma concentration levels and possibly to reduce the occurrence of intolerability from the higher C_{max} in the fasting state.

FORMULATIONS AND ROUTES OF ADMINISTRATION

Tiagabine is available as a film-sealed tablet in the United States in nondivisible strengths of 2, 4, 12, 16, and 20 mg (15). An extended-release formulation has been used in a pilot study of neuropathic pain in patients with diabetes (16). Other formulations, including intravenous and liquid formulations, have been explored but have not been studied clinically. Because tiagabine is water soluble, further development of these formulations should be possible.

DISTRIBUTION
Plasma Protein Binding

In vitro studies have shown that >95% of tiagabine in plasma is bound to protein, primarily to albumin and α_1-acid glycoprotein. In healthy volunteers, approximately 4% to 5% of tiagabine is unbound (17). Tiagabine is not displaced by phenytoin, carbamazepine, or phenobarbital, nor does it displace these drugs in plasma. Valproate reduces tiagabine binding by a small, but statistically significant, amount—from 96.3% to 94.8%; however, tiagabine has no effect on valproate binding. Salicylate and naproxen displace tiagabine, but the clinical implications of these changes are likely to be minimal. Tiagabine binding is not

affected by various other drugs that were studied *in vitro*, including propranolol, verapamil, chlorpromazine, amitriptyline, imipramine, warfarin, ibuprofen, digitoxin, furosemide, tolbutamide, and haloperidol (18).

Central Nervous System

Tiagabine crosses the blood–brain barrier and increases GABA levels in both the extracellular fluid of the brain and the cerebrospinal fluid. An analysis of extracellular GABA levels using microdialysis probes mounted on deeply implanted hippocampal electrodes (in a preoperative evaluation of patients with intractable seizures) showed an increase of approximately 50% in GABA level beginning 1 hour after administration of a tiagabine dose. The increase in GABA level was sustained for several hours, with no observed drug-related adverse events (19).

In a trial for treatment of refractory partial seizures, samples of cerebrospinal fluid were obtained from 10 patients at baseline and after 3 months of treatment with tiagabine or with placebo. The cerebrospinal fluid samples obtained after treatment demonstrated a significant increase in GABA levels, over both baseline levels and levels observed in patients who received placebo (20).

Transporters, Transplacental Passage, and Transmission in Breast Milk

The synaptic action of GABA is terminated by rapid uptake into the presynaptic terminals and adjacent glial cells. The uptake is mediated by the transporters GAT-1, GAT-2, GAT-3, and BGT-1 (21). *In vitro* testing showed tiagabine has the greatest affinity for GAT-1 and relatively low affinity for GAT-2, GAT-3, and BGT-1. GAT-1 is likely to be the transporter responsible for the anticonvulsant action of tiagabine.

No clinical data are available on the transplacental passage or excretion in breast milk. The high protein binding of tiagabine may predict limited crossing of the placenta or into breast milk.

METABOLISM AND ROUTES OF ELIMINATION

Tiagabine is rapidly absorbed and extensively metabolized after oral administration. No active metabolites of tiagabine have been identified. In healthy volunteers receiving 4 mg of ^{14}C-tiagabine, approximately 63% of the total radioactivity was excreted through the feces, and 25% was excreted in the urine. Only 2% of the initial 4-mg dose was excreted unchanged in the urine. Isomers of 5-oxo-tiagabine, the major metabolite, were identified in the urine; these are products of the thiophene ring oxidation pathway (22). The 5-oxo-tiagabine metabolite is inactive.

The metabolism of tiagabine appears to involve primarily the 3A subfamily of cytochrome P450 (CYP) enzymes. Incubation of ^{14}C-tiagabine with human hepatic microsomes and NADPH (the reduced form of nicotinamide-adenine dinucleotide phosphate) demonstrated formation of two 5-oxo-tiagabine isomers, as well as a significant correlation between the disappearance of ^{14}C-tiagabine and CYP3A-mediated activity. Metabolism of tiagabine is inhibited by CYP3A-selective inhibitors, and tiagabine was metabolized slowly by cDNA-expressed CYP3A4. Correlation and selective inhibition studies, along with studies of other cDNA-expressed CYP forms (including CYP2D6, 2E1, 1A2, 2C9, and 2A6), provided little evidence that other CYP isoforms play a significant role in the metabolism of tiagabine (23).

In contrast to several other antiepileptic drugs (AEDs), tiagabine does not appear to induce or inhibit hepatic microsomal enzymes. Analysis of the pharmacokinetics of antipyrine, an indirect measure of hepatic microsomal enzyme activity, revealed no significant differences in clearance or t½ when it was administered before and after 14 days of tiagabine administration (11).

PHARMACOKINETICS IN PATIENTS WITH EPILEPSY

As in healthy volunteers, the pharmacokinetic behavior of tiagabine in patients with epilepsy is linear across all doses. However, the pharmacokinetics of tiagabine in patients with epilepsy is significantly affected by the concomitant administration of enzyme-inducing AEDs (24). The clearance of tiagabine in patients treated with enzyme-inducing drugs is significantly higher than in those treated with tiagabine in combination with noninducing drugs, such as valproate (25,26). This finding suggests that noninduced patients may require a lower dose of tiagabine than induced

patients to produce the same serum concentration and therapeutic effect.

One study examined patients taking tiagabine (dose range, 24 to 80 mg daily) as an add-on to a stable regimen of one to three known enzyme-inducing AEDs. Tiagabine demonstrated linear pharmacokinetics across all dosages, with no significant differences in dose-adjusted C_{max}, trough concentration (C_{min}), and AUC values in induced patients. The harmonic mean t½ ranged from 3.8 to 4.9 hours, in contrast to a harmonic mean t½ of 7.1 hours in 30 historic control subjects not taking enzyme-inducing AEDs (Figure 72.2) (24).

In a population analysis involving 511 patients from clinical studies, age 11 to 77 years (mean age, 32.1±12.3 years), the pharmacokinetics of tiagabine as an add-on therapy was evaluated using a one-compartment model with first-order absorption and elimination (26). No differences were observed in tiagabine pharmacokinetics when patients were analyzed by sex, race or ethnicity, or other selected demographic variables (including age and smoking), and, as in earlier studies, the pharmacokinetics of tiagabine was linear. However, the central clearance value in patients receiving concomitant treatment with enzyme-inducing AEDs was 67% higher than that observed in patients taking only noninducing AEDs (21.4 versus 12.8 L/hr). The effect of enzyme-inducing AEDs on the central clearance value for tiagabine was not additive; the average values for patients receiving a single concomitant enzyme-inducing AED were similar to those for patients receiving multiple enzyme-inducing AEDs.

These findings have important clinical implications. To maintain consistent serum concentrations, tiagabine dosage should be adjusted when either adding or removing adjunctive enzyme-inducing AEDs.

PHARMACOKINETICS IN SPECIAL POPULATIONS

Children

Tiagabine pharmacokinetics in children are similar to those observed in adults. A study of a single tiagabine dose evaluated pharmacokinetics in 25 children (ages 3 to 10 years) who were undergoing epilepsy treatment with either enzyme-inducing or noninducing AEDs (27). The children were given tiagabine at a dose of 0.1 mg/kg. As in the adult population, tiagabine was cleared more quickly in the group of children taking concomitant enzyme-inducing AEDs than in the group taking valproate, a noninducing AED. The harmonic mean t½ in induced pediatric patients was 3.2 hours, consistent with findings in induced adults, whereas the harmonic mean t½ in noninduced children was 5.7 hours, also consistent with adult findings. The plasma concentration–time curves for induced and noninduced pediatric patients are shown in Figure 72.3.

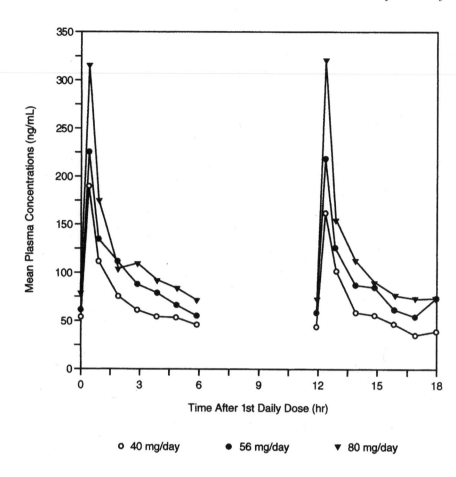

FIGURE 72.2. Mean tiagabine plasma concentrations after a morning dose (6 AM) and an evening dose (6 PM) of tiagabine in 23 patients taking concomitant enzyme-inducing AEDS. (From So EL, Wolff D, Graves NM, et al. Pharmacokinetics of tiagabine as add-on therapy in patients taking enzyme-inducing antiepilepsy drugs. *Epilepsy Res* 1998;22:221–226, with permission.)

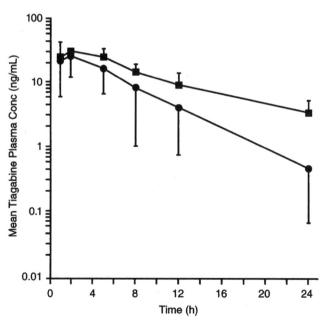

FIGURE 72.3. Plasma concentration-time profiles for tiagabine in pediatric epilepsy patients treated with other antiepileptic drugs (*circles,* induced; *squares,* valproate). (From Gustavson LE, Boellner SW, Granneman GR, et al. A single-dose study to define tiagabine pharmacokinetics in pediatric patients with complex partial seizures. *Neurology* 1997;48:1032–1037, with permission.)

An interesting finding that bears on dosage selection for children is that the pharmacokinetic parameters of volume of distribution over bioavailability (V_{area}/F) and clearance over bioavailability (CL/F) in pediatric patients were more strongly correlated with body surface area than with body weight. At least one study (28) has indicated that liver volume (presumably related to the rate of drug metabolism) correlates more strongly with body surface area than with weight: liver volume (measured by magnetic resonance imaging) normalized to weight decreases with increasing age, whereas liver volume normalized to body surface area remains constant with increasing age. This finding suggests that, at least for certain drugs, body surface area may be a more useful variable than body weight in calculating pediatric doses.

Elderly Patients

Elderly patients are a particularly important population in epilepsy therapy, because 25% of new epilepsy diagnoses are made in people >65 years old, primarily as the result of vascular insult. In addition, age-related changes in metabolism, renal and liver function, and body composition may play a role in the pharmacokinetics of specific drugs. However, tiagabine pharmacokinetics in elderly patients appears similar to that observed in younger adult populations.

In a comparison of healthy elderly volunteers (≥65 years; mean, 70.8; range, 65.9 to 75.7; n = 8), elderly patients with epilepsy who take enzyme-inducing AEDs (≥65 years; mean, 69.4; range, 66.3 to 72.5; n = 8), and healthy young volunteers (mean, 25.6; range, 20.2 to 31.0; n = 8), the pharmacokinetics of tiagabine after single- and multiple-dose administration was similar in healthy young and elderly volunteers (29). The exception was the AUC on the final day of the multiple-dose trial, which was significantly higher (103±29 ng·hr/mL/mg versus 72·20 ng·hr/mL/mg) in the elderly volunteers compared with the younger subjects.

As with other populations, C_{max}, AUC, and $t\frac{1}{2}$ were significantly lower in elderly patients being treated with enzyme-inducing AEDs compared with healthy elderly or young volunteers. The overall pharmacokinetic parameters, for both healthy elderly volunteers and elderly patients with epilepsy who were taking inducing AEDs, were quite similar to those observed in corresponding groups of younger patients. These findings suggest that tiagabine dosage may not need to be adjusted on the basis of age, but as with younger patients, the dosage should be increased in patients receiving inducing AEDs concurrent with tiagabine administration. This study, however, included relatively young elderly patients; very old patients may require dose adjustments if their hepatic function is reduced.

Patients with Hepatic Impairment

The alterations in tiagabine pharmacokinetics that result from the concomitant use of hepatic enzyme-inducing AEDs, in addition to the very small fraction of tiagabine eliminated as unchanged drug in urine, suggest that hepatic function is important in the elimination of tiagabine. This suggestion was confirmed in a pharmacokinetic study comparing healthy subjects and subjects with varying degrees of hepatic impairment.

Volunteers with mild or moderate liver function impairment (Child-Pugh classification) were compared with healthy volunteers in a multiple-dose study with regard to their ability to metabolize tiagabine (30). Four subjects had mild hepatic impairment, three had moderate hepatic impairment, and six were matched healthy subjects. Each study subject received twice-daily oral tiagabine for 5.5 days, and serial blood specimens were obtained for 48 hours after the final dose. The mean AUC and C_{min} values were significantly greater in both hepatic impairment groups compared with values observed in the group of healthy volunteers. The mean C_{max} value was significantly higher in the mild impairment group, and it was higher (but did not reach statistical significance, probably because of the small group size) in the moderate impairment group than in the healthy group. Plasma concentration–time curves for patients with mild and moderate hepatic impairment are compared with the curve from healthy subjects in Figure 72.4.

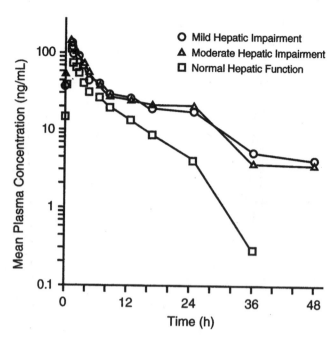

FIGURE 72.4. Mean tiagabine plasma concentrations after a final dose in patients with normal hepatic function, mild hepatic impairment, and moderate hepatic impairment. (From Lau AH, Gustavson LE, Sperelakis R, et al. Pharmacokinetics and safety of tiagabine in subjects with various degrees of hepatic function. *Epilepsia* 1997;38:445–451, with permission.)

The mildly and moderately impaired hepatic function groups exhibited higher plasma tiagabine C_{min} than the normal group, a finding indicating that elimination of tiagabine is slowed in patients with liver function impairment. There were also more adverse events reported by the impaired hepatic function groups. As is generally seen with tiagabine, many of these events involved the central nervous system. The plasma levels of unbound tiagabine were higher in the groups with impaired hepatic function, a finding consistent with the reduced levels of serum albumin and α_1-acid glycoprotein that are typical of liver disease.

These findings strongly suggest that tiagabine should be used with caution in patients with epilepsy and impaired hepatic function, and tiagabine dosage should be reduced or intervals between doses should be increased to maintain safe and effective plasma concentrations. Such patients should be monitored closely for signs of neurologic side effects, and the dosing regimen should be adjusted appropriately.

Patients with Renal Impairment

In contrast to the situation with hepatic function impairment, renal impairment does not appear to alter tiagabine pharmacokinetics. Although drugs such as gabapentin and topiramate are excreted unchanged primarily in the urine, tiagabine is extensively metabolized and removed mostly through fecal elimination. The fraction excreted by the kidneys (~25%) is composed almost completely of inactive metabolites of tiagabine.

A single- and multiple-dose study of tiagabine pharmacokinetics was conducted in 25 nonepileptic adult volunteers stratified according to degree of renal impairment (17). Group I (n = 5) had normal renal function, group II (n = 5) had mild renal impairment (creatinine clearance, 40 to 80 mL/min/1.73 m^2), group III (n = 6) had moderate renal impairment (creatinine clearance, 20 to 39 mL/min/1.73 m^2), group IV had severe renal impairment (creatinine clearance, 5 to 19 mL/min/1.73 m^2), and group V (n = 5) was receiving hemodialysis. For groups I to IV, the study was a 7-day, single- and multiple-dose, one-period, open-label study. These groups received a single 4-mg dose of tiagabine on day 1, 4 mg every 12 hours on days 2 to 4, and a single 4-mg dose on day 5. For group V, the study was a single-dose, two-period, open-label study. In period I, a single 4-mg dose of tiagabine was administered approximately 2 hours before dialysis. In period II, a single 4-mg dose was administered before a dialysis-free period.

Although small differences were observed among the groups, no correlation existed between the degree of renal impairment and the pharmacokinetic parameters. The accumulation ratios were nearly identical (~1.5) in all groups receiving multiple doses, and there was no correlation between the incidence of adverse events and the degree of renal impairment. It can be concluded that renal impairment does not substantially alter the pharmacokinetics of tiagabine; therefore, special dosage adjustment is not necessary for patients with renal impairment.

RELATIONSHIP BETWEEN PLASMA CONCENTRATION AND DOSE

Tiagabine exhibits linear pharmacokinetics for single and multiple doses in both healthy volunteers (11) and enzyme-induced patients with epilepsy (24). The dose-adjusted C_{max} in healthy volunteers is in the range of 15 to 26 ng/mL/mg (11). Persons taking a single 2-mg dose have average C_{max} values of 38 ng/mL, whereas a single 10-mg dose averages 265 ng/mL (Figure 72.5).

As expected, plasma concentrations with concomitant hepatic enzyme-inducing AEDs are lower than in healthy volunteers, but they exhibit linear pharmacokinetics (24). The dose-adjusted C_{max} among 21 patients with epilepsy who were taking enzyme-inducing AEDs in total daily doses of 40, 56, or 80 mg ranged from 15.3 to 18.6 mg/mL/mg in the morning to 15.8 to 15.9 ng/mL/mg in the evening. Dose-adjusted C_{min} values averaged 2.9 to 4.2 ng/mL/mg in the morning and 3.0 ng/mL/mg in the evening. Data from other sources reported with this study indicated the dose-adjusted C_{max} to be 8 to 12 ng/mL/mg and the dose-adjusted C_{min} to be 2 to 4 ng/mL/mg. These data may not reflect the concentrations at the true T_{max}, which is often <1 hour. The diurnal variations are small and are unlikely to have clinical importance.

Extrapolating these data to the clinical setting, a single 8-mg dose should produce a C_{min} concentration of approximately 16 to 32 ng/mL in an enzyme-induced patient. This relationship holds throughout the commonly prescribed dose range for tiagabine, as suggested in a clinical dose-response trial. The concentrations across increasing doses show linear increases at trough and at 1 and 2 hours after administration (Figure 72.6). The dose-adjusted values

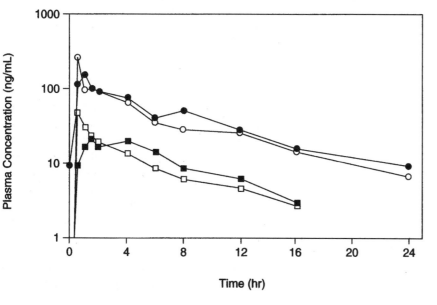

FIGURE 72.5. Tiagabine plasma concentration-time profiles for a subject who received 2 mg tiagabine once daily for 5 days (day 1, *open squares;* day 5, *solid squares*) and for a subject who received 10 mg tiagabine once daily for 5 days (day 1, *open circles;* day 5, *solid circles*). (From Gustavson LE, Mengel HB. Pharmacokinetics of tiagabine, a γ-aminobutyric acid-uptake inhibitor, in healthy subjects after single and multiple doses. *Epilepsia* 1995; 36:605–611, with permission.)

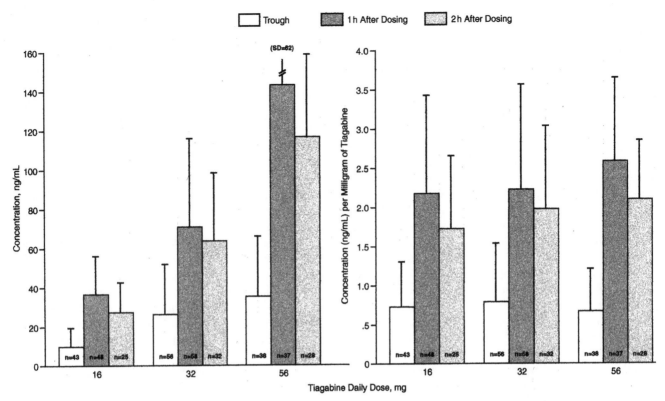

FIGURE 72.6. Mean (±SD) plasma concentrations of tiagabine in patients with complex partial seizures treated with three dose levels of tiagabine, as evaluated after 4 weeks of fixed-dose treatment. **Left,** concentrations by absolute values; **right,** concentration by milligrams of tiagabine administered. (From Uthman BM, Rowan AJ, Ahmann PA, et al. Tiagabine for complex partial seizures: a randomized, add-on, dose-response trial. *Arch Neurol* 1998;55:56–62, with permission.)

from the same dose-response trial were similar for each dosage group (31).

RELATIONSHIP BETWEEN SERUM CONCENTRATION AND EFFECT

Tiagabine has been shown to raise GABA levels in the nervous system, but the increase is transient (19). Serum concentrations of tiagabine may therefore correlate with clinical effects.

The relationship of serum concentrations with adverse events was described in pharmacokinetic studies of healthy volunteers (11). All six subjects given once-daily 6-mg doses of tiagabine for 14 days completed the study, whereas one of three randomly assigned subjects receiving once-daily 12-mg doses discontinued the study because of dizziness, difficulty in concentrating, incoordination, and somnolence. All six subjects receiving once-daily 10-mg doses for 5 days completed the study.

Among healthy subjects receiving single doses of 2, 8, 12, or 24 mg, there were no adverse events with C_{max} concentrations <180 ng/mL (12). Persons with C_{max} values in

the range of 200 to 400 ng/mL had the same incidence of adverse events as those with C_{max} values >400 ng/mL. The adverse events found with concentrations >400 ng/mL were, however, more severe. The adverse events tended to occur at the time of the predicted C_{max} (1 to 2 hours) and generally resolved by 4 to 6 hours after administration.

The relation of serum concentration to efficacy was explored in a United States multicenter, placebo-controlled, add-on trial of 16, 32, and 56 mg/day versus placebo in enzyme-induced patients with partial seizures (31). Serum concentrations in groups with C_{min} values of ≤20 ng/mL, 21 to 40 ng/mL, and >40 ng/mL were compared with placebo, as well as by median reduction and those with ≥50% reduction in 4-week rates of complex partial seizures. Both median reduction and the proportion of those with ≥50% reduction in seizure frequency increased with increasing concentrations of tiagabine. Of the group with the highest concentrations, 45% had a ≥50% reduction in complex partial seizures. This is a better result than the 29% with ≥50% seizure reduction in the group receiving doses of 56 mg/day (Table 72.3). These comparisons are limited, because the timing of C_{min} in multicenter trials is estimated, and the three concentration groups were designated in a *post hoc* analysis. Nevertheless, a

TABLE 72.3. CHANGE IN FREQUENCY OF COMPLEX PARTIAL SEIZURES FROM BASELINE TO TREATMENT PHASE IN PLACEBO- AND TIAGABINE-TREATED PATIENTS BY TROUGH PLASMA CONCENTRATIONS OF TIAGABINE

	Baseline 4-wk Seizure Frequency		Treatment Phase: Change in Seizure Frequency			≥50% Seizure Reduction	
Trough Level, ng/mL	No.	Median (Range)	Median Change	P vs Placebo	Median % Change	No. (%)	P vs Placebo
0 (Placebo)	91	7.4 (2.8–109)	−0.6	...	−9	4 (4)	...
≤20	82	8.6 (2.6–209)	−1.7	.01	−24	11 (13)	.07
21–40	35	10.2 (3.1–136)	−2.0	.36	−17	7 (20)	.02
>40	20	7.5 (2.6–77)	−4.9	<.001	−46	9 (45)	<.001

From Uthman BM, Rowan AJ, Ahmann PA, et al. Tiagabine for complex partial seizures: a randomized, add-on, dose-response trial. *Archives Neurol* 1998;55:56–62, with permission.

significant correlation was found between efficacy in reducing complex partial seizures and increasing C_{min} values.

These data do not provide a definitive therapeutic range of serum C_{min} values. It is not clear whether the pharmacodynamic effects of tiagabine are longer lasting than the pharmacokinetic effects. Another placebo-controlled, multicenter trial in the United States compared tiagabine at daily doses of 32 mg, given either twice or four times daily, with placebo (32). As expected, the average C_{min} values in the twice-daily group were in the range of 14 to 16 ng/mL, whereas values for the group receiving four daily doses were in the range of 29 to 30 ng/mL. There were large standard deviations for both groups, a finding reflecting the nature of these data in multicenter trials. The efficacy of the drug for these two groups was similar; the proportion attaining ≥50% reduction in seizures was 31% in the twice-daily group and 27% in the group receiving four daily doses. The serum concentrations in this study did not correlate as well with efficacy as in the dose-response study. Based on these results, a longer pharmacodynamic than pharmacokinetic effect is possible with tiagabine.

CONCLUSION

The pharmacokinetics of tiagabine are summarized in Table 72.4. Tiagabine is rapidly absorbed. The presence of food slows absorption about twofold; however, administration to fed patients does not alter bioavailability, because the overall AUC is similar to that of the fasting state. Tiagabine penetrates the blood–brain barrier and increases extracellular GABA levels in the central nervous system. Once absorbed, tiagabine is highly protein bound (>95%) and is rapidly and extensively metabolized, primarily through the action of the 3A subfamily of hepatic CYP enzymes; no pharmacologically active metabolites have been identified. Tiagabine and its metabolites are excreted mainly through the feces. About 25% of the total ingested dose is eliminated as metabolites in the urine. Less than 2% of the total administered dose is excreted unchanged. Tiagabine has a relatively short $t\frac{1}{2}$ of 5 to 9 hours, which is reduced to 3 to 5 hours when the drug is given with enzyme-inducing AEDs.

Tiagabine demonstrates linear (non–dose-dependent) pharmacokinetics across the therapeutic dose range ≤80 mg/day. The therapeutic effect does correlate to some extent with plasma C_{min} values, but this relationship is limited by the short $t\frac{1}{2}$. Despite the short $t\frac{1}{2}$, a therapeutic effect has been shown with twice-daily administration. Tiagabine does not induce hepatic enzymes, but its clearance is greater in the presence of enzyme-inducing AEDs. This is the only clinically important drug interaction demonstrated so far. Doses of tiagabine may need to be higher to maintain required concentrations when the agent is given with enzyme-inducing AEDs (e.g., phenytoin, carbamazepine, primidone, and phenobarbital). The pharmacokinetics of tiagabine in elderly patients are similar to that observed in younger adults, although clearance is somewhat lower.

TABLE 72.4. SUMMARY OF KNOWN PHARMACOKINETIC PARAMETERS OF TIAGABINE

Bioavailability	>90%
Tmax (fasting)	0.5–2 hr
Plasma protein binding	>95%
% metabolized	>98% (<2% excreted unchanged in urine)
Metabolic pathway	Primarily via CYP3A subfamily
Liver enzyme induction	None
Liver enzyme inhibition	None
$t\frac{1}{2}$ (enzyme-induced patients)	3–5 hr
$t\frac{1}{2}$ (non-induced patients)	5–9 hr
Effect of renal-function impairment	None
Effect of hepatic-function impairment	Increase in AUC$_{0-12h}$, C_{min}, C_{max}

AUC_{0-12h}, area under the plasma concentration-time curve, a measure of drug exposure; C_{max}, maximum plasma concentration after a dose; C_{min}, minimum plasma concentration after a dose; CYP3A, a subfamily of hepatic enzymes commonly involved in drug metabolism; Tmax(fasting), time to maximum plasma concentration after a dose.

Pediatric pharmacokinetics also appears to be similar to that in adults, although more closely correlated with body surface area than with body weight. Renal impairment does not alter the pharmacokinetics of tiagabine. However, tiagabine should be used with caution, possibly with lower doses or longer dosing intervals in patients, with hepatic impairment, which substantially decreases the rate of metabolism and clearance.

ACKNOWLEDGMENT

We gratefully acknowledge the review of this manuscript by Linda Gustavson, PhD.

REFERENCES

1. Meldrum B. Pharmacology of GABA. *Clin Neuropharmacol* 1982;5:293–316.
2. Krogsgaard-Larsen P, Scheel-Krüger J, Kofoed H. *GABA-neurotransmitters: pharmacochemical, biochemical and pharmacological aspects.* Copenhagen: Munksgaard, 1979.
3. Nielsen EB, Suzdak PD, Andersen KE, et al. Characterization of tiagabine (NO-328), a new potent and selective GABA uptake inhibitor. *Eur J Pharmacol* 1991;196:257–266.
4. Croucher MJ, Meldrum BS, Krogsgaard-Larsen P. Anticonvulsant activity of GABA uptake inhibitors and their prodrugs following central or systemic administration. *Eur J Pharmacol* 1983; 89:217–228.
5. Yunger LM, Fowler PJ, Zarevics P, et al. Novel inhibitors of GABA uptake: anticonvulsant actions in rats and mice. *J Pharmacol Exp Ther* 1984;228:109.
6. Ben-Menachem E. International experience with tiagabine add-on therapy. *Epilepsia* 1995; 36[Suppl 6]:S14–S21.
7. Alarcon G, Binnie CD, Elwes RDC, et al. Monotherapy antiepileptic drug trials in patients undergoing presurgical assessment: methodological problems and possibilities. *Seizure* 1995; 4:293–301.
8. Schachter SC. Tiagabine monotherapy in the treatment of partial epilepsy. *Epilepsia* 1995;32[Suppl 6]:S2–S6.
9. Brodie MJ, Bomhof MAM, Kalviainen R, et al. Double-blind comparison of tiagabine and carbamazepine monotherapy in newly diagnosed epilepsy: preliminary results. Paper presented at the 22nd International Epilepsy Congress, Dublin,1997.
10. Gustavson LE, Chu SY. A high performance liquid chromatographic procedure for the determination of tiagabine concentrations in human plasma using electrochemical detection. *J Chromatogr* 1992;574:313–318.
11. Gustavson LE, Mengel HB. Pharmacokinetics of Tiagabine, a γ-aminobutyric acid-uptake inhibitor, in healthy subjects after single and multiple doses. *Epilepsia* 1995;36:605–611.
12. Jansen JA, Oliver S, Dirach J, et al. Absolute bioavailability of tiagabine. *Epilepsia* 1995;36[Suppl 3]:S159.
13. Mengel HB, Gustavson LE, Soerensen HJ, et al. Bioavailability of tolerability of a tiagabine HCl tablet formulation versus capsules and oral solution in normal subjects. *Epilepsia* 1991;32 [Suppl 3]:S6.
14. Mengel HB, Gustavson LE, Soerensen HJ, et al. Effect of food on the bioavailability of tiagabine HCl. *Epilepsia* 1991;32[Suppl 3]:S6.
15. Gabitril (tiagabine hydrochloride). Package insert. Cephalon, Inc., Westchester, Pennsylvania, 2000.
16. Kirby LC, Collins SD, Deaton RL, et al. Tiagabine (Gabitril) in the management of painful diabetic neuropathy. Poster presented at American Pain Society Meeting, Fort Lauderdale, Florida, 1999.
17. Cato A, Gustavson LE, Qian J, et al. Effect of renal impairment on the pharmacokinetics and tolerability of tiagabine. *Epilepsia* 1998;39:43–47.
18. Bopp BA. *Effect of selected other drugs on the* in vitro protein binding of ^{14}C-tiagabine in human plasma: protocol V93-007. Abbott-70569 drug metabolism report no. 35. Abbott Laboratories Division 46 report no. R&D/94/002. Abbott Park, Illinois: Abbott Laboratories, 1994.
19. During M, Mattson R, Scheyer R, et al. The effect of Tiagabine HCl on extracellular GABA levels in the human hippocampus. *Epilepsia* 1992;33[Suppl 3]:S83.
20. Ben-Menachem E, Hedner T, Hamberger A. Cerebrospinal fluid concentrations of tiagabine and 22 amino acids in patients with refractory partial seizures treated for 3 months with tiagabine. *Epilepsia* 1996;37[Suppl 4]:S59.
21. Borden LA, Miurali Dhar TG, Smith KE, et al. Tiagabine, SK and F 89976-A, Cl-966, and NNC-711 are selective for the cloned GABA transporter GAT-1. *Eur J Pharmacol* 1994;269: 219–224.
22. Bopp BA, Gustavson LE, Johnson M, et al. Pharmacokinetics and metabolism of [^{14}C]tiagabine HCl after oral administration to human subjects. *Epilepsia* 1995;36[Suppl 3]:S158.
23. Bopp BA, Nequist GE, Rodrigues AD. Role of the cytochrome P450 3A subfamily in the metabolism of [^{14}C]tiagabine by human hepatic microsomes. *Epilepsia* 1995;36[Suppl 3]:S159.
24. So EL, Wolff D, Graves NM, et al. Pharmacokinetics of tiagabine as add-on therapy in patients taking enzyme-inducing antiepilepsy drugs. *Epilepsy Res* 1998;22:221–226.
25. Richens A, Gustavson LE, McKelvy JF, et al. Pharmacokinetics and safety of single-dose tiagabine HCl in epileptic patients chronically treated with four other antiepileptic drug regimens. *Epilepsia* 1991;32[Suppl 3]:S12(abst).
26. Samara EE, Gustavson LE, El-Shourbagy T, et al. Population analysis of the pharmacokinetics of tiagabine in patients with epilepsy. *Epilepsia* 1998;39:868–873.
27. Gustavson LE, Boellner SW, Granneman GR, et al. A single-dose study to define tiagabine pharmacokinetics in pediatric patients with complex partial seizures. *Neurology* 1997;48:1032–1037.
28. Murry DJ, Crom WR, Reddick WE, et al. Liver volume as a determinant of drug clearance in children and adolescents. *Drug Metab Dispos* 1995;23:1110–1116.
29. Snel S, Jansen JA, Mengel HB, et al. The pharmacokinetics of tiagabine in healthy elderly volunteers and elderly patients with epilepsy. *J Clin Pharmacol* 1997;37:1015–1020.
30. Lau AH, Gustavson LE, Sperelakis R, et al. Pharmacokinetics and safety of tiagabine in subjects with various degrees of hepatic function. *Epilepsia* 1997;38:445–451.
31. Uthman BM, Rowan AJ, Ahmann PA, et al. Tiagabine for complex partial seizures: a randomized, add-on, dose-response trial. *Arch Neurol* 1998;55:56–62.
32. Sachdeo RC, Leroy RF, Krauss GL, et al. Tiagabine therapy for complex partial seizures: a dose-frequency study. *Arch Neurol* 1997;54:595–601.

TIAGABINE

DRUG INTERACTIONS

KENNETH W. SOMMERVILLE

Tiagabine (Gabitril) is a nipecotic acid derivative that appears to suppress seizures by inhibiting the uptake of γ-aminobutyric acid (GABA) by presynaptic neurons and glial cells. Nipecotic acid, which is unable to cross the blood–brain barrier, was identified as a GABA uptake inhibitor *in vitro;* subsequently, tiagabine was synthesized by adding a lipophilic anchor to the amino acid nitrogen of nipecotic acid. Tiagabine readily crosses the blood–brain barrier, and it demonstrates inhibition of GABA uptake by neurons and glial cells similar to nipecotic acid *in vitro* (1). Tiagabine produces a significant increase in extracellular GABA levels in rat brains at doses that inhibit pentylenetetrazol-induced tonic seizures (2).

In comparison with other antiepileptic drugs (AEDs), tiagabine is well tolerated over a wide range of doses. It appears to have minimal or no effect on the pharmacokinetics of other drugs, in part because it is used therapeutically at low concentrations. The pharmacokinetics of tiagabine are, however, affected by other AEDs. The interactions of tiagabine are limited and predictable, possibly because the drug is active at low concentrations and has a well-defined mechanism of action. In this chapter, studies regarding the effects of other drugs on tiagabine and the effects of tiagabine on other drugs are reviewed.

PHARMACOKINETICS

To understand the interactions between tiagabine and other drugs, it is helpful to review the basics of tiagabine pharmacokinetics. Tiagabine is a drug of high potency and relatively low toxicity: *in vitro* studies have shown it to be the most potent inhibitor of GABA uptake yet identified (1), and therapeutic benefits are observed in the dose range of 24 to 80 mg/day when the agent is coadministered with enzyme-inducing AEDs (3). The median lethal dosage (ED_{50}) of tiagabine in rats and mice is at least 50-fold

Kenneth W. Sommerville, MD: *Medical Director, Neuroscience, Department of Marketed Products, Clinical Research, Abbott Laboratories, Abbott Park, Illinois*

higher than the anticonvulsant ED_{50} (4). In humans, the concentrations of tiagabine associated with clinical use are in the range of nanograms per milliliter. These low concentrations may be a principal reason that the agent has little or no effect on other drugs.

The bioavailability of tiagabine is >90% whether it is administered as tablets, capsules, or oral solution (5). Tiagabine is rapidly absorbed over its complete therapeutic dose range, with the maximum concentration (C_{max}) typically occurring from 0.5 to 1.5 hours of administration under fasting conditions. It also demonstrates linear pharmacokinetics over the dose range of clinical use; both the dose-adjusted C_{max} and the dose-adjusted area under the plasma concentration–time curve (AUC) are independent of dose. The plasma concentration–time curve of tiagabine typically includes secondary peaks, a finding indicating the possibility of enterohepatic recycling; and the harmonic mean half-life is roughly 7 hours (6).

Tiagabine appears to be metabolized principally through the action of the 3A subfamily of cytochrome P450 (CYP) enzymes, a conclusion drawn from *in vitro* experiments involving incubation of tiagabine with hepatic microsomes and studies employing selective CYP3A inhibitors (7). In plasma, tiagabine is highly protein bound (>95%). Tiagabine does not induce hepatic enzymes, as suggested by its lack of effect on antipyrine metabolism (6). No active metabolites of tiagabine have been identified (7). Although food intake slows the rate of tiagabine absorption, it does not appear to affect the extent of absorption; the $AUC_{0-\infty}$ in the fed state is similar to that in the fasting state (5).

EFFECTS OF OTHER ANTIEPILEPTIC DRUGS ON TIAGABINE

By far the most important effect of other AEDs on tiagabine pharmacokinetics is the increased rate of tiagabine metabolism and clearance in the presence of drugs known to induce hepatic metabolism. Because tiagabine is often given in combination therapy or as an add-on to existing AED therapy, this effect is important for dosage recommendations.

The pharmacokinetics of tiagabine was evaluated in an early single-dose trial of safety and tolerability in the presence of other AEDs (8). In this study, a single 8-mg dose of tiagabine was administered to four groups of patients who had been receiving long-term treatment with valproate alone, carbamazepine and phenytoin, carbamazepine and primidone, or carbamazepine and vigabatrin. Previously evaluated normal volunteers, not taking any AEDs, served as historical controls. Carbamazepine, phenytoin, and primidone are known to induce hepatic enzymes, whereas valproate does not. As anticipated, when antipyrine was administered to evaluate enzyme induction, the groups taking known hepatic enzyme-inducing drugs demonstrated elevated antipyrine clearance and decreased half-life. After administration of tiagabine, the mean AUCs for the historical controls and for the valproate group were 754 and 908 ng·hr/mL, respectively. However, the mean AUCs for the other three (enzyme-induced) groups were significantly lower (260, 437, 239 ng·hr/mL, respectively; $p < .05$ for each group). This study suggested the possibility that, in the presence of enzyme-inducing AEDs, the dosage of tiagabine may need to be increased, to provide the same AUC and presumably the same therapeutic effect as when the drug is taken alone or with non–enzyme-inducing AEDs (8).

Another study evaluated the pharmacokinetics of tiagabine when used as add-on therapy in a stable regimen involving one to three enzyme-inducing AEDs, including carbamazepine, phenytoin, phenobarbital, and primidone (9). Patients in this study were enrolled in one of two long-term trials of tiagabine, as add-on therapy to other AEDs. This study confirmed the linear pharmacokinetics of tiagabine in the presence of other AEDs; when groups taking 40, 56, or 80 mg/day of tiagabine were compared, the dose-adjusted C_{max}, trough concentration (C_{min}), and $AUC_{0-6 hr}$ values were independent of dose. The harmonic mean half-life ranged from 3.8 to 4.9 hours in the three dosage groups (individual values ranged from 1.7 to 8.8 hours). When compared with the harmonic mean half-life of 7.1 hours in a group of historical control volunteers who were not taking enzyme-inducing AEDs, these results again demonstrated that tiagabine metabolism and clearance is increased in the presence of enzyme-inducing AEDs (9).

The increased clearance, lower AUC, and shorter half-life of tiagabine in the presence of enzyme-inducing AEDs was further substantiated by a population pharmacokinetic analysis across a large number of patients in two long-term clinical trials of epilepsy. One trial included only patients with partial seizures; the other included patients with any kind of epilepsy. Testing was conducted on a total of 2,147 plasma samples from 511 patients (age range, 11 to 77 years); tiagabine dosage ranged from 2 to 80 mg/day, and the sampling times relative to the previous dose of tiagabine were distributed across a wide range. This study included patients using tiagabine as add-on therapy to enzyme-inducing AEDs (carbamazepine, phenytoin, primidone, or barbiturates), tiagabine as add-on therapy to noninducing AEDs (valproate or clonazepam), and tiagabine monotherapy. The data were analyzed using the NONMEM program (10), which permits the analysis of limited data from large numbers of patients in clinical settings to yield an estimate for oral clearance value (CL/F; intravenous clearance over bioavailability), as well as other pharmacokinetic parameters. In this study, the central oral clearance value CL/*F* was 21.4 L/hr in enzyme-induced patients, compared with 12.8 L/hr in noninduced patients (Figure 73.1). The increased clearance value for tiagabine in enzyme-induced patients is consistent with other studies demonstrating accelerated clearance in such patients. The effect of more than one enzyme-inducing AED on tiagabine pharmacokinetics was not additive: clearance values in patients undergoing stable therapy with more than one inducing AED were similar to those in which tiagabine was used as add-on therapy to a single inducing AED. This study showed that the tiagabine dose should be adjusted (usually increased) when a new enzyme-inducing AED is added to an otherwise noninducing AED regimen that includes tiagabine. The dose of tiagabine should also be adjusted (usually reduced) when inducing AEDs are discontinued as concomitant therapy (11).

After administration, tiagabine in plasma is highly protein bound (>95%), primarily to albumin and α_1-acid glycoprotein. If its pharmacokinetic properties are determined in part by the nature and extent of this binding, they could potentially be affected by drugs that displace tiagabine or otherwise affect its binding. An extensive study of various AEDs and other drugs, however, showed that tiagabine is tightly bound, and little or no change occurs in tiagabine binding in the presence of other drugs. Tiagabine is not displaced by phenytoin, carbamazepine, or phenobarbital, nor is there clinically important displacement of these drugs in plasma. Tiagabine binding is also unaffected by various other drugs that were studied *in vitro,* including propranolol, verapamil, chlorpromazine, amitriptyline, imipramine, warfarin, ibuprofen, digitoxin, furosemide, tolbutamide, and haloperidol (12). Both salicylic acid and naproxen displace tiagabine from protein, but this effect is unlikely to be clinically relevant.

Valproate has been found to affect the binding of tiagabine to plasma proteins, by reducing the bound fraction by a small, but statistically significant, amount—from 96.3% to 94.8% (12). Tiagabine, however, has no effect on valproate binding. Moreover, clinical studies involving concomitant administration of tiagabine and valproate have demonstrated that the clearance values and AUC of tiagabine remain similar to those observed when tiagabine is administered alone (8,11). Therefore, the effect of the minimally reduced binding level with the addition of valproate is clinically unimportant.

The metabolism of tiagabine by the CYP3A family of cytochrome P450 enzymes raises the concern that its pharmacokinetics may be affected by known inhibitors of this

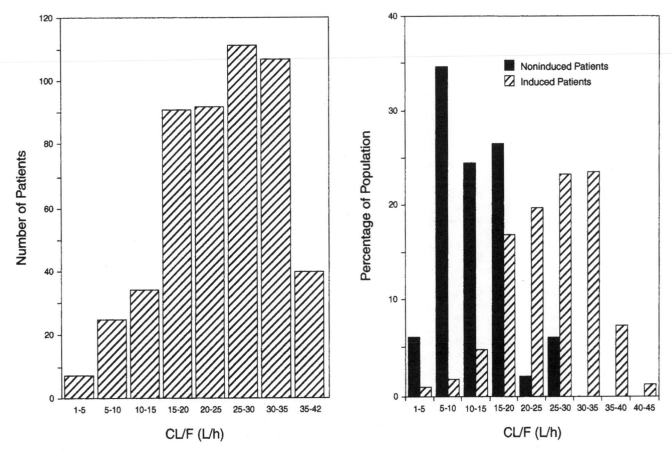

FIGURE 73.1. Distribution of *post hoc* clearance (*CL/F*) estimates in patients included in the NON-MEM analysis. (From Samara EE, Gustavson LE, El-Shourbagy T, et al. Population analysis of the pharmacokinetics of tiagabine in patients with epilepsy. *Epilepsia* 1998;39:868–873, with permission.)

enzyme family (13). Both cimetidine and erythromycin affect cytochrome P450 activity through interaction with its heme moiety; cimetidine itself forms a tight complex with the heme iron, whereas a metabolite of erythromycin is the heme-binding species. In a multiple-dose crossover study, the plasma C_{min} and AUC of tiagabine were slightly increased (~5%) when cimetidine was concurrently administered with tiagabine to healthy volunteers, but the changes were not judged to be clinically important (14).

In a two-period crossover study, erythromycin (500 mg twice daily) was administered to 13 healthy volunteers concurrently with tiagabine (4 mg twice daily) during one period, and placebo was given with tiagabine during the other period. Erythromycin treatment was initiated 12 hours before the initial tiagabine dose and was continued until 24 hours after the final tiagabine dose. The AUC, C_{max}, and half-life of tiagabine were identical in the presence and absence of erythromycin. The only change noted was a decrease in the time to reach maximum plasma level (T_{max}) of tiagabine in the presence of erythromycin (15). These studies indicate that the effects of drugs known to bind to cytochrome P450 on tiagabine metabolism are slight and are of little or no clinical importance.

EFFECT OF TIAGABINE ON OTHER DRUGS

Because tiagabine does not induce hepatic enzymes and is present in small quantities in serum at clinically relevant doses, its effect on pharmacokinetics of other AEDs administered concurrently is expected to be minimal. This has proved to be the case in pharmacokinetic studies. Two single-center open-label studies examined the potential effects of the addition of tiagabine on the pharmacokinetics and safety of carbamazepine or phenytoin at steady state. In adult patients with seizures controlled by a stable fixed dose of either phenytoin (n = 12) or carbamazepine (n = 12), tiagabine was administered in a starting dose of 8 mg/day for 3 days. The doses were then escalated at 3-day intervals to 16, 32, and 48 mg/day (final dose level). Serial blood samples were obtained on day 1 (before tiagabine initiation) and on day 18 (after the final tiagabine dose). Mean C_{max}, T_{max}, C_{min}, and $AUC_{0-\tau}$ values remained unchanged in the presence of tiagabine, both for patients receiving carbamazepine and for those receiving phenytoin (16). The mean plasma concentration–time profiles in the presence and absence of tiagabine are shown for carbamazepine (Figure 73.2A) and for phenytoin (Figure 73.2B).

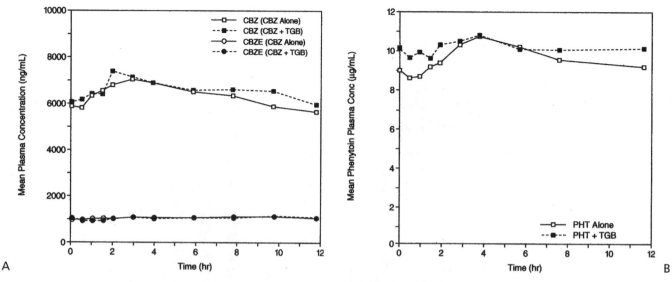

A   B

FIGURE 73.2. A: Mean carbamazepine (CBZ) and carbamazepine epoxide (CBZE) plasma concentrations after treatment with CBZ alone or in combination with tiagabine (TBG). **B:** Mean phenytoin (PHT) plasma concentration–time profiles after treatment with phenytoin alone or in combination with TGB. (A and B, from Gustavson LE, Cato A, Boellner SW, et al. Lack of pharmacokinetic drug interactions between tiagabine and carbamazepine or phenytoin. *Am J Ther* 1998;5:9–16, with permission.)

Another study, of similar design, evaluated the interaction between tiagabine and valproate in patients with seizures controlled by a fixed stable dose of valproate. In this study, the tiagabine dose was started at 8 mg/day, escalating at 3-day intervals to 24 mg/day. Blood samples were obtained on day 1 (before tiagabine initiation) and day 14 (after the final tiagabine dose). The serum concentrations of both valproate and tiagabine were determined; tiagabine pharmacokinetics, as expected, were similar in the presence of valproate (a noninducer) to those observed when tiagabine was administered alone. The mean C_{max} and $AUC_{0-\tau}$ values for valproate were approximately 10% to 12% lower when the drug was coadministered with tiagabine than when it was given alone (Figure 73.3). Much of this variability originated from two patients (out of 12 total) whose valproate values declined >30% during the tiagabine regimen. These patients had a history of missed tiagabine doses, and they may have also missed one or more valproate doses as well; when their values were omitted, the reduction in valproate values fell to ~6%. A possible alternative explanation for these patients' results involved the timing of valproate administration and the use of Depakote, an enteric-coated formulation of valproate. In any case, the small reduction in valproate concentrations was thought to be of limited clinical importance, because valproate has a broad dose range in epilepsy (17).

The effects of tiagabine on other (non-AED) drugs also appear to be minimal. In separate multiple-dose studies, each involving 10 to 23 healthy volunteers, tiagabine did not significantly alter the pharmacokinetics of several other drugs. Twelve healthy male volunteers received

open-label (12 mg/day) tiagabine, alone or with digoxin (0.5 mg/day on day 1, then 0.25 mg/day on days 2 to 9), in a two-period crossover design. Pharmacokinetic parameters measured on day 9 of each period showed no significant differences between the groups (18). Both *(R)*- and *(S)*-warfarin parameters were measured in a parallel-group, double-blind study in 25 healthy male subjects. After achieving a prothrombin time of 14 to 18 seconds for 7 days, tiagabine 12 mg/day or placebo was added for

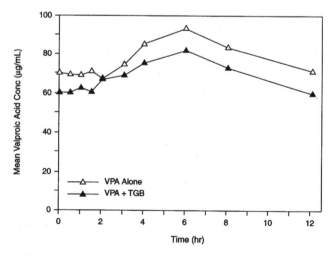

FIGURE 73.3. Mean valproate plasma concentration–time profiles after treatment with valproate (VPA) alone or in combination with tiagabine (TGB). (From Gustavson LE, Sommerville KW, Boellner SW, et al. Lack of a clinically significant pharmacokinetic drug interaction between tiagabine and valproate. *Am J Ther* 1998;5:73–79, with permission.)

5 days, and pharmacokinetic parameters were measured. There were no significant differences between the pharmacokinetics or pharmacodynamics of the *(R)*- and *(S)*-enantiomers with or without the addition of tiagabine. In another double-blind study, 14 healthy male subjects were given theophylline 200 mg every 6 hours for 5 days and a single dose of tiagabine 10 mg or placebo on day 5. Pharmacokinetic parameters of theophylline showed no significant differences with the addition of either tiagabine or placebo. Tiagabine also did not alter the sedative effect or cognitive impairment caused by triazolam or ethanol, although the duration of triazolam-induced effects was observed to be slightly prolonged (14).

The interaction of tiagabine with oral contraceptives was studied in 10 healthy female volunteers taking combination formulations (30 μg ethinyl estradiol with 150 μg of either levonorgestrel or desogestrel) at least 6 months before the study and over two complete pill-taking cycles (28 days) during the study. After a control period (cycle 1, days 1 to 23), 8 mg/day tiagabine was administered for 13 days (cycle 1, days 24 to 28 and cycle 2, days 1 to 7), followed by an evaluation period (cycle 2, days 8 to 28). Plasma hormonal levels were measured throughout both cycles, and bleeding patterns were recorded. The progesterone level on days 19 to 21 of each cycle was used as the indicator of nonovulation; all patients had levels that remained lower than the established threshold level of <13 nmol/L, signaling nonovulation. No induction of hepatic enzymes was observed, based on urinary levels of 6β-hydroxycortisol, an indicator for induction. Two patients experienced breakthrough bleeding, although both remained well below the accepted progesterone threshold for nonovulation. In general, tiagabine was well tolerated, and it demonstrated little or no interaction in combination with oral contraceptives (19).

PHARMACODYNAMIC INTERACTIONS

Because AEDs are usually administered over long periods (often lifelong), it is important to evaluate their interactions with other substances likely to be consumed. The potential interactions between tiagabine and ethanol were investigated using tests selected from the Cognitive Drug Research Computerized Cognitive Assessment System. The selected tests included immediate and delayed word recall and delayed word recognition, digit vigilance (speed and accuracy), choice reaction time, visual tracking, and body sway. Twenty healthy volunteers underwent a double-blind, placebo-controlled, two-period crossover study. The study involved an escalating dose of tiagabine or placebo over 9 days; on the final day, they consumed a standardized ethanol dose (0.7 g/kg for men, 0.6 g/kg for women). Serial cognitive tests were performed, and blood samples obtained, before and after ethanol administration. The

pharmacokinetics of tiagabine and ethanol was not significantly affected by concurrent administration of both. As expected, ethanol caused a significant impairment in performance on the most sensitive assay, the speed and accuracy of digit vigilance. However, concurrent administration of tiagabine did not significantly affect performance on this or any other test, a finding indicating that tiagabine does not potentiate the depressant and cognitive effects of ethanol (20).

The general neuropsychological effects of tiagabine were investigated in 162 adult patients with difficult-to-control seizures (at least six complex partial seizures during the 8 weeks before the initial screening visit). All patients were receiving a stable regimen including at least one enzyme-inducing AED. Patients either received placebo or were stabilized at one of three tiagabine dose levels (16, 32, or 56 mg/day) that were titrated from a starting dose of 8 mg/day. A battery of tests, measuring both abilities (including various cognitive skills) and adjustment (including mood, quality of life, and psychosocial variables), was conducted at baseline and after the stable dose period. The evaluations of abilities and adjustment showed no significant differences between placebo and tiagabine groups at the $p < .01$ level and four differences at the $p < .05$ level. The authors noted that six statistically significant ($p < .05$) differences would have been expected on the basis of chance alone. They concluded that no evidence of a clear drug effect exists; however, the data do not rule out possible small effects that are unlikely to be clinically important. A reduction in complex seizure frequency of >50% was observed in some (16 of 71) of the patients receiving either 32 or 56 mg/day of tiagabine, and this may have been expected to result in significant improvements in measures of adjustment. However, even among patients experiencing such marked improvement, the typical patient would still have had a seizure every 2 weeks on average. This pattern would not alter many of the life-changing attributes of poorly controlled epilepsy (e.g., the inability to drive or the ability to take on new psychosocial roles). Therefore, any improvement may not have been substantial enough to make an important difference in the quality of life (21).

The dose-related effects of tiagabine monotherapy on cognition and mood were studied in 123 adult patients with uncontrolled partial seizures. All patients were treated with only one marketed AED at the time of study entry. The study consisted of an 8-week baseline period, a 6-week withdrawal and titration period, and a 12-week fixed-dose period. At the end of baseline, patients were randomized to 6 mg/day tiagabine monotherapy (n = 66) or to 36 mg/day tiagabine monotherapy (n = 57) under double-blind conditions. Baseline AEDs were tapered beginning at day 15 and were discontinued entirely by 5 weeks after the first dose of the study drug. The 12-week fixed-dose period began after the 6-week withdrawal and titration period. Results showed that few changes in either cognition (abilities) or mood (adjustment) were noted when all patients were considered as a single group. However, analysis of both dose and attainment of tiagabine monotherapy showed that patients able to attain tiagabine monotherapy had improvements compared with the groups at the same dose that failed to achieve monotherapy. The group receiving 6 mg/day improved primarily in the areas of adjustment and mood, and the group receiving 36 mg/day improved in the area of abilities. Failure to attain tiagabine monotherapy was associated with worsening on tests of mood and adjustment in patients receiving 36 mg/day tiagabine. It was suggested that worsening of mood could have been avoided if a slower titration schedule had been used, because there was difficulty in tolerating the 36-mg dose. The investigators concluded that attainment of tiagabine monotherapy at high or low dose was associated with the improvement of varying degree on neuropsychological tests. The withdrawal of the baseline AED may have contributed to improvement in both dose groups (22).

SUMMARY

Tiagabine is an AED with few documented drug–drug interactions. The pharmacokinetic parameters of tiagabine include rapid absorption and virtually complete bioavailability, linear kinetics, and metabolism by the CYP3A family of cytochrome P450 enzymes. Tiagabine does not induce hepatic microsomal enzymes, although its clearance is increased by hepatic enzyme-inducing drugs.

Among other drugs that may be frequently combined with tiagabine, the most clinically important interaction is the increased clearance of tiagabine when it is administered concurrently with hepatic enzyme-inducing AEDs. Because of this interaction, the initial dosage of tiagabine should be considered carefully when it is added to an existing AED regimen. In addition, when tiagabine is part of a stable AED regimen, the dosage should be adjusted on the addition or removal of enzyme-inducing AEDs.

Tiagabine has not been found to have significant effects on the pharmacokinetics of other AEDs or other commonly used drugs, including oral contraceptives and drugs commonly used by elderly patients (digoxin, warfarin). Tiagabine does not potentiate the effects of ethanol. Tiagabine appears to have little or no effect on standardized measures of psychological abilities and adjustment when it is added to other AEDs in patients with refractory partial seizures. Improvement in neuropsychological testing has been noted when tiagabine monotherapy is attained after conversion from other AEDs.

ACKNOWLEDGMENT

I gratefully acknowledge the review of this manuscript by Linda Gustavson, PhD.

REFERENCES

1. Braestrup C, Nielsen EB, Sonnewald U, et al. (*R*)-*N*-[4,4-bis(3-methyl-2-thienyl)-3-buten1yl]nipecotic acid binds with high affinity to the brain γ-aminobutyric acid uptake carrier. *J Neurochem* 1990;54:639–647.
2. Fink-Jensen A, Suzdak PD, Swedberg MDB, et al. The γ-aminobutyric acid (GABA) uptake inhibitor, tiagabine, increases extracellular brain levels of GABA in awake rats. *Eur J Pharmacol* 1992;220:197–201.
3. Ben-Menachem E. International experience with tiagabine add-on therapy. *Epilepsia* 1995;36[Suppl 6]:S14–S21.
4. Østergaard LH, Gram L, Dam M. Tiagabine. In: Levy LH, Mattson RH, Meldrum BS, eds. *Antiepileptic drugs*, 4th ed. New York: Raven Press, 1995:1057–1061.
5. Mengel HB, Gustavson LE, Soerensen HJ, et al. Effect of food on the bioavailability of tolerability of a tiagabine HCl. *Epilepsia* 1991;32[Suppl 3]:S6.
6. Gustavson LE, Mengel HB. Pharmacokinetics of tiagabine, a γ-aminobutyric acid-uptake inhibitor, in healthy subjects after single and multiple doses. *Epilepsia* 1995;36:605–611.
7. Bopp BA, Nequist GE, Rodrigues AD. Role of the cytochrome P450 3A subfamily in the metabolism of [^{14}C]tiagabine by human hepatic microsomes. *Epilepsia* 1995;36[Suppl 3]:S159.
8. Richens A, Gustavson LE, McKelvy JF, et al. Pharmacokinetics and safety of single-dose tiagabine HCl in epileptic patients chronically treated with four other antiepileptic drug regimens. *Epilepsia* 1991;32[Suppl 3]:S12.
9. So EL, Wolff D, Graves NM, et al. Pharmacokinetics of tiagabine as add-on therapy in patients taking enzyme-inducing antiepilepsy drugs. *Epilepsy Res* 1995;22:221–226.
10. Beal SL, Sheiner LB. *NONMEM users' guide.* San Francisco: NONMEM Project Group, University of California, 1989.
11. Samara EE, Gustavson LE, El-Shourbagy T, et al. Population analysis of the pharmacokinetics of tiagabine in patients with epilepsy. *Epilepsia* 1998;39:868–873.
12. Gustavson LE. *Summary and overview of the human pharmacokinetics and bioavailability of tiagabine.* Abbott-70569 drug metabolism report no. 64. Report no. R&D/95/531. Abbott Park, IL: Abbott Laboratories, 1995.
13. Bopp BA, Nequist GE, Rodrigues D. Role of the cytochrome P450 3A subfamily in the metabolism of [^{14}C] tiagabine by human hepatic microsomes. *Epilepsia* 1995;36[Suppl 3] S159.
14. Mengel H, Jansen JA, Sommerville K, et al. Tiagabine: evaluation of the risk of interaction with theophylline, warfarin, digoxin, cimetidine, oral contraceptives, triazolam, or ethanol. *Epilepsia* 1995;36[Suppl 3]:S160.
15. Thompson MS, Groes L, Schwietert HR, et al. An open label sequence listed two period crossover pharmacokinetic trial evaluating the possible interaction between tiagabine and erythromycin during multiple administration to healthy volunteers. *Epilepsia* 1997;38[Suppl 3]:S64.
16. Gustavson LE, Cato A, Boellner SW, et al. Lack of pharmacokinetic drug interactions between tiagabine and carbamazepine or phenytoin. *Am J Ther* 1998;5:9–16.
17. Gustavson LE, Sommerville KW, Boellner SW, et al. Lack of a clinically significant pharmacokinetic drug interaction between tiagabine and valproate. *Am J Ther* 1998;5:73–79.

18. Snel S, Jansen JA, Pedersen PC, et al. Tiagabine, a novel antiepileptic agent: lack of pharmacokinetic interaction with digoxin. *Eur J Clin Pharmacol* 1998;54:355–357.

19. Mengel HB, Houston A, Back DJ. An evaluation of the interaction between tiagabine and oral contraceptives in female volunteers. *J Pharm Med* 1994;4:141–150.

20. Kastburg H, Jansen JA, Cole G, et al. Tiagabine: absence of kinetic or dynamic interactions with ethanol. *Drug Metabol Drug Interact* 1998;14:259–273.

21. Dodrill CB, Arnett JL, Sommerville KW, et al. Cognitive and quality of life effects of differing dosages of tiagabine in epilepsy. *Neurology* 1997;48:1025–1031.

22. Dodrill CB, Arnett JL, Shu V, et al. Effects of tigabine monotherapy on abilities, adjustment, and mood. *Epilepsia* 1998;39:33–42.

TIAGABINE

CLINICAL EFFICACY AND USE IN EPILEPSY

REETTA KÄLVIÄINEN

SPECTRUM OF EFFICACY

Evidence from Randomized Controlled Trials

Tiagabine has proven effective as add-on therapy in patients with refractory partial seizures with or without secondary generalization (Table 74.1). The primary clinical evidence of this efficacy is based on five controlled add-on trials in adults with epilepsy unsatisfactorily controlled with current antiepileptic drugs (AEDs).

The first phase II multicenter trials were two small, placebo-controlled, crossover studies. In an initial titration period lasting ≤8 weeks, patients started with a tiagabine dose of 8 mg/day, and the dose was titrated either to reduce seizures sufficiently or to produce unacceptable adverse events. Patients then entered a 4-week fixed-dose period on the dose attained in titration. The maximal dose allowed in the first study was 52 mg/day (1). Patients were eligible to enter the double-blind crossover phase if their seizure frequency had been reduced by ≥25% during the fixed-dose period. In this two-period crossover study, patients were randomized to placebo or tiagabine or to their previously determined dose of tiagabine or placebo, and they remained on each of these two regimens for 7 weeks. The 7-week treatment periods were separated by a 3-week washout period. The median daily dose of tiagabine in the double-blind phase was 32 mg/day. Of the total 42 patients who contributed data for both periods of the crossover phase, 26% of those with complex partial seizures and 63% with secondarily generalized tonic-clonic seizures (n = 27) experienced a reduction of ≥50% in seizure frequency during the tiagabine period compared with the placebo period. The median seizure rate during the tiagabine treatment period was significantly lower than during the placebo

treatment period for complex partial seizures (p = .05) and for secondarily generalized tonic-clonic seizures (p = .009).

The second phase II study used the same design but allowed a maximal dose of 64 mg/day (2). The intent-to-treat group comprised 36 patients who received a mean total daily dose of 46 mg in the tiagabine treatment periods. Tiagabine was significantly better than placebo in reducing all partial seizures (p = .002), complex partial seizures (p < .001), and partial seizures with secondary generalization (p = .030). A total of 46% of patients with complex partial seizures had a ≥50% reduction in weekly seizure rates.

Altogether, 769 patients took part in the three multicenter, parallel-group, double-blind add-on studies in which tiagabine was compared with placebo: the dose-response study, the dose-frequency study, and the thrice-a-day dosing study (3–5). The dose-ranging multicenter study in the United States had a fixed-dose, placebo-controlled parallel-group design (n = 297) (3). During a 4-week period, tiagabine-treated patients were given increasing doses until the dose level to which they had been randomized was reached (16, 32, or 56 mg/day divided in four equal doses). They then remained on a fixed dose for 12 weeks of double-blind treatment. Median decreases in 4-week complex partial seizure frequency for 32 mg (−2.2) and 56 mg (−2.8) tiagabine groups were significantly greater than for placebo (−0.7) group (p = .03 and p < .03, respectively); 20% and 29% of patients in the 32- and 56-mg groups had a ≥50% reduction in the frequency of complex partial seizures compared with 4% in the placebo group (p = .002 and p < .001, respectively).

The dose-frequency study was also a randomized, double-blind, placebo-controlled United States multicenter study with a parallel-group, add-on design (n = 318) (4). The study lasted for 24 weeks and consisted of an 8-week baseline, a 12-week double-blind treatment phase, and a 4-week termination period. During the first month of treatment, doses were increased weekly to 32 mg/day. The treatment groups were placebo, 16 mg tiagabine twice a day (b.i.d.), and 8 mg tiagabine four times a day (q.i.d.). The

Reetta Kälviäinen, MD, PhD: Head of the Outpatient Clinic, Leader of the Clinical Epilepsy Research Project, Department of Neurology, Kuopio University Hospital and University of Kuopio, Kuopio, Finland

TABLE 74.1. DATA FROM FIVE DOUBLE-BLIND PLACEBO-CONTROLLED TRIALS AND FROM AN INTEGRATED ANALYSIS OF THESE STUDIES SHOWING THE EFFICACY OF TIAGABINE AS ADD-ON THERAPY IN PARTIAL EPILEPSY

Reference	Number of Patients	Daily Dose (mgday)	Responder Rate (>50% Seizure Reduction) for All Partial Seizures	
			Tiagabine	Placebo
Richens et al., 1995	42	33	52%	24%[a]
Crawford et al., 1993	36	46	40%	14%[b]
Uthman et al., 1998	297	16	10%	4%
		32	20%	4%[a]
		56	31%	4%[a]
Sachdeo et al., 1997	318	32 (16 mg b.i.d.)	28%	8%[a]
		32 (8 mg q.i.d.)	23%	8%[a]
Kälviäinen et al., 1998	154	30	10%	5%
Ben-Menachem, 1995	951	16–56	23%	9%

b.i.d., twice daily; q.i.d., four times daily.
[a] $p < .01$.
[b] $p < .05$.

median changes in 4-week complex partial seizure rates were -1.6 ($p = .055$) for the 16 mg b.i.d. group and -1.2 ($p < .05$) for the 8 mg q.i.d. group versus -0.2 for placebo. Statistically significant differences between placebo and two tiagabine groups occurred in the proportion of patients experiencing a >50% rate reduction for complex partial, simple partial, and all partial seizure rates.

The thrice-a-day dosing study was a Northern-European multicenter parallel-group study that compared a dose of 30 mg/day tiagabine with placebo as add-on therapy (n = 154) (5). The study included 12-week baseline, an 18-week double-blind treatment phase, and a 4-week termination period. The median change from baseline in complex partial seizure rates was -1.3 for patients receiving tiagabine, whereas placebo-treated patients had a median increase of 0.1 in complex partial seizure rates ($p < .05$). Tiagabine was significantly more effective than placebo in patients with simple partial seizures with respect to the proportion of patients achieving a seizure reduction of $\geq 50\%$ (21% versus 6%; $p < .05$).

The meta-analysis across all these three trials for 50% responders showed an odds ratio of 3.03 (95% confidence interval [CI], 2.01 to 4.58) (6). The summary odds ratios for each dose indicate increasing efficacy with increasing doses, with no suggestion of a plateauing of effect at the doses examined in these studies. A 16-mg dose has a fairly small effect of 2.40 (95% CI, 0.65 to 8.87). There is a substantial increase with doses of 30 or 32 mg to an odds ratio of 3.17 (95% CI, 2.03 to 4.96) and a smaller additional gain for a dose level 56 mg, with an odds ratio of 7.95 (95% CI, 3.09 to 20.49).

A multicenter, open-label, randomized, parallel group study compared the efficacy, tolerability, and safety of thrice-a-day and twice-a-day administration dosing of tiagabine as adjunctive therapy for the treatment of refractory patients with partial seizures (7). A total of 347 patients were randomized and treated: 175 thrice daily (t.i.d.) and 172 b.i.d. Each group was administered the same daily dose of tiagabine incremented stepwise during a 12-week fixed-schedule titration period to a target 40 mg/day. The patients were followed for a further 12-week flexible continuation phase. A significantly greater number of patients in the thrice-a-day group completed the fixed schedule titration period (81.4% versus 73.1%; 95% CI, .331, .970; $p = .038$). The proportion of responders (patients showing a $\geq 50\%$ decrease in all-seizure frequency from baseline) was similar for both groups (44% for twice-daily and 48% for thrice-daily groups) during last 8 weeks of treatment, and seven (4%) patients in the twice-daily group were seizure free compared with 14 (8%) patients in the thrice-daily group.

A multicenter trial was also performed to determine whether the combination of AEDs with different mechanisms of action was be superior to the combination of AEDs with similar mechanism of action. In this study, patients taking carbamazepine or phenytoin monotherapy with inadequately controlled complex partial seizures were randomized to add-on tiagabine or phenytoin (if previously receiving carbamazepine) or add-on tiagabine or carbamazepine (if previously receiving phenytoin) and were titrated to an optimal dose in a double-blind trial (8). In this trial, tiagabine (n = 170) showed similar efficacy to traditional AED (carbamazepine or phenytoin) (n = 175) adjunctive therapy for complex partial seizures at low average doses of 24 to 28 mg/day. The study also suggested that tiagabine may be better tolerated when it is added to phenytoin or carbamazepine than when carbamazepine and phenytoin are added to each other.

Evidence from Other Studies

Data are available from six long-term open-label trials. More than half the 2,248 patients were treated with tiagabine for >1 year. For each type of partial seizure, 30% to 40% of the patients obtained considerable treatment effect, which was maintained after 12 months of treatment (9). Daily doses in the long-term studies were between 24 and 60 mg in most patients, and mean and median doses were 45 mg/day for most studies. However, ≤15% of patients received a dose of between 80 and 120 mg/day after their first year of treatment (10).

Pragmatic trials use larger patient numbers and a longer follow-up than the trials required for drug registration and more closely mimic routine clinical practice. Three such pragmatic studies—in Germany, Poland, and Spain—were conducted with add-on tiagabine in patients with refractory partial epilepsy (11–13). All had a longer follow-up than that of the pivotal studies, and together these studies included considerably more patients than the studies submitted in the registration dossier. These trials used the newly recommended titration schedule in a total of 1,151 patients, 3 to 93 years old, who were followed-up for ≤6 months. Tiagabine was given thrice daily, at an initial dose of 5 mg/day and following the new titration schedule, with increases of 5 mg/wk. The maintenance dose was titrated individually according to the labeling. The average dose was 30 mg (range, 5 to 90 mg) per day. Rates for 50% responders varied from 41% to 61%, and 8% to 22% of patients became seizure free.

MONOTHERAPY

The efficacy of tiagabine monotherapy in patients with chronic partial epilepsy not satisfactorily controlled by other drugs was studied. A dose-ranging double-blind parallel-group study in 198 patients with refractory epilepsy compared 6 mg/day tiagabine with 36 mg/day after gradual withdrawal of other AEDs over 29 weeks (14). Altogether, 33% of the patients receiving the lower dose completed the study compared with 47% taking the higher dose. For both dose groups, the median complex partial seizure rates decreased significantly during the study compared with baseline ($p < .05$). However, a higher proportion of patients in the 36 mg/day group experienced a reduction in complex partial seizures of ≥50% compared with the 6 mg/day group (31% versus 18%, $p < .05$). In addition to showing a dose-response relationship, this study suggested that even a dose of tiagabine as low as 6 mg/day may be effective when used as monotherapy or with noninducing AEDs.

The second study was a double-blind, randomized comparison of slow and fast switching to tiagabine monotherapy from another type of monotherapy, followed by an open-label evaluation of the safety and efficacy of tiagabine as monotherapy for chronic partial epilepsy (15). When a patient did not tolerate the double-blind titration scheme for tiagabine, even slower open uptitration of tiagabine was used. Thirty-four (85%) of the 40 patients were successfully switched to tiagabine monotherapy in either the double-blind or open-label drug switching scheme. According to this trial, it seems that the open-label uptitration with 5 mg/day, with weekly increments of 5 mg/day, should also be recommended in clinical practice. The retention rate in the study for 12 weeks of tiagabine monotherapy was 63% (25 of 40), and it was 48% for 48 weeks (19 of 40). The initial target dose of tiagabine monotherapy was 10 mg b.i.d., but in the open-label phase, tiagabine could be adjusted upward or downward in individual patients according to clinical adjustment of the investigator up to a maximum daily dose of 70 mg. The median dose was 20 mg/day, and the range was 7.5 to 42.5 mg/day during the first 48 weeks.

Monotherapy in newly diagnosed partial epilepsy was studied by comparing the efficacy and safety of tiagabine versus carbamazepine as monotherapy in a double-blind, randomized, parallel group trial (n = 290) (16). During the 6-week titration, patients were titrated from tiagabine 5 mg/day or carbamazepine 200 mg/day to tiagabine 10 or 15/mg/day or carbamazepine 400 or 600 mg/day in a stepwise fashion. During the 44-week assessment period, the dose could be adjusted within the ranges tiagabine 10 to 20 mg/day or carbamazepine 400 to 800 mg/day. All doses were administered twice daily. The study has so far been published only in abstract form showing a significant difference between the study groups with regard to the end point "time to meeting the exit criterion" ($p < .05$). An exit criterion was either status epilepticus or the occurrence of the second seizure at maximum tolerated or maximum allowed dose level. In the tiagabine-treated group, 41% (77 of 144), and in the carbamazepine-treated group, 53% (77 of 144) completed the assessment period either seizure free or with a single seizure ($p < .05$). Failure of tiagabine monotherapy to show efficacy in this trial may relate to the relatively low maximum dose of tiagabine that was allowed to be used.

PEDIATRIC USE

Use of tiagabine in children was studied as adjunctive therapy in >200 pediatric patients. A European study were carried out at two centers in Denmark and at one center in France (17). This 4-month, single-blind study evaluated the tolerability, safety, and preliminary efficacy of ascending doses (0.25 to 1.5 mg/kg/day) of tiagabine add-on therapy in 52 children over 2 years with different syndromes of refractory epilepsy. Tiagabine appeared to reduce seizures more in localization-related epilepsy syndromes than generalized epilepsy syndromes. Seventeen of the 23 patients with localization-related epilepsy syndromes entered the fourth dosing period. The 17 patients had a median reduction of seizure rate in the fourth month of treatment of 33% compared with baseline. In comparison, 13 of 22 children with seven different generalized epilepsy syndromes entered the fourth dosing period with a median change of seizure rate of 0%. Among generalized seizures, tonic seizures and atypical absences responded best, with median percentage reductions in the weekly seizure rate of 77% and 63%. The overall maximum daily tiagabine dose level received and tolerated (mean ± standard deviation) was 0.65±0.37 mg/kg.

In the United States, the long-term use of tiagabine was also studied in an open-label extension study in 152 children 2 to 11 years old from antecedent double-blind studies (18). Of the 140 evaluable patients, 10 patients were seizure free with tiagabine add-on therapy and 13 patients achieved freedom from seizures with tiagabine monotherapy for periods ranging from 9 to 109 weeks. The shortest seizure-free or monotherapy durations represented patients with recent enrollment dates at the time of the report. The dose range was from 4 to 66 mg/day, and the average dose was 23.5 mg/day. In a preliminary open trial in infantile spasms, six of 12 infants had a ≥50% seizure reduction at dosages of 0.5 to 3.1 mg/kg/day (19).

MODE OF USE

Indications

Tiagabine is recommended as add-on treatment of adults and children >12 years old with partial seizures, with or without secondary generalization, which cannot be satisfactorily controlled with other AEDs.

Dosing Recommendations

Formulation

In preclinical and clinical studies, the tiagabine dose was expressed in terms of milligrams hydrochloride. A conversion factor of 0.91 has been used to calculate the dose as tiagabine free base, which is available everywhere as 5-, 10-, 15-mg tablets, except in the United States, Canada, and Mexico, where 4-, 12-, 16-, and 20-mg tablets of tiagabine hydrochloride are used (Table 74.2).

Initial Dose and Titration Rate

The current labeling with tiagabine free base states that the initial dosage is 7.5 to 15 mg/day, followed by weekly increments of 5 to 15 mg/day. In the United States, Canada, and Mexico, labeling was already modified toward a lower initial dose of 4 mg/day tiagabine hydrochloride, followed by weekly increments of 4 to 8 mg/day. Phase IV trial and clin-

TABLE 74.2. CLINICAL USE OF TIAGABINE

Dosage of current formulation must be titrated slowly (4–5 mg/wk) and individually to avoid dizziness.
Tiagabine should always be taken at the end of the meal (food slows rate of absorption).
In case of adverse events, change easily from twice daily to three or four times daily dosing with higher doses.
The usual initial target maintenance dosage in patients taking enzyme-inducing drugs is 30–32 mg/day and in patients not taking enzyme-inducing drugs 15–16 mg/day.
Usual range of maintenance dosage in patients taking enzyme-inducing drugs is ≤50–56 mg/day and in patients not taking enzyme-inducing drugs ≤30–32 mg/day.
High daily doses of ≥70–80 mg are well tolerated for some individual patients.
After an enzyme-inducing agent is removed, tiagabine clearance will decrease, and tiagabine dosage reduction may be necessary.

ical experience to date would lead one to recommend to start tiagabine with 4 or 5 mg/day and to increase the dose gradually by weekly increments of 4 or 5 mg/day, to minimize side effects related to the central nervous system.

From phase II and III tiagabine trials, it is clear that some central nervous system–related adverse effects are particularly common with tiagabine treatment, especially dizziness. Patients usually describe the dizziness as a lightheaded or unstable feeling. It is a very nonspecific symptom, usually occurring within 1 to 2 hours of taking a tiagabine dose, and it is usually associated with the peak concentration of the drug. Adverse events more common with tiagabine than with placebo are asthenia (lack of energy), nervousness, tremor, concentration difficulties, depressive mood, and language problems (difficulty in finding words or initiation of speech). The increased risk of central nervous system–related adverse events with tiagabine when compared with placebo is evident only in the titration period; the risk levels off during the fixed-dose period (10). Because of these adverse effects, tiagabine should be titrated slowly. Initial doses can be given twice a day, but a change to thrice-daily dosing is recommended, with doses >30 to 32 mg/day. Tiagabine should always be taken with food, and preferably at the end of meals, to avoid rapid rises in plasma concentrations. Individual doses given four times daily may also be helpful, at least with higher doses. Neither somnolence nor drowsiness was seen more frequently in patients receiving tiagabine than in patients receiving placebo.

Maintenance Dosages

Population pharmacokinetic analyses indicate that tiagabine clearance is 60% greater in patients taking enzyme-inducing AEDs. The usual initial target maintenance dose in patients taking enzyme-inducing drugs is 30 to 32 mg/day, and in patients not taking enzyme-inducing drugs, it is 15 to 16 mg/day (20). The usual range of maintenance doses in patients taking enzyme-inducing drugs is ≤50 to 56 mg/day, and in patients not taking enzyme-inducing drugs, it is ≤30 to 32 mg/day; however, high daily doses of ≥70 to 80 mg are well tolerated by some patients. Patients taking a combination of inducing and noninducing drugs (e.g., carbamazepine and valproate) should be considered to be induced.

Stopping of Tiagabine Treatment

No AED should be withdrawn suddenly. Although no clinical data are available, it seems sensible to withdraw tiagabine gradually over ≥2 to 3 weeks (20).

Use in Special Populations

Elderly Patients

The pharmacokinetics of tiagabine in elderly patients is similar to that seen in younger patients, hence there should be no need for dosage modification (21).

Children

Tiagabine has not been investigated in adequate and well-controlled clinical trials in patients <12 years old. The apparent clearance and volume of distribution of tiagabine per unit body surface area or per kilogram were fairly similar in 25 children (age, 3 to 10 years) and in adults taking enzyme-inducing AEDs. In children who were taking a noninducing AED, the clearance of tiagabine, based on body weight and body surface area, was twofold and 1.5-fold higher, respectively, than in uninduced adults with epilepsy, a finding suggesting that dosage requirements (on the basis of milligrams per kilograms) may be higher in children (22). The maximal tolerated doses for children >2 years old used in one study were 0.65±0.37 mg/kg. Patients receiving inducing AEDs had only slightly higher doses than patients receiving noninducing AEDs, but the difference was not significant (0.73±0.44 versus 0.61±0.32 mg/kg) (17).

Patients with Renal Impairment

The pharmacokinetics of tiagabine is unaffected in patients with renal impairment or in patients with renal failure requiring hemodialysis (23).

Patients with Hepatic Impairment

Compared with normal subjects, patients with mild or moderate liver function impairment had higher and more prolonged plasma concentrations of both total and unbound tiagabine after the administration of tiagabine. The patients with hepatic impairment also had more neurologic side effects. Tiagabine should therefore be given with caution to patients with epilepsy who have impaired hepatic function. Patients with impaired liver function may require reduced initial and maintenance doses of tiagabine or longer dosing intervals compared with patients with normal hepatic function. These patients should be monitored closely because of the potential for increased incidence of neurologic side effects (24). Tiagabine should not be used in patients with severely impaired liver function.

Precautions

Pregnancy

Teratogenic effects were seen in the offspring of rats exposed to maternally toxic doses of tiagabine, but not in animals receiving nontoxic dosages. Only limited pregnancy data involving tiagabine, which show no clear teratogenicity, are available (25). Therefore, tiagabine cannot be recommended for women who are pregnant or at risk of becoming pregnant, and it should be used only if the potential benefit justifies the potential risk to the fetus.

Unclassified Seizures or Generalized Epilepsy

Tiagabine should not be used in patients with unclassified epilepsy or in patients with generalized epilepsy, especially those with a history of absence or myoclonic seizures, with a history of spike-and-wave discharges on electroencephalography (EEG), or those with nonconvulsive status epilepticus (20). Tiagabine has not yet been shown to be effective in these patients, and evidence indicates that AEDs that increase γ-aminobutyric acid (GABA)–ergic transmission may exacerbate or induce absences or myoclonus (26). Patients with history of spike-and-wave discharges on EEG have been reported to have exacerbations of their EEG abnormalities associated with cognitive or neuropsychiatric events. In the documented cases of spike-and-wave discharges on EEG with cognitive or neuropsychiatric events, patients usually continued tiagabine, but required dosage adjustment (10).

History of Severe Behavioral Problems and Depression

The addition of tiagabine in clinical trials was associated significantly more often with depression than the use of placebo (5% versus 2%) (27). If the patient has a history of behavioral problems or depression, treatment with tiagabine should be initiated at a low initial dose under close supervision because there may be an increased risk of recurrence of these symptoms during treatment with tiagabine.

CURRENT ROLE OF TIAGABINE IN EPILEPSY TREATMENT

Tiagabine, a selective GABA uptake inhibitor, is effective against all partial seizures and has a relatively favorable safety profile. The frequency of idiosyncratic drug-related reactions, particularly cutaneous reactions, is low with tiagabine, and in rare cases the relationship with tiagabine treatment has been unproven. Moreover, tiagabine has a favorable cognitive profile. The characteristic concentric visual field defect seen with vigabatrin treatment (28) was not observed in two tiagabine monotherapy trials (29,30). These features support the use of tiagabine as add-on treatment in partial epilepsy, for example, after treatment failure with a first-line sodium channel blocking AED or if a first-line AED has caused idiosyncratic reactions. Tiagabine is also suitable in patients for whom it is particularly important that the AED does not cause any deterioration in cognitive performance (31–35). A controlled-released formulation would offset any potential clinical disadvantage stemming from tiagabine's short elimination half-life, particularly in patients receiving enzyme-inducing AEDs (36).

REFERENCES

1. Richens A, Chadwick DW, Duncan JS, et al. Adjunctive treatment of partial seizures with tiagabine: a placebo-controlled trial. *Epilepsy Res* 1995;21:37–42.
2. Crawford PM, Engelsman M, Brown SW. Tiagabine: phase II study of efficacy and safety in adjunctive treatment of partial seizures. *Epilepsia* 1993;34[Suppl 2]:S182.
3. Uthman B, Rowan J, Ahman PA, et al. Tiagabine for complex partial seizures: a randomised, add-on, dose-response trial. *Arch Neurol* 1998;55:56–62.
4. Sachdeo RC, Leroy R, Krauss G, et al. Tiagabine therapy for complex partial seizures: a dose-frequency study. *Arch Neurol* 1997;54:595–601.
5. Kälviäinen R, Brodie MJ, Chadwick D et al. A double-blind, placebo-controlled trial of tiagabine given three-times daily as add-on therapy for refractory partial seizures. *Epilepsy Res* 1998; 30:31–40.
6. Marson AG, Kadir ZA, Hutton JL, et al. The new antiepileptic drugs: a systematic review of their efficacy and tolerability. *Epilepsia* 1997;38:859–880.
7. Biraben A, Beaussart M, Josien E, et al. Tiagabine as adjunctive treatment of partial seizures in patients with epilepsy. A comparison of two dose regimens. *Epilepsia* 2000;40[Suppl]: S96.
8. Biton V, Vasquez KB, Sachdeo RC, et al. Adjunctive tiagabine compared with phenytoin and carbamazepine in the multicenter, double-blind trial of complex partial seizures. *Epilepsia* 1998;39 [Suppl 6]:S125–S126.
9. Ben-Menachem E. International experience with tiagabine add-on therapy. *Epilepsia* 1995;36:14–21.
10. Leppik IE, Gram L, Deaton R. Safety of tiagabine: summary of 53 trials. *Epilepsy Res* 1999;33:235–246.
11. Bergmann A, Bauer J, Stodieck S. Treatment of epilepsy with tiagabine as add-on antiepileptic drug in patients with refractory seizures: experiences in 574 patients. *Epilepsia* 2000;41[Suppl]: S40.
12. Czapinski P, Jedrzejczak J, Kozik A, et al. Open multicentre study of tiagabine as add on treatment in patients with partial seizures. *Epilepsia* 2000;41[Suppl]:S40.
13. Salas-Puig J, Arroyo and the Epilepsy Observational Investigation Group of Spain. Tiagabine adjunctive therapy: an observational study. *Epilepsia* 2000;41[Suppl]:S40.
14. Schachter S. Tiagabine monotherapy in the treatment of partial epilepsy. *Epilepsia* 1995;36[Suppl 6]:S2–S6.
15. Kälviäinen R, Salmenperä T, Jutila L, et al. Slow versus fast drug switch from established AED to tiagabine monotherapy. *Epilepsia* 1998;39:66.
16. Brodie MJ, Bomhof MAM, Kälviäinen R, et al. Double-blind comparison of tiagabine and carbamazepine monotherapy in newly diagnosed epilepsy: preliminary results. *Epilepsia* 1997;38 [Suppl 3]:S66–S67.
17. Uldall P, Bulteau C, Pedersen SA, et al. Tiagabine adjunctive therapy in children with refractory epilepsy: a single-blind dose escalating study. *Epilepsy Res* 2000;42:159–168.
18. Collins SD, Fugate J, Sommerville KW. Long-term use of Gabitril (tiagabine HCl) monotherapy in pediatric patients. *Neurology* 1999;52[Suppl 2]:A392.
19. Kugler SL, Mandelbaum DE, Patel R, et al. Efficacy and tolerability of tiagabine in infantile spasms. *Epilepsia* 1999;40[Suppl 7]:S127.
20. Schmidt D, Gram L, Brodie M, et al. Tiagabine in the treatment of epilepsy: a clinical review with a guide for prescribing physician. *Epilepsy Res* 2000;41:245–251.
21. Snel S, Jansen JA, Mengel HB, et al. The pharmacokinetics of tiagabine in healthy elderly volunteers and elderly patients with epilepsy. *J Clin Pharmacol* 1997;37:1015–1020.
22. Gustavson LE, Boellner SW, Grannemann GR, et al. A single-dose study to define tiagabine pharmacokinetics in pediatric patients with complex partial seizures. *Neurology* 1998;48: 1032–1037.
23. Cato A III, Gustavson LE, Qian J, et al. Effects of renal impairment on the pharmacokinetics and tolerability of tiagabine. *Epilepsia* 1998;39:43–47.
24. Lau AH, Gustavson LE, Sperelakis R, et al. Pharmacokinetics and safety of tiagabine in subjects with various degrees of hepatic function. *Epilepsia* 1997;38:445–451.
25. Collins S, Donnelly J, Krups D, Sommerville KW. Pregnancy and tiagabine exposure. *Neurology* 1997;48[Suppl 2]:P01.039(abst).
26. Loiseau P. Review of controlled trials of tiagabine; a clinician's viewpoint. *Epilepsia* 1999;40[Suppl]:S14–S19.
27. Leppik I. Tiagabine: the safety landscape. *Epilepsia* 1995;36 [Suppl 6]:S10–S13.
28. Kälviäinen R, Nousiainen I. Visual field defects with vigabatrin: epidemiology and therapeutic implications. *CNS Drugs* 2001;15: 217–230.
29. Kälviäinen R, Hache JC, Renault-Djouadi J, et al. A study of visual fields in patients receiving tiagabine as monotherapy and matched controls receiving carbamazepine or lamotrigine monotherapy. *Epilepsia* 2000;41[Suppl]:145.
30. Nousiainen I, Mäntyjärvi M, Kälviäinen R. Visual function in patients treated with the GABAergic anticonvulsant drug tiagabine. *Clin Drug Invest* 2000;20:393–400.
31. Kälviäinen R, Äikiä M, Mervaala E, et al. Long-term cognitive

and EEG effects of tiagabine in drug-resistant partial epilepsy. *Epilepsy Res* 1996;25:291–297.

32. Äikiä M, Kälviäinen R, Salmenperä T, et al. Cognitive effects of tiagabine monotherapy. *Epilepsia* 1997;38:107.

33. Dodrill CB, Arnett JL,Sommerville KW, et al. Cognitive and quality of life effects of differing doses of tiagabine in epilepsy. *Neurology* 1997;48:1025–1031.

34. Dodrill CB, Arnett JL, Shu V, et al. Effects of tiagabine monotherapy on abilities, adjustment and mood. *Epilepsia* 1998;39: 33–42.

35. Dodrill CB, Arnett JL, Deaton R. Tiagabine versus phenytoin and carbamazepine as add-on therapies: effects on abilities, adjustment and mood. *Epilepsy Res* 2000;42:123–132.

36. Leach JP, Brodie MJ. Tiagabine. *Lancet* 1998;351:203–207.

TIAGABINE

CLINICAL EFFICACY AND USE IN NONEPILEPTIC DISORDERS

KENNETH W. SOMMERVILLE

Tiagabine, a derivative of nipecotic acid, is an inhibitor of γ-aminobutyric acid (GABA) uptake that was developed specifically for use as an antiepileptic drug (AED). The drug discovery program for tiagabine was established to identify inhibitors of GABA uptake that were sufficiently lipophilic to cross the blood–brain barrier and to produce anticonvulsive effects in the central nervous system (CNS).

GABA PHARMACOLOGY

Because GABA is the major inhibitory neurotransmitter in the CNS, GABAergic mechanisms have been extensively investigated in research on seizure suppression and epilepsy therapy (1,2). A brief description of GABA-related pharmacology can provide a basis for understanding the role of GABAergic drugs in the treatment of epilepsy and other neuropsychological disorders.

The two principal postsynaptic GABA receptors are the $GABA_A$ and $GABA_B$ receptor complexes. The $GABA_B$ receptor is G-protein coupled; its activation by GABA causes hyperpolarization and resultant inhibition of neurotransmitter release. The $GABA_A$ receptor complex is a pentameric heterooligomer that exists in multiple subtypes in vivo. In addition to binding sites for GABA, the $GABA_A$ receptor has binding sites for benzodiazepines, barbiturates, and neurosteroids, and it is coupled to a chloride ion channel. Activation of the $GABA_A$ receptor induces increased inward chloride ion flux and results in membrane hyperpolarization and neuronal inhibition. Biochemical and clinical evidence indicates that the initiation and spread of seizure activity may involve alterations in the activity of the $GABA_A$ receptor (3). Compounds that directly stimulate the $GABA_A$ receptor complex tend to have anticonvulsant activity, whereas $GABA_A$ receptor antagonists (including bicuculline and pentylenetetrazol) produce convulsions in animals (4).

Kenneth W. Sommerville, MD: Medical Director, Neuroscience, Department of Marketed Products, Clinical Research, Abbott Laboratories, Abbott Park, Illinois

Once released into the synapse, free GABA that does not bind rapidly to the $GABA_A$ or $GABA_B$ receptor complexes may diffuse from the synapse or may be actively taken up by neurons and glial cells. Four different membrane transporter proteins that mediate the uptake of synaptic GABA into neurons and glial cells have been identified, differing in their CNS distribution and localization; they are known as GAT-1, GAT-2, GAT-3, and BGT-1 (5). Tiagabine interacts primarily with the GAT-1 transporter.

TIAGABINE DEVELOPMENT

Because a reduction in GABAergic neuronal activity has been implicated in various neuropsychological disorders, including epilepsy, anxiety, and pain, the enhancement of such activity has been the focus of numerous pharmacologic research initiatives (1,6,7). These have included investigations into the direct stimulation of the $GABA_A$ receptor, the modulation of $GABA_A$ receptor activity (by compounds such as the benzodiazepines), and the inhibition of GABA metabolism (by compounds such as vigabatrin). For the most part, these areas have yielded compounds of only limited utility in the treatment of epilepsy and other disorders, because of side effects caused by generalized GABA receptor stimulation, rapid development of anticonvulsant tolerance (in the case of the benzodiazepines), or other unacceptable effects.

The enhancement of $GABA_A$ receptor activity through the inhibition of GABA uptake represents a promising alternative approach for two principal reasons. First, the inhibition of GABA uptake preferentially accentuates the patterns of endogenous GABA release in the brain, instead of inducing generalized, possibly nonphysiologic, receptor stimulation. Second, the extent to which GABA uptake inhibitors stimulate $GABA_A$ receptors is ultimately limited by the amount of synaptic GABA available, which is presumably under tight physiologic control (8).

Tiagabine was synthesized after the identification of several cyclic amino acids (including nipecotic acid), that

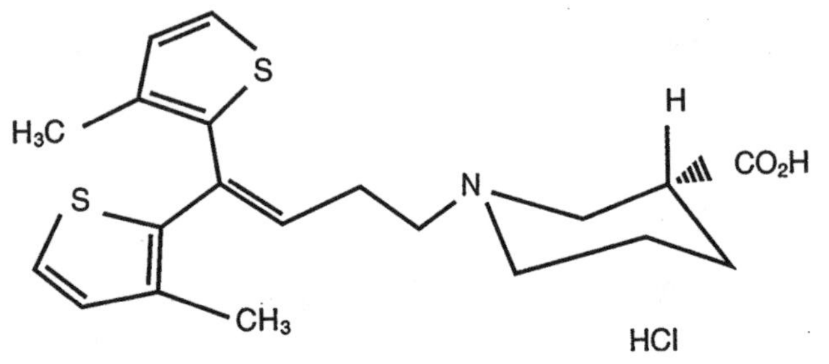

FIGURE 75.1. Chemical structure of tiagabine.

well as inhibiting some chemically induced seizures (10). Tiagabine appears to interact preferentially with the GAT-1 GABA transporter, and this may limit its activity to regions of the CNS in which GAT-1 plays a significant role (the cortex, cerebellum, and hippocampus) (11,12). In clinical trials, tiagabine has been shown to be effective in the treatment of a range of partial seizure types, both as adjunctive therapy (13) and as monotherapy (14–16). A schematic diagram of the synaptic action of tiagabine is shown in Figure 75.2.

POTENTIAL FOR TIAGABINE EFFICACY IN NONEPILEPTIC DISORDERS

The possibility that modulation of GABAergic responses may be useful in therapeutic approaches to conditions other than epilepsy led to the suggestion that tiagabine be considered for clinical evaluation of efficacy in these conditions. Meldrum and Chapman summarized the case for exploring alternate uses for tiagabine (12). The specificity of

inhibit GABA uptake in certain tissues *in vitro.* Tiagabine is a derivative of nipecotic acid with a lipophilic "anchor" covalently attached to the amino nitrogen (Figure 75.1). Tiagabine strongly inhibits GABA uptake in synaptosomal preparations from rat brain and in cultured neurons and glial cells *in vitro* (9). It also generates a dose-dependent increase in extracellular GABA levels in rat brain *in vivo,* as

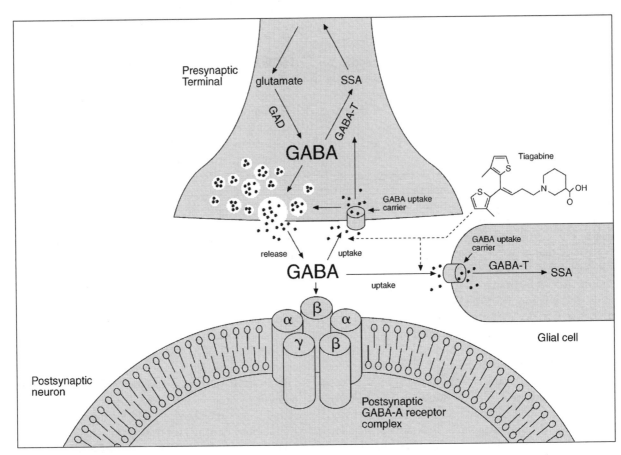

FIGURE 75.2. Schematic diagram of the action of tiagabine at the synapse. GAD, glutamic acid decarboxylase; SSA, succinic semialdehyde. (From Suzdak PD, Jansen JA. A review of the preclinical pharmacology of tiagabine: a potent and selective anticonvulsant GABA uptake inhibitor. *Epilepsia* 1995;36:612–626, with permission.)

tiagabine's antiepileptic activity seems to be related to the importance of GAT-1 as its principal GABA transporter. Tiagabine specifically suppresses various chemically induced and kindled seizures in rats, it is also effective against certain genetic models of reflex epilepsy in other species, and it has some activity against maximal electroshock seizures. Other GABA uptake inhibitors working through transporters different from GAT-1 show a different spectrum of anticonvulsant activity. This specificity may determine how useful tiagabine may be in other conditions possibly responsive to GABAergic treatment (12).

Therapeutic areas for continuing tiagabine research include the following:

- Expansion of epilepsy-related indications (e.g., infantile spasms) (12).
- Suppression of status epilepticus and epileptogenesis (12).
- Exploration of disorders known or suspected to be related to GABAergic mechanisms: sleep disorders (12), pain (including postherpetic neuralgia and diabetic neuropathy) (17–19), movement disorders (particularly those related to basal ganglia disease, e.g., tardive dyskinesia) (20,21), spasticity (22), bipolar disorder (23), and anxiety (24).
- Neuroprotection against ischemia-induced cell loss (25).

EVALUATIONS OF TIAGABINE IN NONEPILEPTIC DISORDERS

Pain

The most extensive area of research with tiagabine outside of epilepsy is neuropathic pain. Tiagabine was evaluated in several standard models of pain in rats and mice (17). Tiagabine demonstrated antinociceptive effects in moderate doses (7.2 and 24.3 μmol/kg) against thermal pain in a mouse hot-plate test, but it was ineffective in rat tail-flick tests at high doses (72.8 μmol/kg). Because the hot-plate test is thought to involve supraspinal processing and the tail-flick test is considered a spinal reflex, these findings suggest that tiagabine selectively modulates supraspinal GABAergic responses. Tiagabine was also effective at moderate doses in reducing the acetic acid–induced abdominal stretching response in mice and the first phase of formalin-induced paw flinches in rats. In the second phase of the formalin paw-flinch test, which involves an active inflammatory component, high doses of tiagabine were required to produce a response, a finding suggesting that tiagabine does not possess significant antiinflammatory activity. Tiagabine was also moderately effective (compared with morphine) in reducing the allodynic response to von Frey filaments in a spinal nerve ligation model of rat neuropathic pain. The specificity of the effects of tiagabine in moderating pain perception suggest that only certain pain pathways may be strongly dependent on GAT-1–mediated GABAergic mechanisms (17).

The effectiveness of tiagabine in the management of diabetic neuropathy was evaluated in a combination open-label and double-blind crossover trial using a once-daily, extended-release formulation. Thirty-five adult patients (≥18 years of age) with painful diabetic polyneuropathy were titrated with tiagabine in the initial open-label phase to determine their maximum tolerated dose and initial pain relief response. The rate of discontinuation for adverse events was higher than expected from earlier evaluations of tiagabine (primarily CNS events thought to be related to too-rapid titration), so only 17 patients completed the open-label phase, and 11 were randomized to the double-blind portion of the study. The high rate of drug discontinuation may also have been related to the lack of extended-release dosage forms other than the 12-mg strength. All adverse events were transient and resolved with tiagabine discontinuation or dose reduction. Pain assessments were based on the Brief Pain Inventory (BPI) and McGill Pain Questionnaire (MPQ). Patients who tolerated a tiagabine dose of at least 12 mg/day, and who demonstrated pain relief of at least three units on the worst/average pain items of the BPI (Figure 75.3), were randomized, underwent drug washout, and were retitrated to their previous dose in a two-period, double-blind placebo-controlled crossover study. Significant differences ($p < .05$) were observed in the treatment group with respect to percentage of pain relief in the last 24 hours and the degree to which pain had interfered with sleep in the last 24 hours. Improvements, although not statistically significant, were noted in other preplanned BPI and MPQ variables, most notably those dealing with the extent to which pain had interfered with social relationships and enjoyment of life on the BPI (Figure 75.3) and the affective subscale of the MPQ. The researchers concluded that the generally favorable results of tiagabine treatment warrant further evaluation in larger-scale studies with greater dosing flexibility (19).

In another small study of neuropathic pain, 17 patients with painful sensory neuropathy received an initial dose of 4 mg tiagabine after a 1-week washout of all previous pain medications. Patients were subsequently titrated to 16 mg/day by increments of 4 mg/wk. Nine patients completed the titration, and eight discontinued for adverse events, mostly nausea, dizziness, or disorientation. In patients who completed the titration, tiagabine reduced symptoms of surface pain (34.2%), skin sensitivity (28%), burning (36%), cold (35.5%), pain sharpness (29%), and discomfort (18.4%). There was no effect on dull or deep pain, or on autonomic tests, although two patients reported less perspiring and four noted improved sleep patterns and skin temperature. The best results were found at doses of 8 to 12 mg/day. The investigators suggested that tiagabine may improve small-fiber neuropathy and recommended further study (18).

Change in Brief Pain Inventory, Mean Group Scores, Double-Blind Period

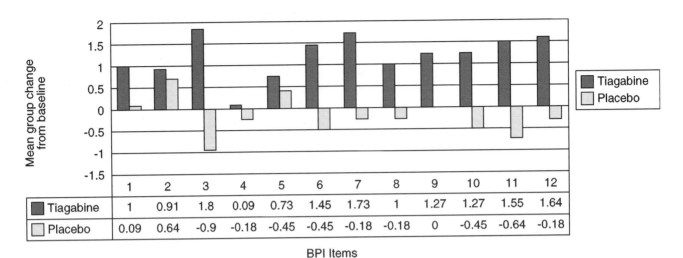

BPI Items	1	2	3	4	5	6	7	8	9	10	11	12
■ Tiagabine	1	0.91	1.8	0.09	0.73	1.45	1.73	1	1.27	1.27	1.55	1.64
□ Placebo	0.09	0.64	-0.9	-0.18	-0.45	-0.45	-0.18	-0.18	0	-0.45	-0.64	-0.18

FIGURE 75.3. Changes in brief pain inventory, mean group scores, double-blind period. [From Kirby LC, Collins SD, Deaton RL, et al. Tiagabine (Gabitril) in the management of painful diabetic polyneuropathy. Presented at the poster session of the American Pain Society meeting, Fort Lauderdale, FL, 1999.]

Spasticity

The use of tiagabine in spasticity was evaluated in a pilot study of 14 children <12 years of age who suffered from both static spastic quadriplegia and epilepsy intractable to treatment by other AEDs. The number of AEDs previously used unsuccessfully for seizures ranged from one to eight, with a mean of 4.5. The children had various seizure types, and all had two or more different types of seizures. Tiagabine was titrated from a starting dose of 0.1 to 0.2 mg/kg/day to seizure abatement, onset of adverse events, or the maximum dose of 1.1 mg/kg/day. Spasticity was assessed by motor function improvements (incorporating gross, fine, and oral motor control) scored by a participating pediatric neurologist on a scale of 0 to 4 (0, no improvement; +1, 25% improvement; +2, 50% improvement; +3, 75% improvement; and +4, 100% improvement). Seizure control was also scored on a scale of 0 to 4 incorporating ranges (0, 0% to 24% reduction; +1, 25% to 49% reduction, etc.). All children demonstrated at least some improvement in motor function (range, +1 to +4), with a mean improvement of +2.3 (~50%). Seizure control improvement scores ranged from 0 to +4, with a mean improvement of +2.4 (reduction of 50% to 74%). The authors noted that the encouraging results in both motor control and seizure control for spasticity and epilepsy of varying origin suggest that longer-term, randomized trials of tiagabine efficacy in spasticity should be undertaken (22).

Migraine

The demonstrated efficacy of divalproex sodium in migraine prophylaxis has led to interest in assessing the ability of other AEDs, including tiagabine, to reduce migraine frequency and severity. In an open-label trial of tiagabine use in 41 patients who had experienced adverse effects (n = 22) or incomplete relief from migraine (n = 14) using divalproex sodium, tiagabine was used at moderate doses (8 to 16 mg/day) over a minimum 3-month period. Because no lead-in baseline phase was monitored, no estimate of reduction in migraine frequency could be reported. However, improvement (measured using global evaluations by both patient and physician) was noted in 28 of 41 patients. They reported improvements of >50%. Twelve patients experienced 14 adverse events, resulting in discontinuation of tiagabine therapy in nine patients. Adverse events included fatigue (n = 9), weight gain (n = 2), confusion (n = 2), and poor memory (n = 1) (26).

Another open-label trial evaluated tiagabine use in 49 patients who were unresponsive to current migraine prophylactic and abortive therapy. Tiagabine dosage was titrated to 16 mg/day. This study allowed the continued use of comedications and abortive treatment. After 6 weeks of treatment, 23% of the patients were headache free; after 12 weeks, 32% were headache free; an additional 34% reported improvement. Five patients discontinued tiagabine because of side effects (sedation, dysphoria, agitation, or tremor). Investigators observed that patients who responded to tiagabine therapy were significantly more likely to have comorbid epilepsy, affective disorder, post-traumatic stress disorder, or fibromyalgia than nonresponders (27).

A case-study report found that tiagabine was effective in four patients with migraine and other types of headache who were refractory to multiple medications, including other AEDs. In two patients with refractory cervicogenic headache, daily headache frequency declined 80% to 90% with relatively high (36 and 80 mg/day) tiagabine doses (28). It was not clear from the report whether these patients were taking concomitant enzyme-inducing drugs, which could account for the high doses.

The apparent efficacy of tiagabine in migraine prophylaxis in small uncontrolled trials led all researchers involved to suggest that larger-scale, well-controlled trials are warranted. The GABAergic mechanism of tiagabine and the frequent comorbidity of migraine and epilepsy suggest that tiagabine has potential in this therapeutic area.

Psychiatry

Tiagabine has also been evaluated in psychiatric disorders, to date, exclusively in a small-scale trial and case studies. A case-study evaluation of three patients reported benefit from tiagabine low-dose (8 mg/day) add-on therapy in all cases. The patient with the most severe case, diagnosed as having schizophrenic disorder (bipolar type), had an extensive history of psychotic episodes and multiple courses of medication, often with significant side effects. Tiagabine was used to replace lamotrigine as an add-on medication to paroxetine and olanzapine and successfully controlled paranoid features that appeared in the absence of lamotrigine. In the other two cases, complete remission of the symptoms of bipolar disorder (severe mania in the first case and a mixed bipolar state with psychotic depressive features in the second) was reported with tiagabine adjunctive to a regimen of valproate, bupropion, and methylphenidate (the first case), and carbamazepine and paroxetine (the second case) (23).

In two patients with refractory bipolar disorder, low-dose tiagabine was evaluated as adjunctive treatment to regimens of lamotrigine and alprazolam (in one patient) and venlafaxine, lithium, and flurazepam (in the other). Both patients showed remission of bipolar symptoms, with improvement in mood. One patient began to experience a manic episode while taking 3 mg/day of tiagabine; he condition apparently was restabilized by an increase to 4 mg/day (29).

A small-scale trial in Europe evaluated the use of tiagabine in bipolar disorder, with relatively rapid titration in eight acutely manic patients. Tiagabine was started at 20 mg/day (described as a loading dose) on day 1 and was further increased in steps of 5 mg/day when tolerated by the patient, up to a maximum of 40 mg/day in two patients.

Tiagabine therapy was adjunctive in all but one patient. There was a slight improvement in three patients, all with moderate manic syndrome, but none of the severely manic patients showed a clear benefit. Side effects were significant in several patients, including a generalized tonic-clonic seizure in one patient that may have been attributable to tiagabine administration. The authors stressed the small scale of the study and compared their results with those reported in the three-patient report cited earlier. The high initial dose and rapid titration may have been a factor in the results and could have contributed to the seizure and other adverse events. These investigators suggest that tiagabine may not be useful as an acute therapy for manic episodes, but it deserves further study in general psychiatric practice (30). The high doses and rapid titration in this study contrast with other, more favorable reports in which drug administration was more cautious. If tiagabine is useful in patients with mania, it would need to be tested at lower doses than in this report and with slower titration.

Tardive dyskinesia is a hyperkinetic motor disorder associated primarily with long-term administration of neuroleptic medications. A double-blind, placebo-controlled trial of γ-vinyl γ-aminobutyric acid (vigabatrin), another GABAergic drug, was carried out in seven schizophrenic patients with tardive dyskinesia. A significant decrease in dyskinetic symptoms (involuntary movements), as measured by Smith Extrapyramidal Scale ratings, occurred with the administration of vigabatrin. This was associated with a twofold increase in cerebrospinal fluid levels of GABA. A significant reduction in cerebrospinal fluid levels of GABA was also observed in the dyskinetic patients with schizophrenia compared with nondyskinetic controls. These results support the view that a GABA deficit plays an important role in the pathophysiology of tardive dyskinesia, and GABA agonists and GABA-receptor potentiators are potentially effective in treating this disorder (21). Although vigabatrin has GABAergic action through a different mechanism than that of tiagabine, these promising data led to preclinical work on tardive dyskinesia with tiagabine.

Haloperidol-induced oral dyskinesias (vacuous chewing movements) in Sprague-Dawley rats have been used in several laboratories as an animal model for tardive dyskinesia. In a study of 48 rats, tiagabine, at a dosage of 75/mg/kg/day, significantly inhibited the onset of vacuous chewing movements and decreased the average severity from 11.2 ± 2.0 vacuous chewing movements per 5 minutes in rats receiving haloperidol alone to 4.4 ± 1.4 in rats receiving haloperidol and tiagabine. By comparison, the placebo rate was 1.3 ± 0.5. The investigators concluded that these data suggest the potential usefulness of tiagabine as a therapeutic agent in the treatment or prophylaxis of tardive dyskinesia (20). Clinical trials of tiagabine in tardive dyskinesia have been initiated, but, at the time of publication, results have not been reported.

CONCLUSION

The relatively specific range of activity of tiagabine in the laboratory and clinic and its ability to be well tolerated at efficacious dose ranges are presumably related to the targeted effect on the uptake of GABA. The important role played by GABAergic mechanisms, in normal and abnormal CNS function, suggests that tiagabine may be of clinical benefit to many patients who are refractory to current therapies for many different disorders.

Both the development of tiagabine and the regulatory approval for tiagabine use in treating epilepsy occurred only recently; therefore, reports on its efficacy in the treatment of other conditions are preliminary. However, the encouraging early results observed in the treatment of pain, spasticity, and migraine and other headaches clearly indicate the need for well-controlled clinical trials. The possibility that tiagabine may be efficacious in the treatment of psychiatric and movement disorders also deserves further study, especially in the promising areas of bipolar disorder and tardive dyskinesia. Further understanding of the pharmacology and specificity of tiagabine, particularly against the background of steadily increasing knowledge about the multiple roles of GABA, should help to guide research into new clinical areas.

REFERENCES

1. Meldrum B. Pharmacology of GABA. *Clin Neuropharmacol* 1982;5:293–316.
2. Krogsgaard-Larsen P, Falch E, Larsson OM, et al. GABA uptake inhibitors: relevance to antiepileptic drug research. *Epilepsy Res* 1987;1:77–93.
3. Tunnicliff G, Raess BU. GABA neurotransmitter activity in human epileptogenic brain. In: Tunnicliff G, Raess BU, eds. *GABA mechanisms in epilepsy.* New York: Wiley–Liss, 1991: 105–120.
4. Schwartz RD. The GABA-A receptor-gated ion channel: biochemical and pharmacological studies of structure and function. *Biochem Pharmacol* 1988;27:3369–3378.
5. Borden LA. GABA transporter heterogeneity: pharmacology and cellular localization. *Neurochem Int* 1996;29:335–356.
6. Krogsgaard-Larsen P. GABA synaptic mechanisms: stereochemical and conformational requirements. *Med Res Rev* 1988;8: 27–56.
7. Krogsgaard-Larsen P, Scheel-Krüger J, Kofoed H. *GABA-neurotransmitters: pharmacochemical, biochemical and pharmacological aspects.* Copenhagen: Munksgaard, 1979.
8. Suzdak PD, Jansen JA. A review of the preclinical pharmacology of tiagabine: a potent and selective anticonvulsant GABA uptake inhibitor. *Epilepsia* 1995;36:612–626.
9. Braestrup C, Nielsen EB, Sonnewald U, et al. (R)-*N*-[4,4-bis(3-methyl-2-thienyl)but-3-en-1-yl]Nipecotic acid binds with high affinity to the brain γ-aminobutyric acid uptake carrier. *J Neurochem* 1990;54:639–647.
10. Fink-Jensen A, Suzdak PD, Swedberg MDB, et al. The γ-aminobutyric acid (GABA) uptake inhibitor, tiagabine, increases extracellular brain levels of GABA in awake rats. *Eur J Pharmacol* 1992;220:197–201.
11. Borden LA, Dhar TGM, Smith KE, et al. Tiagabine, SK&F 89976-A, CI-966, and NNC-711 are selective for the cloned GAB transporter GAT-1. *Eur J Pharmacol Mol Pharmacol* 1994; 269:219–224.
12. Meldrum BS, Chapman AG. Basic mechanisms of gabitril (tiagabine) and future potential developments. *Epilepsia* 1999;40 [Suppl 9]:S52–S56.
13. Ben-Menachem E. International experience with tiagabine add-on therapy. *Epilepsia* 1995;36[Suppl 6]:S14–S21.
14. Alarcon G, Binnie CD, Elwes RDC, et al. Monotherapy antiepileptic drug trials in patients undergoing presurgical assessment: methodological problems and possibilities. *Seizure* 1995;4: 293–301.
15. Schachter SC. Tiagabine monotherapy in the treatment of partial epilepsy. *Epilepsia* 1995;32[Suppl 6]:S2–S6.
16. Brodie MJ, Bomhof MAM, Kalviainen R, et al. Double-blind comparison of tiagabine and carbamazepine monotherapy in newly diagnosed epilepsy: preliminary results. Paper presented at the 22nd International Epilepsy Congress, Dublin, 1997.
17. Giardina WJ, Decker MW, Porsolt RD, et al. An evaluation of the GABA uptake blocker tiagabine in animal models of neuropathic and nociceptive pain. *Drug Dev Res* 1998;44:106–113.
18. Kanard R, Mendell J, Kissel J, et al. Treatment of painful sensory neuropathy with tiagabine hydrochloride. Paper presented at the International Symposium on the Autonomic Nervous System, Rio Grande, Puerto Rico, 2000.
19. Kirby LC, Collins SD, Deaton RL, et al. Tiagabine (Gabitril) in the management of painful diabetic polyneuropathy. Presented at the poster session of the American Pain Society meeting, Fort Lauderdale, FL, 1999.
20. Gao XM, Kakigi T, Friedman MB, et al. Tiagabine inhibits halieridol-induced oral dyskinesias in rats. *J Neurol Transm* 1994; 95:63–69.
21. Thaker GK, Tamminga CA, Alphs LD, et al. Brain γ-aminobutyric acid abnormality in tardive dyskinesia. *Arch Gen Psychiatry* 1987;44:522–529.
22. Holden KR, Titus MO. The effect of tiagabine on spasticity in children with intractable epilepsy: a pilot study. *Pediatr Neurol* 1999;21:728–730(abst).
23. Kaufman KR. Adjunctive tiagabine treatment of psychiatric disorders: three cases. *Ann Clin Psychiatry* 1998;10:181–184.
24. Neilson EB. Anxiolytic effect of NO-328, a GABA-uptake inhibitor. *Psychopharmacology (Berl)* 1988;96:S42(abst).
25. Johansen FF, Diemer NH. Enhancement of GABA neurotransmission after cerebral ischemia in the rat reduces loss of hippocampal CA1 pyramidal cells. *Acta Neurol Scand* 1991;84:1–5.
26. Freitag FG, Diamond S, Diamond ML, et al. An open use trial of tiagabine in migraine. *Headache Q* 2000;11:133–134.
27. Drake ME Jr, Kay AM, Knapp MS, et al. An open-label trial of tiagabine for migraine prophylaxis. *Headache* 1999;39:352(abst).
28. Krusz JC, Belanger J, Scott VB. Tiagabine in the treatment of very refractory migraines and other headaches. *Headache* 1999; 39:363(abst).
29. Schaffer LC, Schaffer CB. Tiagabine and the treatment of refractory bipolar disorder [Letter]. *Am J Psychiatry* 1999;156: 2014–2015.
30. Grunze H, Erfurth A, Marcuse A, et al. Tiagabine appears not to be efficacious in the treatment of acute mania. *J Clin Psychiatry* 1999;60:759–762.

TIAGABINE

ADVERSE EFFECTS

STEVEN C. SCHACHTER

Controlling seizures without intolerable or disabling side effects is the primary goal of seizure therapy. In 1985, Mattson and colleagues found that the development of side effects was often responsible for medication failure in patients with new-onset partial seizures (1). Subsequently, an unprecedented number of antiepileptic drugs (AEDs) as well as a device were developed for treating partial seizures, thus giving renewed hope to patients with suboptimal quality of life resulting from seizures or medication side effects (2–4). This chapter reviews the adverse effects of tiagabine (TGB).

RELEVANT PHARMACOKINETICS

The maximum serum concentration of TGB is reached within 1 to 1.5 hours when the drug is taken without food compared with a mean of 2.6 hours when it is taken with food (5). For this reason, patients should be instructed to take TGB with food, thereby reducing the possibility of peak concentration side effects.

TGB is extensively oxidized in the liver by CYP3A isoform (6). Dosage reductions and less frequent dosing intervals are recommended for patients with hepatic dysfunction to prevent excessive total and unbound TGB concentrations, resulting in symptoms and signs of neurotoxicity (7). However, because only 2% of TGB is excreted unchanged in the urine (8,9), the tolerability of TGB is unchanged in renally impaired patients (10).

Whereas an inducible enzyme metabolizes TGB, concurrently administered drugs that induce CYP3A increase the clearance of TGB, reduce the area under the curve, and decrease its half-life (11–13). Consequently, serum concentrations of TGB are likely to rise if a concomitant enzyme-inducing AED is tapered (14), possibly resulting in side effects.

TGB had no pharmacodynamic interactions with ethanol or triazolam in healthy volunteers (15,16), but a

Steven C. Schachter, MD: Associate Professor, Department of Neurology, Harvard Medical School; and Director of Clinical Trials, Beth Israel Deaconess Medical Center, Boston, Massachusetts

pharmacodynamic interaction with the benzodiazepines diazepam and zolpidem was seen in rats, manifested as behavioral changes (17). The human correlate, if any, has not been well characterized.

CLINICAL STUDIES OF SAFETY AND TOLERABILITY

Controlled Adjunctive Trials

Five multicenter, double-blind, randomized, placebo-controlled studies, including two crossover studies, evaluated TGB for the adjunctive treatment of partial-onset seizures. A total of 951 patients (675 randomly assigned to receive TGB) were enrolled (8,18–20).

Study subjects in the three parallel-design studies received one to three concomitant enzyme-inducing AEDs: carbamazepine (CBZ), phenytoin (PHT), and phenobarbital (21–23). The *dose-response* study compared the efficacy, safety, and tolerability of three different daily doses of TGB—16, 32, and 56 mg/day—with placebo (21). The *dose-frequency* study compared two different TGB dosing schedules of TGB—16 mg twice daily and 8 mg four times daily—with placebo (22). The third trial, a *thrice-daily dosing* study, compared TGB, 10 mg given three times daily, with placebo (23). Patients in both the treatment and placebo groups were well matched in all three studies, they had epilepsy for a median of 23 years, and they had taken a median of six AEDs in the past.

Overall, 90% of TGB-treated patients in the parallel-group, placebo-controlled, add-on trials experienced at least one side effect compared with 86% of patients who received placebo. The side effects that occurred significantly more often with TGB than with placebo were dizziness, asthenia (fatigue or generalized muscle weakness), nervousness, tremor, abnormal thinking (difficulty in concentrating, mental lethargy, or slowness of thought), depression, aphasia (dysarthria, difficulty speaking, or speech arrest), and abdominal pain (24) (Figure 76.1). Most of the side effects were mild or moderate, occurred during titration, and resolved spontaneously.

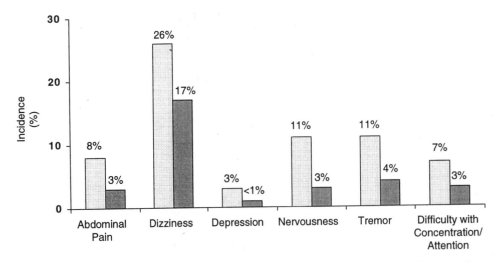

FIGURE 76.1. Tiagabine adverse effects in double-blind, placebo-controlled add-on studies: adverse effects that emerged during treatment with tiagabine and statistically higher than placebo. All patients were also concomitantly receiving one to three enzyme-inducing antiepileptic drugs. *Dark bar,* placebo; *light bar,* tiagabine.

More pronounced side effects were recorded for 9% of patients who received TGB and for 5% of patients who received placebo. The most common of these were somnolence, asthenia, and headache (25). A total of 13% of patients who received TGB withdrew from studies prematurely because of side effects, compared with 5% of those who received placebo. The most common reasons for premature withdrawal were confusion (1.4%), somnolence (1.2%), ataxia (<1%), and dizziness (<1%) (24).

A total of 12% of TGB-treated patients and 13% of placebo-treated patients in the three double-blind, parallel, add-on studies had an increase of ≥50% in their partial seizures (26). Complex or simple partial status epilepticus occurred in 4 of 494 (0.8%) of the TGB recipients and in 4 of 275 (1.5%) of the placebo recipients, findings similar to the expected incidence for the population studied. Convulsive status did not occur (27).

Weakness was noted in 21 of 494 (4%) of the TGB-treated patients as compared with 3 of 275 (1%) of the placebo-treated patients. This effect appeared to be dose related. There were no treatment-related differences with regard to possible psychotic events (1 of 275 placebo; 4 of 494 TGB), rash, hematologic and biochemical test results, electrocardiograms, and vital signs (25). Neuropsychologic testing did not reveal any evidence of worsening in tests of cognitive abilities, adjustment, and mood in the dose-response study (28) or in the thrice-daily dosing study (29). Finally, the incidence of sudden unexpected death resulting from epilepsy was similar among TGB-treated patients compared with incidences reported for the other new AEDs (package insert).

An adjunctive double-blind study compared the efficacy, safety, and tolerability of adding TGB to either CBZ or PHT with the combination of CBZ and PHT. TGB in combination with either CBZ or PHT was better tolerated than the combination of CBZ and PHT and had similar efficacy (30). Adjunctive TGB had no significant effects on total body weight (31) or on abilities, adjustment, and mood compared with adjunctive CBZ or PHT (32). Further, the overall health costs of add-on TGB when calculated with a cost-effectiveness clinical decision analysis model were very favorable when compared with the combination of PHT and CBZ, despite the higher acquisition cost of TGB (33).

Open Adjunctive Trials

Numerous trials have evaluated the long-term tolerability and safety of TGB, including extensions of the placebo-controlled, add-on studies and other trials that enrolled patients with uncontrolled seizures of any type. Leppik et al. reviewed the long-term exposure data for nearly 3,100 patients, including 541 patients with exposures over 36 months and 1,274 patients who had received TGB for at least 12 months (24). Daily TGB doses averaged between 24 and 60 mg. Among patients exposed for at least 12 months, 11% took at least 80 mg daily. Side effects reported by ≥10% patients during long-term treatment included dizziness, somnolence, asthenia, headache, tremor, nervousness, difficulty with concentration or attention, confusion, ataxia, insomnia, nystagmus, depression, amnesia, speech disorder, paresthesia, and incoordination (24). These side effects tended to occur during the first 6 months of treatment and seldom caused patients to withdraw from the study (34). Further, side effects among 674 patients treated for ≤54 months tended to diminish over extended periods (35). No new side effects or laboratory abnormalities occurred in these long-term studies (24,36).

Because of reports of fixed concentric visual field defects occurring in patients treated with vigabatrin, which is another γ-aminobutyric acid (GABA)–ergic AED, though pharmacologically different (37), the preapproval TGB safety database was scanned for adverse events that were suggestive of symptomatic visual field loss. Of the eight patients who had visual symptoms, two had field defects from fixed lesions (temporal lobe resection, cortical infarct), and six had transient visual complaints. Examination did not disclose any fixed visual defects (38).

In a series of infants with infantile spasms, TGB treatment was associated with a >50% seizure reduction in six of 11 (39). Irritability was noted in nine of 11 infants; in seven of the nine, irritability improved with time or with TGB dose reduction.

Monotherapy Trials

A dose-ranging, TGB-substitution study and a high-dose versus low-dose study evaluated the feasibility of converting to TGB monotherapy and the efficacy, safety, and tolerability of TGB as monotherapy, respectively. The dose-ranging study was designed to determine the maximum tolerated dose of TGB as monotherapy for patients with complex partial seizures (median duration, 19.5 years) not adequately controlled with one AED (40). The 31 enrolled patients had taken a mean of 5.1 AEDs in the past. Twelve patients completed the study and were taking a median TGB dose of 38.4 mg/day (range, 24 to 54 mg). Asthenia, dizziness, difficulty in concentrating, insomnia, nervousness, somnolence, and impaired memory were the most common side effects.

The high-dose versus low-dose study was a multicenter, double-blind, randomized, parallel-group trial in which patients with complex partial seizures and with or without secondarily generalized tonic-clonic seizures were randomized to TGB either 6 or 36 mg/day (14). Speech disorder, somnolence, and blurred vision (amblyopia) occurred statistically significantly more often with TGB 36 mg/day than with TGB 6 mg/day (41). Compared with baseline, the neuropsychological tests of adjustment and mood showed improvement in those patients who received TGB 6 mg/day, and tests of abilities showed improvement in patients treated with TGB 36 mg/day (42). However, the relative contributions of TGB, improved seizure control, and discontinuation of baseline AEDs to these improvements could not be determined.

Another randomized, parallel-group monotherapy study compared TGB and CBZ as initial monotherapy in patients with newly diagnosed partial epilepsy. Neuropsychological testing, administered at baseline and after 6 months of treatment, found no evidence of TGB-related worsening of verbal ability, memory performance, attention, or reaction times (43).

POSTMARKETING EXPERIENCE

TGB was approved in France and Denmark in 1996 and in the United States in 1997. As of December, 2000 over 80,000 people had been treated with TGB without any reports of severe, life-threatening reactions attributable to the drug. Clinical experience seems to suggest some patients can tolerate TGB better when a slow titration schedule is used (44).

Two postmarketing studies evaluated visual fields in TGB-treated patients. In one study, eight patients (mean daily dose, 56 mg) treated for at least 1 year (mean duration, 43 months) showed no changes on visual field testing with the Goldmann and Humphrey methods other than changes attributable to previous brain surgery (45). In the other study, none of 40 TGB-treated patients had abnormalities on Goldmann perimetry or ophthalmologic evaluation suggestive of concentric field constriction (44).

Several case reports of serious adverse events possibly attributable to TGB have been published, including one case each of symptomatic thrombocytopenia (46), complex partial status epilepticus (47), and absence status in a patient with a previous history of absence seizures and primary generalized tonic-clonic seizures (48). Other cases of nonconvulsive status epilepticus, with generalized spike–wave electroencephalographic (EEG) abnormalities seen during some of the events, were published (49,50), as well as two cases of partial status epilepticus in a single-blind dose-escalating study (51). In two TGB-treated patients ultimately shown to have nonepileptic seizures, investigation with continuous EEG or EEG-video monitoring during prolonged episodes of stupor was consistent with toxic encephalopathy (52). The incidence of symptoms consistent with nonconvulsive status epilepticus in blinded trials was statistically equivalent among patients who received TGB and those who received placebo, so the clinical importance of isolated reports in patients with partial epilepsy is unclear. Caution appears to be warranted in patients with generalized epilepsy, however.

The safety of TGB during pregnancy is unknown. As of April, 1999, 26 pregnancies in TGB-treated women were reported (*data on file*, Abbott Laboratories, Abbott Park, IL). Eleven patients carried their pregnancies to term: 10 gave birth to healthy babies, and the baby of the eleventh patient had hip displacement resulting from a breech presentation. Of the 15 other patients, seven had elective abortions, five had miscarriages, one had a blighted ovum, one had an ectopic pregnancy, and one died of a cerebral neoplasm that predated the TGB therapy. The outcome of one pregnancy was not determined.

TGB overdoses ≤800 mg were reported in 47 patients as of April, 1999 (*data on file*, Abbott Laboratories, Abbott Park, IL). All patients recovered with supportive care; one patient who took 400 mg developed convulsive status epilepticus that responded to phenobarbital. Others were noted to have somnolence, impaired consciousness, confusion, agitation, hostility, lethargy, weakness, depressed mood, speech difficulty, and myoclonus. As with other AEDs, discontinuation of TGB should be undertaken slowly, although neither pharmacodynamic tolerance to TGB nor withdrawal seizures have been documented.

TGB serum concentrations can be measured by high-performance liquid chromatography (53), but their clinical utility is uncertain because of the short serum half-life of TGB in induced patients and its high protein binding, and the relationship between serum concentration and side effects has not been demonstrated. Routine monitoring of liver, renal, and bone marrow function does not appear to be necessary.

SUMMARY

Controlled studies have established the safety and tolerability of adjunctive TGB, 30 to 56 mg/day. The side effect profile is generally favorable; neurotoxic symptoms typically occur during the early phases of treatment and can be lessened by a slow titration rate and by taking TGB with food. No significant effects of TGB on systemic function or weight have been documented, and the drug has no significant cognitive, affective, and psychiatric effects. Postmarketing reports of nonconvulsive status epilepticus suggest that TGB treatment should be avoided in patients with a history of generalized epilepsy. Long-term TGB therapy does not appear to affect visual fields. There have been too few pregnancies in women treated with TGB to draw any conclusions about its effects, if any, on developing fetuses.

In the future, head-to-head trials that compare the tolerability of TGB with other AEDs as first add-on treatment should be performed to help establish the place of TGB in the overall treatment of seizures for patients who do not achieve optimum results from initial therapy. Although patients who have medically refractory epilepsy can change to TGB monotherapy, more controlled studies are necessary to confirm the side effect profile of TGB as monotherapy.

REFERENCES

1. Mattson RH, Cramer JA, Collins JF, et al. Comparison of carbamazepine, phenobarbital, phenytoin, and primidone in partial and secondarily generalized tonic-clonic seizures. *N Engl J Med* 1985;313:145–151.
2. Schachter SC. Update in the treatment of epilepsy. *Compr Ther* 1995;21:473–479.
3. Schachter SC. Treatment of seizures. In: Schachter SC, Schomer DL, eds. *The comprehensive evaluation and treatment of epilepsy.* San Diego: Academic Press, 1997:61–74.
4. Schachter SC. Antiepileptic drug therapy: general treatment principles and application for special patient populations. *Epilepsia* 1999;40[Suppl 9]:S20–S25.
5. Mengel H, Gustavson LE, Soerensen HJ, et al. Effect of food on the bioavailability of tiagabine HCl. *Epilepsia* 1991;32 [Suppl 3]:S6.
6. Bopp BA, Nequist GE, Rodrigues AD. Role of the cytochrome P450 3A subfamily in the metabolism of [¹⁴C] tiagabine by human hepatic microsomes. *Epilepsia* 1995;36[Suppl 3]:S159.
7. Lau AH, Gustavson LE, Sperelakis R, et al. Pharmacokinetics and safety of tiagabine in subjects with various degrees of hepatic function. *Epilepsia* 1997;38:445–451.
8. Østergaard LH, Gram L, Dam M. Potential antiepileptic drugs: tiagabine. In: Levy RH, Mattson RH, Meldrum BS, ed. *Antiepileptic drugs,* 4th ed. New York: Raven Press, 1995: 1057–1061.
9. Bopp B, Gustavson L, Johnson M, et al. Pharmacokinetics and metabolism of [¹⁴C tiagabine] after oral administration to human subjects. *Epilepsia* 1995;36[Suppl 3]:S158.
10. Cato A, Gustavson LE, Quian J, et al. Effect of renal impairment on the pharmacokinetics and tolerability of tiagabine. *Epilepsia* 1998;39:43–47.
11. Gustavson LE, Mengel HB. Pharmacokinetics of tiagabine, a gamma-aminobutyric acid-uptake inhibitor, in healthy subjects after single and multiple doses. *Epilepsia* 1995;36:605–6l1.
12. Samara EE, Gustavson LE, El-Shourbagy T, et al. Population analysis of the pharmacokinetics of tiagabine in patients with epilepsy. *Epilepsia* 1998;39:868–873.
13. Brodie MJ. Tiagabine pharmacology in profile. *Epilepsia* 1995;36 [Suppl 6]:S7–S9.
14. Schachter SC. Tiagabine monotherapy in the treatment of partial epilepsy. *Epilepsia* 1995;36[Suppl 6]:S2–S6.
15. Kastberg H, Jansen JA, Cole G, et al. Tiagabine: absence of kinetic or dynamic interactions with ethanol. *Drug Metabol Drug Interact* 1998;14:259–273.
16. Mengel H, Jansen IA, Sommerville K, et al. Tiagabine: evaluation of the risk of interaction with theophylline, warfarin, digoxin, cimetidine, oral contraceptives, triazolam, or ethanol. *Epilepsia* 1995;36[Suppl 3]:S160.
17. Schmitt U, Luddens H, Hiemke C. Behavioral effects of GABA(A) receptor stimulation and GABA-transporter inhibition. *Pharmacol Biochem Behav* 2000;65:351–356.
18. Richens A, Chadwick DW, Duncan JS, et al. Adjunctive treatment of partial seizures with tiagabine: a placebo-controlled trial. *Epilepsy Res* 1995;21:37–42.
19. Lassen LC, Sommerville K, Mengel HB, et al. Summary of five controlled trials with tiagabine as adjunctive treatment of patients with partial seizures. *Epilepsia* 1995;36[Suppl 3]:S148.
20. Ben-Menachem E. International experience with tiagabine add-on therapy. *Epilepsia* 1995;36[Suppl 6]:S14–S21.
21. Uthman BM, Rowan AJ, Ahmann PA, et al. Tiagabine for complex partial seizures: a randomized, add-on, dose-response trial. *Arch Neurol* 1998;55:56–62.
22. Sachdeo RC, Leroy RF, Krauss GL, et al. Tiagabine therapy for complex partial seizures. *Arch Neurol* 1997;54:595–601.
23. Kalviainen R, Brodie MJ, Duncan J, et al. A double-blind, placebo-controlled trial of tiagabine given three-times daily as add-on therapy for refractory partial seizures. *Epilepsy Res* 1998; 30:31–40.
24. Leppik LE, Gram L, Deaton R, et al. Safety of tiagabine: summary of 53 trials. *Epilepsy Res* 1999;33:235–246.
25. Schachter SC. Therapeutic choices and decisions. Paper presented at the 22ⁿᵈ International Epilepsy Congress, Dublin, 1997.
26. Somerville E, Sommerville KW, Lyby K. Lack of aggravation of epilepsy by tiagabine. *Epilepsia* 1998;39[Suppl 6]:S146.
27. Shinnar S, Berg AT, Treiman DM, et al. Status epilepticus and tiagabine therapy: review of safety data and epidemiologic comparisons. *Epilepsia* 2001;42:372–379.

28. Dodrill CB, Arnett JL, Sommerville KW, Shu V. Cognitive and quality of life effects of differing dosages of tiagabine in epilepsy. *Neurology* 1997;48:1025–1031.

29. Kalviainen R, Aikia M, Mervaala E, et al. Long-term cognitive and BEG effects of tiagabine in drug-resistant partial epilepsy. *Epilepsy Res* 1996;25:291–297.

30. Biton V, Vasquez B, Sachdeo JC, et al. Adjunctive tiagabine compared to phenytoin and carbamazepine in the multicenter, double-blind trial of complex partial seizures. *Epilepsia* 1998;39 [Suppl 6]:S125–S126.

31. Hogan RE, Bertrand ME, Deaton RL, et al. Total percentage body weight changes during add-on therapy with tiagabine, carbamazepine and phenytoin. *Epilepsy Res* 2000;41:23–28.

32. Dodrill CB, Arnett JL, Deaton R, et al. Tiagabine versus phenytoin and carbamazepine as add-on therapies: effects on abilities, adjustment, and mood. *Epilepsy Res* 2000;42:123–132.

33. Schachter SC, Sommerville KW, Ryan JE. A cost-effectiveness analysis of tiagabine, phenytoin, and carbamazepine adjunctive therapy for patients with complex partial seizures. *Neurology* 1999;52[Suppl 2]:A143.

34. Sommerville KW, Hearell M, Deaton R, et al. Adverse events with long-term tiagabine therapy. *Epilepsia* 1997;38[Suppl 8]:S106.

35. Bergen D, Deaton R, Sommerville KW. The incidence and prevalence of common adverse events in a long-term trial of tiagabine (Gabitril, TGB). *Neurology* 1999;52[Suppl 2]:A236–237.

36. Leppik LE. Tiagabine: the safety landscape. *Epilepsia* 1995;36 [Suppl 6]:S10–S13.

37. Sills GJ, Butler E, Thompson GG, et al. Vigabatrin and tiagabine are pharmacologically different drugs: a pre-clinical study. *Seizure* 1999;8:404–411.

38. Collins SD, Brun S, Kirstein YG, et al. Absence of visual field defects in patients taking tiagabine. *Epilepsia* 1998;39[Suppl 6]:S146–S147.

39. Kugler SL, Mandelbaum DE, Patel R, et al. Efficacy and tolerability of tiagabine in infantile spasms. *Epilepsia* 1999;40[Suppl 7]:S127.

40. Schachter SC, Cahill WT, Wannamaker BB, et al. Open-label dosage and tolerability study of tiagabine monotherapy in patients with refractory complex partial seizures. *Epilepsy* 1998; 11:248–255.

41. Brodie MJ. A monotherapy approach with tiagabine. Paper presented at the 22nd International Epilepsy Congress, Dublin, 1997.

42. Dodrill CB, Arnett JL, Shu V, et al. Effects of tiagabine monotherapy on abilities, adjustment, and mood. *Epilepsia* 1998; 39:33–42.

43. Aikia M, Kalviainen R, Jutila L, et al. Cognitive effects of initial tiagabine monotherapy. *Epilepsia* 1999;40[Suppl 2]:S99.

44. Kalviainen R, Salmenpera T, Jutila L, et al. Tiagabine monotherapy in chronic partial epilepsy. *Epilepsia* 1999;40[Suppl 2]:S258.

45. Fakhoury TA, Abou-Khalil B, Lavin P. Lack of visual field defects with long-term use of tiagabine. *Neurology* 2000;54[Suppl 3]:A309.

46. Willert C, Englisch S, Schlesinger S, et al. Possible drug-induced thrombocytopenia secondary to tiagabine. *Neurology* 1999;52:889–891.

47. Trinka B, Moroder T, Nagler M, et al. Clinical and EEG findings in complex partial status epilepticus with tiagabine. *Seizure* 1999;8:41–44.

48. Knake S, Hamer HM, Schomburg U, et al. Tiagabine-induced absence status in idiopathic generalized epilepsy. *Seizure* 1999;8:314–317.

49. Ettinger AB, Bernal OG, Andriola MR, et al. Two cases of nonconvulsive status epilepticus in association with tiagabine therapy. *Epilepsia* 1999;40:1159–1162.

50. Eckardt KM, Steinhoff BJ. Nonconvulsive status epilepticus in two patients receiving tiagabine treatment. *Epilepsia* 1998;39:671–674.

51. Uldall P, Bulteau C, Pedersen SA, et al. Tiagabine adjunctive therapy in children with refractory epilepsy: a single-blind dose escalating study. *Epilepsy Res* 2000;42:159–168.

52. Abou-Khalil BW. Tiagabine-related stupor: evidence for a nonepileptic origin. *Neurology* 2000;54[Suppl 3]:A194.

53. Gustavson LE, Chu SY. High performance liquid chromatographic procedure for the determination of tiagabine concentrations in human plasma using electrochemical detection. *J Chromatogr* 1992;574:313–318.

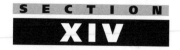

TOPIRAMATE

TOPIRAMATE

MECHANISMS OF ACTION

H. STEVE WHITE

Topiramate, a sulfamate-substituted derivative of D-fructose, has been demonstrated to possess anticonvulsant activity in a battery of well-defined animal models (Table 77.1). Topiramate is highly effective in blocking maximal electroshock seizures in rats and mice (39,50), but it is inactive against clonic seizures induced by subcutaneous administration of the chemoconvulsants pentylenetetrazol, picrotoxin, or bicuculline (39,50). Topiramate does elevate the pentylenetetrazol seizure threshold at low doses; however, this effect is reduced at higher doses of topiramate (57). In addition, topiramate has been shown to be effective against fully kindled seizures in the amygdala-kindled rat model of partial seizures. These findings in animal models support the results of clinical trials in which topiramate has been shown to be effective against both partial and generalized seizures.

Several pharmacologic properties have been identified that may account for the broad anticonvulsant preclinical profile of topiramate in animal models. For example, the drug has been found to modulate voltage-dependent sodium ion (Na^+) channels, to potentiate γ-aminobutyric acid (GABA)–mediated inhibitory neurotransmission, to block excitatory neurotransmission mediated by non–N-methyl-D-aspartate (non-NMDA) receptors, to modulate voltage-gated calcium ion (Ca^{2+}) channels, and to inhibit brain carbonic anhydrase (CA).

This chapter reviews the evidence supporting the multiple mechanisms of action thus far identified for topiramate and briefly considers the therapeutic potential of topiramate in other disease states in which the underlying pathophysiologic features suggest a role for the drug.

H. Steve White, PhD: Professor, Department of Pharmacology and Toxicology, and Director, Anticonvulsant Screening Project, University of Utah, Salt Lake City, Utah

EFFECTS OF TOPIRAMATE IN EXPERIMENTAL MODELS OF EPILEPSY

Maximal Electroshock

Early investigations demonstrated that topiramate, like carbamazepine and phenytoin, possesses the ability to block tonic hind-limb extension seizures induced by maximal electroshock (MES). In the MES test in mice and rats, the potency of topiramate after oral administration was found to be similar to that of carbamazepine, phenytoin, phenobarbitone, and acetazolamide, but it was greater than that of sodium valproate (13,39). Peak anticonvulsant activity was reached within 1 hour in mice and between 1 and 4 hours in the rat, with a duration of activity of >4 and >8 hours in mice and rats, respectively (39). These observations suggest that topiramate acts primarily by blocking the spread of seizures and in this respect shares an anticonvulsant mechanism similar to that of carbamazepine and phenytoin, that is, state-dependent block of voltage-sensitive Na^+ channels (39).

Intravenous Pentylenetetrazol

Early studies found topiramate to be virtually ineffective in preventing seizures induced by *subcutaneous* injection of pentylenetetrazol or other chemicals such as bicuculline, picrotoxin, or metrazol (39,50). However, topiramate was subsequently found to elevate seizure threshold in the *intravenous* pentylenetetrazol test in mice (57), an effect that also indicated possible clinical activity against generalized seizures (55).

Genetic (Spontaneous Epileptic Rat and DBA/2 Mouse) and Amygdala Kindling Models

Studies in the spontaneously epileptic rat demonstrated that topiramate is effective against both tonic extension and spike–wave seizures (30). Topiramate has also been found to

TABLE 77.1. ANTICONVULSANT PROFILE OF TOPIRAMATE IN ANIMAL SEIZURE AND EPILEPSY MODELS

Model	Species	Seizure Stimulus	Seizure Type	Dosing Route	ED50 (mgkg)
MES	Mouse	Electrical	Tonic	i.p.	?
				p.o.	?
MES	Rat	Electrical	Tonic	i.p.	?
				p.o.	?
Spontaneous epileptic rat	Rat	Tactile	Tonic	i.p.	~10
			Spike wave	i.p.	~10
Audiogenic seizures (DBA/2)	Mouse	Auditory	Tonic	p.o.	3.5
			Clonic	p.o.	8.6
Ischemia-induced	Rat	Auditory	Tonic	p.o.	8.2
			Clonic	p.o.	13.0
			Wild running	p.o.	36.1
Amygdala-kindled	Rat	Electrical	Forelimb clonus	p.o.	7.3
			Afterdischarge duration	p.o.	7.1

MES, maximal electroshock; i.p., intraperitoneal; p.o., oral; ED$_{50}$, median effective dose.
From Shank RP, Gardocki IF, Streeter AJ, et al. An overview of the preclinical aspects of topiramate: pharmacology, pharmacokinetics, and mechanisms of action. *Epilepsia* 2000;41[Suppl 1]:S3–S9, with permission.

be effective in blocking audiogenic seizures in the DBA/2 audiogenic seizure-susceptible mouse (30).

In addition, topiramate has been found to be highly effective in various kindling models including mouse (18), rat (18,53), rabbit (18), and cat (29). In the amygdala-kindled rat model, topiramate was found to be more effective than phenytoin (1,53). In this model, topiramate displayed a potent and dose-dependent inhibition of all measured seizure parameters (behavioral seizures, forelimb clonus, amygdala, and cortical afterdischarges). Reissmüller and colleagues (36) evaluated the anticonvulsant efficacy of topiramate in phenytoin-resistant amygdala-kindled rats, a relatively new and unique model of drug resistant partial epilepsy (24). In phenytoin responders, topiramate (40 mg/kg) increased the afterdischarge threshold and decreased seizure severity and duration. Consistent with the proven clinical efficacy of topiramate in patients with refractory partial epilepsy, topiramate also significantly increased the afterdischarge threshold in phenytoin-resistant kindled rats. Finally, topiramate, in addition to blocking the expression of fully kindled seizures, significantly delayed the acquisition of amygdaloid kindling at doses of 100 and 200 mg/kg (1).

PROPOSED MECHANISMS OF ACTION

Topiramate has been evaluated in numerous *in vitro* assays in an attempt to identify the molecular mechanisms of action underlying its broad preclinical and clinical spectrum of activity. These investigations suggest that topiramate possesses activity at various voltage- and receptor-gated ion channels that may account for its *in vivo* activity.

Blockade of Voltage-Sensitive Sodium Channels

The first electrophysiologic studies investigating the mechanisms responsible for the anticonvulsant activity of topiramate were conducted in cultured rat hippocampal neurons (6). At concentrations ranging from 10 to 100 μmol/L, topiramate reversibly reduced the duration and frequency of action potentials within spontaneous epileptiform bursts of neuronal firing. Topiramate, like carbamazepine and phenytoin (26), was also found to block depolarization-induced sustained repetitive firing (SRF), a finding thereby suggesting activity at use-dependent, voltage-sensitive Na$^+$ channels (6,46). Subsequent studies found that topiramate was capable of reducing the duration and frequency of action potentials and of reducing the amplitude of inward voltage-gated Na$^+$ currents in rat cerebellar granule cells (2). Furthermore, topiramate was demonstrated to inhibit neuronal activity in the rat hippocampal slice preparation, in a frequency-dependent manner (58).

A series of whole-cell patch-clamp recordings in a range of preparations provided further evidence of an effect of topiramate on voltage-gated Na$^+$ channels. Zona and colleagues reported reduced amplitude of tetrodotoxin-sensitive, voltage-gated Na$^+$ currents when topiramate was applied to cerebellar granule cells (63). Voltage-gated Na$^+$ conductance was also reduced by topiramate in slice preparations of entorhinal cortex (3), as well as in dissociated neocortical neurons and neocortical slices (48).

Further insight into the modulatory effect of topiramate on voltage-dependent Na$^+$ channels is provided by an investigation using an *in vitro* seizure model of cultured hippocampal neurons wherein spontaneous recurrent seizures are evoked by depolarizing current injection (8). At concentrations of 10 μmol/L, topiramate produced a dose-dependent and partially reversible reduction in the frequency of action potentials induced by a sustained depolarizing current and abolished the late sustained phase of firing. Similarly, topiramate (10 to 100 μmol/L) decreased or abolished spontaneous recurrent seizures, with a marked reduction in both the number of bursts and the duration of epileptiform activity. These observations are consistent with topiramate's ability to modulate voltage-dependent Na^+ and Ca^{2+} (see later) conductances responsible for the generation and propagation of action potentials.

A further study showed that topiramate is capable of producing a voltage-sensitive, use-dependent, and time-dependent suppression of SRF in cultured mouse spinal cord and neocortical cells (28). However, the effect of topiramate in these preparations followed a complex pattern. For example, at concentrations ≥3 μmol/L, limitation of SRF was voltage-sensitive, time-dependent, and associated with a decrease in the rapid inward current during the upstroke of the action potential. At elevated concentrations (30 to 600 μmol/L), topiramate produced a rapid block of SRF in approximately one-third of neurons and did not affect SRF in a further one-third. Of the remaining one-third, SRF was limited in an intermittent fashion or was blocked only after a delay of a few seconds. As pointed out by the authors, the activity of topiramate on Na^+ channels differs from that of other antiepileptic drugs in which a rapid limitation or complete block of SRF occurs. Based on these findings, the authors concluded that although topiramate appears to exert some of its anticonvulsant effects by blocking voltage-sensitive, use-dependent Na^+ channels, it does so by a mechanism that seems to differ from that of classic Na^+ channel blocking antiepileptic drugs such as phenytoin, carbamazepine, and lamotrigine. As such, it has been suggested that Na^+ channel blockade may not be the primary mechanism by which topiramate exerts its anticonvulsant activity (28).

Enhancement of GABA-Evoked Chloride Currents

Topiramate has also been demonstrated to potentiate GABAergic transmission. Topiramate (10 to 100 μmol/L) was originally found to enhance GABA-induced chloride (Cl^-) flux into cultured mouse cerebellar granule cells (5). Subsequent studies demonstrated that topiramate rapidly and reversibly increased the frequency of opening of GABA-mediated Cl^- channels in mouse cortical neurons at 1 to 30 μmol/L (54). At concentrations of 1 to 30 μmol/L, topiramate increased bursting frequency and the frequency of channel opening but did not affect the duration of channel open time. The effects of topiramate on $GABA_A$ channel kinetics suggest that the drug is acting much like a ben-

zodiazepine; however, topiramate's ability to enhance $GABA_A$-mediated Cl^- currents is not blocked by the benzodiazepine antagonist, flumazenil (54). In addition, topiramate has been shown to enhance $GABA_A$-mediated Cl^- currents in clonazepam-insensitive neurons and to be ineffective in some clonazepam-sensitive neuronal populations (57) These findings have suggested that topiramate may exert its positive modulatory effects by binding to a different site on the GABA receptor or to a novel site on the $GABA_A$ receptor complex. Furthermore, clonazepam-induced elevation of pentylenetetrazol seizure threshold was reversed by the benzodiazepine antagonist flumazenil, whereas topiramate-induced elevation of seizure threshold was not.

To investigate the modulatory effects of topiramate on various $GABA_A$ receptor subtypes further, Gordey and colleagues (15) expressed specific subunits of the $GABA_A$ receptor in *Xenopus* oocytes. Topiramate reversibly inhibited GABA-evoked Cl^- currents in oocytes expressing the $GABA_A$ receptor subunits $\alpha1\beta2\gamma2S$ and $\alpha2\beta2\gamma2S$, it potentiated currents in oocytes expressing the $\alpha2\beta2\gamma2S$ subunit combination, but it had no effect on oocytes containing $\alpha4\beta2\gamma2S$ $GABA_A$ receptors. The observed negative modulatory effect of topiramate on Cl^- currents (as mediated by the $\alpha1\beta2\gamma2S$ and $\alpha2\beta2\gamma2S$ receptors) is a novel finding—all other studies reported to date found only a positive modulatory effect whereby topiramate increases GABA-induced Cl^- currents (5,56). Although no obvious explanation exists, the investigators hypothesized that topiramate may modulate GABA activity through desensitization of $GABA_A$ receptors, possibly by effects on secondary messenger systems. Additional findings using the *Xenopus* oocyte expression system have further demonstrated that the effects of topiramate on the $GABA_A$ receptor system are subunit selective. Simeone and colleagues (44) reported that $GABA_A$ receptors containing α_4, β_3, and γ_2S subunits are particularly sensitive to direct activation with topiramate at concentrations as low as 10 μmol/L.

Additional findings that may or may not be associated with the modulatory effects of topiramate on GABAergic transmission relate to the detection of increased GABA concentrations in the brain after topiramate administration. One study, using a low-resolution Tesla magnetic resonance spectrometer, detected increased brain concentrations of GABA in humans after the administration of topiramate (32). However, further investigation in rats failed to support this observation (43). Both single and multiple doses of topiramate were without effect on GABA brain concentration in the rat. The investigators noted that although topiramate was detectable in the brain after a dose of ≥10 mg/kg, there was no accumulation of GABA in the retina or in any of the other brain regions analyzed. Further studies are required to replicate the initial findings in human brains using high-resolution Tesla magnets.

Effects on Glutamate-Mediated Excitatory Neurotransmission

The excitatory neurotransmitter glutamate exerts its excitatory actions by binding to both ionotropic (NMDA, α-amino-3-hydroxy-5-methyl-4-isoxazole propionic acid [AMPA], and kainate) and metabotropic (mGluR$_{1-8}$) glutamate receptors. In addition to the actions described earlier, topiramate has been found to exert a negative modulatory effect on kainate-elicited excitatory currents. This activity was first described after a series of electrophysiologic studies using cultured rat hippocampal neurons. Coulter and colleagues (6,7,38) reported that topiramate (10 to 100 µmol/L) blocked membrane currents evoked by kainate but had no activity at the NMDA-mediated glutamate receptor subtype. Subsequent studies demonstrated that topiramate exerts a biphasic effect on kainate-evoked currents (14). Thus, topiramate was found to produce an initial (phase I), followed by a delayed (phase II), inhibition of kainate currents. The delayed phase II effect was observed after the constant application of topiramate for >10 minutes, and it was not readily reversed during a 2- to 4-hour topiramate washout period. The authors postulated that the delayed effect may be associated with an alteration of the phosphorylation state of kainate-activated channels. Consistent with this hypothesis is the finding that treatment of channels with dibutyryl cyclic adenosine monophosphate enhanced reversal of the phase II topiramate block. In addition, the phase II block, but not the phase I block, was prevented by the nonspecific protein phosphatase inhibitor okadaic acid.

Topiramate was subsequently found to inhibit kainate-evoked inhibition of cobalt (Co^{2+}) flux into cultured cerebellar granule neurons in a concentration- and time-dependent manner (45). In these studies, maximal inhibition of kainate-stimulated Co^{2+} flux was observed after 30-minute pretreatment with topiramate. In addition, the effect of topiramate appeared to depend on the developmental stage of the cerebellar granule cells. For example, topiramate inhibited kainate-stimulated Co^{2+} uptake in cells grown *in vitro* for 9 to 11 days, but it was without effect in older neurons (13 to 14 days). In contrast, the non-NMDA antagonist DNQX was effective at all ages and did not require pretreatment. These findings are of interest because they suggest that topiramate exerts a negative modulatory effect on a Ca^{2+}-permeable non-NMDA receptor that is developmentally regulated.

A further effect of topiramate on glutamate was observed in microdialysis studies in which the drug reduced abnormally high (two- to threefold higher) basal hippocampal concentrations of glutamate and aspartate by approximately 45% in spontaneously epileptic rats (16). In contrast, topiramate had no effect on hippocampal concentrations of other amino acid neurotransmitters, including GABA, taurine, and glycine (16,39).

Negative Modulatory Effect on Neuronal L-Type High-Voltage–Activated Calcium Channels

In addition to the mechanisms outlined earlier, a growing body of evidence suggests that topiramate modulates neuronal Ca^{2+} channels. Activity has been demonstrated at both N- and L-type high-voltage–activated Ca^{2+} channels (HVACCs) in CAl pyramidal neurons using whole-cell patch-clamp techniques in rat dentate gyrus granule cells (61,62). After separation of the different HVACCs into non–L-type and L-type channels, topiramate was tested at concentrations of 1, 10, and 50 µmol/L. Although the drug was without effect at 1 µmol/L, topiramate 10 µmol/L consistently decreased the peak current and area under the curve of L-type Ca^{2+} currents. This effect typically occurred within 10 minutes of perfusion and was partially or fully reversible within 5 minutes of the removal of the drug from the bathing medium. At 50 µmol/L, topiramate was less effective in modifying Ca^{2+} currents, with a greater effect on peak current than area. Topiramate did not affect the voltage sensitivity or the gating properties of the L-type channels. This study provides further evidence of the diverse mechanisms by which topiramate appears to modulate neuronal excitability and suggests that an inhibitory effect on L-type HVACCs is another potential anticonvulsant mechanism.

That topiramate produced a biphasic concentration–response curve, in which a greater reduction in L-type Ca^{2+} currents was seen at l0 µmol/L than at 50µmol/L, suggests a mode of action different from other Ca^{2+} channel blockers. Zhang and colleagues hypothesized that an indirect modulation of L-type HVACCs may occur through effects on intracellular second messenger systems or neurotransmitter receptors. Indeed, emerging evidence suggests that topiramate may bind to phosphorylation sites within AMPA, kainate, GABA$_A$, and voltage-activated Na$^+$ channels (40). Furthermore, HVACCs are partly regulated by protein phosphorylation, and the HVACC phosphorylation site has an amino acid sequence similar to those of the Na$^+$ channel, GABA$_A$ receptor, and AMPA-kainate receptor (40). Whether this accounts for the U-shaped concentration curve observed in these studies is not known at the present time but is currently under investigation.

Inhibition of Carbonic Anhydrase Isoenzymes

At concentrations between 1 and 10 µmol/L, topiramate weakly inhibits the CA isoenzymes CA II and CA IV. When compared with acetazolamide, topiramate is approximately 10 to 100 times less potent as an inhibitor of these isoenzymes (9,39). Topiramate, like the antiepileptic drug and CA inhibitor acetazolamide, contains a sulfamate moiety that is likely to be responsible for its CA-inhibiting properties. Although inhibition of CA is generally not considered

TABLE 77.2. PROPOSED MECHANISMS OF ACTION OF TOPIRAMATE

Site	Action	Consequence
Voltage-activated Na⁺ channels (63)	State-dependent blockade	Stabilizes neuronal membranes and reduces sustained repetitive firing; reduces release of excitatory neurotransmitters
GABA$_A$ receptor subtype(s) (57)	Allosteric modulator of some GABA$_A$ receptors; subunit selective	Potentiates GABA-mediated inhibitory neurotransmission at sites unaffected by benzodiazepines or barbiturates
Glutamate receptor subtypes (kainate and AMPA) (45)	Inhibits kainate-evoked currents	Reduces excitatory neurotransmission through non-NMDA neurons
Ca^{2+} channel subtypes (61,62)	Reduces amplitude of high-voltage–activated Ca^{2+} currents	Reduces neurotransmitter release and inhibits Ca^{2+}-dependent second-messenger systems
Carbonic anhydrase (9)	Inhibits type II and type IV, carbon anhydrase	Modulates pH-dependent activation of voltage- and receptor-gated ion channels

GABA, γ-aminobutyric acid; AMPA, α-amino-3-hydroxy-5-methyl-4-isoxazole propionate; NMDA, N-methyl-D-aspartate.

to represent a significant anticonvulsant mechanism of topiramate, the possibility remains that this inhibition may contribute to its anticonvulsant action by modulation of pH-dependent voltage- and receptor-gated ion channels. For example, the increase in metabolic activity after high-frequency neuronal firing results in an increase in the intracellular concentration of bicarbonate that can alter net current flux and produce membrane depolarization (23,47). Given that the excitatory effect of bicarbonate may occur in the hippocampus, where some forms of epilepsy originate, it can be hypothesized that inhibitors of CA will block the excitation. The proposed mechanisms of action of topiramate are summarized in Table 77.2.

Evidence of Additional, Novel Mechanisms

Interaction with Protein Kinase Phosphorylation Sites

To date, topiramate has demonstrated activity at four main types of protein complex: voltage-activated Na⁺ channels; GABA$_A$ receptors, AMPA, and kainate receptors; and HVACCs and CA. The observed activity of topiramate at a wide range of ion channels and receptors, together with variable responses in different *in vitro* studies and preparations, has led to a hypothesis concerning an underlying common mechanism by which topiramate exerts its effects. Although each of the foregoing effects is reproducible, investigators have also observed a variable response to topiramate. For example, some studies report reversible effects, whereas others fail to observe a readily reversible action of topiramate. Topiramate's action has also been reported to be both immediate and delayed in onset, depending on the preparation studied. One hypothesis that has been proposed to help understand the variability often observed from preparation to preparation and from investigator to investigator suggests that the action of topiramate depends

in part on the phosphorylation state of the receptor or ion channel (40).

In support of this hypothesis is the observation that the AMPA receptor, the GABA$_A$ receptor, the voltage sensitive sodium channel (VSSC), and the voltage-sensitive calcium channel (VSCC) are all regulated by protein phosphorylation mediated by protein kinase A, protein kinase C, and/or Ca^{2+}-CaM–activated kinases (21,37,42,52). Furthermore, the peptide sequence at the protein kinase A–mediated phosphorylation site displays homology among these four molecular targets. According to the hypothesis, topiramate, if bound to the dephosphorylated state of the channel and/or receptor, may shift the channel and/or receptor further toward the dephosphorylated state by preventing protein kinase A from binding to the phosphorylation site. The consequence of this would be a delayed effect on channel conductance. Should this hypothesis prove accurate, the activity of topiramate would be predicted to be inversely related to the degree of phosphorylation of the protein complex (40).

Neurotherapeutic Disease-Modifying Properties

The results of the studies described earlier demonstrate that topiramate exerts either direct or indirect effects on various receptor- and voltage-gated ion channels that control neuronal excitability. In addition to epilepsy, all these molecular targets of topiramate have been associated with the underlying pathologic features of numerous central nervous system (CNS) disorders and insult-induced neuronal damage and death. To date, topiramate has been found effective in models of status epilepticus (31), cerebral ischemia (59,60), hypoxia-induced cell damage and resultant seizures (19), and periventricular leukomalacia (12). These promising results suggest that topiramate may have future utility in conditions other than epilepsy, including cerebral infarction and hemorrhage, CNS trauma, neurodegenerative diseases such as Parkinson's disease and Alzheimer's disease, and neurologic conditions such as multiple sclerosis and encephalopathies. Furthermore, the similarities shared by epilepsy and certain CNS disorders, such as bipolar disorder, essential tremor, and migraine, and the diverse mechanisms of action of topiramate, provide a mechanistic basis supporting ongoing clinical trials in these and other disorders.

Investigators have suggested that GABAergic neurons may play a role in mood disorders, including both major depression and bipolar disorder. Preliminary evidence for this proposition came from a study in which progabide, a GABA agonist, was found to have a marked antidepressant effect (4). Further studies into the disease mechanisms involved in bipolar disorder (33,34) revealed that a kindling process occurs, presumed to be analogous to that seen in epilepsy. Patients initially experience mood-related episodes in response to life events, but eventually the neurologic and biochemical pathways responsible for these episodes are sufficiently reinforced to allow the autonomous initiation of further episodes. Because bipolar disorder and epilepsy are both episodic, it has been hypothesized that the anticonvulsant mechanisms of action of topiramate may also contribute to clinical activity in bipolar disorder. Indeed, results from an open-label study support ongoing clinical evaluation of topiramate in patients with mania (27).

Distinct similarities also exist between the pathophysiologic and biochemical processes responsible for epilepsy and neuropathic pain. In neuropathic pain, a phenomenon known as windup involves an increasing responsiveness to noxious stimuli in the pain-transmitting dorsal horn neurons and results in hyperexcitability of these neurons (49). This hyperexcitability then results in central sensitization, that is, an increased responsiveness of the spinal cord to neuronal pain impulses, which, in turn, leads to chronic pain at normally subthreshold levels of initial stimulation. In part, this hyperexcitability, similarly to kindling in epilepsy, results from activation of both NMDA and non-NMDA glutamate receptors by neuronally released glutamate, which can result from massive membrane depolarization mediated by VSSCs and VSCCs. From a mechanistic perspective, topiramate's demonstrated efficacy in a double-blind controlled study in diabetic neuropathy (10) could result from the drug's ability to normalize glutamate release (17), inhibit VSSCs and VSCCs, and block non-NMDA glutamate receptors.

Two further areas in which topiramate may be useful are essential tremor and migraine prophylaxis. Essential tremor is not yet widely understood at a pathophysiologic level, but it is thought that the illness may result from a dysfunction in GABA neurotransmission (25). Additional evidence suggests that inhibition of CA is a potentially useful strategy in this disorder (20). Because topiramate has distinct GABAergic actions and is also a weak inhibitor of CA, it may prove useful in essential tremor. Patients with migraine are also thought to benefit from drugs that act at GABAer-

gic neurons, a finding suggesting that topiramate may also be useful in this population. In fact, two double-blind trials (11,35) and three open-label studies with topiramate (41, 22,51) have shown that the drug is effective both in the prophylaxis of migraine (with or without aura) and in the treatment of cluster headaches.

SUMMARY

Investigations into the activity of topiramate in experimental epilepsy models and complementary electrophysiologic studies have suggested a range of mechanisms by which topiramate exerts its therapeutic effects. The broad anticonvulsant profile of topiramate that has emerged in both animal studies and clinical use is consistent with the multiple mechanisms of action described. Investigators have suggested that the effects of topiramate against SRF, voltage-sensitive Na^+ channels, and non-NMDA receptors possibly account for an ability to prevent seizure spread and efficacy against secondary generalized partial seizures. Likewise, enhancement of GABA-mediated inhibition by topiramate may contribute to elevation of seizure threshold and possible efficacy against spike–wave seizures and partial epilepsy.

Much of this chapter focuses on the proposed molecular activities relating to the anticonvulsant action of topiramate in children and adults. However, the same mechanisms may also contribute to the growing body of clinical data suggesting efficacy against many different CNS disorders including migraine, bipolar disorder, essential tremor, and diabetic neuropathy. Furthermore, given the similarities that have been identified between the molecular targets of topiramate and the underlying mechanisms of epileptogenesis, focal and global ischemia, and neonatal hypoxia, it seems reasonable, based on the data obtained to date, to suggest that topiramate may have potential disease-modifying properties.

As the specific molecular actions of topiramate are further elucidated and more is understood regarding the relationship that appears to exist among the individual receptor and ion channel effects, protein phosphorylation, and modulation of intracellular second messenger systems, the potential clinical applications of the compound will become increasingly apparent. Early indications are that topiramate will have therapeutic potential in many different disease states in which effective treatment is urgently needed. More important is the potential utility of topiramate as a disease-modifying neurotherapeutic drug that targets the underlying pathologic process contributing to the expression of numerous progressive CNS disorders.

REFERENCES

1. Amano K, Hamada K, Yagi K, et al. Antiepileptic effects of topiramate on amygdaloid kindling in rats. *Epilepsy Res* 1998;31: 123–128.

2. Avoli M, Kawasaki H, Zona C. Effects induced by topiramate on sodium electrogenesis in mammalian central neurons. *Epilepsia* 1996;37[Suppl 4]:S51–S52.

3. Avoli M, Lopantsev V. Topiramate blocks ictal-like discharges in the entorhinal cortex. *Epilepsia* 1997;38[Suppl 8]:S44.

4. Bartholini G. GABA receptor agonists: pharmacological spectrum and therapeutic actions. *Med Res Rev* 1985;5:55–75.

5. Brown SD, Wolf HH, Swinyard EA, et al. The novel anticonvulsant topiramate enhances GABA-mediated chloride flux. *Epilepsia* 1993;34[Suppl 2]:S122.

6. Coulter DA, Sombati S, DeLorenzo RJ. Selective effects of topiramate on sustained repetitive firing and spontaneous bursting in cultured hippocampal neurons. *Epilepsia* 1993;34[Suppl 2]:S123.

7. Coulter DA, Sombati S, DeLorenzo RI. Topiramate effects on excitatory amino acid–mediated responses in cultured hippocampal neurons: selective blockade of kainate currents. *Epilepsia* 1995;36[Suppl 3]:S40.

8. DeLorenzo RI, Sombati S, Coulter DA. Effects of topiramate on sustained repetitive firing and spontaneous recurrent seizure discharges in cultured hippocampal neurons. *Epilepsia* 2000;41 [Suppl I]:S40–S44.

9. Dodgson SJ, Shank RP, Maryanoff BE. Topiramate as an inhibitor of carbonic anhydrase isoenzymes. *Epilepsia* 2000;41 [Suppl 1]:S35–S39.

10. Edwards KR, Glantz MJ, Button J, et al. The evaluation of topiramate in the management of diabetic neuropathy. Paper presented at the 18th annual meeting of the American Pain Society, Fort Lauderdale, FL, 1999.

11. Edwards KR, Glantz MJ, Shea P, et al. A double-blind, randomized trial of topiramate versus placebo in the prophylactic treatment of migraine with and without aura. Paper presented at the 18th annual meeting of the American Pain Society, Fort Lauderdale, FL, 1999.

12. Follett PL, Rosenberg PA, Volpe JJ, et al. Protective effects of topiramate in a rodent model of periventricular leukomalacia. *Ann Neurol* 2000;48:34.

13. Gardocki JF, Labinsky LS, Brown GL, et al. Anticonvulsant activity of McN-4853 (M) 1 ,3:4,5-bis-*O*-(L-methylethylidene)-beta-D-fructopyranose sulfamate in mice and rats. *Epilepsia* 1986;27:648–649.

14. Gibbs JW III, Sombati S, DeLorenzo RI, et al. Cellular actions of topiramate: blockade of kainate-evoked inward currents in cultured hippocampal neurons. *Epilepsia* 2000;41[Suppl 1]:S10–S16.

15. Gordey M, DeLorey TM, Olsen RW. Differential sensitivity of recombinant GABA_A receptors expressed in *Xenopus* oocytes to modulation by topiramate. *Epilepsia* 2000;41[Suppl 1]:S25–S29.

16. Kanda T, Nakamura J, Kurokawa M, et al. Inhibition of excessive releases of excitatory amino acids in hippocampus of spontaneously epileptic rat (SER) by topiramate (KW-6485). *Jpn J Pharmacol* 1992;58[Suppl 1]:592P.

17. Linda T, Kurokawa M, Tamura S, et al. Topiramate reduces abnormally high extracellular levels of glutamate and aspartate in the hippocampus of spontaneously epileptic rats (SER). *Life Sci* 1996;59:1607–1616.

18. Kimishima K, Wang Y, Tanabe T, et al. Anticonvulsant activities and properties of topiramate. *Jpn J Pharmacol* 1992;58[Suppl 1]:S1lP.

19. Koh S, Jensen FE. Topiramate blocks acute and chronic epileptogenesis in a rat model of perinatal hypoxia encephalopathy. *Epilepsia* 1999;40[Suppl 7]:S5.

20. Koller WC, Hristova A, Bin M. Pharmacologic treatment of essential tremor. *Neurology* 2000;54[Suppl 4]:S30–S38.

21. Krebs EG. The growth of research on protein phosphorylation. *Trends Biochem Sci* 1994;19:439.

22. Krusz JC, Scott V. Topiramate in the treatment of chronic migraine and other headaches. *Headache* 1999;39:363.

23. Lee J, Taira T, Pihlaja P, et al. Effects of CO_2 on excitatory transmission apparently caused by changes in intracellular pH in the rat hippocampal slice. *Brain Res* 1996;706:210–216.

24. Loscher W, Reissmuller E, Ebert U. Kindling alters the anticonvulsant efficacy of phenytoin in Wistar rats. *Epilepsy Res* 2000;39:211–220.

25. Louis ED. A new twist for stopping the shakes? Revisiting GABAergic therapy for essential tremor. *Arch Neurol* 1999;56:807–808.

26. Macdonald RL. Antiepileptic drug actions. *Epilepsia* 1989;30 [Suppl 1]:S19–S28.

27. McElroy SL, Suppes T, Keck PE, et al. Open-label adjunctive topiramate in the treatment of bipolar disorders. *Biol Psychiatry* 2000;47:1025–1033.

28. McLean MJ, Bukhari AA, Wamil AW. Effects of topiramate on sodium-dependent action-potential firing by mouse spinal cord neurons in cell culture. *Epilepsia* 2000;41[Suppl 1]:S21–S24.

29. Nakamura J, Tamura S, Kanda T, et al. Anticonvulsant effect of topiramate (2,3:4,5-bis-*O*-(l-methylethylidene)-beta-D-fructopyranose sulfate) on amygdaloid kindled seizures in the cat. *Jpn J Psychiatry Neurol* 1993;47:394–395.

30. Nakamura J, Tamura S, Kanda T, et al. Inhibition by topiramate of seizures in spontaneously epileptic rats and DBAl2 mice. *Eur J Pharmaco* 1994;254:83–89.

31. Niebauer M, Gruenthal M. Topiramate reduces neuronal injury after experimental status epilepticus. *Brain Res* 1999;837:263–269.

32. Petroff QA, Hyder F, Mattson RH, et al. Topiramate increases brain GABA, homocarnosine, and pyrrolidinone in patients with epilepsy. *Neurology* 1999;52:473–478.

33. Post RM, Weiss SRB. Sensitization, kindling, and anticonvulsants in mania. *J Chin Psychiatry* 1989;50[Suppl]:23–30.

34. Post RM. Sensitization and kindling perspectives for the course of affective illness: toward a new treatment with the anticonvulsant carbamazepine. *Pharmacopsychiatry* 1990;23:3–17.

35. Potter DL, Hart DE, Calder CS, et al. A double-blind, randomized, placebo-controlled, parallel study to determine the efficacy of topiramate in the prophylactic treatment of migraine. *Neurology* 2000;54[Suppl 3]:A15.

36. Reissmüller E, Ebert U, Loscher W. Anticonvulsant efficacy of topiramate in phenytoin-resistant kindled rats. *Epilepsia* 2000;41:372–379.

37. Roche KW, O'Brien RI, Mammen AL, et al. Characterization of multiple phosphorylation sites on the AMPA receptor GluR 1 subunit. *Neuron* 1996;16:1179–1188.

38. Severt L, Coulter DA, Sombati S, et al. Topiramate selectively blocks kainate currents in cultured hippocampal neurons. *Epilepsia* 1995;36[Suppl 4]:S38.

39. Shank RP, Gardocki iF, Vaught JL, et al. Topiramate: preclinical evaluation of a structurally novel anticonvulsant. *Epilepsia* 1994;32:450–460.

40. Shank RP, Gardocki iF, Streeter AJ, et al. An overview of the preclinical aspects of topiramate: pharmacology, pharmacokinetics, and mechanisms of action. *Epilepsia* 2000;41[Suppl 1]:S3–S9.

41. Shuaib A, Ahmed F, Muratoglu M, et al. Topiramate in migraine prophylaxis: a pilot study. *Cephalalgia* 1999;19:379.

42. Sigel E. Functional modulation of ligand-gated GABA_A and NMDA receptor channels by phosphorylation. *J Recept Signal Transduct Res* 1995;15:325–332.

43. Sills GJ, Leach JP, Kilpatrick WS, et al. Concentration-effect studies with topiramate on selected enzymes and intermediates of the GABA shunt. *Epilepsia* 2000;41[Suppl 1]:S30–S34.

44. Simeone TA, McClellan AML, Twyman RE, White HS. Direct activation of the recombinant a413~s GABA_A receptor by the

novel anticonvulsant topiramate. *Soc Neurosci Abstr* 2000;26: P237.7(abst).

45. Skradski S, White HS. Topiramate blocks kainate-evoked cobalt influx into cultured neurons. *Epilepsia* 2000;41[Suppl 1]:S45–S47.

46. Sombati S, Coulter DA, DeLorenzo RI. Effects of topiramate on sustained repetitive firing and low Mg^{2+}-induced seizure discharges in cultured hippocampal neurons. *Epilepsia* 1995;36[Suppl 4]:S38.

47. Staley KJ, Soldo BL, Proctor WR. Ionic mechanisms of neuronal excitation by inhibitory $GABA_A$ receptors. *Science* 1995;269: 977–981.

48. Taverna S, Sancini G, Mantegazza M, et al. Inhibition of transient and persistent Na^+ current fractions by the new anticonvulsant topiramate. *J Pharmacol Exp Ther* 1999;288:960–968.

49. Tremont-Lukats LW, Megeff C, Backonja M-M. Anticonvulsants for neuropathic pain syndromes: mechanisms of action and place in therapy. *Drugs* 2000;60:1029–1052.

50. Vaught JL, Maryanoff BE, Shank RI. The pharmacological profile of topiramate: a structurally novel, clinically effective anticonvulsant. *Epilepsia* 1991;32[Suppl 3]:S19.

51. Von Seggern RL, Mannix LK, Adelman JU. Efficacy of topiramate in migraine prophylaxis: a retrospective chart analysis. *Neurology* 2000;54[Suppl 3]:A267.

52. Wang JH, Kelly PT. Postsynaptic injection of Ca^{2+} CaM induces synaptic potentiation requiring CaMKII and PKC activity. *Neuron* 1995;15:443–452.

53. Wauquier A, Thou S. Topiramate: a potent anticonvulsant in the amygdala-kindled rat. *Epilepsy Res* 1996;24:73–77.

54. White HS, Brown D, Skeen GA, et al. The anticonvulsant topiramate displays a unique ability to potentiate GABA-evoked chloride currents. *Epilepsia* 1995;36[Suppl 3]:S39–S40.

55. White HS, Woodhead J, Wolf HH. Effect of topiramate (TPM) on pentylenetetrazol (PTZ) seizure threshold. *Epilepsia* 1996;37 [Suppl 5]:S26.

56. White HS, Brown SD, Woodhead JH, et al. Topiramate enhances GABA-mediated chloride flux and GABA-evoked currents in mouse brain neurons and increases seizure threshold. *Epilepsy Res* 1997;28:167–179.

57. White HS, Brown SD, Woodhead JH, et al. Topiramate modulates GABA-evoked currents m murine cortical neurons by a nonbenzodiazepine mechanism. *Epilepsia* 2000;41[Suppl 1]: S17–S20.

58. Wu SP, Tsai JJ, Gean PW. Frequency-dependent inhibition of neuronal activity by topiramate in rat hippocampal slices. *Br J Pharmacol* 1998;125:826–832.

59. Yang Y, Shuaib A, Li Q, et al. Neuroprotection by delayed administration of topiramate in a rat model of middle cerebral artery embolization. *Brain Res* 1998;804:169–176.

60. Yang Y, Li Q, Shuaib A. Enhanced neuroprotection and reduced hemorrhagic incidence in focal cerebral ischemia of rat by low dose combination therapy of urokinase and topiramate. *Neuropharmacology* 2000;39:881–888.

61. Zhang X, Velumian AA, Jones OT, et al. Topiramate reduces high-voltage activated Ca^{2+} currents in CAl pyramidal neurons *in vitro*. *Epilepsia* 1998;39[Suppl 6]:S44.

62. Zhang X, Velumian AA, Jones OT, et al. Modulation of high-voltage-activated calcium channels in dentate granule cells by topiramate. *Epilepsia* 2000;41[Suppl 1]:S52–S60.

63. Zona C, Ciotti MT. Avoli M. Topiramate attenuates voltage-gated sodium currents in rat cerebellar granule cells. *Neurosci Lett* 1997;231:123–126.

TOPIRAMATE

CHEMISTRY, BIOTRANSFORMATION, AND PHARMACOKINETICS

DENNIS R. DOOSE
ANTHONY J. STREETER

CHEMISTRY

Topiramate is a structurally novel antiepileptic drug (AED) (1–3) marketed in the United States under the brand name Topamax. It is marketed in other countries under the brand names Topimax, Topamac, and Epitomax. Chemically, topiramate is a derivative of D-fructose in the pyranose configuration, and it is identified by the names 2,3:4,5-di-O-isopropylidene-β-D-fructopyranose sulfamate or 2,3:4,5-bis-O-(1-methylethylidene)-β-D-fructopyranose sulfamate. Topiramate has the molecular formula $C_{12}H_{21}NO_8S$ and a molecular weight of 339.4. Its chemical structure is provided in Figure 78.1.

Topiramate drug substance is a white crystalline powder with a bitter taste. Topiramate is most soluble in alkaline solutions containing sodium hydroxide or sodium phosphate and having a pH of 9 to 10. It is freely soluble in acetone, chloroform, dimethylsulfoxide, and ethanol. The solubility in water is 9.8 mg/mL at room temperature. A saturated aqueous solution has a pH of 6.3. Aqueous solubility is increased by the addition of cosolvents, such as propylene glycol or polyethylene glycol 400, 1,500, 4,000, or 6,000 (4).

ABSORPTION

Bioavailability

After oral administration of any commercial formulation, topiramate is rapidly absorbed, with peak plasma concen-

Dennis R Doose, PhD: Associate Director, Global Clinical Pharmacokinetics and Clinical Pharmacology, Johnson & Johnson Pharmaceutical Research and Development, Raritan, New Jersey

Anthony J. Streeter, PhD: Research Fellow, Department of Drug Metabolism, Johnson & Johnson Pharmaceutical Research and Development, Spring House, Pennsylvania

tration occurring at approximately 2 to 4 hours (5). Although oral bioavailability has not been assessed by a classic intravenous-oral crossover comparison in humans, the absolute bioavailability of orally administered topiramate has been estimated to be 81% to 95% based on pharmacokinetic data obtained from a study in subjects with different degrees of renal impairment (6). Absolute bioavailability was calculated as the inverse of the slope of the linear regression curve fit to oral clearance as a function of renal clearance data. The equation for this relationship is:

$$\frac{CL}{F} = CL_R\left(\frac{1}{F}\right) + \frac{CL_{NR}}{F}$$

where Cl is total body clearance, F is bioavailability, Cl_R is renal clearance, and Cl_{NR} is nonrenal clearance.

The extent of absorption estimated pharmacokinetically is consistent with the results obtained after the oral administration of a 100-mg solution dose of [14C]-topiramate, in which 80.6% of the administered radioactivity was excreted in the urine over 10 days (7). Administration with food slightly slows absorption (11% to 13% decreased mean maximum concentration), but with equivalent extent of absorption (−4% to 13% difference in mean area under the curve) (8). These differences in the rate and extent of absorption are not considered clinically significant.

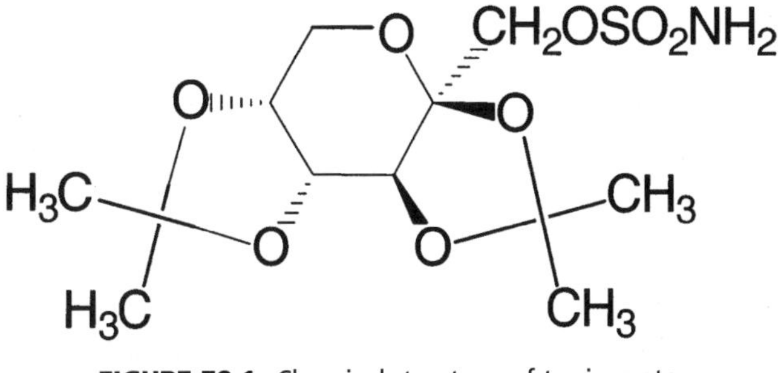

FIGURE 78.1. Chemical structure of topiramate.

Formulations

Topiramate is available commercially as coated tablets and as coated beads (sprinkle) in a gelatin capsule. Coated tablets are available in the following strengths and colors: 25-mg white, 100-mg yellow, 200-mg salmon. Because of the bitter taste of topiramate, it is recommended that tablets not be broken (4).

The encapsulated sprinkle formulation is available for those patients who have difficulty in swallowing tablets, such as pediatric and elderly patients, and it is available in 15- and 25-mg strengths (4). Topiramate sprinkle capsules may be swallowed whole or may be administered by carefully opening the capsule and sprinkling the entire contents on a small amount (teaspoon) of soft food. This drug-food mixture should be swallowed immediately and not chewed. It should not be stored for future use. The tablet and sprinkle formulations are bioequivalent (4). Consuming the sprinkle formulation on food or encapsulated results in bioequivalent exposure. Topiramate tablets and sprinkle capsules should be stored in tightly closed containers at controlled room temperature and protected from moisture (4).

Routes of Administration

Topiramate has been evaluated in humans only after oral administration. There are reports of investigating the use of topiramate after gastric tube and rectal administration. At present, however, no definitive information exists on the therapeutic utility of these routes of administration.

DISTRIBUTION

Plasma Protein Binding

The plasma protein binding of topiramate has been studied *in vitro* using radiotracer methods and microequilibrium dialysis techniques. Topiramate is poorly bound to plasma proteins. Generally, between 9% and 17% of topiramate over a concentration range of 1 to 250 μg/mL is bound to plasma proteins (*unpublished data,* R.W. Johnson Pharmaceutical Research Institute). The clinically relevant topiramate plasma concentration range has been found to extend to ≤33 μg/mL.

Cerebrospinal Fluid, Brain, and Other Tissues

Tissue distribution of topiramate was assessed in the female Wistar rat at 1, 6, 24, and 48 hours after single oral administration of [¹⁴C]-topiramate by quantitative whole-body autoradiography. The amount of radioactivity was determined by densitometry on the exposed autoradiographs, and the results are presented in Figure 78.2 (*unpublished data,* R.W. Johnson Pharmaceutical Research Institute). Validating that this study primarily characterized the tissue distribution of topiramate, parallel studies showed by thin-layer chromatography analysis that most (>83%) of the total radioactivity in plasma, liver, and kidney during the first 24 hours after dosing (*unpublished data,* R.W. Johnson Pharmaceutical Research Institute), and in brain (96%) at 2 hours after administration (9), was unchanged topiramate. Radioactivity was rapidly absorbed and was quickly distrib-

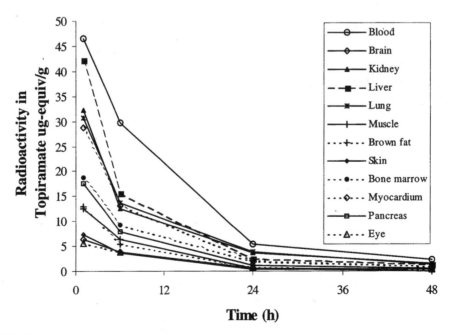

FIGURE 78.2. Mean concentration of total radioactivity in blood and selected tissues and organs of female Wistar rats after a single oral 10 mg/kg dose of ¹⁴C topiramate.

uted into the tissues. The mean concentrations of radioactivity in the brain were less than or equivalent to those in the plasma at 1, 6, 24, and 48 hours after dose administration in both sexes. Exposure of topiramate to the eye was minimal, as evidenced by the low radioactivity detected in this organ. The radioactivity was rapidly eliminated from all tissues, with negligible amounts remaining by 48 hours.

High-affinity, low-capacity binding of topiramate to erythrocytes has been identified. This is postulated to be the result of binding to carbonic anhydrase enzymes present in erythrocytes. In humans, two distinguishable binding sites have been identified, with binding constants of 0.52 and 87 μmol/L (*unpublished data,* R.W. Johnson Pharmaceutical Research Institute). In blood, this binding rapidly becomes saturated and does not significantly influence systemic clearance at clinically relevant concentrations. As indicated, tissue distribution studies showed that topiramate was most highly concentrated in blood, kidney, liver, and lung. Because these tissues are known to be highly enriched with carbonic anhydrase (10), the higher concentrations in these tissues may be explained by binding to carbonic anhydrase.

Transporters

Although topiramate has a chemical structure similar to that of carbohydrates, no carrier-mediated transporters appear to be significantly involved in drug absorption because food appears to have only a dilutional effect on the rate of absorption. Similarly, tissue distribution is rapid, with no evidence of transporter-dependent exposure.

Transplacental Passage

Transplacental distribution of topiramate was assessed as part of the preclinical evaluation of topiramate (*unpublished data,* R.W. Johnson Pharmaceutical Research Institute). A single oral dose of [^{14}C]-topiramate (20 mg/kg) was administered to pregnant female Sprague-Dawley rats on day 11 of gestation. Concentrations of total radioactivity in blood, plasma, fetuses, and selected maternal organs were determined by tissue excision and liquid scintillation spectrometry at 1, 6, 24, and 48 hours after administration. The mean data are presented in Figure 78.3.

Radioactivity was found to distribute rapidly into the fetus and all maternal organs. Concentrations of topiramate and total radioactivity in the fetus and most maternal tissues were found to decline with time in parallel with maternal plasma concentrations.

Breast Milk

Öhman et al. (11) described the excretion of topiramate in human breast milk. Two patients receiving topiramate therapy were evaluated. Simultaneous maternal plasma and breast milk sampling 2 to 3 weeks after delivery was conducted. Reported coincident breast milk/maternal plasma concentrations (mol/L) were 7.6/6.3 and 15/17 in the two patients, respectively. The nursing infant:mother plasma concentration ratio was 0.1 to 0.2. Thus, it appears that infants are exposed to marginal pharmacologically significant amounts of topiramate during nursing.

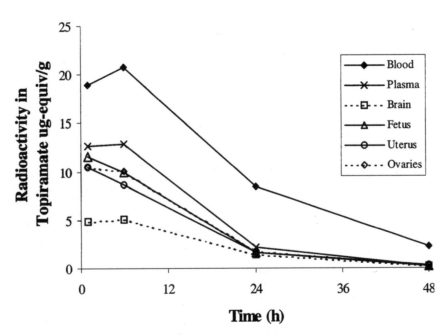

FIGURE 78.3. Mean tissue levels of radioactivity in pregnant female Sprague-Dawley rats after a single oral 20 mg/kg dose of [^{14}C]-topiramate.

ROUTES OF ELIMINATION

Biotransformation

When administered in the absence of enzyme inducers, topiramate is not extensively metabolized. Under this condition, a significant percentage of the dose (~40% in 10 days) is excreted in urine as intact topiramate (7). When it is administered during concomitant therapy with enzyme inducers, the extent of metabolism is significantly greater, but the metabolic profile appears similar. Seven trace metabolites from three types of metabolic pathways—hydroxylation or hydrolysis of the isopropylidene groups, and conjugation (each <3% of the administered radioactivity)—have been identified and characterized (Figure 78.4)

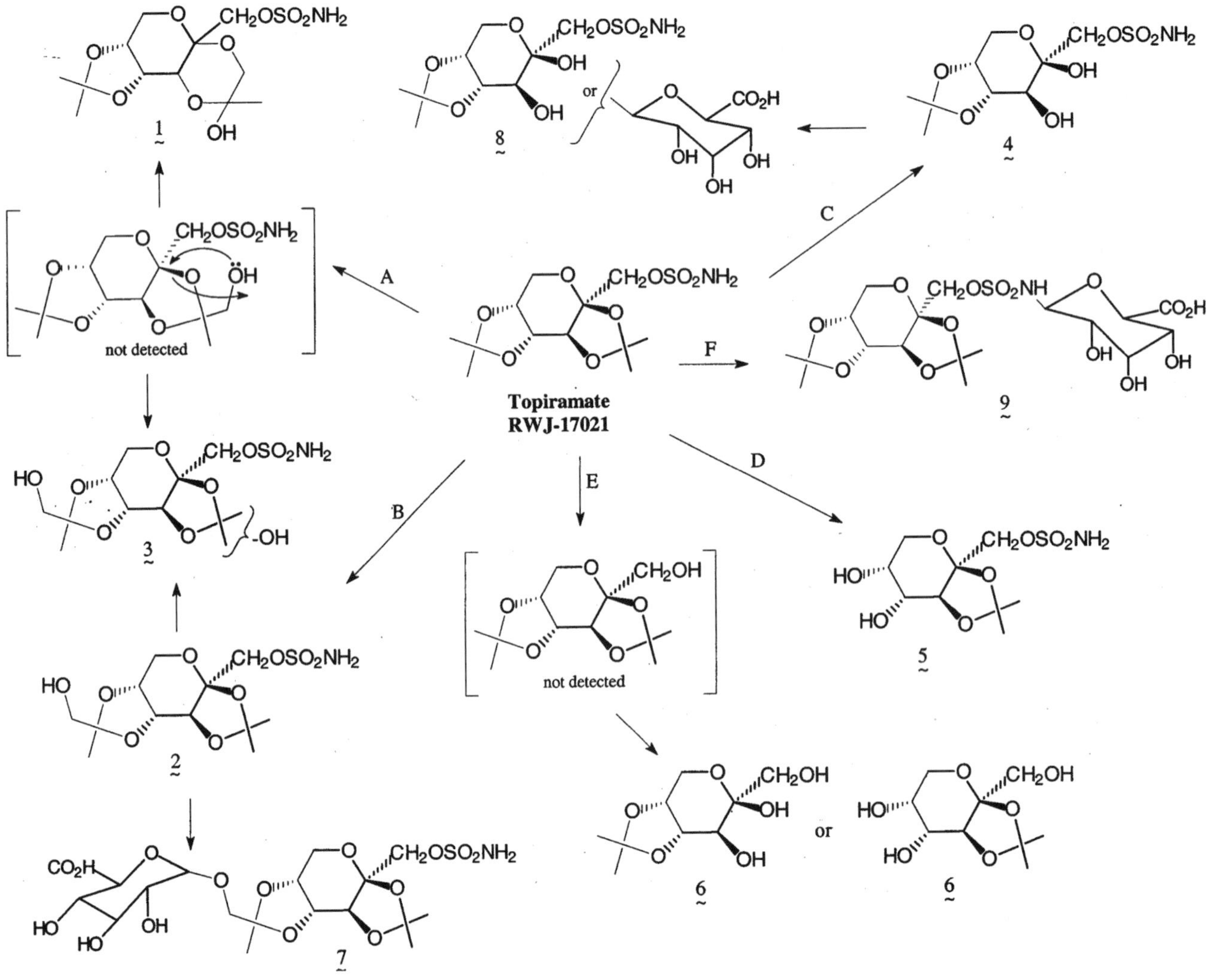

FIGURE 78.4. Metabolites: a rearranged product of a hydroxytopiramate *(1)*; 4,5-*O*-(2-hydroxy-1-methylethylidene)-2,3-*O*-methylethylidene)-β-D-fructopyranose-1-sulfamate *(2)*; 2,3:4,5-bis-*O* -(2-hydroxy-1-methylethylidene)-β-D-fructopyranose sulfamate *(3)*; 4,5-*O*-(1-methylethylidene)-β-D-fructopyranose-1-sulfamate *(4)*; 2,3-*O*-(1-methylethylidene)-β-D-fructo-pyranose-1-sulfamate *(5)*; 2,3- or 4,5-*O*-(1-methylethylidene)-β-D-fructopyranose *(6)*; 4,5-*O*-(2-hydroxy-1-methylethylidene)-2,3-*O*-(1-methyl-ethylidene)-β-D-fructopyranose-1-sulfamate-*O*-glucuronide *(7)*; 4,5-*O*-(1-methylethylidene)-β-D-fructopyranose-1-sulfamate-*O*-glucuronide *(8)*; and 2,3:4,5-bis-*O*-(1-methylethylidene)-β-D-fructopyranose-1-sulfamate-*N*-glucuronide *(9)*. Only metabolites *1, 2, 4, 5, 7, 8,* and *9* have been detected in humans. Proposed pathways: **(A)** hydroxylation at the 7- or 8-methyl group followed by rearrangement to yield metabolite *1;* **(B)** hydroxylation at the 10-methyl group to yield metabolite *2*, followed by glucuronidation to yield metabolite *7;* **(C)** hydrolysis at the 2,3-*O*-isopropylidene group to yield metabolite *4*, followed by glucuronidation to yield metabolite *8;* **(D)** hydrolysis at the 4,5-*O*-isopropylidene group to yield metabolite *5;* **(E)** cleavage at the sulfamate group to yield metabolite *6;* and **(F)** *N*-glucuronidation of topiramate to yield metabolite *9*. Metabolite *3* may be the product of a second hydroxylation of either metabolite *1* or metabolite *2*.

(7,12–14). The two metabolites retaining most of the parent drug structure, metabolites 2 (*unpublished data*, R.W. Johnson Pharmaceutical Research Institute) and 5 (15) (Figure 78.4), show little or no anticonvulsant activity in animal tests. The major route of elimination of unchanged topiramate and its metabolites is by the kidney.

Genetic Factors

There are no reports of genetic factors that influence the pharmacokinetics of topiramate.

Isozymes

The specific metabolic enzymes responsible for the metabolism of topiramate have not been identified. However, it is evident the enzymes induced by phenytoin and carbamazepine play a major role in the clearance of topiramate when the drug is administered with these agents.

Biliary and Renal Excretion

The major route of elimination of unchanged topiramate and its metabolites is by the kidney. A significant percentage of the dose (~40% in 10 days) is excreted in urine as intact topiramate (7).

The dependence of topiramate pharmacokinetics on renal function and hepatic disease was evaluated in separate studies. In two renal impairment studies, patients with moderate and severe renal impairment (creatinine clearance 30 to 60 mL/min/1.73 m^2 and <30 mL/min/1.73 m^2) (16) and patients with end-stage renal disease were studied (17). In a third study, patients with moderate to severe hepatic impairment were investigated (18). The results of these studies are summarized in Table 78.1.

Considering the high renal clearance of topiramate, it is not surprising that renal impairment significantly decreases apparent clearance and increases half-life. Based on these observations, renally impaired patients accumulate topiramate to a greater extent after multiple doses and require a significantly longer time to reach steady state. Therefore, the administration of topiramate to renally impaired patients should be done starting at lower doses and with longer intervals of dose titration.

Topiramate is cleared by hemodialysis at a rate that is four to six times greater than in an otherwise healthy person. Accordingly, a prolonged period of dialysis may cause topiramate concentration to fall significantly. To avoid rapid drops in topiramate plasma concentration during hemodialysis, a supplemental dose of topiramate may be required. The actual adjustment should take into account the duration of dialysis period, the clearance rate of the dialysis system used, and the effective renal clearance of topiramate in the patient undergoing dialysis.

In hepatically impaired patients, topiramate plasma concentrations may be increased. The mechanism is not well understood. The moderate decrease in apparent clearance with hepatic impairment does not appear to warrant adjustment of the topiramate dosing regimen.

No reports have evaluated the extent of biliary excretion in humans. In a study of bile duct-cannulated Wistar rats administered a single oral [^{14}C]-topiramate dose (10 mg/kg), 37.5% and 5.3% of the radioactive dose was excreted in the bile over 24 hours for males and females, respectively (*unpublished data*, R.W. Johnson Pharmaceutical Research Institute). Because the extent of metabolism and clearance in the female rat is closer to that in humans, it is possible that biliary excretion could be a minor elimination pathway in clinical use.

TABLE 78.1. TOPIRAMATE PHARMACOKINETIC PARAMETERS IN DIFFERENT POPULATIONS AFTER ORAL ADMINISTRATION

Type of Subject	T_{max} (h)	F (%)	V/F (L)	Plasma Protein Binding (%)	Half-life (h)	CL/F (mL/min)	CL_R (mL/min)
Healthy subjects and patients with epilepsy without concomitant enzyme inducers	—	—	40–60	—	21	30	18
Patients with epilepsy with concomitant enzyme inducers	—	—	NS	—	NS	60–65	20
	1–3	81–95		9–17			
Severe renal impairment (CL_{CR} <30 mL/min)			NS		58.8	9.2	2.5
Moderate renal impairment (C_{CR}: 30–69 mL/min)	—	—	NS	—	54.6	13.4	6.2
Renal dialysis	—	—	NS	—	78.4	10.8	—
Hepatic disease	—	—	NS	—	33.6	23.5	13.5

C, clearance; C_{CR}, creatinine clearance; CL/F, volume of distribution divided by bioavailability; CL_R, renal clearance; F, bioavailability; NS, not studied; T_{max}, time to maximum plasma concentration, VF, volume of distribution divided by bioavailability.

CLEARANCE AND HALF-LIFE

Healthy Persons

The pharmacokinetics of topiramate is linear, with dose-proportional increases in plasma concentration. The mean plasma elimination half-life is 21 hours after single or multiple doses. Steady state is thus reached in about 4 days in patients with normal renal function. Apparent oral clearance is ~30 mL/min, most of which is renal clearance (~18 mL/min) (19,20).

Comedicated Epileptic Patients

When topiramate is administered to patients as adjunctive therapy with enzyme-inducing drugs, clearance is significantly increased. In controlled pharmacokinetic interaction studies, mean steady-state concentrations were reported to decrease 48% and 40% when topiramate was administrated with phenytoin and carbamazepine, respectively (21,22). The induced clearance appears to be entirely the result of increased nonrenal clearance, because topiramate renal clearance was comparable when administered alone or with carbamazepine.

When topiramate is administered to patients as adjunctive therapy with non–enzyme-inducing drugs, the pharmacokinetics of topiramate is comparable to that in healthy subjects. Valproic acid and lamotrigine appear to have little effect on the plasma clearance of topiramate (23,24).

Children

The pharmacokinetics of topiramate was evaluated in pediatric subjects with epilepsy (ages 4 to 17 years) who were receiving one or two other AEDs (25). Pharmacokinetic profiles were obtained after 1 week at doses of 1, 3, and 9 mg/kg/day. Clearance was independent of dose. Pediatric patients had a 50% higher clearance and consequently shorter elimination half-life than adults. Consequently, the plasma concentration for the same (mg/kg) dose may be lower in pediatric patients compared with adults. As in adults (discussed in the previous section on comedicated epileptic patients), hepatic enzyme-inducing AEDs decreased the steady-state plasma concentrations of topiramate.

In a separate study, unchanged topiramate and six metabolites were quantified from the urine of children with infantile spasms who were between the ages of 9 and 43 months and who were receiving topiramate doses of 7 to 10 mg/kg/day (*unpublished data*, R.W. Johnson Pharmaceutical Research Institute). The relative amounts of topiramate and metabolites found in the urine of children with infantile spasms were similar to those observed in adults. Both infants and adults receiving topiramate adjunctive to enzyme-inducing AEDs had a higher proportion of metabolites to parent topiramate in the urine. Two metabolites, topiramate-*N*-glucuronide and hydroxytopiramate sulfate, were identified in trace amounts (≤8% of total metabolites) in infants but were not detected in adults. Topiramate does not appear to be metabolized significantly differently in infant children compared with adults.

Elderly Patients

The pharmacokinetics of topiramate in elderly subjects (65 to 85 years of age) was evaluated in a controlled clinical study (26). This elderly population had reduced renal function (creatinine clearance of −23%) compared with young adults. After a single oral 100-mg dose, maximum plasma concentrations for elderly and young adults were achieved at approximately 1 to 2 hours. Reflecting the primary renal elimination of topiramate, topiramate plasma concentrations and renal clearance were reduced 21% and 19%, respectively, in elderly subjects, compared with young adults. Similarly, topiramate half-life was longer (13%) in the elderly patients. Reduced topiramate clearance resulted in slightly higher maximum plasma concentration (23%) and area under the curve (25%) in elderly patients than observed in young adults. Topiramate clearance was decreased in the elderly patients only to the extent that renal function was reduced.

Characterized Intersubject Variability and Its Determinants

Aside from the obvious relationship between renal function and elimination pharmacokinetics of topiramate (see the earlier discussion of clearance and half-life in healthy persons), other determinants of pharmacokinetic intersubject variability were evaluated using a population pharmacokinetic analysis (*unpublished data*, R.W. Johnson Pharmaceutical Research Institute). Mixed effects of sex, age, and race were specifically evaluated. Plasma concentration data obtained during the conduct of three multicenter, well-controlled trials in subjects with refractory partial epilepsy who were taking a maximum of two concomitant AEDs were evaluated (see the description of studies discussed in the section on the relationship between plasma concentration and effect). The population pharmacokinetic model was based on a one-compartment model with first-order absorption and elimination. Parameterization of the model included terms for clearance, apparent volume of distribution, and absorption rate. Weight effects were applied to both clearance and volume terms. The database evaluated consisted of 1,239 plasma concentration measurements from 265 patients. This analysis did not reveal any group at risk of altered pharmacokinetics, although sex was found to have an effect on volume of distribution, with values about 50% lower for females. This finding may be attributed to the higher proportion of body fat in women and is of no clinical consequence because the steady-state concentration of a drug is independent of volume of distribution.

RELATIONSHIP BETWEEN PLASMA CONCENTRATION AND DOSE

Generally, the pharmacokinetics of topiramate is linear, with dose-proportional increases in plasma concentration. This has been confirmed by comparing steady-state topiramate plasma concentrations achieved among treatment groups in multicenter, well-controlled trials in patients administered topiramate as adjunctive therapy and as monotherapy (*unpublished data*, R.W. Johnson Pharmaceutical Research Institute). Although the pharmacokinetics is linear, with dose-proportional increases in plasma concentration within the adjunctive and monotherapy regimens, mean steady-state concentrations decreased 40% to 50% when the drug was administrated with concomitant enzyme-inducing AEDs.

RELATIONSHIP BETWEEN PLASMA CONCENTRATION AND EFFECT

The relationship between steady-state topiramate plasma concentration and clinical efficacy and safety was evaluated in three multicenter, well-controlled trials in patients with refractory partial epilepsy who were taking a maximum of two concomitant AEDs (27). Intent-to-treat groups ranged in topiramate dose from 100 to 1,000 mg/day. Patients were titrated in weekly increments to their assigned dose or to their maximum tolerated dose, if less. These patients were maintained at their stable dose for at least 8 weeks. During both the titration period and the stabilization period, single blood samples were taken for topiramate plasma determination at selected clinical visits.

The relationship of clinical efficacy with plasma concentration was evaluated only during the stabilization period. The relationship of clinically relevant adverse events with plasma concentration was evaluated during both the titration and stabilization periods. Although most topiramate-treated patients experienced a decrease in their seizure rates, no consistent relationships were found between this reduction and topiramate plasma concentration. Statistically significantly higher concentrations were observed for the patients who reported central nervous system–related adverse events than for those patients who did not. Despite this correlation, no threshold value could be identified above which central nervous system–related adverse events were more likely to occur.

REFERENCES

1. Shank RP, Gardocki JF, et al. Topiramate: preclinical evaluation of a structurally novel anticonvulsant. *Epilepsia* 1994;35:450–460.
2. Glauser TA. Topiramate. *Epilepsia* 1999;40[Suppl 5]:S71–S80.
3. Reife R, Pledger G, Wu S-C. Topiramate as add-on therapy: pooled analysis of randomized controlled trials in adults. *Epilepsia* 2000;41[Suppl 1]:S66–S71.
4. Walsh P. *Physicians' desk reference*, 54th ed. Montvale, NJ: Medical Economics, 2000.
5. Easterling DE, Zakszewski T, Moyer MD, et al. Plasma pharmacokinetics of topiramate, a new anticonvulsant in humans. *Epilepsia* 1988;29:662(abst).
6. Nayak RK, Gisclon LG, Curtin CA, et al. Estimation of the absolute bioavailability of topiramate in humans without intravenous data. *J Clin Pharmacol* 1994;34:1029.
7. Wu WN, Heebner JB, Streeter AJ, et al. Evaluation of the absorption, excretion, pharmacokinetics and metabolism of the anticonvulsant, topiramate in healthy men. *Pharm Res* 1994;11:S336(abst).
8. Doose DR, Walker SA, Gisclon LG, et al. Single-dose pharmacokinetics and effect of food on the bioavailabilty of topiramate, a novel antiepiletic drug. *J Clin Pharmacol* 1996;36:884–891.
9. Streeter AJ, Wu WN, Stahle PL, et al. An *in vivo* interaction between topiramate and phenytoin in the Sprague-Dawley rat. In: *International Society for the Study of Xenobiotics Proceedings*, Bethesda, Maryland, vol 8., 1996:305.
10. Maren TH. Carbonic anhydrase: chemistry, physiology, and inhibition. *Physiol Rev* 1967;47:595–781.
11. Öhman I, Vitols S, Söderfeldt B, et al. Pharmacokinetics of topiramate in pregnancy and lactation-transplacentar transfer and excretion in breast-milk. Abstract presented at the Fifth Eilat Conference on New Antiepileptic Drugs, Eilat, Israel, 2000.
12. Wu WN, McKown LA, Takacs AR, et al. In: *Proceedings of the 42nd ASMS Conference on Mass Spectrometry and Allied Topics*, Santa Fe, New Mexico, 1994:59.
13. Wu WN, McKown LA, Streeter AJ, et al. In: *Proceedings of the 44th ASMS Conference on Mass Spectrometry and Allied Topics*, Santa Fe, New Mexico, 1996:244.
14. Nortey SO, Wu WN, Maryanoff BE. Synthesis of hydroxylated derivatives of topiramate, a novel antiepileptic drug based on D-fructose: investigation of oxidative metabolites. *Carbohydr Res* 1997;304:29–38.
15. Maryanoff BE, Nortey SO, Gardocki JF, et al. Anticonvulsant O-alkyl sulfamates: 2,3:4,5-bis-O-(1-methylethylidene)-β-D-fructopyranose sulfamate and related compounds. *J Med Chem* 1987;30:880–887.
16. Gisclon LG, Riffts JM, Sica DA, et al. The pharmacokinetics of topiramate in subjects with renal impairment as compared to matched subjects with normal renal function. *Pharm Res* 1993;10[Suppl]:S397(abst).
17. Gisclon LG, Curtin CR. The pharmacokinetics (PK) of topiramate (T) in subjects with end-stage renal disease undergoing hemodialysis. *Clin Pharmacol Ther* 1994;55:196.
18. Doose DR, Walker SA, Venkataramanan R, et al. Topiramate pharmacokinetics in subjects with liver impairment. *Pharm Res* 1994 [Suppl 2]:S446(abst).
19. Easterling DE, Zakszewski T, Moyer MD, et al. Plasma pharmacokinetics of topiramate, a new anticonvulsant in humans. *Epilepsia* 1988;29:662(abst).
20. Doose DR, Scott VV, Margul BL, et al. Multiple-dose pharmacokinetics of topiramate in healthy male subjects. *Epilepsia* 1988;29:662(abst).
21. Gisclon LG, Curtin CR, Kramer LD. The steady-state (SS) pharmacokinetics (PK) of phenytoin (Dilantin) and topiramate (Topamax) in epileptic patients on monotherapy, and during combination therapy. *Epilepsia* 1994;35[Suppl 8]:54(abst).
22. Sachdeo RC, Sachdeo SK, Walker SA, et al. Steady-state pharmacokinetics of topiramate and carbamazepine in patients with epilepsy during monotherapy and concomitant therapy. *Epilepsia* 1996;37:774–780.
23. Rosenfeld WE, Liao S, Kramer LD, et al. Comparison of the

steady-state pharmacokinetics of topiramate and valproate in patients with epilepsy during monotherapy and concomitant therapy. *Epilepsia* 1997;38:324–333.

24. Berry DJ, Besac FMC, Natarajan J, et al. Does topiramate change lamotrigine serum concentrations when added to treatment? An audit of a dose-escalation study. *Epilepsia* 1998;39 [Suppl 6]:56–57(abst).

25. Rosenfeld WE, Doose DR, Walker SA, et al. A study of topira-mate pharmacokinetics and tolerability in children with epilepsy. *Pediatr Neurol* 1999;20:339–344.

26. Doose DR, Larson KL, Natarajan J, et al. Comparative single-dose pharmacokinetics of topiramate in elderly versus young men and women. *Epilepsia* 1998;39[Suppl 6]:56(abst).

27. Reife RA, Pledger G, Doose D, et al. Relationship of steady-state plasma topiramate (TPM) concentration to clinical efficacy and tolerability. *Epilepsia* 1995;36[Suppl 3]:S152(abst).

TOPIRAMATE

DRUG INTERACTIONS

BARRY E. GIDAL

Treatment with the traditional antiepileptic drugs (AEDs) such as phenytoin (PHT), carbamazepine (CBZ), phenobarbital, and sodium valproate (VPA) is complicated by clinically significant, pharmacokinetic interactions. A potential advantage of the newer-generation AEDs is an improved drug interaction profile.

Topiramate (TPM) is a sulfamate-substituted monosaccharide compound. Because TPM is frequently used in combination with other AEDs, it is important to evaluate potentially reciprocal interactions between this drug and the traditional medications. In addition, given the increased use of many of the newer AEDs in conditions other than epilepsy such as bipolar-affective disorder, evaluation of the potential interactions between TPM and various psychiatric medications is also warranted. Although TPM is generally considered to have an improved drug interaction profile, clinically evident pharmacokinetic interactions have been reported.

PHARMACOKINETICS

The clinically relevant pharmacokinetic properties of TPM are summarized here to form a basis for discussion and evaluation of TPM drug interactions. After oral administration, TPM is rapidly (time to maximum concentration or T_{max} of 1.75 to 4.3 hours) and extensively absorbed, with an oral bioavailability of 80% (1,2). Dose-proportionality studies (100 mg to 1,200 mg) carried out in healthy volunteers suggest that increases in maximum concentration (C_{max}) and area under the curve (AUC), although linear, are not dose proportional (3). Although ingestion with a high-fat meal slows TPM absorption (1.4 versus 3 hours at a 100-mg dose and 2.7 versus 4.8 hours at a 400-mg dose), overall completeness of absorption was not impaired (3). Changes in rate of absorption after food ingestion as well as

an apparent prolongation in T_{max} with increasing doses are unlikely to be clinically relevant.

Binding to plasma proteins is minimal for TPM (13% to 17%) (1), thus, one would not predict that TPM would be subject to protein binding displacement interactions. The apparent volume of distribution is 0.6 to 0.8 L/kg. Values for apparent volume of distribution do appear to be inversely related to TPM dose; saturable binding of TPM to erythrocytes may provide a possible explanation for this observation, as well as the apparent lack of dose proportionality seen at higher dose ranges (4).

When TPM is given as monotherapy, the fraction of TPM that is metabolized is relatively low. In this setting, ~70% of an oral TPM dose is excreted unchanged in the urine. The fraction metabolized is substantially increased, however, when TPM is coadministered with enzyme-inducing AEDs, a finding suggesting that, in certain polytherapy settings, significant drug interactions may exist (see later). Metabolites thus far identified include two hydroxy and two diol metabolites, as well as several glucuronide conjugates (1). TPM elimination half-life in monotherapy ranges from 19 to 23 hours, versus 12 to 15 hours when TPM is given with enzyme-inducing drugs.

IN VITRO EVALUATIONS

To characterize the potential inhibitory activity of TPM, *in vitro* studies using human liver microsomes were performed (5). Substrates metabolized by seven specific cytochrome P450 isozymes—GYP1A2, CYP2A6, CYP2C9, CYP2C19, CYP2D6, CYP2E1, and CYP3A4—were incubated with TPM at concentrations ≤1,000 µmol/L. Significant inhibition was not seen for any CYP isoform except CYP2C19. Formation of 4-OH-(S)-mephenytoin was reduced by 29%. Based on these experimental findings, it can therefore be predicted that TPM coadministration would only be expected to result inhibitory interactions for drugs in which CYP2C19 is responsible for a significant fraction of substrate metabolism.

Barry E. Gidal, PharmD: Associate Professor, School of Pharmacy and Department of Neurology, University of Wisconsin, Madison, Wisconsin

INTERACTIONS WITH OTHER ANTIEPILEPTIC DRUGS

The potential for interactions between TPM and CBZ, PHT, and VPA was evaluated in a series of studies in patients receiving one of these three AEDs as monotherapy. Each of these studies was conducted using a common study design (Table 79.1). Determination of pharmacokinetic parameters for each of these traditional AEDs was conducted at baseline and after the introduction of TPM during a stepwise dose escalation over a 6-week period to a maximum possible dose of 800 mg/day. Specifically, pharmacokinetic analysis of the original AED was performed after stabilization at TPM doses of 100, 200, and 400 mg every 12 hours given for 2 weeks at each target dose. Two weeks after the TPM dose escalation period, the background AED was systematically withdrawn in 25% weekly decrements. TPM pharmacokinetic parameters were evaluated before and after withdrawal of the background AED. Using this unique clinical design, evaluation of potential reciprocal interactions between TPM and the background AED could be determined.

Carbamazepine and Topiramate

In an early clinical report, Wilensky et al. (6) noted no significant effects of adjunctive treatment with TPM on CBZ or CBZ-10,11-epoxide (CBZE) plasma concentrations. In a more recent evaluation (7), Sachdeo and coworkers reported that average steady-state plasma concentrations of both total and unbound CBZ and its principal metabolite, CBZE, were unchanged among baseline values, during TPM dose escalation, and after attainment of maximal TPM doses in 11 evaluable patients. Likewise, specific pharmacokinetic parameters including $AUC_{(0-8)}$, C_{max}, T_{max}, and apparent oral clearance (Cl/F) were unchanged by comedication with TPM. Patients in this trial were receiving CBZ in doses of 300 to 800 mg every 8 hours.

Changes in TPM pharmacokinetics were evaluated in 10 of these patients at the beginning and at the end of the CBZ withdrawal. TPM Cl/F was again evaluated in patients in whom TPM monotherapy was successfully maintained. During CBZ dose reduction, TPM Cl/F was reduced by 22%

when CBZ daily dose was reduced by approximately 61%. In the three patients who achieved TPM monotherapy, mean TPM plasma concentrations were substantially altered after withdrawal of CBZ. Specifically, TPM C_{max} (3.4 ± 1.4 versus 5.5 ± 0.6 µg/mL) and C_{min} (2.2 ± 0.4 versus 3.7 ± 0.9 µg/mL) mean concentrations were ~60% to 68% higher during TPM monotherapy as compared with comedication with CBZ. Likewise, TPM apparent Cl/F was reduced by ~50% during monotherapy as compared with baseline polytherapy values (33.2 ± 4.8 versus 63.7 ± 33.5 mL/min). TPM renal clearance was unaffected by comedication with CBZ. In addition, the mean fraction of TPM dose excreted unchanged in urine was approximately 40% less during concomitant treatment with CBZ as compared with monotherapy. These findings suggest that effect of CBZ on TPM apparent Cl/F is the result of enzyme induction.

Phenytoin and Topiramate

In an earlier brief report, Floren et al. (8) reported no apparent change in PHT plasma concentrations in six patients receiving adjunctive treatment with TPM. Conversely, when TPM (200 to 800 mg/day) was added to 12 patients receiving PHT monotherapy (six patients receiving PHT 130 to 300 mg every 12 hours and six patients receiving 360 to 480 mg PHT once daily), using the study design described previously, six of 12 patients had increases in PHT AUC of approximately 25% as compared with baseline values (9,10). This somewhat variable interaction is consistent with TPM ability to inhibit CYP2C19. Although these modest elevations in PHT plasma concentrations are not likely to be clinically significant in most patients, clinicians should nevertheless be alert for signs of PHT intoxication in patients receiving this AED combination.

In this study, the effect of PHT on TPM pharmacokinetics was compared with TPM monotherapy. TPM plasma concentrations are ~48% lower during comedication with PHT. Likewise, TPM apparent Cl/F is ~52% to 59% lower during TPM monotherapy as compared with adjunctive treatment with PHT. Definitive statistical analysis of these data are confounded, however, because only four patients were successfully converted to TPM monotherapy. However, these data suggest that, after discontinuation of PHT, one would expect to see an approximate doubling of TPM plasma concentrations.

Valproate and Topiramate

Rosenfeld and colleagues (11) evaluated VPA and TPM pharmacokinetics in 12 patients receiving monotherapy with VPA after the addition of TPM; the previously described clinical design was used. In this study, all 12 patients achieved the final target TPM dose of 800 mg/day, with data from 10 patients evaluable for VPA pharmacoki-

TABLE 79.1. INTERACTIONS BETWEEN TOPIRAMATE AND TRADITIONAL ANTIEPILEPTIC DRUGS

Antiepileptic Drug	Change in Antiepileptic Drug Plasma Concentration	Change in Topiramate Plasma Concentration
Carbamazepine	None	40% decrease
Phenytoin	0–25% increase	48% decrease
Valproate	13% decrease	14% decrease

netics. VPA doses ranged from 1,000 to 4,500 mg/day. After addition of TPM, statistically significant increases in VPA clearance were noted at all TPM doses. At a daily TPM dose of 800 mg/day, VPA apparent Cl/F was approximately 13% greater and VPA average steady-state concentrations were approximately 12% lower. Although the total percentage of the VPA dose excreted in urine was unaffected by concomitant TPM treatment, the mean formation clearance of the glucuronide conjugate pathway was decreased by 35%, whereas significant increases in the formation clearances of 4-ene VPA (+60%), ω-oxidation (+36%), and β-oxidation (+42%) pathways were seen. Although the overall effects of TPM on VPA pharmacokinetics is only modest, and will most likely not require VPA dosage adjustments, the changes in fractions of VPA metabolic pathways are noteworthy. In particular, 4-ene VPA has been implicated as a potential hepatotoxin (12).

While the clinical significance of these changes is still unclear, however, although the combination of TPM and VPA was implicated in the development of hyperammonemic encephalopathy in several patients (13). With respect to the effect of VPA on TPM pharmacokinetics. Data from eight evaluable patients receiving TPM 800 mg/day suggested that TPM C_{max} (5.8±0.8 versus 6.8±1.1 μg/mL, $p < .05$) and C_{min} (3.9±0.6 versus 4.6±0.9 μg/mL, $p < .05$) values were ~17% to 18% higher during concomitant treatment with VPA as compared with TPM monotherapy. TPM Cl/F was 13% greater during comedication with VPA (29.8±4.2 versus 25.9±4.6 mL/min). TPM renal clearance, however, was unaffected by VPA treatment. These findings taken together suggest induction of TPM metabolism by VPA. These changes are quite modest, however, and would not be expected to be clinically meaningful.

INTERACTIONS WITH PHENOBARBITAL, PRIMIDONE, AND NEWER ANTIEPILEPTIC DRUGS

Evaluation of phenobarbital and primidone plasma concentrations during several placebo-controlled clinical trials suggested no significant pharmacokinetic effect of TPM comedication on these drugs (14). Currently, prospective data are lacking regarding potential pharmacokinetic interactions between TPM and other newer AEDs such as lamotrigine, gabapentin, zonisamide, or oxcarbazepine. Based on TPM's known *in vitro* interaction profile, as well as results from clinical pharmacokinetic trials, one would not predict interactions between TPM and gabapentin, or levetiracetam, drugs that are eliminated by predominantly renal mechanisms and non hepatic metabolism. Preliminary evidence also suggests that no interaction exists between TPM and the investigational agent, retigabine (15). Given that both zonisamide and TPM are modest carbonic anhydrase

inhibitors, the potential for additive adverse effects such as nephrolithiasis exists.

In one case series, 4 of 7 patients comedicated with lamotrigine and topiramate had lamotrigine concentrations 40%–50% lower as compared to monotherapy values (16).

INTERACTIONS WITH PSYCHOTROPIC MEDICATIONS

Increasingly, some AEDs, including TPM, are being used in settings other than epilepsy, including adjunctive treatment of bipolar-affective disorder. At present, however, only limited data exist regarding the potential for pharmacokinetic interactions between TPM and various psychotropic drugs.

Topiramate and Haloperidol

An open-label crossover study evaluated the effect of TPM on haloperidol pharmacokinetics in 12 healthy volunteers (17). Subjects received a single 2-mg dose of haloperidol before and after receiving TPM, titrated to a maximal dose of 200 mg/day over 14 days. Mean haloperidol AUC increased by 15%, with the greatest individual increase in haloperidol AUC being 28%. The authors concluded that this modest increase in haloperidol is unlikely to be of clinical significance in most patients.

Topiramate and Lithium

Results from one study in 12 healthy adults suggest that, after the addition of TPM, serum lithium concentrations declined approximately 11% to 16% (*unpublished data*, Ortho-McNeil Pharmaceutical). In one patient, a 70% reduction in lithium AUC was noted after TPM administration. Mechanistically, these modest reductions in lithium concentrations may reflect TPM's ability to inhibit carbonic anhydrase activity weakly. The administration of acetazolamide has been reported to increase lithium excretion by ~30%, and significantly reduced lithium concentrations have been reported (18). Although the clinical significance of this interaction with TPM is unclear, clinicians using this combination would be advised to monitor lithium concentrations after TPM administration during medication introduction.

INTERACTIONS WITH OTHER MEDICATIONS
Oral Contraceptives

Understanding the potential for interactions between AEDs and oral contraceptive drugs is clinically imperative. Although many of the newer AEDs appear to have a reduced capacity for interactions with oral contraceptives, TPM coadministration may have clinically meaningful effects.

The effect of TPM administration on oral contraceptive kinetics was evaluated in 12 women with epilepsy who were receiving VPA monotherapy (19). Patients received a combination product containing norethindrone 1.0 mg and ethinyl estradiol 35 μg daily for 21 days, followed by inert pills to complete a 28-day cycle. Hormonal concentrations were evaluated on day 20 for four cycles. TPM was coadministered at escalating doses of 200 to 800 mg/day, starting on cycle 2.

Although TPM coadministration had no significant effect on plasma concentrations of norethindrone, norethindrone Cl/F was increased 22% at the highest TPM dose. Plasma concentrations of ethinyl estradiol significantly declined in a dose-related manner. Specifically, at TPM doses of 200, 400, and 800 mg/day, estradiol concentrations declined by 18%, 21%, and 30%. At TPM doses of 200 and 800 mg/day, mean estradiol Cl/F was significantly increased by 14.7% and 33%, respectively, as compared with baseline values.

Although the magnitude of this interaction is substantially less than that seen with either PHT or CBZ, these findings nonetheless suggest that oral contraceptive effectiveness may be compromised in the presence of TPM. Patients receiving preparations with <35 μg estrogenic component should be advised to report changes in bleeding patterns. Alternatively, substitution of an oral contraceptive drug with higher estrogenic dosage may be appropriate in some patients.

Topiramate and Digoxin

Digoxin pharmacokinetics was determined in healthy persons before and after 10-day treatment with TPM at 200 mg/day (20). As compared with baseline values, treatment with TPM resulted in a 13% decline in digoxin Cl/F. There were no significant changes noted in digoxin elimination half-life or renal clearance. Based on this study design, it is unclear whether this interaction is dose dependent or whether it is a result of enhanced digoxin clearance or reduced bioavailability. Although this interaction appears to be modest, because of digoxin's narrow therapeutic index, monitoring of digoxin serum concentrations may be prudent.

CONCLUSIONS

As compared with the traditional AEDs, the drug interaction profile of TPM appears to be relatively modest. In the studies designed to evaluate TPM and CBZ, CBZE, and VPA, TPM comedication had negligible effects. In some patients, treatment with TPM may result in modest elevations in plasma PHT concentrations. Clinical experience would suggest, however, that this inhibitory interaction would seldom require PHT dosage adjustment. In contrast, treatment with the enzyme-inducing AEDs such as PHT or

CBZ can be expected to result in a two- to threefold increase in TPM clearance. These interactions can be clinically significant, and TPM dosage reduction may be required after the removal or reduction of one of these enzyme inducers. Because of the obvious clinically important consequences of oral contraceptive failure, the interaction of these agents with TPM requires close clinical monitoring.

REFERENCES

1. Gamett WR. Clinical pharmacology of topiramate: a review. *Epilepsia* 2000;41[Suppl 1]:S61–S65.
2. Bourgeois BED. Pharmacokinetics and metabolism of topiramate. *Drugs Today* 1999;35:43–48.
3. Doose DR, Scott VV, Margul BL, et al. Multiple-dose pharmacokinetics of topiramate in healthy male subjects. *Epilepsia* 1988; 29:662.
4. Gidal BE, Lensmeyer GL. Therapeutic monitoring of topiramate: evaluation of the saturate distribution using an optimized hill method. *Ther Drug Monit* 1999;21:567–576.
5. Levy RH, Bishop F, Streeter AJ, et al. Explanation and prediction of drug interactions with topiramate using a GYP4SO inhibition spectrum. *Epilepsia* 1995;36[Suppl 4]:47.
6. Wilensky AJ, Ojemann LM, Chmelir T, et al. Topiramate pharmacokinetics in epileptic patients receiving carbamazepine. *Epilepsia* 1989;30:645(abst).
7. Sachdeo RG, Sachdeo SK, Walker SA, et al. Steady-state pharmacokinetics of topiramate and carbamazepine in patients with epilepsy during monotherapy and concomitant therapy *Epilepsia* 1989;30:646(abst).
8. Floren KL, Graves NM, Leppik IE, et al. Pharmakokinetics of topiramate in patients with partial epilepsy receiving phenytoin or valproate. *Epilepsia* 1989;30:646(abst).
9. Gisclon LG, Curtin GR, Kramer LD, et al. The steady-state (SS) pharmacokinetics (PK) of phenytoin (Dilantin) and topiramate (Topamax) in epileptic patients on monotherapy, and during combination therapy. *Epilepsia* 1994;35[Suppl 8]:54.
10. Gisclon LG, Curtin GR, Kramer LD, et al. A comparative study of the steady-state pharmacokinetics of phenytoin (Dilantin) kapseals and topiramate (Topamax) in male and female patients on monotherapy and during combination therapy. *Pharm Res* 1994;11[Suppl 8]:54.
11. Rosenfeld WE, Liao S, Kramer LD, et al. Comparison of the steady-state pharmacokinetics of topiramate and valproate in patients with epilepsy during monotherapy and concomitant therapy. *Epilepsia* 1997;38:324–333.
12. Levy RH, Rettenmeier AW, Anderson GD, et al. Effects of polytherapy with phenytoin, carbamazepine, and stiripentol on formation of 4-ene-valproate, a hepatotoxic metabolite of valproic acid. *Clin Pharmacol Ther* 1990;48:225–235.
13. Hamer HM, Knake S, Schomburg U, et al. Valproate-induced hyperammonemic encephalopathy in the presence of topiramate. Neurology 2000;54:230–232.
14. Doose DR. Walker SA, Pledger G, et al. Evaluation of phenobarbital and primidone/phenobarbital (primidones active metabolite) plasma concentrations during administration of add-on topiramate therapy in five multicenter, double-blind, placebo-controlled trials in outpatients with partial seizures. *Epilepsia* 1995;36[Suppl 3]:158(abst).
15. Sachdeo RG, Ferron GM, Partiot AM, et al. An early determina-

tion of drug-drug interaction between valproic acid, phenytoin, carbamazepine or topiramate and retigabine in epileptic patients. *Neurology* 2001;(abst).

16. Wnuk W, Volanski A, Foletti G. Topiramate decreases lamotrigine concentrations. *Ther Drug Monit* 1999;21:4–449.

17. Doose DR, Kohl KA, Desai-Krieger D, et al. No clinically significant effect of topiramate on haloperidol plasma concentration. *Eur Neuropsychopharmacol* 1999;9[Suppl 5]:S357.

18. Thomsen K, Schou M. Renal lithium excretion in man. *Am J Physiol* 1968;215:823–827.

19. Rosenfeld WE, Doose DR, Walker SA, et al. Effect of topiramate on the pharmacokinetics of an oral contraceptive containing norethindrone and ethinyl estradiol in patients with epilepsy. *Epilepsia* 1997;38:317–323.

20. Liao S, Palmer M. Digoxin and topiramate drug interaction study in male volunteers. *Pharm Res* 1993;10[Suppl]:405.

TOPIRAMATE

CLINICAL EFFICACY AND USE IN EPILEPSY

MICHAEL D. PRIVITERA
ROY E. TWYMAN

Topiramate, a structurally unique anticonvulsant, exhibits multiple mechanisms of action, a feature suggestive of a broad spectrum of antiseizure activity. To characterize the pharmacologic and clinical properties of topiramate further, the agent has been investigated in a comprehensive drug development program. This chapter reviews certain key studies, conducted as part of the clinical development program, together with other investigator-driven studies, that provide evidence for the clinical efficacy of topiramate in epilepsy. This chapter also outlines current recommendations regarding the use of topiramate in clinical practice and lessons learned from the clinical trials program. Many of the studies reviewed in this chapter also investigated the safety and tolerability of topiramate, which are reviewed separately elsewhere in this publication.

Clinical testing was initially carried out with topiramate, administered as adjunctive therapy, in adults with refractory partial-onset seizures. In these controlled regulatory trials, a high starting dose of topiramate was given, and a relatively fast titration schedule was followed. Despite the drug's significant demonstrated efficacy, investigators believed that side effects could be minimized with lower doses and slower titration. In a subsequent study, the benefit of slower titration was substantiated, and dosing recommendations were been adjusted accordingly.

After evaluation as adjunctive therapy in adults with partial-onset seizures, the development program for topiramate followed a traditional route into pediatrics, secondary generalized seizures, primary generalized seizures, and, more recently, monotherapy in adults and children with newly diagnosed or therapy-resistant epilepsy. As reviewed in this chapter, an extensive body of data has accumulated from both clinical trials and postmarketing experience to indicate that topiramate, used adjunctively or as monotherapy, is a highly efficacious, broad-spectrum anticonvulsant in adults and children.

The following sections review the efficacy and clinical use of topiramate in patients with different types of seizures. Special emphasis is placed on randomized controlled trials. When results from long-term follow-up studies are reported, these represent intent-to-treat analyses, with the stipulation that the patient's entry date into open-label treatment had to be at least 3 months or 6 months before data cutoff, depending on whether the analysis called for 3-month data or 6-month data. When a patient's entry into open-label treatment was >3 months before data cutoff, but treatment was discontinued, the patient's last seizure information was carried forward.

SPECTRUM OF EFFICACY

Evidence from Placebo-Controlled Clinical Trials: Adjunctive Therapy

Refractory Partial-Onset Seizures, with or without Secondarily Generalized Seizures, in Adults

Topiramate was evaluated as adjunctive therapy in adults with refractory partial-onset seizures, with or without secondary generalization, in eight double-blind, randomized, placebo-controlled trials (2,11,23,29,34,39,41,44). These trials investigated a single target dose (2,34,39,41) or a range of target doses (11,29) of topiramate. In addition, several pooled analyses and meta-analyses further examined the efficacy of topiramate in treating partial-onset seizures in adults. In all trials, topiramate was administered on a twice-daily schedule, and concomitant medication was kept unchanged.

Michael D. Privitera, MD: Professor and Vice Chair, Department of Neurology, University of Cincinnati Medical Center, Cincinnati, Ohio

Roy E. Twyman, MD: Senior Director, Department of Clinical Development, Neurology, R. W. Johnson Pharmaceutical Research Institute, Raritan, New Jersey

Trials Exploring One Target Dosage

Six double-blind, placebo-controlled trials studied a single target dosage of topiramate as adjunctive therapy in patients with partial-onset seizures (Table 80.1). In the study reported by Rosenfeld et al. (34), 167 of 209 patients received topiramate at doses up to 1,000 mg/day (or maximum tolerated dose) over an 11-week titration period, followed by an 8-week maintenance period. The mean actual dose achieved was 799 mg/day. The median reduction in seizure frequency versus baseline was 51% after topiramate treatment compared with 1% reduction after placebo (*p* < .001). Freedom from seizures was achieved in 6% of topiramate-treated patients but in none of the placebo recipients. These findings were corroborated by five subsequent single-dosage trials, studying different target dosages of 300, 400, 600 (two studies), or 800 mg/day.

TABLE 80.1. MEDIAN PERCENTAGE REDUCTION IN SEIZURE FREQUENCY AND RESPONSE RATES (INTENT-TO-TREAT ANALYSIS) IN EIGHT MULTICENTER, RANDOMIZED, DOUBLE-BLIND, PLACEBO-CONTROLLED TRIALS OF ADJUNCTIVE TOPIRAMATE (SINGLE AND MULTIPLE DOSE) IN ADULTS WITH REFRACTORY PARTIAL-ONSET SEIZURES, WITH OR WITHOUT SECONDARY GENERALIZED SEIZURES[a]

Reference	Variable	Placebo	Target Topiramate Dosage (mg/day)					
			200	300	400	600	800	1,000
Studies exploring a single target dosage								
Rosenfeld et al., 1996 (34)	n	42						167
	Median % reduction	1						51[b]
	≥50% reduction	19						52[b]
	≥75% reduction	5						25
	100% reduction	0						6
Sharif et al., 1996 (39)	n	24			23			
	Median % reduction	1			41			
	≥50% reduction	8			35[b]			
	≥75% reduction	4			22			
	100% reduction	0			9			
Tassinari et al., 1996 (41)	n	30				30		
	Median % reduction	12 (increase)				46[b]		
	≥50% reduction	10				47[b]		
	≥75% reduction	3				23[b]		
	100% reduction	0				0		
Ben-Menachem et al., 1996 (2)	n	28					28	
	Median % reduction	18 (increase)					36[b]	
	≥50% reduction	0					43[b]	
	≥75% reduction	0					36[b]	
	100% reduction	0					7	
Korean et al., 1999 (23)	n	86				91		
	Median % reduction	9				51		
	≥50% reduction	13				51		
	100% reduction	1				8		
Yen et al., 2000 (44)	n	23	23					
	Median % reduction	7	44					
	≥50% reduction	13	48[b]					
Studies exploring a range of target dosages								
Faught et al., (1996) (11)	n	45		45	45	46		
	Median % reduction	13		30	48[b]	45[b]		
	≥50% reduction	18		27	47[b]	46[b]		
	≥75% reduction	9		9	27	25		
	100% reduction	0		0	4	4		
Privitera et al., 1996 (29)	n	47				48	48	47
	Median % reduction	1				41[b]	41[b]	38[b]
	≥50% reduction	9				44[b]	40[b]	38[b]
	≥75% reduction	0				23	13	13
	100% reduction	0				10	2	0

[a]Responder rates are expressed as percentage of patients showing the indicated degree of seizure reduction compared with a prospective baseline.
[b]Significantly different from placebo (*p* ≤ .05).

In a small trial conducted in Taiwan (44), 46 patients were randomized to receive topiramate (300 mg/day) or placebo, using a 6-week titration and an 8-week maintenance period. Mean reduction in seizure frequency was 44% in the topiramate group and 7% in the placebo group (p < .01), and 48% of patients receiving topiramate compared with 13% receiving placebo (p = .01) had a >50% seizure reduction.

Topiramate, 400 mg/day, resulted in a median percentage reduction in seizure rate of 40.7% versus 1.1% in those receiving placebo in a similarly small European trial (39). In this trial, the titration period was 3 weeks, and the maintenance period was 8 weeks. There were significantly more responders ($\geq$50% reduction in seizure rate relative to baseline) in the topiramate-treated group than in the placebo group (35% versus 8%, p < .05). Seizures were eliminated in 9% of those receiving topiramate but in none of those receiving placebo.

Tassinari et al. (41) reported a European comparison of topiramate (n = 30; patients titrated up to a target dose of 600 mg/day, or maximum tolerated dose, over a 4-week period) with placebo (n = 30). Again, the maintenance period was 8 weeks, and the actual mean dosage of topiramate achieved was 519 mg/day. The median percentage reduction in seizure rate was 46.4% in topiramate-treated patients. This compared with a rise of 12.2% among placebo recipients (p < .005). There were more treatment responders ($\geq$50% reduction) in the topiramate group (47%) than in the placebo group (10%; p < .001). A trial in Korea compared 600 mg topiramate (or highest tolerated dose) with placebo in 177 patients. Titration and maintenance periods were 10 and 8 weeks, respectively, and the actual mean achieved dose was 449 mg/day, with only 51 of 91 patients randomized to topiramate achieving the target dose. Median reduction in seizure frequency was 51% in patients receiving topiramate and 9% in those receiving placebo, and 51% of patients receiving topiramate (versus 13% receiving placebo, p < .01) achieved a $\geq$50% seizure reduction (23).

Ben-Menachem and colleagues studied a topiramate target dose of 800 mg/day (n = 8) versus placebo (n = 28) (2). Titration and maintenance periods were 5 and 8 weeks, respectively. The mean daily dose of topiramate achieved was 568 mg/day. There was a significant reduction in average monthly seizure rate in the topiramate group compared with placebo (35.8% versus 17.8%, respectively; p < .001). In addition, 43% of topiramate recipients were rated as responders ($\geq$50% reduction), whereas none of the placebo-treated patients achieved this level of response (p < .001).

Trials Exploring Multiple Target Dosages

Two dose-ranging trials were included in the topiramate clinical development program. Each evaluated three doses

of topiramate: 200, 400, and 600 mg/day with 4-week titration (11); and 600, 800, and 1,000 mg/day with 6-week titration (29). Maintenance periods were 12 versus in both studies. In the study by Faught et al., mean doses achieved in the three treatment arms were 200, 391, and 556 mg/day. Results are summarized in Table 80.1. The median percentage reduction in seizure rate, relative to baseline, was significantly greater with topiramate than placebo in the 400 and 600 mg/day groups, and it was of borderline significance in the 200 mg/day group (p = .051). There were significantly more responders ($\geq$50% reduction) in the topiramate 400 and 600 mg/day groups than in the placebo recipients. A significant dose–response relationship was observed for both seizure reduction (p < .005 excluding the placebo group) and the percentage of treatment responders (p < .05 excluding the placebo group).

Privitera and colleagues (29) extended the highest dosage (600 mg/day) studied by Faught et al. (11) to 800 and 1,000 mg/day and thereby covered the full anticipated dosage range encountered in clinical practice. The mean daily doses achieved in the three topiramate arms of the study were 544, 739, and 799 mg. There were statistically significant differences between each topiramate group and placebo with respect to median percentage reduction in seizure rate relative to baseline. A significantly higher percentage of patients in each topiramate group than placebo were considered responders ($\geq$50% reduction): 44%, 40%, and 38% for the 600, 800, and 1,000 mg/day groups, respectively, compared with 9% in placebo recipients (p < .001 for all groups versus placebo). Although statistical comparisons were reported between the three treatment groups, the authors commented that doses >600 mg/day did not appear to be associated with any significant efficacy advantage.

Meta-Analyses and Pooled Analyses

Additional information on the efficacy of topiramate has been provided by pooled analyses of the data generated in the six trials conducted in Europe and the United States. Because the studies involved similar protocols, patient populations, and efficacy end points, the pooled data are an important source of information on treatment response in different patient subgroups. Overall, 527 patients were treated with topiramate and 216 with placebo (31). Seizures were reduced by $\geq$50% from baseline in 43% of topiramate-treated patients and in 12% of placebo-treated patients (p < .001). Freedom from seizures was achieved in 5% of topiramate recipients but in none of the placebo-treated patients during the 11 to 19 weeks of double-blind therapy (p < .001) (Figure 80.1). The therapeutic effect of topiramate was consistent regardless of gender, age, baseline seizure frequency, and concomitant antiepileptic drug therapy.

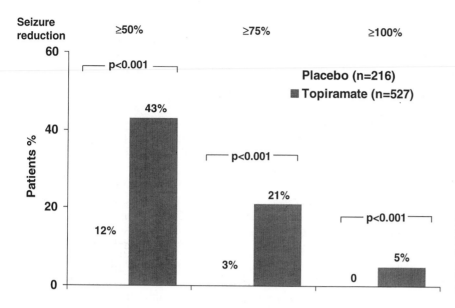

FIGURE 80.1. Response rates (≥50%, ≥75%, and 100% reduction in seizures compared with baseline) in the pooled analysis of six multicenter trials of adjunctive topiramate conducted in Europe and the United States; all dosage groups are combined (topiramate 200 to 1,000 mg/day).

Refractory Partial-Onset Seizures, with or without Secondarily Generalized Seizures, in Children

Topiramate has also been studied in children with epilepsy. A multicenter, double-blind, adjunctive-therapy, 16-week placebo-controlled trial was conducted to study the efficacy of topiramate in children ≤16 years of age with refractory partial-onset seizures, with or without secondarily generalized seizures (10). Of a total of 86 patients, 41 were randomized to topiramate and 45 to placebo. Topiramate was titrated upward to a target dose of 125 to 400 mg/day, depending on the patient's body weight (125 mg/day for 16 to 24.9 kg; 175 mg/day for 25 to 33.9 kg; 225 mg/day for 34 to 42.9 kg; 400 mg/day for ≥43 kg). Topiramate treatment was associated with a 33.1% reduction in the median percentage seizure frequency relative to baseline, compared with a 10.5% reduction in the placebo group ($p < .05$). More topiramate than placebo recipients achieved ≥50% reduction in seizure frequency (39% versus 20%, respectively). This difference was of borderline statistical significance. However, topiramate was associated with a statistically superior response when evaluated against the higher response rate of ≥75% reduction (17% versus 2%; $p < .05$), and it was also favored over placebo by the patients' parents; 69% of patients were rated by parents as showing improvement with topiramate compared with 33% with placebo ($p < .05$).

Children who participated in this double-blind trial were eligible for entry into a long-term open-label extension study in which the dose of topiramate could be raised to a maximum of 30 mg/kg/day and concomitant medication adjusted according to patient response (32). The mean topiramate dose was 9 mg/kg/day. Open-label topiramate was received by a total of 83 patients for ≥3 months and by 73 patients for ≥6 months. The median percentage reduction in seizures at ≥3 and ≥6 months was 65% and 71%, respectively. Of those who received ≥6 months treatment, seizure reductions of ≥50%, ≥75%, and 100% were achieved by 64%, 40%, and 14% of patients, respectively. Ritter and colleagues (32) noted that seizure control in this open-label extension, in which the mean dose was 9 mg/kg/day, was greater than that observed during double-blind treatment, in which topiramate was given at a mean dose of 4.8 mg/kg/day. The increase in seizure control appears to reflect the dosage adjustment. Ritter and colleagues (32) pointed out that the magnitude of the therapeutic effect observed in the double-blind trial may have been underestimated because of the higher plasma clearance of topiramate (~50% higher) in children compared with adults (35). This would imply that the mean target dose of topiramate in the controlled trial (6 mg/kg/day) would actually be equivalent to an adult dose of approximately 270 mg/day. In adults, however, maximum control of partial-onset seizures was achieved at 400 mg/day (11,39).

Refractory Primary Generalized Tonic-Clonic Seizures in Adults and Children

A multicenter, randomized, placebo-controlled, double-blind trial was conducted in 80 patients to evaluate the efficacy of topiramate in adults and children with primary generalized tonic-clonic seizures (GTCS) (4–6). Patients were required to have previously experienced tonic-clonic seizures (or at least three over an 8-week baseline) with or without other generalized seizure types and electroencephalographic (EEG) recordings consistent with generalized-onset seizures (normal or generalized epileptiform abnormalities). Patients with Lennox-Gastaut syndrome were excluded from the study. Enrolled patients were therefore most likely to present with idiopathic generalized epilepsy syndromes. However, some patients with partial-onset epilepsy often present with normal EEG readings or with what appear to be generalized epileptiform abnormalities (sometimes called secondary bilateral synchrony), and seizures in these patients may rapidly generalize into tonic-clonic seizures. It is therefore probable that a few patients with symptomatic generalized epilepsy syndromes or partial-onset seizures with rapid secondary generalization were also included in the study. In this trial, >70% of patients had at least one other type of generalized seizure (absence, myoclonic, or tonic), a finding indicating that the proportion of patients with misdiagnosed partial seizures was probably small.

Of the 80 patients enrolled, 39 were assigned to treatment with topiramate (mean age, 26.8 years) and 41 to placebo (mean age, 25.6 years), with titration and maintenance periods of 8 and 12 weeks, respectively. The study included a wide age range, with some very young children (3 to 59 years). Titration and target doses (175, 225, or 400 mg/day) were determined by patient body weight (25 to 33.9, 34 to 42.9, and ≥43 kg, respectively). Treatment with topiramate resulted in a median percentage reduction in the frequency of primary GTCS of 56.7% compared with 9.0% after placebo (*p* < .05). For all generalized seizure types, the difference between topiramate and placebo response was further increased (42.1 % reduction for topiramate and 0.9% reduction for placebo; *p* < .005). A statistically significantly higher number of topiramate-treated patients than placebo recipients were rated as responders on both ≥50% (*p* < .001) and ≥75% (*p* < .05) reduction of tonic-clonic and all generalized seizures (based on analysis of double-blind completers). The data generated in this study were further analyzed to determine whether any differences in treatment effect existed with regard to patient age, that is, ≤16 years or >16 years. The superiority of topiramate to placebo in terms of median percentage reduction in seizure frequency and percentage of patients with ≥50% reduction in seizures was maintained, regardless of patient age, for both tonic-clonic and all generalized seizure types. Despite the relative limitations of the inclusion criteria, this was the first trial to demonstrate under double-blind, placebo-controlled conditions a statistically significant therapeutic effect of an antiepileptic drug against primary GTCS.

Twelve patients who participated in the double-blind study were selected to continue topiramate treatment in a 20-week open extension (37). Compared with baseline, the frequency of GTCS was reduced by ≥50% in 11 of 12 patients (91%). Freedom from seizures was achieved by seven of 12 patients (58.3%).

An additional open-label extension of the double-blind study (4–6) was conducted to investigate the effect of long-term topiramate in children with primary GTCS without focal onset. Adjunctive topiramate was given to 33 patients for ≥3 months (18). Compared with baseline of the double-blind trial, 67% of patients showed a reduction in seizure frequency of ≥50%, whereas 6% were seizure free during the 3-month period.

A second double-blind trial of topiramate in patients with GTCS was completed, but the results have not been published. The study protocol and patient entry criteria were essentially identical to those of the trial published by Biton et al. (6).

A long-term open-label investigation of topiramate in GTCS was also undertaken as a pooled extension of both of the double-blind, placebo-controlled trials discussed earlier (3, 6). Adults and children who completed these trials (n = 131) entered the open-label extension (25). The mean duration of open-label topiramate treatment was 387 days, and the mean dose was 7 mg/kg/day. Long-term adjunctive topiramate was effective in controlling GTCS; of those patients who received open-label topiramate for ≥6 months (n = 96), GTCS were reduced ≥50% from baseline in 63% of patients and ≥75% from baseline in 44%. Although they had previously had a median pretreatment seizure rate of one GTCS a week, 16% of patients became free of GTCS over a period of ≥6 months.

Juvenile Myoclonic Epilepsy

Biton et al. reported data on a subset of 22 patients from the two primary generalized epilepsy trials noted above (4,6) who likely had juvenile myoclonic epilepsy. These data are the only comparative data of an antiepileptic drug and placebo given as adjunctive therapy in juvenile myoclonic epilepsy. Primary GTCS were reduced by at least half in 73% of topiramate-treated patients and in 18% of placebo-treated patients (*p* = .03). Although the patient populations were not sufficiently large to detect statistically significant differences in other seizure types, myoclonic seizure frequency was also reduced with topiramate. The number of weeks free of myoclonic seizures increased by 171% in topiramate-treated patients and by 130% in placebo-treated patients. For absence seizures, the median percentage increase in seizure-free weeks was 15% for topiramate-treated patients, whereas in placebo-treated patients, there was a decrease of 7%.

Lennox-Gastaut Syndrome

Topiramate was also evaluated as an adjunctive treatment for patients with Lennox-Gastaut syndrome. In this trial, Lennox-Gastaut syndrome was confirmed by EEG (i.e., slow spike-and-wave pattern) and multiple seizure types including drop attacks and a history of atypical absence seizures. A multicenter, double-blind, placebo-controlled trial enrolled patients with multiple seizure types (tonic or atonic drop attacks) and atypical absence seizures plus an

EEG pattern typical of Lennox-Gastaut syndrome and a history of ≥60 seizures in the month before baseline (38). Overall, 98 patients were enrolled in the trial (48 randomized to topiramate and 50 to placebo). Age ranged from 2 to 42 years, with a mean age of 11 years in each group. The average topiramate dose during the double-blind treatment phase was 4.8 mg/kg/day. The median percentage reduction in drop attacks relative to baseline in topiramate-treated patients was 14.5%, whereas the placebo group experienced a median increase of 5% ($p < .05$). A combined measure of drop attacks and tonic-clonic seizures was reduced by 26% with topiramate, but it increased by 5% with placebo ($p = .015$). Of the parents or guardians of patients in the topiramate group, 53% believed there had been some degree of improvement in seizure severity compared with baseline. This finding compared with 28% in the placebo group ($p < .05$). The study continued into a long-term open-label extension phase. Topiramate effectiveness in Lennox-Gastaut syndrome compared favorably to that reported in a controlled trial of lamotrigine (27). The placebo-adjusted responder rate for drop attacks was 14% for topiramate and 15% for lamotrigine; that for major motor seizures was 25% with topiramate and 17% with lamotrigine.

Ninety-seven patients (mean age, 11 years) continued open-label topiramate for a mean treatment duration of 539 days at a mean dose of 10 mg/kg/day (21). Of those patients who received topiramate for ≥6 months and who experienced drop attacks (n = 82), 55% had a reduction in drop attacks of ≥50%. A reduction of ≥75% was experienced by 35% of these patients, and 15% were free of drop attacks for at least 6 months. Of those patients who started open-label topiramate treatment, 71% continued therapy for at least 3.4 years.

Evidence from Randomized Controlled Clinical Trials: Monotherapy

As the clinical development program for topiramate has evolved, the drug has been increasingly evaluated as monotherapy. Two randomized controlled trials established the efficacy of topiramate monotherapy in patients with partial-onset seizures with or without secondary generalized seizures: (a) a multicenter trial in patients with recently diagnosed epilepsy (14) and (b) a single-center study in patients with chronic, refractory epilepsy (36).

Monotherapy trials of antiepileptic drugs are typically designed either to demonstrate superiority of the tested drug over some alternative treatment or to demonstrate equivalence of the newer medication to an established standard. The United States Food and Drug Administration has made it clear that it will not accept as evidence of efficacy the latter type of study showing that a new antiepileptic drug is equivalent to a standard antiepileptic drug. This regulatory requirement is based on the possibility that, in the particular study being evaluated, both treatments could

have been equally ineffective. In epilepsy monotherapy trials, in which a placebo control would usually be considered unethical, novel trial designs have evolved to demonstrate superiority of a new antiepileptic drug over a control treatment. The control treatment is typically a lower dose of the test drug or a relatively low dose of a standard drug. The ethical issues related to this trial design have been discussed (8). For patients and their clinicians, however, the most relevant type of monotherapy study is one that compares clinical outcomes, such as freedom from seizures, retention time in the study, and intolerable adverse events, with a new versus an old antiepileptic drug both used at optimal dosages. Such studies are designed to establish equivalence, rather than differences, as an outcome, and they require large numbers of patients with a prior definition of equivalence based on confidence intervals. The approach increasingly being taken by European regulatory authorities is to license antiepileptic drugs for monotherapy after the demonstration of equivalence, with the active control used in clinical situations for which it is approved and known to be effective. The optimal monotherapy trial design that satisfies both regulatory requirements in Europe and in the United States and provides ethically acceptable "best treatment" for patients remains a topic of discussion.

Recently Diagnosed Epilepsy

This multicenter trial was conducted at 76 sites throughout North America and Europe (14). Topiramate was administered at a low dose (25 or 50 mg/day) or a high dose (200 or 500 mg/day) according to body weight, so those patients weighing ≤50 kg received either 25 or 200 mg/day and those weighing >50 kg received either 50 or 500 mg/day (or highest tolerated dose). A total of 252 patients (aged 6 to 85 years) with recently diagnosed (within 3 years) partial-onset epilepsy or GTCS were randomized to either the low- or high-dose arm of the trial. Forty-five percent of patients received anticonvulsant medication at the time of recruitment, and this medication was discontinued over the initial 6 weeks (titration period) of the trial. Virtually all patients randomized to the low-dose group achieved the target dose, compared with 72% of patients randomized to the high-dose group.

A significant difference was observed between the low- and high-dose groups with respect to seizure frequency. After achieving the target dose of topiramate, 65% of the high-dose group compared with 39% of the low-dose group became seizure free ($p = .001$).

The median time to first seizure was greater in the high-dose group (317 days) than in the low-dose group (108 days; $p = .06$). The median time to exit because of a second seizure was also longer in the high-dose group (422 days) than in the low-dose group (293 days), although this did not reach statistical significance. However, using a bivariate analysis taking into account the dependence of the time to

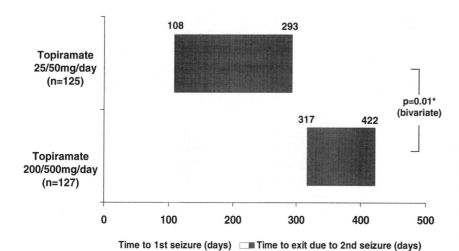

FIGURE 80.2. Median time to first seizure and to exit resulting from second seizure after high-dose (200/500 mg/day) and low-dose (25/50 mg/day) topiramate monotherapy in patients with recently diagnosed partial epilepsy. Data are based on bivariate analysis allowing for the dependence of the occurrence of a second seizure on the occurrence of a first seizure.

second seizure on the occurrence of a first seizure, the difference in time to exit resulting from a second seizure was significant and favored the higher dose ($p = .01$) (Figure 80.2).

A correlation between plasma level of topiramate and time to first seizure was observed; those patients who had the highest plasma concentrations (>9.91 μg/mL) had the longest time to first seizure. The median time to first seizure was 451 days in patients with a plasma topiramate concentration of >9.91 μg/mL, 194 days in patients with a plasma topiramate concentration of 1.77 to 9.91 μg/mL, and 84 days in those with a plasma topiramate concentration of ≤1.76 μg/mL ($p = .015$).

Chronic Refractory Epilepsy

Sachdeo and colleagues (36) reported a double-blind, single-center study comparing high (1,000 mg/day; n = 24) and low (100 mg/day; n = 24) doses of topiramate in patients ≥14 years of age with refractory partial-onset seizures, with or without secondary GTCS. Preexisting treatment was gradually tapered and was finally withdrawn over a 5-week conversion period as the dose of topiramate was titrated upward to 1,000 mg/day (or the maximum tolerated dose) or 100 mg/day. Topiramate monotherapy was subsequently stabilized at the high- or low-dose level for a further 11 weeks. The primary efficacy variable was time to exit, mainly resulting from seizure deterioration. Patients in the high-dose group remained in the study significantly longer than those in the low-dose group ($p = .002$). Of those patients who received high-dose topiramate, 13 of 24 (54%) did not leave the study for any of the predefined reasons for exit, whereas four of 24 (17%) patients in the low-dose group did not leave the study ($p = .015$).

A reduction in seizure frequency of ≥50% was achieved in 46% of patients who received 1,000 mg/day topiramate compared with 13% of those receiving 100 mg/day. Freedom from seizures was achieved in 13% of the high-dose

group compared with none of the low-dose group. Patient and investigator global ratings also confirmed the greater efficacy of the high-dose treatment, with marked improvement noted in 46% of high-dose compared with 8% of low-dose patients.

In an open-label extension phase, 19 of 20 patients experienced a reduction in seizures of ≥50% at an average dose of 555 mg/day (range, 100 to 800 mg/day). Freedom from seizures was achieved in 14 patients for periods ranging from 3 months to >2 years (37).

Topiramate Monotherapy versus Standard Monotherapy in Newly Diagnosed Epilepsy

Monotherapy is the preferred treatment choice in patients presenting with newly diagnosed epilepsy. However, the exact classification of seizure type and syndromes in this patient population can be difficult and relies on clear information at the time of diagnosis. Over time, the initial classification can be found to be incomplete or inaccurate, and thus, treatment of this patient group represents a particular clinical problem. Topiramate represents a good candidate for use in patients with newly diagnosed epilepsy because it has demonstrated efficacy in many seizure types and syndromes, as well as proven effectiveness as monotherapy.

A uniquely designed, double-blind study was conducted to compare the efficacy of topiramate monotherapy with the physician's preferred choice of initial standard antiepileptic drug monotherapy (carbamazepine or valproate) in patients with newly diagnosed epilepsy, regardless of seizure type or syndrome (30). At study entry, patients were assigned to either a carbamazepine or a valproate comparative treatment arm, based on the investigator's assessment of the best treatment choice. These patients were subsequently randomized to receive topiramate under double-blind conditions, either 100 or 200 mg/day, or the investigator's choice at doses effective for patients with newly diagnosed epilepsy (600 mg/day carbamazepine or

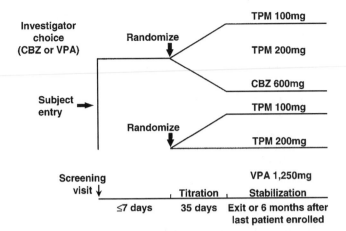

FIGURE 80.3. Patients with newly diagnosed epilepsy were assigned to either a carbamazepine or valproate comparative treatment arm according to the investigator's "best choice" of treatment and were then randomized to receive under double-blind conditions topiramate (100 or 200 mg/day) or the investigator's best choice of carbamazepine (600 mg/day) or valproate (1,250 mg/day). After a 35-day titration period, patients received their assigned treatment until exit or for 6 months after the last patient was enrolled.

1,250 mg/day valproate). After a 35-day titration period, patients received their assigned treatment until exit or for 6 months after the last patient was enrolled (Figure 80.3).

A total of 623 patients aged 6 to 84 years entered the trial, with 395 assigned to the carbamazepine-topiramate arm and 228 assigned to the valproate-topiramate arm. In total, 52% and 49% of patients in the carbamazepine and valproate treatment arms, respectively, completed the study. There were no statistically significant between-group differences for topiramate and carbamazepine or valproate in terms of time to exit, time to first seizure, and the proportion of patients who were free of seizures during the last 6 months of treatment. Discontinuation rates because of adverse events were not different among the three treatments. These results suggest that topiramate is at least as effective as carbamazepine or valproate in patients with newly diagnosed epilepsy. Topiramate, at a dose of 100 mg/day, had comparable efficacy but tended to be better tolerated than 200 mg/day, and it was at least as well tolerated as 600 mg/day carbamazepine and 1,250 mg/day valproate (30). In addition, topiramate monotherapy was associated with a lower incidence of cognitive effects such as speech disorders, related speech problems, and psychomotor slowing than reported in trials using adjunctive topiramate therapy

Evidence from Other Studies—Open Trials and Case Reports: Adjunctive Therapy

In addition to the randomized controlled trials described earlier, the clinical efficacy of topiramate has been evaluated in numerous open investigator studies and case reports. Several of these are summarized in the following discussion.

A series of open-label studies investigated the efficacy of topiramate against refractory partial seizures. The combined results of nine of these studies suggest that 80 of 173 patients who received topiramate were responders (46.2%). In seven of the studies, response was defined as median percentage reduction in seizure frequency ≥50%. This was achieved by 94 of 123 patients (76.4%). The remaining two studies defined response as percentage reduction in seizure frequency for the whole group, and the investigators reported response rates of 47% and 69% (28).

Several open-label studies have also been conducted to evaluate the therapeutic effect of topiramate as long-term adjunctive therapy further and thereby to obtain a more accurate indication of the drug's likely effectiveness as maintenance therapy. Abou-Khalil and colleagues (1) reported an open-label study in which topiramate was given to 292 adult patients with previously refractory partial and/or generalized seizures. Seizure reductions were calculated for two subsets of patients: (a) those completing ≥84 days (3 months of topiramate therapy; n = 241); and (b) those completing ≥168 days (6 months of therapy; n = 196). Overall, the mean treatment duration was 413 days, and the mean topiramate dose was 503 mg/day.

A reduction in seizure frequency of ≥50% was experienced by 54% of patients, and a reduction of ≥75% was experienced by 36% of patients. In those patients receiving adjunctive topiramate for ≥3 months, freedom from seizures was achieved in 11%, 10%, and 34% for all seizures, partial seizures, and generalized seizures, respectively. Seizure control was sustained at 6 months, with seizure reductions almost identical to findings at 3 months (10%, 9%, and 35%, respectively).

Other studies provide support for the use of topiramate in the long-term treatment of patients with partial-onset seizures. For example, Canger and colleagues (7) observed continued efficacy in the treatment of partial-onset epilepsy over a 4-year period. Michelucci et al. (24) noted that the response to topiramate was sustained for at least 5 years in those patients who previously had refractory partial seizures but who experienced an initial response.

These results are consistent with data from long-term extensions of randomized clinical trials in which 467 patients received topiramate for >6 months (*unpublished data*, Ortho-McNeil Pharmaceutical). In these trials, the percentage of patients discontinuing because of the drug's lack of effectiveness peaked at 6% in those patients who received topiramate for between 6 and 18 months. In patients who received topiramate for longer still (some patients received topiramate for >48 months), the percentage who discontinued treatment because of ineffectiveness declined to between 3% and 4%. These results suggest fairly convincingly that tolerance to topiramate does not develop over time.

Evidence from Other Studies—Open Trials and Case Reports: Monotherapy in Adults

Several investigators have reported continued good response rates to topiramate in patients with refractory partial-onset seizures after the withdrawal of concomitant antiepileptic medication (17,33,42). Some studies have subsequently investigated these observations in larger patient groups. A retrospective analysis of combined open extension data from randomized controlled trials (35) identified 45 patients from a total of 136 (33%) who had successfully been converted to monotherapy with topiramate for a mean duration of 22 months (3 to 44 months). Of these, 28 (62%) were seizure free during the last 3 months of observation.

Further long-term monotherapy data were generated in a prospective observational study of 170 patients with refractory localization-related or idiopathic generalized epilepsy (40). Thirty patients had concomitant medication discontinued, 12 had established topiramate monotherapy, and eight remained seizure free at 6 months. The authors concluded that topiramate was "efficacious as add-on and monotherapy in patients with refractory partial and generalized seizures in everyday clinical use." They also pointed out that, in many patients, good response rates were achieved with topiramate doses that were considerably lower than those used in the regulatory clinical trials; of the total study population, 16 responders and 13 seizure-free patients were receiving ≤100 mg/day topiramate.

Evidence from Other Studies—Open Trials and Case Reports: Monotherapy in Pediatrics

Refractory Partial-Onset and Primary Generalized Seizures

To date, studies investigating the use of topiramate as monotherapy in children have followed an open-label design. A pilot trial was conducted by Glauser and colleagues (19) to investigate topiramate monotherapy for partial-onset seizures in five children (3 to 12 years of age). Two patients, who were titrated up to 3 mg/kg/day over a 3-week period, remained seizure free at the time the report was published.

Further studies conducted by Moreland et al. (26) found topiramate monotherapy to be effective in children with complex partial seizures over a dose range of 2.5 to 5.0 mg/kg/day. Efficacy was also demonstrated in children with generalized epilepsy. However, the study population was too small for statistical analysis.

West's Syndrome (Infantile Spasms)

In a pilot study of West's syndrome, 11 children, aged 3 to 48 months, received topiramate (up to a target level of 24 mg/kg/day) with tapering of other antiepileptic drugs (20). Topiramate monotherapy was achieved in seven patients. A ≥50% reduction in seizure frequency was achieved by nine patients (82%), and five (45%) children became spasm free. All 11 children who participated in this study entered a long-term extension phase. The mean duration of treatment was 18 months, and the mean topiramate dosage was 29 mg/kg/day (22). At data analysis (October, 1998), eight patients (73%) were continuing topiramate treatment. Of these, four (50%) remained spasm free, and seven (88%) continued to experience a ≥50% reduction in spasm frequency. Three of the eight children (38%) who continued to take topiramate at data analysis were able to receive topiramate monotherapy (all were spasm free).

Other Childhood Epilepsies

Two small, open-label reports documented topiramate's effect in some less common syndromes. In five patients diagnosed with Angelman's syndrome and treated with topiramate (12,13), two patients were seizure free, one for 8 months and the other for 12 months. Two patients had resolution of GTCS. On patient discontinued treatment because of adverse effects. Of 14 patients with tuberous sclerosis who were treated with topiramate (12,13), nine patients had a ≥50% reduction in seizures, and three remained seizure free, whereas five were considered nonresponders. Some, but not all, of these patients had infantile spasms at some time in the past, but none of the reported cases of tuberous sclerosis or Angelman's syndrome had active spasms at the time of these studies.

Additional Studies in the Topiramate Clinical Development Program

In addition to the randomized controlled trials and long-term open-label studies described earlier, several other investigations were conducted to evaluate other aspects of topiramate—for example, optimal dose and titration rate; tolerability profile—as clinical development has evolved through adjunctive therapy, monotherapy, and, more recently, low-dose monotherapy.

To determine the optimal dose and titration rate of topiramate in the treatment of epilepsy, a multicenter, randomized, double-blind, parallel group trial was conducted in 188 patients (9). Patients were randomized to either slow titration of topiramate (n = 95) or a faster titration rate (n = 93), similar to that used in the regulatory trials of adjunctive therapy in adults. Patients in the slow-titration group received starting doses of 50 mg/day that were increased by weekly increments of 50 mg/day over an 8-week period to a maximum dose of 400 mg/day. The faster-titration group received starting doses of 100 mg/day that were increased to 200 mg/day and then to 400 mg/day over a 3-week period. Although the efficacy of topiramate was similar in the two dosage groups (according to median percentage reduction from baseline in seizure rate, percentage of responders, and percentage seizure free), the proportion of patients who discontinued treatment because of adverse events was significantly lower in the slower-titration group than in the faster-titration group (10 of 95 versus 20 of 93, respectively; *p* = .036). These data suggest that some of the adverse events reported in the controlled clinical trials may have been caused by excessively fast titration. Clinical experience certainly indicates that an initial low dose and slower titration to clinical response (which may be achieved with doses as low as 100 mg/day monotherapy) is associated with a good tolerability profile.

In addition, preliminary results of a recently completed trial of topiramate monotherapy in newly diagnosed epilepsy suggest that a dose of 100 mg/day is at least as effective and as well tolerated as the investigator's choice of standard antiepileptic drugs for this population (600 mg/day carbamazepine or 1,250 mg/day valproate) (30). The tolerability and safety of topiramate are discussed elsewhere in this publication.

MODE OF USE

Indications

Topiramate is indicated as adjunctive therapy for adults and children (≥2 years of age) with partial-onset seizures in 86 countries, for GTCS in 20 countries, and as monotherapy in eight countries. Topiramate is also indicated in 15 countries as adjunctive therapy in adults and children for seizures associated with Lennox-Gastaut syndrome.

Dosing Recommendations

Based on clinical experience and randomized, controlled trials, clinicians and investigators appear to agree that topiramate produces equal seizure control and is better tolerated when it is given at a low starting dose and is titrated slowly to clinical response.

Adults

Monotherapy. In adults, it is recommended that topiramate be given at a starting dose of 25 mg nightly for 1 week. Dosage should then be increased at 1- or 2-week intervals by increments of 25 or 50 mg/day, administered in two divided doses. The dose and titration rate should be guided by clinical outcome. Smaller increments or longer intervals between increments may be used if the patient is unable to tolerate the titration regimen. The initial target dose range for monotherapy appears to be 100 to 200 mg/day, and the maximum recommended daily dose is 500 mg. These recommendations apply to all adults, including the elderly, in the absence of underlying renal disease.

Adjunctive Therapy. As for monotherapy, it is recommended that titration be initiated at 25 mg nightly for 1 week and increased at 1- or 2-week intervals by 25 mg/day in two divided doses. The minimum effective dose is 200 mg/day, and the usual total daily dose as adjunctive therapy is 200 to 400 mg/day in two divided doses.

Children (≥2 Years)

Monotherapy. It is recommended that topiramate be given at a starting dose of 1 to 3 mg/kg nightly for the first week and then increased at 1- or 2-week intervals by increments of 1 to 3 mg/kg/day, administered in two divided doses.

Adjunctive Therapy. The recommended total daily dosage of adjunctive topiramate for children is 5 to 9 mg/kg/day in two divided doses. Titration should begin at 15 to 25 mg (or less, based on a range of 1 to 3 mg/kg/day) nightly for the first week. Dosage may then be increased by increments of 1 to 3 mg/kg/day (in two divided doses) at 1- or 2-week intervals.

In both adults and children, the tolerability of topiramate is significantly improved by slower titration without compromising clinical efficacy (9). Tolerability is therefore improved by using lower doses or by extending the time interval between dose increments in the upward titration period.

Current Role in Epilepsy Management

The clinical trial program for topiramate in epilepsy has generated a large body of data (approximately 2,600 patients, including >350 children) regarding the efficacy and safety of the anticonvulsant across a broad range of seizure types and in a wide age range. These epilepsy trials have provided some important insights into the optimal use of topiramate in clinical practice. For example, efficacy has been demonstrated with topiramate at a wide range of doses, including doses that are substantially lower than those initially employed in the controlled regulatory trials of adjunctive therapy in adults. Likewise, further investigation indicates that the titration rates used in these first controlled trials were not optimal for many patients. By using a slower titration schedule, fewer side effects are reported without compromising efficacy. Data from monotherapy trials have indicated that some side effects previously associated with adjunctive topiramate use may reflect, at least in part, pharmacodynamic interactions with other antiepileptic drugs. When topiramate is administered as monotherapy, the incidence of several adverse events, including psychomotor slowing, speech disorders, memory difficulty, and confusion, is reduced. Further investigation of topiramate use as monotherapy has also revealed that a 100 mg/day dose of topiramate had similar efficacy to 200 mg/day in newly diagnosed epilepsy, and it was better tolerated.

There is now considerable postmarketing experience with topiramate. As of October 1, 2000, 750,000 patients with epilepsy had been treated with topiramate, representing more than 400,000 patient-years of exposure. The efficacy seen in clinical practice appears to reflect the results of the clinical trials.

Use in Special Populations

The pharmacokinetics of topiramate may be affected by individual patient characteristics, such as age and coexisting medical conditions. Dosage and titration should follow the recommended guidelines, but they should also be guided by clinical outcome. In patients with renal impairment, a few additional considerations apply, as outlined in the next section.

Impaired Renal Function

Decreased renal function can alter the pharmacokinetics of drugs such as topiramate that are renally eliminated. The clearance of topiramate has been found to be reduced by 42% in patients with moderate renal impairment and 54% in those with severe renal impairment (15). It is therefore recommended that the usual topiramate dose be halved in such patients.

In contrast, a supplemental dose of topiramate is recommended for patients undergoing hemodialysis. The mean hemodialysis plasma clearance of topiramate in patients with end-stage renal disease was found to be four to six times greater than in persons with normal renal function (16). It is suggested that the supplemental dose be equivalent to one-half of the daily dose, administered in divided doses at beginning and completion of hemodialysis.

Precautions

Nephrolithiasis

Some patients who receive topiramate may be at increased risk of renal stone formation. Adequate hydration is recommended to reduce this risk, particularly in patients with a family history of nephrolithiasis, prior stone formation, or hypercalciuria.

The incidence of nephrolithiasis observed with topiramate in clinical trials was 1.5%, approximately two to four times higher than expected in a similar untreated population. Stones passed spontaneously in two-thirds of those affected, and 75% of patients decided to continue topiramate therapy despite this occurrence (31,43).

Pregnancy

Insufficient data exist at this time to assess accurately whether topiramate is more or less teratogenic than the standard antiepileptic drugs. Topiramate is teratogenic in mice, rats, and rabbits, and it leads primarily to craniofacial defects as well as limb and vertebral malformations. Teratogenic effects associated with carbonic anhydrase inhibitors are not, however, seen in humans, based on information provided to the Food and Drug Administration, but exposure to these drugs has been limited. To date, there have been no studies of topiramate in pregnant women. It is therefore recommended that topiramate be used in pregnancy only if the potential benefit outweighs the potential risk to the fetus.

The current data on pregnancies in women receiving topiramate include some retrospective and some prospective cases. Retrospective data should always be evaluated with caution, because substantial selection bias may overestimate malformation rates. For pregnancies reported prospectively, information on birth status and outcome have been collected on 27. Of these, there were no major anomalies, one minor anomaly (harelip with exposure to phenytoin and topiramate), 11 births with no anomalies, seven spontaneous abortions (consistent with the incidence of spontaneous abortion report in other data in epilepsy), one ectopic pregnancy, and seven therapeutic abortions (dysmorphic features on autopsy). Of the retrospective data, there are 40 cases with information. Of these, there were five major anomalies, three minor anomalies, 16 live births with no anomalies, eight spontaneous abortions, six therapeutic abortions (one with an abnormal finding of spina bifida and hydrocephalus; the mother had received valproate and topiramate), one fetal death, one "blighted ovum," and one not specified in terms of outcome.

Women with epilepsy who become pregnant and the physicians who treat these women should be encouraged to report and enroll in the Antiepileptic Drug Pregnancy Register of North America, a pharmaceutical company–driven registry, or in the European Registry of Antiepileptic Drugs and Pregnancy (EURAP), set up by a consortium of independent research groups and now extended to several non-European countries. The aim of both of these registries is to improve the analysis and assessment of pregnancy outcome, in terms of fetal risk, after prenatal antiepileptic drug exposure.

Oral Contraception

Topiramate has been found to increase the clearance of the estrogenic component of oral contraceptives in a dose-related manner. Therefore, the efficacy of low-dose (i.e., 20 or 30 μg) oral contraceptives may be reduced in the presence of topiramate. This effect is currently under further investigation in an ongoing steady-state monotherapy oral contraceptive study. Women receiving topiramate should be warned of the possibility of oral contraceptive failure. Clinicians should recommend that additional contraceptive measures be taken.

Contraindications

Topiramate is contraindicated in patients with a history of hypersensitivity to any component of the product.

SUMMARY

The clinical trials program for topiramate in epilepsy and considerable postmarketing experience (750,000 patients treated for ≤400,000 patient-years of exposure) indicate that topiramate is an efficacious, broad-spectrum anticonvulsant. Efficacy has been demonstrated in partial-onset seizures and primary GTCS in adults and children, as both monotherapy and adjunctive therapy. Topiramate has also demonstrated efficacy in treating the refractory and multiple seizure types of Lennox-Gastaut syndrome. Preliminary data are promising for use in treatment-resistant infantile spasms of West's syndrome. The multiple mechanisms of action exhibited by the drug (Chapter 77) may help to explain the agent's apparent broad activity in epilepsy, in both the short term and the longer term. Good clinical responses to topiramate (~10% to 30% of previously treatment-refractory patients becoming seizure free) have now been maintained in some patients for periods of ≤5 years, both as adjunctive treatment and as monotherapy.

Topiramate is currently indicated in 19 countries as adjunctive therapy for children as young as 2 years of age, the lowest child age approval of all antiepileptic agents. Use of topiramate across such a wide age range has provided valuable information, not only about efficacy and tolerability, but also about pharmacokinetics, dosing, and titration. Because of increased plasma clearance of topiramate in children compared with adults, it has been suggested that suboptimal doses were given to children under double-blind conditions (4.8 to 6 mg/kg/day). Higher dose levels (>9 mg/kg/day, as administered during open-label extension trials) are now preferred to achieve optimal clinical outcome in children.

Use of topiramate in clinical practice and subsequent clinical testing has also provided valuable information about optimal dosing in adults. The benefit of a lower starting dose and slower titration than that used in the initial regulatory trials has been substantiated.

Finally, preliminary findings of one study suggest that topiramate monotherapy is no less effective than standard carbamazepine or valproate monotherapy in patients with newly diagnosed epilepsy. Furthermore, the optimal monotherapy dose in this patient population was reported to be 100 mg/day. This dosage was as efficacious but better tolerated than 200 mg/day topiramate and at least as well tolerated as 600 mg/day carbamazepine monotherapy or 1,250 mg/day valproate monotherapy, with a notable lack of cognitive side effects reported with topiramate add-on therapy.

Although additional studies are required to investigate and define the role of topiramate further as monotherapy for adults and children with epilepsy, early indications are promising. Optimal dosing and titration as employed in recent clinical trials may substantially improve the agent's tolerability without compromising efficacy.

REFERENCES

1. Abou-Khalil B, Topiramate YOL Study Group. Topiramate in the long-term management of refractory epilepsy. *Epilepsia* 2000; 41[Suppl 1]:S72–S76.
2. Ben-Menachem E, Henriksen O, Dam M, et al. Double-blind, placebo-controlled trial of topiramate as add-on therapy in patients with refractory partial epilepsy. *Epilepsia* 1996;37: 539–543.
3. Ben-Menachem E, Topiramate YTC-E Study Group. A double-blind trial of topiramate in patients with generalized tonic-clonic seizures of non-focal origin. *Epilepsia* 1997;38[Suppl 3]:S60.
4. Biton V, Montouris GD, Riviello JD, et al. Efficacy and safety of topiramate in generalized seizures of non-focal origin. *Epilepsia* 1997;38[Suppl 8]:206–207.
5. Biton V, Chadwick D, Montouris GD, et al. Topiramate as long-term therapy in patients with generalized tonic-clonic seizures without focal onset. *Neurology* 1998;50:A311–A312.
6. Biton V, Montouris GD, Ritter F, et al. A randomized, placebo-controlled study of topiramate in primary generalized tonic-clonic seizures. *Neurology* 1999;52:1330–1337.
7. Canger R, Avanzini G, Tartara A, et al. Long-term efficacy and tolerability of topiramate add-on therapy: interim analysis after four years of treatment. *Epilepsia* 1997;38[Suppl 3]:S59.
8. Chadwick D, Privitera M. Placebo-controlled studies in neurology: where do they stop? *Neurology* 1999;52:682–685.
9. Edwards KR, Kamin M, Topiramate TPS-TR Study Group. The beneficial effect of slowing the initial titration rate of topiramate. *Neurology* 1997;48[Suppl 2]:A39.
10. Elterman RD, Glauser TA, Wyllie E, et al. A double-blind, randomized trial of topiramate as adjunctive therapy for partial-onset seizures in children. *Neurology* 1999;52:1338–1344.
11. Faught E, Wilder BJ, Ramsay RE, et al. Topiramate placebo-controlled dose-ranging trial in refractory partial epilepsy using 200-, 400-, and 600- mg daily dosages. *Neurology* 1996;46: 1684–1690.
12. Franz DN, Glauser TA, Tudor C, et al. Topiramate therapy of epilepsy associated with Angelman's syndrome. *Neurology* 2000; 54:1185–1188.
13. Franz DN, Tudor C, Leonard J. Topiramate as therapy for tuberous sclerosis complex–associated seizures. *Epilepsia* 2000;41 [Suppl 7]:87.
14. Gilliam FG, Reife R, Shu-Chen W. Topiramate monotherapy: randomized controlled trial in patients with recently diagnosed localization-related epilepsy. *Neurology* 1999;52[Suppl 2]:A248.
15. Gisclon LG, Riffitts JM, Sica DA, et al. The pharmacokinetics (PK) of topiramate (T) in subjects with renal impairment (RI) as compared to matched subjects with normal renal function (NRF). *Pharm Res* 1993;10[Suppl]:S397.
16. Gisclon LG, Curtin CR. The pharmacokinetics (PK) of topiramate (T) in subjects with end-stage renal disease undergoing hemodialysis. *Clin Pharmacol Ther* 1994;55:196.
17. Glauser TA, Olberding L, Clark P, et al. Topiramate monotherapy substitution in children with partial epilepsy. *Epilepsia* 1996; 37[Suppl 4]:S98.
18. Glauser TA. Topiramate. *Semin Pediatr Neurol* 1997;4:34–42.

19. Glauser TA, Elterman R, Wyllie E, Topiramate YP Study Team. Open-label topiramate in paediatric partial epilepsy. *Epilepsia* 1997;38[Suppl 3]:S94.

20. Glauser TA, Clark PO, Strawburg R. A pilot study of topiramate in the treatment of infantile spasms. *Epilepsia* 1998;39:1324–1328.

21. Glauser TA, Levisohn PM, Ritter F, et al. Topiramate in Lennox-Gastaut syndrome: open-label treatment of patients completing a randomized controlled trial. *Epilepsia* 2000;41[Suppl 1]:S86–S90.

22. Glauser TA, Clark PO, McGee K. Long-term response to topiramate in patients with West syndrome. *Epilepsia* 2000;41[Suppl 1]:S91–S94.

23. Korean Topiramate Study Group. Topiramate in medically intractable partial epilepsies: double-blind placebo-controlled randomized parallel group trial. *Epilepsia* 1999;40:1767–1774.

24. Michelucci R, Passarelli D, Riguzzi P, et al. Long-term follow-up of TPM in refractory partial seizures. *Epilepsia* 1998;39[Suppl 2]:S67.

25. Montouris GD, Biton V, Rosenfeld WE, et al. Nonfocal generalized tonic-clonic seizures: response during long-term topiramate treatment. *Epilepsia* 2000;41[Suppl 1]:S77–S81.

26. Moreland EC, Griesemer DA, Holden KR. Topiramate for intractable childhood epilepsy. *Seizure* 1999;8:38–40.

27. Motte J, Trevathan E, Arvidsson JF, et al. Lamotrigine for generalized seizures associated with the Lennox-Gastaut syndrome. *N Engl J Med* 1997;337:1807–1812.

28. Perucca E. A phamacological and clinical review on topiramate, a new antiepileptic drug. *Pharmacol Res* 1997;35:241–256.

29. Privitera M, Fincham R, Penry J, et al. Topiramate placebo-controlled dose-ranging trial in refractory partial epilepsy using 600-, 800-, and 1000- mg daily dosages. *Neurology* 1996;46:1678–1683.

30. Privitera MD, Brodie MJ, Neto W, et al. Monotherapy in newly diagnosed epilepsy: topiramate versus investigator choice of carbamazepine or valproate. *Epilepsia* 2000;41[Suppl F]:138.

31. Reife R, Pledger G, Shu-Chen W. Topiramate as add-on therapy: pooled analysis of randomized controlled trials in adults. *Epilepsia* 2000;41[Suppl 1]:S66–S71.

32. Ritter F, Glauser TA, Elterman RD, et al. Effectiveness, tolerability and safety of topiramate in children with partial-onset seizures. *Epilepsia* 2000;41[Suppl 1]:S82–S85.

33. Rosenfeld WE, Sachdeo RC, Wood R. Topiramate can be a successful monotherapy drug. *Epilepsia* 1995;36[Suppl 4]:S56.

34. Rosenfeld W, Abou-Khalil B, Morrell M, et al. Double-blind placebo-controlled trial of topiramate adjunctive therapy for partial onset epilepsy. *Epilepsia* 1996;37[Suppl 4]:S5.

35. Rosenfeld WE, Sachdeo RC, Faught RE, et al. Long-term experience with topiramate as adjunctive therapy and as monotherapy in patients with partial onset seizures: retrospective survey of open-label treatment. *Epilepsia* 1997;38[Suppl 1]:S34–S36.

36. Sachdeo RC, Reife RA, Lim P, et al. Topiramate monotherapy for partial onset seizures. *Epilepsia* 1997;38:294–300.

37. Sachdeo RC, Patel R, Rehman KU. Long-term experience with topiramate monotherapy. *Epilepsia* 1997;38[Suppl 8]:S97.

38. Sachdeo RC, Glauser TA, Ritter F, et al. A double-blind randomized trial of topiramate in Lennox-Gastaut syndrome: Topiramate YL Study Group. *Neurology* 1999;52:1881–1887.

39. Sharief M, Viteri C, Ben-Menachem E, et al. Double-blind, placebo-controlled study of topiramate in patients with refractory epilepsy. *Epilepsy Res* 1996;25:217–224.

40. Stephen LJ, Sills GJ, Brodie MJ. Topiramate in refractory epilepsy: a prospective observational study. *Epilepsia* 2000;41:977–980.

41. Tassinari CA, Michelucci R, Chauvel P, et al. Double-blind, placebo-controlled trial of topiramate (600 mg daily) for the treatment of refractory partial epilepsy. *Epilepsia* 1996;37:763–768.

42. Tigaran S, Dam M. Topiramate monotherapy: patient with refractory complex partial seizures becomes seizure-free. *Epilepsia* 1996;37[Suppl 4]:S62.

43. Wasserstein A, Reife R, Rak I. Topiramate and nephrolithiasis. *Epilepsia* 1995;36[Suppl 3]:S153.

44. Yen D-J, Yu H-Y, You Y-C, et al. A double-blind, placebo controlled study of topiramate in adult patients with refractory partial epilepsy. *Epilepsia* 2000;61:1162–1166.

TOPIRAMATE

CLINICAL EFFICACY AND USE IN NONEPILEPTIC DISORDERS

MARC KAMIN

For many agents effective against seizures, the term *anticonvulsant* or *antiepileptic drug* (AED) does not reflect the full scope of their potential therapeutic effects in paroxysmal and other neuropsychiatric disorders. Beginning with the initial use of carbamazepine in trigeminal neuralgia to the now routine use of valproate in bipolar disorder and migraine prophylaxis and the more recent use of gabapentin in managing various pain syndromes, AEDs are proving to be of benefit in many disorders characterized by neuronal hyperexcitability centrally and peripherally. Thus, the broader label *neuronal stabilizing agent* may be a more accurate depiction of their therapeutic activity. Topiramate appears to be one of the newer AEDs to join the ranks of neuronal stabilizing agents with potential usefulness beyond antiseizure effects.

Topiramate is a structurally novel AED used in the treatment of partial-onset seizures and primary generalized tonic-clonic seizures. Electrophysiologic and biochemical studies have identified various mechanisms of action of topiramate, including sodium channel blockade, inhibition of kainate–α-amino-3-hydroxy-5-methyl-4-isoxazole priopionate (AMPA) glutamate receptors, and potentiation of γ-aminobutyric acid (GABA)–related neuroinhibition at GABA$_A$ receptors (1). In addition, topiramate is a weak carbonic anhydrase inhibitor (2), and it may have an inhibitory effect on certain calcium channels (3). Preliminary data suggest that, in addition to its use in epilepsy, topiramate may have therapeutic effects in various chronic pain syndromes, migraine and cluster headache prophylaxis, tremor, and certain psychiatric disorders.

DIABETIC NEUROPATHY AND OTHER PAIN SYNDROMES

Peripheral neuropathy is common in patients with diabetes. Altered nerve conduction and axonal structural alterations as a result of long-standing disease can produce acute, disabling pain in the legs and feet that is often resistant to treatment with nonsteroidal antiinflammatory drugs and opioids. Agents that block sodium channels or potentiate GABAergic inhibition may also be able to ameliorate neuropathic pain.

Animal studies suggest an effect of topiramate on neuropathic pain. In a spinal nerve ligation model (4), rats received 3, 10, or 30 mg/kg doses of topiramate (5). Topiramate exhibited a long-lasting dose-dependent antiallodynic effect that peaked at 1 to 2 hours and was maintained with long-term treatment. These experimental observations are supported by findings from open-label and double-blind clinical studies. In a pilot study of eight patients with painful diabetic neuropathy, topiramate was added to baseline therapy of gabapentin, opioids, benzodiazepines, and/or tricyclic antidepressants (6). Topiramate treatment for ≤6 months at doses of 50 to 600 mg/day (mean, 258 mg/day) resulted in decreased pain intensity at the final study visit (*p* < .005). Topiramate was generally well tolerated and provided pain relief sufficient to discontinue concomitant gabapentin and benzodiazepine in all patients.

A subsequent double-blind, placebo-controlled study was conducted in 27 diabetic patients whose pain had persisted for >6 months (7). Baseline pain scores were recorded using the 45-point Short-Form McGill Pain Questionnaire (SF-MPQ) and the 100-mm visual analog scale of the SF-MPQ (Table 81.1). Topiramate was added to stable doses of existing therapy (serotonin reuptake inhibitors, tricyclic antidepressants, clonazepam) in 18 patients and was titrated over 9 weeks to the target dose of 400 mg/day. After 4 weeks of maintenance treatment, pain scores were again recorded. Patients on topiramate showed significant pain reduction in both SF-MPQ (*p* < .05) and visual analog scale

Marc Kamin, MD: Director, Clinical Research, Ortho-McNeil Pharmaceutical, Raritan, New Jersey

TABLE 81.1. MEAN PAIN SCORES IN PATIENTS WITH DIABETIC NEUROPATHY

	SF-MPQ			VAS		
	Baseline	Final Visit	% Change	Baseline	Final Visit	% Change
Topiramate (n = 18)	14.3	11.1	−22%	69.2	40.7	−41%
Placebo (n = 9)	22.7	25.1	+11%	64.6	70.4	+9%
		p < .05			*p* < .01	

SF-MPQ, Short-Form McGill Pain Questionnaire; VAS, 100-mm visual analog scale of SF-MPQ.
From White HS. Comparative anticonvulsant and mechanistic profile of the established and newer antiepileptic drugs. *Epilepsia* 1999; 40(suppl 1):S52-S60, with permission.

scores (*p* < .01), whereas patients receiving placebo had no pain reduction. Topiramate was generally well tolerated; four topiramate-treated patients and one placebo recipient withdrew because of side effects. The most common adverse events in patients receiving topiramate were asthenia, confusion, and weight loss. Average weight loss at the final visit was 9 pounds for 14 topiramate-treated patients versus 1 pound for eight placebo recipients.

Topiramate-related weight loss has been associated with improvements in metabolic parameters such as glucose, insulin, and lipid levels (8). Further studies are needed to document whether topiramate has dual benefits in patients with diabetic neuropathy.

Anecdotal reports of topiramate use in other pain syndromes suggest that it may be a reasonable alternative treatment for patients in whom other therapies have failed. Open-label topiramate administered to 14 patients with histories of painful neuropathic symptoms resulted in significant pain reduction (9). Neuropathic pain syndromes included reflex sympathetic dystrophy in five patients and other forms of painful neuritis in nine (diabetic neuropathies were excluded). Before topiramate treatment, all patients reported substantial pain on a 10-point scale (mean, 8.8). After ≤6 months of topiramate treatment at doses of 100 to 800 mg/day, pain scores were significantly improved (mean, 3.1; *p* < .0001). Patients reported that pain relief first became apparent at doses of 50 to 600 mg/day (mean, 214 mg/day).

Patients undergoing thoracic surgery often develop an intense intercostal neuralgia that is refractory to treatment with antidepressants, AEDs, and opioid and nonopioid analgesics. In a case report of a 60-year-old patient with chronic postthoracotomy pain syndrome, various therapies failed to alleviate burning pain, either because of intolerable side effects (oral amitriptyline, mexiletine, carbamazepine, phenytoin, lidocaine, capsaicin) or because of suboptimal analgesia (nortriptyline, desipramine, paroxetine, gabapentin, lamotrigine) (10). A bedtime dose of 75 mg/day topiramate provided sufficient pain relief to allow the patient to sleep through the night. An additional morning dose of 75 mg/day provided consistent pain relief throughout the day and was maintained for >6 months without intolerable side effects.

In case reports of patients with chronic regional pain syndrome type 1, low doses of topiramate (50 to 125 mg/day) added to existing opioid analgesic therapy produced marked pain reduction, which was sustained for >1 year even though previous treatment with nonsteroidal antiinflammatory drugs, acetaminophen, tricyclic antidepressants, carbamazepine, gabapentin, and other pain therapies had failed to provide effective pain relief for these patients (6). Topiramate appeared to be especially helpful in relieving allodynia and improving sleep. A patient with postherpetic neuralgia also had persisting pain relief at a topiramate dose of 50 mg/day but discontinued treatment after 7 months because of dizziness and unsteadiness. A patient with atypical facial pain did not respond to topiramate at 400 mg/day.

Topiramate may also be effective against trigeminal neuralgia. Because this pain syndrome is more common in patients with multiple sclerosis than in the general population, open-label topiramate was administered to six patients with multiple sclerosis who had long-standing trigeminal neuralgia resistant to carbamazepine and other conventional therapy (11). Patients typically reported pain relief within the first week of topiramate therapy. Five patients reported complete disappearance of pain at 100 mg taken twice daily, and these patients were able to discontinue their concomitant medications. Pain also resolved completely for one patient who required 150 mg topiramate twice daily plus adjunctive carbamazepine. After 6 months, the therapeutic effect of topiramate was maintained with only minor side effects (mild nausea and dizziness) and no discontinuation of therapy.

MIGRAINE PROPHYLAXIS AND OTHER HEADACHE SYNDROMES

Migraine is a chronic neurologic disorder characterized by episodic attacks, occurring most frequently in women. Migraine therapy encompasses avoidance of triggers to prevent attacks, symptomatic treatment of acute attacks, and long-term prophylactic treatment.

Two relatively small, double-blind, placebo-controlled studies have evaluated topiramate prophylaxis in patients with migraine. In one trial, 40 patients (39 female patients) were randomized to treatment with topiramate (n = 19) or placebo (n = 21) for 16 weeks (12). All patients had migraine, with or without aura, for >1 year and were experiencing at least two episodes every month. After a 4-week baseline phase, topiramate was started at 25 mg/day and was gradually increased over 8 weeks to a mean dose of 125 mg/day. Concomitant migraine prophylaxis was permitted at prestudy doses. After an 8-week maintenance phase, the mean 28-day headache rate calculated for the entire double-blind phase was compared with baseline. Topiramate prophylaxis significantly reduced headache frequency versus placebo (*p* < .005) (Figure 81.1). Mean headache frequency was reduced by 36% in topiramate-treated patients and by 12% in placebo recipients. In addition, 26% of topiramate-treated patients responded to treatment with a ≥50% reduction in headache frequency versus 10% of placebo recipients. Adverse events were generally mild and included paresthesia, taste alteration, weight loss, anorexia, memory impairment, dysarthria, abnormal vision, emotional lability, and urinary frequency. Two topiramate-treated patients discontinued the study because of adverse events (nausea, emotional lability).

A second double-blind, placebo-controlled study used a similar design with a slightly shorter titration phase (4-week baseline, 6-week titration, 12-week maintenance) (13). In this study, 30 patients (29 female patients) were randomized to topiramate prophylaxis (n = 15) or placebo (n = 15). Abortive migraine medication was permitted. Eleven patients reached a topiramate dose of 200 mg/day (mean, 173 mg/day). After 18 weeks of treatment, mean 28-day headache frequency was reduced by 29% in topiramate-treated patients and by 7% in placebo recipients (Figure 81.1). In addition, 47% of topiramate-treated patients had a ≥50% reduction in headache frequency versus 7% of placebo recipients. Topiramate also significantly reduced migraine severity and migraine disability. Therapy was well

tolerated, and discontinuation rates were similar between study groups. Adverse events included paresthesia, diarrhea, altered taste, and somnolence. Weight loss was significantly greater with topiramate treatment (*p* = .01). Mean body weight in placebo-treated patients did not change, whereas topiramate-treated patients lost an average of 6.2 pounds; weight loss tended to correlate with baseline body weight.

Anecdotal reports also support a prophylactic effect of topiramate in migraine management. In a retrospective chart review, 69 patients with migraine (56 female patients) who received topiramate prophylaxis ranging from 25 to 500 mg/day were followed-up for ≤24 weeks (14). Topiramate treatment significantly reduced the frequency of moderate to severe headaches by 30%. A subset analysis of 38 treatment-refractory patients in whom nine or more migraine preventive medications had previously failed showed that topiramate reduced moderate to severe headaches by 23%. Fifty patients experienced side effects, most commonly paresthesia, drowsiness, diarrhea, and decreased appetite. Twenty-seven patients discontinued topiramate, 21 because of adverse events.

A chart review of 34 patients (31 female patients) with intractable chronic migraine also found topiramate to be effective prophylaxis (15). All patients had chronic migraine (median, 20 years) unresponsive to various acute and preventive therapies, with at least three episodes of migraine per week and daily or near-daily migraines in 29 patients. Topiramate was added to existing therapy and was increased to a mean dose of 98 mg/day; patients were maintained on topiramate for ≤18 weeks (mean, 9 weeks). At the end of the maintenance period, 19 patients were improved or much improved with topiramate treatment, and 15 reported no change. Common adverse events were fatigue, paresthesia, and anorexia or weight loss. Fourteen patients lost between 1 and 26 pounds. Seven patients discontinued treatment because of adverse events.

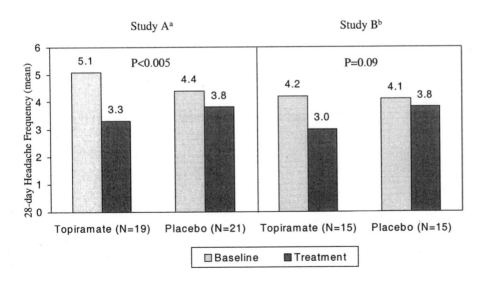

FIGURE 81.1. Effect of topiramate prophylaxis in patients with migraine. Frequency of migraine episodes in a 28-day period was reduced from baseline by 36% and 29% with topiramate treatment versus 12% and 7% with placebo. (Data from Potter DL, Hart DE, Calder CS, et al. A double-blind, randomized, placebo-controlled, parallel study to determine the efficacy of topiramate in the prophylactic treatment of migraine. *Neurology* 2000;54[Suppl 3]:A15(abst); and Edwards KR, Glantz MJ, Norton JA, et al. Topiramate in the prevention of episodic migraine: a double-blind, placebo-controlled trial. Abstract presented at the 42nd annual meeting of the American Headache Society, Montreal, 2000.)

In an open-label study of topiramate as migraine prophylaxis in patients with refractory migraine or chronic daily headache, Shuaib et al. found that low-dose topiramate reduced the frequency and severity of severe migraines or chronic daily headaches (16). Topiramate was administered to 68 patients with frequent (more than seven) headaches each month and in whom previous prophylaxis with two or more agents had failed. Patients received topiramate for ≤18 months, starting at 25 mg twice daily and increasing to a maximum of 200 mg/day over 6 to 8 weeks. A treatment effect was apparent within 8 to 10 weeks; 38% reported significant improvement (>60% reduction in headaches) and 24% reported moderate improvement (40% to 60% reduction). Headache severity was also reduced in most patients reporting improvement. Topiramate was well tolerated, with a few patients reporting drowsiness, concentration difficulty, paresthesia, and dizziness.

Small, open-label investigations of topiramate in other headache syndromes have also been reported. Cluster headache, a relatively uncommon condition that is easily misdiagnosed, is characterized by episodes of severe pain several times a day for weeks or months, followed by long periods of remission. Low-dose topiramate was administered to 10 patients in an open-label study of cluster headache, including two patients with chronic cluster headache unremitting from onset and one patient with a cluster-tic syndrome (17). Topiramate treatment at doses of ≤125 mg/day (mean, 85 mg/day) was associated with rapid improvement in all patients, with remission of cluster episodes in nine patients within 1 to 3 weeks. Side effects of drowsiness, paresthesia, and word-finding difficulty were mild and were reported by only three patients.

ESSENTIAL TREMOR

Essential tremor is one of the most common movement disorders, but it is often confused with Parkinson's disease.

Drug treatment strategies include propranolol and primidone, but adverse effects and drug interactions limit the usefulness of these agents in the elderly. Although results with GABAergic agents, carbonic anhydrase inhibitors, and calcium channel blockers have been inconsistent (18–20), topiramate's multiple mechanisms may offer a different approach to treatment. In a pilot, placebo-controlled crossover study (6), 24 patients received either 2 weeks of topiramate (≤400 mg/day) or placebo in addition to stable doses of existing therapy. After a 2-week washout period, patients were crossed over to the other study arm. Tremor rating scores that quantified tremor location/severity, specific motor tasks/functional disabilities, and tremor-resultant functional disabilities showed significant reduction with topiramate treatment (Table 81.2). The most common adverse events were appetite suppression or weight loss and paresthesia.

Two open-label studies of topiramate in essential tremor also suggested a treatment benefit. Eleven patients received 75 to 400 mg/day topiramate for ≤21 months (21). Results showed significant improvement in patients in whom who previous treatment with propanolol, primidone, and/or gabapentin had failed. Ten patients had ≥50% improvement and seven ≥75% improvement in tremors. Five patients were able to reduce or discontinue concomitant treatment with primidone, propanolol, and/or clonazepam. No serious adverse events occurred. Three patients reported weight loss, two experienced paresthesia, and one reported memory difficulty that resolved when the topiramate dose was reduced.

In another open-label study, nine patients in whom previous standard therapy for essential tremor had failed received an average topiramate dose of 144 mg/day (22). The study population included eight patients age ≥68 years, seven patients with long-standing tremor (>10 years), three with associated head tremor, and two with associated voice tremor. With topiramate treatment, there was a 60% improvement in the Archimedes Spiral average scores and a

TABLE 81.2. MEAN CHANGE IN NORMALIZED TREMOR RATING SCORES

	Intent-to-Treat (n = 24)[a]		Study Completers (n = 15)	
	Topiramate	Placebo	Topiramate	Placebo
Overall score	−0.88 p < .05	−0.15	−1.38 p = .001	−0.07
Location/severity	−0.42 p = .010	−0.09	−0.68 p < .001	−0.09
Motor tasks/function	−0.19 p < .05	−0.01	−0.29 p < .003	−0.03
Functional disability	−0.27 p = .06	−0.06	−0.45 p < .05	−0.08

[a]Imputed intent-to-treat analysis with baseline observation carried forward for subjects discontinuing treatment.
From Dodgson SJ, Shank RP, Maryanoff BE. Topiramate as an inhibitor of carbonic anhydrase isozymes. *Epilepsia* 2000; 41(suppl 1):S35-S39, with permission.

53% improvement in the Activities of Daily Living average scores. Eight patients rated themselves as better and with less disability on a visual analog scale. There was no improvement in head or voice tremors. Topiramate was generally well tolerated, with fatigue and paresthesia as the most common side effects. One patient reported increased diuresis, and two patients discontinued treatment because of fatigue, despite improvements in tremor.

BIPOLAR DISORDER

Bipolar disorder affects about 1% of the general population. Standard treatment for manic episodes includes lithium and the anticonvulsants valproate, which potentiates neuroinhibition by GABA, and carbamazepine, a sodium channel blocker. Alternative treatments include clonazepam and lorazepam, which enhance GABAergic neurotransmission by binding to the $GABA_A$ receptor, and acetazolamide, a carbonic anhydrase inhibitor. Topiramate has been used as an alternative treatment for bipolar disorder because of similar mechanisms, including potentiation of GABA-related neuroinhibition at $GABA_A$ receptors, sodium channel blockade, and weak carbonic anhydrase inhibition (1–3).

In an open-label study, 56 outpatients with bipolar disorder who did not respond to or could not tolerate lithium, valproate, or carbamazepine therapy had topiramate added to their existing therapy (23). At baseline, 32 patients had manic, mixed, or rapidly cycling mood symptoms, 11 were depressed, and 13 were relatively euthymic. Topiramate was started at 25 to 50 mg/day and increased gradually over the course of treatment to a maximum dose of 1,200 mg/day. Mean dose was 291 mg/day at 6 months and 425 mg/day at 1 year. Two patients with manic symptoms at the start of treatment discontinued topiramate in the first week because of dizziness and hallucinations. Overall, patients with mania at baseline showed significant response to topiramate, but depressed and euthymic patients showed no significant changes. Clinical Global Impression scores showed that 55% of 30 initially manic patients were much or very much improved in their manic symptoms after a mean of 312 days of treatment; these patients also had significant decreases in Young Mania Rating scores. Topiramate was generally well tolerated, with mild and transient central nervous system– or gastrointestinal-related adverse effects, including reduced appetite, cognitive impairment, fatigue, and sedation.. Weight and body mass index were significantly reduced with topiramate treatment. Ten patients discontinued treatment because of side effects, including two because of weight loss.

In another open-label study, 45 patients with bipolar disorder, in all of whom previous treatment with at least two mood stabilizers had failed, were treated with topiramate for 6 months (24). Before topiramate treatment, all patients had moderately severe depression according to Hamilton Depression Rating scores (range, 18 to 29). Topiramate was added to existing therapy of mood stabilizers, antidepressants, and/or benzodiazepines and was increased every 2 days to a mean dose of 275 mg/day. Of the 31 patients completing the trial, 19 had a full response to treatment (scores of 3 to 7), and 12 responded partially (scores of 8 to 12). Response was seen within the first 4 weeks of therapy, with further mood stabilization after 8 weeks. Transient paresthesia and numbness occurred in three patients, which resolved with dose reduction. Fourteen patients discontinued treatment, nine because of adverse events of headache, tremor, dizziness, nausea, incoordination, sedation, or paresthesia. Seven patients lost weight previously gained while they were taking lithium and valproate.

An open-label trial of topiramate included 20 patients, including 18 patients with bipolar disorder and two patients with schizoaffective disorder, treated for an average of 142 days (25). All patients had responded poorly or not at all to combination therapy with mood stabilizers and/or antipsychotic agents, including recent treatment with lithium, valproate, carbamazepine, and gabapentin. Topiramate was added to stable doses of psychotropic drugs and was increased every 5 to 7 days to a maximum of 300 mg/day; mean dose at week 5 was 210 mg/day. Twelve patients responded positively to topiramate treatment, including one patient who discontinued treatment temporarily because of confusion and was successfully restarted on the drug after 2 weeks. Four patients had no response, and one patient worsened. Topiramate was generally well tolerated, with adverse events in nine patients during the first month of treatment. Three diabetic patients achieved good glycemic control with topiramate. All patients lost weight with topiramate treatment, with an average loss of 9 pounds over 5 weeks.

Open-label topiramate was given as a treatment for acute mania in 11 patients with bipolar disorder type 1 who were unresponsive to lithium and/or valproate (26). Topiramate was administered (with or without adjunctive lorazepam) for ≤29 days (mean dose, 313 mg/day). Mania was reduced in half of patients, with increased level of functioning and global improvement. Three patients had a >50% reduction in mania scores, and five patients had improved global impression scores. Treatment was generally well tolerated, with paresthesia as the most common side effect. Three of four patients completing the study lost weight.

Retrospective chart reviews also showed the potential of topiramate in bipolar disease. A chart review of 58 consecutive patients treated with open-label topiramate for various psychiatric disorders showed improvement in more than half (27). Diagnoses included 44 patients with rapidly cycling bipolar disorder, nine patients with schizoaffective disorder, three patients with dementia, and two patients with psychosis. In 18 patients, treatment with lamotrigine and/or gabapentin plus conventional mood stabilizers had previously failed. Topiramate was added to concomitant medications and was gradually increased to doses ≤400 mg/day; 12 patients with rapidly cycling bipolar disorder had concomitant medications discontinued. Positive response to treatment—changes in sleep, appetite, mood, and concentration—were seen in 36 patients, often within 72 hours of the first dose and usually within days to weeks of topiramate initiation. Six patients were worse during topiramate therapy. Topiramate produced marked or moderate improvement in all five patients with dementia and psychosis, a finding suggesting an antipsychotic effect. Of the 18 patients in whom lamotrigine and/or gabapentin had previously failed, 50% had marked or moderate improvement with topiramate. Adverse events included delirium in one bipolar patient with a history of psychosis (the patient overmedicated with topiramate, tranylcypromine sulfate, and alcohol). One patient with epilepsy and mixed bipolar with panic attacks had an increase in panic attacks and a generalized tonic-clonic seizure. Other adverse events were generally minor gastrointestinal or central nervous system effects, including paresthesia, somnolence, fatigue, and concentration or memory difficulty; six patients treatment because of adverse events.

Twenty-seven women with rapidly cycling bipolar disorder were treated with open-label topiramate (28). Patients had long-standing disease (≤41 years) and were refractory to at least two previous mood stabilizers for >12 months; all 27 had significant weight gain from previous therapy. Patients received a mood stabilizer (lithium or valproate) for 3 weeks, then topiramate was added at 25 mg/day and was increased to a maximum of 150 mg/day. Fifteen of 23 treatment completers showed significant improvement in mood in <12 weeks. Therapy was well tolerated, with four discontinuations resulting from side effects, all before week 3 of treatment. One patient who discontinued treatment at week 3 had significant improvement in mood. Fourteen patients lost weight during the 16-week study (>5% body weight in nine), and 12 patients maintained baseline weight.

These preliminary observations suggest that topiramate may be an effective treatment for acute manic and mixed episodes associated with bipolar disorder. Pharmacokinetic studies show that topiramate has no clinically significant effect on haloperidol serum concentrations (29) and results in a modest decrease in lithium serum concentrations (30), findings suggesting that topiramate can be added to existing therapy without complication.

Anecdotal reports of topiramate use in other psychiatric conditions include patients with posttraumatic stress disorder (31) and binge-eating disorder (32). Topiramate was added to existing therapy in 17 patients with posttraumatic stress disorder (31). Symptoms included nightmares in 13 patients and flashbacks involving reexperience of trauma in all 17. Six patients also had bipolar disorder (including two with hallucinations), and 10 patients had major depressive disorder. Topiramate was started at 25 mg/day and was

increased by 25 to 50 mg every 3 to 4 days. Nightmares were suppressed in 12 of 13 patients (completely in nine), and flashbacks were suppressed in 16 of 17 (completely in 10). All patients with nonhallucinatory disorder responded, usually within 2 to 3 days of reaching an effective dose. Three patients had a full response within the first week of treatment. Five patients discontinued treatment because of adverse events or the patient's choice. For those continuing treatment, topiramate remained effective, with no evidence of developing tolerance.

Topiramate was used as an open-label treatment for binge-eating disorder, characterized by recurrent episodes of binge eating not associated with compensatory behavior (e.g., bulimia) (32). Thirteen female patients with binge-eating disorder received ≤1,400 mg/day topiramate added to existing psychotropic therapy. The improved response in nine patients was maintained for 3 to 30 months. One patient had a mild response, one had no response, and two were lost to follow-up. Mean weight decreased from 99 to 88 kg, and mean body mass index dropped from 36.5 to 32.2. However, only seven patients accounted for this weight loss; one patient lost <5 kg, three patients lost no weight, and two patients gained weight. Mean topiramate dose for all 13 patients was 492 mg/day, but the mean dose in the seven patients losing >5 kg was 725 mg/day, significantly higher than in the six who lost <5 kg (mean, 221 mg/day). Of seven patients electing to continue topiramate after the study because of improvement of binge eating, response has continued for 21 months. Topiramate was well tolerated, with transient central nervous system side effects.

CONCLUSION

Topiramate has multiple mechanisms of action that may be important both in controlling seizures and in treating other neurologic conditions. Results of pilot controlled trials and open-label studies suggest that topiramate is a potential therapy for numerous disorders other than epilepsy. In patients with neuropathic pain, including painful diabetic neuropathy and trigeminal neuralgia, topiramate appears to provide consistent pain relief to patients in whom other analgesics, including other AEDs, have failed. At low doses, side effects are minor and tolerable. Initial experience in patients with chronic headache and migraine suggest that low-dose topiramate may be an effective prophylactic therapy, reducing the monthly frequency of episodes. Topiramate may be effective in controlling essential tremor in some patients, perhaps because of the combination of GABAergic and carbonic anhydrase inhibitory effects. Topiramate also appears to be effective in controlling manic episodes in bipolar patients and may find application as a neuronal stabilizing agent in other neurologic disorders as well. Further study in randomized controlled trials is needed to document these initial observations.

REFERENCES

1. White HS. Comparative anticonvulsant and mechanistic profile of the established and newer antiepileptic drugs. *Epilepsia* 1999; 40[Suppl 1]:S52–S60.
2. Dodgson SJ, Shank RP, Maryanoff BE. Topiramate as an inhibitor of carbonic anhydrase isozymes. *Epilepsia* 2000;41 [Suppl 1]:S35–S39.
3. Zhang X-I, Velumian AA, Jones OT, et al. Modulation of high-voltage-activated calcium channels in dentate granule cells by topiramate. *Epilepsia* 2000;41[Suppl 1]:S52–S60.
4. Kim SH, Chung JM. An experimental model for peripheral neuropathy produced by segmental spinal nerve ligation in the rat. *Pain* 1992;50:355–363.
5. Wild KD, Yagel SK, Codd EE, et al. The anticonvulsant topiramate is anti-allodynic in a rat model of neuropathic pain. *Soc Neurosci Abstr* 1997;23:2358(abst).
6. Ortho-McNeil Pharmaceutical. Data on file. Raritan, NJ.
7. Edwards KR, Glantz MJ, Button J, et al. Efficacy and safety of topiramate in the treatment of painful diabetic neuropathy: a double-blind, placebo-controlled study. *Neurology* 2000;54 [Suppl 3]:A81(abst).
8. Ben-Menachem E, Smith U, Hellstrom K, et al. Prospective study on metabolism and weight changes in patients with epilepsy treated with topiramate. *Epilepsia* 2000;41[Suppl 7]:222(abst).
9. Potter D, Edwards KR. Potential role of topiramate in relief of neuropathic pain. *Neurology* 1998;50[Suppl 4]:A255(abst).
10. Bajwa ZH, Sami N, Warfield CA, et al. Topiramate relieves refractory intercostal neuralgia. *Neurology* 1999;52:1917.
11. Zvartau-Hind M, Din MU, Gilani A, et al. Topiramate relieves refractory trigeminal neuralgia in MS patients. *Neurology* 2000;55:1587–1588.
12. Potter DL, Hart DE, Calder CS, et al. A double-blind, randomized, placebo-controlled, parallel study to determine the efficacy of topiramate in the prophylactic treatment of migraine. *Neurology* 2000;54[Suppl 3]:A15(abst).
13. Edwards KR, Glantz MJ, Norton JA, et al. Topiramate in the prevention of episodic migraine: a double-blind, placebo-controlled trial. Abstract presented at the 42nd annual meeting of the American Headache Society, Montreal, 2000.
14. Von Seggern RL, Mannix LK, Adelman JU. Efficacy of topiramate in migraine prophylaxis: a retrospective chart analysis. *Neurology* 2000;54[Suppl 3]:267–268(abst).
15. Wilson MC. Efficacy of topiramate in the prophylactic treatment of intractable chronic migraine: a retrospective chart analysis. *Cephalagia* 2000;20:301(abst).
16. Shuaib A, Ahmad F, Kochanski P, et al. Efficacy of topiramate in prophylaxis of frequent severe migraines or chronic daily headaches: experience with 70 patients over 18 months. *Cephalalgia* 2000;20:423(abst).
17. Wheeler SD, Carrazana EJ. Topiramate-treated cluster headache. *Neurology* 1999;53:234-236.
18. Gironell A, Kulisevsky J, Barbanoj M, et al. A randomized placebo-controlled comparative trial of gabapentin and propanolol in essential tremor. *Arch Neurol* 1999;56:475–480.
19. Busenbark K, Pahwa R, Hubble J, et al. Double-blind controlled study of methazolamide in the treatment of essential tremor. *Neurology* 1993;43:1045–1047.
20. Biary N, Bahou Y, Sofi MA, et al. The effect of nimodipine on essential tremor. *Neurology* 1995;45:1523–1525.
21. Connor GS. Topiramate as a novel treatment for essential tremor. Poster abstract presented at Headache World 2000, London, 2000.
22. Galvez-Jimenez N, Hargreave M. Topiramate and essential tremor. *Ann Neurol* 2000;47:837–838.
23. McElroy SL, Suppes T, Keck PE, et al. Open-label adjunctive topiramate in the treatment of bipolar disorders. *Biol Psychiatry* 2000;47:1025–1033.
24. Hussain MZ, Chaudhry ZA. Treatment of bipolar depression with topiramate. *Eur Neuropsychopharmacol* 1999;9[Suppl 5]: S222(abst).
25. Chengappa KNR, Rathore D, Levine J, et al. Topiramate as add-on treatment for patients with bipolar mania. *Bipolar Disord* 1999;1:42–53.
26. Calabrese JR, Shelton MD, Keck PE, et al. Topiramate in severe treatment-refractory mania. Paper presented at the 151st annual meeting of the American Psychiatric Association, Toronto, 1998.
27. Marcotte D. Use of topiramate, a new anti-epileptic as a mood stabilizer. *J Affect Disord* 1998;50:245–251.
28. Kusumaker V, Yatham LN, O'Donovan C, et al. Topiramate augmentation in women with refractory rapid cycling bipolar disorder and significant weight gain from previous treatment. *Bipolar Disord* 1999;1[Suppl 1]:38–39(abst).
29. Doose DR, Kohl KA, Desai-Krieger D, et al. No clinically significant effect of topiramate on haloperidol plasma concentration. Poster presented at the 1999 World Congress of Psychiatry, Hamburg, Germany, 1999.
30. Doose DR, Kohl KA, Desai-Krieger D, et al. No significant effect of topiramate on lithium serum concentration. Poster presented at the 1999 World Congress of Psychiatry, Hamburg, Germany, 1999.
31. Berlant J. Open-label trial of topiramate in post-traumatic stress disorder. Poster presented at the 1999 World Congress of Psychiatry, Hamburg, Germany, 1999.
32. Shapira NA, Goldsmith TD, McElroy SL. Treatment of binge-eating disorder with topiramate: a clinical case series. *J Clin Psychiatry* 2000;61:368–372.

Antiepileptic Drugs, 5th Edition. Edited by R.H. Levy, R.H. Mattson, B.S. Meldrum, and E. Perucca. Lippincott Williams & Wilkins, Philadelphia © 2002.

TOPIRAMATE

ADVERSE EFFECTS

RAJESH C. SACHDEO
ROOPAL M. KARIA

New antiepileptic drugs (AEDs) are approved on the basis of controlled clinical trials in a limited number of patients. Although these types of trials do enable us to see the most common emerging side effects of the new medication, it is really with postmarketing surveillance, when the drug has had a large patient population exposure, that we can begin to appreciate its full adverse potential.

Most second-generation anticonvulsants are fairly well tolerated; nonetheless, there are certain well-recognized side effects. Topiramate, currently in use in 750,000 patients worldwide, is no exception. As is the case with most AEDs, most adverse events are related to the central nervous system, although the spectrum of potential toxicities associated with topiramate use is quite broad. Other systems affected include renal, metabolic, and endocrine.

CENTRAL NERVOUS SYSTEM

The most common and most important central nervous system side effect is cognitive slowing. A prospective study designed to evaluate cognition was performed in a group of healthy adults who were randomized to one of three drug groups: topiramate, lamotrigine, and gabapentin (1). The subjects were assessed for attention, psychomotor speed, memory, language, mood, concentration, and cognition. After single doses, topiramate (5.7 mg/kg) decreased performance in attention and word fluency tests, whereas lamotrigine (3.5 mg/kg) and gabapentin (35 mg/kg) had no effect. After 4 weeks of multiple doses, topiramate (5.7 mg/kg) was still associated with impairment in verbal memory and psychomotor speed, whereas lamotrigine (7.1 mg/kg) and

Rajesh C. Sachdeo, MD: Clinical Professor of Neurology, Department of Neurology, University of Medicine and Dentistry of New Jersey, Robert Wood Johnson Medical School; and Director, Comprehensive Epilepsy Center, Robert Wood University Hospital, New Brunswick, New Jersey

Roopal M. Karia, MD: Fellow and Instructor, Department of Neurology, University of Medicine and Dentistry of New Jersey, Robert Wood Johnson Medical School, New Brunswick, New Jersey

gabapentin (35 mg/kg) did not cause any impairment. In an add-on study conducted in patients receiving carbamazepine comedication, topiramate was also titrated rapidly by 50 mg/day, at weekly intervals up to 400 mg/day and compared with valproate, which was titrated up to 2, 250 mg/day (2). In this study, the topiramate-treated group had slightly more psychomotor slowing, speech problems, confusion, and mood problems in comparison with the valproate-treated group, but after 20 weeks, the effects of the two drugs did not differ significantly in most patients. Another study with a more gradual dose-escalation (25 mg weekly) paradigm demonstrated a higher dropout rate in the topiramate group compared to the valproate group because of side effects. At the end of the maintenance phase of this trial, changes in one of 10 cognitive function variables (short-term verbal memory) were significantly worse for the topiramate-treated group (3).

Patients taking topiramate may have word-finding difficulty as well as difficulties using words, and they tend to repeat themselves. In a meta-analysis on the safety of topiramate based on double-blind controlled studies, many of which used target doses higher than those currently recommended, "abnormal thinking" was noted in 25% to 33% of patients (4). This term encompassed slowed thoughts, difficulty in calculating, dulled thinking, difficulty with calculation, slowness in response, and blunted mental reaction. Burton et al. (5) studied topiramate's effects specifically on attention, which was assessed by way of digit span. Subjects were tested at weekly intervals over a 3-month period, and results were compared with those of the control group. These investigators found that four of nine patients had problems with attention, especially at higher drug doses (5). Most of these side effects are seen during the first 2 months of initial titration period, they are often transient, or they abate after dosage reduction (6). Although their incidence can be reduced with a low starting dose and a slower dose-escalation rate, these effects continue to be seen in everyday practice, and their importance cannot be overemphasized.

Other side effects of topiramate include somnolence, fatigue, and slurred speech (7). These effects were notably seen in a double-blind, randomized trial studying the use of topiramate in Lennox-Gastaut syndrome (8). In the initial randomized placebo-controlled trials (9–13) in adults with refractory partial-onset seizures, topiramate doses of 100 mg/day were added to the other AEDs and were titrated at 100 to 200 mg/day on a weekly basis, which is faster than currently recommended. The most common adverse effects seen with a 10% higher rate than in the placebo-treated group were dizziness, somnolence, psychomotor slowing, ataxia, and memory difficulty. Treatment withdrawals were more commonly seen in the higher-dosage groups. In a pooled analysis of data from 527 patients treated with top-iramate and 216 patients taking placebo, the central nervous system side effects associated with topiramate were mild to moderate and included speech problems, memory difficulty, somnolence, fatigue, and dizziness (14).

The use of topiramate in children is also associated with significant side effects. In a 3-year retrospective analysis of 51 children and adolescents ranging in age from 3 to 16 years, most of the patients had the drug withdrawn because of adverse effects. Of the 51 patients, 57% experienced side effects including cognitive difficulties (15). Other adverse events noted in children include dizziness, fatigue, ataxia, and confusion (16). Moreland et. al. followed-up 49 children with intractable epilepsy. In these patients, the most efficacious dose of topiramate was between 2.5 and 7.5 mg/kg/day. More then 50% of the children experienced side effects that could interfere with their learning ability at school. Hence, the authors recommended that although topiramate may be efficacious, patients taking the drug should be closely watched for a possible decline in cognitive function (17).

Adverse events emerging when topiramate is added to other AEDs are not likely to reflect pharmacokinetic interactions because topiramate does not significantly alter plasma levels of concomitant AEDs. With topiramate, pharmacodynamic interactions appear to be a major contributor to treatment-related adverse events. This is demonstrated by the observation of a lower incidence of side effects with topiramate monotherapy (18,19).

Because topiramate is a carbonic anhydrase inhibitor, this mechanism may be the explanation for the occurrence of paresthesias, which have been reported in ≤15% of the patients who participated in the controlled clinical trials. The symptoms are mild and are often transient (20). However, in a monotherapy study involving 48 patients with partial seizures who were randomized to topiramate at 100 mg/day, topiramate at 1,000 mg/day, or placebo, paresthesias were present in 63% of the 100 mg/day group and 58% in the 1,000 mg/day group (21). In a another monotherapy study comparing topiramate with standard AEDs such as carbamazepine and valproate, the incidence of paresthesia was 25% in the topiramate-treated group (20).

Development of hemiparesis was reported in two patients during the first few weeks of topiramate therapy (22). The condition cleared after drug withdrawal. Both patients had preexisting cerebral damage, which may have facilitated the appearance of this unusual side effect.

Alterations in mood and behavior are common in patients with epilepsy, and AEDs may play a significant role in the pathogenesis of these disorders. In the already discussed study in health volunteers in whom topiramate was compared with lamotrigine and gabapentin, subjects allocated to topiramate had a higher incidence of depression 4 weeks after starting the drug (1). The topiramate-treated group also had more anger and hostility when these patients were evaluated for mood profile compared with the lamotrigine group. Overall analysis showed that the patients treated with topiramate had higher scores for depression, anger, and hostility at 4 weeks of starting treatment in comparison to baseline. As discussed earlier, however, the applicability of these data to the therapeutic situation is uncertain.

Psychotic episodes are not uncommon in patients with refractory epilepsy (23,24). The incidence of psychosis in patients taking topiramate was 0.8% in randomized controlled trials. In a separate cohort of ≤1,000 patients treated for ≤5.3 years, an incidence of 3% was reported (25,26). A retrospective chart review of 80 patients taking topiramate (50 to 400 mg/day) showed a 6% incidence of acute psychotic symptoms (25). A postmarketing study of 787 patients revealed an incidence of 1.3% (27). A prior history of psychotic symptoms was a risk factor in some, but certainly not all, of the patients. Symptoms of psychosis in most instances were thought to be related to topiramate, because rapid resolution occurred once topiramate was discontinued.

RENAL CALCULI

Renal calculi are a well-recognized concern with the use of topiramate. The reported incidence is about 1.5% (21), representing a two- to fourfold increase over the estimated occurrence in the general population. Most patients faced with this problem do not need surgery and go on to continue treatment with topiramate once the stone is passed (21). Renal calculi may be more common in men (28). The proposed mechanism for the calculus formation is the inherent action of topiramate as a carbonic anhydrase inhibitor. The result is reduced urinary citrate excretion, which, in turn, raises the urinary pH. It is proposed that the risk of stone formation from this process can be reduced with proper hydration. The concomitant administration of other carbonic anhydrase inhibitors such as acetazolamide and the use of diuretics may increase the risk.

CENTRAL HYPERVENTILATION

As a carbonic anhydrase inhibitor, topiramate reduces serum bicarbonate levels. This, in turn, can lead to reversible metabolic acidosis in some patients (29–33). The clinical expression of this in a pediatric population has been described as the central hyperventilation syndrome (33). Other reports of dyspnea on exertion were described in the context of topiramate use as migraine prophylaxis (34). In these otherwise healthy migraineurs, respiratory symptoms resolved with discontinuation of the drug, and these patients were not found to have any cardiopulmonary problems to account for the symptoms. Another clinical manifestation of reversible metabolic acidosis is encephalopathy. Such encephalopathies have been reported in patients taking topiramate and also receiving adjunctive therapy with valproate (35,36). Once again, the symptoms resolve when topiramate or valproate is discontinued.

WEIGHT LOSS

That patients taking topiramate actually lose weight rather than experiencing weight gain, as with some other AEDs, has been widely observed. The average body weight decreases 2% to 7% (1.6 to 6.5 kg) (14). The mechanism by which this phenomenon happens is unclear, although an attempt has been made to investigate it through the use of animal models. Rats given topiramate showed decreased body fat as well as acutely reduced food intake and an increased metabolic rate. These animals also had decreased levels of total insulin, leptin, and corticosterone (37). The precise mechanism for all these changes remains to be determined.

Other investigators suggest that topiramate inhibits fat deposition. The activity of lipoprotein lipase is reduced in adipose tissue in topiramate-treated rats (38).

The reasons for the observed weight loss may, in fact, be mulifactorial and remain to be properly characterized. In patients taking topiramate, weight loss occurs early in the treatment and is maximal by 15 to 18 months. It appears to be the greatest in patients who are heavier at the onset and is most commonly seen in female patients (39).

HORMONAL EFFECTS

As with most AEDs, topiramate may reduce the effects of oral contraceptive medications. Rosenfeld et al. (40) gave topiramate to 12 women who were taking valproate and a contraceptive containing a combination of norethindrone 1.0 mg/ethinyl estradiol 35 μg. Serum norethindrone, ethinyl estradiol, and progesterone levels were measured first with the patient taking valproate and the oral contraceptive pill alone (cycle 1). Once topiramate was added at three different doses (200, 400, and 800 mg/day over cycles 2, 3, and 4, respectively), the same tests were repeated. Ethinyl estradiol concentration decreased in a dose-dependent fashion during topiramate administration, with a 30%

reduction seen at the highest topiramate dose (800 mg/day). Hence, in women taking topiramate who are also taking oral contraceptive medication, an oral contraceptive medication with a higher estrogen content should be preferably used (41).

PREGNANCY AND BREAST-FEEDING

It is estimated that approximately 1 million women with epilepsy are of childbearing age in the United States (42). In the postmarketing experience, cases of hypospadias have been seen in male infants exposed to topiramate *in utero*. This has been observed in monotherapy as well as with the use of other concomitant anticonvulsants; however, a causal relationship has yet to be determined, and overall available data remain insufficient to assess potential risks for the human embryo (43). Teratogenicity has been described in experimental animals. Problems include craniofacial malformations, low fetal body weight, and limb malformations such as ectrodactyly, micromelia, and amelia. Rats who were exposed to topiramate in late pregnancy and during lactation had offspring with poor physical development. Although AEDs have been implicated as a major cause of teratogenesis, the clinician should be aware that uncontrolled epilepsy is also a risk to the mother as well as to the infant (44).

In animal studies, topiramate was found to be secreted in breast milk (45). Most authorities advise weighing the risk:benefit ratio in patients taking topiramate who wish to breast-feed their infants.

HEMATOLOGIC EFFECTS

Topiramate binds to erythrocytes more so than to plasma proteins, even though binding to red blood cells has been shown to be saturable (46). Nonetheless, there have not been any well-described changes in hematologic parameters with the use of this AED (47).

HYPERSENSITIVITY AND IDIOSYNCRATIC REACTIONS

The so-called anticonvulsant hypersensitivity syndrome can manifest as a rash, lymphadenopathy, fever, hepatitis, and/or eosinophilia. To date, this kind of a reaction has not been observed with the use of topiramate (48). In controlled clinical trials, the incidence of rash was similar in topiramate-treated groups when compared with placebo-treated groups.

In controlled trials, no clinically significant changes in the mean values of clinical laboratory tests, including liver and renal function, were observed. In addition, there were no treatment-related changes in electrocardiographic, ophthalmologic, or audiometric parameters.

Since then, a few case reports have described problems in clinical use. A brief case report (49) described the development of liver failure requiring a transplant in a female patient receiving topiramate (300 mg/day) who was also receiving carbamazepine (800 mg/day). More data and observation will be needed to ascertain a causal relationship.

CONCLUSION

Thus far, the most important adverse effect of topiramate is cognitive dysfunction, as evidenced by mental slowing and word-finding difficulty, which can be quite significant. The other significant side effects are renal calculi, weight loss, paresthesias, and a pharmacokinetic interaction with steroid oral contraceptives. Significant effects on cardiovascular function, as well as effects on bone density, bone marrow cells, and thyroid function, have not been reported so far. With the exception of the rather high incidence of troublesome central nervous system problems, topiramate appears otherwise to be a relatively well-tolerated and reasonably safe addition to our antiepileptic armamentarium.

REFERENCES

1. Martin R, Kuzniecky R, Ho S, et al. Cognitive effects of topiramate, gabapentin, and lamotrigine in healthy young adults. *Neurology* 1999;52:321–327.
2. Loring D, Kamin M, Karim R. Topiramate (TPM) or valproate (VPA) added to carbamazepine (CBZ) in adults with epilepsy: effects on subjective and objective measure of cognitive function. *Epilepsia* 2000;41[Suppl F]:113.
3. Aldenkamp AP, Baker G, Mulder OG, et al. A multicenter, randomized clinical study to evaluate the effect on cognitive function of topiramate compared with valproate as add-on therapy to carbamazepine in patients with partial-onset seizures. *Epilepsia* 2000;41:1167–1178.
4. Jones MW. Topiramate. *Epilepsia* 1999;40[Suppl 5]:S71–S80.
5. Burton LA, Harden C. Effect of topiramate on attention. *Epilepsy Res* 1997;27:29–32.
6. Sachdeo RC. Topiramate. *Clin Pharm* 1998;34:335–346.
7. Genton P, Biraben A. Topiramate in clinical practice. Part 20. Multicentric retrospective evaluation of its tolerability. *Rev Neurol* 2000;156:1120–1125.
8. Sachdeo RC, Glauser TA, Ritter F, et al. A double-blind, randomized trial of topiramate in Lennox-Gestaut syndrome. *Neurology* 1999;52:1882–1887.
9. Faught E, Wilder BJ, Ramsy RE, et al. Topiramate placebo-controlled dose ranging trial in refractory partial epilepsy using 200-, 400-, and 600 mg daily dosages. *Neurology* 1996;46:1684–1690.
10. Privitera M, Fincham R, Penry J, et al. Topiramate placebo-controlled dose-ranging trial in refractory partial epilepsy using 600-, 800-, and 1000-mg daily dosages. *Neurology* 1996;46:1678–1683.
11. Sharief M, Viteri C, Ben-Menachem E, et al. Double-blind, placebo-contoleed trial of topiramate in patients with refractory partial epilepsy. *Epilepsy Res* 1996;25:217–224.
12. Tassinri CA, Michelicci R, Chauvel P, et al. Double-blind,

placebo-controlled trial of topiramate (600 mg daily) for the treatment ofrefractory partial epilepsy. *Epilepsia* 1996;37:763–768.
13. Ben-Menachem E, Henrisken O, Dam M, et al. Double-blind, placebo-controlled trial of topiramate as add-on therapy in patients with refractory partial seizures. *Epilepsia* 1996;37:539–543.
14. Reife R, Pledger G, Wu SC. Topiramate as add-on therapy: pooled analysis of randomized controlled trials in adults. *Epilepsia* 2000;41[Suppl 1]:S66–S71.
15. Mohamed K, Appleton R, Rosenbloom L. Efficacy and tolerability of topiramate in childhood and adolescent epilepsy: a clinical experience. *Seizure* 2000;9:137–141.
16. Glauser TA. Topiramate. *Epilepsia* 1999;40[Suppl 5]:S71–S80.
17. Moreland EC, Griesemer DA, Holden KR. Topiramte for intractable childhood epilepsy. *Seizure* 1999;8:38–40.
18. Gilliam FG, Veloso F. Tolerability of topiramate as monotherapy in patients with recently diagnosed partial epilepsy. *Epilepsia* 1998;39[Suppl 6]:56.
19. Privitera MD, Brodie MJ, Neto S, et al. Monotherapy in newly diagnosed epilepsy: topiramate vs. investigator choice of carbmazepine orvalproate. *Epilepsia* 2000;41[Suppl F]:138.
20. Krauss G, Crone N. Non-CNS side effects of antiepileptic drugs. *Neurol Neurosurg* 2000;1–12.
21. Sachdeo RC, Reife RA, Lim P, Pledger G. Topiramate monotherapy for partial onset seizures. *Epilepsia* 1997;38:294–300.
22. Stephen LJ, Maxwell JE, Brodie MJ. Transient hemiparesis with topiramate. *BMJ* 1999;318:845.
23. Trimble MR. *The psychosis of epilepsy.* New York: Raven Press, 1991.
24. Mendez MF. Grau R, Doss RC, Taylor JL. Schizophrenia in epilepsy: seizure and psychosis variables. *Neurology* 1993;43:1073–1077.
25. Khan A, Faught E, Gilliam F, et al. Acute psychotic symptoms induced by topiramate. *Seizure* 1999;8:235–237.
26. Shorvon SD. Safety of topiramate: adverse events and relationships to dosing. *Epilesia* 1996;37[Suppl 2]:S18–S22.
27. Kanner AM, Faufght E, French JA, et al. Psychiatric adverse events caused by topiramate and lamotrigine: a postmarketing prevalence and risk-factor study. *Epilepsia* 2000; 41[Suppl 7]:169.
28. Wasserstein AG, Rak I, Reife RA. Nephrolithiasis during treatment with topiramate. *Epilepsia* 1995;36[Suppl 3]:S153.
29. Stowe CD, Bolliger T, James LP, et al. Acute mental status changes and hyperchloremic metabolic acidosiswith long-term topiramate therapy. *Pharmacotherapy* 2000;20:105–109.
30. Wilner A, Raymond K, Pollard R. Topiramate and metabolic acidosis. *Epilepsia* 1999;40:792–795.
31. Sethi PP, Tulyapronchote R, Faught E, et al. Topiramate-induced metabolic acidosis. *Epilepsia* 1999;40[Suppl 7]:148.
32. Takeoka M, Holmes GL, Thiele E, et al. Topiramate andmetabolic acidosis in pediatric epilepsy. *Epilepsia* 1999;40[Suppl 7]:127.
33. Laskey AL, Korn DE, Moorjani BI, et al. Central hyperventilation related to administration of topiramate. *Pediatr Neurol* 2000;22:305–308.
34. Waterhouse X, et al. *Neurology* 2000;54[Suppl 3]:XX(abst).
35. Hamer HM, Knake S, Schomburg U, et al. Valproate-induced hyperammonemic encephalopathy in the presence of topiramate. *Neurology* 2000;54:230–232.
36. Solomon GE. Valproate-induced hyperammonemic encephalopathy in the presence of topiramate [Letter]. *Neurolgy* 2000;55:606.
37. York DA, Singer L, Thomas S, et al. Effect of topiramate on body weight and body composition of Osborne-mendel rats fed a high-fat diet: alterations in hormones, neuropeptide, and uncoupling-protein mRNAs. *Nutrition* 2000;16:967–975.

38. Richard D, Ferland J, Lalonde J, et al. Influence of topiramate in the regulation of energy balance. *Nutrition* 2000;16:961–966.

39. Greenwood RS. Adverse effects of antiepileptic drugs. *Epilepsia* 2000;41[Suppl 2]:S42–S51.

40. Rosenfeld WE, Doose DR, Walker SA, et al. Effect of topiramate on the pharmacokenetics of an oral contraceptive containing norethindrone and ethinyl estradiol in patients with epilepsy. *Epilepsia* 1997;38:317–323.

41. Wilbur K, Ensom MH. Pharmacokenetic drug interactions between oral contraceptives and second-generation anticonvulsants. *Clin Pharmcotherapy* 2000;38:355–365.

42. Chang SI, Mcauley JW. Pharmacotherapeutic issues for women of childbearing age with epilepsy. *Ann Pharmacother* 1998;32:794–801.

43. *Topamax product labeling.* Raritan, NJ: Ortho-McNeil Pharmaceutical, 2000.

44. Zahn C. Neurologic care of pregnant women with epilepsy. *Epilepsia* 1998;39[Suppl 8]:S26–S31.

45. Bar-Oz B, Nulman I, Koren G, et al. Anticonvulsants and breast feeding: a critical review. *Paediatr Drugs* 2000;2:113–126.

46. Gidal BE, Lensmeyer GL. Therapeutic monitoring of topiramate: evaluation of the saturable distribution between erythrocytes and plasma of whole blood using an optimized high-pressure liquid chromatography method. *Ther Drug Monit* 1999;21:567–576.

47. Harden C. Therapeutic safety monitoring: what to look for and when to look for it. *Epilepsia* 2000;41[Suppl 8]:S37–S43.

48. Hamer HM, Morris HH. Hypersensitivity syndrome to antiepileptic drugs: a review including new anticonvulsants. *Cleve Clin J Med* 1999;66:239–245.

49. Bjoro K, Gjerstad L, Bentdal O, et al. Topiramate and fulminant liver failure. *Lancet* 1998;352:119.

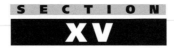

VALPROIC ACID

VALPROIC ACID

MECHANISMS OF ACTION

WOLFGANG LÖSCHER

Valproic acid or valproate (VPA) is the common name for 2-propylpentanoic acid (also called *n*-dipropylacetic acid). As a simple branched-chain carboxylic acid, it differs markedly in structure from all other antiepileptic drugs in clinical use. VPA was first synthesized in 1882 by Burton (1), but there was no known clinical use until its anticonvulsant activity was fortuitously discovered by Pierre Eymard in 1962 in the laboratory of G. Carraz, a discovery published by Meunier et al. (2). The first clinical trials of the sodium salt of VPA were reported in 1964 by Carraz et al. (3). The drug was marketed in France in 1967 and was released subsequently in more than 100 other countries (in the United States in 1978) for the treatment of epilepsy. Since then, VPA has established itself worldwide as a major antiepileptic drug for patients with several types of epileptic seizures, including both partial and generalized seizures. Clinical experience with VPA has continued to grow, including the use of VPA for diseases other than epilepsy, such as in bipolar disorders and migraine.

Although limitations of space do not permit a detailed review of the numerous effects of VPA in diverse experimental preparations, this chapter summarizes the drug's major properties and effects on nervous tissue, with particular emphasis on VPA's actions that appear to be of importance for its anticonvulsant effect. For a more comprehensive survey of the multiple effects of VPA, several previous reviews and monographs are available (4–7).

MULTIPLE ACTIONS OF VALPROIC ACID AND ITS METABOLITES

Experimentally, VPA exerts anticonvulsant effects in almost all animal models of seizure states examined in this respect,

including models of different types of generalized seizures as well as focal seizures (6). The anticonvulsant potency of VPA strongly depends on the species, the type of seizure induction, the seizure type, the route of administration, and the time interval between drug administration and seizure induction. Because of the rapid penetration into the brain but the short half-life of VPA in most species (6), the most marked effects are obtained shortly (i.e., 2 to 15 minutes) after intraparenteral (i.p.) injection. Depending on the preparation, the onset of action after oral administration may be slower. In most laboratory animal species, the duration of anticonvulsant action of VPA is short, so high doses of VPA are needed to suppress long-lasting or recurring seizures in animal models. In general, the anticonvulsant potency of VPA increases in parallel with the size of the animal. In rodents, the highest anticonvulsant potencies are obtained in genetically seizure-susceptible species, such as gerbils, with an anticonvulsant median effective dose (ED_{50}) of 73 mg/kg i.p., and rats with spontaneously occurring spike–wave discharges (ED_{50} 80 mg/kg i.p.), and against seizures induced by the inverse benzodiazepine receptor agonist DMCM in mice (ED_{50} 60 mg/kg i.p.), whereas ED_{50} doses in other rodent models of generalized or focal seizures are usually substantially higher, in the range of 200 to 400 mg/kg (6).

In addition to animal models of generalized or focal seizures, VPA also has been evaluated in models of status epilepticus. As shown by Hönack and Löscher (8) in a mouse model of generalized convulsive (grand mal) status epilepticus, VPA, by intravenous injection, was as rapid as benzodiazepines in suppressing generalized tonic-clonic seizures; this effect was related to the instantaneous entry of VPA into the brain after this route of administration. In view of the different mechanisms presumably involved in anticonvulsant activity of VPA against different seizure types, the situation may be different for other types of status epilepticus, because not all cellular effects of VPA occur rapidly after administration. This finding is substantiated by accumulating clinical experience with parenteral formu-

Wolfgang Löscher, PhD: Professor and Chairman, Department of Pharmacology, Toxicology and Pharmacy, School of Veterinary Medicine, Hannover, Germany

lations of VPA in treatment of different types (e.g., convulsive versus nonconvulsive) of status epilepticus.

Whereas most reports dealing with VPA's anticonvulsant activity in animal models examine the *acute* short-lasting anticonvulsant effects after single-dose administration, several studies have evaluated the anticonvulsant efficacy of VPA during *long-term* administration. During the first days of treatment of amygdala-kindled rats, a marked increase in anticonvulsant activity was observed that was not related to alterations in brain or plasma drug or metabolite levels (9,10). Similarly, when anticonvulsant activity was measured by means of timed intravenous infusion of pentylenetetrazol (PTZ), prolonged treatment of mice with VPA resulted in marked increases in anticonvulsant activity on the second day of treatment and thereafter compared with the acute effect of VPA, although plasma levels measured at each seizure threshold determination did not differ significantly (11). This late effect of VPA developed irrespective of the administration protocol (once per day, three times per day, continuous infusion) used for treatment with VPA in the animals. Such an increase in anticonvulsant activity during long-term treatment was also observed in epileptic patients and should be considered when *acute* anticonvulsant doses or concentrations of VPA in animal models are compared with effective doses or concentrations in epileptic patients during *long-term* treatment. In other words, doses or plasma levels that are ineffective after acute administration can become effective during long-term administration. The possible mechanisms involved in early (i.e., occurring immediately after first administration of an effective dose) and late (i.e., developing during long-term administration) anticonvulsant effects of VPA are discussed later in this chapter. Early and late effects of VPA have been also observed in *in vitro* preparations (12,13).

In addition to short- or long-term anticonvulsant effects in animal models of seizures or epilepsy, data from the kindling model indicate that VPA may exert antiepileptogenic effects (14).

The active concentrations of VPA in the brain or plasma strongly depend on the model examined. When a VPA-sensitive model, such as the threshold for clonic seizures determined by intravenous infusion of PTZ in mice, is used, the drug concentrations in brain tissue after administration of effective doses are close to the range of effective concentrations determined in brain biopsies of epileptic patients, which are in the range of 40 to 200 μmol/L (6). However, because of the marked differences in pharmacokinetics of VPA between rodents and humans (rodents eliminate VPA about 10 times more rapidly than humans), the doses that have to be administered to reach these brain concentrations in mice or rats are much higher (~100 to 200 mg/kg) than respective doses in humans (~20 mg/kg). Such determinations of effective brain concentrations are important for interpretation of *in vitro* data on VPA, because the neurochemical or neurophysiologic effects of VPA found *in vitro*

are only of interest if they occur in concentrations that are reached *in vivo* at anticonvulsant (nontoxic) doses.

In addition to its anticonvulsant activity, VPA exerts several other pharmacodynamic effects in animal models, including anxiolytic, antiaggressive, anticonflict, antidystonic, antinociceptive, sedative-hypnotic, immunostimulating, and antihypertensive actions (6). Several of these preclinical actions are in line with VPA's therapeutic potential in indications other than epilepsy (7,15).

Because VPA is rapidly metabolized to various pharmacologically active metabolites *in vivo* (16), these substances have to be considered when mechanisms of action of VPA are discussed. One of the major active metabolites of VPA in plasma and central nervous system (CNS) of different species, including humans, is the *trans* isomer of 2-en-VPA (E-2-en-VPA). This compound is the most potent and most extensively studied active metabolite of VPA (6,17,18). *Trans*-2-en-VPA is effective in the same seizure models as VPA, often with higher potency than the parent drug. Accordingly, in most neurochemical and neurophysiologic experiments with *trans*-2-en-VPA, the compound exerted more potent effects than VPA (6).

The precise mechanism of action of VPA or its active metabolites, like that of many other antiepileptic drugs, is unknown. Much attention has focused on VPA's effects on γ-aminobutyric acid (GABA), one of the principal inhibitory neurotransmitters in the CNS. However, given VPA's various experimental and clinical effects and its numerous effects on neuronal tissue, no single action of VPA can completely account for these effects.

EFFECTS ON EPILEPTIFORM DISCHARGES

Various *in vitro* preparations were used to study the anticonvulsant action of VPA on epileptiform discharges. In slices prepared from guinea pig brain, VPA was shown to prevent the appearance of penicillin-induced epileptiform spikes (19). In contrast, VPA was either ineffective or caused an increase in both burst frequency and amplitude when epileptiform activity was induced by PTZ in the CA3 region of the *in vitro* hippocampus, a finding indicating that these chemically induced hippocampal epileptiform activities may be differentially sensitive to antiepileptic drugs (20). Epileptiform bursting induced by bicuculline in rat amygdala slices was decreased by VPA (21). When epileptiform discharges were induced by combined application of bicuculline and 4-aminopyridine in combined entorhinal cortex–hippocampal slices from rats, these discharges were resistant to VPA and other standard anticonvulsants (22), whereas epileptiform discharges induced by 4-aminopyridine alone were potently suppressed by VPA (23). In studies on the age-dependency of VPA's anticonvulsant effect on 4-aminopyridine–induced epileptiform discharges in hippocampal slices, VPA blocked the ictal discharges in slices from both young and adult rats, whereas interictal epileptiform activity was blocked by VPA only in slices from young rats (24). In young rat hippocampus, extracellular magnesium was shown to influence the effects of VPA on 4-aminopyridine–induced epileptiform events (25).

When epileptiform discharges were induced in the combined entorhinal cortex–hippocampal slice by removing magnesium ions from the perfusion fluid, early clonic-tonic discharges in the entorhinal cortex and the interictal-like activity in area CA3 were effectively suppressed by VPA, whereas the late recurrent tonic discharge state in the entorhinal cortex was unaffected by the drug (26). This late epileptiform activity was, however, still sensitive to an *N*-methyl-D-aspartate (NMDA) receptor antagonist. Subsequent experiments showed that the late recurrent discharges produced in the entorhinal cortex by prolonged exposure to low magnesium are resistant to all major anticonvulsants, a finding suggesting that they may represent a model of difficult-to-treat status epilepticus (27). In addition to induction of epileptiform events by reducing extracellular magnesium, such events can be produced in the entorhinal cortex and hippocampus by reducing extracellular calcium (Ca^{2+}) or increasing extracellular potassium, but the patterns of epileptiform activity differ between these extracellular ion manipulations (28). VPA and its major active metabolite, *trans*-2-en-VPA, were shown to block all these forms of epileptiform activity, except the late recurrent discharges in the entorhinal cortex (28). The metabolite appeared to be more effective than VPA in these experiments. Analogous to entorhinal cortex–hippocampal slices, in rodent thalamocortical slices, different types of spontaneous epileptiform activity can be elicited by a medium containing no added magnesium. VPA was found to be effective in this *in vitro* model of primary generalized epilepsy (29).

Like phenytoin and carbamazepine, therapeutic concentrations of VPA were shown to limit the ability of cultured mouse CNS (cortical and spinal cord) neurons to fire sodium (Na^+)-dependent action potentials at high frequency (30). Such high-frequency firing has, for instance, been detected along subcortical pathways from a penicillin-induced cortical epileptogenic focus (31). Limitation of such firing may be important in preventing the spread of seizures. More recently, the effects of VPA on high-frequency sustained repetitive firing (SRF) in mouse central neurons in cell culture was compared with those of its major active metabolite *trans*-2-en-VPA (13). Both compounds limited firing in a concentration-, voltage-, rate-, and time-dependent fashion. The concentration dependence of limitation by both drugs markedly shifted to the left with duration of exposure; VPA was slightly more potent than *trans*-2-en-VPA after prolonged exposure (13). Although the precise biophysical mechanism underlying the ability of VPA (and its metabolite) to reduce SRF has not been elucidated, it was suggested that this effect proba-

bly relates to a phenytoinlike use- and voltage-dependent blockade of voltage-dependent Na^+ channels (30). Detailed voltage clamp experiments of VPA actions on Na^+ currents are described later in this chapter.

With respect to *in vivo* studies, VPA suppressed electrically induced afterdischarges in the hippocampus of cats (32) and significantly elevated the afterdischarge threshold and decreased the afterdischarge duration in the rat amygdala (33). VPA also raised the threshold for thalamic afterdischarges induced by electrical stimulation of the cat nucleus centralis lateralis and the rat nucleus reticularis without changing the duration of the afterdischarges in both species (34). With respect to focal seizures, VPA suppressed the epileptiform activity generated by a cobalt focus in the cat hippocampus and blocked the spreading of spontaneous as well as electrically induced seizure discharge from the hippocampus to the neocortex (32). Mutani and Fariello (35) noted that VPA suppressed the ictal and interictal seizure discharges in cats with an epileptogenic cobalt focus in the cruciate cortex. After administration of the drug, electrical stimulation of the cobalt focus failed to produce seizure activity. The same authors (36) observed that subcortical injection of aluminium gel into the sensorimotor cortex of cats produced focal cortical seizure discharges and myoclonic jerks of the head; this focal seizure activity could generalize, and VPA prevented this secondary generalization without influencing the epileptogenic focus. Moreover, van Duijn and Beckmann (37) noted that VPA did not decrease the focal discharge in the sensorimotor cortex of the awake cat produced by topical cobalt administration, but it effectively inhibited the spread of seizure activity from the focus. When two epileptogenic foci were formed in homotopic areas of the sensorimotor cortex of rats by application of penicillin, VPA blocked the focal discharges and secondary generalization of these discharges (38). In the amygdala-kindling model in rats, VPA was found to increase the threshold for electrical induction of afterdischarges and to reduce seizure severity, seizure duration, and afterdischarge duration recorded at the elevated threshold, findings indicating that VPA suppresses both the initiation and propagation of focal seizures in this model (39).

When cortical self-sustained afterdischarges were induced by rhythmic electrical stimulation of subcortical structures as a model of primary generalized seizures of the absence type, these epileptiform discharges were almost completely blocked by VPA (40). Similarly, VPA suppressed spontaneous spike–wave discharges in a genetic rat model of absencelike seizures (41). The major metabolite of VPA, *trans*-2-en-VPA, was more potent than VPA in blocking the spontaneous spike–wave discharges in these rats (42). Taken together, with few exceptions, VPA proved to be effective in suppressing epileptiform discharges in all *in vitro* and *in vivo* models tested in this respect, a finding in line with its broad spectrum of anticonvulsant activity against different seizure types in patients.

PHYSIOLOGIC EFFECTS

The well-documented effects of VPA on seizure discharge and the spread of neuronal excitability set the stage for studying the physiologic mechanisms underlying these effects. However, whether VPA acts through postsynaptic effects on neurotransmitter functions or ion channels or by presynaptic biochemical effects is still a matter of debate.

Effects on Excitability or Inhibition

Macdonald and Bergey (43) were the first to describe that VPA potentiates neuronal responses to GABA by a postsynaptic effect. However, VPA was examined after microiontophoretic application, so the local (extracellular) drug concentration was unknown. Subsequent *in vitro* studies showed that increased postsynaptic GABA responses are only obtained with very high VPA concentrations (6). To my knowledge, only one report demonstrated GABA potentiation at therapeutically relevant concentrations of VPA *in vitro* (44). The authors, using locus coeruleus neurons for their experiments, suggested that the difference between their data and those of other groups may result from the different brain regions examined in these studies. Indeed, based on neurophysiologic data, a regionally specific action of VPA in the brain was also suggested by Baldino and Geller (45).

In *in vivo* experiments, VPA was shown to lead to a potentiation of postsynaptic GABA responses at doses of 200 to 400 mg/kg (6). Because brain concentrations of VPA after these doses are much lower than the concentrations that potentiate GABA responses *in vitro*, the *in vivo* effect of VPA was likely not related to a direct postsynaptic action but more probably was the result of VPA's presynaptic effects, that is, enhanced GABA turnover (see later).

Experiments on central mouse neurons in culture indicated that neuronal responses to glycine or excitatory amino acids, such as glutamate, are not altered by VPA at relevant concentrations (6). However, one study showed that VPA suppresses glutamate responses and, much more potently, NMDA-evoked transient depolarizations in rat neocortex (46). The authors suggested that attenuation of NMDA receptor–mediated excitation is an essential mode of action for the anticonvulsant effect of VPA. This view is substantiated by numerous reports, using different preparations to study synaptic responses mediated by the NMDA subtype of glutamate receptors (6). In all studies, VPA blocked these responses, a finding indicating that antagonism of NMDA receptor–mediated neuronal excitation may be an important mechanism of VPA. VPA, but not phenobarbital, phenytoin, or ethosuximide, blocked seizures induced by *N*-methyl-DL-aspartate in rodents (47). In contrast to NMDA receptors, VPA had no effect on membrane responses mediated by kainate or quisqualate (α-amino-3-hydroxy-5-methyl-4-isoxazole propionate; AMPA) receptors (48).

The spontaneous firing of neurons is usually inhibited only by high doses or concentrations of VPA (49). However, in substantia nigra pars reticulata (SNR) of rats, a rapid and sustained reduction in the firing rate of GABAergic neurons was found *in vivo* after intraparenteral administration of doses as low as 50 to 100 mg/kg (50–52). This inhibitory effect on SNR neurons may result from the selective increase in GABA turnover induced by VPA in the nigra of rats (53) rather than from the direct effects of VPA on GABAergic neurons in SNR. Reduction of SNR firing as found with VPA has been shown effectively to suppress different types of seizures in diverse animal models of epilepsy, and this effect is explained by the important role of the SNR in seizure propagation (54,55). The inhibitory effect of VPA on SNR firing could therefore be crucially involved in its mechanisms of anticonvulsant action.

Effects on Ion Channels

At much lower concentrations than those depressing normal neuronal cell activity, VPA has been shown to diminish high-frequency repetitive firing of action potentials of central neurons in culture (30). It has been suggested that this effect may be critically involved in the anticonvulsant action of VPA on generalized tonic-clonic seizures (30). The effect of VPA on SRF was similar to limitation of SRF produced by phenytoin and carbamazepine (30). The most likely explanation for this effect of VPA would be a use-dependent reduction of inward Na$^+$ current (30). However, in most studies carried out to date, effects on Na$^+$ channels were inferred indirectly from changes in the maximal rate of increase of Na$^+$-dependent action potentials. In an electrophysiologic study using cultured rat hippocampal neurons, VPA indeed strongly delayed the recovery from inactivation of Na$^+$ channels, a finding that would be consistent with reduction of Na$^+$ conductance (56). Studies using nonvertebrate preparations also indicated that VPA has a direct inhibitory effect on voltage-sensitive Na$^+$ channels (6). However, the concept that VPA mediates its main anticonvulsant effect by slowing the recovery from inactivation of voltage-dependent Na$^+$ channels has been questioned because, in contrast to cultured neurons, VPA has no effects on the refractory period and, consequently, the bursting behavior of neurons when rat hippocampal slice is used for studying the neurophysiologic effects of VPA (57). The latter authors concluded that, at least in the hippocampal slice, the drug's principal anticonvulsant effect cannot be explained by an action on voltage-dependent Na$^+$ channels.

When phenytoin-sensitive Na$^+$ channels in cultured neuroblastoma cells and rat brain synaptosomes were studied, VPA did not affect the Na$^+$ influx (58). Furthermore, VPA had no effect on the phenytoin binding site on voltage-dependent Na$^+$ channels (59). In rat neocortical neurons in culture, VPA (0.2 to 2 mmol/L) was reported to reduce voltage-dependent Na$^+$ currents (60). More recent whole-voltage clamp measurements of Na⁺ currents in acutely isolated CA1 neurons from rats and patients with pharmacoresistant temporal lobe epilepsy showed that VPA induced a shift of the voltage dependence of inactivation in a hyperpolarizing direction with an EC_{50} of 2.5 mmol/L (rats) or 1.6 mmol/L (patients), respectively (61,62). In view of these high concentrations, the fatty acid VPA may modulate the Na⁺ channel by influencing the biophysical properties of the membrane surrounding the channel, as has been proposed for free polyunsaturated fatty acids (63). Indeed, when using therapeutically relevant VPA concentrations, VPA (≤400 μmol/L) was found to be ineffective on the fast Na⁺ current in acutely dissociated neocortical rat neurons (64). In contrast, VPA potently reduced the persistent fraction of the Na⁺ current with an EC_{50} of 14 μmol/L (64). Whether this highly potent effect of VPA can explain its action on SRF remains to be determined. Apart from interference with Na⁺ channels, VPA's effect on SRF could be the result of activation of Ca²⁺-dependent potassium conductance (65).

An activating effect on potassium conductance has been repeatedly discussed as a potential mechanism for the action of VPA (65–67), although such an effect has been demonstrated only at high drug concentrations. Previous experiments using various potassium channel subtypes from vertebrate brain expressed in oocytes of *Xenopus laevis* substantiated that the effects of VPA on potassium currents are too small to be significant in its mechanism of anticonvulsant action (68).

In regard to Ca²⁺ channels, the antiabsence drugs ethosuximide and dimethadione (the major active metabolite of trimethadione) have been shown to block use-dependent activation of T-type Ca²⁺ channels in thalamic neurons, which have been implicated in the generation of spike–wave activity associated with absence epilepsy (69). However, VPA did not affect this T current in thalamic neurons, although VPA is as effective as ethosuximide in blocking absence seizures. In contrast to thalamic neurons, VPA was shown to block low-threshold T Ca²⁺ channels in peripheral ganglion neurons (70). Veratrine-stimulated Ca²⁺ influx in brain slices was not altered by VPA, whereas the drug reduced NMDA- or quisqualate-stimulated Ca²⁺ influx at 5 mmol/L (67,71). In such high, millimolar concentrations of VPA, this lipophilic compound interferes with membrane functions by partition into cell membranes (72,73), and this may explain many of the neurochemical or neurophysiologic effects of the drug in studies involving this high concentration range.

BIOCHEMICAL EFFECTS

As a consequence of early reports establishing that VPA leads to an elevation of cerebral GABA levels in rodents (74), and that the period of GABA elevation coincides with the protection against seizures (75,76), numerous subsequent studies dealt with the effects of VPA on the GABA system (6). However, unlike GABAmimetic drugs, which selectively affect the GABA system, VPA certainly acts through more than one mechanism in providing its broad anticonvulsant activity. Furthermore, despite the clear effects of VPA on GABA metabolism, the role of these effects in VPA's anticonvulsant action is a matter of ongoing controversy.

Effects on the GABA System

It seems generally accepted that impairment of GABAergic inhibitory neurotransmission can lead to convulsions, whereas potentiation of GABAergic transmission results in anticonvulsant effects (77). Several clinically used antiepileptic drugs are GABAmimetic drugs, that is, they act by potentiating GABAergic neurotransmission either by increasing GABA concentrations through inhibition of GABA degradation (vigabatrin) or GABA uptake (tiagabine) or by directly acting at the postsynaptic GABA_A receptor complex (e.g., benzodiazepines, barbiturates). It is thus not astonishing that the initial reports on brain GABA increase by VPA (74,78) led to the assumption that enhancement of GABAergic neurotransmission is the mechanism of anticonvulsant action of VPA. Since it was first postulated in 1968, this GABA hypothesis has been the matter of ongoing dispute in the literature. For instance, it has been claimed that increases of GABA levels in the brain of rodents are seen only after high doses of VPA, whereas lower doses, which still exert anticonvulsant effects, do not change GABA levels (65,66). Furthermore, the finding that in some seizure models the rise in brain GABA by VPA lags behind the earlier appearance of the anticonvulsant effect led to questions about the relevance of the GABA increases by VPA (65). However, these apparent discrepancies result because most studies on VPA's effects on brain GABA levels used GABA determination in whole brain or whole tissue of few brain regions, thus ignoring the marked differences in GABA metabolism between brain regions and the cellular compartmentation of GABA within a brain region (6). Regional brain studies in rats showed marked differences in VPA's effects on GABA levels across brain areas, with significant GABA increases in midbrain regions, such as substantia nigra (SN), which are thought to be critically involved in seizure generation and propagation (79,80). In the SNR, the GABA increases induced by VPA occurred predominantly in nerve terminals, that is, in the "neurotransmitter pool" of GABA (80–82). The onset of VPA's effects on presynaptic (synaptosomal) GABA levels in brain regions was very rapid (significant increases were already observed after 5 minutes), and the time course of anticonvulsant activity correlated with that of the nerve terminal alterations in GABA levels (80). In *in vivo* experiments in dogs, in which VPA was infused continuously to obtain plasma levels in the range known from long-term oral treatment in humans, GABA increases were determined in cerebral cortex and cerebrospinal fluid (CSF) at an infusion rate of 25 mg/kg/hr (83). Accordingly, significant increases in CSF GABA levels were also found during treatment with VPA in patients with epilepsy or schizophrenia (6). Furthermore, significant GABA increases were determined in plasma of dogs and humans under VPA treatment (6). In dogs, the plasma GABA increases paralleled those in CSF and brain tissue and thus indicated that plasma GABA determination may be an indirect indicator of alteration in CNS GABA levels in response to VPA (83).

Although there is substantial evidence that VPA increases GABA concentrations at clinically relevant doses, the mechanism and functional meaning of the increase in brain GABA levels are still matters of debate. The increase of presynaptic GABA levels induced by VPA could be explained by three different mechanisms: (a) an inhibitory effect of VPA on GABA degradation; (b) an enhancement of GABA synthesis; or (c) no direct effects of VPA on synthesis or degradation of GABA, but an indirect effect on presynaptic GABA levels by direct potentiation of postsynaptic GABAergic function leading to feedback inhibition of GABA turnover and thereby to increases in nerve terminal GABA.

Shortly after the initial reports on the GABA-elevating effect of VPA, several groups examined the action of this drug on GABA degradation. GABA is synthesized in GABAergic nerve terminals by decarboxylation of glutamate and is degraded in nerve terminals, glia cells, and postsynaptic neurons (after diffusion) by transamination to succinic semialdehyde (SSA). SSA can either be oxidized by SSA dehydrogenase to succinate or it can be reduced by SSA reductase to γ-hydroxybutyrate (GHB). The relative importance of these two degradative pathways *in vivo* is unclear, although it appears that the reduction to GHB is generally a minor route of metabolism. The GABA-elevating effect of VPA was originally attributed to inhibition of GABA transaminase (GABA-T), which catalyses the degradation of GABA to SSA (74). Yet most studies on *in vitro* inhibition of GABA-T by VPA found inhibitory effects only at very high (millimolar) concentrations that are not reached *in vivo* (6). Indeed, when VPA was administered to rodents and GABA-T was determined in brain homogenates *ex vivo*, no inhibition of the enzyme was found (74,84–86). However, a significant reduction of GABA-T activity was found in synaptosomes prepared from brain tissue after VPA administration in mice (84,85). Similarly, in rats, VPA treatment induced a significant inhibition of synaptosomal GABA-T activities in several brain regions, including SN, hippocampus, hypothalamus, pons, and cerebellum (87). These data may be explained by assuming that the presynaptic (nerve terminal) GABA-T is different from glial GABA-T (which predominates in whole tissue homogenates) in terms of susceptibility to VPA. Alternatively, the significant reduction in

synaptosomal GABA-T observed *in vivo* is not the result of a direct inhibition of GABA-T by VPA but is a secondary effect caused by alterations in the subsequent steps of GABA metabolism. The first assumption was substantiated by experiments showing that VPA is much more potent to inhibit GABA-T in neurons (mean inhibitory concentration, 630 μmol/L) than in astrocytes or whole-tissue homogenates (88). The second assumption has been extensively discussed, and it has been concluded that it is not possible to raise brain GABA levels by inhibition of SSADH (6). Thus, the GABA-T reduction observed in synaptosomes but not in whole-tissue homogenates of rodents after treatment with VPA is most certainly the result of a higher susceptibility of nerve terminal GABA-T compared with the enzyme outside nerve terminals. Inhibition of nerve terminal GABA-T could explain the increase of presynaptic GABA levels by VPA, although the reduction of synaptosomal GABA-T activity was not marked (6).

Besides effects of VPA on GABA degradation, activation of GABA synthesis could be another likely explanation for the GABA-elevating action of this drug (6). Godin et al. (74) measured the relative incorporation of carbon-14 (^{14}C) into GABA in rat brain after the subcutaneous injection of [^{14}C]glucose. Thirty minutes after administration of VPA 400 mg/kg i.p., the incorporation of ^{14}C into the GABA molecule was increased by 30%, but this was not significant on account of the small number of animals studied. In similar experiments in mice, Taberner et al. (89) found that VPA, 80 mg/kg i.p., produced a significant increase in the rate of production of GABA by 90%. Studies on GABA turnover in various rat brain regions demonstrated that the most marked increase in GABA synthesis by VPA is found in the SN (53); the reason for this finding could be that the SN is one of the regions with the highest rates of GABA synthesis. Indeed, the increase in GABA synthesis by VPA most likely relates to an activation of the GABA-synthesizing enzyme glutamic acid decarboxylase (GAD). Increase of GAD activity by VPA has been demonstrated *ex vivo* after administration in mice and rats in several independent studies (6). In rats, GAD was not activated in all regions, a finding indicating a regional specificity of VPA's effects (86). Increase of GAD by VPA is rapid in onset, and the time course of GAD activation matches that of the GABA increase and the anticonvulsant effect (90). The rapid activation of GAD by VPA may indicate that VPA converts the inactive apoenzyme to the active holoenzyme (86). However, at high, toxic doses, VPA has been shown to inhibit GAD activity and to reduce GABA synthesis (91).

Activation of GAD by VPA has also been reported *in vitro* (6). GAD from neonatal rats was more sensitive to activation by VPA than GAD from adult animals (92). In neonatal rat brain slices, VPA significantly increased the activity of the GABA shunt, which was related to an increase of GAD activity (93). However, high (toxic) concentrations of VPA (7 mmol/L) significantly decrease GAD (94).

Neurochemical experiments in beef brain preparations have shown that the coenzyme A ester of VPA, which is rapidly formed from VPA *in vivo,* is a potent inhibitor of α-ketoglutarate dehydrogenase complex (95). Because decreased activity of this complex would reduce substrate flux through the citric acid cycle and may increase flux into GABA synthesis, this finding adds to the accumulating evidence that VPA increases GABA levels predominantly by enhancing the synthesis of this amino acid (95).

An increase of presynaptic GABA levels by VPA would potentiate GABAergic neurotransmission only if the release of GABA into the synaptic cleft would be also increased. The first direct evidence of enhanced GABA release by VPA came from studies on cortical slices prepared from VPA-treated animals and from studies in neuronal culture (96,97). Thus, in the cortical slice from VPA-treated rats, the potassium-induced release of GABA was increased, and this was potentiated further by the GABA$_B$ receptor antagonist phaclofen (97). Similarly, VPA increased the potassium-induced release of GABA from cortical neurons in culture in clinically relevant concentrations (96). Similar to the biphasic effects of VPA on GABA synthesis (i.e., increase at low doses but decrease at high doses), high concentrations of VPA seem to inhibit GABA release. The uptake of GABA from the synaptic cleft is not affected by VPA (6). However, in a study on GABA transporter proteins in rats with spontaneous recurrent seizures induced by amygdala injection of ferric chloride, VPA caused downregulation of GABA transporters (98).

Indirect evidence of enhanced GABA release by VPA comes from *in vivo* studies in rats in which microdialysis was used to measure extracellular GABA levels in the hippocampus (99,100). Biggs et al. (99) reported biphasic effects of VPA on extracellular GABA levels, which depended on the dose used. At 100 mg/kg, VPA transiently reduced GABA concentrations by 50% when compared with basal levels, and 200 mg/kg VPA had virtually no effect, whereas 400 mg/kg VPA raised extracellular GABA levels to 200% of basal levels. Such biphasic effects of VPA on extracellular GABA levels were also found by Wolf et al. (101), using local application of VPA into the rat preoptic area through push-pull cannulae. Similar to the study of Biggs et al. (99), Rowley et al. (100) reported that VPA, 400 mg/kg, significantly increased extracellular levels of GABA measured by microdialysis in the hippocampus of freely moving rats. Furthermore, VPA prevented decreases in GABA in response to maximal electroshock seizures in these animals (100). Using the push-pull technique to measure extracellular GABA in the SN of rats, Farrant and Webster (51) found no effect of VPA, 200 mg/kg, on the spontaneous release of GABA into the perfusate. However, as pointed out by Timmermann and Westerink (102), none of these techniques of measuring extracellular GABA allow investigators to draw direct conclusions on drug effects on GABA release, because of the marked compartmentalization of this neurotransmitter.

An enhancement of GABA release at clinically relevant concentrations of VPA is indirectly indicated by the increase in CSF GABA levels observed in different species, including humans (6). In view of the different reports demonstrating an increase of GABA turnover and release by VPA (6), the previous hypothesis that the increased brain GABA concentrations induced by VPA treatment are only secondary as a result of feedback inhibition of GABA turnover because of direct postsynaptic effects of the drug has to be rejected.

In contrast to VPA's effects on GABA synthesis and degradation, the drug does not exert direct effects on the major components of the postsynaptic GABA$_A$ receptor complex. Thus, *in vitro,* VPA did not alter GABA binding, benzodiazepine binding, or the binding of the selective chloride ionophore ligand [^{35}S]*t*-butylbicyclophosphorothionate (TBPS) (6). Therefore, the previous assumption that VPA could potentiate GABA$_A$ receptor function by a barbituratelike effect on the picrotoxinin site, which was based on low-potency inhibition by VPA of [^{3}H]α-dihydropicrotoxinin binding (103), could not be substantiated by subsequent experiments with the more suitable ligand [^{35}S]TBPS. However, *in vivo* VPA has been shown to reduce TPBS binding and to increase benzodiazepine binding, which is most likely secondary, as a result of the increase in GABA levels produced by VPA *in vivo* (104). The functional meaning of the alteration in benzodiazepine receptor binding is not clear, because benzodiazepine receptor antagonists do not reduce the anticonvulsant potency of VPA (105). Conversely, prolonged pretreatment of mice with benzodiazepines reduced the anticonvulsant potency of VPA and thus demonstrated the development of cross-tolerance between benzodiazepines and VPA (106). Furthermore, the anticonflict action of VPA was reversed by benzodiazepine antagonists (107), a finding indicating that enhanced binding of benzodiazepines to the GABA$_A$ receptor complex may be involved in this pharmacodynamic effect of VPA.

Two groups independently reported increase of GABA$_B$ receptor binding by long-term treatment of rats with VPA (108,109). In a study by Motohashi (109), short-term treatment with VPA had no effect on [^{3}H]baclofen binding in frontal cortex, hippocampus, and thalamus, whereas long-term treatment enhanced binding in the hippocampus. [^{3}H]muscimol binding to the GABA$_A$ receptor did not change after VPA administration in any region (109). Because similar effects were observed with lithium and carbamazepine, Motohashi (109) concluded that one common mechanism of action of mood stabilizers may be mediated by GABA$_B$ receptors in the hippocampus.

Taken together, the numerous neurochemical reports of VPA's effects on the GABA system indicate that increases in GABA function may be involved in several pharmacodynamic effects of this drug, including the anticonvulsant, anticonflict, and antimanic actions (6). Furthermore, in view of the role of GABA in antinociception (110), increased GABAergic function by VPA may be involved in its antinociceptive effects. However, the effects of VPA on GABA alone are not sufficient to explain its broad anticonvulsant activity, and several of VPA's effects on neuronal tissue, such as on acutely dissociated neurons, have been demonstrated not to be related to GABA potentiation (29).

Effects on γ-Hydroxybutyrate, Glutamate, and Aspartate

Compared with the numerous studies on VPA's effects on the GABA system, only relatively few neurochemical studies were done on other transmitter amino acids (6). Several of these studies dealt with VPA's effects on GHB metabolism. VPA was shown to be a potent inhibitor of NADPH (reduced form of nicotinamide-adenine dinucleotide phosphate)–dependent aldehyde reductase (111). Aldehyde reductase is presumably identical to nonspecific SSA reductase (SSAR) (112). Whereas the specific SSAR is thought to reduce SSA to GHB, the nonspecific SSAR is thought to be responsible for the catabolism of GHB to SSA (112). In contrast to the potent effect of VPA on nonspecific SSAR, specific SSAR is not affected by the drug (112). However, Whittle and Turner (113), using rat brain homogenates, demonstrated that VPA inhibited the formation of GHB *in vitro,* a finding indicating that the specific SSAR is not exclusively responsible for GHB formation but the nonspecific (VPA sensitive) aldehyde reductase may also contribute to a significant extent to this metabolic pathway. Inhibition of GHB formation by VPA could be of considerable interest because this amino acid has been shown to produce epileptogenic (absencelike) effects in several species (114). Administration of VPA to rats has been shown to increase (rather than decrease) the brain level of GHB *in vivo* (115). This increase in GHB levels by VPA is time and dose dependent and appears to result from a reduction in synaptic release of GHB (112). Because GHB produces absencelike epileptic seizures in animals (114), reduction of GHB release could be an important factor in the antiabsence action of VPA (112).

Glutamate concentrations in regional brain homogenates or in extracellular fluid obtained by microdialysis from hippocampus or SN were not significantly altered by systemic administration of VPA (51,99,100). However, Dixon and Hokin (116) reported that VPA stimulates glutamate release in mouse cerebral cortex slices at therapeutic concentrations. This effect may be involved in the antimanic action of VPA (116). Nilsson et al. (117) reported that VPA inhibits the transport of glutamate and aspartate in astroglial cells in primary cultures from newborn rat cerebral cortex. In adult rats, VPA treatment decreased the expression of glutamate transporter-1 in the hippocampus (98).

With respect to aspartate, VPA was shown to reduce the concentration and release of this excitatory amino acid in rat and mouse brain (6). Furthermore, some reports found that concentrations of glycine and taurine increased in brain tissue (6). However, there is as yet no evidence that these effects on amino acids other than GABA are relevant to the anticonvulsant effect of VPA.

Effects on Serotonin and Dopamine

VPA induces in rats a behavioral syndrome with "wet dog shakes" and other symptoms reminiscent of the "serotonin syndrome" induced by serotonin precursors or receptor agonists in rodents. Indeed, microdialysis studies in rats have demonstrated that VPA enhances the extracellular concentration of serotonin (5-hydroxytryptamine or 5-HT) in hippocampus and striatum of rats (118). However, in contrast to the increase in anticonvulsant efficacy during prolonged treatment, the wet-dog-shake behavior induced by VPA is markedly diminished within some days of treatment, thus indicating that activation of serotonergic transmission is not related to the anticonvulsant action of the drug (9). Accordingly, Horton et al. (119) showed that pretreatment of mice with *p*-chloro-phenylalanine, which blocked serotonin synthesis and prevented the increase in serotonin metabolism by VPA, did not diminish the anticonvulsant action of VPA.

As with serotonin, microdialysis studies have demonstrated an increased extracellular level of dopamine in response to VPA (118,120). Thus, the initial assumption (119) that VPA does not exert effects on serotonin or dopamine levels but only blocks outward transport of their metabolites from the CNS has to be rejected. As with serotonin, the alterations in dopamine levels seem not associated with VPA's anticonvulsant effect, because pretreatment of mice with α-methyl-*p*-tyrosine to inhibit dopamine synthesis did not diminish the anticonvulsant action of VPA (119). However, alterations of dopaminergic functions by VPA may be important for the antipsychotic effects of the drug (6). Ichikawa and Meltzer (120) showed that the increase in prefrontal dopamine release by VPA can be blocked by a selective 5-HT$_{1A}$ receptor antagonist, a finding indicating that VPA's effect on dopamine release is mediated by this 5-HT receptor subtype.

Other Biochemical Effects

Guanosine 3',5'-monophosphate (cGMP) has been implicated as a second messenger in a variety of cellular events (121). For instance, the levels of cGMP in the cerebellum and cortex are known to increase sharply at the onset of experimentally induced seizures, and it has been proposed that an elevated cerebellar cGMP level is involved in initiating or maintaining seizure activity through the regulation of Purkinje cell activity (122,123). VPA was shown to decrease the cerebellar cGMP level during the time of anticonvulsant activity, whereas the cortical cGMP level was elevated

(122,123). In contrast to cGMP, cyclic adenosine monophosphate levels were not altered by VPA. Because levels of cGMP in the CNS are altered by several neurotransmitters, including amino acids (121), the effects of VPA on cGMP may be secondary, resulting from the various alterations of neurotransmitter systems described earlier.

VPA was reported to downregulate the myristoylated alanine-rich C kinase substrate (MARCKS) in an immortalized hippocampal cell line, which is thought to be a property of protein kinase C–mediated mood stabilizers (124). MARCKS is a prominent and preferential substrate in the brain for protein kinase C and has been implicated in cellular processes associated with neuroplasticity (e.g., neurotransmitter release and transmembrane signaling) and cytoskeletal restructuring (125). Long-term exposure of hippocampal cells with VPA (for ≥3 days) at therapeutic concentrations produced a decrease in MARCKS protein levels, whereas short-term exposure produced no significant change (124). This retarded onset of action is in line with the delay of several days in the onset of VPA's antimanic effects seen in patients. MARCKS was also downregulated by lithium, whereas other psychotropic drugs, including carbamazepine, haloperidol, diazepam, and fluoxetine, did not affect levels of the MARCKS protein (124). These data thus indicate that the property of regulating MARCKS is shared by the mood stabilizers lithium and VPA, which may be specific to a class of drugs effective in the treatment of bipolar disorders (124).

VPA, lithium, and carbamazepine were shown to inhibit at therapeutically relevant concentrations the high-affinity myoinositol transport in astrocytelike cells *in vitro* (126). When rats were treated on a long-term basis with VPA or lithium, the brain concentrations of myoinositol and inositol monophosphates significantly increased (127). It was suggested that both lithium and VPA may share a common mechanism of action in the treatment of bipolar disorder through actions on the phosphoinositol cycle.

PUTATIVE MECHANISMS INVOLVED IN THE EARLY AND LATE ANTICONVULSANT EFFECTS OF VALPROIC ACID

As described earlier in this chapter, depending on the seizure model or seizure type, VPA's anticonvulsant effect may either occur immediately (early) or late, that is, with some lag time after acute administration or only during long-term administration, a finding suggesting that these early and late effects of VPA are mediated by different cellular mechanisms. As outlined in this chapter, VPA has both extracellular (e.g., ion channels) and intracellular (e.g., GABA synthesis) sites of action. The access to these sites will determine how rapidly VPA acts after systemic action. Frey and Löscher were the first to describe that VPA enters and leaves the brain by active, carrier-mediated transport at

the blood–brain barrier (128). Whereas it was initially thought that this probenecid-sensitive transport is mediated by the monocarboxylic acid carrier (128), more recent experiments have revealed that the bidirectional movement of VPA across the blood–brain barrier is mediated jointly by passive diffusion and carrier transport, with different transporters responsible for each direction of transport (129). The uptake of VPA from blood into brain is facilitated by a medium- and long-chain fatty acid selective anion exchanger at the brain capillary epithelium, which accounts for two-thirds of the barrier permeability, whereas the mechanism governing the efficient transport of VPA in the reverse direction, that is, from brain to blood, appears to involve a probenecid-sensitive, active transport system (129). Huai-Yun et al. (130) showed that VPA is a potent inhibitor of the adenosine triphosphate–dependent probenecid-sensitive transporters of the multidrug resistance-associated protein (MRP) family in the blood–brain barrier, which raises the possibility that MRPs may serve as the efflux transporters of VPA. This active transport at the blood–brain barrier explains why VPA, despite its physicochemical properties (highly ionized at physiologic pH, highly plasma protein bound), enters the brain so quickly (91,129). Assuming that VPA has to enter neurons by passive diffusion, its rapid anticonvulsant effect in some seizure models after parenteral administration of a single dose is most likely explained by an effect on extracellular sites. The late anticonvulsant effects observed both preclinically and clinically are more likely explained by slow access to intracellular sites of action. This view is corroborated by neurophysiologic experiments. Thus, in the buccal ganglia *Helix pomatia* preparation, extracellular application of VPA decreased frequency of occurrence of PTZ-induced epileptic depolarizations immediately (early effect) and, with a delay, led to a decay in paroxysmal depolarizations (late effect) (12). This late effect was obtained immediately when VPA was applied intracellularly (E.-J. Speckmann, *personal communication*), a finding substantiating that the delay in this effect after extracellular application was the result of slow penetration of VPA into the neuron. Slow diffusion into and out of neurons could also be involved in carryover effects observed both preclinically and clinically, because whereas extracellular levels of VPA will rapidly leave brain or CSF by active outward transport, elimination from neurons may be retarded. More recent microdialysis experiments by Shen's group in rabbits suggested that VPA does not solely enter neurons by passive diffusion, but that another set of transporters at the neural cell membrane is involved (129). The putative parenchymal cell transport system is able to concentrate VPA within the cellular compartment, and this finding has important implications in our understanding of the intracellular mechanisms versus membrane actions of VPA (129). The efflux component from the cellular compartment is inhibited by probenecid (129), and this could indicate that MRPs are involved.

CONCLUSION

No single action of VPA can completely account for the drug's numerous effects on neuronal tissue and its broad clinical activity in epilepsy and other brain diseases. In view of the diverse molecular and cellular events that underlie different seizure types, the combination of several neurochemical and neurophysiologic mechanisms in a single drug molecule may explain the broad antiepileptic efficacy of VPA. Furthermore, by acting on diverse regional targets thought to be involved in the generation and propagation of seizures, VPA may antagonize epileptic activity at several steps of its organization. The finding that VPA exerts not only anticonvulsant but also several other pharmacodynamic and pharmacotherapeutic effects, including antimanic and migraine-prophylactic efficacy, certainly relates to the multiplicity of VPA's effects on neuronal functions (6,110,117,131,132). Because of the different pharmacodynamic effects of VPA, it is difficult to ascertain which specific neurochemical or neurophysiologic actions are related to the anticonvulsant activity of the drug. There is now ample evidence that VPA increases GABA turnover and thereby potentiates GABAergic functions in some specific brain regions thought to be involved in the control of seizure generation and propagation. Furthermore, the effect of VPA on neuronal excitation mediated by the NMDA subtype of glutamate receptors may be important for its anticonvulsant effects. In contrast, the relevance of the often-cited effect of VPA on SRF in cultured neurons remains debatable, because there is no convincing evidence that VPA—at therapeutically relevant concentrations—blocks voltage-dependent Na^+ currents and SRF in more conventional preparations (57). Whereas the GABA potentiation and glutamate-NMDA inhibition could be a likely explanation for the anticonvulsant action on focal and generalized motor seizures, they do not explain the effect of VPA on nonconvulsive seizures, such as absences. In this respect, the reduction of GHB release reported for VPA could be of interest.

Despite considerable discussion about the possible mechanisms of action of VPA, no definite answer has gained general acceptance so far, and much remains to be learned at numerous different levels of VPA's actions. In view of the advances in molecular neurobiology and neuroscience, future studies will undoubtedly further our understanding of the mechanisms of action of this major antiepileptic drug.

REFERENCES

1. Burton BS. On the propyl derivatives and decomposition products of ethylacetoacetate. *Am Chem J* 1882;3:385–395.
2. Meunier H, Carraz G, Meunier Y, et al. Propriétés pharmacodynamiques de l'acide *n*-dipro-pylacétique. 1er mémoire: propriétés antiépileptiques. *Therapie* 1963;18:435–438.
3. Carraz G, Fau R, Chateau R, et al. Communication à propos des premiers essais cliniques sur l'activité anti-épileptique de l'acide *n*-dipropylacétiques (sel de Na). *Ann Med Psychol (Paris)* 1964;122:577–585.
4. Cotariu D, Zaidman JL, Evans S. Neurophysiological and biochemical changes evoked by valproic acid in the central nervous system. *Prog Neurobiol* 1990;34:343–354.
5. Davis R, Peters DH, Mctavish D. Valproic acid: a reappraisal of its pharmacological properties and clinical efficacy in epilepsy. *Drugs* 1994;47:332–372.
6. Löscher W. Valproate: a reappraisal of its pharmacodynamic properties and mechanisms of action. *Prog Neurobiol* 1999;58: 31–59.
7. Löscher W, ed. *Valproate.* Basel: Birkhäuser, 1999.
8. Hönack D, Löscher W. Intravenous valproate: onset and duration of anticonvulsant activity against a series of electroconvulsions in comparison with diazepam and phenytoin. *Epilepsy Res* 1992;13:215–221.
9. Löscher W, Fisher JE, Nau H, et al. Marked increase in anticonvulsant activity but decrease in wet-dog shake behaviour during short-term treatment of amygdala-kindled rats with valproic acid. *Eur J Pharmacol* 1988;150:221–232.
10. Löscher W, Fisher JE, Nau H, et al. Valproic acid in amygdala-kindled rats: alterations in anticonvulsant efficacy, adverse effects and drug and metabolite levels in various brain regions during chronic treatment. *J Pharmacol Exp Ther* 1989;250: 1067–1078.
11. Löscher W, Hönack D. Comparison of anticonvulsant efficacy of valproate during prolonged treatment with one and three daily doses or continuous ("controlled release") administration in a model of generalized seizures in rats. *Epilepsia* 1995; 36:929–937.
12. Altrup U, Gerlach G, Reith H, et al. Effects of valproate in a model nervous system (buccal ganglia of *Helix pomatia.* I. Antiepileptic actions. *Epilepsia* 1992;33:743–752.
13. Wamil AW, Löscher W, Mclean MJ. *Trans*-2-en-valproic acid limits action potential firing frequency in mouse central neurons in cell culture. *J Pharmacol Exp Ther* 1997;280: 1349–1356.
14. Silver JM, Shin C, McNamara JO. Antiepileptogenic effects of conventional anticonvulsants in the kindling model of epilepsy. *Ann Neurol* 1991;29:356–363.
15. Balfour JA, Bryson HM. Valproic acid: a review of its pharmacology and therapeutic potential in indications other than epilepsy. *CNS Drugs* 1994;2:144–173.
16. Nau H, Löscher W. Valproic acid and metabolites: pharmacological and toxicological studies. *Epilepsia* 1984;25:14–22.
17. Semmes RLO, Shen DD. Comparative pharmacodynamics and brain distribution of E-Δ^2-valproate and valproate in rats. *Epilepsia* 1991;32:232–341.
18. Löscher W. Pharmacological, toxicological and neurochemical effects of $\Delta^{2(E)}$-valproate in animals. *Pharm Weekblad* 1992;14: 139–143.
19. Voskuyl RA, Ter Keurs HE, Meinardi H. Actions and interactions of dipropylacetate and penicillin on evoked potentials of excised prepiriform cortex of guinea pig. *Epilepsia* 1975;16: 583–592.
20. Piredda S, Yonekawa W, Whittingham TS, et al. Effects of antiepileptic drugs on pentylenetetrazole-induced epileptiform activity in the in vitro hippocampus. *Epilepsia* 1986;27: 341–346.
21. Tian LM, Alkadhi KA. Valproic acid inhibits the depolarizing rectification in neurons of rat amygdala. *Neuropharmacology* 1994;33:1131–1138.
22. Bruckner C, Stenkamp K, Meierkord H, et al. Epileptiform discharges induced by combined application of bicuculline and 4-

aminopyridine are resistant to standard anticonvulsants in slices of rats. *Neurosci Lett* 1999;268:163–165.

23. Bruckner C, Heinemann U. Effects of standard anticonvulsant drugs on different patterns of epileptiform discharges induced by 4-aminopyridine in combined entorhinal cortex-hippocampal slices. *Brain Res* 2000;859:15–20.

24. Fueta Y, Avoli M. Pattern- and age-dependency of the antiepileptic effects induced by valproic acid in the rat hippocampus. *Can J Physiol Pharmacol* 1991;69:1301–1304.

25. Fueta Y, Siniscalchi A, Tancredi V, et al. Extracellular magnesium and anticonvulsant effects of valproate in young rat hippocampus. *Epilepsia* 1995;36:404–409.

26. Dreier JP, Heinemann U. Late low magnesium-induced epileptiform activity in rat entorhinal cortex slices becomes insensitive to the anticonvulsant valproic acid. *Neurosci Lett* 1990;119:68–70.

27. Zhang CL, Dreier JP, Heinemann U. Paroxysmal epileptiform discharges in temporal lobe slices after prolonged exposure to low magnesium are resistant to clinically used anticonvulsants. *Epilepsy Res* 1995;20:105–111.

28. Sokolova S, Schmitz D, Zjang CL, et al. Comparison of effects of valproate and *trans*-2-en-valproate on different forms of epileptiform activity in rat hippocampal and temporal cortex slices. *Epilepsia* 1998;39:251–258.

29. Zhang YF, Gibbs JW 3rd, Coulter DA. Anticonvulsant drug effects on spontaneous thalamocortical rhythms *in vitro*: valproic acid, clonazepam, and alpha-methyl-alpha-phenylsuccinimide. *Epilepsy Res* 1996;23:37–53.

30. McLean MJ, Macdonald RL. Sodium valproate, but not ethosuximide, produces use- and voltage-dependent limitation of high frequency repetitive firing of action potentials of mouse central neurons in cell culture. *J Pharmacol Exp Ther* 1986;237:1001–1011.

31. Sypert GW, Reynolds AF. Single pyramidal-tract fiber analysis of neocortical propagated seizures with reference to inactivation responses. *Exp Neurol* 1974;45:228–240.

32. Mutani R, Doriguzzi T, Fariello R, et al. Azione antiepilettica del sale di sodio dell'acido *N*-dipropilacetico: studio sperimentale sul gatto. *Riv Patol Nerv Ment* 1968;89:24–33.

33. Salt TE, Tulloch IF, Walter DS. Anti-epileptic properties of sodium valproate in rat amygdaloid kindling. *Br J Pharmacol* 1980;68[Suppl]:134P.

34. Ito T, Hori M, Yoshida K, et al. Effect of anticonvulsants on thalamic afterdischarge in rats and cats. *Jpn J Pharmacol* 1977;27:823–831.

35. Mutani R, Fariello R. Effetti dell'acido n-dipropilacetico (Depakine) sull'attività del focus epilettogeno da cobalto. *Riv Patol Nerv Ment* 1969;90:40–49.

36. Fariello R, Mutani R. Modificazioni dell'attività del focus epilettogeno cortico-monotorio da alluminia indotte dal sale di sodio n-dipropilacetico (DPA). *Acta Neurol (Napoli)* 1970;25:116–122.

37. van Duijn H, Beckmann MK. Dipropylacetic acid (Depakine) in experimental epilepsy in the alert cat. *Epilepsia* 1975;16:83–90.

38. Maresova D, Mares P. Influence of valproate and carbamazepine on symmetrical cortical penicillin foci in the rat. *Physiol Bohemoslov* 1985;34:562–566.

39. Löscher W, Hönack D. Effects of the competitive NMDA receptor antagonist, CGP 37849, on anticonvulsant activity and adverse effects of valproate in amygdala-kindled rats. *Eur J Pharmacol* 1993;234:237–245.

40. Mares P, Maresova D, Pohl M, et al. Effect of anticonvulsant drugs on thalamo-cortical and hippocampo-cortical self-sustained after-discharges in the rat. *Physiol Bohemoslov* 1984;33:179–187.

41. Marescaux C, Micheletti G, Vergnes M, et al. A model of chronic spontaneous petit mal-like seizures in the rat: comparison with pentylenetetrazol-induced seizures. *Epilepsia* 1984;25:326–331.

42. Löscher W, Nau H, Marescaux C, et al. Comparative evaluation of anticonvulsant and toxic potencies of valproic acid and 2-en-valproic acid in different animal models of epilepsy. *Eur J Pharmacol* 1984;99:211–218.

43. Macdonald RL, Bergey GK. Valproic acid augments GABA-mediated postsynaptic inhibition in cultured mammalian neurons. *Brain Res* 1979;170:558–562.

44. Olpe HR, Steinmann MW, Pozza MF, et al. Valproate enhances GABA-A mediated inhibition of locus coeruleus neurons *in vitro. Naunyn Schmiedebergs Arch Pharmacol* 1988;338:655–657.

45. Baldino F, Geller HM. Effect of sodium valproate on hypothalamic neurons *in vivo* and *in vitro. Brain Res* 1981;219:231–237.

46. Zeise ML, Kasparaow S, Zieglgansberger W. Valproate suppresses *N*-methyl-D-aspartate evoked, transient depolarizations in the rat neocortex in vitro. *Brain Res* 1991;544:345–348.

47. Czuczwar SJ, Frey H-H, Löscher W. Antagonism of *N*-methyl-D,L-aspartic acid-induced convulsions by antiepileptic drugs and other agents. *Eur J Pharmacol* 1985;108:273–280.

48. Musshoff U, Madeja M, Düsing R, et al. Valproate affects glutamate but not GABA receptors. *Eur J Neurosci* 1996;9[Suppl]:205.

49. Chapman A, Keane PE, Meldrum BS, et al. Mechanism of anticonvulsant action of valproate. *Prog Neurobiol* 1982;19:315–359.

50. Kerwin RW, Olpe H-R, Schmutz M. The effect of sodium-*n*-dipropylacetate on γ-aminobutyric acid-dependent inhibition in the rat cortex and substantia nigra in relation to its anticonvulsant activity. *Br J Pharmacol* 1980;71:545–551.

51. Farrant M, Webster RA. Neuronal activity, amino acid concentration and amino acid release in the substantia nigra of the rat after sodium valproate. *Brain Res* 1989;504:49–56.

52. Rohlfs A, Rundfeldt C, Koch R, et al. A comparison of the effects of valproate and its major active me tabolite E-2-en-valproate on single unit activity of substantia nigra pars reticulata neurons in rats. *J Pharmacol Exp Ther* 1996;277:1305–1314.

53. Löscher W. Valproate enhances GABA turnover in the substantia nigra. *Brain Res* 1989;501:198–203.

54. Gale K. Progression and generalization of seizure discharge: anatomical and neurochemical substrates. *Epilepsia* 1988;29 [Suppl 2]:S15–S34.

55. Löscher W, Ebert U. Basic mechanisms of seizure propagation: targets for rational drug design and rational polypharmacy. *Epilepsy Res Suppl* 1996;11:17–44.

56. Van den Berg RJ, Kok P, Voskuyl RA. Valproate and sodium currents in cultured hippocampal neurons. *Exp Brain Res* 1993;93:279–287.

57. Albus H, Williamson R. Electrophysiologic analysis of the actions of valproate on pyramidal neurons in the rat hippocampal slice. *Epilepsia* 1998;39:124–139.

58. Willow M, Kuenzel EA, Catterall WA. Inhibition of voltage-sensitive sodium channels in neuroblastoma cells and synaptosomes by the anticonvulsant drugs diphenylhydantoin and carbamazepine. *Mol Pharmacol* 1984;25:228–234.

59. Francis J, Burnham WM. [³H]Phenytoin identifies a novel anticonvulsant-binding domain on voltage-dependent sodium channels. *Mol Pharmacol* 1992;42:1097–1103.

60. Zona C, Avoli M. Effects induced by the antiepileptic drug valproic acid upon the ionic currents recorded in rat neocortical neurons in cell culture. *Exp Brain Res* 1990;81:313–317.

61. Vreugdenhil M, Vanveelen CWM, Vanrijen PC, et al. Effect of valproic acid on sodium currents in cortical neurons from

patients with pharmaco-resistant temporal lobe epilepsy. *Epilepsy Res* 1998;32:309–320.

62. Vreugdenhil M, Wadman WJ. Modulation of sodium currents in rat CA1 neurons by carbamazepine and valproate after kindling epileptogenesis. *Epilepsia* 1999;40:1512–1522.

63. Vreugdenhil M, Bruehl C, Voskuyl RA, et al. Polyunsaturated fatty acids modulate sodium and calcium currents in CA1 neurons. *Proc Natl Acad Sci USA* 1996;93:12559–12563.

64. Taverna S, Mantegazza M, Franceschetti S, et al. Valproate selectively reduces the persistent fraction of Na^+ current in neocortical neurons. *Epilepsy Res* 1998;32:304–308.

65. Fariello RG, Varasi M, Smith MC. Valproic acid: mechanisms of action. In: Levy RH, Mattson RH, Meldrum BS, eds. *Antiepileptic drugs,* 4th ed. New York: Raven Press, 1995:581–604.

66. Morre M, Keane PE, Vernières JC, et al. Valproate: recent findings and perspectives. *Epilepsia* 1984;25[Suppl 1]:S5–S9.

67. Franceschetti S, Hannon B, Heinemann U. The action of valproate on spontaneous epileptiform activity in the absence of synaptic transmission and on evoked changes in $[Ca^{2+}]_0$ and $[K^+]_0$ in the hippocampal slice. *Brain Res* 1986;386:1–11.

68. Roderfeld H-J, Altrup U, Düsing R, et al. Effects of the antiepileptic drug valproate on cloned voltage-dependent potassium channels. *Pflugers Arch* 1994;426[Suppl]:R32.

69. Coulter DA, Huguenard JR, Prince DA. Characterization of ethosuximide reduction of low-threshold calcium current in thalamic neurons. *Ann Neurol* 1989;25:582–593.

70. Kelly KM, Gross RA, Macdonald RL. Valproic acid selectively reduces the low-threshold (T) calcium current in rat nodose neurons. *Neurosci Lett* 1990;116:1–2.

71. Crowder JM, Bradford HF. Common anticonvulsants inhibit Ca^{2+} uptake and amino acid neurotransmitter release in vitro. *Epilepsia* 1987;28:378–382.

72. Perlman BJ, Goldstein DB. Membrane-disordering potency and anticonvulsant action of valproic acid and other short-chain fatty acids. *Mol Pharmacol* 1984;26:83–89.

73. Rumbach L, Mutet C, Cremel G, et al. Effects of sodium valproate on mitochondrial membranes: electron paramagnetic resonance and transmembrane protein movement studies. *Mol Pharmacol* 1986;30:270–273.

74. Godin Y, Heiner L, Mark J, et al. Effects of di-*n*-propylacetate, an anticonvulsive compound, on GABA metabolism. *J Neurochem* 1969;16:869–873.

75. Simler S, Ciesielski L, Maitre M, et al. Effect of sodium *n*-dipropylacetate on audio genic seizures and brain γ-aminobutyric acid level. *Biochem Pharmacol* 1973;22:1701–1708.

76. Schechter PJ, Tranier Y, Grove J. Effect of *n*-dipropylacetate on amino acid concentrations in mouse brain: correlations with anti-convulsant activity. *J Neurochem* 1978;31:1325–1327.

77. Löscher W. GABA and the epilepsies: experimental and clinical considerations. In: Bowery NG, Nisticò G, eds. *GABA: basic research and clinical applications.* Rome: Pythagora Press, 1989: 260–300.

78. Simler S, Randrianarisoa H, Lehman A, et al. Effects du di-*n*-propylacétate sur les crises audiogènes de la souris. *J Physiol (Paris)* 1968;60:547.

79. Iadarola MJ, Raines A, Gale K. Differential effects of *n*-dipropylacetate and aminooxyacetic acid on γ-aminobutyric acid levels in discrete areas of rat brain. *J Neurochem* 1979; 33:1119–1123.

80. Löscher W, Vetter M. *In vivo* effects of aminooxyacetic acid and valproic acid on nerve terminal (synaptosomal) GABA levels in discrete brain areas of the rat: correlation to pharmacological activities. *Biochem Pharmacol* 1985;34:1747–1756.

81. Iadarola MJ, Gale K. Dissociation between drug-induced increases in nerve terminal and non-nerve terminal pools of GABA *in vivo. Eur J Pharmacol* 1979;59:125–129.

82. Iadarola MJ, Gale K. Cellular compartments of GABA in brain and their relationship to anticonvulsant activity. *Mol Cell Biochem* 1981;39:305–330.

83. Löscher W. GABA in plasma, CSF and brain of dogs during acute and chronic treatment with γ-acetylenic GABA and valproic acid. In: Okada Y, Roberts E, eds. *Problems in GABA research: from brain to bacteria.* Amsterdam: Exerpta Medica, 1982:102–109.

84. Löscher W. Valproate induced changes in GABA metabolism at the subcellular level. *Biochem Pharmacol* 1981;30:1364–1366.

85. Löscher W. Effect of inhibitors of GABA aminotransferase on the metabolism of GABA in brain tissue and synaptosomal fractions. *J Neurochem* 1981;36:1521–1527.

86. Phillips NI, Fowler LJ. The effects of sodium valproate on γ-aminobutyrate metabolism and behavior in naive and ethanolamine-*O*-sulphate pretreated rats and mice. *Biochem Pharmacol* 1982;31:2257–2261.

87. Löscher W. *In vivo* administration of valproate reduces the nerve terminal (synaptosomal) activity of GABA aminotransferase in discrete brain areas of rats. *Neurosci Lett* 1993;160:177–180.

88. Larsson OM, Gram L, Schousboe I, et al. Differential effects of gamma-vinyl GABA and valproate on GABA-transaminase from cultured neurons and astrocytes. *Neuropharmacology* 1986;25:617–625.

89. Taberner PV, Charington CB, Unwin JW. Effects of GAD and GABA-T inhibitors on GABA metabolism *in vivo. Brain Res Bull* 1980;5[Suppl 2]:621–625.

90. Nau H, Löscher W. Valproic acid: brain and plasma levels of the drug and its metabolites, anticonvulsant effects and GABA metabolism in the mouse. *J Pharmacol Exp Ther* 1982;220: 654–659.

91. Löscher W. Valproic acid. In: Frey H-H, Janz D, eds. *Antiepileptic drugs.* Berlin: Springer-Verlag, 1985:507–536.

92. Wikinski SI, Acosta GB, Rubio MC. Valproic acid differs in its *in vitro* effect on glutamic acid decarboxylase activity in neonatal and adult rat brain. *Gen Pharmacol* 1996;27:635–638.

93. Bolanos JP, Medina JM. Evidence of stimulation of the gamma-aminobutyric acid shunt by valproate and E-delta-2-valproate in neonatal rat brain. *Mol Pharmacol* 1993;43:487–490.

94. Löscher W, Frey H-H. Zum Wirkungsmechanismus von Valproinsäure. *Arzneimittelforschung* 1977;27:1081–1082.

95. Luder AS, Parks JK, Frerman F, et al. Inactivation of beef brain α-ketoglutarate dehydrogenase complex by valproic acid and valproic acid metabolites. *J Clin Invest* 1990;86:1574–1581.

96. Gram L, Larsson OM, Johnsen AH, et al. Effects of valproate, vigabatrin and aminooxyacetic acid on release of endogenous and exogenous GABA from cultured neurons. *Epilepsy Res* 1988;2:87–95.

97. Ekwuru MO, Cunningham JR. Phaclofen increases GABA release from valproate treated rats. *Br J Pharmacol* 1990;99 [Suppl]:251P.

98. Ueda Y, Willmore LJ. Molecular regulation of glutamate and GABA transporter proteins by valproic acid in rat hippocampus during epileptogenesis. *Exp Brain Res* 2000;133:334–339.

99. Biggs CS, Pearce BR, Fowler LJ, et al. The effect of sodium valproate on extracellular GABA and other amino acids in the rat ventral hippocampus: an *in vivo* microdialysis study. *Brain Res* 1992;594:138–142.

100. Rowley HL, Marsden CA, Martin KF. Differential effects of phenytoin and sodium valproate on seizure-induced changes in gamma-aminobutyric acid and glutamate release *in vivo. Eur J Pharmacol* 1995;294:541–546.

101. Wolf R, Tscherne U, Emrich HM. Suppression of preoptic GABA release caused by push-pull-perfusion with sodium valproate. *Naunyn Schmiedebergs Arch Pharmacol* 1988;338: 658–663.

102. Timmermann W, Westerink BHC. Brain microdialysis of GABA and glutamate: what does it signify? *Synapse* 1997;27:242–261.

103. Ticku MK, Davis WC. Effect of valproic acid on [³H]diazepam and [³H]dihydroxypicrotoxinin binding sites at the benzodiazepine-GABA receptor ionophore complex. *Brain Res* 1981;223:218–222.

104. Miller LG, Greenblatt DJ, Barnhill JG, et al. "GABA shift" *in vivo*: enhancement of benzodiazepine binding in vivo by modulation of endogenous GABA. *Eur J Pharmacol* 1988;148:123–130.

105. Nutt DJ, Cowen PJ, Little HJ. Unusual interactions of benzodiazepine receptor antagonists. *Nature* 1982;295:436.

106. Gent JP, Bentley M, Feely M, et al. Benzodiazepine cross-tolerance in mice extends to sodium valproate. *Eur J Pharmacol* 1986;128:9–15.

107. Liljequist S, Engel JA. Reversal of anticonflict action of valproate by various GABA and benzodiazepine antagonists. *Life Sci* 1984;34:2525–2531.

108. Lloyd KG, Thuret F, Pilc A. Upregulation of gamma-aminobutyric (GABA) B binding sites in rat frontal cortex: a common action of repeated administration of different classes of antidepressants and electroshock. *J Pharmacol Exp Ther* 1985;235:191-199.

109. Motohashi N. GABA receptor alterations after chronic lithium administration: comparison with carbamazepine and sodium valproate. *Prog Neuropsychopharmacol Biol Psychiatry* 1992;16:571–579.

110. DeFeudis FV. Gamma-aminobutyric acid-ergic analgesia: implications for gamma-aminobutyric acid–ergic therapy for drug addiction. *Drug Alcohol Depend* 1984;14:101–111.

111. Whittle SR, Turner AJ. Effects of the anticonvulsant sodium valproate on γ-aminobutyrate and aldehyde metabolism in ox brain. *J Neurochem* 1978;31:1453–1459.

112. Vayer P, Cash CD, Maitre M. Is the anticonvulsant mechanism of valproate linked to its interaction with the cerebral γ-hydroxybutyrate system? *Trends Pharmacol Sci* 1988;9:127–129.

113. Whittle SR, Turner SJ. Effects of anticonvulsants on the formation of γ-hydroxybutyrate from γ-aminobutyrate in rat brain. *J Neurochem* 1982;38:848–851.

114. Snead OC. γ-Hydroxybutyrate model of generalized absence seizures: further characterization and comparison with other absence models. *Epilepsia* 1988;29:361–377.

115. Snead OCI, Bearden LJ, Pegram V. Effect of acute and chronic anticonvulsant administration on endogenous γ-hydroxybutyrate in rat brain. *Neuropharmacology* 1980;19:47–52.

116. Dixon JF, Hokin LE. The antibipolar drug valproate mimics lithium in stimulating glutamate release and inositol 1,4,5-trisphosphate accumulation in brain cortex slices but not accumulation of inositol monophosphates and bisphosphates. *Proc Natl Acad Sci USA* 1997;94:4757–4760.

117. Nilsson M, Hansson E, Ronnback L. Interactions between valproate, glutamate, aspartate, and GABA with respect to uptake in astroglial primary cultures. *Neurochem Res* 1992;17:327–332.

118. Biggs CS, Pearce BR, Fowler LJ, et al. Regional effects of sodium valproate on extracellular concentrations of 5-hydroxytryptamine, dopamine, and their metabolites in the rat brain: an *in vivo* microdialysis study. *J Neurochem* 1992;59:1702–1708.

119. Horton RW, Anlezark GM, Sawaya MCB, et al. Monoamine and GABA metabolism and the anticonvulsant action of di-*n*-propylacetate and ethanolamine-*O*-sulphate. *Eur J Pharmacol* 1977;41:387–397.

120. Ichikawa J, Meltzer HY. Valproate and carbamazepine increase prefrontal dopamine release by 5-HT1A receptor activation. *Eur J Pharmacol* 1999;380:R1–R3.

121. Nathanson JA. Cyclic nucleotides and nervous system function. *Physiol Rev* 1977;57:157–256.

122. Lust WD, Kupferberg HJ, Yonekawa WD, et al. Changes in brain metabolites induced by convulsants or electroshock: effects of anticonvulsant agents. *Mol Pharmacol* 1978;14:347–356.

123. McCandless DW, Feussner GK, Lust WD, et al. Metabolite levels in brain following experimental seizures: the effects of isoniazid and sodium valproate in cerebellar and cerebral cortical layers. *J Neurochem* 1979;32:755–760.

124. Watson DG, Watterson JM, Lenox RH. Sodium valproate down-regulates the myristoylated alanine-rich C kinase substrate (MARCKS) in immortalized hippocampal cells: a property of protein kinase C–mediated mood stabilizers. *J Pharmacol Exp Ther* 1998;285:307–316.

125. Blackshear PJ. The MARCKS family of cellular protein kinase C substrates. *J Biol Chem* 1993;268:1501–1504.

126. Lubrich B, van Calker D. Inhibition of the high affinity myo-inositol transport system: a common mechanism of action of antibipolar drugs? *Neuropsychopharmacology* 1999;21:519–529.

127. O'Donnell T, Rotzinger S, Nakashima TT, et al. Chronic lithium and sodium valproate both decrease the concentration of myo-inositol and increase the concentration of inositol monophosphates in rat brain. *Brain Res* 2000;880:84–91.

128. Frey H-H, Löscher W. Distribution of valproate across the interface between blood and cerebrospinal fluid. *Neuropharmacology* 1978;17:637–642.

129. Shen DD. Valproate: absorption, distribution, and excretion. In: Löscher W, ed. *Valproate*. Basel: Birkhäuser, 1999.

130. Huai-Yun H, Secrest DT, Mark KS, et al. Expression of multidrug resistance–associated protein (MRP) in brain microvessel endothelial cells. *Biochem Biophys Res Commun* 1998;243:816–820.

131. Cutrer FM, Limmroth V, Moskowitz MA. Possible mechanisms of valproate in migraine prophylaxis. *Cephalalgia* 1997;17:93–100.

132. Maes M, Calabrese J, Jayathilake K, et al. Effects of subchronic treatment with valproate on L-5-HTP-induced cortisol responses in mania: evidence for increased central serotonergic neurotransmission. *Psychiatry Res* 1997;71:67–76.

VALPROIC ACID

CHEMISTRY, BIOTRANSFORMATION, AND PHARMACOKINETICS

RENÉ H. LEVY
DANNY D. SHEN
FRANK S. ABBOTT
K. WAYNE RIGGS
HOUDA HACHAD

The branched-chain fatty acid structure of valproic acid (VPA) explains some of its disposition characteristics. VPA is highly bound to plasma albumin, and this property tends to keep most of the drug within the vascular compartment. In common with endogenous fatty acids, VPA undergoes phase I biotransformation mediated by both β-oxidative enzymes in the mitochondria and cytochrome P450 enzymes in the smooth endoplasmic reticulum. Early on, it was assumed that VPA, being lipophilic like the endogenous long-chain fatty acids, readily permeates the blood–brain barrier. However, more recent studies suggest that specialized transport mechanisms may be involved in the distribution of VPA into the brain, as well as its transfer across the placenta to reach the fetus. These unique features of VPA disposition represent an important aspect of the clinical pharmacology of this widely used and versatile antiepileptic and mood-stabilizing agent.

CHEMISTRY AND METABOLIC SCHEME

VPA (2-propylpentanoic acid, dipropylacetic acid) (1) (Figures 84.1 and 84.2) is an achiral C-8 branched-chain

René H. Levy, PhD: Professor and Chair, Department of Pharmaceutics, Professor of Neurological Surgery, University of Washington School of Pharmacy and Medicine, Seattle, Washington

Danny D. Shen, PhD: Professor, Department of Pharmacy and Pharmaceutics, University of Washington, Seattle, Washington

Frank S. Abbott, BSP, MS, PhD: Professor and Dean, Faculty of Pharmaceutical Sciences, University of British Columbia, Vancouver, British Columbia, Canada

K. Wayne Riggs, PhD: Associate Professor of Pharmaceutical Sciences, University of British Columbia, Vancouver, British Columbia, Canada

Houda Hachad, MD: Research Associate, Department of Pharmaceutics, University of Washington, Seattle, Washington

fatty acid having a molecular weight of 144.2 g mol^{-1}. The pure acid, a colorless liquid (boiling point, 221 to 222°C) with a characteristic odor, is only slightly soluble in water but is highly soluble in organic solvents (log p = 2.72 – 2.75) (1,2). The white crystalline sodium salt is very soluble in water and in some organic solvents (e.g., methanol and acetone), whereas the calcium and magnesium salts are insoluble in water. A common therapeutic form of the drug is divalproex sodium (Depakote, Epival), a stable coordination compound derived from sodium VPA and VPA in a 1:1 molar ratio. The free acid (negative log of dissociation constant = 4.56 – 4.8) (2) and sodium salt forms are also stable compounds. Further details of physical constants and spectroscopic details of VPA can be found in the monograph by Chang (3). Key references on assays of VPA and its metabolites can be found in the previous edition of this book (4) and in a book on VPA (5). Of the chemical forms of VPA, the amide analog valpromide is an active anticonvulsant and is readily converted *in vivo* to VPA. As such, it can be considered to be a prodrug form of VPA, although it has effects of its own, such as being a selective inhibitor of human microsomal epoxide hydrolase (6). Other amides and chemical analogs of VPA including metabolites of VPA have been studied for anticonvulsant activity in the search for an alternative drug to VPA. Much of that work has been reviewed (5).

ABSORPTION

Bioavailability

The gastrointestinal absorption of VPA from all its oral formulations appears to be almost complete. The absolute bioavailability of a divalproex sodium extended-release

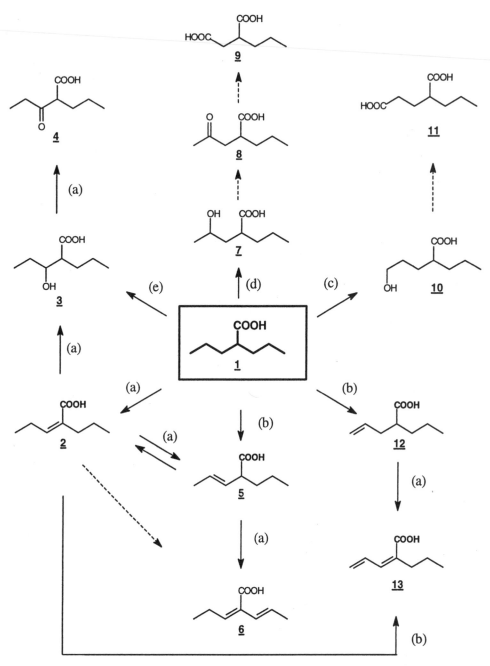

FIGURE 84.1. Valproic acid *(1)* and metabolites involved in phase I metabolic pathways observed in humans: *2*, 2-ene-VPA (E- and Z-isomers); *3*, 3-OH-VPA; *4*, 3-keto-VPA; *5*, 3-ene-VPA (E- and Z-isomers); *6*, 2,3′-diene-VPA (E,E- and E,Z-isomers); *7*, 4-OH-VPA; *8*, 4-keto-VPA; *9*, 2-PSA; *10*, 5-OH-VPA; *11*, 2-PGA; *12*, 4-ene-VPA; *13*, 2,4-diene-VPA (E- and Z-isomers). The putative characterized enzymatic pathways are as follows: *(a)* β-oxidation; *(b)* P450-dependent desaturation; *(c)* P450-dependent ω-hydroxylation; *(d)* P450-dependent (ω-1)-hydroxylation; *(e)* P450-dependent (ω-2)-hydroxylation. The *broken lines* indicate a metabolic route in which the details are not yet confirmed.

tablet administered as a single dose after a meal was ~90% (product information, Depakote ER, 2000). Several bioequivalence studies have shown comparable bioavailability (>90 %) for all dose formulations (7,8). Controlled-released formulations of VPA given once daily were shown to be bioequivalent to enteric-coated formulations given twice daily, with respect to area under the curve (AUC) (9). The sprinkle formulation of sodium hydrogen divalproex (coated particles in capsules) exhibited the same extent of absorption as enteric-coated tablets (10).

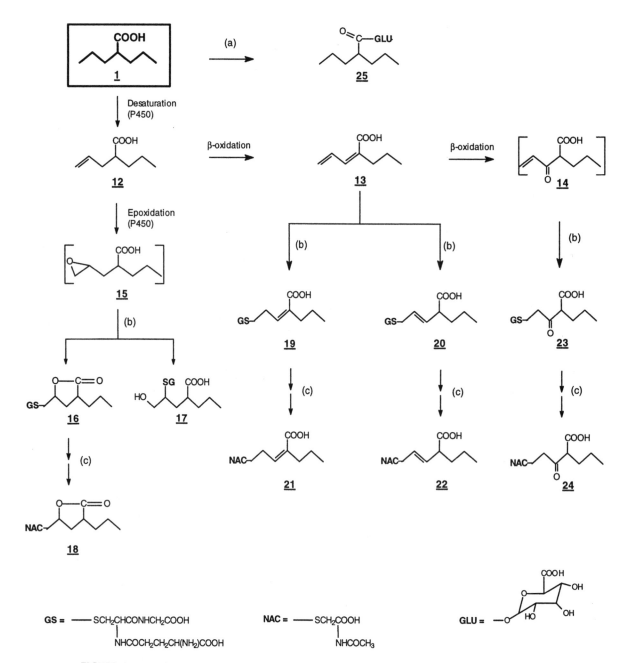

FIGURE 84.2. Valproate *(1)* and phase I metabolites *(12, 13)* involved in phase II metabolic pathways: *12,* 4-ene-VPA; *13,* 2,4-diene-VPA; *14,* 3-keto-4-ene-VPA; *15,* 4,5-epoxy-VPA; *16,* 5-GS-4-OH-VPA-γ-lactone; *17,* 4-GS-5-OH-VPA; *18,* 5-NAC-4-OH-VPA-γ-lactone; *19,* 5-GS-2-ene-VPA; *20,* 5-GS-3-ene-VPA; *21,* 5-NAC-2-ene-VPA; *22,* 5-NAC-3-ene-VPA; *23,* 5-GS-3-keto-VPA; *24,* 5-NAC-3-keto-VPA; *25,* VPA glucuronide. The putative enzymatic pathways are as follows: *(a)* glucuronidation; *(b)* glutathione conjugation; *(c)* mercapturic acid pathway. Postulated intermediate compounds are shown in *square brackets.*

The rate of absorption of VPA depends on the dosage form; the rapid-release formulations (syrup, capsule, and uncoated tablet) are absorbed with peak times (T_{max}) between 0.5 and 2 hours. T_{max} increases in the following order: dragée > tablet > solution (11). Enteric-coated tablets exhibit variable absorption rates (12–16), and peak times range between 3 and 8 hours. Compared with enteric-coated tablets, sprinkle capsules have a slightly slower absorption rate, with a T_{max} value of 4.0 versus 3.4 hours (10).

The AUC and maximum concentration resulting from intravenous administration of VPA (500 mg as a single 1-hour infusion) and a single oral (500-mg) dose of VPA syrup to healthy volunteers were equivalent. T_{max} occurred at the end of the infusion, whereas T_{max} after oral administration in this study occurred at ~4 hours (product information, Depacon, 2000).

Food intake had no significant effect on the bioavailability of VPA in soft gelatin capsules (17) or in a sustained-release preparation (18). However, multiple-dose administration of enteric-coated VPA tablets with meals in patients was associated with a delay in absorption; T_{max} was increased from 2.0 to 5.8 hours. Meals had no effect on the extent of absorption (19).

The plasma VPA concentration time course after rectal administration of VPA syrup is comparable to that observed after the oral capsule (20). The absorption of VPA from suppositories is generally slower than that from rectal solutions (21–25).

Formulations

Three different chemical forms of VPA are most commonly used: the free acid, the sodium salt, and divalproex sodium, which is a coordinated 1:1 complex of sodium VPA and VPA. VPA is available as a *capsule* (Deproic) or as *soft gelatin capsules* (Depakene) of 250 mg. It is also available as a *syrup* containing the equivalent of 250 mg/5 mL as the sodium salt.

An *intravenous* formulation of VPA sodium is available in 5-mL single-dose vials available in trays of 10 vials (Depacon). Each milliliter contains VPA sodium equivalent to 100 mg VPA.

Divalproex sodium *tablets* are supplied in three dosage strengths containing divalproex sodium equivalent to 125 mg, 250 mg, or 500 mg of VPA. It is also available as coated particles in capsules (Depakote Sprinkle capsules), delayed-release tablets, or extended-release tablets. *The Springle capsule* form contains specially coated particles of divalproex sodium equivalent to 125 mg of VPA in a hard gelatin capsule. Depakote *delayed-release tablets* are supplied in three dosage strengths containing divalproex sodium equivalent to 125 mg, 250 mg, or 500 mg of VPA. Depakote *extended-release tablets* contain divalproex sodium in a once-a-day extended release formulation equivalent to 500 mg of VPA.

Routes of Administration

Oral Administration. The rapid-release, enteric-coated, and slow-release formulations of VPA are administered orally with food to minimize gastrointestinal irritation.

Intravenous Administration. The intravenous formulation of VPA should be administered as 60-minute infusion at a rate not exceeding 20 mg/min. Because the use of VPA sodium injection for more than 14 days has not been studied, patients should be switched to oral formulations as soon as clinically feasible.

Rectal Administration. Rectal administration of VPA has been successful in the treatment of intractable status epilep-

ticus in children (26). Commercially available VPA syrup (250 mg/5 mL) was diluted 1:1 with tap water and was given as a retention enema in a loading dose of 10 to 20 mg/kg. Maintenance doses (10 to 15 mg/kg every 8 hours) were started 8 hours after the initial loading dose.

DISTRIBUTION

Plasma Protein Binding

VPA has a rather small distribution volume (slightly larger than extracellular fluid volume) that reflects its high binding affinity for plasma proteins relative to its binding or sequestration at extravascular sites. VPA binds mainly to albumin in human plasma (27). Early studies established that ~90% of VPA in plasma is bound to albumin at therapeutic concentrations (28).

A significant feature of VPA binding to plasma albumin is the dependence of free fraction on drug concentration. Detailed studies on VPA binding in plasma obtained from patients with epilepsy and receiving long-term VPA therapy have shown that the equilibrium dissociation constant of VPA for albumin is in the range of 90 to 200 µmol/L or 13 to 29 µg/mL (29,30). Because the therapeutic concentrations of free VPA in plasma (i.e., 5 to 15 µg/mL) are close to the dissociation constant for the VPA-albumin complex, the serum free fraction of VPA is expected to vary with total drug concentration. Cramer et al. (31) reported that the average plasma unbound fraction in adult patients receiving VPA monotherapy ranged between 7% and 9% at total concentrations <75 µg/mL; it increased to 15% at 100 µg/mL, 22% at 125 µg/mL, and 30% at 150 µg/mL. Similar concentration-dependent changes in the plasma free fraction of VPA have also been observed in children and infants with seizure disorders (32–35).

Concentration dependence in the plasma free fraction of VPA leads to differing degrees of fluctuation between total and unbound VPA concentrations at steady state. Numerous studies have shown that fluctuations in unbound concentration were generally 50% to 100% greater than fluctuations in total concentrations (35–40). Aside from concentration dependence in plasma protein binding, elevated free fatty acid levels in early morning samples and true diurnal differences in metabolic clearance can also explain the apparent difference in total and free VPA kinetics.

Diminished plasma protein binding of VPA has been observed in numerous pathophysiologic states, notably those associated with hypoalbuminemia, for example, pregnancy (41,42), aging (37,43), head trauma, liver diseases (44), uremia (45,46), and advanced disease with human immunodeficiency virus (47). In uremia, the increase in free fraction is the result, at least in part, of displacement from protein binding sites by endogenous compounds. The concentration dependence in plasma free fraction of VPA becomes more pronounced at low serum albumin (48). The effects of lowering of plasma protein binding on VPA clearance kinetics are discussed later, in the section on elimination and half-life.

As expected, other drugs bound to albumin can competitively reduce the plasma protein binding of VPA. Such is the case for sulfamethoxazole (47), salicylates (49), and naproxen (50). A similar binding displacement is observed when plasma endogenous fatty acid levels are raised (51,52). An elevation in free fatty acid level also explains the decrease in VPA binding to plasma proteins in the sera of patients with insulin-dependent diabetes mellitus (53).

The merits of monitoring free, rather than total, VPA concentrations, an approach that assumes that only free drug is available for distribution into the brain, have been debated in the literature with no clear resolution (42,54–56). Lenn and Robertson (57) reported the results of a retrospective analysis of clinical records and unbound and total plasma concentrations of VPA that were collected from 395 epileptic patients over a 13-month period. Unbound VPA concentration was considered clinically meaningful when (a) an unbound fraction fell outside the normal range of 5% to 15%, (b) unbound and total concentrations appeared discordant (not both high or both low), and (c) current seizures or side effects such that a change in antiepileptic drug regimen was indicated. About 15% of unbound values from 18% of patients fit clinically significant criteria. Most of these patients had unsatisfactory control of current seizures. The authors advocated monitoring of plasma free VPA regardless of total plasma VPA concentration when there is an unresolved clinical problem. Anecdotal reports attest to the usefulness of unbound VPA levels in diagnosing side effect problems in patients with hypoalbuminemia (58,59), and during removal of an enzyme-inducing anticonvulsant from VPA polytherapy when monitoring total VPA concentration may lead to underestimate the rise in free VPA concentration, because of concentration-dependent change in plasma free fraction (60).

Central Nervous System

VPA enters the central nervous system very rapidly. Tissue distribution studies in mice and rats (61,62) showed that peak concentration in brain was reached within minutes after either intravenous or intraperitoneal injection of VPA. The subsequent decline of drug concentration in brain paralleled that in plasma, a finding indicating a facile equilibration of VPA between brain and capillary blood. In rhesus monkeys equipped with a chronically implanted ventricular catheter, the upswing and decline of VPA in cerebrospinal fluid (CSF) followed closely the time course of plasma concentration during and after the cessation of intravenous VPA infusion (63). A reasonably rapid penetration of VPA into brain also occurs in humans, as evidenced by the effective treatment of status epilepticus, acute manic

episodes, and severe refractory migraine with rectal or intravenous VPA (26,64–68).

Much of the early information on the extent of VPA distribution into the central nervous system of humans was obtained indirectly through CSF sampling studies in patients with epilepsy (69). In general, a good correlation was observed between lumbar CSF and total plasma concentration of VPA. The CSF:total plasma concentration ratio averaged about 0.1 to 0.15, with notable variation among subjects within any given study. VPA concentrations in CSF tended to be lower than unbound VPA concentrations in plasma. The reported CSF:free plasma concentration ratio varied from 0.6 to near 1.

There are three available reports of VPA concentrations in the human brain (70–72). All three studies reveal an exceptionally low and variable presence of VPA in the brain. In the most recent study, by Shen et al. (70), cortical (gray matter) samples were obtained in 13 patients receiving long-term VPA therapy who underwent surgical treatment for intractable seizures. The respective mean brain:plasma concentration ratios based on total and free drug in serum were 0.11 and 0.54. This finding stands in contrast to the older aromatic or heterocyclic antiepileptics such as phenytoin and phenobarbital, which typically concentrate in brain tissue and exhibit brain:CSF concentration ratios well exceeding unity. The brain:total serum concentration ratio varied over a fourfold range. Some of this variability was related to interpatient variability in serum protein binding, as indicated by a modest correlation between the distribution ratio and serum free fraction ($r^2 = 0.47$, $p < .01$). However, the brain-to-unbound concentration ratio still showed a threefold variation. Two conclusions were reached. First, the unusually low distribution ratio of VPA explains the relatively high plasma levels of VPA (usually >350 µmol/L or 50 µg/mL) that are needed for effective seizure control. A brain:unbound concentration ratio less than the brain water content indicates a more rapid removal rate of VPA from the brain than its entry rate into the brain at steady state. Using the tissue-sampling, carotid artery-injection method (i.e., the Oldendorf technique), Cornford et al. (73) showed that the kinetic rate constant for the efflux of VPA from rat brain exceeded the rate constant for uptake into the brain, a finding that confirms the apparent asymmetry in the transport kinetics of VPA between blood and brain. Second, the variability in distribution of VPA between brain and blood may be one underlying factor for the lack of a clearly definable therapeutic range of serum VPA concentrations in epileptic patients. Hence, there is a need to elucidate the mechanisms for the transport of VPA into and out of the brain as well as the physiologic factors that regulate those transport processes.

Animal studies have revealed that the bidirectional movement of VPA across the blood–brain barrier is mediated jointly by passive diffusion and carrier transport. The entry of VPA from blood into the brain is mediated by a medium-

and long-chain fatty acid selective anion exchanger at the brain capillary epithelium, which accounts for two-thirds of the barrier permeability. The mechanism governing the efficient clearance of VPA from the brain into blood appears to involve a probenecid-sensitive, active transport system at the brain capillary endothelium.

A brain microdialysis study in rabbits suggests that another set of transporters exists within the brain parenchyma that shuttles VPA between the interstitial fluid and intracellular compartments. The putative parenchymal cell transport system appears to concentrate VPA within the cellular compartments (i.e., those of neurons and glia). This, coupled with the efficient removal process at the blood–brain barrier, results in a very low interstitial concentration of VPA. During intravenous VPA infusion, the average steady-state concentration in the interstitial fluid was 36% of that in the intracellular compartment and 17% of that in plasma water. The high intracellular:interstitial concentration gradient suggests that intraneuronal mechanisms of VPA may be more important than its actions at the plasma membrane with respect to anticonvulsant and neuropsychiatric effects.

One other important aspect of the blood–brain barrier transport mechanism is the effect of plasma protein binding on the uptake of VPA. The traditional notion that drug molecules bound to plasma proteins and blood cells do not diffuse readily across the capillary endothelium appears to hold true in the blood:brain distribution behavior of certain anticonvulsants. It was previously mentioned that Shen et al. (70) found that the interpatient variation in brain:serum distribution ratio of VPA is in part related to variation in serum free fraction, a finding consistent with limitation of brain uptake by serum protein binding. However, Cornford et al. (73) showed that VPA uptake into rat brain is not entirely restricted to the equilibrium free fraction. These investigators estimated that as much as 18% of VPA that was extracted during a single pass through the capillaries is derived from protein-bound VPA in serum-containing injectate. It was also shown that although brain extraction increased with increasing serum concentration of VPA as a result of saturation in serum drug binding, the extraction of the bound moiety remained constant. The mechanism by which protein-bound drug is released for uptake across the capillary endothelium is not understood.

Aside from the obvious need for studies relating to the brain distribution of VPA, questions have been raised on the central nervous system uptake and accumulation of VPA metabolites (discussed in the section on biotransformation). Some of the mono-ene and di-ene metabolites of VPA have been shown to possess anticonvulsant activity at a dose potency near that of VPA (74,75). Earlier attention had focused on the role of the predominant unsaturated metabolite in circulation –(E)-2-ene-VPA in the pharmacodynamics of VPA. However, the circulating levels of the unsaturated metabolites are typically lower than those of the parent drug (see the later section on biliary and renal excretion). Moreover, studies have shown that, in epileptic patients, the brain cortical and CSF concentrations of these pharmacologically active metabolites are much lower than their plasma concentrations and are low relative to VPA concentrations at the respective sites (76,77). Although sequestration of active metabolites at the critical target sites in the brain has been proposed (78), there is no firm evidence that the unsaturated metabolites play a quantitatively significant role in the pharmacodynamics of VPA.

Transplacental Passage

VPA has been implicated as a teratogen causing neural tube defects, especially spina bifida aperta. Consequently, transplacental transfer and fetal accumulation of VPA in pregnant mouse and rats have been investigated extensively, as reviewed by Nau (79). More recently, maternal-to-fetal distribution of VPA was studied in a chronically catheterized late-term pregnant sheep model (80,81). Collectively, these studies found that VPA crosses the placental barrier readily, resulting in significant fetal exposure. A study by Utoguchi and Audus (82) in a human trophoblast cell line (BeWo) suggested that the transplacental transfer of VPA from the maternal to the fetal side may be mediated by the proton-coupled monocarboxylic acid transporters. Nau and Scott (83) observed higher VPA concentrations in early mouse embryos than the corresponding free VPA concentration in maternal serum. These investigators attributed the accumulation of VPA to "ion trapping" resulting from the remarkably high intracellular pH of the rodent embryo during organogenesis. The same investigative team also reported preferential accumulation of VPA in embryonic neuroepithelium of the mouse during early stages of organogenesis (84).

Information on distribution of VPA into human fetus has been gathered through amniocentesis in pregnant women and by sampling of umbilical and maternal blood at birth. Omtzigt et al. (85) gathered maternal serum and amniotic fluid data from 52 pregnant women during the late first trimester and early second trimester of pregnancy. VPA concentrations in the amniotic fluid correlated better with total than unbound concentrations in maternal serum. The median amniotic fluid:total serum concentration ratio was 0.09. All unsaturated and hydroxylated metabolites of VPA present in the serum were detected in the amniotic fluid, although at very low concentrations.

Some studies have been performed during delivery of newborns from mothers who received VPA throughout pregnancy. VPA concentration is 1.5 to 2 times higher in umbilical cord serum than in maternal serum (86–89). Several investigators examined the possible contribution of protein binding to this phenomenon and consistently found that the unbound fraction of VPA is lower in umbilical cord serum than in maternal serum: 9.1% versus 15% in one study (86) and 6% versus 12% in another study (90).

A longitudinal study in fetus-mother pairs throughout pregnancy was performed by Nau and Krauer (41). In fetal serum, unbound fractions were 40% to 80% during weeks 13 through 16 of gestation, they decreased to 20% around week 20, and they continued to decrease to 10% at the end of gestation. This behavior of unbound fraction was explained by the increase in fetal serum albumin concentrations from 3 to 12 g/L during early gestation to 30 to 40 g/L at term. Maternal unbound fractions, conversely, increased during pregnancy from 10% to 20%, a finding that correlates with the decline in maternal serum albumin (91). Thus, whereas the extent of serum protein binding is higher in fetus than in mother at term, the opposite is true during gestation.

Breast Milk

Literature reports on excretion of VPA into breast milk and consumption by the suckling infant were summarized in two reviews (92,93). The concentrations of VPA in breast milk were found to range from >1% to 10% of the maternal serum concentration. Serum concentrations of VPA in the nursing infants were mostly between 4% and 12% of the corresponding maternal serum level. The estimated dose to the suckling infant is <6% of the recommended initial pediatric therapeutic dose of 20 mg/kg/day. Therefore, exposure of newborn to VPA through ingestion breast milk is generally not an issue. Stahl et al. (94) reported an incidence of thrombocytopenia purpura and anemia in a breast-fed infant whose mother was treated with VPA. These authors suggested that significant transfer of VPA metabolites, some of which may be toxic, could be a cause of this adverse event.

ROUTES OF ELIMINATION

Biotransformation

Figures 84.1 and 84.2 summarize the metabolic scheme for VPA. Figure 84.1 is not inclusive but for the most part describes the phase I metabolites of VPA most commonly found in human plasma and urine (4,95–97). Five metabolic pathways of VPA are illustrated, with at least three—β-oxidation, cytochrome P450 (P450)–dependent (ω)- and (ω-1)-hydroxylation—being shared by endogenous fatty acids (98). Complexity in the metabolism of VPA arises because several of the metabolites are formed by more than one pathway. For example, mitochondrial β-oxidation transforms VPA to 2-ene-VPA (2-*n*-propyl-2-pentenoic acid; *2* in Figure 84.1), 3-OH-VPA (2-*n*-propyl-3-hydroxypentanoic acid; *3* in Figure 84.1), and 3-keto-VPA (2-*n*-propyl-3-oxopentanoic acid; *4* in Figure 84.1) (99), whereas P450-dependent (ω-, (ω-1)-, and (ω-2)-hydroxylation produces 5-OH-VPA (2-*n*-propyl-

5-hydroxypentanoic acid; *10* in Figure 84.1), 4-OH-VPA (2-*n*-propyl-4-hydroxypentanoic acid; *7* in Figure 84.1), and 3-OH-VPA (2-*n*-propyl-3-hydroxypentanoic acid; *3* in Figure 84.1), respectively (100–102). Evidence suggests that the 3-OH-VPA detected in serum is largely of P450 origin (103,104). Of the unsaturated metabolites, 2-ene-VPA (*2* in Figure 84.1), 3-ene-VPA (2-*n*-propyl-3-pentenoic acid; *5* in Figure 84.1), 2,3'-diene-VPA (2-[1'-propenyl]-2-pentenoic acid; *6* in Figure 84.1), and 2,4-diene-VPA (2-*n*-propyl-2,4-pentadienoic acid; *13* in Figure 84.1) are products of β-oxidation (103–105). The 2,4-diene-VPA (*13* in Figure 84.1), a metabolite implicated in the hepatotoxicity of VPA (105–111), is a product of the mitochondrial β-oxidation pathway that converts 4-ene-VPA (2-*n*-propyl-4-pentenoic acid; *12* in Figure 84.1) as the coenzyme A (CoA) ester to the corresponding 2,4-diene-VPA-CoA (105). The 2,4-diene metabolite is also the product of endoplasmic reticulum P450 transformation of the primary serum metabolite 2-ene-VPA (*2* in Figure 84.1) (110). The route by which 2,4-diene-VPA (*13* in Figure 84.1) is formed is thought to have significance with respect to the hepatotoxicity of VPA (105).

A novel discovery of VPA biotransformation was the finding that terminal desaturation of VPA to 4-ene-VPA (*12* in Figure 84.1) is catalyzed by P450 (112,113) and is common to certain animal species including human (113). This reaction is unique to VPA metabolism in showing a high degree of specificity, with the *(R)*-isomer of 4-ene-VPA (*12* in Figure 84.1) being the preferred product (114). Mechanistic studies using stable isotopes and mass spectrometry illustrated that an intermediate carbon-centered radical at C-4 is an essential common rate-limiting step for the formation of both 4-ene-VPA (*12* in Figure 84.1) and 4-OH-VPA (*7* in Figure 84.1) (113). Initial studies on subcellular fractions demonstrated that rat (112) and rabbit (113) CYP2B (cytochrome P450, CYP) isoforms as well as rabbit lung CYP4B1 significantly catalyze the biotransformation of VPA to 4-ene-VPA (115). More recent experiments with human cDNA-expressed P450 isoforms have demonstrated that multiple human P450 enzymes are involved in the desaturation of VPA. These include CYP2C9 and CYP2A6 (116) as well as CYP2B6 (117). In an elegant experiment using stable isotopes, this type of P450 desaturation was also shown to be true for the formation of 3-ene-VPA (*5* in Figure 84.1) (102). In female rat microsomes induced by triacetyloleandomycin and pregnenolone-16α-carbonitrile and in baculovirus expressed P450, CYP3A1 was determined to mediate the direct dehydrogenation of VPA to E (*trans*) and Z (*cis*)-3-ene-VPA. Based on the deuterium isotope effects, the metabolite most likely arises from partitioning of the intermediate C-3 or C-4 radicals between olefin formation and hydroxyl radical rebound to form 3-OH-VPA and 4-OH-VPA, respectively. The significance of this pathway to the formation of 3-ene-VPA is uncertain because this route is highly specific to the rat in that neither human CYP3A4 nor rabbit CYP3A6 forms significant quantities of the metabolite. Control microsomes (noninduced) did not produce detectable levels of the metabolite (102). *In vivo* in rats, 3-ene-VPA is a secondary metabolite of VPA that is formed by isomerization of the primary mitochondrial product 2-ene-VPA (*2* in Figure 84.1) (103,104). Because (E,E)-2,3′-diene-VPA (*6* in Figure 84.1) is a β-oxidation product of 3-ene VPA (*5* in Figure 84.1) (103) and is also a major serum metabolite of VPA in rats and human (4,95), it is likely that most of the 3-ene-VPA seen in the human arises from 2-ene-VPA.

Of the ketone metabolites, 3-keto-VPA (*4* in Figure 84.1) is a major metabolite of VPA in most species (4,118) and is derived largely from (E)-2-ene-VPA (*2* in Figure 84.1) in the β-oxidation pathway (99,104). Enzymes involved in the β-oxidation of VPA may differ from those reported for endogenous straight chain fatty acids (99,119). For example, in mitochondrial studies, 3-OH-VPA-CoA was not a substrate for mitochondrial or peroxisomal *L*-3-hydroxyacyl-CoA dehydrogenases but was oxidized to 3-keto-VPA (*4* in Figure 84.1) by a novel membrane oxidized nicotinamide-adenine dinucleotide (NAD+)-specific 3-hydroxyacyl-CoA dehydrogenase (99). The resulting 3-keto-VPA-CoA appeared to be resistant to hydrolysis by 3-keto-acyl-CoA thiolase, an enzyme that catalyzes the final step of fatty acid CoA hydrolysis in the β-oxidation pathway (99). The corresponding 4-keto-VPA (2-*n*-propyl-4-oxopentanoic acid; *8* in Figure 84.1) is formed from 4-OH-VPA (*7* in Figure 84.1) and is subsequently oxidized to the dicarboxylic acid 2-PSA (2-*n*-propylsuccinic acid; *9* in Figure 84.1) (120). The 2-PGA (2-*n*-propylglutaric acid; *11* in Figure 84.1) metabolite is the primary dicarboxylic acid derived from VPA biotransformation that is found in the urine of patients on VPA therapy (4) and is thought to be an oxidation product of 5-OH-VPA (*10* in Figure 84.1) (120).

The phase II metabolism of VPA is described in Figure 84.2. Glucuronidation is the major route of VPA metabolism and results in the formation of the 1-*O*-acyl-β-D-ester-linked glucuronide in most animals (121) and humans (122–124). Because of continuing interest in reactive metabolites of VPA that may contribute to the hepatotoxicity and teratogenicity of VPA, the glutathione (GSH) and mercapturic acid (NAC, *N*-acetylcysteine) conjugates arising from reactive intermediates are also summarized in Figure 84.2. Other acyl conjugates of VPA such as valproyl-L-carnitine, VPA-CoA, VPA adenosine monophosphate (VPA-AMP) and amino acid conjugates of VPA are known and have been described previously (4).

Conjugation of VPA with glucuronic acid is mediated by hepatic microsomal UDPGT (uridine diphosphate glucuronosyltransferase) enzymes (125), although the specific UDPGT isoforms involved in VPA conjugation have yet to be reported. A high metabolic capacity was observed in this *in vitro* system for VPA glucuronidation, which, in fact, inhibited the conjugation of other drugs in a competitive

fashion (125). Like other acyl glucuronide conjugates, VPA glucuronide (*25* in Figure 84.2) is intrinsically reactive and is capable of undergoing numerous reactions including hydrolysis, rearrangement, and covalent binding to proteins (126). Rearrangement of the acyl moiety of VPA glucuronide occurs in a pH-dependent fashion to yield the β-glucuronidase–resistant 2-, 3-, and 4-*O* positional isomers (127). Although VPA glucuronides may give rise to covalent adducts with proteins (128), these conjugates appear to be only weakly immunogenic in humans (129). One example of a reactive VPA glucuronide comes from liquid chromatography-tandem mass spectrometry (LC/MS/MS) analysis of (*E*)-2,4-diene-VPA (*13* in Figure 84.2) metabolites in rats that indicated the presence of novel di-conjugates characterized as 5-GS-3-ene-VPA glucuronide and the corresponding 5-NAC-3-ene-VPA glucuronide (106). This study provided direct evidence for the reactivity of a VPA acyl glucuronide with GSH through a Michael addition mechanism, a result that may partially reflect the large propensity of the rat for the glucuronidation of VPA (121). Conversely, no 5-NAC-3-ene-VPA glucuronide or its 2-ene isomer could be found in the urine of patients receiving VPA therapy (130). Other metabolites of VPA also undergo phase II glucuronidation (4,5).

Numerous investigators have sought evidence for the bioactivation of VPA to reactive metabolites as a mechanism of VPA-induced hepatotoxicity. The detection of GSH conjugates (mostly in bile) and their corresponding mercapturate conjugates in urine is strong evidence of the reactivity of metabolic intermediates in the biotransformation of VPA. Figure 84.2 summarizes some of the key findings. Not surprisingly, 4-ene-VPA (*12* in Figure 84.2) and (E)-2,4-diene-VPA (*13* in Figure 84.2), the two metabolites shown to be hepatotoxic in rats (44), give rise to GSH conjugates 16, 17, 19, 20, 23 seen in rat bile and NAC conjugates 18, 21, 22, and 24 isolated from rat urine (105,106, 109). The NAC conjugates 21 and 22 derived from (E)-2,4-diene-VPA (*13* in Figure 84.2) have also been isolated from patient urine (109,130). When 4-ene-VPA (*12* in Figure 84.2) was administered to rats, the predominant GSH conjugate was that of 4-OH-VPA-γ-lactone (*16* in Figure 84.2), a product of the reactive epoxide intermediate (*15* in Figure 84.2) (105). Further β-oxidation of 4-ene-VPA (*12* in Figure 84.2) generates the metabolites (E)-2,4-diene-VPA (*13* in Figure 84.2) and 3-keto-4-ene-VPA (*14* in Figure 84.2) that in mitochondria are present as their CoA thioester derivatives, a necessary form to react with GSH (105,109). In support of this, when 4-ene-VPA was substituted with a fluoro atom at the α position to block β-oxidation, no thiol conjugates from the biotransformation of α-fluoro-4-ene-VPA could be detected in either bile or urine of rats (108). Significantly reduced levels of thiol conjugates in urine were evident when either VPA or (E)-2-ene-VPA was administered to rats with only the NAC conjugate 22 (in Figure 84.2) being detected (105). This finding is consistent with VPA patient urine samples in which NAC conjugates 21 and 22 (in Figure 84.2) were the only GSH-derived conjugates of VPA to be identified (130,131). The enzyme glutathione-S-transferase is implicated in these conjugation reactions (132), although the specific isozymes to catalyze the reactions involving VPA metabolites have yet to be characterized. The case to link the formation of GSH conjugates of VPA metabolites with the toxicity of the drug can be found in several references (4,105,109,132), but other mechanisms may equally apply.

Plasma concentrations of VPA metabolites exhibit extremely high interindividual variability. The major VPA metabolites in plasma are generally (E)-2-ene-VPA, (E,E)-2,3'-diene-VPA, and 3-keto-VPA (4,95–97,124), with plasma concentrations of these metabolites usually within the range of 1 to 10 μg/mL, that is, well less than 20% of parent drug. Other metabolites such as 3-ene-VPA, 4-keto-VPA, and the hydroxylated metabolites are present at concentrations of 0.5 to 2 μg/mL (4). The 4-ene-VPA, (E)-2,4-diene-VPA, 2-PSA, and 2-PGA metabolites in plasma are usually present only in trace amounts; however, plasma concentrations of 4-ene-VPA may be elevated in patients taking enzyme-inducing comedication (133).

Genetic Aspects and Isoenzymes

Conjugation of VPA with glucuronic acid is catalyzed by the action of hepatic microsomal UDPGT enzymes (125) that may be responsible for the wide variation in the excretion of VPA glucuronide. Although much of this variability likely arises from the dose-dependent increase in glucuronide formation (124,134), pharmacogenetic factors could also be a contributor because some of these enzymes are polymorphically expressed (135). Specific UDGPT isoforms responsible for VPA conjugation have yet to be identified. Similarly, the specific P450 isozymes involved in phase I metabolism of VPA have not been fully characterized. As described previously, studies using subcellular fractions have shown that rat and rabbit liver CYP2 isoforms (112,113), as well as rabbit lung CYP4B1 (115), are capable of catalyzing the formation of 4-ene-VPA. In contrast, the lauric acid ω-hydroxylases, CYP4A1 and CYP4A3, do not result in 4-ene-VPA formation (115). More recent work using individual human cDNA-expressed isoforms indicate that CYP2C9, CYP2A6, and CYP2B6 (116,117) contribute to the terminal desaturation of VPA, and rat microsomal CYP3A1 catalyzes the oxidative formation of 3-, 4-, and 5-hydroxy-VPA, plus 3- and 4-ene-VPA (102). Based on known interactions of VPA with other antiepileptic drugs, CYP2C19 may also be involved in the oxidative metabolism of VPA (136). Of these P450 isozymes, CYP2A6, CYP2C9, and CYP2C19 are polymorphically expressed (137,138) and may therefore contribute to patient-to-patient variability in the metabolism of VPA. In the case of VPA biotransformation to 4-ene-VPA, genetic polymorphisms may contribute to the occur-rence of hepatotoxicity associated with this metabolite in certain individuals.

Urinary Excretion

In humans, VPA undergoes extensive hepatic metabolism ,and on average only 1% to 3% of the total dose is excreted unchanged in urine (122, 134). The major urinary metabolites of VPA are VPA glucuronide (10% to 70% of the dose) and 3-keto-VPA (6% to 60% of the dose) (97,122,124,133). Other metabolites such as (E,E)-2,3'-diene-VPA, 3-OH-VPA, 4-OH-VPA, 5-OH-VPA, 4-keto-VPA, and 2-PGA may account for 1% to 5% of the administered VPA dose (122,124,133,134). The 4-ene-VPA, (E)-2,4-diene-VPA, (E)-2-ene-VPA, 3-ene-VPA, and 2-PSA metabolites are very minor urinary products, and each accounts for 0% to 0.5% of the total VPA dose (122,133). The urinary excretion of 2-ene-VPA and 3-keto-VPA have been observed to increase after 200 mg twice daily administration of VPA over a 3-week period, apparently as a consequence of autoinduction of the β-oxidation pathway (118). This is accompanied by a small (~18%) decrease in the plasma AUC of VPA. As in humans, an increase in the urinary excretion of VPA and products of β-oxidation has also been observed in long-term VPA administration studies in rats, again apparently the result of autoinduction (139). Contribution of the glucuronide pathway to total VPA metabolism increases as a function of increasing VPA dose because of saturation of the β-oxidation pathway (120,122,124,134,140); the elimination of (ω) and (ω-1) cytochrome P450 oxidation products, however, appears to be relatively independent of dose. The percentage of VPA dose recovered in urine as 4-ene-VPA and its sequential metabolites has been observed to increase with increasing doses of VPA (141).

CLEARANCE AND HALF-LIFE

It has long been recognized that the level–dose relationship for VPA is highly variable among patients. Results from therapeutic monitoring studies (142–144) have shown that, at a given daily dose of VPA, the plasma drug level could vary as much as six- to eightfold among individual patients. Variation in VPA level:dose ratio largely reflects variability in the clearance characteristics of the drug.

The reported plasma (or metabolic) clearance in healthy volunteers (Table 84.1) is in the range of 6 to 8 mL/hr/kg, which is much lower than (≤0.03) the average hepatic blood flow (1,500 mL/min). Thus, VPA may be classified as a low-extraction drug, whose clearance is independent of blood flow and is positively dependent on its plasma free fraction (145). Consequently, factors affecting drug plasma protein binding and hepatic drug-metabolizing enzyme activities are important determinants of VPA clearance. A review of the relevant factors is presented in the following sections.

TABLE 84.1. PHARMACOKINETIC PARAMETERS OF VALPROIC ACID IN ADULT VOLUNTEERS AND PATIENTS WITH EPILEPSY

Populations	Study	Antiepileptic Drug Therapy	Valproic Acid Regimen	$V_d{}^a$ (L/Kg)	$T_{1/2\beta}$ (hr)	Free Fraction[b] (%)	Clearance (mL/hr/kg)[a]	
							Total	Free
Healthy adults (16–60 yrs)[c]	Perucca et al.[d] (43) n = 6	None	Single dose: 800 mg p.o.	0.14 ± 0.02[e]	13.0 ± 2.4	6.6 ± 1.2	7.7 ± 1.5	127 ± 29
	Bialer et al. (202,203) n = 6	None	Single dose: 1,000 mg p.o.	0.14 ± 0.02	14.9 ± 2.4	4.1 ± 1.2	6.7 ± 1.4	170 ± 46
	Gugler et al. (14) n = 6	None	Steady state: 1,200 mg/day p.o.	0.15 ± 0.02	15.9 ± 2.6	—	6.4 ± 1.1	—
	Bowdle et al. (152) n = 6	None	Steady state (p.o.): 500 mg/day	0.13 ± 0.02	13.6 ± 2.8	6.4 ± 2.1	6.7 ± 1.3	89 ± 71
			1,000 mg/day	0.15 ± 0.04	13.9 ± 3.4	9.8 ± 3.1	6.7 ± 1.5	72 ± 21
			1,500 mg/day	0.18 ± 0.03	14.5 ± 4.3	9.1 ± 0.7	8.2 ± 1.6	91 ± 18
	Bauer et al.[d,g] (36) n = 6	None	Steady state: 500 g/day p.o. Morning	—	—	6.4 ± 0.8	6.7 ± 0.9	106 ± 19
			Evening	—	—	6.1 ± 1.3	7.4 ± 1.0	123 ± 18
Adults with epilepsy (16–60 yrs)	Miljkovic et al. (204) n = 10	Monotherapy	Single dose: 900 mg p.o.	0.20 ± 0.04	15.0 ± 4.0	—	9.4 ± 2.9	125 ± 69
	Herngren et al. (34) n = 7	Monotherapy	Steady state: ???	0.15 ± 0.10	11.9 ± 5.9	7.2 ± 1.6	9.2 ± 4.8	126 ± 44
	Sundqvist et al. (149) n = 16	Monotherapy	Steady state (p.o.): 500 mg b.i.d.	—	—	8.8 ± 1.4	10.7 ± 2.8	118 ± 67
			1,000 mg b.i.d.	—	—	13.4 ± 3.3	14.5 ± 4.3	—
	Perucca et al. (205) n = 6	Polytherapy[g]	Single dose: 800 mg i.v.	0.18 ± 0.03	9.0 ± 1.4	—	15.1 ± 5.8	—
			800 mg p.o.	0.18 ± 0.03	9.0 ± 1.2	—	17.6 ± 2.8	—
	Schapel et al. (206) n = 17	Polytherapy[g]	Single dose: 600 mg p.o.	0.19 ± 0.09	9.3 ± 2.0	—	14.8 ± 5.8	—
	Hoffmann et al. (207) n = 6	Polytherapy[g]	Steady state: ???	0.14 ± 0.03	5.2 ± 2.7	—	14.7 ± 8.0	—
	Eadie et al. (208) n = 8	Polytherapy[g]	Steady state: ???	0.19 ± 0.05	8.5 ± 3.3	—	18.1 ± 10.8	—
Healthy elderly (>60 yrs)	Perucca et al. (43) n = 6	None	Single dose: 800 mg p.o.	0.16 ± 0.02	15.3 ± 1.7	9.5 ± 1.4	7.5 ± 2.2	78 ± 15
	Bauer et al.[f] (37) n = 6	None	Steady state: 500 mg/day p.o. Morning	—	—	10.7 ± 1.6	6.6 ± 0.5	64 ± 12
			Evening	—	—	9.7 ± 1.1	7.3 ± 0.7	75 ± 11

VD, volume of distribution; $T_{1/2}\beta$, half-life; p.o., oral; i.v., intravenous [a] In the calculation of V_d and clearance after oral administration of various dosage forms, complete absorption is assumed.

[b] Because plasma protein binding of valproic acid is concentration dependent and hence varies over time, a time-averaged free fraction based on the ratio of free area under the curve (AUC) to total AUC is quoted.

[c] Literature reports on single-dose pharmacokinetics of valproic acid in healthy adult volunteers are too numerous to be individually listed in this table. There is general agreement among studies. Therefore, only data from single dose studies that provide free drug measurements or steady-state studies are presented.

[d] Control data in young adults to be compared with the data in elderly subjects from the same study listed below.

[e] Data are presented as mean ± standard deviation.

[f] Diurnal variation in valproic acid clearance was examined. Morning and evening doses were administered at 8 AM and 8 PM.

[g] Polytherapy generally refers to enzyme-inducing comedication.

789

Nonlinear Kinetics

One complicating factor that contributes to the reported interindividual variability in the elimination kinetics of VPA is its dependence on dose. During long-term drug administration, a curvilinear relationship between plasma VPA level and dose has been noted in numerous studies (142,146–151). Above a daily dose of 500 mg/kg, the steady-state plasma concentration of VPA increased *less* than proportionally with an increase in dose (i.e., a convex plot of concentration *versus* dose). A population kinetic study (150) in Japanese patients found that dose dependence in clearance was more pronounced in patients receiving carbamazepine than in patients receiving monotherapy or polytherapy with phenobarbital.

The mechanism of nonlinearity in VPA clearance was examined earlier by Bowdle et al. (152) in a multiple-dose study in healthy volunteers. Each volunteer received 500, 1,000, and 1,500 mg/day of oral VPA in three consecutive steps. The nonlinearity in clearance was attributed principally to an increase in free fraction (as plasma VPA concentration increased). No consistent change in the clearance of unbound VPA was observed. Comparable findings were reported by Gómez-Bellver et al. (153) in a single-dose study at 1,000, 2,000, and 3,000 mg of orally administered VPA. These investigators noted a trend toward a decrease in the clearance of unbound VPA with the increase in dose, a finding consistent with the hypothesis of a saturation in β-oxidation as mentioned earlier in the discussion of urinary excretion.

Hussein et al. (154) investigated the effect of infusion duration on the pharmacokinetics of intravenous VPA in a group of healthy volunteers. Each subject received an intravenous infusion of 1,000 mg sodium VPA over 5, 10, 30, and 60 minutes on four separate occasions. A biphasic postinfusion decline in plasma VPA concentration was observed. A more rapid initial decline occurred as the infusion duration was shortened; that is, initial half-life varied from 48 minutes for the 60-minute infusion to 8 minutes for the 5-minute infusion. The plasma clearance of VPA for the 5-minute infusion study was consistently lower than those for the longer infusion durations (0.56 L/hr versus ≥0.64 L/hr). These investigators proposed that the more rapid extravascular distribution of VPA with the 5-minute infusion duration was the result of saturation of plasma protein binding. The lower plasma clearance, conversely, reflected a partial saturation of intrinsic metabolic clearance that more than compensated for the effect from the increase in plasma free fraction.

Gender and Body Size

In a population pharmacokinetic study in a large cohort of Japanese patients, Yukawa et al. (150) reported that female patients on average had a slightly (~10%) lower weight-normalized clearance than male patients. This and another study by Suemaru et al. (155) in moderately obese Japanese patients also showed that apparent oral clearance correlated better with ideal body weight than either total body weight or body mass index. Hence, VPA should be given according to ideal body weight, rather than total body weight, in overweight patients.

Concomitant Antiepileptic Medications

VPA clearance is on average twofold higher in adult epileptic patients who are taking enzyme-inducing comedication than in patients receiving VPA monotherapy or in nonepileptic, healthy volunteers (Table 84.1). This increase in VPA clearance is attributed to induction of liver drug-metabolizing enzymes caused by concurrent antiepileptic medications (Chapter 85). An approximate 40% to 100% increase in VPA clearance has also been observed in epileptic children receiving multiple enzyme-inducing antiepileptic medications as compared with children receiving VPA monotherapy (Table 84.2). The increase in VPA clearance is seen in patients taking the older antiepileptic drugs, including phenobarbital, phenytoin, carbamazepine, or a combination thereof. Thus, higher doses of VPA may be required to maintain therapeutic concentrations in patients receiving polytherapy. Some reports indicate that, in some patients, these interactions are so pronounced that therapeutic levels of VPA are barely maintained or are not achievable even at extraordinary high doses (156–158). There is also evidence that the magnitude of metabolic interaction may depend on the VPA dose (150).

The reported plasma half-life of VPA in healthy adult volunteers ranged from 12 to 16 hours (Table 84.1). The half-life of VPA is typically shorter in comedicated epileptic patients, and this is attributable to induction of VPA metabolism by other antiepileptic drugs. The mean half-life in epileptic adults taking enzyme-inducing comedication is ~9 hours (Table 84.1). However, elimination half-life values as short as 5 hours have been documented (34).

The half-life values in Tables 84.1 and 84.2 are all based on total VPA in plasma. When the plasma concentration of VPA ranges over 75 μg/mL during a dosage interval, the half-life of unbound drug will be shorter than that of total drug, as a result of the diminishing free fraction as the total drug concentration declines (see the earlier section on plasma protein binding). For example, in a group of young adult epileptic patients, Herngren and Nergardh (34) found that the mean terminal half-life of free VPA was 6.4±3.9 hours as compared with 11.9±5.9 hours for the mean half-life of total VPA. The relatively short plasma half-life of free VPA argues for the use of sustained-release formulations.

Development

Physiologic changes occurring during childhood development are known to affect the disposition of many

TABLE 84.2. PHARMACOKINETIC PARAMETERS FOR VALPROIC ACID IN PEDIATRIC PATIENTS

Populations	Study	Antiepileptic Drug Therapy	Valproic Acid Regimen[a]	$V_d{}^a$ (L/Kg)	$T_{\frac{1}{2}\beta}$ (hr)	Free Fraction[b] (%)	Clearance (mL/hr/kg)[a] Total	Clearance (mL/hr/kg)[a] Free
Neonates (0–2 mo)	Brachet-Lierman and Demarquez (161)	Monotherapy n = 5	Single dose: 100 mg/kg p.o.	0.43	40 ± 21[b]	—	18.0	—
	Irvine-Meek et al. (163)	Polytherapy[e] n = 1	Single dose: 7.5 mg/kg p.o.	0.28	17.2	—	10.8	—
	Gal et al. (162)	Polytherapy[e] n = 5	Steady state: 20–25 mg/kg p.o.	0.39 ± 0.04	26.4 ± 16.1	13.1 ± 1.9[c]	14.4 ± 9.3	109 ± 96
Infants (2–36 mo)	Herngren et al. (33) 11 ± 4 mo	Monotherapy[e] n = 7	Steady state: 21–54 mg/kg p.o.	0.32	12.5 ± 2.8	14.6 ± 2.5[c]	17.8 ± 5.6	128 ± 38
	Hall et al. (164) 16 ± 6 mo	Monotherapy n = 5	Steady state: 10–100 mg/kg p.o.	0.22 ± 0.05	8.4 ± 2.1	—	19.6 ± 8.2	—
		Polytherapy[e] n = 9	Steady state: 10–100 mg/kg p.o.	0.28 ± 0.07	5.9 ± 2.1	—	35.6 ± 10.5	—
Children (3–18 yr)	Cloyd et al. (32) 6.9 ± 2.7 yr	Monotherapy n = 21	Steady state: 28 ± 10 mg/kg p.o.	0.22 ± 0.05	11.6 ± 3.9	12.2 ± 2.1[c]	14.0 ± 4.7	119 ± 44
	Farrell et al. (49) 8.2 ± 3.5 yr	Monotherapy n = 4	Steady state: 35 ± 12 mg/kg p.o.	—	—	12.0 ± 2.0[d]	17.5 ± 5.4	130 ± 40
	Hall et al. (164) 9 ± 3 yr	Monotherapy n = 8	Steady state: 13 ± 6 mg/kg p.o.	0.18 ± 0.04	8.6 ± 1.4	—	14.3 ± 4.3	—
	Chiba et al. (209) 9.4 ± 2.9 yr	Monotherapy n = 21	Steady state: 28 ± 7 mg/kg p.o.	0.22 ± 0.05	12.3 ± 3.1	—	13.0 ± 4.7	—
	Steinborn and Galas-Zgorzalewicz 9 ± 3 yr	Monotherapy n = 18	Single dose: 13 ± 4 mg/kg p.o.	0.16 ± 0.06	9.6 ± 2.2	—	13.9 ± 4.4	—
	Herngren and Nergårdh (34) 17 ± 4 yr	Monotherapy n = 7	Steady state: 19 ± 6 mg/kg p.o.	0.15 ± 0.10	11.9 ± 5.9	7.3 ± 3.8	9.2 ± 4.8	125 ± 69
	Schobben et al. (210) 6.8 ± 3.4 yr	Polytherapy[e] n = 6	Steady state: 12 ± 4 mg/kg p.o.	0.25 ± 0.10	9.4 ± 1.4	—	19.1 ± 9.8	—
	Cloyd et al. (32) 7.0 ± 3.2 yr	Polytherapy[e] n = 27	Steady state: 47 ± 26 mg/kg p.o.	0.26 ± 0.10	7.0 ± 2.5	12.5 ± 2.3[c]	27.7 ± 14.9	219 ± 84
	Hall et al. (164) 9 ± 3 yr	Polytherapy[e] n = 23	Steady state: 13 ± 6 mg/kg p.o.	0.20 ± 0.05	7.4 ± 2.4	—	20.6 ± 7.8	—
	Chiba et al. (209) 10.7 ± 3.1 yr	Polytherapy[e] n = 16	Steady state: 27 ± 9 mg/kg p.o.	0.30 ± 0.10	9.4 ± 2.9	—	23.5 ± 6.6	—
	Otten et al. (145) 14.8 ± 5.8 yr	Polytherapy[e] n = 4	Steady state: 12 ± 4 mg/kg p.o.	0.18 ± 0.04	7.2 ± 2.0	9.9 ± 4.8[c]	18.5 ± 4.9	228 ± 151

VD, volume of distribution; $T_{1/2}\beta$, half-life; p.o., oral.
[a] The indicated steady-state dosages are per day.
[b] Data are presented as mean ± standard deviation.
[c] Time-averaged free fraction calculated from ratio of free arm under the curve (AUC) to total AUC.
[d] Plasma free fraction at a total plasma level of 70–85 μg/mL.
[e] Polytherapy generally refers to enzyme-inducing comedication.

antiepileptic drugs (159,160). A compilation from available literature of data on VPA pharmacokinetics in pediatric patients (Table 84.2) revealed marked changes in drug clearance throughout the early stages of development.

VPA is not used routinely in the treatment of neonatal seizures; therefore, pharmacokinetic data on newborns are scanty. Most of the literature reports were anecdotal observations in infants exposed to VPA *in utero,* which provide information on elimination half-life but do not afford clearance estimates. Pronounced changes in VPA half-life were observed during the postnatal period (Table 84.2). Within the first 10 days after birth, half-lives ranging between 10 and 67 hours were observed (161). Longer half-lives appeared to be associated with low birth weight (<1,000 g) and prematurity. Clearance data from a study of six neonates with intractable seizures were reported by Gal et al. (162). VPA was added to an existing regimen of anticonvulsants (mainly phenobarbital), and clearance kinetics were studied at steady state. Although highly variable, the steady-state clearance per kilogram of body weight for total drug in serum appeared to be within the range of values reported for adult epileptic patients receiving multiple anticonvulsants. The estimates were also consistent with results from two earlier case studies (161,163). The free fractions of VPA in neonatal serum are significantly higher than those reported for adult serum at comparable drug levels (an area average free fraction of $14.4\pm9.3\%$ in the neonates versus $\leq10\%$ in adults). Consequently, clearance for unbound VPA was in the low range of expected values for adult epileptic patients, a finding suggesting that the intrinsic metabolic clearance of VPA may be low because of immature drug-metabolizing enzyme activities.

A remarkable increase in plasma clearance, a decrease in extravascular distribution volume, and a corresponding shortening in half-life of VPA occur from 10 days to 2 months of infancy. The increase in clearance presumably reflects maturation in drug-metabolizing function.

Data from the studies by Hall et al. (164) showed that in older infants between the ages of 3 to 36 months, clearance values exceeding 30 mL/min/kg are often observed in patients receiving enzyme-inducing comedication. In such patients, daily doses much higher than the usually recommended range of 15 to 30 mg/kg/day would be required to achieve plasma VPA levels >50 μg/mL. During this middle to late period of infancy, mean elimination half-lives of 8 to 12 hours and 6 hours have been reported for patients receiving monotherapy and for patients receiving enzyme-inducing comedication, respectively (Table 84.2).

Studies detailing age-related changes in VPA glucuronidation and β-oxidation, which appear to represent the primary pathways for VPA elimination in all species, have been described in postnatal lambs (165,166). Similar to human newborns and children <2 years of age, plasma concentrations of β-oxidation metabolites, 2-ene-VPA and 3-keto-VPA, and the P450-mediated hydroxylation

metabolite, 4-OH-VPA were approximately five- to 10-fold higher in newborn lambs (1 day, 10 day, and 1 month of age) compared with the ewe, whereas glucuronide formation was considerably reduced (approximately threefold) (165,166). Urinary excretion of the major urinary metabolite, VPA glucuronide, accounted for ~28% of the dose in 1- and 10-day-old lambs but increased to adult levels (~75% of the dose) by 2 months of age. In agreement with very limited data available in infants and children, these studies suggest that β-oxidation activity is substantially developed early in life, whereas glucuronidation activity increases significantly with increasing age.

Ample data are available on VPA clearance in school-age children (3 to 16 years). Overall, the mean clearance estimates from numerous studies (Table 84.2) are in the range of 13 to 18 and 19 to 28 mL/hr/kg for patients receiving monotherapy and for patients taking enzyme-inducing comedication, respectively. These estimates are intermediate between those reported for the infants and young adults. It appears that VPA clearance normalized to per kilogram of body weight begins to decline after infancy and continues on throughout childhood, reaching adult values by adolescence. This pattern of continual decline in clearance relative to body weight over the first decade or so of childhood has been verified in more recent large-scale plasma VPA monitoring studies coupled with sophisticated population pharmacokinetic modeling (150,151,167,168). The pattern of development in the metabolic clearance of VPA is similar to the general trend observed with other antiepileptic drugs that are subject to oxidative metabolism, such as phenytoin and phenobarbital (159,160), and it can be attributed to prepubertal changes in cytochrome P450–mediated drug metabolism in the liver.

The elimination half-life of VPA begins to assume adult values during the early years of childhood. The average half-lives for school-age children and young adolescents are within the range of adult values (Table 84.2).

Aging

The pharmacokinetics of VPA in elderly subjects has been studied by several groups of investigators (Table 84.1). Both Perucca et al. (43) and Bauer et al. (37) reported that the clearance of total VPA in serum did not appear to differ between young and elderly volunteers. However, a decrease in serum protein binding of VPA associated with hypoalbuminemia was observed in the elderly group. Consequently, the mean clearance of free VPA was 40% lower in the elderly than in the young control subjects. This decrease in free drug clearance is consistent with the generally recognized age-related decline in hepatic function, notably with respect to oxidative drug metabolism (169). The results of these studies suggest that monitoring free, rather than total, serum VPA concentration may be more meaningful in elderly patients.

Pregnancy

Alterations in VPA clearance may be observed during pregnancy and after parturition. Plasse et al. (170) reported the level:dose ratio of VPA in one pregnant mother. The level:dose ratio began to decline in the latter part of the second trimester and continued through the early part of the third trimester; it finally reached nadir within 3 weeks of delivery. After parturition, VPA levels rose rapidly and regained prepregnancy values within 2 to 3 weeks. In a review article, Philbert and Dam (171) cited similar experience in five pregnant patients. Other studies confirmed that a gradual and marked decrease in total plasma VPA concentration occurs during pregnancy, followed by a rapid rise after delivery; however, the concentration of free VPA in plasma was found not to be markedly altered during pregnancy compared with preconception levels, and therefore a need for dosage adjustments would not be anticipated (171a). Overall, these data suggest that the apparent increase in total VPA clearance during late gestation is largely caused by the previously recognized decrease in maternal serum protein binding of VPA, as a result of elevated nonesterified fatty acids and hypoalbuminemia (41). Although the question remains whether there is an actual change in the intrinsic metabolic clearance of VPA during pregnancy, monitoring of free, rather than total, serum VPA concentration may be more meaningful throughout the entire period of pregnancy and postpartum.

Disease States

Orr et al. (46) reported the disposition kinetics of VPA in a 9-year-old uremic epileptic child. Total serum clearance was 23.6 mL/hr/kg after the first dose and increased to 40.8 mL/hr/kg after 5 months of therapy. The observed steady-state clearance was higher than reported estimates in polytherapy patients of comparable age (19 to 28 mL/hr/kg). Serum free fractions were higher than normal, at 22.4% and 27.2%, respectively, for the single-dose and steady-state studies. The corresponding free serum clearances of VPA were calculated to be 149 and 152 mL/hr/kg, in line with estimates for children with normal renal function. Thus, the primary effect of uremia is a decrease in serum protein binding resulting in an apparent increase in total drug clearance. Because free drug clearance and, therefore, the average free drug concentration at steady state is not altered, adjustment in VPA dosage may not be necessary in uremic patients. The elimination half-life of VPA after 5 months of treatment was 10.2 hours, a finding that agrees with expected values for epileptic children of this age. The rise in serum free fraction induced by uremia had no apparent effect on half-life, because there was a comparable increase in both clearance and apparent volume of distribution.

Only a limited fraction of the VPA dose (<20%) is removed by either hemodialysis (172) or peritoneal dialysis (46), probably because of the significant degree of binding of VPA to plasma protein. Therefore, there is no need to supplement the VPA dose in uremic patients who receive maintenance dialysis treatment. Hemodialysis for detoxification in VPA overdose, however, should be considered, because the plasma free fraction is elevated (>30%) at toxic concentrations (173).

VPA pharmacokinetics has been examined in patients with alcoholic liver cirrhosis and in patients recovering from acute hepatitis (44). VPA free fraction in serum was increased by more than twofold in patients with liver disease. However, the clearance of total VPA in serum was not significantly different from that in healthy volunteers because intrinsic clearance (reflecting drug-metabolizing activity) of VPA was also reduced, presumably as a consequence of hepatocellular damage. Thus, hepatic disease causes two opposing effects resulting in no apparent change in total clearance. Accordingly, AUC of plasma total VPA at steady state would not change, whereas that of plasma free VPA would increase in such a situation. The increase in unbound concentrations of VPA may warrant a downward adjustment in daily dose. The mean half-life in seven patients with alcoholic cirrhosis was 18.9±5.1 hours, and in patients recovering from acute hepatitis it was 17.0±3.7 hours. The prolongation in half-life reflects the decrease in intrinsic metabolic clearance of VPA in hepatic diseases.

Metabolic clearance of some drugs is known to increase in critically ill patients suffering from acute head injury (174,175). Anderson et al. (176) reported pharmacokinetic data on intravenously administered VPA in 35 patients with head trauma as part of a clinical trial to evaluate the efficacy of VPA in preventing posttraumatic seizures. The clearance of total VPA in plasma showed a steady increase over the next 2 weeks of treatment. By 1 month, the VPA clearance had returned to baseline level. Part of the apparent increase in plasma clearance was attributed to hypoalbuminemia in response to trauma. In addition, clearance of unbound VPA also showed a significant rise. The mechanism underlying the apparent induction in VPA metabolism is not known.

RELATIONSHIP BETWEEN SERUM CONCENTRATION AND DOSE

In patients receiving VPA monotherapy, doses between 10 and 20 mg/kg/day will usually achieve a good clinical response and will result in concentrations within the therapeutic range (50 to 100 μg/mL) (177–180). The dose may be increased as necessary and as tolerated by 5 to 10 mg/kg/day at weekly intervals. Because of age-dependent kinetics, younger children may require a higher dose (181,182). However the level–dose relationship is highly variable among patients.

During long-term drug administration, a nonlinear relationship between plasma VPA levels and dose has been observed in numerous studies, as mentioned earlier in the section on clearance and half-life. Above a daily dose of 500 mg, the steady-state plasma concentration of VPA increased less than proportionately with an increase in dose. The non-linearity in clearance was attributed principally to an increase in the unbound fraction as plasma VPA concentration increased (152). However, dose proportionality was observed for doses >500 mg/day in other studies; Davis et al. (183) reported that peak plasma concentrations after oral administration of VPA (capsule, uncoated tablet, liquid formulation) increased dose proportionally, ranging from 24.5 µg/mL after a 250-mg dose to 108.5 µg/mL after a 1,000-mg dose. In another study, Wangemann et al. (184), investigated the proportionality of low doses, 100 to 300 mg, and the pharmacokinetics of sustained-release sodium VPA in healthy persons. Parameters determining the extent and rate of absorption, AUC, and maximum concentration increased proportionally with the dose.

Loading and maintenance intravenous doses necessary to achieve and maintain therapeutic serum VPA concentrations were determined by Hovinga et al. in a study in children (185). A 20 mg/kg loading dose and maintenance infusions of 4 and 6 mg/kg/hr produced steady-state total concentrations of 66 and 92.4 mg/L, respectively. In neonates, Alfonso et al. reported that each 1 mg/kg loading dose of intravenous VPA increased the 45-minute and 3-hour postinfusion serum VPA concentrations by approximately 4 and 3 µg/mL, respectively (186).

RELATIONSHIP BETWEEN SERUM CONCENTRATION AND EFFECT

Interpretation of VPA levels obtained in patients is difficult given that VPA levels fluctuate considerably during the 24-hour period because of a short half-life. No clear correlation between VPA levels and clinical effects at any given time has been demonstrated so far.

Epilepsy

In epilepsy, several studies found clinical response, in term of seizure control or reduction in electroencephalographic seizure discharge, at VPA concentrations ranging from 43 to 109.5 µg/mL (146,179,181,187–191). In children, complete seizure control was obtained at lower VPA levels, between 20.2 and 50.5 µg/mL (192). The therapeutic range in epilepsy is considered to be between 50 and 100 µg/mL of total VPA. High concentration (80 to 150 µg/mL) may be needed in patients with epilepsy that is difficult to control (193).

Although no relationship could be established between the incidence of side effects and plasma VPA levels, patients with side effects had usually received significantly higher doses and exhibited higher serum VPA concentrations (194, 195). Lethargy and drowsiness were observed at mean levels of 80.4 and 94.5 µg/mL (195).

Other Indications

VPA is also currently used for treatment of psychiatric disorders, including acute mania, bipolar disorders, and schizophrenic disorders. A marked antimanic response may require plasma levels to be >50 µg/mL (196). However, Grunze et al. reported a drastic remission of mania in depressed patients with bipolar I disorder with VPA levels at or only slightly >50 µg/mL, when blood was drawn 12 hours after VPA intravenous infusion (66). In other psychiatric disorders, the therapeutic range is unknown, although 60 to 90 mg/L was cited on the basis of retrospective studies in patients with mania (197). In uncontrolled studies of VPA in bipolar and schizophrenic disorders, significant response occurred within 1 to 2 weeks of achieving serum VPA concentrations >50 mg/L (198).

VPA has also been used in the prophylaxis of migraine headaches. Lenaerts et al. assessed the prophylactic effect of VPA (mean daily dose, 928.5 mg) over 6 months in 56 patients with migraine or tension type-headaches. In the migraine group, 60% of the patients had a 75% to 100% improvement. This clinical improvement correlated with VPA levels, and the authors suggested aiming for VPA plasma levels between 70 and 90 µg/mL (199). Another clinical trial studied VPA in migraine prophylaxis and found no correlation between VPA levels and the therapeutic response (200). Erdemoglu et al. showed that a mean average daily dose of 1,250 mg VPA produced improvement in headache frequency in 67% of patients, with plasma levels ranging from 27 to 128 µg/mL (average, 74 µg/mL). In that study, no clear correlation between VPA levels and either treatment efficacy or side effects was found (201).

REFERENCES

1. Keane PE, Simiand J, Morre M. Comparison of the pharmacological and biochemical profiles of valproic acid (VPA) and its cerebral metabolite (2-en-VPA) after oral administration in mice. *Methods Find Exp Clin Pharmacol* 1985;7:83–86.
2. Palaty J, Abbott FS. Structure-activity relationships of unsaturated analogues of valproic acid. *J Med Chem* 1995;38:3398–3406.
3. Chang ZL. Sodium valproate and valproic acid. In: Florey K, ed. *Analytical profiles of drug substances.* New York: Academic Press, 1979:529–556.
4. Baillie TA, Sheffels PR. Valproic acid: chemistry and biotransformation. In: Levy RH, Mattson RH, Meldrum BS, eds. *Antiepileptic drugs,* 4th ed. New York: Raven Press, 1995:589–604.
5. Abbott FS, Anari MR. Chemistry and biotransformation. In: Löscher W, ed. *Milestones in drug therapy: valproate.* Basel: Birkhauser, 1999:47–75.
6. Robbins DK, Wedlund PJ, Elsberg S, et al. Interaction of valproic acid and some analogues with microsomal epoxide hydrolase. *Biochem Pharmacol* 1992;43:775–783.

7. Anderson P, Elwin CE. Single-dose kinetics and bioavailability of sodium-hydrogen divalproate. *Clin Neuropharmacol* 1985;8: 156–164.

8. Glazko AJ, Chang T, Daftsios AC, et al. Bioavailability of calcium valproate in normal men compared with the free acid and sodium salt. *Ther Drug Monit* 1983;5:409–417.

9. Roberts D, Easter D, O'Bryan-Tear G. Epilim chrono: a multi-dose, crossover comparison of two formulations of valproate in healthy volunteers. *Biopharm Drug Dispos* 1996;17:175–182.

10. Carrigan PJ, Brinker DR, Cavanaugh JH, et al. Absorption characteristics of a new valproate formulation: divalproex sodium-coated particles in capsules (Depakote Sprinkle). *J Clin Pharmacol* 1990;30:743–747.

11. Franke G, Diletti E, Hoffmann C, et al. Relative bioavailability of different valproic acid formulations. *Int Clin Pharmacol Ther* 1995;33:653–657.

12. Bialer M, Rubinstein A, Raz I, et al. Pharmacokinetics of valpromide after oral administration of a solution and a tablet to healthy volunteers. *Eur J Clin Pharmacol* 1984;27:501–503.

13. Albani F, Riva R, Contin M, et al. Valproic acid binding to human serum albumin and human plasma: effects of pH variation and buffer composition in equilibrium dialysis. *Ther Drug Monit* 1984;6:31–33.

14. Gugler R, Schell A, Eichelbaum M, et al. Disposition of valproic acid in man. *Eur J Clin Pharmacol* 1977;12:125–132.

15. Klotz U, Antonin KH. Pharmacokinetics and bioavailability of sodium valproate. *Clin Pharmacol Ther* 1977;21:736–743.

16. Levy RH, Cenraud B, Loiseau P, et al. Meal-dependent absorption of enteric-coated sodium valproate. *Epilepsia* 1980;21: 273–280.

17. Hamilton RA, Garnett WR, Kline BJ, et al. Effects of food on valproic acid absorption. *Am J Hosp Pharm* 1981;38: 1490–1493.

18. Retzow A, Vens-Cappell B, Wangemann M. Influence of food on the pharmacokinetics of a new multiple unit sustained release sodium valproate formulation. *Arzneimittelforschung* 1997;47:1347–1350.

19. Fischer JH, Barr AN, Paloucek FP, et al. Effect of food on the serum concentration profile of enteric-coated valproic acid. *Neurology* 1988;38:1319–1322.

20. Cloyd JC, Kriel RL. Bioavailability of rectally administered valproic acid syrup. *Neurology* 1981;31:1348–1352.

21. Holmes GB, Rosenfeld WE, Graves NM, et al. Absorption of valproic acid suppositories in human volunteers. *Arch Neurol* 1989;46:906–909.

22. Issakainen J, Bourgeois BF. Bioavailability of sodium valproate suppositories during repeated administration at steady state in epileptic children. *Eur J Pediatr* 1987;146:404–407.

23. Johannessen SI, Henriksen O, Munthe-Kaas AW, et al. Serum concentration profile studies of tablets and suppositories of valproate and carbamazepine in healthy subjects and patients with epilepsy. In: Levy RH, Pitlick WH, Eichelbaum M, et al., eds. *Metabolism of antiepileptic drugs.* New York: Raven Press, 1984: 61–71.

24. Moolenaar F, Greving WJ, Huizinga T. Absorption rate and bioavailability of valproic acid and its sodium from rectal dosage forms. *Eur J Clin Pharmacol* 1980;17:309–315.

25. Scanabissi E, Dal Pozzo D, Franzoni E, et al. Rectal administration of sodium valproate in children. *Ital J Neurol Sci* 1984;5:189–193.

26. Snead OCd, Miles MV. Treatment of status epilepticus in children with rectal sodium valproate. *J Pediatr* 1985;106:323–325.

27. Kober A, Olsson Y, Sjoholm I. Binding of drugs to human serum albumin. XIV. The theoretical basis for the interaction between phenytoin and valproate. *Mol Pharmacol* 1980;18: 237–242.

28. Levy RH, Lai AA. Valproate: absorption, distribution, and excretion. In: Woodbury DM, Penry JK, Pippenger C, eds. *Antiepileptic drugs.* New York: Raven Press, 1982:555–565.

29. Scheyer RD, Cramer JA, Toftness BR, et al. *In vivo* determination of valproate binding constants during sole and multi-drug therapy. *Ther Drug Monit* 1990;12:117–123.

30. Yu HY. Clinical implications of serum protein binding in epileptic children during sodium valproate maintenance therapy. *Ther Drug Monit* 1984;6:414–423.

31. Cramer JA, Mattson RH, Bennett DM, et al. Variable free and total valproic acid concentrations in sole- and multi-drug therapy. *Ther Drug Monit* 1986;8:411–415.

32. Cloyd JC, Fischer JH, Kriel RL, et al. Valproic acid pharmacokinetics in children. IV. Effects of age and antiepileptic drugs on protein binding and intrinsic clearance. *Clin Pharmacol Ther* 1993;53:22–29.

33. Herngren L, Lundberg B, Nergardh A. Pharmacokinetics of total and free valproic acid during monotherapy in infants. *J Neurol* 1991;238:315–319.

34. Herngren L, Nergardh A. Pharmacokinetics of free and total sodium valproate in adolescents and young adults during maintenance therapy. *J Neurol* 1988;235:491–495.

35. Riva R, Albani F, Franzoni E, et al. Valproic acid free fraction in epileptic children under chronic monotherapy. *Ther Drug Monit* 1983;5:197–200.

36. Bauer LA, Davis R, Wilensky A, et al. Diurnal variation in valproic acid clearance. *Clin Pharmacol Ther* 1984;35:505–509.

37. Bauer LA, Davis R, Wilensky A, et al. Valproic acid clearance: unbound fraction and diurnal variation in young and elderly adults. *Clin Pharmacol Ther* 1985;37:697–700.

38. Marty JJ, Kilpatrick CJ, Moulds RF. Intra-dose variation in plasma protein binding of sodium valproate in epileptic patients. *Br J Clin Pharmacol* 1982;14:399–404.

39. Riva R, Albani F, Cortelli P, et al. Diurnal fluctuations in free and total plasma concentrations of valproic acid at steady state in epileptic patients. *Ther Drug Monit* 1983;5:191–196.

40. Roman EJ, Ponniah P, Lambert JB, et al. Free sodium valproate monitoring. *Br J Clin Pharmacol* 1982;13:452–455.

41. Nau H, Krauer B. Serum protein binding of valproic acid in fetus-mother pairs throughout pregnancy: correlation with oxytocin administration and albumin and free fatty acid concentrations. *J Clin Pharmacol* 1986;26:215–221.

42. Perucca E. Free level monitoring of antiepileptic drugs: clinical usefulness and case studies. *Clin Pharmacokinet* 1984;9[Suppl 1]:71–78.

43. Perucca E, Grimaldi R, Gatti G, et al. Pharmacokinetics of valproic acid in the elderly. *Br J Clin Pharmacol* 1984;17:665–669.

44. Klotz U, Rapp T, Muller WA. Disposition of valproic acid in patients with liver disease. *Eur J Clin Pharmacol* 1978;13: 55–60.

45. Dasgupta A, Jacques M. Reduced *in vitro* displacement of valproic acid from protein binding by salicylate in uremic sera compared with normal sera: role of uremic compounds. *Am J Clin Pathol* 1994;101:349–353.

46. Orr JM, Farrell K, Abbott FS, et al. The effects of peritoneal dialysis on the single dose and steady state pharmacokinetics of valproic acid in a uremic epileptic child. *Eur J Clin Pharmacol* 1983;24:387–390.

47. Dasgupta A, McLemore JL. Elevated free phenytoin and free valproic acid concentrations in sera of patients infected with human immunodeficiency virus. *Ther Drug Monit* 1998;20: 63–67.

48. Anderson GD, Gidal BE, Hendryx RJ, et al. Decreased plasma protein binding of valproate in patients with acute head trauma. *Br J Clin Pharmacol* 1994;37:559–562.

49. Farrell K, Orr JM, Abbott FS, et al. The effect of acetylsalicylic

acid on serum free valproate concentrations and valproate clearance in children. *J Pediatr* 1982;101:142–144.

50. Grimaldi R, Lecchini S, Crema F, et al. *In vivo* plasma protein binding interaction between valproic acid and naproxen. *Eur J Drug Metab Pharmacokinet* 1984;9:359–363.

51. Patel IH, Venkataramanan R, Levy RH, et al. Diurnal oscillations in plasma protein binding of valproic acid. *Epilepsia* 1982;23:283–290.

52. Bowdle TA, Patel IH, Levy RH, et al. The influence of free fatty acids on valproic acid plasma protein binding during fasting in normal humans. *Eur J Clin Pharmacol* 1982;23:343–347.

53. Gatti G, Crema F, Attardo-Parrinello G, et al. Serum protein binding of phenytoin and valproic acid in insulin-dependent diabetes mellitus. *Ther Drug Monit* 1987;9:389–391.

54. Barre J, Didey F, Delion F, et al. Problems in therapeutic drug monitoring: free drug level monitoring. *Ther Drug Monit* 1988;10:133–143.

55. Levy RH, Schmidt D. Utility of free level monitoring of antiepileptic drugs. *Epilepsia* 1985;26:199–205.

56. Pugh CB, Garnett WR. Current issues in the treatment of epilepsy. *Clin Pharm* 1991;10:335–358.

57. Lenn NJ, Robertson M. Clinical utility of unbound antiepileptic drug blood levels in the management of epilepsy. *Neurology* 1992;42:988–990.

58. Gidal BE, Collins DM, Beinlich BR. Apparent valproic acid neurotoxicity in a hypoalbuminemic patient. *Ann Pharmacother* 1993;27:32–35.

59. Haroldson JA, Kramer LE, Wolff DL, et al. Elevated free fractions of valproic acid in a heart transplant patient with hypoalbuminemia. *Ann Pharmacother* 2000;34:183–187.

60. Battino D, Croci D, Granata T, et al. Changes in unbound and total valproic acid concentrations after replacement of carbamazepine with oxcarbazepine. *Ther Drug Monit* 1992;14:376–379.

61. Hariton C, Ciesielski L, Simler S, et al. Distribution of sodium valproate and GABA metabolism in CNS of the rat. *Biopharm Drug Dispos* 1984;5:409–414.

62. Löscher W, Esenwein H. Pharmacokinetics of sodium valproate in dog and mouse. *Arzneimittelforschung* 1978;28:782–787.

63. Levy RH. CSF and plasma pharmacokinetics: relationship to mechanisms of action as exemplified by valproic acid in monkey. In: Lockard JS, Ward AA, eds. *Epilepsy: a window to brain mechanism.* New York: Raven Press, 1980:191–200.

64. Vajda FJ, Mihaly GW, Miles JL, et al. Rectal administration of sodium valproate in status epilepticus. *Neurology* 1978;28:897–899.

65. Rosenfeld WE, Leppik IE, Gates JR, et al. Valproic acid loading during intensive monitoring. *Arch Neurol* 1987;44:709–710.

66. Grunze H, Erfurth A, Amann B, et al. Intravenous valproate loading in acutely manic and depressed bipolar I patients. *J Clin Psychopharmacol* 1999;19:303–309.

67. Mathew NT, Kailasam J, Meadors L, et al. Intravenous valproate sodium (Depacon) aborts migraine rapidly: a preliminary report. *Headache* 2000;40:720–723.

68. Uberall MA, Trollmann R, Wunsiedler U, et al. Intravenous valproate in pediatric epilepsy patients with refractory status epilepticus. *Neurology* 2000;54:2188–2189.

69. Levy RH, Shen DD. Valproate: absorption, distribution, excretion. In: Levy RH, Mattson R, Meldrum BS, et al., eds. *Antiepileptic drugs,* 3rd ed. New York: Raven Press, 1989:583–599.

70. Shen DD, Ojemann GA, Rapport RL, et al. Low and variable presence of valproic acid in human brain. *Neurology* 1992;42:582–585.

71. Vajda FJ, Donnan GA, Phillips J, et al. Human brain, plasma, and cerebrospinal fluid concentration of sodium valproate after 72 hours of therapy. *Neurology* 1981;31:486–487.

72. Wieser HG. Comparison of valproate concentrations in human plasma, CSF and brain tissue after administration of different formulations of valproate or valpromide. *Epilepsy Res* 1991;9:154–159.

73. Cornford EM, Diep CP, Pardridge WM. Blood–brain barrier transport of valproic acid. *J Neurochem* 1985;44:1541–1550.

74. Abbott FS, Acheampong AA. Quantitative structure-anticonvulsant activity relationships of valproic acid, related carboxylic acids and tetrazoles. *Neuropharmacology* 1988;27:287–294.

75. Löscher W, Nau H. Pharmacological evaluation of various metabolites and analogues of valproic acid: anticonvulsant and toxic potencies in mice. *Neuropharmacology* 1985;24:427–435.

76. Adkison KD, Ojemann GA, Rapport RL, et al. Distribution of unsaturated metabolites of valproate in human and rat brain: pharmacologic relevance? *Epilepsia* 1995;36:772–782.

77. Löscher W, Nau H, Siemes H. Penetration of valproate and its active metabolites into cerebrospinal fluid of children with epilepsy. *Epilepsia* 1988;29:311–316.

78. Löscher W, Fisher JE, Nau H, et al. Valproic acid in amygdala-kindled rats: alterations in anticonvulsant efficacy, adverse effects and drug and metabolite levels in various brain regions during chronic treatment. *J Pharmacol Exp Ther* 1989;250:1067–1078.

79. Nau H. Valproic acid-induced neural tube defects. *Ciba Found Symp* 1994;181:144–152.

80. Gordon JD, Riggs KW, Rurak DW, et al. The pharmacokinetics of valproic acid in pregnant sheep after maternal and fetal intravenous bolus administration. *Drug Metab Dispos* 1995;23:1383–1389.

81. Kumar S, Wong H, Yeung SA, et al. Disposition of valproic acid in maternal, fetal, and newborn sheep. I. Placental transfer, plasma protein binding, and clearance. *Drug Metab Dispos* 2000;28:845–856.

82. Utoguchi N, Audus KL. Carrier-mediated transport of valproic acid in BeWo cells, a human trophoblast cell line. *Int J Pharm* 2000;195:115–124.

83. Nau H, Scott WJ. Teratogenicity of valproic acid and related substances in the mouse: drug accumulation and pHi in the embryo during organogenesis and structure-activity considerations. *Arch Toxicol Suppl* 1987;11:128–139.

84. Dencker L, Nau H, D'Argy R. Marked accumulation of valproic acid in embryonic neuroepithelium of the mouse during early organogenesis. *Teratology* 1990;41:699–706.

85. Omtzigt JG, Nau H, Los FJ, et al. The disposition of valproate and its metabolites in the late first trimester and early second trimester of pregnancy in maternal serum, urine, and amniotic fluid: effect of dose, co-medication, and the presence of spina bifida. *Eur J Clin Pharmacol* 1992;43:381–388.

86. Froescher W, Gugler R, Niesen M, et al. Protein binding of valproic acid in maternal and umbilical cord serum. *Epilepsia* 1984;25:244–249.

87. Nau H, Rating D, Koch S, et al. Valproic acid and its metabolites: placental transfer, neonatal pharmacokinetics, transfer via mother's milk and clinical status in neonates of epileptic mothers. *J Pharmacol Exp Ther* 1981;219:768–777.

88. Nau H, Helge H, Luck W. Valproic acid in the perinatal period: decreased maternal serum protein binding results in fetal accumulation and neonatal displacement of the drug and some metabolites. *J Pediatr* 1984;104:627–634.

89. Philbert A, Pedersen B, Dam M. Concentration of valproate during pregnancy, in the newborn and in breast milk. *Acta Neurol Scand* 1985;72:460–463.

90. Albani F, Riva R, Contin M, et al. Differential transplacental binding of valproic acid: influence of free fatty acids. *Br J Clin Pharmacol* 1984;17:759–762.

91. Riva R, Albani F, Contin M, et al. Mechanism of altered drug binding to serum proteins in pregnant women: studies with valproic acid. *Ther Drug Monit* 1984;6:25–30.

92. Hagg S, Spigset O. Anticonvulsant use during lactation. *Drug Saf* 2000;22:425–440.

93. Chaudron LH, Jefferson JW. Mood stabilizers during breast-feeding: a review. *J Clin Psychiatry* 2000;61:79–90.

94. Stahl MM, Neiderud J, Vinge E. Thrombocytopenic purpura and anemia in a breast-fed infant whose mother was treated with valproic acid. *J Pediatr* 1997;130:1001–1003.

95. Kassahun K, Farrell K, Zheng JJ, et al. Metabolic profiling of valproic acid in patients using negative-ion chemical ionization gas chromatography-mass spectrometry. *J Chromatogr* 1990; 527:327–341.

96. Siemes H, Nau H, Schultze K, et al. Valproate (VPA) metabolites in various clinical conditions of probable VPA-associated hepatotoxicity. *Epilepsia* 1993;34:332–346.

97. Sugimoto T, Muro H, Woo M, et al. Metabolite profiles in patients on high-dose valproate monotherapy. *Epilepsy Res* 1996;25:107–112.

98. Guan X, Fisher MB, Lang DH, et al. Cytochrome P450-dependent desaturation of lauric acid: isoform selectivity and mechanism of formation of 11-dodecenoic acid. *Chem Biol Interact* 1998;110:103–121.

99. Li J, Norwood DL, Mao LF, et al. Mitochondrial metabolism of valproic acid. *Biochemistry* 1991;30:388–394.

100. Prickett KS, Baillie TA. Metabolism of valproic acid by hepatic microsomal cytochrome P-450. *Biochem Biophys Res Commun* 1984;122:1166–1173.

101. Rettie AE, Rettenmeier AW, Beyer BK, et al. Valproate hydroxylation by human fetal tissues and embryotoxicity of metabolites. *Clin Pharmacol Ther* 1986;40:172–177.

102. Fisher MB, Thompson SJ, Ribeiro V, et al. P450-catalyzed in-chain desaturation of valproic acid: isoform selectivity and mechanism of formation of Delta 3-valproic acid generated by baculovirus-expressed CYP3A1. *Arch Biochem Biophys* 1998; 356:63–70.

103. Bjorge SM, Baillie TA. Studies on the beta-oxidation of valproic acid in rat liver mitochondrial preparations. *Drug Metab Dispos* 1991;19:823–829.

104. Rettenmeier AW, Gordon WP, Barnes H, et al. Studies on the metabolic fate of valproic acid in the rat using stable isotope techniques. *Xenobiotica* 1987;17:1147–1157.

105. Kassahun K, Hu P, Grillo MP, et al. Metabolic activation of unsaturated derivatives of valproic acid. Identification of novel glutathione adducts formed through coenzyme A-dependent and -independent processes. *Chem Biol Interact* 1994;90: 253–275.

106. Tang W, Abbott FS. Bioactivation of a toxic metabolite of valproic acid, (E)-2-propyl-2,4-pentadienoic acid, via glucuronidation. LC/MS/MS characterization of the GSH-glucuronide diconjugates. *Chem Res Toxicol* 1996;9:517–526.

107. Tang W, Abbott FS. Characterization of thiol-conjugated metabolites of 2-propylpent-4-enoic acid (4-ene VPA), a toxic metabolite of valproic acid, by electrospray tandem mass spectrometry. *J Mass Spectrom* 1996;31:926–936.

108. Tang W, Borel AG, Fujimiya T, et al. Fluorinated analogues as mechanistic probes in valproic acid hepatotoxicity: hepatic microvesicular steatosis and glutathione status. *Chem Res Toxicol* 1995;8:671–682.

109. Kassahun K, Farrell K, Abbott F. Identification and characterization of the glutathione and *N*-acetylcysteine conjugates of (E)-2-propyl-2,4-pentadienoic acid, a toxic metabolite of valproic acid, in rats and humans. *Drug Metab Dispos* 1991; 19:525–535.

110. Kassahun K, Baillie TA. Cytochrome P-450-mediated dehydro-genation of 2-*n*-propyl-2(E)-pentenoic acid, a pharmacologically-active metabolite of valproic acid, in rat liver microsomal preparations. *Drug Metab Dispos* 1993;21:242–248.

111. Kassahun K, Abbott F. *In vivo* formation of the thiol conjugates of reactive metabolites of 4-ene VPA and its analog 4-pentenoic acid. *Drug Metab Dispos* 1993;21:1098–1106.

112. Rettie AE, Rettenmeier AW, Howald WN, et al. Cytochrome P-450—catalyzed formation of delta 4-VPA, a toxic metabolite of valproic acid. *Science* 1987;235:890–893.

113. Rettie AE, Boberg M, Rettenmeier AW, et al. Cytochrome P-450–catalyzed desaturation of valproic acid *in vitro:* species differences, induction effects, and mechanistic studies. *J Biol Chem* 1988;263:13733–13738.

114. Porubek DJ, Barnes H, Meier GP, et al. Enantiotopic differentiation during the biotransformation of valproic acid to the hepatotoxic olefin 2-*n*-propyl-4-pentenoic acid. *Chem Res Toxicol* 1989;2:35–40.

115. Rettie AE, Sheffels PR, Korzekwa KR, et al. CYP4 isozyme specificity and the relationship between omega-hydroxylation and terminal desaturation of valproic acid. *Biochemistry* 1995; 34:7889–7895.

116. Sadeque AJM, Fisher MB, Korzekwa KR, et al. Human CYP2C9 and CYP2A6 mediate formation of the hepatotoxin 4-ene-valproic acid. *J Pharmacol Exp Ther* 1997;283:698–703.

117. Anari MR, Burton RW, Gopaul S, et al. Metabolic profiling of valproic acid by cDNA-expressed human cytochrome P450 enzymes using negative-ion chemical ionization gas chromatography-mass spectrometry. *J Chromatogr B Biomed Appl* 2000; 742:217–227.

118. McLaughlin DB, Andrews JA, Hooper WD, et al. Apparent autoinduction of valproate beta-oxidation in humans. *Br J Clin Pharmacol* 2000;49:409–415.

119. Ito M, Ikeda Y, Arnez JG, et al. The enzymatic basis for the metabolism and inhibitory effects of valproic acid: dehydrogenation of valproyl-CoA by 2-methyl-branched-chain acyl-CoA dehydrogenase. *Biochim Biophys Acta* 1990;1034: 213–218.

120. Granneman GR, Wang SI, Machinist JM, et al. Aspects of the metabolism of valproic acid. *Xenobiotica* 1984;14:375–387.

121. Dickinson RG, Harland RC, Lynn RK, et al. Transmission of valproic acid (Depakene) across the placenta: half-life of the drug in mother and baby. *J Pediatr* 1979;94:832–835.

122. Dickinson RG, Hooper WD, Dunstan PR, et al. Urinary excretion of valproate and some metabolites in chronically treated patients. *Ther Drug Monit* 1989;11:127–133.

123. Kuhara T, Hirohata Y, Yamada S, et al. Metabolism of sodium dipropylacetate in humans. *Eur J Drug Metab Pharmacokinet* 1978;3:171–177.

124. Yoshida H, Hirozane K, Kimoto H, et al. Valproic acid elimination rate and urinary excretion of its glucuronide conjugate in patients with epilepsy. *Biol Pharm Bull* 1999;22:716–720.

125. Taburet AM, Aymard P. Valproate glucuronidation by rat liver microsomes: interaction with parahydroxyphenobarbital. *Biochem Pharmacol* 1983;32:3859–3861.

126. Spahn-Langguth H, Benet LZ. Acyl glucuronides revisited: is the glucuronidation process a toxification as well as a detoxification mechanism? *Drug Metab Rev* 1992;24:5–47.

127. Dickinson RG, Hooper WD, Eadie MJ. pH-dependent rearrangement of the biosynthetic ester glucuronide of valproic acid to beta-glucuronidase-resistant forms. *Drug Metab Dispos* 1984;12:247–252.

128. Bailey MJ, Dickinson RG. Chemical and immunochemical comparison of protein adduct formation of four carboxylate drugs in rat liver and plasma. *Chem Res Toxicol* 1996;9:659–9 66.

129. Williams AM, Worrall S, de Jersey J, et al. Studies on the reac-

tivity of acyl glucuronides. III. Glucuronide-derived adducts of valproic acid and plasma protein and anti-adduct antibodies in humans. *Biochem Pharmacol* 1992;43:745–755.

130. Gopaul SV, Farrell K, Abbott FS. Identification and characterization of N-acetylcysteine conjugates of valproic acid in humans and animals. *Drug Metab Dispos* 2000;28:823–832.

131. Gopaul SV, Farrell K, Abbott FS. Gas chromatography/negative ion chemical ionization mass spectrometry and liquid chromatography/electrospray ionization tandem mass spectrometry quantitative profiling of N-acetylcysteine conjugates of valproic acid in urine: application in drug metabolism studies in humans. *J Mass Spectrom* 2000;35:698–704.

132. Tang W, Borel AG, Abbott FS. Conjugation of glutathione with a toxic metabolite of valproic acid, (E)-2-propyl-2,4-penta-dienoic acid, catalyzed by rat hepatic glutathione-S-transferases. *Drug Metab Dispos* 1996;24:436–446.

133. Levy RH, Rettenmeier AW, Anderson GD, et al. Effects of polytherapy with phenytoin, carbamazepine, and stiripentol on formation of 4-ene-valproate, a hepatotoxic metabolite of valproic acid. *Clin Pharmacol Ther* 1990;48:225–235.

134. Katayama H, Watanabe M, Yoshitomi H, et al. Urinary metabolites of valproic acid in epileptic patients. *Biol Pharm Bull* 1998;21:304–307.

135. Guillemette C, Ritter JK, Auyeung DJ, et al. Structural heterogeneity at the UDP-glucuronosyltransferase 1 locus: functional consequences of three novel missense mutations in the human UGT1A7 gene. *Pharmacogenetics* 2000;10:629–644.

136. Tanaka E. Clinically significant pharmacokinetic drug interactions with benzodiazepines. *J Clin Pharm Ther* 1999;24:347–355.

137. Brockmoller J, Kirchheiner J, Meisel C, et al. Pharmacogenetic diagnostics of cytochrome P450 polymorphisms in clinical drug development and in drug treatment. *Pharmacogenomics* 2000;1:125–151.

138. Miller MS, McCarver DG, Bell DA, et al. Genetic polymorphisms in human drug metabolic enzymes. *Fundam Appl Toxicol* 1997;40:1–14.

139. Fisher JE, Nau H, Löscher W. Alterations in the renal excretion of valproate and its metabolites after chronic treatment. *Epilepsia* 1991;32:146–150.

140. Pollack GM, McHugh WB, Gengo FM, et al. Accumulation and washout kinetics of valproic acid and its active metabolites. *J Clin Pharmacol* 1986;26:668–676.

141. Anderson GD, Acheampong AA, Wilensky AJ, et al. Effect of valproate dose on formation of hepatotoxic metabolites. *Epilepsia* 1992;33:736–742.

142. Baruzzi A, Bordo B, Bossi L, et al. Plasma levels of di-no-propylacetate and clonazepam in epileptic patients. *Int J Clin Pharmacol Biopharm* 1977;15:403–408.

143. McQueen JK, Blackwood DH, Minns RA, et al. Plasma levels of sodium valproate in childhood epilepsy. *Scott Med J* 1982;27:312–317.

144. Sackellares JC, Sato S, Dreifuss FE, et al. Reduction of steady-state valproate levels by other antiepileptic drugs. *Epilepsia* 1981;22:437–441.

145. Otten N, Hall K, Irvine-Meek J, et al. Free valproic acid: steady-state pharmacokinetics in patients with intractable epilepsy. *Can J Neurol Sci* 1984;11:457–460.

146. Gram L, Flachs H, Wurtz-Jorgensen A, et al. Sodium valproate, serum level and clinical effect in epilepsy: a controlled study. *Epilepsia* 1979;20:303–311.

147. Gidal BE, Pitterle ME, Spencer NW, et al. Relationship between valproic acid dosage, plasma concentration and clearance in adult monotherapy patients with epilepsy. *J Clin Pharm Ther* 1995;20:215–219.

148. May T, Rambeck B. Serum concentrations of valproic acid: influence of dose and comedication. *Ther Drug Monit* 1985;7:387–390.

149. Sundqvist A, Tomson T, Lundkvist B. Pharmacokinetics of valproic acid in patients with juvenile myoclonic epilepsy on monotherapy. *Ther Drug Monit* 1997;19:153–159.

150. Yukawa E, To H, Ohdo S, et al. Population-based investigation of valproic acid relative clearance using nonlinear mixed effects modeling: influence of drug-drug interaction and patient characteristics. *J Clin Pharmacol* 1997;37:1160–1167.

151. Blanco-Serrano B, Otero MJ, Santos-Buelga D, et al. Population estimation of valproic acid clearance in adult patients using routine clinical pharmacokinetic data. *Biopharm Drug Dispos* 1999;20:233–240.

152. Bowdle AT, Patel IH, Levy RH, et al. Valproic acid dosage and plasma protein binding and clearance. *Clin Pharmacol Ther* 1980;28:486–492.

153. Gomez-Bellver MJ, Garcia-Sanchez MJ, Alonso-Gonzalez AC, et al. Plasma protein binding kinetics of valproic acid over a broad dosage range: therapeutic implications. *J Clin Pharm Ther* 1993;18:191–197.

154. Hussein Z, Patterson KJ, Lamm JE, et al. Effect of infusion duration on valproate pharmacokinetics. *Biopharm Drug Dispos* 1993;14:389–399.

155. Suemaru K, Kawasaki H, Yasuhara K, et al. Steady-state serum concentrations of carbamazepine and valproic acid in obese and lean patients with epilepsy. *Acta Med Okayama* 1998;52:139–142.

156. Henriksen O, Johannessen SI. Clinical observations of sodium valproate in children: an evaluation of therapeutic serum levels. In: Johannessen SI, Morselli PL, Pippenger C, et al., eds. *Antiepileptic therapy: advances in drug monitoring.* New York: Raven Press, 1980:253–261.

157. Johannessen SI, Henriksen O. Pharmacokinetic observations of dipropylacetate in children. In: Wada JA, Penry JK, eds. *Xth International Symposium on Epilepsy.* New York: Raven Press, 1980:353.

158. Kriel RL, Fischer JH, Cloyd JC, et al. Valproic acid pharmacokinetics in children. III. Very high dosage requirements. *Pediatr Neurol* 1986;2:202–208.

159. Battino D, Estienne M, Avanzini G. Clinical pharmacokinetics of antiepileptic drugs in paediatric patients. II. Phenytoin, carbamazepine, sulthiame, lamotrigine, vigabatrin, oxcarbazepine and felbamate. *Clin Pharmacokinet* 1995;29:341–369.

160. Battino D, Estienne M, Avanzini G. Clinical pharmacokinetics of antiepileptic drugs in paediatric patients. I. Phenobarbital, primidone, valproic acid, ethosuximide and mesuximide. *Clin Pharmacokinet* 1995;29:257–286.

161. Brachet-Liermain A, Demarquez JL. Pharmacokinetics of dipropylacetate in infants and children. *Pharm Weekbl* 1977;112:293–297.

162. Gal P, Oles KS, Gilman JT, et al. Valproic acid efficacy, toxicity, and pharmacokinetics in neonates with intractable seizures. *Neurology* 1988;38:467–471.

163. Irvine-Meek JM, Hall KW, Otten NH, et al. Pharmacokinetic study of valproic acid in a neonate. *Pediatr Pharmacol* 1982;2:317–221.

164. Hall K, Otten N, Johnston B, et al. A multivariable analysis of factors governing the steady-state pharmacokinetics of valproic acid in 52 young epileptics. *J Clin Pharmacol* 1985;25:261–268.

165. Kumar S, Wong H, Yeung SA, et al. Disposition of valproic acid in maternal, fetal, and newborn sheep. II. Metabolism and renal elimination. *Drug Metab Dispos* 2000;28:857–864.

166. Wong H, Kumar S, Rurak DW, et al. Ontogeny of valproic acid

disposition and metabolism: a developmental study in postnatal lambs and adult sheep. *Drug Metab Dispos* 2000;28:912–919.

167. Botha JH, Gray AL, Miller R. A model for estimating individualized valproate clearance values in children. *J Clin Pharmacol* 1995;35:1020–1024.

168. Sanchez-Alcaraz A, Quintana MB, Lopez E, et al. Valproic acid clearance in children with epilepsy. *J Clin Pharm Ther* 1998; 23:31–34.

169. Bernus I, Dickinson RG, Hooper WD, et al. Anticonvulsant therapy in aged patients: clinical pharmacokinetic considerations. *Drugs Aging* 1997;10:278–289.

170. Plasse J-C, Revol M, Chabert G. Neonatal pharmacokinetics of valproic acid. In: Schaaf D, Van de Kleijn E, eds. *Progress in clinical pharmacy.* Amsterdam: Elsevier/North-Holland Biomedical Press, 1979:247–252.

171. Philbert A, Dam M. The epileptic mother and her child. *Epilepsia* 1982;23:85–99.

171a. Yerby MS, Friel PN, McCormick K. Antiepileptic drug disposition during pregnancy. *Neurology* 1992;42[Suppl 5]:12–16.

172. Marbury TC, Lee CS, Bruni J. Hemodialysis of valproic acid in uremic patients. *Dial Transpl* 1980;9:961–964.

173. Franssen EJ, van Essen GG, Portman AT, et al. Valproic acid toxicokinetics: serial hemodialysis and hemoperfusion. *Ther Drug Monit* 1999;21:289–292.

174. Boucher BA, Rodman JH, Jaresko GS, et al. Phenytoin pharmacokinetics in critically ill trauma patients. *Clin Pharmacol Ther* 1988;44:675–683.

175. Boucher BA, Kuhl DA, Fabian TC, et al. Effect of neurotrauma on hepatic drug clearance. *Clin Pharmacol Ther* 1991;50: 487–497.

176. Anderson GD, Awan AB, Adams CA, et al. Increases in metabolism of valproate and excretion of 6beta-hydroxycortisol in patients with traumatic brain injury. *Br J Clin Pharmacol* 1998; 45:101–105.

177. Bourgeois BF, Beaumanoir A, Blajev B, et al. Monotherapy with valproate in primary generalized epilepsies. *Epilepsia* 1987;28 [Suppl 2]:S8–S11.

178. Feuerstein J, Revol M, Roger J, et al. Monotherapy with sodium valproate in generalized primary epilepsy—2d phase: study of long-term efficacy and tolerance. *Sem Hop* 1983;59: 1263–1274.

179. Henriksen O, Johannessen SI. Clinical and pharmacokinetic observations on sodium valproate: a 5-year follow-up study in 100 children with epilepsy. *Acta Neurol Scand* 1982;65: 504–523.

180. Wilder BJ, Ramsay RE, Murphy JV, et al. Comparison of valproic acid and phenytoin in newly diagnosed tonic-clonic seizures. *Neurology* 1983;33:1474–1476.

181. Covanis A, Gupta AK, Jeavons PM. Sodium valproate: monotherapy and polytherapy. *Epilepsia* 1982;23:693–720.

182. Redenbaugh JE, Sato S, Penry JK, et al. Sodium valproate: pharmacokinetics and effectivensss in treating intractable seizures. *Neurology* 1980;30:1–6.

183. Davis R, Peters DH, McTavish D. Valproic acid: a reappraisal of its pharmacological properties and clinical efficacy in epilepsy. *Drugs* 1994;47:332–372.

184. Wangemann M, Retzow A, Mazur D, et al. Study on the dose proportionality of the pharmacokinetics of sustained release sodium valproate. *Int Clin Pharmacol Ther* 2000;38:395–401.

185. Hovinga CA, Chicella MF, Rose DF, et al. Use of intravenous valproate in three pediatric patients with nonconvulsive or convulsive status epilepticus. *Ann Pharmacother* 1999;33:579–584.

186. Alfonso I, Alvarez LA, Gilman J, et al. Intravenous valproate dosing in neonates. *J Child Neurol* 2000;15:827–829.

187. Braathen G, Theorell K, Persson A, et al. Valproate in the treat-ment of absence epilepsy in children: a study of dose-response relationships. *Epilepsia* 1988;29:548–552.

188. Ishikawa T, Ogino C, Furuyama M, et al. Serum valproate concentrations in epileptic children with favourable responses. *Brain Dev* 1987;9:283–287.

189. Sato S, White BG, Penry JK, et al. Valproic acid versus ethosuximide in the treatment of absence seizures. *Neurology* 1982; 32:157–163.

190. Klotz U, Schweizer C. Valproic acid in childhood epilepsy: anticonvulsive efficacy in relation to its plasma levels. *Int Clin Pharmacol Ther Toxicol* 1980;18:461–465.

191. Villarreal HJ, Wilder BJ, Willmore LJ, et al. Effect of valproic acid on spike and wave discharges in patients with absence seizures. *Neurology* 1978;28:886–891.

192. Farrell K, Abbott FS, Orr JM, et al. Free and total serum valproate concentrations: their relationship to seizure control, liver enzymes and plasma ammonia in children. *Can J Neurol Sci* 1986;13:252–255.

193. Beydoun A, Sackellares JC, Shu V. Safety and efficacy of divalproex sodium monotherapy in partial epilepsy: a double-blind, concentration-response design clinical trial. Depakote Monotherapy for Partial Seizures Study Group. *Neurology* 1997; 48:182–188.

194. Herranz JL, Armijo JA, Arteaga R. Effectiveness and toxicity of phenobarbital, primidone, and sodium valproate in the prevention of febrile convulsions, controlled by plasma levels. *Epilepsia* 1984;25:89–95.

195. Herranz JL, Arteaga R, Armijo JA. Side effects of sodium valproate in monotherapy controlled by plasma levels: a study in 88 pediatric patients. *Epilepsia* 1982;23:203–214.

196. Keck PE Jr, McElroy SL, Tugrul KC, et al. Valproate oral loading in the treatment of acute mania. *J Clin Psychiatry* 1993;54:305–308.

197. Janicak PG. The relevance of clinical pharmacokinetics and therapeutic drug monitoring: anticonvulsant mood stabilizers and antipsychotics. *J Clin Psychiatry* 1993;54[Suppl]:35-41, 55—56.

198. Guay DR. The emerging role of valproate in bipolar disorder and other psychiatric disorders. *Pharmacotherapy* 1995;15: 631–647.

199. Lenaerts M, Bastings E, Sianard J, et al. Sodium valproate in severe migraine and tension-type headache: an open study of long-term efficacy and correlation with blood levels. *Acta Neurol Belg* 1996;96:126–129.

200. Coria F, Sempere AP, Duarte J. Low dose sodium valproate in the prophylaxis of migraine. *Clin Neuropharmacol* 1994;17: 568–573.

201. Erdemoglu AK, Ozbakir S. Valproic acid in prophylaxis of refractory migraine. *Acta Neurol Scand* 2000;102:354–358.

202. Bialer M, Hussein Z, Dubrovsky J, et al. Pharmacokinetics of valproic acid obtained after administration of three oral formulations to humans. *Isr J Med Sci* 1984;20:46–49.

203. Bialer M, Hussein Z, Raz I, et al. Pharmacokinetics of valproic acid in volunteers after a single dose study. *Biopharm Drug Dispos* 1985;6:33–42.

204. Miljkovic B, Pokrajac M, Varagic V, et al. Single dose and steady state pharmacokinetics of valproic acid in adult epileptic patients. *Int J Clin Pharmacol Res* 1991;11:137–141.

205. Perucca E, Gatti G, Frigo GM, et al. Disposition of sodium valproate in epileptic patients. *Br J Clin Pharmacol* 1978;5: 495–499.

206. Schapel GJ, Beran RG, Doecke CJ, et al. Pharmacokinetics of sodium valproate in epileptic patients: prediction of maintenance dosage by single-dose study. *Eur J Clin Pharmacol* 1980; 17:71–77.

207. Hoffmann F, von Unruh GE, Jancik BC. Valproic acid disposi-

tion in epileptic patients during combined antiepileptic maintenance therapy. *Eur J Clin Pharmacol* 1981;19:383–385.

208. Eadie MJ, Heazlewood V, McKauge L, et al. Steady-state valproate pharmacokinetics during long term therapy. *Clin Exp Neurol* 1983;19:183–191.

209. Chiba K, Suganuma T, Ishizaki T, et al. Comparison of steady-state pharmacokinetics of valproic acid in children between monotherapy and multiple antiepileptic drug treatment. *J Pediatr* 1985;106:653–658.

210. Schobben F, van der Kleijn E, Gabreels FJ. Pharmacokinetics of di-*n*-propylacetate in epileptic patients. *Eur J Clin Pharmacol* 1975;8:97–105.

VALPROIC ACID

DRUG INTERACTIONS

RICHARD D. SCHEYER

Valproic acid (VPA) frequently interacts with other drugs, especially other antiepileptic drugs (AEDs). The extent of such interactions is often sufficient to alter the pharmacokinetics of both VPA and the interacting drug in clinically significant ways. Endogenous substances and disease states also may alter VPA pharmacokinetics.

MECHANISMS

An understanding of the mechanisms of drug–drug interactions is gradually replacing our reliance on a laundry list of interactions to an understanding of mechanistically based principles.

Metabolism

VPA is metabolized through multiple metabolic pathways, including cytochrome P450 (CYP) CYP2A6, CYP2C9, and CYP2C19. In addition, glucuronidation by uridine diphosphate glucoronosyltransferase (UGT) plays a major role in VPA metabolism. Details may be found in Chapter 84.

Metabolism of VPA is subject to induction by drugs that induce these pathways, including many AEDs. As described later, this enzyme induction may take days or weeks to manifest itself. VPA causes little or no induction of the metabolism of itself or of other drugs (1–3).

VPA may also affect the metabolism of other compounds. Although effects may be seen on CYP-mediated reactions, the most prominent effects have been noted on compounds whose metabolism is through UGT-mediated glucuronidation or through epoxide hydrolase. These inhibitory effects are typically faster than enzyme induction, but they may take time to manifest, especially if the half-life of the affected drug (e.g., phenobarbital) is quite long.

Protein Binding

VPA is highly protein bound, and thus small changes in protein binding may cause large changes in unbound VPA fraction. Binding is subject to displacement not only by other drugs, but also by endogenous substances or even by VPA itself.

Transport

VPA exists in the body primarily ionized as valproate. In the ionized form, its lipophilicity is relatively low, and its ability to enter the brain by diffusion across the blood–brain barrier is limited. To enter the brain, VPA depends, at least in part, on transport processes. These transporters may be inhibited by other drugs or by endogenous substances.

SPECIFIC DRUG INTERACTIONS

Changes in Valproic Acid Pharmacokinetics Induced by Other Drugs

Enzyme-Inducing Antiepileptic Drugs. Carbamazepine, phenytoin, and phenobarbital are capable of inducing VPA clearance. Coulthard noted increasing serum levels of VPA and improved seizure control in one patient after discontinuation of phenytoin (4). When administered with VPA, carbamazepine, phenobarbital, and phenytoin lower VPA concentrations (5–8). Very large VPA doses may be needed to achieve therapeutic levels and efficacy with concomitant use of enzyme-inducting drugs.

The timing of induction or deinduction of VPA metabolism has received little study. Miller showed evidence of deinduction beginning within 2 days of carbamazepine discontinuation (9). Mattson and coworkers found the rise in VPA levels to begin in some patients while they were still receiving 100 to 200 mg phenytoin. In others, no change occurred for 1 to 2 weeks after phenytoin was discontinued (10,11). Battino found that when carbamazepine was replaced by oxcarbazepine, an antiepileptic prodrug with less propensity for drug interactions, unbound VPA concentrations rose, followed by a rise in total VPA concentra-

Richard D. Scheyer, MD: Director, Clinical Discovery and Human Pharmacology, Aventis Pharmaceuticals, Bridgewater, New Jersey

tions (12). Maximal deinduction was not apparent for ≥2 weeks after completion of the crossover.

As mentioned earlier, VPA binding is saturable. Hence a reduction in VPA concentration by enzyme-inducing drugs can result in a decreased unbound fraction of VPA and an even greater decrease in unbound VPA concentration. There is no evidence of alteration in the number of VPA binding sites or in the binding dissociation constant in patients receiving concomitant AEDs (13).

The coadministration of enzyme-inducing drugs not only increases the clearance of VPA but also may change metabolic pathways (14). Increases in the putative hepatotoxic 4-en-VPA and 2-4-en-VPA may be one reason for greater incidence of VPA hepatotoxicity in patients treated with polytherapy (15–18).

Ethosuximide. Ethosuximide may lower VPA levels, but the effect is modest, with a decrease in VPA concentration of ~28% when ethosuximide was added to VPA in two children (19).

Felbamate. The addition of felbamate (2,400 mg/day) increases total VPA area under the curve by approximately 50% (20). A reduction in VPA dosage may be necessary.

Lamotrigine. Lamotrigine may cause a modest increase in VPA clearance. Anderson and coworkers reported a 25% decrease in VPA concentration with the addition of lamotrigine (21).

Tiagabine. The addition of tiagabine results in a 10% to 12% decrease in VPA area under the curve. This is unlikely to be clinically significant (22).

Topiramate. Topiramate may modestly reduce VPA levels. This effect is also unlikely to be clinically significant (23).

Investigational Antiepileptic Drugs. Stiripentol may inhibit ω-oxidation of VPA and may decrease the formation clearance of 4-en-VPA, a hepatotoxic metabolite of VPA (24).

Nonantiepileptic Drugs. Salicylic acid displaces VPA from protein and results in higher unbound VPA levels (25). Schobben (26) noted a significant rise in urinary excretion of VPA after administration of 1 to 2 g of aspirin daily. Aspirin also competes with VPA for mitochondrial oxidation. This leads to an increase in microsomal metabolism with production of 4-en-VPA (27). With the exception of aspirin, changes in VPA protein binding caused by exogenous displacers are relatively small.

The enzyme-inducing antibiotic rifampin increases VPA clearance by 40% (28). This effect may be expected to be clinically significant. Conversely, isoniazid may increase VPA concentration, with resulting clinical VPA toxicity

(29). Probenecid increases systemic and especially central nervous system concentrations by blockade of the organic anion transporter in rats (30); the effect in humans is unknown. Case reports suggest that fluoxetine may significantly increase VPA concentrations, possibly through inhibition of CYP2C19 (31–33).

Valproic Acid–Induced Changes in the Pharmacokinetics of Other Drugs

Benzodiazepines. The combined use of VPA with benzodiazepines is not unusual. VPA inhibits the clearance of lorazepam, a drug eliminated primarily through glucuronide conjugation (34). A total daily dose of VPA of 1,000 mg raised lorazepam area under the curve 20% in healthy male volunteers but did not result in increased sedation (35). VPA displaces diazepam from plasma protein binding sites in a manner similar to its effects on phenytoin, as detailed later (36). With these exceptions, there is little evidence of pharmacokinetic interactions of benzodiazepines with VPA.

Carbamazepine. Some patients develop sedation, nausea, diplopia, or a confusional state when VPA is added to carbamazepine therapy (37–40). These case reports suggest an interaction, but has been proven with blood level changes. The considerable variation in carbamazepine levels between doses makes analysis difficult unless determinations are consistently made both before drug administration and at times of clinical toxicity.

Inhibition of clearance of carbamazepine-10,11-epoxide may contribute to toxicity (41–44). However, direct administration of carbamazepine epoxide to patients with seizures, with drug levels in excess of those usually achieved with the combination of VPA and carbamazepine, did not produce significant neurotoxicity (45).

When VPA is added *in vitro* to plasma samples containing carbamazepine, the pharmacologically active unbound fraction of carbamazepine increases 25% (46). Because carbamazepine is only moderately bound, with a baseline unbound fraction of about 25%, this binding interaction is unlikely to be of major clinical significance (47–51). Carbamazepine toxicity tends to occur at times of peak concentration. Ideally, samples of total and unbound carbamazepine and epoxide should be obtained both at trough and at times of clinical toxicity (52). A more marked inhibition of carbamazepine epoxide clearance is seen with coadministration of valpromide, a prodrug of VPA (53).

Ethosuximide. Ethosuximide levels may increase as much as 53% when VPA is added, but there appears to be substantial interindividual variability (54,55).

Felbamate. Felbamate concentrations are increased in patients receiving VPA compared with those receiving enzyme-inducing AEDs. This effect appears to be the result of a felbamate-mediated inhibition of VPA clearance as well as the effect of the val of enzyme-inducing AEDS (20).

Lamotrigine. VPA blocks the glucuronidation of lamotrigine and results in increased concentrations of lamotrigine (56). This effect appears to be maximal even at subclinical concentrations of VPA (57,58). Perhaps as a result of the more rapid rise in lamotrigine concentrations in patients receiving VPA, or by increased formation of reactive metabolites (e.g., arene oxides) through other pathways (59), patients receiving VPA are at greater risk of lamotrigine-related rashes and possibly hepatic toxicity (60).

Phenobarbital. Serum phenobarbital levels rise when VPA is added (61,62). Loiseau noted an elevation of serum phenobarbital levels and an increase in phenobarbital half-life from a mean of 83 to 105 hours after administering VPA. At the same time, urinary phenobarbital excretion is unchanged or increases, but urinary hydroxyphenobarbital decreases (62,63).

High concentrations of VPA may compete with phenobarbital for microsomal oxidation. At low to moderate levels of VPA, the major metabolite is 3 OXO-VPA created by oxidation in the mitochondria. Higher levels of VPA saturate this pathway and lead to microsomal smooth endoplasmic reticulum production of metabolites 4-OH-VPA, 5-OH VPA, and conjugates to D-glucuronide (14). These latter actions compete with phenobarbital metabolism.

Other Barbiturates. Primidone concentrations, as well as the derived phenobarbital concentrations, increase when VPA is added. The magnitude is unclear, ranging from a 17% to a >100% increase in primidone (37,64).

Phenytoin. Most reports note an initial fall in phenytoin levels after initiation of VPA. VPA is highly bound to plasma albumin and displaces phenytoin from binding sites (1). The acute displacement of phenytoin from plasma proteins produces an increase in the concentration of unbound phenytoin. Redistribution of unbound drug to tissues (including brain) may lead to the paradox of neurotoxicity despite a lower total serum phenytoin concentration (65,66).

As the liver removes the increased unbound phenytoin, unbound levels decrease to their initial levels, with a corresponding further decrease in total levels (2,67). Changes in phenytoin dosage to bring total levels back to the usual therapeutic range may raise unbound phenytoin to toxic levels. Even in the absence of dose adjustment, total phenytoin concentrations may return to pre-VPA baseline, and unbound phenytoin levels exceed baseline (68,69). This may be caused by a noncompetitive metabolic inhibition of phenytoin metabolism (70,71), possibly resulting from inhibition of CYP2C9 or CYP2C19.

Interdose fluctuations in VPA concentration may cause fluctuation in phenytoin protein binding and transient phenytoin toxicity. This effect may be estimated using one of several regression equations that permit calculation of unbound phenytoin concentrations from measured total phenytoin and VPA levels. These equations include those described by Haidukewych—% unbound phenytoin = 9.5 + .1 × VPA (µg/mL)—and Scheyer—% unbound phenytoin = 8.0 + .07 × VPA (µg/mL) (49,66). These equations were based on studies in which unbound phenytoin concentrations were determined after ultrafiltration at 20° to 25°C. The unbound fraction of phenytoin would be expected to be greater at 37°C (72).

Investigational Antiepileptic Drugs. Unlike carbamazepine and phenytoin, VPA does not appear to decrease concentrations of the investigational drug remacemide (73). The extensive glucuronidation of retigabine suggests a potential for VPA to inhibit its metabolism (74).

Nonantiepileptic Drugs. VPA may be a weak displacer of warfarin binding (75). VPA has been reported to inhibit the clearance of the antiviral drug zidovudine, presumably by inhibition of glucuronidation (76).

Unlike enzyme-inducing AEDs such as carbamazepine, VPA does not appear to decrease concentration of the antipsychotic drug haloperidol (77), and it has no clinically significant effects on clozapine concentration (78). Concentrations of amitriptyline (and its active metabolite nortriptyline) increase by about one-third with the addition of VPA 1,000 mg/day (79).

Unlike enzyme-inducing AEDs, VPA does not decrease cyclosporine concentration, a property that may be useful in patients with seizures after organ transplantation (80). Likewise, VPA does not increase clearance of female sex hormones used in oral contraceptives. Consequently, birth control failures are less likely in women taking VPA (81).

Antiepileptic Drugs Believed Not to Interact with Valproic Acid. VPA has been reported not to interact with the renally eliminated drugs vigabatrin (82) or gabapentin (83). VPA also does not appear to have a significant interaction with clobazam (84) or zonisamide (85). *In vitro* data suggest that there is no significant interaction with levetiracetam (86). As noted earlier, oxcarbazepine has less propensity to interact with VPA than does carbamazepine.

INTERACTIONS WITH ENDOGENOUS COMPOUNDS

Endogenous free fatty acids can displace VPA binding (87). Because free fatty acids are acutely affected by food intake, this may confound assessments of unbound VPA concentration (13). Free fatty acids may also compete with VPA

TABLE 85.1. EFFECTS OF OTHER DRUGS ON VALPROIC ACID

Compound	Effect on Valproic Acid	Mechanism
Antiepileptic drugs		—
Carbamazepine	↓ C_{total} and $C_{unbound}$	Enzyme induction
Felbamate	↑ C_{total} and $C_{unbound}$	Enzyme inhibition
Phenytoin	↓ C_{total} and $C_{unbound}$	Enzyme induction
Phenobarbital	↓ C_{total} and $C_{unbound}$	Enzyme induction
Non antiepileptic drugs		—
Acetylsalicylic acid	↑ $f_{unbound}$	—
Fluoxetine	↑ C_{total}	Inhibition of metabolism (↑ $C_{unbound}$ also anticipated)

C, concentration; $f_{unbound}$, fraction unbound.

for transport through the medium-chain fatty acid transporter across the blood–brain barrier (88). The clinical relevance of this interaction is unknown.

Decreased binding is found in uremia and can only partly be attributed to decreased protein concentration. Allosteric changes in plasma protein may explain increased unbound fraction (71). Endogenous "toxic" uremic displacers also may be responsible (89). The result is a lower total serum VPA concentration and an increase percentage of unbound VPA with no change in the concentration of unbound drug.

PHARMACODYNAMIC INTERACTIONS

Few data indicate a supraadditive (synergistic) or infraadditive (antagonistic) pharmacodynamic interaction when VPA is coadministered with other drugs (10) (Tables 85.1 and 85.2). A combination of drugs, such as phenytoin or carbamazepine with VPA, may provide additive efficacy with infraadditive toxicity resulting from different dose-limiting neurotoxicity and may yield an improved therapeutic index for the combination. This has not been established in clinical trials. Reports have described instances of profound sedation with addition of VPA to a regimen of phenobarbital in excess of what may be expected from the

pharmacokinetic interaction and the additive effect of their sedative properties (90). Some cases may be explained by increased ammonia concentration caused by hepatic dysfunction (91).

Jeavons and Clark reported absence status in five of 12 patients who were given the two drugs (92). The observation is unexplained, and it appears to be uncommon.

CONCLUSIONS AND CLINICAL IMPLICATIONS

Pharmacokinetic interactions between VPA and other drugs are frequent. Many AEDs induce hepatic enzymatic activity to accelerate VPA metabolism. This results in lower plasma VPA concentrations and a shorter VPA half-life. The effect of metabolic interactions may be underestimated when total VPA concentrations are measured, because the saturable nature of VPA binding means that modest changes in total VPA concentration may be associated with greater changes in unbound VPA concentration, and the short half-life makes a consistent sampling schedule critical. Newer AEDs may be associated with fewer interactions, but any advantages of combining these agents with VPA remains to be demonstrated clinically.

TABLE 85.2. EFFECTS OF VALPROIC ACID ON OTHER DRUGS: INTERACTIONS WITH PROBABLY CLINICAL RELEVANCE

Compound	Effect of Valproic Acid	Mechanism
Antiepileptic drugs		
Carbamazepine	↑ $f_{unbound}$ (±), ↑ $C_{unbound}$ (±), ↑ Epoxide	Protein binding displacement Inhibition of epoxide hydrolase
Ethosuximide	↑ Concentration	Inhibition of metabolism
Lamotrigine	↑ Concentration	Inhibition of metabolism
Phenytoin	↓ C_{total}, ↑ $f_{unbound}$, ↑ $C_{unbound}$	Protein binding displacement Inhibition of metabolism
Phenobarbital	↑ Concentration	Inhibition of metabolism
Nonantiepileptic drugs		
Amitriptyline	↑ Amitriptyline and nortriptyline	Inhibition of metabolism
Zidovudine	↑ Concentration	Inhibition of metabolism

C, concentration; $f_{unbound}$, fraction unbound.

VPA is metabolized almost completely in the liver and can interfere with the biotransformation of other AEDs. VPA slows hydroxylation and glucuronidation of some drugs and thus causes a rise of serum levels of, for example, carbamazepine epoxide, phenobarbital, and lamotrigine. A similar effect on phenytoin metabolism may be masked by changes in protein binding that produce opposite effects on the usually measured total concentration. These interactions may lead to toxicity and may require adjustment of dosage.

The frequency of VPA interactions calls for clinical awareness and appropriate determinations of blood levels of both VPA and other drugs, at times including unbound levels. Although the conversion to VPA monotherapy requires special effort, the benefits of avoiding interactions with other drugs are worthwhile (93).

ACKNOWLEDGMENT

This work was supported in part by the United States Department of Veterans Affairs.

REFERENCES

1. Jordan BJ, Shillingford JS, Steed KP. Preliminary observations on the protein binding and enzyme-inducing properties of sodium valproate (Epilim). In: Legg NJ, ed. *Clinical and pharmacological aspects of sodium valproate (Epilim) in the treatment of epilepsy.* Tunbridge Wells, UK: MCS Consultants, 1976:112–116.
2. Mattson RH, Cramer JA, Williamson PD, et al. Valproic acid in epilepsy: clinical and pharmacological effects. *Ann Neurol* 1978; 3:20–25.
3. McLaughlin DB, Andrews JA, Hooper WD, et al. Apparent autoinduction of valproate beta-oxidation in humans. *Br J Clin Pharmacol* 2000;49:409–415.
4. Coulthard MG. Sodium valproate in the treatment of intractable childhood epilepsy. *Dev Med Child Neurol* 1975;17:534.
5. Bowdle TA, Levy RH, Cutler RE. Effects of carbamazepine on valproic acid kinetics in normal subjects. *Clin Pharmacol Ther* 1979;26:629–634.
6. Mihaly GW, Vajda FJ, Miles JL, et al. Single and chronic dose pharmacokinetic studies of sodium valproate in epileptic patients. *Eur J Pharmacol* 1979;15:23–29.
7. Sackellares JC, Sato S, Dreifuss FE, et al. Reductions of steady state valproate levels by other antiepileptic drugs. *Epilepsia* 1981; 22:437–441.
8. Richens A, Scoular IT, Ahmad S, et al. Pharmacokinetics and efficacy of Epilim in patients receiving long-term therapy with other antiepileptic drugs. In: Legg NJ, ed. *Clinical and pharmacological aspects of sodium valproate (Epilim) in the treatment of epilepsy.* Tunbridge Wells, UK: MCS Consultants, 1976: 78–88.
9. Miller ML, Graves NM, Leppik IE, et al. Time course for resolution of carbamazepine-valproate interaction. *Epilepsia* 1989;30: 640–641(abst).
10. Mattson RH, Cramer JA. Antiepileptic drug interactions in clinical use: summary. In: Pitlick W, ed. *Drug interactions.* New York: Demos, 1989:75–85.
11. Mattson RH, Cramer JA, Scheyer RD, et al. Disinduction of valproate metabolism: timing and magnitude of change. *Proc R Soc Med* 1990:138–142.
12. Battino D, Croci D, Granata T, et al. Changes in unbound and total valproic acid concentrations after replacement of carbamazepine with oxcarbazepine. *Ther Drug Monit* 1992;14: 376–379.
13. Scheyer RD, Cramer JA, Toftness BR, et al. *In vivo* determinations of valproate binding constants during sole and multi-drug therapy. *Ther Drug Monit* 1990;12:117–123.
14. Baillie TA. Metabolic activation of valproic acid and drug-mediated hepatotoxicity: role of the terminal olefin, 2-*n*-propyl-4-pentenoic acid. *Chem Res Toxicol* 1988;1:195–199.
15. Dreifuss FE, Langer DH, Moline KA, et al. Valproic acid hepatic fatalities. II. US experince since 1984. *Neurology* 1989;39: 201–207.
16. Scheffner D, St. Konig IR-R, Kochen W, et al. Fatal liver failure in 16 children with valproate therapy. *Epilepsia* 1988;29: 530–542.
17. McLaughlin DB, Eadie MJ, Parker-Scott SL, et al. Valproate metabolism during valproate-associated hepatotoxicity in a surviving adult patient. *Epilepsy Res* 2000;41:259–268.
18. Tennison MB, Miles MV, Pollack GM, et al. Valproate metabolites and hepatotoxicity in an epileptic population. *Epilepsia* 1988;29:543–547.
19. Salke-Kellermann RA, May T, Boenigk HE. Influence of ethosuximide on valproic acid serum concentrations. *Epilepsy Res* 1997;26:345–349.
20. Wagner ML, Graves NM, Leppik IE, et al. The effect of felbamate on valproate disposition. *Epilepsia* 1991;32[Suppl 3]:15 (abst).
21. Anderson GD, Yau MK, Gidal BE, et al. Bidirectional interaction of valproate and lamotrigine in healthy subjects. *Clin Pharmacol Ther* 1996;60:145–156.
22. Curran S, Wattis J. Critical flicker fusion threshold: a potentially useful measure for the early detection of Alzheimer's disease. *Hum Psychopharmacol* 2000;15:103–112.
23. Bougeois BF. Drug interaction profile of topiramate. *Epilepsia* 1996;37[Suppl 2]:S14–S17.
24. Levy RH, Rettenmeier AW, Anderson GD, et al. Effects of polytherapy with phenytoin, carbamazepine, and stiripentol on formation of 4-ene-valproate, a hepatotoxic metabolite of valproic acid. *Clin Pharmacol Ther* 1990;48:225–235.
25. Fleitman JS, Bruni J, Perrin JH, et al. Albumin-binding interactions of sodium valproate. *J Clin Pharmacol* 1980;20:514–517.
26. Schobben F, Vree TB, van der Kleijn D. Pharmacokinetics, metabolism and distribution of 2-*N*-proply pentanoate (sodium valproate) and the influence of salicylate comedication. In: Meinardi H, Rowan AJ, eds. *Advances in epileptology.* Amsterdam: Swets & Zeitlinger, 1978:271–277.
27. Abbott FS, Kassam J, Orr JM, et al. The effect of aspirin on valproic acid metabolism. *Clin Pharmacol Ther* 1986;40:94–100.
28. *Physician's desk reference.* Montvale, NJ: Medical Economics Company, 2000.
29. Jonville AP, Gauchez AS, Autret E, et al. Interaction between isoniazid and valproate: a case of valproate overdosage. *Eur J Clin Pharmacol* 1991;40:197–198.
30. Adkison KDK, Artru AA, Powers KM, et al. Contribution of probenecid-sensitive anion transport processes at the brain capillary endothelium and choroid plexus to the efficient efflux of valproic acid from the central nervous system. *J Pharmacol Exp Ther* 1994;94:797–805.
31. Sovner R, Davis JM. A potential drug interaction between fluoxetine and valproic acid. *J Clin Psychopharmacol* 1991;11:389.
32. Lucena MI, Blanco E, Corrales MA, et al. Interaction of fluoxetine and valproic acid. *Am J Psychiatry* 1998;155:575.
33. Jeppesen U, Gram LF, Vistisen K, et al. Dose-dependent inhibi-

tion of CYP1A2, CYP2C19 and CYP2D6 by citalopram, fluoxetine, fluvoxamine and paroxetine. *Eur J Clin Pharmacol* 1996; 51:73–78.

34. Lancman ME, Asconape JJ, Penry JK. Choreiform movements associated with the use of valproate. *Arch Neurol* 1994;51: 702–704.

35. Samara EE, Granneman RG, Witt GF, et al. Effect of valproate on the pharmacokinetics and pharmacodynamics of lorazepam. *J Clin Pharmacol* 1997;37:442–450.

36. Dhillon S, Richens A. Valproate acid and diazepam interaction *in vivo*. *Br J Clin Pharmacol* 1982;13:553–560.

37. Adams DJ, Luders H, Pippenger C. Sodium valproate in the treatment of intractable seizure disorders: a clinical and electroencephalographic study. *Neurology* 1978;28:152–157.

38. Hassan MN, Laljee HCK, Parsonage MJ. Sodium valproate in the treatment of resistant epilepsy. *Acta Neurol Scand* 1976;54: 209–218.

39. Jeavons PM, Clark JE, Maheswari MC. Treatment of generalized epilepsies of childhood and adolescence with sodium valproate (Epilim). *Dev Med Child Neurol* 1977;19:9–25.

40. L'Hermitte F, Marteau R, Serdaru M. Dipropylacetate (valproate de sodium) et carbamazepine: Une association antiepileptique suspecte. *Presse Med* 1978;7:3780.

41. Levy RH, Moreland TA, Morselli PL, et al. Carbamazepine/valproic acid interaction in man and rhesus monkey. *Epilepsia* 1984; 25:338–345.

42. Pisani F, Caputo M, Fazio A, et al. Interaction of carbamazepine-10,11-epoxide, an active metabolite of carbamazepine, with valproate: a pharmacokinetic study. *Epilepsia* 1990;31:339–342.

43. Robbins DK, Wedlund PJ, Kuhn R, et al. Inhibition of epoxide hydrolase by valproic acid in epileptic patients receiving carbamazepine. *Br J Clin Pharmacol* 1990;29:759–762.

44. Tomson T, Bertilsson L. Potent therapeutic effect of carbamazepine-10,11 epoxide in trigeminal neuralgia. *Arch Neurol* 1984; 41:598–601.

45. Tomson T, Almkvist O, Nilsson BY, et al. Carbamazepine-10,11-epoxide in epilepsy. *Arch Neurol* 1990;47:888–892.

46. Mattson GF, Mattson RH, Cramer JA. Interaction between valproic acid and carbamazepine: an *in vitro* study of protein binding. *Ther Drug Monit* 1982;4:181–184.

47. Disalle E, Pacifici GM, Morselli PL. Studies on plasma protein binding of carbamazepine: studies on plasma protein binding of carbamazepine. *Pharmacol Res Commun* 1974;6:193–202.

48. Hooper WD, Dubetz DK, Bochner F, et al. Plasma protein binding of carbamazepine. *Clin Pharmacol Ther* 1975;17:433–440.

49. Haidukewych D, Zielinski JJ, Rodin EA. Derivation and evaluation of an equation for prediction of free carbamazepine concentration in patients comedicated with valproic acid. *Ther Drug Monit* 1989;11:528–532.

50. Mckee PJW, Blacklaw J, Butler E, et al. Variability and clinical relevance of the interaction between sodium valproate and carbamazepine in epileptic patients. *Epilepsy Res* 1992;11:193–198.

51. Rambeck B, Salke-Treumann A, May T, et al. Valproic acid-induced carbamazepine-10,11-epoxide toxicity in children and adolescents. *Eur Neurol* 1990;30:79–83.

52. Levy RH, Koch KM. Drug interactions with valproic acid. *Drugs* 1982;24:543–556.

53. Pisani F, Fazio A, Oteri G, et al. Sodium valproate and valpromide: differential interactions with carbamazepine in epileptic patients. *Epilepsia* 1986;27:548–552.

54. Mattson RH, Cramer JA. Valproic acid and ethosuximide interaction. *Ann Neurol* 1980;7:583–584.

55. Pisani F, Narbone MC, Trunfio C, et al. Valproic acid–ethosuximide interaction: a pharmacokinetic study. *Epilepsia* 1984;25: 229–233.

56. Binnie CD, van Emde Boas W, Kasteleijn-Nolste-Trenite DGA,

et al. Acute effects of lamotrigine (BW430C) in persons with epilepsy. *Epilepsia* 1986;27:248–254.

57. Kanner AM, Frey M. Adding valproate to lamotrigine: a study of their pharmacokinetic interaction. *Neurology* 2000;55:588–591.

58. Gidal BE, Anderson GD, Rutecki PR, et al. Lack of an effect of valproate concentration on lamotrigine pharmacokinetics in developmentally disabled patients with epilepsy. *Epilepsy Res* 2000;42:23–31.

59. Maggs JL, Naisbitt DJ, Tettey JNA, et al. Metabolism of lamotrigine to a reactive arene oxide intermediate. *Chem Res Toxicol* 2000;13:1075–1081.

60. Fayad M, Choueiri R, Mikati M. Potential hepatotoxicity of lamotrigine. *Pediatr Neurol* 2000;22:49–52.

61. Bruni J, Wilder BJ, Perchalski RJ, et al. Valproic acid and plasma levels of phenobarbital. *Neurology* 1980;30:94–97.

62. Kapetanovic I, Kupferberg HJ, Porter RJ, et al. Valproic acid-phenobarbital interaction: a systematic study using stable isotopically labeled phenobarbital in an epileptic patient. In: Morselli PL, Pippenger CE, Richens A, et al., eds. *Antiepileptic therapy: advances in drug monitoring*. New York: Raven Press, 1980:373–380.

63. Loiseau P, Orgogozo JM, Centaud B, et al. Further pharmacokinetic observations on the interaction between phenobarbital and valproic acid in epileptic patients. In: Wada JA, Penry JK, eds. *Advances in epileptology: the Xth Epilepsy International Symposium*. New York: Raven Press, 1980:353–354.

64. Windorfer A, Sauer W, Gadeke R. Elevation of diphenylhdantoin and primidone serum concentration by addition of dipropylacetate, a new anticonvulsant drug. *Acta Paediatr Scand* 1972; 64:771–772.

65. Patsalos PN, Lascelles PT. Effect of sodium valproate on plasma protein binding of diphenylhydantoin. *J Neurol Neurosurg Psychiatry* 1977;50:570–574.

66. Scheyer RD, Cramer JA, Mattson RH. Valproate induced variable phenytoin binding. *Epilepsia* 1989;30:647(abst).

67. Bruni J, Wilder BJ, Willmore LJ, et al. Valproic acid and plasma levels of phenytoin. *Neurology* 1979;29:904–905.

68. Bruni J, Gallo JM, Lee CS, et al. Interactions of valproic acid with phenytoin. *Neurology* 1980;30:1233–1236.

69. Lai ML, Huang JD. Dual effect of valproic acid on the pharmacokinetics of phenytoin. *Biopharm Drug Dispos* 1993;14:365–370.

70. Wang S-L, Lai M-L, Huang J-D. Increased microsomal irreversible binding of phenytoin by valproic acid. *Biochem Pharmacol* 1991;42:1143–1144.

71. Perucca E, Gatti G, Frigo GM, et al. Sodium valproate in epileptic patients. *Br J Pharmacol* 1978;5:495–499.

72. Schottelius DD. Exogenous and endogenous factors influencing unbound antiepileptic drug concentrations. *Clin Pharmacokinet* 1984;9[Suppl 1]:88–89.

73. Scheyer RD, Cramer JA, Leppik IE, et al. Remacemide elimination after initial and chronic dosing. *Clin Pharmacol Ther* 1992; 51:189(abst).

74. Hempel R, Schupke H, McNeilly PJ, et al. Metabolism of retigabine (D-23129), a novel anticonvulsant. *Drug Metab Dispos* 1999;27:613–622.

75. Panjehshahin MR, Bowmer CJ, Yates MS. Effect of valproic acid, its unsaturated metabolites and some structurally related fatty acids on the binding of warfarin and dansylsarcosine to human albumin. *Biochem Pharmacol* 1991;41:1227–1233.

76. Lertora JJ, Greenspan DL al, Rege AB, et al. Valproic acid inhibits glucuronidation of zidovudine (AZT) in HIV-infected patients. *Clin Pharmacol Ther* 1993;53:197(abst).

77. Hesslinger B, Normann C, Langosch JM, et al. Effects of carbamazepine and valproate on haloperidol plasma levels and on psychopathologic outcome in schizophrenic patients. *J Clin Psychopharmacol* 1999;19:310–315.

78. Facciola G, Avenoso A, Scordo MG, et al. Small effects of valproic acid on the plasma concentrations of clozapine and its major metabolites in patients with schizophrenic or affective disorders. *Ther Drug Monit* 1999;21:341–345.

79. Wong SL, Cavanaugh J, Shi H, et al. Effects of divalproex sodium on amitriptyline and nortriptyline pharmacokinetics. *Clin Pharmacol Ther* 1996;60:48–53.

80. Robinson RO. What is the appropriate management, including drug therapy, for epilepsy in a child with a renal transplant. *Pediatr Nephrol* 1993;7:364.

81. Mattson RH, Cramer JA, Darney PD, et al. Use of oral contraceptives by women with epilepsy. *JAMA* 1986;256:238–240.

82. Armijo JA, Arteaga R, Valdiz EM, et al. Coadministration of vigabatrin and valproate in children with refractory epilepsy. *Clin Neuropharmacol* 1992;15:459–469.

83. Basim M, Uthman EI, Hammond EJ, et al. Absence of gabapentin and valproate interaction: an evoked potential and pharmacokinetic study. *Epilepsia* 1990;31:645.

84. Wang JJ, Hug D, Gautschi K, et al. Clobazam for treatment of epilepsy. *J Epilepsy* 1993;6:180–184.

85. Tasaki K, Minami T, Ieiri I, et al. Drug interactions of zonisamide with phenytoin and sodium valproate: serum concentrations and protein binding. *Brain Dev* 1995;17:182–185.

86. Nicolas JM, Collart P, Gerin B, et al. *In vitro* evaluation of potential drug interactions with levetiracetam, a new antiepileptic agent. *Drug Metab Dispos* 1999;27:250–254.

87. Patel IH, Levy RH. Valproic acid binding to human serum albumin and determination of free fraction in the presence of anticonvulsants and free fatty acids. *Epilepsia* 1979;20:85–90.

88. Adkison KDK, Shen DD. Uptake of valproic acid into rat brain is mediated by a medium-chain fatty acid transporter. *J Pharmacol Exp Ther* 1996;276:1189–1200.

89. Bruni J, Wang LH, Marburt TC, et al. Protein binding of valproic acid in uremic patients. *Neurology* 1980;30:557–559.

90. Sackellares JC, Lee SI, Dreifuss FE. Stupor following administration of valproic acid to patients receiving other antiepileptic drugs. *Epilepsia* 1979;20:697–703.

91. Loscher W, Nau H, Wahnschaffe U, et al. Effects of valproate and e-2-en-valproate on functional and morphological parameters of rat liver .II. Influence of phenobarbital comedication. *Epilepsy Res* 1993;15:113–131.

92. Jeavons PM, Clark JE. Sodium valproate in treatment of epilepsy. *BMJ* 1974;2:584–586.

93. Mattson RH, Cramer JA. Crossover from polytherapy to monotherapy in primary generalized epilepsy. *Am J Med* 1988;84 [Suppl]:23–28.

86

VALPROIC ACID

CLINICAL EFFICACY AND USE IN EPILEPSY

BLAISE F. D. BOURGEOIS

Since its first clinical use in France in 1964 (20), valproate, or valproic acid (VPA), rapidly established itself worldwide as a major antiepileptic drug against several types of seizures. It was soon recognized as a highly effective first-line drug against the generalized seizures encountered in idiopathic or primary generalized epilepsies: absence, generalized tonic-clonic, and myoclonic seizures (58). Clinical experience with VPA has continued to grow and is still the subject of numerous studies and publications. Antiepileptic therapy with VPA has been the subject of several reviews (14,42,79,91).

SPECTRUM OF EFFICACY

Evidence from Randomized Controlled Clinical Trials

Absence Seizures

When VPA was released for clinical use in North America in 1978, the primary indication was the treatment of absence seizures. The efficacy of VPA and ethosuximide in the treatment of absence seizures was found to be equal in at least two comparison studies (19,86). In a double-blind, crossover study of 16 patients not previously treated for absence seizures and in 29 treatment-refractory patients, the measure of efficacy was based on the frequency and duration of 3/sec generalized spike-and-wave bursts on 12-hour telemetered electroencephalographic (EEG) recordings (86). In the patients who had not previously received antiepileptic therapy, VPA and ethosuximide were equally effective.

Partial Seizures

The most comprehensive assessment of VPA in the treatment of partial and secondarily generalized seizures was car-

ried out by Mattson et al. (70), in what can be qualified as a landmark study. In a multicenter, double-blind trial, 480 adults with complex partial or secondarily generalized tonic-clonic seizures were randomly assigned to monotherapy with carbamazepine or VPA. Targeted serum levels were 7 to 8 µg/mL for carbamazepine and 80 to 100 µg/mL for VPA. The following efficacy indicators were determined at 12 and 24 months of treatment: seizure count per 12 months, seizure rate per month, percentage of patients without seizure, seizure rating score, the time to first seizure, and a seizure rating score representing a weighted sum of generalized tonic-clonic, complex partial, and simple partial seizures. Systemic toxicity and neurotoxicity were also quantified, and they were combined with the efficacy variables into a composite score (0 to 20 representing a good clinical outcome, and >50 representing an unacceptable outcome). No difference in efficacy between carbamazepine and VPA was found for secondarily generalized tonic-clonic seizures. In the treatment of complex partial seizures, four of five efficacy indicators were significantly in favor of carbamazepine. The composite score for efficacy and toxicity was the same for both drugs in patients with generalized tonic-clonic seizures. In the group of patients with complex partial seizures, the composite score was significantly better for carbamazepine (6.8) than for VPA (16.0) at 12 months, but not at 24 months. From these results, it appears that VPA is one of the drugs of choice in the treatment of secondarily generalized tonic-clonic seizures, and it is a valuable alternative in the treatment of complex partial seizures. Although the composite score is an excellent indicator of efficacy for the comparison of drugs, it is difficult to attribute a relative weight to different side effects, and this relative weight can vary from one patient to another.

These additional randomized studies confirmed that VPA is a valuable first-line treatment for newly diagnosed partial epilepsy in adults. Callaghan et al. (18) compared monotherapy with carbamazepine, phenytoin, and VPA in 181 previously untreated patients, with a median follow-up

Blaise F. D. Bourgeois, MD: Professor of Neurology, Harvard Medical School; and Director, Division of Epilepsy and Clinical Neurophysiology, Children's Hospital Boston, Boston, Massachusetts

ranging from 14 to 24 months. In the 79 patients with simple or complex partial seizures, there was no significant difference among the three drugs with regard to both seizure reduction and complete control of seizures. In another series of 140 adults with previously untreated seizures, monotherapy with phenytoin and VPA was compared in a randomized design; 76 patients had tonic-clonic seizures only, and 64 patients had predominantly complex partial seizures (99). Using time to 2-year remission and time to first seizure as the measures of efficacy, the authors could find no difference between the two drugs in either group. Among patients with partial seizures, 27% had a 2-year remission while they were receiving VPA, and 29% had a similar remission while they were taking phenytoin. In the trial by Richens et al. (81a), conducted in 300 patients with primarily generalized tonic-clonic seizures or partial seizures, with or without secondary generalization, VPA was equally effective as carbamazepine, regardless of seizure type; however, carbamazepine was associated with a higher withdrawal rate because of adverse events (15% versus 5% on VPA), and therefore more patients taking VPA than carbamazepine (90% versus 75%) remained on the allocated treatment for at least 6 months.

Two comparative studies of VPA were carried out in children (30,103); 260 children with newly diagnosed primary generalized or partial epilepsy were randomized to VPA or carbamazepine and were followed-up for 3 years (103). The doses were titrated as needed and as tolerated according to clinical response. Equal efficacy was found for the two drugs against generalized and partial seizures, and adverse events were mostly mild for both drugs. Four drugs—phenobarbital, phenytoin, carbamazepine, and VPA—were compared in 167 children with untreated tonic-clonic or partial seizures entered into a randomized, unblinded study (30). Based on time to first seizure and to 1-year remission, there was no difference in efficacy at 1, 2, or 3 years. Unacceptable side effects necessitating withdrawal occurred in six of 10 patients receiving phenobarbital, which was prematurely eliminated from the study; such side effects occurred in 9% of children receiving phenytoin and in 4% each of children taking carbamazepine or VPA.

More recently, VPA was evaluated in 143 adult patients with poorly controlled partial epilepsy who were randomized to monotherapy with VPA at low levels (25 to 50 mg/L) or high levels (80 to 150 mg/L) (8). The reduction in the frequency of both complex partial and secondarily generalized tonic-clonic seizures was significantly higher among patients in the high-level group.

In a study of patients with complex partial seizures not controlled by carbamazepine or phenytoin, patients were randomized to add-on VPA or add-on placebo (110). In the intent-to-treat analysis of 137 patients, those treated with VPA experienced a median reduction of 7.9 complex partial seizures per 8 weeks, and 38% of them had a seizure reduction of ≥50%. The corresponding numbers for the placebo group were 2.5 and 19%, respectively, both differences being statistically significant.

Evidence from Other Studies

Absence Seizures

A reduction of spike-and-wave discharges was demonstrated repeatedly when VPA was administered to patients with typical and atypical absences (1,6,11,67,71). In a group of 25 patients with absence seizures who were treated with VPA for 10 weeks, 19 patients experienced a reduction in seizure frequency, and 21 had a reduction in the total time of spike-and-wave discharge (105). The reduction was >75% in 11 patients. In various series, complete control of simple absence seizures was achieved with VPA monotherapy in 10 of 12 patients (46), 11 of 12 patients (26), 14 of 17 patients (37), and 20 of 21 patients (10). Complete control of absence seizures appears to be more likely when they occur alone than when they occur in combination with another seizure type (10,46). When atypical or "complex" absences are included, results are generally less favorable than in patients with simple absences only (26,35). Absence seizures refractory to VPA and ethosuximide given alone may respond well to a combination of these drugs (85a). VPA and lamotrigine in combination have also been reported to be valuable in refractory absence seizures (36a). Oral VPA was also found to be highly effective in the prevention of recurrent absence status epilepticus (7). In an open evaluation of 25 patients, the yearly frequency of attacks of absence status was decreased from an average of 5.7 to 0.6. The results were clearly better in the 18 patients who had primary generalized epilepsy. Experience has also suggested that VPA is a useful drug in the treatment of myoclonic absence epilepsy (104).

Generalized Tonic-Clonic Seizures

Although it was initially used for the treatment of absences, VPA has since been recognized to be effective in convulsive seizures as well (34, 80, 93, 100). Therapy with VPA as the only drug was used in 36 patients with primary tonic-clonic seizures, of whom 24 had been previously treated with other antiepileptic drugs (26). Complete seizure control was achieved in 33 patients. In a series of 100 children with intractable epilepsy, grand mal seizures were completely controlled by the addition of VPA in 14 of 42 patients (46). Wilder et al. (109) compared VPA with phenytoin in 61 previously untreated patients with generalized tonic-clonic, clonic, or tonic seizures in a randomized fashion. No seizures recurred in 73% of patients treated with VPA and in 47% of patients treated with phenytoin. These percentages increased to 82% for VPA and 76% for phenytoin when seizures that had occurred at a time when therapeutic plasma drug levels had not yet been reached were discounted. In another randomized study of the relative efficacy of VPA and phenytoin, a 2-year remission was used as the end point (99). In patients with previously untreated tonic-clonic seizures, this remission was achieved in 27 of 37 cases with VPA and in 22 of 39 cases with phenytoin. In the 3-year randomized trial carried out by Richens et al. (81a), patients with primarily generalized tonic-clonic seizures achieved higher 12-month remission rates with VPA than with carbamazepine (76% versus 62%). The average dosage of VPA required to control primarily generalized tonic-clonic seizures was also lower than that required to control partial seizures (821 versus 1,066 mg/day). In two studies of monotherapy for primary (or idiopathic) generalized epilepsies with VPA, complete control of generalized tonic-clonic seizures was achieved in 51 of 70 patients (37) and in 39 of 44 patients (10) in whom only these types of seizures occurred. Excellent results for generalized tonic-clonic seizures were also obtained with VPA monotherapy in children (33).

Myoclonic Seizures

VPA is the drug of first choice against myoclonic seizures occurring in patients with primary or idiopathic generalized epilepsies (10,26,37). Sixteen of 23 patients with myoclonic epilepsy of adolescence had complete seizure control with VPA monotherapy (26). Among 22 patients with myoclonic epilepsy of adolescence and abnormality on intermittent photic stimulation, 17 had complete seizure control, although 17 patients had not responded to previous medications (26). In general, photosensitivity is easily controlled by VPA, whether it is associated with tonic-clonic, absence, or myoclonic seizures (57). A good response to VPA in the treatment of juvenile myoclonic epilepsy was reported by Delgado-Escueta and Enrile-Bacsal (29). In a study of VPA monotherapy for primary generalized epilepsies, myoclonic seizures were suppressed in 18 of 22 patients (10). Twenty of these 22 patients had another type of seizure (either absence or tonic-clonic) in addition to the myoclonic seizures. Good results with VPA monotherapy were also obtained in children with the so-called benign myoclonic epilepsy of infancy (33). VPA has also been used successfully against the postanoxic intention myoclonus (15,83) and, in conjunction with clonazepam, against the myoclonic and tonic-clonic seizures occurring in patients with severe progressive myoclonic epilepsy (51).

Lennox-Gastaut Syndrome and Infantile Spasms

Like all other antiepileptic therapies that have been used so far, therapy with VPA has been less successful for the generalized seizures encountered in the symptomatic generalized epilepsies (e.g., Lennox-Gastaut syndrome) and for the prevention of infantile spasms occurring as part of West's syndrome. There is also much less information available on

the use of VPA in these forms of epilepsy than in the treatment of the primary generalized epilepsies. In the series by Covanis et al. (26), myoclonic absence seizures were fully controlled in three of six patients, but none of the patients was treated with VPA alone. Among their 38 patients with myoclonic astatic epilepsy (a term used by the authors synonymously with Lennox syndrome), only seven patients became and remained seizure free with VPA. However, the addition of VPA was associated with a 50% to 80% improvement in one-third of the patients, and other antiepileptic drugs could be withdrawn or reduced after the introduction of VPA. In their series of 100 children treated with VPA, Henriksen and Johannessen (46) reported that 12 of 27 children with "absences and other seizures" and nine of 39 children with atonic seizures became seizure free.

Several studies on the use of VPA for the prevention of infantile spasms were based either on small numbers of patients (5,76,82) or on a combination of VPA and corticotropin given simultaneously (12,112). In a series of 19 babies with infantile spasms (3), VPA was not used simultaneously with corticotropin. Good spasm control was achieved with VPA as a first drug in eight patients, and these patients therefore did not require corticotropin. The doses of VPA ranged from 20 to 60 mg/kg/day. An analysis of the cases of initial failure with either corticotropin or VPA and subsequent treatment with the other drug revealed a tendency toward a better response to corticotropin. However, treatment with VPA was associated with a lower incidence and severity of side effects. In another study, VPA was given at a dosage of 20 mg/kg/day to 18 infants with infantile spasms who were never treated with corticotropin (78). Short-term results were good to excellent in 12 patients. Follow-up revealed that seven patients still had residual seizures, and 16 had either moderate or severe mental retardation. The results were judged to be similar to those obtained with corticotropin or steroids, but VPA was found to have fewer side effects.

Partial Seizures

Additional information on the effect of VPA against partial seizures is derived in part from small numbers of patients in studies not dealing primarily with partial seizures. In the series by Covanis et al. (26), nine patients with simple partial seizures responded poorly to VPA, and five of 11 patients with complex partial seizures were seizure free while they were taking VPA, mostly in combination with carbamazepine. Among the 100 children with uncontrolled epilepsy reported by Henriksen and Johannessen (46), 13 had simple partial seizures. Of those, only one became seizure free after the addition of VPA, and a seizure reduction of >75% and 50% to 75% was observed in three patients each. Among 19 patients with complex partial seizures, four became seizure free, five experienced a seizure reduction of 75%, and five experienced a seizure reduction of 50% to

75%. In 24 adults with poorly controlled complex partial seizures, Bruni and Albright (13) added VPA to the existing regimen. A >50% seizure reduction was initially achieved in 12 patients, but in seven patients this improvement was temporary. Thus, a long-term benefit was obtained in only five of 24 patients. Better results were observed when VPA was compared with carbamazepine in an open study of 31 previously untreated patients with partial seizures (65). Seizures were completely controlled by VPA in 11 patients and by carbamazepine in eight patients. However, only 19 patients were followed for a period of 1 year.

Gupta and Jeavons (44) compared 40 patients with complex partial seizures who responded to carbamazepine monotherapy with 45 patients who were not seizure free while receiving carbamazepine monotherapy and in whom VPA was added as a second drug. Their response to therapy was analyzed as a function of the side of the interictal EEG abnormality. Carbamazepine alone fully controlled the seizures in 24 of 47 patients who had a left temporal EEG abnormality exclusively and in only seven of 33 patients with a right-sided abnormality. Among those patients whose seizures were not controlled by carbamazepine alone, the addition of VPA was associated with full seizure control in 18 of the 26 patients with a right temporal abnormality and in only one of the 13 patients with a left temporal abnormality. Although these results suggest a better response to carbamazepine alone in patients with a left temporal abnormality and a better response to the addition of VPA to carbamazepine in patients with a right temporal abnormality, a control group with VPA as the only drug was not included in the study. VPA monotherapy in partial seizures was evaluated retrospectively in 30 patients with simple and complex partial seizures who had not tolerated or had not responded to conventional initial drugs (27). Change to VPA monotherapy was associated with surprisingly good results. Twelve patients became seizure free, 10 experienced reduced seizure frequency by more than 50%, and nine were not improved. All generalized components of partial seizures were controlled in these patients. In patients with refractory partial seizures, as in other types of refractory seizures, the combination of VPA and lamotrigine has been found to produce more favorable results than other antiepileptic drug combinations (79a).

Other Uses

The effectiveness of VPA in the prevention of febrile convulsions is well documented (21,75). In a group of 196 children with febrile seizures of whom 69 received prolonged treatment with phenobarbital, 32 with primidone, and 95 with VPA, Minagawa and Miura (72) found no statistical difference in the recurrence rate in the three groups. In other series of children with febrile seizures, VPA was found to be more effective than phenobarbital, placebo, or no treatment (47,60,68).

Although VPA is effective in the prophylaxis of febrile seizures, its use cannot be recommended for this indication. The use of long-term prophylactic treatment in patients with febrile seizures has declined markedly in recent years. This has been mainly the result of a reassessment of the risk:benefit ratio and of the increasing use of intermittent diazepam during febrile episodes. The latter approach was found to be as effective as prophylactic treatment with VPA in a group of children with a high risk of recurrence of febrile seizures (61).

VPA has also been used for the treatment of seizures during the neonatal period. Two newborns whose seizures were not controlled by conventional antiepileptic drugs responded well to a rectal infusion of VPA (95). In a more recent trial, VPA was administered orally as syrup to six neonates who had persistent seizures despite levels of phenobarbital of >40 µg/mL and despite the administration of an additional anticonvulsant in five of the six infants (38). The loading dose of VPA was 20 to 25 mg/kg, and the initial maintenance dose was 5 to 10 mg/kg every 12 hours. The seizures were controlled in all but one infant, a 30-week gestational age newborn with meningitis. An elevation of serum ammonia was observed in all patients. This elevation was reversible despite continuation of the VPA therapy in three cases. Seizures recurred in two cases after VPA was discontinued because of hyperammonemia. The mean VPA elimination half-life in five of these newborns was 26.4 hours, a value considerably higher than in children and adults.

Since it became available for intravenous administration, VPA has been administered for the treatment of status epilepticus. Among 23 patients treated with an intravenous bolus of 15 mg/kg followed by 1 mg/kg/hr, status epilepticus resolved in 19 (39). Eight patients had tonic-clonic status, and the remainder had absence, myoclonic, focal motor, and focal myoclonic status. Intravenous VPA was also used successfully in two patients with juvenile myoclonic epilepsy who were in myoclonic status epilepticus (90). In a group of 41 children with various forms of status epilepticus, intravenous VPA was successful in 78% overall (101). None of the patients with epilepsia partialis continua responded, but the success rate was 67% to 90% in the other groups.

MODE OF USE

Indications and Current Role in Epilepsy Management

VPA is the prime example of a broad-spectrum antiepileptic drug. It has been shown to be potentially effective against every known type of seizure, including neonatal seizures, febrile seizures, and status epilepticus. VPA is clearly the drug of first choice in idiopathic (primary) generalized epilepsies, including juvenile myoclonic epilepsy, juvenile absence epilepsy, childhood absence epilepsy, myoclonic absence epilepsy, and myoclonic astatic epilepsy. It is also often used as a drug of first choice in cryptogenic or symptomatic generalized epilepsies such as Lennox-Gastaut syndrome, as well as in most cases of myoclonic seizures, regardless of the syndrome. In patients with infantile spasms, VPA is often used as a drug of second choice, occasionally as a first drug. VPA is used as a drug of first or second choice against generalized tonic-clonic seizures without evidence of focal onset. Against simple or complex partial seizures without or with secondary generalization, VPA is commonly used as a drug of second choice, in certain countries as a first drug. VPA is often used in patients with benign focal epilepsies of childhood. It is currently uncommon for VPA to be used in neonatal seizures. Risk:benefit considerations preclude VPA from being used in the prophylaxis of febrile seizures.

Dosing Recommendations

In various parts of the world, the drug is marketed as VPA, sodium VPA, magnesium VPA, sodium hydrogen divalproate, or valpromide, the amide of VPA. VPA is available as oral syrup, immediate-release formulations, and enteric-coated tablets or sprinkles. Slow-release oral preparations and intravenous formulations are available in certain countries. Although VPA syrup has been used for rectal administration (24,98), sodium VPA suppositories are available in certain countries. In volunteers, the relative bioavailability of VPA suppositories was 80% compared with oral syrup, and the time to maximal concentration was longer (3.1 hours versus 1.0 hour) (50). In another study, suppositories were found to be well tolerated, even when administered for several days, and to have the same bioavailability as the oral preparations (56). Comparison of enteric-coated sprinkles with syrup in 12 children showed no difference in overall bioavailability, but the absorption of VPA was slower from sprinkles. The time to maximal concentration was 4.2 hours with sprinkles and 0.9 hour with syrup (23). Divalproex sodium extended-release tablets have become available, which are intended for once-a-day oral administration. Compared with delayed-release tablets given twice daily, these tablets were found to have a relative bioavailability of 81% to 89%, and they produced fluctuations of serum levels that were 10% to 20% lower (*unpublished data,* Abbott Laboratories, North Chicago, IL).

The question of the appropriate daily dose of VPA has been addressed in numerous reports. The recommended initial dose is 10 to 15 mg/kg/day. The dose may be increased as necessary, and as tolerated, by 5 to 10 mg/kg/day at weekly intervals. Because of pronounced pharmacokinetic interactions, the dose of VPA will differ markedly between patients receiving VPA monotherapy and patients receiving combination therapy, if similar concentrations are to be achieved. Furthermore, the adequate VPA dose or concentration can be a function of the patient's seizure type (66,81a). In patients receiving VPA monotherapy, doses between 10 and 20 mg/kg/day usually achieve a good clinical response and result in concentrations within the generally accepted therapeutic range (10,37, 46,109). Because of age-dependent kinetics, younger children may require higher doses (26,81). Patients receiving combination therapy will almost invariably need higher doses if the same concentrations are to be obtained, usually between 30 and 60 mg/kg/day. This effect of comedication is particularly pronounced in children, in whom VPA concentrations in the accepted therapeutic range often cannot be achieved, even with doses >100 mg/kg/day (46).

If the therapeutic levels of VPA are to be achieved rapidly or in patients who are unable to take oral medications, VPA can be administered intravenously (31). This route has also been suggested for the treatment of status epilepticus, with a loading dose of 15 mg/kg (given at a rate of 20 mg/min) followed by 1 mg/kg/hr (39). An alternative loading dose of 20 mg/kg a rate of 33.3 to 555 mg/min (62), or ≤6 mg/kg/min (108), has been advocated. Overall, such rapid intravenous loading with VPA has been well tolerated (74,92). In those receiving intravenous replacement therapy or bolus administration, subsequent doses should be given within 6 hours because of the precipitous fall in VPA levels.

A curvilinear relationship between VPA dose and concentration was reported by Gram et al. (43), with relatively smaller increases in concentrations at higher doses. Among the different possible explanations, the most likely seems to be a higher free fraction at higher concentrations, resulting in a higher total drug clearance. This explanation implies that the relationship between dosage and concentration of free, pharmacologically active drug is in fact linear. When therapeutic levels of VPA are to be achieved rapidly, a loading dose of 12.5 mg/kg given orally has been shown to be adequate (84). Although it is a common practice to divide the daily dose of VPA into two or three single doses because of the short elimination half-life, equally good results were obtained when VPA was administered as a single daily dose (26,40,94). In patients with primary generalized epilepsy, a mean VPA dose of 15.6 mg/kg/day administered once daily was adequate (94). Even though maximal concentrations were about twice as high as minimal concentrations, side effects were rare. Sixteen patients with juvenile myoclonic epilepsy were randomized in a double-blind fashion to monotherapy with VPA at 1,000 and 2,000 mg/day (96,97). The higher dose, with a mean level of 700 μmol/L, did not result in better seizure control than 1,000 mg/day with a mean level of 470.4 μmol/L.

What is the concentration–effect relationship for VPA, and what is the value of determining plasma or serum concentrations? There are two main reasons for the difficulties associated with interpretation of VPA levels obtained in patients: first, VPA levels fluctuate considerably during a 24-hour period because of the short half-life; and second, no good correlation between VPA levels and clinical effects at a given time has been demonstrated so far. Studying the photoconvulsive response in humans, Rowan et al. (85) found that reduction or abolition of photosensitivity in the EEG occurred on the average 3 hours after peak serum VPA levels had been achieved and persisted for hours as the levels continued to decrease. Burr et al. (17) measured the course of spike-and-wave discharge rate in the EEG and analyzed its relationship with fluctuations in VPA levels. They found no significant correlation, whether they analyzed the actual discharge profile or the profile of changes in discharge rate. During long-term VPA therapy, a continued reduction of spike-and-wave activity or seizure frequency occurred even after a steady state had been reached (10, 12,14). This phenomenon is probably not the result of delayed brain penetration, selective concentration, or slow elimination of VPA from the brain, because a good correlation between the brain and cerebrospinal fluid concentration and free plasma concentrations could be demonstrated in patients undergoing neurosurgery (102). In a more recent report, VPA was found to have the lowest brain: blood ratio of all major antiepileptic drugs, with a fourfold range among patients (89).

In a group of 25 patients with absence seizures, Villareal et al. (105) found no correlation between plasma VPA concentrations and EEG changes, but these investigators observed a clinical response when levels reached 50 to 60 μg/mL (347 to 417 μmol/L). Among children with absence seizures, those who became seizure free during VPA monotherapy had a mean plasma concentration of 83.1 μg/mL (VPA as a first drug) and 59.6 μg/mL (patients previously refractory to ethosuximide) (86). In a group of 28 children whose seizures were completely controlled by VPA monotherapy, the mean plasma level was 65.1 μg/mL (452 μmol/L) (59). Farrell et al. (36) found serum levels of 140 to 420 μmol/L (20.2 to 50.5 μg/mL) by gas chromatography and 210 to 560 μmol/L (30.2 to 80.6 μg/mL) by enzyme-multiplied immunoassay test (EMIT) in 80% of children with complete seizure control. Ishikawa et al. (52) reported mean levels of 47.8 to 85.2 μg/mL (322 to 592 μmol/L) in children whose seizures were well controlled. Younger children had lower average concentrations, and half of them had their seizures controlled with levels of <50 μg/mL (350 μmol/L). In the series by Covanis et al. (26), mean serum levels in seizure-free patients ranged from 82 to 109.5 μg/mL (569 to 760 μmol/L), and these authors recommend a therapeutic range of 60 to 120 μg/mL (417 to 833 μmol/L). In seven children with absence epilepsy, VPA concentrations of 440 to 660 μmol/L (63 to 95 μg/mL) were necessary to achieve a reduction of EEG seizure discharges by ≥50% (11). There is no evidence in any of the studies cited earlier that VPA was actually increased to the minimally effective dose or concentration. In the series by Henriksen and Johannessen (46), clinical effect was observed only after the fasting serum VPA levels had reached values of about 300 μmol/L (43.2 μg/mL), and

seizure control was frequently achieved only after these levels had persisted for 2 to 4 weeks. Lethargy and drowsiness were noticed at levels >600 μmol/L in almost all cases. In previously untreated adults, adverse effects were common when plasma VPA levels were >100 μg/mL (700 μmol/L) during monotherapy, and primarily generalized tonic-clonic seizures did not occur at levels of >50 μg/mL (350 μmol/L) (98). A lower limit for the prevention of partial seizures could not be determined in this study.

Based on their finding of a good linear correlation between VPA dose and level in patients receiving monotherapy, Lundberg et al. (66) considered that monitoring VPA levels was not necessary in these patients. In a group of 88 children receiving VPA monotherapy, those with certain side effects had received significantly higher doses than patients without side effects (48). However, a relationship between the incidence of side effects and plasma VPA levels could not be established, except for children presenting with lassitude and drowsiness, whose levels were significantly higher (mean values of 94.5 and 80.4 μg/mL, respectively). In their study on the prevention of febrile seizures, Herranz et al. (47) found no difference in doses or plasma levels among patients with or without recurrence of seizures or side effects. However, patients with side effects were receiving a higher VPA dose. Schobben et al. (87) also found that the therapeutic effect correlated better with the VPA dose in milligrams per kilogram of body weight than with the plasma concentration. Gram et al. (43) concluded that seizure control was better at serum levels of 300 to 350 μmol/L (43 to 50 μg/mL) than at lower values, but they found no correlation between VPA levels and side effects. The value of a single trough level of VPA was questioned by Loiseau et al. (64), based on the observation that the mean fluctuation in concentrations was 113% during a 24-hour period, and consecutive fasting levels were not reproducible.

In conclusion, although VPA levels can be valuable in selected cases, and particularly during combination therapy, a single measurement is often of limited value, and results should be interpreted cautiously (22). Rigid adherence by the physician to the indicated therapeutic range, usually 50 to 100 μg/mL (350 to 700 μmol/L), is not likely to be beneficial to the patient. Saliva VPA levels are of little use because they do not seem to correlate well with plasma levels (41).

Contraindications and Precautions

VPA is contraindicated in patients with hepatic disease, significant hepatic dysfunction, metabolic disorders associated with an increased susceptibility to liver toxicity, or known hypersensitivity to VPA. Box warnings included in the package insert include potentially fatal hepatotoxicity, pancreatitis, and teratogenicity (e.g., spina bifida). The possible adverse effects of VPA are discussed in Chapter 89 and are not reviewed here. However, the risk of some of these adverse effects can be reduced if certain precautions are taken in patients treated with VPA.

Because infants <3 years old who were taking VPA with other antiepileptic drugs were found to have the highest risk of fatal hepatotoxicity (16), VPA therapy should be preferably avoided in this age group. Benign elevation of liver enzymes can be seen with VPA, and severe hepatotoxicity is usually not preceded by elevation of liver enzymes. Although routine monitoring of liver enzymes during VPA therapy is a common practice, the diagnosis of hepatotoxicity depends mostly on early recognition of the clinical features, which include nausea, vomiting, anorexia, lethargy, and at times loss of seizure control, jaundice, or edema. Similarly, the occurrence of abdominal pain, nausea, vomiting, or anorexia requires evaluation for the possibility of pancreatitis.

Supplementation with L-carnitine may be beneficial in certain patients taking VPA (32,73). Currently, intravenous L-carnitine supplementation is indicated for VPA-induced hepatotoxicity, overdose, or other acute metabolic crisis associated with carnitine deficiency (32). L-Carnitine supplementation is also indicated for the primary plasmalemmal carnitine transporter defect. L-Carnitine supplementation is suggested in the following circumstances: patients with certain secondary carnitine deficiency syndromes, symptomatic VPA-associated hyperammonemia, multiple risk factors for VPA hepatotoxicity or renal-associated syndromes, infants and young children taking VPA, patients with epilepsy using the ketogenic diet who have hypocarnitinemia, patients receiving dialysis, and premature infants who are receiving total parenteral nutrition. The recommended oral L-carnitine dosage is 100 mg/kg/day up to a maximum of 2 g/day. It does not appear that VPA lowers carnitine levels in otherwise healthy and well-nourished children (49). Investigators have suggested that comedication with topiramate represents a risk factor for VPA-induced hypoammonemic encephalopathy (45). Similarly, an association between treatment with VPA and complications of the ketogenic diet has been suggested (4).

One should routinely monitor blood count, including the platelet count, in patients taking VPA. Thrombocytopenia is by far the most frequently diagnosed hematologic adverse effect of VPA, and it is much more common at higher VPA levels (28). Some physicians discontinue VPA therapy before surgical intervention because of VPA-mediated disturbances of hemostasis, although no objective evidence of excessive operative bleeding has been found (2,106,111).

In women, VPA can cause menstrual irregularities (69), hormonal changes, (53–55), and pubertal arrest (25). One concern has been the increasing recognition of the frequent association between VPA therapy and polycystic ovaries (53–55,88). Treatment with VPA during the first trimester of pregnancy has been found to be associated with an estimated 1% to 2% risk of neural tube defect in the newborn

(9,63,77). Folate supplementation may reduce the risk (107), and a daily dose of at least 1 mg should be recommended to all female patients of childbearing age who are taking VPA. The possible endocrinologic and teratogenic adverse effects of VPA should be discussed with every woman of childbearing age in whom treatment with VPA is being considered.

REFERENCES

1. Adams DJ, Lüders H, Pippenger CE. Sodium valproate in the treatment of intractable seizure disorders: a clinical and electroencephalographic study. *Neurology* 1978;28:152–157.
2. Anderson GD, Lin YX, Berge C, et al. Absence of bleeding complications in patients undergoing cortical surgery while receiving valproate treatment. *J Neurosurg* 1997;87:252–256.
3. Bachman DS. Use of valproic acid in treatment of infantile spasms. *Arch Neurol* 1982;39:49–52.
4. Ballaban-Gil K, Callahan C, O'Dell C, et al. Complications of the ketogenic diet. *Epilepsia* 1998;39:744–748.
5. Barnes SE, Bower BD. Sodium valproate in the treatment of intractable childhood epilepsy. *Dev Med Child Neurol* 1975;17:175–181.
6. Bergamini L, Mutani R, Fulan PM. The effect of sodium valproate (Epilim) on the EEG. *Electroencephalogr Clin Neurophysiol* 1975;39:429.
7. Berkovic SF, Andermann F, Guberman A, et al. Valproate prevents the recurrence of absence status. *Neurology* 1989;39:1294–1297.
8. Beydoun A, Sackellares JC, Shu V. Safety and efficacy of divalproex sodium monotherapy in partial epilepsy: a double-blind, concentration-response design clinical trial. Depakote monotherapy for partial seizures study group. *Neurology* 1997;48:182–188.
9. Bjerkedal T, Czeizel A, Goujard J, et al. Valproic acid and spina bifida. *Lancet* 1982;2:1096.
10. Bourgeois B, Beaumanoir A, Blajev B, et al. Monotherapy with valproate in primary generalized epilepsies. *Epilepsia* 1987;28 [Suppl 2]:S8–S11.
11. Braathen G, Theorell K, Persson A, et al. Valproate in the treatment of absence epilepsy in children. *Epilepsia* 1988;29:548–552.
12. Brachet-Liermain A, Demarquez JL. Pharmacokinetics of dipropylacetate in infants and young children. *Pharm Week* 1977;112:293–297.
13. Bruni J, Albright P. Valproate acid therapy for complex partial seizures: its efficacy and toxic effects. *Arch Neurol* 1983;40:135–137.
14. Bruni J, Wilder BJ. Valproic acid: review of a new antiepileptic drug. *Arch Neurol* 1979;36:393–398.
15. Bruni J, Willmore LJ, Wilder BJ. Treatment of postanoxic intention myoclonus with valproic acid. *Can J Neurol Sci* 1979;6:39–42.
16. Bryant A, Dreifuss FE. Valproic acid hepatic fatalities. III. U.S. experience since 1986. *Neurology* 1996;46:465–469.
17. Burr W, Fröscher W, Hoffmann F, et al. Lack of significant correlation between circadian profiles of valproic acid serum levels and epileptiform electroencephalographic activity. *Ther Drug Monit* 1984;6:179–181.
18. Callaghan N, Kenny RA, O'Neill B, et al. A prospective study between carbamazepine, phenytoin and sodium valproate as monotherapy in previously untreated and recently diagnosed patients with epilepsy. *J Neurol Neurosurg Psychiatry* 1985;48:639–644.

19. Callaghan N, O'Hare J, O'Driscoll D, et al. Comparative study of ethosuximide and sodium valproate in the treatment of typical absence seizures (petit mal). *Dev Med Child Neurol* 1982; 24:830–836.

20. Carraz G, Gau R, Chateau R, et al. Communication à propos des premiers essais cliniques sur l'activité anti-épileptique de l'acide *n*-dipropylacétique (sel de Na⁺). *Ann Med Psychol (Paris)* 1964;122:577–585.

21. Cavazzutti GB. Prevention of febrile convulsions with dipropylacetate (Depakine). *Epilepsia* 1975;16:645–648.

22. Chadwick DW. Concentration-effect relationships of valproic acid. *Clin Pharmacokinet* 1985;10:155–163.

23. Cloyd J, Kriel R, Jones-Saete C, et al. Comparison of sprinkle versus syrup formulations of valproate for bioavailability, tolerance, and preference. *J Pediatr* 1992;120:634–638.

24. Cloyd JC, Kriel RL. Bioavailability of rectally administered valproic acid syrup. *Neurology* 1981;31:1348–1352.

25. Cook JS, Bale JF, Hoffman RP. Pubertal arrest associated with valproic acid therapy. *Pediatr Neurol* 1992;8:229–231.

26. Covanis A, Gupta AK, Jeavons PM. Sodium valproate: monotherapy and polytherapy. *Epilepsia* 1982;23:693–720.

27. Dean JC, Penry JK. Valproate monotherapy in 30 patients with partial seizures. *Epilepsia* 1988;29:140–144.

28. Delgado MR, Riela AR, Mills J, et al. Thrombocytopenia secondary to high valproate levels in children with epilepsy. *J Child Neurol* 1994;9:311–314.

29. Delgado-Escueta AV, Enrile-Bacsal F. Juvenile myoclonic epilepsy of Janz. *Neurology* 1984;34:285–294.

30. deSilva M, MacArdle B, McGowan M, et al. Randomised comparative monotherapy trial of phenobarbitone, phenytoin, carbamazepine, or sodium valproate for newly diagnosed childhood epilepsy. *Lancet* 1996;347:709–713.

31. Devinsky O, Leppik I, Willmore LJ, et al. Safety of intravenous valproate. *Ann Neurol* 1995;38:670–674.

32. DeVivo D, Bohan T, Coulter D, et al. L-Carnitine supplementation in childhood epilepsy: current perspectives. *Epilepsia* 1998;39:1216–1225.

33. Dulac O, Steru D, Rey E, et al. Sodium valproate monotherapy in childhood epilepsy. *Brain Dev* 1986;8:47–52.

34. Dulac O, Steru D, Rey E, et al. Monothérapie par le valproate de sodium dans les épilepsies de l'enfant. *Arch Fr Pediatr* 1982;39:347–352.

35. Erenberg G, Rothner AD, Henry CE, et al. Valproic acid in the treatment of intractable absence seizures in children: a single-blind clinical and quantitative EEG study. *Am J Dis Child* 1982; 136:526–529.

36. Farrell K, Abbott FS, Orr JM, et al. Free and total serum valproate concentrations: their relationship to seizure control, liver enzymes and plasma ammonia in children. *Can J Neurol Sci* 1986;13:252–255.

36a. Ferrie CD, Robinson RO, Knott C, et al. Lamotrigine as an add-on drug in typical absence seizures. *Acta Neurol Scand* 1995; 91:200–202.

37. Feuerstein J. A long-term study of monotherapy with sodium valproate in primary generalized epilepsy. *Br J Clin Pract* 1983; 27[Suppl 1]:17–23.

38. Gal P, Oles KS, Gilman JT, et al. Valproic acid efficacy, toxicity and pharmacokinetics in neonates with intractable seizures. *Neurology* 1988;38:467–471.

39. Giroud M, Gras D, Escousse A, et al. Use of injectable valproic acid in status epilepticus: a pilot study. *Drug Invest* 1993;5: 154–159.

40. Gjerloff I, Arentsen J, Alving J, et al. Monodose versus 3 daily doses of sodium valproate: a controlled trial. *Acta Neurol Scand* 1984;69:120–124.

41. Gorodischer R, Burtin P, Verjee Z, et al. Is saliva suitable for therapeutic monitoring of anticonvulsants in children: an elevation in the routine clinical setting. *Ther Drug Monit* 1997;19: 637–642.

42. Gram L, Bentsen KD. Valproate: an update review. *Acta Neurol Scand* 1985;72:129–139.

43. Gram L, Flachs H, Würtz-Jorgensen A, et al. Sodium valproate, serum level and clinical effect in epilepsy: a controlled study. *Epilepsia* 1979;20:303–312.

44. Gupta AK, Jeavons PM. Complex partial seizures: EEG foci and response to carbamazepine and sodium valproate. *J Neurol Neurosurg Psychiatry* 1985;45:131–138.

45. Hamer HM, Knake S, Schomburg U, et al. Valproate-induced hyperammonemic encephalopathy in the presence of topiramate. *Neurology* 2000;54:230–232.

46. Henriksen O, Johannessen SI. Clinical and pharmacokinetic observations on sodium valproate - a 5–year follow-up study in 100 children with epilepsy. *Acta Neurol Scand* 1982;65:504–523.

47. Herranz JL, Armijo JA, Arteaga R. Effectiveness and toxicity of phenobarbital, primidone and sodium valproate in the prevention of febrile convulsions, controlled by plasma levels. *Epilepsia* 1984;25:89–95.

48. Herranz JL, Arteaga R, Armijo JA. Side effects of sodium valproate in monotherapy controlled by plasma levels: a study in 88 pediatric patients. *Epilepsia* 1982;23:203–214.

49. Hirose S, Mitsudome A, Yasumoto S, et al. Valproate therapy does not deplete carnitine levels in otherwise healthy children. *Pediatrics* 1998;101:E9.

50. Holmes GB, Rosenfeld WE, Graves NM, et al. Absorption of valproic acid suppositories in human volunteers. *Arch Neurol* 1989;46:906–909.

51. Iivanainen M, Himberg JJ. Valproate and clonazepam in the treatment of severe progressive myoclonus epilepsy. *Arch Neurol* 1982;39:236–238.

52. Ishikawa T, Ogino C, Furuyama M, et al. Serum valproate concentrations in epileptic children with favorable responses. *Brain Dev* 1987;9:283–287.

53. Isojarvi JI, Laatikainen TJ, Knip M, et al. Obesity and endocrine disorders in women taking valproate for epilepsy. *Ann Neurol* 1996;39:579–584.

54. Isojarvi JI, Laatikainen TJ, Pakarinen AJ, et al. Polycystic ovaries and hyperandrogenism in women taking valproate for epilepsy. *N Engl J Med* 1993;19:1383–1388.

55. Isojarvi JI, Rattya J, Myllyla VV, et al. Valproate, lamotrigine, and insulin-mediated risks in women with epilepsy. *Ann Neurol* 1998;43:446–451.

56. Issakainen J, Bourgeois BFD. Bioavailability of sodium valproate suppositories during repeated administration of steady-state in epileptic children. *Eur J Pediatr* 1987;146:404–407.

57. Jeavons PM, Bishop A, Harding GFA. The prognosis of photosensitivity. *Epilepsia* 1986;27:569–575.

58. Jeavons PM, Clark JE, Maheshwari MC. Treatment of generalized epilepsies of childhood and adolescence with sodium valproate (Epilim). *Dev Med Child Neurol* 1977;19:9–25.

59. Klotz U, Schweizer C. Valproic acid in childhood epilepsy: anticonvulsant efficacy in relation to its plasma levels. *Int J Clin Pharmacol Ther Toxicol* 1980;18:461–465.

60. Lee K, Melchoir JC. Sodium valproate versus phenobarbital in the prophylactic treatment of febrile convulsions in childhood. *Eur J Pediatr* 1981;137:151–153.

61. Lee K, Taudorf K, Hvorslev V. Prophylactic treatment with valproic acid or diazepam in children with febrile convulsions. *Acta Paediatr Scand* 1986;75:593–597.

62. Limdi NA, Faught E. The safety of rapid valproic infusion. *Epilepsia* 2000;41:1342–1345.

63. Lindhout D, Meinardi H. Spina bifida and *in utero* exposure to valproate. *Lancet* 1984;2:396.

64. Loiseau P, Cenraud B, Levy RH, et al. Diurnal variations in steady-state plasma concentrations of valproic acid in epileptic patients. *Clin Pharmacokinet* 1982;7:544–552.

65. Loiseau P, Cohadon S, Jogeix M, et al. Efficacité du valproate de sodium dans les épilepsies partielles. *Rev Neurol (Paris)* 1984;140:434–437.

66. Lundberg B, Nergardh A, Boreus LO. Plasma concentrations of valproate during maintenance therapy in epileptic children. *J Neurol* 1982;228:133–141.

67. Maheshwari MC, Jeavons PM. The effect of sodium valproate (Epilim) on the EEG. *Electroencephalogr Clin Neurophysiol* 1975;39:429.

68. Mamelle N, Mamelle JC, Plasse JC, et al. Prevention of recurrent febrile convulsions—a randomized therapeutic assay: sodium valproate, phenobarbital and placebo. *Neuropediatrics* 1984;15:37–42.

69. Margraf JW, Dreifuss FE. Amenorrhea following initiation of therapy with valproic acid. *Neurology* 1981;31:159.

70. Mattson RH, Cramer JA, Collins JF, et al. A comparison of valproate with carbamazepine for the treatment of complex partial seizures and secondarily generalized tonic-clonic seizures in adults. *N Engl J Med* 1992;327:765–771.

71. Mattson RH, Cramer JA, Williamson PD, et al. Valproic acid in epilepsy: clinical and pharmacological effects. *Ann Neurol* 1978;3:20–25.

72. Minagawa K, Miura H. Phenobarbital, primidone and sodium valproate in the prophylaxis of febrile convulsions. *Brain Dev* 1981;3:385–393.

73. Murakami K, Sugimoto T, Woo M, et al. Effect of L-carnitine supplementation on acute valproate intoxication. *Epilepsia* 1996;37:687–689.

74. Naritoku DK, Mueed S. Intravenous loading of valproate for epilepsy. *Clin Neuropharmacol* 1999;22:102–106.

75. Ngwane E, Bower B. Continuous sodium valproate or phenobarbital in the prevention of "simple" febrile convulsions. *Arch Dis Child* 1980;55:171–174.

76. Olive D, Tridon P, Weber M. Action du dipropylacétate de sodium sur certaines variétés d'encéphalopathies épileptogènes du nourrisson. *Schweiz Med Wochenschr* 1969;99:87–92.

77. Omtzigt JGC, Los FJ, Grobbee DE, et al. The risk of spina bifida aperta after first-trimester exposure to valproate in a prenatal cohort. *Neurology* 1992;42[Suppl 5]:119–125.

78. Pavone L, Incorpora G, LaRosa M, et al. Treatment of infantile spasms with sodium dipropylacetic acid. *Dev Med Child Neurol* 1981;23:454–461.

79. Pinder RM, Brodgen RN, Speight TM. Sodium valproate: a review of its pharmacological properties and therapeutic efficacy in epilepsy. *Drugs* 1977;13:81–123.

79a. Pisani F, Oteri G, Russo MF, et al. The efficacy of valproate-lamotrigine comedication in refractory complex partial seizures: evidence for a pharmacodynamic interaction. *Epilepsia* 1999;40:1141–1146.

80. Ramsay RE, Wilder BJ, Murphy JV, et al. Efficacy and safety of valproic acid versus phenytoin as sole therapy for newly diagnosed primary generalized tonic-clonic seizures. *J Epilepsy* 1992;5:55–60.

81. Redenbaugh JE, Sato S, Penry JK, et al. Sodium valproate: pharmacokinetics and effectiveness in treating intractable seizures. *Neurology* 1980;30:1–6.

81a. Richens A, Davidson DLW, Cartlidge NEF, et al. A multicentre comparative trial of sodium valproate and carbamazepine in adult onset epilepsy. *J Neurol Neurosurg Psychiatry* 1996;57:682–687.

82. Rohmann E, Arndi R. The efficacy of Ergenyl (dipropyl acetate) in clonic-, jackknife-, and salaam spasms. *Kinderaerztl Prax* 1976;44:109–113.

83. Rollinson RD, Gilligam BS. Post-anoxic action myoclonus (Lance-Adams syndrome) responding to valproate. *Arch Neurol* 1979;36:44–45.

84. Rosenfeld WE, Leppik IE, Gates JR, et al. Valproic acid loading during intensive monitoring. *Arch Neurol* 1987;44:709–710.

85. Rowan AJ, Binnie CD, Warfield CA, et al. The delayed effect of sodium valproate on the photoconvulsive response in man. *Epilepsia* 1979;20:61–68.

85a. Rouan AJ, Meijer JWA, de Beer Pawlikowski N, et al. Valproate-ethosuximide combination therapy for refractory absence seizures. *Arch Neurol* 1983;40:797–802.

86. Sato S, White BG, Penry JK, et al. Valproic acid versus ethosuximide in the treatment of absence seizures. *Neurology* 1982;32:157–163.

87. Schobben F, van der Kleijn E, Vree TB. Therapeutic monitoring of valproic acid. *Ther Drug Monit* 1980;2:61–71.

88. Sharma S, Jacobs HS. Polycystic ovary syndrome associated with treatment with the anticonvulsant sodium valproate. *Curr Opin Obstet Gynecol* 1997;9:391–392.

89. Shen DD, Ojemann GA, Rapport RL, et al. Low and variable presence of valproic acid in human brain. *Neurology* 1992;42:582–585.

90. Sheth RD, Gidal BE. Intravenous valproic acid for myoclonic status epilepticus. *Neurology* 2000;54:1201–1202.

91. Simon D, Penry JK. Sodium di-*n*-propylacetate (DPA) in the treatment of epilepsy: a review. *Epilepsia* 1975;22:1701–1708.

92. Sinha S, Naritoku DK. Intravenous valproate is well tolerated in unstable patients with status epilepticus. *Neurology* 2000;55:722–724.

93. Spitz MC, Deasy DN. Conversion to valproate monotherapy in nonretarded adults with primary generalized tonic-clonic seizures. *J Epilepsy* 1991;4:33–38.

94. Stefan H, Burr W, Fichsel H, et al. Intensive follow-up monitoring in patients with once daily evening administration of sodium valproate. *Epilepsia* 1974;25:152–160.

95. Steinberg A, Shaley RS, Amir N. Valproic acid in neonatal status convulsion. *Brain Dev* 1986;8:278–279.

96. Sundqvist A, Nilsson BY, Tomson T. Valproate monotherapy in juvenile myoclonic epilepsy: dose-related effects on electroencephalographic and other neurophsyiologic tests. *Ther Drug Monit* 1999;21:91–96.

97. Sundqvist A, Tomson T, Lundkvist B. Valproate as monotherapy for juvenile myoclonic epilepsy: dose-effect study. *Ther Drug Monit* 1998;20:149–157.

98. Thorpy MJ. Rectal valproate syrup and status epilepticus. *Neurology* 1980;30:1113–1114.

99. Turnbull DM, Howel D, Rawlins MD, et al. Which drug for the adult epileptic patient: phenytoin or valproate? *BMJ* 1985;290:816–819.

100. Turnbull DM, Rawlins MD, Weightman D, et al. A comparison of phenytoin and valproate in previously untreated adult epileptic patients. *J Neurol Neurosurg Psychiatry* 1982;45:55–59.

101. Uberall MA, Trollmann R, Wunsiedler U, et al. Intravenous valproate in pediatric epilepsy patients with refractory status epilepticus. *Neurology* 2000;54:2188–2189.

102. Vajda FJE, Donnan GA, Phillips J, et al. Human brain, plasma and cerebrospinal fluid concentration of sodium valproate after 72 hours of therapy. *Neurology* 1981;31:486–487.

103. Verity CM, Hosking G, Easter DJ. A multicentre comparative trial of sodium valproate and carbamazepine in pediatric epilepsy: the Paediatric EPITEG Collaborative Group. *Dev Med Child Neurol* 1995;37:97–108.

104. Verrotti A, Greco R, Chiarelli F, et al. Epilepsy with myoclonic absences with early onset: a follow-up study. *J Child Neurol* 1999;14:746–749.

105. Villareal HJ, Wilder BJ, Willmore LJ, et al. Effect of valproic

acid on spike and wave discharges in patients with absence seizures. *Neurology* 1978;28:886–891.

106. Ward MM, Barbaro NM, Laxer KD, et al. Preoperative valproate administration does not increase blood loss during temporal lobectomy. *Epilepsia* 1996;37:98–101.

107. Wegner C, Nau H. Alteration of embryonic folate metabolism by valproic acid during organogenesis. *Neurology* 1992;42 [Suppl 5]:17–24.

108. Wheless J, Venkataraman V. Safety of high intravenous valproate loading doses in epilepsy patients. *J Epilepsy* 1998;11:319–324.

109. Wilder BJ, Ramsey RE, Murphy JV, et al. Comparison of valproic acid and phenytoin in newly-diagnosed tonic-clonic seizures. *Neurology* 1983;33:1474–1476.

110. Willmore LJ, Shu V, Wallin B, et al. Efficacy and safety of add-on divalproex sodium in the treatment of complex partial seizures. *Neurology* 1996;46:49–53.

111. Winter SL, Kriel RL, Novachec TF, et al. Perioperative blood loss: the effect of valproate. *Pediatr Neurol* 1996;15:19–22.

112. Yokoyama S, Kodama S, Ogini H. Study of the treatment of infantile spasms. *Brain Dev* 1976;8:447–453.

Antiepileptic Drugs, 5th Edition. Edited by R.H. Levy, R.H. Mattson, B.S. Meldrum, and E. Perucca. Lippincott Williams & Wilkins, Philadelphia © 2002.

VALPROIC ACID

CLINICAL EFFICACY AND USE IN OTHER NEUROLOGICAL DISORDERS

STEPHEN D. SILBERSTEIN

Valproic acid is commercially available in the United States in three preparations: valproic acid, sodium valproate (Depakene syrup; Abbott Laboratories, Abbott Park, IL), and divalproex sodium (Depakote; Abbott Laboratories), an enteric-coated, stable coordination compound that contains equal proportions of valproic acid and sodium valproate (1). In this chapter, the term *valproate* is used for these formulations (2). An extended-release form (Depakote-ER; Abbott Laboratories), which allows once-daily dosing and decreased peak related side effects has just become available. The amide of valproic acid, valpromide (Depamide), is available in Europe.

Valproate is an anticonvulsant agent that shows broad-spectrum efficacy against partial and generalized seizure types (3). It is useful and well tolerated as a mood stabilizer in patients with bipolar and schizoaffective disorder, even those who have been unable to tolerate lithium or have failed to respond to this medication (4). Valproate is approved by the U.S. Food and Drug Administration for mania and migraine in the United States. Its use in psychiatric disorders is discussed in Chapter 88.

Five double-blind, placebo-controlled studies (5–9) have confirmed that valproate is an effective migraine treatment. Some investigators have suggested that valproate is especially useful for treating migraineurs who also have mania, seizures, aggressive behavior, or an anxiety disorder (4,10). In addition, studies have shown that it is effective for chronic daily headaches (11) and cluster headaches (12). This chapter reviews the evidence concerning the effectiveness of valproate in migraine and other headache disorders, and provides recommendations on its clinical use in these conditions.

MIGRAINE TREATMENT

The pharmacologic treatment of migraine may be acute (abortive, symptomatic) or preventive (prophylactic) (13, 14), and patients who are experiencing frequent, severe headaches often require both approaches. Acute treatment attempts to abort (reverse or stop the progression of) a headache once it has started. Preventive therapy is given, even in the absence of a headache, to reduce the frequency and severity of anticipated attacks.

The United States Headache Consortium Guidelines (15) recommend preventive treatment under the following circumstances: (a) recurring migraines that, in the patient's opinion, significantly interfere with their daily routines, despite acute treatment; (b) frequent headaches (more than two per week); (c) contraindication, or failure or overuse of acute therapies; (d) use of acute medication more than twice a week; or (e) presence of uncommon migraine conditions, including hemiplegic migraine, basilar migraine, migraine with prolonged aura, or migrainous infarction (to prevent neurologic damage—as based on expert consensus). Medications for prophylactic treatment are more restricted during pregnancy, during which time severe, disabling attacks accompanied by nausea, vomiting, and possibly dehydration are required for chronic treatment to be prescribed (16).

The major medication groups of preventive migraine treatment include β-adrenergic blockers, antidepressants, calcium channel antagonists, serotonin [5-hydroxytryptamine (5-HT)] antagonists, anticonvulsants, and nonsteroidal antiinflammatory drugs (NSAIDs) (13,14). If preventive medication is indicated, the agent should be chosen from one of the major categories, based on side effect profiles and coexistent comorbid conditions (13,14).

MIGRAINE MECHANISMS

There is no certainty about how migraine medications work. Although there are no true animal models for

Stephen D. Silberstein, MD, FACP: Professor of Neurology, Department of Neurology, Jefferson Medical College; and Director, Jefferson Headache Center, Thomas Jefferson University, Philadelphia, Pennsylvania

migraine, a number of innovative models are available for the development of drugs for acute migraine treatment. These models were developed based on either the presumed pathophysiology of the migraine attack or the presumed mechanism of action of an existing migraine drug. Most migraine preventive medications were designed to treat other disorders. Methysergide, however, was developed as a migraine preventive agent, based on the concept that migraine is a serotonin excess disorder and methysergide is a serotonin antagonist. It has been suggested that downregulating the 5-HT$_2$ receptor or modulating the discharge of serotonergic neurons may be involved in migraine prevention (17,18).

Antidromic stimulation of the trigeminal nerve releases substance P, calcitonin gene–related peptide, and neurokinin A from the sensory C-fibers and results in neurogenic inflammation (NI). The released neuropeptides interact with the blood vessel wall, producing dilation, plasma extravasation, and sterile inflammation. Platelet activation is seen on electron micrographs of the interior of these blood vessels (19).

The development of NI results in the breakdown of the blood–brain barrier in the dura mater. Sumatriptan and dihydroergotamine, drugs that are agonists at the presynaptic inhibitory 5-HT$_{1D}$ heteroreceptor, prevent leakage. Neither drug blocks the production of inflammation induced by direct application of neuropeptides to the dural vessels. Methysergide, after long-term, but not acute, administration, worked in this model, consistent with its clinical usefulness as a migraine preventive (20).

NI can be prevented by blocking neuronal transmission. Acute specific headache medications may work by blocking nerve fiber transmission in the trigeminal system rather than by vascular constriction. Elevated calcitonin gene–related peptide levels have been found in the jugular blood during a human migraine attack. The headache is aborted and calcitonin gene–related peptide reduced to control levels by 5-HT$_{1D}$ receptor agonists (21). Other drugs that block NI include valproate, neurosteroids, NSAIDs, and neuropeptide Y.

Diener's group reported brainstem activation in spontaneous migraine attacks (22). Using positron emission tomography to measure regional cerebral blood flow, nine patients who had migraine without aura and right-sided headaches were studied within hours of migraine onset. High regional cerebral blood flow values (compared with the headache-free interval) were found in the cerebrum in the cingulate cortex, the auditory association cortex, and the visual association cortex bilaterally, and in the inferior anterocaudal cingulate cortex on the left side only. There was increased regional cerebral blood flow lateralized to the left in the brainstem anterior to the aqueduct and posterior to the corticospinal tract. Sumatriptan relieved the headache and associated symptoms and reversed the cerebral increase in regional cerebral blood flow, but not the brainstem increase.

This is the first report of brainstem activation during a spontaneous attack of migraine without aura and is most likely a result of brainstem gray matter activation, including the dorsal raphe nucleus (a serotonergic nucleus) and the locus ceruleus (a noradrenergic nucleus).

Migraine may be due to abnormal activation of a network that has normal physiologic functions. The strong familial association of migraine and the association of some varieties of migraine with chromosome 19 suggest an underlying genetic basis with an unknown biologic basis. It is uncertain if migraine with aura and migraine without aura are distinct entities.

A preventive migraine drug could raise the threshold to activation of the migraine process either centrally or peripherally. Drugs could decrease activation of the migraine generator, enhance central antinociception, raise the threshold for spreading depression, or stabilize the more sensitive migrainous nervous system by changing sympathetic or serotonergic tone. Preventive drugs probably work by more than one mechanism. The drugs could, in part, have a peripheral mechanism of action, similar to specific acute medications. Because the prolonged use of most acute medications can cause daily headache and block the effect of preventive drugs, a theoretical problem is created. A clue to this problem may be found in the exceptions, long-acting NSAIDs and dihydroergotamine, which are both acute and preventive medications. Saxena (23) has postulated a primary peripheral mechanism for methysergide, which may work by closing cerebral AVAs, and Moskowitz (24) has shown that both methysergide and valproate block the development of NI in his model.

Valproate's mechanism of action in migraine prophylaxis may be related to facilitation of GABAergic neurotransmission (25–27). Valproate also attenuates plasma extravasation in the Moskowitz model of NI (24) by interacting with the γ-aminobutyric acid type A (GABA$_A$) receptor. The relevant receptor may be on the parasympathetic nerve fibers that project from the sphenopalatine ganglia, where it attenuates nociceptive neurotransmission (28). Valproate-induced increased central enhancement of GABA$_A$ activity may enhance central antinociception (24). Valproate also interacts with the central 5-HT system and reduces the firing rate of midbrain serotonergic neurons (24).

PLACEBO-CONTROLLED, DOUBLE-BLIND TRIALS IN PATIENTS WITH MIGRAINE

In 1992, Hering and Kuritzky (5) evaluated sodium valproate's efficacy in migraine treatment in a double-blind, randomized, crossover study (Table 87.1). Thirty-two patients were divided into two groups and given either 400 mg of sodium valproate or placebo twice a day for 8 weeks. The patients were then crossed over to the opposite treatment for an additional 8 weeks. Three patients dropped out. Sodium valproate was effective in preventing migraine

TABLE 87.1. DOUBLE-BLIND PLACEBO-CONTROLLED CLINICAL TRIALS OF VALPROIC ACID IN MIGRAINE

Study	Patient Population (Diagnostic Criteria)	No.	Design	Dosage (mg/d) Medication	Plasma Valproic Acid Levels	Duration	Responder Rates
Hering and Kuritzky (1992)(5)	Migraine	29	crossover	800mg (400 mg bid)/ sodium valproate	31.1 to 91.9µg /ml	8 Weeks each; total of 16 weeks	86.2% of patients responded better to valproate
Jensen et al. (1994)(6)	Migraine without aura	43	crossover	1,000 to 1,500 mg/ sodium valproate	Mean 73.4µg /ml	32 Weeks	50% valproate 18% placebo
Mathew et al. (1995)(7)	Migraine with/ without aura	107	Parallel-group	500 to 1,500mg/ Divalproex	70 to 120µg /ml	16 Weeks	48% divalproex 14% placebo
Klapper (1995)(8)	Migraine with/ without aura	176	Parallel-group	500 to 1,600 or 1,500 mg/Divalproex	??	10 Weeks	43% divalproex 21% placebo
Silberstein et al. (2000)(9)	Migraine with/ without aura	237	Parallel-group	500 to 1,000 mg/ Divalproex ER		12 Weeks	41% divalproex 28% placebo

or reducing the frequency, severity, and duration of attacks in 86.2% of the remaining 29 patients, whose attacks were reduced from 15.6 to 8.8 a month. The drug was a well tolerated, effective migraine treatment.

Jensen et al., in 1994 (6), studied 43 patients with migraine without aura in a triple-blind, placebo- and dose-controlled, crossover study of slow-release sodium valproate. After a 4-week, medication-free, run-in period, the patients were randomized to sodium valproate (n = 22) or placebo (n = 21). Thirty-four patients completed the trial. Patients randomized to sodium valproate received 1,000 mg/day for the first week. Patients with serum levels below 50 µg/mL were blindly adjusted to 1,500 mg of sodium valproate a day and those with serum levels above 50 µg/mL were continued on 1,000 mg/day. The number of migraine days was 3.5 per 4 weeks during sodium valproate treatment and 6.1 during placebo (*p* = 0.002) treatment. The severity and duration of the migraine attacks that did occur were not affected by sodium valproate when compared with placebo. Fifty percent of the patients had a reduction in migraine frequency to 50% or less for the sodium valproate group, compared with 18% for placebo. During the last 4 weeks of valproate treatment, 65% of patients responded. The mean serum sodium valproate concentration was 73.4 µg/mL after 8 days and 64.2 µg/mL after 12 weeks of treatment. The most common side effects (33% valproate, 16% placebo) were intensified nausea and dyspepsia, tiredness, increased appetite, and weight gain; these usually were mild or moderate. Fifty-eight percent of the patients had no side effects. It was concluded that sodium valproate was an effective and well tolerated prophylactic medication for migraine without aura.

In 1995, in a multicenter, double-blind, randomized, placebo-controlled investigation, Mathew et al. (7) compared the effectiveness and safety of divalproex sodium and placebo in migraine prophylaxis. A 4-week, single-blind, placebo-baseline phase was followed by a 12-week treatment phase (4-week dose adjustment, 8-week mainte-

nance). One-hundred seven patients were randomized to divalproex sodium or placebo (2:1 ratio), with 70 receiving divalproex sodium and 37 receiving placebo. Divalproex sodium and placebo dosages were titrated in blinded fashion during the dose adjustment period to achieve actual/sham trough valproate sodium concentrations of approximately 70 to 120 µg/mL. During the treatment phase, the mean migraine headache frequency per 4 weeks was 3.5 in the divalproex sodium group and 5.7 in the placebo group (*p* ≤ .001), compared with 6.0 and 6.4, respectively, during the baseline phase. Forty-eight percent of the divalproex sodium–treated patients and 14% of the placebo-treated patients showed a 50% or greater reduction in migraine headache frequency from the baseline phase (*p* < .001). Among those with migraine headaches, the divalproex sodium–treated patients reported significantly less functional restriction than the placebo-treated patients and used significantly less symptomatic medication per episode. No significant treatment-group differences in average peak severity or duration of individual migraine headaches were observed. (A nonsignificant decrease in duration was noted.) Treatment was stopped in 13% of the divalproex sodium–treated patients and 5% of the placebo-treated patients because of intolerance, a statistically nonsignificant difference. The authors concluded that divalproex sodium is an effective prophylactic drug for patients with migraine headaches and is generally well tolerated.

Klapper et al. (8) evaluated the efficacy and safety of divalproex sodium as prophylactic monotherapy in a multicenter, double-blind, randomized, placebo-controlled study. During the 4-week, single-blind, baseline-placebo phase, patients completed a headache diary. Patients with two or more migraine attacks during the baseline phase were randomized to a daily divalproex sodium dose of 500, 1,000, or 1,500 mg, or placebo. The experimental phase lasted 12 weeks, the first 4 weeks for dose escalation and the remaining 8 weeks for dose maintenance. The primary efficacy variable was 4-week headache frequency during the experimental phase.

During the experimental phase, the mean reduction in the combined daily divalproex sodium groups was 1.8 migraines per 4 weeks, compared with a mean reduction of 0.5 attacks per 4 weeks in the placebo group. Overall, 43% of divalproex sodium–treated patients achieved ≥50% reduction in their migraine attack rates, compared with 21% of placebo-treated patients. A statistically significant ($p ≤ .05$) dose–response effect across the dose range placebo, 500, 1,000, and 1,500 mg, was observed for both overall reduction in attack frequency and a ≥50% reduction in attack frequency. A nonsignificant decrease in headache duration was noted. With the exception of nausea, whose frequency was 24% in the divalproex groups combined (compared with 7% on placebo; $p = .015$), adverse events were similar in all groups, and most adverse effects were mild or moderate in severity. This study showed divalproex sodium to be an effective migraine prophylactic agent.

Silberstein et al. (9) recruited 237 patients with migraine 12 years of age or older. A 14-day washout period was followed by a 28-day baseline period. Divalproex sodium-extended release (DVS-ER) 500 mg once daily or placebo was administered for 7 days, then titrated up to 1,000 mg for an additional 7 days. After 14 days of treatment, patients could be reduced to 500 mg. During the next 70 days, 98 patients took 1,000 mg DVS-ER and 16 patients took 500 mg DVS-ER. After a total of 84 days of treatment, all patients were tapered to 500 mg, and all medication was stopped at 91 days.

There was a significant reduction in the 4-week headache rate from baseline in those taking DVS-ER compared with placebo (1.2 versus 0.6, $p = .006$; the primary efficacy measure). The secondary efficacy measure (reduction in the number of migraine headache days from baseline) showed a significant benefit for those in the DVS-ER group compared with those in the placebo group (1.7 versus 0.7, $p = .009$). The reduction in the number of migraine headache days during the last 4 weeks of the experimental phase also was substantially greater for the treatment group (2.0 versus 0.7, $p = .001$), and the percentage of patients with at least a 50% reduction in headaches was also greater in the treatment group (41% versus 28%, $p = .024$).

DVS-ER was well tolerated. There was no difference in premature discontinuation and abdominal pain between the two groups. Patients on placebo reported more asthenia, but there was more dyspepsia, nausea, vomiting, tremor, and rash in the DVS-ER group. However, none of the differences was significant.

DVS-ER had twice the efficacy in 4-week headache rate and produced a reduction in the number of 4-week headache days. There were significant decreases in migraine headache rate, migraine headache days, and patients with at least a 50% reduction in migraine headache rate in those who completed the study. DVS-ER is safe and well tolerated at dosages up to 1,000 mg once daily.

OTHER TRIALS IN PATIENTS WITH MIGRAINE

In 1988, in a prospective open trial of valproate, Sorenson (29) studied 22 patients who had severe migraine resistant to previous prophylactic treatment (Table 87.2). Seventeen patients had migraine without aura and five had migraine with aura. The attack frequency ranged from 4 to 16 per month in 21 patients (one had daily headache). The dose of valproate was 600 mg twice a day adjusted upward to a serum level of approximately 700 μmol/L. Follow-up in 3 to 12 months revealed that 11 patients were migraine free, 6 had had a significant reduction in frequency, 1 had had no change, and 4 had dropped out.

In 1991, Viswanathan et al. (30) conducted an open study of 16 patients who had resistant migraine and paroxysmal electroencephalographic changes. The patients were treated with sodium valproate, 200 mg three times a day as an add-on medication. After 2 weeks, 12 patients were headache free and the rest had 50% relief. The drug was continued for 3 months in the totally headache-free patients, whereas the other four patients increased their dose to 800 to 1,000 mg/day. Two of these dropped out, and the other two had complete relief.

Moore, in 1992 (31), reported a retrospective analysis of 207 patients with refractory headache who were treated with valproate 750 to 2,000 mg/day. Patients with either migraine (n = 125) or chronic daily headache (n = 82) were treated with the drug. Sixty-five percent of patients with migraine without aura and 50% of patients with migraine with aura had a good or excellent response (criteria not defined). Patients with mixed headache had a 52% response, whereas those with chronic tension-type headache (TTH) had a 73% response. The average duration of treatment was 246 days.

In 1993, Sianard-Gainko et al. (32) assessed the prophylactic effects of sodium valproate over 6 months in 56 patients with severe primary headaches. Thirty-two patients had migraine without aura, 3 had migraine with aura, 14 had both frequent migraine attacks and TTH, and 7 had only chronic TTH. Twenty-nine percent of the patients overused analgesics or ergotamine. The mean daily dose of sodium valproate (given twice a day) was 928.5 mg. Efficacy was assessed by comparing the number of headache days before treatment and during the sixth month of therapy. In the migraine-only group (n = 35), 60% had a 75% to 100% reduction and 20% had a 50% to 75% reduction in headache days. In the mixed or TTH group, only 33% had a >50% reduction in headache days. Clinical improvement significantly correlated with serum valproic acid levels. These results confirmed that sodium valproate is an effective prophylactic treatment for severe migraine, but is of limited value for TTH, at least when compounded by overuse of symptomatic medication. This study suggested aiming for a valproic acid plasma level between 70 and 90 μg/mL.

TABLE 87.2. OTHER CLINICAL TRIALS OF VALPROIC ACID IN MIGRAINE

Study	Patient Population (Diagnostic Criteria)	No.	Design	Dosage (mg/d)/Other Medication	Plasma Levels	Duration	Responder Rates
Sorensen (1988)(29)	Resistant common or classic migraineurs	22	Open; prospective	600mg Valproate bid adjusted to serum level	100 µg/ml	3 to 12 Months	11 Headache free; 6 significant improvement; 4 dropped out; 1 no effect
Viswanathan et al. (1991)(30)	Migraine with EEG changes	16	Open	600mg/Valproate	??	14 Days	12 Headache-free
Moore (1992) (31)	Migraine; CDH	207	Retrospective review	750 to 2,000mg Divalproex	??	Average 246 days	Migraine with aura 50%; migraine 65%; CDH, mixed 52%; CTTH 73%
Sianard-Gainko et al. (1993)(32)	Migraine with/ without aura	35	Open	928.5mg/ Valproate mean dosage	70 to 90µg/ml	6 Months	60%: 75–100% reduction; 20%: 50–75% Reduction; improvement correlated to plasma level
Coria et al. (1994)(33)	Migraine with/ without aura	62	Open	400mg/ Valproate	Mean 30µg/ml	12 Weeks	69.8% Substantial benefit; no correlation to plasma level
Rothrock (1994)(34)	Intractable headache; migraine; TM; TTH	75	Prospective; open	500mg bid/ Divalproex titrate	<150µg/ml	10 Weeks	TTH 27%; TM 61%; Frequent migraine 85%
Czapinski (1995)(35)	Migraine without aura	32	Open; two groups	600mg,* titrate to 1,422mg**/ Valproate	*<50µg/ml **70 to 100µg/ml	26 Weeks	Better results with higher dose
Klapper (1995)(37)	Migraine with/ without aura	12	Open, crossover	Highest dose tolerated	??	4.5 Months	92% had fewer headache on divalproex compared to propranolol
Kaniecki (1995)(36)	Migraine without aura	37	Single blind crossover comparison to propranolol	Mean dose divalproex 1,414mg; propranolol 168mg	Mean 68.5µg/ml	28 Weeks	Placebo 19%; propranolol 66%; divalproex 66%
Ghose and Niven (1998)(39)	Migraine with/ without aura	27	Open	600 to 2,000 Valproate	<106µg/ml	12 to 24 Moths	50% reduction; 59% at 12 weeks

EEG, electroencephalogram; TM, transformed migraine; CDH, chronic daily headache; CTTH, chronic tension-type headache.
*, Patients with serum levels less than 50 mcgr/ml remained on 600 mg/day.
**, Patients with serum levels above 50 mcgr/ml were titrated up to levels in range of 70 to 100 mcgr/ml (mean dose after titration 1,422 mg/day).

Coria et al., in 1994 (33), conducted an open-label trial of sodium valproate in which they assessed migraine prophylaxis in 62 consecutive patients with severe migraine with and without aura. The patients were given 200 mg of sodium valproate twice a day for 3 months and then asked to withdraw the drug for 3 months. The therapeutic response was measured with a scale of 15 items, which included the frequency and severity of migraine attacks. Substantial benefit was obtained by 69.8% of patients; it lasted 3 months after drug withdrawal in 67.6% of cases, perhaps because of a positive carry-over effect. No significant correlation was found between valproate levels and the

therapeutic response as measured by the migraine assessment scale.

Rothrock et al., in 1994 (34), consecutively recruited 75 patients with intractable headache syndromes. They divided these patients into three groups [frequent migraine (FM; n = 18], transformed migraine (n = 43), and TTH (n = 14)] and treated all 75 with divalproex sodium. Thirty-six patients (48%) reported a ≥50% reduction in headache frequency. Significantly different treatment response rates were found in the three groups: patients with FM improved the most (61%); patients with transformed migraine less (51%); and patients with TTH the least (21%). They concluded that prophylactic treatment with divalproex sodium may be effective in selected patients with intractable headache syndromes and that identification of clinically distinct headache subtypes may assist in predicting response to treatment.

Czapinski, in 1995 (35), assessed the effect of valproic acid in a six-month open study of 32 patients (24 women and eight men) with migraine without aura. For the first month, valproate was slowly increased to a total divided dose of 600 mg/day. Serum valproic acid levels were obtained, and the patients were divided into two groups: (A) those with valproic acid levels below 50 µg/mL (n = 14); and (B) those with levels above 50 µg/mL (n = 18). In group B, the valproate dose was increased until the concentration reached 70 to 100 µg/mL (mean dose, 1,422 mg), whereas group A received the original dose. The outcome measure was the number of days with migraine before and after 2, 4, and 6 months of treatment. Valproate was found to be effective, with its beneficial effect increasing during the course of therapy. Efficacy correlated to serum valproic acid concentrations. Adverse events occurred in 10 patients (gastrointestinal complaints, loss of hair, weight gain), but did not necessitate the discontinuation of therapy.

In 1995, Kaniecki (36) enrolled 37 patients with International Headache Society–diagnosed migraine without aura in a randomized, single-blind, placebo-controlled, crossover study comparing divalproex sodium (mean dosage, 1,414 mg/day) and propranolol prophylaxis. After a 4-week baseline phase followed by a 4-week placebo phase, patients were randomized to either divalproex sodium or propranolol for 12 weeks. After a 4-week washout phase, they were crossed over to the opposite treatment. Thirty-two patients completed the study. Responders were defined as those patients who achieved a greater than 50% reduction in either mean migraine frequency (events per month) or mean number of days with migraine (days per month). Assessment of migraine frequency revealed a significant response to divalproex sodium in 66% of patients, to propranolol in 63% of patients, and to placebo in 19% of patients (compared with baseline). Similar results were seen in assessment of migraine days per month.

Klapper (37) compared divalproex sodium with propranolol in an open-label crossover study in which migraineurs randomly received either divalproex sodium or propranolol. The dose was titrated to the highest level tolerated, and the patients recorded their headaches for 2 months. They were then withdrawn from their first medication over a period of 2 weeks and the process was repeated for the second drug. Twelve patients completed both arms of the study. The number of headaches in the divalproex sodium arm was 10.9 per 2 months compared with 20.4 per 2 months in the propranolol arm, with 92% having fewer headaches when taking divalproex sodium. Nine of the patients who took divalproex sodium (38%) did not complete the study owing to side effects, compared with three patients (13%) who took propranolol. In this study, patients with migraine had significantly fewer headaches when taking divalproex

sodium than when taking propranolol. However, the dropout rate was higher in the divalproex sodium group.

Silberstein and Collins (38) reported on 163 patients who (8) were enrolled in an open-label extension study after completion of either of the two placebo-controlled divalproex sodium trials (7). This represented 198 patient-years of divalproex exposure, with an average dosage of 974 mg/day. Forty-nine percent of patients experienced a ≥50% reduction in migraine headache rates from days 1 to 90. This increased to 70% from days 901 to 1,080, in part because of selective dropout.

A subset of patients who were treated for at least 12 months was analyzed. Patients who discontinued divalproex after 1 year failed to show this improvement up to days 361 to 500, in contrast to patients who remained in the study. Overall, 67% of the patients discontinued divalproex. Reasons included administrative problems (31%), drug intolerance (21%), and treatment ineffectiveness (15%). The most common adverse events were nausea (42%), infection (39%), alopecia (31%), tremor (28%), asthenia (25%), dyspepsia (25%), and somnolence (25%).

Ghose and Niven (39) studied 37 patients from a headache clinic who had a diagnosis of migraine with or without aura. They treated the patients with sodium valproate for 3 months. Response to therapy was defined as a ≥50% reduction in headache frequency. Four noncompliers were identified by plasma drug level monitoring and were excluded from the study. Seventeen (71%) patients improved within 4 to 6 weeks and maintained the improvement for 12 weeks. Between 12 and 24 months, two patients withdrew because of side effects and one because of non–drug-related problems. Twelve of the original 27 patients maintained their response for 12 months or longer. At 13 to 24 months, clinical improvement (percentage reduction in the frequency of migraine attacks) correlated inversely with the plasma drug levels and daily valproate dose among the responders. In this study, patients who did not respond to low-dose (600 mg) valproate were unlikely to benefit from higher doses.

Divalproex has been used in the acute treatment of migraine. Small open studies have suggested that intravenous (i.v.) valproic acid is effective in acute migraine treatment. Fourteen consecutive patients with moderate to severe headaches of 24 to 72 hours' duration were given 500 mg of valproate i.v. over 15 to 30 minutes or 10 mg metoclopramide with 1 mg DHE intramuscularly. In the i.v. valproate group, 71.4% of patients improved to a state of mild or no headache at 1 hour, 85.7% at 2 hours, and 71.4% at 4 hours. Migraine-associated symptoms of nausea, photophobia, and phonophobia showed similar improvement. In the DHE group, 42.8% of patients improved to a state of mild or no headache at 1 and 2 hours and 57.1% at 4 hours (40).

Czapinski and Motyl (41) studied 25 patients (18 women and 7 men) with an acute migraine attack, with or without aura, within 6 hours of onset. They were given either valproate i.v. for 5 minutes at the dosage of 15 mg/kg of body weight, or 0.9% NaCl according to the same protocol. Ten of 13 patients treated with valproate showed a decrease or subsidence of pain, in contrast to 4 of 12 patients in the placebo group. Complete pain relief occurred as soon as 10 minutes, with a range of 10 to 25 minutes (40–42).

STUDIES IN PATIENTS WITH OTHER HEADACHE TYPES

Some of these trials in patients with migraine also included patients with other headache types (31,32,34), and results are discussed in the previous section. Additional studies examined in greater detail the potential usefulness of valproate in other headache types. In 1989, Hering and Kuritzky (12) treated 15 patients with cluster headache (2 chronic and 13 episodic) with sodium valproate in an open pilot study (Table 87.3). The dosage ranged from 600 to 2,000 mg/day. Eleven patients (73.3%) improved: nine reported complete cessation of attacks and two reported marked improvement. There was no correlation between efficacy and valproate plasma levels.

Freitag et al. (43) enrolled 26 patients in a long-term, open-label, flexible-dose study of divalproex sodium for cluster headache prevention. Patients had an inadequate response or had experienced adverse events from preventive therapy. Twenty-one patients had chronic cluster and five had episodic cluster headache. Ten of 15 men and 5 of 6 women with chronic cluster headache had a ≥50% response. Six patients had a complete response and were able to discontinue treatment without recurrence of their cluster headache attacks. The mean degree of improvement was 53.9% for patients with chronic cluster headache and

58.6% for patients with episodic cluster headache. The mean dose of divalproex sodium was 850 mg for episodic cluster headaches and 826 mg for chronic cluster headaches. Five patients had adverse events: one each with a rash, hair breakage, tiredness, nausea, and tremor.

In 1991, Mathew and Ali (11) reported on 32 patients with chronic daily headache who were unresponsive to prior treatment. After a baseline observation period of 1 month, the patients were given divalproex sodium 1,000 to 2,000 mg/day for 3 months. Serum valproic acid levels were between 75 and 100 µg/mL. Two thirds of the patients showed a significant improvement in headache index and headache-free days. The most common side effects were weight gain, tremor, hair loss, and nausea. No liver function abnormalities were noted.

Delva et al. (44) suggested in a case report that valproate was useful to treat migraine induced by selective serotonin reuptake inhibitors.

Freitag et al. (45) assessed the safety and efficacy of divalproex sodium in the long-term treatment of chronic daily headache through a retrospective chart review with data extraction from headache diaries. Six hundred forty-two current patients under treatment with divalproex for chronic daily headache were reviewed; 132 were being treated with divalproex alone. The mean improvement was 47%, with migraine improving approximately 65%. Ninety-three of 132 patients had at least a 50% reduction in headache frequency. In patients who could differentiate their migraine from TTHs, the response of the migraine was better than the TTH component in 33 patients; in 47 patients, both changed at the same rate. Nine patients had an improved response for their TTH compared with their migraines. The remainder of the patients' headaches could not be differentiated clearly into migraine or TTHs, but

TABLE 87.3. CLINICAL TRIALS OF VALPROIC ACID IN OTHER HEADACHE TYPES

Study	Patient Population (Diagnostic Criteria)	No.	Design	Dosage (mg/d)/ Other Medication	Plasma Levels	Duration	Responder Rates
Hering and Kuritzky (1989)(12)	Cluster, chronic episodic	15	Open	600 to 2,000 mg/Valproate	31 to 94 µg/ml	Until end of cluster	73.3% responded; 9/15 complete disappearance; 2/15 marked improvement
Mathew and Ali (1991)(11)	Chronic daily headache	30	Open	1,000 to 2,000mg Divalproex	75 to 100µg/ml	3 Months	2/3 Significant improvement
Freitag et al. (43)	Cluster, chronic and episodic	26 21-chronic 5-episodic	Open	Mean dose Divalproex 800mg— chronic 850mg— episodic		Until end of cycle or mean? Of 11.1 months	Chronic: 15/21 significantly improved Episodic: 3/3 men improved; 2/2 women partially responded
Freitag et al.(45)	Chronic daily headache	132	Open				~75% had at least a 50% reduction in headache frequency

met Silberstein's criteria for transformed migraine. The mean improvement in the migraine-differentiated component was 65.2%, whereas the patients with TTH demonstrated a mean improvement of 45.4% from baseline frequency. There was no correlation between response and age, sex, duration of treatment, and the dose of divalproex sodium given. Adverse events occurred in approximately 31% of patients; none was severe. Women were more likely to experience adverse events than men, but their weight gain was less (average weight gain was 1.9 pounds for women and 7 pounds for men). Divalproex sodium could be used for a long time as the sole drug for the successful treatment of chronic daily headache. Nearly three-fourths of patients had at least a 50% reduction in headache frequency; adverse events occurred in approximately one-third.

TREATMENT CHOICES FOR MIGRAINE

The goals of migraine preventive therapy are to (a) reduce attack frequency, severity, and duration; (b) improve responsiveness to treatment of acute attacks; and (c) improve function and reduce disability. The medications used to treat migraine have been put into the following treatment groups based on their established clinical efficacy, tolerability and safety profile, and the clinical experience of the United States Headache Consortium participants (15):

Group 1. Medications with proven high efficacy and mild to moderate adverse effects.

Group 2. Medications with lower efficacy (i.e., limited number of studies, studies reporting conflicting results, efficacy suggesting only "modest" improvement) and mild to moderate adverse effects.

Group 3. Medication use based on opinion, not randomized, controlled trials.

a. Low to moderate adverse effects

b. Frequent or severe adverse effects (or safety concerns) or complex management issues.

Group 4. Medication with proven efficacy but frequent or severe adverse effects (or safety concerns), or complex management issues

Group 5. Medications proven to have limited or no efficacy.

When deciding on a preventive drug, the clinician should choose a drug from one of the high-efficacy alternatives based on the patient's profile and the presence or absence of coexisting or comorbid disease. The clinician should use the drug with the best risk-to-benefit ratio for the individual patient, and take advantage of the side effect profile of the drug. An underweight patient would be a candidate for one of the medications that commonly produce weight gain; in contrast, one would avoid these drugs in the overweight patient. Sedating tertiary tricyclic antidepressants (TCAs) would be useful at bedtime for patients with insomnia. The older patient with cardiac disease may not be able to use TCAs, calcium channel blockers, or β blockers, but could easily use valproate. The athletic patient should not be prescribed β blockers. Patients who are dependent on their wits should not take medication that can impair cognitive functioning.

Comorbid and coexistent diseases have important implications for treatment. The presence of a second illness provides therapeutic opportunities but also imposes certain therapeutic limitations. In some instances, two or more conditions may be treated with a single drug (13,46). For example, valproate is a drug of choice for the patient with migraine and epilepsy (5,7) or migraine and manic-depressive illness (47,48). When individuals have more than one disease, certain categories of treatment may be relatively contraindicated. For example, β blockers should be used with caution in the depressed migraineur, whereas TCAs, neuroleptics, or sumatriptan may lower the seizure threshold and should be used with caution in the epileptic migraineur.

CONCLUSIONS AND RECOMMENDATIONS ON THE USE OF VALPROATE IN MIGRAINE

In all of the clinical studies, whether open, retrospective, or placebo-controlled and double-blind, valproate was an effective preventive treatment for migraine. There was a reduction in the number of migraine attacks, and migraine duration and intensity also were reduced in some instances. There was some evidence that symptomatic medication use could be decreased. Some studies (6,32), but not all (39), suggested that clinical efficacy is correlated to serum concentration. Preliminary reports (36,49) suggest that divalproex sodium is as effective as the β blocker propranolol. The data from two multicenter, double-blind, placebo-controlled studies were combined and demonstrated that divalproex sodium was equally as effective in migraine with aura as in migraine without aura (49). It also appears to be effective in cluster headache and chronic daily headache, but it does not seem to be as effective for pure TTH. It is equally as effective in patients with severe, frequent migraines as in those with less severe migraines (50). The following recommendations can be made for the optimal use of valproate in migraine.

1. Before initiating treatment, perform a physical examination and take a thorough medical history, with special attention to hepatic, hematologic, and bleeding abnormalities. Inform the patient about possible hair loss, weight gain, and teratogenic effects and the signs and symptoms of hepatic and hematologic dysfunction. Obtain screening baseline laboratory studies to help identify risk factors that could influence drug selection.

Suggested studies include complete blood count, differential, and platelets; prothrombin time and partial thromboplastin time; serum chemistry, including glucose, blood urea nitrogen, electrolytes, calcium, potassium, magnesium, creatinine, urate, cholesterol, bilirubin, alkaline phosphatase, aspartate aminotransferase, alanine aminotransferase, total protein, and albumin (SMA profile).

2. To minimize gastrointestinal side effects, use enteric-coated formulations of valproate. Begin with a dose of 250 mg at bedtime. If nausea still occurs, use the sprinkle formulation (125 mg) and increase the dose very slowly. Slowly increase the dosage to 500 to 750 mg/day (in two to three divided dose) to limit gastrointestinal side effects. Higher doses are needed at times.

3. Obtain follow-up serum valproic acid levels to test for compliance, toxicity, and drug reactions as needed. Rigid adherence to the suggested optimal range for epilepsy (50 to 100 μg/mL) is not likely to benefit the patient; we occasionally push to trough levels of 125 μg/mL.

4. See the patient on a regular basis (every 1 to 2 months) during the first 6 to 9 months of therapy.

5. It is not necessary to monitor blood and urine in healthy and asymptomatic patients who are on monotherapy, despite the manufacturer's recommendation that liver function tests be performed at frequent intervals, especially during the first 6 months. Identify patients who belong to one of the high-risk groups at the inception of treatment. Obtain follow-up chemistry, if needed, particularly in patients on polypharmacy.

6. If mild elevation of serum hepatic aminotransferase levels occurs, continue valproate at the same dose or a lower dose until the enzymes normalize. If the hepatic aminotransferase elevations are much higher (e.g., two to three times the upper limit of normal), discontinue valproate. If severe, abnormal pain suggestive of pancreatitis occurs, check serum amylase and lipase.

7. Avoid valproate for headache in children younger than 10 years of age unless routine treatments have failed, in which case use it as monotherapy. Avoid valproate in patients with preexisting liver disease and metabolic disorders predisposing to liver toxicity. Avoid valproate for headache when women are pregnant or attempting to become pregnant.

8. Ten percent of treated patients may experience tremor. If this is bothersome, decrease the dose of valproate or use propranolol, a β blocker that also is an effective migraine-preventive agent (51).

9. Excessive weight gain can occur. Advise the patient to exercise regularly, obtain a dietary consultation, and avoid using other medications, such as TCAs, that can produce weight gain. The incidence of hair loss is 2.6% to 12% (25). Anecdotally, multivitamins and zinc supplements have been reported to control hair loss. We have our patients take 220 mg/day of zinc (mega zinc) and a multivitamin.

REFERENCES

1. Medical Economics Company. *Physicians' desk reference*, 54th ed. Medical Economics Company, 2000.
2. McElroy SL, Keck PE, Pope HG. Valproate in psychiatric disorders: literature review and clinical guidelines. *J Clin Psychiatry* 1989;50:23–29.
3. Bourgeois FD. Valproic acid. In: Levy RH, Mattson RH, Meldrum BS, eds. *Antiepileptic drugs*, 4th ed. New York: Raven Press, 1995:633–639.
4. Balfour JA, Bryson HM. Valproic acid: a review of its pharmacology and therapeutic potential in indications other than epilepsy. *CNS Drugs* 1994;2:144–173.
5. Hering R, Kuritzky A. Sodium valproate in the prophylactic treatment of migraine: a double-blind study versus placebo. *Cephalalgia* 1992;12:81–84.
6. Jensen R, Brinck T, Olesen J. Sodium valproate has a prophylactic effect in migraine without aura. *Neurology* 1994;44:647–651.
7. Mathew NT, Saper JR, Silberstein SD, et al. Prophylaxis of migraine headaches with divalproex sodium. *Arch Neurol* 1995;52:281–286.
8. Klapper JA. Divalproex sodium in migraine prophylaxis: a dose-controlled study. *Cephalalgia* 1997;17:103–108.
9. Silberstein SD, Collins SD, Carlson H, and the Depakote ER Migraine Study Group. Safety and efficacy of once-daily, extended-release divalproex sodium monotherapy for the prophylaxis of migraine headaches. *Cephalalgia* 2000;20:269(abstr).
10. Roy-Byrne P, Ward NG, Donnelly PJ. Valproate in anxiety and withdrawal syndromes. *J Clin Psychiatry* 1989;50:44–48.
11. Mathew NT, Ali S. Valproate in the treatment of persistent chronic daily headache: an open label study. *Headache* 1991;31:71–74.
12. Hering R, Kuritzky A. Sodium valproate in the treatment of cluster headache: an open clinical trail. *Cephalalgia* 1989;9:195–198.
13. Silberstein SD, Lipton RB, Goadsby PJ. *Headache in clinical practice*. Oxford: Isis Medical Media, 1998.
14. Silberstein SD, Saper JR, Freitag F. Migraine: diagnosis and treatment. In: Silberstein SD, Lipton RB, Dalessio DJ, eds. *Wolff's headache and other head pain*, 7th ed. New York: Oxford University Press, 2001.
15. Silberstein SD. Practice parameter: evidence-based guidelines for migraine headache (an evidence-based review). Report of the Quality Standards Subcommittee of the American Academy of Neurology for the United States Headache Consortium. *Neurology* 2000;55:754–762.
16. Silberstein SD. Migraine and pregnancy. *Neurol Clin* 1997;15:209–231.
17. Silberstein SD. Review: serotonin (5-HT) and migraine. *Headache* 1994;34:408–417.
18. Peroutka SJ. Developments in 5-hydroxytryptamine receptor pharmacology in migraine. *Neurol Clin* 1990;8:829–838.
19. Moskowitz MA. Neurogenic versus vascular mechanisms of sumatriptan and ergot alkaloids in migraine. *Trends Pharmacol Sci* 1992;13:307–311.
20. Goadsby PJ. The pathophysiology of headache. In: Silberstein SD, Lipton RB, Dalessio DJ, eds. *Wolff's headache and other head pain*, 7th ed. New York: Oxford University Press, 2001.
21. Goadsby PJ, Edvinsson L. Sumatriptan reverses the changes in calcitonin gene-related peptide seen in the headache phase of migraine. *Ann Neurol* 1993;33:48–56.

22. Weiller C, May A, Limmroth V, et al. Brainstem activation in spontaneous human migraine attacks. *Nat Med* 1995;1: 658–660.

23. Saxena PR. Cranial arteriovenous shunting: an in vivo animal model for migraine. In: Olesen J, Moskowitz MA, eds. *Experimental headache models*. Philadelphia: Lippincott–Raven, 1995: 189.

24. Limmroth V, Lee WS, Cutrer FM, et al. Meningeal GABA$_A$ receptors located outside the blood brain barrier mediate sodium valproate blockade of neurogenic and substance P-induced inflammation: possible mechanism in migraine. Proceedings of the 7th International Headache Congress, Canada, September 16–20. *Cephalalgia* 1995;15:102.

25. Rimmer EM, Richens A. An update on sodium valproate. *Pharmacotherapy* 1985;5:171–184.

26. Rall TW, Schleifer LS. Drugs effective in the therapy of epilepsies. In: Gilman AG, Rall TW, Nies AS, et al., eds. *Goodman and Gilman's the pharmacologic basis of therapeutics*, 8th ed. New York: Pergamon Press, 1990:436–462.

27. Chapman A, Keane PE, Meldrum BS. Mechanisms of anticonvulsant action of valproate. *Prog Neurobiol* 1982;19:315–359.

28. Cutrer FM, Limmroth V, Moskowitz MA. Possible mechanisms of valproate in migraine prophylaxis. *Cephalalgia* 1997;17:93–100.

29. Sorensen KV. Valproate: a new drug in migraine prophylaxis. *Acta Neurol Scand* 1988;78:346–348.

30. Viswanathan KN, Sundraram N, Rajendiran C. Sodium valproate in therapy of intractable headaches with EEG changes. *Cephalalgia* 1995;11:282–283.

31. Moore KL. Valproate in the treatment of refractory recurrent headaches: a retrospective analysis of 207 patients. *Headache* 1992;3:323–325.

32. Sianard-Gainko J, Lenaerts M, Bastings E, et al. Sodium valproate in severe migraine and tension-type headache: clinical efficacy and correlations with blood levels. *Cephalalgia* 1993;13:252.

33. Coria F, Sempere AP, Duarte J. Low-dose sodium valproate in the prophylaxis of migraine. *Clin Neuropharmacol* 1994;17: 569–573.

34. Rothrock JF, Kelly NM, Brody ML. A differential response to treatment with divalproex sodium in patients with intractable headache. *Cephalalgia* 1994;14:241–244.

35. Czapinski P. Valproic acid in preventive treatment of migraine. *Cephalalgia* 1995;15:283.

36. Kaniecki RG. A comparison of divalproex with propranolol and placebo for the prophylaxis of migraine without aura. *Arch Neurol* 1995;54:1141–1145.

37. Klapper JA. An open label crossover comparison of divalproex sodium and propranolol HCl in the prevention of migraine headaches. *Headache Q* 1995;5:50–53.

38. Silberstein SD, Collins SD. Safety of divalproex sodium in migraine prophylaxis: an open-label, long-term study (for the Long-Term Safety of Depakote in Headache Prophylaxis Study Group). *Headache* 1999;39:633–643.

39. Ghose K, Niven B. Prophylactic sodium valproate therapy in patients with drug-resistant migraine. *Methods Find Exp Clin Pharmacol* 1998;20:353–359.

40. Edwards K, Santarcangelo V, Shea P, et al. Intravenous valproate for acute treatment of migraine headaches. *Cephalalgia* 1999;19: 356(abstr).

41. Czapinski P, Motyl R. Randomized comparative placebo-controlled assessment of intravenous valproic acid effectiveness and safety in patients with acute migraine. *Cephalalgia* 1999;19: 372–373(abstr).

42. Mathew NT, Kailasam J, Meadors L, et al. Intravenous valproate sodium (Depacon®) aborts migraine rapidly: a preliminary report. *Cephalalgia* 1999;19:373(abstr).

43. Freitag FG, Diamond S, Diamond M, et al. Divalproex sodium in the preventive treatment of cluster headache. *Headache* 2000;40:408(abstr).

44. Delva NJ, Horgan SA, Hawken ER. Valproate prophylaxis for migraine induced by selective serotonin reuptake inhibitors. *Headache* 2000;40:248–251.

45. Freitag FG, Diamond S, Diamond M, et al. Divalproex in the long-term treatment of chronic daily headache. *Headache* 2001 (*in press*).

46. Silberstein SD, Lipton RB, Breslau N. Migraine: association with personality characteristics and psychopathology. *Cephalalgia* 1995;15:337–369.

47. Bowden CL, Brugger AM, Swann AC. Efficacy of divalproex vs lithium and placebo in the treatment of mania. *JAMA* 1994;271: 918–924.

48. Curran DA, Hinterberger H, Lance JW. Methysergide. *Res Clin Stud Headache* 1967;1:74–122.

49. Deaton RL, Thomas JR. The efficacy of divalproex sodium prophylactic treatment in patients experiencing migraine with or without aura. Proceedings of the 7th International Headache Congress. *Cephalalgia* 1995;15:268(abstr).

50. Silberstein SD. Divalproex sodium in headache: literature review and clinical guidelines. *Headache* 1996;36:547–555.

51. Karas BJ, Wilder BJ. Treatment of valproate tremors. *Neurology* 1983;33:1380–1382.

Antiepileptic Drugs, 5th Edition. Edited by R.H. Levy, R.H. Mattson, B.S. Meldrum, and E. Perucca. Lippincott Williams & Wilkins, Philadelphia © 2002.

VALPROIC ACID

CLINICAL EFFICACY AND USE IN PSYCHIATRIC DISORDERS

ALAN C. SWANN

Valproic acid preparations have been used in manic episodes, depressive episodes, and maintenance treatment of bipolar disorder in children, adolescents, and the elderly. Other psychiatric uses of valproate have included treatment of personality disorders, anxiety disorders, psychotic disorders, posttraumatic stress disorder, and impulsive aggression. The quantity and rigor of evidence vary widely. We discuss reported uses of valproic acid and their supporting evidence.

ACUTE MANIA

Efficacy of Monotherapy

Based on early case reports of its effectiveness in mania, Emrich et al. gave valproate, using a placebo-controlled design, to five patients experiencing manic episodes. Four of the five improved substantially (1). Subsequently, the same investigators observed positive responses to valproate in seven lithium-resistant patients (2).

These and similar reports led other investigators to use double-blind, parallel-group study designs to assess the effectiveness of valproate. Freeman et al. compared valproate with lithium in 27 hospitalized patients, finding that overall response was similar but that valproate was more effective in patients who also had depressive symptoms (3). Valproate was reported more effective than carbamazepine in a study of 30 patients.

Pope et al. assessed the efficacy of valproate in patients who were either resistant to lithium or unable to tolerate it. Valproate was substantially more effective than placebo; the reductions in Young Mania Rating Scale scores were 54% for valproate and 5% for placebo (4). This strikingly low placebo response rate probably was a result of selecting previously treatment-resistant patients.

Bowden et al. subsequently carried out a larger study comparing valproate with lithium or placebo. Effectiveness

of valproate was similar to that of lithium, and both were more effective than placebo (5). Interestingly, this was the first parallel-group, placebo-controlled study of lithium in manic episodes; earlier lithium studies had used crossover designs. The results of this study demonstrated also that optimal effectiveness of valproate required a blood level of at least 45 µg/mL, with a point of diminishing return at approximately 100 to 120 µg/mL (6).

It may be a fortunate patient whose manic episode responds optimally to a single agent. In the aforementioned studies, as usually is the case with structured, controlled efficacy studies, "responders" whose mania scores had improved substantially were still symptomatic, on average, at the end of the study period.

Subtypes of Mania

Manic episodes associated with mixed states or with rapid cycling appear relatively resistant to lithium and to have poorer overall outcomes than episodes without these features. Neither mixed states nor rapid cycling appear to have adverse effects on response to valproate. Two controlled studies found valproate to be at least as effective in manic episodes with depressive features as it was in pure mania (3,7). A prospective, open-label study found divalproex to be effective in treating manic and mixed states associated with rapid cycling (8). There also are case reports of effectiveness in 48-hour cycling (9,10). One study showed that, in addition to preventing affective cycling, valproate prevented the associated changes in norepinephrine excretion, plasma cortisol, and growth hormone in a patient with 48-hour mood cycles (9).

Combination Treatments

A review of treatment combinations in bipolar disorder showed that the most frequently reported, effective, and practical combination appeared to be lithium and valproate (11). Ketter et al. found an apparent synergy between valproate and carbamazepine in a blinded study of a patient

Alan C. Swann, MD: Pat R. Rutherford, Jr. Professor and Vice Chair for Research, Department of Psychiatry, University of Texas Health Science Center, Houston, Texas

responding to neither agent alone (12). This was later confirmed in 12 patients with bipolar disorder, although the combination was not as effective in patients with schizoaffective disorder (13). Similarly, lithium and valproate in combination were reported to be more effective than either agent alone, although there also were more side effects (14–16).

The role of antipsychotic treatments relative to other treatments in manic episodes requires critical examination. Muller-Oerlinghausen et al. carried out an important study in which patients undergoing manic episodes were treated with an antipsychotic drug (17). The patients were randomized to receive, in addition, valproate or placebo. The treating physician periodically was given the option of reducing the dose of antipsychotic medicine if the patient's clinical status allowed. Patients randomized to receive valproate required lower doses of antipsychotic and yet had superior symptomatic improvement compared with those given antipsychotic medicine alone (17).

Economics of Treatment

Practical benefits of lithium, valproate, and carbamazepine have been compared using meta-analysis and pharmacoeconomic studies. Interpretation of these studies is strongly affected by the quality of data and accuracy of underlying assumptions. Meta-analysis showed similar antimanic effects for valproate, lithium, and carbamazepine, but the authors found valproate or carbamazepine to be better tolerated than lithium (18). Pharmacoeconomic studies found valproate had the benefit of shorter hospital stays because of the feasibility of rapid dose escalation and better response in mixed states. Length of hospital stay was similar in divalproex and in the combination of lithium plus carbamazepine, whereas either lithium or carbamazepine alone was associated with longer hospitalizations (19). Cost of treatment was approximately 9% per year less overall with divalproex than with lithium (19).

Biology of Antimanic Response

Acute administration of valproate to rats was shown to decrease hyperactivity associated with combined administration of chlordiazepoxide and amphetamine, proposed as a model for mania; this effect was reduced by γ-aminobutyric acid (GABA) receptor antagonists (20). Valproate also reduces motor responses to acute methylphenidate in doses that do not have independent effects on motor behavior (21). These effects are consistent with reported enhancement of GABA function by valproate (22–24). In clinical studies, low plasma GABA was shown to predict positive antimanic outcome in women (25), and pretreatment plasma GABA was shown to correlate negatively with symptom change (26). Based partly on effects of valproate, it has been proposed that bipolar disorder was associated with deficient GABAergic function (27).

DEPRESSION

Although evidence from animal models suggests that valproate may be effective in treating depressive episodes, the published experience with valproate in depression is relatively small, and there are no published conventional placebo-controlled studies. A review of early experience with valproate revealed a response rate of approximately 30% in depressive episodes, but this consisted largely of patients whose depressions had been refractory to other treatments or combinations, so cannot be compared realistically with other response rates (28). More recent reports found valproate to be effective in depression with atypical features (largely hypersomnia) (29) and in treating residual depression in partial responders to other treatments (30). A prospective, open-label study in major depressive disorder, based on the idea that GABA-mimetic agents would have general antidepressant activity, reported most patients responding to valproate (based on >50% improvement in Hamilton Depression scores) at 4 weeks and two-thirds responding at 8 weeks (31).

There is a surprising lack of data in acute bipolar depression, but two randomized studies suggest effectiveness under maintenance conditions. Young et al. found that, for breakthrough depression in patients receiving either lithium or divalproex, addition of the other mood-stabilizing agent was as effective as adding paroxetine (32). Although patients appeared to tolerate the combination of mood stabilizer plus paroxetine better than combined mood stabilizers, combined mood stabilizers may be the better long-term choice because of the potential for better protection against relapse. During a 12-month controlled maintenance study, Bowden et al. found that subjects randomized to divalproex had a lower rate of relapse to depression than did those given placebo, and had a significantly lower rate of interepisode depressive symptoms than did subjects given lithium (33).

Biology of Antidepressant Response

Valproate appears effective in reducing immobilization in the forced swim test, an animal model of depression (34,35). This appears to be a combination of direct $GABA_A$- (34) and indirect 5-hydroxytryptamine ($5-HT_{1A}$)-mediated effects (35). The latter is consistent with other observations that valproate administration increased brain 5-hydroxyindoleacetic acid, a possible indicator of serotonin utilization, in stressed rats (36).

MAINTENANCE IN BIPOLAR DISORDER

Early open-label studies suggested that valproate might have prophylactic effectiveness in bipolar disorder (37–39). These studies included series of patients with frequent recurrence and schizoaffective characteristics (40). Calabrese and Delucchi carried out a prospective, open-label study of divalproex in 78 patients with rapid cycling and found that, over an average of approximately 16 months, this treatment was effective in preventing recurrences of manic, mixed, or depressive states (8). A randomized, open-label comparison of lithium with valpromide maintenance found that patients given valpromide had slightly fewer episodes and significantly better toleration of treatment, and that lithium nonresponders improved when switched to valpromide, but valpromide nonresponders did not improve when switched to lithium (41).

In a continuation of their study of lithium and carbamazepine as maintenance treatments, Denicoff et al. reported that those not stable on lithium or on lithium plus carbamazepine improved when valproate was added (42).

These results encouraged Bowden et al. to conduct a controlled maintenance study of divalproex in bipolar disorder, the first placebo-controlled maintenance study of this illness in over 20 years (33). Subjects were treated for acute manic episodes and were converted, if possible, to monotherapy with lithium or divalproex. Those able to meet recovery criteria on monotherapy (approximately two-thirds of those originally entering the study) were randomized to receive divalproex, lithium, or placebo. Perhaps because of cautious study design and exclusion of severely ill subjects, placebo performed better than it had in the early lithium–placebo studies. Despite a low overall rate of relapse into mania, subjects randomized to divalproex fared better than those receiving placebo in outcome measures, including retention in the study and relapse into depression, and better than those given lithium in retention in the study and in interepisode depressive symptoms (33).

Biology of Maintenance Effects in Bipolar Disorder

Behavioral sensitization to stimulants may be related to the recurrent course of bipolar disorder and to its association with substance abuse. Repeated treatment with valproate, at a dose having no direct effects on motor behavior, prevented the induction of behavioral sensitization to methylphenidate (21). Repeated valproate given after sensitization to methylphenidate had developed prevented the expression of the sensitized motor response (43). These effects may be consistent with the effectiveness of divalproex in subjects who had a large number of previous episodes of illness (44).

COMORBIDITIES, BIPOLAR SPECTRUM, OR RELATED CONDITIONS

Bipolar Disorder and Substance Abuse

Substance abuse is a troubling aspect of bipolar disorder, occurring in as many as 60% of patients and complicating treatment (45). Perhaps because of its association with mixed

states (46), which frequently are lithium resistant (7,47–49), treatment outcome in these patients is believed to be relatively poor. A group of 20 patients with bipolar disorder and substance abuse experienced a decrease in "craving" during open-label divalproex treatment (50). A retrospective chart review study suggested that valproate treatment was associated with a reduction in severity of substance abuse (51). A small, prospective, open-label study suggested that patients with substance abuse and dysphoric mania experienced marked improvement in both mania and substance abuse with divalproex treatment (52). None of these studies compared valproate with other treatments. More recently, Goldberg et al. investigated the effect of substance abuse on outcome in a large group of patients hospitalized for treatment of mania (53). Patients with substance abuse were twice as likely to achieve remission with divalproex or carbamazepine than with lithium treatment. The differential effect appeared to result from substance abuse rather than the associated mixed states, and combinations of lithium with anticonvulsant were no more effective than anticonvulsant alone (53).

Anxiety Disorders

Valproate has anxiolytic effects in some, but not all, animal models of anxiety (54–56). These effects may involve GABA because they usually are prevented by GABA$_A$ receptor antagonists (55,56). In a group of 13 patients with mood instability and panic attacks that had been refractory to other treatments, 10 achieved substantial improvement in mood instability, depressive symptoms, anxiety, and frequency of panics with 8 weeks' divalproex treatment (57).

Personality and Bipolar Spectrum Disorders

Valproate may be effective in patients whose presentation lies on the fringes of bipolar disorder. In a group of "bipolar spectrum" patients with cyclothymia or "hyperthymia," valproate treatment was associated with reduction in mood symptoms and in "noxious personality traits." Another open-label study found divalproex to be effective in improving mood symptoms, impulsivity, and anxiety in four of eight patients with borderline personality disorder (58). More recently, Hollander et al. (59) reported that valproate was more effective than placebo in treating affective and behavioral symptoms of borderline personality disorder over a 10-week period. Low doses (125 to 500 mg) were reported to be effective in milder forms of illness, including cyclothymic and "mild rapid cycling"; patients not responding to these doses improved with conventional doses (60).

Posttraumatic Stress Disorder

Valproate reduces catecholamine and behavioral changes in animals exposed to stress, suggesting that it may be effective in stress-related disorders. Two open-label studies and one case report suggest that valproate preparations may be effective in reducing hyperarousal, intrusive symptoms, affective symptoms including depression, and impulsivity in patients with posttraumatic stress disorder (61–63).

Impulsive Aggression

Valproate has been used extensively as a treatment for impulsive aggression. One review found 17 studies involving 164 subjects, approximately three-fourths of whom had at least 50% reductions in the target symptom (64). Anti-aggressive effects of valproate may be complementary to those of serotonin-enhancing treatments because a group of patients with assorted personality disorders whose aggressive behavior did not improve during treatment with fluoxetine at up to 60 mg/day had a marked reduction during 4 weeks of divalproex treatment (65).

Until recently, there were no placebo-controlled studies of valproate in aggression. Donovan et al. found valproate to reduce aggression symptom scores and mood lability in a series of 10 adolescent subjects who had explosive aggression and labile mood severe enough to disturb major life areas but who did not meet criteria for bipolar disorder (66). They then carried out a placebo-controlled crossover study in similar subjects. Eight of 10 subjects initially given divalproex improved, compared with 0 of 10 randomized to placebo; when subjects were crossed to the other treatment, valproate was effective in 6 of 7 who initially had not responded to placebo, whereas placebo was effective in 2 of 8 who previously had responded to valproate (67).

PSYCHOTIC DISORDERS

Schizoaffective Disorder

The diagnosis of schizoaffective disorder is very unstable, and many patients with this diagnosis ultimately receive a diagnosis of schizophrenia or bipolar disorder (68). Use of valproate in treating schizoaffective disorder, usually in combination with antipsychotic treatments, has increased markedly since 1994 (69). Retrospective reviews suggest effectiveness in up to 75% of these patients (70,71), especially if they have seizures or other neurologic problems (72). We know of no prospective, controlled studies in these patients.

Schizophrenia

The use of mood stabilizers, especially valproate, has increased substantially in patients with schizophrenia, essentially doubling between 1994 and 1998 in the New York State psychiatric hospital system (73). Evidence supporting effectiveness of valproate has been mixed but includes some tantalizing studies. Unlike carbamazepine,

valproate has little or no effect on haloperidol levels (74). A review of previous studies, essentially all open-label, suggested that GABAergic treatments like valproate and benzodiazepines were useful adjunctive treatments in schizophrenia (75). An early study comparing addition of valproate or placebo with haloperidol treatment found improvement in hostile belligerence but not in psychotic symptoms (76). More recently, Wassef et al. carried out an open-label study in which divalproex added to haloperidol, either early or late in treatment, resulted in substantial improvement in psychosis symptoms and a briefer hospitalization (77). On this basis, the same authors carried out a small (n = 12), randomized clinical trial comparing haloperidol combined with placebo or with divalproex; improvement was significantly greater in the group receiving divalproex despite the small sample (78).

Tardive Dyskinesia

Largely because it increases GABA function, there have been multiple trials of valproate in tardive dyskinesia. As with other treatments, results have varied, likely in part because of heterogeneity of subjects and of other medicines that they were receiving. Randomized placebo-controlled trials have produced both positive (79) and negative (80) results. Valproate may be more effective when antipsychotic treatments are continued (81). A meta-analysis of randomized clinical trials in tardive dyskinesia found valproate to be more effective than placebo, although the effect size was not large (82).

Interestingly, valproate is effective in animal models of tardive dyskinesia (83). Valproate reduces prolactin levels in schizophrenic patients with tardive dyskinesia, but not in those without it (84). It was shown to decrease cerebrospinal fluid (CSF) homovanillic acid (a dopamine metabolite) and to increase CSF cyclic guanosine monophosphate in patients with tardive dyskinesia, interpreted as consistent with redressing a dopamine–acetylcholine imbalance (85). These data suggest that, at least in certain patients or under proper conditions, valproate may be a useful adjunct in tardive dyskinesia. No data have been published specifically addressing tardive dyskinesia in bipolar disorder.

CHILDREN AND ADOLESCENTS

The diagnosis and treatment of bipolar disorder or of bipolar-like conditions in children is not yet well defined. Results of treatment studies are very preliminary. A group of 59 children with "manic-like" presentations previously not responding to stimulant, antidepressive, or antipsychotic treatments responded to divalproex (86). A comparison of treatment studies in children or adolescents (mean age, 11.2 years) revealed that valproate, lithium, and carbamazepine were all potentially effective, with effect sizes of 1.63, 1.06, and 1, respectively (87). In a group of 15 adolescents with mania, divalproex treatment was associated with greater than 75% reduction in mania rating scores in 10 (88).

VALPROATE IN GERIATRIC PSYCHIATRY

There are many reports that valproate was effective in open trials involving geriatric patients, but few data from controlled studies. A case series reported impressive effectiveness and good tolerability in seven patients with mean age of 66 years, most of whom had multiple other medical illnesses and treatments (89).

Valproate has been used extensively to treat behavioral problems associated with dementia in the elderly; many of the symptoms treated resemble those of mania or include impulsive aggression (90). One comparison with lithium treatment in nursing home residents found that lithium treatment was substantially more expensive, largely because of a higher cost of medical adverse events and monitoring (91). A comparison of efficacy found that valproate and lithium were similarly effective if drug levels were adequate (92). Doses and drug levels in case series demonstrating successful treatment have ranged from 375 to 750 mg/day in one prospective series of patients 71 to 94 years of age (93), to 743 mg/day (52.9 mg/L) in a series of patients averaging 71 years of age who were treated for 3 years (94), to 1,650 mg/day (64 mg/L) in a series of 25 patients whose age averaged 77 years (95). When response to a lower dose is inadequate, a higher dose should be considered, if tolerable (90). The incidence of cognitive, hepatic, or other side effects with valproate treatment has been low (94,96,97).

Although overall rates of toxicity are low, a small number of older patients treated with valproate have developed reversible drug-induced parkinsonian symptoms (98,99). These symptoms were reported to resolve with L-DOPA treatment (99) or discontinuation of valproate (98,99).

PREDICTORS OF RESPONSE

Characteristics of classic bipolar disorder predict good response to lithium, and departure from these characteristics predicts unfavorable outcome. The same is not true for valproate: Presence of substance abuse (53), manic-depressive symptoms (7), neurologic abnormalities (72), and poor course of illness with many previous episodes or rapid cycling all predict better outcome with valproate than with lithium treatment. Substance abuse is associated with depressive features in manic episodes, but effects of substance abuse and depressive features on response to lithium versus valproate may be independent (7,53). There is no clear evidence that presence or absence of these characteris-

tics alters response to valproate; outcome with this drug may be independent of them. Apparent improved outcome in patients with many episodes (44) is consistent with effects of valproate on behavioral sensitization to stimulants (21,43).

Other than data on response in acute mania, there is little evidence about predictors of treatment outcome in bipolar disorder. Information on relative predictors of response among anticonvulsants, or among predictors in maintenance treatment or treatment of depressive episodes, would be valuable.

USE AND PREPARATIONS OF VALPROATE

Treatments in bipolar disorder are more effective if therapeutic levels of medicine are achieved quickly (100). Keck et al. showed that subjects responding to divalproex started at 20 mg/kg/day had a 50% improvement in mania rating scores within 48 hours after achieving a threshold valproate level of 50 μg/mL (101). The same group found 20 mg/kg/day divalproex to be equivalent, in improvement of mania and psychosis scores, to haloperidol at 0.2 mg/kg/day (102). More rapid oral loading with an initial dose of 30 mg/kg/day for 2 days appears feasible in some patients, producing a wide range of valproate levels (56 to 124 μg/mL) at 3 days, but additional clinical benefit of this method remains to be demonstrated (103,104).

Intravenous valproate may be an even more efficient way to achieve effective tissue concentrations quickly. Three "neuropsychiatric" patients with mania-like states tolerated and responded to intravenous valproate (105). In a series of patients with severe bipolar disorder, intravenous valproate was tolerated well and was effective for mania but not for depression. One patient improved who had not responded to oral divalproex loading (106).

Oral treatment may be given as valproic acid, as sodium valproate, or as its divalproex complex. In a series of 150 patients with bipolar disorder, those treated with valproate were twice as likely as those given divalproex to have gastrointestinal side effects, and three times as likely to discontinue treatment because of side effects (107). Among 12 patients who discontinued valproate treatment because of gastrointestinal side effects and were placed on divalproex, all but 2 were able to remain in treatment. The oral loading and placebo-controlled studies described previously were all carried out using divalproex. In this review, we have used the term *valproate* to refer to any of its preparations, including divalproex and valpromide, although in the United States divalproex is the form most commonly used.

Based on the preceding considerations, the best method of instituting treatment depends on the clinical context. When time is of the essence, because of severity of manic symptoms or other behavioral disturbances, it may be most efficient to start divalproex at 20 to 30 mg/kg/day followed by adjustments as indicated by symptomatic response and side effects (101,102). Under other circumstances, more gradual dose escalation starting at 750 mg/day (or less in elderly patients) may produce better toleration. Lower doses may be indicated in patients with liver disorders or who are taking medicines that can inhibit the oxidative metabolism of valproate; higher doses may be needed if the patient is taking a drug, like carbamazepine or other aromatic anti-convulsants, that can induce oxidation of valproate. In any case, the final dose depends on the balance between symptomatic improvement and side effects. Although a threshold valproate level of at least 45 µg/mL appears to be required for effectiveness (6), the actual optimal level will be different for every patient, usually within a range of 50 to 125 µg/mL. The valproate blood level therefore is a secondary consideration relative to response and side effects, but is useful as a pharmacokinetic benchmark.

CONCLUSION

Valproate preparations appear effective for acute mania and a range of possibly related problems. Studies in bipolar disorder are summarized in Table 88.1. The strongest supporting evidence is for acute mania and in maintenance for depression, with somewhat less supporting evidence in acute depression or as maintenance for mania. There also is evidence for effects in behavioral problems associated with affective lability, aggression, and impulsivity across a range of clinical contexts, as shown in Table 88.2. Valproate often may be optimally effective as part of judicious combination treatments. Although no single treatment is effective for all patients or circumstances, and controlled studies in bipolar depression and maintenance are sparse, valproate has a substantial breadth of use in bipolar and related disorders.

TABLE 88.1. STUDIES OF VALPROATE PREPARATIONS IN BIPOLAR DISORDER[a]

	Mono-therapy vs. Placebo	Other Randomized Trials	Nonrandomized, Prospective
Acute mania	1,4,5	3,5,16,17	2
Acute depression	—	32	28–30
Mixed/rapid cycling	7	3	8–10
Maintenance	33	33	37–42
Child-adolescent	—	87	88

[a]The table gives reference numbers of the relevant studies. Other randomized trials include comparisons to treatments other than placebo, or nonmonotherapy randomized trials. References in the third column include reviews.

TABLE 88.2. PSYCHIATRIC STUDIES OF VALPROATE PREPARATIONS OUTSIDE BIPOLAR DISORDER[a]

	Monotherapy vs. Placebo	Other Randomized Trials	Non-randomized, Prospective
Substance abuse	—	—	50,52,53
Personality disorder	59	—	58
Impulsive aggression	67	—	64–66
Resembling posttraumatic skin disorder	—	—	61–63
Agitation-dementia	—	91	92–95
Anxiety-panic	—	—	57
Psychosis	—	78	70,71,75–77
Tardive dyskinesia	79,80	82	—

[a]Definitions are as in Table 88.1.

REFERENCES

1. Emrich HM, Dose M, von Zerssen D. The use of sodium valproate, carbamazepine and oxcarbazepine in patients with affective disorders. *J Affect Disord* 1985;8:243–250.
2. Emrich HM, Wolf R. Valproate treatment of mania. *Prog Neuropsychopharmacol Biol Psychiatry* 1992;16:691–701.
3. Freeman TW, Clothier JL, Pazzaglia P, et al. A double-blind comparison of valproate and lithium in the treatment of acute mania. *Am J Psychiatry* 1992;149:108–111.
4. Pope HG Jr, McElroy SL, Keck PE Jr, et al. Valproate in the treatment of acute mania: a placebo-controlled study. *Arch Gen Psychiatry* 1991;48:62–68.
5. Bowden CL, Brugger AM, Swann AC, et al. Efficacy of divalproex vs lithium and placebo in the treatment of mania. *JAMA* 1994;271:918–924.
6. Bowden CL, Janicak PG, Orsulak PJ, et al. Relation of serum valproate concentration to response in mania. *Am J Psychiatry* 1996;153:765–770.
7. Swann AC, Bowden CL, Morris D, et al. Depression during mania: treatment response to lithium or divalproex. *Arch Gen Psychiatry* 1996.
8. Calabrese JR, Delucchi GA. Spectrum of efficacy of valproate in 55 patients with rapid-cycling bipolar disorder. *Am J Psychiatry* 1990;147:431–434.
9. Juckel G, Hegerl U, Mavrogiorgou P, et al. Clinical and biological findings in a case with 48-hour bipolar ultrarapid cycling before and during valproate treatment. *J Clin Psychiatry* 2000; 61:585–593.
10. Lepkifker E, Iancu I, Dannon PN, et al. Valproic acid in ultrarapid cycling: a case report. *Clin Neuropharmacol* 1995;18:72–75.
11. Freeman MP, Stoll AL. Mood stabilizer combinations: a review of safety and efficacy. *Am J Psychiatry* 1998;155:12–21.
12. Ketter TA, Pazzaglia PJ, Post RM. Synergy of carbamazepine and valproic acid in affective illness: case report and review of the literature. *J Clin Psychopharmacol* 1992;12:276–281.
13. Tohen M, Castillo J, Pope HG, et al. Concomitant use of valproate and carbamazepine in bipolar and schizoaffective disorders. *J Clin Psychopharmacol* 1994;14:67–70.

14. Solomon DA, Ryan CE, Keitner GI, et al. A pilot study of lithium carbonate plus divalproex sodium for the continuation and maintenance treatment of patients with bipolar I disorder. *J Clin Psychiatry* 1997;58:95–99.

15. Sharma V, Persad E, Mazmanian D, et al. Treatment of rapid cycling bipolar disorder with combination therapy of valproate and lithium. *Can J Psychiatry* 1993;38:137–139.

16. Vasudev K, Goswami U, Kohli K. Carbamazepine and valproate monotherapy: feasibility, relative safety and efficacy, and therapeutic drug monitoring in manic disorder. *Psychopharmacology (Berl)* 2000;150:15–23..

17. Muller-Oerlinghausen B, Retzow A, Henn FA, et al. Valproate as an adjunct to neuroleptic medication for the treatment of acute episodes of mania: a prospective, randomized, double-blind, placebo-controlled, multicenter study. European Valproate Mania Study Group. *J Clin Psychopharmacol* 2000;20: 195–203.

18. Emilien G, Maloteaux JM, Seghers A, et al. Lithium compared to valproic acid and carbamazepine in the treatment of mania: a statistical meta-analysis. *Eur Neuropsychopharmacol* 1996;6: 245–252.

19. Frye MA, Altshuler LL, Szuba MP, et al. The relationship between antimanic agent for the treatment of classic or dysphoric mania and length of hospital stay. *J Clin Psychiatry* 1996; 57:17–21.

20. Cao BJ, Peng NA. Magnesium valproate attenuates hyperactivity induced by dexamphetamine–chlordiazepoxide mixture in rodents. *Eur J Pharmacol* 1993;237:177–181.

21. Yang P, Beasley A, Swann A, et al. Valproate modulates the expression of methylphenidate (Ritalin) sensitization. *Brain Res* 2000;874:216–220.

22. Fowler LJ, Beckford J, John RA. An analysis of the kinetics of the inhibition of rabbit brain gamma-aminobutyrate aminotransferase by sodium n-dipropylacetate and some other simple carboxylic acids. *Biochem Pharmacol* 1975;24:1267–1270.

23. Gent JP, Phillips NI. Sodium di-n-propylacetate (valproate) potentiates responses to GABA and muscimol on single central neurons. *Brain Res* 1980;197:275–278.

24. Loscher W. Valproate enhances GABA turnover in the substantia nigra. *Brain Res* 1989;501:198–203.

25. Swann AC, Petty F, Bowden CL, et al. Mania: gender, transmitter function, and response to treatment. *Psychiatry Res* 1999; 88:55–61.

26. Petty F, Rush AJ, Davis JM, et al. Plasma GABA predicts response to divalproex in mania. *Biol Psychiatry* 1996;39: 278–284.

27. Emrich HM, von Zerssen D, Kissling W, et al. Effect of sodium valproate on mania: the GABA-hypothesis of affective disorders. *Arch Psychiatr Nervenkr* 1980;229:1–16.

28. Brown R. U.S. experience with valproate in manic depressive illness: a multicenter trial. *J Clin Psychiatry* 1989;50:13–16.

29. Pies R, Adler DA, Ehrenberg BL. Sleep disorders and depression with atypical features: response to valproate. *J Clin Psychopharmacol* 1989;9:352–357.

30. Kemp LI. Sodium valproate as an antidepressant. *Br J Psychiatry* 1992;160:121–123.

31. Davis LL, Kabel D, Patel D, et al. Valproate as an antidepressant in major depressive disorder. *Psychopharmacol Bull* 1996; 32:647–652.

32. Young LT, Joffe RT, Robb JC, et al. Double-blind comparison of addition of a second mood stabilizer versus an antidepressant to an initial mood stabilizer for treatment of patients with bipolar depression. *Am J Psychiatry* 2000;157:124–126.

33. Bowden CL, Calabrese JR, McElroy SL, et al. A randomized, placebo-controlled 12-month trial of divalproex and lithium in treatment of outpatients with bipolar I disorder. Divalproex

34. Fernandez TA, Boix F, Escorihuela RM, et al. Sodium valproate reduces immobility in the behavioral "despair" test in rats. *Eur J Pharmacol* 1988;152:1–7.

35. Redrobe JP, Bourin M. Evidence of the activity of lithium on 5-HT1B receptors in the mouse forced swimming test: comparison with carbamazepine and sodium valproate. *Psychopharmacology (Berl)* 1999;141:370–377.

36. Mitsikostas D, Sfikakis A, Papadopoulou-Daifoti Z, et al. The effects of valproate in brain monoamines of juvenile rats after stress. *Prog Neuropsychopharmacol Biol Psychiatry* 1993;17: 295–310.

37. Puzynski S, Klosiewicz L. Valproate amide as a prophylactic agent in affective and schizoaffective disorders. *Psychopharmacol Bull* 1984;20:151–159.

38. Tariot PN, Patel SV, Cox C, et al. Age-related decline in central cholinergic function demonstrated with scopolamine. *Psychopharmacology (Berl)* 1996;125:50–56.

39. Solomon DA, Keitner GI, Miller IW, et al. Course of illness and maintenance treatments for patients with bipolar disorder. *J Clin Psychiatry* 1995;56:5–13.

40. Schaff MR, Fawcett J, Zajecka JM. Divalproex sodium in the treatment of refractory affective disorders. *J Clin Psychiatry* 1993;54:380–384.

41. Lambert PA, Venaud G. Comparative study of valpromide vs lithium in the treatment of affective disorders. *Nervure* 1992; 5:57–65.

42. Denicoff KD, Smith-Jackson EE, Bryan AL, et al. Valproate prophylaxis in a prospective clinical trial of refractory bipolar disorder. *Am J Psychiatry* 1997;154:1456–1458.

43. Yang P, Beasley A, Eckermann K, et al. Valproate prevents the induction of sensitization to methylphenidate (Ritalin) in rats. *Brain Res* 2000;887:276–284.

44. Swann AC, Bowden CL, Calabrese JR, et al. Differential effect of number of previous episodes of affective disorder on response to lithium or divalproex in acute mania. *Am J Psychiatry* 1999; 156:1264–1266.

45. Regier DA, Farm ME, Rae DS. Comorbidity of mental disorders with alcohol and other drug abuse: results from the Epidemiologic Catchment Area (ECA) study. *JAMA* 1990;264: 2511–2518.

46. Himmelhoch JM, Mulla D, Neil JF, et al. Incidence and severity of mixed affective states in a bipolar population. *Arch Gen Psychiatry* 1976;33:1062.

47. Himmelhoch JM, Garfinkel ME. Sources of lithium resistance in mixed mania. *Psychopharmacol Bull* 1986;22:613–620.

48. Swann AC, Secunda SK, Katz MM, et al. Lithium treatment of mania: clinical characteristics, specificity of symptom change, and outcome. *Psychiatry Res* 1986;18:127–141.

49. Licht RW. Drug treatment of mania: a critical review. *Acta Psychiatr Scand* 1998;97:387–397.

50. Albanese MJ, Clodfelter RC, Khantzian EJ. Divalproex sodium in substance abusers with mood disorder. *J Clin Psychiatry* 2000;61:916–921.

51. Hertzman M. Divalproex sodium to treat concomitant substance abuse and mood disorders. *J Subst Abuse Treat* 2000;18:371–372.

52. Brady KT, Sonne SC, Anton R, et al. Valproate in the treatment of acute bipolar affective episodes complicated by substance abuse: a pilot study. *J Clin Psychiatry* 1995;56:118–121.

53. Goldberg JF, Garno JL, Leon AC, et al. A history of substance abuse complicates remission from acute mania in bipolar disorder. *J Clin Psychiatry* 1999;60:733–740.

54. Vellucci SV, Webster RA. The role of GABA in the anti-conflict action of sodium valproate and chlordiazepoxide. *Pharmacol Biochem Behav* 1984;21:845–851.

55. Liljequist S, Engel J. Reversal of the anticonflict action of valproate by various GABA and benzodiazepine antagonists. *Life Sci* 1984;34:2525–2533.

56. Misslin R, Ropartz P, Mandel P. The effects of n-dipropylacetate on the acquisition of conditioned behaviour with negative reinforcement in mice. *Psychopharmacologia* 1975;44:263–265.

57. Baetz M, Bowen RC. Efficacy of divalproex sodium in patients with panic disorder and mood instability who have not responded to conventional therapy. *Can J Psychiatry* 1998;43:73–77.

58. Stein DJ, Simeon D, Frenkel M, et al. An open trial of valproate in borderline personality disorder. *J Clin Psychiatry* 1995;56:506–510.

59. Hollander E, Allen A, Lopez RP, et al. A preliminary double-blind, placebo-controlled trial of divalproex sodium in borderline personality disorder. *J Clin Psychiatry* 2001;62:199–203.

60. Jacobsen FM. Low-dose valproate: a new treatment for cyclothymia, mild rapid cycling disorders, and premenstrual syndrome. *J Clin Psychiatry* 1993;54:229–234.

61. Ford N. The use of anticonvulsants in posttraumatic stress disorder: case study and overview. *J Trauma Stress* 1996;9:857–863.

62. Clark RD, Canive JM, Calais LA, et al. Divalproex in posttraumatic stress disorder: an open-label clinical trial. *J Trauma Stress* 1999;12:395–401.

63. Fesler FA. Valproate in combat-related posttraumatic stress disorder. *J Clin Psychiatry* 1991;52:361–364.

64. Lindenmayer JP, Kotsaftis A. Use of sodium valproate in violent and aggressive behaviors: a critical review. *J Clin Psychiatry* 2000;61:123–128.

65. Kavoussi RJ, Coccaro EF. Divalproex sodium for impulsive aggressive behavior in patients with personality disorder. *J Clin Psychiatry* 1998;59:676–680.

66. Donovan SJ, Susser ES, Nunes EV, et al. Divalproex treatment of disruptive adolescents: a report of 10 cases. *J Clin Psychiatry* 1997;58:12–15.

67. Donovan SJ, Stewart JW, Nunes EV, et al. Divalproex treatment for youth with explosive temper and mood lability: a double-blind, placebo-controlled crossover design. *Am J Psychiatry* 2000;157:818–820.

68. Chen YR, Swann AC, Johnson BA. Stability of diagnosis in bipolar disorder. *J Nerv Ment Dis* 1998;186:17–23.

69. Fenn HH, Robinson D, Luby V, et al. Trends in pharmacotherapy of schizoaffective and bipolar affective disorders: a 5-year naturalistic study. *Am J Psychiatry* 1996;153:711–713.

70. Bogan AM, Brown ES, Suppes T. Efficacy of divalproex therapy for schizoaffective disorder. *J Clin Psychopharmacol* 2000;20:520–522.

71. DelBello MP, Lopez-Larson MP, Getz GE, et al. Treatment of schizoaffective disorder with divalproex sodium. *Schizophr Res* 2000;46:77–79.

72. Stoll AL, Banov M, Kolbrener M, et al. Neurologic factors predict a favorable valproate response in bipolar and schizoaffective disorders. *J Clin Psychopharmacol* 1994;14:311–313.

73. Citrome L, Levine J, Allingham B. Changes in use of valproate and other mood stabilizers for patients with schizophrenia from 1994 to 1998. *Psychiatr Serv* 2000;51:634–638.

74. Hesslinger B, Normann C, Langosch JM, et al. Effects of carbamazepine and valproate on haloperidol plasma levels and on psychopathologic outcome in schizophrenic patients. *J Clin Psychopharmacol* 1999;19:310–315.

75. Wassef AA, Dott SG, Harris A, et al. Critical review of GABA-ergic drugs in the treatment of schizophrenia. *J Clin Psychopharmacol* 1999;19:222–232.

76. Dose M, Hellweg R, Yassouridis A, et al. Combined treatment of schizophrenic psychoses with haloperidol and valproate. *Dig Dis Sci* 1998;31:122–125.

77. Wassef AA, Hafiz NG, Hampton D, et al. Divalproex sodium augmentation of haloperidol in hospitalized patients with schizophrenia: clinical and economic implications. *J Clin Psychopharmacol* 2001;21:21–26.

78. Wassef AA, Dott SG, Harris A, et al. Randomized, placebo-controlled pilot study of divalproex sodium in the treatment of acute exacerbations of chronic schizophrenia. *J Clin Psychopharmacol* 2000;20:357–361.

79. Linnoila M, Viukari M, Kietala O. Effect of sodium valproate on tardive dyskinesia. *Br J Psychiatry* 1976;129:114–119.

80. Fisk GG, York SM. The effect of sodium valproate on tardive dyskinesia: revisited. *Br J Psychiatry* 1987;150:542–546.

81. Nair NP, Lal S, Schwartz G, et al. Effect of sodium valproate and baclofen in tardive dyskinesia: clinical and neuroendocrine studies. *Adv Biochem Psychopharmacol* 1980;24:437–441.

82. Soares KV, McGrath JJ. The treatment of tardive dyskinesia: a systematic review and meta-analysis. *Schizophr Res* 1999;39:1–16.

83. Takeuchi H, Ishigooka J, Kobayashi K, et al. Study on the suitability of a rat model for tardive dyskinesia and the preventive effects of various drugs. *Prog Neuropsychopharmacol Biol Psychiatry* 1998;22:679–691.

84. Monteleone P, Maj M, Ariano MG, et al. Prolactin response to sodium valproate in schizophrenics with and without tardive dyskinesia. *Psychopharmacology (Berl)* 1988;96:223–226.

85. Ogawa T, Nagao T, Kashiwabara K, et al. Tardive dyskinesia and neurotransmitters: effects of sodium valproate, cyproheptadine, oxypertine, hydroxyzine pamoate and Ca-hopantenate on monoamine metabolites, cyclic nucleotides and gamma-aminobutyric acid in human cerebrospinal fluid. *Clin Ther* 1984;7 [Spec No]:1–17.

86. Biederman J, Mick E, Bostic JQ, et al. The naturalistic course of pharmacologic treatment of children with maniclike symptoms: a systematic chart review. *J Clin Psychiatry* 1998;59:628–637.

87. Kowatch RA, Suppes T, Carmody TJ, et al. Effect size of lithium, divalproex sodium, and carbamazepine in children and adolescents with bipolar disorder. *J Am Acad Child Adolesc Psychiatry* 2000;39:713–720.

88. Papatheodorou G, Kutcher SP, Katic M, et al. The efficacy and safety of divalproex sodium in the treatment of acute mania in adolescents and young adults: an open clinical trial. *J Clin Psychopharmacol* 1995;15:110–116.

89. McFarland BH, Miller MR, Straumfjord AA. Valproate use in the older manic patient. *J Clin Psychiatry* 1990;51:479–481.

90. Niedermier JA, Nasrallah HA. Clinical correlates of response to valproate in geriatric inpatients. *Ann Clin Psychiatry* 1998;10:165–168.

91. Conney J, Kaston B. Pharmacoeconomic and health outcome comparison of lithium and divalproex in a VA geriatric nursing home population: influence of drug-related morbidity on total cost of treatment. *Am J Manag Care* 1999;5:197–204.

92. Chen ST, Altshuler LL, Melnyk KA, et al. Efficacy of lithium vs. valproate in the treatment of mania in the elderly: a retrospective study. *J Clin Psychiatry* 1999;60:181–186.

93. Lott AD, McElroy SL, Keys MA. Valproate in the treatment of behavioral agitation in elderly patients with dementia. *J Neuropsychiatry Clin Neurosci* 1995;7:314–319.

94. Kando JC, Tohen M, Castillo J, et al. The use of valproate in an elderly population with affective symptoms. *J Clin Psychiatry* 1996;57:238–240.

95. Narayan M, Nelson JC. Treatment of dementia with behavioral disturbance using divalproex or a combination of divalproex and a neuroleptic. *J Clin Psychiatry* 1997;58:351–354.

96. Wroblewski BA, Joseph AB, Kupfer J, et al. Effectiveness of valproic acid on destructive and aggressive behaviours in patients with acquired brain injury. *Brain Inj* 1997;11:37–47.

97. Grossman F. A review of anticonvulsants in treating agitated demented elderly patients. *Pharmacotherapy* 1998;18: 600–606.

98. Masmoudi K, Gras-Champel V, Bonnet I, et al. Demence et troubles extra-pyramidaux sous acide valproique au long cours. [Dementia and extrapyramidal problems caused by long-term valproic acid]. *Therapie* 2000;55:629–634.

99. Onofrj M, Thomas A, Paci C. Reversible parkinsonism induced by prolonged treatment with valproate. *J Neurol* 1998;245: 794–796.

100. Goldberg JF, Garno JL, Leon AC, et al. Rapid titration of mood stabilizers predicts remission from mixed or pure mania in bipolar patients [published erratum appears in *J Clin Psychiatry* 1998;59:320]. *J Clin Psychiatry* 1998;59:151–158.

101. Keck PE Jr, McElroy SL, Tugrul KC, et al. Valproate oral loading in the treatment of acute mania. *J Clin Psychiatry* 1993; 54:305–308.

102. McElroy SL, Keck PE Jr, Stanton SP, et al. A randomized comparison of divalproex oral loading versus haloperidol in the initial treatment of acute psychotic mania. *J Clin Psychiatry* 1996; 57:142–146.

103. Hirschfeld RM, Allen MH, McEvoy JP, et al. Safety and tolerability of oral loading divalproex sodium in acutely manic bipolar patients. *J Clin Psychiatry* 1999;60:815–818.

104. Martinez JM, Russell JM, Hirschfeld RM. Tolerability of oral loading of divalproex sodium in the treatment of acute mania. *Depress Anxiety* 1998;7:83–86.

105. Norton JW, Quarles E. Intravenous valproate in neuropsychiatry. *Pharmacotherapy* 2000;20:88–92.

106. Grunze H, Erfurth A, Amann B, et al. Intravenous valproate loading in acutely manic and depressed bipolar I patients. *J Clin Psychopharmacol* 1999;19:303–309.

107. Zarate CA, Tohen M, Narendran R, et al. The adverse effect profile and efficacy of divalproex sodium compared with valproic acid: a pharmacoepidemiology study. *J Clin Psychiatry* 1999;60:232–236.

VALPROIC ACID

ADVERSE EFFECTS

PIERRE GENTON
PHILIPPE GELISSE

Valproate (VPA), which was first marketed in France over 30 years ago, and in North America over 20 years ago, has become one of the leading drugs for the treatment of various forms of epilepsy. It was recently approved in other indications, including mood disorders and migraine. Patient-years of treatment are numbered in millions and are steadily increasing; VPA now is probably the antiepileptic drug (AED) with the best-investigated array of adverse effects (AEs), some frequent, sometimes predictable and mostly benign, others rare and potentially severe. AEs of VPA have been extensively collected, studied, and reported; over 2,000 peer-reviewed papers have been published on this topic, with a new interest triggered by the new indications, especially in psychiatry. There remains much controversy over the prevalence, severity, and clinical significance of most of these AEs, as well as over their mechanisms. This reflects in part unresolved questions pertaining to the multiple mechanisms of action of VPA, and to its complex metabolic pathways. A specific, genetically determined sensitivity may play a major part in the occurrence of many of these AEs.

The successful career of VPA has been punctuated by three major "scares." The first concern was raised in the 1970s after observations of acute liver toxicity. The second serious concern was raised in the early 1980s and focused on the occurrence of major malformations (e.g., spina bifida) in children born to mothers treated with VPA. A third problem came to the foreground in the 1990s with regard to the risk of reproductive disorders [specifically, of polycystic ovary syndrome (PCOS)] in girls and young women treated with VPA. At the onset of the 21st century, these concerns can be put into perspective, but need to be discussed in detail.

Using a clinician's perspective, we review the acute and chronic dose-related AEs, the allergic and idiosyncratic AEs,

Pierre Genton, MD: Neurologist, Center of Saint Paul, Merseilles, France
Philippe Gelisse, MD: Chief of Clinic, Laboratory of Experimental Medicine, Institute of Biology; and Chief of Clinic, Epilepsy Unit, Gui de Chauliac Hospital, Montpellier, France

the risks involved in reproduction and pregnancy, and some special situations, including the coprescription of VPA with some of the newer AEDs. The AEs of VPA are considered globally here, but the availability of several presentations of VPA, including chemical variants (valproic acid, valproate salts, divalproex sodium, valpromide) and a solution for intravenous (i.v.) use, also may raise some specific questions. The issue of paradoxical aggravation of epilepsy by AEDs also is worth considering. This review thus adds a significant amount of recent data to the extensive review written by F. Dreifuss in the previous edition of this volume (52).

GLOBAL TOLERABILITY PROFILE

Clinical trials easily detect the common, dose-related AEs that are seen most often during the early days or weeks of treatment, especially during uptitration The most recent studies were performed in patients treated for psychiatric disorders or for migraine; very few recent studies have evaluated valproate in the context of epilepsy, either in comparison with placebo or with other AEDs.

Divalproex sodium has been used as adjunctive therapy for complex partial seizures in patients who were not adequately controlled with either carbamazepine (CBZ) or phenytoin monotherapy (Abbott Laboratories, data on file). The adverse events occurring significantly more often with divalproate versus placebo (>5% of patients) were nausea, asthenia, somnolence, vomiting, tremor, abdominal pain, and anorexia (Table 89.1). Table 89.2 reports the most common AEs in a trial comparing high-dose (mean valproic acid level = 123 μg/mL) versus low-dose (mean valproic acid level = 71 μg/mL) divalproex sodium monotherapy in patients with refractory complex partial seizures (16). The main AEs related to high-dose therapy were asthenia, nausea, diarrhea, vomiting, tremor, somnolence, alopecia, and thrombocytopenia. Headache was the only adverse event that occurred with a higher incidence in the low-dose group. The probability of thrombocytopenia increased significantly at total trough valproic acid plasma

TABLE 89.1. ADVERSE EVENTS REPORTED BY ≥5% OF PATIENTS TREATED WITH DIVALPROEX SODIUM DURING PLACEBO-CONTROLLED TRIAL OF ADJUNCTIVE THERAPY FOR COMPLEX PARTIAL SEIZURES[a]

Body System/Event	Divalproex Sodium (n = 77)	Placebo (n = 70)
Body as a whole		
Headache	31%	21%
Asthenia	27%	7%
Fever	6%	4%
Gastrointestinal system		
Nausea	48%	14%
Vomiting	27%	7%
Abdominal pain	23%	6%
Diarrhea	13%	6%
Anorexia	12%	0
Dyspepsia	8%	4%
Constipation	5%	1%
Nervous system		
Somnolence	27%	11%
Tremor	25%	6%
Dizziness	25%	13%
Diplopia	16%	9%
Amblyopia/blurred vision	12%	9%
Ataxia	8%	1%
Nystagmus	8%	1%
Emotional lability	6%	4%
Mental slowing	6%	0
Amnesia	5%	1%
Respiratory system		
Flu syndrome	12%	9%
Infection	12%	6%
Bronchitis	5%	1%
Rhinitis	5%	4%
Other		
Alopecia	6%	1%
Weight loss	6%	0

[a]The dosage of divalproex sodium was increased gradually over 8 weeks. At the maintenance period, the mean daily dose and serum valproic acid concentration were respectively, 31.4 mg/kg/day and 59.1 μg/mL.
Data from Abbott Laboratories.

TABLE 89.2. ADVERSE EVENTS DURING DIVALPROEX SODIUM MONOTHERAPY IN PARTIAL EPILEPSIES, IN A TRIAL COMPARING HIGH- AND LOW-DOSE GROUPS

	Divalproex Sodium, High-dose, 80–150 μg/mL (n = 96)	Divalproex Sodium, Low-dose, 25–50 μg/mL (n = 47)
Tremor	61%	6%
Thrombocytopenia	31%	0%
Alopecia	28%	4%
Diarrhea	21%	4%
Asthenia	17%	0%
Vomiting	17%	0%
Headache	16%	32%
Weight gain	15%	4%
Anorexia	15%	0%
Exit rate from adverse events	32%	2%

Adapted from Beydoun A, Sackellares JC, Shu V, and the Depakote Monotherapy for Partial Seizures Study Group. Safety and efficacy of divalproex sodium monotherapy in partial epilepsy: a double-blind, concentration-response designed clinical test. *Neurology* 1997;48:182–188, with permission.

TABLE 89.3. INCIDENCE OF SIDE EFFECTS AND RATE OF WITHDRAWAL RESULTING FROM SIDE EFFECTS IN RANDOMIZED CONTROLLED TRIALS COMPARING MONOTHERAPY IN ADULTS WITH NEWLY DIAGNOSED EPILEPSY

Reference	Duration (mo)		Valproate	Carbamazepine	Phenytoin
Richens et al., 1994 (141)	36	Number of patients	n = 149	n = 151	
		Average dose	924 mg/day	516 mg/day	
		Withdrawal rate	5% (first 6 mo)	15% (first 6 mo)	
			5% (between 6 and 36 mo)	5% (between 6 and 36 mo)	
		Incidence of side effects	49.4% (at 36 mo)	48.9% (at 36 mo)	
Heller et al., 1995 (77)	30	Number of patients	n = 61	n = 61	n = 63
		Average dose	NS	NS	NS
		Withdrawal rate	5%	11%	3%
		Incidence of side effects	NS	NS	NS
Callaghan et al., 1985 (28)	14–18[a]	Number of patients	n = 64	n = 59	n = 58
		Average dose	15.6 mg/kg/day	10.9 mg/kg/day	5.4 mg/kg/day
		Withdrawal rate[b]	14%	14%	9%
		Incidence of side effects	10.9%	8.5%	10.3%
Turnbull et al., 1985 (164)	24	Number of patients	n = 70		n = 70
		Average dose	NS		NS
		Withdrawal rate	23%		23%
		Incidence of side effects	NS		NS

NS, not stated in published trial data.
[a]Median follow-up for patients with partial and generalized seizures was 14 and 15 months, respectively, for carbamazepine, 18 and 24 months, respectively, for phenytoin, and 24 and 24 months, respectively, for valproate.
[b]Withdrawal resulting from all causes.
Adapted from Heaney DC, Shorvon SD, Sander JW. An economic appraisal of carbamazepine, lamotrigine, phenytoin and valproate as initial treatment in adults with newly diagnosed epilepsy. *Epilepsia* 1998;39[Suppl 3]:S19–S25, with permission.

concentrations >110 µg/mL in women and >135 µg/mL in men. In this trial, 27% of patients receiving approximately 50 mg/kg/day on average had at least one platelet count value ≤75 × 10^9/L. Approximately half of these patients discontinued treatment, with return of platelet counts to normal. In the remaining patients, platelet counts normalized with continued treatment (Abbott Laboratories, data on file). Table 89.3 compares the global incidence of AEs and of withdrawal from study in head-to-head comparisons between VPA and other AEDs.

From these data, a global tolerability profile of VPA as it is used in clinical practice becomes apparent. These findings, however, must be discussed in detail.

DOSE-RELATED ADVERSE EFFECTS

Overdosage

Toxic doses are greater than 3 g in adults and 50 mg/kg in children. The main risks of overdosage are calm hypotonic coma, convulsions, and respiratory depression at very high doses (17). Doses less than 100 mg/kg are associated with minor toxicity. Profound coma usually occurs only at doses greater than 200 mg/kg; otherwise, the presence of coingestants should be suspected. Overdosage with VPA may result in gastrointestinal disturbances, drowsiness, mental confu-

sion, and encephalopathy. At high doses, heart block, hypotension, hypophosphatemia, deep coma, cerebral edema, muscular hypotonia, hyporeflexia, myosis, respiratory depression, convulsions, and metabolic disorders (metabolic acidosis, hypernatremia, hypoglycemia, hyperammonemia) can arise. Reversible methemoglobinemia also has been reported (113). Fatalities have been described (15,35,94) but are rare. Mortensen et al. (120) reported the case of 20-year-old woman who was comatose for several days after intoxication with 75 g VPA (peak serum VPA of a 2,120 µ/mL 8.5 hours after drug intake) and who recovered. Treatment must be symptomatic and supportive, with particular attention to the maintenance of adequate urinary output. Gastric lavage and activated charcoal should be performed as soon as possible. Because the drug is rapidly absorbed, gastric lavage may be of limited value excepted for delayed-release formulations. Multiple dosing of activated charcoal may be effective. In overdosage, the fraction of drug not bound to protein is high, and in severe intoxication with coma, hemodialysis or hemoperfusion may be beneficial (96,120,156). Naloxone has been reported to reverse the central nervous system–depressant effects of VPA overdosage (2,118). L-Carnitine (100 mg/kg loading dose, then 250 mg every 8 hours for 4 days, or 150 to 500 mg/kg/day, up to 3 g/day) may be useful to prevent hepatic dysfunction after VPA overdose (44,84,122).

Acute Dose-Related Adverse Effects

Gastrointestinal

Nausea with or without vomiting and gastrointestinal distress are common AEs, often noted at the initiation of VPA therapy, in up to 25% of patients. Their incidence is maximal with the oral solutions, and has been markedly decreased by the availability of enteric-coated and controlled release preparations. Tolerance to these symptoms usually develops within weeks, but in many cases it is necessary to recommend drug intake during or after meals, and a slowing of uptitration (49). Their persistence beyond the initial period of treatment or their occurrence during long-term treatment should raise specific concerns about metabolic, hepatic, or pancreatic complications.

Tremor

Although patients exhibit a specific sensitivity to this AE, tremor clearly is a dose-related symptom that is associated with high blood levels of VPA (97). It usually appears as fast, low-amplitude tremor resembling adrenergic tremor, or it resembles essential tremor; it rarely appears as asterixis (21), which is mostly a symptom of hepatopathy with or without hyperammonemia in VPA-treated patients. VPA-induced tremor always responds to dose reduction, but propranolol may be useful in some patients (97).

Encephalopathy and Coma

Acute encephalopathy or coma may occur early in the course of VPA treatment with or without evident metabolic changes such as hyperammonemia and low carnitine (see later), with or without interactions with other AEDs, especially phenobarbital (146), and without overdosage (171). This makes its categorization as a dose-related AE uncertain. However, many such cases cannot be fully explained by coexisting metabolic disturbances, and their pathogenesis remains unclear. They are characterized by marked alterations of the electroencephalogram (EEG), mostly in the form of continuous slow waves, and are rapidly reversible on discontinuation of VPA. In clinical practice, this complication should be rapidly diagnosed using the EEG, overdosage and major metabolic changes quickly evaluated, and VPA discontinued.

Chronic Dose-Related Adverse Effects

Weight Gain

In clinical practice, weight gain is significantly associated with VPA (47). It may be particularly difficult to control in younger patients and in patients with mental handicap. Girls are particularly at risk (127), as are persons with normal or below-normal baseline weight (38): In the latter study, 70% of patients on VPA monotherapy gained at least 4 kg. Patients tend to report increased appetite, and to increase both the number and the size of daily food intakes. Several mechanisms have been proposed that may be based on a genetic predisposition to obesity, and weight gain may be associated with decreased β-oxidation of fatty acids (23), increased insulin and insulin/glucose ratios (42), and increased leptin and insulin levels (169). A direct central effect on hunger or satiety is not excluded. Carnitine levels do not seem to play a significant part (42). However, weight gain may occur owing to other factors, and the causal role of VPA in the genesis of weight gain in children receiving VPA has been challenged recently (53). In a randomized trial comparing VPA with CBZ in 260 children aged 4 to 15 years with newly diagnosed epilepsy, it was shown that there was no statistical difference in weight increase between the two groups, and that three-fourths of subjects who gained weight on VPA continued to do so if they were switched to CBZ. Weight gain and related metabolic disturbances may play a major part in the genesis of reproductive disorders in women (see later), and also may lead to social problems. Patients therefore should be warned about this risk, and dietary measures should be proposed whenever necessary.

Hair Changes

Some patients may report thinning of hair, alopecia (95), change of hair color, or regrowth of curly hair. Such changes have been seen with many psychotropic drugs (116), and their incidence has not been established. These changes usually are benign and transient, and may remit even under continuing therapy. There is no explanation for this phenomenon, which may be related to hypothyroidism in a minority of cases. The therapeutic value of vitamin or mineral supplements has not been documented, although most patients receive such treatment in case of hair changes induced by VPA.

Cognitive and Other Chronic Central Nervous System-Related Side Effects

The negative effects of VPA on cognition usually are considered minimal (162). A study compared the effects of newly prescribed VPA (low-dose and high-dose) and CBZ on motor speed and coordination, memory, concentration, and mental flexibility (137). There were no significant differences compared with pretreatment levels at 6 and 12 months. However, subtle cognitive dysfunctions may be present, especially in children who receive high doses of VPA, and should be monitored (106). If present, cognitive AEs are nonspecific and quickly and completely reversible after withdrawal (62). There are some rare cases of severe cognitive disturbances. In a 21-year-old man with a 3-year history of dementia, dementia was reversed within 2 months on discontinuation of VPA (185). In another case report, an 11-year-old girl with normal intelligence experienced marked mental deterioration after 2 years and 6 months of continuing VPA treatment (72). There were no metabolic changes, and magnetic resonance imaging (MRI) findings mimicked diffuse brain atrophy; both MRI changes and cognitive dysfunctions disappeared within 4 months after drug reduction and discontinuation. A similar case of reversible cognitive dysfunction was reported in a patient in whom cognitive decline and "pseudoatrophy" of the brain appeared within 2 weeks of initiation of VPA (153). Reversible pseudoatrophy also may be associated with parkinsonism (149), but the latter may occur in an isolated manner, or in association with cognitive decline (10); it remits within weeks after discontinuation of VPA (129). Reversible hearing loss was reported but not confirmed by other observations (9).

Endocrine (Excluding Reproduction) and Metabolic Changes

Subclinical peripheral hypothyroidism (i. e., elevated serum levels of thyroid-stimulating hormone) has been reported in children (56,181). These changes were reversed in selected cases after discontinuation of VPA, and never were associated with overt thyroid dysfunction. Coadministration of VPA with enzyme-inducing AEDs may cause a decrease in serum levels of the thyroid hormones triiodothyronine and thyroxine (86). The occurrence of a dose-related inappropriate secretion of antidiuretic hormone–like syndrome has been reported in a patient on VPA who also had nephritis (22). Subclinical hyperglycemia and hyperglycinemia also have been reported (91). An unfavorable lipid profile has been associated with the use of VPA in women who gained weight and in whom polycystic ovaries also developed (89), and the metabolic changes were partially reversed after substitution of VPA by lamotrigine (LTG), with an increase in the high-density lipoprotein cholesterol/total cholesterol ratio.

However, the major metabolic changes associated with VPA concern hyperammonemia and the metabolism of carnitine. Hyperammonemia appears to occur in as much as 50% of patients treated with VPA, especially in polytherapy, and is a subclinical change in most cases, without signs of hepatic dysfunction (5,124,158,184). Serum valproic acid levels above 100 μg/mL and age younger than 2 years may be risk factors for development of hyperammonemia (5). It also may appear in the form of marked encephalopathy with or without coma, and in association with overt liver toxicity. It is clearly enhanced in the presence of polytherapy with hepatic cytochrome P450 (CYP) inducers (182). Hyperammonemia has been ascribed to increased renal production of ammonia, to inhibition of nitrogen elimination due to inhibition of urea synthesis, or to a combination of these factors (80). Hyperammonemia also

might be secondary to increased glycine and propionic acid concentrations (39). Similarly, lowered carnitine levels have been reported in patients receiving VPA (125), but whether these changes are clinically significant remains debatable. Carnitine deficiency has been related to the occurrence of malignant, fatal cerebral edema without liver dysfunction in a young woman (161). In many instances, the occurrence of encephalopathy related to hyperammonemia and carnitine deficiency has been ascribed to a preexisting, unrecognized metabolic defect such as ornithine transcarbamylase deficiency (81,82,128,159). Carnitine deficiency may predispose to the occurrence of otherwise unexplained coma (160). Hence, carnitine supplementation, which is highly recommended in the presence of liver toxicity, also may be useful as a preventive measure in some cases (115). However, otherwise healthy children treated with VPA apparently do not exhibit carnitine deficiency, and supplementation therefore may not be necessary (138) except in those who are exposed to low-carnitine diets because of associated handicaps (79).

Other Uncommon Chronic Adverse Effects

Diffuse peripheral edema may be associated with long-standing VPA therapy (26,57). This occurs without associated liver toxicity, and the mechanisms are unknown. Gingival hyperplasia, which is a very common AE of phenytoin, has been ascribed to VPA in a 9-year-old girl who had not been treated with other AEDs (6,8). VPA has also been reported to provoke an increase in sister-chromatid exchange and in chromosomal abnormalities in peripheral lymphocytes in patients on VPA monotherapy who were compared with age-matched control subjects (83); such acquired changes also were found after short-term, 6-month VPA treatment, and in lymphocytes of control subjects exposed *in vitro* to VPA. However, these interesting findings have not been duplicated. Facilitation of bone fractures also has been reported in children on long-term VPA treatment, without any speculation on possible mechanisms (132). Renal toxicity, in the form of Fanconi's syndrome, was reported in two children (104). Both recovered normal proximal tubular function within 4 months of discontinuing VPA therapy.

ALLERGIC AND IDIOSYNCRATIC SIDE EFFECTS

Allergic Reactions

Because of the simple, nonaromatic structure of VPA, allergic reactions are uncommon, and less frequent than with other AEDs (24). In a retrospective study, there were 8 serious adverse skin reactions in 8,888 new phenytoin users, 6 in 9,768 new CBZ users, and none in 1,504 new VPA users (157). As with other AEDs, skin reactions develop early in the course of VPA treatment. A 28-year old woman who had a generalized skin eruption associated with marked eosinophilia and altered liver function was reported (134); the responsibility of VPA was confirmed by a positive patch test. A case of Stevens-Johnson syndrome was ascribed to VPA in another case report (163). Two cases of systematic lupus erythematosus possibly induced by VPA have been reported (20), but the causal relationship was unclear because one of these patients clearly had other predisposing factors. A case of acute, near-fatal multiorgan system failure that probably was of allergic origin also has been reported (135).

Blood Dyscrasias

Blood dyscrasias due to AEDs are rare, although all classic agents have been implicated in their occurrence (19). Thrombocytopenia and inhibition of platelet aggregation are the most common hematologic abnormalities associated with VPA (111). VPA may reduce the activity of the arachidonate cascade in platelets and inhibit the cyclooxygenase pathway and synthesis of the platelet aggregator thromboxane (98). Thrombocytopenia can be tolerated as long as the platelet count is stable in the range of 100,000/mm^3 and there are no signs of an increased bleeding tendency, the risk of which is low (3,170). Thrombocytopenia with a platelet count below 80,000/mm^3 requires close monitoring. This condition is correlated with both dosage and serum concentration of VPA (69), and responds to dosage reduction or discontinuation of the drug. Occasionally, severe bleeding, hematoma, epistaxis, and petechiae have been observed (111). May and Sunder (115a) reported that 33% of 60 patients receiving long-term VPA monotherapy (mean, 14.6 years) exhibited at least one prominent hematologic abnormality (i.e., thrombocytopenia, macrocytosis, leukopenia, and anemia). The incidence was 55% in the subset of patients whose VPA plasma concentrations exceeded 100 mg/L. However, these abnormalities were not severe enough to discontinue therapy and always responded to small decrements in VPA therapy. Neutropenia, macrocytosis, bone marrow suppression leading to aplastic anemia or peripheral cytopenia affecting one or more cell lines, myelodysplasia, and a clinical picture resembling acute promyelocytic leukemia are extremely rare but all have been associated with VPA therapy [review in Acharya and Bussel (1)] (63,172). Valproic acid also may be associated with abnormal coagulation factors such as low fibrinogen levels (14, 75,114) and acquired von Willebrand's disease type I. Kreuz et al. (103) investigated bleeding disorders in a group of children receiving VPA and observed a reduction in fibrinogen concentration and platelet count, and a significant decrease in factor VII complex. The effect of VPA on bleeding time and coagulation factors can lead to hemorrhage. It is recommended that a complete blood count, thrombocyte count, and coagulation parameters be performed before initiation of treatment, after initiation, and before elective surgery. However, a surgical series has shown no increase in bleeding complications or blood loss in patients who underwent cortical surgery (6).

Hepatotoxicity

A minor increase in serum aminotransferases is common. It is observed in 30% to 50% of patients (154), appears to be dose related, is transient, and is observed more commonly during initial therapy and in patients comedicated with phenobarbital or phenytoin (73). When this increase remains moderate (lower than two or three times baseline values), asymptomatic, and without any abnormal changes in other liver function test results, the treatment may be continued. More rarely, results of other liver tests, such as alkaline phosphatase, lactate dehydrogenase, and bilirubin, may be increased. Occasionally, γ-glutamyl transferase activity may be slightly increased (70). If the level is higher than expected, alcoholism or hepatitis may be suspected.

VPA has been linked to serious hepatotoxicity. It is a rare, typically idiosyncratic side effect. In a retrospective study of patients treated between 1978 and 1984, the overall incidence was approximately 1 in 10,000 cases (50). Children younger than 2 years of age appear to be at higher risk, particularly those receiving multiple AEDs, those with genetic disorders of metabolism, and those with mental retardation or organic brain disease. The overall risk of fatal hepatic dysfunction was approximately 1/500 in children younger than 2 years of age receiving VPA in polytherapy. The risk declined with age, with a rate of 1/12,000 if receiving polytherapy and 1/37,000 in monotherapy (51). From 1987 through 1993, over 1 million patients were newly treated with VPA. Fatal hepatotoxicity was observed in 29 patients (25). This apparent decrease in fatal liver toxicity appears to be due to changes in prescribing patterns and to physician awareness of high-risk factors for hepatic failure. Adult patients are considered to have a lower risk than children. However, they can be affected as well. König et al. (102) conducted a thorough review of the medical literature and identified 26 cases of adult fatalities published since 1980: The age range was from 17 to 62 years, 3 had received VPA in monotherapy, and 23 in combination. Twelve (46%) had no significant underlying disease. Thus, VPA should be used with extreme caution in higher-risk groups and should be avoided in patients with preexisting hepatotoxicity and inborn errors of metabolism such as carnitine deficiency. Such disorders, however, may be subclinical, as was the case in a fatal hepatopathy of a child after 4 months of VPA treatment; fibroblast culture showed the presence of a medium-chain acyl-CoA dehydrogenase deficiency (52,101,126). Dreifuss (52) and König et al. (101) provided guidelines to minimize the risk of serous VPA-related hepatotoxicity, which are summarized in Table 89.4.

Severe hepatotoxic effects of VPA typically occur during the first 6 months of treatment, but can occur later (100). A

TABLE 89.4. RECOMMENDATIONS TO MINIMIZE THE RISKS OF VALPROATE-INDUCED HEPATIC TOXICITY

1. Avoid the use of valproate in patients with preexisting liver disease and/or elevated baseline liver and/or pancreatic enzymes at least three times the normal upper limit and/or significant coagulopathies.
2. Avoid the use of valproate in patients with a personal or a family history of metabolic diseases implying β-oxidation, mitochondrial and peroxisomal functions, or unclear liver diseases with or without previous toxicity of valproate.
3. Specially careful monitoring should be provided when valproate is given in children aged less than 2 years, in association with enzyme-inducing drugs and in patients with mental retardation of unexplained origin, neurometabolic diseases or hereditary metabolic disorders. Administration of valproate in these situations should be done only after careful evaluation of the risk/benefit ratio.
4. Liver enzymes, amylase, platelets, bilirubin, and prothrombin time should be assessed prior to initiation of valproate in all patients, and reassessed after 1 month. They should then be reassessed only in the presence of significant clinical symptoms and (concerning coagulation parameters) prior to surgical procedures.
5. If possible, use valproate only in monotherapy under the age of 3 years, and at the lowest possible dosage in all.
6. Patients and parents should be advised to report immediately vomiting, anorexia, headache, edema, jaundice, or seizure breakthrough, especially after a febrile illness and/or other symptoms suggestive of possible hepatic dysfunction.
7. Administration of salicylates should be done cautiously, and high doses of salicylates should be avoided.

Adapted from Dreifuss FE, Langer DH, Moline KA, et al. Valproic acid hepatic fatalities: II. US experience since 1984. *Neurology* 1989;39:201–207; and König SA, Elger CE, Vassella F, et al. Empfehlungen zu Blutuntersuchungen und klinischer Überwachung zur Früherkennung des Valporat-associierten Leberversagens. *Nervenarzt* 1998;69:835–840, with permission.

baseline liver evaluation usually is recommended before starting therapy and at regular intervals thereafter. However, hepatic failure may occur after repeatedly normal measurements of liver enzymes. Laboratory tests have a poor predictive value for serious hepatotoxicity. In most cases, changes in laboratory values were preceded by clinical signs such as vomiting, anorexia, lethargy, facial edema, weakness, abdominal pain, and sudden and inexplicable increases in seizure frequency, especially in the presence of febrile disorders. Thus, clinical symptoms appear to be more reliable indicators of hepatotoxicity. The histologic findings in VPA hepatotoxicity differ from those observed with other AEDs such as CBZ, phenytoin, and phenobarbital, where liver damage is associated with inflammatory changes. The typical liver histology of VPA toxicity includes microvesicular steatosis, cellular ballooning, and single- or multiple-cell necrosis (102). The histologic features resemble those found in Jamaican vomiting sickness and Reye's syndrome. Young et al. (180) reported a case described as a fatal Reye's-like syndrome. The pathogenesis of hepatotoxicity remains unclear, and different theories

have been proposed. A breakdown of β-oxidation is considered to be the main mechanism of VPA-related hepatotoxicity (102). The 4-ene metabolite may be play a role in hepatotoxicity by inhibiting enzymes involved in β-oxidation (40). This metabolite depends on CYP, which may explain in part the higher risk of liver toxicity in cotherapy with enzyme-inducing AEDs (52). However, the CYP3A4 isoform usually associated with induction by anticonvulsants is not responsible for the enhanced 4-ene-VPA formation that occurs during polytherapy; instead, enhanced 4-ene-VPA formation *in vivo* likely results from induction of CYP2A6 or CYP2C9 (147). Triggs et al. (160) also hypothesized that VPA may sequester coenzyme A, which leads to impairment of β-oxidation enzymes. Metabolic defects, polytherapy, or infections probably contribute by depleting intracellular coenzyme A (100). VPA therapy often is associated with decreased carnitine levels (125,166). L-Carnitine is an essential cofactor in the β-oxidation of fatty acids (138). It was suggested that the carnitine deficiency induced by VPA leads to impairment of mitochondrial β-oxidation enzymes. Neurologic handicap, age younger than 2 years, or multiple AEDs are risk factors for carnitine deficiency (138). L-Carnitine supplementation helps restore β-oxidation. Carnitine supplementation clearly is indicated in case of hepatotoxicity, overdosage, and other acute metabolic events associated with carnitine deficiency (i.v. carnitine 150 to 500 mg/kg/day, up to 3 g/day) (44).

Pancreatitis

Potentially fatal acute hemorrhagic pancreatitis has been reported (4,11,18,27,29,58,130,174,177). Reexposure to VPA after recovery may lead to recurrence of pancreatitis. This complication is rare, with an incidence estimated at 1/40,000 (101). In their survey of 39 cases identified from personal files, literature, and a survey of physicians with a special interest in treatment of epilepsy, Asconapé et al. (11) noted that 14.5% of the 366 physicians who participated in the survey had seen at least 1 case. Acute pancreatitis may occur at any age, but is more common in patients younger than 20 years of age, in polytherapy, and in patients with chronic encephalopathy (58). Patients on hemodialysis, particularly children, may represent a group at greater risk (60). It can appear at any stage of treatment, although nearly half of the cases occur during the first 3 months, and 70% during the first year, secondary either to a recent dosage increase or to initiation of treatment. Most patients in whom acute pancreatitis develops have serum VPA levels within the therapeutic range. Abdominal pain, nausea, vomiting, or anorexia are the initial symptoms, and prompt medical attention should be sought if they appear while on VPA therapy. In patients treated with VPA who experience severe abdominal pain, amylase or lipase levels should be systematically performed before a surgical decision. Wyllie et al. (177) reported two patients who underwent exploratory laparotomy before diagnosis of pancreatitis. Complications include pseudocyst, pericardial effusion, laparotomy wound infection, and coagulopathy. If pancreatitis is diagnosed, VPA should be discontinued and pancreatitis may be rapidly reversed. The mortality rate has been estimated at 21% (18). The prognosis is worse in patients with associated liver failure (18). Systematic measurement of amylase levels is not recommended because mild, transient, and asymptomatic elevations are not uncommon, and at least one case of pancreatitis has been reported in which the plasma amylase level was normal but the other pancreatic enzymes (lipase, elastase, trypsin) were elevated (130).

REPRODUCTION

Puberty

Pubertal arrest has been reported to occur during VPA therapy (37), but a prospective study of eight boys and four girls treated with VPA and followed throughout puberty failed to detect any significant clinical or biologic change (36,112). Recently, the focus has been shifted to the occurrence of hyperandrogenism in peripubertal girls on VPA (165): compared with a control population, testosterone levels exceeding the mean plus two standard deviations were seen in 38% of prepubertal, 36% of pubertal, and 57% of postpubertal girls. However, there were no definite clinical consequences of these changes, although the authors suggest that they might be related to development of polycystic ovaries in later life. Such changes might be at least partially related to weight gain in the population treated with VPA.

Polycystic Ovaries and Polycystic Ovary Syndrome

Studies have focused on the occurrence of polycystic ovaries (PCO) and PCOS in women treated with VPA. In a retrospective study (87), 238 women with epilepsy (9 treated with VPA, 120 with CBZ, 12 with a combination of these, and 62 with other AEDs, whereas 15 were untreated) and 51 healthy control subjects were compared. Menstrual disturbances were present in 45% of the VPA group, 19% of the CBZ group, 25% of the combination group, 13% of the group receiving other drugs, 0% of the untreated group, and 16% of control group. Vaginal ultrasonographic examination was performed in all patients with menstrual disturbances and in some of the others, as well as in the control subjects. Ultrasonography revealed PCO in 43%, 22%, 50%, and 11%, respectively, in the four treatment groups and in 5% in the regularly menstruating control subjects; elevated serum testosterone levels occurred in 17%, 0%, 38%, and 0% of patients, respectively, in the four treatment groups. Eighty percent of women treated with VPA before

the age of 20 years had PCO or elevated testosterone; this compared with 27% of women treated with other AEDs. The mechanism involved was suggested to be related to hyperinsulinism and lowered insulin-like growth factor–binding protein 1 (88,89). These ovarian, hormonal, and metabolic changes were partly reversed after substitution of VPA with LTG. More recent studies, however, have questioned the reproducibility of these findings.

In a study of 65 women with epilepsy, including 21 women treated with VPA, 21 with phenobarbital, and 23 with CBZ, and 20 healthy control subjects, there was no difference in hirsutism score, ovary volume, or in the prevalence of PCO, although the VPA group had higher body weight and body mass index (123). Herzog, although acknowledging the possibility of increased incidence of PCO, pointed to the increased incidence of menstrual disorders and possibly PCO in women with epilepsy, and suggested that enzyme-inducing AEDs might protect against the effects of hyperandrogenism by increasing the level of sex hormone binding globulin (78). In a review on PCO, PCOS, and anticonvulsant therapy, it was stressed that many factors were involved in this very common disorder, and that the prevalence of VPA-induced changes was not as high as suggested by the aforementioned studies (68). In practice, there are limited data suggesting that VPA increases the incidence of reproductive disorders in young women, but clinicians should be aware of this possibility and monitor patients accordingly, with special attention given to the occurrence of weight gain (32,68). There are, however, no data that contraindicate the use of VPA in young women with epilepsy (12).

Male Reproduction

No major effects of VPA have been reported on male sexual and reproductive function. Follicle-stimulating hormone levels were shown to be slightly increased in men on VPA (65), whereas levels of other sex hormones (pituitary, adrenal, and gonadal) were unchanged (61,85). A recent comparison of monotherapies with VPA, CBZ, and oxcarbazepine showed that VPA increases the serum concentrations of androgens, whereas CBZ decreases their free fractions (139). The clinical significance of these findings is unclear. However, treatment with VPA has been associated with abnormal sperm mobility and count. In a 32-year-old man, a low sperm count of 50,000/mL was improved to >16 million with subsequent fertility after a switch from VPA to felbamate (179). Indeed, long-term treatment with VPA and with other AEDs [i.e., CBZ and phenytoin (but not phenobarbital)] has been associated with lower sperm mobility (34), but others failed to find any such abnormality with VPA (155).

Teratogenicity

The first case of spina bifida related to fetal exposure to VPA were seen in France approximately 20 years ago (143), where nine cases were reported in infants born to mothers who had received VPA during pregnancy. There had been isolated reports before this impressive series (41,71), and further cases afterward (64,108). These findings were confirmed by prospective studies (48), and later studies (both prospective and retrospective) showed that the incidence of neural tube defects is approximately of 1% to 2% in children born to mothers treated with VPA, which is approximately the risk of recurrence of neural tube defects in case of previous occurrence in a sibling. In a multicenter survey, the prevalence of neural tube defects was 2.5% in offspring of mothers treated with VPA monotherapy during the first trimester of pregnancy, which compared with 0.35% when other AEDs were used, and 0% in nonepileptic control subjects (109). The risk appears to be related to dose and peak VPA blood levels, but does not depend on seizure frequency during pregnancy (110). Additional risk factors include family history of neural tube defects, and association with CBZ.

A fetal VPA syndrome has been described that is characterized by minor craniofacial abnormalities with possible subsequent developmental delay, with or without occurrence of major organ malformations (46). Congenital defects associated with exposure to VPA include lung hypoplasia (three cases, including two siblings) (93), abnormal pulmonary artery origin (117), autism (175), other types of developmental delays (119), and limb deficiencies (131,144), especially bilateral radial hypoplasia (99). Although exposure to the AED is thought to play the predominant role in the incidence of malformations, other factors, such as genetic predisposition, appear to play a major role (30). Prevention of major malformation associated with intrauterine exposure to VPA is based:

In case of a planned pregnancy, on the use of alternative treatments or on a reappraisal of the necessity of VPA

Whenever VPA treatment appears unavoidable, on the lowest possible dosage and on fragmentation of intake (or use of controlled-release forms) to avoid high peak plasma VPA concentrations

Prophylactic administration of folic acid is recommended (121), although its effectiveness in preventing VPA-induced neural tube defects is unproven. Diagnostic ultrasonography (18th to 20th week of gestation) is indicated whenever there has been exposure to VPA in early pregnancy and pregnancy termination is an option. Amniocentesis at week 15 to 16 for the determination of α-fetoprotein also may be considered, but its use has declined after advances in ultrasonography (including specialized applications such as transvaginal ultrasonography).

Pregnancy and Lactation

The course of pregnancy usually is not affected by VPA (178). Specific problems such as bleeding, toxemia, preterm delivery, spontaneous abortion, intrauterine growth retardation, or mortality may be increased in women with epilepsy, but have not been associated specifically with VPA. However, a study of pregnancy outcome in women on VPA monotherapy showed a higher rate of infant distress at birth and of low Apgar scores compared with control subjects (92). Other mechanisms of toxicity may occur during pregnancy: A fatal case of liver toxicity has been reported in infants exposed during gestation (107). Newborns may experience withdrawal symptoms and hypoglycemia (54). Because only 3% to 5% of VPA diffuses in maternal milk, breast-feeding is not contraindicated. However, an infantile case of thrombocytopenic purpura that remitted after cessation of breast-feeding was reported recently (150).

DRUG COMBINATIONS

Because of a clear potentiation of their respective anticonvulsant activities, VPA and LTG are now increasingly used in combination for the treatment of resistant forms of generalized and focal epilepsies. This combination, however, poses several problems of tolerability that are due mostly to pharmacokinetic interactions (i.e., to the marked increase in half-life and plasma levels of LTG in the presence of VPA). Most AEs attributed to LTG (i.e., dizziness, headache, insomnia) are increased by this combination, and tremor may occur at comparatively low plasma levels values of VPA. However, the increased risk of LTG-induced skin rash and of more severe forms of cutaneous allergy after the addition of LTG in patients already receiving VPA represents the major risk, and titration of LTG should be particularly slow in this situation, with increments as small as 5 mg/day at intervals of 2 weeks in children, and 25 mg in adults (59). A lupus anticoagulant developed in a 5-year old boy, which eventually disappeared after discontinuation of VPA (55). Disseminated intravascular coagulation and multiorgan dysfunction, including rhabdomyolysis, was reported in two other children (33).

Although the combination of VPA and CBZ also is useful, it produces significant interactions. VPA decreases the clearance of CBZ-10,11-epoxide (CBZ-E) and increases CBZ-E blood levels (142), sometimes resulting in the appearance of CBZ-related AEs (dizziness, ataxia, diplopia, fatigue) that may be wrongly ascribed to VPA. The amide derivative of VPA, valpromide, is a much stronger inhibitor of CBZ-E metabolism, and CBZ-E–related side effects are seen much more commonly when valpromide is combined with CBZ (136).

The combination of VPA with topiramate (TPM) may be useful, and pharmacokinetic interactions do not pose specific problems (145). However, this combination occasionally has been associated with a hyperammonemic encephalopathy with mental confusion and slowing of the EEG (74), which clearly is related to the combination because its clinical, EEG, and biologic symptoms and signs remit after dose reduction or discontinuation of either VPA or TPM.

Pharmacokinetic interactions may have accounted for the occurrence of status epilepticus in a patient who received clomipramine in addition to VPA: Serum clomipramine concentrations were markedly elevated (43). Hepatic encephalopathy was precipitated by the addition of clozapine in a patient treated with VPA (176). A case of catatonia, which recurred after rechallenge with VPA and remitted definitively after withdrawal of VPA, occurred in a patient treated for schizoaffective disorder with risperidone and sertraline, and might represent a very uncommon interaction (105).

SPECIFIC ADVERSE EFFECTS ACCORDING TO PRESENTATION AND ADMINISTRATION ROUTE

Except for the aforementioned interactions between valpromide and CBZ-E, there are very few indications that chemical variants of VPA may produce different AEs. Divalproex sodium may be marginally better tolerated than VPA with regard to gastrointestinal side-effects, especially anorexia, nausea, and dyspepsia, and patients are less likely to stop medication because of AEs (183). Diarrhea has been ascribed to the excipient of a VPA solution (i.e., to glycerin and sorbitol) rather than to the drug itself because it

TABLE 89.5. ADVERSE EVENTS REPORTED BY AT LEAST 0.5% OF PATIENTS AFTER INTRAVENOUS VALPROATE[a]

Type of Event	Percentage of Patients (%)
Any event	17
Body as a whole	
Headache	2.4
Injection site inflammation	0.9
Injections site reaction	2.4
Injection site pain	0.9
Pain (unspecified)	0.6
Digestive system	
Abdominal pain	0.6
Diarrhea	0.6
Nausea with or without vomiting	2.8
Vomiting alone	1.6
Nervous system	
Dizziness	
Taste perversion	1.3
Hiccup	0.6
Somnolence	1.9
Tremor	0.6

[a]This study includes 318 patients (22 children and 296 adults). Adapted from Devinsky O, Leppik I, Willmore LJ, et al. Safety of intravenous valproate. *Ann Neurol* 1995;38:670–674, with permission.

resolved with another VPA preparation (167). Although most patients now receive either enteric-coated or controlled-release preparations of VPA, which were marketed with the aim of decreasing dose-related, acute AEs, an increasing number of generic preparations of VPA now are used around the world. Change to generic forms has caused gastrointestinal AEs to appear (148).

Intravenous VPA has been evaluated in clinical trials involving 318 patients with epilepsy, given at doses of 50 to 1,500 mg (45) (Table 89.5). The mean rate of infusion studied was 6.3 mg/min (range, 0.8 to 25 mg/min). Nausea, headache, and injection site reactions were the AEs most often reported, but their incidence was very low. There are, however, numerous, often contradictory reports on the tolerability of i.v. VPA. In 21 patients who received 24 infusions of VPA, there were no AEs on blood pressure and ECG parameters, and local reactions were seen only twice (168). In another study, however, reactions at peripheral injection sites occurred in 21% of patients (versus 30% of patients receiving i.v. phenytoin) (7). Other AEs have been reported in isolated cases or very small series of patients—significant hypotension (173), pathologic laughter (90), and metabolic acidosis (140).

PARADOXICAL AGGRAVATION OF SEIZURES

Aggravation of epilepsy due to AED therapy may have several causes, among which a specific adverse pharmacodynamic effect of the drug on a specific seizure type is the most troublesome (66). This type of aggravation occurs without overdosage, encephalopathy, or other metabolic side effects. Many AEDs can produce this type of aggravation, resulting in increased seizure frequency and occurrence of new seizure types (13,67,133). Among currently prescribed AEDs, VPA stands out with a very low potential for seizure exacerbation. There are only very isolated reports mentioning this possibility: somnolence and increased spike-and-wave activity in a patient with hypothalamic hamartoma when VPA was added to CBZ and phenobarbital (151); and induction of tonic status epilepticus in a patient when VPA was added to phenobarbital (31). In both cases, pharmacodynamic interactions may help explain this apparent aggravating effect, which may not be due to a direct effect of VPA. A further case report described the reversing effect of flumazenil on impairment of consciousness considered to be due to VPA-induced nonconvulsive status epilepticus (152); however, these authors apparently mistake slow-wave stupor, which was probably a marker of VPA-induced encephalopathy, for nonconvulsive status. Exacerbation of seizure in the context of VPA-induced hepatotoxicity, encephalopathy, or metabolic disturbances is described earlier in this chapter.

CONCLUSION

As an established anticonvulsant, with expanding indications in various fields of neurology and psychiatry, VPA has fared well. If the success of a given drug is a measure of its usefulness and tolerability, it appears that VPA has withstood the test of time. Although its common, benign, dose-related undesired side effects usually are easily managed, its comparatively long history has been marked by a succession of more severe, well advertised, and intensively scrutinized AEs. The possibility of their occurrence in patients treated for epilepsy should be kept in mind by practitioners, who also should be aware of their true incidence and clinical signification. Honest and comprehensive information should be given to patients who are treated with VPA for epilepsy, and preventive measures should be taken whenever possible to limit the extent and severity of AEs. In daily clinical practice, weight gain probably is the most troublesome AE, but aggravation of epilepsy by VPA is not an issue. Hepatic and pancreatic toxicity, teratogenicity, and reproductive dysfunctions are rare but significant problems. Abnormal laboratory values are not always associated with clinically significant problems. Overall, however, benefit/cost and benefit/risk ratios still appear to be quite favorable for the continuing and even increasing use of VPA in the treatment of epilepsy.

REFERENCES

1. Acharya S, Bussel JB. Hematologic toxicity of sodium valproate. *J Pediatr Hematol Oncol* 2000;22:62–65.
2. Alberto G, Erickson T, Popiel R, et al. Central nervous system manifestations of a valproic acid overdose responsive to naloxone. *Ann Emerg Med* 1989;18:889–891.
3. Allarakhia IN, Garofalo EA, Komarynski MA, et al. Valproic acid and thrombocytopenia in children: a case-controlled retrospective study. *Pediatr Neurol* 1996;14:303–307.
4. Allen RJ, Coulter DL. Valproic acid induced pancreatitis in children. *Pediatrics* 1980;65:1194–1195.
5. Altunbasak S, Baytok V, Tasouji M, et al. Asymptomatic hyperammonemia in children treated with valproic acid. *J Child Neurol* 1997;12:461–463.
6. Anderson GD, Lin YX, Berge C, et al. Absence of bleeding complications in patients undergoing cortical surgery while receiving valproate treatment. *Neurosurgery* 1997;87:252–256.
7. Anderson GD, Lin Y, Temkin NR, et al. Incidence of intravenous site reactions in neurotrauma patients receiving valproate or phenytoin. *Ann Pharmacother* 2000;34:697–702.
8. Anderson HH, Rapley JW, Williams DR. Gingival overgrowth with valproic acid: a case report. *J Dent Child* 1997;64:294–297.
9. Armon C, Brown E, Carwile S, et al. Sensorineural hearing loss: a reversible effect of valproic acid. *Neurology* 1990;40:896–898.
10. Armon C, Shin C, Miller P, et al. Reversible parkinsonism and cognitive impairment with chronic valproate use. *Neurology* 1996;47:626–635.
11. Asconapé JJ, Penry JK, Dreifuss FE, et al. Valproate-associated pancreatitis. *Epilepsia* 1993;34:177–183.
12. Balen A, Genton P. Valproate for girls with epilepsy. *Ann Neurol* 2000;47:550–552.
13. Bauer J. Seizure-inducing effect of antiepileptic drugs: a review. *Acta Neurol Scand* 1996;94:367–377.
14. Bavoux F, Fournier-Perhilou AI, Wood C, et al. Neonatal fibrinogen depletion caused by sodium valproate. *Ann Pharmacother* 1994;28:1307.
15. Berthelot-Moritz F, Chadda K, Chanavaz I, et al. Fatal sodium valproate poisoning. *Intensive Care Med* 1997;23:599.
16. Beydoun A, Sackellares JC, Shu V, and the Depakote Monotherapy for Partial Seizures Study Group. Safety and efficacy of divalproex sodium monotherapy in partial epilepsy: a double-blind, concentration-response designed clinical test. *Neurology* 1997;48:182–188.
17. Bigler D. Neurological sequelae after intoxication with sodium valproate. *Acta Neurol Scand* 1985;72:351–352.
18. Binek J, Hany A, Heer M. Valproic-acid-induced pancreatitis: case report and review of the literature. *J Clin Gastroenterol* 1991;13:690–693.
19. Blackburn SC, Oliart AD, Garcia Rodriguez LA, et al. Antiepileptics and blood dyscrasias: a cohort study. *Pharmacotherapy* 1998;18:1277–1283.
20. Bleck TP, Smith MC. Possible induction of systemic lupus erythematosus by valproate. *Epilepsia* 1990;31:343–345.
21. Bodensteiner JB, Morris HH, Golden GS. Asterixis associated with sodium valproate. *Neurology* 1981;31:186–190.
22. Branten AJ, Wetzels JF, Weber AM, et al. Hyponatremia due to sodium valproate. *Ann Neurol* 1998;43:265–267
23. Breum L, Astrup A, Gram L, et al. Metabolic changes during treatment with valproate in humans: implications for weight gain. *Metabolism* 1992;41:666–670.
24. Bruni J, Albright P. Valproic acid therapy for complex partial seizures. Its efficacy and toxic effects. *Arch Neurol* 1983;40:135–137.
25. Bryant AE 3rd, Dreifuss FE. Valproic acid hepatic fatalities: III. U.S. experience since 1986. *Neurology* 1996;46:465–469.
26. Buchanan N, Hayden M. Sodium valproate and edema. *Med J Aust* 1992;156:68.
27. Buzan RD, Firestone D, Thomas M, et al. Valproate-associated pancreatitis and cholecystitis in six mentally retarded adults. *J Clin Psychiatry* 1995;56:529–532.
28. Callaghan N, Kenny RA, O'Neill B, et al. A prospective study between carbamazepine, phenytoin and sodium valproate as monotherapy in previously untreated and recently diagnosed patients with epilepsy. *J Neurol Neurosurg Psychiatry* 1985;48:639–644.
29. Camfield PR, Bagnell P, Camfield CS, et al. Pancreatitis due to valproic acid. *Lancet* 1979;1:1198–1199.
30. Canger R, Battino D, Canevini MP, et al. Malformations in offspring of women with epilepsy: a prospective study. *Epilepsia* 1999;40:1231–1236.
31. Capocchi G, Balducci A, Cecconi M, et al. Valproate-induced epileptic tonic status. *Seizure* 1998;7:237–241.
32. Chappell KA, Markowitz JS, Jackson CW. Is valproate pharmacotherapy associated with polycystic ovaries? *Ann Pharmacother* 1999;33:1211–1216.
33. Chattergoon DS, McGuigan MA, Koren G, et al. Multiorgan dysfunction and disseminated intravascular coagulation in children receiving lamotrigine and valproic acid. *Neurology* 1997;49:1442–1444.
34. Chen SS, Shen MR, Chen TJ, et al. Effects of antiepileptic drugs on sperm motility of normal controls and epileptic patients with long-term therapy. *Epilepsia* 1992;33:149–153.
35. Connacher AA, Macnab MS, Moody JP, et al. Fatality due to massive overdose of sodium valproate. *Scott Med J* 1987;32:85–86.

36. Conran MJC, Kearney PJ, Callaghan MN, et al. Hypothalamic pituitary function testing in children receiving carbamazepine or sodium valproate. *Epilepsia* 1985;26:585–588.

37. Cook JS, Bale JF, Hoffmann RP. Pubertal arrest associated with valproic acid therapy. *Pediatr Neurol* 1992;8:229–231.

38. Corman CL, Leung NM, Guberman AH. Weight gain in epileptic patients during treatment with valproic acid: a retrospective study. *Can J Neurol Sci* 1997;24:240–244.

39. Coulter DL, Allen RJ. Pancreatitis associated with valproic acid therapy for epilepsy. *Ann Neurol* 1980;7:92.

40. Coulter DL. Carnitine, valproate, and toxicity. *J Child Neurol* 1991;6:7–14.

41. Dalens B, Raynaud EJ, Gaume J. Teratogenicity of valproic acid. *J Pediatr* 1980;97:332–333.

42. Demir E, Aysun S. Weight gain associated with valproate in childhood. *Pediatr Neurol* 2000;22:361–364.

43. DeToledo JC, Haddad H, Ramsay RE. Status epilepticus associated with the combination of valproic acid and clomipramine. *Ther Drug Monit* 1997;19:71–73.

44. De Vivo DC, Bohan TP, Coulter DL, et al. L-carnitine supplementation in childhood epilepsy: current perspectives. *Epilepsia* 1998;39:1216–1225.

45. Devinsky O, Leppik I, Willmore LJ, et al. Safety of intravenous valproate. *Ann Neurol* 1995;38:670–674.

46. DiLiberti JH, Farndon PA, Dennis NR, et al. The fetal valproate syndrome. *Am J Med Genet* 1984;19:473–481.

47. Dinesen H, Gram L, Anderson T, et al. Weight gain during treatment with valproate. *Acta Neural Scand* 1984;70:65–69.

48. Dravet C, Julian C, Legras C, et al. Epilepsy, antiepileptic drugs and malformations in children of epileptic women: a French prospective cohort study. *Neurology* 1992;42[Suppl 5]:75–82.

49. Dreifuss FE, Langer DH. Side effects of valproate. *Am J Med* 1988;84[Suppl IA]:39–41.

50. Dreifuss FE, Santilli N, Langer DH, et al. Valproic acid hepatic fatalities: a retrospective review. *Neurology* 1987;37:379–385.

51. Dreifuss FE, Langer DH, Moline KA, et al. Valproic acid hepatic fatalities: II. US experience since 1984. *Neurology* 1989;39:201–207.

52. Dreifuss FE. Valproate: toxicity. In: Levy RH, Mattson RH, Meldrum BS, eds. *Antiepileptic drugs*, 4th ed. New York: Raven Press, 1995:641–648.

53. Easter D, O'Bryan-Tear CG, Verity C. Weight gain with valproate or carbamazepine: a reappraisal. *Seizure* 1997;6:121–125.

54. Ebbesen F, Joergensen A, Hoseth E, et al. Neonatal hypoglycaemia and withdrawal symptoms after exposure in utero to valproate. *Arch Dis Child Fetal Neonatal Ed* 2000;83:F124–F129.

55. Echaniz-Laguna A, Thiriaux A, Ruolt-Olivesi I, et al. Lupus anticoagulant induced by the combination of valproate and lamotrigine. *Epilepsia* 1999;40:1661–1663

56. Eiris-Punal J, Del Rio-Garma M, Del Rio-Garma MC, et al. Long-term treatment of children with epilepsy with valproate or carbamazepine may cause subclinical hypothyroidism. *Epilepsia* 1999;40:1761–1766.

57. Ettingr A, Moshe S, Shinnar S. Edema associated with longterm valproate therapy. *Epilepsia* 1990;32:211–213.

58. Evans RJ, Miranda RN, Jordan J, et al. Fatal acute pancreatitis caused by valproic acid. *Am J Forensic Med Pathol* 1995;16:62–65.

59. Faught E, Morris G, Jacobson M, et al. Adding lamotrigine to valproate: incidence of rash and other adverse effects. Postmarketing Antiepileptic Drug Survey (PADS) Group. *Epilepsia* 1999;40:1135–1140.

60. Ford DM, Portman RJ, Lum GM. Pancreatitis in children on chronic dialysis treated with valproic acid. *Pediatr Nephrol* 1990;4:259–261.

61. Franceschi M, Perego L, Cavagnini F, et al. Effects of long-term antiepileptic therapy on the hypothalamic-pituitary axis in man. *Epilepsia* 1984;25:46–52.

62. Gallassi R, Morreale A, Lorusso S, et al. Cognitive effects of valproate. *Epilepsy Res* 1990;5:160–164.

63. Ganick DJ, Sunder T, Finley JL. Severe hematologic toxicity of valproic acid: a report of four patients. *Am J Pediatr Hematol Oncol* 1990;12:80–85.

64. Garden AS, Benzie RJ, Hutton EM, et al. Valproic acid therapy and neural tube defects. *CMAJ* 1985;132: 933–936.

65. Geisler J, Engelsen BA, Berntsen H, et al. Differential effect of carbamazepine and valproate monotherapy on plasma levels of oestrone sulphate and dehydroepiandrosterone sulphate in male epileptic patients. *J Endocrinol* 1997;153:307–312.

66. Genton P. When antiepileptic drugs aggravate epilepsy. *Brain Dev* 2000;22:75–80.

67. Genton P, McMenamin J. Can antiepileptic drugs aggravate epilepsy ? *Epilepsia* 1998;39[Suppl 3]:1–28.

68. Genton P, Bauer J, Duncan S, et al. On the association of valproate and polycystic ovaries. *Epilepsia* 2001;42:295–304.

69. Gidal B, Spencer N, Maly M, et al. Valproate-mediated disturbances of hemostasis: relationship to dose and plasma concentration. *Neurology* 1994;44:1418–1422.

70. Giroud M, D'Athis P, Guard O, et al. Elevation of gamma-glutamyltransferase levels in treated epileptic patients. *Presse Med* 1986;15:791–794.

71. Gomez M. Possible teratogenicity of valproic acid. *J Pediatr* 1981;98:508–509.

72. Guerrini R, Belmonte A, Canapicchi R, et al. Reversible pseudoatrophy of the brain and mental deterioration associated with valproate treatment. *Epilepsia* 1998;39:27–32.

73. Haidukewych D, John G. Chronic valproic acid and coantiepileptic drug therapy and incidence of increases in serum liver enzymes. *Ther Drug Monit* 1986;8:407–410.

74. Hamer HM, Knake S, Schomburg U, et al. Valproate-induced hyperammonemic encephalopathy in the presence of topiramate. *Neurology* 2000;54:230–232.

75. Hauser E, Seidl R, Freilinger M, et al. Hematologic manifestations and impaired liver synthetic function during valproate monotherapy. *Brain Dev* 1996;18:105–109.

76. Heaney DC, Shorvon SD, Sander JW. An economic appraisal of carbamazepine, lamotrigine, phenytoin and valproate as initial treatment in adults with newly diagnosed epilepsy. *Epilepsia* 1998;39[Suppl 3]:S19–S25.

77. Heller AJ, Chesterman P, Elwes RD, et al. Phenobarbitone, phenytoin, carbamazepine, or sodium valproate for newly diagnosed adult epilepsy: a randomised comparative monotherapy trial. *J Neurol Neurosurg Psychiatry* 1995;58:44–50.

78. Herzog AG. Polycystic ovarian syndrome in women with epilepsy: epileptic or iatrogenic? *Ann Neurol* 1996;39:559–560.

79. Hirose S, Mitsudome A, Yasumoto S, et al. Valproate therapy does not deplete carnitine levels in otherwise healthy children. *Pediatrics* 1998;101:E9.

80. Hjelm M, Oberholzer V, Seakins J, et al. Valproate-induced inhibition of urea synthesis anemia in healthy subjects. *Lancet* 1986;2:859.

81. Hjelm M, de Silva LV, Seakins JW, et al. Evidence of inherited urea cycle defect in valproate toxicity. *BMJ* 1986;292:23–24.

82. Honeycutt D, Callahan K, Rutledge L, et al. Heterozygous ornithine transcarbamylase deficiency presenting as symptomatic hyperammonemia during initiation of valproate treatment. *Neurology* 1992;42:666.

83. Hu LJ, Lu XF, Lu BQ, et al. The effect of valproic acid on SCE and chromosome aberrations in epileptic children. *Mutat Res* 1990;243:63–66.

84. Ishikura H, Matsuo N, Matsubara M, et al. Valproic acid overdose and L-carnitine therapy. *J Anal Toxicol* 1996;20:55–58.

85. Isojärvi JI, Pakarinen AJ, Ylipalosaari PJ, et al. Serum hormones in male epileptic patients receiving anticonvulsant medication. *Arch Neurol* 1990;47:670–676.

86. Isojärvi JIT, Pakarinen AJ, Myllylä VV. Thyroid function with antiepileptic drugs. *Epilepsia* 1992;33:142–148.

87. Isojärvi JI, Laatikainen TJ, Knip M, et al. Polycystic ovaries and hyperandrogenism in women taking valproate for epilepsy. *N Engl J Med* 1993;329:1383–1388.

88. Isojärvi JI, Laatikainen TJ, Knip M, et al. Obesity and endocrine disorders in women taking valproate for epilepsy. *Ann Neurol* 1996;39:579–584.

89. Isojärvi JI, Rattya J, Myllyla VV, et al. Valproate, lamotrigine, and insulin-mediated risks in women with epilepsy. *Ann Neurol* 1998;43:446–551.

90. Jacob PC, Chand RP. Pathological laughter following intravenous sodium valproate. *Can J Neurol Sci* 1998;25:252–253.

91. Jaeken J, Casaer P, Corbeel L. Valproate, hyperglycemia and hyperglycinaemia. *Lancet* 1980;2:260.

92. Jäger-Roman E, Deichl A, Jakob S, et al. Fetal growth, major malformations and minor anomalies in children born to women receiving valproic acid. *J Pediatr* 1986;108:997–1004.

93. Janas MS, Arroe M, Hansen SH, et al. Lung hypoplasia: a possible teratogenic effect of valproate. Case report. *APMIS* 1998;106:300–304.

94. Janssen F, Rambeck B, Schnabel R. Acute valproate intoxication with fatal outcome in an infant. *Neuropediatrics* 1985;16:235–238.

95. Jeavons PM. Non-dose-related side effects. *Epilepsia* 1984;25 [Suppl 1]:S50–S55.

96. Johnson LZ, Martinez I, Fernandez MC, et al. Successful treatment of valproic acid overdose with hemodialysis. *Am J Kidney Dis* 1999;33:786–789.

97. Karas BJ, Wilder BJ, Hammond EJ, et al. Treatment of valproate tremors. *Neurology* 1983;33:1380–1382.

98. Kis B, Szupera Z, Mezei Z, et al. Valproate treatment and platelet function: the role of arachidonate metabolites. *Epilepsia* 1999;40:307–310.

99. Koch S, Göpfert-Geyer J, Jäger-Roman E, et al. Antiepileptika während der Schwangerschaft. *Dtsch Med Wochenschr* 1083;108:250–257.

100. Konig SA, Siemes H, Blaker F, et al. Severe hepatotoxicity during valproate therapy: an update and report of eight new fatalities. *Epilepsia* 1994;35:1005–1015.

101. König SA, Elger CE, Vassella F, et al. Empfehlungen zu Blutuntersuchungen und klinischer Überwachung zur Früherkennung des Valporat-associierten Leberversagens. *Nervenarzt* 1998;69:835–840.

102. Konig SA, Schenk M, Sick C, et al. Fatal liver failure associated with valproate therapy in a patient with Friedreich's disease: review of valproate hepatotoxicity in adults. *Epilepsia* 1999;40:1036–1040.

103. Kreuz W, Linde R, Funk M, et al. Valproate therapy induces von Willebrand disease type I. *Epilepsia* 1992;33:178–184.

104. Lande MB, Kim MS, Bartlett C, et al. Reversible Fanconi syndrome associated with valproate therapy. *Pediatr Pathol* 1993;13:863–868.

105. Lauterbach EC. Catatonia-like events after valproic acid with risperidone and sertraline. *Neuropsychiatry Neuropsychol Behav Neurol* 1998;11:157–163.

106. Legarda SB, Booth MP, Fennell EB, et al. Altered cognitive functioning in children with idiopathic epilepsy receiving valproate monotherapy. *J Child Neurol* 1996;11:321–330.

107. Legius E, Jaecken J, Eggermont E. Sodium valproate, pregnancy and infantile fatal liver failure. *Lancet* 1987;2:1518–1519.

108. Lindhout D, Meinardi H. Spina bifida and in utero exposure to valproate. *Lancet* 1984;2:396.

109. Lindhout D, Schmidt D. In-utero exposure to valproate and neural tube defects. *Lancet* 1986;1:1392–1393.

110. Lindhout D, Meinardi H, Meijer JWA, et al. Antiepileptic drugs and teratogenesis in two consecutive cohorts: changes in prescription policy paralleled by changes in pattern of malformations. *Neurology* 1992;[Suppl.5]:94–110.

111. Loiseau P. Sodium valproate platelet dysfunction and bleeding. *Epilepsia* 1981;22:141–146.

112. Lundberg B, Nergardh A, Ritzen EM, et al. Influence of valproic acid on the gonadotropin-releasing hormone test in puberty. *Acta Paediatr Scand* 1986;75:787–792.

113. Lynch A, Tobias JD. Acute valproate ingestion induces symptomatic methemoglobinemia. *Pediatr Emerg Care* 1998;14:205–207.

114. Majer RV, Green PJ. Neonatal afibrinogenaemia due to sodium valproate. *Lancet* 1987;2:740–741.

115. Melegh B, Kerner J, Acsadi G, et al. L-carnitine replacement therapy in chronic valproate treatment. *Neuropediatrics* 1990;21:40–43.

115a. Nay RB, Snuder TR. Hematologic manifestations of long-term valproate therapy. *Epilepsia* 1993;34:1098–1101.

116. Mercke Y, Sheng H, Khan T, et al. Hair loss in psychopharmacology. *Ann Clin Psychiatry* 2000;12:35–42.

117. Mo CN, Ladusans EJ. Anomalous right pulmonary artery origins in association with the fetal valproate syndrome. *J Med Genet* 1999;36:83–84.

118. Montero FJ. Naloxone in the reversal of coma induced by sodium valproate. *Ann Emerg Med* 1999;33:357–358.

119. Moore SJ, Turnpenny P, Quinn A, et al. A clinical study of 57 children with fetal anticonvulsant syndromes. *J Med Genet* 2000;37:489–497.

120. Mortensen PB, Hansen HE, Pedersen B, et al. Acute valproate intoxication: biochemical investigations and hemodialysis treatment. *Int J Clin Pharmacol Ther Toxicol* 1983;21:64–68.

121. MRC Vitamin Study Research Group. Prevention of neural tube defects: results of the Medical Research Council Vitamin Study. *Lancet* 1991;338:131–137.

122. Murakami K, Sugimoto T, Woo M, et al. Effect of L-carnitine supplementation on acute valproate intoxication. *Epilepsia* 1996;37:687–689.

123. Murialdo G, Galimberti CA, Gianelli MV, et al. Effects of valproate, phenobarbital and carbamazepine on sex steroid setup in women with epilepsy. *Clin Neuropharmacol* 1998;21:52–58.

124. Murphy JV, Marquard K. Asymptomatic hyperammonemia in patients receiving valproic acid. *Arch Neurol* 1982;39:591–592.

125. Murphy JV, Marquardt KM, Shug AL. Valproic acid associated abnormalities of carnitine metabolism. *Lancet* 1985;1:820–821.

126. Njolstad PR, Skjeldal OH, Agsteribbe E, et al. Medium chain acyl-CoA dehydrogenase deficiency and fatal valproate toxicity. *Pediatr Neurol* 1997;16:160–162.

127. Novak GP, Maytal J, Alshansky A, et al. Risk of excessive weight gain in epileptic children treated with valproate. *J Child Neurol* 1999;14:490–495.

128. Oechsner M, Steen C, Sturenburg HJ, et al. Hyperammonaemic encephalopathy after initiation of valproate therapy in unrecognised ornithine transcarbamylase deficiency. *J Neurol Neurosurg Psychiatry* 1998;64:680–682.

129. Onofrj M, Thomas A, Paci C. Reversible parkinsonism induced by prolonged treatment with valproate. *J Neurol* 1998;245:794–796.

130. Otusbo S, Huruzono T, Kobae H, et al. Pancreatitis with nor-

mal serum amylase associated with sodium valproate: a case report. *Brain Dev* 1995;17:219–221.

131. Pandya NA, Jani BR. Post-axial limb defects with maternal sodium valproate exposure. *Clin Dysmorphol* 2000;9: 143–144.

132. Pavlakis SG, Chusid RL, Roye DP, et al. Valproate therapy: predisposition to bone fracture? *Pediatr Neurol* 1998;19:143–144.

133. Perucca E, Gram L, Avanzini G, et al. Antiepileptic drugs as a cause of worsening seizures. *Epilepsia* 1998;39: 5–17.

134. Picart N, Periole B, Mazereeuw J, et al. Drug hypersensitivity syndrome to valproic acid. *Presse Med* 2000;29:648–650.

135. Pinkston R, Walker LA. Multiorgan system failure caused by valproic acid toxicity. *Am J Emerg Med* 1997;15:504–506.

136. Pisani F, Fazio A, Oteri G, et al. Sodium valproate and valpromide: differential interactions with carbamazepine in epileptic patients. *Epilepsia* 1986;27:568–552.

137. Prevey ML, Delaney RC, Cramer JA, et al. Effect of valproate on cognitive functioning: comparison with carbamazepine. *Arch Neurol* 1996;53:1008–1016.

138. Raskind JY, El-Chaar GM. The role of carnitine supplementation during valproic acid therapy. *Ann Pharmacother* 2000;34: 630–638.

139. Rattya J, Turkka J, Pakarinen AJ, et al. Reproductive effects of valproate, carbamazepine, and oxcarbazepine in men with epilepsy. *Neurology* 2001;56:31–36.

140. Riche H, Salord F, Marti-Flich J, et al. Metabolic acidosis caused by injectable sodium valproate: 6 postoperative cases in neurosurgery. *Presse Med* 1996;25:642.

141. Richens A, Davidson DL, Cartlidge NE, et al. A multicentre comparative trial of sodium valproate and carbamazepine in adult onset epilepsy: Adult EPITEG Collaborative Group. *J Neurol Neurosurg Psychiatry* 1994;57:682–687.

142. Robbins DK, Wedlund PJ, Kuhn R, et al. Inhibition of epoxide hydrolase by valproic acid in epileptic patients receiving carbamazepine. *Br J Clin Pharmacol* 1990;29:759–762.

143. Robert E, Guiband P. Maternal valproic acid and congenital neural tube defects. *Lancet* 1982;2:937.

144. Rodriguez-Pinilla E, Arroyo I, Fondevilla J, et al. Prenatal exposure to valproic acid during pregnancy and limb deficiencies: a case-control study. *Am J Med Genet* 2000;90:376–381

145. Rosenfeld WE, Liao S, Kramer LD, et al. Comparison of the steady-state pharmacokinetics of topiramate and valproate in patients with epilepsy during monotherapy and concomitant therapy. *Epilepsia* 1997;38:324–333.

146. Sackellares JC, Lee SI, Dreifuss FE. Stupor following administration of valproic acid to patients receiving other antiepileptic drugs. *Epilepsia* 1979;20:697–703.

147. Sadeque AJM, Fisher MB, Korzekwa KR, et al. Human CYP2C9 and CYP2A6 mediate formation of the hepatotoxin 4-ene-valproic acid. *J Pharmacol Exp Ther* 1997;283:698–703.

148. Sherwood Brown E, Shellhorn E, Suppes T. Gastrointestinal side-effects after switch to generic valproic acid. *Pharmacopsychiatry* 1998;31:114.

149. Shin C, Gray L, Armon C. Reversible cerebral atrophy: radiologic correlate of valproate-induced Parkinson-dementia syndrome. *Neurology* 1992;42[Suppl 3]:277.

150. Stahl MM, Neiderud J, Vinge E. Thrombocytopenic purpura and anemia in a breast-fed infant whose mother was treated with valproic acid. *J Pediatr* 1997;130:1001–1003.

151. Stecker MM, Kita M. Paradoxical response to valproic acid in a patient with a hypothalamic hamartoma. *Ann Pharmacother* 1998;32:1168–1672.

152. Steinhoff BJ, Stodieck SR. Temporary abolition of seizure activity by flumazenil in a case of valproate-induced non-convulsive status epilepticus. *Seizure* 1993;2:261–265.

153. Straussberg R, Kivity S, Weitz R, et al. Reversible cortical atrophy and cognitive decline induced by valproic acid. *Eur J Paediatr Neurol* 1998;2:213–218.

154. Sussman NM, McLain LW Jr. A direct hepatotoxic effect of valproic acid. *JAMA* 1979;242:1173–1174.

155. Swanson BN, Harland RC, Dickinson RG, et al. Excretion of valproic acid in semen in rabbits and man. *Epilepsia* 1978;19: 541–546.

156. Tank JE, Palmer BF. Simultaneous "in series" hemodialysis and hemoperfusion in the management of valproic acid overdose. *Am J Kidney Dis* 1993;22:341–344.

157. Tennis P, Stern RS. Risk of serious cutaneous disorders after initiation of use of phenytoin, carbamazepine, or sodium valproate: a record linkage study. *Neurology* 1997;49:542–546.

158. Thom H, Carter PE, Cole GF, et al. Ammonia and carnitine concentrations in children treated with sodium valproate compared with other anticonvulsant drugs. *Dev Med Child Neurol* 1991;33:795–802.

159. Tokatli A, Coskun S, Cataltepe S, et al. Valproate-induced lethal hyperammonemic coma in a carrier of ornithine transcarbamylase deficiency. *J Inherit Metab Dis* 1991;14: 836–837.

160. Triggs WJ, Bohan TP, Lin SN, et al. Valproate-induced coma with ketosis and carnitine insufficiency. *Arch Neurol* 1990; 47:1131–1133.

161. Triggs WJ, Gilmore RL, Millington DS, et al. Valproate-associated carnitine deficiency and malignant cerebral edema in the absence of hepatic failure. *Int J Clin Pharmacol Ther* 1997;35: 353–356.

162. Trimble MR, Thompson PJ. Sodium valproate and cognitive function. *Epilepsia* 1984;25[Suppl 1]:S60–S64.

163. Tsai SJ, Chen YS. Valproic acid-induced Stevens-Johnson syndrome. *J Clin Psychopharmacol* 1998;18:420.

164. Turnbull DM, Howel D, Rawlins MD, et al. Which drug for the adult epileptic patient: phenytoin or valproate? *BMJ* 1985; 290:815–819.

165. Vainionpaa LK, Rattya J, Knip M, et al. Valproate-induced hyperandrogenism during pubertal maturation in girls with epilepsy. *Ann Neurol* 1999;45:444–450.

166. Van Wouwe JP. Carnitine deficiency during valproic acid treatment. *Int J Vitam Nutr Res* 1995;65:211–214.

167. Venkataraman V, Wheless JW. Safety of rapid intravenous infusion of valproate loading doses in epilepsy patients. *Epilepsy Res* 1999;35:147–153.

168. Veerman MW. Excipients in valproic acid syrup may cause diarrhea: a case report. *DICP* 1990;24:832–833.

169. Verrotti A, Basciani F, Morresi S, et al. Serum leptin changes in epileptic patients who gain weight after therapy with valproic acid. *Neurology* 1999;53:230–232.

170. Verrotti A, Greco R, Matera V, et al. Platelet count and function in children receiving sodium valproate. *Pediatr Neurol* 1999;21: 611–614.

171. Wason S, Savitt D. Acute valproic acid toxicity at therapeutic concentrations. *Clin Pediatr* 1985;24:466–467.

172. Watts RG, Emanuel PD, Zuckerman KS, et al. Valproic acid-induced cytopenias: evidence for a dose-related suppression of hematopoiesis. *J Pediatr* 1990;117:495–499

173. White JR, Santos CS. Intravenous valproate associated with significant hypotension in the treatment of status epilepticus. *J Child Neurol* 1999;14:822–823.

174. Williams LH, Reynolds RP, Emery JL. Pancreatitis during sodium valproate treatment. *Arch Dis Child* 1983;58:543–544.

175. Williams PG, Hersh JH. A male with fetal valproate syndrome and autism. *Dev Med Child Neurol* 1997;39:632–634.

176. Wirshing WC, Ames D, Bisheff S, et al. Hepatic encephalopa-

thy associated with combined clozapine and divalproex sodium treatment. *J Clin Psychopharmacol* 1997;17:120–121.

177. Wyllie E, Wyllie R, Cruse RP, et al. Pancreatitis associated with valproic acid therapy. *Am J Dis Child* 1984;138:912–914.

178. Yerby MS, Koepsell T, Daling J. Pregnancy complications and outcomes in a cohort of women with epilepsy. *Epilepsia* 1985;26:631–635.

179. Yerby MS, McCoy GB. Male infertility: possible association with valproate exposure. *Epilepsia* 1999;40:520–521.

180. Young RS, Bergman I, Gang DL, et al. Fatal Reye-like syndrome associated with valproic acid. *Ann Neurol* 1980;7:389.

181. Yüksel A, Katal A, Cenani A, et al. Serum thyroid hormones and pituitary response to thyrotropin-releasing hormone in epileptic children receiving anti-epileptic medication. *Acta Pediatr Jpn* 1993;35:108–112.

182. Zaccara G, Paganini M, Campostrini R, et al. Effect of associated antiepileptic treatment on valproate-induced hyperammonemia. *Ther Drug Monit* 1985;7:185–190.

183. Zarate CA Jr, Tohen M, Narendran R, et al. The adverse effect profile and efficacy of divalproex sodium compared with valproic acid: a pharmacoepidemiology study. *J Clin Psychiatry* 1999;60:232–236.

184. Zaret BS, Becker RR, Marini AM, et al. Sodium valproate induced hyperammonemia without clinical hepatic dysfunction. *Neurology* 1982;32:206–208.

185. Zaret BS, Cohen RA. Reversible valproic acid-induced dementia: a case report. *Epilepsia* 1986;27:234–240.

VIGABATRIN

VIGABATRIN

ELINOR BEN-MENACHEM

The first proposal that γ-aminobutyric acid (GABA) might be an inhibitory neurotransmitter came from Elliot and van Gelder (1) in 1958. Several compounds have since been successfully developed for the treatment of epilepsy that affect GABA$_A$-mediated inhibition. Vigabatrin (γ-vinyl-GABA), however, is unique because it is the only antiepileptic drug that is a selective, irreversible GABA-transaminase (GABA-T) inhibitor that greatly increases whole-brain levels of GABA, presumably making it more available to its receptor site. As a secondary effect, there is some evidence that it may even stimulate GABA release (2).

Vigabatrin was first synthesized specifically as a substrate for GABA-T (3). It is now available worldwide for use as an anticonvulsant except in the United States, and is effective in the treatment of partial seizures and infantile spasms (IS). Vigabatrin has not been approved for use by the U.S. Food and Drug Administration (FDA) because of the discovery of visual peripheral field defects occurring in a substantial number of patients.

CHEMICAL CHARACTERISTICS

Vigabatrin (4-amino-5-hexenoic acid; γ-vinyl GABA) is a structural analog of GABA with a vinyl appendage (Figure 90.1) rationally designed as an enzyme-activated, irreversible, specific inhibitor of GABA-T (4,5). Vigabatrin is highly soluble in water, only slightly soluble in ethanol and methanol, and insoluble in hexane and toluene. It is a white to off-white, crystalline solid with a melting point of 171° to 177°C. The molecular weight is 129.16.

The drug exists as a racemic mixture of $R(-)$ and $S(+)$ enantiomers in equal proportions and does not have optical activity. Pharmacologic activity and toxic effects are associated only with the $S(+)$ enantiomer; the $R(-)$ enantiomer is entirely inactive (6,7). No chiral inversion exists in humans.

The major pharmacologic effects seem to be determined by the half-life of the enzyme, GABA-T, rather than by the drug. This can be explained because GABA-T, which is the target enzyme irreversibly inhibited by vigabatrin, has a much longer half-life than the drug itself (3,8).

PHARMACOLOGIC ACTIVITY AND MECHANISMS OF ACTION

Animal Studies

Vigabatrin causes specific effects in the brain. The brain content of GABA, GABA-T, and glutamic acid decarboxylase (GAD) have been determined after single intraperitoneal injections of 1,500 mg/kg vigabatrin in mice. By 4 hours, whole-brain GABA increased fivefold, whereas GABA-T activity declined sharply. Recovery to 60% of baseline concentrations occurred after 5 days. A 30% decrease in GAD, demonstrated only at the high dose used, most likely results from a feedback mechanism after the sudden increase in GABA concentration (3).

At high doses, vigabatrin increases concentrations of β-alanine (an alternative substrate to GABA-T), homocarnosine (GABA and histidine combined), and hypotaurine while decreasing glutamine and threonine levels (9). Concentrations of free and total GABA and homocarnosine in both the brain and cerebrospinal fluid (CSF) increase in parallel with increasing doses of vigabatrin (10).

Anticonvulsant Effects in Animals

Vigabatrin is inactive in maximal electroshock (MES), bicuculline-induced (GABA antagonist), and pentylenetetrazol-induced seizures unless injected directly into the midbrain of rats (11); however, an intravenous injection provided seizure protection against bicuculline-induced

Elinor Ben-Menachem, MD, PhD: Associate Professor, Department of Clinical Neuroscience, Neurology Section, Sahlgrenska University Hospital, Goteborg, Sweden

Adapted from Chapter 67 in *The Treatment of Epilepsy: Principles and Practice*, 3rd edition, by Elaine Wylie. New York: Lippincott Williams & Wilkins, 2001, ISBN: 0-7817-2374-4.

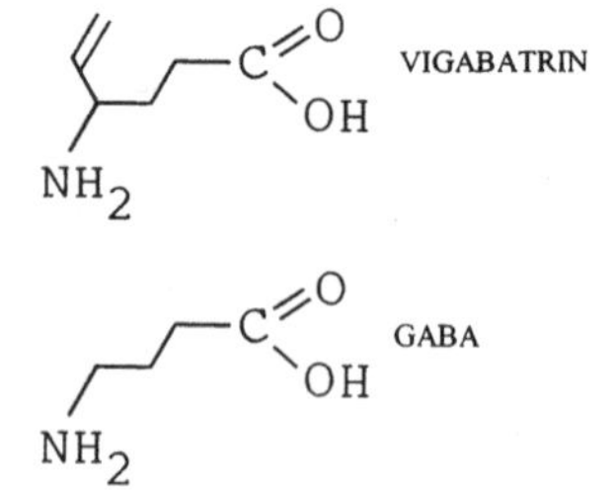

FIGURE 90.1. Structures of vigabatrin and GABA.

myoclonic activity (12), strychnine-induced tonic seizures (5), isoniazid-induced generalized seizures (5), audiogenic seizures in mice (13), photic-induced seizures in the baboon (14), and amygdala-kindled seizures in the rat (15,16).

Stereotaxic injections of small amounts of vigabatrin into certain areas of rat brain provided seizure protection probably by causing locally increased GABA levels (11). Seizure protection against MES was most prominent with local GABA increases in the midbrain tegmentum, including substantia nigra and midbrain reticular formation, but vigabatrin injected into the thalamus, hippocampus, and cortex was not protective in this model.

Human Studies

Grove et al. (17) were the first to investigate the relationship between vigabatrin and GABA in the CSF in humans. Patients were given 0.5 to 6 g of vigabatrin daily for 3 days. Free and total concentrations of GABA, β-alanine, homocarnosine, and vigabatrin increased in a dose-responsive manner. In another study (18), patients were given 0.5 g of vigabatrin twice daily followed by 1 g twice daily for 2 weeks and 2 weeks on placebo. At the end of the treatment, dose-related increases were seen in free and total GABA and homocarnosine. By the end of the placebo period, GABA and homocarnosine levels had decreased to baseline. In CSF, concentrations of acetylcholine, somatostatin, β-endorphins, prolactin, and cyclic adenosine or guanine monophosphate were unchanged during long-term treatment (19,20). No consistent changes have been found in amino acids, homovanillic acid (HVA), or 5-hydroxyindoleacetic acid (5-HIAA) with vigabatrin 50 mg/kg for up to 3.5 years in brain tissue and CSF (20,21). In a single-dose study, however, HVA and 5-HIAA concentrations in the CSF increased initially up to 100% but returned to baseline levels or slightly below after 1 month (8). At 50 mg/kg, vigabatrin caused a 200% to 300% increase in CSF and brain levels of GABA (22). A reduction in dose from 3 to 1.5 g/day proportionally decreased GABA levels in CSF (21). Dose and percentage increases in CSF GABA concentrations show a linear relationship, but that between dose and efficacy is more complex and may depend on the type of epilepsy. Kälviäinen et al. (23) suggested that responders to vigabatrin

monotherapy have higher initial glutamate levels (14%) in the CSF than do nonresponders. Recently, nuclear magnetic resonance spectroscopy in patients treated with vigabatrin added to conventional antiepileptic drugs confirmed results of GABA analysis in CSF (20,24); however, increased levels of glutamine and corresponding decreased levels of glutamate (by 9%) were noted.

Vigabatrin also changes blood GABA and platelet GABA-T levels. At therapeutic doses, platelet GABA-T is markedly reduced. In fact, 2 g/day maximally inhibits platelet GABA-T, with mean inhibition at approximately 70% (25). The concentration of plasma vigabatrin is almost 10-fold that in the CSF. Because platelets cannot regenerate GABA-T, the effect of vigabatrin on this system also is influenced by platelet regeneration.

ABSORPTION, DISTRIBUTION, AND METABOLISM

Absorption

Peak vigabatrin concentration is reached within 2 hours after administration (6,26,27). Absorption half-life ranges from 0.18 to 0.59 hour and the mean terminal half-life is between 5 and 7 hours. Peak concentration and area under the curve (AUC) values of the (*S*)-enantiomer are lower than those of the (*R*)-enantiomer, possibly because of irreversible binding of the active (*S*)-enantiomer to the substrate (6). Approximately 60% to 80% of the drug is recovered unchanged in a 24-hour urine collection, indicating a bioavailability of at least 60% to 80%. There are no metabolites, but the remaining amount of vigabatrin probably disappears when it binds to GABA-T.

Effect of Food

The AUC for fasted and fed volunteers is not significantly different, indicating that food does not affect the extent of absorption (28,29).

Distribution

The apparent volume of distribution is 0.8 L/kg (total body water is 0.6 L/kg) in volunteers. The half-life of distribution is 1 to 2 hours. Between 50% and 75% of the drug is outside the central compartment at steady state (2).

In patients with epilepsy, the concentration of vigabatrin in CSF was approximately 10% of plasma levels (8). After a single oral dose, the highest vigabatrin concentrations were found in the CSF after the 6 hours. By 24 hours, only a trace was detectable in the CSF, and no vigabatrin was found at 72 hours or thereafter. The peak concentration in plasma was reached by 1 hour, decreasing to only small amounts by 72 hours. The mean elimination half-life was

4.5 hours and the AUC was 310 nmol/mL/hr. The vigabatrin CSF:plasma ratio was 0.10. After a 3-year follow-up, CSF vigabatrin levels were not significantly increased compared with the 6-month levels (20).

Vigabatrin does not bind to plasma proteins (25,30).

There is a low level of transfer from maternal to fetal blood of vigabatrin across the placenta. This is comparable with other α-amino acids. An estimate of the maximum amount of vigabatrin that an infant would ingest per day during breast-feeding is 3.6 % of the R (−) and 1% of the S(+) enantiomer of the vigabatrin dose that the mother takes. Therefore, the quantity of vigabatrin that a nursing infant would receive from a mother taking vigabatrin is very small (31).

Elimination

The elimination half-life is 5 to 8 hours and the total clearance is approximately 1.7 to 1.9 mL/min/kg, with renal clearance accounting for 70% of the total oral clearance. Elimination is not influenced by dose or duration of treatment (32). The biologic half-life for vigabatrin, however, is measured in days, not hours.

Both renal and total-body clearance are slower in the elderly. Terminal half-life shows an inverse relationship to renal function (26). Patients with renal impairment, therefore, have higher plasma concentrations of vigabatrin. The AUC in the elderly with reduced creatinine clearance is increased up to 10-fold compared with normal healthy volunteers, which may explain the poorer tolerability of conventional doses of vigabatrin in the elderly (26).

Children demonstrate a lower AUC than adults (7). Children therefore need higher doses of vigabatrin to achieve the plasma levels seen in adults.

EFFICACY

Vigabatrin is an effective drug for partial seizures as well as other specific seizure types. Many randomized, controlled studies have confirmed this statement.

Adults

Double-Blind Adjunctive Therapy Studies

Six double-blind, placebo-controlled, adjunctive-therapy, crossover studies published in the late 1980s provided the basis for registration of the drug in most countries, excluding the United States (33–38). In two of the studies, some patients were included who had primary generalized tonic-clonic seizures instead of partial seizures only (35,38). Their inclusion in the efficacy analysis caused these two studies to show no significant difference between the treatment groups. When the patients with primary generalized

seizures were excluded, both studies showed significant efficacy results favoring vigabatrin over the placebo groups, as did the remaining four studies, which included patients with partial seizures only. Doses ranged in the trials from 2 to 3 g/day as add-on therapy to standard antiepileptic drugs. Between 0% and 7% of patients became seizure free and between 33% and 64% had >50% seizure reduction.

Two large, multicenter, double-blind trials in the United States (39,40) using a parallel design included a total of 356 patients with complex partial seizures with or without secondary generalization. Patients were treated with vigabatrin at doses of 1, 3, and 6 g/day or placebo. There was a statistically significant reduction in seizures in all dosage groups compared with placebo, but there were more seizure-free patients in the 6 g/day treatment group.

Monotherapy

A single-center, open-label, randomized, parallel-group study from Finland (41) compared carbamazepine and vigabatrin as the initial drug for new-onset seizures regardless of seizure type. Most patients had partial seizures during the 1-year follow-up; seizures were completely controlled in 16 of 50 patients taking vigabatrin and in 26 of 50 taking carbamazepine. More carbamazepine-treated patients dropped out as a result of adverse events (12 versus 0 with vigabatrin), and more vigabatrin-treated patients discontinued therapy because of lack of efficacy (13 versus 3 with carbamazepine).

A large, double-blind, multicenter trial in adults with new-onset partial seizures with or without secondary generalization (n = 459) showed that vigabatrin was less effective than carbamazepine in time to first seizure after the first 6 weeks after randomization (42). All other efficacy outcomes tended to favor carbamazepine. As in the Finnish study, patients reported fewer side effects in the vigabatrin group compared with the carbamazepine group, but patients on vigabatrin more frequently experienced psychotic symptoms (25% versus 15% on carbamazepine) and weight gain (10% versus 3%).

Tanganelli et al. (43) performed a randomized, response-conditioned, crossover study comparing vigabatrin and carbamazepine in 51 patients with new-onset seizures. Slightly more patients became seizure free on carbamazepine as the first drug (51% versus 46% for vigabatrin), whereas vigabatrin was better tolerated than carbamazepine. Visual field testing was not performed during any of the aforementioned studies.

Long-Term Studies

Numerous long-term follow-up studies have been published, some reporting efficacy and safety results over more than 10 years. Approximately 60% of initial responders showed continued long-term benefits (44–51). Tolerance, although reported, does not seem to be a major factor in view of the long-maintained efficacy results.

Children

Partial Seizures

In an open, randomized study, 70 children were treated with either carbamazepine (n = 32) or vigabatrin (n = 38) for new-onset partial seizures and followed for 2 years. Vigabatrin was dosed at 50 to 60 mg/kg/day and carbamazepine at 15 to 30 mg/kg/day. The results showed no significant difference between efficacy variables, but side effects were less with vigabatrin than carbamazepine (52).

In one open-label trial (53), 135 children with varied refractory seizure types received vigabatrin at dosages of 40 to 80 mg/kg/day. Eleven patients became seizure free, and 37% had >50% reduction in seizures, similar to results in the adult studies. Patients with partial seizures responded best. In another study (54), 16 children with refractory epilepsy of various types were treated, and again those with partial seizures had the most favorable response. Myoclonic epilepsy tended to be aggravated.

Infantile Spasms

The first report that vigabatrin could be effective in IS dates from 1991 (55). In this open-label, prospective study of 70 children, 37 had a significant reduction in spasms. Most impressive were the patients with symptomatic IS; 71% with tuberous sclerosis became completely seizure free. In a 2-year follow-up in the United Kingdom (56), 20 patients (aged 3 to 11 months) were treated with vigabatrin as the initial drug; 14 of the 20 had symptomatic IS. The starting dosages were 50 to 80 mg/kg/day, and some reached a maximum daily dosage of 150 mg/kg. Of these 20 patients, 13 were free of seizures for 30 months, 4 showed no response, and 3 experienced reductions of >75% but were not seizure free. Response to vigabatrin was rapid and occurred within 72 hours of the initiation of therapy. No adverse side effects were seen in any of the 20 patients.

One randomized, placebo-controlled trial of vigabatrin in IS has been published (57). Forty children with newly diagnosed IS were given either placebo or vigabatrin for 5 days. Afterward, all children were treated with vigabatrin for 24 weeks. Patients on vigabatrin had a significant reduction in spasms (78% compared with 26% on placebo, $p = .02$). By the end of the open-label follow-up, 38% of the original 40 patients were spasm free on vigabatrin. No patient stopped because of adverse events. The conclusion was, in this study and all the previous ones, that vigabatrin should be considered the drug of first choice for this patient category.

Another randomized, controlled trial compared vigabatrin (100 to 150 mg/kg/day) with adrenocorticotropic hormone (ACTH) depot (0.1 mL/day) in 39 infants with newly diagnosed IS of various origins (58). Vigabatrin was associated with complete control of spasms in 9 of 21 patients (43%), whereas ACTH was effective in 14 of 18 (78%). However, severe side effects were more common with ACTH than with vigabatrin (33% versus 19%), and it was concluded that vigabatrin can be a valuable first-line agent for the treatment of spasms. Interestingly, all three patients with spasms secondary to tuberous sclerosis responded well to vigabatrin.

The value of vigabatrin in spasms associated with tuberous sclerosis was confirmed in open studies (59) and in a randomized trial by Chiron and coworkers (60). Vigabatrin (150 mg/kg/day) or hydrocortisone (15 mg/kg/day) was given to 22 infants with tuberous sclerosis as first-line therapy. Spasms disappeared in all of the 11 infants randomized to vigabatrin, and in only 4 of the 11 randomized to hydrocortisone; moreover, all nonresponders to hydrocortisone responded when they were switched to vigabatrin. Mean time to disappearance of spasms also was shorter with vigabatrin than with hydrocortisone (3.5 versus 13 days, respectively). Three patients on vigabatrin and one on hydrocortisone showed late emergence of partial seizures.

In other long-term follow-up studies (61,62), children with IS treated with vigabatrin responded favorably. Sixty-two percent became seizure free, especially those with cryptogenic seizures. In the report by Fejerman et al. (61), all seizure-free cryptogenic cases showed normal neuropsychological development. The most effective dosage seemed to be 150 mg/k/day. After 5 years of follow-up in Siemes and colleagues' study (62), 72% of 18 evaluable patients were seizure free for at least 1 year. Side effects were present in only 10% of patients. However, other types of seizures eventually developed in 55% of the children. The results are comparable with those of long-term ACTH treatment, but patients report less side effects.

Lennox-Gastaut Syndrome

Only a few published reports have described the use of vigabatrin in this disorder. Some noted increases in seizure frequency after initiating vigabatrin therapy in patients with Lennox-Gastaut syndrome and myoclonic epilepsy (63,64), whereas other studies described significant improvement (65,66), perhaps reflecting the dose administered. Patients with Lennox-Gastaut syndrome require lower doses than patients with other seizure types. Myoclonic jerks may develop during vigabatrin treatment especially in this patient category.

INTERACTIONS WITH OTHER DRUGS

Because vigabatrin is not metabolized, it is excreted unchanged in the urine, does not cause enzyme induction, and does not interact significantly with most drugs (25,30). Only phenytoin seems to be significantly affected. Phenytoin levels have been reported to be reduced by up to 20% (36,67). The cause of this decrease (25,68) has never been explained. There are no changes in protein binding or changes in phenytoin absorption, metabolism, or clearance (48). Importantly, the dosage of phenytoin seldom requires adjustment. In a study of healthy women, vigabatrin has not been found consistently to affect the plasma levels of steroid oral contraceptives (69).

ADVERSE EFFECTS

Reports of adverse events are based on 18 years of clinical trials as well as marketed use for 11 years. In the double-blind, placebo-controlled studies, sedation and fatigue were the most commonly reported side effects. Weight gain also may be a significant problem with vigabatrin (42). Several studies on the cognitive effects of vigabatrin treatment confirm no deterioration in performance scores and even improvement in certain test scores (70–74).

Psychosis and depression have been noted in some studies and have been the topic of heated discussion. A description of severe psychiatric reactions in 14 of 210 patients (75,76) was followed by published case reports and warnings. However, the two multicenter, placebo-controlled, double-blind studies (39,40) from the United States analyzed the occurrence and nature of psychiatric side effects and thereby clarified the issues raised by the various non-blinded, nonprospective reports in the literature. The studies, which excluded patients with severe brain damage or psychiatric disorders, reported that 2.2% in the 1-g treatment group (n = 45), 6.6% in the 3-g group (n = 135), and 7.3% in the 6-g group (n = 41) stopped treatment because of a psychiatric adverse event. These results found that severe psychiatric adverse events occur in approximately 5% of the patients treated with vigabatrin who have not previously had severe psychiatric disease. An unpublished but large postmarketing surveillance study (data on file, Aventis Behring, Pennsylvania) reported manifest psychosis, hallucinations, paranoia, or delusions in 88 (0.64%) of more than 6,000 patients. This rate is not greater than that seen with other antiepileptic drugs (77,78), psychiatric problems being common in patients with intractable epilepsy, especially those with focal seizures. Although these data suggest that vigabatrin may not elicit psychosis more frequently than other antiepileptic drugs, a large, multicenter, randomized monotherapy trial did identify a more common occurrence of psychiatric symptoms with vigabatrin than with carbamazepine (25% versus 15%, respectively) (42). In the same trial, psychiatric disturbances classified as serious occurred in 5 of 229 patients randomized to vigabatrin and in none of 230 patients randomized to carbamazepine.

Nevertheless, patients with a history of severe psychiatric disturbances or very severe brain damage should be treated with caution. A good rule is to give low doses initially, and titrate with caution. Even sudden withdrawal of vigabatrin can lead to postictal psychosis.

Chronic Toxicity

Vigabatrin has been tested in clinical trials since 1981. After 1989, it has been given as a registered drug in most parts of the world, excluding the United States. Initially, there were concerns about the finding of intramyelinic edema in the brains of mice, rats, and dogs treated with vigabatrin, but there is no evidence that a similar effect occurs in humans receiving therapeutic doses of the drug (79). The greatest concern about the safety of vigabatrin at present is related to the potential for adverse effects on vision, which has been a pressing issue after alarming reports began to appear in 1997 about irreversibly impaired visual fields in some patients on chronic vigabatrin therapy. This is now the most important safety issue and the primary reason why the FDA has not approved vigabatrin. The nature and cause of the visual field defects are still obscure, but there is some indication that there may be a reduction in cones, which in turn may be due to dysfunction of GABAergic cells of the inner retina (80). The retina is outside the blood–brain barrier and has its own blood–brain barrier and a blood–aqueous barrier. This raises the possibility that vigabatrin concentrations and inhibition of GABA-T in the GABAergic cells in the retina could be higher than in the central nervous system (81).

One of the initial reports about the visual field defects was from Mackenzie and Klistoner in 1998 (82). They found that although some patients reported the visual defects as a problem, most were asymptomatic. This can explain why this serious side effect was not noticed earlier.

One of the best studies done to date to examine this issue was by Kalvianen et al. (83) In the monotherapy trial previously cited in this chapter (41), 19 patients on carbamazepine and 32 patients on monotherapy vigabatrin were analyzed with visual field testing. Forty-one percent of patients on vigabatrin and none on carbamazepine showed asymptomatic concentric visual field defects. The deficits seemed to be irreversible when vigabatrin was stopped.

The appearance of vigabatrin-induced visual field loss in the central field out to 30° eccentricity is typically that of a localized bilateral nasal loss, particularly with static threshold perimetry, extending in an annulus over the horizontal midline, together with a relative sparing of the temporal field (84,85). Overall prevalence is approximately 20% to 40% and is twice as high in men than in women (84,86). The prevalence of symptomatic cases, however, is much lower, possibly around 1%.

More recently, there have been reports of children with concentric visual field defects similar to those seen in adults

(87–89). Small children, however, are not able to perform perimetry tests, so the results must be interpreted accordingly. When tested with visual evoked potentials and electroretinography, as well as perimetry when appropriate, there was some relationship to length of vigabatrin treatment and pathologic findings on these three measurements (89).

Several studies, although not prospective, report that the concentric contractions of the visual fields due to vigabatrin treatment seem to be irreversible even when the drug has been stopped (84,90,91) [although preliminary reports suggest that recovery may occur after early withdrawal (92,93)]. There seems to be a relationship of visual changes with time on vigabatrin and with cumulative dose of vigabatrin taken (94,95). There is suggestive evidence, however, that visual field loss is less likely to occur after the first 4 years of continuous treatment (84).

Many questions remain. We still do not really know precisely when the problem occurs in the course of treatment. Are the deficits progressive or do they occur abruptly, although there is some indication that they may be progressive (90)? Are certain combinations with other antiepileptic drugs more likely to cause these changes? What shall we do with patients who are currently taking vigabatrin, who have asymptomatic visual field deficits and who are seizure free?

Teratogenicity

No serious teratogenic effects in animals have been reported except for an increased incidence of cleft palate in rabbits receiving high doses. Vigabatrin has a class warning against use in pregnancy because of inadequate evidence for or against teratogenic effects. Information on 100 pregnancies during vigabatrin therapy shows the concomitant use of at least one other antiepileptic drug in almost all patients (96). No pattern of abnormalities reported to date suggests that vigabatrin has a specific teratogenic effect, but the results are inconclusive. No other reports have been forthcoming about the effects of vigabatrin on the unborn child, but there currently are large pregnancy registries in progress around the world to monitor the possible teratogenic effects of the new antiepileptic drugs.

CLINICAL USE

Indications

Vigabatrin is indicated primarily for the treatment of partial seizures, with or without secondary generalization, refractory to other antiepileptic drugs. Vigabatrin also is indicated for the treatment of IS, where it may be considered as one of the first-line agents.

Administration

Most clinical trials have used dosages between 2 and 3 g/day. In U.S. double-blind studies (39,40), the 6-g dose produced more seizure-free patients, but more side effects were reported. Today, 2 to 3g/day is considered to be the effective dosage range in adults. In children, the dosage is between 45 and 150 mg/kg. If 150 mg/kg is not effective, the dosage should be tapered and the drug discontinued. Vigabatrin can be given once or twice daily.

Titration

Gradual increases are recommended to prevent side effects and, especially, to reduce the possible occurrence of psychiatric or behavioral reactions such as confusion or depression. Also, some patients with milder forms of epilepsy may respond to lower doses, thereby decreasing the need to titrate upward to a full dosage of 3 g/day. For patients with severe brain damage, as in Lennox-Gastaut syndrome, low dosages probably are best. Therapy should be initiated with 500 mg/day, increasing no faster than one 500-mg tablet each week.

Discontinuation

To avoid rebound seizures, which can elicit postictal behavioral abnormalities or even status epilepticus, vigabatrin therapy never should be stopped abruptly. It is a good rule to taper the dosage no faster than 500 mg every fifth day. According to animal and human CSF studies (3,97), this should stabilize the GABA level at a lower level for each reduction.

Clinical Monitoring

Visual field testing should be carried out at regular intervals after initiation of vigabatrin therapy.

It is not necessary to monitor blood levels of vigabatrin because there is no clear relationship between the drug concentration in plasma and clinical response. Blood levels are not appropriate even for determining compliance because a full dose of vigabatrin taken in the morning before an appointment yields a "clinically acceptable" blood level.

CONCLUSION

Vigabatrin has proven to be an important antiepileptic drug for the treatment of complex partial seizures and IS. Unfortunately, this drug can cause irreversible visual field deficits and retinal changes with chronic use in as many as 40% of patients. Therefore, the place of vigabatrin in the treatment of patients with epilepsy is being reevaluated. Except for IS, where vigabatrin may be used as the first-line drug, this antiepileptic drug should be used with caution, and repeated ophthalmologic examinations, including visual fields, should be conducted regularly.

REFERENCES

1. Elliot KAC, van Gelder NM. Occlusion and metabolism of gamma-aminobutyric acid by brain tissue. *J Neurochem* 1958;3: 28–40.
2. Schechter PJ. Vigabatrin. In: Meldrum B, Porter RJ, eds. *New anticonvulsant drugs.* London: John Libbey, 1986:265–275.
3. Jung MF, Lippert B, Metcalf BW, et al. Gamma-vinyl GABA (4-amino-hex-5-enoic acid), a new selective irreversible inhibitor of GABA-T: effects on brain GABA metabolism in mice. *J Neurochem* 1977;29:797–802.
4. Lippert B, Metcalf B, Jung MJ, et al. 4-Amino-hex-5-enoic acid, a selective catalytic inhibitor of 4-aminobutyric acid aminotransferase in mammalian brain. *Eur J Biochem* 1977;74:441–445.
5. Schechter PJ, Tranier Y, Grove J. Attempts to correlate alterations in brain GABA metabolism by GABA-T inhibitors with their anticonvulsant effects. In: Mandel P, DeFeudes FV, eds. *GABA—biochemistry and CNS functions.* New York: Plenum Press, 1979: 43–45.
6. Haegele KD, Schechter PJ. Kinetics of the enantiomers of vigabatrin after an oral dose of the racemate or the active S-enantiomer. *Clin Pharmacol Ther* 1986;40:581–586.
7. Rey E, Pons G, Richard MO, et al. Pharmacokinetics of the individual enantiomers of vigabatrin (gamma-vinyl GABA) in epileptic children. *Br J Clin Pharmacol* 1990;30:253–257.
8. Ben-Menachem E, Persson LI, Schechter PJ, et al. Effects of single doses of vigabatrin on CSF concentrations of GABA, homocarnosine, homovanillic acid and 5- hydroxyindoleacetic acid in patients with complex partial epilepsy. *Epilepsy Res* 1988;2: 96–101.
9. Perry TL, Kish SJ, Hansen S. Gamma-vinyl GABA: effects of chronic administration on the metabolism of GABA and other amino compounds in rat brain. *J Neurochem* 1979;32: 1641–1645.
10. Palfreyman MG, Böhlen P, Huot S, et al. The effect of gamma-vinyl GABA and gamma-acetylenic GABA on the concentration of homocarnosine in brain and CSF of the rat. *Brain Res* 1980; 190:288–292.
11. Gale K. Role of the substantia nigra in GABA-mediated anticonvulsant actions. *Adv Neurol* 1986;44:343–364.
12. Kendall DA, Fox DA, Enna SJ. Effects of gamma-vinyl GABA on bicuculline-induced seizures. *Neuropharmacology* 1981;20: 351–355.
13. Schechter PJ, Tranier Y. Effect of elevated brain GABA concentrations of the actions of bicuculline and picrotoxin in mice. *Psychopharmacology* 1977;54:145–148.
14. Meldrum BS, Horton R. Blockade of epileptic responses in the photosensitive baboon, *Papio papio,* by two irreversible inhibitors of GABA-transaminase, gamma-acetylenic GABA (4-amino-hex-5-ynoic acid) and gamma-vinyl GABA (4-amino-hex-5-enoic acid). *Psychopharmacology* 1978;59:47–50.
15. Piredda S, Lim CR, Gale K. Intracerebral site of convulsant action of bicuculline. *Life Sci* 1985;56:1295–1298.
16. Stevens JR, Phillips I, de Beaurepaire R. Gamma-vinyl GABA in endopiriform area suppresses kindled amygdala seizures. *Epilepsia* 1988;29:404–411.
17. Grove J, Fozard JR, Mamont PS. Assay of alpha-difluoromethylornithine in body fluids and tissues by automatic amino acid analysis. *J Chromatogr* 1981;223:409–416.
18. Schechter PJ, Hanke NF, Grove J, et al. Biochemical and clinical effects of gamma-vinyl GABA in patients with epilepsy. *Neurology* 1984;34:182–186.
19. Pitkänen A, Halonen T, Ylinen A, et al. Somatostatin, β-endorphin, and prolactin levels in human cerebrospinal fluid during the gamma-vinyl GABA treatment of patients with complex partial seizures. *Neuropeptides* 1987;9:185–195.
20. Ben-Menachem E, Persson LI, Mumford JP. Effect of long term vigabatrin therapy on selected CSF neurotransmitter concentrations. *J Child Neurol* 1991;6[Suppl 2]:11–16.
21. Sivenius MRJ, Ylinen A, Murros K, et al. Double-blind dose-reduction study of vigabatrin in complex partial epilepsy. *Epilepsia* 1987;28:688–692.
22. Ben-Menachem E, Mumford J, Hamberger A. Effect of long-term vigabatrin therapy on GABA and other amino acid concentrations in the central nervous system: a case study. *Epilepsy Res* 1993;16:241–243.
23. Kälviäinen R, Halonen T, Pitkänen A, et al. Amino acid levels in the cerebrospinal fluid of newly diagnosed epileptic patients: effect of vigabatrin and carbamazepine monotherapy. *J Neurochem* 1993;60:1244–1250.
24. Petroff OA, Rothman DL. Measuring human brain GABA in vivo: effects of GABA- transaminase inhibition with vigabatrin. *Mol Neurobiol* 1998;16:97–121.
25. Richens A. Pharmacology and clinical pharmacology of vigabatrin. *J Child Neurol* 1991;6:2S7–2S10.
26. Haegele KD, Huebert ND, Ebel M, et al. Pharmacokinetics of vigabatrin: implications of creatinine clearance. *Clin Pharmacol Ther* 1988;44:558–565.
27. Saletu B, Grunberger J, Linzmayer L, et al. Psychophysiological and psychometric studies after manipulating the GABA system by vigabatrin, a GABA-transaminase inhibitor. *Int J Psychophysiol* 1986;4:63–80.
28. Frisk-Holmberg M, Kerth P, Meyer P. Effect of food on the absorption of vigabatrin. *Br J Clin Pharmacol* 1989;27:23S–25S.
29. Hoke JF, Chi EM, Antony K, et al. Effect of food on the bioavailability of vigabatrin tablets. *Epilepsia* 1991;32[Suppl 3]:7.
30. Mumford JP. A profile of vigabatrin. *Br J Clin Pract* 1988; 42[Suppl 61]:7–9.
31. Tran A, O'Mahoney T, Rey E, et al. Vigabatrin: placental transfer in vivo and excretion into breast milk of the enantiomers. *Br J Clin Pharmacol* 1998;45:409–411.
32. Grant SM, Heel RC. Vigabatrin: a review of its pharmacodynamic and pharmacokinetic properties and therapeutic potential in epilepsy and disorders of motor control. *Drugs* 1991;4: 889–926.
33. Gram L, Klosterskov P, Dam M. Gamma-vinyl GABA: a double-blind, placebo-controlled trial in partial epilepsy. *Ann Neurol* 1985;17:262–266.
34. Loiseau P, Hardenberg JP, Pestre M, et al. Double-blind, placebo-controlled study of vigabatrin (gamma-vinyl GABA) in drug resistant epilepsy. *Epilepsia* 1986;27:115–120.
35. Remy C, Favel P, Tell G. Double-blind, placebo-controlled, crossover study of vigabatrin in drug resistant epilepsy of the adult. *Boll Lega Ital Epil* 1986;54/55:241–243.
36. Rimmer EM, Richens A. Double-blind study of gamma-vinyl GABA in patients with refractory epilepsy. *Lancet* 1984;1: 189–190.
37. Tartara A, Manni R, Galimberti CA, et al. Vigabatrin in the treatment of epilepsy: a double-blind, placebo controlled study. *Epilepsia* 1986;27:717–723.
38. Tassinari CA, Michelucci R, Ambrossetto G, et al. Double-blind study of vigabatrin in the treatment of drug resistant epilepsy. *Arch Neurol* 1987;44:907–910.
39. Dean C, Mosier M, Penry K. Dose-response study of vigabatrin as add-on therapy in patients with uncontrolled complex partial seizures. *Epilepsia* 1999;40:74–82.
40. French JA, Mosier M, Walker S, et al., and the Vigabatrin Protocol 024 Investigative Cohort . A double-blind, placebo-controlled study of vigabatrin three g/day in patients with uncontrolled complex partial seizures. *Neurology* 1996;46:54–61.
41. Kälviäinen R, Aikia M, Saukkonen AM, et al. Vigabatrin versus carbamazepine monotherapy in patients with newly diagnosed

epilepsy: a randomized controlled study. *Arch Neurol* 1995; 52:989–996.

42. Chadwick D. Safety and efficacy of vigabatrin and carbamazepine in newly diagnosed epilepsy: a multicentre randomised double-blind study. Vigabatrin European Monotherapy Study Group. *Lancet* 1999;354:13–19.

43. Tanganelli P, Regesta G. Vigabatrin vs carbamazepine monotherapy in newly diagnosed focal epilepsy: a randomized response conditioned cross-over study. *Epilepsy Res* 1996;25:257–262.

44. Browne TR, Mattson RH, Penry JK, et al. Multicenter long-term safety and efficacy study of vigabatrin for refractory complex partial seizures: an update. *Neurology* 1991;41:363–364.

45. Cocito L, Maffini M, Perfumo P, et al. Vigabatrin in complex partial seizures: a long-term study. *Epilepsy Res* 1989;3:160–166.

46. Michelucci R, Veri L, Passarelli D, et al. Long-term follow-up study of vigabatrin in the treatment of refractory epilepsy. *J Epilepsy* 1994;7:88–93.

47. Remy C, Beaumont D. Efficacy and safety of vigabatrin in the long-term treatment of refractory epilepsy. *Br J Clin Pharmacol* 1989;27[Suppl 1]:125S–129S.

48. Reynolds EH, Ring HA, Farr IN, et al. Open, double-blind and long-term study of vigabatrin in chronic epilepsy. *Epilepsia* 1991; 32:530–538.

49. Sivenius J, Ylinen A, Murros K, et al. Efficacy of vigabatrin in drug-resistant partial epilepsy during a 6-year follow-up period. *Epilepsia* 1991;32[Suppl 1]:11.

50. Tartara A, Manni R, Galimberti CA, et al. Vigabatrin in the treatment of epilepsy: a long-term follow-up study. *J Neurol Neurosurg Psychiatry* 1989;52:467–471.

51. Ylinen A, Salmenoera T, Mumford JP, et al. Long-term treatment with vigabatrin-10 years of clinical experience. *Seizure* 1999;8: 181–183.

52. Zamponi N, Cardinai C. Open comparative long-term study of vigabatrin vs carbamazepine in newly diagnosed partial seizures in children. *Arch Neurol* 1999;56:605–607.

53. Livingston JH, Beaumont D, Arzimanoglou A, et al. Vigabatrin in the treatment of epilepsy in children. *Br J Clin Pharmacol* 1989;27[Suppl 1]:109S–112S.

54. Luna D, Dulac O, Pajot N, et al. Vigabatrin in the treatment of childhood epilepsies: a single-blind placebo controlled study. *Epilepsia* 1989;30:430–437.

55. Chiron C, Dulac O, Beaumont D, et al. Therapeutic trial of vigabatrin in refractory infantile spasms. *J Child Neurol* 1991;6 [Suppl 2]:S52–S59.

56. Appelton R. Vigabatrin in the management of generalized seizures in children. *Seizure* 1995;4:45–48.

57. Appelton RE, Peters AC, Mumford JP, et al. Randomised, placebo-controlled study of vigabatrin as first-line treatment of infantile spasms. *Epilepsia* 1999;40:1627–1633.

58. Vigevano F, Cilio MR. Vigabatrin versus ACTH as first-line treatment for infantile spasms: a randomized, prospective study. *Epilepsia* 1997;38:1270–1274.

59. Aicardi J, Sabril IS Investigators and Peer Review Groups, Mumford JP, et al. Vigabatrin as initial therapy for infantile spasms: a European retrospective survey. *Epilepsia* 1996;37:638–642.

60. Chiron C, Dumas C, Jambaque I, et al. Randomized trial comparing vigabatrin and hydrocortisone in infantile spasms due to tuberous sclerosis. *Epilepsy Res* 1997;26:389–395.

61. Fejerman N, Cersosimo R, Caraballo R, et al. Vigabatrin as a first-choice drug in the treatment of West syndrome. *J Child Neurol* 2000;15:161–165.

62. Siemes H, Brandl U, Spohr HL, et al. Long-term follow-up study of vigabatrin in pretreated children with West syndrome. *Seizure* 1998;7:293–297.

63. Lortie A, Chiron C, Mumford J, et al. The potential for increasing seizure frequency, relapse, and appearance of new seizure types with vigabatrin. *Neurology* 1993;43[Suppl 5]:S24–S27.

64. Michelucci R, Tassinari CA. Response to vigabatrin in relation to seizure type. *Br J Clin Pharmacol* 1989;27[Suppl 1]:119S–124S.

65. Feucht M, Brantner-Inthaler S. Gamma-vinyl GABA (vigabatrin) in the therapy of Lennox-Gastaut syndrome: an open study. *Epilepsia* 1994;35:993–998.

66. Herranz JL, Arteaga R, Farr IN, et al. Dose-response study of vigabatrin in children with refractory epilepsy. *J Child Neurol* 1991;6[Suppl 2]:S45–S51.

67. Browne TR, Mattson RH, Penry JK, et al. Vigabatrin for refractory complex partial seizures: multicenter single-blind study with long-term follow-up. *Neurology* 1987;37:184–189.

68. Rimmer EM, Richens A. Interaction between vigabatrin and phenytoin. *Br J Clin Pharmacol* 1989;27:27S–33S.

69. Bartoli A, Gatti G, Cipolla G, et al. A double-blind, placebo-controlled study on the effect of vigabatrin on in vivo parameters of hepatic microsomal enzyme induction and on the kinetics of steroid oral contraceptive in healthy female volunteers. *Epilepsia* 1997;38:702–707.

70. de Bittencourt PRM, Mazer S, Marcourakis T, et al. Vigabatrin: clinical evidence supporting rational polytherapy in management of uncontrolled seizures. *Epilepsia* 1994;35:373–380.

71. JB, McGuire AM, Trimble MR. The effect of vigabatrin on cognitive function and mood. *Hum Psychopharmacol* 1992;7:329.

72. Dodrill CB, Arnett JL, Sommerville KW, et al. Evaluation of the effects of vigabatrin on cognitive abilities and quality of life. *Neurology* 1993;43:2501–2507.

73. Grunewald RA, Thompson PJ, Corcoran R, et al. Effects of vigabatrin on partial seizures and cognitive function. *J Neurol Neurosurg Psychiatry* 1994;57:1057–1063.

74. Provinviali L, Bartolini M, Mari F, et al. Influence of vigabatrin on cognitive performance and behaviour in patients with drug resistant epilepsy. *Acta Neurol Scand* 1996;94:12–18.

75. Sander JWAS, Hart YM. Vigabatrin and behavior disturbances. *Lancet* 1990;335:57.

76. Sander JWAS, Hart YM, Trimble MR, et al. Behavioral disturbances associated with vigabatrin therapy. *Epilepsia* 1991;34 [Suppl 1]:12.

77. Matsuo F, Bergen D, Faught E, et al. Placebo-controlled study of efficacy and safety of lamotrigine in patients with partial seizures. *Neurology* 1993;43:2284–2291.

78. Wolf P. The use of antiepileptic drugs in epileptology with respect to psychiatry. *Neuropsychobiology* 1993;27:127–131.

79. Cohen JA, Fisher RS, Grigell MG, et al. The potential for vigabatrin-induced intramyelinic edema in humans. *Epilepsia* 2000; 41:148–157.

80. Krauss GL, Johnson MA. Miller NR. Vigabatrin-associated retinal cone system dysfunction: electroretinogram and ophthalmologic findings. *Neurology* 1998;50:614–618.

81. Cunha-Vaz JG. The blood-ocular barriers: past, present and future. *Doc Ophthalmol* 1997;93:149–157.

82. Mackenzie R, Klistoner A. Severe persistent visual field constriction associated with vigabatrin: asymptomatic as well as symptomatic defects occur with vigabatrin. *BMJ* 1998;316:233.

83. Kälviäinen R, Nousiainen I, Mantyjarvi M. Initial vigabatrin monotherapy is associated with increased risk of visual field constriction: a comparative follow-up study with patients on initial carbamazepine monotherapy and healthy controls. *Epilepsia* 1998;39[Suppl 6]:72.

84. Wied JM, Martinez C, Reinshagen G, et al. Characteristics of a unique visual field defect attributed to vigabatrin. *Epilepsia* 1999;40:1786–1794.

85. Harding GFA, Wied JM, Robertson UA, et al. Electro-oculography, electroretinography, visual evoked potentials, and multifocal

electroretinography in patients with vigabatrin-attributed visual field constriction. *Epilepsia* 2000;41:1420–1431.

86. Hardus P, Verduin WM, Postma G, et al. Concentric contraction of the visual field in patients with temporal lobe epilepsy and its association with the use of vigabatrin medication. *Epilepsia* 2000; 41:581–587.

87. Vanhatalo S, Pääkkonen L. Visual field constriction in children treated with vigabatrin. *Neurology* 1999;52:1713–1714.

88. Russell-Eggitt IM, Mackey DA, Taylor DS, et al. Vigabatrin-associated visual field defects in children. *Eye* 2000;14:334–339.

89. Gross-Tsur V, Banin E, Shahar E, et al. Visual impairment in children with epilepsy treated with vigabatrin. *Ann Neurol* 2000; 48:60–64.

90. Hardus P, Verduin WM, Postma G, et al. Long term changes in the visual fields of patients with temporal lobe epilepsy using vigabatrin. *Br J Ophthalmol* 2000;84:788–790.

91. Johnson MA, Krauss GI, Miller NR, et al. Visual function loss from vigabatrin: effect of stopping the drug. *Neurology* 2000;15:40–45.

92. Krakow K, Polizzi G, Riordan-Eva P, et al. Recovery of visual field constriction following discontinuation of vigabatrin seizure. *Seizure* 2000;9:287–290.

93. Kraumer G, Ried S, Landau K, et al. Vigabatrin: reversibility of severe concentric visual field defects after early detection and drug withdrawal: a case report. *Epilepsia* (*in press*).

94. Manuchehri K, Goodman S, Siviter L, et al. A controlled study of vigabatrin and visual abnormalities. *Br J Ophthalmol* 2000;84: 499–505.

95. Lawden MC, Eke T, Degg C, et al. Visual field defects associated with vigabatrin treatment. *J Neurol Neurosurg Psychiatry* 1999;67: 716–722.

96. Mumford JP. Epilepsy, pregnancy and vigabatrin. *Int Med News-lett* 1994;2:2–4.

97. Ben-Menachem E, Persson LI, Schechter PJ, et al. The effect of different vigabatrin treatment regimens on CSF biochemistry and seizure control in epileptic patients. *Br J Clin Pharmacol* 1989;27:79S–85S.

ZONISAMIDE

ZONISAMIDE

MECHANISMS OF ACTION

ROBERT L. MACDONALD

CLINICAL ANTIEPILEPTIC ACTIONS OF ZONISAMIDE

Zonisamide (Zonegran; Elan Pharmaceuticals, Gainesville, GA) is a 1,2-benzisoxazole compound with a sulfonamide side chain (1,2-benzisoxazole-3-methanesulfonamide) that is structurally different from other marketed antiepileptic drugs (AEDs). Zonisamide was shown to be an effective AED in patients with refractory partial seizures (1–6) and generalized seizures (4,7–13). Based on these clinical trials, therapeutic plasma levels were determined to be 15 to 25 µg/mL (approximately 70 to 120 µmol/L) (14) or 20 to 30 µg/mL (85 to 140 µmol/L) (15), and zonisamide is 50% to 60% bound to plasma proteins (14).

ANTICONVULSANT ACTIONS OF ZONISAMIDE IN EXPERIMENTAL ANIMALS

Zonisamide is an effective anticonvulsant drug in experimental animal models of seizures and has an anticonvulsant profile that is similar but not identical to that of phenytoin and carbamazepine. Zonisamide was effective against maximal electroshock (MES) seizures at nontoxic doses in mice [median effective dose (ED$_{50}$), 19.6 mg/kg orally (p.o.)] and rats (ED$_{50}$, 7.9 mg/kg p.o.) and was more potent that phenytoin or carbamazepine. Similar to phenytoin and carbamazepine, zonisamide was not active against subcutaneous pentylenetetrazol (PTZ)-induced seizures (16,17). With MES seizures, effective nontoxic plasma levels ranged from 10 to 70 µg/mL (47 to 330 µmol/L) in rats (18). Zonisamide was effective against partial seizures in experimental animals, reducing hippocampus-kindled seizures in rat (19) and amygdala-kindled seizures in rat (20) and cat (21). Zonisamide also reduced kindled generalized seizures to partial seizures in the cat (22). In addition, zonisamide was effective against tonic-clonic and myo-clonic seizures in the genetic animal model of reflex epilepsy in the Mongolian gerbil (23) and suppressed tonic, but not absence-like, seizures in spontaneously epileptic rats (SER) and sound-induced seizures in DBA/2 mice (24). However, zonisamide did not completely suppress spontaneous seizures in the EL mouse (25). Although not always predictive of efficacy against seizures in patients with epilepsy, this anticonvulsant profile suggests that zonisamide would be effective against partial seizures and secondarily generalized seizures and may have some efficacy against tonic and myoclonic seizures. The lack of effect against PTZ seizures and seizures in SER suggests that zonisamide would not be effective in the treatment of generalized absence seizures.

ZONISAMIDE ACTIONS ON EPILEPTIFORM DISCHARGES *IN VIVO* AND *IN VITRO*

Zonisamide prevented spread of epileptiform activity in the cortex of experimental animals. Zonisamide suppressed focal seizure activity induced by direct electrical stimulation of the cat visual cortex and increased afterdischarge threshold (22), and after unilateral injection of kainic acid into the amygdala of rat, zonisamide reduced spread of seizures to the contralateral side (26). Zonisamide also suppressed epileptogenic focal activity induced in the cortex of experimental animals. Zonisamide suppressed spiking activity induced by cortical freezing in cat cortex and interictal spikes induced by tungstic acid gel in rat cortex (27,28).

ZONISAMIDE MECHANISMS OF ACTION

Multiple mechanisms of action for zonisamide have been proposed. However, these can be divided into three basic mechanisms of drug action: an action on neuronal sodium channels to reduce sustained, high-frequency repetitive firing of action potentials, on T-type voltage-dependent calcium channels, and on synaptic transmission. Although evidence has been reported supporting all of these mechanisms, the weight of current experimental evidence

Ronald L. Macdonald, MD, PhD: Professor and Chairman, Department of Neurology, Vanderbilt University, Nashville, Tennessee

suggests that the major mechanisms of action of zonisamide are to modify the ability of neurons to fire at high frequency by producing an enhancement of sodium channel inactivation and to reduce T-type calcium current. These mechanisms and the others are discussed in the following sections.

Reduction of Sustained, High-Frequency Repetitive Firing by Zonisamide

In an early study, zonisamide was shown to reduce the excitability of *Myxicola* giant axons by reducing sodium current (29). This effect was specific for sodium currents because voltage-dependent potassium currents were unaffected. Zonisamide had no effect on sodium channel activation, but produced a shift in the steady-state fast inactivation curve to more negative voltages and slowed recovery from both fast and slow inactivation. The effect of zonisamide was produced only with intracellular zonisamide; extracellular zonisamide did not affect sodium channel inactivation. The zonisamide effect on fast inactivation occurred at relatively low zonisamide concentrations (1 to 100 μmol/L), with a half-maximal concentration of 12 μmol/L producing a 20-mV shift in the steady-state inactivation curve. The effect of zonisamide to slow recovery from slow inactivation occurred at even lower concentrations (0.1 to 10 μmol/L). Slow inactivation was slowed from 4.4 seconds to 11.5 and 16 seconds by 1 and 12 μmol/L zonisamide, respectively. Thus, this early study demonstrated that zonisamide directly affected sodium channels at clinically relevant concentrations.

The effect of zonisamide on repetitive firing was not limited to axonal preparations. Zonisamide reduced high-frequency repetitive firing of action potentials recorded from fetal mouse spinal cord neurons grown in primary dissociated cell culture (30). When depolarized, spinal cord neurons fire high-frequency repetitive discharges (31). In the presence of zonisamide at or below therapeutic free serum concentrations (35 to 60 μmol/L), there was a concentration-dependent reduction in sustained repetitive firing [above 2 μmol/L; median therapeutic serum concentration (IC$_{50}$) of 17 μmol/L]. Thus, zonisamide limited sustained, high-frequency repetitive firing of action potentials at therapeutic free serum concentrations.

These results suggested that zonisamide was affecting sodium channels, and that the effect was likely on the inactivation process of sodium channels. It was proposed that zonisamide produced limitation of high frequency repetitive firing by binding to sodium channels in the inactive state and by slowing the rate of recovery of these channels from inactivation. The effect appeared to be selective for the inactive form of the closed channel. Thus, it is likely that zonisamide binds preferentially to the inactive form of the sodium channel to produce use- and voltage-dependent block of sodium channels, an action consistent with the modulated receptor hypothesis of local anesthetic drug action proposed by Hille (32). Zonisamide therefore would be more effective in reducing high-frequency repetitive firing when neurons were depolarized because more channels would be in the inactive state. Under normal physiologic conditions, it is likely that vertebrate myelinated and unmyelinated axons have a large negative membrane potential, and therefore propagated action potentials would be relatively resistant to the action of zonisamide. In contrast, the cell body of neurons is subject to synaptic depolarization and inward currents that produce burst firing. This is particularly true in neurons undergoing epileptic discharge. Zonisamide would be effective, therefore, in limiting high-frequency action potentials generated in bursting neurons.

In addition to altering neuronal excitability, zonisamide may alter the process of synaptic transmission by affecting presynaptic sodium channels. It has been demonstrated that [³H]BTX-B binding sites are not restricted to cell bodies and axons but are present in synaptic zones with a heterogeneous distribution in the nervous system (33). In the hippocampal slice, stimulation of stratum radiatum elicited extracellular field potentials recorded from the CA1 pyramidal cell layer. The field potentials consisted of a fiber spike, which reflects axonal propagation, and a population spike, which reflects effective synaptic transmission. Veratridine, which displaces [³H] BTX-B binding, produced a specific reduction in the synaptically evoked population spike without affecting the fiber spike. This effect of veratridine was antagonized by carbamazepine. It is likely, therefore, that zonisamide would block presynaptic sodium channels and the firing of action potentials; this would secondarily reduce voltage-dependent calcium entry and synaptic transmission.

In summary, zonisamide is likely to act both presynaptically to block release of neurotransmitter by blocking firing of action potentials and postsynaptically by blocking the development of high-frequency repetitive discharge initiated at cell bodies. This combined presynaptic and postsynaptic effect is likely to form the basis for the anticonvulsant actions of zonisamide. It appears that zonisamide blocks sustained, high-frequency repetitive firing of action potentials and spontaneous burst discharges by enhancing voltage-dependent sodium channel inactivation in both mature and immature neuronal preparations, which suggests that the mechanism of action of zonisamide is the same in both mature and immature animals. In addition to zonisamide, several other AEDs that are effective against generalized tonic-clonic and partial seizures have a similar mechanism of action and also block high-frequency repetitive firing (34–38), including phenytoin (31), carbamazepine (39,40), and valproic acid (41), possibly by a similar mechanism. Thus, zonisamide may share this mechanism of action with several currently used AEDs.

Reduction of T-Type Calcium Current by Zonisamide

Zonisamide did not alter calcium-dependent action potentials in mouse spinal cord neurons that are primarily composed of high-threshold calcium currents (30). However, low-threshold, T-type calcium currents in cultured fetal rat cortical neurons were reduced by zonisamide in a concentration-dependent manner (42). The reduction in T current was maximal at 500 μmol/L (60% reduction), and reductions of 10% to 25% were produced by therapeutic concentrations of zonisamide (10 to 50 μmol/L). In contrast, the high-threshold L-type calcium current was unaffected by zonisamide at concentrations up to 500 μmol/L. In these experiments, zonisamide was dissolved in 50% dimethylsulfoxide (DMSO), which produced an 18% reduction in T current but did not affect L current. Thus, the reductions in T current were reported as reductions above 18%. The 7-methylated analog of zonisamide reduced T current only by 13.5%, similar to that of the DMSO control, suggesting that this effect was specific for zonisamide. Zonisamide also reduced the T-type calcium current recorded from cultured neuroblastoma cells (43). Zonisamide reduced T current by 38% at 50 mmol/L and shifted the inactivation curve to more negative potentials by 20 mV.

In addition to zonisamide, several other AEDs that are effective against generalized absence seizures also reduce T-type calcium currents, including ethosuximide (44,45), the active metabolite of trimethadione, dimethadione (44,45), and valproic acid (46). Generalized absence epilepsy is characterized clinically by brief periods of loss of consciousness and electrically by a generalized 3-Hz spike-and-wave discharge recorded on the electroencephalogram. Thalamic relay neurons play a critical role in the generation of the abnormal thalamocortical rhythmicity that underlies the 3-Hz spike-and-wave discharge. Low-threshold T-type and high-threshold calcium currents are present in rat thalamic neurons (47), and T-current activation was necessary and sufficient to cause the generation of low-threshold calcium spikes in thalamic relay neurons. Ethosuximide and dimethadione, the active metabolite of trimethadione, both reduced the T-type current of thalamic neurons isolated from guinea pigs and rats at clinically relevant concentrations (44,45). Valproic acid also decreased T-type current in rat nodose ganglion neurons (46). Thus, zonisamide may share this mechanism of action with several currently used AEDs.

Actions of Zonisamide on Neurotransmitter Systems

Zonisamide has been reported to alter neurotransmitter metabolism and levels and to modify neurotransmitter receptor function. The primary neurotransmitter systems studied include monoamine, γ-aminobutyric acid (GABA)-ergic, glutamatergic, and cholinergic neurotransmitter systems.

It has been suggested that alteration of monoamine neurotransmission may be involved in the actions of zonisamide. The threshold for inducing electroshock seizures was shown to be reduced after administration of drugs that deplete brain monoamines (48–52). In contrast, the threshold for inducing electroshock seizures was elevated by administration of monoamine precursors or inhibitors of monoamine catabolism (50,53,54). The anticonvulsant effect of zonisamide was reduced but not abolished by reserpine, and zonisamide had increased potency in reserpinized rats (16), suggesting that its anticonvulsant effect may be mediated, at least in part, by altered monoaminergic function. Zonisamide has been shown to increase both total and extracellular levels of striatal and hippocampal dopamine (DA) (55–57) and serotonin [(5-hydroxytryptamine (5-HT)] (55,56,58,59).

Administration of therapeutic doses of zonisamide (20 and 50 mg/kg) altered DA metabolism in rat striatum and hippocampus (55,57). Acute administration of zonisamide increased striatal extracellular dihydroxyphenylalanine (DOPA) levels and intracellular striatal and hippocampal 3,4-DOPA levels, and stimulated DOPA accumulation in both striatum and hippocampus; zonisamide also increased striatal and hippocampal intracellular and extracellular DA and homovanillic acid (HVA) levels and decreased 3,4-dihydroxyphenylacetic acid (DOPAC) levels (57). Acute administration of zonisamide had no effect on calcium-dependent dopamine release in rat striatum (55) or DA reuptake in rat striatum or hippocampus (57), but did weakly inhibit monoamine oxidase B (MAOB) activity more than MAOA activity (57). Chronic (3 weeks) administration of zonisamide increased intracellular and extracellular DA, DOPA, DOPAC, and HVA levels in striatum and hippocampus (57). Acute and chronic high-dose (100 mg/kg) administration of zonisamide decreased intracellular levels of all compounds and inhibited DOPA accumulation (57). These data suggest that acute administration of therapeutic doses of zonisamide enhances DA function by enhancing DA synthesis and inhibiting DA degradation, resulting in an increase in intracellular DA. Chronic administration of therapeutic doses of zonisamide also enhances DA function by increasing DA synthesis without altering DA degradation, leading to increased intracellular DA. Administration of supratherapeutic doses of zonisamide inhibits DA function by reducing intracellular DA, suggesting that zonisamide inhibits DA synthesis and degradation, leading to decreased DA turnover. Thus, zonisamide has biphasic effects on DA function, with therapeutic doses enhancing and supratherapeutic doses decreasing DA function. Acute and chronic therapeutic and supratherapeutic administration of carbamazepine had effects on DA metabolism that were similar to those of zonisamide (60).

Zonisamide also altered 5-HT turnover (55,56,58,59). Both acute and chronic administration of therapeutic doses of zonisamide increased striatal and hippocampal levels of 5-HT, its precursor 5-hydroxytryptophan (5-HTP), and its metabolite 5-hydroxyindoleacetic acid (5-HIAA), thus increasing 5-HT turnover (56,59). In contrast, supratherapeutic doses of zonisamide had the opposite effect of either decreasing or not changing 5-HT, 5-HTP, and 5-HIAA levels. Thus, zonisamide has biphasic effects on 5-HT function, with therapeutic doses enhancing and supratherapeutic doses decreasing 5-HT function.

Administration of therapeutic doses of zonisamide (20 mg/kg) altered acetylcholine (ACh) metabolism in rat striatum (61). Acute or chronic administration of zonisamide increased ACh release and metabolism, thus increasing ACh turnover, without affecting acetylcholinesterase or butyrylcholinesterase activities. Supratherapeutic doses of zonisamide decreased ACh turnover and extracellular ACh levels without affecting cholinesterase activity. Similar experiments with carbamazepine demonstrated similar acute and chronic effects. However, the relationship of this effect of zonisamide on ACh metabolism in rat striatum to its antiepileptic effects is unclear.

A number of anticonvulsant drugs have been demonstrated to enhance GABA$_A$ receptor function (62). Zonisamide inhibited [^{3}H]flunitrazepam and [^{3}H]muscimol binding in rat brain (63). Zonisamide reduced [^{3}H]flunitrazepam to 65% (1 mmol/L) and 92% (100 μmol/L) of control by increasing K$_d$ but not altering B$_{max}$. Zonisamide also reduced [^{3}H]muscimol binding to 28% (1 mmol/L) and 68% (100 μmol/L) of control. In addition, [^{3}H]zonisamide was found to bind to a crude synaptosomal fraction of whole rat brain with a K$_d$ of 90 nmol/L (64,65). Clonazepam reduced and GABA increased [^{3}H]zonisamide binding, suggesting that the zonisamide binding site was coupled to benzodiazepine receptors. However, on spinal cord neurons in cell culture, no effect of zonisamide was found on postsynaptic responses to iontophoretically applied GABA (30). Thus, there is no direct evidence that zonisamide modifies GABA$_A$ receptor currents.

Zonisamide has been reported to modify excitatory amino acid receptor function (66). The effects of zonisamide and carbamazepine administration on extracellular levels of glutamate in the hippocampus were studied using *in vivo* microdialysis. Perfusion of the microdialysis probe with zonisamide (1 mmol/L) or carbamazepine (100 μmol/L) reduced glutamate release evoked by KCl and the enhanced glutamate release evoked by KCl and Ca^{2+}. No affect of zonisamide was observed, however, on glutamate responses evoked on spinal cord neurons in cell culture (30). These data suggest that zonisamide may inhibit excitatory glutamatergic synaptic transmission by reducing the presynaptic release of glutamate. However, whether this is a direct action of zonisamide on the release or an indirect action on voltage-gated sodium or calcium channels is

unclear. Therefore, there is no compelling evidence that zonisamide acts directly on glutamatergic synaptic transmission to produce an antiepileptic effect.

Thus, zonisamide appears to alter DA, 5-HT, and ACh metabolism but not directly to affect GABA$_A$ receptor or glutamate receptor function. These actions of zonisamide are shared by carbamazepine. It is unclear, however, if these effects on DA, 5-HT, and ACh metabolism have any relationship to the antiepileptic actions of zonisamide or carbamazepine.

Carbonic Anhydrase Inhibitory Activity of Zonisamide

Zonisamide has a sulfonamide side chain that is common to the carbonic anhydrase inhibitor acetazolamide, and zonisamide has been shown to have activity as a carbonic anhydrase inhibitor (67). Acetazolamide inhibited rat red blood cell carbonic anhydrase with an IC$_{50}$ of 15 μmol/L, and although zonisamide and 7-methylated zonisamide also inhibited carbonic anhydrase, they were much less potent carbonic anhydrase inhibitors, with IC$_{50}$s 200 times higher than that of acetazolamide (68). Furthermore, although both zonisamide and 7-methyated zonisamide inhibited carbonic anhydrase, only zonisamide had anticonvulsant activity in the MES test in mice, and the anti-MES activity of zonisamide was dose dependent and correlated with increasing brain levels of zonisamide (68). These data suggest that the anticonvulsant action of zonisamide against MES seizures or against seizures in humans is unrelated to inhibition of carbonic anhydrase.

CONCLUSION

Zonisamide has been shown to limit sustained, high-frequency repetitive firing of sodium-dependent action potentials and reduce T-type calcium currents at clinically effective free serum concentrations. In addition, zonisamide appears to alter DA, 5-HT, and ACh metabolism but not directly to affect GABA$_A$ receptor or glutamate receptor function. These data are consistent with the human and animal data suggesting that zonisamide has multiple mechanisms of action. Carbamazepine produces similar effects, except that it does not alter T-type calcium currents. Phenytoin also alters sustained, high-frequency repetitive firing of sodium-dependent action potentials, but does not have the reported effects on T-type calcium currents or neurotransmitter metabolism. Although it is unclear if the effects on DA, 5-HT, and ACh metabolism have any relationship to the anticonvulsant actions of zonisamide, it has been well established that AEDs act on sodium and T-type calcium channels to block simple partial, generalized tonic-clonic, and absence seizures. Zonisamide appears to have "broad-spectrum" antiepileptic activity using similar mechanisms of action, and thus would be expected to have actions on simple partial, generalized tonic-clonic, and absence seizures.

REFERENCES

1. Sackellares JC, Donofrio PD, Wagner JG, et al. Pilot study of zonisamide (1,2-beziosoxazole-3-methanesulfonamide) in patients with refractory partial seizures. *Epilepsia* 1985;26:206–211.
2. Wilensky AJ, Friel PN, Ojemann LM, et al. Zonisamide in epilepsy: a pilot study. *Epilepsia* 1985;26:212–220.
3. Seino M. Efficacy evaluation of AD-810 (zonisamide): double-blind study comparing with carbamazepine. *J Clin Exp Med* 1988;144:275–291.
4. Kumagai N, Seki T, Yamawaki H, et al. Monotherapy for child-hood epilepsies with zonisamide. *Jpn J Psychiatry Neurol* 1991; 45:357.
5. Leppik IE, Wilmore LJ, Homan RW, et al. Efficacy and safety of zonisamide: result of a multicenter study. *Epilepsy Res* 1993;14: 165–173.
6. Schmidt D, Jacob R, Loiseau P, et al. Zonisamide for add-on treatment of refractory partial epilepsy: a European double-blind trial. *Epilepsy Res* 1993;15:67–73.
7. Ono T, Yagi K, Seino M. Clinical efficacy and safety of a new antiepileptic drug, zonisamide: a multi-institutional phase three study. *Clin Psychiatry* 1988;30:471–482.
8. Oguni I, Hayashi K, Yoshida K, et al. Phase III study of a new antiepileptic AD-810, zonisamide, in childhood epilepsy. *Jpn J Pediatr* 1988;41:439–450.
9. Yamatogi Y, Ohtahara S. Current topics of treatment. In: Ohtahara S, Roger J, eds. *Proceedings of the international symposium, new trends in pediatric epileptology.* Okayama University Medical School, 1991:136–148.
10. Yagi K, Seino M. Open clinical trial of new antiepileptic drug, zonisamide (ZNA) on 49 patients with refractory epileptic seizures. *Clin Psychiatry* 1992;29:111–119.
11. Kyllerman M, Ben-Menachem E. Long-term treatment of pro-gressive myoclonic epilepsy syndromes with zonisamide and n-acetylcysteine. *Epilepsia* 1996;37:172.
12. Seino M, Miyazaki H, Ito T. Zonisamide. *Epilepsy Res Suppl* 1997;3:169–174.
13. Henry T, Leppik IE, Gumnit RJ, et al. Progressive myoclonus epilepsy treated with zonisamide. *Neurology* 1998;38:928–931.
14. Bialer M, Johannessen SI, Kupferberg HJ, et al. Progress report on new antiepileptic drugs: a summary of the Fourth Eilat Con-ference (EILAT IV). *Epilepsy Res* 1999;34:1–41.
15. Leppik I. Zonisamide. *Epilepsia* 1999;40[Suppl 5]:S23–S29.
16. Masuda Y, Karasawa T, Shiraishi Y, et al. 3-Sulfamoylmethyl-1,2-benz-isoxazole, a new type of anticonvulsant drug: pharmacolog-ical profile. *Arzneimittelforschung* 1980;30:477–483.
17. Taylor CP, McLean JR, Bockbrader HN, et al. Zonisamide (A-810, CI-912). In: Meldrum BS, Porter RJ, eds. *New anticonvul-sant drugs.* London: Libbey, 1986:277–294.
18. Masuda Y, Utsui Y, Shiraishi Y, et al. Relationships between plasma concentrations of diphenylhydantoin, phenobarbital, car-bamazepine, and 3-sulfamoylmethly-1,2-benzisoxazole (AD-810), a new anticonvulsant agent, and their anticonvulsant or neurotoxic effects in experimental animals. *Epilepsia* 1979;20: 623–633.
19. Kamei C, Oka M, Masuda Y, et al. Effects of 3-sulfamoylmethyl-1,2-benzisoxazole (AD-810) and some antiepileptics on the kin-dled seizures in the neocortex, hippocampus and amygdala in rats. *Arch Int Pharmacodyn* 1981;249:164–176.
20. Hamada K, Ishida S, Yagi K, Seino M. Anti-convulsant effects of zonisamide on amygdaloid kindling in rats. *Neurosciences* 1990; 16:407–412.
21. Kakegawa N. An experimental study on the modes of appearance and disappearance of suppressive effect of antiepileptic drugs on kindled seizure. *Psychiatr Neurol Jpn* 1986;88:81–98.
22. Wada Y, Hasegawa H, Okuda A, et al. Anticonvulsant effects of zonisamide and phenytoin on seizure activity of the feline visual cortex. *Brain Dev* 1990;12:206–210.
23. Bartoszyk GD, Hamer M. The genetic animal model of reflex epilepsy in the Mongolian gerbil: differential efficacy of new anti-convulsive drugs and prototype antiepileptics. *Pharmacol Res Commun* 1987;19:429–440.
24. Nakamura J, Tamura S, Kandra T, et al. Inhibition by topiramate of seizures in spontaneously epileptic rats and DBA/2 mice. *Eur J Pharmacol* 1994;11:83–89.
25. Nagatomo I, Akasaki Y, Nagase F, et al. Relationships between convulsive seizures and serum and brain concentrations of phe-nobarbital and zonisamide in mutant inbred strain EL mouse. *Brain Res* 1996;26:190–198.
26. Takano K, Tanaka T, Fujita T, et al. Zonisamide: electrophysio-logical and metabolic changes in kainic acid-induced limbic seizures in rats. *Epilepsia* 1995;36:644–648.
27. Ito T, Hori M, Masuda Y, et al. 3-Sulfamoylmethyl-1,2-ben-zisoxazole, a new type of anticonvulsant drug: electroencephalo-graphic profile. *Arzneimittelforschung* 1980;30:603–609.
28. Ito T, Hori M, Kadokawa T. Effects of zonisamide (AD-810) on tungstic acid gel-induced thalamic generalized seizures and con-jugated estrogen-induced cortical spikewave discharges in cats. *Epilepsia* 1986;27:367–374.
29. Schauf CL. Zonisamide enhances slow sodium inactivation in *Myxicola. Brain Res* 1987;413:185.
30. Rock DM, Macdonald RL, Taylor CP. Blockade of sustained repetitive action potentials in cultured spinal cord neurons by zonisamide (AD 810, CI 912), a novel anticonvulsant. *Epilepsy Res* 1989;3:138–143.
31. McLean MJ, Macdonald RL. Multiple actions of phenytoin on mouse spinal cord neurons in cell culture. *J Pharmacol Exp Ther* 1983;227:779–789.
32. Hille B. Local anesthetics: hydrophilic and hydrophobic path-ways for the drug-receptor reaction. *J Gen Physiol* 1977;69: 497–515.
33. Worley PF, Baraban JM. Site of anticonvulsant action on sodium channels: autoradiographic and electrophysiological studies in rat brain. *Neurobiology* 1987;84:3051–3055.
34. Macdonald RL. Mechanisms of anticonvulsant drug action. In: Meldrum BS, Pedley TA, eds. *Recent advances in epilepsy.* New York: Churchill Livingston, 1983:1–23.
35. Macdonald RL, McLean MJ, Skerritt JH. Anticonvulsant drug mechanisms of action. *Fed Proc* 1985;44:2634–2639.
36. Macdonald RL, McLean MJ. Anticonvulsant drugs: mechanisms of action. *Adv Neurol* 1986;44:713–735.
37. Macdonald RL, Meldrum BS. Principles of antiepileptic drug action. In: Levy RH, Mattson RH, Meldrum B, eds. *Antiepilep-tic drugs,* 4th ed. New York: Raven Press, 1995:61–77.
38. Macdonald RL. Cellular effects of antiepileptic drugs. In: Engel J, Pedley TA, eds. *Epilepsy: a comprehensive textbook.* New York: Raven Press, 1997:1383–1392.
39. McLean MJ, Macdonald RL. Carbamazepine and 10, 11-epoxy-carbamazepine produce use- and voltage-dependent limitation of rapidly firing action potentials of mouse central neurons in cell culture. *J Pharmacol Exp Ther* 1986;238:727–738.
40. Macdonald RL. Carbamazepine: mechanisms of action. In: Levy RH, Mattson RH, Meldrum B, eds. *Antiepileptic drugs,* 4th ed. New York: Raven Press, 1995:491–498.
41. McLean MJ, Macdonald RL. Sodium valproate, but not etho-suximide, produces use- and voltage-dependent limitation of

high frequency repetitive firing of action potentials of mouse central neurons in cell culture. *J Pharmacol Exp Ther* 1986;237:1001–1011.

42. Suzuki S, Kawakami K, Nishimura S, et al. Zonisamide blocks T-type calcium channel in cultured neurons of rat cerebral cortex. *Epilepsy Res* 1992;12:21–27.

43. Kito M, Maehara M, Watanabe K. Mechanisms of T-type calcium channel blockade by zonisamide. *Seizure* 1996;5:115–119.

44. Coulter DA, Hugenard JR, Prince DA. Specific petit mal anticonvulsants reduce calcium currents in thalamic neurons. *Neurosci Lett* 1989;98:74–78.

45. Coulter DA, Hugenard JR, Prince DA. Characterization of ethosuximide reduction of low-threshold calcium current in thalamic neurons. *Ann Neurol* 1989;25:582–593.

46. Kelly KM, Gross RA, Macdonald RL. Valproic acid selectively reduces the low-threshold (T) calcium in rat nodose neurons. *Neurosci Lett* 1990;116:233–238.

47. Coulter DA, Hugenard JR, Prince DA. Calcium currents in rat thalamocortical relay neurones: kinetic properties of the transient low-threshold current. *J Physiol (Lond)* 1989;414:587–604.

48. Chen G, Ensor CR, Bohner B. A facilitation action of reserpine on the central nervous system. *Proc Soc Exp Biol Med* 1954;86:507–510.

49. Koe BK, Weissman A. The pharmacology of para-chloro-phenylalanine, a selective depletor of serotonin stores. *Adv Pharmacol* 1968;6B:29–47.

50. Kilian M, Frey H-H. Central monoamines and convulsive thresholds in mice and rats. *Neuropharmacology* 1973;12:681–692.

51. Azzaro AJ, Wenger GR, Craig CR, et al. Reserpine-induced alterations in brain amines and their relationship to changes in the incidence of minimal electro-shock seizures in mice. *J Pharmacol Exp Ther* 1972;180:558–568.

52. Quattrone A, Samanin R. Decreased anticonvulsant activity of carbamazepine in 6-hydroxydopamine-treated rats. *Eur J Pharmacol* 1977;41:333–336.

53. Prockop DJ, Shore PA, Brodie BB. An anticonvulsant effect of monoamine oxidase inhibitors. *Experientia* 1959;15:145–147.

54. Chen G, Ensor CR, Bohner B. Studies of drug effects on electrically induced extensor seizures and clinical implications. *Arch Int Pharmacodyn Ther* 1968;172:183–218.

55. Okada M, Kaneko S, Hirano T, et al. Effects of zonisamide on extracellular levels of monoamine and its metabolites, and on Ca^{2+} dependent dopamine release. *Epilepsy Res* 1992;13:113–119.

56. Kaneko S, Okada M, Hirano T, et al. Carbamazepine and zonisamide increase extracellular dopamine and serotonin levels in vivo, and carbamazepine does not antagonize adenosine effect in vitro: mechanisms of blockade of seizure spread. *Jpn J Psychiatry Neurol* 1993;47:371–373.

57. Okada M, Kaneko S, Hirano T, et al. Effects of zonisamide on dopaminergic system. *Epilepsy Res* 1995;22:193–205.

58. Mizuno K, Okada M, Kaneko S, et al. Effects of zonisamide, carbamazepine and valproate on monoamine metabolism in rat striatum and hippocampus. *Jpn J Psychiatry Neurol* 1994;48:406–408.

59. Okada M, Hirano T, Kawata Y, et al. Biphasic effects of zonisamide on serotonergic system in rat hippocampus. *Epilepsy Res* 1999;34:187–197.

60. Okada M. Effects of carbamazepine and zonisamide on monoaminergic system in rat striatum and hippocampus. *Jpn J Psychopharmacol* 1994;14:337–354.

61. Mizuno K. Effects of carbamazepine and zonisamide on acetylcholine levels in rat striatum. *Nihon Shinkei Seisin Yakurigaku Zasshi* 1997;17:17–23.

62. Macdonald RL. Cellular actions of antiepileptic drugs. In: Eadie MJ, Vajda FJE, eds. *Antiepileptic drugs: pharmacology and therapeutics.* Berlin: Springer-Verlag, 1999:123–150.

63. Mimaki T, Suzuki Y, Tagawa T, et al. Interaction of zonisamide with benzodiazepine and GABA receptors in rat brain. *Med J Osaka Univ* 1990;39:13–17.

64. Mimaki T, Suzuki Y, Tagawa T, et al. [³H]Zonisamide binding in rat brain. *Jpn J Psychiatr Neurol* 1988;42:640–642.

65. Mimaki T, Suzuki Y, Tagawa T, et al. [³H]zonisamide binding in rat brain. *Med J Osaka Univ* 1990;39:19–22.

66. Okada M, Kawada Y, Mizuna K, et al. Interaction between Ca^{2+}, K^+, carbamazepine and zonisamide on hippocampal extracellular glutamate monitored with a microdialysis electrode. *Br J Pharmacol* 1998;124:1277–1285.

67. Masuda Y, Karasawa T. Inhibitory effect of zonisamide on human carbonic anhydrase in vitro. *Arzneimittelforschung* 1993;43:416–418.

68. Masuda Y, Noguchi H, Karasawa T. Evidence against a significant implication of carbonic anhydrase inhibitory activity of zonisamide in its anticonvulsive effects. *Arzneimittelforschung* 1994;44:267–269.

ZONISAMIDE

CHEMISTRY, BIOTRANSFORMATION, AND PHARMACOKINETICS

JAYMIN SHAH
KENT SHELLENBERGER
DANIEL M. CANAFAX

CHEMISTRY

Zonisamide (1,2-benzisoxazole-3-methanesulfonamide) is a broad-spectrum antiepileptic drug (AED) marketed in Japan and South Korea for more than 10 years as Excegran (Dainippon Pharmaceuticals, Osaka, Japan). Zonisamide (Zonegran; Elan Pharmaceuticals, Gainesville, GA) has been approved since March 2000 for marketing in the United States. Zonisamide was first synthesized by Uno and collaborators (1) in 1972. The chemical structure of zonisamide (molecular formula: $C_8H_8N_2O_3S$; molecular weight, 212.23) is shown in Figure 92.1. The drug appears as nonhygroscopic, white to pale yellow crystals or as a crystalline powder with a slightly bitter taste, and has a melting point of 164°C to 168°C. The pK_a value of zonisamide is 9.66 and its solubility in water (25°C) is pH dependent; at neutral pH, the solubility is approximately 0.78 mg/mL. The drug is undisassociated at acidic pH up to approximately 8, but becomes dissociated above pH 8, leading to increased solubility as the pH increases. Zonisamide is soluble in acetone (1 g/8 mL), but has low solubility in methanol, ethanol, ether, and chloroform (range, 1 g/60 mL to 1 g/1.7 L). The partition coefficient ratio of zonisamide at neutral pH is 1.04 in chloroform/water and 3.24 in 1-octanol/water.

The commercial formulation contains 100 mg of zonisamide and 200 mg total of excipients such as microcrystalline cellulose and sodium lauryl sulfate in a hard gelatin capsule. The encapsulated materials are chemically stable and exhibit no change in dissolution rate unless stored in high humidity and excessive light conditions in a nonprotective package. The commercial product is packaged in a high-density polyethylene bottle and has a documented shelf life of 2 years.

MECHANISM OF ACTION

Voltage-dependent Na^+ and Ca^{2+} channels have a critical role in neural membrane excitability (2). *In vitro* pharmacology studies suggest that zonisamide blocks both Na^+ channels and T-type Ca^{2+} channels, thereby reducing voltage-dependent, transient inward currents. These effects promote stabilizing of neuronal membranes and suppression of neuronal hypersynchronization. Given these effects, it has been suggested that zonisamide disrupts synchronized neu-

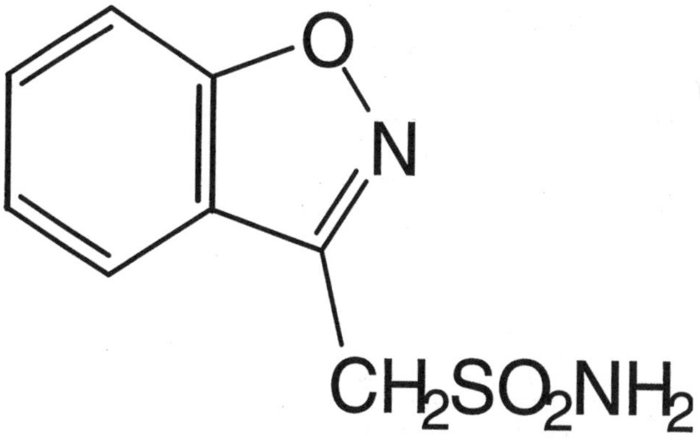

Jaymin Shah, PhD: Director, Clinical Pharmacology, Elan Pharmaceuticals, South San Francisco, California

Kent Shellenberger, PhD: Vice President, Clinical Affairs, Elan Pharmaceuticals, South San Francisco, California

Daniel M. Canafax, PharmD: Director, Clinical Affairs, Elan Pharmaceuticals, South San Francisco, California

FIGURE 92.1. Chemical structure of zonisamide.

ronal firing in the seizure forms, thereby limiting the spread of seizures (3). Zonisamide also inhibits carbonic anhydrase activity, but this effect is not thought to be a major contributing factor in producing antiepilepsy activity.

PHARMACOKINETIC OVERVIEW

The pharmacokinetics of zonisamide have been evaluated in numerous studies with volunteers recruited in Japan and the United States. Zonisamide's pharmacokinetic parameters are summarized in Table 92.1. In general, zonisamide has rapid absorption, good bioavailability that is not affected by food, and a long terminal half-life from mixed hepatic (70%) and renal (30%) routes of elimination. The metabolites produced by cytochrome P450 (CYP) 3A4 and 2D6 microsomal enzymes are inactive. After dosing between 200 and 600 mg/day in adults with epilepsy, the resulting zonisamide concentrations are approximately 10 to 30 μg/mL and have a modest relationship between efficacy and adverse events. Drug interactions with zonisamide and the other AEDs are uncommon and of minor clinical significance, except for phenytoin (decreased clearance from zonisamide and increases zonisamide clearance), and phenobarbital and carbamazepine (both increase zonisamide clearance).

In these pharmacokinetic studies, methods for measuring zonisamide levels in various biologic matrices, such as, plasma, serum, and tissue were developed using high-performance liquid chromatography and enzyme-linked assay techniques. These assays were optimized to avoid interference from zonisamide metabolites and other AEDs and their metabolites (4–6). Usual monitoring of zonisamide levels is performed using plasma or serum samples.

ABSORPTION AND BIOAVAILABILITY

After oral doses of radiolabeled zonisamide given in experimental models, absorption from the gastrointestinal tract is rapid and complete as determined by measurement of radioactive drug excretion in bile and urine (7). In a dose escalation study, single oral zonisamide doses of 200, 400, and 800 mg were given to 12 healthy volunteers with a 3-week washout period between doses. Moderately rapid absorption was observed, with the time to maximal plasma concentration (T_{max}) ranging from 2.4 to 3.6 hours, which was independent of dose size (8). The maximum concentration (C_{max}) in plasma increases as the dose increases from 200 to 800 mg and ranged from 2.3 to 12 μg/mL (Table 92.1). The elimination half-life is long and appears to be independent of the zonisamide dose, ranging from 49.7 to 62.5 hours. The mean area under the zonisamide concentration–time curve (AUC) is proportional to the dose administered and ranged from 170 to 863 μg/hr/mL.

A multiple dose pharmacokinetic study was conducted in two groups of healthy subjects receiving 400 mg/day dose either as 200 mg twice daily or 400 mg once daily for 35 days in a gradual dose escalation design. At steady state, mean C_{max} was 30.3 (twice-daily group) and 28.0 μg/mL (once-daily group), reached in 2.1 and 1.8 hours, respectively. The bioavailability of zonisamide with the once-daily regimen is approximately 84% of the twice-daily dosing regimen. At steady state, the fluctuation between peak and trough zonisamide concentrations was 14% for twice-daily (12-hour) dosing and 27% for once-daily (24-hour) dosing (9).

Administration of a single 400-mg dose to patients with refractory epilepsy receiving concomitant AEDs results in

TABLE 92.1. MEAN PHARMACOKINETIC PARAMETERS OF ZONISAMIDE IN HEALTHY VOLUNTEERS AND IN PATIENTS WITH EPILEPSY

Dose (mg)	n	Fluid	C_{max} (μg/mL)	T_{max} (h)	$T_{1/2}$	AUC (m/mL)	CLp/F (mL/min/kg)	Vd/F (L/kg)	Reference
200	12[a]	Plasma	2.3	2.4	63	170	0.315	1.8	8
		Blood	11.6	2.8	80	1,324	0.041	0.28	
400	12[a]	Plasma	5.2	2.8	52	347	0.316	1.5	8
		Blood	17.4	2.5	81	2,062	0.052	0.37	
800	12[a]	Plasma	12.2	3.6	50	863	0.252	1.09	8
		Blood	26.5	3.8	88	3,477	0.061	0.47	
400	10[b]	Plasma	5.5	2.7	—	193	—	—	35
		Blood	6.7	5.8	—	389	—	—	
200 b.i.d.	11[c]	Serum	30.3	2.1	69	339	0.514		9

AUC, area under the curve; b.i.d., twice daily; C_{max}, maximum concentration; CLp, plasma clearance; F, bioavailability; T_{max}, time to maximum plasma concentration; $T_{1/2}$, half-life; V_d, volume of distribution.
[a]Single dose, healthy volunteers.
[b]Single dose, patients with epilepsy.
[c]Multiple dose, healthy volunteers.

mean C_{max} of 5.9 µg/mL that is reached in 3.3 hours and a mean AUC of 213 µg/hr/mL. It is noteworthy that these pharmacokinetic parameters from patient studies are similar to values observed in healthy subjects.

Pharmacokinetic studies of zonisamide have been conducted using either capsule or tablet formulations. At present, an intravenous formulation of zonisamide is not available; therefore, any potential first-pass metabolism has not been assessed. As an indirect measure of bioavailability, [14C]-zonisamide was given to humans and 65% of the administered radioactivity was recovered in 10 days, indicating that the oral bioavailability of the zonisamide capsule is high (10). The systemic availability of zonisamide is similar with or without administration of the drug with food, except for a slight delay in T_{max} to 4 to 6 hours (11).

DISTRIBUTION

Tissue distribution studies of 14C-zonisamide after single and multiple doses show that the drug is distributed evenly throughout the entire body. The concentrations of radioactivity in various tissues, as a function of time, are similar to the plasma concentrations, except for the liver, kidney, and adrenal concentrations, which are approximately twofold greater than the plasma concentrations. The distribution pattern in the body after repeated doses is similar to that after a single dose. A drug distribution study in the rat brain model shows high concentrations in the cerebral cortex and midbrain (12). Peak radioactivity occurs in most tissues within 3 hours after administering zonisamide and decreases in parallel to the decline in plasma radioactivity. No measurable accumulation of zonisamide is found in the central nervous system. Brain uptake is not through a saturable, carrier-mediated mechanism, but is attributable to lipid-mediated transport (13).

Zonisamide is approximately 40% to 60% bound to human serum albumin. Erythrocytes have a higher affinity than serum albumin for binding zonisamide. There is a dynamic equilibrium between free zonisamide and the drug concentrations in red cells and tissue and on plasma protein binding sites.

The binding capacity of zonisamide in erythrocytes is limited to a maximum of approximately 450 µmol/L (14). Also, saturation of erythrocyte binding occurs at a concentration of approximately 5 µg/mL. These characteristics of zonisamide create a dose–erythrocytes and dose–whole blood concentration relationship that in the therapeutic range (10 to 30 µg/mL) appears to be nonlinear, whereas the dose–plasma concentration relationship is linear.

Estimates of the plasma Vd/F (apparent oral volume of distribution) after single oral doses range from 1.09 to 1.77 L/kg, indicating that zonisamide is widely distributed outside the plasma compartment. At steady state, the mean plasma Vd for zonisamide is significantly lower than the Vd/F observed for single-dose administration (0.91 versus 1.45 L/kg). The changes observed in the single-dose plasma Vd/F as a function of dose and those observed at steady state are likely produced by the concentration-dependent binding of zonisamide to erythrocytes.

Zonisamide readily penetrates across lipid membranes into various body fluid compartments. The drug also crosses the blood–brain barrier and, in animal studies, the concentration in cerebrospinal fluid is similar to the free fraction in serum (15). Zonisamide crosses the placenta and enters breast milk. Fetal rat concentrations are similar to those in the plasma of the mother, and concentrations in the breast milk are similar to maternal plasma concentrations (16,17). Zonisamide appears to be actively secreted into saliva because saliva levels are higher than the free fraction in serum. It is possible this is the cause of a metallic taste that occasionally is reported by patients taking zonisamide.

Red Blood Cell Binding

Zonisamide, like other sulfonamides, has a high affinity for binding carbonic anhydrase and other red cell components, as opposed to extracellular serum albumin (14); therefore, zonisamide is highly concentrated in erythrocytes (14,18). This results in higher drug concentrations in whole blood than in the plasma. Erythrocyte uptake is best described by the sum of linear passive diffusion and a saturable binding to carbonic anhydrase. Because of this saturable binding, a greater proportion of whole blood to plasma drug concentration is bound to erythrocytes at low concentrations (<5 µg/mL) compared with higher concentrations. Therefore, the erythrocyte to plasma concentration ratio is concentration dependent and produces a degree of apparent concentration nonlinearity at low plasma concentrations. For example, at plasma concentrations of 1 µg/mL, the predicted erythrocyte–plasma ratio is >15, and as plasma concentration increases, this ratio decreases (Table 92.2). The ratio of erythrocyte to plasma drug concentration at steady-state levels of 15 to 20 µg/mL is approximately 4. The erythrocyte uptake of zonisamide has minimal effect on the pharmacokinetic characteristics of the drug at therapeutic steady-state concentrations between 10 and 30 µg/mL.

BIOTRANSFORMATION AND EXCRETION

Zonisamide undergoes significant biotransformation, with various metabolites identified in animal urine. The main

TABLE 92.2. ZONISAMIDE ERYTHROCYTE-TO-PLASMA DRUG CONCENTRATION RATIO FOR PHARMACOKINETIC PARAMETERS AFTER A SINGLE DOSE

Dose (mg)	N	C_{max}	$T_{1/2}$	AUC	CL/F
200	12	10.8	1.4	17.2	0.594
400	12	6.45	1.7	12.6	0.784
800	12	3.79	2.0	8.5	0.117

AUC, area under the curve; C_{max}, maximum concentration; CL/F, clearance; F, bioavailability; N, number of subjects; $T_{1/2}$, half-life.
From Taylor C, McLean J, Bockbrader H, et al. Zonisamide. In: Meldrum B, Porter R, eds. *New anticonvulsant drugs*. London: John Libbey, 1986:277–294, with permission.

metabolic pathways in animals include glucuronide conjugation, acetylation, hydroxylation followed by oxidation of the methylene carbon of the sulfamoylmethyl group, finally resulting in loss of the sulfamoylmethyl group, and N–O bond cleavage of the isoxazole ring to produce two ring-cleft metabolites. The hydroxylation and ring-cleft products subsequently are excreted as sulfate or glucuronide conjugates (16,19). The metabolite composition in various body fluids and tissues has been studied in young and adult animal models (12,19). ^{14}C-zonisamide administered to healthy subjects showed that most of the activity was associated with the intact drug and no appreciable metabolites were present in the plasma (10).

The two primary metabolites identified from human urine are the glucuronide of the open-ring metabolite [2-(sulfamoylacetyl)-phenol-glucuronide] (SMAP) and the *N*-acetylzonisamide (Figure 92.2). These metabolites, along with unchanged zonisamide in the urine, account for almost all the radioactivity administered. *In vitro* human liver microsomal studies (20) indicate that CYP is involved in the reductive metabolism of zonisamide. The metabolism of zonisamide to SMAP is almost completely inhibited by anti-CYP3A4 antibody, whereas the anti-CYP2D6 antibody has no effect. Therefore, the 3A subfamily includes the major isoenzymes of the CYP enzymes responsible for the formation of SMAP from zonisamide. These results closely parallel the findings in the rat model, which indicate that CYP3A4 mediates the formation of SMAP (21). At concentrations of 200 μmol/L, which is approximately 40 μg/mL or at the high end of the therapeutic concentration,

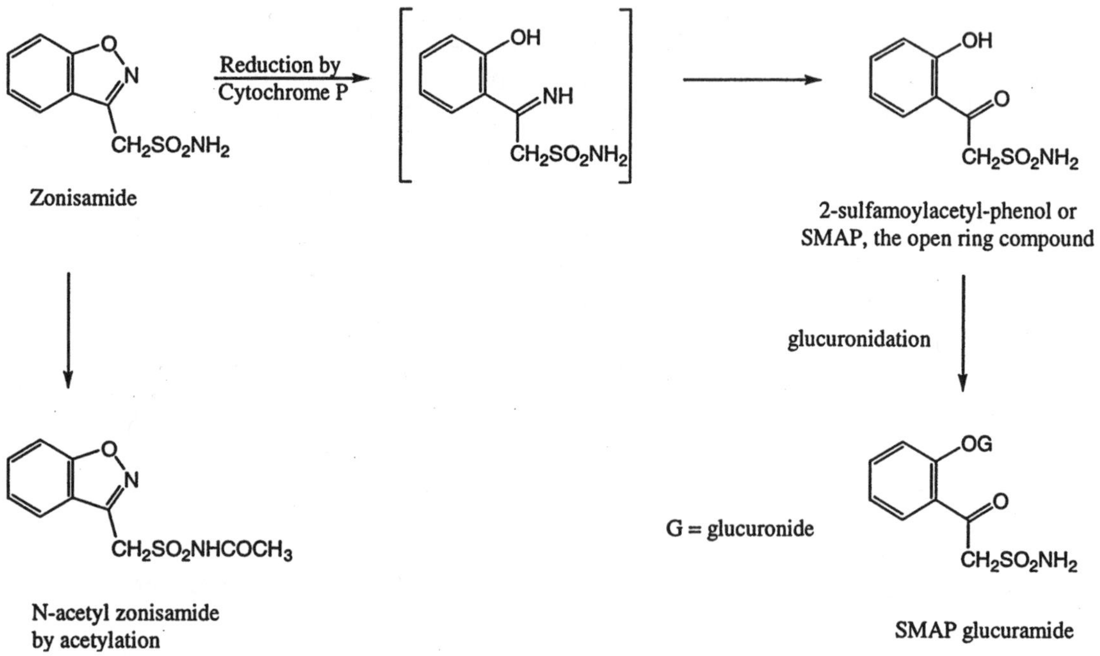

FIGURE 92.2. Metabolic pathway of zonisamide in humans.

zonisamide had less than a 10% inhibitory effect on several of the CYP isozymes, including CYP3A4 (*unpublished data*). This inhibition of enzymatic activity is not concentration dependent because the inhibition does not exceed 14% of control levels at concentrations up to 1,000 µmol/L of zonisamide. In humans, repeated administration of the drug does not alter the pharmacokinetic characteristics; therefore, autoinduction of zonisamide metabolism apparently does not occur (18,22).

After a single dose of ^{14}C-zonisamide in animal models, most (>80%) of the parent drug is eliminated in urine, with a minor fraction (approximately 15% in rats and dogs, 4% in monkeys) eliminated in the feces. Biliary excretion accounts for approximately 22% in rats, a portion of which was eventually eliminated in the feces (7). This suggests that the major route of excretion of zonisamide and its metabolite is by the kidney in animal models. In humans, unchanged zonisamide comprises approximately 30% of total urine radioactivity, *N*-acetyl-zonisamide approximately 20%, and the glucuronide of the open-ring metabolite (SMAP) approximately 50% of the total dose administered (10,18). The total excretion of unchanged zonisamide and the conjugated open-ring metabolite of zonisamide accounts for 48% to 60% of the administered dose, suggesting that renal elimination is a major route of excretion in humans and the feces is a minor route of elimination.

CLEARANCE AND HALF-LIFE

Healthy Subjects

In healthy subjects after single zonisamide doses of 200, 400, and 800 mg on three separate occasions with an adequate washout period, the mean half-life of the drug in plasma ranged from 49.7 to 62.5 hours and the apparent oral clearance ranged from 0.25 to 0.32 mL/min/kg (8). In a multiple-dose study with healthy subjects, the mean half-life of zonisamide ranged from 63.0 to 68.6 hours, with apparent oral clearance from 0.143 to 0.17 mL/min/kg (9). The higher plasma clearance from a single dose could be attributable to the nonlinear binding to erythrocytes at low concentrations.

Epileptic Patients Taking Other Antiepileptic Drugs

Studies using pretreatment with phenobarbital or carbamazepine in rats demonstrate a decrease in zonisamide half-life (23). Similarly in humans, an increase in zonisamide plasma clearance and a decrease in half-life is observed with concomitant administration of zonisamide with phenytoin, carbamazepine, phenobarbital, and valproic acid (24). The half-life of zonisamide when given concomitantly with phe-

nobarbital is 38 hours, and is 27 hours when administered concomitantly with phenytoin (25). A similar reduction in the zonisamide half-life to 36 hours is produced by carbamazepine administration (25). These interactions were found after the administration of single zonisamide doses to patients receiving stable doses of the other AEDs. In steady-state drug interaction studies performed in patients with epilepsy receiving stable doses of commonly used AEDs, we observed that in the presence of phenytoin and carbamazepine, the half-life of zonisamide is approximately 27 and 36 hours, respectively, whereas the clearance was increased by 40% to 50%. In contrast to the previous reports, no reduction in the zonisamide half-life (approximately 50 hours) was observed in presence of lamotrigine and valproic acid (26).

Children

Unfortunately, formal zonisamide pharmacokinetic studies have not been conducted in children as yet. Many Japanese trials in children with epilepsy included monitoring steady-state zonisamide blood or serum concentrations. Recent studies showed that serum zonisamide concentrations increased linearly with increasing doses of less than 10 mg/kg/day, and when stabilized at effective doses of 5 to 8 mg/kg/day, the resulting serum zonisamide concentrations were approximately in the range of 10 to 30 µg/mL (27). In addition, dose titration in small increments of 0.5 to 1 mg/kg every 2 weeks is well tolerated, and serum concentrations above 40 µg/mL are more likely to produce adverse effects. It appears that larger zonisamide doses (milligrams per kilogram) are required in children than in adults to achieve equivalent serum drug concentrations, possibly because of increased zonisamide clearance in this population, as seen with the other AEDs (28).

Elderly

The mean plasma C_{max} for an equivalent dose of zonisamide in elderly subjects (mean age, 69 years; range, 65 to 71 years) is 32.4% higher than that for young adult subjects (mean age, 28 years; range, 21 to 40 years). Conversely, mean AUCs for young and elderly are not different, indicating that the extent of zonisamide absorption is similar for both of these age groups. The mean (standard deviation) zonisamide elimination half-life in the elderly subjects is observed to be 51.9 (23.6) hours, and is somewhat shorter than that in young subjects, 65.7 (11.1) hours (29). The mean Vd is lower in elderly subjects and could account for the decreased plasma half-life in the elderly group. Mean plasma clearance, renal clearance, and the percentage dose excreted unchanged in urine are similar in both age groups, indicating that zonisamide distribution and elimination are not affected by age (30).

ZONISAMIDE INTERSUBJECT VARIABILITY AND ITS DETERMINANTS

Low (<30%) intersubject zonisamide pharmacokinetic parameter variability occurs in healthy subjects and children with epilepsy (9,31). A somewhat higher degree of variability (approximately 45%) is observed in patients with epilepsy who are concurrently taking other AEDs. This results from effects by the other AEDs combined with the innate interpatient differences in microsomal enzyme activity. Most of the interpatient zonisamide pharmacokinetic variability likely is due to metabolic differences between patients with epilepsy.

The primary metabolites formed from zonisamide degradation in humans are 2-(sulfamoylacetyl)-phenol-glucuronide and N-acetylzonisamide, produced from CYP enzyme alteration of the molecule. Significant genetic polymorphism is observed in both N-acetylation and P450 oxidation (32). For example, N-acetyltransferase activity has a bimodal or possibly trimodal distribution in humans. Similarly, distribution of other P450 hepatic isoenzymes is known to vary across racial groups, such as the variation seen in the frequency of slow and rapid metabolizers for isoenzymes CYP3A4, CYP2D6, and CYP2C19 (33). Predominant intersubject variability commonly is observed for most other AEDs, especially those drugs that have poor aqueous solubility, long elimination half-lives, and CYP-mediated metabolism, and are given concomitantly with medications metabolized by the same pathways.

RELATIONSHIP BETWEEN CONCENTRATION AND DOSE

Clinical studies conducted in adult (34) and pediatric patients (27,31) have demonstrated that steady-state serum drug concentrations increase linearly with increasing dosages above 3 mg/kg/day. Zonisamide concentrations after single doses are not predictive of the eventual steady-state concentrations (35). This appears to result from saturable uptake of zonisamide by red blood cells at approximately 5 µg/mL. The apparent nonlinearity possibly is due to saturable binding of zonisamide to erythrocytes at low concentrations.

A recent report on nonlinear kinetics of zonisamide in patients receiving other AEDs fails to consider this unique red cell binding saturation characteristic of zonisamide (36). Population pharmacokinetic analysis of zonisamide data from clinical studies in patients demonstrates dose-dependent pharmacokinetics of zonisamide with first-order clearance (37). The reported V_{max} value of 27.6 mg/kg/day is well above the daily maintenance dose of 400 to 600 mg for adults. This dose results in serum drug levels in the desired range of 10 to 30 µg/mL. For clinical purposes, steady-state concentrations can be regarded empirically to be proportional to the dose of zonisamide administered in patients with epilepsy.

RELATIONSHIP BETWEEN CONCENTRATION AND EFFECT

The assessment of zonisamide pharmacodynamic characteristics suggests that both antiepilepsy and drug-related adverse events occur over a wide range of drug concentrations. Zonisamide concentrations greater than 20 µg/mL are associated with reduced seizure rates. Most adverse events occur during the initiation of zonisamide therapy, usually disappearing within the first 4 weeks of treatment. This accommodation or tolerance to zonisamide side effects (mostly neurologic) guided the creation of the current gradual dose titration method that is performed over approximately a 4-week period. It also makes defining a concentration–adverse event relationship difficult.

When the dose of zonisamide is titrated to individual patient requirements based on efficacy and tolerability, the optimal dosage for most adult patients is between 400 and 600 mg/day. These dosages result in serum levels that range from 15 to 30 µg/mL. In contrast, results from a parallel-design study that administered fixed zonisamide doses of 100, 200, and 400 mg/day found no statistically significant relationship between plasma concentrations and clinical response (38). However, in this study, antiepilepsy effects and serum levels did increase as the dose increased (400 > 200 > 100 mg/day). Therefore, patients with low zonisamide levels are more likely to have less antiepilepsy benefits and, conversely, higher drug levels produce more drug-related adverse effects. The interpretation of zonisamide concentrations for each patient should be done in conjunction with their clinical response to the pharmacotherapy.

REFERENCES

1. Uno H, Kurokawa M, Natsuka K, et al. Studies on substituted 1,2-benzisoxazole derivatives. *Chem Pharm Bull (Tokyo)* 1976;24: 632–643.
2. Adams PR, Galvin M. Voltage-dependent current of vertebrate neurons and their role in membrane excitability. *Adv Neurol* 1986;44:137–170.
3. Suzuki S, Kawakami K, Nishimura S, et al. Zonisamide blocks T-type calcium channel in cultured neurons in rat cerebral cortex. *Epilepsy Res* 1992;12:21–27.
4. Berry DJ. Determination of zonisamide in plasma therapeutic concentrations by high performance liquid chromatography. *J Chromatogr* 1990;534:173–181.
5. Juergens U. HPLC analysis of antiepilepsy drugs in blood samples: microbore separation of fourteen compounds. *J Liquid Chromatogr* 1987;10:507–532.
6. Kaibe K, Nishimura S, Ishii H, et al. Competitive binding enzyme immunoassay for zonisamide, a new antiepilepsy drug, with selected paired-enzyme labelled antigen and antibody. *Clin Chem* 1990;36:24–27.

7. Matsumoto K, Miyazaki H, Fujii T, et al. Absorption, distribution and excretion of 3-(sulphamoyl[^{14}C]methyl)-1,2-benzisoxazole (AD-810) in rats, dogs and monkeys and of AD-810 in men. *Arzneimittelforschung* 1983;33:961–968.

8. Taylor C, McLean J, Bockbrader H, et al. Zonisamide. In: Meldrum B, Porter R, eds. *New anticonvulsant drugs*. London: John Libbey, 1986:277–294.

9. Kochak G, Page J, Buchanan R, et al: Steady-state pharmacokinetics of zonisamide, an antiepilepsy agent for treatment of refractory complex partial seizures. *J Clin Pharmacol* 1998;38:166–171.

10. Buchanan R, Bockbrader H, Chang T, et al. Single- and multiple- dose pharmacokinetics of zonisamide. *Epilepsia* 1996;37 [Suppl 5]:172.

11. Siedlik P, Brockbader H, Chang T, et al. Effect of food on the oral absorption of zonisamide in normal healthy volunteers. *Pharm Res* 1986;3[Suppl]:158S.

12. Stiff D, Zemaitis M. Metabolism of the anticonvulsant agent zonisamide in the rat. *Drug Metab Dispos* 1990;18:888–894.

13. Cornford E, Landon K. Blood-brain barrier transport of CI-912: single passage equilibration of erythrocyte-borne drug. *Ther Drug Monit* 1985;7:247–254.

14. Matsumoto K, Miyazaki H, Fujii T, et al. Binding of sulfonamides to erythrocytes and their components. *Chem Pharm Bull (Tokyo)* 1989;37:1913–1915.

15. Kumagai N, Seki T, Yamada T, et al. Concentrations of zonisamide in serum, free fraction, mixed saliva and cerebrospinal fluid in epileptic children treated with monotherapy. *Jpn J Psychol Neurol* 1993;47:291–292.

16. Seino M, Naruto S, Ito T, et al. Other antiepilepsy drugs. In: Levy R, Mattson R, Meldrum B, eds. *Antiepilepsy drugs*, 4th ed. New York: Raven Press, 1995:1011–1023.

17. Kimura S: Distribution of zonisamide to placenta and breast milk and its biological half-life in a neonate. *Brain Dev* 1998;30:350–351.

18. Ito T, Yamaguchi T, Miyizaki H, et al. Pharmacokinetic studies of AD-810, a new antiepilepsy compound. *Arzneimittelforschung* 1982;32:1581–1586.

19. Matsumoto K, Yoshida K, Fujii T, et al. Metabolism of ^{14}C-zonisamide in rats, dogs and monkeys [in Japanese]. *Xenobiot Metab Dispos* 1989;4:411–418.

20. Nakasa H, Komiya M, Ohmori S, et al. Characterization of human liver microsomal cytochrome P450 involved in the reductive metabolism of zonisamide. *Mol Pharmacol* 1993;44:216–221.

21. Nakasa H, Komiya M, Ohmori S, et al. Formation of reductive metabolite, 2-sulfamoylacetylphenol, from zonisamide in rat liver microsomes. *Res Commun Chem Pathol Pharmacol* 1992;77:31–41.

22. Nakasa H, Nakamura H, Ono S, et al. Prediction of drug-drug interactions of zonisamide metabolism in humans from in vitro data. *Eur J Clin Pharmacol* 1998;54:177–183.

23. Kimura M, Tanaka N, Kimura Y, et al. Pharmacokinetic interaction of zonisamide in rats: effect of other antiepileptics on zonisamide. *J Pharmacobiodyn* 1992;15:631–639.

24. Sackellares J, Donofrio P, Wagner J. Pilot study of zonisamide (1,2-benzisoxazole-3-methanesulfonamide) in patients with refractory partial seizures. *Epilepsia* 1985;26:206–211.

25. Ojemann L, Shastri R, Wilensky A, et al. Comparative pharmacokinetics of zonisamide (CI-912) in epileptic patients on carbamazepine or phenytoin monotherapy. *Ther Drug Monit* 1986;8:293–296.

26. Shellenberger K, Shah J, Hawkes D, et al. Multiple dose pharmacokinetics of antiepileptic drugs in presence of zonisamide. Presented at 24th IEC Congress, Argentina, May, 2001.

27. Oguni H, Hayashi K, Fukuyama Y, et al. Phase III study of a new antiepilepsy drug AD-810, zonisamide in childhood epilepsy [in Japanese]. *Jpn J Pediatr* 1988;41:439–450.

28. Perucca E, Bialer M. The clinical pharmacokinetics of the newer antiepileptic drugs. *Clin Pharmacokinet* 1996;31:29–46.

29. Wallace J, Shellenberger K, Groves L. Pharmacokinetics of zonisamide in young and elderly subjects. *Epilepsia* 1998;39:190–191.

30. Kaku M, Jono K, Ishitsu T, et al. Pharmacokinetics of zonisamide. *J Kyushu Pharm Soc* 1992;46:17–20.

31. Kaku M, Ishitsu T, Chikazawa S, et al. Serum concentrations of zonisamide in children with epilepsy. *J Kyushu Pharm Soc* 1991;45:2–30.

32. West W, Knight E, Pradhan S, et al. Interpatient variability: genetic predisposition and other genetic factors. *J Clin Pharmacol* 1997;37:635–648.

33. Ahsan C, Renwick A, Macklin B, et al. Ethnic differences in the pharmacokinetics of oral nifedipine. *Br J Clin Pharmacol* 1991;31:399–403.

34. Shimizu A, Yamamoto J, Yamada Y, et al. The antiepilepsy effect of zonisamide in patients with refractory seizures. *Curr Ther Res* 1987;42:147–155.

35. Wagner J, Sackellares J, Donofrio P, et al. Nonlinear pharmacokinetics of CI-912 in adult epileptic patients. *Ther Drug Monit* 1984;6:277–283.

36. McJilton J, Ramsay E, Vasquez D, et al. Pharmacokinetics of zonisamide: results from randomized, double-blind, multicenter, placebo-controlled study. *AES mtg*, 2001.

37. Hashimoto Y, Odani A, Tanigawara Y, et al. Population analysis of the dose-dependent pharmacokinetics of zonisamide in epileptic patients. *Biol Pharm Bull* 1994;17:323–326.

38. Buchanan R, Montouris G, Ayala R, et al. Zonisamide efficacy and dose response. *Epilepsia* 1998;39:39.

ZONISAMIDE

DRUG INTERACTIONS

GARY G. MATHER
JAYMIN SHAH

Zonisamide [3-(sulfamoylmethyl)-1,2-benzisoxazole] is a new antiepileptic drug (AED) with a novel mechanism of action and a broad spectrum of activity. Although zonisamide was approved in the United States only recently, it has been prescribed in Japan for over 10 years. Experience with zonisamide suggests that clinical responses can be achieved at a targeted steady-state plasma concentration close to 20 μg/mL, with individual patients maintained successfully throughout a range of 10 to 40 μg/mL (1). This range is approximately equivalent to 45 to 200 μmol/L zonisamide.

Zonisamide has proven to be useful in the treatment of several types of seizures (2,3) in combination with other AEDs and thus has the potential to interact with AEDs. Zonisamide also is used in the treatment of patients with manic disorders (4) and thus can interact with a variety of other drugs.

ZONISAMIDE METABOLISM

Zonisamide metabolism has been described in detail in Chapter 92, and metabolic features relevant to drug interactions are reviewed here. The largest portion of an oral dose of zonisamide is excreted in the urine as unchanged zonisamide, 2-sulfamoylacetylphenol (SMAP), and SMAP conjugates (5). The open-ring metabolite SMAP is formed by enzyme-dependent reductive cleavage of the 1,2-benzisoxazole ring catalyzed largely by cytochrome P450 (CYP) isoenzyme CYP3A4 (6). The *in vitro* K_m describing this reaction has been estimated at approximately 312 μmol/L (7). It recently has been reported that the expressed enzymes CYP2C19 and CYP3A5 also are capable of catalyzing zonisamide reduction (8). However, the intrinsic clearance of CYP3A4 is much higher than those of CYP2C19 and CYP3A5. Therefore, from the point of view

Gary G. Mather, PhD, DABT: Program Director, Preclinical ADME/TOX, Myriad Pharmaceuticals Inc., Salt Lake City, Utah
Jaymin Shah, PhD: Director, Clinical Pharmacology, Elan Pharmaceuticals, South San Francisco, California

of enzyme quantity and relative intrinsic clearances, it appears that CYP3A4 is the primary enzyme responsible for zonisamide metabolism *in vivo*. The enzyme aldehyde oxidase in the cytosol of several mammalian species also has been shown to catalyze formation of SMAP *in vitro* (9). Similar studies with enzymes of human origin have not been reported.

Based on the *in vitro* data, it can be anticipated that inhibitors of CYP3A4-mediated formation of SMAP may decrease zonisamide clearance and increase its plasma concentrations. The degree of interaction depends not only on the potency of the inhibitor but also on the extent to which this metabolic pathway contributes to the overall clearance of zonisamide. Conversely, inducers of CYP3A4 may increase zonisamide clearance and reduce half-life and plasma concentrations. It also can be inferred that the percentage of zonisamide dose cleared by reductive metabolism to SMAP will be increased in patients also treated with drugs known to induce CYP3A4, such as phenytoin, carbamazepine, and phenobarbital. Therefore, the pharmacokinetic effects of CYP3A4 inhibitors are expected to be greatest in patients treated with polytherapy.

EFFECTS OF ANTIEPILEPTIC DRUGS AND OTHER DRUGS ON THE PLASMA CONCENTRATION OF ZONISAMIDE

Phenytoin

The average zonisamide half-life was 26.8 hours in eight patients also treated with phenytoin (n = 7) or phenytoin and carbamazepine (n = 1) (10), a time considerably shorter than the 60 hours reported in untreated volunteers (11). A half-life of 27.1 hours, lower zonisamide maximum plasma concentration (C_{max}), and decreased area under the concentration–time curve (AUC) were accompanied by increased clearance in a similar study in patients treated with phenytoin (12). These data are consistent with the knowledge that phenytoin increases the clearance of other substrates of CYP3A4 such as oral contraceptives and carbamazepine

(13). Most recently, zonisamide was added in a stepwise fashion to therapy of patients maintained at steady state with phenytoin. After 2 weeks of treatment with 200 mg twice daily, the zonisamide half-life was 27.3 hours (14). Protein binding characteristics of zonisamide in human serum are not altered by phenytoin treatment, and therefore no changes in zonisamide clearance are anticipated due to altered levels of unbound zonisamide (15).

Carbamazepine

In a recent study, zonisamide was added in a stepwise manner to therapy of patients taking only carbamazepine. After maintaining treatment with zonisamide at 200 mg twice daily for at least 2 weeks, its half-life was 39 hours (16). This is consistent with earlier studies, where the average zonisamide half-life was 36.4 hours in patients also treated with carbamazepine and the oral clearance was 20.6 mL/hr/kg (12). The extent of the reduction of zonisamide half-life by carbamazepine appears to be less than that observed with phenytoin. In a population pharmacokinetics study, the clearance of zonisamide was found to be increased by 13% in 37 patients also treated with carbamazepine (17).

Lamotrigine

McJilton et al. (18) reported two patients treated with zonisamide whose serum levels became elevated when lamotrigine was introduced. Both patients had been treated with zonisamide for approximately 3 years and had a history of stable zonisamide serum concentrations. After introduction of lamotrigine with incremental doses of 25 mg/wk, signs and symptoms of toxicity appeared as lamotrigine doses reached 400 mg/day. Trough zonisamide levels were increased from approximately 27 or 33 μg/mL to 61.8 or 64.6 μg/mL, respectively, for the two patients. Toxicities subsided as lamotrigine was withdrawn and recurred when the patients were rechallenged. The mechanism for this interaction is unclear but would be consistent with reduction of zonisamide clearance. Conversely, Brodie et al. (19) has reported a zonisamide half-life of 51 hours in healthy epileptic patients also treated with lamotrigine, a value shorter than estimated after extended treatment with 400 mg/day (63 to 69 hours) in a group of 24 healthy volunteers (20).

Phenobarbital

In a study of volunteers treated with phenobarbital, the C_{max} and time to maximal plasma concentration (T_{max}) of a single dose of zonisamide were unaffected, but clearance was increased and half-life was decreased to 38 hours (21). These data are similar to previous reports demonstrating

that clearance of zonisamide is significantly increased and half-life reduced in subjects also treated with phenobarbital (22).

Valproic Acid

The free fraction of zonisamide was slightly but significantly increased *in vitro* when measured in the presence of valproic acid. Although the increase was small (approximately 3%), a similar increase in free fraction was noted in patients also treated with valproic acid (23). In a separate study, steady-state pharmacokinetics were determined after administration of zonisamide to patients also treated with valproate. The observed zonisamide half-life was 52 hours, similar to previously reported data (24).

Sulfonamides

The high concentration of zonisamide in erythrocytes suggests that a drug–drug interaction with other sulfonamides may be possible. Although binding to serum proteins is not altered by other sulfonamides (15), zonisamide bound to erythrocyte membranes can be readily displaced by other sulfonamides *in vitro* (25), with a potency similar to their dissociation constants for carbonic anhydrase. In a study performed in rats, plasma and tissue levels of zonisamide did not change significantly even though erythrocyte levels of zonisamide decreased in the presence of other sulfonamides (25). This is most likely because the tissue and plasma compartments of zonisamide are large compared with the erythrocyte compartment at therapeutic dose levels.

Cimetidine

The formation of SMAP was inhibited by approximately 40% by high concentrations of cimetidine (1 mmol/L) in human liver microsomes *in vitro* (6), suggesting the possibility of interaction. However, no significant differences were reported in a recent study (26). The zonisamide AUC, mean elimination half-life, and C_{max} were all similar in groups administered a single 300-mg dose of zonisamide either with or without coadministration of cimetidine 300 mg four times daily. Although cimetidine is known to elevate phenytoin plasma concentrations, the interaction with phenytoin is most likely mediated through inhibition of CYP2C19, an enzyme inhibited by cimetidine at plasma concentrations.

Other Drugs

The *in vitro* formation of SMAP was inhibited by ketoconazole, cyclosporine, dihydroergotamine, itraconazole, miconazole, triazolam, and fluconazole, in order of potency, with inhibition constants (K_i) ranging from 0.18 to 61.4

μmol/L (8). Using these data and the maximal unbound concentration of each inhibitor, these investigators predicted that only ketoconazole, cyclosporine, and miconazole would decrease zonisamide clearance by more than 10%. Because the degree of inhibition estimated was based on the assumption that zonisamide is eliminated entirely by metabolism, these predictions estimate maximum levels of inhibition. However, "tight binders" (inhibitors) of CYP3A4 may exhibit more significant inhibition than can be predicted *in vitro* by their unbound concentrations (27). Although clinical interactions have not been reported to date, it seems prudent to be aware of this possibility whenever potent inhibitors of CYP3A4 are added to zonisamide treatment regimens.

EFFECTS OF ZONISAMIDE ON THE PLASMA CONCENTRATION OF OTHER DRUGS

Carbamazepine

Reports of the interaction between zonisamide and carbamazepine have been conflicting. Early studies suggested that average serum concentrations of carbamazepine after addition of zonisamide (300 to 600 mg/day for 2, 4, 8 and 12 weeks) were not significantly different from baseline values in a group of 10 patients (28). Mean carbamazepine concentrations during zonisamide treatment were unchanged in one, increased in three, and decreased in six patients. In other preliminary studies, initiation of zonisamide therapy was accompanied by higher carbamazepine plasma concentrations. Sackellares et al. (29) reported a significant elevation in carbamazepine plasma concentration as zonisamide was added. Carbamazepine levels increased from a mean of 6.8 to 11.7 μg/mL in seven patients treated concomitantly with two, three, or four other AEDs. However, one additional AED (phenytoin for four patients, phenobarbital for two patients, and primidone for one patient) was eliminated over the same period. Thus, the increases in carbamazepine levels may have resulted from withdrawal of an inducing drug rather than from introduction of zonisamide. Minami et al. (30) reported that the average level-to-dose ratio of carbamazepine in 16 pediatric patients receiving zonisamide was lower than that in patients treated with carbamazepine alone. In the same study, the ratio of carbamazepine epoxide to carbamazepine nearly doubled as zonisamide dosages increased from zero to 8.1 ± 3.8 mg/kg/day and zonisamide serum levels increased to 27.7 ± 7.8 μg/mL. Conversely, the epoxide-to-carbamazepine ratio was decreased significantly and the carbamazepine level-to-dose ratio was slightly increased in 15 patients when zonisamide was added to their treatment regimen (31). The reasons for these discrepancies are unclear but may result from differences in the time between drug administration and sample collection. Carbamazepine is metabolized by enzymes found in the gastrointestinal mucosa. It is conceivable that the local concentration of zonisamide in the gastrointestinal tract may affect the rate of carbamazepine metabolism during the absorption phase.

Lamotrigine

In a study of 18 patients whose seizures were controlled with lamotrigine, zonisamide was added after two baseline measurements of plasma lamotrigine (7 days apart). Zonisamide was titrated from initial dosages of 100 mg/day to 200 mg twice daily within 3 weeks. After 2 weeks of stable treatment, the mean lamotrigine C_{max}, T_{max}, and AUC were similar to baseline measurements, with no statistically significant differences detected (19).

Phenytoin

The effect of zonisamide on plasma concentrations of phenytoin is unclear. Zonisamide initially was reported to increase the serum concentrations of phenytoin. Indeed, phenytoin levels were higher after addition of zonisamide in two of three patients also treated with phenytoin and at least one additional AED (29); however, phenobarbital was withdrawn from one patient and carbamazepine from the other over the same period. Thus, the change in phenytoin may have resulted from withdrawal of an inducing drug rather than introduction of zonisamide. Consistent with this hypothesis, a study conducted in 10 patients revealed that the average serum concentration of phenytoin was not significantly different from baseline values after addition of zonisamide (300 to 600 mg/day for 2, 4, 8, and 12 weeks). Mean phenytoin concentrations increased in three patients, decreased in six patients, and remained unchanged in the remaining patient (28). A population pharmacokinetics study revealed a significant effect of zonisamide on the disposition of phenytoin. Slight but significant increases in the serum phenytoin concentrations were observed in patients receiving zonisamide. The apparent clearance of phenytoin at a given dose was decreased by 14% by zonisamide. Moreover, the apparent K_m for phenytoin was increased by 16% in the presence of zonisamide (32). Phenytoin protein binding in human serum was not changed significantly in the presence of zonisamide (21.3 μg eq/mL) *in vitro* (15); therefore, no changes in phenytoin clearance due to changes in unbound phenytoin should be anticipated.

Valproic Acid

In one study, zonisamide was added to the therapy of 16 patients with epilepsy controlled with valproic acid alone. Zonisamide doses were titrated to 200 mg twice daily within 3 weeks. The mean C_{max}, T_{max}, and AUC of valproic acid at 35 days were similar to baseline measurements without zonisamide (24). Similar results were reported in previous studies (21).

Oral Contraceptives

Numerous studies have shown that induction of metabolism and specifically induction of CYP3A4 increases the metabolic clearance of contraceptive compounds. This leads to reductions in their plasma concentrations and ultimately decreased efficacy. Enzyme induction by zonisamide is unclear. Zonisamide administration has been accompanied by either a slight increase or a slight decrease in the level of carbamazepine, a drug also cleared predominantly by CYP3A4 (33). There also is limited evidence of autoinduction with chronic zonisamide treatment. Although zonisamide clearance decreased with increasing dose, the V_{max} (maximum velocity) increased in six patients from a mean of 0.36783 L/kg/hr to 0.59588 L/kg/hr with chronic dosing (34). No change was noted in two additional patients. In a more recent study, single-dose pharmacokinetic parameters of levonorgestrel and ethinylestradiol were measured in a randomized, two-way crossover study in 12 healthy volunteers. Volunteers were given a single dose of Eugynon 50 (Schering AG, Montville, NJ) (50 μg ethinylestradiol and 250 μg levonorgestrel) alone or after approximately 4 weeks of zonisamide treatment. Zonisamide was initiated at 100 mg/day and escalated to 200 mg twice daily over 15 days. The AUC and C_{max} for both ethinylestradiol and levonorgestrel were similar regardless of zonisamide treatment (unpublished data). These data suggest that zonisamide does not increase the clearance of these compounds. Therefore, it appears that zonisamide can be used without decreasing the efficacy of these oral contraceptives.

REFERENCES

1. Oommen KJ, Mathews S. Zonisamide: a new antiepileptic drug. *Clin Neuropharmacol* 1999;22:192–200.
2. Leppik IE. Zonisamide. *Epilepsia* 1999;40:S23–S29.
3. Perucca E. The clinical pharmacokinetics of the new antiepileptic drugs. *Epilepsia* 1999;40[Suppl 9]:S7–S13.
4. Kanba S, Yagi G, Kamijima K, et al. The first open study of zonisamide, a novel anticonvulsant, shows efficacy in mania. *Prog Neuropsychopharmacol Biol Psychiatry* 1994;18:707–715.
5. Ito T, Yamaguchi T, Miyazaki H, et al. Pharmacokinetic studies of AD-810, a new antiepileptic compound. *Arzneimittelforschung* 1982;32:1581–1586.
6. Nakasa H, Komiya M, Ohmori S, et al. Characterization of human liver microsomal cytochrome P450 involved in the reductive metabolism of zonisamide. *Mol Pharmacol* 1993;44:216–221.
7. Mather GG, Carlson S, Trager WF, et al. Prediction of zonisamide interactions based on metabolic isozymes. *Epilepsia* 1997;38[Suppl 8]:108.
8. Nakasa H, Nakamura H, Ono S, et al. Prediction of drug-drug interactions of zonisamide metabolism in humans from in vitro data. *Eur J Clin Pharmacol* 1998;54:177–183.
9. Sugihara K, Kitamura S, Tatsumi K. Involvement of mammalian liver cytosols and aldehyde oxidase in reductive metabolism of zonisamide. *Drug Metab Dispos* 1996;24:199–202.
10. Browne TR, Szabo GK, Kres J. Elimination half-life of zon-

11. Seino M, Miyazaki H, Ito T. Zonisamide. *Epilepsy Res* 1991; [Suppl 3].
12. Ojemann LM, Shastri RA, Wilensky AJ, et al. Comparative pharmacokinetics of zonisamide (CI-912) in epileptic patients on carbamazepine or phenytoin monotherapy. *Ther Drug Monit* 1986; 8:293–296.
13. Mather GG, Levy RH. Anticonvulsants. In: Levy RH, Thummel KE, Trager WF, et al., eds. *Metabolic drug interactions.* Philadelphia: Lippincott Williams & Wilkins, 2000:217–243.
14. Garnett WR, Towne AR, Rosenfeld WE, et al. Steady-state pharmacokinetic interaction study of zonisamide (Zonegran) and phenytoin in subjects with epilepsy. American Academy of Neurology, 2000.
15. Matsumoto K, Miyazaki H, Fujii T, et al. Absorption, distribution and excretion of 3-(sulfamoyl[^{14}C]methyl)-1,2-benzisoxazole (AD-810) in rats, dogs and monkeys and of AD-810 in men. *Arzneimittelforschung* 1983;33:961–968.
16. Rosenfeld WE, Bergen D, Garnett W, et al. Steady state drug interaction study of zonisamide and carbamazepine in epileptic patients. American Academy of Neurology, 2000.
17. Hashimoto Y, Odani A, Tanigawara Y, et al. Population analysis of the dose-dependent pharmacokinetics of zonisamide in epileptic patients. *Biol Pharm Bull* 1994;17:323–326.
18. McJilton J, DeToledo J, DeCerce J, et al. Cotherapy of lamotrigine/zonisamide results in significant elevation of zonisamide levels. *Epilepsia* 1996;37[Suppl 5]:173.
19. Brodie M, Wilson E, Smith D, et al. Steady state drug interaction study of zonisamide and lamotrigine in epileptic patients. American Academy of Neurology, 2000.
20. Kochak GM, Page JG, Buchanan RA, et al. Steady-state pharmacokinetics of zonisamide, an antiepileptic agent for treatment of refractory complex partial seizures. *J Clin Pharmacol* 1998; 38:166–171.
21. Buchanan RA, Page JG, French JA, et al. Zonisamide drug interactions. *Epilepsia* 1997;38[Suppl 9]:107.
22. Schentag JJ, Bengo FM, Wilton JH, et al., Influence of Phenobarbital, cimetidine, and renal disease on zonisamide kinetics. *Pharm Res* 1987;4(S):S79.
23. Kimura M, Tanaka N, Kimura Y, et al. Factors influencing serum concentration of zonisamide in epileptic patients. *Chem Pharm Bull (Tokyo)* 1992;40:193–195.
24. Smith D, Brodie M, Dunkley D, et al. Steady state drug interaction study of zonisamide and sodium valproate in epileptic patients. American Academy of Neurology, 2000.
25. Matsumoto K, Miyazaki H, Fujii T, et al. Binding of sulfonamides to erythrocyte proteins and possible drug-drug interaction. *Chem Pharm Bull (Tokyo)* 1989;37:2807–2810.
26. Groves L, Wallace J, Shellenberger K. Effect of cimetidine on zonisamide pharmacokinetics in healthy volunteers. *Epilepsia* 1996;39[Suppl 6]:191.
27. Thummel KE, Wilkinson GR. In vitro and in vivo drug interactions involving human CYP3A. *Annu Rev Pharmacol Toxicol* 1998;38:389–430.
28. Browne TR, Szabo GK, Kres J, et al. Drug interactions of zonisamide (CI-912) with phenytoin and carbamazepine. *J Clin Pharmacol* 1986; 26:555.
29. Sackellares JC, Donofrio PD, Wagner JG, et al. Pilot study of zonisamide (1,2-benzisoxazole-3-methanesulfonamide) in patients with refractory partial seizures. *Epilepsia* 1985; 26: 206–211.
30. Minami T, Ieiri I, Ohtsubo K, et al. Influence of additional therapy with zonisamide (Excegran) on protein binding and metabolism of carbamazepine. *Epilepsia* 1994; 35:1023–1025.
31. Shinoda M, Akita M, Hasegawa M, et al. The necessity of adjust-

isamide (CI-912) after chronic administration. *J Clin Pharmacol* 1986;26:555.

ing the dosage of zonisamide when coadministered with other anti-epileptic drugs. *Biol Pharm Bull* 1996;19:1090–1092.

32. Odani A, Hashimoto Y, Takayanagi K, et al. Population pharmacokinetics of phenytoin in Japanese patients with epilepsy: analysis with a dose-dependent clearance model. *Biol Pharm Bull* 1996;19:444–448.

33. Kerr BM, Thummel KE, Warden CJ, et al. Human liver carbamazepine metabolism: role of CYP3A4 and CYP2C8 in 10,11-epoxide formation. *Biochem Pharmacol* 1994;47:1969–1979.

34. McJilton JS, Ramsay RE, Vasquez D, et al. Pharmacokinetics of zonisamide: results from a randomized double-blind multi-center placebo controlled study. *Epilepsia* 2000;41[Suppl 7]:224.

Antiepileptic Drugs, 5th Edition. Edited by R.H. Levy, R.H. Mattson, B.S. Meldrum, and E. Perucca. Lippincott Williams & Wilkins, Philadelphia © 2002.

ZONISAMIDE

CLINICAL EFFICACY AND USE IN EPILEPSY

MASAKAZU SEINO
BUICHI FUJITANI

EVIDENCE FROM RANDOMIZED, CONTROLLED CLINICAL TRIALS

Although in the United States zonisamide (ZNS) was not approved for treatment of epilepsy until 2000, initial use in Japan in 1989 has allowed more experience concerning many aspects of efficacy than is available for most new antiepileptic drugs (AEDs) at the time of licensing.

Five randomized, controlled trials on ZNS were performed: three placebo-controlled studies and two comparative studies with active reference drugs, either carbamazepine (CBZ) or valproate (VPA). All of the three placebo-controlled studies were evaluated ZNS for add-on treatment for patients with refractory partial or generalized epileptic seizures. The designs and results of these studies are summarized in Table 94.1.

Schmidt et al. (1) reported the European multicenter, placebo-controlled study of ZNS in adult patients who had four or more partial or generalized seizures per month and were refractory to other existing AEDs, either in monotherapy or in bitherapy. One hundred thirty-nine patients were randomly allocated to the ZNS group (n = 71) or the placebo (PLC) group (n = 68). ZNS was given once a day for 12 weeks in an add-on manner at an average maintenance dosage of 430 mg/day after a 1-month baseline period. Although the study involved patients with either partial or generalized seizures, most of the patients were having complex partial seizures. In patients with complex partial seizures, the median seizure frequency decreased by 27.7% in the ZNS group and increased by 3.9% in the PLC group from baseline ($p < .05$). Responder rates, defined as percentage of patients whose seizure frequency decreased by 50% or more, decreased by 30.3% in the ZNS

Masakazu Seino, MD: Honorary President, National Epilepsy Center, Shizuoka, Medical Institute of Neurological Diseases, Shizuoka, Japan

Buichi Fujitani, PhD: Department of International Affairs, Dainippon Pharmaceutical Company, Limited, Osaka, Japan

group and 12.7% in the PLC group ($p < .05$). The median daily doses and plasma concentrations of ZNS did not differ between responders and nonresponders (7.8 versus 6.8 mg/kg/day; 17.0 versus 15.2 µg/mL).

A multicenter, double-blind, placebo-controlled study was conducted by Sackellares et al. (2) in the United States under a protocol similar to that used in the study described previously (1). One hundred fifty-two patients (ZNS group, n = 78; PLC group, n = 74) with refractory partial seizures were enrolled in the study, and efficacy was evaluated in 141 patients (ZNS group, n = 69; PLC group, n = 72). After a 2- to 3-month baseline period, ZNS was given twice a day for 12 weeks in an add-on manner, with an average maintenance dosage of 530 mg/day. The median seizure frequency decreased by 29.5% in the ZNS group (n = 69) and increased by 0.8% in the PLC group (n = 72). The difference was statistically significant ($p < .05$). Responder rates were 26.1% in the ZNS group and 16.7% in the PLC group ($p < .05$). The final median plasma concentrations of ZNS were 16.9 µg/mL and 13.0 µg/mL in responders and nonresponders, respectively.

The third ZNS trial, a randomized, double-blind, placebo-controlled study, was conducted to assess the efficacy and dose–response characteristics of ZNS as adjunctive therapy for refractory partial seizures (3). After a 4-week baseline period, 203 patients enrolled were randomly allocated to group A (n = 85), group B1 (n = 60), and group B2 (n = 58). Group A patients received placebo, along with their concomitant AEDs, for 12 weeks. At week 13, they were then crossed over to ZNS treatment, starting at a 100-mg/day increment per week to 400 mg/day for the final 5 weeks (weeks 16 to 20). Group B1 patients received 100 mg/day of ZNS for weeks 1 to 5, 200 mg/day during week 6, 300 mg/day during week 7, and 400 mg/day for weeks 8 to 20. Group B2 patients received 100 mg/day of ZNS for week 1, 200 mg/day for weeks 2 to 6, 300 mg/day during week 7, and 400 mg/day for weeks 8 to 20. This unique study protocol allowed parallel comparisons with placebo

TABLE 94.1. SUMMARY OF PLACEBO-CONTROLLED STUDIES OF ZONISAMIDE IN PATIENTS WITH REFRACTORY PARTIAL SEIZURES (ADJUNCTIVE THERAPY)[a]

Reference	Number of Patients	Duration (mo)	Dose (mg/day)	Responder Rate (%)	Median Reduction of Seizure Frequency (%)
1	66 (63)	5–12	100–600	30.3 (12.7)	27.7 (−3.9)
2	69 (72)	5–12	100–600	26.1 (16.7)	29.5 (−1.8)
3	98 (72)	8–12	400	41.8 (22.2)	40.5 (9.0)

[a]Data were analyzed for all types of partial seizures. Numbers in parentheses are patient numbers, responder rate, and median reduction of seizure frequency in placebo-control group, respectively.

for three fixed doses and a final crossover to 400 mg/day for all patients. During weeks 8 to 12, median seizure frequency in patients treated with ZNS at 400 mg (n = 98) decreased by 40.5% from baseline, compared with a 9.0% decrease in the PLC group (n = 72; $p < .01$). During these weeks, the responder rate for all seizures was 41.8% in patients treated with 400 mg/day of ZNS, compared with 22.2% in the PLC group ($p < .05$). As for the dose–efficacy relation for ZNS, the median reduction of seizure frequency in patients treated with ZNS at 100 mg/day for weeks 1 to 5 was 24.7%, compared with 8.3% in the PLC group during the same period ($p < .05$). The median reduction in patients given 200 mg/day ZNS for weeks 2 to 6 was 20.4%, compared with 4.0% in the PLC group ($p < .05$), and that in patients given 400 mg/day ZNS (weeks 8 to 12) was 40.5%, compared with 9.0% in the PLC group ($p < .01$). The significant reduction of seizure frequency with ZNS was consistent at dosages of 100, 200, and 400 mg/day.

CONTROLLED, COMPARATIVE STUDY WITH ACTIVE REFERENCE DRUGS

The design and results of two controlled, comparative studies with active reference drugs are summarized in Table 94.2. A double-blind, controlled, comparative study of ZNS with CBZ was carried out by Seino et al. (4). One hundred twenty-three patients with partial seizures, two

seizures per month or more, who had been untreated with other AEDs or were refractory to one to three other AEDs, were assigned to the ZNS group (n = 59) or the CBZ group (n = 64). Based on a preclinical study (5) and a preliminary clinical study (6), 100 mg ZNS was equated with 200 mg CBZ. The patients were placed on ZNS (mean dosage = 330 mg/day) or CBZ (mean dosage = 600 mg/day) for 16 weeks. After the 16-week-treatment period, the average frequency of simple or complex partial seizures was reduced by 68.4% in the ZNS group and 46.6% in the CBZ group from baseline. The average frequency of secondarily generalized tonic-clonic seizures also was markedly reduced in the ZNS group (69.7%) and in the CBZ group (70.2%). There were no statistical differences in the reduction of seizure frequency between the two groups. Responder rates were 81.8% in the ZNS group and 70.7% in the CBZ group (not statistically significant). Overall improvement rates in terms of seizure frequency and interseizure condition also were similar for the ZNS group (66.1%) and the CBZ group (65.4%).

GENERALIZED SEIZURES

A controlled study in pediatric patients with generalized seizures was carried out and the efficacy of ZNS was compared with that of VPA (7). Thirty-four patients with convulsive or nonconvulsive generalized seizures, four seizures or more per month, and who were refractory to one to three

TABLE 94.2. SUMMARY OF CONTROLLED COMPARATIVE STUDIES OF ZONISAMIDE WITH ACTIVE REFERENCE DRUGS[a]

Reference	Subjects	Test Drug	Number of Patients	Duration (wk)	Dose (mg/day)	Overall Improvement (%)
4	Adults with partial seizures	Zonisamide	59	16	330	66.1
		Carbamazepine	64	16	600	65.4
7	Children with generalized seizures	Zonisamide	18	8	2–8	50.0
		Valproate	16	8	400–1,200	43.8

[a]Overall improvement rate was assessed by seizure frequency, electroencephalographic findings, and interseizure condition.

other AEDs, were allocated to the ZNS group (n = 18) or the VPA group (n = 16). The patients were on medication for 8 weeks with ZNS or VPA at the mean daily dosage of 7.3 mg/kg/day or 27.6 mg/kg/day, respectively. Overall improvements rates based on assessment of seizure frequency, electroencephalographic (EEG) findings, and interseizure condition were 50.0% in the ZNS group and 43.8% in the VPA group. The efficacy of ZNS was at least comparable with that of VPA for children with convulsive or nonconvulsive generalized seizures.

EVIDENCE FROM OTHER CLINICAL STUDIES

Noncomparative, Multicenter Studies

Leppik et al. (8) studied the efficacy of ZNS in a noncomparative, multicenter study in the United States. In this study, 167 patients with simple or complex partial seizures, including secondarily generalized tonic-clonic seizures, who were refractory to one to two other AEDs and were having four or more seizures per month, were enrolled. After 12-week baseline period, patients were given ZNS, 50 to 1,100 mg/day, for 16 weeks in an add-on manner. Treatment of patients with ZNS resulted in a significant reduction in seizure frequency per month from 11.5 during baseline to 5.5, or a 51.8% reduction during the final month. At least a 50% reduction in seizure frequency was noted in 41% of all patients, 43.2% of those with complex partial seizures, and 67.5% of those with secondarily generalized tonic-clonic seizures.

Ono et al. (9) conducted a multicenter, noncomparative clinical study in 538 adult patients with partial seizures (n = 433) or secondarily generalized tonic-clonic seizures (n = 105). ZNS was given in an add-on manner with daily dosage of 6.08 ± 2.89 mg/kg for at least 3 months. The mean duration of administration was 273 days. At the completion of the trial, at least a 50% reduction of seizure frequency was obtained in 254 of 506 patients (50.2%). Overall improvement rates based on assessment of severity and duration of seizures, interseizure condition, and EEG findings were 41.4% (213/514) in all patients, 48.1% (13/27) in those with simple partial seizures, 38.3% (23/60) in those with simple followed by complex partial seizures, 41.2% (98/238) in those with complex partial seizures, and 50% (45/90) in those with secondarily generalized tonic-clonic seizures. There were no statistically significant differences in the overall improvement rates between patients with these seizure types.

Oguni et al. (7) carried out an open-label trial in 393 patients with partial or generalized epilepsies. Patients, either adults or children who were refractory to previous AEDs and in whom the average number of AEDs concomitantly used was 2.8, were given ZNS at a dosage of 2 to 8 mg/kg/day, with an average final dosage at 7.3 mg/kg/day. The overall responder rate was 44.4%. The

overall improvement rate based on assessment of severity and duration of seizures, interseizure condition, and EEG findings was 51.0% in all patients. According to seizure types, the overall improvement rates were 50% to 70% in patients with simple or complex partial seizures or secondarily generalized tonic-clonic seizures. Improvement rates in patients with generalized seizures were lower than in those with partial seizures: 47% in patients with generalized tonic-clonic seizures, 31.3% in those with generalized tonic seizures, and 20.0% in those with myoclonic seizures.

Yagi and Seino (10) analyzed the clinical efficacy of ZNS in a total of 1,008 adult and pediatric patients with various epilepsies (605 adults and 403 children), who were enrolled in controlled studies and noncomparative, multicenter studies already cited (4,7,9). Mean daily dosages of ZNS ranged between 5.9 and 8.8 mg/kg, and their mean serum concentrations ranged between 19.6 and 20.7 μg/mL at steady state. The efficacy was assessed by the percentage of patients whose seizure frequency decreased by 50% or more from the baseline with simple or complex seizures, and secondarily generalized tonic-clonic seizures. It also was beneficial for the treatment of convulsive and nonconvulsive generalized seizures and combined seizures, although efficacy rates varied between 26% and 100% by the seizure type (Table 94.3). The responder rate for ZNS also was analyzed according to epileptic syndromes in this study (Table 94.4). ZNS showed efficacy in more than 50% of patients with symptomatic partial epilepsies, including temporal lobe epilepsy, extratemporal lobe epilepsy, and unclassified symptomatic partial epilepsies. As for generalized epilepsies, responder rates to ZNS were 66% in patients with idiopathic generalized epilepsy, 32% in those with Lennox-Gas-

TABLE 94.3. CLINICAL EFFICACY OF ZONISAMIDE BY SEIZURE TYPES WITH 1,008 PATIENTS IN CONTROLLED AND OPEN-LABEL STUDIES IN JAPAN

Seizure Type	Number of Patients	Responder Rate (%)
Partial		
Simple partial	63	57
Simple partial followed by complex partial	82	50
Complex partial	362	50
Partial-onset generalized tonic-clonic	168	60
Generalized		
Generalized tonic-clonic	46	59
Generalized tonic	74	26
Atypical absences	9	67
Typical absences	4	50
Atonic	10	50
Myoclonic	7	43
Clonic	1	100
Combination	129	41

TABLE 94.4. CLINICAL EFFICACY OF ZONISAMIDE BY EPILEPSY CLASSIFICATION WITH 1,008 PATIENTS IN CONTROLLED AND OPEN-LABEL STUDIES

Epilepsies	Number of Patients	Responder Rate (%)
Partial		
Temporal lobe	428	54
Extratemporal lobe	224	51
Unclassified	21	57
Generalized		
Idiopathic generalized	41	66
Lennox-Gastaut syndrome	132	32
West syndrome	9	22
Other symptomatic generalized	100	47

taut syndrome, 22% in those with West's syndrome, and 47% in those with other symptomatic generalized epilepsies. This study suggested that ZNS had a wide spectrum of efficacy for the treatment of patients with various seizure types and syndromes. Supporting the analysis, more than 20 open-label studies demonstrated the efficacy of ZNS in the treatment of adults and children with partial, generalized, or combined seizures in the late 1980s and early 1990s in Japan (11).

Long-Term Efficacy

Seino and Yagi (10) also analyzed the efficacy of ZNS in 155 patients who were treated for at least 1 year with ZNS in controlled, comparative studies and noncomparative studies conducted in Japan. The responder rates were 75% in patients with simple partial seizures (n = 4), 65% in those with simple partial followed by complex partial seizures (n = 26), 64% in those with complex partial seizures (n = 47), 61% in those with secondarily generalized tonic-clonic seizures (n = 28), 67% in those with generalized tonic-clonic seizures (n = 6), 40% in those with tonic seizures (n = 20), and 50% in those with combined seizures (n = 24). The analysis demonstrated the long-term efficacy of ZNS.

Three open-label trials were completed for assessment of the long-term efficacy of ZNS in the United States. One of these trials, a multicenter study, enrolled 103 patients with partial seizures who were refractory to other AEDs (12). Patients were given ZNS (usually 400 to 600 mg/day) for less than 24 months. The median reduction of seizure frequency and responder rate were 37.6% and 36.4% (35/96) after 5- to 16-week treatment, and those after 5- to 24-month treatment were 45.5% and 42.3% (33/78), respectively.

In the second trial (13), long-term efficacy was investigated in 137 patients with partial seizures who were refractory to other AEDs. ZNS was given for at least 5 months in an add-on fashion, and the dosage did not exceed the smaller of 20 mg/kg/day or the amount producing a plasma

concentration of 40 μg/mL. Forty patients were treated with ZNS for longer than 16 months. The overall median seizure frequency was reduced by 64.9% (n = 129). Responder rates were consistently higher than 40% throughout the study period, at 44% (53/120), 46% (44/95), 51% (38/74), and 49% (31/63) during 5- to 7-, 8- to 10-, 11- to 13-, and 14- to 16-month periods, respectively, and 40% (16/40) for more than 16 months.

The third trial (14) was an extension of a U.S. placebo-controlled study (2). A total of 123 patients having documented refractory partial seizures with or without secondary generalization received open-label ZNS therapy (median dosage = 450 mg/day). Of the 123 patients who began open-label therapy, 47 patients received ZNS for at least 12 months, and 40 patients received ZNS for 15 months or more before the study terminated. The median percentage reduction in seizure frequency from the baseline was 50.1% for patients with any kind of partial seizures and 50.8% for those with complex partial seizures only. The responder rate, the percentage of patients who showed a reduction in seizure frequency of at least 50%, ranged from 42.1% to 55.0% according to the treatment period.

Long-term efficacy of ZNS also was shown by Ota et al. (15), Kohsaka et al. (16), Nishiura and Oiwa (17), Kanazawa et al. (18), Wilder et al. (19), Shimizu et al. (20), and Sugahara et al. (21).

ZONISAMIDE MONOTHERAPY

Analysis of 1,008 epileptic patients recruited in controlled studies and multicenter, open-label studies in Japan included 55 patients who were treated with ZNS alone (10). Seventy-two percent of these 55 patients showed at least a 50% reduction of seizure frequency. Kumagai et al. (22) investigated the efficacy and safety of ZNS monotherapy in 44 pediatric patients. ZNS was given for 4 months to 4.5 years (mean treatment period = 1.1 years). The starting dosages were 2 to 4 mg/kg/day and increased to 12 mg/kg/day; unless a satisfactory response was obtained at a previous dose. The seizures completely disappeared in 30 of 38 patients (78.9%) whose efficacy could be evaluated (5/5 in patients with idiopathic generalized epilepsy, 7/8 in those with symptomatic generalized epilepsy, 1/1 in those with idiopathic partial epilepsy, and 17/24 in those with symptomatic partial epilepsy). Hosoda et al. (23) also investigated the efficacy of ZNS monotherapy in 72 pediatric patients with cryptogenic localization-related epilepsies. ZNS at 2 to 8 mg/kg/day was given once daily for 6 to 43 months. During this period, complete seizure control was achieved in 57 of 72 patients (79%), including 8 patients whose dosage was increased at an early stage of the treatment because of seizure recurrence with the initial maintenance dosage. The efficacy of ZNS monotherapy for infantile spasms was reported by Suzuki et al. (24). Eleven newly diagnosed children with infantile spasms who failed to respond to vitamin B_6 were treated with ZNS at 3 to 10 mg/kg/day. Four of the 11 infants had cessation of spasms and disappearance of hypsarrhythmia within a few days after starting treatment, although two of them relapsed into spasms several weeks after cessation of seizures. Two other patients showed reduction of seizure frequencies, but seizure frequency did not change in the remaining five patients.

ZONISAMIDE THERAPY FOR SPECIFIC SYNDROMES

Progressive Myoclonus Epilepsy and the Antioxidant Effect of Zonisamide

Progressive myoclonus epilepsies (PME) are a group of syndromes mainly consisting of generalized convulsive seizures, fragmentary myoclonus, status epilepticus, ataxia, and progressive dementia. In 1988, Henry et al. (25) first reported dramatic improvement of seizures after treatment with ZNS (8.8 and 10.5 mg/kg/day, respectively) in two patients with PME of the Unverricht- Lundborg type. Later, Kyllerman and Ben-Menachem (26) treated seven cases of PME with ZNS at 100 to 600 mg/day. They demonstrated that it dramatically reduced the number of myoclonus and generalized convulsive seizures in six of seven cases, although the initial effect on myoclonus wore off after 2 to 4 years of the treatment in three of these cases. Yagi and Seino (10) also reported that ZNS monotherapy resulted in the complete disappearance of seizures in one patient having mitochondrial encephalopathy with ragged-red fibers, and a significant improvement in two pediatric patients with other PMEs.

ZNS has been thought to exert its antiepileptic effect through the blockade of the sodium channel (27) and the T-type calcium channel (28). Because other sodium channel blocking agents, such as phenytoin or CBZ, do not improve PME seizures, ZNS seems to exhibit its improving effect on PMEs through its blockade of the T-type calcium channel or some unknown mechanisms. In relation to the therapeutic effect of ZNS on PME, it should be noted that ZNS has a free radical scavenging action, because treatment with *N*-acetylcysteine, an antioxidant, markedly decreased the frequency of seizures and normalized somatosensory evoked potentials in patients with PME of the Unverricht-Lundborg type (29). ZNS scavenged 1,1-diphenyl-2-picrylhydroxy radicals [DPPH] (30), hydroxyl radicals, and nitric oxide in a concentration-dependent manner *in vitro* (31), but phenytoin, phenobarbital (PB), VPA, and CBZ did not show DPPH-scavenging action (32). In an *in vivo* experiment, treatment of rats with ZNS (20 and 100 mg intraperitoneally) prevented the increase of lipid peroxides in the cerebral cortex induced by topical injection of iron solution (30). Taking these findings into consideration,

ZNS may, at least partly, exert therapeutic effects on PMEs and other symptomatic generalized epilepsies through its free radical scavenging action in addition to its blocking action on the T-type calcium channel.

Prevention of Postsurgical Seizures

After demonstrating the cerebral protective effect of ZNS in animal models of cerebral ischemia or traumatic head injury, Fukuda and Masuda (33) first tried to treat six craniotomy patients with ZNS and showed its efficacy in five of these patients. Later, Nakamura et al. (34) conducted a randomized, controlled study of ZNS in postoperative seizures using PB as an active placebo. Patients at high risk for seizures (n = 278) who underwent craniotomy for their brain tumors, cerebrovascular diseases, or head injuries were recruited in this study and were randomly assigned to the ZNS group (n = 141) or the PB group (n = 137). ZNS (100 to 400 mg/day) or PB (40 to 160 mg/day) was given from 1 week before to 1 year after the surgery, after which the patients were followed up for 3 years. Occurrence of seizures was recorded in 255 patients (ZNS group, 129; PB group, 126) during the treatment period and in 219 patients (ZNS group, 112; PB group, 107) during follow-up. The incidences of development of epileptic seizures during medication were 5.4% (7/129) and 6.3% (8/126) in the ZNS group and the PB group, respectively (not significant), and during the follow-up period, they were 7.1% (8/112) and 12.1% (13/107), respectively (not significant). Although six patients (5.6%) in the PB group experienced partial seizures during follow-up, none in the ZNS group experienced such seizures (Fisher test; $p = .013$). In addition to its antiepileptic action, the free radical scavenging action of ZNS may, at least in part, contribute to its preventive effect on postsurgical seizures.

MODE OF USE

Indications

ZNS has been commercially available since 1989 in Japan and since 1992 in Korea. It was approved in the United States in March 2000. Based on its wide-spectrum clinical antiepileptic efficacy as demonstrated by controlled and open-label trials in Japan (4,7,9,10), ZNS monotherapy or adjunctive therapy is approved in adults and children with the following types of seizures in Japan and Korea:

1. Partial seizures: simple or complex partial seizures, and secondarily generalized tonic-clonic seizures
2. Generalized seizures: tonic-clonic seizures, tonic seizures, and atypical absence seizures
3. Mixed seizures: combinations of the aforementioned generalized seizures

On the other hand, in the United States, ZNS is indicated as adjunctive therapy in partial seizures in adults (16 years of age or older) based on efficacy demonstrated by the placebo-controlled studies in the United States and Europe (1–3). Efficacy of ZNS as monotherapy or in pediatric patients is being evaluated in the United States and Europe. As mentioned previously, ZNS improved seizures in patients with PMEs (10,25,26).

Dosing Recommendations

ZNS is available in a 100-mg tablet and a 200-mg/g powder formulations in Japan, a 100-mg tablet formulation in Korea, and a 100-mg capsule formulation in the United States. The drug can be used for treatment in children and adults in Japan and Korea, but its use is limited to adults in the United States. Safety in infants younger than 1 year of age has not been established. As for the elderly, 328 patients older than 65 years of age were recorded in postmarketing surveillance in Japan (35), but no systematic studies have been performed in the elderly patient population. Treatment should be started in elderly patients at the lowest dosage of the therapeutic range.

Initial Dosage

The recommended initial adult dosage is 100 mg/day in the United States and 100 to 200 mg/day in Japan and Korea. For children older than 1 year of age, the recommended initial dosage is 2 to 4 mg/kg/day in Japan and Korea.

Titration Rate

In adult patients, the dosage should be increased if necessary to 200 to 400 mg/day, with every 100-mg increase at an interval of 2 weeks or longer in the United States, whereas a 1- to 2-week interval is acceptable in Japan and Korea because it requires approximately 2 weeks to attain a new steady-state plasma concentration of ZNS (36). In children, the dosage should be increased to 4 to 8 mg/kg/day at the interval of 1 to 2 weeks in Japan and Korea. A gradual increase of dosage may reduce adverse drug events.

Maintenance Dosage

The usual maintenance dosage of ZNS is 200 to 400 mg/day for adults and 4 to 8 mg/kg/day for children. Therapeutic plasma concentrations were reported to be 10 to 20 µg/mL or approximately 20 µg/mL (1,2,7,10).

Maximum Dosage

The approved highest dosage is 600 mg/day for adults and 12 mg/kg/day for children in Japan.

CURRENT ROLE IN EPILEPSY MANAGEMENT

ZNS is an important addition to the ranks of available AEDs. It has proven efficacy in adults and children for a wide variety of partial and generalized seizures since it was launched in 1989 in Japan. Many studies demonstrated the efficacy of ZNS in the treatment of simple and complex partial seizures, and secondarily generalized tonic-clonic seizures. For generalized seizures, efficacy was demonstrated in patients with atypical absence tonic, atonic, myoclonic, or clonic seizures. It also is effective in the treatment of infantile spasms or West's syndrome, and tonic and atypical absence seizures in Lennox-Gastaut syndrome. Some investigators reported the dramatic improvement of seizures in patients with PME.

Although the indications for ZNS are limited to adjunctive therapy for adult patients with refractory partial epilepsy in the United States, studies on its use as monotherapy and in pediatric patients are under way.

Seizure Relapse on Withdrawal

Because an abrupt reduction or discontinuation of dosage may precipitate relapse of seizures or even status epilepticus in patients who have taken the drug for a prolonged period, the dosage should be reduced gradually, with particular caution in patients with intractable seizures.

REFERENCES

1. Schmidt D, Jacob R, Loiseau P, et al. Zonisamide for add-on treatment of refractory partial epilepsy: a European double-blind trial. *Epilepsy Res* 1993;15:67–73.
2. Sackellares CJ, Ramsay RE, Wilder BJ, et al. Controlled clinical trial of zonisamide: an effective adjunctive treatment for refractory partial seizures. Files of Dainippon Pharmaceutical Co., Ltd. (#912 US) Osaka, Japan, 1997.
3. Faught E, Ayala R, Montouris GG, et al. Randomized controlled trial of zonisamide for the treatment of refractory partial onset seizures. *Neurology* 2001;7:1777–1779.
4. Seino M, Ohkuma T, Miyasaka M, et al. Efficacy evaluation of AD-810: results of a double blind comparison with carbamazepine [in Japanese]. *J Clin Exp Med* 1988;144:275–291.
5. Kakegawa N. An experimental study on the modes of appearance and disappearance of suppressive effect of antiepileptic drugs on kindled seizure [in Japanese]. *Psychiatr Neurol Jpn* 1986;88:81–98.
6. Wilensky AJ, Friel PN, Ojemann L, et al. Zonisamide in epilepsy: a pilot study. *Epilepsia* 1985;26:212–220.
7. Oguni H, Hayashi K, Fukuyama Y, et al. Phase III clinical study of the new antiepileptic drug, AD-810 (zonisamide), in patients with childhood epilepsy [in Japanese]. *Jpn J Pediatr* 1988;42:439–450.
8. Leppik IE, Willmore LJ, Homan RW, et al. Efficacy and safety of zonisamide: results of a multicenter study. *Epilepsy Res* 1993;14:165–173.
9. Ono T, Yagi K, Seino M. Clinical efficacy and safety of a new

antiepileptic drug, zonisamide: a multi-institutional phase three study [in Japanese]. *Clin Psychiatry* 1988;30:471–482.

10. Yagi K, Seino M. Methodological requirement for clinical trials in refractory epilepsies: our experience with zonisamide. *Prog Neuropsychopharmacol Biol Psychiatry* 1992;16:79–85.

11. Peters DH, Sorkin EM. Zonisamide, a review of its pharmacodynamic and pharmacokinetic properties, and therapeutic potential in epilepsy. *Drugs* 1993;45:760–787.

12. Arlt G, Barkley GL, Bergen D, et al. Baseline controlled safety and efficacy evaluation of zonisamide in the treatment of seizures in medically refractory patients. Files of Dainippon Pharmaceutical Co., Ltd., (#810-920). Osaka, Japan.

13. Dinner S, Fromm G, Homan R, et al. Efficacy and safety report of the extended phase of a baseline-controlled 16-week multicenter study of the efficacy and safety of zonisamide (CI-912) in medically refractory patients with seizures. Files of Dainippon Pharmaceutical Co., Ltd., (#Baseline Contr-Ext). Osaka, Japan.

14. Sackellares CJ, Donofrio PD, Berent S, et al. Overall report of the extended phase of multicenter placebo-controlled double blind study of the efficacy and safety of zonisamide (CI-912) in the complex partial seizures in medically refractory patients (USA). Files of Dainippon Pharmaceutical Co., Ltd., (#912-US-Ext). Osaka, Japan.

15. Ota Y, Nakane Y, Hironaka I, et al. Therapeutic effect of zonisamide (AD-810, ZNS) on refractory partial epilepsy [in Japanese]. *J Clin Ther Med* 1987;3[Suppl]:1079–1087.

16. Kohsaka M, Sumi T, Hiba T, et al. The long term treatment of zonisamide for epileptic patients with intractable epilepsy [in Japanese]. *J Clin Ther Med* 1987;3[Suppl]:1343–1352.

17. Nishiura N, Oiwa N. Clinical study of a new antiepileptic drug, AD-810 (zonisamide): long-term use in intractable patients [in Japanese]. *Jpn Pharmacol Ther* 1987;15:4217–4223.

18. Kanazawa O, Sengoku A, Kawai I. Experiences of zonisamide treatment on adults and children with refractory epilepsy: follow up for more than 1 year. *J Jpn Epilept Soc* 1990;8:29–38.

19. Wilder BJ, Sackellares JC, Wilensky AJ, et al. Zonisamide as long-term treatment for refractory partial and generalized tonic-clonic seizures. *Neurology* 1987;37[Suppl 1]:351–352.

20. Simizu A, Ikoma R, Shimizu T. Effects and side effects of zonisamide during long-term medication. *Curr Ther Res Clin Exp* 1990;47:696–706.

21. Sugihara H, Yoneyama K, Kamo C, et al. Long-term clinical efficacy of zonisamide in patients with symptomatic epilepsies [in Japanese]. *Jpn Pharmacol Ther* 1992;20:4657–4661.

22. Kumagai N, Seki T, Yamawaki H, et al. Monotherapy for childhood epilepsies with zonisamide. *Jpn J Psychiatr Neurol* 1991;45:357–359.

23. Hosoda N, Miura H, Takanashi S, et al. Once-daily dose of zonisamide monotherapy in the control of partial seizures in children with cryptogenic localization-related epilepsies: clinical efficacy and their pharmacokinetic basis. *Jpn J Psychiatr Neurol* 1994;48:335–337.

24. Suzuki Y, Nagai T, Ono J, et al. Zonisamide monotherapy in newly diagnosed infantile spasms. *Epilepsia* 1997;38:1035–1038.

25. Henry TR, Leppik IE, Robert J, et al. Progressive myoclonus epilepsy treated with zonisamide. *Neurology* 1988;38:928–931.

26. Kyllerman M, Ben-Menachem E. Zonisamide for progressive myoclonus epilepsy: long-term observations in seven patients. *Epilepsy Res* 1998;29:109–114.

27. Schauf CL. Zonisamide enhances slow sodium inactivation in *Myxicola*. *Brain Res* 1987;413:185–188.

28. Suzuki S, Kawakami K, Nishimura S, et al. Zonisamide blocks T-type calcium channel in cultured neurons of rat cerebral cortex. *Epilepsy Res* 1992;12:21–27.

29. Hurd RW, Wilder BJ, Wendell R, et al. Treatment of four siblings with progressive myoclonus epilepsy of the Unverricht-Lundborg type with N-acetylcysteine. *Neurology* 1996;47:1264–1268.

30. Komatsu M, Okamura Y, Hiramatu M. Free radical scavenging activity of zonisamide and its inhibitory effect on lipid peroxide formation in iron-induced epileptogenic foci of rats. *Neuroscience* 1995;21:23–29.

31. Mori A, Noda Y, Packer L. The anticonvulsant zonisamide scavenges free radicals. *Epilepsy Res* 1998;30:153–158.

32. Hiramatsu M, Komatsu M, Shi M. Free radical scavenging activity of anti-convulsants on in vivo study of iron-induced epileptogenic foci of rats [in Japanese]. *Annu Rep Jpn Epilepsy Res Found* 1997;9:91–96.

33. Fukuda M, Masuda Y. Cerebral protective effect of zonisamide and its clinical experience on post operative seizures [in Japanese]. *Jpn Pharmacol Ther* 1991;19:2011–2018.

34. Nakamura N, Ishijima B, Mayanagi Y. A randomized controlled trial of zonisamide in postoperative epilepsy: a report of the cooperative group study. *Jpn J Neurosurg* 1999;8:647–656.

35. Report of post marketing surveillance of excegran: II general survey. Dainippon Pharmaceutical Co., Ltd., Osaka, Japan, 1997.

36. Ito T, Yamaguchi T, Miyazaki H, et al. Pharmacokinetic studies of AD-810, a new antiepileptic compound: phase I trials. *Arzneimittelforschung* 1982;32:1581–1586.

95

ZONISAMIDE

ADVERSE EFFECTS

BYUNG IN LEE

Zonisamide (ZNS) is a broad-spectrum antiepileptic drug (AED) that was first synthesized by Uno et al. (1). ZNS became commercially available for use in Japan in 1989 and in Korea in 1993. However, its development in the United States and Europe was prematurely terminated because of a high incidence of renal stones (2). In Japan, ZNS was not associated with a higher incidence of renal stones and continued its successful development. Clinical studies of ZNS were reinstituted in the United States in 1992, and ZNS was approved for clinical use in 1999.

Most of the clinical experience with ZNS is from Japan. The European and U.S. experience with ZNS has been limited to a few clinical studies conducted during its early stage of development (2–6). One of two controlled clinical trials performed in the United States (6,7) have not been published yet, but their results are available through the data files of Dainippon Pharmaceutical Co., Ltd., Osaka, Japan (8).

MOST COMMONLY OBSERVED ADVERSE EFFECTS

In the European double-blind, placebo-controlled study of ZNS add-on therapy (5), the incidence of adverse effects (AEs) was 59% in the ZNS group and 27% in the placebo group. Most common AEs reported in the ZNS group were fatigue (22.5%), dizziness (16.9%), somnolence (14.1%), anorexia (12.7%), psychomotor slowing (11.3%), ataxia (11.3%), nervousness (9.9%), abdominal pain (7.0%), and confusion (5.6%). Among those, dizziness, anorexia, psychomotor slowing, ataxia, and confusion were more common in the ZNS group than the placebo group. In one U.S. trial (6), the incidence of AEs was higher for both ZNS and placebo groups, 92% and 58%, respectively. However, in the other U.S. trial (7), the incidence of AEs was lower and comparable between the two groups, which might be related to the adoption of a slower dose escalation of ZNS in this study.

The incidences of AEs in the pooled data of these three double-blind, placebo-controlled trials (8) were 78.1% for ZNS and 61.3% for placebo. Somnolence, ataxia, anorexia, dizziness, fatigue, nausea and vomiting, and irritability were the most common AEs (Table 95.1). AEs that occurred more than twice as often in the ZNS than in the placebo group were ataxia, anorexia, irritability, diplopia, impaired concentration, insomnia, abdominal pain and discomfort, and depression. Premature dropout from the placebo-controlled trials because of AEs occurred in 31 of 269 patients (11.5%) treated with ZNS and 15 of 230 patients (6.5%) on placebo. Among 84 AEs reported from 31 patients prematurely withdrawn from the trials during ZNS treatment, psychiatric or behavioral symptoms were the most common (28.6%), followed by cognitive impairment (10.7%), fatigability (10.7%), anorexia (9.5%), and headache (7.1%). Skin rash and asymptomatic renal calculi were found in one patient each.

In a comparative trial of ZNS and carbamazepine (CBZ) conducted in Japan (9), the incidence of AEs was 52% in the ZNS group and 57% in the CBZ group. Common AEs with ZNS were similar to those in the placebo-controlled trials, with a significantly higher incidence of anorexia in the ZNS group and ataxia in the CBZ group (Table 95.2).

A double-blind, comparative trial of ZNS and CBZ in newly diagnosed epilepsies was conducted in Korea (10). The design of the study was basically similar to the monotherapy trial of lamotrigine conducted by Brodie et al. (11). The incidence of AEs was 67.1% in the ZNS group and 53.7% in the CBZ group, which was not significantly different. Common AEs in the ZNS group in order of frequency were anorexia, abdominal pain or discomfort, dizziness, weight loss, and fatigue, compared with dizziness, somnolence, skin rash, headache, and fatigue in the CBZ group (Table 95.2). Most AEs were reported during the dose-escalation phase (ZNS, 54.8%; CBZ, 46.3%). After the dose-escalation phase, AEs were reported in 50.0% of the ZNS group and 27.1% of the CBZ group ($p = .006$), but in only 13.2% of the ZNS group and 8.6% of the CBZ group were these AEs newly reported ones ($p = .4$). The results suggested that the AEs related to ZNS treatment

Byung In Lee, MD: Professor, Department of Neurology, Yonsei University College of Medicine; and Chief, Department of Neurology, Severance Hospital, Seoul, Korea

TABLE 95.1. TREATMENT-RELATED EMERGENCY ADVERSE EVENTS OCCURRED IN >5% OF PATIENTS IN DOUBLE-BLIND PLACEBO-CONTROLLED CLINICAL TRIALS (POOLED DATA)

Adverse Events	Placebo (n = 230)	Zonisamide				
		Total (n = 269)	<200 (n = 249)	200–399 (n = 258)	400–599 (n = 256)	≥600 (n = 92)
All Events	61.3	78.1	33.3	47.3	51.2	29.3
Somnolence	12.2	19.3	7.6	8.9	8.2	2.2
Ataxia	5.7	16.7	4.4	6.6	9.8	7.6
Anorexia	6.1	15.6	2.8	5.0	7.0	1.1
Dizziness	10.9	15.6	3.6	5.0	5.9	7.6
Fatigue	10.4	14.1	2.0	4.7	7.4	5.4
Nausea and/or vomiting	11.7	11.5	2.4	4.7	4.7	6.5
Irritability	5.2	11.5	2.0	4.3	5.9	2.2
Diplopia	4.3	8.9	2.0	4.3	5.5	2.2
Headache	8.3	8.6	2.4	4.3	2.0	1.1
Decreased concentration	0.9	8.2	0.4	2.3	5.9	7.6
Insomnia	3.5	7.8	2.8	1.9	1.2	1.1
Abdominal pain or discomfort	1.7	7.4	0.8	3.5	3.1	2.2
Depression	3.0	7.4	0.8	1.9	4.7	1.1
Forgetfulness	2.2	7.1	0.8	2.3	3.1	5.4
Rhinitis	6.1	6.7	2.8	3.1	1.2	0
Confusion	1.3	5.6	0.8	1.9	2.7	2.2
Anxiety	2.6	5.6	0.4	2.3	2.3	0
Nystagmus	2.6	5.2	0.8	0.8	3.1	2.2

lasted longer than the AEs associated with CBZ (*p* = .02). Premature withdrawal from the study due to AEs occurred in 11 patients from each group. However, the AE-precipitated premature withdrawals from the study were quite different between the two groups: for the ZNS group, AEs were gastrointestinal (GI) symptoms (four patients), anorexia (three patients), renal stone (two patients), psychomotor slowing (one patient), and skin rash (one patient), compared with skin rash (eight patients), somnolence (two patients), and exacerbation of seizures (one patient) in the CBZ group.

Three large-scale open trials are worth mention. In the Japanese series of 1,008 adult patients (12), AEs were reported by 51.3%, and 185 patients (18%) discontinued ZNS. The most common AEs were drowsiness (24%), ataxia (13%), anorexia (11%), GI symptoms (7%), decrease

TABLE 95.2. ADVERSE EFFECTS DEVELOPED IN >5% OF PATIENTS IN THE COMPARATIVE CLINICAL TRIALS BETWEEN ZONISAMIDE AND CARBAMAZEPINE

Adverse Effects	Adjunctive Therapy (Reference 9)		Monotherapy (Reference 10)	
	Zonisamide (n = 58)	Carbamazepine (n = 58)	Zonisamide (n = 73)	Carbamazepine (n = 82)
Somnolence	21%	28%	8.2%	19.5%
Dizziness	—	—	16.4%	22.0%
Anorexia	12%[a]	0%	30.1%[a]	2.4%
Headache	—	—	13.7%	9.8%
Psychomotor slowing	—	—	8.2%[a]	1.2%
Nemory impairment	10%	3%	11.0%[b]	3.7%
Nausea or vomiting	9%	2%	9.6%	3.7%
Abdominal discomfort	—	—	16.4%[a]	2.4%
Indigestion	—	—	6.8%[a]	0.0%
Visual disturbance	3%	12%	5.5%	4.9%
Rash	2%	10%	4.2%	12.2%[b]
Weight loss	—	—	45.1%[a]	0.0%
Fatigue	—	—	15.1%	7.3%
Irritability	9%	2%	—	—
Ataxia	9%	35%[a]	—	—

[a]*p* < .05.
[b]*p* < .1.

in spontaneity (6%), and psychomotor slowing (5%). In 55 patients given ZNS monotherapy, the incidence of AEs was 29%, compared with 41% in patients taking one concomitant drug and 55% in patients taking two or more concomitant drugs. Another Japanese open trial of ZNS that recruited 393 pediatric patients (13) revealed that the incidence of AEs was 43.8%. Somnolence was the most common AE (26.2%), followed by ataxia (10.2%), anorexia (9.2%), decreased mental activity (7.1%), and enervation (6.9%). In the open trial of ZNS conducted in the United States (2), 136 of 167 patients (81.4%) reported adverse events and 21 patients (12.6%) were prematurely withdrawn from the study due to AEs. Common AEs were anorexia, asthenia, ataxia, confusion, fatigue, and psychomotor slowing. Most AEs were reported during the first 4 weeks after introduction.

From these clinical studies, the common AEs related to ZNS treatment could be identified: symptoms related to the central nervous system (somnolence, dizziness, ataxia, fatigue, anorexia), GI symptoms (abdominal discomfort or pain, nausea and vomiting), and cognitive dysfunction (psychomotor slowing, decreased concentration, and memory impairment).

Dose-Dependent Incidence and Prevalence

An earlier clinical study (2) suggested a higher incidence of AEs in patients taking doses above 5 mg/kg or greater than 300 mg/day. AEs that were more common at the highest doses and may be dose related included amnesia, ataxia, visual disturbances, headache, confusion, dysarthria, and somnolence.

From the pooled data of controlled trials (8) (Table 95.1), the incidence of AEs was lower at lower doses (<200 mg/day) and peaked at doses of 400 to 599 mg/day, which were the most common doses used in the trials, and then leveled off at doses greater than 600 mg/day. This leveling-off of AEs might reflect the duration of exposure (adaptation effect). The importance of adaptation effects on AEs was more apparent in the analysis of the blood level–AE relationship of the pooled data (8). The incidence of patients reporting AEs was higher at lower plasma levels of ZNS: 55.7% at a concentration of 0 to 10 μg/mL, 51.1% at 10 to 20 μg/mL, 39.9% at 20 to 30 μg/mL, 35.8% at 30 to 40 μg/mL, and 19.0% at >40 μg/mL. This is consistent with the fact that the highest incidence of AEs was found during the first month of treatment, when initial doses were low and being titrated upward. Mimaki (14) also reported a poor relationship between dose or blood level of ZNS and the emergence of AEs. The effects of ZNS on cognition were assessed in nine patients with refractory epilepsy (15). At minimal steady-state plasma concentrations of >30 μg/mL, ZNS adversely affected acquisition and concentration of new information in the absence of clinical signs and symptoms of toxicity. How-

ever, repeated tests after 24 weeks of ZNS therapy revealed improvement in cognitive AEs.

All these findings suggest that most of the common AEs emerge in a dose-related manner at the start of ZNS treatment but that an adaptation process takes place over 4 to 8 weeks. Thus the prevalence of AEs decreases as the duration of exposure increases.

Time Dependency

From the pooled data of placebo-controlled trials (8), the prevalence of AEs was highest (60.2%) during the first month of ZNS treatment and decreased to 34.4% during the third month of treatment, which was a gradual reduction rather than an abrupt change. However, the incidence of first occurrence of most common AEs dropped sharply after the first month to become similar in both ZNS- and placebo-treated patients from the second month, with a few exceptions. Anorexia and GI symptoms became less frequent during the second month, but still were more frequent than with placebo. The incidence of first occurrence of depression and anxiety did not decrease during the first 2 months. These features also were noticed in the ZNS monotherapy trial in newly diagnosed patients (10), in which the prevalence of AEs was significantly higher in ZNS than CBZ group during the maintenance phase, but the number of patients reporting the first occurrence of AEs was comparable between the two groups after the first 4 weeks of dose escalation. Therefore, common AEs usually appear during the first month of ZNS therapy, but patients appear to adapt to most untoward side effects over 1 to 2 months of treatment, and they do not represent a major clinical concern after prolonged treatment. According to the pooled data of Dainippon Pharmaceutical Co. (8), the incidence of first occurrence of AEs after 6 months of ZNS treatment did not exceed 5% for any specific AE except rhinitis.

Risk Factors

Analysis of clinical data revealed that the incidence of common AEs was higher in cases of rapid dose escalation, higher doses of ZNS, and two or more concomitant AEDs. From the pooled data of controlled trials, the incidence of AEs was slightly higher in patients aged 40 to 65 years than in patients younger than 40 years of age: 85.5% and 74.9%, respectively. The number of patients aged 65 years and older was too small to be adequately analyzed; however, the trend of higher incidences of AEs in patients older than 40 years of age certainly suggests a need for caution with ZNS therapy in older patients. Because ZNS is metabolized in the liver and mainly excreted through the kidneys, patients with hepatic or renal diseases may require special caution. No specific studies have been conducted to evaluate the safety of ZNS in these groups of patients.

Advice Concerning Precaution and Management

ZNS is available in tablet (100 mg/tablet) and powder (200 mg/g) forms. The recommended initial dosage is 100 to 200 mg/day for adults and 2 to 4 mg/day for children. Because the elimination half-life is long (60 hours or 27 to 36 hours in patients taking enzyme-inducing AEDs), the steady-state blood level is reached 7 to 14 days after drug administration, and the peak-to-trough difference in plasma concentration is small (27% in once-daily dosing and 14% in twice-daily dosing) (16). Therefore, ZNS is administered once or twice a day and doses should be titrated at 2-week intervals while efficacy and tolerability are carefully monitored. Maintenance dosages of ZNS in adults and children are 200 to 400 mg/day and 4 to 8 mg/day, respectively, and the usual maximum dosage is 600 mg/day for adults and 12 mg/day for children. However, in the author's opinion, the current recommendation for ZNS titration may be too fast to avoid the common AEs that usually occur during the first 4 to 8 weeks of drug initiation. Given a slow process of adaptation to most of the common AEs, it seems preferable to start with an initial dosage of 50 mg/day and escalate the dose by 50 mg every 2 weeks until the initial target dosage of 200 mg/day.

It usually is recommended to monitor the blood level of ZNS. Therapeutic blood level ranges have been reported to be 20 to 30 μg/mL, and the plasma concentration of >30 μg/mL has been associated with the emergence of AEs (3,15,17). However, a recent investigation (14) and the analysis of pooled data (8) did not demonstrate any clear concentration–response relationships. Therefore, dose adjustment and therapeutic blood level monitoring should be based on clinical judgment. Further clinical studies on the schedules of dose escalation and dose–response or concentration–response relationships are needed. Withdrawal of ZNS may cause aggravation of seizures (5.1%) or status epilepticus (1.3%) (8). Among nine patients who were confirmed to have withdrawal effects, status epilepticus developed in two after abrupt discontinuation of ZNS, but in none after gradual tapering. Therefore, a gradual tapering of ZNS is recommended.

LESS COMMON BUT CLINICALLY RELEVANT ADVERSE EFFECTS

Renal Calculi

Earlier ZNS development in the United States and Europe was stopped because of a high incidence of renal stones (2). Overall, 13 of 505 subjects (2.6%) in the U.S. and European series had symptomatic kidney stones. Four stones have been analyzed; one was mostly urate and the others were primarily calcium oxalate and calcium phosphate (18). Yagi and colleagues (19) measured 24-hour urine calcium, magnesium, citrate, and phosphate excretion and found a significant decrease in urine citrate excretion, but no change in the other substances. Compared with the Western trials, the incidence of renal stones was very low in Japan. Only 2 of 1,008 patients (0.2%) treated with ZNS were found to have renal stones, and both patients had a history nephrolithiasis in one parent (12).

In 1992, Dainippon Pharmaceutical Co. restarted clinical trials of ZNS in partnership with the Institute of Biological Research and Development–Rostrum Global (IRG). Renal ultrasound examinations were conducted at baseline, after 12 weeks of treatment, annually, and at discontinuation of therapy to determine whether ZNS is associated with an increased incidence of renal calculi. Thirteen of 429 (3.0%) ZNS-treated patients and 2 of 85 (2.4%) placebo-treated patients developed calculi (either symptomatic or asymptomatic) in the IRG studies (8). The duration of ZNS therapy was ≤6 months in four patients, 7 to 12 months in four patients, and ≥12 months in five patients. ZNS dosages for these patients were 400 to 600 mg/day in 11 patients and >600 mg/day in 2 patients. One additional healthy volunteer who did not have an ultrasound study had symptoms of renal colic after 24 days of ZNS administration while participating in a clinical pharmacology study. Follow-up assessment of seven patients who remained in the study despite the occurrence of renal calculi revealed that three had no evidence of calculi, two patients had evidence of calculi on follow-up examination, and two other patients developed symptoms of renal colic and passed calculi. In summary, the incidence of renal calculi in ZNS-treated patients was 3.3%, compared with 2.4% in placebo-treated patients (8).

Reasons for the lower incidence of real calculi related to ZNS treatment in Japan still are unclear but may be related to racial, dietary, or other environmental factors. In fact, the incidence of renal calculi in the general population seems lower in Japan than in Western countries (20–22), which might be related to the lower incidence of ZNS-induced renal calculi in Japan. However, there is evidence to suggest a causal relationship between ZNS and renal calculi even in Japan. Recently, Kubota et al. (23) reported that renal calculi developed in three patients, and the ZNS monotherapy trial in Korea found development of renal calculi in two patients (2.7%) (10). Kubota et al. (23) suggested alkaline urine and hypercalciuria were risk factors for development of renal calculi during ZNS treatment. It is reasonable to perform routine urinalysis before and during ZNS treatment in daily practice.

Cognitive Dysfunction

From the analysis of pooled data of controlled trials, ZNS was found to cause cognitive dysfunctions more frequently than placebo: difficulty concentrating (8.2% versus 0.9%), slowed thought (3.3% versus 1.7%), and forgetfulness (7.1% versus 2.2%). Berent et al. (15) conducted serial neuropsychological assessments in nine patients with refractory epilepsies under polypharmacy. ZNS adversely affected memory quotient (MQ) scores at the end of 12 weeks of treatment, and there was a linear relationship between the change in MQ and plasma levels of ZNS. However, repeated tests at the end of 24 weeks of ZNS treatment revealed a significant recovery of MQ and a loss of relationship between MQ and plasma levels of ZNS. In the subtest analysis, ZNS appeared to affect specific cognitive functions such as acquisition and consolidation of new information and verbal learning at 12 weeks of ZNS treatment. Previously learned material, psychomotor performance, and visual-perceptual learning were not affected.

These results suggest that ZNS adversely affects specific cognitive dysfunctions, especially verbal learning, in a dose- or concentration-dependent manner during the acute stage, but an adaptation process occurs subsequently with a gradual recovery of cognitive function. The cognitive effects of ZNS require further investigation, and it seems likely that a lower starting dose and slower dose escalation of ZNS may help decrease the emergence of cognitive dysfunction.

Oligohidrosis

Oligohidrosis or a heat stroke–like episode was found to occur in children taking ZNS. Shimizu et al. (24) reported a child who presented with a heat stroke–like episode during ZNS treatment. A sweating test using pilocarpine iontophoresis revealed a marked reduction in the sweat response, which suggested a postganglionic sweating dysfunction. A skin biopsy did not show any abnormalities of sweat glands, and oligohidrosis resolved within 2 weeks of withdrawal from ZNS. Okumura et al. (25) reported that 12 of 70 epileptic children treated with ZNS had oligohidrosis. Although none of them presented with heat stroke–like episodes, reversible oligohidrosis was confirmed by either heat-loading tests or acetylcholine-loading tests. Although oligohidrosis has not been reported in adults yet, the a presence of hyperpyrexia in patients taking ZNS needs to be carefully investigated for the possibility of oligohidrosis.

Weight Loss

In the placebo-controlled trials, weight loss was found in only 3.3% (8); however, a greater than 5% loss of baseline body weight has been shown in 15% of patients taking ZNS in the monotherapy trial conducted in Korea (10), and a U.S. controlled trial (7) reported that 21.6% of ZNS-treated patients lost more than 2.3 kg. It is likely that weight loss is related to anorexia, which is one of the most common AEs related to ZNS treatment.

Teratogenicity

ZNS has teratogenic effects in mice, rats, and dogs at a higher dosage than the human maximal daily dosage (26),
and it causes a higher incidence of spontaneous abortions at the maximal human daily dose (10 mg/kg) (27).

Kondo et al. (28) assessed the risk of teratogenicity of ZNS in humans. They found 26 pregnancies from 22 mothers between 1989 and 1994; 4 were exposed to ZNS alone and the others to multiple drugs. Artificial abortions were performed in 4 mothers and congenital malformations were found in 2 of 24 offspring, anencephaly in one and atrial septal defect in the other. All mothers exposed to ZNS alone delivered normal infants. The authors concluded that the risk of ZNS teratogenicity is no greater than that of other conventional AEDs. However, such a risk cannot be neglected because of the small sample size of this study. ZNS currently is classified as category C.

ZNS is recovered in breast milk in an almost equal concentration to that in plasma, with the ratio of 0.93 ± 0.09 (29), which needs to be considered in the nursing mother. Interactions between ZNS and oral contraceptive pills have not been investigated.

Abnormal Laboratory Test Results

ZNS usually does not alter clinical laboratory test results, and no patients were withdrawn from the controlled clinical trials because of abnormal results on such tests. In one Japanese open trial (13), abnormal values, based solely on deviation from the normal range, were found in 5% to 10% of patients during the 2-year study period, but all were insignificant, and ZNS was discontinued in only 5 of 393 patients (1.3%); they consisted of anemia in 1 patient, elevated alanine aminotransferase (ALT) in 3, and neutropenia in 1. In the other open trial (9), clinical laboratory testing conducted in 909 patients revealed elevated values for r-gamma glutamyl transpeptidase (4.9%), alkaline phosphatase (2.6%), ALT (2.3%), and aspartate aminotransferase (1.4%). A mild degree of hypocalcemia was found in 5.9% of patients in the pooled data of Dainippon Pharmaceutical Co. (8).

Decreased immunoglobulin A (IgA), and sometimes of other immunoglobulins as well, was reported in 14 patients during postmarketing surveillance in Japan (8). Hypoimmunoglobulinemia is well known to occur in patients taking other conventional AEDs, especially phenytoin (30,31). Maneoka et al. (32) reported a patient in whom IgA and IgG2 subclass deficiency developed associated with ZNS therapy. After cessation of ZNS, the serum IgA level was rapidly recovered and the IgG2 level gradually increased but remained subnormal. They recommended that serum immunoglobulins be checked in patients having recurrent infections.

POTENTIALLY LIFE-THREATENING ADVERSE EFFECTS

Life-threatening AEs related to ZNS treatment were rare, and their causal relationships have not been well established.

Hematologic Disorders

Serious, irreversible hematologic disorders have not been reported. However, Leppik et al. (2) reported a case of severe leukopenia that resolved after withdrawal of ZNS. In a Japanese open trial (9), leukopenia was found in 18 patients (2%). According to the Dainippon serious AE reports (8), 22 hematologic adverse events were reported in 19 patients: pancytopenia in 2, leukopenia in 11, and thrombocytopenia in 5. In 7 of 19 patients, clinicians considered it unlikely that ZNS was causally related to the AEs. Aplastic anemia was reported in two patients; one had multiple myeloma and the other recovered after withdrawal of ZNS.

Skin Disorders

The incidence of skin rash from the pooled data of placebo-controlled trials (8) of ZNS was 3.0% in the ZNS group and 1.3% in the placebo group, with only one patient taking ZNS being withdrawn from the controlled trials. In Japanese open trials, skin rash/itching occurred in 2% (9) and 1.3% (13) of patients. Twenty-six instances of serious skin disorders were reported during postmarketing surveillance in Japan (8). Nineteen were Stevens-Johnson syndrome and seven were toxic epidermal necrolysis. However, most patients were taking multiple drugs, and a causal relationship between the skin disorder and ZNS theory could be established in only one case.

Psychiatric Disorders

Psychiatric symptoms such as depression, irritability, mania, paranoia, hallucinations, or psychosis have been reported in association with ZNS treatment. In the pooled data of placebo-controlled trials (8), the incidences of irritability (11.5% ZNS versus 5.2% placebo), depression (7.4% versus 3.0%), anxiety (5.6% versus 2.6%), paranoia (1.9% versus 0.4%) and hallucination (1.5% versus 0.0%), were more than twice those with placebo. Psychiatric symptoms were reported as serious AEs in four patients (1.5%) in ZNS groups, compared with two patients (0.9%) in placebo groups.

Several authors in Japan reported psychotic episodes or behavioral abnormalities in patients taking ZNS (33,34). One case each of ZNS-induced paranoia (4) and mania (35) were reported from the U.S. trial. Kimura (36) reported two children in whom ZNS-induced severe behavioral disturbances developed that resolved after withdrawal of ZNS. Recently, Miyamoto et al. (37) reported 14 patients in whom psychotic episodes developed that met the International Classification of Diseases, 10th edition criteria for organic delusional disorder and organic hallucinosis. Most patients made a good recovery with antipsychotic medications and discontinuation of ZNS. They estimated that the incidence of psychotic symptoms in their patient population was 13%, which was higher than the previously reported prevalence of epileptic psychosis (38). Five of the 14 patients who experienced psychosis were mentally retarded.

These findings suggest that ZNS may be implicated in the genesis of various psychiatric disturbances. However, most patients who experienced psychiatric disturbances were taking multiple drugs because of refractory epilepsies, and clear documentation of their causal relationship to ZNS was difficult except in a few cases. ZNS affects the synthesis and degradation of monoamine neurotransmitters (39), especially dopamine and norepinephrine, and its binding sites are related to the γ-aminobutyric acid/benzodiazepine receptor ionophore complex (40), which might be responsible for the induction of psychiatric disturbances in some vulnerable patients.

Sudden Unexplained Death in Epilepsy

Review of sudden unexplained death in epilepsy (SUDEP) associated with ZNS revealed an incidence of approximately 3.1 deaths per 1,000 patients (8), which was similar to the incidence of SUDEP of 4 per 1,000 associated with lamotrigine and gabapentin. The incidence of SUDEP in patients with epilepsy varied widely, but was higher in patients with refractory epilepsies. The incidence of SUDEP in ZNS trials was considered within the range described for the epileptic patient population as a whole.

MANIFESTATIONS AND MANAGEMENT OF OVERDOSE

Naito et al. (41) reported a patient who attempted suicide by taking 7,400 mg of ZNS, 126 mg of clonazepam, and 4,000 mg of CBZ. She was found comatose and was hospitalized. In the hospital, she was comatose with bradycardia and depressed respirations. A mild mydriasis, sluggish light reflexes, and mild hypotension were observed. Gastric lavage, saline infusion, and oxygen inhalation were performed, with a gradual recovery of respiration and blood pressure. She became conscious 10 hours after drug ingestion. Focal myoclonus and nystagmus appeared approximately 13 hours after the ingestion and lasted for approximately 8 hours, with spontaneous improvement. The blood concentration of ZNS was 100.1 μg/mL, that of clonazepam, 376.3ng/mL, and that of CBZ, 3.6 μg/mL at 31 hours after the drug ingestion. Considering that the elimination half-life of ZNS is 36 hours in the presence of CBZ, the peak serum concentration of ZNS might have been approximately 200 μg/mL in this patient. She eventually recovered fully without any sequelae. Based on this case report, ZNS overdose may be managed by gastric lavage and general supportive care, adequate hydration, respiratory support, and frequent monitoring of vital signs. Because of the low protein binding of ZNS (40% to 50%), renal dialysis may not be effective.

REFERENCES

1. Uno H, Kurokawa M, Natsuka K, et al. Studies on 3- substituted 1,2-benzisoxazole derivatives. *Chem Pharmacol Bull* 1972;24:632–643.
2. Leppik IE, Willmore LJ, Homan RW, et al. Efficacy and safety of zonisamide: results of a multicenter study. *Epilepsy Res* 1993;14:165–173.
3. Wilensky AJ, Friel PN, Ojeman LM, et al. Zonisamide in epilepsy: a pilot study. *Epilepsia* 1985;26:212–212.
4. Sackellares JC, Donofrio PD, Wagner JG, et al. Pilot study of zonisamide (1,2-benzisoxazole-3-methanesulfomide) in patients with refractory partial seizures. *Epilepsia* 1985;26:206–211.
5. Schmidt D, Jacob R, Loiseau P, et al. Zonisamide for add-on treatment of refractory partial epilepsy: a European double-blind trial. *Epilepsy Res* 1993;15:67–73.
6. Wilder BJ, Ramsay RE, Guterman A, et al. A double-blind multicenter placebo-controlled study of the efficacy and safety of zonisamide in the treatment of complex partial seizures in medically refractory patients. Internal report of Dainippon Pharmaceutical Co., Ltd., Osaka, Japan: Dainippon Pharmaceutical Co., 1986.
7. Faught E, Ayata R, Montouris GG, et al. Randomized controlled trial of zonisamide for the treatment of refractory partial onset seizures. *Neurology* 2001;1774–1779.
8. Dainippon Pharmaceutical U.S.A. Corporation. Integrated summary of safety in NDA of zonisamide in the U.S. Dainippon Pharmaceutical U.S.A. Corporation, Teaneck, New Jersey, 1997.
9. Seino M, Okuma T, Miyasaka M, et al. Efficacy evaluation of AD-810 (zonisamide): double-blind study comparing with carbamazepine [in Japanese]. *J Clin Exp Med* 1988;144:275–291.
10. Korean Zonisamide Study Group. Double-blind comparative clinical trial of zonisamide and carbamazepine as initial monotherapy in newly diagnosed epilepsy. *J Kor Epilepsy Soc* 1999;3:50–57.
11. Brodie MJ, Richens A, UK Lamotrigine/Carbamazepine Monotherapy Trial Group. Lamotrigine versus carbamazepine: a double blind comparative study in newly diagnosed epilepsy. *Lancet* 1995;345:476–479.
12. Yagi K, Seino M. Methodological requirements for clinical trials in refractory epilepsies-our experience with zonisamide. *Prog Neuropsychopharmacol Biol Psychiatry* 1992;16:79–85.
13. Oguni H, Hayashi K, Fukuyama Y, et al. Phase III study of a new antiepileptic AD-810, zonisamide in childhood epilepsy [in Japanese]. *Jpn J Pediatr* 1988;41:439–450.
14. Mimaki T. Clinical pharmacology and therapeutic drug monitoring of zonisamide. *Ther Drug Monit* 1998;20:593–597.
15. Berent S, Sackellares JC, Giordani B, et al. Zonisamide (CI-912) and cognition: results from preliminary study. *Epilepsia* 1987;28:61–67.
16. Kochak GM, Page JG, Buchanan RA, et al. Steady state pharmacokinetics of zonisamide, an antiepileptic agent for treatment of refractory complex partial seizures. *J Clin Pharmacol* 1998;38:166–171.
17. Miura H, Hosoda N, Takanashi S, et al. Once-daily dose of zonisamide monotherapy in the control of partial seizures in children: clinical effects and their pharmacokinetic basis [in Japanese]. *Jpn J TDM* 1993;10:240–241.
18. Seino M, Naruto S, Ito T, et al. Other antiepileptic drugs: zonisamide. In: Levy RH, Mattson RH, Meldrum BS, eds. *Antiepileptic drugs*, 4th ed. New York: Raven Press, 1995:1011–1023.
19. Yagi K, Seino M, Watanabe Y, et al. Change of urine volume and urinary components in patients with epilepsy before and after zonisamide treatment. Internal report of Dainippon Pharmaceutical Co., Ltd., Osaka, Japan: Dainippon Pharmaceutical Co., 1992.
20. Hiatt RA, Dales LG, Friedman GD, et al. Frequency of urolithiasis in a prepaid medical care program. *Am J Epidemiol* 1982;115:255–265.
21. Vahlensieck EW, Bach D, Heses A. Incidence, prevalence and mortality of urolithiasis the German Federal Republic. *Urol Res* 1982;10:161
22. Yoshida O, Okada Y. Epidemiology of urolithiasis in Japan: a chronological and geographical study. *Urol Int* 1990;45:104–111.
23. Kubota M, Nishi-Nagase M, Sakakihara, et al. Zonisamide-induced urinary lithiasis in patients with intractable epilepsy. *Brain Dev* 2000;22:230–233.
24. Shimizu T, Yamashita Y, Satoi M, et al. Heat stroke-like episode in a child caused by zonisamide. *Brian Dev* 1997;19:366–368.
25. Okumura A, Hayakawa F, Kuno K, et al. Oligohidrosis caused by zonisamide [in Japanese]. *No To Hattatsu (Tokyo)* 1996;28:44–47.
26. Terada Y, Fukagawa S, Shigematsu K, et al. Reproduction studies of zonisamide: 4. teratogenicity study in mice, dogs and monkeys [in Japanese]. *Jpn Pharmacol Ther* 1987;15:4435–4451.
27. Terade Y, Ichikawa H, Nishimura K, et al. Reproduction studies of zonisamide: 2. teratogenicity study in rats [in Japanese]. *Jpn Pharmacol Ther* 1987;15:4399–4416.
28. Kondo T, Kaneko S, Amano Y, et al. Preliminary report on teratogenic effects of zonisamide in the offspring of treated women with epilepsy. *Epilepsia* 1996;37:1241–1244.
29. Shimoyama R, Ohkuto T, Sugawara K. Monitoring of zonisamide in human breast milk and maternal plasma by solid-phase extraction HPLC method. *Biomed Chromatogr* 1999;13:370–372.
30. Seager J, Jameson DL, Wilson J, et al. IgA deficiency, epilepsy and phenytoin treatment. *Lancet* 1975;2:632–635.
31. Gihus NE, Lea T. Carbamazepine: effect on IgG subclasses in epileptic patients. *Epilepsia* 1988;29:317–320.
32. Maneoka Y, Hara T, Dejima S, et al. IgA and IgG 2 deficiency associated with zonisamide therapy: a case report. *Epilepsia* 1997;38:611–613.
33. Matsuura M, Senzaki A, Okubo Y, et al. Eight epileptic patients showing delusional-hallucinatory state during zonisamide administration [in Japanese]. *Seishin Igaku* 1993;35:413–419.
34. Mayahara K, Kanemoto K, Kawasaki J, et al. Zonisamide and episodic psychosis [in Japanese]. *J Jpn Epilepsy Soc* 1995;13:177–183.
35. Charles CL, Stoesz L, Tollefson G. Zonisamide-induced mania. *Psychosomatics* 1990;31:214–217.
36. Kimura S. Zonisamide-induced behavior disorder in two children. *Epilepsia* 1994;35:403–405.
37. Miyamoto T, Kohsaka M, Koyama T. Psychotic episodes during zonisamide treatment. *Seizure* 2000;9:65–70.
38. Toone B. Psychoses of epilepsy. In: Reynolds EH, Trimble MR, eds. *Epilepsy and psychiatry*. London: Churchill-Livingstone, 1981:113–137.
39. Okada M, Kaneko S, Hirano T, et al. Effects of zonisamide on dopaminergic system. *Epilepsy Res* 1995;22:193–205.
40. Mimaki T, Suzuki Y, Tagawa T, et al. Interaction of zonisamide with benzodiazepine and GABA receptors in rat brain. *Med J Osaka Univ* 1990;39:19–22.
41. Naito H, Itoh N, Matsui N, et al. Monitoring plasma concentrations of zonisamide and clonazepam in an epileptic attempting suicide by an overdose of the drugs. *Curr Ther Res* 1988;43:463–467.

Antiepileptic Drugs, 5th Edition. Edited by R.H. Levy, R.H. Mattson, B.S. Meldrum, and E. Perucca. Lippincott Williams & Wilkins, Philadelphia © 2002.

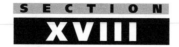
DRUGS IN DEVELOPMENT

DRUGS IN DEVELOPMENT

PREGABALIN

ELINOR BEN-MENACHEM
ALAN R. KUGLER

PRECLINICAL

Pregabalin (CI-1008; S-(+)-3-isobutyl-GABA; Pfizer, Inc., New York, NY) is a novel central nervous system (CNS)–active compound with anticonvulsant activity. It is a white solid and is stable for >18 months at 25°C. It is currently being developed as an anticonvulsant as well as an analgesic and an anxiolytic. Although it is similar in action to the antiepileptic drug (AED) gabapentin, it is more potent in animal models of pain and seizures. In general, the effective doses are lower and the duration of effect longer than with gabapentin. The isomer of S-pregabalin is the R-isobutyl γ-aminobutyric acid (GABA), but it is more than 10-fold weaker in animal models of epilepsy and pain than the isomer being developed (1).

Pregabalin, like gabapentin, is a structural analog of GABA; however, neither pregabalin nor gabapentin is active at $GABA_A$ or $GABA_B$ receptors. In fact, the mechanism of action of both gabapentin and pregabalin remains elusive. Pregabalin competes with [^{3}H]-gabapentin at its specific binding site (α2δ protein) in brain tissues, and the R- isomer has a 10 times lower affinity. Radioligand binding studies show that pregabalin has little affinity to GABA (2), and it exhibits a high affinity and selectivity to the α2δ subunit of voltage-dependent calcium channels.

There are conflicting results if gabapentin and pregabalin in fact alter calcium currents. In a recent study (3), pregabalin, like gabapentin, reduced paired-pulse inhibition in the dentate gyrus in rats. Pregabalin caused a dose-dependent loss of paired-pulse inhibition and blocked the lengthening of the duration of the seizure discharge. Nimodipine, however, could not mimic this response, so

the conclusion was that the reduction in paired-pulse inhibition was not due to the L-type calcium channel mechanism.

In other studies, there is an indication that pregabalin can modulate norepinephrine and glutamate release by inhibiting K^+-evoked release of the neurotransmitters (4,5).

In animal models of epilepsy, pregabalin has a greater potency than gabapentin in all models tested, although it has a similar profile (6). In the maximal electric shock (MES) model, pregabalin prevented tonic extensor seizures in mice at similar dosages for both oral (p.o.) and intravenous (i.v.) delivery, suggesting high bioavailability [median effective dosage (ED_{50}), 20 mg/kg p.o.]; the same was true in rats (ED_{50}, 1.5 mg/kg p.o.). Maximal effect on MES was seen 2 to 4 hours after dosing. This test suggests that pregabalin would be effective for generalized tonic-clonic seizures.

Pentylenetetrazol administration causes clonic seizures and is a model of primary generalized seizures. Pregabalin prevented threshold clonic seizures (ED_{50}, 97 mg/kg p.o. in mice and >125 mg/kg p.o. in rats). For the bicuculline, picrotoxin, and strychnine seizure models, pregabalin only partially blocked the response. Less than 100% of the mice were protected with dosages up to 500 mg/kg. These three seizure models reflect an effect on the GABAergic system in the brain. Therefore, it is proposed that pregabalin might have some effect on GABA neurotransmitter systems, although so far there is no evidence to suggest that it affects GABA receptors or metabolism.

In the hippocampal kindling rat model, pregabalin at dosages of 9.5 mg/kg reduced behavioral seizures, and higher dosages still prevented both behavioral seizures and afterdischarges. This suggests that pregabalin might be effective for the treatment of focal seizures (7).

There was no effect of pregabalin on genetically susceptible rats with spontaneous absence seizures [genetic absence epilepsy in rats from Strasbourg (GAERS)] with dosages of up to 100 mg/kg. Dosages over 200 mg/kg

---

Elinor Ben-Menachem, MD, PhD: Associate Professor, Department of Clinical Neuroscience, Neurology Section, Sahlgrenska University Hospital, Goteborg, Sweden

Alan R. Kugler, PhD: Pfizer Global Research and Development, Ann Arbor Laboratories, Ann Arbor, Michigan

intraperitoneally increased the amount of absence seizures (1). This dosage is over 20-fold higher than the highest recommended dosage in humans (600 mg/day). Pregabalin also prevented audiogenic seizures in DBA/2 mice at 3 and 10 mg/kg p.o. (1).

PHARMACOKINETICS

Pregabalin exhibits predictable linear pharmacokinetics. It has been tested in two phase 1 studies to determine its pharmacokinetics after single and rising multiple oral doses (8). The studies entailed single rising doses of 1 to 300 mg and multiple rising doses of 25 to 300 mg given every 8 hours and 300 mg given every 12 hours for 14 days. A total of 86 healthy volunteers between 19 and 50 years of age participated (47 men and 39 women). Concentrations of pregabalin were determined using specific, sensitive, and validated high-performance liquid chromatography-UV methodology (8).

Given orally to healthy volunteers, pregabalin was rapidly absorbed [mean time to maximal concentration (T_{max}) approximately 1 hour], with a bioavailability ≥90%, independent of dose. The plasma pregabalin half-life was approximately 6 hours, which was independent of dose and with repeated administration. Maximal plasma pregabalin concentrations (C_{max}) and total exposures (area under the concentration–time curve) were dose-proportional after either single or multiple dosing. The concentration–time profiles of pregabalin were similar after twice-daily or three-times–daily administration.

Metabolism and Elimination

Pregabalin is not metabolized to any extent in humans, nor does it bind to plasma proteins. This also is similar to gabapentin. Approximately 98% of the drug can be recovered unchanged in the urine. The percentage excreted was similar with single or multiple dosing and was independent of dose.

Drug Interactions

No drug interactions have been reported clinically and none are anticipated since pregabalin is neither metabolized nor bound to plasma proteins. Population pharmacokinetic analyses (9) demonstrated that pregabalin could be administered with carbamazepine, lamotrigine, phenobarbital, phenytoin, topiramate, and valproate without concern for clinically significant changes in their pharmacokinetics.

Effects on Renal and Liver Disease

Pregabalin is not expected to affect the liver because it is not metabolized at therapeutic dosages. In the rat, pregabalin

induced the cytochrome P450 (CYP) isoenzymes CYP2B1/2 and CYP2E1 only at extreme dosages >1,250 mg/kg/day (approximately 145-fold higher than the highest recommended dose in humans). Because pregabalin is excreted by the kidney, dose adjustments may need to be considered in patients with renal insufficiency.

Elderly

A population pharmacokinetics analysis (9) showed that the only factor with a clinically significant impact on pregabalin pharmacokinetics was renal function; age was not an independent covariate. The safety and efficacy of pregabalin in the elderly are being assessed.

Pregnancy

There is no information available on the effect of pregabalin on pregnancy because the drug is still undergoing clinical trials. However, pregabalin is not teratogenic in mice or rabbits. Teratogenicity was observed in rats at very high dosages of 1,250 to 2,500 mg/kg. These dosages were much higher than those used in humans (usually <10 mg/kg) (data on file; Pfizer, Ann Arbor, MI).

CLINICAL EFFICACY

Randomized, Controlled Trials

Pregabalin has been evaluated in more than 1,500 patients with epilepsy (10). Even more patients have been involved in clinical trials for other indications, mainly analgesic and psychiatric.

One monotherapy study (1008-007) (11) has been completed in patients with refractory partial epilepsy admitted for surgical evaluation. Using a typical presurgical inpatient monotherapy protocol, patients were randomized either to 600 mg/day pregabalin (n = 42) or 300 mg/day gabapentin (n = 51) for 8 days. There was a positive trend in favor of pregabalin in time to exit and a significantly higher study completion rate for the pregabalin group.

Three major outpatient randomized, controlled trials for adjunctive therapy in patients with partial seizures with or without secondary generalization have been reported in abstract form. Patients in these three studies had received anticonvulsant therapy for many years before randomization, with a mean duration of epilepsy of 25 years. At entry, 30% of patients were receiving one AED, 50% were receiving two AEDs, and 20% were receiving three AEDs. Despite this treatment, patients remained refractory at baseline with a median of 10 partial seizures per month and a mean of 24 seizures per month. Over 83% of patients entered open-label extensions (12).

Analyses used an intent-to-treat population, defined as those randomized to treatment and taking at least one dose of study medication. Two end points were evaluated in each study, response ratio and responder rate. Response ratio (RRatio), the primary efficacy parameter, is a measure of the percentage change from baseline in seizure frequency during treatment, such that:

$$[(T - B)/(T + B)] \times 100$$

where B = baseline seizure frequency and T = seizure frequency during treatment. RRatio, using parametric statistical methods, reflects a direct transformation of the difference in percentage of seizures that occur during treatment compared with baseline. Results are distributed normally in the range of −100 to +100. A zero value would indicate no change in seizure frequency and a −100 value would indicate complete elimination of seizures. A 50% reduction would result in an RRatio of −33. For display purposes (Figure 96.1), mean RRatio values were converted to seizure reductions. Responder rate, a secondary efficacy parameter, is defined as the percentage of patients with ≥50% reduction in seizure frequency during treatment compared with baseline.

The first study (1008-009) (13) was a 43-center, double-blind, placebo-controlled, parallel-group, randomized trial of pregabalin as add-on therapy in patients with refractory partial epilepsy not controlled on one to three drugs. A total of 312 patients with at least 6 seizures during an 8-week baseline were given pregabalin 300 mg twice daily (bid), pregabalin 200 mg three times daily (tid), or placebo for 12 weeks. Baseline AEDs were not changed during the study time. Of the 312 patients, 76% completed the study. RRatio was significantly better for pregabalin bid and tid groups than placebo (*p* ≤ .0001). The mean RRatio for the various treatment groups was −28 (600 mg/day administered bid), -36 (600 mg/day administered tid), and 0.6 (placebo). Responder rates were 43%, 49%, and 9%, respectively for the bid, tid, and placebo groups. Seizure freedom (last 28

days of the study) rates were 3% for placebo, 3% for pregabalin 600 mg/day bid, and 14% for pregabalin 600 mg/day tid. The most common side effects reported were dizziness, somnolence, and ataxia. The dropout rate due to adverse events was 26% in the bid group, 19% in the TID group, and 7% in the placebo group.

In the second randomized, controlled trial (1008-034) (14), the efficacy and tolerability of pregabalin in 453 patients with refractory partial seizures was determined. This study included 80 centers and was a double-blind, parallel-group study with an 8-week baseline and a 12-week treatment period. Patients were taking one to three other AEDs and were randomized to one of five groups: pregabalin 50, 150, 300, or 600 mg/day bid or placebo with no titration phase. RRatio was significantly better for pregabalin 150, 300, and 600 mg/day groups than placebo (*p* ≤ .0001). The mean RRatio for the various treatment groups was −4 (placebo), −6 (50 mg/day), −21 (150 mg/day), −28 (300 mg/day), and −37 (600 mg/day). Responder rates were 14%, 15%, 31%, 40%, and 51%, respectively. Seizure freedom (last 28 days of the study) rates were 8%, 5%, 6%, 11%, and 17%, respectively. Withdrawal rates due to adverse events were 5%, 7%, 1%, 14%, and 24%, respectively. The most common adverse events were dizziness and somnolence, and both were dose related. Pharmacokinetics were found to be dose proportional, low variability, and predictable. The conclusion of the abstract was that pregabalin treatment can be initiated at a dosage of 150 mg/day, administered in two divided doses, and can be increased based on individual response both to efficacy and tolerability.

In the third multicenter, double-blind, placebo-controlled study (1008-011) (15), 287 patients with severe refractory partial seizures were given the study drug. After an 8-week baseline phase, patients were given either placebo, pregabalin 150 mg/day tid, or pregabalin 600 mg/day tid for 12 weeks, with only 1 week of titration. RRatio was significantly better for the pregabalin 150 mg/day (*p* = .0007) and 600 mg/day (*p* ≤ .0001) groups than for placebo. The mean RRatio for the various treatment groups was −12 (150 mg/day), −31 (600 mg/day), and 0.9 (placebo). Responder rates were 6.2% for the placebo group, 14.1% for the 150 mg/day group, and 43.5% for the 600 mg/day group. Seizure freedom (last 28 days of the study) rates were 1% for the placebo group, 7% for the 150 mg/day group, and 12% for the 600 mg/day group. Adverse events were judged to be transient, mild to moderate in intensity, and CNS related.

Figure 96.1 shows the RRatio values converted to seizure reductions for all three adjunctive studies. There was a statistically significant increase in efficacy with increasing dose in studies 1008-034 and 1008-011 (linear dose–response; *p* ≤ .0001 for both studies) (12,16). In all three controlled studies, statistically significant efficacy was present by week 1 (17).

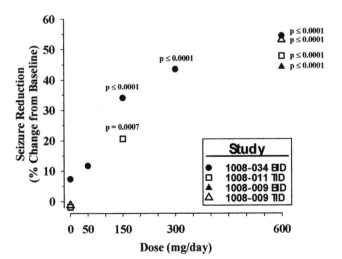

FIGURE 96.1. Seizure reduction by study, regimen, and daily dose.

Adverse Events

Data from all three studies also were pooled to assess safety (12). The most frequently occurring adverse events were dizziness and somnolence. Some of the adverse events appeared to be dose related. However, in general, events were mild to moderate in intensity. Withdrawal rates due to adverse events ranged from 1.2% to 25% and also appeared to be dose related. Studies are ongoing to determine whether a longer titration to the higher doses would result in fewer dropouts and an improved safety profile. Serious adverse events were infrequent, and no deaths occurred during these studies. There were some mild, transient increases in hepatic enzymes in the multiple-dose study in healthy volunteers at 900 mg/day (8). The highest recommended dose in clinical trials is 600 mg/day. Overall, pregabalin was well tolerated as reflected by the fact that 83% of pregabalin-treated patients enrolled in open-label extensions to the double-blind studies.

Two epilepsy investigators have published their single-site observations of myoclonus. Huppertz et al. (18) reported myoclonus in 21% (4 of 19 pregabalin-treated patients) and Asconape et al. (19) reported myoclonus in 33% (2 of 6 pregabalin-treated patients). However, myoclonus has been reported in only 1.2% (60 of 5,026 patients) of all patients treated with pregabalin in 29 controlled and uncontrolled epilepsy and analgesia studies, and led to withdrawal in 0.12% (6 of 5,026) of patients (Data on file; Pfizer, Ann Arbor, MI). Of the 60 cases, 56 had epilepsy and were receiving 1 to 3 other AEDs. The overall incidence of myoclonus in epilepsy trials was 3.5% (56 of 1,160 patients). Electroencephalograms were obtained in six of the cases and none showed visible correlates, thus indicating that the myoclonus did not appear to be cortical in origin.

CLINICAL THERAPEUTICS

Place of the Drug in Therapy

So far, pregabalin has been tested in patients with refractory partial seizures and has been found to be efficacious and well tolerated. Preliminary preclinical studies indicate that this drug might not be as effective in idiopathic epilepsy forms, but this has not been tested in humans yet. Monotherapy trials for new-onset partial seizures, as well as pediatric studies, comparative studies, and studies in patients with other seizure types, are in the planning stages.

Dose and Titration Rates

From the randomized clinical trials, there is evidence that the starting dosage of pregabalin should be 150 mg/day given in two divided doses. Efficacy and tolerability should then be evaluated before further titration is contemplated.

Titration should depend on individual tolerability and response to the drug. In the clinical studies, titration was either over 1 week, or therapy was initiated without titration at dosages up to 600 mg/day.

Therapeutic Ranges

In clinical trials, the drug has been tested at dosages between 50 and 600 mg/day. Studies 1008-034 (14) and 1008-011 (15) demonstrate a significant dose–response relationship up to the maximum dosages tested of 600 mg/day. Because the pharmacokinetics of pregabalin are linear and predictable, the benefit of therapeutic drug monitoring to guide dosing is thought to be minimal.

SUMMARY

Several clinical studies demonstrate the effectiveness and safety of pregabalin for the treatment of focal epilepsy (all partial seizures with or without secondary generalization). The efficacy data appear very encouraging considering the refractory nature of patients enrolled in studies to date. More details on the safety and tolerability of pregabalin are required to understand more fully the position of pregabalin in the therapy of patients with epilepsy.

REFERENCES

1. Bryans JS, Wustrow DJ. 3-Substituted GABA analog with central nervous system activity: a review. *Med Res Rev* 1999;19: 149–177.
2. Gee NS, Brown JP, Dissanayake VU, et al. The novel anticonvulsant drug gabapentin (Neurontin) binds to the alpha2delta subunit of a calcium channel. *J Biol Chem* 1996;271:5768–5776.
3. Stringer JL, Taylor CP. The effects of gabapentin in the rat hippocampus are mimicked by two structural analogs, but not by nimodipine. *Epilepsy Res* 2000;41:155–162.
4. Dooley DJ, Donovan CM, Pugsley TA. Stimulus-dependent modulation of (^{3}H) norepinephrine release from rat neocortical slices by gabapentin and pregabalin. *Pharmacology* 2000;295: 1086–1093.
5. Dooley DJ, Mieske CA, Borosky SA. Inhibition of K (+)-evoked glutamate release from rat neocortical and hippocampal slices by gabapentin. *Neurosci Lett* 2000;18:107–110.
6. Taylor CP, Vartanian MG, Profile of the anticonvulsant activity of CI-1008 (pregabalin) in animal models. *Epilepsia* 1997;38 [Suppl 8]:8.
7. Williamson J, Lothman CTE, Bertran E. Comparison of S(+)-3 isobutyl GABA and gabapentin against kindled hippocampal seizures. *Epilepsia* 1997;38[Suppl 8]:29.
8. Bockbrader HN, Hunt T, Strand J, et al. Pregabalin pharmacokinetics and safety in healthy volunteers: results from two phase 1 studies. *Neurology* 2000;54[Suppl 3]:421.
9. Bockbrader HN, Burger PJ, Kugler AR, et al. Population pharmacokinetic (PK) analyses of commonly prescribed antiepileptic drugs (AEDs) coadministered with pregabalin (PGB) in adult patients with refractory partial seizures. *Epilepsia* 2001;42[Suppl 7]:84.

10. Bialer M, Johannessen SI, Kupferberg HJ, et al. Progress report on new antiepileptic drugs: a summary of the Fifth Eilat Conference (EILAT V). *Epilepsy Res* 2001;43:11–58.

11. Abou-Khalil BW, Vazquez BR, Beydoun AA, et al., and the Pregabalin 7/8 Study Group. Pregabalin in-patient monotherapy trial: study results and impact of seizure frequency on efficacy evaluations. *Epilepsia* 1999;40[Suppl 7]:109.

12. Kugler AR, Robbins JL, Strand JC, et al. Pregabalin overview: a novel CNS-active compound with anticonvulsant activity. Presented at the meeting of the American Epilepsy Society, Philadelphia, 2001.

13. Beydoun AA, Uthman BM, Ramsay RE, et al., and the Pregabalin 1008-009/010 Study Group. Pregabalin add-on trial: double-blind, multicenter study in patients with partial epilepsy. *Epilepsia* 2000;41[Suppl 7]:253–254.

14. French JA, Malicsi MJR, Kugler AR, et al., and the Pregabalin 1008-034/-035 Study Group. Dose-response trial of pregabalin add-on therapy in patients with partial seizures. *Epilepsia* 2000;41[Suppl 7]:254.

15. Arroyo S, Anhut H, Messmer S, et al. Pregabalin double-blind add-on study in patients with partial seizures. *Epilepsia* 2001;43.

16. French JA, Kugler AR, Garofalo EA, et al. Pregabalin dose-response in patients with partial seizures as evaluated in two add-on trials. Presented at the International Epilepsy Congress, Buenos Aires, Argentina, May 14, 2001.

17. Robbins JL, Kugler AR, Anhut H, et al. Pregabalin shows anticonvulsant activity onset by second day. *Epilepsia* 2001;42[Suppl 7]:211.

18. Huppertz H-J, Feuerstein TJ, Schulze-Bonhage A. Myoclonus in epilepsy patients with anticonvulsive add-on therapy with pregabalin [Brief communication]. *Epilepsia* 2001;42: 790–792.

19. Asconape JJ, Hartman LM, Salanova V. Pregabalin-associated myoclonus. *Epilepsia* 1999;40[Suppl 7]:143.

DRUGS IN DEVELOPMENT

RUFINAMIDE

MARY ANN KAROLCHYK
DIETER SCHMIDT

Rufinamide (CGP33101; RUF331) is a triazole derivative synthesized by Novartis Pharma AG (Basel, Switzerland). It is structurally unrelated to other anticonvulsant drugs. The compound's effectiveness as an anticonvulsant was evaluated in standard animal screening models. It was chosen for further preclinical testing from a number of related compounds based on its favorable efficacy and side effect profile. Controlled clinical studies have shown rufinamide to be an effective and safe anticonvulsant in the treatment of inadequately controlled partial seizures in adults.

CHEMISTRY AND METHODS OF DETERMINATION

Rufinamide, 1-(2,6-difluorophenyl)methyl-1H-1,2,3-triazole-4-carboxamide, is a triazole derivative (Figure 97.1). This neutral compound has a molecular weight of 238.20, exists as a white to practically white crystalline powder, and melts at 240°C to 242°C. The solubility of rufinamide in water as well as in gastric and intestinal fluids is low (approximately 60 mg/L at 37°C).

Plasma and urine levels of rufinamide are determined by high-performance liquid chromatography. Concentrations down to 0.1 μg/mL can be detected with this methodology (1,2).

PRECLINICAL PHARMACOLOGY AND MECHANISM OF ACTION

Anticonvulsant Activity

The anticonvulsant spectrum of activity and the side effect profile of rufinamide were evaluated internally by Novartis

Mary Ann Karolchyk, DO: Global Head, Epilepsy Section, Department of Clinical Research and Development, Novartis Pharmaceuticals Corporation, Basel, Switzerland

Dieter Schmidt, MD: Head, Epilepsy Research Group Section, Berlin, Germany

and externally through the National Institutes of Health–sponsored Antiepileptic Drug Development program. In this program, a compound's efficacy in electrically and chemically induced seizures in rodent species was evaluated in a blinded manner. In addition to measures of anticonvulsant activity, the Rotorod test was performed to assess toxicity. The protective index, the median toxic dose divided by the median effective dose (TD_{50}/ED_{50}), of the compound was then calculated. As a reference, four prototype antiepileptic drugs (AEDs), ethosuximide, phenobarbital, phenytoin, and valproic acid, were tested in the same manner. Results from these tests in mice are shown in Table 97.1 (3,4).

Kindled seizures can be regarded as an animal model of partial seizures evolving to generalized seizures (5). In fully kindled cats, oral rufinamide at doses of 100 and 300 mg/kg delayed kindling development and suppressed afterdischarges, as did carbamazepine (40 mg/kg) and sodium valproate (180 mg/kg). Unlike these two AEDs, however, rufinamide antagonized kindling without provoking motor disturbances. Another animal model of chronically recurring partial seizures (with or without generalization) is the rhesus monkey with an aluminum hydroxide implant in the motor cortex. Subchronic treatment with oral rufinamide (30 to 50 mg/kg/day for 15 days) reduced seizure frequency by 75% to 100%, without producing limiting side effects.

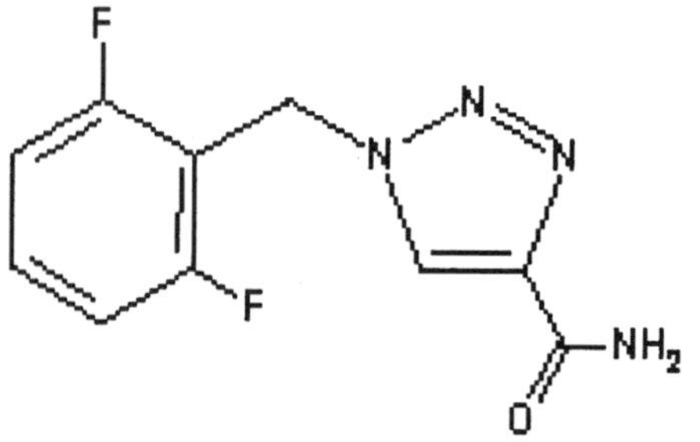

FIGURE 97.1. Chemical structure of rufinamide, 1-(2,6-difluorophenyl)methyl-1H-1,2,3-triazole-4-carboxamide.

TABLE 97.1. ANTICONVULSANT ACTIVITY AND PROTECTIVE INDEX IN ELECTRICALLY AND CHEMICALLY INDUCED SEIZURES IN MICE

Convulsant	TD_{50} (mgkg), i.p.	ED_{50} (mgkg) and PI, i.p.				
	Rotarod Test	MES	s.c. PTZ	s.c. BIC	s.c. PIC	s.c. STR
Rufinamide	>500, >1000	15.5, >32.2	54, >9.3	50.5, >9.9	76.3, >6.6	Max 37.5%[b]
Ethosuximide	441	—[a]	130, 3.4	459, 1	243, 1.8	Max 62.5%[b]
Phenobarbital	69	21.8, 3.2	13.2, 5.2	37.7, 1.8	27.5, 2.5	95.3, 0.7
Phenytoin	65.5	9.5, 6.9	—[a]	—[a]	—[a]	Max 50%[b]
Sodium valproate	426	272, 1.6	149, 2.9	360, 1.2	387, 1.1	293, 1.5

[a]No protection.
[b]Indicates percentage protected at maximum dose; values cannot be calculated as not all animals were protected at the maximum dose.
BIC, bicuculline; ED_{50}, median effective dose; i.p., intraperitoneally; MES, maximal electroshock; PI, protective index; PIC, picrotoxin; PTZ, pentylenetetrazol; s.c., subcutaneous; STR, strychmine; TD_{50}, median toxic dose.

Rufinamide also has been evaluated in genetic animal models of epilepsy. All components of sound-induced seizures in the audiogenic seizure–susceptible DBA/2 mouse were suppressed at oral rufinamide doses of 7 to 45 mg/kg. Rufinamide was ineffective, however, in preventing absence seizures in WAG/Rij rats.

Proposed Mechanism of Action

The anticonvulsant activity of rufinamide is mediated, at least in part, through prolongation of the inactivation phase of voltage-dependent sodium channels. In cultured mouse neurons, rufinamide limited the frequency of firing of sodium-dependent action potentials at a median inhibitory concentration of 2×10^{-7} g/mL. This effect could contribute to blocking the spread of seizure activity from an epileptogenic focus (6,7). Radioligand studies were performed to assess binding to other neurotransmitter sites. Concentrations of 10 μmol/L rufinamide showed no affinity for 5-hydroxytryptophan type 1 (5-HT$_1$), 5-HT$_2$, α_1-, α_2-, and β-adrenergic receptors; histamine-1 and cholinergic muscarinic agonist and antagonist sites also were not affected at this concentration. Rufinamide at concentrations of 10 to 100 μmol/L had no effect on [³H]flunitrazepam and [³H]γ-aminobutyric acid receptor binding. No binding to the N-methyl-D-aspartate, strychnine-insensitive glycine, and α-amino-3-hydroxy-5-methyl-4-isoxazole propionate (AMPA)/kainate receptors was detected at rufinamide concentrations up to 100 μmol/L.

General Pharmacology

Rufinamide at doses up to 10 mg/kg intravenously in dogs did not significantly affect cardiovascular or respiratory function, as assessed by changes in systolic and diastolic blood pressure, blood flow, respiratory rate, and tidal volume. In these animals, rufinamide produced a slight increase in heart rate that was apparent at 1 and 10 mg/kg, but not at 3 mg/kg.

In mice, sedation was noted at oral rufinamide doses of 900 mg/kg and 1,200 mg/kg. Rufinamide was effective in enhancing learning and memory in mice at and below effective anticonvulsant doses. At doses between 0.3 and 30 mg orally and intraperitoneally, learning performance in the stepdown passive avoidance paradigm was enhanced and electroshock-induced amnesia was partially counteracted.

There is neither physical nor psychological dependence liability associated with rufinamide. In a test of physical dependence, cynomolgus monkeys given 400 mg/kg/day oral rufinamide did not have withdrawal signs when the benzodiazepine antagonist Ro15-1788 was administered. No drug-seeking behavior was seen when increasing doses of rufinamide (5, 10, and 20 mg/kg) were administered to monkeys with implanted intragastric cannulae connected to injection devices to assess psychological dependence.

TOXICOLOGY

The acute (single-dose) toxicology of orally administered rufinamide was evaluated in the mouse, rat, and dog. In mice and rats, rufinamide was well tolerated after administration of doses up to 5,000 mg/kg. There was a 200- to 800-fold separation between the LD$_{50}$ (median lethal dose) and ED$_{50}$ in mice and rats, respectively. Doses up to 2,000 mg/kg were well tolerated in the dog; further dose increases were limited by emesis.

During chronic (≥6 months) oral rufinamide administration in the mouse, rat, dog, and monkey, several findings involving the bone, biliary system, and thyroid axis were reported. All findings occurred in a species-specific manner and were not considered to be relevant to humans.

Rufinamide showed no evidence of teratogenicity in mice, rats, or rabbits at oral doses of 300 to 1,000 mg/kg, administered during the period of organogenesis. There was no impairment of general reproductive performance and fertility when rufinamide was orally administered to rats doses up to 150 mg/kg. Increased postnatal pup mortality rates were seen in some rat reproductive studies. This finding was further investigated with two cross-fostering studies. Both studies suggested the mortality rates to be related to late *in utero* effects secondary to maternal toxicity. This perinatal effect was not noted in other animals, including the mouse, thus confirming a species-specific finding.

The mutagenic potential of rufinamide was evaluated in a battery of *in vitro* and *in vivo* studies. Neither rufinamide nor its metabolites showed mutagenic potential in any study.

In a 104-week mouse carcinogenicity study, species-specific findings of an increased incidence of benign and malignant liver tumors and benign osteomas were noted at rufinamide doses of 400 mg/kg. The pathogenesis of both findings are linked to metabolism specific to the mouse: In particular, the liver findings are consistent with those produced by phenobarbital-type microsomal enzyme inducers, whereas the bone findings result from latent retrovirus activation by fluoride released from the rufinamide molecule during oxidative metabolism. In a rat carcinogenicity study of identical duration, a species-specific finding of an increased incidence of thyroid follicular adenomas at rufinamide doses of 60 mg/kg was noted. Liver tumors were not present in the rat.

Phase I investigations included approximately 85 healthy subjects who received oral rufinamide at doses up to 2,100 mg/day in single-dose and multiple-dose, double-blind, placebo-controlled studies. The most common adverse events in the rufinamide-treated subjects were headache, fatigue, and concentration difficulties. There were no clinically relevant abnormalities of laboratory parameters, electrocardiogram (ECG), and vital signs in rufinamide-treated subjects.

PHARMACOKINETICS

Absorption, Distribution, Metabolism, and Elimination Profile

Absorption of orally administered [^{14}C]-labeled rufinamide was determined in the mouse, rat, dog, monkey, and baboon (8). In all species, absorption was near complete at low doses and decreased with the highest doses tested. The rate of absorption usually was slow in all species, with the exception of the immature rat. The absolute bioavailability of the compound in dogs and baboons was assessed using a [^{14}C]-labeled intravenous formulation of the compound; plasma concentrations between the intravenous and oral formulations were comparable, indicating little or no first-pass metabolism.

The distribution of the radiolabel in most organs of the mouse and rat was similar to that in the blood and plasma, with the highest levels in the liver and the lowest levels in white fat. Serum protein binding was low (23% to 29%) in all species tested.

In all investigated animal species, the radiolabel excreted with the urine was predominantly due to inactive metabolites; less than 13% was the parent compound. No active metabolites were identified. The major urinary metabolite in all species, accounting for 50% to 90% of urinary radioactivity, was CGP47292, formed by hydrolysis of the carboxylamide group. Prominent (10% to 40% of urinary radioactivity) in the mouse and rat was 2,6-difluorobenzoic acid, CGP47291, a metabolite formed by oxidative cleavage at the benzylic carbon atom. Fifty percent to 65% of systemically available radioactivity was excreted within 7 days in the urine of tested animals. Rufinamide and it metabolites were eliminated predominantly renally, with low biliary/fecal elimination.

A single 600-mg dose of radiolabeled rufinamide was administered to three healthy human subjects (9). Thirty-four percent of rufinamide was protein bound, predominantly to albumin. The parent compound accounted for approximately 80% of the total plasma radioactivity. Less than 2% of the dose was recovered unchanged in urine, indicating extensive metabolism. As in animal studies, the major biotransformation pathway was hydrolysis of the carboxylamide group to CGP47292. This metabolite accounted for approximately 78% of the urinary radioactivity. There was no indication for involvement of oxidizing cytochrome P450 (CYP) enzymes or glutathione in the biotransformation process. Renal excretion was predominant, accounting for 84.7% of the dose.

Human Pharmacokinetic Studies

The onset of rufinamide absorption was rapid under both fed and fasted conditions in single-dose studies in healthy subjects and patients with epilepsy. Pharmacokinetic profiles in healthy volunteers were similar under both single- and multiple-dose (28 days) administration. In multiple-dose studies in patients with epilepsy, the plasma area under the curve (AUC) increased less than proportionally with individual doses greater than 400 mg, probably because of dose-limited absorption behavior. In one large population pharmacokinetics study in patients with epilepsy, the AUC at a dose of 1,600 mg/day (800 mg twice daily) was 73% greater than that of 800 mg/day (400 twice daily) (10). Food increased the extent of rufinamide absorption by approximately 40%.

A formulation change from dry compaction to the final market image (FMI) was made during the course of development. Twenty-four healthy volunteers participated in a three-way, crossover bioavailability/food effect study comparing the dry compaction tablet in the fed state and the FMI tables in both the fed and the fasting states. The FMI tablet had a 22% higher AUC and 34% higher maximal

TABLE 97.2. PHARMACOKINETIC PARAMETERS AFTER SINGLE ORAL ADMINISTRATION OF 400 MG RUFINAMIDE IN HEALTHY VOLUNTEERS

	Dry Compaction Formulation, Fed State (n = 24)	FMI Formulation, Fed State (n = 24)	FMI Formulation, Fasting State (n = 24)
Mean AUC (γg/mL · h)	69.9	84.3	63.3
Mean half-life (h)	10.7	10.6	10.8
Mean C_{max} (γg/mL)	3.3	4.4	2.9
Median T_{max} (h)	6	4	6

AUC, area under the curve; C_{max}, maximum concentration; FMI, final market image; T_{max}, time to maximum plasma concentration.

plasma concentration (C_{max}) than the dry compaction tablet. Similar to the dry compaction tablet, administration of the FMI tablet with food increased the AUC, although to a lesser extent (34%). Plasma parameters from this study are shown in Table 97.2.

Neither sex nor age (14 to 64 years) had a significant influence on steady-state $AUC_{(0-12h)}$, C_{max}, and minimum plasma concentration (C_{min}) of rufinamide (10). To evaluate the profile in pediatric patients with epilepsy, 16 children aged 2 through 17 years were enrolled in a 2-week, open-label, ascending-dose study stratified by age (2 to 6 years, 7 to 12 years, and 13 to 17 years) (11). Rufinamide was administered orally in equally divided twice-daily doses of 10 mg/kg/day in week 1 and 30 mg/kg/day in week 2. There were no significant differences in plasma pharmacokinetic parameters as a function of age. On a milligram per kilogram per day basis, the $AUC_{(0-12h)}$, C_{max}, and C_{min} of rufinamide in this study were similar to data from adult pharmacokinetic studies.

The pharmacokinetic profile of rufinamide in the elderly was assessed in nine healthy elderly subjects and nine sex-matched younger adult subjects under both single- (400 mg) and multiple-dose (800 mg/day × 4 days) conditions (12,13). No significant pharmacokinetic differences were found between the groups.

Drug Interactions

In vitro, rufinamide demonstrated little or no competitive or mechanism-based inhibition of the following human CYP enzymes: CYP1A2, CYP2A6, CYP2C9, CYP2C19, CYP2D6, CYP2E1, CYP3A4/5, and CYP4A9/11 (14). The K_i values were ≥450 μmol/L and at least 40 times the trough plasma levels (10.6 μmol/L) after daily administration of 800 mg rufinamide for 12 weeks.

In vivo interaction studies were conducted to assess any potential pharmacokinetic effect of rufinamide on concomitant drug administration. The effect of repeated-dose rufinamide on the AUC, C_{max}, and time to maximum plasma concentration (T_{max}) of hormonal components [ethinyl estradiol (EE) and norethindrone (NED)] of the low-dose contraceptive Ortho-Novum 1/35 (Ortho

McNeil, Raritan., NJ) was determined in an open-label study in healthy subjects (15). Rufinamide, 1,600 mg/day, was administered for 14 consecutive days; 24-hour NED and EE levels were measured at the end of the rufinamide dosing cycle and compared with baseline values. Coadministration of rufinamide resulted in an approximately 22% and 14% decrease in EE and NED AUCs, respectively. A decrease in the C_{max} of 31% (NED) and 18% (EE) also was seen; there was no significant difference in T_{max}. There were no reported cases of breakthrough bleeding during coadministration of rufinamide. Although this interaction was statistically significant, the clinical significance is unknown because markers of ovulation were not assessed.

Two healthy-subject, open-label interaction studies were performed with the specific CYP substrates olanzapine (CYP1A2) (16) and triazolam (CYP3A4). In both studies, pharmacokinetic parameters were assessed after single-dose administration of the substrate and again after 11 days of rufinamide (800 mg/day) dosing. Pretreatment with rufinamide had no effect on the pharmacokinetic parameters of olanzapine; however, the triazolam $AUC_{(0-\infty)}$ and C_{max} were decreased by approximately 37% and 23%, respectively. This interaction may be significant only for those concomitantly administered drugs that are metabolized predominantly through the CYP3A4 pathway.

Potential interactions with concomitantly administered AEDs were assessed in 471 rufinamide-treated patients who participated in the trials described by Stefan et al. (17). All patients had inadequately controlled partial seizures and were taking one, two, or three fixed-dose concomitant AEDs. In this population pharmacokinetics analysis, valproate and lamotrigine decreased the plasma clearance of rufinamide by 22% (10), whereas any combination of phenytoin, phenobarbital, and primidone increased the clearance by approximately 25% (10). Because rufinamide has a wide therapeutic window, these changes are not expected to be clinically significant. Although it is known that valproate is a broad-spectrum inhibitor of hepatic metabolism and phenytoin and phenobarbital/primidone are known inducers of CYP isoenzymes, the mechanism of these interactions with rufinamide have not been fully elucidated. Other AEDs, including carbamazepine, vigabatrin, oxcarbazepine, and clobazam, did not modify the plasma pharmacokinetics of rufinamide. Similarly, rufinamide did not influence the trough levels of the most commonly coadministered AEDs in this study, including carbamazepine, valproate, phenytoin, clobazam, phenobarbital, primidone, oxcarbazepine, and clonazepam.

CLINICAL EFFICACY AND SAFETY

Efficacy

To date, more than 1,500 patients with epilepsy have been treated with rufinamide during the course of clinical studies. Table 97.3 lists the completed efficacy studies in adult patients.

The study of Pålhagen et al. provided the first proof of anticonvulsant effect in humans (18). It was a multicenter, double-blind, placebo-controlled, weekly rising dose study in patients with epilepsy on one or two fixed-dose concomitant AEDs to investigate the pharmacokinetic and safety profile of rufinamide in single- (open-label) and multiple-dose (double-blind) administration. Fifty patients with inadequately controlled partial or generalized seizures were equally randomized to rufinamide or placebo treatment groups. Weekly ascending doses of 400, 800, 1,200, and 1,600 mg/day of rufinamide or matching placebo were administered in a twice-daily dosing regimen.

The efficacy analyses used the following standard parameters: seizure frequency ratio, as defined as the seizure frequency per 28 days during treatment divided by the baseline seizure frequency, as the primary variable; and the 25% and 50% responder rates as secondary variables. Patients who received rufinamide had a statistically significant decrease in seizure frequency ratio relative to the placebo treatment group ($p = .0397$; Wilcoxon rank-sum test). The 25% responder rate was significantly higher in rufinamide-treated patients than in placebo-treated patients (52% versus 16%, $p = .014$; chi-square test); the 50% responder rate also showed a trend toward significance in rufinamide-treated patients (39% versus 16%, $p = .096$; chi-square test) despite the small sample size.

After this proof-of-concept study, a large, double-blind, placebo-controlled, dose-ranging study was conducted in patients with partial seizures inadequately controlled with one, two, or three fixed-dose concomitant AEDs (17). Six hundred forty-seven patients with inadequately controlled partial seizures were randomized to one of the four rufinamide treatment groups (200, 400, 800, or 1,600 mg/day administered twice daily) or placebo. After a prospective 12-week baseline phase, patients entered a 13-week treatment phase; study drug was initiated at the randomized dose without titration. The primary outcome, the linear trend of dose response for seizure frequency per 28 days in the treatment phase, was statistically significant in favor of rufinamide ($p = .003$; linear regression). A secondary efficacy variable compared the seizure frequency ratio of each treatment group with that of placebo (Wilcoxon rank-sum tests). The seizure frequency ratio was statistically significantly lower for the 400, 800, and 1,600 mg/day treatment groups compared with placebo (all $p \leq .0274$). These significant differences corresponded to a reduction in median seizure frequency ratio of 12%, 17%, and 18%, respectively, relative to placebo (Figure 97.2). A key secondary variable, the linearity of dose response of 50% responders, was statistically significant ($p = .0319$; logistic regression). At daily doses of 400 to 1,600 mg, the 50% responder rates ranged between 11.6% and 16.0%, relative to a placebo rate of 9.0%.

A second double-blind, placebo-controlled study was conducted in a similar population. A total of 313 adult patients with inadequately controlled partial seizures receiving one to two fixed-dose concomitant AEDs were randomized to rufinamide treatment (3,200 mg/day, administered twice daily) or placebo. After a prospective 8-week

TABLE 97.3. DOUBLE-BLIND, PLACEBO-CONTROLLED, PARALLEL GROUP, RANDOMIZED STUDIES OF RUFINAMIDE AS ADJUNCTIVE THERAPY IN ADULT PATIENTS WITH INADEQUATELY CONTROLLED SEIZURES

Reference	Study Description/ Population	Number of Patients Per Treatment	RFA Dose (mg/day)	Results of Primary Analysis
Pålhagen et al., 2001 (18)	4-week rising-dose study in adults with partial/generalized seizures	RFA: n = 25 PLB: n = 25	Week 1: 400 Week 2: 800 Week 3: 1,200 Week 4: 1,600	Decrease in seizure frequency ratio relative to PLB ($p = .0397$)
Stefan et al., 2000 (17)	12-week, 5-arm dose-ranging study in adults with partial seizures	RFA: n = 514 PLB: n = 133	Four treatment arms: 200, 400, 800, 1,600	Significant linear trend of dose-response for seizure frequency ($p = .003$)
Vazquez et al., 2000 (19)	13-week study in adults with partial seizures	RFA: n = 156 PLB: n = 157	3,200	Decrease in partial seizure frequency relative to PLB ($p = .0158$)

PLB, placebo; RFA, rufinamide.

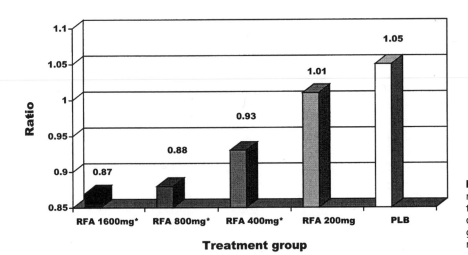

FIGURE 97.2. Median seizure frequency ratios. The results of Wilcoxon rank-sum tests were used to compare the seizure frequency ratio of each rufinamide treatment group with placebo; significant values are marked with an asterisk (all $p \leq .0274$).

baseline phase, patients entered a 13-week treatment phase; study drug was titrated to 3,200 mg/day over a 1- to 2-week period. The primary efficacy variable, percentage change in partial seizure frequency during the treatment phase relative to the baseline phase, was statistically significant in favor of the rufinamide treatment group ($p = .0158$; Wilcoxon rank-sum test). Rufinamide-treated patients had a 20.4% median reduction in partial seizure frequency, whereas placebo-treated patients had a 1.6% median increase. The percentage of patients who responded to treatment was significantly greater in the rufinamide treatment group than in the placebo treatment group. Of the rufinamide-treated patients, 28.2% experienced at least a 50% reduction in seizure frequency per 28 days relative to baseline, compared with 18.6% of the placebo-treated patients ($p = .0381$; logistic regression).

Two addition double-blind, placebo-controlled, adjunctive-therapy studies, one in primary generalized tonic-clonic seizures (n = 153, rufinamide dose 800 mg/day) and one in partial seizures in children 4 to 16 years of age (n = 269, rufinamide dose approximately 45 mg/kg/day), assessed rufinamide's safety and efficacy. The primary efficacy variable in both studies was the percentage change in seizure frequency (primary, generalized, tonic-clonic, and partial, respectively) during treatment relative to baseline. Although rufinamide decreased the respective seizure frequency in both studies, the primary efficacy analyses did not reach statistical significance.

Safety

Rufinamide as adjunctive therapy in patients with epilepsy was safe and well tolerated.

In the study of Stefan et al. (17), the most frequently reported adverse events were related to the nervous system; these events were more common in patients who received

rufinamide than placebo (52.9 % versus 40.6%, respectively). The most frequent (incidence of ≥10% in any treatment group) were headache, fatigue, dizziness, viral infection, somnolence, nausea, and diplopia. Most adverse events were mild to moderate in severity and were transient; there was no evidence of a dose–response relationship for any adverse event. The incidence of adverse events was generally similar in patients who received rufinamide 200, 400, and 800 mg/day and placebo. At the 1,600-mg/day dose, only dizziness, somnolence, and diplopia occurred with a frequency at least twice that with placebo. Rufinamide had no significant adverse effects on pulse rate or blood pressure compared with placebo, and there were no clinically relevant changes in laboratory parameters. The percentage of patients who discontinued the study prematurely because of adverse events was similar between treatments (10.3% rufinamide all doses; 6.8% placebo), although slightly higher at the top dose of rufinamide (12.0%). The incidence of serious adverse events (SAEs) was low and similar in the rufinamide-treated (n = 21; 4.1%) and the placebo-treated (n = 5; 3.8%), patients, and there were no fatal or life-threatening events.

The rufinamide dose (3,200 mg/day) in the subsequent study of Vazquez et al. (18) was twice that of the highest dose in the Stefan et al. study (17); in addition, the more bioavailable FMI formulation was used in this study. As in the Stefan et al. study (17), the most frequently reported adverse events (serious and nonserious) were central nervous system related and were more common in rufinamide-than in placebo-treated patients (80.8% versus 58.6%). Adverse events with an incidence of at least 10% were similar to the previous study; the only additional adverse events occurring with a frequency of at least 10% were ataxia, vomiting, and abnormal vision. Most adverse events in the rufinamide-treatment group were transient and mild to moderate in severity, and had onset in the titration period of the study. Although the adverse event rates were in general higher than those in the previous study, the percentage of patients who discontinued the study prematurely because of adverse events (13.5%) was similar to that in the highest dose group (12%) in the Stefan et al. study (17). The incidence of SAEs was low in both the rufinamide-treated (n = 8; 5.1%) and the placebo-treated (n = 4; 2.5%) patients. Three fatal adverse events occurred during the study: two of the patients received rufinamide and one received placebo. None of these events was suspected to be related to the study drug. As in the previous study, no treatment-emergent changes in laboratory parameters, vital signs, ECG, or physical examination results were evident.

In the two additional adjunctive therapy studies conducted in patients with primary generalized tonic-clonic seizures and in children, the most common treatment-emergent adverse events were related to the nervous system (headache and somnolence) and the gastrointestinal system (vomiting). The overall safety profile was similar to that seen in previous studies.

In all studies, rufinamide did not have a significant effect on the levels of concomitantly administered AEDs.

To date, patients have been treated with rufinamide for greater than 5 years in ongoing extension studies. No new safety findings have been noted with long-term therapy.

SUMMARY

Well controlled studies completed to date show rufinamide to be efficacious as an adjunctive treatment of partial seizures in adults. Rufinamide was effective over the dose range of 400 to 3,200 mg/day in patients with partial seizures inadequately controlled with one, two, or three concomitantly administered AEDs. Rufinamide was safe and well tolerated over the entire dose range. Although adverse events increased in frequency at the highest doses tested, the types of adverse events were similar over the entire dose range. At the highest dose (3,200 mg/day), most adverse events occurred during titration, were mild to moderate in severity, and were transient.

Based on its favorable preclinical pharmacologic, toxicologic, and pharmacokinetic profiles in humans, and proven efficacy and safety in patients with inadequately controlled partial seizures, rufinamide may be considered to be a valuable addition to currently available therapies.

REFERENCES

1. Rouan MC, Souppart C, Alif L, et al. Automated analysis of a novel antiepileptic compound, CGP33101, and its metabolite, CGP 49292, in body fluids by high-performance liquid chromatography and liquid-solid extraction. *J Chromatogr B* 1995; 667:307–313.

2. Rouan MC, Le Duigou F, Campestrini J, et al. Fast liquid chromatography for the determination of drugs in plasma and combination with liquid-solid extraction in a fully automated system. *J Chromatogr B* 1992;573:59–64.

3. White HS. Preclinical anticonvulsant profile of rufinamide (CGP33101). Presented at the 8th International Bethel-Cleveland Clinical Epilepsy Symposium, Bielefeld, Germany, 1997.

4. Schmutz M, Allgeier H, Pozza MF, et al. Rufinamide (CGP33101): broad anticonvulsant spectrum and excellent tolerability in rodents. *Epilepsia* 2000;41[Suppl Florence]:159 (abstr).

5. Löscher W. Basic aspects of epilepsy. *Curr Opin Neurol Neurosurg* 1993;6:223–232.

6. Schmutz M, Allgeier H, Jeker A, et al. Anticonvulsant profile of CGP33101 in animals. *Epilepsia* 1993;34[Suppl 2]:122(abstr).

7. Wamil AW, Schmutz M, Portet CH, et al. Effects of oxcarbazepine and 10-hydroxycarbamazepine on action potential firing and generalized seizures. *Eur J Pharmacol* 1994;271: 301–308.

8. Schütz J, Gschwind HP, Pfaar U, et al. Absorption and disposition of CGP33101 in mice, rats, dogs and baboons. Presented at the 14th European Drug Metabolism Workshop, Paris, 1994.

9. Waldmeier F, Gschwind HP, Rouan MC, et al. Metabolism of the new anticonvulsive trial drug rufinamide (CGP 33101) in healthy male volunteers. *Epilepsia* 1996;37[Suppl 5]:167(abstr).

10. Racine A, Rouan MC, Chang SW, et al. Population pharmacokinetics and drug-drug interactions of rufinamide in a multicenter, double-blind, randomized, placebo-controlled, 5-arm parallel trial in patients with partial seizures on up to three concomitant antiepileptic drugs. *Epilepsia* 2000;41[Suppl Florence]:149(abstr).

11. Sachdeo R, Rosenfeld WE, Choi L, et al. Pharmacokinetic and safety of adjunctive rufinamide therapy in pediatric patients with epilepsy. *Epilepsia* 1998;39[Suppl 6]:166–167(abstr).

12. Chang SW, Choi L, Karolchyk MA. A pharmacokinetic evaluation of rufinamide in elderly and younger subjects. *Epilepsia* 1998;39[Suppl 6]:59(abstr).

13. Chang SW, Yeh CM, Van Logtenberg M, et al. A geriatric pharmacokinetic evaluation of rufinamide. *Clin Pharmacol Ther* 2000;67(2):54(abstr).

14. Kapeghian JS, Madan A, Parkinson A, et al. Evaluation of rufinamide (CGP33101), a novel anticonvulsant, for potential drug interactions *in vitro*. *Epilepsia* 1996;37[Suppl 5]:26(abstr).

15. Svendsen K, Choi L, Chen BC, et al. Single-center, open-label, multiple-dose pharmacokinetic trial investigating the effect of rufinamide administration on Ortho-Novum 1/35 in healthy women. *Epilepsia* 1998;39[Suppl 6]:59(abstr).

16. Kalbag JB, White-VanLogtenberg M, Yeh CM, et al. Rufinamide, a novel antiepileptic drug, does not alter the pharmacokinetics of CYP1A2 substrate, olanzapine, in healthy adults. *Epilepsia* 2000;41[Suppl Florence]:150(abstr).

17. Stefan H, Remy C, Guberman A, et al. A multicenter, double-blind, randomized, placebo-control, 5-arm, parallel-group trial of rufinamide in patients with therapy-resistant partial seizures. *Epilepsia* 2000;41[Suppl Florence]:39(abstr).

18. Pålhagen S, Canger R, Henriksen O, et al. Rufinamide: a double-blind, placebo-controlled proof of principle trial in patient with epilepsy. *Epilepy Res* 2001;43:115–124.

19. Vazquez B, Sachdeo R, Maxoutova A, et al. Efficacy and safety of rufinamide as adjunctive therapy in adult patients with therapy-resistant partial-onset seizures. *Epilepsia* 2000;41[Suppl 7]:255 (abstr).

DRUGS IN DEVELOPMENT

DRUGS IN EARLY CLINICAL DEVELOPMENT

EMILIO PERUCCA
HARVEY J. KUPFERBERG

Although it is acknowledged that the second-generation antiepileptic drugs introduced in the 1990s represent a valuable addition to the therapeutic armamentarium, these drugs are far from ideal for a number of reasons. First of all, they fail to achieve the ultimate goal of producing complete seizure freedom in most patients with epilepsy refractory to older agents (33,83). Second, many of these drugs exhibit significant shortcomings in terms of adverse side effects, limited activity spectrum against different seizure types, and drug–drug interactions.

Development of newer drugs with an improved safety and efficacy profile depends to a large extent on expanding knowledge about the pathogenesis and neurobiology of epilepsy. In addition, basic science findings need to be translated into applied research because understanding the neurobiology of seizures does not necessarily mean that an effective therapy can be developed immediately through rational drug design. An example of this problem can be demonstrated by progress in knowledge about glutamate's action in the central nervous system (CNS). Although a large amount of basic research has been generated describing the glutamate receptor, its subtypes, and the channels that are influenced by it, none of the strategies aimed at counteracting specifically glutamatergic responses in the brain has as yet yielded a clinically effective treatment (84).

The persistence of major clinical needs provides a powerful driving force for continuous investment toward discovery of better antiepileptic drugs and, as a result of this, during the last few years a number of new chemical entities have been identified and tested in preclinical and clinical

Emilio Perucca, MD, PhD, FRCP (Edin): Professor of Medical Pharmacology, Clinical Pharmacology Unit, Department of Internal Medicine and Therapeutics, University of Pavia; and Consultant Clinical Pharmacologist, Institute of Neurology, C. Mondino Foundation, Pavia, Italy

Harvey J. Kupferberg, MD: Epilepsy Branch, National Institute of Neurological Disorders and Stroke, National Institutes of Health, Bethesda, Maryland

models. The compounds described in this chapter are among the latest to enter clinical development. Although history has demonstrated that only 1 of 10 compounds initially submitted for human testing will find its way to approval for clinical use, it is hoped that many of these agents will in fact fulfill their promises and eventually be of help to the multitude of patients whose seizures are not controlled by currently available anticonvulsants.

ANTIEPILEPSIRINE

Antiepilepsirine (3,4-methylendioxycynnamoylpiperine) is a potential antiepileptic drug that originally was extracted from a Chinese folk remedy, and subsequently chemically characterized and synthesized at Beijing Medical University. In preclinical studies, antiepilepsirine has been found to be effective against pentylenetetrazole (PTZ)-induced seizures at dosages of 150 to 500 mg/kg in rats (123–125). The compound also is active against audiogenic seizures in genetically epilepsy-prone rats, with a median effective dose (ED_{50}) of approximately 65 mg/kg (22,127). It is, however, ineffective in protecting against amygdaloid-kindled seizures (123). Neurochemical studies suggest that its anticonvulsant activity may be related to an increase in extracellular serotonin concentration (22,127).

A double-blind, add-on, crossover trial has been conducted in children with refractory partial or generalized epilepsies who were given antiepilepsirine (10 mg/kg/day) or placebo each for 3-month periods (125). Only 34 patients completed the study because the parents of 24 children refused permission to cross over to the alternate treatment at the completion of the first 3 months. In those patients who completed the 6-month study, seizures were fewer during the antiepilepsirine period than during the placebo period. There were no changes in serum levels of concomitant antiepileptic drugs, and no serious acute side effects were recorded.

AWD 131-138

AWD 131-138 [1-(4-chlorophenyl)-4-morpholino-imida-zolin-2-one] was selected for development by Asta Medica (Radebeul, Germany) because of its broad-spectrum anti-convulsant effects and its potency in tests predictive of anx-iolytic activity. It is currently in phase I clinical development.

Anticonvulsant Activity in Animal Models. In rats and mice, AWD 131-138 protects against seizures induced by maximal electroshock (MES) and supramaximal stimulation with PTZ and bicuculline (9,91,113). It also is effective in seizure threshold tests with intravenous (i.v.) PTZ and elec-trical stimulation in mice. Audiogenic seizures in DBA/2 and Frings mice are potently inhibited, with intraperitoneal (i.p.) ED_{50} values of 2.6 and 5.0 mg/kg, respectively (9,114). AWD 131-138 increases dose dependently the threshold for induction of afterdischarges in amygdala-kindled rats, the effect being already detectable at 1 mg/kg i.p., the lowest dose tested. Secondary generalization of the kindled seizures is completely inhibited at 20 mg/kg i.p., and at doses of 20 and 30 mg/kg i.p., kindling acquisition also is significantly delayed. In WAG rats, a model for absence epilepsy, AWD 131-138 suppresses dose dependently spontaneous spike–wave discharges, with almost complete suppression at 30 mg/kg orally (p.o.) (114).

Activities in Other Models. AWD 131-138 is active in several mouse and rat models of anxiolytic activity (92). In rats, the ratio between the median toxic dose (TD_{50}) in the Rotorod test and the dose inducing anticonvulsant and anx-iolytic activity (~3 mg/kg) is 333 after p.o. administration

Mechanism of Action. The mechanism of action of AWD 131-138 appears to involve, at least in part, dose-dependent blockade of voltage-activated calcium channels (9). An inhibiting action on the increase in action potentials firing induced by corticotropin-releasing factor in locus ceruleus neurons of murine brainstem slices also may be relevant for anxiolytic activity. AWD 131-138 shows very low affinity [median inhibitory concentration (IC_{50}) ~5.8 μmol/L] and very low intrinsic activity at benzodiazepine receptor sites (91,97), and it is not identified as a benzodiazepine-like drug in discrimination tests in primates (128).

GANAXOLONE

Ganaxolone (3α-hydroxy-3β-methyl-5α-pregnan-20-one, CCD 1042) is a member of a new class of neuroactive steroids called epalons, which allosterically modulate the type A γ-aminobutyric acid (GABA_A) receptor. The synthe-sis and development of this compound at CoCensys, Inc. (Irvine, CA) was stimulated by the observation that endoge-nously occurring metabolites of progesterone and deoxycor-ticosterone exhibit significant anticonvulsant activity in ani-mal models (18). Ganaxolone has already undergone early phase II trials in patients with epilepsy.

Anticonvulsant Activity in Animal Models. In rodents, ganaxolone shows potent protective activity against seizures induced by PTZ, bicuculline, aminophylline, t-butyl-bicy-clo-phosphorothionate, fluorothyl, and corneal kindling, whereas its activity in the MES test is comparatively weak (5,15,32,65).

Mechanism of Action. The anticonvulsant effects of gana-xolone are considered to be mediated by stereoselective, high-affinity positive modulation of the GABA_A receptor through an interaction with a specific recognition site (34). Although ganaxolone retains some structural similarity with progesterone, it has no detectable hormonal activity (6).

Pharmacokinetics. After oral administration with a high-fat meal in healthy volunteers, peak plasma ganaxolone concentrations are achieved within 1 to 3 hours and decline thereafter biexponentially, with a terminal half-life of 37 to 70 hours (75).

Drug Interactions. In preliminary studies, add-on use of ganaxolone in patients with epilepsy did not result in changes in the plasma concentration of concomitant anti-convulsants (59).

Clinical Trial Data. Tolerability studies in healthy volun-teers used dosages up to 1,500 mg/day in three divided daily administrations for treatment periods up to 3 weeks. The most commonly observed adverse events were seda-tion, dizziness, headache, gastrointestinal disturbances, fatigue, unsteady gait, and impaired concentration (74,75). Side effects were more common in women than in men, despite similar plasma ganaxolone concentrations in both sexes. In a small trial in children given dosages up to 12 mg/kg three times daily, adverse events included somno-lence, sleep disturbances, nervousness, constipation and, in one case, disturbed behavior and cognition (59). In another open-label, add-on trial in 20 children with refractory infantile spasms, ganaxolone given at dosages up to 36 mg/kg/day was well tolerated, and a 50% or greater improvement in seizure frequency was observed in one-third of the patients (47).

A proof-of-concept, double-blind, monotherapy study has been completed in which 52 patients undergoing assess-ment for epilepsy surgery were withdrawn from preexisting medication and randomized to receive ganaxolone (500 mg three times daily on day 1 and 625 mg three times daily on days 2 to 8) or placebo (55). Patients were required to exit the study if seizure control was deemed unacceptable. Fifty percent of patients randomized to ganaxolone completed the treatment period, compared with 25% of those randomized to placebo. Although intent-to-treat analysis just failed to reach statistical significance, secondary analyses did suggest that ganaxolone had antiepileptic activity in these patients. In this study, the tolerability of ganaxolone was similar to that observed with placebo.

HARKOSERIDE

Harkoseride (*R*-2-acetamido-*N*-benzyl-3-methoxypropionamide) belongs to a series of propionamides synthesized at Schwarz Pharma in Manheim, Germany. These compounds have substitutions that generate an asymmetric carbon atom, giving rise to *R*- and *S*-enantiomers. Stereoselectivity for anticonvulsant activity resides only in the *R* configuration. Harkoseride can be termed a *functional amino acid* because it is an optical antipode of the naturally occurring amino acid L-serine. Its amphiphilic character imparts water solubility and transmembrane passage.

Anticonvulsant Activity in Animal Models. Harkoseride is active in primary screening tests for anticonvulsant activity in mice and rats using electrically induced seizures. After i.p. administration, ED_{50} in the MES test is 4.5 mg/kg in mice and 3.9 mg/kg in rats (9). In the audiogenic seizure susceptible Frings mouse model, i.p. ED_{50} is 0.63 mg/kg. The protective indices in these models are excellent, being 6, >500, and 46, respectively. Harkoseride does not attenuate the clonic seizures induced by subcutaneous (s.c.) administration of PTZ, bicuculline, or picrotoxin. Hippocampal-kindled seizures in rats were suppressed after i.p. administration of harkoseride. Both the behavioral expressions of seizures and seizure afterdischarge duration decreased in a dose-dependent manner, and the ED_{50} for harkoseride's ability to block the generalized kindled seizures was 13.5 mg/kg. The focal seizures (e.g., twitching of the vibrissae and automatisms) were attenuated at the higher doses.

Harkoseride is effective in blocking repetitive seizures in various models of status epilepticus, including the status induced by stimulation of the perforant pathway, the cobalt–homocysteine thiolactone model, and the lithium–pilocarpine model (9). In the focal model of status epilepticus induced by cobalt–homocysteine thiolactone, harkoseride blocks the secondarily generalized seizures (ED_{50}, 45.4 mg/kg), but focal seizures are unaffected.

Mechanism of Action. Receptor binding studies have revealed an interaction at the strychnine-insensitive glycine site of the N-methyl-D-aspartate (NMDA) receptor complex. At this site, harkoseride displaces the radioligand 5,7-dichlorokynurenic acid, with an IC_{50} of 5.2 μmol/L. To test the hypothesis that harkoseride modulates the strychnine-insensitive glycine receptor, the glycine agonist D-serine was administered intracerebroventricularly. The dose–response curve for harkoseride anticonvulsant activity in the MES test was shifted to the right when D-serine was combined (ED_{50} for harkoseride alone 1.0 mg/kg, versus 2.7 mg/kg when combined with D-serine).

In electrophysiologic experiments, harkoseride did not affect NMDA-evoked currents at nonsaturating or saturating glycine concentrations. At −90mV, harkoseride (100 μmol/L) had no effect at the voltage-sensitive sodium channel, whereas phenytoin (100 μmol/L) produced a marked inhibition.

Pharmacokinetics. In early studies to determine safety, tolerability, and pharmacokinetics, harkoseride was given to healthy male volunteers as single i.v. doses up to 300 mg, single oral doses up to 600 mg, and multiple oral doses up to 200 mg twice daily for 7 days. Absorption from the gastrointestinal tract was rapid (9). The plasma half-life was approximately 12 hours and plasma protein binding was less than 1%. The areas under the curve (AUC) after a 100-mg dose administered p.o. and i.v. were nearly identical, indicating virtually complete oral bioavailability. Plasma concentrations and AUCs were proportional to the administered dose.

Tolerability Data in Humans. The most frequently observed adverse events in tolerability studies were headache, dizziness, and lightheadedness.

LOSIGAMONE

Losigamone, or threo (±)5(*R,S*),α(*S,R*)-5-[(2-chlorophenyl) hydroxy-methyl)]-4-methoxy(5H)-furanone, is a racemic mixture of two enantiomers synthesized at the Willmar Schwabe Company in Karlsruhe, Germany. The *S*(+)-enantiomer (AO-242) is more potent than the *R*(−)-enantiomer (AO-294) in most pharmacologic tests (130).

Anticonvulsant Activity in Animal Models. In experiments conducted in rodents, losigamone inhibits in a dose-dependent manner the tonic hindleg extension produced by electroshock, PTZ, bicuculline, nicotine, and 4-aminopyridine (108). It also attenuates the clonic seizures induced by PTZ, bicuculline, and picrotoxin, whereas it has no effect on the hindleg extension caused by strychnine and picrotoxin or the clonic seizures induced by NMDA. Five- to 7-day administration of 7 mg/kg losigamone to rats produced no evidence of tolerance to anticonvulsant activity (108). Losigamone has been found to protect against audiogenic seizures in rats and gerbils, and against PTZ-induced kindling in mice (84).

Mechanism of Action. Losigamone reduces the frequency of spontaneous and stimulus-induced epileptiform discharges in the presence of picrotoxin (48) or low Ca^{2+} or low Mg^{2+} in rat hippocampal slices (49). Similar results were observed in experiments using high potassium, low magnesium, and low calcium concentrations in hippocampal slices, and in experiments with low magnesium concentrations in the CA1 and CA3 region of the hippocampus and in the entorhinal cortex (84). In the entorhinal cortex, losigamone reduces repetitive spike firing elicited by depolarizing current and depresses moderately stimulus-induced excitatory postsynaptic potentials, whereas monosynaptic fast and slow inhibitory postsynaptic potentials are unaffected (103). Losigamone also has been found to decrease 4-aminopyridine–induced epileptiform activity in rat hippocampal slices (129). A primarily presynaptic mode of action dependent on functional sodium channels was suggested by experiments in cultured rat hippocampal neurons (26). Postsynaptic mechanisms also have been suggested for losigamone. A direct binding of losigamone with the GABA, picrotoxin, or benzodiazepine receptors has not been demonstrated. Losigamone does enhance chloride uptake in mouse spinal cord neurons in the absence of GABA, and potentiates the effects of GABA (23). In separate studies, racemic losigamone suppressed depolarizations induced by NMDA, but not those induced by α-amino-3-hydroxy-5-methyl-4-isoxazole propionate (AMPA) (106). In another study, $S(+)$ losigamone 100 μmol/L and 200 μmol/L significantly reduced both potassium- and veratridine-elicited release of glutamate and aspartate from cortical slices, whereas $R(-)$ losigamone had no effect on release of the amino acids at 400 μmol/L (42). The conclusions from the latter study were that the mechanism of anticonvulsant activity was partly due to effects on glutamate release.

Pharmacokinetics. In healthy volunteers, losigamone pharmacokinetics are linear after single oral doses ranging from 100 to 700 mg, or multiple doses up to 600 mg three times daily for 28 days (10,108). Losigamone is absorbed rapidly from the gastrointestinal tract, with peak plasma concentrations usually observed after 2 to 3 hours. The compound is approximately 60% bound to plasma proteins (109), and its apparent volume of distribution is approximately 1.5 L/kg (108). Mean apparent oral clearance (Cl/F) after single doses in healthy volunteers is approximately 300 to 400 mL/min, whereas mean half-life and mean residence time are approximately 4 and 7 hours, respectively. Although these estimates are based on measurement of racemic drug concentrations, there are important pharmacokinetic differences between enantiomers. A single-step liquid–liquid extraction followed by a reverse-phase high-performance liquid chromatography on a chiral column was used to separate and quantitate the enantiomers of losigamone in human plasma after oral administration of racemic losigamone (115,116). The apparent oral clearance of the $R(-)$-enantiomer was found to be approximately 10-fold higher than that of the $S(+)$-enantiomer (84,115). In

healthy volunteers, the half-life of the $R(-)$-enantiomer was approximately 2.2 hours, compared with 4.8 hours for the $S(+)$-enantiomer. Studies based on recording of auditory evoked potentials in healthy volunteers suggest that the duration of effect may be longer than anticipated from the plasma half-life (101).

Only traces of unchanged losigamone are detected in urine. Approximately 15% of an orally administered dose is excreted in urine as a glucuronide conjugate. A conjugate also accounts for 11% to 32% of the total concentration of the drug in plasma (118). Losigamone undergoes oxidative biotransformation. Of five metabolites identified from human liver microsomes, M1 and M5 were identified as phenolic analogues, with M5 probably corresponding to 5'-hydroxy-($\pm$)-losigamone (115). Two additional metabolites, M3 and M4, were considered to be precursors of M5, whereas the fifth metabolite, M2, appeared to be a nonphenolic substance. Metabolism is stereoselective, with M1 being primarily produced from the $S(+)$-enantiomer and M3, M4, and M5 being formed preferentially from the $R(-)$-enantiomer. The main cytochrome P450 (CYP) isoenzyme involved in the metabolism of both enantiomers appeared to be CYP2A6. *In vitro*, the formation of the M1 metabolite was markedly inhibited by $R(-)$-losigamone.

Drug Interactions. Losigamone elimination is accelerated by concomitant administration of enzyme-inducing anticonvulsants. Cl/F values slightly in excess of 500 to 600 mL/min and mean half-lives of approximately 3.8 hours have been described in patients comedicated with carbamazepine and phenytoin, resulting in plasma losigamone levels that are reduced by approximately one-third compared with those observed in non-comedicated healthy volunteers receiving comparable doses (24,51,53). Losigamone pharmacokinetics do not appear to be affected by valproic acid (52) and lamotrigine (24).

In clinical studies, losigamone did not affect the serum concentration of phenytoin, carbamazepine, carbamazepine-10,11-epoxide, and lamotrigine (52,99,108). Likewise, losigamone has not been found to affect the metabolism of antipyrine and caffeine (10). At a dosage of 1,000 mg/day, losigamone may reduce slightly the plasma concentration of valproic acid (52,53).

Clinical Trial Data. Open pilot studies suggested that the optimal dosage of losigamone, added to preexisting anticonvulsant medication, may be in the order of 1,500 mg/day in three divided doses (84). In a randomized, double-blind, parallel-group, add-on trial completed in 203 patients with refractory partial epilepsy (27), median reduction in seizure frequency in the group allocated to losigamone (500 mg three times daily) was significantly greater than that in the placebo group, but the magnitude of the effect was relatively modest (15% versus 7%, *p* < .005).

Adverse events most commonly associated with losigamone include dizziness and fatigue. Headache, sedation, diplopia, ataxia, dysarthria, restlessness, nausea, vomiting, and palpitations have been reported with a lower frequency (10,84). Although an elevation of liver enzymes has been described, none of over 400 patients included in clinical trials at dosages up to 1,500 mg/day dropped out because of hepatic toxicity (10).

NPS 1776

Many carboxylic acids and their ester and amide derivatives are known to have CNS activity and to protect experimental animals against PTZ-induced seizures (54). NPS 1776 (3-methylbutanamide, or isovaleramide) is a branched-chain aliphatic amide originally discovered by NPS Pharmaceuticals, Inc. (Salt Lake City, UT) Exclusive worldwide rights to the development and marketing of this compound have been acquired by Abbott Laboratories (Abbott Park, IL).

Anticonvulsant Activity in Animal Models. NPS 1776 possesses in animal models an activity profile comparable with that of valproic acid, with a range of findings predictive of broad-spectrum efficacy against partial and generalized seizures (126). The p.o. ED_{50} against MES-induced tonic extension seizures is 76 mg/kg in rats and 913 mg/kg in mice. The ED_{50} in blocking PTZ-induced clonic seizures after p.o. administration is 205 and 748 mg/kg in rats and mice, respectively (9). In the i.v. PTZ seizure threshold test, NPS 1776 elevates seizure threshold. NPS 1776 also is active in attenuating the tonic phase of sound-induced seizures in the Frings mouse, with an ED_{50} of 207 mg/kg after p.o. administration. NPS 1776 also protects against clonic seizures induced by s.c. picrotoxin (ED_{50}, 103 mg/kg), and is partially effective against clonic seizures induced by s.c. bicuculline in mice. In experiments conducted in Frings mice, no evidence of tolerance to the anticonvulsant effect was observed when animals were treated daily with NPS 1776 for 4 consecutive weeks.

In animal models of partial seizures, NPS1776 blocks the fully generalized kindled seizures in corneal- and amygdala-kindled rats, with ED_{50} values of 127 and 140 mg/kg, respectively (9). The effects of NPS 1776 are comparable with those of valproate on both behavioral effects and electrographic seizure duration. NPS1776 also has been found to delay the acquisition of kindling in the amygdala-kindled rat, suggesting that it may exhibit antiepileptogenic effects.

Mechanism of Action. As is the case with valproic acid, the mechanism of the anticonvulsant action of NPS 1776 has not been clarified. NPS 1776 does not interact in any *in vitro* receptor assay at concentrations up to 300 µmol/L.

Pharmacokinetics. When administered as an oral solution to healthy volunteers at doses ranging between 100 and 1,600 mg, NPS 1776 is absorbed rapidly from the gastrointestinal tract and peak plasma concentrations are achieved in 30 to 45 minutes (9). NPS 1776 does not bind to plasma proteins and shows a relatively short half-life of approximately 2.5 hours. Although half-life values were similar across the explored dose range, there was a trend for apparent oral clearance and volume of distribution to decrease slightly with increasing single oral doses. Renal excretion does not appear to play a major role in NPS 1776 elimination, with only 2% to 4% of the administered dose being excreted in urine within 24 hours.

After treatment with total daily doses of 1,200 to 2,400 mg, given in three divided administrations, pharmacokinetic parameters are essentially the same as those observed after a single dose. Because of the short half-life, steady-state plasma levels are achieved in 2 days. Intersubject variability in pharmacokinetic parameters appears to be relatively low, and peak plasma concentrations and AUC values are proportional to dose.

Drug Interactions. NPS 1776 does not inhibit any of the major CYP drug-metabolizing enzymes in experiments performed *in vitro*.

Tolerability Data in Humans. Dosages up to 2,400 mg/day in three divided daily administrations have been tolerated well in healthy volunteers (9).

NW-1015

NW-1015, formerly known as PNU-151774E, was originally discovered by the Pharmacia-Upjohn group (Milan, Italy) (85), and currently is being developed by the Newron company in Gerenzano, Italy. Chemically, it corresponds to (S)-(+)-2-4-[(3-fluorobenzyloxy) benzylamino] propanamide methansulfonate. Pharmacologically, it combines multiple mechanisms of action, including blockade of voltage-dependent sodium channels, modulation of calcium channels, and inhibition of monoamine oxidase B (MAO-B) activity.

Anticonvulsant Activity in Animal Models. NW-1015 prevents seizure spread in a wide variety of animal models, with a potency similar to or greater than that of most classic antiepileptic drugs (28). The oral ED_{50} in the MES test is 8.2 mg/kg in mice and 12.8 mg/kg in rats; these dosages are much lower than neurotoxic doses, the protective index (MES ED_{50}/Rotorod TD_{50}, p.o.) being 76 in rats (9). NW-1015 is effective against seizures induced by bicuculline, picrotoxin, 3-methyl-aspartate, strychnine, and NMDA, as well as against seizures induced by amygdaloid kindling in rats (9,28,71). In the kainate model in rats, NW-1015 protects against convulsions and the resulting neuronal dam-

age, with an approximately 40% reduction in number of animals experiencing status epilepticus observed at 10 mg/kg i.p. (70). In a model of partial complex seizures in the conscious monkey, NW-1015 25 mg/kg p.o. reduces the behavioral paroxysms associated with afterdischarge-generating stimuli to the amygdala; plasma levels associated with this effect are in the order of 5 μg/mL, and at plasma levels of 9 μg/mL, local afterdischarge also is significantly reduced (29).

Activity in Other Models. A neuroprotectant activity of NW-1015 has been documented in its ability to prevent neuronal cell loss induced by kainic acid in rats and by cerebral ischemia in gerbils (84).

Mechanisms of Action. NW-1015 binds to the batrachotoxin recognition site of the sodium channel with an IC_{50} of 8.2 μmol/L, and it is more potent than carbamazepine, phenytoin, and lamotrigine as a blocker of voltage-dependent sodium channels (100). In rat hippocampal slices, NW-1015 inhibits the release of aspartate and glutamate evoked by veratridine and KCl stimulation. Additional properties include modulation of calcium channels (100), affinity for the sigma-1 receptor in receptor ligand assays (84), and selective inhibition of MAO-B (IC_{50}, 0.08 μmol/L) in rat and human brain tissue. It has been claimed that the latter effect, through reduction of free radical formation (111), might play a role in preventing epileptogenesis after trauma and cerebrovascular accident (9).

Pharmacokinetics. NW-1015 shows linear pharmacokinetics. After single oral doses ranging from 1 to 10 mg/kg and multiple doses ranging from 1.25 to 5.0 mg/kg/day in healthy volunteers, peak plasma concentrations proportional to dose were reached in approximately 2 hours, and the elimination half-life was in the order of 21 to 23 hours (9). After multiple dosing, steady-state plasma levels were achieved at approximately day 5.

Drug Interactions. *In vitro*, NW-1015 exerts no inducing or inhibiting activity on the main CYP isoenzymes known to be involved in the metabolism of other antiepileptic drugs (9).

Pharmacodynamic Studies in Humans. In healthy volunteers, doses of NW-1015 as low as 75 and 150 μg/kg have been found to inhibit platelet MAO-B activity by up to 75%. Higher doses resulted in complete and long-lasting MAO-B inhibition, whereas MAO-A was unaffected even at the highest dose tested (10 mg/kg) (9).

In tolerability studies in healthy volunteers, NW-1015 was in general well tolerated. Headache, somnolence, and lightheadedness were transiently reported by a few subjects at the highest doses tested (10 mg/kg single dose and 5 mg/kg/day repeated dosing).

REMACEMIDE

The discovery of remacemide, or (±)2-amino-*N*-(1-methyl-1,2-diphenylethyl)-acetamide monohydrochloride, resulted from a screening program for new anticonvulsants and neuroprotectants conducted by Fisons (currently Astra-Zeneca Loughborough, England) (17). Remacemide has undergone extensive clinical studies, but development plans are being reassessed after the compound was found to be inferior to carbamazepine in a recent monotherapy trial (9).

Anticonvulsant Activity in Animal Models. In mice, remacemide is active against seizures induced by MES (ED_{50}, 48 mg/kg p.o., versus 22 mg/kg p.o. in the rat), NMDA (ED_{50}, 57 mg/kg. i.p.), kainic acid (ED_{50}, 60 mg/kg), and 4-aminopyridine (ED_{50}, 18 mg/kg i.p.) (9,17,31,79,107). It also is effective in antagonizing audiogenic seizures in mice and status epilepticus induced by injection of homocysteine thiolactone in rats with a cortical cobalt focus (17,119), whereas it shows no protection against seizures induced by PTZ, bicuculline, picrotoxin, or strychnine (17). Remacemide is ineffective in preventing kindled seizures induced by subthreshold bicorneal stimulation in rats (31,80), but at doses of 50 to 240 mg/kg s.c. it protects against kindled seizures induced by hippocampal stimulation in the same species (17).

In most animal models, the desglycinyl metabolite is more potent than remacemide, but it also is more toxic (17,79). Some differences in activity have also been detected between the (*S*)- and (*R*)-enantiomers of both parent drug and metabolite, with the (*S*)-forms being slightly more potent both in terms of anticonvulsant effect and neurotoxicity (31,79). These differences, however, were considered insignificant in biologic terms.

Activities in Other Models. Remacemide exerts protective activity against neuronal damage caused by hypoxia and ischemia in rodents, cats, and dogs (3,79,84). In addition, remacemide potentiates the antiparkinsonian activity of levodopa in animal models of Parkinson's disease (36), an observation that led to exploratory trials in parkinsonian patients (84).

Compared with more potent noncompetitive NMDA receptor antagonists, remacemide lacks abuse potential (40) and produces fewer adverse behavioral effects (84). In toxicology studies, large acute doses of remacemide (≥160 mg s.c.), similar to other NMDA antagonists, cause neuronal vacuolation in various brain regions. This effect is thought to be due to exposure to high concentrations of the desglycinyl metabolite and has not been considered relevant to human safety issues (17).

Mechanism of Action. Remacemide and its desglycinyl metabolite are low-affinity, noncompetitive antagonists of NMDA receptors, with $IC_{50}s$ for inhibition of MK801 binding in the order of 68 μmol/L and 0.48 μmol/L, respectively (81). *In vivo*, the difference in potency between remacemide and its metabolite in inhibiting NMDA-induced seizures and death are less marked than expected from *in vitro* studies, presumably because *in vivo*, the metabolite contributes to the effects of the parent drug (17). In addition to blocking NMDA receptors, remacemide and its desglycinyl metabolite exhibit a blocking action on voltage-dependent sodium channels, with the metabolite again more potent in this effect (84,121).

Pharmacokinetics. At dosages in the clinically used range, remacemide exhibits linear pharmacokinetics. Remacemide is absorbed rapidly from the gastrointestinal tract and reaches peak plasma concentration in 1 hour, whereas the desglycinyl metabolite takes 2 to 3 hours to reach maximum concentration (9). Concomitant ingestion of food may delay the time to peak concentration without affecting the extent of absorption. A volume of distribution of 5 to 6 L/kg, calculated after i.v. dosing in healthy subjects, indicates extensive penetration into tissues (17). The extent of binding to plasma proteins is 75% for remacemide and approximately 90% for the desglycinyl metabolite. In noncomedicated subjects, the half-life of remacemide is 3 to 4 hours, whereas the half-life of the desglycinyl metabolite is approximately 12 to 15 hours (17,77,80). In subjects dosed with 300 mg twice daily, mean peak and trough levels of remacemide were 1,069 and 124 ng/mL, respectively, compared with 143 and 89 ng/mL, respectively, for the metabolite (17). Remacemide is virtually entirely metabolized. In addition to cleavage of the glycine group by aminopeptidases in hepatic and extrahepatic tissues, biotransformation routes include CYP-mediated oxidation and glucuronidation to a carbamoyl glucuronide (17).

Drug Interactions. Enzyme-inducing anticonvulsants such as carbamazepine, phenytoin, and barbiturates increase the clearance of both remacemide and its desglycinyl metabolite. In enzyme-induced patients, the AUCs of remacemide and desglycinyl remacemide are reduced by 25% to 50% and 70%, respectively, compared with values recorded in healthy subjects (17,56,57,102). Valproate, on the other hand, has no major effects on remacemide pharmacokinetics (84).

Remacemide inhibits CYP3A4 and by this mechanism increases the plasma concentration of carbamazepine by approximately 30% (56,58,88). Some increase in plasma phenytoin levels has been observed in occasional patients, probably due to concomitant inhibition of CYP2C9 (17,88), whereas plasma valproic acid levels usually are unaffected.

Antiepileptic Efficacy and Adverse Effects. An initial double-blind, add-on, crossover trial in 23 patients with refractory partial epilepsy showed a median 33% seizure reduction during 4 weeks of treatment with remacemide, 150 mg four times daily, compared with placebo, but interpretation of the findings was complicated by a concomitant increase in serum carbamazepine levels (19). Two subsequent parallel-group, placebo-controlled, dose-ranging studies in similar populations of patients evaluated total daily doses of 300, 600, or 1,200 mg/day in a four times daily regimen, and 300, 600, or 800 mg/day in a twice daily regimen. Each treatment lasted for 8 weeks, there were approximately 60 patients per treatment arm, and changes in plasma levels of concomitantly administered carbamazepine and phenytoin were minimized by adjusting dosage of comedication. In the four times daily study, the proportion of patients showing at least 50% seizure reduction compared with baseline was 23% at the highest dosage, compared with 7% on placebo (pairwise comparison *p* = .03) (7). The twice daily study also demonstrated a greater responder rate at the highest dose than on placebo (30 versus 15%, pairwise comparison *p* = .05) (41).

Two monotherapy studies have been completed. The first involved treatment at 600 mg/day for up to 10 days in 61 patients undergoing neurosurgical evaluation and showed a longer time to fourth seizure with remacemide (6.8 days) than with placebo (3.8 days; *p* = .045), as well as a halving of median seizure counts (6.2 versus 12.8, *p* = .033) (8). The second was a multicenter, double-blind, flexible-dose comparison of remacemide (approximately 600 mg/day) with carbamazepine in 570 patients with newly diagnosed epilepsy, using sequential analysis of time to seizure recurrence. Preliminary results of this trial indicate that the efficacy of remacemide is inferior to that of carbamazepine (9).

To date, more than 1,400 patients have been exposed to remacemide in doses up to 2,400 mg/day, which corresponds to a safety database of over 1,200 patient-years. Most commonly observed adverse experiences include dizziness, ataxia, somnolence, abdominal pain, dyspepsia, nausea, vomiting, fatigue, and diplopia. These usually are mild and transient, but they have been a cause of discontinuation in approximately 15% of patients.

RETIGABINE

Retigabine, or *N*-[2-amino-4-(4-fluorobenzyl-amino)-phenyl] carbamic acid ethyl ester, formerly know as D23129, is a flupirtine derivative endowed with broad-spectrum anticonvulsant activity and low neurotoxic potential in a wide variety of animal models. It is being developed by Wyeth-Ayerst (Philadelphia, PA) and is undergoing phase IIb clinical trials.

Anticonvulsant Activity in Animal Models.
Retigabine protects against seizures in the threshold and supramaximal electroshock test, and it also is effective in inhibiting seizures induced by PTZ, picrotoxin, penicillin,

kainate, and intracerebroventricular NMDA (43,89,90,94), as well as audiogenic seizures in GEPR-3 and GEPR-9 rats (21) and DBA/2 mice (89). Retigabine exhibits considerable potency in delaying epileptogenesis and in protecting against focal and generalized seizures in the amygdala-kindled model (43,112). At a dosage of 5 mg/kg i.p., retigabine blocks status epilepticus induced by systemic administration of homocysteine thiolactone in rats with actively epileptogenic cortical cobalt lesions (120).

The electrophysiologic effects of retigabine have been investigated in a number of models. In 4-aminopyridine–treated rat hippocampal slices, retigabine suppresses spontaneous bursts in CA1 and CA3 areas, and eliminates afterdischarge-like trains of population spikes induced by a single electrical stimulation pulse without interfering with the normal evoked potentials (129). In other brain slice models of drug-resistant epileptiform discharges, retigabine was the only compound to produce a concentration-dependent inhibition of paroxysmal activity (1,2). In human brain slices obtained from surgical specimens, retigabine suppressed the epileptiform discharges that appear at low magnesium concentrations, and abolished spontaneous field potentials at concentrations that were without effect on evoked field potentials (110). Suppression of epileptiform discharges in a low-calcium hippocampal slice model suggests an extrasynaptic site of action (25).

Activities in Other Models. Retigabine improves learning and memory in rat models of cerebral ischemia and electroshock-induced amnesia (89,90). Retigabine also has been found to exert dose-dependent activity in two models of neuropathic pain, the formalin test and a spinal nerve injury test (93).

Mechanisms of Action. Retigabine is considered to act, at least in part, through selective activation of neuronal potassium channels. Enhancement of potassium conductance by retigabine has been demonstrated in a hippocampal slice preparation (39), in cortical neurons, in neuron growth factor–differentiated PC12 cells, and in oocytes expressing the KCNQ2 and KCNQ3 potassium channels, but not in glial and undifferentiated PC12 cells (69,95,96). Studies designed to characterize the mode of interaction with potassium channels showed that retigabine behaves as an M-channel agonist, possibly through a preferential interaction with the KCNQ2 channel, without interacting with the cyclic adenosine monophosphate modulatory site (69,98,122). Alterations in potassium channels have been implicated among causes of epilepsy (104). In addition to its action on potassium channels, retigabine may enhance GABAergic transmission through stimulation of GABA synthesis and amplification of GABA-induced currents (43–45,89).

Pharmacokinetics. Retigabine exhibits linear pharmacokinetics, at least within the range of 50 to 600 mg as single doses or 50 to 200 mg twice daily as multiple doses (9). After oral administration, absorption is rapid and peak plasma concentrations usually are achieved within 1 hour. Retigabine is eliminated predominantly by *N*-glucuronidation and acetylation.

The elimination half-life in healthy volunteers is 9 to 11 hours on average, and it is similar after single or multiple doses. After a single 200-mg dose, retigabine half-life has been found to be slightly longer in elderly men (12.2 ± 4.2 hours) than in young men (8.5 ± 2.2 hours) or elderly women (8.9 ± 1.4 hours). In the same study, however, peak concentrations were higher in elderly women than in elderly men (717 ± 409 versus 354 ± 119 ng/mL) (9).

Drug Interactions. In a pharmacokinetic study in healthy subjects, treatment with retigabine, 300 mg twice daily had no effect on the pharmacokinetics of a single 200-mg oral dose of lamotrigine. Likewise, administration of lamotrigine, 25 mg/day, did not affect the pharmacokinetics of a single dose of retigabine (9).

Clinical Trial Data. In a safety and tolerability add-on study, a total of 46 patients with refractory partial seizures were divided into three groups and received mean maintenance retigabine dosages of 360, 800, and 950 mg/day, given in two divided doses for approximately 3 months. The most commonly observed adverse events included ataxia, blurred vision, and vertigo, which were of mild to moderate intensity in most cases. There were no abnormalities in laboratory data, vital signs, and ECGs. Eighteen patients entered a long-term extension study, and 13 are still on treatment at dosages between 600 and 1,400 mg/day (9).

SORETOLIDE

Soretolide [2,6-dimethyl *N*-(5-methyl-3-isoxazolyl) benzamide, ADD169026, D-2916] is a benzamide derivative being developed for the treatment of partial seizures with or without secondary generalization. Its preclinical anticonvulsant profile was established in collaboration with Biocodex (Paris, France) and the Antiepileptic Drug Development (ADD) Program, Epilepsy Branch, National Institute of Neurological Disorders and Stroke. In general, benzamides have been used for several clinical applications, and agents as pharmacologically distinct as anticholinergics, anesthetics, and antiarrhythmics are known to possess a benzamide structure. None of the approved anticonvulsants, however, belongs to this chemical class.

Anticonvulsant Activity in Animal Models. Soretolide is active in preventing the tonic phase after MES stimulation in rodents. In the MES test, the ED_{50} is 19.2 mg/kg p.o. in rats and 61.8 mg/kg i.p. in mice. Soretolide is metabolized in several species to an active hydroxylated derivative, 2,6 dimethyl *N*-(5-hydroxymethy-3-isoxazolyl) benzamide (D-3187), which is twice as potent as the parent compound in animal models of anticonvulsant activity. In the MES, the ED_{50} of D3187 in rats and mice is 10.1 and 33.8 mg/kg, respectively (35,60). Both soretolide and its metabolite are inactive in protecting against the clonic seizures induced by PTZ, bicuculline, and picrotoxin, and in blocking the generalized or focal seizures in the hippocampal-kindled rat model after i.p. administration.

Mechanism of Action. *In vitro* experiments failed to detect any interactions with the glutamate receptors, GABA receptors, and sodium receptors or channels.

Pharmacokinetics. In clinical pharmacology studies, soretolide was given to healthy volunteers in oral doses ranging from 50 to 3,000 mg. Absorption was relatively rapid, with peak plasma levels usually observed in approximately 90 minutes. The peak concentration of the hydroxylated active metabolite, D-3187, was reached in approximately 3 hours and was consistently greater than that of the parent drug. Of the different formulations tested, the tablet and the suspension forms were found to be superior to the originally used capsules, and to produce peak plasma concentrations and AUC values proportional to dose within the dose range 125 to 1,000 mg. Soretolide is approximately 75% bound to plasma proteins, and studies in experimental animals indicate that it distributes uniformly throughout body tissues. In healthy volunteers, the half-life of soretolide is 3 to 9 hour, whereas the half life of D-3187 is 5 to 14 hours (84). Soretolide is not excreted unchanged in urine to any significant extent. It undergoes extensive oxidative metabolism by hydroxylation of the 5-methyl group of the isoxazole moiety, through intervention of the microsomal enzymes CYP1A2 and CYP2C19 (38,61). D3187 is further metabolized to the carboxylic acid (D-3269).

Drug Interactions. Interaction studies *in vitro* showed that both soretolide and D-3187 inhibit the enzyme isoform CYP2C19. Although this may suggest a potential for inhibiting the metabolism of phenytoin, the inhibition constant for this reaction leads to the prediction that soretolide should cause little or no changes in serum phenytoin concentration.

Tolerability Data in Humans. Soretolide has been given to patients with uncontrolled epilepsy in a tolerability study at dosages of 500 to 3,000 mg/day for up to 17 days. Fatigue, drowsiness, and headache were the most common adverse events observed at the highest dosage.

SPD 421

SPD 421, also known as DP16 or DP-VPA, is an interesting valproate prodrug that is intended selectively to deliver the active principle directly to the site of epileptic activity. It was originally developed by D-Pharm in Israel, and later acquired by Shire Pharmaceuticals in Andover, United Kingdom.

Mechanism of Action and Anticonvulsant Activity in Animal Models. Based on a drug delivery technology known as Regulated Activation of Prodrugs (D-RAP, D-Pharm, Rehovot, Israel), SPD 421 is a complex consisting of one molecule of valproic acid chemically linked to a phospholipid carrier. Although the complex *per se* is considered to be pharmacologically inert, cleavage and the consequent release of valproic acid occurs after exposure to phospholipase A2 (PlA2), an enzyme that is released preferentially at the site of paroxysmal neuronal activity. The concept behind SPD 421 development is that seizure activity should trigger the local release of valproic acid, which would then selectively suppress the epileptic discharges. Exposure to the active principles outside the site(s) of epileptic activity should be minimized, with consequent reduction of the potential for adverse effects.

In animals subjected to convulsant stimuli, a first seizure usually is required to activate phospholipase A2. Therefore, as expected from its mode of action, SPD 421 protects preferentially against occurrence of a second seizure, whereas activity against a first seizure is absent or greatly reduced. In the PTZ test in mice, the ED_{50} of SPD 421 for protection against a second seizure is 12 mg/kg (expressed as valproic acid equivalents), with a protective index of 6, compared with an ED_{50} of 150 mg/kg and a protective index of 1.8 for valproic acid itself (9). Similar results were found using the s.c. picrotoxin test in mice and rats.

Using the audiogenic seizures model in Frings mice, SPD 421 given i.p. 1 hour before stimulus application shows an ED_{50} of 4.5 mg/kg (valproic acid equivalents), compared with 220 mg/kg for valproic acid. In the same model, the duration of activity of SPD 421 is much longer when animals are stimulated every 2 hours compared with animals exposed to a single stimulation (9). Again, this is considered to be related to the greater local release of the active principle after repeated stimulation. SPD 421 is ineffective in the genetic absence epilepsy in rats from Strasbourg (GAERS) model of absence seizures, possibly because the mechanisms triggering seizures in this model may not result in the activation of phospholipase A2.

Drug Interactions. In animal experiments, enzyme induction by phenobarbital has no effect on plasma SPD 421 levels, probably because SPD 421 is minimally metabolized by CYP enzymes. SPD 421 itself does not cause induction of carbamazepine metabolism.

Tolerability Data in Humans. In a double-blind, placebo-controlled tolerability study in a total of 56 healthy volunteers, SPD 421 (up to 5 g as single doses and up to 1.25 g/day as multiple dose, was well tolerated in general. The only adverse event reported was transient epigastric pain, and no dropouts were reported in any of the dosage groups (9).

STIRIPENTOL

Stiripentol is 4,4-dimethyl-1-[(3,4 methylenedioxy)phenyl]-1-penten-3-ol, an allyl alcohol that occurs in two enantiomeric forms. Its anticonvulsant properties were discovered by the Biocodex Laboratories in Paris, France over 20 years ago, and the compound still is being used clinically on a named basis despite the fact that its development was hampered by interactions with concomitant antiepileptic drugs.

Anticonvulsant Activity in Animal Models. Stiripentol exhibits broad-spectrum activity against seizures induced by MES, PTZ, and bicuculline (68,86), spike-and-wave discharges in a genetic model of petit mal epilepsy in Wistar rats (73), and interictal electroencephalogram spike discharges in an alumina gel rhesus monkey model of focal epilepsy (66).

Mechanisms of Action. The mode of action is poorly understood, but it may involve inhibition of the synaptosomal uptake of glycine and GABA (68,86), enhanced β-hydroxybutyrate dehydrogenase activity, and inhibition of GABA-transaminase (84).

Pharmacokinetics. After oral administration, peak plasma concentrations usually are achieved within 2 hours. Stiripentol is 99% bound to plasma proteins and is eliminated according to capacity-limited, Michaelis-Menten kinetics (62). In one study in patients receiving concomitant anticonvulsants, the steady-state stiripentol concentration increased by approximately 250% with a dose increase from 600 to 1,200 mg/day, and a further doubling of the dose to 2,400 mg/day caused an almost 400% rise in serum concentration (63). Identified metabolic pathways include glucuronide conjugation (20% to 30% of the dose), opening of the methylenedioxy ring (11% to 14%), and *O*-methylation of catechol metabolites at positions 3 and 4 (17% to 24%) (68,76).

Drug Interactions. Enzyme-inducing anticonvulsants accelerate stiripentol metabolism. At a dosage of 1,200 mg/day, stiripentol clearance in enzyme-induced patients is on average threefold higher than in non-comedicated subjects (63).

Stiripentol is an inhibitor of oxidative drug metabolism, leading to increased serum concentrations of phenytoin (63,68), carbamazepine (46), phenobarbital (63,68), primidone (4), clobazam, norclobazam (16,82,87), and valproic acid (64). Most of these interactions are clinically relevant and may require reduction in dosage of associated drugs.

Antiepileptic Efficacy and Adverse Effects. In open studies, stiripentol has been reported to improve the frequency of both partial and generalized seizures, including typical and atypical absences, at maintenance dosages in the range of 1,000 to 3,000 mg/day in adults and 20 to 100 mg/kg/day in children (30,68,82). In a recent, open-label, pediatric add-on trial in a total of 212 children, 49% of patients showed a 50% reduction in seizure frequency, the best results being observed in partial epilepsies (82). Particularly good responses also were obtained in combination with clobazam in patients with severe myoclonic epilepsy of infancy, a finding subsequently confirmed in a double-blind, placebo-controlled trial in 40 children (16). Despite the fact that the appearance of adverse effects (or a predefined treatment protocol) often led to a reduction in the dosage of comedication in these studies, serum levels of concomitant anticonvulsants were almost invariably higher during stiripentol treatment than at baseline, and therefore it has been difficult to establish to what degree pharmacokinetic interactions contributed to clinical improvement. Chiron et al. (16) suggested that patients on stiripentol may tolerate higher concentrations of concomitant anticonvulsants, particularly clobazam and norclobazam, compared with patients not receiving stiripentol, leading to an improved therapeutic index of associated therapy. When attempts were made to discontinue comedication and stabilize patients on stiripentol monotherapy, most patients showed a deterioration in seizure control (68).

The most commonly reported adverse effects include gastrointestinal disturbances (nausea, vomiting, gastric/abdominal discomfort, anorexia), weight loss, neurobehavioral disorders, insomnia, and drowsiness (68,82). Leukopenia also has been reported. Many CNS adverse effects may be managed through reduction in the dosage of concomitant antiepileptic drugs.

TALAMPANEL

Talampanel (LY 300164, GYKI 53773) is the *R*(−)-enantiomer of 7-acetyl-5-(4-aminophenyl)-8,9-dihydro-8-methyl-7H-1,3-dioxolo(4,5H)-2,3-benzodiazepine. This compound, discovered by Eli Lilly Co. (Indianapolis, IN) and currently being developed by Ivax, Miami, Florida, acts as a stereoselective noncompetitive antagonist of the AMPA subtype of the glutamate receptor (11). Although it is structurally considered a benzodiazepine, its affinity for the benzodiazepine receptor and spectrum of anticonvulsant activity differ from those of 1,4-benzodiazepines such as diazepam. Because of their specific AMPA antagonist activity, 2,3-benzodiazepines have been considered as potential therapeutic agents in a variety of neurologic disorders, including amyotrophic lateral sclerosis (ALS) (117) and levodopa-induced dyskinesias in patients with Parkinson's disease (50).

Anticonvulsant Activity in Animal Models. Talampanel is effective in protecting against electrically and chemically induced seizures in rodents. The threshold for electrically induced seizures is increased dose dependently at doses above 2 mg/kg (20). In mice, talampanel is effective in inhibiting seizure spread in the MES test (ED_{50}, 4.6 mg/kg) and in raising seizures threshold in the s.c. PTZ test (ED_{50}, 16.8 mg/kg). Talampanel suppresses chemically kindled seizures at a dose of 12.5 mg/kg and electrically kindled seizures in mice at a dose of 20 mg/kg. When administered i.p. at a dose of 5 mg/kg, talampanel significantly reduces the seizure and afterdischarge duration, but it has minor activity in suppressing both generalized and focal seizures in fully kindled rats (13). Talampanel also has been found to antagonize seizures in a dose-related manner in a mouse model of phenytoin-resistant status epilepticus (9).

At doses that by themselves are inactive against electrically induced seizures (0.75 to 2 mg/kg), talampanel potentiates the anticonvulsant activity of carbamazepine, valproic acid, and diazepam (13,14,20).

Activity in Other Models. The neuroprotective efficacy of talampanel *in vitro* was investigated in an embryonic rat hippocampal culture model of non–NMDA receptor-mediated excitotoxicity using kainic acid as an agonist at the AMPA/kainate receptor (72). Using lactate dehydrogenase efflux as a biomarker for cellular toxicity, talampanel attenuated kainate effects in a dose-dependent manner, with an IC_{50} of 4 µmol/L. The (*S*)-enantiomer was inactive in this model. *In vivo*, talampanel has been found to be effective in protecting against the excitation of spinal neurons induced by electrophoretic application of NMDA and AMPA in anesthetized rats (67,78). Talampanel also protects against damage induced by bilateral carotid occlusion in gerbils, inhibits flexor reflexes in cats, and protects mice from memory-impairing effects of cerebral ischemia (9). Talampanel decreases contusion volume in a rat fluid percussion model of head trauma when given 30 minutes after the trauma.

In nonhuman primates, talampanel has been found to exert a modest antiparkinsonian activity when given alone, to potentiate the antiparkinsonian effect of levodopa in 1-methyl-4-phenyl-1,2,3,b-tetra hydropyridine (MPTP)-lesioned animals, and to attenuate levodopa-induced dyskinesias. These effects are seen at doses as low as 1 mg/kg and increase in magnitude at the well-tolerated dose of 10 mg/kg (50).

Talampanel induces microsomal drug-metabolizing enzymes in rats and mice (9).

Mechanism of Action. Talampanel is a noncompetitive antagonist at AMPA receptor sites. In binding assays, talampanel does not appear to interact (>100 mmol/L K_i) with α_1- and β-adrenergic receptors or with dopamine type 1 (D_1), D_2, histamine type 1, GABA, 5-hydroxytryptamine type 2, and muscarinic receptors (9).

Pharmacokinetics. Talampanel is well absorbed from the gastrointestinal tract, with peak plasma concentrations being observed at approximately 2.5 hours after an oral dose (84). Plasma protein binding ranges from 67% to 88%. Nonlinear kinetics have been observed after single and multiple doses in healthy volunteers, and evidence has been provided that elimination occurs by a combination of a first-order and a capacity-limited process, with the latter becoming saturated at plasma levels of approximately 200 ng/mL. At dosages producing plasma levels higher than these (single doses above 50 mg and multiple doses above 20 mg three times daily), the half-life is approximately 7 to 8 hours and plasma concentrations are expected to increase linearly with increasing dosages.

Talampanel is eliminated primarily by biotransformation, and one of the metabolic pathways involves acetylation. The apparent oral clearance at steady state has been found to be approximately 50% lower in slow acetylators than in fast acetylators (84).

Drug Interactions. Talampanel is an irreversible inhibitor of CYP3A4 and therefore it may increase the plasma concentration of CYP3A4 substrates such as carbamazepine (9). On the other hand, the plasma levels of the cholesterol-lowering drug lovastatin were unchanged after 10 days of treatment with talampanel, 60 mg three times daily.

There is evidence that talampanel metabolism is partly mediated through inducible pathways. In fact, microsomal enzyme inducers such as phenytoin and carbamazepine were found to increase the clearance of talampanel in a 1-week drug interaction study in patients with epilepsy (9). On the other hand, valproic acid decreases the clearance of talampanel.

Antiepileptic Efficacy and Adverse Effects. In a randomized, double-blind, add-on, crossover trial in 49 patients with refractory partial seizures, talampanel treatment was associated with a median 21% reduction in seizure frequency compared with placebo treatment, and 80% of patients had fewer seizures on talampanel than on placebo (9). The protocol required that the plasma concentrations of concomitant anticonvulsants be maintained within 30% of baseline, which led to a reduction in carbamazepine dose in six patients The 16 patients who did not receive carbamazepine comedication showed a similar (21%) seizure reduction. Most patients were receiving concomitant enzyme inducers, and the median dose of talampanel in these patients was 52 mg three times daily (versus a maximum allowable dose in this group of 75 mg three times a day), resulting in a mean plasma level of 125 ng/mL. The most commonly encountered adverse events were dizziness and ataxia, which occurred in 52% and 26%, respectively, of talampanel-treated patients. Discontinuation rates were 13% during the talampanel period and 11% during the placebo period.

Trials in Other Indications. Forty patients with ALS who had been symptomatic for 2 years or less were included in a randomized, parallel-group, placebo-controlled trial (9). Eighty-five percent of patients assigned to talampanel achieved the maximum dosage of 50 mg three times daily, with a mean plasma level of 400 ng/mL. Talampanel-treated patients showed a 15% decrease in rate of decline on the Tufts Quantified Neuromuscular Examination scale and showed less deterioration than placebo patients on the ALS functional rating scale, although differences were not statistically significant. Dizziness and somnolence were the two most commonly observed adverse events in this study.

VALROCEMIDE

Valrocemide (*N*-valproyl glycinamide, TV 1901) is a *N*-acetyl derivative of valproic acid, selected for clinical development by Teva Pharmaceuticals (Petach Tikva, Israel) among a series of valproyl derivatives of GABA and glycine (12).

Anticonvulsant Activity in Animal Models. Valrocemide shows broad-spectrum protective activity against electrically and chemically induced seizures (7,9,37,105). The ED_{50} in the MES test is 73 mg/kg p.o. in rats and 152 mg/kg i.p. in mice. Valrocemide also raises seizure threshold, with an ED_{50} of 127 mg/kg i.p. in the s.c. PTZ test in mice. The neurotoxic oral TD_{50}, determined by the gait and stance test in rats, is greater than 1,000 mg/kg, whereas the i.p. TD_{50}, determined by the Rotorod test, is 332 mg/kg in mice. In two separate types of kindling models, corneal and hippocampal kindling, valrocemide was capable of suppressing both generalized and focal seizures at doses below the TD_{50}. Valrocemide is effective in antagonizing seizure activity in two genetic models of epilepsy, the audiogenic seizure-prone Frings mouse and the lethargic mouse.

Mechanism of Action. In animal models, the activity profile of valrocemide resembles that of valproic acid. Its precise mechanism of action remains to be defined.

Pharmacokinetics. After administration of single doses up to 4,000 mg and multiple daily doses between 250 and 1000 mg three times daily in healthy volunteers, valrocemide is absorbed rapidly and is eliminated with a half-life of 6.4 to 9.4 hours (8,9). The Cl/F is in the range of 4.3 to 6.8 L/h, and the volume of distribution (Vss/F) is 48 to 83 L. The pharmacokinetics of valrocemide appears to be linear over the explored dose range.

Approximately 40% of an orally administered dose is excreted in urine as valproyl glycine. During multiple dosing, the renal clearance of unchanged drug is in the order of 1.2 to 1.4 L/h and the formation clearance of valproyl glycine is approximately 2.4 to 2.7 L/h. The fraction of valrocemide metabolized to valproic acid in healthy subjects, assessed by calculating the ratio between the plasma valproic acid AUC after oral administration of valrocemide and the plasma valproic acid AUC (derived from literature data) after direct administration of valproate, has been estimated to be approximately 4% to 6% (9).

Drug Interactions. Epileptic patients comedicated with phenytoin, carbamazepine, and other anticonvulsants show higher Cl/F values (mean, 8.2 L/h) and shorter half-lives (mean, 4.7 hours) compared with healthy subjects. This suggests that valrocemide metabolism is stimulated by enzyme-inducing antiepileptic comedication. In patients not receiving enzyme-inducing anticonvulsants, valrocemide kinetics are similar to those observed in healthy volunteers (9).

In human liver microsomes, clinically relevant concentrations of valrocemide and valproyl glycine have no inhibitory effect on the activity of CYP1A2, CYP2C9, CYP2C19, CYP2D6, CYP2E2, CYP3A4, and epoxide hydrolase.

Tolerability Data in Humans. In a 13-week tolerability study in 22 epileptic patients, valrocemide was well tolerated in general (9). Twenty-one patients completed the study, with 14 patients achieving the maximum allowed dose of 2,000 mg twice daily. Most commonly observed adverse effects affected the CNS or the gastrointestinal system. Of 15 patients with three or more seizures per month at baseline, 2 remained seizure free for the duration of the study.

REFERENCES

1. Armand V, Rundfeldt C, Heinemann U. Effects of retigabine (D-23129) on different patterns of epileptiform activity induced by low magnesium in rat entorhinal cortex hippocampal slices. *Epilepsia* 2000;41;28–33.
2. Armand V, Rundfeldt C, Heinemann U. Effects of retigabine (D-23129) on different patterns of epileptiform activity induced by 4-aminopyridine in rat entorhinal cortex hippocampal slices. *Naunyn Schmiedebergs Arch Pharmacol* 1999; 359:33–39.
3. Bannan PE, Graham DI, Lees KR, et al. Neuroprotective effect of remacemide hydrochloride in focal ischaemia in the cat. *Brain Res* 1994;664:271–275.
4. Bebin M, Black TP. New anticonvulsant drugs: focus on flunarizine, fosphenytoin, midazolam and stiripentol. *Drugs* 1994;48:153–171
5. Beekman M, Ungard JT, Gasior M, et al. Reversal of behavioral effects of pentylenetetrazole by the neuroactive steroid ganaxolone. *J Pharmacol Exp Ther* 1998;285:868–877.
6. Belelli D, Bolger MB, Gee KW. Antiepileptic profile of the progesterone metabolite, 5α-pregnan-3α-ol-20-one. *Eur J Pharmacol* 1989;166:325–329.
7. Bialer M, Johannessen SI, Kupferberg HJ, et al. Progress report on new antiepileptic drugs: A summary of the Third Eilat Conference. *Epilepsy Res* 1996;25:299–319.
8. Bialer M, Johannessen SI, Kupferberg HJ, et al. Progress report

on new antiepileptic drugs: A summary of the Fourth Eilat Conference (EILAT IV). *Epilepsy Res* 1999;34:1–41.

9. Bialer M, Johannessen SI, Kupferberg HJ, et al. Progress report on new antiepileptic drugs: A summary of the fifth Eilat conference (EILAT IV). *Epilepsy Res* 2001;43:11–58.

10. Biber A, Dienel A. Pharmacokinetic of losigamone, a new antiepileptic drug, in healthy male volunteers. *Int J Clin Pharmacol Ther* 1996;34:6–11.

11. Bleakman D, Ballyk BA, Schoepp DD, et al. Activity of 2,3-benzodiazepines at native rat and recombinant human glutamate receptors in vitro: stereospecificity and selectivity profiles. *Neuropharmacology* 1996;35:1689–1702.

12. Blotnick S, Bergman F, Bialer M. The disposition of valproyl glycinamide and valproyl glycine in rats. *Pharm Res* 1997;14:873–878.

13. Borowicz KK, Luszczki J, Szadkowski M, et al. Influence of LY 300164, an antagonist of AMPA/kainate receptors, on the anticonvulsant activity of clonazepam. *Eur J Pharmacol* 1999;380:67–72

14. Borowicz KK, Kleinrok Z, Czuczwar SJ. The AMPA/kainate receptor antagonist, LY 300164, increases the anticonvulsant effects of diazepam. *Naunyn Schmiedebergs Arch Pharmacol* 2000;361:629–635.

15. Carter RB, Wood PL, Wieland S, et al. Characterization of the anticonvulsant properties of ganaxolone (CCD 1042; 3α-hydroxy-3β-methyl-5α-pregnan-20-one), a selective high-affinity steroid modulator of the GABA$_A$ receptor. *J Pharmacol Exp Ther* 1997;280:1284–1295.

16. Chiron C, Marchand MC, Tran A, et al. Stiripentol in severe myoclonic epilepsy in infancy A randomized placebo-controlled syndrome-dedicated trial. *Lancet* 2000;356:1638–1642.

17. Clark B, Hutchison JB, Jamieson V, et al.. Potential antiepileptic drugs: remacemide hydrochloride. In: Levy RH, Mattson RH, Meldrum B, eds. *Antiepileptic drugs*, 4th ed. New York: Raven Press, 1995:1035–1044.

18. Craig CR. Antiepileptic activity of steroids: separability of antiepileptic from hormonal effects. *J Pharmacol Exp Ther* 1966;153:337–343.

19. Crawford P, Richens A, Mawer G, et al. A double-blind placebo controlled cross-over study of remacemide hydrochloride as adjunctive therapy in patients with refractory epilepsy. *Epilepsy Res* 1992;1[Suppl A]:7–13.

20. Czuczwar SJ, Swiader M, Kuzniar H, et al. LY 300164, a novel antagonist of AMPA/kainate receptors, potentiates the anticonvulsive activity of antiepileptic drugs. *Eur J Pharmacol* 1998;359:103–109.

21. Dailey JW, Cheong JH, Ko KH, et al. Anticonvulsant properties of D-20443 in genetically epilepsy-prone rats: prediction of clinical response. *Neurosci Lett* 1995;195:77–80.

22. Dailey JW, Adams-Curtis LE, Ryu JR, et al. Neurochemical correlates of antiepileptic drugs in the genetically epilepsy-prone rat (GEPR). *Life Sci* 1996;58:259–266.

23. Dimpfel W, Chatterjee SS, Noldner M, et al. Effects of the anticonvulsant losigamone and its isomers on the GABAA receptor system. *Epilepsia* 1995;36:983–989.

24. Dienel A, Biber A. Losigamone: comprehensive summary of safety and tolerability in volunteers. *Epilepsia* 1996;37[Suppl 4]:63–64.

25. Dost R, Rundfeldt C. The anticonvulsant retigabine potently suppresses epileptiform discharges in the low Ca++ and low Mg++ model in the hippocampal slice preparation. *Epilepsy Res* 1999;38:53–66.

26. Draguhn A, Jungclaus M, Sokolowa S, et al. Losigamone decreases the spontaneous synaptic activity in cultured hippocampal neurons. *Eur J Pharmacol* 1997;325:245–251.

27. Elger CE, Stefan H, Runge U, et al. Losigamone, double-blind study of 1,500 mg/day versus placebo in patients with focal epilepsy. *Epilepsia* 1996;37[Suppl 4]:64.

28. Fariello RG, McArthur RA, Bonsignori A, et al. Preclinical evaluation of PNU-151774E as a novel anticonvulsant. *J Pharmacol Exp Ther* 1998;285:397–403.

29. Fariello RG, Maj R, Marrari P, et al. Acute behavioral and EEG effects of NW-1015 on electrically-induced afterdischarge in conscious monkeys. *Epilepsy Res* 2000;39:37–46.

30. Farwell JR, Anderson GD, Kerr B, et al. Stiripentol in atypical absence seizures in children: an open trial. *Epilepsia* 1993;34:305–311.

31. Garske GE, Palmer GC, Napier JJ, et al. Preclinical profile of the anticonvulsant remacemide and its enantiomers in the rat. *Epilepsy Res* 1991;9:161–174.

32. Gasior M, Carter RB, Goldberg SR, et al. Anticonvulsant and behavioural effects of neuroactive steroids alone and in conjunction with diazepam. *J Pharmacol Exp Ther* 1997;282:543–553.

33. Gatti G, Bonomi I, Jannuzzi G, et al. The new antiepileptic drugs: pharmacological and clinical aspects. *Curr Pharm Design* 2000;6:839–860.

34. Gee KW, McCauley LD, Lan NC. A putative receptor for neurosteroids on the GABA receptor complex: the pharmacological properties and therapeutic potential of epalons. *Crit Rev Neurobiol* 1995;9:207–227.

35. Gillardin JM, Verleye M, Ralambosoa C, et al. Anticonvulsant profile and plasma-brain concentrations of a new 2,6-dimethyl-benzamide-N-(5-methyl-3-isoxazolyl)(D2916) in rats. *Epilepsia* 1993;34[Suppl 6]:38.

36. Greenamyre JT, Eller RV, Zhang Z, et al. Antiparkinsonian effects of remacemide hydrochloride, a glutamate antagonist, in rodent and primate models of Parkinson's disease. *Ann Neurol* 1994;35:655–661.

37. Hadad S, Bialer M. Pharmacokinetic analysis and antiepileptic activity of N-valproyl derivatives of GABA and glycine. *Pharm Res* 1995;12:1160–1163.

38. Harr JE, Maher GG, Kunze KL, et al. Predictions of drug interactions based on identification of CYP450 isoforms which metabolize and are inhibited by D2916, a novel anticonvulsant. Presented at the Meeting of the American Association of Pharmaceutical Scientists, Seattle, WA, October 28–31, 1996.

39. Hetka R, Rundfeldt C, Heinemann U, et al. Retigabine (D-23129) strongly reduces repetitive firing in rat entorhinal cortex. *Eur J Pharmacol* 1999;386:165–171.

40. Hudzik TJ, Freedman L, Palmer GC. Remacemide hydrochloride and ARL 15896AR lack abuse potential: additional differences from other uncompetitive NMDA antagonists. *Epilepsia* 1996;37:544–550.

41. Jones MW, Blume W, Guberman A, et al. Remacemide hydrochloride (300mg, 600mg, 800 mg/day) efficacy and safety versus placebo in patients with refractory epilepsy. *Epilepsia* 1996;37[Suppl 5]:166.

42. Jones FA, Davies JA. The anticonvulsant effects of the enantiomers of losigamone. *Br J Pharmacol* 1999;128:1223–1228.

43. Kapetanovic IM, Rundfeldt C. D-23129: A new anticonvulsant compound. *CNS Drug Rev* 1996;2:308–321.

44. Kapetanovic IM, Yonekawa WD, Kupferberg HJ. The effect of anticonvulsant compounds on 4-aminopyridine-induced *de novo* synthesis of neurotransmitter amino acids in rat hippocampus *in vitro*. *Epilepsy Res* 1995;20:113–120.

45. Kapetanovic IM, Yonekawa WD, Kupferberg HJ. D-23129 stimulated *de novo* synthesis of GABA in rat hippocampal slices is blocked by an inhibitor of the Na+/K+ antiporter. *Epilepsia* 1996;37[Suppl 5]:81

46. Kerr BM, Martinez-Lage JM, Viteri C, et al. Carbamazepine dose requirements during stiripentol therapy: influence of cytochrome P450 inhibition by stiripentol. *Epilepsia* 1991;32:267–274

47. Kerrigan JF, Shields WD, Nelson TY, et al. Ganaxolone for treating intractable infantile spasms: a multicentre, open-label, add-on trial. *Epilepsy Res* 2000;42:133–139.

48. Kohr G, Heinemann U. Anticonvulsant effects of tetronic acid derivatives on picrotoxin-induced epileptiform activity in rat hippocampal slices. *Neurosci Lett* 1990;112:43–47.

49. Kohr G, Heinemann U. Effects of tetronic acid derivatives AO-33 (losigamone) and AO-78 on epileptiform activity and on stimulus-induced calcium concentration changes in rat hippocampal slices. *Epilepsy Res* 1990;7:49–55.

50. Konitsiotis C, Blanchet PJ, Verhagen L, et al. AMPA receptor blockade improves levodopa-induced dyskinesia in MPTP monkey. *Neurology* 2000;54:1589–1595.

51. Krämer G, Wad N, Bredel-Geissler A, et al. Losigamone-phenytoin interaction: a placebo-controlled, double-blind study in healthy volunteers. *Epilepsia* 1995;36[Suppl 3]:S163.

52. Krämer G, Wad N, Bredel-Geissler, et al. Losigamone-valproate interaction: a placebo-controlled, double-blind study in healthy volunteers. *Epilepsia* 1995;36[Suppl 4]:53.

53. Krämer G, Wad N, Bredel-Geissler A, et al. Losigamone interactions with antiepileptic drugs in healthy volunteers. *Epilepsia* 1996;37[Suppl 4]:89.

54. Kupferberg HJ. Sodium valproate. *Adv Neurol* 1980;27:643–654.

55. Laxer K, Blum D, Abou-Khalil B, et al. Assessment of ganaxolone's anticonvulsant activity using a randomized, double-blind, presurgical trial design. *Epilepsia* 2000;41:1187–1194

56. Leach JP, Blacklaw J, Jamieson V, et al. Mutual interaction between remacemide hydrochloride and carbamazepine: two drugs with active metabolites. *Epilepsia* 1996;37:1100–1106.

57. Leach JP, Girvan J, Jamieson V, et al. Mutual interaction between remacemide hydrochloride and phenytoin. *Epilepsy Res* 1997;26:381–388.

58. Leach JP, Blacklaw J, Jamieson V, et al. Mutual interaction between remacemide hydrochloride and carbamazepine: two drugs with active metabolites. *Epilepsia* 1996;37:1100–1106.

59. Lechtenberg R, Villeneuve N, Monagham EP, et al. An open-label dose-escalation study to evaluate the safety and tolerability of ganaxolone in the treatment of refractory epilepsy in pediatric patients. *Epilepsia* 1996;37[Suppl 5]:204.

60. Lepage F, Tombret F, Cuvier G, et al. New N-aryl isoxazolecarboxamides and N-isoxazolylbenzamides as anticonvulsant agents. *Eur J Med Chem* 1992;27:581–593.

61. Lepage F, Gillardin JM, Tombret F, et al. Human and rat metabolism of D2916 and anticonvulsant properties of its metabolites. *Epilepsia* 1995;36[Suppl 4]:49.

62. Levy RH, Lin HS, Blehaut H, et al. Pharmacokinetics of stiripentol in normal man: evidence of nonlinearity. *J Clin Pharmacol* 1983;23:523–533.

63. Levy RH, Loiseau P, Guyot M, et al. Stiripentol kinetics in epilepsy: nonlinearity and interactions. *Clin Pharmacol Ther* 1984;36:661–669.

64. Levy RH, Loiseau P, Guyot M, et al. Effects of stiripentol on valproate plasma level and metabolism. *Epilepsia* 1987;28:605.

65. Liptakova S, Velisek L, Veliskova J, et al. Effect of ganaxolone on fluorothyl seizures in developing rats. *Epilepsia* 2000;41:788–793.

66. Lockard JS, Levy RH, Rhodes PH, et al. Stiripentol in acute/chronic efficacy tests in monkeys model. *Epilepsia* 1985;26:704–712.

67. Lodge D, Bond A, O'Neill MJ, et al. Stereoselectivity effects of 2,3-benzodiazepines in vivo: electrophysiology and neuroprotection studies. *Neuropharmacology* 1996;35:1681–1688.

68. Loiseau P, Duche B. Potential antiepileptic drugs: stiripentol. In: Levy RH, Mattson RH, Meldrum BS, eds. *Antiepileptic drugs*, 4th ed. New York: Raven Press, 1995:1045–1056.

69. Main MJ, Cryan JE, Dupere JR, et al. Modulation of KCNQ2/3 potassium channels by the novel anticonvulsant retigabine. *Mol Pharmacol* 2000;58:253–262.

70. Maj R, Fariello RG, Ukmar G, et al. PNU-151774E protects against kainate-induced status epilepticus and hippocampal lesions in the rat. *Eur J Pharmacol* 1998;359:27–32.

71. Maj R, Fariello RG, Pevarello P, et al. Anticonvulsant activity of PNU-151774E in the amygdala kindled model of complex partial seizures. *Epilepsia* 1999;40:1523–1528.

72. May PC, Robison PM, Fuson KS. Stereoselective neuroprotection by novel 2,3 benzodiazepine non-competitive AMPA antagonist against non-NMDA receptor-mediated excitotoxicity in primary rat hippocampal cultures. *Neurosci Lett* 1999; 262:219–221. .

73. Micheletti G, Vergnes M, Lannes B, et al. Effect of stiripentol on petit-mal like epilepsy in Wistar rats. *Epilepsia* 1988;29:709.

74. Monagham EP, Densel MB, Lechtenberg R. Gender differences in sensitivity to ganaxolone, a neuroactive steroid under investigation as an antiepileptic drug. *Epilepsia* 1996;37[Suppl 5]:171.

75. Monagham EP, Navalta LA, Shum L, et al. Initial human experience with ganaxolone, a neuroactive steroid with antiepileptic activity. *Epilepsia* 1997;38:1026–1031.

76. Moreland TA, Astoin J, Lepage F. The metabolic fate of stiripentol in man. *Drug Metab Dispos* 1986;14:654–662.

77. Muir KT, Palmer GC. Remacemide. In: Pisani F, Perucca E, Avanzini G, et al., eds. *New antiepileptic drugs*. Amsterdam: Elsevier Science, 1991:147–152.

78. Nakao N, Grasbon-Frodl EM, Widner H, et al. DARPP-32-rich zones in grafts of lateral ganglionic eminence govern the extent of functional recovery in skilled paw reaching in an animal model of Huntington's disease. *Neuroscience* 1996;74:959–970.

79. Palmer GC, Stagnitto ML, Ordy JM, et al. Preclinical profile of stereoisomers of the anticonvulsant remacemide in mice. *Epilepsy Res* 1991;8:36–48.

80. Palmer GC, Murray RJ, Wilson TCM, et al. Biological profile of the metabolites and potential metabolites of the anticonvulsant remacemide. *Epilepsy Res* 1992;12:9–20.

81. Palmer GC, Harris EW, Ray R, et al. Classification of compounds for prevention of NMDLA-induced seizures/mortality or maximal electroshock and pentylenetetrazol seizures in mice and antagonism of MK-801 binding *in vitro*. *Arch Int Pharmacodyn Ther* 1992;317:16–34.

82. Perez J, Chiron C, Musial C, et al. Stiripentol: efficacy and tolerability in epileptic children. *Epilepsia* 1999;40:1618–1626.

83. Perucca E. The new generation of antiepileptic drugs: advantages and disadvantages. *Br J Clin Pharmacol* 1996;42:531–543.

84. Perucca E. Drugs under clinical trial. In: Eadie MJ, Vajda FJE, eds. *Antiepileptic drugs: pharmacology and therapeutics. Handbook of experimental pharmacology*, vol 138. Berlin: Springer-Verlag, 1999:515–551.

85. Pevarello P, Bonsignori A, Dostert P, et al. Synthesis and anticonvulsant activity of a new class of 2-[(arylalkyl)amino]alkanamide derivatives. *J Med Chem* 1998;41:579–590.

86. Poisson M, Huguet F, Savatier A, et al. A new type of anticonvulsant, stiripentol. *Arzneimittelforschung* 1984;34:199–204.

87. Rey E, Tran A, D'Athis P, et al. Stiripentol potentiates clobazam in childhood epilepsy: a pharmacological study. *Epilepsia* 1999;40[Suppl 7]:112–113.

88. Riley RJ, Slee D, Martin CA, et al. *In vitro* evaluation of pharmacokinetic interactions between remacemide hydrochloride and established anticonvulsants. *Br J Clin Pharmacol* 1996;41:461P.

89. Rostock A, Tober G, Rundfeldt C, et al. D-23129: a new anticonvulsant with a broad spectrum of activity in animal models of epileptic seizures. *Epilepsy Res* 1996;23:211–223.

90. Rostock A, Bartsch R, Engel J. D-23129, a new anticonvulsant improves learning and memory in rat models of cerebral deficiency. *Epilepsia* 1996;37[Suppl 4]:140.

91. Rostock A, Tober C, Dost R., et al. AWD 131-138. *Drugs Future* 1998;23:253–255.

92. Rostock A, Tober C, Dost R, et al. AWD 131-138 is a potential novel anxiolytic without sedation and amnesia: a comparison with diazepam and buspirone. *Naunyn Schmiedebergs Arch Pharmacol* 1998;358[Suppl 1]:R68.

93. Rostock A, Rundfeldt C, Bartsch R. Effect of the anticonvulsant retigabine in neuropathic pain models. *Naunyn Schmiedebergs Arch Pharmacol* 2001 (*in press*).

94. Rostock A., Tober C, Rundfeldt C, et al. D-23129: a new anticonvulsant with a broad spectrum activity in animal models of epileptic seizures. *Epilepsy Res* 2000;23:211–223.

95. Rundfeldt C. The new anticonvulsant retigabine (D-23129) acts as an opener of K+ channels in neuronal cells. *Eur J Pharmacol* 1997;336:243–249.

96. Rundfeldt C. Characterization of the K+ channel opening effect of the anticonvulsant retigabine in PC12 cells. *Epilepsy Res* 1999;35:99–107.

97. Rundfeldt C, Roeper J, Netzer R. AWD 131-138 antagonizes the effect of corticotrophin releasing factor in locus coeruleus neurones in murine brain stem slices. *Naunyn Schmiedebergs Arch Pharmacol* 1999;359[Suppl 3]:R97.

98. Rundfeldt C, Netzer R. The novel anticonvulsant retigabine activates M-currents in chinese hamster ovary-cells transfected with human KCNQ2/3 subunits. *Neurosci Lett* 2000;282:73–76.

99. Runge U, Rabending G, Dienel A. Losigamone: preliminary efficacy with 1,500 mg fixed daily dose for >6 months in patients with focal epilepsy. *Epilepsia* 1996;37[Suppl 4]:75.

100. Salvati P, Maj R, Caccia C, et al. Biochemical and electrophysiological studies on the mechanism of action of PNU-151774E, a novel antiepileptic compound. *J Pharmacol Exp Ther* 1999; 288:1151–1159.

101. Schaffler K, Wauschkuhn CH, Dienel A, et al. Losigamone has a longer CNS bioavailability in volunteers than is expected from pharmacokinetics. *Epilepsia* 1996;37[Suppl 4]:159.

102. Scheyer RD, Cramer JA, Leppik IE, et al. Remacemide elimination after initial and chronic dosing. *Clin Pharmacol Ther* 1992;51:189.

103. Schmitz D, Gloveli T, Heinemann U. Effects of losigamone on synaptic potentials and spike frequency habituation in rat entorhinal cortex and hippocampal CA1 neurons. *Neurosci Lett* 1995;200:141-143.

104. Schroeder BC, Kubisch C, Stein V, et al. Moderate loss of function of cyclic-AMP modulated KCNQ2/KCNQ3 K+ channels causes epilepsy. *Nature* 1998;396,687–690.

105. Spiegelstein O, Yagen B, Bialer M. Structure-pharmacokinetic-pharmacodynamic relationships of the new antiepileptic drug valproyl glycinamide. *Epilepsia* 1999;40:545–552.

106. Srivanasan J, Richens A, Davies JA. Losigamone reduces glutamate and aspartate release from mouse cortex. *Br J Pharmacol* 1996;117[Suppl]:164P.

107. Stagnitto ML, Palmer GC, Ordy JM, et al. Preclinical profile of remacemide: a novel anticonvulsant effective against maximal electroshock seizures in mice. *Epilepsy Res* 1990;7:11–28.

108. Stein U. Potential antiepileptic drugs: losigamone. In: Levy RH, Mattson RH, Meldrum BS, eds. *Antiepileptic drugs*, 4th ed. New York: Raven Press, 1995:1025–1034.

109. Stein U, Klessing K, Chatterjee SS. Losigamone. In: Pisani F, Perucca E, Avanzini G, et al., eds. *New antiepileptic drugs*. Amsterdam: Elsevier Science, 1991:129–133.

110. Straub H, Köhling R, Speckmann E-J, et al. Retigabine suppresses epileptiform activity in human neocortical slice preparations. *Epilepsia* 1999;40[Suppl 2]:38.

111. Strolin Benedetti M, Marrari P, Colombo M, et al. The anticonvulsant FCE 26743 is a selective and short-acting MAO-B inhibitor devoid of inducing properties towards cytochrome

P450-dependent testosterone hydroxylation in mice and rats. *J Pharm Pharmacol* 1994;46:814–819.

112. Tober C, Rostock A, Rundfeldt C, et al. D-23129: a potent anticonvulsant in the amygdala kindling model of complex partial seizures. *Eur J Pharmacol* 1996;303:163–169.

113. Tober C, Rostock A, Bartsch R. AWD 131-138: a derivative of a series of imidazolinones with anticonvulsant activity. *Naunyn Schmiedebergs Arch Pharmacol* 1998;358[Suppl 1]:R68.

114. Tober C, Rostock A, White HS, et al. Anticonvulsant activity of AWD 131-138 in genetic animal models of epilepsy. *Naunyn Schmiedebergs Arch Pharmacol* 1999;359[Suppl 3]:R97.

115. Torchin CD, McNeilly PJ, Kapetanovic IM, et al. Stereoselective metabolism of a new anticonvulsant drug candidate, losigamone, by human liver microsomes. *Drug Metab Dispos* 1996; 24:1002–1008.

116. Torchin CD, Yonekawa WD, Kapetanovic IM, et al. Chiral high-performance liquid chromatographic analysis of enantiomers of losigamone, a new candidate antiepileptic drugs. *J Chromatogr B Biomed Sci Appl* 1999;724:101–108.

117. Van den Bosch L, Vandenberghe W, Klaassen H, et al. Ca++ permeable AMPA receptors and selective vulnerability of motor neurons. *J Neurosci* 2000;180:290–334.

118. Wad N, Kramer G. Losigamone: detection of its glucuronide in serum. *Epilepsia* 1997;38[Suppl 3]:148.

119. Walton NY, Treiman DM. Remacemide versus phenytoin for treatment of experimental status epilepticus. *Epilepsia* 1997;37 [Suppl 5]:212.

120. Walton NY, Jaing Q, Hyun B, et al. Lamotrigine vs phenytoin for treatment of status epilepticus: comparison in an experimental model. *Epilepsy Res* 1996;24:19–28.

121. Wamil AW, Cheung H, Harris EW, et al. Remacemide HCl and its metabolite, AR-C 12495AA, limit action potential firing frequency and block NMDA responses of mouse spinal cord neurons in cell culture. *Epilepsy Res* 1996;23:1–14.

122. Wang HS, Pan Z, Shi W, et al. KCNQ2 and KCNQ3 potassium channel subunits: molecular correlates of the M-channel. *Science* 1998;282:1890–1893.

123. Wang L, Vieth R, Landes RC, et al. Antiepileptic effect of antiepilepsirine in pentylenetetrazol and amygdala kindled rats. *Epilepsy Res* 1993;15:1–5.

124. Wang L, Walson PD, Zuo CH. Clinical and experimental evaluation of anti-epilepsirine. *Epilepsia* 1997;38[Suppl 3]:101.

125. Wang L, Zhao D, Zhang Z, et al. Trial of antiepilepsirine in children with epilepsy. *Brain Dev* 1999;21:36–40.

126. White HS, Armstrong H, Barton M, et al. Anticonvulsant profile of NPS 1776: a broad-spectrum anticonvulsant. *Epilepsia* 1999;40[Suppl 7]:28.

127. Yan QS, Mishra PK, Burger RL, et al. Evidence that carbamazepine antiepilepsirine may produce a component of their anticonvulsant effects by activating serotonergic neurons in genetically epilepsy-prone rats. *J Pharmacol Exp Ther* 1992;261:652–659.

128. Yasar S, Paronis C, Munzar P, et al. Evaluation of the antiepileptic drug AWD 131-138 for reinforcing and discriminative stimulus effects. *Behav Pharmacol* 1999;10[Suppl 1]:103.

129. Yonekawa WD, Kapetanovic IM, Kupferberg HJ. The effects of anticonvulsant agents on 4-aminopyridine induced epileptiform activity in rat hippocampus *in vitro*. *Epilepsy Res* 1995;20: 137–150.

130. Zhang CL, Chatterjee SS, Stein U, et al. Comparison of the effects of losigamone and its isomers on maximal electroshock-induced convulsions in mice and on three different patterns of low magnesium induced epileptiform activity in slices of the rat temporal cortex. *Naunyn Schmiedebergs Arch Pharmacol* 1992; 345:85–92.

SUBJECT INDEX

Page numbers ending in f *refers to figures; those ending in* t *to tables.*